Clinical
MEDICINE

For W. B. Saunders:

Commissioning Editors: Ellen Green, Margaret Macdonald
Project Manager: Jennifer Bew
Design: Sarah Cape
Typesetting and Illustrations: Hardlines, Oxford
Production Controller: Frances Affleck
Project Editors: Louise Cook, Carol Parr
Indexer: Jan Ross

Clinical MEDICINE

Fourth Edition

A textbook for medical students and doctors

Edited by

Parveen Kumar
BSc MD FRCP FRCP(Edin)
Reader
St Bartholomew's and the Royal London School of Medicine and Dentistry
Queen Mary and Westfield College
Honorary Consultant Physician
The Royal Hospitals NHS Trust (St Bartholomew's and the Royal London Hospitals) and Homerton Hospital
London

Michael Clark
MD FRCP
Honorary Senior Lecturer
St Bartholomew's and the Royal London School of Medicine and Dentistry
Queen Mary and Westfield College
London

Benjamin Black
Bart's & The London

W. B. SAUNDERS

Edinburgh • London • Philadelphia • Toronto • Sydney • Tokyo

W. B. Saunders
An imprint of Harcourt Publishers Limited

First edition 1987
Second edition 1990
Third edition 1994
Fourth edition 1998
Reprinted 1999
Reprinted 2001

Standard edition ISBN 0 7020 2019 2
International edition ISBN 0 7020 2458 9

British Library Cataloguing in Publication Data
A catalogue record for this book is available from the British Library.

Library of Congress Cataloging in Publication Data
A catalog record for this book is available from the Library of Congress.

Medical knowledge is constantly changing. As new information becomes available, changes in treatment, procedures, equipment and the use of drugs become necessary. The editors, the contributors and the publishers have, as far as it is possible, taken care to ensure that the information given in this text is accurate and up to date. However, readers are strongly advised to confirm that the information, especially with regard to drug usage, complies with current legislation and standards of practice.

Printed in China

The publisher's policy is to use **paper manufactured from sustainable forests**

Contents

Contents in detail

13 Intensive care medicine 829

14 Adverse drug reactions and poisoning 861

15 Environmental medicine 885

16 Endocrinology 895

17 Diabetes mellitus and other disorders of metabolism 959

18 Neurological disease 1007

Contributors

Jane Anderson PhD MB BS FRCP
Senior Lecturer in HIV Medicine
Honorary Consultant Physician
Department of Immunology
St Bartholomew's and the Royal London School of Medicine and Dentistry
London

Sexually transmitted diseases

John V. Anderson MA MD MBBS FRCP
Consultant Physician
The Royal Hospitals NHS Trust and Homerton Hospital
Honorary Senior Lecturer
St Bartholomew's and the Royal London School of Medicine and Dentistry
London

Diabetes mellitus and lipids

Larry R.I. Baker MA MD FRCP FRCP(Edin)
Consultant Physician and Nephrologist
Department of Nephrology
The Royal Hospitals NHS Trust
St Bartholomew's Hospital
London

Renal disease

N. Benjamin DM FRCP(Edin)
Professor of Clinical Pharmacology
St Bartholomew's and the Royal London School of Medicine and Dentistry
London

Adverse drug reactions and poisoning

A. John Camm MD FRCP
Professor of Clinical Cardiology
St George's Hospital and Medical School
London

Cardiovascular disease

Anthony W. Clare MD FRCPI FRCP FRCPsych MPhil
Clinical Professor of Psychiatry
Trinity College
Dublin
Medical Director
St Patrick's Hospital
Dublin

Psychological medicine

Michael Clark MD FRCP
Honorary Senior Lecturer
St Bartholomew's and the Royal London School of Medicine and Dentistry
Queen Mary and Westfield College
London

Nutrition; gastroenterology; liver, biliary tract and pancreatic diseases; environmental medicine

Charles R.A. Clarke MA MB BCh FRCP
Consultant Neurologist
National Hospital for Neurology and Neurosurgery
Queen Square and Whipps Cross Hospital
London

Environmental medicine; neurological disease

Robert J. Davies MA MD FRCP
Professor of Respiratory Medicine
St Bartholomew's and the Royal London School of Medicine and Dentistry
London Chest Hospital
London

Respiratory disease

Paul L. Drury MA MB BCh FRCP
Medical Director
Auckland Diabetes Centre
Physician
Auckland Hospital
Auckland
New Zealand

Endocrinology; bone disease

Michael J.G. Farthing MD FRCP
Professor of Gastroenterology
St Bartholomew's and the Royal London School of Medicine and Dentistry
London

Infectious diseases and tropical medicine

Edwin A.M. Gale MB FRCP
Professor of Diabetic Medicine
Diabetes and Metabolism
Southmead Hospital
Bristol

Diabetes and other disorders of metabolism

Charles J. Hinds FRCP FRCA
Consultant Anaesthetist, Senior Lecturer and Director of Intensive Care
Department of Anaesthesia and Intensive Care
St Bartholomew's Hospital
London

Intensive care

Trevor A. Howlett MD FRCP
Consultant Physician and Endocrinologist
Leicester Royal Infirmary
Leicester

Endocrinology

Ray K. Iles BSc MSc PhD CBiol MIBiol
Senior Lecturer (non-clinical) in Obstetrics and Gynaecology
Director of the Willliamson Laboratory
St Bartholomew's and the Royal London School of Medicine and Dentistry
St Bartholomew's Hospital
London

Cell and molecular biology and genetic disorders

Donald J. Jeffries BSc MB BS FRCPath
Professor and Head of Department of Virology
St Bartholomew's and the Royal London School of Medicine and Dentistry
London

Virology

Parveen Kumar BSc MD FRCP FRCP(Edin)
Reader
St Bartholomew's and the Royal London School of Medicine and Dentistry
Queen Mary and Westfield College
Honorary Consultant Physician
The Royal Hospitals NHS Trust (St Bartholomew's and the Royal London Hospitals) and Homerton Hospital
London

Genetics and molecular biology; gastroenterology; liver, biliary tract and pancreatic diseases

Irene M. Leigh MD FRCP
Professor of Dermatology
Head of Department
Centre for Cutaneous Research
St Bartholomew's and the Royal London School of Medicine and Dentistry
Queen Mary and Westfield College
Clinical Sciences Research Centre
London

Dermatology

W. John W. Morrow BSc PhD
Senior Lecturer in Immunopathology
Department of Immunology
St Bartholomew's and the Royal London School of Medicine and Dentistry
London

Immunology

Michael F. Murphy MD FRCP FRCPath
Consultant Haematologist
National Blood Service and Department of Haematology
John Radcliffe Hospital
Oxford
Honorary Senior Clinical Lecturer in Blood Transfusion
Oxford University
Oxford

Diseases of the blood

David G. Paige MA MRCP
Consultant Dermatologist
The Royal Hospitals NHS Trust
Royal London Hospital
London
Honorary Senior Lecturer
Centre for Cutaneous Research
St Bartholomew's and the Royal London School of Medicine and Dentistry
Queen Mary and Westfield College
Clinical Sciences Research Centre
London

Dermatology

Jacqueline M. Parkin PhD MRCP
Senior Lecturer and Honorary Consultant in Clinical Immunology
St Bartholomew's and the Royal London School of Medicine and Dentistry
London

Immunology

Richard M. Pearson MB FRCP
Senior Lecturer in Clinical Pharmacology
St Bartholomew's and the Royal London School of Medicine and Dentistry
London
Consultant Physician
Harold Wood and Oldchurch Hospitals
Romford

Poisoning

Anthony J. Pinching DPhil FRCP
Louis Freedman Professor of Immunology
St Bartholomew's and the Royal London School of Medicine and Dentistry
London

Immunology

Ama Z.S. Rohatiner MD FRCP
Reader and Consultant Physician in Medical Oncology
St Bartholomew's Hospital
London

Medical oncology

Michael Shipley MA MD FRCP
Consultant Rheumatologist
University College London Hospitals
London

Rheumatology and bone disease

Maurice L. Slevin MBChB MD FRCP
Consultant Physician and Medical Oncologist
St Bartholomew's and the Royal London School of Medicine and Dentistry
London

Medical oncology

Teresa Tate FRCP FRCR
Consultant in Palliative Medicine
Whipps Cross Hospital
London
Consultant and Honorary Senior Lecturer in Palliative Medicine
St Bartholomew's Hospital
London

Medical oncology

Magdi Yaqoob MD MRCP
Consultant Nephrologist
St Bartholomew's and the Royal London Hospitals
London

Water, electrolytes and acid–base homeostasis

Preface to the Fourth Edition

We started this textbook of medicine in the mid-1980s with no real expectation that we would still be writing just prior to the millennium. We now, however, face this historic milestone with great enthusiasm because this new fourth edition is, we believe, even better than previous editions. This is partly because there have been many exciting recent advances in both our knowledge and the management of medical problems, and partly because modern book design and printing have ensured a book pleasing to the eye. We have of course stuck rigidly to the tried-and-tested formula of previous editions, as this has proved popular with our readers. We have added to this new drawings, figures and boxes to make *Clinical Medicine* even more user-friendly.

Four chapters have been completely rewritten by new, enthusiastic, young authors, who have made sure that everything is up to date and that complacency does not creep in. All other chapters have been extensively revised and brought up to date.

The views expressed in the book are, we believe, high-standard 'best practice' medicine open to peer review. In order to be 'evidence based' we have included recent key references so that the reader can examine the evidence for a particular viewpoint in detail in the latest article or review.

This book continues to be one of the standard medical textbooks consulted throughout the world. Our readers often write to us with suggestions, and we would like to thank them for their help and continuing support.

The book is widely read by undergraduate and postgraduate students, practising physicians, nurses, professionals allied to medicine, and many other groups who find it useful to have available in the clinic or hospital. We know that undergraduate students sometimes find the size and detail of the book daunting. For this reason *Pocket Essentials of Clinical Medicine*, by A. Ballinger and S. Patchett, and *MCQs in Clinical Medicine*, by R.R. Baliga, have also been revised. These are specifically designed to accompany *Clinical Medicine* and to help undergraduates pass their final examinations. *Clinical Medicine* itself should always be the constant companion throughout a long medical career.

We would, again, like to thank everyone who has supported us in this endeavour, in particular our families, who have put up with many late nights and lost weekends!

Parveen Kumar
Michael Clark

Preface to the First Edition

There must be a good reason to write a new textbook of medicine when there are already a number on the market. It seemed to us that none of those currently available adequately conveyed the detail and background needed for medical practice in the late 1980s and 1990s. We have tried to strike a balance between exciting new developments in medical research and the vast quantity of established fact that needs to be absorbed by today's student. For this reason each chapter attempts to link scientific advances with clinical practice so that the management of disease can be based on sound physiological concepts.

This book is designed for both medical students and practising doctors, and we have tried to produce a detailed but comprehensible text that bridges the gap between the purely introductory and the larger reference works. Tropical diseases have been included, and because the book will have a worldwide distribution we have discussed the presentation of disease as seen in developing countries. Disorders seen only in childhood have been excluded as these are well covered in other texts and would make this book too large. However, there are chapters on intensive care, nutrition, adverse drug reactions, poisoning and environmental medicine, which are often neglected yet play an important role in modern medical practice. There is inevitably an enormous chapter on infectious diseases, but we felt that a description of all infectious agents should be included for quick reference; this chapter also contains basic information on antibiotic chemotherapy and a section on epidemiology and host resistance. A short chapter on genetics, molecular biology and immunology provides the basic principles of these subjects. Today's clinical students will have covered much of this in their preclinical course, but we hope that established practitioners will find it a useful introduction. Specific genetic and immunological disorders are covered in appropriate chapters.

We have concentrated on the management of disease, but within the text have highlighted details of practical procedures and emergency therapy so that this book will be an invaluable companion in clinical practice. The practising clinician can use the book for reference or as a quick and easy guide to the management of an individual patient. Each chapter contains many tables and figures as an aid to learning. There are many cross-references, so that it is easy to move through different parts of the book to pursue different aspects of a particular topic, and repetition has been minimized.

The contributors are all actively engaged in both clinical and research work, so the text has been written by clinicians who are not only in the forefront of medical advance but who also do ward rounds and outpatient clinics. At the time of writing all the contributors were working at St Bartholomew's Hospital, London, and thus combine a unified teaching approach with high academic standards.

We would like to thank all our colleagues for their hard work and co-operation and also our families and the many friends who have supported us during the preparation of this book.

Parveen Kumar
Michael Clark

Acknowledgements

We would like to thank all of our colleagues who have helped us in the preparation of this edition. These include Alison McLean, David Leaver, Steve Patchett, Anne Ballinger, Peter Fairclough, Paul Kelly, Paola Domizio, David Silk, Hugh Mulcahy, Tim Hodgson, Donal Shanahan, Cathy Laversuch, Nigel Stephens, Judy Webb, Rodney Reznik, Peter White and Brian Colvin. Many others have offered valuable advice by correspondence from all over the world. Our daily ward rounds are a source of continuing evidence-based education and we are grateful to our specialist registrars, senior house officers, house officers and our own medical students who continue to ask penetrating questions. We would like to thank our previous contributors for their invaluable contributions: Ted Huskisson, Charles Tomson, John Kirby, Elizabeth Fisher and the late Paul Turner.

We would particularly like to acknowledge the help of our two secretaries, Wendy Draper and Victoria Hollings. The illustrations for Chapter 20 Dermatology were prepared by Medical and Dental Media Resources of St Bartholomew's and the Royal London School of Medicine and Dentistry.

We are grateful for the skill and support of our publishers. Ellen Green and Jennifer Bew have taken us through the final preparations for this edition with patience and unfailing good humour. The hard work of the publishing team, including Sarah Cape, Louise Cook, Carol Parr, Jan Ross and Margaret Macdonald, as well as all of those at Hardlines, has ensured the success of this project. Lastly, we would like to acknowledge the generous help, advice and friendship of Seán Duggan, who saw us through the previous two editions and the beginning of this one.

P.J.K.
M.L.C.

Acknowledgements

Important note

Every effort has been made to check the drug dosages given in this book. However, as it is possible that dosage schedules have been revised, the reader is strongly urged to consult the drug companies' literature before administering any of the drugs listed.

Please see the Appendices, page 1197 — *British National Formulary*.

Key features

Readers will appreciate the following helpful features incorporated into the text:

To help you find your way around the book:

- Contents listed in detail at the beginning of the book
- Colour coding of chapters carried onto each page

To help you find your way around each chapter:

- Contents summary lists at the beginning of each chapter
- Headings at the top of each page:
  - to identify the chapter (left-hand page)
  - to indicate the main topic under discussion (right-hand page)

To help you identify key information:

- Information boxes
- Emergency boxes
- Practical boxes

To make learning easier and more enjoyable:

- colourful line drawings and tables
- text broken up with headings and lists
- further reading incorporated at the appropriate place in the chapter.

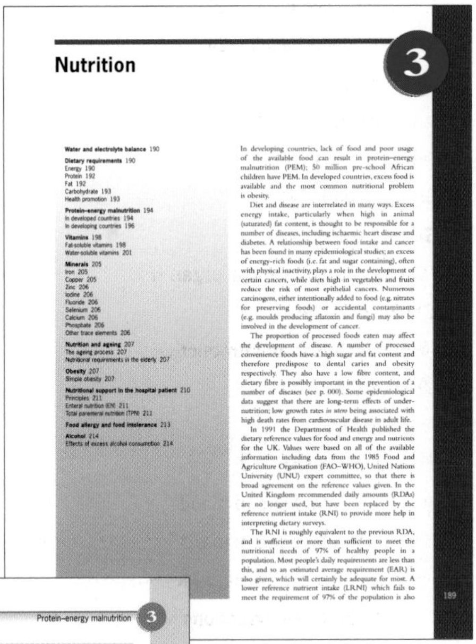

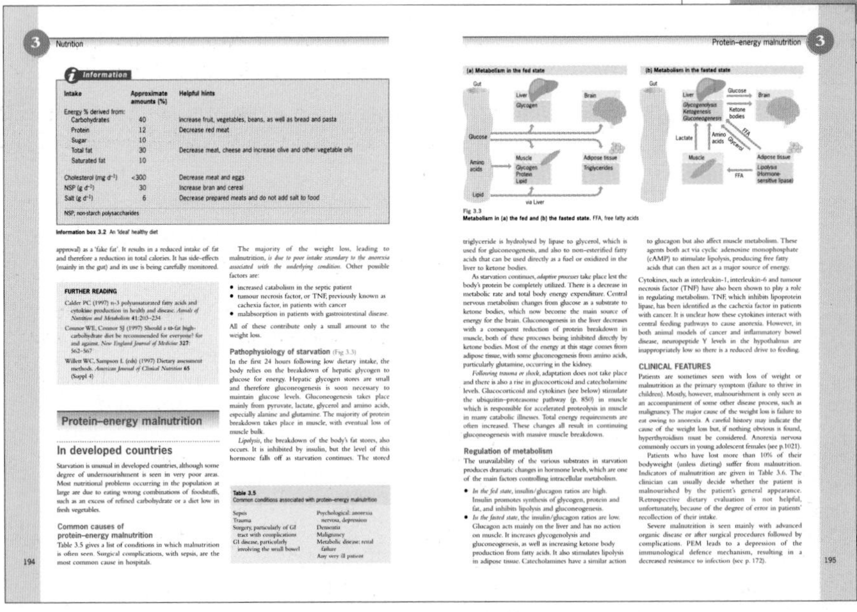

Infectious diseases, tropical medicine and sexually transmitted diseases

1

Epidemiology

Infectious diseases are the most common afflictions of humans and are a major source of morbidity and mortality in both developed and developing countries. Table 1.1 shows estimated morbidity and mortality figures for the common infectious diseases. The prevalence of infectious diseases varies markedly throughout the world and depends on climatic conditions, sanitation, the quality of the water supply, and to some extent the specific disease resistance of the indigenous population at risk. The continuance of infectious diseases in a human population requires:

- reservoirs of infection
- effective modes of transmission.

Reservoirs

Human reservoirs

Human reservoirs are necessary for the agents of those diseases that (under natural conditions) exclusively afflict humans. Specific examples of such diseases are hepatitis A and B, cholera and shigellosis. Many sites in the body act as permanent reservoirs for micro-organisms:

- skin (e.g. *Staphylococcus epidermidis*)
- nasopharynx (e.g. meningococci)
- intestinal tract (e.g. *Giardia*, *Entamoeba histolytica* – both can continue to colonize after clinical recovery).

Viruses may remain in the body for many months or years, notable examples being hepatitis B virus and the herpes viruses.

Table 1.1
League table of infectious diseases worldwide

Disease	Estimated morbidity (cases in thousands per year)	Estimated mortality (deaths in thousands per year)
Diarrhoeal disease	3 000 000–5 000 000	10 000
Respiratory infection	?	5 000
Malaria	270 000	1 500
Measles	80 000	1 000
Schistosomiasis	20 000	1 000
Whooping cough	20 000	400
Neonatal tetanus	?	150

Helminths may remain in the circulation (e.g. schistosomes in the portal vein) or lymphatic system (e.g. filarial worms) for many years, the former constantly producing millions of ova, a high proportion of which are deposited back into the environment.

Animal reservoirs

Animal reservoirs of human disease are important in both the developed and developing worlds. The following are common examples of zoonoses (infections that can be transmitted from animals, except via arthropods, to man):

- from battery-farmed chickens – *Salmonella* or *Campylobacter jejuni* infection
- from domestic cats – *Toxoplasma gondii* infection
- from domestic and wild animals – *Giardia* infection
- from cattle – *Cryptosporidium parvum*, enterohaemorrhagic *E. coli* O157:H7 infection, and prions such as Creutzfeld-Jacob disease (CJD).

Diseases that rely on arthropods for their transmission include malaria, many viruses (e.g. yellow fever and Dengue fever) and rickettsial infections.

Environmental reservoirs

These may also act as a temporary lodging place for some bacteria, viruses and parasites. Water is an important vehicle for enteropathogens in the tropics and in the developed world; water may also be a reservoir of hepatitis A virus. Cysts and oocysts of some protozoa, notably *Giardia* and *Cryptosporidium parvum*, may remain viable despite apparently effective water-purification procedures.

Soil is another source of the agents of human disease, particularly spore-forming bacteria such as *Clostridium* spp. and *Bacillus anthracis*, whose spores can remain viable under suitable climatic conditions for many months.

Transmission

Airborne spread

Some viruses, bacteria and bacterial spores can be carried directly by the wind. Some are generally spread by droplets in the air (e.g. influenza viruses), and other micro-organisms such as *Legionella* are spread by aerosol, characteristically from air-conditioning units.

Spread by direct contact

This includes:

- person-to-person spread, such as through skin infections (impetigo, ringworm and scabies) and sexually transmitted diseases
- faecal–oral spread, particularly amongst children in residential institutions (e.g. shigellosis, giardiasis and hepatitis A)
- inoculation of infection, such as transfusion of blood or blood products containing hepatitis B, C or HIV, or by contaminated needles (drug abusers, medical and paramedical personnel)
- insect bites, such as by mosquitoes (malaria), sandfly (leishmaniasis), Tsetse fly (African trypanosomiasis), ticks (babesiosis, Lyme disease) and bugs (Chagas' disease)
- entry through the skin, which occurs with the larval forms of some helminths that can survive in soil or water (e.g. *Schistosoma*, *Strongyloides* and hookworm).

Spread by food and water

Contaminated food and water are the usual mode of transmission of enteropathogens. Some bacteria, such as *Shigella*, require as few as 100 organisms to initiate infection, whereas others like *Vibrio cholerae* require approximately 10^8 organisms. Preformed bacterial toxins such as Staphylococcal enterotoxin may contaminate food causing 'food poisoning'. Cysts of parasites such as *Giardia* and *Entamoeba histolytica* can survive in water for many months and are relatively resistant to water-treatment procedures. Swimming pools are also recognized to be a source of these parasites.

Spread by fomites

Transmission of infection can occur between persons via an inanimate object, such as bed linen or a book.

FURTHER READING

Hart CA, Trees AJ, Duerden BI (1997) Zoonoses. *Journal of Medical Microbiology* **46**: 4–33.

Principles and basic mechanisms

Pathogenesis

Fig 1.1 summarizes the important steps that occur during the pathogenesis of infection.

Specificity

Some infectious agents are strictly species-selective. Amoebiasis, for example, only naturally affects humans. Even within a species, relative resistance is apparent, such as the decreased susceptibility of Duffy blood group-negative individuals to *Plasmodium vivax* malaria.

Micro-organisms are also highly specific with respect to the organ or tissue they infect. This predilection for specific sites in the body relates partly to the *milieu exterieur* – the immediate environment in which the organism finds itself; for example, anaerobic organisms colonize the highly anaerobic colon, whereas aerobic organisms are generally found in the mouth, pharynx and proximal intestinal tract. Other organisms that clearly show selectivity are:

- *Streptococcus pneumoniae* (respiratory tract)
- *Escherichia coli* (urinary and alimentary tract).

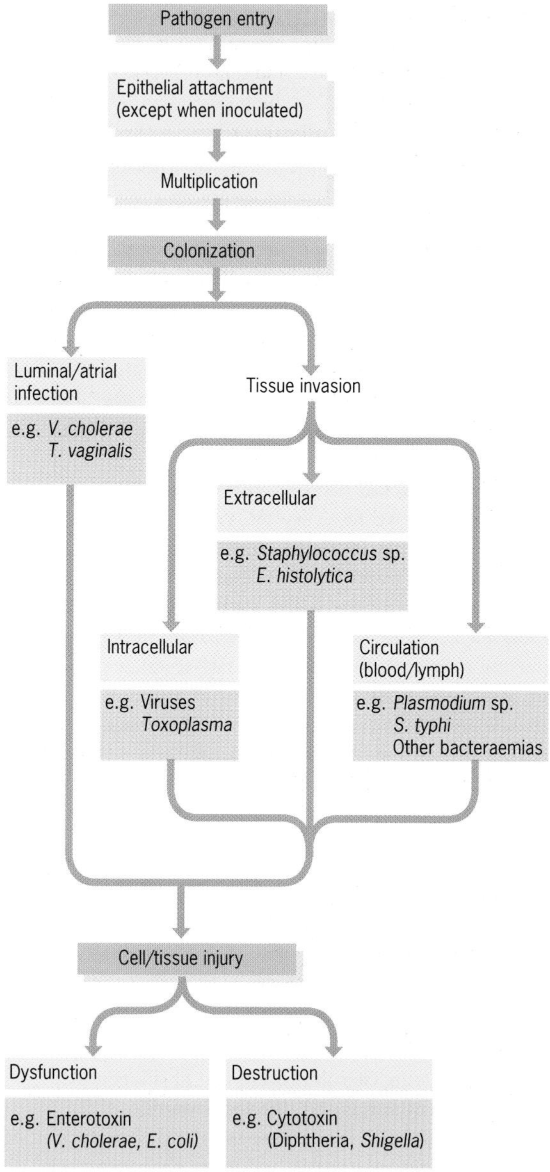

Fig 1.1
The pathogenesis of infection

Even within a species of bacterium such as *E. coli*, different strains will show selectivity towards a particular organ. For example, the enterotoxigenic *E. coli* causes acute diarrhoeal disease, whereas the uropathogenic *E. coli* is responsible for urinary tract infection.

Within an organ a pathogen may show selectivity for a particular cell type. In the intestine, for example, rotavirus predominantly invades and destroys intestinal epithelial cells on the upper portion of the villus, whereas reovirus selectively enters the body through the specialized epithelial cells, known as M cells, that cover the Peyer's patches (see p. 250).

Epithelial attachment

Many bacteria attach to the epithelial substratum by specific organelles called *pili* (or *fimbriae*) that contain a surface lectin(s) – a protein or glycoprotein that recognizes specific sugar residues on the host cell. This family of adhesion molecules is known as *adhesins* (see p. 163). Such is the specificity of this attachment mechanism that it limits enterotoxigenic *E. coli* infection, for example, to certain species. Following attachment some bacteria grow, divide and recruit additional bacteria, which cluster together in pillar or mushroom-like structures (biofilms) etc. These pillars have water channels between for the flow of nutrients and the excretion of waste products. Bacteria in these biofilm communities communicate with each other. These biofilms can be difficult to eradicate, for example, in indwelling catheters.

Some viruses and protozoa (*Plasmodium*, *Entamoeba histolytica*) also interact with their target-cell surface membrane by a similar adhesive mechanism. Other parasites such as hookworm have specific attachment organelles (buccal plates) that firmly grip the intestinal epithelium.

Multiplication and colonization

These follow epithelial attachment. Pathogens may then either remain within the lumen of the organ that they have colonized or invade the tissues.

Invasion

Invasion may result in:

- an *intracellular* location for the pathogen (e.g. viruses, *Toxoplasma*, *Leishmania*, *Plasmodium*)
- an *extracellular* location for the pathogen (e.g. mycobacteria, staphylococci and *Entamoeba histolytica*)
- invasion directly into the blood or lymph circulation (e.g. schistosome larvae, trypanosomes, *Leishmania* and *Plasmodium*)

Once the pathogen is firmly established in its target tissue, a series of events follows that usually culminates in damage to the host.

Tissue dysfunction or damage

The mechanism by which micro-organisms produce disease has been the subject of intensive investigation and a number of well-defined mechanisms have been described.

Exotoxins and endotoxins

Exotoxins have many diverse activities including inhibition of protein synthesis (diphtheria toxin), neurotoxicity (*Clostridium perfringens*, *C. tetani* and *C. botulinum*) and enterotoxicity, which results in intestinal secretion of water and electrolytes (*E. coli*, *V. cholerae*).

Endotoxin is a lipopolysaccharide (LPS) in the cell wall of Gram-negative bacteria. It is responsible for many of the features of septicaemic shock (see p. 838), namely hypotension, fever, intravascular coagulation and, at high doses, death. The effects of endotoxin are mediated predominantly by release of tumour necrosis factor.

Tumour necrosis factor (TNF)

TNF-α is released from a variety of phagocytic cells (macrophages/monocytes) and TNF-β from non-phagocytic cells (lymphocytes, natural killer cells) in response to infections and inflammatory stimuli (Fig 1.2). TNF itself then stimulates the release of a cascade of other mediators involved in inflammation and tissue remodelling, such as interleukin (IL-1 and IL-6), prostaglandins, leukotrienes and corticotrophin. TNF is therefore responsible for many of the effects of an infection.

Tissue invasion

Staphylococcus aureus has tissue-invasive qualities, such as abscess formation and bacteraemia, as well as producing toxins causing diarrhoea and a toxin responsible for a widespread erythema (staphylococcal scalded skin syndrome). Similarly, some pathogenic *E. coli* can produce tissue invasion without production of a specific toxin.

Secondary immunological phenomena

All organisms can initiate secondary immunological mechanisms, such as complement activation, immune complex formation and antibody-mediated cytolysis of cells. The immunological response to infection is described in Chapter 2.

Many infections are self-limiting, and immune and non-immune host defence mechanisms will eventually clear the pathogens. This is generally followed by tissue repair, which may result in complete resolution or leave residual damage.

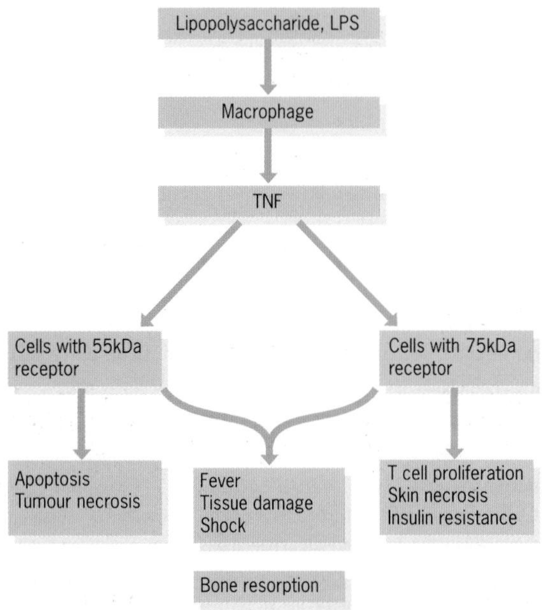

Fig 1.2
Biology of tumour necrosis factor in infection LPS acts on macrophages to stimulate TNF. TNF acts on its two receptors (55 kDa and 75 kDa), producing the effects shown. Both receptors mediate the general effects of fever, tissue damage, shock and bone resorption

Metabolic consequences

Infection not only causes local damage but also has important generalized effects.

Fever

Body temperature is controlled by the thermoregulatory centre in the anterior hypothalamus in the floor of the third ventricle. This centre is sensitive to IL-1 which is released from a variety of cells involved in host defence, primarily blood monocytes and phagocytes, under the influence of microbial exogenous pyrogens such as lipopolysaccharide (LPS). IL-1 acts on the thermoregulatory centre by increasing prostaglandin synthesis. The antipyretic effect of salicylates is brought about, at least in part, through its inhibitory effects on prostaglandin synthetase.

Fever production has a positive effect on the course of infection. However, for every 1°C rise in temperature, there is a 13% increase in resting metabolic rate and oxygen consumption. Fever therefore leads to increased energy requirements at a time when anorexia leads to decreased food intake. The normal compensatory mechanisms in starvation (e.g. mobilization of fat stores) are inhibited in acute infections. This leads to an increase in skeletal muscle breakdown, releasing amino acids, which, via gluconeogenesis, are used to provide energy.

In chronic infection there is time for adaptation. The body is able to utilize fat stores more effectively, and thus weight loss is much slower.

Protein metabolism

During acute infection three major changes occur in protein metabolism:

- There is a diversion of synthesis away from somatic and circulating proteins such as albumin towards acute-phase proteins such as C-reactive protein, haptoglobin, α_1-antitrypsin, caeruloplasmin and fibrinogen.
- Protein synthesis is also directed towards immunoglobulin production and there is production of lymphocytes, neutrophils and other phagocytic cells.
- There is a marked increase in nitrogen losses due to tissue breakdown (see p. 195), which may reach 10–15 g per day.

Mineral metabolism and acid–base balance

Mineral metabolism and acid–base balance are disturbed during acute infection. In general, sodium and water are retained, principally owing to the effects of increased levels of aldosterone and inappropriate secretion of antidiuretic hormone. During the convalescent period after acute infection, a diuresis may occur. Acid–base balance disturbance is common and causes include respiratory alkalosis following tachypnoea related to fever, respiratory acidosis and hypoxaemia associated with pneumonia, and metabolic acidosis associated with septicaemia.

In acute infection these changes are mild and resolve promptly without specific intervention. However, in situations where infections are prolonged and resolution is slow, supportive care may be necessary, particularly with respect to managing nutritional deficits and electrolyte and acid–base disturbances.

Interaction between nutrition and infection

Undernutrition impairs host defence (Fig 1.3). Natural resistance to infection is lowered by alterations in the integrity of body surfaces, the reduced ability to repair epithelia, and the reduction in gastric acid production. In addition, with malnutrition immunological abnormalities are found:

- *Macrophage function* (both tissue and circulating) is impaired.
- *T lymphocyte* function is depressed.
- *Total lymphocyte count* is below 1×10^9 cells/L, which is indicative of a relatively immunocompromised host.
- *Cell-mediated immunity* is in a state of anergy, i.e. the body fails to respond to a recall antigen such as the Mantoux test.
- *Antibody production* is less sensitive to undernutrition, but in severe malnutrition depression in both circulating and secretory immunity are detectable. This is of importance clinically in that vaccination (e.g. against polio) may have to be more aggressive in malnutrition before protective immunity is achieved.
- *Complement levels* fall rapidly in severe acute malnutrition and remain low during long periods of established suboptimal nutritional status. Complement levels have been used as a biochemical marker of nutritional status.

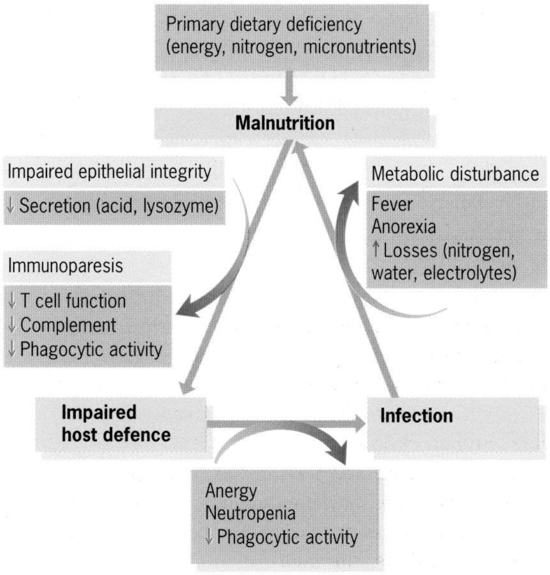

Fig 1.3
Nutrition–infection–host defence: a complex interaction

Host defence and susceptibility

There are a number of normal immune defence mechanisms against pathogens – innate and specific responses are discussed on p. 160.

FURTHER READING

Falkow S (1997) Invasion and intracellular sorting of bacteria: searching for bacterial genes expressed during host/pathogen interactions. *Journal of Clinical Investigations* **100**: 239-243.

Diagnosis (Fig 1.4)

HISTORY

Particular attention should be paid to the following:

- Age of the patient.
- Foreign travel – certain diseases can exist both in the tropics and in Europe (e.g. leishmaniasis, giardiasis). Causes of a fever in the returning traveller to the UK are shown in Table 1.2.
- Immigrants – country of origin.

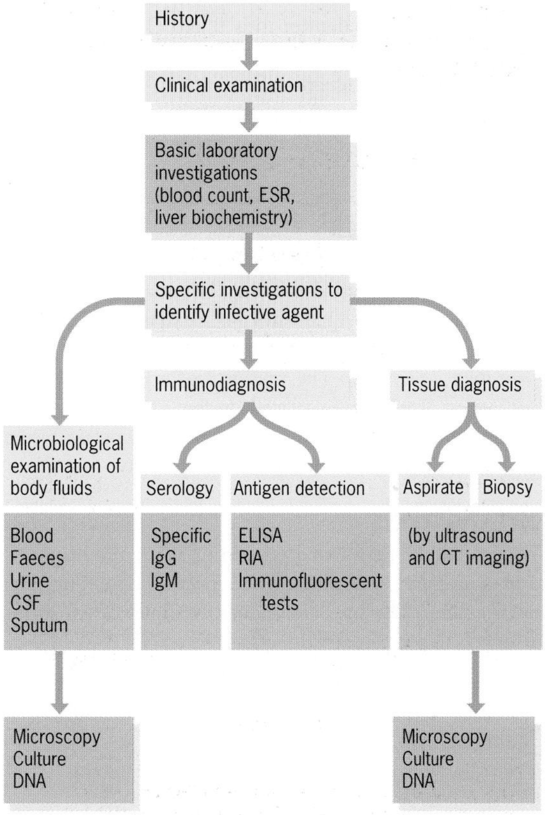

Fig 1.4
An approach to the diagnosis of infectious diseases

Table 1.2
Fever in the traveller returning to the UK

Protozoal infection	Viral infection
Malaria*	Unproven 'viral' infection*
Toxoplasmosis	Hepatitis A**
Amoebic liver abscess	Hepatitis B**
Visceral leishmaniasis	Human immunodeficiency
	Dengue fever
Bacterial infection	Viral meningitis
Pneumonia**	
Dysentery**	**Helminth infection**
Typhoid**	Acute schistosomiasis (Katayama fever)
Urinary tract infection**	
Brucellosis	
Tuberculosis	

* Common; ** frequent.

- Food and water consumed – food poisoning is extremely common.
- Occupation (e.g. sheep farmers – hydatid disease; sewer workers – leptospirosis; leather workers – anthrax)
- Domestic pets (e.g. budgerigars – psittacosis; cats – toxoplasmosis; dogs – *Toxocara canis* infection, rabies).
- Sexual activity – hepatitis B, mixed enteric infections and HIV should be particularly considered in male homosexuals.
- Intravenous drug addiction – consider hepatitis B and C, HIV and pyogenic infections (e.g. staphylococcal).
- Tattooing – consider hepatitis B and C, HIV.
- Injections and transfusions – may act as a route of transmission for infections.
- Immunization history (e.g. BCG).
- Leisure activities (e.g. hunting, watersports – leptospirosis).

CLINICAL FEATURES

A general examination should be performed with particular attention to skin rashes, lymphadenopathy and hepatosplenomegaly. In cases of sexually transmitted diseases the perineum, rectum and vagina should be examined (see p. 98). The presence of a fever is helpful, but less emphasis is now placed on fever patterns because of improved laboratory diagnosis. High swinging fevers are characteristically seen with localized pus.

INVESTIGATIONS

Tests should be performed as appropriate. If the diagnosis is obvious, such as when a measles rash is present, no tests are necessary. The list below gives examples of situations in which tests are useful.

- **Full blood count and film** are usually performed and often give a guide to the type of infection, although the changes are not invariable:
  (a) Polymorphonuclear leucocytosis – bacterial infections
  (b) Neutropenia – viral infections, brucellosis, typhoid, overwhelming septicaemia
  (c) Lymphocytosis – viral infections, whooping cough
  (d) Atypical lymphocytes – infectious mononucleosis
  (e) Eosinophilia – parasitic infections, helminths
  The erythrocyte sedimentation rate (ESR) and C-reactive protein are usually raised.
- **Liver biochemistry** is often slightly abnormal in infections but this is a nonspecific finding. The serum transferases are also raised in hepatitis and other liver infections.
- **Urinanalysis and chest X-ray** should be performed, even in the absence of symptoms and signs.

Further investigations are often required to make the specific diagnosis:

- **Blood culture** is always worthwhile before giving antibiotics.
- **Microscopic examination and culture** of appropriate body fluids (e.g. urine, faeces, CSF, sputum).
- **Viruses** can be identified in the above body fluids by:
  (a) Electron microscopy
  (b) Tissue culture
  (c) Immunological antigen detection techniques (rotavirus)
  (d) Molecular genetic techniques, e.g. polymerase chain reaction.
- **Immunodiagnosis**. Immunological techniques are now available for the identification of:
  (a) *Pathogen-specific antigens* which can be detected in body fluids using polyvalent antisera or monoclonal antibodies
  (b) *Specific serological responses* to infection using indirect immunofluorescence or enzyme-linked immunosorbent assay (ELISA).

A high titre of IgM specific to a pathogen (e.g. hepatitis A or B virus, cytomegalovirus) is diagnostic of a recent infection. In infection a single raised IgG is unhelpful as this indicates only a previous rather than a current infection. However, a rising titre can confirm the diagnosis (e.g. in brucellosis or *Mycoplasma* infection).

These immunological techniques are particularly useful in the identification of pathogens that are difficult to culture by standard microbiological techniques or intracellular pathogens that require tissue culture.

- **Tissue diagnosis** – biopsy/aspiration with isolation of pathogen:
  (a) Bone marrow/liver biopsy for generalized infections such as tuberculosis, leishmaniasis
  (b) Rarely, if the above technique is negative, splenic aspiration for leishmaniasis
  (c) Transbronchial biopsy for *Pneumocystis carinii*, tuberculosis.
- **DNA/RNA-based techniques**. Many genes encoding virulence factors and other specific proteins of pathogenic micro-organisms have been cloned and sequenced. From this information DNA probes have been constructed and used for the detection of pathogen-specific DNA in body fluids or tissue. The use

of amplification techniques like the polymerase chain reaction has increased the sensitivity of this approach.

- **Imaging procedures** – ultrasound and CT scan (with needle aspiration) for abscesses in liver, lung, brain or abdomen. Magnetic resonance imaging may assist abscess localization in the central nervous system and bone. Abscesses can also be imaged by radionuclide scanning using radiolabelled neutrophils or radiolabelled ciprofloxacin.

Pyrexia of unknown origin (PUO)

A major diagnostic problem is the patient who has a pyrexia, either intermittent or continuous, that lasts for three weeks or more and in whom routine investigations have failed to reveal a cause. PUO (or FUO – fever of unknown origin) may merely be an unusual presentation of a common disease. Information box 1.1 shows some of the common causes of PUO.

Age is an important pointer, since cancer and the connective tissue diseases are more common in the elderly.

Immunocompromised individuals are at particular risk of infectious disease and often present with a particularly unusual spectrum of infections.

An aggressive approach to the diagnosis of PUO is justified since there is a good chance that determination of a specific diagnosis will influence management and result in curative treatment. It is always worth repeating the history and examination because new signs may have evolved since the patient's initial admission to hospital. All drug therapy should be reassessed and, if possible, stopped.

INVESTIGATIONS

First-line investigations such as a full blood count, blood culture, urinalysis, routine blood chemistry and chest X-ray should be repeated.

Other investigations

- **Imaging** with ultrasound, CT or MRI is particularly valuable in revealing primary and secondary neoplastic diseases and for showing occult abscesses.
- **Aspiration or needle biopsy** under imaging control provides a cyto/histological diagnosis.
- **Laparoscopy** may be required to confirm a gynaecological cause, such as pelvic inflammatory disease, multiple peritoneal metastases or tuberculous peritonitis.
- **Needle biopsy of the liver** (histology and culture) may be required to confirm granulomatous hepatitis, tuberculosis or metastatic cancer.
- **Radionuclide scanning** gallium-59 or ciprofloxacin-labelled polymorphs, or indium-111 or technetium-labelled leucocytes, can localize an abscess.

Septicaemia (sepsis syndrome)

The term *bacteraemia* refers to the transient presence of organisms in the blood (generally without causing symptoms) as a result of local infection or penetrating injury.

The term *septicaemia*, on the other hand, is usually reserved for when bacteria or fungi are actually multiplying in the blood, usually with the production of severe systemic symptoms such as fever and hypotension.

Information

Infection (40%)
Pyogenic abscess (e.g. liver)
Tuberculosis
Urinary infection
Biliary infection
Subacute infective endocarditis
EBV infection
CMV infection
Q fever
Toxoplasmosis
Brucellosis
Septic arthritis in prosthetic joint

Cancer (30%)
Lymphomas
Leukaemia
Solid tumours; e.g.
  Renal carcinoma
  Hepatocellular carcinoma
  Pancreatic carcinoma

Immunogenic (20%)
Drugs
Connective tissue and autoimmune diseases; e.g.
  Rheumatoid disease
  Systemic lupus erythematosus
  Polyarteritis nodosa
  Polymyalgia/cranial arteritis
Sarcoidosis

Miscellaneous
Thyrotoxicosis
Chronic liver disease
Inflammatory bowel disease
Familial Mediterranean fever
Kawasaki disease

Factitious (1–5%)
Switching thermometers
Injection of pyrogenic material

Remain unknown (5–9%)

Information box 1.1 Some causes of pyrexia of unknown origin (PUO)

Pyaemia describes the serious situation when, in a septicaemia, organisms and neutrophil polymorphs embolize to many sites in the body, causing abscesses, notably in the lungs, liver and brain.

Severe septicaemia (septic shock) has an extremely high mortality and demands immediate attention. It is discussed on p. 833.

CAUSES

In many cases of septicaemia the focus of infection is not apparent. Such patients are generally elderly, undernourished or suffering from chronic disease, particularly alcoholic cirrhosis and diabetes.

The common sites of infection and infective agents responsible for septicaemia are shown in Tables 1.3 and 1.4. Pneumococcus is a common cause of septicaemia in children, whereas in neonates Gram-negative rods and group B streptococci are the most likely aetiological agents. *Neisseria gonorrhoeae* is a common cause of septicaemia in young adults, but it is usually mild without serious effects. Intravenous drug abusers frequently suffer bacteraemia and septicaemia often caused by *Staph. aureus*, *Pseudomonas* and *Serratia*.

Table 1.3
Septicaemia in a previously healthy adult

Site of origin	Usual pathogen(s)
Skin	*Staphylococcus aureus* and other Gram-positive cocci
Urinary tract	*Escherichia coli* and other aerobic Gram-negative rods
Respiratory tract	*Streptococcus pneumoniae*
Gallbladder or bowel	*Streptococcus faecalis*, *Escherichia coli* and other Gram-negative rods
	Bacteroides fragilis
Pelvic organs	*Neisseria gonorrhoeae*, anaerobes

Table 1.4
Septicaemia in hospitalized patients

Clinical problem	Usual pathogen(s)
Urinary catheter	*Escherichia coli*, *Klebsiella*, *Proteus*, *Serratia*, *Pseudomonas*
Intravenous catheter	*Staphylococcus aureus* and *Staphylococcus epidermidis*, *Klebsiella*, *Pseudomonas*, *Candida albicans*
Peritoneal catheter	*Staphylococcus epidermidis*
Post surgery:	
Wound infection	*Staphylococcus aureus*, *Escherichia coli*, *anaerobes* (depending on site)
Deep infection	Depends on anatomical location
Burns	Gram-positive cocci, *Pseudomonas*, *Candida albicans*
Immunocompromised patients	Any of the above

CLINICAL FEATURES

Fever, rigors and hypotension are the cardinal features of septic shock. However, the illness may be preceded by less specific symptoms such as headache, lethargy, apprehension and subtle changes in conscious level. Other clinical features and their pathogenesis are shown in Table 1.5.

INVESTIGATIONS

Septicaemia is almost always treated initially on the basis of a clinical diagnosis after appropriate specimens have been sent to the laboratory. Probable origins of infection and likely pathogens must be sought on the basis of a careful history and examination. The type of infection will clearly differ in hospitalized and otherwise previously healthy adults (see Tables 1.3 and 1.4). Body fluids or other specimens (blood, urine, CSF, tissue or abscess aspirates) should be submitted to full microbiological examination. Imaging investigations such as ultrasonography and CT scan may be required.

Catheters or cannulae, which might be sources of infection, should be removed and sent for culture.

TREATMENT

Management of septic shock is discussed on p. 842. Antibiotic therapy should be commenced immediately. If the organism and its antibiotic sensitivities are unknown, a combination of drugs should be chosen to cover the likely pathogens. If there is an obvious site of skin sepsis, drugs such as flucloxacillin (1 g i.v. six-hourly) plus benzylpenicillin (to cover β-haemolytic streptococci) should be used. In severe sepsis with osteomyelitis or endocarditis, an aminoglycoside to cover *Staph. aureus* should be used. If bowel sepsis is suspected, then a broader-spectrum drug of the cephalosporin group (e.g. cefuroxime/cefotaxime/ceftazidime) would be advisable. In the absence of any helpful clinical guidelines, a combination of a penicillin drug that is active against *Pseudomonas* such as piperacillin (200–300 mg kg^{-1} daily) with an aminoglycoside such as gentamicin (3–5 mg kg^{-1} daily in divided doses every eight hours) should be given. Metronidazole (1 g per rectum every eight hours) is often

Table 1.5
Special features of septic shock

Clinical feature	Cause and effect
Hypotension	Liberation of bacterial endotoxin (cell-wall lipopolysaccharide) that reduces vascular tone and increases permeability
Pulmonary oedema and acute respiratory distress syndrome (ARDS)	Increased permeability of the alveolar capillary endothelium, impaired gas exchange and hypoxia
Disseminated intravascular coagulation (DIC)	Activation of blood coagulation by endothelial damage, endotoxins and immune complexes

added to provide additional cover against anaerobic organisms. Steroids should not be used for the treatment of septic shock.

FURTHER READING

Arnow PM, Flaherty JP (1997) Fever of unknown origin. *Lancet* **350**: 575–580.

Humar A, Keystone J (1996) Evaluating fever in travellers returning from tropical countries. *British Medical Journal* **312**: 953-956.

Antimicrobial chemotherapy

Principles

Widespread and often inappropriate use of antibiotics has led to increasing numbers of organisms with multiple drug resistance. Antibiotics are not required for minor infections.

Although the majority of antibiotics are relatively safe drugs, hypersensitivity reactions can occur and important toxic effects are seen with incorrect dosages and in the presence of other disease states, notably renal disease. In addition, antibacterial therapy may result in secondary yeast or fungal infection or may facilitate the growth of a second bacterial pathogen, such as *Clostridium difficile*, an important cause of antibiotic-associated colitis.

Choice of drug

Blind therapy

Antimicrobial therapy is often begun before the organism is identified and its antibiotic sensitivities known. The choice of drug(s) is therefore dependent on a clinical diagnosis and a knowledge of the organisms likely to be involved in a given situation. Before beginning 'blind' therapy it is essential to obtain appropriate body fluids or other specimens for microbiological examination. Adjustments to the antibiotic regimen can then be made, if necessary, when antibiotic sensitivities are available. Consultation with microbiologists is helpful.

Spectrum of activity

The spectrum of antibacterial activity of the drug chosen should ideally be as narrow as possible, as it will then have fewer detrimental effects on the normal bacterial flora of the host. 'Blind' therapy, however, by necessity generally covers a broader spectrum than required.

Bactericidal versus bacteriostatic

In the majority of infections there is no firm evidence that bactericidal drugs (penicillins, cephalosporins, aminoglycosides) are more effective than bacteriostatic drugs, but it is generally considered important to use the former in the treatment of bacterial endocarditis and in patients in whom host defence mechanisms are compromised, particularly in those with neutropenia.

Patient factors

In addition to age and pregnancy, the following factors should be considered.

- *The site of infection.* The chosen drug must be able to gain access to the part of the body involved. The brain, eye, biliary tract, prostate and loculated abscesses are inaccessible to many drugs.
- *Renal and hepatic function.* Impaired renal or hepatic function necessitates a major modification of the dose regimen or even complete avoidance of certain drugs. Care should be taken when using aminoglycosides, ticarcillin, flucytosine and some antimycobacterial agents in patients with renal impairment. Other drugs, such as nalidixic acid and tetracycline, should be avoided altogether.

Dose and duration of therapy

This is influenced by the type of infection to be treated and the age of the patient. Bacterial endocarditis and deep-seated abscesses (e.g. in brain or lung) generally require high-dose therapy for several weeks.

With the more potent drugs, only short courses or even single doses may be required. Examples are uncomplicated urinary tract infection or gonorrhoea.

Route of administration

Some drugs (e.g. some of the cephalosporins) are available only as intravenous preparations, but many antibiotics are well absorbed by the oral route and in the absence of severe infection such as septicaemia there is no advantage to the patient for therapy to be administered by the more expensive parenteral route. Patient compliance must, however, be taken into account.

Monitoring

In serious infections (e.g. infective endocarditis), monitoring of circulating drug concentrations is routinely performed for assessing efficacy of treatment. Drug concentrations can be measured directly in serum, but the efficacy of therapy is usually determined by serum bactericidal assay just before and at a standard time after administration of antibiotics. The highest dilution of serum that completely kills the causative organism can then be determined. The clinical value of serum bactericidal assays is still debated.

Monitoring for toxicity is particularly relevant for the aminoglycoside antibiotics. Concentrations are determined immediately before ('trough' levels) and usually one hour after ('peak' levels) of the drug. High 'trough' levels of >2 mg mL^{-1} are considered to be the most important factor in causing the ototoxicity and nephrotoxicity commonly seen with these agents. The 'peak' level should be 5–10 g mL^{-1} to be therapeutically effective.

Antibiotic chemoprophylaxis

This is required in certain disease states (Table 1.6).

Mechanisms of resistance to antimicrobial agents

Antibiotics act at different sites of the bacterium. For example penicillins, cephalosporins and vancomycin act on the cell wall, erythromycin and aminoglycosides affect protein synthesis, rifampicin affects RNA synthesis, and the quinolones affect DNA synthesis; sulphonamides and trimethoprin are folic acid anatagonists; polymyxins disrupt the cell membrane and amphotericin inhibits sterol synthesis.

Resistance to an antibiotic can be the result of:

- failure to reach the target site, for example because impaired permeability causes a failure to penetrate the outer bacterial membrane (e.g. penicillins in Gram-negative bacteria)
- enzyme inactivation (e.g. β-lactamase enzymes – see p. 11)
- alteration of the target site (e.g. single point mutations in *E. coli* lead to acquired resistance – see below).

The development or acquisition of resistance to an antibiotic by bacteria invariably involves a mutation at a single point in a gene or transfer of genetic material from another organism (Fig 1.5).

Larger fragments of DNA may be introduced into a bacterium either by transfer of 'naked' DNA or via a bacteriophage (a virus) DNA vector. Both the former (transformation) and the latter (transduction) are dependent on integration of this new DNA into the recipient chromosomal DNA. This requires a high degree of homology between the donor and recipient chromosomal DNA.

Finally, antibiotic resistance can be transferred from one bacterium to another by conjugation, when extrachromosomal DNA (a plasmid) containing the resistance factor (R factor) is passed from one cell into another during direct contact. Transfer of such R factor plasmids can occur between unrelated bacterial strains and involve large amounts of DNA.

Table 1.6
Antibiotic chemoprophylaxis (see *British National Formulary*)

Clinical problem	Aim	Drug regimen
Rheumatic fever	To prevent recurrence and further cardiac damage	Phenoxymethylpenicillin 250 mg twice-daily, or sulphadiazine 1 g when penicillin-allergic
Infective endocarditis	To prevent infection on abnormal, prosthetic or homograft heart valves, patent ductus or septal defect (see 'special' risk patients)	*Dental/upper respiratory tract procedures* (LA) Oral amoxycillin 3 g one hour before procedure For penicillin-allergic individuals, clindamycin 600 mg one hour before procedure Chlorhexidine mouthwash may also be used *Dental under GA* At induction: i.v. amoxycillin 1 g Six hours later: oral amoxycillin 500 mg **'Special' risk patients only** (prosthetic valves and/or previous endocarditis): *Gastrointestinal, obstetric or gynaecological, dental (GA) and genito-urinary procedures* At induction i.v. amoxycillin 1 g i.v. gentamicin 120 mg Six hours after procedure, amoxycillin 500 mg (vancomycin for penicillin-allergic patient)
Splenectomy/spleen malfunction	To prevent serious pneumococcal sepsis	Phenoxymethyl penicillin 500 mg 12 hourly
Meningitis:		
Due to meningococci	To prevent infection in close contacts	Adults: rifampicin 600 mg twice-daily for 2 days Children < 1 month: 5 mg kg^{-1} Children > 1 month: 10 mg kg^{-1}
Due to *H. influenzae* type b	To reduce nasopharyngeal carriage and prevent infection in close contacts	Adults: rifampicin 100 mg daily for 4 days Children: 20 mg kg^{-1}
Tuberculosis	To prevent infection in exposed (close contacts) tuberculin-negative individuals, infants of infected mothers and immunosuppressed patients	Oral isoniazid 5 mg kg^{-1} daily for 6–12 months
Malaria	To prevent infection	Oral chloroquine 400–500 mg as a single dose each week, and/or proguanil 200 mg daily 2 weeks before and for 4 weeks after leaving endemic area Where chloroquine resistance occurs, mefloquine 250 mg once a week – but get advice

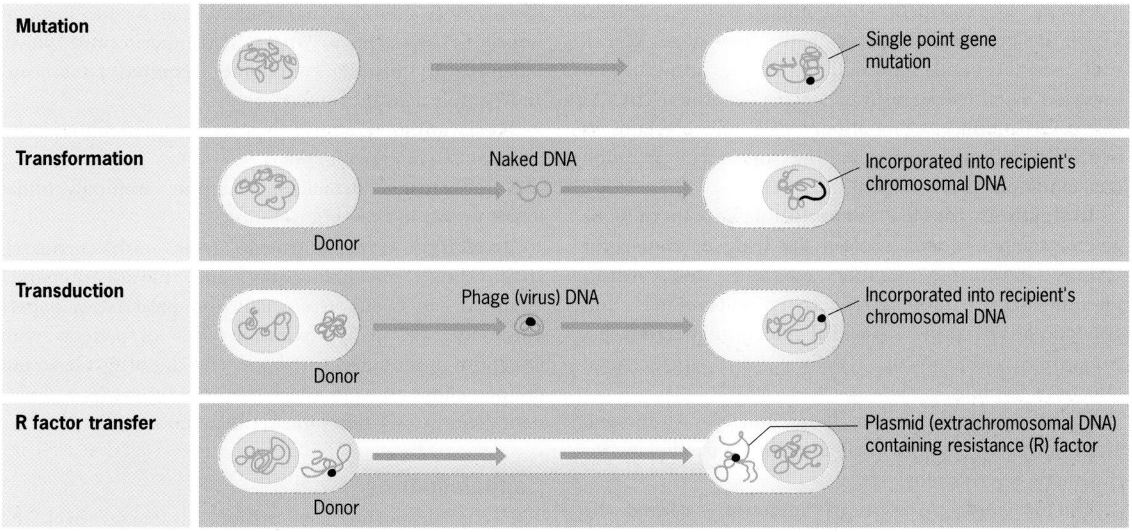

Fig 1.5
Some mechanisms for the development of resistance to antimicrobial drugs. These involve either a single point mutation or transfer of genetic materials from another organism (transformation, transduction or R factor transfer)

Transformation is probably the least clinically important mechanism, whereas transduction and R factor transfer are probably the most important for the sudden emergence of multiple antibiotic resistance in a single bacterium. Increasing resistance to many antibiotics has developed (Table 1.7)

Antibacterial drugs

β-Lactams

Penicillins (Table 1.8)

Structure. Penicillins, like cephalosporins, have a β-lactam ring. Penicillins are fused to a thiazolidine ring (Fig 1.6).

Relatively minor changes to the side-chain of benzylpenicillin render the phenoxymethyl derivative acid resistant and allow it to be absorbed well when given orally. The presence of an amino group in the phenyl radical of benzylpenicillin increases the antimicrobial spectrum of the native penicillin and makes it active against both Gram-negative and Gram-positive organisms. More extensive modification of the side-chain (e.g. as in flucloxacillin) renders the drug insensitive to bacterial penicillinase. This is useful in treating infections caused by penicillinase also called β-lactamase-producing staphylococci.

Mechanisms of action. Penicillins block the terminal cross-linking reaction (between alanine and glycine) of bacterial cell wall mucopeptide formation. Penicillins and other β-lactam antibiotics bind to and

Table 1.7 Some bacteria that have developed resistance to common antibiotics

Pathogen	Previously sensitive to:
Streptococcus pneumoniae	Penicillin, erythromycin, tetracycline
Streptococcus pyogenes	Erythromycin, tetracycline
Streptococcus aureus	Penicillin, methicillin, ciprofloxacin
Neisseria gonorrhoeae	Penicillin, ciprofloxacin
Haemophilus influenzae	Amoxycillin, chloramphenicol
Enterobacteria	Amoxycillin, trimethoprim vancomycin
Salmonella spp.	Amoxycillin, sulphonamides
Shigella spp.	Amoxycillin, trimethoprim, tetracycline
Pseudomonas aeruginosa	Gentamicin

Table 1.8
Classification of penicillins

GROUP 1: Benzylpenicillin and its long-acting parenteral relatives
Benzylpenicillin*
Benethamine penicillin*
Benzathine penicillin*
Clemizole penicillin*
Procaine penicillin

GROUP 2: Oral alternatives of benzylpenicillin
Azidocillin*
Phenoxymethylpenicillin (penicillin V)

GROUP 3: β-lactamase-stable penicillins
Cloxacillin
Flucloxacillin
Oxacillin*
Methicillin*
Nafcillin*

GROUP 4: Extended-spectrum penicillins
Ampicillin, pivampicillin, talampicillin*
Amoxycillin
Mecillinam*, pivmecillinam*

GROUP 5: Pencillins active against *Pseudomonas*
Azlocillin, mezlocillin*, piperacillin, ticarcillin

GROUP 6: β-lactamase-resistant penicillins
Temocillin**

* not available in the UK; ** for Gram-negative bacilli only

inactivate specific penicillin-binding proteins (PBPs) which are peptidases involved in the final stages of cell wall assembly and remodelling during growth and division. Methicillin-resistant *Staph. aureus* (MRSA) (see p. 21) produce a low-affinity PBP which retains its peptidase activity even in the presence of high concentrations of methicillin.

Indications for use. Benzylpenicillin can only be given parenterally and is often the drug of choice for serious infections, notably infective endocarditis, pneumococcal, meningococcal, streptococcal and gonococcal infections, clostridial infections (tetanus, gas gangrene), actinomycosis, anthrax, and spirochaetal infections (syphilis, yaws).

Phenoxymethylpenicillin (penicillin V) is an oral preparation that is chiefly used as maintenance therapy for rheumatic fever prophylaxis.

Flucloxacillin is used in infections caused by penicillinase-producing staphylococci.

Ampicillin is susceptible to penicillinase, but its antimicrobial activity includes Gram-negative organisms such as *Salmonella, Shigella, E. coli, H. influenzae* and *Proteus*. It is useful in the treatment of urinary tract and upper respiratory tract infections. Amoxycillin has a similar sphere of activity to ampicillin, but is better absorbed when given by mouth.

Clavulanic acid is a powerful inhibitor of many bacterial β-lactamases and when given in combination with an otherwise susceptible agent such as amoxycillin (co-amoxiclav) or ticarcillin can broaden the spectrum of activity of the drug.

The extended-spectrum penicillin ticarcillin is active against *Pseudomonas* infection and the acylureidopenicillin derivatives (azlocillin and pipera-cillin) have increased activity against Gram-negative organisms, including *Pseudomonas*, compared with other penicillins. However, they are susceptible to staphylococcal β-lactamases and are therefore not reliable for treating staphylococcal disease. The combination of piperacillin with tazobactam

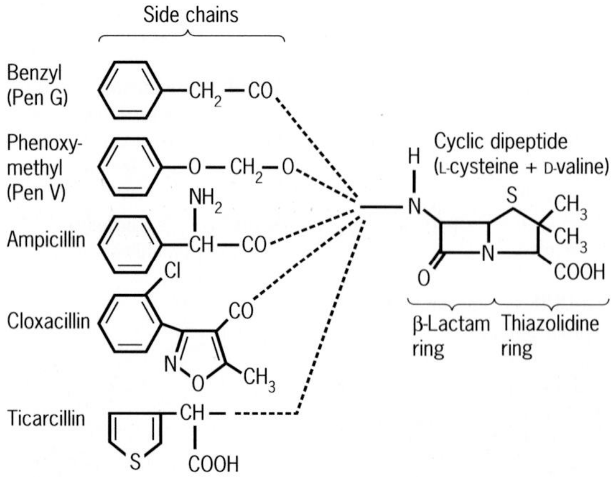

Fig 1.6
The structure of penicillins

(β-lactamase inhibitor) has resulted in an agent (Tazocin) which is effective in appendicitis, peritonitis, pelvic inflammatory disease, community acquired pneumonia and complicated skin infections.

Resistance. Bacteria producing penicillinase are resistant to some penicillins.

Interactions. Penicillins inactivate aminoglycosides when mixed in the same solution.

Toxicity. Hypersensitivity (skin rash, urticaria, anaphylaxis), encephalopathy and tubulo-interstitial nephritis can occur. Ampicillin also produces a hypersensitivity rash in approximately 90% of patients with infectious mononucleosis who receive this drug. Generally, the penicillins are very safe. Co-amoxiclav causes a cholestatic jaundice six times greater than amoxycillin.

Cephalosporins (Fig 1.7)

The cephalosporins have major advantages over the penicillins in that they are innately resistant to staphylococcal penicillinases and have a broader range of activity that includes both Gram-negative and Gram-positive organisms.

Mechanism of action. Like penicillins, cephalosporins inhibit bacterial cell wall synthesis.

Indications for use (Table 1.9). These potent broad-spectrum antibiotics are useful for the treatment of serious systemic infections, particularly when the precise nature of the infection is unknown. They are commonly used for serious postoperative sepsis and in immunocompromised patients, particularly during treatment of leukaemia and other malignancies.

Resistance. Cephalosporins generally resist the action of β-lactamase-producing bacteria. Penicillin-resistant pneumococci are developing and will be resistant to oral cephalosporins. Ceftazidime (and cefpirome) are active against *Pseudomonas aeruginosa*.

Interactions. Increased nephrotoxicity is seen when cephalosporins are used in conjunction with other nephrotoxic antibiotics such as aminoglycosides and some diuretics.

Toxicity. The toxicity is the same as with penicillin. Some patients (about 10%) are allergic to both groups of drugs. The early cephalosporins caused proximal tubule damage, although the newer derivatives have fewer nephrotoxic effects.

Monobactams

Aztreonam is the only member of this class currently available.

Structure. Aztreonam is a synthetic analogue of an antibiotic found in soil bacteria (Fig 1.8), with a novel structure containing a β-lactam ring in the core configuration.

Its mechanism of action is by inhibition of bacterial cell wall synthesis. It is resistant to most β-lactamases and does not induce β-lactamase production.

Cephalosporin

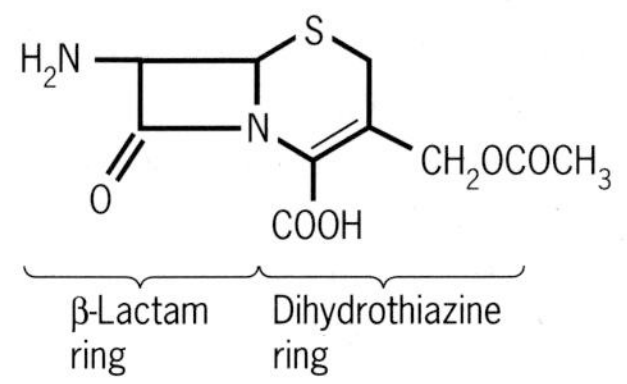

Fig 1.7
The structure of a cephalosporin

Monobactams

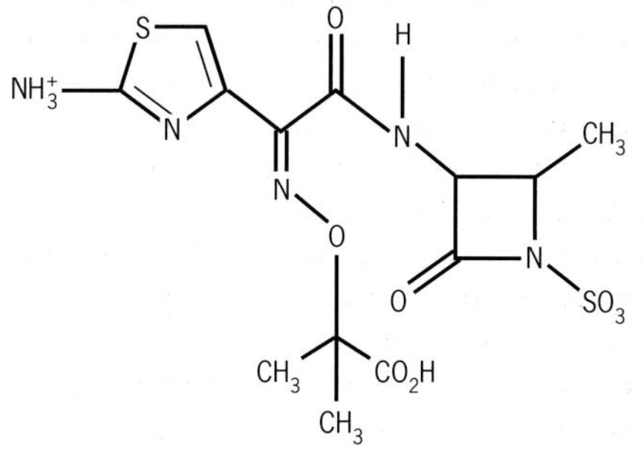

Aztreonam

Fig 1.8
The structure of monobactams

Indications for use. Aztreonam's spectrum of activity is limited to aerobic Gram-negative bacilli, including *Pseudomonas aeruginosa* – thus to some extent resembling aminoglycosides. With the exception of urinary tract infections, aztreonam should be used in combination with metronidazole (for anaerobes) and an agent active against Gram-positive cocci (a penicillin or erythromycin). It is a useful alternative to aminoglycosides in combination therapy.

Toxicity is as for β-lactam antibiotics.

Carbapenems

N-Formimidoyl thienamycin (imipenem) and two other semi-synthetic carbapenems, biapenem and meropenem, are available for clinical use.

Structure. Imipenem has a novel structure with a carbon replacing the sulphur in the five-membered ring (Fig 1.9). Meropenem has a unique side-chain which increases its activity against Gram-positive bacteria as well as *Ps. aeruginesa*. All are highly resistant to β-lactamases.

Mechanism of action. This is by inhibition of bacterial cell wall synthesis. Imipenem is partially inactivated in the kidney by enzymatic inactivation and is therefore administered in combination with cilastatin.

Indications for use. The carbapenems have the broadest spectrum of activity of all known antibiotics.

Table 1.9
Some examples of cephalosporins

	Activity	Use
First generation		
Cephalexin (oral)	Gram-positive cocci and Gram-negative organisms	Urinary tract infections
Cephradine (oral)		Penicillin allergy
Second generation		
Cefuroxime	Extended spectrum	Prophylaxis and treatment of Gram-negative infections and mixed aerobic-anaerobic infections
Cephamandole	More effective than first-generation against *E. coli*, *Klebsiella* spp. and *Proteus mirabilis*, but less effective against Gram-positive organisms	
Cefoxitin		
Cefaclor (oral)		
Cefuroxime (oral)		
Third generation		
Cefotaxime	Broad-spectrum	Especially severe infection with Enterobacteriaceae, *Pseudomonas aeruginosa* (ceftazidime), cefpirome, and *Neisseria gonorrhoeae*, Lyme disease (ceftriaxone)
Ceftazidime	More potent against aerobic Gram-negative bacteria than first or second generation	
Cefpirome		
Cefodizime		
Ceftriaxone		
Cefpodoxime (oral)		
Cefixime (oral)		
Ceftibutin (oral)		

They are active against Gram-positive cocci (with a similar potency to penicillins), Gram-negative organisms and anaerobes (similar potency to metronidazole and clindamycin). They should only rarely be used for community-acquired infection; the main indications being nosocomial infections when multiple-resistant Gram-negative bacilli or mixed aerobe and anaerobe infections are suspected.

Toxicity. This is similar to that of β-lactam antibiotics. Nausea, vomiting and diarrhoea occur in less than 5% of cases. There is no evidence of nephrotoxicity or coagulation abnormalities.

Aminoglycosides

Structure. These antibiotics are derived from *Streptomyces spp.* and are polycationic compounds of amino sugars (Fig 1.10).

Mechanism of action. Aminoglycosides interrupt bacterial protein synthesis by inhibiting ribosomal function (messenger and transfer RNA).

Indications for use. Streptomycin is bactericidal for susceptible organisms but is not often used except for tuberculosis. Neomycin is used only for the topical treatment of eye and skin infections and orally for preoperative 'bowel sterilization' and in the management of portosystemic encephalopathy. Even though it is poorly absorbed, prolonged oral administration can produce toxic effects such as ototoxicity.

Gentamicin and tobramycin are given parenterally. They are highly effective against many Gram-negative organisms including *Pseudomonas*. They are synergistic with a penicillin against *Streptococcus faecalis*. The newer aminoglycosides, netilmicin and amikacin, have a similar spectrum of antibacterial activity but are generally resistant to the aminoglycoside-inactivating enzymes produced by some bacteria. Their use should be restricted to gentamicin-resistant organisms.

Resistance. Some bacteria produce phosphorylating, adenylating or acetylating enzymes that inactivate aminoglycoside antibiotics. These enzymes are coded for and transferred by R factors (extrachromosomal DNA).

Interactions. Enhanced nephrotoxicity occurs with other nephrotoxic drugs, ototoxicity with some diuretics, and neuromuscular blockade with curariform drugs.

Toxicity. This is dose-related. Aminoglycosides are nephrotoxic and ototoxic (vestibular and auditory), particularly in the elderly. Blood levels must be checked.

Tetracyclines

Structure. These are bacteriostatic drugs possessing a four-ring hydronaphthacene nucleus (Fig 1.11). Variation of the native compound is obtained by different substitutions to give, for example, oxytetracycline and chlortetracycline, or doxycycline.

Mechanism of action. Tetracyclines inhibit bacterial protein synthesis by interrupting ribosomal function (transfer RNA).

Indications for use. Tetracyclines are active against Gram-positive and Gram-negative bacteria but their use is now limited partly owing to increasing bacterial resistance. A tetracycline is used for the treatment of acne and rosacea. Tetracyclines are also active against *V. cholerae*, *Rickettsia*, *Mycoplasma*, *Coxiella burnetii*, *Chlamydia* and *Brucella*.

Resistance. Some bacteria possess reduced cell permeability to tetracycline, which is coded for by an R factor (see Fig 1.5). Resistance is now found with *S. pneumoniae* and *Shigella* spp.

Interactions. The efficacy of tetracyclines is reduced by antacids and oral iron-replacement therapy.

Toxicity. Tetracyclines are generally safe drugs, but they may enhance established or incipient renal failure, although doxycycline is safer than others in this group. They cause brown discoloration of growing teeth, and thus these drugs are not given to children or pregnant women. Photosensitivity can occur.

N-formimidoyl thienamycin (imipenem)

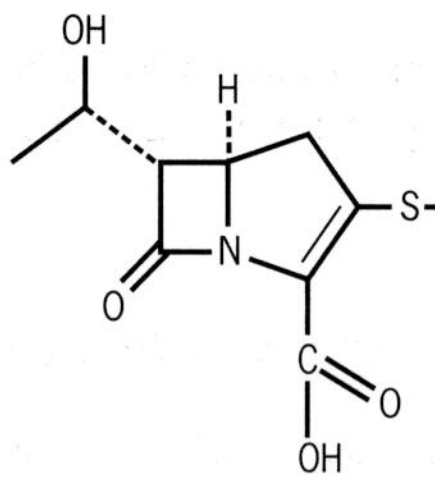

Fig 1.9
The structure of imipenem

Aminoglycoside

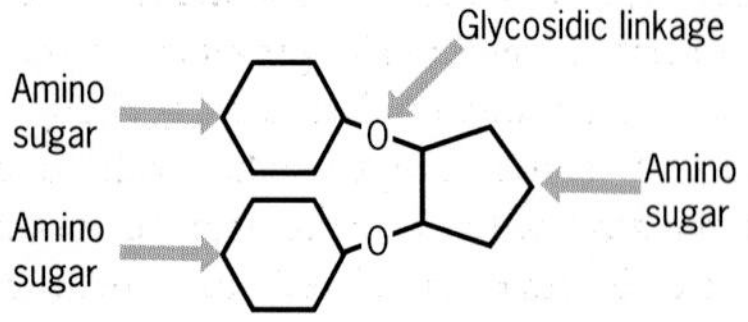

Fig 1.10
The structure of an aminoglycoside

Tetracycline

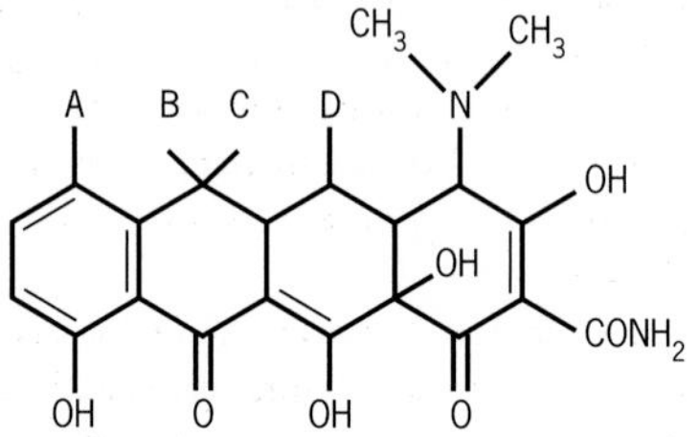

Fig 1.11
The structure of tetracycline. Substitution of CH_3, OH or H at positions A to D produces variants of tetracycline

Macrolides

Erythromycin

Structure. Erythromycin consists of a lactone ring with unusual sugar side-chains.

Mechanism of action. Erythromycin inhibits protein synthesis by interrupting ribosomal function.

Indications for use. Erythromycin has a similar (but not identical) antibacterial spectrum to penicillin and is useful in individuals with penicillin allergy. It can be given orally or parenterally. It is included in the treatment regimen of all pneumonias as many are due to *Mycoplasma*. It is also effective in the treatment of infections due to *Bordetella pertussis* (whooping cough), *Legionella*, *Campylobacter*, *Chlamydia*, *Coxiella* and *Listeria*.

Other macrolides

These include azithromycin, clarithromycin and roxithromycin. They have a broad spectrum of activity that includes Gram-negative organisms, mycobacteria and *Toxoplasma gondii*. Compared with erythromycin, they have superior pharmacokinetic properties with enhanced tissue and intracellular penetration and longer half-life that allows once or twice daily dosage. Clarithromycin is now widely recommended as a component of triple therapy regimens (usually with a proton pump inhibitor and metronidazole) for the eradication of *H. pylori*.

Azithromycin is now used for trachoma (see p. 49).

Toxicity. Diarrhoea, vomiting and abdominal pain are the main side-effects of erythromycin (less with clarithromycin). It may also rarely produce cholestatic jaundice after prolonged treatment.

Chloramphenicol

Structure. Chloramphenicol is the only naturally occurring antibiotic containing nitrobenzene (Fig 1.12). This structure is probably important for its toxicity in humans and for its activity against bacteria.

Mechanism of action. Chloramphenicol is structurally similar to uridine-5-phosphate and competes with messenger RNA for ribosomal binding. It also inhibits peptidyl transferase.

Indications for use. Despite its toxicity, chloramphenicol is indicated for the treatment of severe infection that is due to *Salmonella typhi* and *S. paratyphi* (enteric fevers) and severe infections due to *H. influenzae* (meningitis and acute epiglottitis) which are still prevalent in areas not receiving Hib vaccination. It is also active against *Yersinia pestis* (plague) and is used topically for purulent conjunctivitis.

Resistance. Bacterial R factors code for acetylating enzymes that can inactivate chloramphenicol and also reduce bacterial cell permeability to this agent.

Interactions. Chloramphenicol enhances the activity of anticoagulants, phenytoin and oral hypoglycaemic agents.

Chloramphenicol

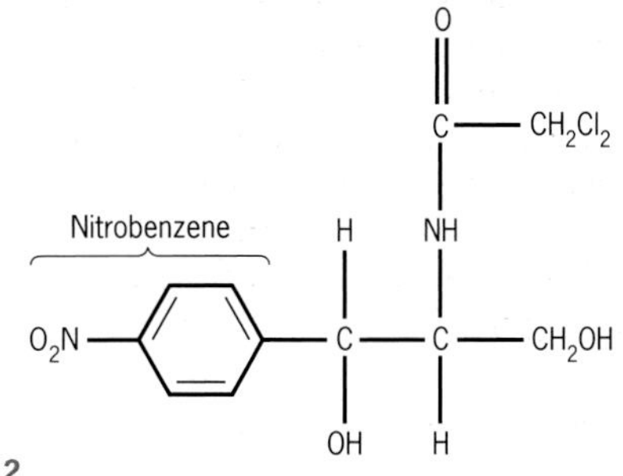

Fig 1.12
The structure of chloramphenicol

Toxicity. Severe irreversible bone marrow suppression is rare but nevertheless restricts the usage of this drug to the indications above and for ill patients. Chloramphenicol should not be given to premature infants or neonates because of their inability to conjugate and excrete this drug; high blood levels lead to circulatory collapse and the often fatal 'grey baby syndrome'.

Fusidic acid

Structure. Fusidic acid has a structure resembling that of bile salts (see p. 291).

Mechanism of action. It is a potent inhibitor of bacterial protein synthesis. Its entry into cells is facilitated by the detergent properties inherent in its structure.

Indications for use. Fusidic acid is mainly used for penicillinase-producing *Staph. aureus* infections such as osteomyelitis (it is well concentrated in bone) or endocarditis, and for other staphylococcal infections accompanied by septicaemia. The drug is well absorbed orally but is relatively expensive.

Resistance. Resistance may occur rapidly and is the reason why fusidic acid is given in combination with another antibiotic.

Toxicity. Fusidic acid may occasionally be hepatotoxic but is generally a safe drug and if necessary can be given during pregnancy.

Sulphonamides and trimethoprim

Structure. The sulphonamides are all derivatives of the prototype sulphanilamide (Fig 1.13). Trimethoprim is a 2,4-,diaminopyrimidine.

Mechanism of action. Sulphonamides block thymidine and purine synthesis by inhibiting microbial folic acid synthesis. Trimethoprim prevents the reduction of dihydrofolate to tetrahydrofolate (see Fig 6.10).

Indications for use. Sulphamethoxazole is mainly used in combination with trimethoprim (as co-trimoxazole). Its use is now restricted for treatment of *P. carinii* infection, for toxoplasmosis and nocardiosis. It may also be used in acute exacerbations of chronic bronchitis

Sulphonamide

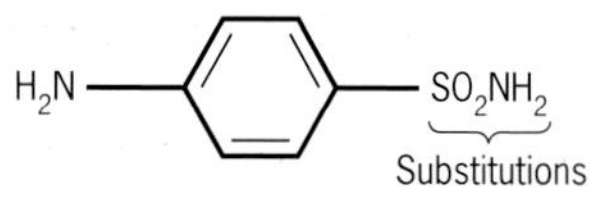

Fig 1.13
The structure of a sulphonamide

and in urinary tract infections when other antibiotics would be less effective as a result of sensitivity testing. Trimethoprim alone is now used for other infections such as urinary tract infections and acute-on-chronic bronchitis, as the side-effects of co-trimoxazole are most commonly due to the sulphonamide component. Sulphapyridine in combination with 5-aminosalicylic acid (i.e. sulphasalazine) is used in inflammatory bowel disease.

Resistance. Bacteria may become resistant to sulphonamides by production of sulphonamide-resistant dihydropteroate synthetase and by altering bacterial cell permeability to these agents.

Interactions. Sulphonamides potentiate oral anticoagulants and hypoglycaemic agents.

Toxicity. Sulphonamides cause thrombocytopenia, folate deficiency and megaloblastic anaemia and haemolysis in individuals with glucose-6-phosphate dehydrogenase deficiency, and therefore should not be used in such people. Co-trimoxazole should be avoided in the elderly if possible, as deaths have been recorded, probably owing to the sulphonamide component.

Quinolones

The quinolone antibiotics, such as ciprofloxacin, norfloxacin, cinoxacin and olfloxacin are useful oral broad-spectrum antibiotics, related structurally to nalidixic acid. The latter achieves only low serum concentrations after oral administration and its use has been limited to the urinary tract where it is concentrated. Newer quinolones, including sparfloxacin and grepafloxacin, have greater activity against Gram-positive pathogens. The *structure* is shown in Fig 1.14.

A new class of antimicrobial agents, the 2-pyridones, are related to the quinolones. They also inhibit DNA gyrase and have broad-spectrum activity, particularly against resistant Gram-positive organisms.

Mechanism of action. The quinolone group of bactericidal drugs inhibit bacterial DNA synthesis by inhibiting DNA gyrase, the enzyme responsible for maintaining the superhelical twists in DNA.

Indications for use. The 4-fluoroquinolones should be reserved for infections caused by organisms resistant to standard drugs. The extended-spectrum quinolones such as ciprofloxacin have activity against Gram-negative and some Gram-positive bacteria. They are useful in Gram-negative

Quinolone

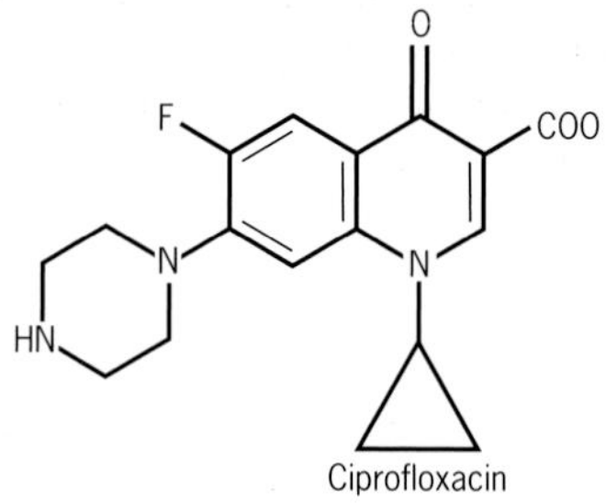

Fig 1.14
The structure of a quinolone

septicaemia, skin and bone infections, gastro-intestinal, urinary and respiratory tract infections, meningococcal carriage and in some sexually transmitted diseases such as gonorrhoea and nonspecific urethritis due to *Chlamydia trachomatis*. The newer quinolones are the only orally effective anti-pseudomonal antibiotics currently available. They are probably the drugs of choice for treatment of traveller's diarrhoea (see Table 1.22).

Toxicity. Gastrointestinal disturbances, photosensitive rashes and occasional neurotoxicity can occur.

Nitroimidazoles

Structure. These agents are active against anaerobic organisms, notably anaerobic bacteria and some pathogenic protozoa. The most widely used drug is metronidazole (Fig 1.15). Minor modifications in the structure of nitroimidazole have produced other related compounds such as tinidazole and nimorazole.

Mechanism of action. After reduction of their nitro group to a nitrosohydroxyl amino group by microbial enzymes, nitroimidazoles cause strand breaks in microbial DNA.

Indications for use. Metronidazole is of major importance in the treatment of anaerobic bacterial infection, particularly that due to *Bacteroides*. It is also used prophylactically in colonic surgery. It may be given orally, by suppository (entirely satisfactory blood levels can be obtained by this route) or intravenously (very expensive). It is also the treatment of choice for amoebiasis, giardiasis and infection with *Trichomonas vaginalis*.

Interactions. Nitroimidazoles can produce a disulfiram-like reaction with ethanol.

Metronidazole

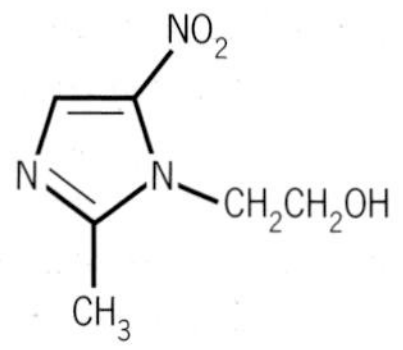

Fig 1.15
The structure of metronidazole, a nitroimidazole

Toxicity. Nitroimidazoles are tumorigenic in animals and mutagenic for bacteria, although carcinogenicity has not been described in humans. They cause a metallic taste, and polyneuropathy with prolonged use. They should be avoided in pregnancy.

Glycopeptides

Vancomycin

Vancomycin is produced by *Streptomyces orientalis*.

Structure. Vancomycin is a complex and unusual glycopeptide active against Gram-positive bacteria.

Mechanism of action. Vancomycin inhibits cell wall synthesis and is bactericidal.

Indications for use. Vancomycin is given orally for *Clostridium difficile*-related pseudomembranous enterocolitis and intravenously for methicillin-resistant *Staph. aureus* and other multiresistant Gram-positive organisms. It is also used for treatment and prophylaxis against Gram-positive infections in penicillin-allergic patients. It has recently been recommended for *S. pneumoniae* meningitis because of penicillin resistance.

Toxicity. Vancomycin can cause ototoxicity and nephrotoxicity and thus serum levels should be monitored. Care must be taken to avoid extravasation at the injection site as this causes necrosis and thrombophlebitis.

Resistance. Vancomycin-resistant enterococci (VRE) are increasingly being recognized as the result of changes in bacterial cell wall glycopeptides.

Teicoplanin

This is another glycopeptide antibiotic which is less nephrotoxic than vancomycin. It has more favourable pharmacokinetic properties, allowing once-daily dosage.

Anti-tuberculosis drugs

These are described on p. 805. Rifampicin is also used in other infections apart from tuberculosis.

Antifungal drugs (Table 1.10)

Polyenes

The most potent of these is amphotericin B, which is used intravenously in severe systemic fungal infections. Nephrotoxicity is a major problem and dosage levels must take background renal function into account. Liposomal amphotericin B is less toxic but very expensive. Nystatin is not absorbed through mucous membranes and is therefore useful for the treatment of oral and enteric candidiasis and for vaginal infection. It can only be given orally or as pessaries. Polyenes react with the sterols in fungal membranes, increasing permeability and thus damaging the organism.

Azoles

Imidazoles such as miconazole (Fig 1.16), ketoconazole and clotrimazole are broad-spectrum antifungal drugs.

- *Clotrimazole* is used topically for the treatment of ringworm.
- *Miconazole* is a potent systemic antifungal and is active both orally and parenterally. It is not as effective as amphotericin B and has been superseded by the triazoles, fluconazole and itraconazole.
- *Ketoconazole* is active orally but can produce liver damage. It is effective in candidiasis and deep mycoses including histoplasmosis and blastomycosis but not in aspergillosis and cryptococcosis.

Triazoles

- *Fluconazole* is noted for its ability to enter CSF and is used for candidiasis and for the treatment of central nervous system (CNS) infection with *Cryptococcus neoformans*.
- *Itraconazole* fails to penetrate CSF. The indications are as for ketoconazole but it may also be effective in cryptococcosis and aspergillosis. Toxicity is mild.

Allylamines

Terbinafine has antifungal and anti-inflammatory activity orally and is useful for the treatment of superficial mycoses such as tinea infections, onychomycosis and cutaneous candidiasis.

Other antifungals

The fluorinated pyridine derivative, *flucytosine*, is usually used in combination with amphotericin B for systemic fungal infection. Side-effects are uncommon, although it may cause bone marrow suppression. It is active when given orally or parenterally.

Griseofulvin, a naturally occurring antifungal, is widely used for the treatment of more extensive superficial mycoses.

Amorolfine is a new antifungal available for topical use.

Table 1.10
Antifungal agents

Polyenes Amphotericin B, nystatin	**Allylamines** Terbinafine
Azoles Miconazole, ketoconazole, fluconazole, itraconazole, clotrimazole	**Other antifungals** Amorolfine (topical only) Fluorinated pyrimidizine 5-Flucytosine Griseofulvin

Miconazole

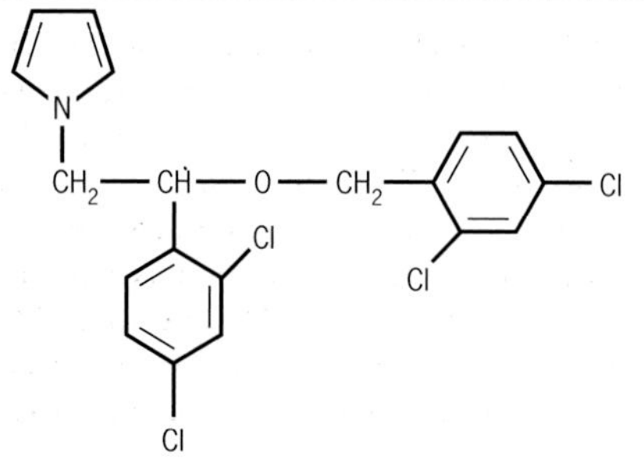

Fig 1.16
The structure of miconazole, an imidazole

Antiviral drugs

Drugs for HIV infection are discussed on p. 120.

Acyclovir

A nucleoside analogue, acyclovir (Fig 1.17), is a chain terminator of viral DNA synthesis following phosphorylation by a virus-encoded thymidine kinase produced by certain herpesviruses. Acyclovir mono-phosphate is converted to the triphosphate by cellular enzymes. The triphosphate competes with deoxyguanine triphosphate and the drug is incorporated into the growing chains of herpesvirus DNA. This highly specific mode of activity, targeted only to virus-infected cells, means that acyclovir has very low toxicity. Intravenous, oral and topical preparations are available for the treatment of herpes simplex types I and II and varicella-zoster virus infections (Table 1.11).

A prodrug of acyclovir, *valaciclovir*, has recently been introduced. Coupling of the amino acid valine to the acyclic side-chain of acyclovir allows better intestinal absorption. The valine is removed by enzymic action and acyclovir is released into the circulation. A similar prodrug of a related nucleoside analogue (penciclovir) is the antiherpes drug, *famciclovir*. The mode of action and efficacy of famiclovir are similar to those of acyclovir.

Ganciclovir

This guanine analogue is structurally similar to acyclovir, with extension of the acyclic side-chain by a carboxymethyl group. It is active against herpes simplex viruses and varicella zoster virus by the same mechanism as acyclovir. In addition, phosphorylation by a protein kinase encoded by the UL97 region of cytomegalovirus renders it potently active against this virus. Thus ganciclovir is currently the first-line treatment for cytomegalovirus disease. Intravenous and oral preparations are available although the latter has poor bio-availability. Unlike acyclovir, ganciclovir has a significant toxicity profile including neutropenia, thrombo-cytopenia and the likelihood of sterilization by inhibiting spermatogenesis. For this reason, it is reserved for the treatment or prevention of life- or sight-threatening cytomegalovirus infection.

Acyclovir

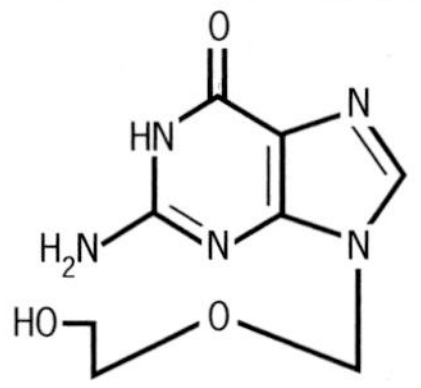

Fig 1.17
The structure of acyclovir

Table 1.11
Antiviral agents (for drugs against HIV see Table 1.49)

Drug	Use
Nucleosides	
Acyclovir	Topical – HSV infection Oral – VZV and HSV
Famciclovir	VZV and HSV-2
Valaciclovir	VZV and HSV
Ganciclovir	CMV
Idoxuridine	HSV (topical eye treatment)
Trifluorothymidine	HSV (topical eye treatment)
Vidarabine	Topical-HSV (eye) Parental-severe VZV and HSV
Phosphonates	
Foscarnet	CMV
Adamantanes	
Amantidine	Influenza A
α-Interferon	HBV, HCV, some malignancies (e.g. renal cell carcinomas)

Foscarnet

Foscarnet (sodium phosphonoformate) is a simple pyrophosphate analogue which inhibits viral DNA polymerases. It is active against herpesviruses and its main roles are as a second-line treatment for severe cytomegalovirus disease and for the treatment of acyclovir-resistant herpes simplex infection. It is given intravenously and the potential for severe side-effects, particularly renal damage, limits its use.

Idoxuridine

This is a nucleoside analogue with activity against herpesviruses (mainly HSV-1). Its use is nowadays confined mainly to the topical treatment of ophthalmic herpes simplex infection.

Amantadine

Amantadine is a synthetic symmetrical amine which is active prophylactically and therapeutically against influenza A virus (it is inactive against influenza B virus). Although its prophylactic efficacy is similar to that of influenza vaccine, it is occasionally used to prevent the spread of influenza A in institutions such as nursing homes. Although CNS side-effects such as insomnia, dizziness and headache may occur (it is also used as a treatment for Parkinson's disease) these are not usually produced by the lower doses currently recommended.

Interferons (see also p. 166)

These are naturally occurring proteins produced by virus-infected cells, macrophages and lymphocytes. Interferons are stimulated by a number of factors, including viral nucleic acid, and render uninfected cells resistant to infection with the same – or in some circumstances different – viruses. They have been synthesized commercially by either culture of lymphoblastoid cells or by recombinant DNA technology and are licensed for therapeutic use. Currently, infection with hepatitis viruses B and C (and certain malignancies) are treated with regular injections of α-interferon).

FURTHER READING

Anyes SGB, Gemmell CG (1997) Antibiotic resistance. *Journal of Medical Microbiology* **33**: 436–470.

Gold HS, Hoellering RC (1996) Antimicrobial drug resistance. *New England Journal of Medicine* **335**: 1445–1450.

Prevention

Although effective antimicrobial chemotherapy is available for many diseases, the ultimate aim of any infectious disease control programme is to prevent infection occurring. This may be achieved either by:

- eliminating the source or mode of transmission of an infection, or
- reducing host susceptibility to environmental pathogens.

Control of sources and transmission

Water and food supplies constitute a major reservoir of infection, so careful surveillance of supplies reduces the incidence of many diseases (e.g. acute diarrhoeal disease, bovine tuberculosis). For many diseases, vector control (e.g. mosquitoes) is essential to control disease.

Screening of blood donors has proved essential to control the spread of hepatitis and HIV. Defining high-risk carrier populations, such as male homosexuals and immigrants from endemic areas of infectious disease, is also important.

Reduction of host susceptibility

Immunization has changed the course and natural history of many infectious diseases. Passive immunization by administering preformed antibody, either in the form of immune serum or purified gamma globulin, provides short-term immunity and has been effective in both the prevention and treatment of a number of bacterial and viral diseases (Table 1.12). The active immunization schedule currently recommended is summarized in Information box 1.2.

Long-lasting immunity is achieved only by active immunization with a live attentuated or an inactivated organism (Table 1.13). Active immunization may also be performed with microbial toxin (either native or modified) – that is, a toxoid. Immunization should be kept up to date with booster doses throughout life. Travellers to developing countries, especially if visiting rural areas, should in addition enquire about further specific immunizations.

In 1974 the World Health Organization introduced the Expanded Programme on Immunization (EPI). Twenty years later more than 80% of the world's children had been immunized against tuberculosis, diphtheria, tetanus, pertussis, polio and measles. Introduction of conjugate vaccines against *Haemophilus influenzae* type b (Hib) has proved to be a major advance in vaccine development (see p. 30).

Table 1.12
Examples of passive immunization available

Infection	Antibody	Indication	Efficacy
Bacterial			
Tetanus	Human tetanus immune globulin	Prevention and treatment	+
Diptheria	Horse serum	Prevention and treatment	±
Botulism	Horse serum	Treatment	+
Viral			
Hepatitis A, Measles	Human normal immune globulin	Prevention	+
Hepatitis B	Human hepatitis B immune globulin	Prevention	+
Varicella zoster	Human varicella zoster immune globulin	Prevention	+
Rabies	Human rabies immune globulin	Prevention	+

Information

Year of life	Vaccines	Dose schedule
1	DPT plus OPV plus Hib or DT Hib (if P contraindicated)	At 2, 3 and 4 months
After 1	MMR	Single dose
3–5	Booster DT plus OPV + MMR (2nd dose)	Single dose
10–14 (females)	BCG (tuberculin-negative individuals)	Single dose[a]
13–18	DT plus OPV	Single dose
Developing countries		
Birth or first contact	BCG + OPV	
6, 10 and 14 weeks	DPT, OPV	
9 months	Measles	
12 months	Yellow fever (in endemic areas)	
12–24 months	DPT, OPV	
5 years	DT, OPV	

Other vaccines (e.g. Hib and MMR are being introduced)

BCG, Bacille Calmette–Guérin; DTP, diphtheria (D)/tetanus (T)/pertussis (P) (triple vaccine); Hib, *Haemophilus influenzae* b; MMR, measles, mumps and rubella (single antigen measles vaccine still available if MMR refused); OPV, oral polio vaccine.

[a] Interval of three weeks between rubella and BCG.

Information box 1.2 Immunization schedule recommended in the UK and developing countries (WHO)

Table 1.13
Preparations available for active immunization

Live attenuated vaccines
Oral polio (Sabin)
Measles
Mumps
Rubella
Yellow fever
BCG
Typhoid (TY 21a)
Inactivated
Hepatitis A
Pertussis
Typhoid – whole cell and Vi antigen
Polio (Salk)
Influenza
Cholera
Meningococci (groups A and C)
Rabies
Pneumococcal
Haemophilus influenza type B
Toxoids
Diphtheria
Tetanus
Recombinant vaccines
Hepatitis B

BCG, Bacille Calmette–Guérin

FURTHER READING

Salisbury DM, Begg NT (eds) (1996) *Immunization Against Infectious Disease*. London: HMSO.

'Vaccine Series' (1997) *Lancet* **350**.

Gram-positive cocci

Staphylococcal infections

Staphylococci are aerobic, facultatively anaerobic, Gram-positive cocci. They contain a number of cellular antigens and produce enzymes such as coagulase as well as toxins such as enterotoxin. Their pathogenicity correlates most closely with the production of the coagulase enzymes.

Table 1.14 Examples of host factors that increase susceptibility to staphylococcal infections (predominantly *Staph. aureus*)

Injury to skin or mucous membranes	**Abnormal leucocyte function**
Abrasions	Job's syndrome
Trauma (accidental or surgical)	Chediak–Higashi syndrome
Burns	Steroid therapy
Insect bites	Drug-induced leucopenia
Metabolic abnormalities	**Postviral infections**
Diabetes mellitus	Influenza
Uraemia	
Foreign bodies[a]	**Miscellaneous conditions**
Intravenous and other indwelling catheters	Excess alcohol consumption
Cardiac and orthopaedic prostheses	Malnutrition
Tracheostomies	Malignancies
	Old age

[a] Often *Staphylococcus epidermidis*

Table 1.15
Clinical conditions produced by *Staphylococcus aureus*

Due to invasion	**Bones and joints**
Skin	Osteomyelitis, arthritis
Furuncles	**Miscellaneous**
Cellulitis	Parotitis
Impetigo	Pyomyositis
Carbuncles	Septicaemia
Lungs	Enterocolitis
Pneumonia	
Lung abscesses	**Due to toxin**
Heart	Staphylococcal food poisoning
Endocarditis	Scalded-skin syndrome
Pericarditis	Bullous impetigo
Central nervous system	Staphylococcal scarlet fever
Meningitis	Toxic shock syndrome
Brain abscesses	

Three pathogenic species are recognized. *Staph. aureus* is coagulase-positive and *Staph. epidermidis* and *Staph. saprophyticus* are coagulase-negative. Staphylococci are part of the normal microflora of the human skin, the upper respiratory tract, especially the nasopharynx, and the intestinal tract. Twenty-five per cent of the population are permanent carriers of *Staph. aureus*.

Approximately 20% of all human staphylococcal infections are autogenous. Transmission is most frequently by direct contact with an infected individual but may be by air or via fomites. Several predisposing host factors have been identified (Table 1.14).

The organism can cause a wide clinical spectrum of diseases. These are usually localized causing an abscess, but infection may spread, resulting in bacteraemia or metastatic infection. Table 1.15 shows a list of conditions due to *Staph. aureus*; discussed below are those conditions not discussed in other chapters.

Food poisoning (see Table 1.21 and p. 32)

This results from ingestion of food contaminated with preformed heat-stable enterotoxins A, B, C, D and E in varying combinations. *Staph. aureus* accounts for approximately 5% of all food poisoning in the UK. Contamination is usually from an infected individual.

Foodstuffs such as canned food, processed meats, milk and cheese favour the growth of *Staph. aureus*. The illness is manifest within six hours of ingestion of contaminated food and affects virtually all individuals who have eaten such food. In contrast to food poisoning that is due to other organisms, staphylococcal food poisoning is characterized by the presence of persistent vomiting. Fever, when present, is usually below 38°C. Abdominal discomfort, diarrhoea or dysentery may be present. No specific treatment is necessary as the illness usually lasts just 12–24 hours; however, supportive treatment with fluids and electrolytes is occasionally indicated.

Acute staphylococcal enterocolitis

This presents as a more severe fulminant clinical syndrome, typically following broad-spectrum antibiotics. Pseudomembranes may be seen at sigmoidoscopy.

Toxic shock syndrome (TSS)

Staphylococci that produce the toxic shock syndrome toxin-1 (TSST-1) are responsible for this syndrome. TSS is seen most frequently in menstruating women below the age of 30 years who use high-absorbancy polyacrylate-containing tampons. However, it can occur in other situations, such as with the use of female barrier contraceptives. Men and children are not exempt. It is characterized by the abrupt onset of fever, a diffuse macular erythema, vomiting, diarrhoea, severe myalgia and shock. Blood cultures are negative and anti-TSST-1 antibodies are present in low concentrations in serum. Treatment is supportive. Antibiotics are usually given, although the syndrome is produced by the exotoxin. Mortality is about 10%.

A toxic shock-like syndrome has also been described in association with group A streptococcal infection.

Scalded skin syndrome (SSS)

Scalded skin syndrome is caused by staphylococci which elaborate the toxin exfoliatin. It is seen in neonates and is characterized by a painful macular skin rash followed by bullae and generalized shedding of the epidermis.

TREATMENT OF STAPHYLOCOCCAL INFECTIONS

Any local lesion, such as an abscess, should be drained. Systemic infection is treated with antibiotics. Hospital-acquired infections are usually resistant to penicillin, so treatment is with flucloxacillin often together with fusidic acid. Of infections acquired outside the hospital 75% are penicillin-sensitive and then a penicillin is the drug of choice. Increasing antibiotic resistance is still a problem, and most hospitals have restrictions on the use of single antibiotics. The control of staphylococcal cross-infection as discussed below is important.

Methicillin-resistant *Staph. aureus* (MRSA) were detected in 1961 soon after methicillin was introduced. Such strains were only resistant to β-lactam antibiotics and never caused serious problems. The MRSA strains that emerged first in Australia in the late 1970s and that have spread worldwide are resistant to many other antibiotics, including aminoglycosides. These are now referred to as MARSA (methicillin–aminoglycoside-resistant *Staph. aureus*). There have been many outbreaks of infection, particularly in patients in tertiary referral centres, in the seriously ill and in those with surgical wounds and venous access sites. The origin of infection is often 'another hospital' or from healthy staff carriers. Control is essential and involves:

- close and constant microbiological surveillance both before and during attacks
- immediate isolation of infected individuals
- appropriate management of the carrier state

Although topical antibiotics have been used to eradicate nasal colonization their efficacy is still in doubt. Careful handwashing with chlorhexidine solution is still widely recommended. MARSA can be treated with vancomycin, but teicoplanin and the quinolones are also effective.

Streptococcal infections

Streptococci are round or ovoid Gram-positive bacteria. Virulence is attributed to the cell-wall M protein and the production by some streptococci of hyaluronidase, DNAses or streptokinase. The spread of streptococci is mediated by direct contact, fomites or airborne droplet infection. Group A β-haemolytic streptococci (*Strep. pyogenes*) are responsible for over 95% of human infections, the most common being pharyingitis and tonsilitis (Table 1.16).

Necrotizing fasciitis and myositis is a deep-seated aggressive infection of subcutaneous tissue and skin which requires surgical bridement of infected tissue in addition to antibiotics. There may be progressive destruction of the tissue which is life-threatening. Group B streptococci frequently produce neonatal sepsis and meningitis, group C, F and G organisms occasionally cause pharyngitis, and group D endocarditis and septicaemia. Three-quarters of all streptococcal endocarditis is caused either by α-haemolytic streptococci found commonly in the mouth (known collectively as *Strep. viridans* – e.g. *Strep. sanguis* and *Strep. mitior*) or by *Strep. mutans*, a non-haemolytic streptococcus.

Strep. pneumoniae is the most common cause of pneumonia (see p. 795).

Table 1.16
Diseases caused by streptococci

Suppurative	**Infections confined to women**
Skin	Puerperal sepsis
Impetigo	Endometritis
Pyoderma	Toxic shock-like syndrome
Erysipelas	
Cellulitis	
Pharyngeal	**Non-suppurative**
Pharyngitis	Rheumatic fever
Tonsillitis	Glomerulonephritis
Peritonsillar abscess	Scarlet fever
Pulmonary	
Pneumonia	
Empyema	
Others	
Osteomyelitis	
Infective endocarditis	
Meningitis	
Peritonitis	
Necrotizing fasciitis and myositis	
Lymphangitis	
Bacteraemia	

Scarlet fever

Scarlet fever occurs when the infectious organism (usually a group A streptococcus) produces erythrogenic toxin in an individual who does not possess neutralizing antitoxin antibodies. This is a notifiable disease in the UK.

CLINICAL FEATURES

The incubation period of this relatively mild disease, which mainly affects children, is 2–4 days following a streptococcal infection, usually in the pharynx. Regional lymphadenopathy, fever, rigors, headache and vomiting are present. The rash, which blanches on pressure, usually appears on the second day of illness; it initially occurs on the neck but rapidly becomes punctate, erythematous and generalized. It is typically absent from the face, palms and soles, and is prominent in the flexures. The rash usually lasts about five days and is followed by extensive desquamation of the skin (Fig 1.18). The face is flushed with characteristic circumoral pallor. Early in the disease the tongue has a white coating through which prominent bright red papillae can be seen ('strawberry tongue'). Later the white coating

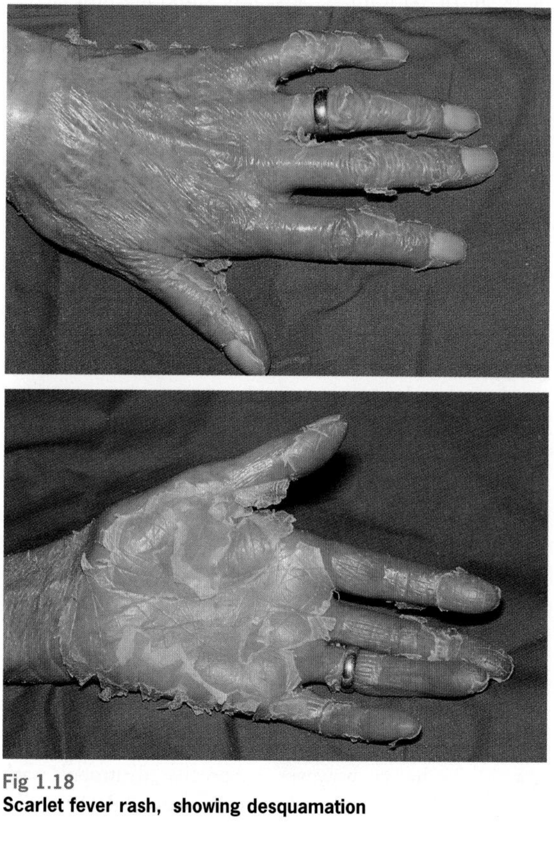

Fig 1.18
Scarlet fever rash, showing desquamation

disappears, leaving a raw-looking, bright red colour ('raspberry tongue'). The patient is infective for 10–21 days after the onset of the rash unless treated with penicillin.

Scarlet fever may be complicated by the development of peritonsillar or retropharyngeal abscesses and otitis media.

DIAGNOSIS

The diagnosis is established by the typical clinical features and culture of throat swabs, where the organisms are usually found in abundance, or more rapidly by latex agglutination of throat swab extracts. Elevated antistreptolysin O and anti-DNAse B levels in the serum are indicative of streptococcal infection.

TREATMENT OF STREPTOCOCCAL INFECTIONS

Treatment is directed at preventing the non-suppurative complications of streptococcal infections (see Table 1.16).

Penicillin is the drug of choice and may be given orally as phenoxymethylpenicillin 125 mg four times daily for 10 days, or as a single intramuscular injection of benzathine penicillin 916 mg in adults. Individuals allergic to penicillin can be treated effectively with erythromycin 250 mg four times daily for 10 days.

PREVENTION

Chemoprophylaxis with penicillin or erythromycin should be given in epidemics.

Erysipelas

Erysipelas is an acute, rapidly progressive infection of the skin that is almost always due to group A streptococci. It usually occurs in the very young, the elderly, the debilitated or the immunosuppressed. The onset is abrupt; fever, headache and vomiting are common. The erythematous skin lesion, which is usually on the face, enlarges rapidly and has a sharply demarcated raised edge. Vesicles and bullae appear within this lesion, which then rupture, leaving crusts on the surface. Regional lymphadenopathy is common. Bacteraemia, when present, is associated with a high mortality rate. Treatment with penicillin is rapidly effective.

Rheumatic fever

This is discussed on p. 699.

Acute glomerulonephritis

This is discussed on p. 531.

FURTHER READING

Bisno AL, Stevens DL (1995) Streptococcal infections of skin and soft tissue. *New England Journal of Medicine* **334**: 240–246.

Gram-negative cocci

Neisserial infections

Neisseria are Gram-negative diplococci. *N. meningitidis* and *N. gonorrhoeae* are the only two bacteria in this group that are commonly pathogenic to humans. They are notifiable diseases in the UK.

Meningococcal infection

Meningococci (*N. meningitidis*) are ubiquitous. However, group A is commonly found in Africa and group B on the European and American continents. The incidence of groups C, Y and W135 infections is steadily rising worldwide. Group A is responsible for epidemics of meningitis and group B and C for sporadic infections. Its virulence is attributed to the polysaccharide capsule (which resists phagocytosis) and the lipopolysaccharide-endotoxin complex (which is responsible for its clinical toxicity). Transmission is by droplet infection or direct contact. Humans are the only known reservoirs. Following transmission, *N. meningitidis* colonize the nasopharynx preferentially because of the humidity, increased carbon dioxide tension and specific receptor substances synthesized by the nasopharynx to which they adhere. Invasiveness of the organism appears to be almost solely dependent on the amount of specific antimeningococcal bactericidal antibody in the host. A history of a recent viral respiratory infection is common.

CLINICAL FEATURES

Four major clinical syndromes due to meningococci are recognized.

Meningococcaemia

This may occur alone or in association with meningitis. It is characterized by the presence of headache, fever, malaise and myalgia. The patient looks toxic, and has tachycardia and tachypnoea. Skin manifestations occur early and consist of a purpuric rash and/or petechiae that also affect the conjunctivae (Fig 1.19).

Fulminant meningococcaemia (Waterhouse–Friderichsen syndrome)

This occurs in about 10% of cases. It is characterized by an extremely rapid downhill clinical course, with extensive haemorrhage into the skin, hypotension, shock, confusion, coma and death within a few hours of the onset of symptoms. Disseminated intravascular coagulation (DIC), due to activation of the complement system, may further complicate the clinical picture. Haemorrhage into the adrenal glands may or may not be present. Without prompt treatment, the mortality rate approaches 100%.

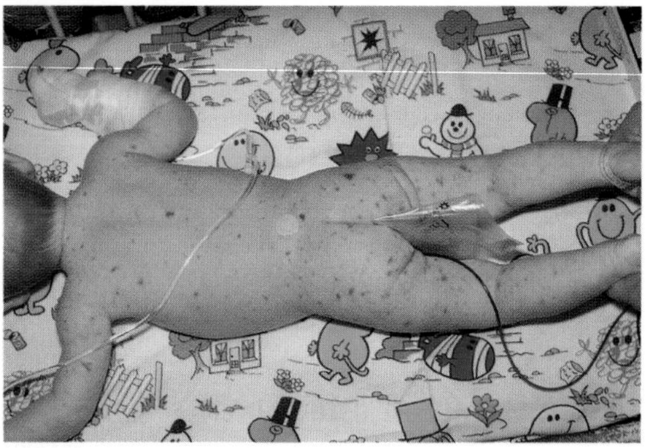

Fig 1.19
Meningococcal infections, showing a purpuric rash

Meningococcal meningitis

This presents with fever, nausea, vomiting, headache, photophobia, altered consciousness and neck rigidity. The clinical presentation is indistinguishable from other acute bacterial meningitides (see p. 1071).

Chronic meningococcaemia

This condition is rare. It is characterized by intermittent fever, a maculopapular rash, arthralgia and splenomegaly. Blood cultures are positive during bacteraemic episodes.

N. meningitidis may also rarely result in polyarthritis, pericarditis and glomerulonephritis.

DIAGNOSIS

This is established by demonstrating meningococci in body fluids such as blood, CSF, petechial or joint aspirates. The CSF is turbid with an increase in neutrophils and protein. Counterimmunoelectrophoresis and latex agglutination to the polysaccharide antigen of group A, C, D and Y have been found useful.

TREATMENT OF MENINGOCOCCAL INFECTIONS

Benzylpenicillin is the treatment of choice, the dose being 1.2–2.4 g i.v. four-hourly for adults started immediately on suspicion of diagnosis. Cefotaxime is equally effective. Chloramphenicol (75–100 mg kg^{-1}) is the drug of choice in individuals allergic to penicillin. Resistance to penicillin has been reported. Treatment for shock and DIC should be instituted. Steroids should not be used in meningococcal meningitis. On discharge from hospital, rifampicin should be given – see below.

PREVENTION AND CONTROL

Penicillin does not affect the carrier state. Family and school contacts of patients are protected effectively by rifampicin 600 mg twice-daily for two days. Immunoprophylaxis with a quadrivalent vaccine against group A, C, Y and W135 organisms is effective and is recommended when travelling to high-risk places – Africa, Asia, South America, Middle and Far East.

Gonorrhoea

Gonorrhoea is caused by *N. gonorrhoeae*. It is discussed further on p. 99.

Gram-positive bacilli

Corynebacteria infection

Corynebacterium diphtheriae is a Gram-positive, club-shaped bacillus. Three morphological varieties are recognized – *mitis*, *intermedius* and *gravis*. Of these, *mitis* is generally associated with mild infections. Only corynebacteria exposed to the bacteriophage β, which carries the *tox*$^{+}$ gene, are capable of toxin production. The toxin has two subunits, A and B. Subunit A is responsible for clinical toxicity. Subunit B serves only to transport the toxin component to specific receptors, present chiefly on the myocardium and in the peripheral nervous system. Humans are the only natural hosts.

Diphtheria

Diphtheria caused by *C. diphtheriae* occurs worldwide. Its incidence in the West has fallen dramatically following widespread active immunization, but it is epidemic in Russia and Eastern Europe. Transmission is mainly through airborne droplet infection and rarely through fomites.

CLINICAL FEATURES

The incubation period is 2–7 days. Diphtheria is essentially a disease of childhood. The manifestations may be regarded as local (due to the membrane) or systemic (due to exotoxin). The presence of a membrane, however, is not essential to the diagnosis. The illness is insidious in onset and is associated with tachycardia but only low-grade fever. If complicated by infection with other bacteria such as *Strep. pyogenes*, fever is high and spiking.

Nasal diphtheria is characterized by the presence of a unilateral, serosanguinous nasal discharge that crusts around the external nares.

Pharyngeal diphtheria is associated with the greatest toxicity and is characterized by marked tonsillar and pharyngeal inflammation and the presence of a membrane. This tough greyish yellow membrane is formed by fibrin, bacteria, epithelial cells, mononuclear cells and polymorphs, and is firmly adherent to the underlying tissue. Regional lymphadenopathy, often tender, is prominent and produces the so-called 'bull-neck'.

Laryngeal diphtheria is usually a result of extension of the membrane from the pharynx. A husky voice, a brassy cough, and later dyspnoea and cyanosis due to respiratory obstruction are common features.

Clinically evident myocarditis occurs, often weeks later, in patients with pharyngeal or laryngeal diphtheria. Acute circulatory failure due to myocarditis may occur in convalescent individuals around the tenth day of illness and is usually fatal. Neurological manifestations may occur either early in the disease (palatal and pharyngeal wall paralysis) or several weeks after its onset (cranial nerve palsies, paraesthesiae, polyneuropathy or, rarely, encephalitis).

Cutaneous diphtheria is increasingly being seen in association with burns and in individuals with poor personal hygiene. Typically the ulcer is punched-out with undermined edges and is covered with a greyish white to brownish adherent membrane. Constitutional symptoms are uncommon.

DIAGNOSIS

This must be made on clinical grounds since therapy is usually urgent and bacteriological results of culture studies and toxin production cannot be awaited.

TREATMENT OF DIPHTHERIA

The patient should be isolated and bedrest advised. Antitoxin therapy is the only specific treatment. It must be instituted rapidly to prevent further fixation of toxin to tissue receptors, since fixed toxin is not neutralized by antitoxin. Depending on the severity, 20 000–100 000 units of horse-serum antitoxin should be administered intramuscularly after an initial test dose to exclude any allergic reaction. Intravenous therapy may be required intramusclulatory in a very severe case. There is a risk of anaphylaxis immediately after antitoxin administration and of serum sickness 2–3 weeks later (Information box 1.3). However, the risk of death outweighs the problems of anaphylaxis. Antibiotics should be administered concurrently to eliminate the organisms and thereby remove the source of toxin production. Benzylpenicillin 2–4 g daily is given for one week.

The cardiac and neurological complications need intensive therapy, as described on p. 20.

PREVENTION

Diphtheria can be effectively prevented by active immunization in childhood (see p. 20).

All contacts of the patient should have throat swabs sent for culture; those with a positive result should be treated with penicillin or erythromycin and active immunization or a booster dose of toxoid given.

Listerial infection

Listeria monocytogenes is a non-spore-forming, facultatively anaerobic bacillus that is motile at 20–25°C. It grows optimally at 30–37°C but can multiply at 4°C and survive heating to 60°C. It is found worldwide and is widely disseminated in the environment. Listeriosis predominantly occurs perinatally but may occasionally occur in adults, particularly the immunocompromised and elderly. It causes abortions, septicaemia and meningitis (see p. 1070). The mortality rate is high. Concern has arisen because of the increasing number of foodborne outbreaks in the past 15 years. Foods most commonly implicated are raw vegetables, coleslaw, milk, non-pasteurized soft cheeses, undercooked chicken and paté. The organism can multiply in a refrigerator if temperatures are not kept below 4°C

Diagnosis is established by blood or CSF culture. Treatment is with ampicillin and gentamicin. Erythromycin, co-trimoxazole or rifampicin are alternatives.

i Information

- Many antitoxins are heterologous and therefore dangerous.
- Hypersensitivity reactions are common.

Prior to treatment:

Question patient about:
(a) allergic conditions (e.g. asthma, hayfever)
(b) previous antitoxin administration.

Read instructions on antitoxin package carefully.

Always give a subcutaneous test dose.

Information box 1.3 Antitoxin administration

Clostridial infections

Clostridium is a Gram-positive, spore-forming, obligatory anaerobic bacillus. Some species, such as *C. botulinum* and *C. tetani*, produce potent neurotoxins, whereas *C. perfringens* produces numerous enzymes and only occasionally an enterotoxin (see Table 1.21). All clostridia that are pathogenic to humans produce exotoxins and require a low redox potential for growth. They are normal commensals of human and animal gastrointestinal tracts, and are widely distributed in soil where, as spores, they may survive for many years in adverse conditions.

Tetanus

Tetanus occurs when a wound is contaminated by *C. tetani* in non-immunized individuals. The wound may be trivial and disregarded by the individual. In the UK the patient is often elderly having sustained a mild injury whilst gardening. The clinical manifestations of the disease are due to the potent neurotoxin, tetanospasmin. Tetanospasmin acts on both the α and γ motor systems at synapses, resulting in disinhibition. It also produces neuromuscular blockade and skeletal muscle spasm, and acts on the sympathetic nervous system. The end result is marked flexor muscle spasm and autonomic dysfunction. The organism is not invasive.

CLINICAL FEATURES

The incubation period varies from a few days to several weeks. Four clinical varieties are recognized.

Generalized tetanus

This is the most common form. Initially the patient complains of feeling unwell. This is followed by trismus (lockjaw) due to masseter muscle spasm. Spasm of the facial muscles produces the characteristic grinning expression known as risus sardonicus. If the disease is severe, painful reflex spasms develop, usually within 24–72 hours of the initial symptoms. The interval between the first symptom and the first spasm is referred to as the 'onset time'. The spasms may occur spontaneously but are easily precipitated by noise, handling of the patient or by light. The frequency of spasms usually increases and respiration becomes impaired because of laryngeal spasm. Oesophageal and urethral spasm lead to dysphagia and urinary retention, respectively. Arching of the neck and back muscles (opisthotonus) occurs. Autonomic dysfunction is evidenced by tachycardia, a labile blood pressure, sweating and cardiac arrhythmias. Patients with tetanus are mentally alert.

Death results from aspiration, hypoxia, respiratory failure, cardiac arrest or exhaustion. Mild cases with rigidity usually recover. Poor prognostic indicators are:

- short incubation period
- short onset time
- cephalic tetanus
- extremes of age
- 'skin poppers' (narcotic addicts who inject drugs subcutaneously).

Localized tetanus

Pain and stiffness is confined to the site of the wound. The tone of the surrounding muscles is increased. Recovery usually occurs.

Cephalic tetanus

This form is uncommon but invariably fatal. It usually occurs when the portal of entry of *C. tetani* is the middle ear. Cranial nerve abnormalities, particularly of the seventh nerve, are usual. Generalized tetanus may or may not develop.

Neonatal tetanus

This occurs in neonates owing to infection of the umbilical stump caused by dressing it with dung or dusting powder. Failure to thrive, poor sucking, grimacing and irritability are followed by rapid development of intense rigidity and spasms. Mortality approaches 100%. The goal of the WHO Expanded Programme on Immunization (EPI) is to eliminate this condition by immunizing all women of childbearing age, providing clean delivery facilities and strengthening surveillance in high-risk areas.

DIAGNOSIS

Few diseases resemble tetanus in its fully developed form. The diagnosis is therefore a clinical one. Rarely, *C. tetani* may be isolated from wounds. However, phenothiazine overdosage, strychnine poisoning, meningitis and tetany can mimic tetanus.

TREATMENT OF TETANUS

For a suspected case. The wound is cleaned and debrided if necessary. Human tetanus antitoxin 250 units should be given along with an intramuscular injection of toxoid. If the patient is already protected a booster dose of the toxoid is given. If the immunization status is unknown, the full three-dose course of absorbed vaccine is given (see below).

For an established case. Improvement in nursing-care techniques has contributed more than any other single measure to the decrease in the mortality rate from 60% to nearer 20%. Patients are nursed in a quiet, isolated, well-ventilated, darkened room. Intragastric feeds may be necessary; bladder and bowel care are also important.

Antibiotics and antitoxin. Both antibiotics and antitoxin should be administered, even in the absence of an obvious wound. Intravenous penicillin 2.4 g daily is the drug of choice. Human antitetanus immunoglobulin 150 IU kg^{-1} i.m. in multiple sites should be given to neutralize any circulating toxin; it has no effect on fixed toxin. The intravenous route is used in very severe cases. In developing countries, if human antitetanus immunoglobulin is not available, immune equine tetanus immunoglobulin 10 000–20 000 units i.m. should be given, after excluding allergy to this product (see Information box 1.3).

Control of spasms. Diazepam is the drug of choice. Up to 120 mg per 24 hours may be required to control spasm and rigidity in adults. β-Blocking drugs may be useful to control autonomic dysfunction.

The role of corticosteroids is controversial. Curarization and artificial respiratory support is best left to specialist units. The judicious use of a tracheostomy may be helpful in averting death.

Active immunization. Once recovery has occurred, active immunization should be instituted, as immunity following tetanus is incomplete.

PREVENTION

Tetanus is an eminently preventable disease and all persons should be immunized regardless of age. Those who work in a contaminated environment, such as farmers, are particularly at risk and should have regular booster injections. Active immunization with the alum-adsorbed toxoid should be given. Initially two doses of 0.5 mL of the toxoid are given intramuscularly at eight-week intervals. The third dose is given 6–12 months later as a booster. Subsequent boosters are required at five-year intervals. Infant immunization schedules in all countries include tetanus (see Information box 1.2 on p. 20).

Protection by passive immunization with either the equine or human antitetanus toxin is short-lived, lasting only about two weeks.

Botulism

Botulism is caused by *C. botulinum*. This organism is found in the soil and food is easily contaminated with the spores, which can survive heating to 100°C. The organisms proliferate in preserved canned foods and produce toxins. Only three types of neurotoxin – A, B and E – have been shown consistently to produce disease in humans. The toxins, which are the most potent known to man, result in marked neuromuscular blockade. They are heat-labile and are inactivated by heating at 80°C for 30 minutes or at 100°C for 10 minutes. Three clinical forms are recognized:

- foodborne: ingestion of preformed toxin usually in home canned or bottled food
- infant botulism: toxin production *in vivo*
- wound botulism.

CLINICAL FEATURES

Nausea, vomiting and diarrhoea are early symptoms and usually occur 18–20 hours after ingesting contaminated food. Neurological symptoms dominate the clinical picture and include blurred vision and diplopia. Laryngeal and pharyngeal paralysis occur, and later generalized paralysis; consciousness is not altered. Respiratory insufficiency may occur. The marked cholinergic blockade results in urinary retention and constipation. Fever is unusual.

A strabismus occurs owing to lateral rectus weakness and the pupil is fixed mid position or dilated and unresponsive to light or accommodation.

DIAGNOSIS

The presence of toxin in faeces, serum or suspected food items is demonstrated by injecting the material into mice. The differential diagnosis includes the Guillain-Barré syndrome and myasthenia gravis.

TREATMENT OF BOTULISM

Treatment is supportive and should be directed at maintaining adequate respiration, with assisted ventilation if necessary. Intravenous administration of 20 mL of antitoxin is followed by 10 mL 2–4 hours later and then every 12–24 hours as necessary. The role of antibiotics has not been adequately evaluated. Guanidine hydrochloride in doses of 15–40 mg kg^{-1} improves botulism-induced paralysis by reversing the intramuscular blockage.

PROGNOSIS

The overall mortality rate for botulism is high (50–70%) but patients who survive the acute paralysis can recover completely.

Gas gangrene

Gas gangrene (clostridial myonecrosis) is commonly caused by *C. perfringens*; *C. novyi* and *C. septicum* are less frequently implicated. Gas gangrene occurs in lacerated wounds associated with fractures or retained foreign bodies particularly if there is a decreased vascular supply and anaerobic conditions. It is characterized by the onset of inordinately severe pain, with thickened induration and oedema at the injury site. When gas gangrene occurs in a limb, the part distal to the injury becomes cold and pulseless. Blebs occur and discharge a watery fluid, which later becomes haemorrhagic. The involved muscles at first appear pale and oedematous, but later they become beefy-red in colour and then brownish black and frankly gangrenous. The characteristic crepitus of gas gangrene is a late feature. Systemic signs of toxicity are prominent. The patient is febrile, tachypnoeic and has a marked tachycardia. Hypotension, renal failure and hepatic failure develop as terminal events. Consciousness remains unaltered.

TREATMENT OF GAS GANGRENE

Treatment consists of adequate surgical debridement, with parenteral penicillin or chloramphenicol combined with another antibiotic to cover aerobic and anaerobic organisms that are frequent wound contaminants. The role of anti-gas gangrene toxin and hyperbaric oxygen is controversial.

Pseudomembranous colitis

Pseudomembranous colitis is caused by the A and B toxins produced by *C. difficile*. It usually occurs a few days after institution of antibiotic therapy, although it has been known to occur even a month after discontinuing antibiotics. All broad spectrum antibiotics have been causally related to some extent. Diarrhoea (rarely with blood) and abdominal cramps are usual; elderly hospitalized patients are most frequently affected. Sigmoidoscopic examination may reveal a markedly erythematous, ulcerated mucosa covered by a membrane-like material, although in about 20% of patients only the ascending colon is involved. A normal sigmoidoscopy therefore does not exclude infection. The presence of this membrane is not essential to the diagnosis.

DIAGNOSIS

Identification of the toxin (by observing its cytopathic effect on cells in tissue culture or by ELISA) in stool specimens is usually diagnostic but the test can be unreliable. Culture of the organism alone is insufficient as 5% of healthy adults carry *C. difficile*. Both the organism and its toxin are commonly found in healthy neonates in whom it has no pathological significance.

TREATMENT OF PSEUDOMEMBRANOUS COLITIS

All suspected antibiotics should be discontinued and this alone may result in the diarrhoea stopping. Vancomycin

125 mg orally, four times daily, for 10 days is often used but metronidazole is also effective and considerably less expensive. Relapses are common and toxic dilatation can rarely occur. There is no evidence that changing chemotherapy helps. Patients should be isolated to try to prevent spread to other susceptible individuals.

Bacillus infections

Anthrax

Anthrax is caused by *Bacillus anthracis*. Its spores are extremely hardy and withstand extremes of temperature and humidity. The organism is capable of toxin production and this property correlates most closely with its virulence. The disease occurs worldwide. Epidemics have been reported in The Gambia, in both North and South America and in southern Europe. Transmission is through direct contact with an infected animal and is seen in farmers, butchers and dealers in wool and animal hides. Spores can also be ingested or inhaled.

CLINICAL FEATURES

The incubation period is 1–5 days.

The cutaneous form

This is the most common mode of presentation and is seen most frequently in the tropics. It is self-limiting in the majority of patients. Typically, a small erythematous, maculopapular relatively painless lesion is present that subsequently vesiculates and undergoes ulceration, with formation of a central black eschar. Occasionally the perivesicular oedema is marked and toxaemia may be present.

Respiratory involvement (Woolsorter's disease)

Inhalation of spores results in a non-productive cough, fever and retrosternal discomfort. Pleural effusions are common. In some patients there is apparent clinical improvement followed by the abrupt onset of dyspnoea, marked cyanosis and death.

Gastrointestinal anthrax

This presents as severe gastroenteritis. Haematemesis and bloody diarrhoea may occur.

DIAGNOSIS

The diagnosis is established by demonstrating the organism in smears or by culture. Detection of a fourfold increase in antibodies measured by indirect micro-haemagglutination or ELISA in paired sera (i.e. acute and convalescent samples) is diagnostic.

TREATMENT OF ANTHRAX

Penicillin is the drug of choice. In mild cutaneous infections, phenoxymethylpenicillin 500 mg four times daily for two weeks is adequate. In more severe infections, such as when septicaemia is present, up to 2.4 g of intravenous penicillin is required daily. Erythromycin, chloramphenicol and tetracycline have also been used successfully. The role of steroids in fulminant anthrax infections is questionable.

Any infected animal that dies should be burned and the area in which it was housed disinfected. Where animal husbandry is poor, mass vaccination of animals may prevent widespread contamination.

Vaccination of exposed workers is effective.

Bacillus cereus infection

This Gram-positive, aerobic, spore-forming bacillus can cause food poisoning (see Table 1.21) often from contaminated rice. It produces a toxin called 'cerulide' which causes liver failure (see p. 335). It also causes wound sepsis.

Gram-negative bacilli

Brucella infections

Brucella is a Gram-negative coccobacillus. Three species are recognized: *B. abortus*, *B. melitensis* and *B. suis*.

Brucellosis (Malta fever, undulant fever)

Brucellosis is a zoonosis and has a worldwide distribution (Table 1.17), although it has been virtually eliminated from cattle in the UK. The organism does not withstand pasteurization.

The *Brucella* endotoxin (a cell-wall lipopolysaccharide) is responsible for systemic symptoms and host hypersensitivity accounts for formation of granulomas. The organisms usually gain entry into the human body via the mouth, though less frequently they may enter via the respiratory tract, genital tract or abraded skin. The bacilli travel in the lymphatics and infect lymph nodes. This is followed by haematogenous spread with ultimate localization of the bacilli in the reticuloendothelial system. Spread is largely by the ingestion of raw milk from infected cattle or goats. The disease often occurs in workers in close contact with animals or carcasses.

CLINICAL FEATURES

The incubation period is 1–3 weeks.

Acute brucellosis

The onset is insidious, with malaise, headache, weakness, generalized myalgia and night sweats. The fever pattern is classically undulant, although continuous and intermittent

Table 1.17 Main geographical distribution and natural hosts of the *Brucella* species

Organism	Geographical distribution	Natural host
B. abortus	Worldwide, except northern Europe, Japan	Cattle
B. melitensis	Mediterranean region especially Malta	Goats, sheep and camels
B. suis	Far East, USA	Pigs
B. canis[a]		Beagles

[a] Rarely causes disease in humans.

patterns are frequent. Lymphadenopathy, hepatomegaly and spinal tenderness may also be present. The presence of splenomegaly is indicative of severe infection. Arthritis, spondylitis, bursitis, osteomyelitis, orchitis, epididymitis, meningo-encephalitis and endocarditis have all been described, especially in infections with *B. melitensis* or *B. suis*.

Chronic brucellosis

This is characterized by easy fatiguability, myalgia, occasional bouts of fever and depression, which may persist for several months. Splenomegaly is present. It needs to be distinguished from other causes of prolonged fever.

Localized brucellosis

This condition is uncommon. Bones and joints, spleen, endocardium, lungs, urinary tract and nervous system may be involved. Systemic symptoms occur in less than one-third. Antibody titres are low. Diagnosis is established by culturing the organisms from the involved site.

DIAGNOSIS

Blood (or bone marrow) cultures are positive during the acute phase of illness in 50% of patients. This is less helpful in more chronic disease where serological tests are of greater value. The *Brucella* agglutination test, which demonstrates a fourfold or greater rise in titre over a four-week period, is highly suggestive of brucellosis. A single titre greater than 1 in 160 is also suggestive of brucellosis in the appropriate clinical setting. An elevated serum IgG level detected by extraction with 2-mercaptoethanol (2-ME) is evidence of current or recent infection. A negative 2-ME test excludes chronic brucellosis. Specific *Brucella* antibodies can be detected by ELISA. Occasionally serology is negative when blood cultures are positive.

TREATMENT OF BRUCELLOSIS

Doxycycline 200 mg daily is given combined with rifampicin 600–900 mg once-daily for six weeks, but relapses occur. Alternatively, tetracycline can be combined with streptomycin, which is usually given for only the first two weeks of treatment.

PREVENTION AND CONTROL

Prevention and control involves careful attention to hygiene when handling infected animals, eradication of infection in animals, and pasteurization of milk. No vaccine is available for use in humans.

Bordetella infections

Bordetella is a Gram-negative coccobacillus. *B. pertussis* causes pertussis and is notifiable in the UK. *B. parapertussis* and *B. bronchiseptica* produce milder infections.

Pertussis (whooping cough)

Pertussis occurs worldwide. Humans are both the natural hosts and reservoirs of infection. Pertussis is highly contagious and is spread by droplet infection. In its early stages it is indistinguishable from other types of upper respiratory tract infection and hence spread occurs easily. Epidemics were common in the UK because the safety of the whooping cough vaccine was questioned. By 1995, however, 94% of the population under the age of two years had been vaccinated and the number of cases dropped dramatically.

CLINICAL FEATURES

The incubation period is 7–10 days. It is a disease of childhood, with 90% of cases occurring below five years of age. However, no age is exempt.

During the *catarrhal stage* the patient is highly infectious, and cultures from respiratory secretions are positive in over 90% of patients. Malaise, anorexia, mucoid rhinorrhoea and conjunctivitis are present.

The *paroxysmal stage*, so called because of the characteristic paroxysms of coughing, begins about a week later. Paroxysms with the classic inspiratory whoop are seen only in younger individuals in whom the lumen of the respiratory tract is compromised by mucus secretion and mucosal oedema. The whoop results from air being forcefully drawn through the narrowed tract. These paroxysms usually terminate in vomiting. Conjunctival suffusion and petechiae and ulceration of the frenulum of the tongue are usual. Lymphocytosis due to the elaboration of a lymphocyte-promoting factor by *B. pertussis* is characteristic; lymphocytes may account for over 90% of the total white blood cell count. This stage lasts approximately two weeks and may be associated with several complications, including pneumonia, atelectasis, rectal prolapse and inguinal hernia. Cerebral anoxia may occur, especially in younger children, resulting in convulsions. Bronchiectasis is a rare sequel.

DIAGNOSIS

The diagnosis is suggested clinically by the characteristic whoop and a history of contact with an infected individual. It is confirmed by growing the organism in culture. Cultures of swabs of nasopharyngeal secretions result in a higher positive yield than cultures of 'cough plates'.

TREATMENT OF PERTUSSIS

If the disease is recognized in the catarrhal stage, erythromycin will abort or decrease the severity of the infection. In the paroxysmal stage antibiotics have little role to play in altering the course of the illness.

PREVENTION AND CONTROL

Affected individuals should be isolated to prevent contact with others. This is particularly important in hostels and boarding schools. Pertussis is an easily preventable disease and effective active immunization is available (see Table 1.13). Convulsions and encephalopathy have been reported as rare complications of vaccination but they are probably less frequent than after whooping cough itself. Any exposed susceptible infant should receive prophylactic erythromycin.

Haemophilus infections

Haemophilus is a Gram-negative, pleomorphic, coccobacillus. Those pathogenic to humans include *H. influenzae*, *H. ducreyi* and *H. parainfluenzae*. In general, non-encapsulated forms produce luminal infections (e.g. bronchitis) and encapsulated organisms produce invasive disease (e.g. meningitis). *Haemophilus* is a normal commensal of the upper respiratory tract and is found in about 80% of healthy individuals.

Of the six antigenic types of *H. influenzae* identified, type b is the most important in humans and demonstrates the greatest pathogenicity, especially in children below five years of age. Fortunately an effective vaccine is now available (see below). In developed countries all children are vaccinated. Many developing countries (e.g. The Gambia) also have instituted mass immunization programmes. Patients undergoing splenectomy or those with hyposplenism (e.g. with sickle cell disease) and patients who are HIV-positive should receive vaccination. *H. influenzae* can produce disease in several human organs (Table 1.18). Infection is generally autogenous and hence sporadic cases are common.

There is evidence of increasing immunity to *Haemophilus* with age. This is related to the presence of anticapsular and specific bactericidal antibodies. Cross-reacting antibodies to other Gram-negative bacteria can also contribute to immunity.

Infections with *Haemophilus influenzae*

H. influenzae infections have a worldwide distribution, but have fallen dramatically since vaccination.

Table 1.18
Major clinical syndromes associated with *Haemophilus influenzae*

Respiratory system	**Cardiac system**
Sinusitis	Endocarditis
Bronchitis	Pericarditis
Pneumonia	
	Miscellaneous
Central nervous system	Septic arthritis
Meningitis	Cellulitis
Brain abscess	Epiglottitis
	Otitis media

Meningitis

H. influenzae is now a rare cause of meningitis where the vaccine is available. The clinical features are described on p. 1071.

Epiglottitis

This has been virtually eliminated in the UK. The clinical features are described on p. 772.

DIAGNOSIS AND TREATMENT

This is made by isolation and culture of the organism. Counterimmunoelectrophoresis can be used to detect type b capsular antigen in 75% of patients.

Treatment is urgent, as delay may result in a high mortality, especially in patients with meningitis and epiglottitis. In these conditions the drug of choice is intravenous chloramphenicol 50–100 mg kg^{-1} per day for children and 4 g per day for 7–10 days for adults. Cefuroxime can be given orally or, for meningitis, 3 g eight-hourly. Ampicillin can be used for less severe cases, but resistance to this drug is increasing.

PREVENTION

Children in close contact with an infected individual are at an increased risk of developing the disease. Rifampicin 20 mg kg^{-1} for four days is helpful. Conjugate vaccines have been developed in which a purified capsular polysaccharide is linked to a protein to improve immunogenicity. They are highly effective; 99% of children have protective levels after three days. Primary vaccination is recommended in the UK and in many countries in the first year of life (see Information box 1.2).

Cholera

Cholera is caused by the curved, actively motile, flagellated Gram-negative bacillus, *Vibrio cholerae*. The organism is killed by temperatures of 100°C in a few seconds but can survive in ice for up to six weeks. The major pathogenic strain possesses a somatic antigen (O1) with two biotypes – classical and El Tor. The El Tor biotype has replaced the classical biotype as the major cause of cholera. This is because the El Tor *V. cholerae* is a hardier organism. Infection with the El Tor biotype is frequently unrecognized because it produces milder clinical symptoms; a chronic gallbladder carrier state can result in about 3% of all infected adults. All three strains (Inaba, Ogawa and Hikojima) are pathogenic.

The fertile, humid Gangetic plains of West Bengal have traditionally been regarded as 'the home of cholera'. However, the seventh pandemic of cholera, which was caused by the El Tor biotype, affected large areas of Asia, North Africa, Kenya and southern Europe. The pandemic has spread to South and Central America in recent years, claiming thousands of lives. It has been suggested that the eighth cholera pandemic has begun and is due to a non-O1 *V. cholerae* (*V. cholerae* 0139) which may be an El Tor mutant. However, this organism has as yet not been found extensively outside the Indian subcontinent and South East Asia. Humans are the only known natural hosts. Contaminated water plays a major role in the dissemination of cholera, although contaminated foodstuffs and contact carriers may contribute in epidemics.

Transmission is by the faecal–oral route. Achlorhydria or hypochlorhydria facilitates passage of the cholera bacilli into the small intestine, where they proliferate and elaborate an exotoxin with A and B subunits. The B subunit binds to specific GM1 ganglioside receptors and the A subunit activates the intracellular enzyme adenylate cyclase. This produces elevation of 3,5-cyclic-AMP, which in turn produces massive secretion of isotonic fluid into the intestinal lumen (see p. 277). Cholera toxin also releases serotonin (5-HT) from enterochromaffin cells in the gut which activates a neural secretory reflex in the enteric nervous system. This may account for at least 50% of cholera toxins' secretory activity.

V. cholerae has been shown to produce a second toxin known as 'zonula occludens toxin' (ZOT). This impairs the integrity of the 'tight junctions' between enterocytes, allowing escape of water and electrolytes. A third toxin, 'accessory cholera toxin' (ACE), which also produces intestinal secretion, has been identified.

CLINICAL FEATURES

The incubation period varies from a few hours to six days. The majority of patients with cholera have a mild illness that cannot be distinguished clinically from diarrhoea owing to other infective causes. Classically, however, three phases are recognized in the untreated disease.

The *evacuation phase* is characterized by the abrupt onset of painless, profuse, watery diarrhoea, associated with vomiting in the severe forms. 'Rice water' stools, so called because of mucus flecks floating in the watery stools, are characteristic of this stage.

If appropriate supportive treatment is not given, the patient passes on to the *collapse phase*. This is characterized by features of circulatory shock (cold clammy skin, tachycardia, hypotension and peripheral cyanosis) and dehydration (sunken eyes, hollow cheeks and a diminished urine output). The patient, though apathetic, is usually lucid. Muscle cramps may be severe. Children may, in addition, present with convulsions owing to hypoglycaemia. At this stage renal failure and aspiration of vomitus present major problems.

If the patient survives the collapse stage, then the *recovery phase* starts, with a gradual return to normal of clinical and biochemical parameters in 1–3 days.

Cholera sicca is an uncommon but severe form of cholera. It presents with massive outpouring of fluid and electrolytes into dilated intestinal loops. Diarrhoea and vomiting do not occur and hence the disease is frequently not recognized. The mortality rate is high.

DIAGNOSIS

Diagnosis is largely clinical. Examination of freshly passed stools may demonstrate rapidly motile organisms. This is not diagnostic, as *Campylobacter jejuni* may also give a similar appearance. However, demonstration of the rapidly motile vibrios by dark-field illumination and subsequent inhibition of their movement with type-specific antisera is diagnostic.

Stool and rectal swabs should be taken for culture.

TREATMENT OF CHOLERA

With appropriate and effective rehydration therapy, mortality has decreased to less than 1%. Rehydration is mainly oral, but intravenous therapy is occasionally required.

Oral rehydration. For maintenance therapy or for correction of mild to moderate dehydration, oral rehydration is best carried out by giving a glucose–electrolyte solution. The World Health Organization's oral rehydration solution (ORS) is shown in Table 1.19.

Mildly dehydrated individuals are given ORS 50 mL kg^{-1} in the first four hours, followed by a maintenance solution of 100 mL kg^{-1} daily until the diarrhoea stops. For moderate dehydration, ORS 100 mL kg^{-1} is given within the first four hours, followed by 10–15 mL kg^{-1} per hour. Rice-based and other cereal-based electrolyte solutions have been found to be as effective and actually reduce stool volume as well as rehydrating, so that they are replacing the WHO's ORS.

Intravenous rehydration. This is required only for severely dehydrated individuals with features of collapse. Intravenous solutions recommended by the WHO include Ringer's lactate solution and the 'Diarrhoea Treatment Solution' (sodium chloride 4.0 g, sodium acetate 6.5 g, potassium chloride 1.0 g, and glucose 9.0 g, all per litre). Several litres of intravenous fluid are usually required to overcome the features of shock. Maintenance of hydration is effectively carried out by oral rehydration solutions.

Antibiotics. Antibiotics such as tetracycline 250 mg four times daily for three days, or doxycycline, help to eradicate the infection, decrease stool output and shorten the duration of the illness dramatically. Drug resistance is becoming an increasing problem, and ciprofloxacin is now being used more frequently.

Table 1.19
Oral rehydration solutions

	Sodium (mmol L^{-1})	Potassium (mmol L^{-1})	Chloride (mmol L^{-1})	Bicarbonate (mmol L^{-1})	Glucose (mmol L^{-1})	Citrate (mmol L^{-1})	Rice (g L^{-1})
WHO/UNICEF[a]	90	20	80	–	111	10	–
Cereal-based ORS[a]	90	20	80	–	–	10	50–80
UK/Europe ORS[b]	35–60	20	37	18–30	90–200	10	–

[a] Used in cholera.
[b] ORS composition currently recommended for children in UK and Europe.

PREVENTION AND CONTROL

Immunization with currently available parenteral vaccines results in poor immunity and is no longer recommended. Attenuated live oral cholera vaccines are under intensive evaluation. Chemoprophylaxis with tetracycline 500 mg twice-daily for three days for adults, or 125 mg daily for children, is effective. The most effective preventive measures, however, are good hygiene and improved sanitation.

Table 1.20 compares the pattern of infection caused by *V. cholerae* with the patterns of infection caused by other gut organisms.

Food poisoning

'Food poisoning' is a general term used to describe acute illnesses that are related to food ingestion. Most are infective and Table 1.21 shows the common bacterial causes. Viral causes are shown in Table 1.33.

Traveller's diarrhoea is also transmitted by water and contaminated food and the causes are shown in Table 1.22.

Diarrhoea, vomiting and abdominal pain occur after ingestion of food contaminated with a variety of enteropathogens or with preformed enterotoxins. These infections are usually self-limiting and antibiotics are generally not required. Oral rehydration therapy may be required to replace fluid and electrolyte losses. Samples of candidate foods and faecal specimens should be sent for bacteriological culture. This is especially important in tracking the source of major foodborne outbreaks of diarrhoeal disease. Individual causes of food poisoning are described under the causative agents.

Escherichia coli infection

E. coli is one of a group of aerobic Enterobacteria and is commonly responsible for urinary tract infections, bacteraemia, neonatal meningitis, and peritoneal and biliary infections. Such infections are indistinguishable from similar clinical conditions caused by other bacteria.

E. coli responsible for enteric disease have different serotype characteristics from those that cause disease elsewhere in the body. The main categories of *E. coli* capable of producing human diarrhoeal disease are given in Table 1.23.

Table 1.20
Patterns of gut infection

	Non-inflammatory	Inflammatory	Penetrating
Major location	Jejunum	Colon	Ileum
Clinical presentation	Watery diarrhoea	Dysentery	Enteric fever
Common pathogens	*Vibrio cholerae* *Escherichia coli:* ETEC EHEC	*Shigella* spp. *Escherichia coli:* EPEC EIEC *Salmonella* sp. *Clostridium difficile* *Campylobacter jejuni* *Entamoeba histolytica* (see p. 81)	*Salmonella typhi* *Yersinia enterocolitica*
Pathogenic mechanisms	Enterotoxin (CT, LT, ST) production causing intestinal secretion of water and electrolytes	Invasion of gut epithelium ± cytotoxin release	Invasion and bacteraemia

CT, cholera toxin; LT and ST, *Escherichia coli* heat-labile and heat-stable toxins.

Table 1.21
Bacterial causes of food poisoning

Organism	Source	Incubation period	Symptoms	Diagnosis	Recovery
Staphylococcus aureus	Contaminated food, usually by humans	2–6 h	Diarrhoea, vomiting and dehydration	Culture organism in vomitus or remaining food	Rapid (few hours)
E. Coli O157:H7	Undercooked beef; raw cow's milk	12–48 h	Watery diarrhoea ± haemorrhagic colitis, HUS	Stool culture	10–12 days
Bacillus cereus	Spores in food (often rice) survive boiling	1–6 h	Diarrhoea, vomiting and dehydration	Culture organism in faeces and food	Rapid
Clostridium perfringens	Spores in food survive boiling	8–22 h	Watery diarrhoea and cramping pain	Culture organism in faeces and food	2–3 days
Clostridium botulinum	Spores survive cooking but only germinate in anaerobic conditions, e.g. canned or bottled food	18–36 h	Brief diarrhoea and paralysis due to neuromuscular blockade	Demonstrate toxin in food or faeces	10–14 days
Salmonella enteritidis/ typhimurium	Bowels of animals, especially fowl	12–24 h	Abrupt diarrhoea, fever and vomiting	Stool culture	Usually 2–5 days, but may be up to 2 weeks
Campylobacter jejuni	Bowels of animals, especially fowl; also milk	48–96 h	Diarrhoea ± blood, fever, malaise and abdominal pain	Stool culture	3–5 days
Shigella sp.	Contaminated food	28 h	Acute watery, bloody diarrhoea	Stool culture	Few days

Non-microbial toxins such as dinoflagellate plankton toxin in shellfish ('red tide'), scrombotoxin from some varieties of spoiled fish and red kidney bean toxin (haemagglutinin) from partially cooked beans also cause acute diarrhoea.
HUS, haemorrhagic uraemia syndrome.

Enterotoxigenic *E. coli* (ETEC)

ETEC produces a diarrhoeal illness that is mediated through a heat-labile toxin (LT) and/or a heat-stable toxin (ST). Toxin production is genetically encoded by transferable DNA plasmids. LT resembles cholera toxin in its mode of action since it also acts on the enterocyte via cyclic AMP and is associated with massive secretion of water and electrolytes into the intestinal lumen. ST activates guanylate cyclase with elevation of cyclic GMP levels and subsequent secretion of water and electrolytes (see Fig 4.36). Clinically, ETEC produces three syndromes:

- an illness indistinguishable from severe cholera
- 'traveller's diarrhoea', an acute but milder disease (Table 1.22)
- diarrhoea of varying severity in children, especially in developing countries.

Enteroinvasive *E. coli* (EIEC)

EIEC produces an illness similar to that produced by *Shigella* (see below).

Enteropathogenic *E. coli* (EPEC)

EPEC attaches to and damages intestinal epithelium, producing diarrhoea, primarily in children below two years of age. Toxins have not been demonstrated. Epidemics are common, especially in nurseries.

Enterohaemorrhagic *E. coli* (EHEC)

EHEC produces a shiga-like cytotoxin which kills Vero cells – called verotoxin-producing *E. coli* (VTEC) or shiga-toxin producing *E. coli* (STEC). It causes bloody diarrhoea and colitis. Fever is unusual. Outbreaks due to EHEC O157:H7 have been linked with contaminated food, particularly hamburgers. Infection may be complicated by the haemolytic–uraemic syndrome and fatalities occur in the elderly. Screening of stools for *E. coli* O157:H7 is now included in the culture protocols of most laboratories.

TREATMENT OF *E. COLI* INFECTIONS

Oral administration of fluids and electrolytes is the mainstay of therapy for *E. coli* gut infections as many are self-limiting and require no specific antimicrobial therapy. For severe infection, particularly with colitis and a systemic illness, ciprofloxacin 500 mg twice-daily is often used as resistance to ampicillin and co-trimoxazole is widespread. Gentamicin 2–5 mg kg^{-1} daily or tobramycin 3–5 mg kg^{-1} daily in divided eight-hourly doses are used in severe illness with septicaemia. Urinary tract infection is discussed on p. 545.

Trimethoprim and doxycycline have been used in the prophylaxis of ETEC traveller's diarrhoea, but early treatment rather than prophylaxis is preferred.

Table 1.22
Causes of traveller's diarrhoea

Pathogen	Proportion of cases (%)
Enterotoxigenic *Escherichia coli*	40–75
Shigella spp.	0–15
Salmonella spp.	0–10
Rotavirus, Norwalk family of viruses	0–10
Giardia lamblia, Entamoeba histolytica	0–3
Unknown	22–25

Table 1.23
Escherichia coli infections of the intestine

	Site	Disease
Enterotoxigenic *E. coli* (ETEC)	SI	Acute watery diarrhoea
Enteropathogenic *E. coli* (EPEC)	SI	Acute/persistent diarrhoea (especially in children)
Enteroadherent *E. coli* (EAEC)	SI	Acute/ persistent diarrhoea
Enteroinvasive *E. coli* (EIEC)	Colon	Dysentery
Enterohaemorrhagic *E. coli* (EHEC)	Colon	Haemorrhagic colitis Haemolytic uraemic syndrome

SI, small intestine.

Salmonella infections

Salmonellae are a Gram-negative, generally motile bacillus. Clinically they can be divided into two groups:

- *S. enteritidis* and *S. typhimurium* cause acute gastroenteritis (food poisoning)
- *S. typhi* and *S. paratyphoid* cause typhoid and paratyphoid fever.

Salmonellae have a worldwide distribution and withstand freezing and dry conditions for prolonged periods.

Gastroenteritis (food poisoning)

Transmission occurs by ingestion of contaminated foods (particularly eggs and poultry products) or water. The organism is found in the alimentary tract and the oviducts of poultry and within the egg itself. The increase of food poisoning in the UK has been related to modern mechanized processing of battery chickens causing cross-contamination. The *Salmonella* serotypes *S. enteritidis* phage type 4 caused 43% of cases of food poisoning, but this is decreasing whereas *S. typhimurium* dt 104 is on the increase. *S. agona* has been spread around the world by contaminated Peruvian fishmeat used as chickenfeed.

Person-to-person infection is uncommon except in people in confined communities, such as nursing homes for the elderly. The organisms predominantly affect the small bowel with invasion causing inflammation. A typical attack of diarrhoea lasts 2–3 days and is usually accompanied by malaise, nausea and headache. Many infected patients remain asymptomatic. Occasionally an enterocolitis with bloody diarrhoea occurs.

Treatment is asymptomatic. Antibiotic therapy is required only for severe disease and resistance is becoming a major problem. Notification is necessary in the UK.

Prevention involves improved animal husbandry and care with slaughtering and processing of animals for human consumption. Careful handling of food and hand-washing by shopkeepers and cooks is also required.

Typhoid fever

This is caused by *S. typhi*. Humans are the only known reservoirs and spread is via the faeco-oral route. In developing countries milllions develop the disease and the mortality is as high as 30%. The incubation period is usually 10–14 days following the ingestion of contaminated food, milk or water.

Carriers

Carriers can be divided into *chronic* carriers, defined as individuals who excrete *Salmonella* for at least one year, and *convalescent* carriers. The presence of Vi agglutinin in the serum in a dilution greater than 1:10 is suggestive of a carrier state. Since the gallbladder is frequently the focus of infection, duodenal aspirates for culture of the bile-containing duodenal juice may yield useful information.

CLINICAL FEATURES

The onset is insidious, with headache being a prominent symptom. The fever is remittent and gradually increases in severity in a stepladder fashion over 3–4 days. Cough, sore throat and altered behaviour may also be present. Constipation is usually present initially and diarrhoea occurs only late in the disease.

Physical examination during the first week reveals a toxic individual with a relative bradycardia. During the second week several physical signs can be elicited. An erythematous maculopapular rash that blanches on pressure and is referred to as 'rose spots' appears, chiefly on the upper abdomen and thorax, and lasts for only 2–3 days. These spots are not easily visible on dark-skinned patients. A soft splenomegaly occurs in about 75% of patients. Cervical lymphadenopathy, hepatosplenomegaly (present in about 30% of patients) and right iliac fossa tenderness are other physical signs that may be present.

The third week of illness, aptly referred to as 'the week of complications', is the time when the majority of complications occur. These include lobar pneumonia, haemolytic anaemia, meningitis, polyneuropathy, acute cholecystitis, urinary tract infection and osteomyelitis. Intestinal perforation occurs in 2–3% and intestinal haemorrhage in 2–8% of cases.

The fourth week of illness ('the week of convalescence') is characterized by a gradual return to health.

INVESTIGATIONS AND DIAGNOSIS

Leucopenia is present. Blood cultures are positive in about 80% during the first week and 30% in the third week. Urine cultures are helpful during the second week and stool cultures during the second to fourth week. Marrow cultures are occasionally helpful. Of the serological tests, the Widal test, which measures serum agglutinins against the O and H antigens, is most helpful; but high antibody levels are seen in some populations. A fourfold increase in titre in sequential blood samples is suggestive of *Salmonella* infection.

TREATMENT OF *SALMONELLA* INFECTIONS

Chloramphenicol, co-trimoxazole and amoxycillin are all effective but increasing resistance is becoming widespread. Ciprofloxacin 500 mg twice-daily is therefore used but is expensive. The temperature may take 4–6 days before settling, although subjective improvement is noted earlier. Treatment should be continued for two weeks. Complications such as intestinal perforation or haemorrhage may occur despite adequate treatment. These complications can often be managed conservatively.

Eradication of a carrier state can be difficult, but ciprofloxacin for four weeks may be effective. Chemotherapy does not effect a cure in about 40% of cases. In such individuals cholecystectomy remains the only mode of treatment.

PREVENTION AND CONTROL

This includes provision of safe drinking water, sanitary disposal of excreta and proper attention to hygiene by those who handle food. The parenteral monovalent typhoid vaccine is used as it is less likely to produce local and systemic reactions, but protection is incomplete and relatively short-lived (one year). An improved parenteral vaccine based on the Vi polysaccharide antigen gives protection for about three years. An attenuated strain of *S. typhi* (Ty 21a) is available as a live oral vaccine and gives a similar efficacy, although the length of protection is less; it should be repeated after one year.

Paratyphoid fever

Paratyphoid fever is due to *S. paratyphi* A, B or C. They result in an illness clinically indistinguishable from typhoid fever. However, paratyphoid fever is a milder illness. Treatment is with co-trimoxazole 960 mg daily for two weeks.

Shigella infections

Shigellosis (bacillary dysentery)

Shigellosis is an acute self-limiting intestinal infection caused by one of four species of Gram-negative non-spore-forming bacilli. These include *Shigella dysenteriae*, *Sh. flexneri*, *Sh. boydii* and *Sh. sonnei*. While all of them are enteroinvasive, *Sh. dysenteriae* type 1 and some strains of *Sh. flexneri* and *Sh. sonnei* have been demonstrated to elaborate a toxin that is enterotoxic, neurotoxic and cytotoxic (see Fig 4.36).

Like salmonellosis, shigellosis is found worldwide and is more prevalent in areas with poor hygiene and overcrowding. Transmission is by the faecal-oral route and a very low dose is sufficient to produce the disease.

CLINICAL FEATURES

Children usually under five years are predominantly affected. The incubation period is short, usually two days. The onset is acute, with fever, malaise, abdominal pain and watery diarrhoea. As the disease increases in intensity, bloody diarrhoea with mucus, tenesmus, faecal urgency and severe cramping abdominal pain becomes prominent. Nausea, vomiting, headache and convulsions (in children) may occur and have been attributed to the neurotoxin. When the disease is due to *Sh. dysenteriae*, which is responsible for the more fulminant forms of shigellosis, a cholera-like picture is occasionally seen.

Sigmoidoscopy shows the presence of a markedly hyperaemic and inflamed mucosa, with transversely distributed ulcers with ragged undermined edges. The appearances are often indistinguishable from other dysenteric infections and from nonspecific inflammatory bowel disease.

Complications may be mild (arthritis, conjunctivitis, morbilliform rash) or life-threatening, such as colonic perforation, septicaemia and the haemolytic uraemic syndrome.

DIAGNOSIS

The diagnosis is made on the basis of a stool culture.

TREATMENT AND PREVENTION

Treatment is symptomatic with oral fluid replacement as necessary. In severe cases, trimethoprim 200 mg twice-daily or ciprofloxacin 500 mg twice-daily are used.

Public health measures, particularly the disposal of excreta and the provision of potable water, prevent infection. Outbreaks in schools can be controlled only by good hygiene.

Campylobacter infections

Campylobacter jejuni is a Gram-negative, motile, curved spiral rod that is microaerophilic and thus fails to multiply under aerobic or strict anaerobic conditions. It invades the mucosa of both the small and large bowel causing inflammation and sometimes ulceration. *C. jejuni* causes acute diarrhoea, sometimes with blood, and is one of the most common causes of acute gastroenteritis in adults in the UK. In developing countries asymptomatic carriers occur in young children.

CLINICAL FEATURES

Symptoms begin 2–5 days after eating infected material (usually chicken or milk), the most common being fever, headache and malaise. These are followed rapidly by diarrhoea, often with blood, and quite severe cramping abdominal pain. The patient generally appears unwell.

Sigmoidoscopy can show the changes of acute colitis, which may be indistinguishable from those of ulcerative colitis. Complications include cholecystitis, pancreatitis, a reactive arthritis, the Guillain–Barré syndrome and the haemolytic uraemic syndrome.

DIAGNOSIS

Direct phase microscopy of a wet mount of stool may reveal the motile curved rods resembling 'flying birds'. The organism may be cultured on special media within 48 hours. In severe infections the organism may be cultured from the blood.

TREATMENT OF *CAMPYLOBACTER* INFECTIONS

In the majority of cases, *Campylobacter* enteritis is a self-limiting illness, resolving in 5–7 days. Although the organism is sensitive to erythromycin, there is no evidence that treatment with this antibiotic alters the natural history of the infection. However, if systemic symptoms continue in association with persistent bacteraemia, antibiotics are usually administered.

Helicobacter infections

(see also p. 235)

Helicobacter pylori, a curved Gram-negative organism, colonizes the gastric epithelium beneath the mucus layer and in areas of gastric metaplasia such as occur in the duodenum. *H. pylori* is noted for its ability to produce urease, which is thought to be involved in the pathogenesis of disease.

Yersinia infections

The only three major human pathogens are *Y. pseudotuberculosis* and *Y. enterocolitica*, which respectively cause mesenteric lymphadenitis and enterocolitis, and *Yersinia pestis*, which causes plague.

Y. enterocolitica and *Y. pseudotuberculosis* infections

These result in a number of clinical syndromes depending on the host's age and immune status. Patients may present with enterocolitis, acute mesenteric lymphadenitis or terminal ileitis. Enterocolitis is characterized by the presence of fever, diarrhoea and severe abdominal pain, which may lead to a mistaken diagnosis of appendicitis. Arthritis (sometimes with Reiter's syndrome – see p. 264) and erythema nodosum are seen and are immunologically mediated.

This is usually a self-limiting disease and no treatment is required. In very severe cases, tetracycline 1 g daily may be given.

Plague

Plague is caused by *Y. pestis*, a Gram-negative bacillus. Sporadic cases of plague, as well as occasional epidemics, occur worldwide in humans. From 1980 to 1994 approximately 19 000 cases were reported to the WHO with a 10% mortality. Cases have occurred in developed countries in people undertaking outdoor pursuits. The major reservoirs are woodland rodents, which transmit infection to domestic rats (*Rattus rattus*). The vector is the rat flea, *Xenopsylla cheopis*. These fleas bite humans when there is a sudden decline in the rat population. Occasionally, spread of the organisms may be through infected faeces being rubbed into skin wounds or through inhalation of droplets.

Virulence is attributed to the presence of the endotoxin, exotoxin and fraction I (a soluble protein that prevents phagocytosis of the organism). Clinical manifestations are attributed to the lipopolysaccharide endotoxin.

CLINICAL FEATURES

Four clinical forms are recognized: bubonic, pneumonic, septicaemic and cutaneous.

Bubonic plague

This is the most common form and occurs in about 90% of infected individuals. The incubation period is about one week. The onset of illness is acute, with high fever, chills, headache, myalgia, nausea, vomiting and, when severe, prostration. This is rapidly followed by the development of lymphadenopathy, most commonly involving the inguinal lymph nodes (buboes). Characteristically these are matted and tender, and suppurate in 1–2 weeks. Petechiae, ecchymoses and bleeding from the gastrointestinal tract, the respiratory tract and the genitourinary tract may occur. Mental confusion follows the development of toxaemia.

Pneumonic plague

This is characterized by the abrupt onset of features of a fulminant pneumonia with bloody sputum, marked respiratory distress, cyanosis and death in almost all affected patients.

Septicaemic plague

This presents as an acute fulminant infection with evidence of shock and DIC. If left untreated, death usually occurs in 2–5 days. Lymphadenopathy is unusual.

Cutaneous plague

This presents either as a pustule, eschar or papule or an extensive purpura, which can become necrotic and gangrenous.

DIAGNOSIS

The diagnosis is easily established by demonstrating the organism in lymph node aspirates, in blood cultures or on examination of sputum.

TREATMENT OF PLAGUE

Treatment is urgent and should be instituted before the results of culture studies are available. Several antimicrobial drugs are effective, including streptomycin 0.5 g i.m. every four hours for 48 hours, followed by 0.5 g every six hours for five days, or tetracycline 2–3 g daily for 14 days. Isolated antibiotic resistance has been reported and recently multidrug resistance was found in Madagascar.

PREVENTION AND CONTROL

Prevention of plague is largely dependent on the control of the flea population and the use of potent antiflea agents such as 2% aldrin. Outhouses, or huts, should be sprayed with insecticides that are effective against the local flea. Rodents should not be killed until the fleas are under control as the fleas will leave dead rodents to bite humans. Tetracycline 500 mg four times daily or sulphonamides 2–4 g daily for seven days are effective chemoprophylactic agents.

Patients themselves can be infective when the buboes break down; patients with pneumonic plague can spread the organism by droplets. A partially effective formalin-killed vaccine is available for use by travellers to plague-endemic areas.

Other infections

Tularaemia

Tularaemia is due to infection by *Francisella tularensis*, a Gram-negative organism. It is primarily a zoonosis, affecting mainly rodents, including rabbits and squirrels. Vectors are ticks and blood-sucking flies. Humans are infected by handling infected animals or from vector bites. The micro-organisms enter through the skin or through minor abrasions in the mouth or conjunctivae. Occasionally infection occurs from contaminated water or from eating uncooked meat. The disease occurs worldwide and is frequently seen in the USA, particularly in hunters and butchers.

CLINICAL FEATURES

The incubation period of 2–7 days is followed by a generalized illness. A number of clinical syndromes can be seen:

The *ulceroglandular form* is the most common. A papule occurs at the site of inoculation. This ulcerates and is followed by tender, suppurative lymphadenopathy. Infected material entering the eye is followed by a purulent conjunctivitis with periauricular lymphadenopathy.

Pneumonic forms present with cough, chest pain and eventually a pneumonia, sometimes accompanied by a pericarditis.

The *septicaemic form* is very rare and presents with the sudden onset of a fever, myalgia, headache and shock.

Diagnosis is by culture of the organism or by a rising titre seen on a bacterial agglutination test.

TREATMENT AND PREVENTION

Treatment is with gentamicin. The patient should be isolated.

In endemic areas all wild animals should be handled using gloves. Infected meat and water should be adequately cooked. A vaccine is available for laboratory staff handling possibly infected animals.

Glanders

Glanders is caused by a Gram-negative bacillus, *Pseudomonas mallei*. It affects mainly horses but can very rarely be transmitted to humans, mainly horse handlers. The disease is acquired by inhalation or inoculation of infected material. In the acute state, the patient is toxic with a high fever and delirium. There is an ulceration of the upper respiratory tract with eventual pneumonia, empyema and lung abscess. Septicaemia develops. Treatment is with intravenous broad-spectrum antibiotics.

Melioidosis

Melioidosis is due to the Gram-negative bacillus, *Pseudomonas pseudomallei*, which is a soil saprophyte. It infects humans (particularly diabetics or traumatized patients) by penetrating through skin abrasions in, for example, barefoot farmers in paddy-fields. Rarely it can be aquired by inhalation. It is found worldwide, but occurs mainly in South East Asia.

Septicaemia with abscesses in the lung, kidney, liver and spleen may occur and here the prognosis is poor. With localized lesions the prognosis is excellent with appropriate therapy. A chronic form, usually presenting with an unresolved pneumonia, also occurs. Relapses following therapy are common.

Diagnosis is by culture of the organism. An indirect haemagglutination test is positive after one week. The chest X-ray may resemble tuberculosis.

TREATMENT OF MELIOIDOSIS

Treatment is with ceftazidime 120 mg kg^{-1} for 2–4 weeks, followed by oral amoxycillin/clavulanic acid (amoxiclav) for six months.

Pasteurellosis

Pasteurelloses are infections primarily of animals. Three species are known to infect humans, the most common being *Pasteurella multocida*, which is also the most virulent. All these organisms are commensal in the nasopharynx and gastrointestinal tract of a number of domestic and wild mammals. Transmission to humans may occur through a bite or scratch.

CLINICAL FEATURES

Focal soft tissue infection with marked erythema, severe tenderness and regional lymphadenopathy may be present. These organisms are also responsible for chronic respiratory infections, bacteraemia, and brain and renal abscesses.

TREATMENT OF PASTEURELLOSIS

Penicillin is the drug of choice and should be given parenterally as benzylpenicillin 1–2 g every four hours.

Legionnaires' disease

This is caused by the fastidious *Legionella pneumophila*, a weakly Gram-negative, catalase-positive bacillus. It is described on p. 797.

Bacteroides infection

Bacteroides is an obligate anaerobic, Gram-negative bacillus. *B. fragilis* is the most important anaerobic human pathogen and is a normal commensal in the human large gut. It does not produce an endotoxin and because of its polysaccharide capsule it resists phagocytosis. *B. fragilis* also produces heparinase, which may be involved in the development of thrombophlebitis, and β-lactamases, which inhibit the action of penicillin. It is not a highly invasive organism and grows best in necrotic tissues.

CLINICAL FEATURES

Seventy-five per cent of all intra-abdominal infections, particularly postoperative infections, are caused by anaerobes. *Bacteroides* is a frequent cause of hepatic, subhepatic, pelvic and splenic abscesses. The pus has a characteristic putrid smell. *Bacteroides* also causes pelvic infections and may result in endometritis, Bartholin's abscess and pelvic peritonitis. Fournier's gangrene is also caused by *B. fragilis*.

DIAGNOSIS

This depends on strict anaerobic culture with special media. Gas–liquid chromatography has been used to detect the volatile fatty acids produced by anaerobic bacteria.

TREATMENT OF *BACTEROIDES* INFECTION

Surgery is usually required as well as chemotherapy. Metronidazole (1–2 g daily by mouth or 1 g eight-hourly per rectum) is the drug of choice. It is also used prophylactically in colorectal surgery, with a dramatic reduction in postoperative infections.

Bartonella infections

These are due to Gram-negative bacilli (Table 1.24).

Bartonellosis (Carrión's disease)

Caused by *B. bacilliformis*, this is restricted mainly to the habitat of its main vector, the sandfly, in the river valleys of the Andes mountains at an altitude of 500–3000 m. Two to six weeks following the bite, the patient develops 'oroya fever' with myalgia, arthralgia, severe headache and confusion followed by a haemolytic anaemia. Four to five weeks later reddish-purple haemangiomatous nodules develop and persist for 3–4 months. Superinfection can occur particularly with *Salmonella*.

DIAGNOSIS AND TREATMENT

Diagnosis is by finding bacilli in erythrocytes or blood culture. Serological tests have been developed but are not widely available.

Treatment is with chloramphenicol, tetracycline, penicillin, co-trimoxazole or a fluoroquinolone.

Cat-scratch disease

The cause is *B. henselae*. Between 7 and 14 days after a scratch or bite, a small red papule appears at the site associated with regional lymph-node enlargement. Lymphadenopathy may persist for several weeks and suppurate in up to 40% of cases. The disease may occasionally progress systemically with encephalitis, neuroretinitis, arthritis, hepatitis, osteolytic bone lesions and pleurisy. *B. henselae* is sensitive to erythromycin, doxycycline, some cephalosporins (cefoxitin, cefotaxime) and aminoglycosides (gentamicin, tobramycin).

Trench fever

The cause is *B. quintana*. Trench fever is characterized by cyclical fever (every five days), chills, and headaches, accompanied by postorbital and pretibial pain. The

Table 1.24
Bartonella infections

Bacillus	Disease
B. bacilliformis	Bartonellosis (Carrión's disease)
B. elizabethae	? Endocarditis
B. henselae	Cat-scratch disease, bacillary angiomatosis, peliosis hepatis and CNS and eye infections
B. quintana	Trench fever, cutaneous bacillary angiomatosis, bacteraemia and endocarditis in HIV infection

condition is now occurring in the homeless population. The disease is self-limiting but is usually treated with erythromycin or doxycycline.

FURTHER READING

Dennis DT, Hughes JM (1997) Multidrug resistance in plague. *New England Journal of Medicine* **337**:702-705.

Parry SM, Salmon RL, Willshaw GA, Cheasty T (1998) Risk factors for and prevention of sporadic infections with verocytotoxin (Shiga toxin) producing E. coli O157. *Lancet* **351**: 1019-1022.

Steinhoff MC (1997) Hib infections are preventable everywhere. *Lancet* **349**: 1186–1187

Actinomycetes

Actinomycetes (*Actinomyces* and *Nocardia*) are Gram-positive, branching higher bacteria and include *Actinomyces israelii* which is the most common pathogen.

Actinomyces is a normal mouth and intestine commensal particularly associated with poor mouth hygiene. It produces an illness characterized by chronicity and poor infectivity. It has a worldwide distribution but is a rare cause of disease in the West.

Actinomycosis

Three clinical forms of disease are recognized. Occasionally actinomycosis becomes disseminated to involve any site.

- The *cervicofacial variety* usually occurs following dental infection or extraction. It is often indolent and slowly progressive, associated with little pain, and results in induration and localized swelling of the lower part of the mandible ('lumpy jaw'). Lymphadenopathy is uncommon. Occasionally acute inflammation occurs. Sinuses and tracts develop with discharge of 'sulphur' granules.
- The *thoracic variety* follows inhalation of these organisms usually into a previously damaged lung. The clinical picture is not distinctive and is often mistaken for malignancy or tuberculosis. Symptoms such as fever, malaise, chest pain and haemoptysis are present. Empyema occurs in 25% of patients and local extension produces chest-wall sinuses with discharge of 'sulphur' granules.
- *Abdominal actinomycosis* most frequently affects the caecum. Characteristically, a hard indurated mass is felt in the right iliac fossa. Later, sinuses develop. The differential diagnosis includes malignancy, tuberculosis, Crohn's disease and amoeboma. Pelvic actinomycosis appears to be increasing with wider use of intrauterine contraceptive devices.

DIAGNOSIS AND TREATMENT

Diagnosis is by microscopy and culture of the organism.

Treatment involves surgery, and penicillin is the drug of choice. High-dose intravenous penicillin 2.4 g four-hourly is given for 4–6 weeks, followed by oral penicillin for some weeks after clinical resolution. Tetracyclines are also effective.

Nocardiosis

Nocardia is a Gram-positive, filamentous branching bacterium, of which *N. asteroides* and less often *N. Brasiliensis* and *N. caviae* produce mycetomas.

CLINICAL FEATURES

Nocardia gives rise to two distinct clinical entities although widespread dissemination can occur in the immunocompromised patient.

- *Pulmonary disease* presents with cough, fever, and haemoptysis. Pleural involvement and empyema may occur.
- *Mycetoma* is the result of local invasion by *Nocardia* and presents as a painless swelling, usually on the sole of the foot (madura foot). The swelling of the affected part of the body continues inexorably. Nodules gradually appear from which purulent fluid containing characteristic 'grains' of the organisms are discharged. Systemic symptoms and regional lymphadenopathy are distinctly uncommon. Sinuses may occur several years after the onset of the first symptom.

Mycetoma may also be produced by several other members of actinomycetes, including *Actinomadura* and *Streptomyces*. It is then referred to as an 'actinomycetoma'. When caused by true fungi belonging to Eumycetes (e.g. *Madurella mycetomi* or *Petriellidium boydii*) it is referred to as 'eumycetoma'. The clinical presentation, with the exception of differently coloured 'grains', is similar to that of mycetoma.

DIAGNOSIS AND TREATMENT

The diagnosis is often difficult to establish, as *Nocardia* is not easily detected in sputum cultures or on histological section.

Treatment consists of adequate surgical drainage of the pus combined with prolonged chemotherapy. The drug of choice is sulphadiazine in doses of up to 9 g daily.

FURTHER READING

Lerner PL et al. (1992) Actinomyces. In: Gorbach SL, Barlett JG, Blacklow NR (eds) *Infectious Diseases*. WB Saunders, Philadelphia.

Table 1.25 Classification of *Mycobacterium* species based on their capacity to produce disease

Species	Disease produced
Obligate intracellular bacteria:	
M. leprae	Leprosy
Facultative intracellular bacteria: *M. tuberculosis*	Most cases of human tuberculosis
M. bovis	Cattle and rarely human tuberculosis
Other forms:	
M. avium intracellulare	Fowl and human tuberculosis, particularly in HIV infection
M. paratuberculosis	Johne's disease (chronic granulomatous enteritis) in cattle
M. scrofulaceum	Lymph node infection
M. kansasii	Human tuberculosis (occasionally)

Mycobacteria

Mycobacteria are acid-fast, aerobic bacilli that grow extremely slowly. The cell wall contains complex lipids and glycolipids, such as trehalose dimycolate which is responsible for producing granulomas. No extracellular enzyme or toxins have been identified. The capacity of mycobacteria to produce disease is therefore attributed to their ability to multiply within phagocytic cells and to withstand intracellular enzymatic digestion.

A clinical classification of mycobacteria is shown in Table 1.25.

Tuberculosis

Tuberculosis is due largely to *Mycobacterium tuberculosis*.

EPIDEMIOLOGY

Tuberculosis is present worldwide with an extremely high prevalence in Asian countries, where 60–80% of children below the age of 14 years are infected. Tuberculosis is spread predominantly by droplet infection.

The prevalence of tuberculosis increases with poor social conditions, inadequate nutrition and overcrowding.

PATHOLOGY

The characteristic lesion is a granuloma with central caseation and Langhans' giant cells. The primary infection usually involves the lungs, but can involve other areas such as the ileocaecal region of the gastrointestinal tract. It is almost always accompanied by lymph node involvement.

In most people the primary infection heals leaving some surviving tubercle bacilli. With a lowering of host resistance these are reactivated, producing local spread as well as haematogenous spread to all organs of the body, including the lungs, bones and kidneys. This particularly occurs in the elderly, in alcohol abusers, in patients with diabetes mellitus, lung disease, or after gastrectomy, as well as in patients who are on corticosteroids or are immunosuppressed. There is a high incidence in patients infected with HIV.

Occasionally the primary infection progresses locally to a more widespread lesion. Haematogenous spread can also occur, giving miliary tuberculosis.

Tuberculosis in the adult is therefore usually the result of reactivation of old disease, occasionally a primary infection or, more rarely, reinfection.

CLINICAL FEATURES

Pulmonary tuberculosis is the most common form; this is described on p. 801, along with the chemotherapeutic regimens.

Tuberculosis also affects other parts of the body:

- The *gastrointestinal tract* – mainly the ileocaecal area, but occasionally the peritoneum, producing ascites (see p. 284).
- The *genitourinary system* – the kidneys are mainly involved, but tuberculosis is also the cause of painless, craggy swellings in the epididymis and salpingitis, tubal abscesses and infertility in females.
- The *central nervous system* – tuberculous meningitis and tuberculomas.
- The *skeletal system* – arthritis and osteomyelitis, with cold abscess formation.
- The *skin* – lupus vulgaris.
- The *eyes* – signs of choroiditis, iridocyclitis or phlyctenular keratoconjunctivitis.
- The *pericardium* – producing constrictive pericarditis.
- The *adrenal glands* – causing destruction and producing Addison's disease.
- *Lymph nodes* This is a common mode of presentation, especially in young adults and children. Any group of lymph nodes may be involved, but hilar and paratracheal lymph nodes are the most common. Initially the nodes are firm and discrete but later they become matted and can suppurate and form sinuses.

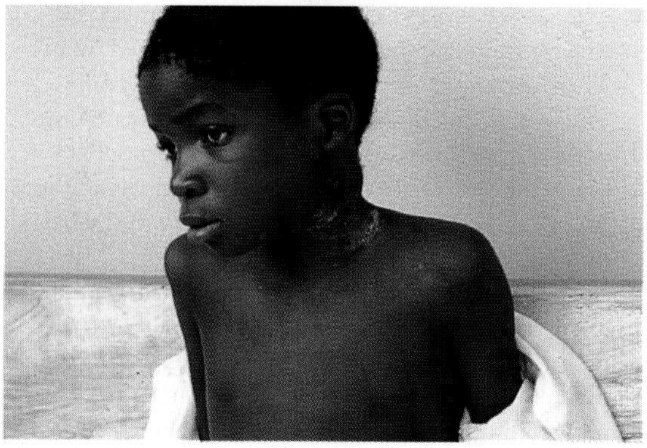

Fig 1.20
Scrofula, showing enlarged cervical lymph nodes

Scrofula is the term used to describe massive cervical lymph node enlargement with discharging sinuses (Fig 1.20). It is most often due to *M. tuberculosis*, and rarely to *M. scrofulaceum* or *M. kansasi*. Signs of acute inflammation are absent.

Leprosy (Hansen's disease)

The causative organism is the acid-fast bacillus *M. leprae*. Unlike other mycobacteria, it does not grow in artificial media or even in tissue culture. While inability to culture the organism obtained from lesions and secretions is suggestive of *M. leprae*, it is not diagnostic. The following additional properties have been found to be useful in its identification:

- loss of acid-fastness following pyridine extraction
- the ability of the organism to grow slowly in the footpad of mice (other mycobacteria also grow in the footpad of mice, but these produce distinct histological changes)
- the ability of *M. leprae* to oxidize 3,4-dihydroxyphenylalanine to pigmented products
- the ability of this organism to invade peripheral nerves, a property not demonstrated by other mycobacteria.

Leprosy occurs in all tropical and warm temperate climate regions, particularly in Asia and Africa (Fig 1.21). Endemic foci are still present in Southern Europe and parts of the USA. Of the 15 million people with leprosy worldwide, about two-thirds are in Asia. The precise mode of transmission is still uncertain but it is likely that nasal secretions play an important role.

Once an individual has been infected, subsequent progression to clinical disease appears to be dependent on several factors:

- *Sex* – males appear to be more susceptible than females. In India, the ratio of affected males to females is 2:1.
- *Genetic susceptibility* – studies in twins have shown a concordance in identical but not in non-identical twins.
- *Immunological response* – the clinical course will depend on the host's cell-mediated immunity (CMI).

CLASSIFICATION

Two polar types of leprosy are recognized:

- *tuberculoid leprosy* – a localized disease that occurs in individuals with a high degree of CMI
- *lepromatous leprosy* – a generalized disease that occurs in individuals with impaired CMI.

Two subdivisions of lepromatous leprosy are included in the classification. The patient is said to have the 'subpolar' lepromatous (LL_S) form when he has passed through a borderline phase before becoming lepromatous, and the polar lepromatous (LL_P) form when the patient is lepromatous throughout.

Indeterminate leprosy is characterized by one or more hypopigmented, sometimes erythematous, ill-defined macules of variable size. Sensation, sweating and hair growth over the macules are usually normal. This form of leprosy is usually seen in children.

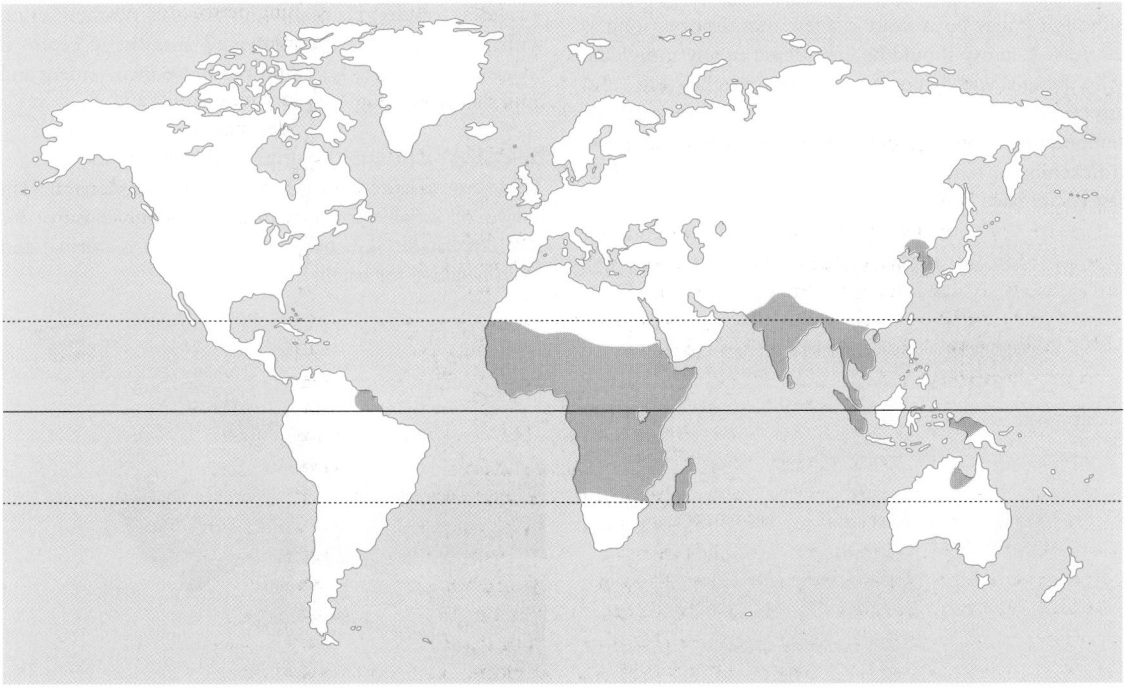

Fig 1.21
Geographical distribution of leprosy, showing areas where the prevalance is 5 in 1000 or greater

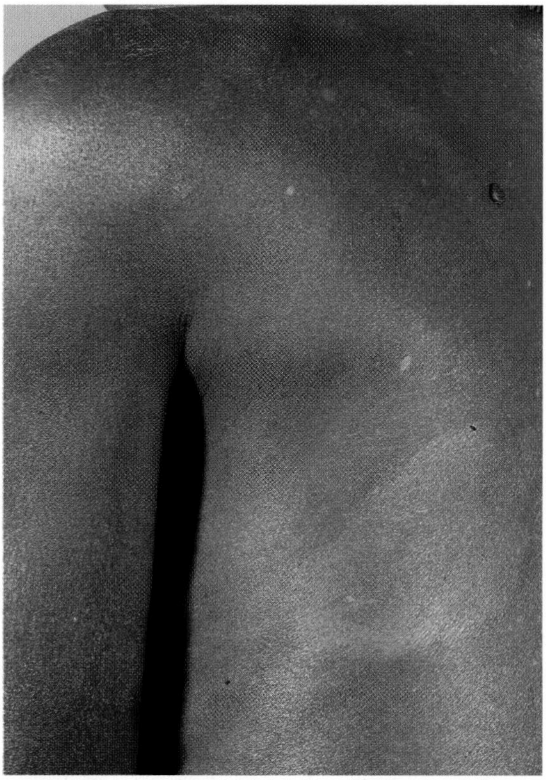

Fig 1.22
Multiple asymmetrical hypopigmented anaesthetic patches (courtesy of Dr P. Matondo, Zambia)

CLINICAL FEATURES

The incubation period varies from two to six years, although it may be as short as a few months or as long as 20 years. Leprosy should be considered in any individual who presents with hypopigmented skin patches (Fig 1.22) associated with loss of sensation, especially to touch or temperature, and evidence of nerve involvement (thickening or tenderness), in whom non-cultivable acid-fast bacilli have been identified in skin smears.

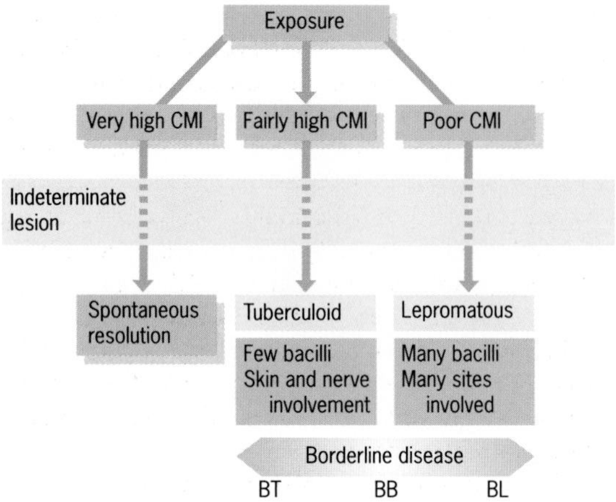

Fig 1.23
Clinical spectrum of leprosy

The onset of leprosy is generally insidious. However, acute onset is known to occur and patients may present with a transient rash, with features of an acute febrile illness, with evidence of nerve involvement, or with any combination of these.

CLINICAL SPECTRUM (Fig 1.23)

Five clinical groups are recognized which cover the spectrum of disease.

Tuberculoid leprosy (TT)

In tuberculoid leprosy the infection is localized because the patient has unimpaired cell-mediated immunity. The characteristic, usually single, skin lesion is a hypopigmented, anaesthetic patch with thickened, clearly demarcated edges, central healing and atrophy. The face, gluteal region and extremities are most commonly affected. Frequently the nerve leading to this hypopigmented patch and the regional nerve trunk are thickened and tender. Unlike other parts of the body, a tuberculoid patch on the face is not anaesthetic. Nerve involvement leads to marked muscle atrophy. Tuberculoid lesions are known to heal spontaneously.

Borderline-tuberculoid (BT) leprosy

This resembles TT but skin lesions are usually more numerous, smaller and may be present as small 'satellite' lesions around larger ones. Peripheral but not cutaneous nerves are thickened, leading to deformity of hands and feet.

Borderline (BB) leprosy

Skin lesions are numerous, varying in size and form (macules, papules, plaques). The annular, rimmed lesion with punched-out, hypopigmented anaesthetic centre is characteristic. There is widespread nerve involvement and limb deformity (Fig 1.24).

Borderline lepromatous (BL) leprosy

There are a large number of florid asymmetrical skin lesions of variable form, which are strongly positive for acid-fast bacilli. Skin between the lesions is normal and often negative for bacilli.

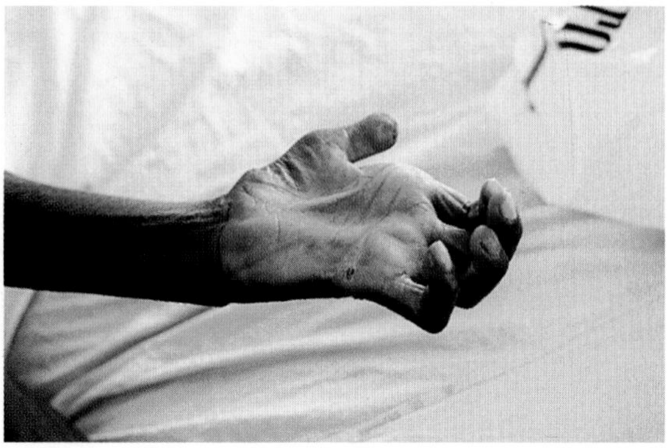

Fig 1.24
Leprosy – claw hand due to median and ulnar nerve damage

Lepromatous leprosy (LL)

Although practically every organ can be involved, the changes in the skin are the earliest and most obvious manifestation. Peripheral oedema and rhinitis are the earliest symptoms. The skin lesions predominantly occur on the face, the gluteal region and the upper and lower limbs. They may be macules, papules, nodules or plaques. Of these, the macule is the earliest lesion. Infiltration is most noticeable in the ear lobes. Thinning of the lateral margins of the eyebrows is characteristic. The mucous membranes are frequently involved, resulting in nasal stuffiness, laryngitis and hoarseness of the voice. Nasal septal perforation with collapse of the nasal cartilages produces a saddle-nose deformity. With progression of the disease, the typical leonine facies due to infiltration of the skin becomes apparent. Glove and stocking anaesthesia, gynaecomastia, testicular atrophy, ichthyosis and nerve palsies (facial, ulnar, median and radial) develop late in the disease. Neurotrophic atrophy affecting the phalanges leads to the gradual disappearance of fingers. Nerve involvement is less pronounced than in TT.

Lucio's phenomenon is seen only in Mexico and Central America, where LL is associated with an endarteritis which results in skin ulceration. The ulcers are large, with undermined edges and markedly necrotic bases. Smears from the base generally reveal numerous acid-fast bacilli. Healing is by scar formation. Treatment is wide surgical excision with skin grafts. Chemotherapy alone is ineffective in healing ulcers.

The lepromin test

This is a measure of host resistance to leprosy and not a test for detecting leprosy: 0.1 mL of a suspension of dead bacilli (either Mitsuda lepromin or the Dharmendra lepromin) is injected intradermally. Two types of reaction are observed:

- The early (Fernandez) reaction becomes positive in 48 hours and reflects the sensitivity of the tissue to the leprosy bacilli protein.
- The late (Mitsuda) reaction develops in 4–5 weeks and reflects the resistance of the host to the bacteria. This reaction is strongly positive in TT and is negative in LL.

Lepra reactions

Lepra reactions are immunologically mediated acute reactions that occur in patients with the borderline or lepromatous spectrum of disease usually during treatment. Two forms are recognized.

Non-lepromatous lepra reaction (type I lepra reaction). This is seen following treatment of patients with borderline disease; it is a type IV delayed hypersensitivity reaction. Both upgrading or reversal reactions (i.e. a clinical change towards a more tuberculoid form) and downgrading reactions (i.e. a change towards the lepromatous form) can occur. The borderline reaction is characterized by acute inflammation of pre-existing borderline lesions. Skin lesions become swollen and erythematous. Neurological deficits such as an ulnar nerve palsy may occur abruptly.

Erythema nodosum leprosum (ENL; type II lepra reaction). This is a humoral antibody response to an antigen–antibody complex (i.e. a type III hypersensitivity reaction). It is seen in 50% of patients with treated LL. It is characterized by fever, arthralgia and crops of painful, subcutaneous erythematous nodules, iridocyclitis and other systemic manifestations. It may last from a few days to several weeks.

DIAGNOSIS

The diagnosis of leprosy is essentially clinical. Patients should be examined in adequate natural light. The demonstration of acid-fast bacilli in smears from the skin or nasal mucosa is highly suggestive. Occasionally nerve biopsies are helpful. The definitive diagnosis is established by cultivating the organisms in the footpads of mice. Detection of *M. leprae* DNA is possible in all forms of leprosy using the polymerase chain reaction and can be used to assess the efficacy of treatment.

Two indices are currently in use to evaluate the response to treatment of patients in whom the skin-smear test for acid-fast bacilli is positive:

- The *bacteriological index* (BI) is an objective way of evaluating the response to treatment. The skin-smear is graded from 1+ to 6+ depending upon the number of bacilli present per high-power field. The BI is calculated by taking the mean result of four slide examinations. For example, a decrease in BI from 6 to 3.5 on therapy indicates a good response to treatment.
- The *morphological index* (MI) is the percentage of solid staining acid-fast bacilli on smears (solid bacilli represent viable bacteria). A patient with an MI of 0% is not infectious.

TREATMENT

Leprosy should be treated in specialist centres with adequate physiotherapy and occupational therapy support. Multidrug therapy is now essential because of developing drug resistance (up to 20% of cases are resistant to dapsone).

Dapsone (di-amino-di-phenyl sulphone, DDS), a folate synthetase inhibitor, is bacteriostatic. It has the advantage of being cheap and well tolerated. Side-effects are few and include haemolytic anaemia and sulphaemoglobinaemia. In 1982 the World Health Organization recommended that for multibacillary forms of leprosy (BB, BL and LL types) it should be taken on a daily basis (100 mg) along with rifampicin 600 mg once-monthly and clofazimine 50 mg daily with an extra dose of 300 mg monthly. The monthly doses are given under supervision. This triple therapy should be given for a minimum of two years or continued until a patient's skin smears become negative for acid-fast bacilli. However, in paucibacillary forms (TT or BT) six months' therapy with DDS 100 mg daily and rifampicin 600 mg monthly is recommended.

The major disadvantage with clofazimine is that it is a dye and causes a generalized reddish brown pigmentation in light-skinned individuals and a slate-grey pigmentation in dark-skinned individuals. Ethionamide is a suitable alternative. Acedapsone (DADDS), a depot sulphone, has been used with some success.

Three new groups of drugs have been identified to be active against *M. lepra* and are currently under evaluation in human infection: (i) the 4-fluoroquinolones, ofloxacin and perfloxacin; (ii) minocycline; and (iii) the erythromycin derivative, clarithromycin. It is likely that use of these drugs will substantially reduce the duration of treatment in the future.

Surgery and physiotherapy play an important role in the management of trophic ulcers and deformities of the hands, feet and face.

Treatment of lepra reactions

Treatment of lepra reactions is urgent, as irreversible eye and nerve damage can occur with amazing rapidity. Antileprosy therapy must be continued. Type II lepra reactions (ENL) are effectively treated with analgesics, chloroquine, clofazimine and antipyretics. Thalidomide, a drug known for its potent teratogenic effects, is by far the most effective in the ENL reaction, but must be used with caution. Prednisolone 30–40 mg daily for a few weeks is effective in type I reactions.

PREVENTION AND CONTROL

This depends on rapid treatment of infected patients, particularly those with LL and BL, to decrease the bacterial reservoir. It is spread by close contact, but only a small proportion of contacts – approximately 1% – develop the disease. Antileprosy vaccines are under clinical trial; the efficacy of the BCG vaccine against leprosy is debatable. Mass chemoprophylaxis is impracticable and its efficacy in household contacts has not been established.

Mycobacterial ulcer

Also known as Buruli ulcer, after the Buruli region in Uganda, this condition occurs in tropical, rural areas near rivers (e.g. in Zaire, Nigeria and Malaysia). It is caused by *M. ulcerans*. The disease is contracted by swimming in infected water. Initially a small subcutaneous nodule develops. This undergoes ulceration that involves the subcutaneous tissue, muscle and fascial planes. The ulcers are usually large, with undermined edges and markedly necrotic bases. Smears taken from necrotic tissue generally reveal numerous acid-fast bacilli. Treatment is wide surgical excision with skin grafts. Antituberculous therapy is ineffective.

FURTHER READING

Grzybowski S, Allen EA (1995) History and importance of scrofula. *Lancet* **346**: 1472–1474.

WHO Expert Committee on Leprosy (1994) Chemotherapy of leprosy. Technical Report Series WHO, **847**.

Mycoplasma

Mycoplasma is a small, free-living, motile bacterium that lacks a cell wall. *Mycoplasma pneumoniae* is found worldwide and may cause up to 20% of pneumonias. Infection is endemic but epidemics also occur, the infection being spread by airborne droplets between close contacts. *M. pneumoniae* infection is found most commonly in childhood, adolescence and early adulthood.

The oropharynx, trachea and bronchi are commonly involved, but there is frequently infiltration into the lung, causing pneumonia. The clinical features and treatment are described on p. 796.

M. hominis and *Ureaplasma urealyticum* cause nonspecific urethritis and cervicitis.

Spirochaetes

Spirochaetal infections include those due to *Treponema*, *Leptospira* and *Borrelia* (Table 1.26).

Syphilis

This is described on p. 101.

Bejel (endemic non-venereal syphilis), yaws and pinta

These diseases are endemic throughout the tropical and subtropical regions of the world (Fig 1.25). The WHO treated over 50 million cases in the 1950s and 60s, reducing the prevalence of these diseases, but subsequently there has been a resurgence of infection. Improvements in sanitation and an increase in living standards will be required to eradicate the diseases completely as organisms are transmitted by bodily contact, usually in children.

Yaws

Apart from syphilis, yaws is the most widespread of the treponemal diseases worldwide but particularly in Africa, South America and Asia. It is spread by direct contact often in overcrowded huts at night, usually in children; the organism enters through damaged skin. After an incubation period of weeks or months, a primary inflammatory reaction occurs at the inoculation site, from which organisms can be isolated. Dissemination of the organism leads to multiple papular lesions containing treponemes; these skin lesions usually involve the palms and soles. There may also be bone involvement, particularly the long bones and those of the hand.

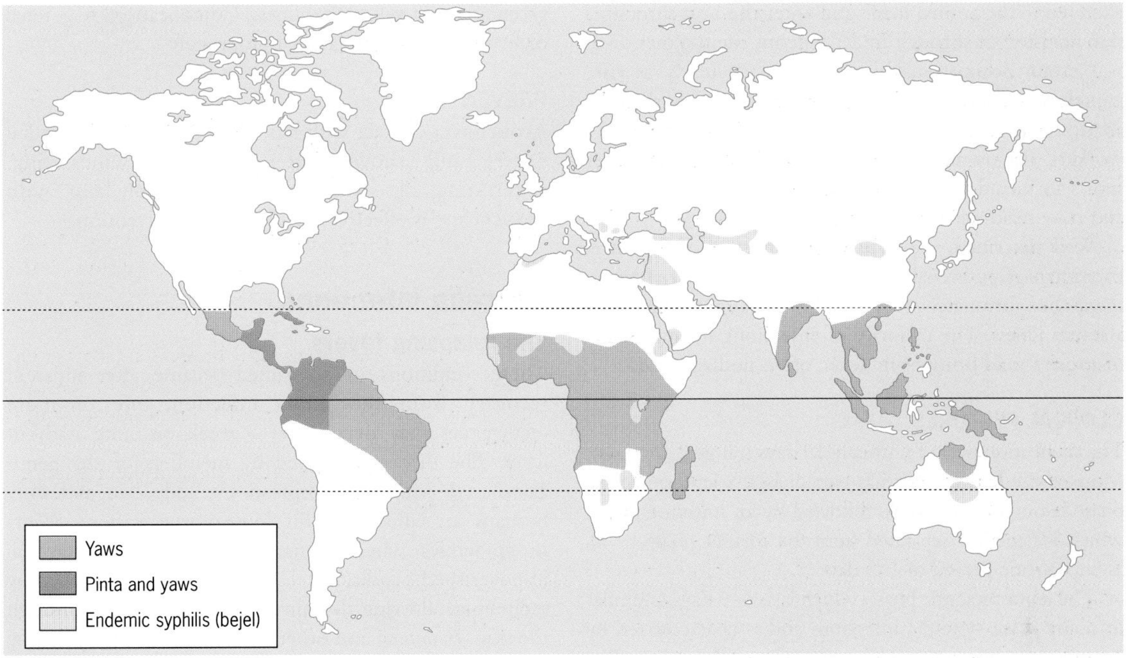

Fig 1.25
Bejel, yaws and pinta – geographical distribution

In late yaws bony gummatous lesions may progress to cause gross destruction and disfigurement, particularly of the skull and facial bones, the interphalangeal joints and the long bones. Plantar hyperkeratosis is characteristic. Like syphilis, there may be a latent period between the early and late phases of the disease, but visceral, neurological and cardiovascular problems do not occur

Bejel (endemic syphilis)

Bejel is seen in Africa and the Middle East. The organism enters through abrasions in the skin or from contaminated drinking vessels. It is interfamilial and occurs in children. It differs from venereal syphilis in that a primary lesion is not commonly seen, although the late stages are indistinguishable from syphilis.

Table 1.26
Spirochaetal infections

Disease	Organism
Syphilis	*Treponema pallidum*
Yaws	*Treponema pertenue*
Bejel (endemic non-venereal syphilis)	*Treponema pallidum* variant
Pinta	*Treponema carateum*
Leptospirosis	*Leptospira interrogans icterohaemorrhagiae, canicola, hardjo, pomona*
Louse-borne relapsing fever	*Borrelia recurrentis*
Tick-borne relapsing fever	*Borrelia duttonii* and others
Cancrum oris	*Borrelia vincenti*
Lyme disease	*Borrelia burgdorferi*
Rat-bite fever	*Spirillum minus* *Streptobacillus moniliformis*

Pinta

Pinta is restricted mainly to Central and South America but otherwise closely resembles endemic syphilis. The primary lesion is a pruritic red papule, usually on the hand or foot. It may become scaly but never ulcerates and is generally associated with regional lymphadenopathy. In the later stages similar lesions can continue to occur for up to one year associated with generalized lymphadenopathy. Eventually the lesions heal, leaving hyperpigmented or depigmented patches.

DIAGNOSIS AND TREATMENT

Under dark-ground microscopy the causative organism can be identified from the exudative lesions. Serological tests for syphilis are positive but do not differentiate between the conditions.

The treatment is with long-acting penicillin (e.g. benzathine), 1.2 g given intramuscularly as a single dose.

Leptospirosis

This zoonosis is caused by the Gram-negative organism *Leptospira interrogans*. There are over 200 serotypes; the main types affecting humans are *L. interrogans icterohaemorrhagiae* (from rodents and other wild animals), *L. interrogans canicola* (from dogs and pigs) and *L. interrogans hardjo* and *L. interrogans pomona* from cattle. Leptospires are excreted in the animal urine and enter the host through a skin abrasion or through intact mucous membranes.

Certain occupational groups are particularly at risk, namely veterinarians, those involved in animal husbandry, abattoir workers and, in the past, miners and sewer workers. Pet owners and those who take part in water sports in inland waters are also exposed to the infection and now make up over 50% of all reported cases.

Weil described a disease that consisted of jaundice, haemorrhage and renal impairment due to *L. icterohaemorrhagiae* but, fortunately, only 10–15% of patients suffer such a severe illness. The majority of infections are subclinical or cause a mild nonspecific fever, often undiagnosed.

CLINICAL FEATURES

The incubation period is usually 10 days (range 2–20 days). More severe leptospirosis has two phases: a leptospiraemic phase lasting up to a week, followed by an immune phase, which is generally separated from the former phase by an asymptomatic period of 1–3 days.

The leptospiraemic phase, which lasts 4–9 days, is similar to many acute systemic infections and is characterized by severe headache, fever, malaise, anorexia and myalgia. The majority of patients have suffusion of the conjunctivae. Infrequently there is arthralgia, hepatosplenomegaly, lymphadenopathy and various skin rashes.

During the immune phase of the illness 50% of patients have meningism, about one-third of whom have CSF lymphocytosis and a modest elevation of CSF protein concentration. The majority recover uneventfully at this stage. However, a small proportion go on to develop tender hepatomegaly, jaundice, haemolytic anaemia and oliguric renal failure with microscopic haematuria. Occasionally cardiac involvement develops, characterized by atrial and ventricular dysrhythmias and congestive cardiac failure. The mortality of leptospirosis is very variable but with a severe infection in the elderly it can be as high as 15–20%.

The diagnosis is most often made clinically.

INVESTIGATIONS

- **Blood tests** show a polymorpholeucocytosis and a raised ESR.
- **Culture**. Leptospires can be cultured from blood or CSF during the first week of the illness. A minority of patients excrete the organism in the urine during the second week of the illness and may continue to do so for a further 2–4 weeks. They can also be detected by the polymerase chain reaction (PCR).
- **Specific IgM leptospiral antibodies** appear by the end of the first week.
- Other laboratory investigations may be abnormal, depending on the organs involved.

TREATMENT

Leptospires are sensitive to penicillins, erythromycin, tetracycline and chloramphenicol. Penicillin is most commonly used (2.4 g daily for one week) and should be given at any stage of the illness. Complications (e.g. renal or liver failure) are treated appropriately.

PREVENTION

Avoid direct contact with rats, avoid immersion in natural waters and shower after canoeing, windsurfing, waterskiing or swimming. Chemoprophylaxis with doxycycline is effective for short-term prevention.

Borrelia infections

The relapsing fevers

These conditions are so named because, after apparent recovery from the initial infection, one or more recurrences may occur after a week or more without fever. The disease is caused by members of the genus *Borrelia*. *B. recurrentis* is spread by body lice and only humans are affected. This louse-borne variety occurs in epidemics when humans live in close contact in impoverished conditions; the infected louse is crushed by scratching, allowing the spirochaete to penetrate through the skin. *B. duttoni* and other *Borrelia* species are spread by soft (Argasid) ticks. Rodents are also infected, and humans are incidental hosts, acquiring the spirochaete from the saliva of the infected tick. This disease is found where traditional mud huts are the form of shelter but is also found in old houses and in camp sites in the USA.

These diseases are, however, found mainly in Africa, India, the Middle East, Mediterranean Europe and South America.

CLINICAL FEATURES

Symptoms begin 7–10 days after infection and consist of a high fever of abrupt onset with rigors, generalized myalgia and headache. A petechial or ecchymotic rash may be seen. The general condition then deteriorates, with delirium, hepatosplenomegaly, jaundice, haemorrhagic problems and circulatory collapse. Although complete recovery may occur at this time, the majority experience one or more relapses of diminishing severity approximately a week after the initial illness. Without specific treatment, approximately one-third of patients will die.

Louse- and tick-borne relapsing fevers are clinically similar, although louse-borne fever tends to have a shorter initial illness with more frequent relapses.

DIAGNOSIS AND TREATMENT

Spirochaetes can be demonstrated microscopically in the blood during febrile episodes.

Tetracycline or erythromycin are most commonly used. A severe Jarisch–Herxheimer reaction (see p. 103) occurs in many patients, often requiring intensive nursing care and intravenous fluids.

PREVENTION

Ticks live for years and remain infected, passing the infection to their progeny. These reservoirs of infection should be controlled by spraying houses with insecticides such as 2% benzene hexachloride and by reducing the number of rodents. In contrast, patients infested with lice should be deloused by washing with 1% Lysol or dusting with 10% dicophane (DDT). All clothes must be thoroughly disinfected.

Cancrum oris

Cancrum oris is caused by *Borrelia vincenti* in association with anaerobic bacteria, commonly a member of the fusobacteria. The disease occurs in deprived and undernourished individuals with poor hygiene.

Cancrum oris usually occurs in children who are recovering from a debilitating illness, commonly measles. Rapidly progressive gangrenous destruction of the inner aspect of the mouth and cheek occurs, which may continue to progress even after treatment with penicillin. The mortality is high, probably reflecting the underlying poor physical state of the patient.

Lyme disease

This disease is caused by *Borrelia burgdorferi sensu lato*. The disease is transmitted by *Ixodes dammini* or related ixodid ticks (*Ixodes ricinus* in Europe). It was originally described in Lyme, Connecticut, but is now known to occur in many parts of the USA, in Europe and in Australia. In the UK, 300–500 cases are reported annually. Ticks (on deer and sheep) are widespread in the UK, particularly in forests and woodland. Prompt removal of any tick is essential as infection is unlikely to take place until the tick begins to engorge. Ticks should be removed by grasping them with forceps near to the point of attachment to the skin and then withdrawn by gentle traction.

CLINICAL FEATURES

The first stage of the illness (within 7–10 days) consists of the unique and characteristic skin lesion – erythema chronicum migrans, often accompanied by headache, fever, malaise, myalgia, arthralgia and lymphadenopathy. The second stage follows weeks or months later, when some patients develop neurological (meningo-encephalitis, cranial or polyneuropathies) or cardiac problems (conduction disorders, myocarditis). Finally, the third stage of the disease consists of arthritis (see p. 486), which recurs in attacks for several years, often with associated erosion of cartilage and bone.

The 'agent' causing human granulocytic erlichiosis is also transmitted by the same ticks. It produces a similar clinical picture and can be co-transmitted.

DIAGNOSIS AND TREATMENT

The clinical features and epidemiological considerations are usually strongly suggestive of infection with this spirochaete. The diagnosis can only rarely be confirmed by isolation of the organisms from blood, skin lesions or CSF. IgM antibodies are detected in the first month; IgG antibodies are invariably present late in the disease. IgM antibodies can also be found in CSF.

Amoxycillin, doxycycline and cephalosporins given early in the course of the disease shortens the duration of the illness in approximately 50% of patients. Intravenous benzylpenicillin (2 g daily for 10 days) should be given for the later stages.

PREVENTION

In tick-infested areas, repellants and protective clothing should be worn. If a bite occurs the tick should be identified if possible. Antibiotic prophylaxis is being tried.

Rat bite fevers

Two spirochaetes, *Spirillum minus* and *Streptobacillus moniliformis*, produce similar febrile illnesses following rat bites. With *S. minus*, the bite usually heals but a local inflammatory response occurs 1–3 weeks later and is associated with swelling, ulceration (sodoku) and lymphadenopathy. A dark maculopapular rash is present during the febrile period and arthralgia occurs.

S. moniliformis infection can also occur after drinking infected milk (Haverhill fever). The incubation period is short (1–3 days), the rash is morbilliform and petechiae and arthritis is common.

Systemic sequelae of generalized infection occur with both conditions and periodic fever may continue for several weeks. *S. minus* usually causes a milder illness with a shorter incubation period and has less prolonged sequelae.

DIAGNOSIS, TREATMENT AND PREVENTION

Spirochaetes can be identified in aspirates from the inflammatory site, from a regional lymph node (*S. minus*), or from the blood (*S. moniliformis*). Serological tests are available and may be helpful in diagnosis. Remember that rat bites can also cause other illness, such as leptospirosis or murine typhus.

Both organisms are sensitive to penicillin and tetracycline. Rodent control is vital.

FURTHER READING

Pfister H-W, Wilske B, Weber K (1994) Lyme borreliosis: basic science and clinical aspects. *Lancet* **343**: 1013-1016.

Spach DM *et al.* (1993) Tick-borne disease in the United States. *New England Journal of Medicine* **329**: 936-947.

Rickettsiae and similar organisms

Rickettsiae are small bacteria that are spread to humans by arthropod vectors, namely human body lice, fleas, ticks and larval mites. Rickettsiae inhabit the alimentary tract of these arthropods and the disease is spread to the human host by

Table 1.27
Infections due to *Rickettsia* and *Rickettsia*-like organisms

Disease	Organism	Reservoir	Vector
Typhus fevers:			
Epidemic typhus	*Rickettsia prowazekii*	Man	Human lice
Endemic (murine) typhus	*Rickettsia typhi* (*R. mooseri*)	Rat	Flea
Rocky Mountain spotted fever	*Rickettsia ricketsii*	Rodents, dog	Tick
Tick typhus (*fièvre boutonneuse*)	*Rickettsia conori*	Rodents, dog	Tick
Scrub typhus	*Rickettsia tsutsugamushi*	Rodents	Larval mite
Rickettsial pox	*Rickettsia akari*	House mice	Mite
Q fever	*Coxiella burnetii*	Domestic animals	None (airborne)

inoculation of their faeces through human skin, generally by irritation and scratching. Rickettsiae multiply intracellularly and can enter most mammalian cells, although the main lesion produced is a vasculitis due to invasion of endothelial cells of small blood vessels. Thus multisystem involvement is usual. The causative organisms and arthropod vectors for rickettsial infections are shown in Table 1.27.

CLINICAL FEATURES

Epidemic typhus

This is the most important rickettsial infection. Major outbreaks of typhus fever have occurred, mainly during famines and wars. It is found in Africa, Mexico, South America and Asia.

The incubation period is 1–3 weeks followed by an abrupt febrile illness associated with profound malaise and generalized myalgia. After two or three days the fever remains constant at around 40°C. Headache is severe and there may be conjunctivitis with orbital pain. A measles-like eruption appears around the fifth day, the macules increasing in size and eventually becoming purpuric in character. At the end of the first week, signs of meningo-encephalitis are evident and CNS involvement may progress to stupor or coma, sometimes with extrapyramidal involvement. At the height of the illness, splenomegaly, pneumonia, myocarditis and gangrene at the peripheries may be evident. Oliguric renal failure occurs in fulminating disease, which is usually fatal. Recovery begins in the third week but is generally slow.

The disease may recur many years after the initial attack owing to rickettsiae that lie dormant in lymph nodes. The recrudescence is known as Brill–Zinsser disease. The factors that precipitate recurrence are not clearly defined, although other infections may be important.

Endemic (murine) typhus

This is a rat infection that is inadvertently spread to humans by a rickettsiae-carrying rat flea. The disease closely resembles epidemic typhus but is much milder and rarely fatal.

Rocky Mountain spotted fever and other tick-borne typhus fevers

Infected hard ticks transmit this infection to humans, the same arthropod vector being responsible for other tick-borne typhus fevers in Africa, India and the Mediterranean (*Rickettsia conori* causing '*fièvre boutonneuse*'), in Central Asia and the Far East (*Rickettsia siberica*), and in Australia (*Rickettsia australis*).

Rocky Mountain spotted fever is limited to North and South America. As in other tick-borne typhus fevers, many patients will be able to give an account of tick bites or exposure to ticks. Clinical features closely resemble those of epidemic typhus, although the incubation period may be shorter and an eschar (crusted necrotic papule) may develop at the site of the bite in association with regional lymphadenopathy. The typical, generalized maculopapular rash occurs, which includes the palms and soles of the feet. The rash eventually becomes petechial. Neurological, haematological and cardiovascular complications occur as in epidemic typhus.

Scrub typhus

Found throughout Asia and the Western Pacific, this disease is spread by larval trombiculid mites (chiggers). As with tick-borne typhus, an eschar can often be found. Again the clinical illness resembles that of epidemic typhus, with an abrupt-onset febrile illness, rash and severe toxaemia. Bronchitis and interstitial pneumonia occur commonly but physical findings in the chest are minimal. The infection may recur despite treatment with antibiotics.

Rickettsial pox

Rickettsial pox is an urban disease described initially in New York City in 1946. A rodent mite was responsible for the spread of the infection to humans, the epidemic being related to massive expansion of the mouse community in large apartment buildings. The disease is mild, but similar in character to other rickettsial infections.

DIAGNOSIS

The diagnosis is generally made on the basis of the history and clinical course of the illness. Although the causative organisms can be isolated by inoculation of infected blood into laboratory animals, this is laborious and a biohazard and may take several weeks.

Serodiagnosis is by the indirect fluorescent antibody test (the most sensitive and specific), the indirect immunoperoxidase antibody test and the latex agglutination test. The Weil–Felix agglutination test is not specific or sensitive.

TREATMENT

Tetracycline 500 mg four times daily for seven days is given and improvement generally occurs in 48 hours. Ciprofloxacin is also effective. Doxycycline 200 mg weekly protects against scrub typhus; it is reserved for highly endemic areas. Resistance is developing to chloramphenicol, and doxycycline in Thailand.

CONTROL

This is achieved by control of vectors, namely lice, fleas, mites and ticks. Lice and fleas can be eradicated from clothing by insecticides (0.5% malathion or DDT). Chemical repellants are also useful. Control of rodents is vital. Short-term prophylaxis for travellers with doxycycline is effective.

Bites from ticks and mites should be avoided by wearing protective clothing on exposed areas of the body. In high-risk regions the body should be inspected for ticks twice a day. Mites can also be destroyed by chemical spraying from the air.

Q fever

Q fever is a zoonosis due to the rickettsial-like organism *Coxiella burnetii*. This organism is smaller than true rickettsiae and more resistant to physical and chemical injury. Clinically, Q fever differs from rickettsial illnesses as the rash is not a major feature and transmission of the disease to humans is independent of an arthropod vector. Important modes of spread to humans are thought to be dust, aerosols and unpasteurized milk from infected cows. *C. burnetii* is widespread in domestic and farm animals. It is spread between them by ticks, which constitute an important arthropod reservoir of the disease.

CLINICAL FEATURES

Fever begins insidiously, together with other symptoms of an influenza-like illness, 1–2 weeks after exposure. The acute illness often resolves spontaneously without treatment, but in a few persistent, symptoms and signs of pneumonia may develop, followed by endocarditis. A petechial rash may be apparent at this stage. Occasionally epididymo-orchitis, myocarditis, uveitis and osteomyelitis may be present. Untreated chronic infection is usually fatal.

DIAGNOSIS AND TREATMENT

Serodiagnosis is by complement fixation tests. *C. burnetii* is an obligate intracellular organism and does not grow on standard microbiological culture media. The organism possesses two classes of antigens, phase I and phase II. Antibodies to the phase I antigens appear later in the illness than antibodies to the phase II antigens; high titres are diagnostic in endocarditis. A rising titre or persistently high titres of both antibodies confirm chronic infection.

Tetracycline 500 mg four times daily is the treatment of choice for acute infection. For endocarditis a prolonged course of treatment is required, clindamycin often being given in association with tetracycline. Rifampicin may also be useful.

FURTHER READING

Dennis DT, Meltzer MI (1997) Editorial: Prophylaxis for tick bites. *Lancet* **350**: 1191–1192.

Chlamydiae

Chlamydiae are obligate intracellular organisms. They are ubiquitous and found in almost every avian and mammalian species; it has been estimated that up to 20% of the human population is infected. They are highly infectious, but rarely kill their host. Three species cause disease in humans: *Chlamydia trachomatis*, *C. psittaci* and *C. pneumoniae*. Table 1.28 shows the diseases produced.

Trachoma

This is the most common cause of blindness in the world and is found in the tropics and the Middle East. It is entirely preventable. It commonly occurs in children and is probably spread by direct transmission or possibly by flies.

Infection is bilateral and begins in the conjunctiva, with marked follicular inflammation and subsequent scarring. Scarring of the upper eyelid causes entropion, leaving the cornea exposed to further damage with the eyelashes rubbing against it (trichiasis). The corneal scarring that eventually occurs leads to blindness. The changes in the eye are sometimes accompanied by an upper respiratory tract infection.

Trachoma may also occur as an acute ophthalmic infection in the neonate.

Table 1.28
Chlamydia infections

Disease	Organism
Trachoma	*C. trachomatis*
Lymphogranuloma venereum	*C. trachomatis* (serotypes L1, L2 and L3)
Urethritis, cervicitis, proctitis	*C. trachomatis*
Psittacosis	*C. psittaci*
Respiratory	*C. pneumoniae*

DIAGNOSIS, TREATMENT AND PREVENTION

The diagnosis is generally established by:

- the typical clinical picture
- the presence of intracytoplasmic inclusion bodies in a conjunctival cell scraping stained with species-specific fluorescent monoclonal antibodies.

Tetracycline ointment applied locally each day for 2–3 months is effective, as is systemic therapy with oral tetracycline or sulphonamide. In endemic areas repeated courses of therapy are necessary. Once infection has been controlled, surgery may be required for eyelid reconstruction and for treatment of corneal opacities.

Community health education with respect to hygiene and earlier case reporting could make a substantial impact on disease prevalence. Data suggest that eradication of the disease may be possible with azithromycin.

Genital infections

Lymphogranuloma venereum is caused by *C. trachomatis* serotypes L1, L2 and L3 and is described on p. 101. Genital infections are also caused by other strains of *C. trachomatis*.

Psittacosis (ornithosis)

Although originally thought to be limited to the psittacine birds (parrots, parakeets and macaws), it is now known that the disease is widely spread amongst many species of birds, including pigeons, turkeys, ducks and chickens. Hence the broader term 'ornithosis'. Human infection is related to exposure to infected birds and is therefore a true zoonosis. The causative organism, *C. psittaci*, is excreted in avian secretions; it can be isolated for prolonged periods from birds who have apparently recovered from infection. The organism gains entry to the human host by inhalation.

CLINICAL FEATURES AND TREATMENT

These are discussed on p. 797.

Respiratory infection (see also p. 797)

C. pneumoniae strain TWAR causes relatively mild pneumonias in young adults, clinically resembling *Mycoplasma* pneumonia. Infection occurs in outbreaks. Diagnosis can be confirmed by specific IgM serology. Treatment is with erythromycin or tetracycline.

FURTHER READING

Dolin PJ *et al.* (1997) Reduction of trachoma in a sub-Saharan village in absence of a disease control programme. *Lancet* **349**: 1511-1512

Viral infections: an introduction

Viruses are much smaller than other infectious agents (viruses are not, by definition, micro-organisms), and contain either DNA or RNA. Since they are metabolically inert, they must live intracellularly, using the host cell for synthesis of viral proteins and nucleic acid. Viruses have a central nucleic acid core surrounded by a protein coat that is antigenically unique for a particular virus. The protein coat (capsid) imparts a helical or icosahedral structure to the virus. Some viruses also possess an envelope consisting of lipid and protein (Fig 1.26).

Hepatitis viruses are discussed on p. 303.

DNA viruses

Details of the structure, size and classification of human DNA viruses are shown in Table 1.29.

Adenoviruses

Adenovirus infection commonly presents as an acute pharyngitis, and extension of infection to the larynx and trachea in infants may lead to croup. By school age the majority of children show serological evidence of previous infection. Certain subtypes produce an acute conjunctivitis associated with pharyngitis. In adults, adenovirus causes acute follicular conjunctivitis and rarely pneumonia that is clinically similar to that produced by *Mycoplasma* (see p. 796). Adenoviruses have also been implicated as a cause of gastroenteritis (see p. 58) without respiratory disease and may be responsible for acute mesenteric lymphadenitis in children and young adults. Mesenteric adenitis that is due to adenoviruses may lead to intussusception in infants.

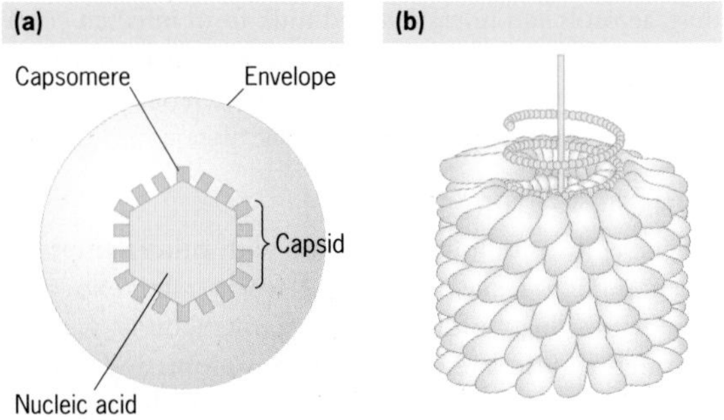

Fig 1.26
Viruses.
(a) Schematic diagram of a virus structure (icosahedral)
(b) Helical symmetry, showing capsomers arranged along the helical nucleic acid molecule

Herpesviruses

Members of the herpesviruses are important causes of a wide range of human diseases. Details are summarized in Table 1.30. The hallmark of all herpes virus infections is the ability of the virus to establish latent (or silent) infections that then persist for the life of the individual.

Herpes simplex virus (HSV) infection

(Fig 1.27)

Two types of HSV have been identified: HSV-1 is the major cause of herpetic stomatitis, herpes labialis ('cold sore'), keratoconjunctivitis and encephalitis, whereas HSV-2 causes genital herpes and may also be responsible for systemic infection in the immunocompromised host. These divisions, however, are not rigid, for HSV-1 can give rise to genital herpes and HSV-2 can cause pharyngitis.

The portal of entry of HSV-1 infection is usually via the mouth or occasionally the skin. The primary infection may go unnoticed or may produce a severe inflammatory reaction with vesicle formation leading to painful ulcers (gingivostomatitis; see Fig 1.28). The virus then remains latent, most commonly in the trigeminal ganglia, but may be reactivated by stress, trauma, febrile illnesses and ultraviolet radiation, producing the recurrent form of the disease

Table 1.29
Human DNA viruses

Structure				
Symmetry	**Envelope**	**Approximate size**	**Family**	**Viruses**
Icosahedral	–	80 nm	Adenovirus	Adenoviruses
Icosahedral	+	100 nm (160 nm with envelope)	Herpesvirus	Herpes simplex virus types 1 and 2 Varicella zoster virus Cytomegalovirus Epstein–Barr virus Human herpes virus type 6 (HHV6) Human herpes virus type 7 (HHV 7) Human herpes virus type 8 (HHV 8)
Icosahedral	+	42 nm	Hepadnavirus	Hepatitis B virus
Icosahedral	–	50 nm	Papovavirus	Human papillomavirus Polyomavirus
Icosahedral	–	23 nm	Parvovirus	Parvovirus B19
Complex	+	300 nm × 200 nm	Poxvirus	Variola virus Vaccinia virus Monkeypox Cowpox Orf Molluscum contagiosum

Table 1.30
Major diseases caused by human herpesviruses

Subfamily	Virus	Children	Adults	Immunocompromised
α-Herpesvirus	Herpes simplex type 1	Stomatitis*	Cold sores Keratitis Erythema multiforme	Dissemination
	Herpes simplex type 2		Primary genital herpes* Recurrent genital herpes	Dissemination
	Varicella zoster virus	Chickenpox*	Shingles	Dissemination
β-Herpesvirus	Cytomegalovirus	Congenital*		Pneumonitis Retinitis Gastrointestinal
	Human herpes virus type 6	Roseola infantum*		Pneumonitis
	Human herpes virus type 7	Roseola infantum*		
γ-Herpesvirus	Epstein–Barr virus		Infectious mononucleosis* Burkitt's lymphoma Nasopharyngeal carcinoma	Lymphoma
	Human herpesvirus type 8		Kaposi's sarcoma	Kaposi's sarcoma

* Signifies primary infections.

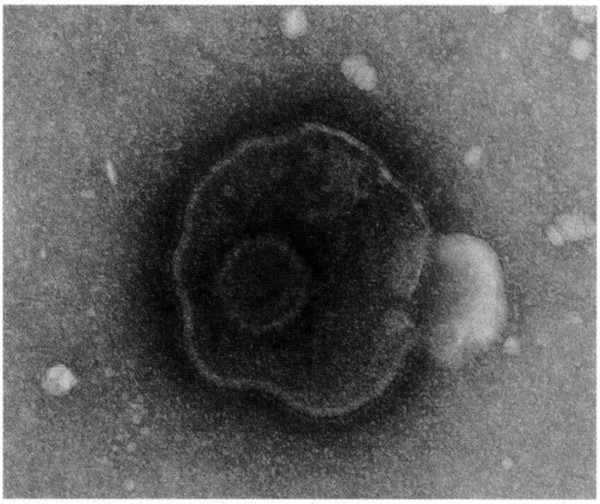

Fig 1.27
Electronmicrograph of herpes simplex virus

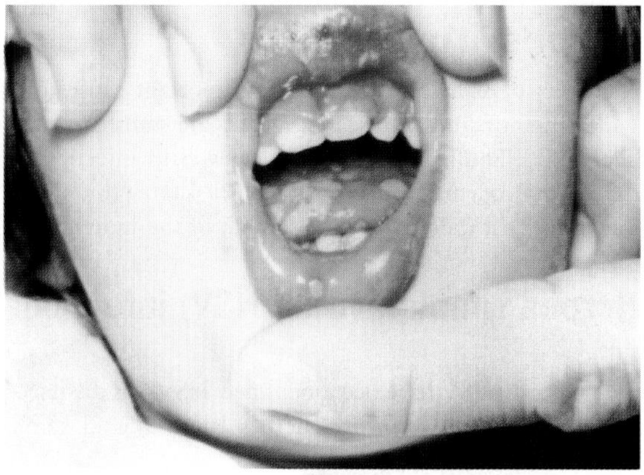

Fig 1.28
Primary herpes simplex type I (gingivostomatitis)

known as herpes labialis ('cold sore'). Approximately 70% of the population are infected with HSV-1 and recurrent infections occur in one-third of individuals. Reactivation often produces localized paraesthesiae in the lip before the appearance of a cold sore.

Complications of HSV-1 infection include transfer to the eye (dendritic ulceration, keratitis), acute encephalitis (p. 1073), skin infections such as herpetic whitlow, and erythema multiforme (see p. 1174).

In genital herpes the primary infection is usually more severe and recurrences are common. The virus remains latent in the sacral ganglia and during recurrence can produce a radiculomyelopathy, with pain in the groin, buttocks and upper thighs. Primary anorectal herpes infection is common in male homosexuals (see p. 104).

Immunocompromised patients such as those receiving intensive cancer chemotherapy or those with the acquired immunodeficiency syndrome (AIDS) may develop disseminated HSV infection involving many of the viscera. In severe cases death may result from severe hepatitis and encephalitis.

Neonates may develop primary HSV infection following vaginal delivery in the presence of active genital HSV infection in the mother. The disease in the baby varies from localized skin lesions to widespread visceral disease often with encephalitis. Caesarean section should therefore be considered if active genital HSV infection is present during labour.

Humoral antibody develops following primary infection, but mononuclear cell responses are probably more important in preventing dissemination of disease.

The clinical picture, diagnosis and treatment are described on p. 1154.

Varicella zoster virus (VZV) infection

VZV produces two distinct diseases, varicella (chickenpox) and herpes zoster (shingles). The primary infection is chickenpox. It usually occurs in childhood, the virus entering through the mucosa of the upper respiratory tract. It should be noted that, in some countries (e.g. the Indian subcontinent) a different epidemiological pattern exists with most infections occurring in adulthood. Chickenpox almost never occurs twice in the same individual. Infectious virus is spread from fresh skin lesions by direct contact or airborne transmission and the period of infectivity in chickenpox extends from two days before the appearance of the rash until the skin lesions are all at the crusting stage. Following recovery from chickenpox the virus then remains latent in dorsal root and cranial nerve ganglia.

CLINICAL FEATURES OF CHICKENPOX

Fourteen to twenty-one days after exposure to VZV, a brief prodromal illness of fever, headache and malaise heralds the eruption of chickenpox, characterized by the rapid progression of macules to papules to vesicles to pustules in a matter of hours (Fig 1.29). In young children the prodromal illness may be very mild or absent. The illness tends to be more severe in older children and can be debilitating in adults. The lesions occur on the face, scalp and trunk, and to a much lesser extent on the extremities. It is characteristic to see skin lesions at all stages of development on the same area of skin. Fever subsides as soon as new lesions cease to appear. Eventually the pustules crust and heal without scarring.

Important complications of chickenpox include pneumonia, which generally begins 1–6 days after the skin eruption, and bacterial superinfection of skin lesions. Pneumonia is more common in adults than children and cigarette smokers are at particular risk. Pulmonary symptoms are usually more striking than the physical findings, although a chest radiograph usually shows diffuse changes throughout both lung fields. CNS involvement occurs in about 1 per 1000 cases and most commonly presents as an acute truncal cerebellar ataxia. The immunocompromised are susceptible to disseminated infection with multiorgan involvement.

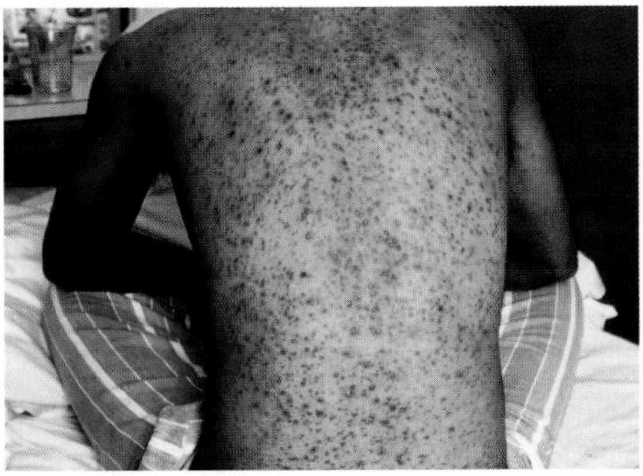

Fig 1.29
Chickenpox in an adult

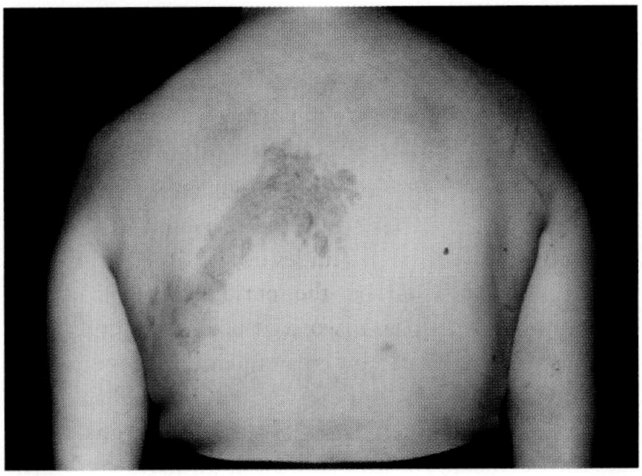

Fig 1.30
Shingles. HZV affecting a dermatome

CLINICAL FEATURES OF SHINGLES

Shingles (see p. 1155) occurs at all ages but is most common in the elderly, producing similar skin lesions to chickenpox, although classically they are unilateral and restricted to a sensory nerve (dermatomal) distribution (Fig 1.30). Shingles never occurs as a primary infection but results from reactivation of latent VZV from dorsal root and/or cranial nerve ganglia. The onset of the rash of shingles is usually preceded by severe dermatomal pain, indicating the involvement of sensory nerves in its pathogenesis. Virus is disseminated from freshly formed vesicles and may cause chickenpox in susceptible contacts.

DIAGNOSIS

The diseases are usually recognized clinically but can be confirmed by electronmicroscopy, immunofluorescence or culture of vesicular fluid and by serology.

PROPHYLAXIS AND TREATMENT

Chickenpox usually requires no treatment in healthy children and infection results in lifelong immunity. However, the disease may be fatal in the immunodeficient or the immunosuppressed, when it is reasonable to use passive immunization for prophylaxis, with zoster immune immunoglobulin (ZIG). In the immunocompromised host it is important to give acyclovir as early as possible to prevent serious complications.

Anyone with chickenpox who is over the age of 16 years should be considered for antiviral therapy with acyclovir if they present within 72 hours of onset. Women in pregnancy are prone to severe chickenpox and, in addition, there is a risk of intrauterine infection with structural damage to the fetus (mainly in the mid trimester – risk rate 2%). For these reasons ZIG is recommended for prophylaxis of women in pregnancy exposed to varicella zoster virus and, if chickenpox develops, acyclovir treatment is considered. If a woman has chickenpox at term, her baby should be protected by ZIG if delivery occurs within five days of the onset of the mother's illness.

Shingles is also treated with acyclovir and the duration of lesion formation and time to healing can be reduced by early treatment. Acyclovir, valaciclovir and famciclovir have all been shown to reduce the burden of zoster-associated pain when treatment is given at the acute phase. Shingles involving the ophthalmic division of the trigeminal nerve has an associated incidence of acute and chronic ophthalmic complications of 50%. Early treatment with acyclovir reduces this to 20% or less. As for chickenpox, all immunocompromised individuals should be given acyclovir at the onset of shingles.

Cytomegalovirus (CMV) infection

Infection with CMV is found worldwide and has its most profound effects as an opportunistic infection in the immunocompromised, particularly in recipients of bone-marrow and solid organ transplants and in patients with AIDS – 90% of patients with AIDS are infected with CMV and 95% of this population have disseminated CMV at autopsy. Over 50% of the adult population have serological evidence of latent infection with the virus, although infection is generally symptomless. As with all herpesviruses, the virus persists for life, usually as a latent infection in which the naked DNA is situated extrachromosomally in the nuclei of the cells in the endothelium of the arterial wall and in T lymphocytes.

CLINICAL FEATURES

In healthy adults CMV infection is usually asymptomatic but may cause an illness similar to infectious mononucleosis, with fever, occasionally lymphocytosis with atypical lymphocytes, and hepatitis with or without jaundice. The Paul–Bunnell test for heterophile antibody is negative. Infection may be spread by kissing, sexual intercourse or blood transfusion, and transplacentally to the fetus. Disseminated fatal infection with widespread visceral involvement occurs in the immunocompromised (see p. 114) and may cause encephalitis, retinitis, pneumonitis and diffuse involvement of the gastro-intestinal tract.

Intrauterine infection usually occurs in primary infection acquired during pregnancy and may have serious consequences on the fetus; CNS involvement may cause microcephaly and motor disorders. Jaundice and hepatosplenomegaly are common and thrombocytopenia and haemolytic anaemia also occur. Evidence of CNS involvement may be provided by demonstration of periventricular calcification on X-ray.

DIAGNOSIS

Serological tests can identify latent (IgG) or primary (IgM) infection. The virus can also be identified in tissues by the presence of characteristic intranuclear 'owl's eye' inclusions (Fig 1.31) on histological staining and by direct immunofluorescence. Culture in human embryo fibroblasts is usually slow but diagnosis can be accelerated by immunofluorescent detection of antigen in the cultures. Polymerase chain reaction, which can be quantitative, provides a sensitive way of detecting CMV in blood and other body fluids.

TREATMENT

In the immunocompetent, infection is usually self-limiting and no specific treatment is required. In the immunosuppressed, ganciclovir (5 mg kg^{-1} daily for 14–21 days) reduces retinitis and gastrointestinal damage and can eliminate CMV from blood, urine and respiratory secretions. It is less effective against pneumonitis. In patients with continuing immunocompromise, particularly AIDS, maintenance therapy may be necessary. Drug resistance has been reported and bone marrow toxicity is common. No antiviral drugs are currently recommended for treatment of CMV in neonates and the toxicity of ganciclovir prohibits its use in most cases.

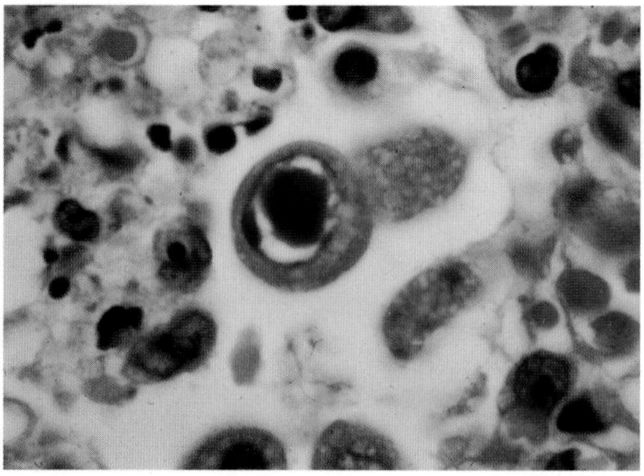

Fig 1.31
Typical 'owl-eye' inclusion bearing cell infected with cytomegalovirus

Epstein–Barr virus (EBV) infection

This virus causes an acute febrile illness known as infectious mononucleosis (glandular fever), which occurs worldwide in adolescents and young adults. EBV is probably transmitted in saliva and by aerosol.

CLINICAL FEATURES

The predominant symptoms are fever, headache, malaise and sore throat. Palatal petechiae and a transient macular rash are common, the latter occurring in 90% of patients who have received ampicillin (inappropriately) for the sore throat. Cervical lymphadenopathy, particularly of the posterior cervical nodes, and splenomegaly are characteristic. Mild hepatitis is common, but other complications such as myocarditis, meningitis, encephalitis, mesenteric adenitis and splenic rupture are rare.

Although some young adults remain debilitated and depressed for some months after infection, the evidence for reactivation of latent virus in healthy individuals is controversial, although this is thought to occur in immunocompromised patients. Following primary infection, EBV remains latent in B lymphocytes. Severe, often fatal infectious mononucleosis may result from a rare X-linked immunoproliferative syndrome affecting young boys. Those who survive have an increased risk of hypogammaglobulinaemia and/or lymphoma.

DIAGNOSIS

EBV infection should be strongly suspected if atypical mononuclear cells (glandular fever cells) are found in the peripheral blood. It can be confirmed during the second week of infection by a positive Paul–Bunnell reaction, which detects heterophile antibodies (IgM) that agglutinate sheep erythrocytes. False-positives can occur in other conditions such as viral hepatitis, Hodgkin's disease and acute leukaemia. The Monospot test is a sensitive and easily performed screening test. Specific EBV IgM antibodies indicate recent infection by the virus. Clinically similar illnesses are produced by CMV and toxoplasmosis but these can be distinguished serologically.

TREATMENT

The majority of cases require no specific treatment and recovery is rapid. Corticosteroid therapy is advised when there is neurological involvement (e.g. encephalitis, meningitis, Guillain–Barré syndrome) or when there is marked thrombocytopenia or haemolysis.

EBV is also considered to be the cause of oral hairy leukoplakia in AIDS patients and to be the major aetiological agent responsible for Burkitt's lymphoma, nasopharyngeal carcinoma, post-transplant lymphoma and the immunoblastic lymphoma of AIDS patients.

Human herpesvirus type 6 (HHV-6)

This human herpesvirus infects CD4+ T lymphocytes, occurs worldwide, and exists as a latent infection in over 85% of the adult population. The virus causes roseola infantum (exanthem subitum) which presents as a high fever followed by generalized macular rash in infants. HHV-6 is a common cause of febrile convulsions, and aseptic meningitis or encephalitis may occur as rare complications. Reactivation in the immunocompromised may lead to severe pneumonia.

TREATMENT

Supportive management only is recommended for the common infantile disease. Ganciclovir can be used in the immunocompromised.

Human herpesvirus type 7 (HHV-7)

This virus is similar to HHV-6 in being a T lymphotropic herpesvirus. It is also present as a latent infection in over 85% of the adult population and it is known to infect CD4+ helper T cells by using the CD4 antigen (the main receptor employed by HIV). The full spectrum of disease due to HHV-7 has not yet been fully characterized, but, like HHV-6, it is known to cause roseola infantum in infants.

Human herpesvirus type 8 (Kaposi's sarcoma virus)

This recently discovered human herpesvirus is strongly associated with the aetiology of classical and AIDS-related Kaposi's syndrome. Antibody prevalence is high in those with tumours but relatively low in the general population. HHV-8 RNA transcripts have been detected in Kaposi's sarcoma cells and in circulating mononuclear cells from patients with the tumour.

Papovaviruses

These small viruses tend to produce chronic infections, often with evidence of latency. They are capable of inducing neoplasia in some animal species and were among the first viruses to be implicated in tumorigenesis. Human papillomaviruses, of which there are at least 70 types, are responsible for the common wart and have been implicated in the aetiology of carcinoma of the cervix (mainly types 16 and 18). The human BK virus, a polyomavirus, is generally found in immunosuppressed individuals and may be detected in the urine of 15–40% of renal transplant patients, in patients receiving cytotoxic chemotherapy, and in those with immunodeficiency states. A related virus, JC, is the cause of progressive multifocal leukoencephalopathy (PML) which presents as dementia in the immunocompromised and is due to progressive cerebral destruction resulting from accumulation of the virus in brain tissue (see p. 1076).

For genital warts see p. 104.

Human parvovirus B19

Human parvovirus B19 produces erythema infectiosum (fifth disease), a common infection in schoolchildren. The rash is typically on the face (the 'slapped-cheek' appearance). The patient is well and the rash can recur over weeks or months. Asymptomatic infection occurs in 20% of children. Moderately severe self-limiting arthropathy (see p. 486) is common if infection occurs in adulthood. Aplastic crisis may occur in patients with chronic haemolysis (e.g. sickle cell disease). Chronic infection with anaemia may occur in immunocompromised subjects. Hydrops fetalis and/or fetal death occurs in about 10% of cases of infection occurring during the first and second trimesters of pregnancy.

Poxviruses

Smallpox (variola)

This disease has been eradicated following an aggressive vaccination policy and careful detection of new cases coordinated by the World Health Organization.

Monkeypox

This is a rare zoonosis that occurs in small villages in the tropical rainforests in several countries of western and central Africa. Its clinical effects, including a generalized vesicular rash, are indistinguishable from smallpox, but person-to-person transmission is unusual. Serological surveys indicate that several species of squirrel are likely to represent the animal reservoir.

Cowpox

Cowpox produces large vesicles which are classically on the hands in those in contact with infected cows. The lesions are associated with regional lymphadenitis and fever. Cowpox virus has been found in a range of species including domestic and wild cats, and the reservoir is thought to exist in a range of rodents.

Vaccinia virus

This is a laboratory virus and does not occur in nature in either humans or animals. Its origins are uncertain but it has been invaluable in its use as the vaccine to prevent smallpox. Vaccination is now not recommended except for laboratory personnel handling certain poxviruses for experimental purposes. It is being assessed experimentally as a possible carrier for new vaccines.

Orf

This poxvirus causes contagious pustular dermatitis in sheep and hand lesions in humans (see p. 1156).

Molluscum contagiosum

This is discussed on p. 1156.

RNA viruses (Table 1.31)

Picornaviruses

Poliovirus infection (poliomyelitis)

Poliomyelitis occurs when a susceptible individual is infected with poliovirus type 1, 2 or 3. These viruses have a propensity for the nervous system, especially the anterior horn cells of the spinal cord and cranial nerve motor neurones. Poliomyelitis is found worldwide but its incidence has decreased dramatically following improvements in sanitation, hygiene and the widespread use of polio vaccines. Spread is usually via the faecal–oral route, as the virus is excreted in the faeces.

CLINICAL FEATURES

The incubation period is 7–14 days. Although polio is essentially a disease of childhood, no age is exempt. The clinical manifestations vary considerably.

Inapparent infection

Inapparent infection is common and occurs in 95% of infected individuals.

Abortive poliomyelitis

Abortive poliomyelitis occurs in approximately 4–5% of cases and is characterized by the presence of fever, sore throat and myalgia. The illness is self-limiting and of short duration.

Non-paralytic poliomyelitis

Non-paralytic poliomyelitis has features of abortive poliomyelitis as well as signs of meningeal irritation, but recovery is complete.

Paralytic poliomyelitis

Paralytic poliomyelitis occurs in approximately 0.1% of infected children (1.3 % of adults). Several factors predispose to the development of paralysis:

- male sex
- exercise early in the illness
- trauma, surgery or intramuscular injection which localize the paralysis
- recent tonsillectomy (bulbar poliomyelitis).

This form of the disease is characterized initially by features simulating abortive poliomyelitis. Symptoms subside for 4–5 days, only to recur in greater severity with signs of meningeal irritation and muscle pain, which is most prominent in the neck and lumbar region. These symptoms persist for a few

Table 1.31
Human RNA viruses

Structure				
Symmetry	**Envelope**	**Approximate size**	**Family**	**Viruses**
Icosahedral	–	30 nm	Picornavirus	Poliovirus Coxsackievirus Echovirus Enterovirus 68–72 Rhinovirus
Icosahedral	–	80 nm	Reovirus	Reovirus Rotavirus
Icosahedral	+	50–80 nm	Togavirus	Rubella virus Alphaviruses Flaviviruses
Spherical	+	80–100 nm	Bunyavirus	Congo–Crimean haemorrhagic fever Hantavirus
Spherical	–	35–40 nm	Calicivirus	Norwalk agent Hepatitis E
Spherical	–	28–30 nm	Astrovirus	Astrovirus
Helical	+	80–120 nm	Orthomyxovirus	Influenza viruses A, B and C
Helical	+	100–300 nm	Paramyxovirus	Measles virus Mumps virus Respiratory syncytial virus
Helical	+	60–175 nm	Rhabdovirus	Rabies virus
Helical	+	100 nm	Retrovirus	Human immunodeficiency viruses (HIV 1 and 2)
Helical	+	100–300 nm	Arenavirus	Lassa virus Lymphocytic choriomeningitis virus
Pleomorphic	+	Filaments or circular forms; 100 × 130–2600 nm	Filovirus	Marburg virus Ebola virus

days and are followed by the onset of asymmetric paralysis without sensory involvement. The paralysis is usually confined to the lower limbs in children under five years of age and the upper limbs in older children, whereas in adults it manifests as paraplegia or quadriplegia.

Bulbar poliomyelitis

Bulbar poliomyelitis is characterized by the presence of cranial nerve involvement and respiratory muscle paralysis. Soft palate, pharyngeal and laryngeal muscle palsies are common.

Aspiration pneumonia, myocarditis, paralytic ileus and urinary calculi are late complications of poliomyelitis.

DIAGNOSIS

The diagnosis is a clinical one. Distinction from the Guillain–Barré syndrome is easily made by the absence of sensory involvement and the asymmetrical nature of the paralysis in poliomyelitis. Laboratory confirmation and distinction between the wild virus and vaccine strains is achieved by virus culture, neutralization and temperature marker tests.

TREATMENT

Treatment is supportive. Bedrest is essential during the early course of the illness. Respiratory support with intermittent positive pressure respiration is required if the muscles of respiration are involved. Once the acute phase of the illness has subsided, occupational therapy, physiotherapy and occasionally surgery have important roles in patient rehabilitation.

PREVENTION AND CONTROL

Immunization has dramatically decreased the prevalence of this disease worldwide. Trivalent oral poliovaccine (OPV) (active virus) is used (see Information box 1.2); occasionally, inactivated poliovirus vaccine is used intramuscularly for the immunocompromised and their family contacts and to women in pregnancy.

Coxsackievirus, echovirus and enterovirus infection

These viruses are spread by the faecal–oral route. They each have a number of different types and are responsible for a broad spectrum of disease involving the skin and mucous membranes, muscles, nerves, the heart (Table 1.32), and rarely other organs, such as the liver and pancreas. They are frequently associated with pyrexial illnesses and are the most common cause of aseptic meningitis.

Skin and oropharyngeal disease

There is a vesicular eruption on the fauces, palate and uvula (herpangina). The lesions eventually evolve into aphthous ulcers. The illness is usually associated with fever and headache but is short-lived, recovery occurring within a few days.

Hand, foot and mouth disease

This disease is mainly caused by coxsackievirus A16 or A10. Oral lesions are similar to those seen in herpangina but may be more extensive in the oropharynx. Vesicles and a maculopapular eruption also appear, typically on the palms of the hands and the soles of the feet, but also on other parts of the body. This infection commonly affects children. Recovery occurs within a week.

Neurological disease

Other enteroviruses in addition to poliovirus can cause a broad range of neurological disease, including meningitis, encephalitis, and a paralytic disease characteristic of poliomyelitis.

Heart and muscle disease

Enteroviruses are an important cause of acute myocarditis and pericarditis, from which, in general, there is complete recovery. However, these viruses can also cause chronic congestive cardiomyopathy and, rarely, constrictive pericarditis.

Skeletal muscle involvement, particularly of the intercostal muscles, is an important feature of Bornholm disease, a febrile illness usually due to Coxsackievirus B. The pain may be of such an intensity as to mimic pleurisy or an acute abdomen. The infection affects both children and adults and may be complicated by meningitis or cardiac involvement.

Rhinovirus infection

Rhinoviruses are responsible for the common cold (see p. 163). Chimpanzees and humans are the only species to develop the common cold. ICAM-1 is the cellular receptor (p. 769) for rhinovirus and it is only in these two species that the specific binding domain is present. Peak incidence rates occur in the colder months, especially spring and autumn. There are multiple rhinovirus immunotypes, which makes vaccine control impracticable. In contrast to enteroviruses which replicate at 37°C, rhinoviruses grow at 33°C (the temperature of the upper respiratory tract), which explains the localized disease characteristic of common colds.

Reoviruses

Reovirus infection

Reovirus infection occurs mainly in children, causing mild respiratory symptoms and diarrhoea. A few deaths have been reported following disseminated infection of brain, liver, heart and lungs.

Rotavirus infection

Rotavirus (Latin *rota* = wheel) is so named because of its electronmicroscopic appearance with a characteristic circular outline with radiating spokes (Fig 1.32). It is responsible

Table 1.32
Picornavirus infections (excluding poliovirus and rhinovirus)

	Coxsackievirus			
Disease	**A (types A_1–A_{22}, A_{24})**	**B (types B_1–B_6)**	**Echovirus (types 1–9, 11–27, 29–33)**	**Enterovirus (types 68–71)**
Cutaneous and oropharyngeal				
Herpangina	+++	+	+	
Hand, foot and mouth	+++	+		+
Erythematous rashes	+	+	+++	
Neurological				
Paralytic	+		±	+
Meningitis	++	++	+++	+
Encephalitis	++	++	±	+
Cardiac				
Myocarditis and pericarditis	+	+++	+	
Muscle				
Myositis (Bornholm disease)	+	+++	+	

+++, often causes; ++, sometimes causes; +, rarely causes; ±, possibly causes.

worldwide for both sporadic cases and epidemics of diarrhoea, and is currently one of the most important causes of childhood diarrhoea. More than 870 000 children under the age of five years are estimated to die annually in developing countries, compared with 75–150 in the USA. The prevalence is higher during the winter months. Asymptomatic infections are common, and bottle-fed babies are more likely to be symptomatic than breast-fed.

Adults may become infected with rotavirus but symptoms are usually mild or absent. The virus may, however, cause outbreaks of diarrhoea in patients on geriatric wards.

CLINICAL FEATURES

The illness is characterized by vomiting, fever, diarrhoea, and the metabolic consequences of water and electrolyte loss. Histology of the jejunal mucosa in children shows shortening of the villi, with crypt hyperplasia and mononuclear cell infiltration of the lamina propria.

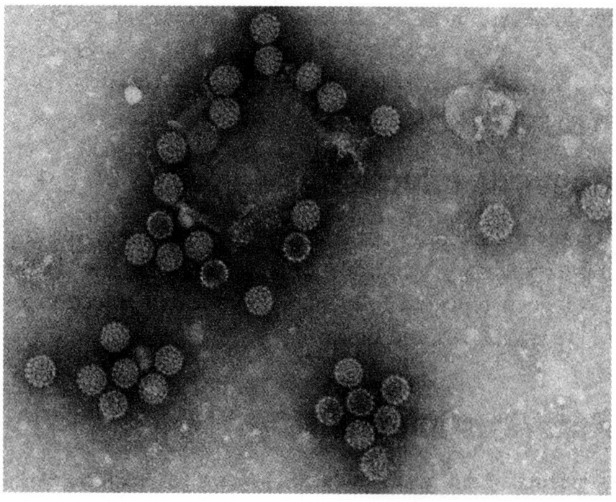

Fig 1.32
Electronmicrograph of human rotavirus

DIAGNOSIS AND TREATMENT

The diagnosis can be established by ELISA for the detection of rotavirus antigen in faeces and by electronmicroscopy of faeces.

Treatment is directed at overcoming the effects of water and electrolyte imbalance with adequate oral rehydration therapy and, when indicated, intravenous fluids (see Table 1.19). Antibiotics should not be prescribed.

Rhesus-human reassortant vaccines have been developed whereby a human rotavirus VP7 is expressed on the surface of a rhesus rotavirus. The tetravalent vaccine contains three reassortants for human rotavirus G-types 1, 2 and 4 plus the rhesus rotavirus (G-type 3). This vaccine (IRRV-TV Rhesus (human) RotaVirus – Tetravalent Vaccine) has been shown to give high levels of protection in children in developing countries. This vaccine is likely to have a major impact.

Other viruses associated with gastroenteritis are shown in Table 1.33. These include members of two major families which can be recognized by their electron-microscopic appearance. Caliciviruses include the Norwalk agents and are responsible for winter vomiting. Astroviruses produce watery diarrhoea and vomiting. The small round structured viruses are not, as yet, fully characterized.

Table 1.33
Viruses associated with gastroenteritis

Rotavirus (groups A, B, C, D and E)
Enteric adenovirus (types 40 and 41)
Calicivirus (Norwalk and related viruses)
Astrovirus
Small rounded structured viruses (SRSV)

Togaviruses

This family comprises two genera: the rubiviruses, which include rubellavirus; and the arboviruses, which include some of the arthropod-borne viruses.

Rubella

Rubella ('German measles') is caused by a spherical, enveloped fragile RNA virus that is easily killed by heat and ultraviolet light. While the disease can occur sporadically, epidemics are not uncommon. It has a worldwide distribution. Spread of the virus is via droplets; maximum infectivity occurs before and during the time the rash is present.

CLINICAL FEATURES

The incubation period is 14–21 days, averaging 18 days. The clinical features are largely determined by age, with symptoms being mild or absent in children under five years

During the prodrome the patient complains of malaise and fever. Mild conjunctivitis and lymphadenopathy may be present. The distribution of the lymphadenopathy is characteristic and involves the suboccipital, postauricular and posterior cervical groups of lymph nodes. Small petechial lesions on the soft palate (Forchheimer spots) are suggestive but not diagnostic. Splenomegaly may be present.

The eruptive or exanthematous phase usually occurs within the first seven days of the initial symptoms. The rash first appears on the forehead and then spreads to involve the trunk and the limbs. It is pinkish red, macular and discrete, although some of these lesions may coalesce (Fig 1.33). It usually fades by the second day and rarely persists beyond the third day after its appearance.

COMPLICATIONS

Complications are rare. They include superadded pulmonary bacterial infection, arthralgia, haemorrhagic manifestations due to thrombocytopenia, encephalitis and the *congenital rubella syndrome*. Rubella affects the fetuses of up to 80% of all women who contract the infection during the first trimester of pregnancy. The incidence of congenital abnormalities diminishes in the second trimester and no ill-effects result from infection in the third trimester.

Fig 1.33
Rubella rash

Congenital rubella syndrome is characterized by the presence of fetal cardiac malformations, especially patent ductus arteriosus and ventricular septal defect, eye lesions (especially cataracts), microcephaly, mental retardation and deafness.

The *expanded rubella syndrome* consists of the manifestations of the congenital rubella syndrome plus hepatosplenomegaly, myocarditis, interstitial pneumonia and metaphyseal bone lesions.

DIAGNOSIS AND TREATMENT

The diagnosis may be suspected clinically, but laboratory diagnosis is essential to distinguish the illness from other virus infections (e.g. echovirus) and drug rashes. This is achieved by demonstrating a rising antibody titre (measured using the sensitive haemagglutination inhibition test or ELISA) in two successive blood samples taken 14 days apart or by the detection of rubella-specific IgM. The virus can be cultured from throat swabs, urine and, in the case of intrauterine infection, the products of conception.

Treatment is symptomatic.

PREVENTION

Prevention of rubella is important. Human immunoglobulin can decrease the symptoms of this already mild illness, but does not prevent the teratogenic effects. Several live attenuated rubella vaccines have been used with great success in preventing this illness and these have been successfully combined with the measles and mumps (MMR) vaccine. The side-effects of vaccination have been dramatically decreased by using vaccines prepared in human embryonic fibroblast cultures (RA 27/3 vaccine). Use of the vaccine is contraindicated during pregnancy or if there is a likelihood of pregnancy within three months of immunization. Inadvertent use of the vaccine during pregnancy has not, however, revealed a risk of teratogenicity.

Arbovirus (arthropod-borne) infection

Arboviruses are zoonotic viruses, with the possible exception of the *O'nyong-nyong fever* virus of which humans are the only known vertebrate hosts. They are transmitted through the bites of insects, especially mosquitoes and ticks. Over 385 viruses are classified as arboviruses. *Culex*, *Aedes* and *Anopheles* mosquitoes account for the transmission of the majority of these viruses.

Although most arbovirus diseases are generally mild, epidemics are frequent and when these occur the mortality is high. In general, the incubation period is less than 10 days. The illness tends to be biphasic and, as in other viral fevers, pyrexia, conjunctival suffusion, a rash, retro-orbital pain, myalgia and arthralgia are common.

Table 1.34
Viral infections associated with haemorrhagic manifestations[a]

Flavivirus
Yellow fever (urban and sylvan)
Dengue haemorrhagic fever
Kyasanur Forest disease
Omsk haemorrhagic fever
Rift Valley fever
Bunyavirus
Congo–Crimean haemorrhagic fever
Hantavirus infections
Arenavirus
Argentinian haemorrhagic fever
Bolivian haemorrhagic fever
Lassa fever
Epidemic haemorrhagic fever
Togavirus
Chikungunya
Filovirus
Marburg
Ebola

[a]Most of these are arboviruses. Some (e.g. Hantavirus, lassa fever) have a rodent vector. The source and transmission route of filoviruses is not known.

Lymphadenopathy is seen in dengue. Lifelong immunity to a particular virus is usual. In some of these viral fevers, haemorrhage is a feature (Table 1.34). Increased vascular permeability, capillary fragility and consumptive coagulopathy have been implicated as causes of the haemorrhage. Encephalitis resulting from cerebral invasion may be prominent in some fevers.

Alphaviruses

The 24 viruses of this group are all transmitted by mosquitoes; eight result in human disease. These viruses are globally distributed and tend to acquire their names from the location where they were first isolated (such as Ross River, Eastern Venezuelan, and Western encephalitis viruses) or by the local expression for a major symptom caused by the virus (such as chikungunya, meaning 'doubled up'). Infection is characterized by fever, skin rash, arthralgia, myalgia and sometimes encephalitis.

Flaviviruses

There are 60 viruses in this group, some of which are transmitted by ticks and others by mosquitoes. Hepatitis G virus is discussed on p. 308.

Yellow fever

Yellow fever, caused by a flavivirus, results in an illness of widely varying severity so that the disease is under-reported. It is a disease confined to Africa (90% of cases) and South America between latitudes 15°N and 15°S of the equator. For poorly understood reasons, yellow fever has not been reported from Asia, despite the fact that climatic conditions are suitable and the vector, *Aedes aegypti*, is common. The infection is transmitted in the wild by *A. africanus* in Africa and the *Haemagogus* species in South and Central America. Extension of infection to humans (via the mosquito or from monkeys) leads to the occurrence of 'jungle' yellow fever. *A. aegypti*, a domestic mosquito which lives in close relationship to humans, is responsible for human-to-human transmission in urban areas (urban yellow fever). Once infected, a mosquito remains so for its whole life.

CLINICAL FEATURES

The incubation period is 3–6 days. When the infection is mild, the disease is indistinguishable from other viral fevers such as influenza or dengue.

Three phases in the severe (classical) illness are recognized. Initially the patient presents with a high fever of acute onset, usually 39–40°C, which then returns to normal in 4–5 days. During this time, headache is prominent. Retrobulbar pain, myalgia, arthralgia, a flushed face and suffused conjunctivae are common. Epigastric discomfort and vomiting are present when the illness is severe. Relative bradycardia (Faget's sign) is present from the second day of illness. The patient then makes an apparent recovery and feels well for several days. Following this 'phase of calm' the patient again develops increasing fever, deepening jaundice and hepatomegaly. Ecchymosis, bleeding from the gums, haematemesis and melaena may occur. Coma, which is usually a result of uraemia or haemorrhagic shock, occurs for a few hours preceding death. The mortality rate is up to 40% in severe cases. The pathology of the liver shows mid-zone necrosis, and eosinophilic degeneration of hepatocytes (Councilman bodies).

DIAGNOSIS AND TREATMENT

The diagnosis is established by a careful history of travel and vaccination status, and by isolation of the virus (when possible) from blood during the first three days of illness. Serodiagnosis is possible, but in endemic areas cross-reactivity with other flaviviruses is a problem.

Treatment is supportive. Bedrest (under mosquito nets), analgesics, and maintenance of fluid and electrolyte balance are important.

PREVENTION AND CONTROL

Yellow fever is an internationally notifiable disease. It is easily prevented using the attenuated 17d chick embryo vaccine. Vaccination is not recommended for children under 9 months and immunosuppressed patients unless there are compelling reasons. For the purposes of international certification, immunization is valid for 10 years, but protection lasts much longer than this and probably for life. The WHO Expanded Programme of Immunization now includes yellow fever vaccination in endemic areas.

Dengue

This is the commonest arthropod-borne viral infection in humans: 50–100 million cases occur every year in the tropics, with over 10 000 deaths from dengue haemorrhagic fever. Dengue is caused by a flavivirus and is found mainly in Asia, South America and Africa, although it has been reported from the USA. Four different antigenic varieties of the dengue virus are recognized and all are transmitted by the daytime-biting *A. aegypti*. Humans are infective during the first three days of the illness (the viraemic stage). Mosquitoes become infective about two weeks after feeding on an infected individual, and remain so for the rest of their lives. The disease is usually endemic. Immunity after the illness is partial.

CLINICAL FEATURES

The incubation period is 5–6 days. Asymptomatic or mild infections are common. Two clinical forms are recognized.

Classic dengue fever

Classic dengue fever is characterized by the abrupt onset of fever, malaise, headache, facial flushing, retrobulbar pain which worsens on eye movements, conjunctival suffusion and severe backache, which is a prominent symptom. Lymphadenopathy, petechiae on the soft palate and skin rashes may also occur. The rash is transient and morbilliform. It appears on the limbs and then spreads to involve the trunk. Desquamation occurs subsequently. Cough is uncommon. The fever subsides after 3–4 days, the temperature returns to normal for a couple of days, and then the fever returns, together with the features already mentioned, but milder. This biphasic or saddleback pattern is considered characteristic. Severe fatigue, a feeling of being unwell and depression are common for several weeks after the fever has subsided.

Dengue haemorrhagic fever

Dengue haemorrhagic fever is a severe form of dengue fever and is believed to be the result of two or more sequential infections with different dengue serotypes. It is a disease of children and has been described almost exclusively in South East Asia. The disease has a mild start, often with symptoms of an upper respiratory tract infection. This is then followed by the abrupt onset of shock and haemorrhage into the skin and ear, epistaxis, haematemesis and melaena known as the *dengue shock syndrome*. Serum complement levels are depressed and there is laboratory evidence of a consumptive coagulopathy.

DIAGNOSIS AND TREATMENT

Isolation of the dengue virus by tissue culture in sera obtained during the first few days of illness is diagnostic. Demonstration of rising antibody titres by neutralization (most specific), haemagglutination inhibition or complement-fixing antibodies in sequential serum samples is evidence of dengue virus infection.

Treatment is supportive.

PREVENTION

Travellers should be advised to sleep under impregnated nets and to use topical insect repellants. Adult mosquitoes should be destroyed by sprays and breeding sites should be eradicated.

Rift Valley fever

Rift Valley fever is primarily an acute febrile illness of livestock – sheep, goats and camels. It is found in southern and eastern Africa. The vector in East Africa is *Culex pipiens* and in southern Africa, *Aedes caballus*. Following an incubation period of 3–6 days, the patient has an acute febrile illness that is difficult to distinguish clinically from other viral fevers. The temperature pattern is usually biphasic. The initial febrile illness lasts 2–4 days and is followed by a remission and a second febrile episode. Complications are indicative of severe infection and include retinopathy, meningo-encephalitis, haemorrhagic manifestations and hepatic necrosis. Mortality approaches 50% in severe forms of the illness. Treatment is supportive.

Japanese encephalitis

Japanese encephalitis is a mosquito-borne encephalitis caused by a flavivirus. It has been reported most frequently from the rice-growing countries of South East Asia and the Far East. *Culex tritaeniorhynchus* is the most important vector and feeds mainly on pigs as well as birds such as herons and sparrows. Humans are accidental hosts.

As with other viral infections, the clinical manifestations are variable. The onset is heralded by severe rigors. Fever, headache and malaise last 1–6 days. Weight loss is prominent. In the acute encephalitic stage the fever is high (38–41°C), neck rigidity occurs and neurological signs such as altered consciousness, hemiparesis and convulsions develop. Mental deterioration occurs over a period of 3–4 days and culminates in coma. Mortality varies from 7 to 40% and is higher in children. Residual neurological defects such as deafness, emotional lability and hemiparesis occur in about 70% of patients who have had CNS involvement. Convalescence is prolonged. Antibody detection in serum and CSF by IgM capture ELISA is a useful rapid diagnostic test. An inactivated mouse brain vaccine is effective and available. Treatment is supportive.

Bunyaviruses

Bunyaviruses belong to a large family of more than 200 viruses, most of which are arthropod-borne.

Congo–Crimean haemorrhagic fever

This is found mainly in Asia and Africa. The primary hosts are cattle and hares and the vectors are the Hyalomma ticks.

Following an incubation period of 3–6 days there is an influenza-like illness with fever and haemorrhagic manifestations. The mortality is 10–50%.

Hantaviruses

Hantaviruses are enzootic viruses of wild rodents which are spread by aerosolized excreta and not by insect vectors. The disease was first recognized in 1951 in United Nations soldiers in Korea. The most severe form of this infection is Korean haemorrhagic fever (or haemorrhagic fever with renal syndrome – HFRS). This condition has a mortality of 5–10% and is characterized by fever, shock and haemorrhage followed by an oliguric phase. Milder forms of the disease are associated with related viruses (e.g. Puumala virus) and may present as nephropathia epidemica, an acute fever with renal involvement. This has been recognized for many years in Scandinavia (and recently in other European countries in people who have been in contact with bank voles). In the USA, a new Hantavirus (transmitted by the deer mouse) causes the acute respiratory distress syndrome (ARDS).

Diagnosis is made by an ELISA technique for specific antibodies.

Orthomyxoviruses

Influenza

Three types of influenza virus are recognized: A, B and C. The influenza virus is a spherical or filamentous enveloped virus. Haemagglutinin, a surface glycopeptide, aids attachment of the virus to the wall of susceptible host cells at specific receptor sites. Cell penetration, probably by pinocytosis, and release of replicated viruses from the cell surface is effected by budding through the cell membrane facilitated by the action of the enzyme neuraminidase which is also present on the viral envelope.

- Influenza A is generally responsible for pandemics and epidemics.
- Influenza B often causes smaller or localized and milder outbreaks, such as in camps or schools.
- Influenza C rarely produces disease in humans.

Antigenic shift (major antigenic change within an influenza A subtype) usually heralds the onset of a pandemic. This results from genetic recombination of the RNA of the virus with that of an animal orthomyxovirus.

Antigenic drift (minor changes in influenza A and B viruses) results from point mutations leading to amino acid changes in the two surface glycoproteins, haemagglutinin and neuraminidase, which are important in inducing humoral immunity.

Thus, changes due to antigenic shift or drift render the individual's immune response less able to combat the new variant. Purified haemagglutin and neuraminidase from recently circulating strains of influenza A and B viruses are incorporated in current vaccines.

Sporadic cases of influenza and outbreaks among groups of people living in a confined environment are frequent. The incidence increases during the winter months, when crowding is common. Spread is mainly by droplet infection but fomites and direct contact have also been implicated.

The clinical features, diagnosis, treatment and prophylaxis of influenza are discussed on p. 773.

Paramyxoviruses

These are a heterogeneous group of enveloped viruses of varying size that are responsible for parainfluenza, mumps, measles and other respiratory infections (Fig 1.34).

Parainfluenza

Parainfluenza is caused by the parainfluenza viruses types I-IV; these have a worldwide distribution and cause acute respiratory disease. Type IV appears to be less virulent than the other types and has been linked only to mild upper respiratory diseases in children and adults.

Parainfluenza is essentially a disease of children and presents with features similar to the common cold. When severe, a brassy cough with inspiratory stridor and features of laryngotracheobronchitis (croup) are present. Fever is usually present for 2–3 days and may be more prolonged if pneumonia develops. The development of croup is due to submucosal oedema and consequent airway obstruction in the subglottic region. This may lead to cyanosis, subcostal and intercostal recession and progressive airway obstruction. Infection in the immunocompromised is usually prolonged and may be severe. Treatment is supportive with oxygen, humidification and sedation when required. The role of steroids is controversial.

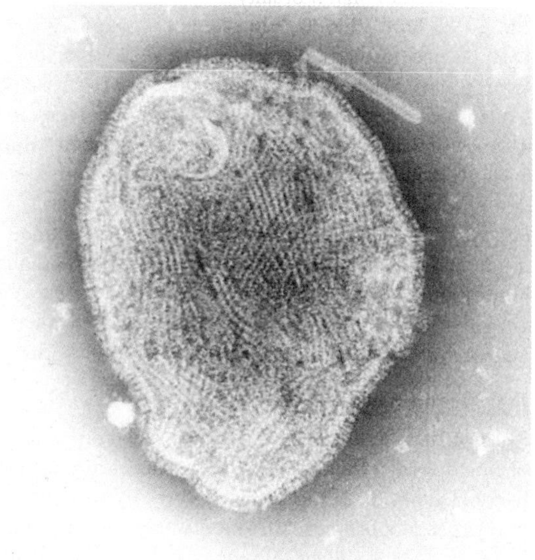

Fig 1.34
Electronmicrograph of a paramyxovirus (parainfluenza)

Measles (rubeola)

Measles is a highly communicable disease that occurs worldwide. With the introduction of aggressive immunization policies, the incidence of measles has fallen dramatically in the West, but it still remains one of the most common childhood infections in the developing countries, where it is associated with a high morbidity and mortality. It is spread by droplet infection and the period of infectivity is from four days before until two days after the onset of the rash.

CLINICAL FEATURES

The incubation period is 8–14 days. Two distinct phases of the disease can be recognized.

Typical measles

- *The pre-eruptive and catarrhal stage.* This is the stage of viraemia and viral dissemination. Malaise, fever, rhinorrhoea, cough, conjunctival suffusion and the pathognomonic Koplik's spots are present during this stage. Koplik's spots are small, greyish, irregular lesions surrounded by an erythematous base and are found in greatest numbers on the mucous membrane opposite the second molar tooth. They occur a day or two before the onset of the rash.
- *The eruptive or exanthematous stage.* This is characterized by the presence of a maculopapular rash that initially occurs on the face, chiefly the forehead, and then spreads rapidly to involve the rest of the body (Fig 1.35). At first the rash is discrete but later it may become confluent and patchy, especially on the face and neck. It fades in about one week and leaves behind a brownish discoloration.

Although measles is a relatively mild disease in the healthy child, it carries a high mortality in the malnourished and in those who have other diseases. Complications are common in such individuals and include bacterial pneumonia, bronchitis, otitis media and gastroenteritis. Less commonly, myocarditis, hepatitis and encephalomyelitis may occur. The virus has also been implicated in the rare condition, *subacute sclerosing panencephalitis*, which may follow measles infection occurring early in life (<18 months of age). Persistence of the virus with reactivation pre-puberty results in accumulation of virus in the brain, progressive mental deterioration and a fatal outcome (see p. 1076).

Maternal measles, unlike rubella, does not cause congenital fetal abnormalities. It is, however, associated with spontaneous abortions and premature delivery.

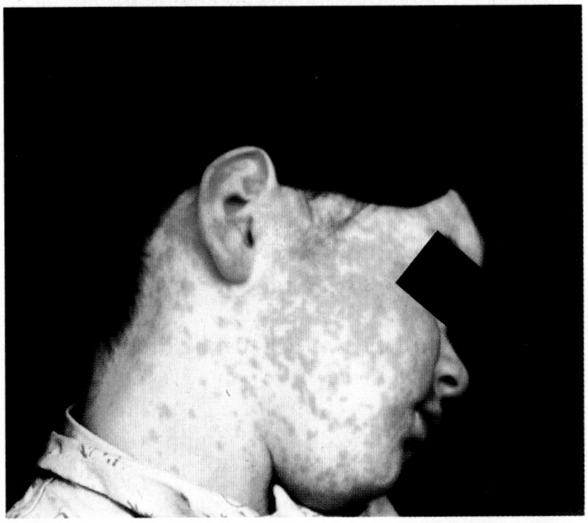

Fig 1.35
Measles

Atypical measles

Atypical measles is a severe illness that usually occurs in individuals who have previously received an inactivated vaccine (now withdrawn) and are exposed to wild measles virus. The high fever (>40°C), myalgia, abdominal pain and cough are followed by vesicles, petechiae and purpura. Skin lesions may be mistaken for scarlet fever, meningococcaemia or varicella. Pneumonia invariably occurs and the pulmonary infiltrates may persist for years.

DIAGNOSIS AND TREATMENT

Most cases are diagnosed clinically but, if necessary, immunofluorescence, virus culture and serological tests (complement fixation test (CFT), haemagglutination inhibition tests) are used to confirm the diagnosis.

Treatment is supportive. Antibiotics are indicated only if secondary bacterial infection occurs.

PREVENTION

A previous attack of measles confers a high degree of immunity and second attacks are uncommon.

Human immunoglobulin 0.25 mL kg^{-1} given within five days of exposure effectively aborts an attack of measles. It is indicated for previously unimmunized children below three years of age, during pregnancy, and in those with debilitating disease.

Active immunization Children are immunized with the combined mumps–measles–rubella (MMR) vaccine (Information box 1.2). A measles vaccine is available.

Mumps

Mumps is the result of infection with a paramyxovirus. It is spread by droplet infection, by direct contact or through fomites. Humans are the only known natural hosts. The peak period of infectivity is 2–3 days before the onset of the parotitis and for three days afterwards.

CLINICAL FEATURES

The incubation period averages 18 days. Although no age is exempt, it is primarily a disease of school-aged children and young adults; it is uncommon before the age of two years. The prodromal symptoms are nonspecific and include fever, malaise, headache and anorexia. This is usually followed by severe pain over the parotid glands, with either unilateral or bilateral parotid swelling. The enlarged parotid glands obscure the angle of the mandible and may elevate the ear lobe, which does not occur in cervical lymph node enlargement. Trismus due to pain is common at this stage. Submandibular gland involvement occurs less frequently.

COMPLICATIONS

CNS involvement is the most common extrasalivary-gland manifestation of mumps. Clinical meningitis occurs in 5% of all infected patients, and 30% of patients with CNS involvement have no evidence of parotid gland involvement.

Epididymo-orchitis develops in about one-third of patients who develop mumps after puberty. Bilateral testicular involvement results in sterility in only a small percentage of these patients.

Pancreatitis, oophoritis, myocarditis, mastitis, hepatitis and polyarthritis may also occur.

DIAGNOSIS AND TREATMENT

The diagnosis of mumps is on the basis of the clinical features. In doubtful cases, serological demonstration of a fourfold rise in antibodies detected by complement fixation or indirect haemagglutination or neutralization tests on acute and convalescent sera is diagnostic. Virus can be isolated in cell culture from saliva, throat swab, urine and CSF and identified by immunofluorescence or haemadsorption.

Treatment is supportive. Attention should be given to adequate nutrition and mouth care. Analgesics should be used to relieve pain.

PREVENTION

Active immunization Children are immunized with the MMR (Information box 1.2). A live attenuated mumps virus vaccine given as a single 0.5 mL intramuscular dose is also available. Vaccination is contra-indicated in immunosuppressed individuals, during pregnancy, or in those with severe febrile illnesses.

Respiratory syncytial virus infection

Respiratory syncytial virus is a paramyxovirus that causes many respiratory infections in epidemics each winter. It is a common cause of bronchiolitis in infants, which is complicated by pneumonia in approximately 10% of cases. The infection normally starts with upper respiratory symptoms. After an interval of 1–3 days a cough and low-grade fever may develop. The onset of bronchiolitis is characterized by dyspnoea, hyperexpansion of the chest with subcostal and intercostal recession. The disease may be severe and potentially fatal in babies with underlying cardiac or respiratory disease. RSV infection has been associated with the occurrence of sudden infant death syndrome (SIDS). Immunity is short-lived and consequently reinfection can occur throughout life. RSV is occasionally the cause of outbreaks of pneumonia in the elderly and in the immunocompromised.

Transfer of infection between children in hospital commonly occurs unless infected patients are isolated or cohorted. Meticulous attention to handwashing and other infection control measures reduces the risk of transmission by staff members.

DIAGNOSIS AND TREATMENT

Immunofluorescence on nasopharyngeal aspirates, virus culture and serology are the usual ways of confirming the diagnosis.

Treatment is generally supportive, but aerosolized ribavirin can be given to severe cases, particularly those with underlying cardiac or respiratory disease. No vaccine is available.

Rhabdoviruses

Rabies

Rabies is a major problem in some countries and established infection is invariably fatal. The rabies virus is bullet-shaped and has spike-like structures arising from its surface containing glycoproteins that cause the host to produce neutralizing, haemagglutination-inhibiting antibodies. The virus has a marked affinity for nervous tissue and the salivary glands. It exists in two major epidemiological settings:

- *Urban rabies* is most frequently transmitted to humans through rabid dogs and, less frequently, cats.
- *Sylvan (wild) rabies* is maintained in the wild by a host of animal reservoirs such as foxes, skunks, jackals, mongooses and bats.

With the exception of Australia, New Zealand and the Antarctic, human rabies has been reported from all continents. Transmission is usually through the bite of an infected animal. However, the percentage of rabid bites leading to clinical disease ranges from 10% (on the legs) to 80% (on the head). Rabies has been transferred by corneal grafting, but anecdotal reports of human-to-human spread by kissing, biting and sexual intercourse have not been confirmed. Rabid animals can also transmit the disease by licking abraded skin or mucosa. Rarely, airborne droplet infection occurs from exposure to infected bats in caves or in laboratory workers handling concentrated virus.

Having entered the human body, the virus replicates in the muscle cells near the entry wound. It penetrates the nerve endings and travels in the axoplasm to the spinal cord and brain. In the CNS the virus again proliferates before spreading to the salivary glands, lungs, kidneys and other organs via the autonomic nerves.

There have been only two recorded cases of survival from clinical rabies.

CLINICAL FEATURES

The incubation period is variable and may range from a few weeks to several years; on average it is 1–3 months. In general, bites on the head, face and neck have a shorter incubation period than those elsewhere. In humans, two distinct clinical varieties of rabies are recognized:

- *furious rabies* – the classic variety
- *dumb rabies* – the paralytic variety.

Furious rabies

The only characteristic feature in the prodromal period is the presence of pain and tingling at the site of the initial wound. Fever, malaise and headache are also present. About 10 days later, marked anxiety and agitation or depressive features develop. Hallucinations, bizarre behaviour and paralysis may also occur. Hyperexcitability, the hallmark of this form of rabies, is precipitated by auditory or visual stimuli. Hydrophobia (fear of water) is present in 50% of patients and is due to severe pharyngeal spasms on attempting to eat or drink. Aerophobia (fear of air) is considered pathognomonic of rabies. Examination reveals hyperreflexia, spasticity, and evidence of sympathetic overactivity indicated by pupillary dilatation and diaphoresis.

The patient goes on to develop convulsions, respiratory paralysis and cardiac arrhythmias. Death usually occurs in 10–14 days.

Dumb rabies

Dumb rabies, or paralytic rabies, presents with a symmetrical ascending paralysis resembling the Guillain–Barré syndrome. This variety of rabies commonly occurs after bites from rabid bats.

DIAGNOSIS

The diagnosis of rabies is generally made clinically. Fluorescent antibody has been used to detect rabies antigen in corneal impressions or in salivary secretions; this is a useful test. The classic Negri bodies are detected at postmortem in 90% of all patients with rabies; these are eosinophilic, cytoplasmic, ovoid bodies, 2–10 nm in diameter, seen in greatest numbers in the cells of the hippocampus and the cerebellum. The diagnosis should be made pathologically on the biting animal.

TREATMENT

Once the disease is established, therapy is symptomatic as death is inevitable. The patient should be nursed in a quiet, darkened room. Nutritional, respiratory and cardiovascular support may be necessary.

Drugs such as morphine, diazepam and chlorpromazine should be used liberally in patients who are excitable.

PREVENTION

The vaccine is the human diploid cell strain vaccine (HDCSV).

Postexposure prophylaxis. Five 1.0 mL doses of HDCSV should be given intramuscularly: the first dose is given on day 0 and is followed by injections on days 3, 7, 14 and 28. Reaction to the vaccine is uncommon. The wound should be cleaned carefully with soap and water, adequately debrided and left open. Human rabies immunoglobulin should be given immediately (20 IU kg^{-1}); half should be injected around the area of the wound and the other half should be given intramuscularly.

Pre-exposure prophylaxis. This is given to individuals with a high risk of contracting rabies, such as laboratory workers, animal handlers and veterinarians. Two doses of HDCSV 1.0 mL deep subcutaneously or intramuscularly given four weeks apart should provide effective immunity. A reinforcing dose is given after 12 months and additional reinforcing doses are given every 1–3 years depending on the risk of exposure. Vaccines of nervous-tissue origin are still used in some parts of the world. These, however, are associated with significant side-effects and are best avoided if HDCV is available.

Control of rabies Domestic animals should be vaccinated if there is any risk of rabies in the country. In the UK, control is by quarantine of imported animals and no indigenous case of rabies has been reported for many years. Wild animals in 'at risk' countries must be handled with great care.

Retroviruses

Retroviruses (Table 1.35) are distinguished from other RNA viruses by their ability to replicate through a DNA intermediate using an enzyme, reverse transcriptase. HIV-1 and the related virus, HIV-2, are further classified as lentiviruses ('slow' viruses) because of their slowly progressive clinical effects.

HIV-1 and HIV-2 are discussed on p. 107.

HTLV-1 causes adult T cell leukaemia/lymphoma and tropical spastic paraparesis (see p. 1029).

Arenaviruses

Arenaviruses are pleomorphic, round or oval viruses with diameters ranging from 50 to 300 nm. The virion surface has club-shaped projections, and the virus itself contains a

Table 1.35
Human lymphotropic retroviruses

Subfamily	Virus	Disease
Lentivirus	HIV-1	AIDS
	HIV-2	AIDS
Oncovirus	HTLV-1[a]	Adult T-cell leukaemia/lymphoma
		Tropical spastic paraparesis
	HTLV-2	not defined

[a] HTLV, human T-cell leukaemia virus.

variable number of characteristic electron-dense granules that represent residual, non-functional host ribosomes. The prototype virus of this group is lymphocytic choriomeningitis virus, which is a natural infection of mice. Arenaviruses are also responsible for Argentinian and Bolivian haemorrhagic fevers and Lassa fever.

Lassa fever

This illness was first documented in the town of Lassa, Nigeria, in 1969 and is confined to sub-Saharan West Africa (Nigeria, Liberia and Sierra Leone). The multimammate rat, *Mastomys natalensis*, is known to be the reservoir. Humans are infected by ingesting foods contaminated by rat urine or saliva containing the virus. Person-to-person spread by body fluids also occurs. Only 10–30% of infections are symptomatic.

CLINICAL FEATURES

The incubation period is 7–18 days. The disease is insidious in onset and is characterized by fever, myalgia, severe backache, malaise and headache. A transient maculopapular rash may be present. A sore throat, pharyngitis and lymphadenopathy occur in over 50% of patients. In severe cases epistaxis and gastrointestinal bleeding may occur – hence the classification of Lassa fever as a viral haemorrhagic fever. The fever usually lasts 1–3 weeks and recovery within a month of the onset of illness is usual. However, death occurs in 15–20% of hospitalized patients, usually from irreversible hypovolaemic shock.

DIAGNOSIS

The diagnosis is established by serial serological tests (including the Lassa-specific IgM titre) or by culturing the virus from the throat, serum or urine. Great care should be taken in handling the specimens.

TREATMENT

Treatment is supportive. In addition, clinical benefit and reduction in mortality can be achieved with ribavirin therapy, if given in the first week.

In non-endemic countries, strict isolation procedures should be used, the patient ideally being nursed in a flexible-film isolator. Specialized units for the management of Lassa fever and other haemorrhagic fevers have been established in the UK.

Lymphocytic choriomeningitis (LCM)

This infection is a zoonosis, the natural reservoir of the LCM virus being the house mouse. Infection is characterized by:

- non-nervous system illness, with fever, malaise, myalgia, headache, arthralgia and vomiting
- aseptic meningitis in addition to the above symptoms.

Occasionally, a more severe form occurs, with encephalitis leading to disturbance of consciousness.

This illness is generally self-limiting and requires no specific treatment.

Marburg virus disease and Ebola virus disease

These severe, haemorrhagic, febrile illnesses are discussed together because their clinical manifestations are similar. The diseases are named after Marburg in Germany and the Ebola river region in the Sudan and Zaire where these viruses were first isolated. The natural reservoir for these viruses has not been identified and the precise mode of spread from one individual to another has not been elucidated.

Epidemics have occurred periodically in recent years, mainly in sub-Saharan Africa. The mortality from Marburg and Ebola has ranged from 25% to 90% and recovery is slow in those who survive.

The illness is characterized by the acute onset of severe headache, severe myalgia and high fever, followed by prostration. On about the fifth day of illness a non-pruritic maculopapular rash develops on the face and then spreads to the rest of the body. Diarrhoea is profuse and is associated with abdominal cramps and vomiting. Haematemesis, melaena or haemoptysis may occur between the seventh and sixteenth day. Hepatosplenomegaly and facial oedema are usually present. In Ebola virus disease, chest pain and a dry cough are prominent symptoms.

Treatment is symptomatic. Convalescent human serum appears to decrease the severity of the attack.

Postviral/chronic fatigue syndrome (see also p. 1112)

Viral illnesses have been implicated aetiologically, including those due to EBV, Coxsackie B viruses, echoviruses, CMV and hepatitis A virus. Non-viral causes such as allergy to *Candida* spp. have also been proposed.

The proportion of patients with 'organic' diagnoses remains uncertain. Studies have suggested that two-thirds of patients with a symptom duration of more than six months may have an underlying psychiatric disorder.

Prion disease

A number of diseases of humans and animals have been loosely termed 'slow virus' diseases. These are now known as *transmissible spongiform encephalopathies* and are thought to be caused by the accumulation in the nervous system of a unique protein, termed a prion, which is an abnormal isoform of a normal, host protein.

Although familial forms of prion disease are known to exist, these conditions can be transmissible, particularly if brain tissue enters another host. There is no convincing evidence for the presence of nucleic acid in association with prions; thus these agents cannot be considered orthodox viruses and the current view is that the abnormal prion protein itself is infectious and can trigger a conversion of the normal protein into the atypical isoform. After infection a long incubation period is followed by CNS degeneration associated with dementia or ataxia which invariably leads to death. Histology of the brain reveals spongiform change with an accumulation of the abnormal prion protein in the form of amyloid plaques.

The human prion diseases are Creutzfeldt–Jakob disease, Gerstmann–Straussler–Scheinker syndrome, and Kuru.

- *Creutzfeldt–Jakob disease* usually occurs sporadically at an annual rate of one per million of the population. Although, in most cases, the epidemiology remains obscure, transmission to others has occurred as a result of administration of human cadaveric growth hormone or gonadotrophin, from dura mater and corneal grafting, and in neurosurgery from reuse of contaminated electrodes.
- *Gerstmann–Straussler–Scheinker syndrome* is a prion disease usually occurring in families with a positive history. The pattern of inheritance is an autosomal dominant with some degree of variable penetrance.
- *Kuru* was described and characterized in the Fore highlanders in NE New Guinea. Transmission was associated with ritualistic cannibalism of deceased relatives. With the cessation of cannibalism by 1960, the disease has gradually diminished and recent cases had all been exposed to the agent before 1960.

Concern has been publicized in the UK with the description of the appearance of a small number of cases of a new variant of Creutzfeldt–Jakob disease in people under the age of 50 years. Fears that these cases have resulted from consumption of bovine brain and other offal contaminated with the bovine prion disease, bovine spongiform encephalopathy (BSE), have resulted in a decision to cull large numbers of potentially infected cattle.

The infectious agent of prion disease has remarkable characteristics. In the infected host there is no evidence of inflammatory, cytokine or immune reactions. The agent is highly resistant to decontamination, and infectivity is not destroyed by standard autoclaving or by treatment with formaldehyde and most other gas or liquid disinfectants. It is very resistant to γ irradiation. Autoclaving at a high temperature (134–137°C for 18 minutes) is used for decontamination of instruments, and hypochlorite (20 000 ppm available chlorine) is used for liquid disinfection.

FURTHER READING

Haywood AM (1997) Transmissible spongiform encephalopathies. *New England Journal of Medicine* **337**: 1821–1828.

Center for Disease Control and Prevention (1995) Update: Management of patients with suspected haemorrhagic fever. United States *MMWR* **44**: 475-479.

The BMA guide to rabies (1995) Radcliffe Medical Press, Oxford.

Robertson SE, Hull BP, Tomori O *et al.* (1995) Yellow fever. A decade of resurgence. *Journal of the American Medical Association* **276**: 1157-1162.

Fungal infections

Morphologically, fungi can be grouped into three major categories.

- *Yeasts* reproduce by budding.
- *Moulds* grow by branching and longitudinal extension of hyphae.
- *Dimorphic fungi* behave as yeasts in the host but as moulds *in vitro* (e.g. *Histoplasma* and *Sporothrix*).

Despite the fact that fungi are ubiquitous, systemic fungal infections are uncommon. Fungal infections are transmitted by inhalation of spores or by contact with the skin. Opportunistic mycoses can cause disease in immunocompromised patients.

Fungi do not produce endotoxin, but exotoxin (e.g. aflatoxin) production has been documented *in vitro*. Fungi may also produce allergic pulmonary disease.

In general, human fungal infections are indolent and respond poorly to treatment. Some fungi such as *Candida albicans* are human commensals. Diseases are usually divided into *systemic*, *subcutaneous* or *superficial* (Table 1.36).

Systemic fungal infections

Candidiasis

Candidiasis is the most common fungal infection in humans and is caused by *Candida albicans*. *Candida* are small asexual fungi. All the species that are pathogenic to humans are normal oropharyngeal and gastrointestinal commensals. Candidiasis is found worldwide.

CLINICAL FEATURES

Practically any organ in the body can be invaded by *Candida*, but vaginal infection and oral thrush are the most common forms. This latter is seen in the very young, in the elderly, following antibiotic therapy and in those who are immunosuppressed. Candidal oesophagitis may present with painful dysphagia. Cutaneous candidiasis typically occurs in intertriginous areas. It is also an important cause of paronychia. Balanitis and vaginal infection are also common (see p. 105).

Table 1.36
Common fungal infections

Systemic	Subcutaneous
Histoplasmosis	Sporotrichosis
Cryptococcosis	Subcutaneous zygomycosis
Coccidiomycosis	Chromomycosis
Blastomycosis	Mycetoma
Zygomycosis (mucomycosis)	
Candidiosis	**Superficial**
Aspergillosis	Dermatophytosis
Pneumocystic carinii (previously classed as a protozoa)	Superficial candidiasis
	Malassezia infections

Chronic mucocutaneous candidiasis

This is a rare manifestation, usually occurring in children, and is associated with a T-cell defect. It presents with hyperkeratotic plaque-like lesions on the skin, especially the face, and on the fingernails. It is associated with several endocrinopathies, including hypothyroidism and hypoparathyroidism. Less commonly dissemination of candidiasis may lead to haematogenous spread, with meningitis, pulmonary involvement, endocarditis or osteomyelitis.

DIAGNOSIS AND TREATMENT

The fungi can be demonstrated in scrapings from infected lesions or in tissue secretions.

Treatment varies depending on the site and severity of infection. Oral lesions respond to nystatin, oral amphotericin or miconazole. For more severe systemic infections, parenteral therapy with amphotericin or ketoconazole, or oral therapy with flucytosine 50–75 mg kg^{-1} daily for 2–3 weeks may be required.

Histoplasmosis

Histoplasmosis is caused by *Histoplasma capsulatum*, a non-encapsulated, dimorphic fungus. Spores can survive in moist soil for several years, particularly when it is enriched by bird and bat droppings. Histoplasmosis occurs worldwide and is commonly seen in Ohio and the Mississippi river valley where over 80% of the population have been subclinically exposed. Transmission is mainly by inhalation of the spores.

CLINICAL FEATURES

Fig 1.36 summarizes the pathogenesis, main clinical forms and sequelae of Histoplasma infection.

Primary pulmonary histoplasmosis is usually asymptomatic. The only evidence of infection is conversion of a histoplasmin skin test from negative to positive, and radiological features similar to those seen with the Ghon primary complex of tuberculosis (see p. 802). Calcification in the lungs, spleen and liver occurs in patients from areas of high endemicity. When symptomatic, primary pulmonary histoplasmosis generally presents as a mild influenza-like illness, with fever, chills, myalgia and cough. The systemic symptoms are pronounced in severe disease.

Complications such as atelectasis, secondary bacterial pneumonia, pleural effusions, erythema nodosum and erythema multiforme may also occur.

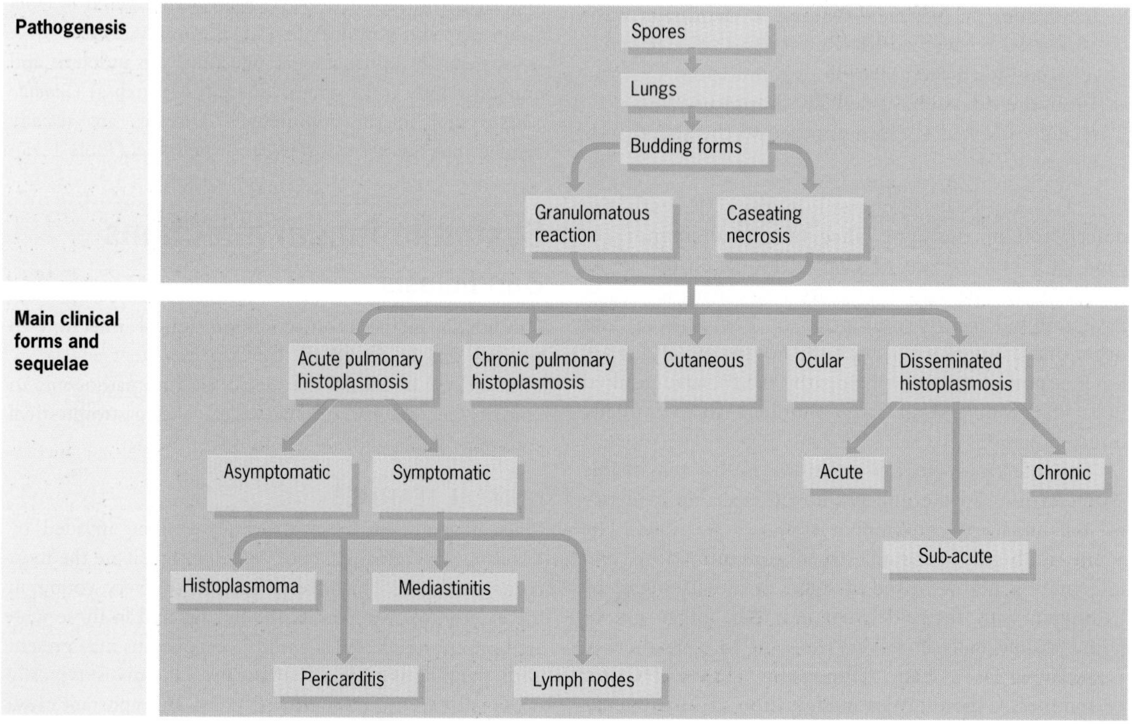

Fig 1.36
Histoplasma infection Summary of pathogenesis, main clinical forms and sequelae

Chronic pulmonary histoplasmosis is clinically indistinguishable from pulmonary tuberculosis (see p. 803). It is usually seen in white males over the age of 50 years. Radiologically, pulmonary cavities, infiltrates and characteristic fibrous streaking from the periphery towards the hilum are seen.

Disseminated histoplasmosis resembles disseminated tuberculosis clinically. Fever, lymphadenopathy, hepatosplenomegaly, weight loss, leucopenia and thrombocytopenia are common. Rarely, features of meningitis, hepatitis, Addison's disease, endocarditis and peritonitis may dominate the clinical picture.

DIAGNOSIS

Definitive diagnosis is possible only by culturing the fungi or by demonstrating them on histological sections. The histoplasmin skin test is usually positive but can be negative in acute disseminated disease.

Antibodies usually develop within three weeks of the onset of illness and are best detected by the complement-fixation immunodiffusion or the counter immunoelectrophertic tests.

TREATMENT

Only severe acute pulmonary histoplasmosis, chronic histoplasmosis and acute disseminated histoplasmosis require therapy. Intravenous amphotericin 0.5–0.6 mg kg^{-1} daily or 1.0–1.2 mg kg^{-1} on alternate days for 10 weeks has been the mainstay of therapy. The less toxic antifungal agents itraconazole and ketoconazole are now preferred as first-line therapy in some countries. Patients with AIDS still require treatment with amphotericin. Surgical excision of histoplasmomas (pulmonary granuloma due to *H. capsulatum*) or chronic cavitatory lung lesions and release of adhesions following mediastinitis is often required.

African histoplasmosis

African histoplasmosis is caused by *Histoplasma duboisii*, the spores of which are larger than those of *H. capsulatum*. Skin lesions (e.g. abscesses, nodules, lymph node involvement and lytic bone lesions) are prominent. Pulmonary lesions do not occur. Treatment is similar to that for *H. capsulatum* infection.

Aspergillosis

Aspergillosis is caused by several species of dimorphic fungi of the genus *Aspergillus*. Of these, *A. fumigatus* is the most common cause of disease in humans, although *A. flavus* and *A. niger* have also been implicated as pathogens. These fungi are ubiquitous in the environment and are commonly found on decaying leaves and trees. Humans are infected by inhalation of the spores. Disease manifestation depends on the dose of the spores inhaled as well as the immune response of the host. Three major forms of the disease are recognized:

- *Bronchopulmonary allergic aspergillosis* (see p. 811) shows symptoms suggestive of bronchial asthma.
- *Aspergilloma* (see p. 812) is sometimes referred to as a pulmonary mycetoma.
- *Fulminant disease*, which occurs in immunosuppressed patients, presents as acute pneumonia, meningitis or an intracerebral abscess, lytic bone lesions, and granulomatous lesions in the liver; less commonly endocarditis, paranasal *Aspergillus* granuloma or keratitis may occur. Urgent treatment with intravenous amphotericin is required.

The diagnosis and treatment are described in more detail on p. 811.

Cryptococcosis

Cryptococcosis is caused by the yeast-like fungus, *Cryptococcus neoformans*. It has a worldwide distribution and appears to be spread by birds, especially pigeons, in their droppings. The spores gain entry into the body through the respiratory tract, where they elicit a granulomatous reaction. Pulmonary symptoms are, however, uncommon; meningitis, which is clinically indistinguishable from bacterial meningitis, is the usual mode of presentation.

Lung cavitation, hilar lymphadenopathy, pleural effusions and occasionally pulmonary fibrosis occur. Less commonly, the skin and bones are involved.

DIAGNOSIS AND TREATMENT

This is established by demonstrating the organisms in appropriately stained tissue sections. A positive latex cryptococcal agglutinin test performed on the CSF is diagnostic of cryptococcosis.

Amphotericin (0.3–0.5 mg kg^{-1} daily i.v.) alone or in combination with flucytosine (100–200 mg kg^{-1} daily) has reduced the mortality of this once always fatal condition. Therapy should be continued for three months if meningitis is present. Fluconazole has greater CSF penetration and is used when toxicitity is encountered with amphotericin and flucytosine and as maintenance therapy in immunocompromised patients.

Coccidioidomycosis

Coccidioidomycosis is caused by the non-budding spherical form (spherule) of *Coccidioides immitis*. This is a soil saprophyte and is found in the southern USA, Central America and parts of South America.

Humans are infected by inhalation of the thick-walled barrel-shaped spores called arthrospores. Occasionally epidemics of coccidioidomycosis have been documented following dust storms.

CLINICAL FEATURES

The majority of patients are asymptomatic. Infection is detected by the conversion of a skin test using either coccidioidin (extract from a culture of mycelial growth of *C. immitis*) or spherulin (the soluble fraction from a culture of *C. immitis* spherules) from negative to positive.

Acute pulmonary coccidioidomycosis presents, after an incubation period of about 10 days, with fever, malaise, cough and expectoration. Erythema nodosum, erythema multiforme, phlyctenular conjunctivitis and, less commonly, pleural effusions may occur. Complete recovery is usual.

Pulmonary cavitation with haemoptysis, pulmonary fibrosis, meningitis, lytic bone lesions, hepatosplenomegaly, and skin ulcers and abscesses may occur in severe disease.

DIAGNOSIS

Because of the high infectivity of this fungus, and consequent risk to laboratory personnel, serological tests (rather than culture of the organism) are widely used for diagnosis. These include the highly specific latex agglutination and precipitin tests (IgM) which are positive within two weeks of infection and decline thereafter. A positive complement-fixation test (IgG) performed on the CSF is diagnostic of coccidioidomycosis meningitis within 4–6 weeks and may remain positive for many years.

TREATMENT

Mild pulmonary infections are self-limiting and require no treatment, but progressive and disseminated disease requires urgent therapy. Fluconazole 400 mg daily for 3–6 months is the treatment of choice for primary pulmonary disease with more prolonged courses for cavitating or fibronodular disease. Higher doses are given for meningitis (600–1000 mg daily). Amphotericin is still indicated for life-threatening infection and is used intrathecally for severe meningitis. Surgical excision of cavitatory pulmonary lesions or localized bone lesions may be necessary. For meningitis, intrathecal amphotericin may be required; the role of steroids remains controversial. Ketoconazole or miconazole can be of value.

Blastomycosis

Blastomycosis is a systemic infection caused by the biphasic fungus *Blastomyces dermatitidis*. Although initially believed to be confined to certain parts of North America, it has been reported in Canada, Africa, Israel, Eastern Europe and Saudi Arabia.

CLINICAL FEATURES

Blastomycosis primarily involves the skin, where it presents as non-itchy papular lesions that later develop into ulcers with red verrucous margins. The ulcers are initially confined to the exposed parts of the body but later involve the unexposed parts as well. Atrophy and scarring may occur. Pulmonary involvement presents as a solitary lesion resembling a malignancy or gives rise to radiological features similar to the primary complex of tuberculosis. Systemic symptoms such as fever, malaise, cough and weight loss are usually present. Bone lesions are common and present as painful swellings.

DIAGNOSIS AND TREATMENT

The diagnosis is confirmed by demonstrating the organism in histological sections or by culture, although results can be negative in 30–50% of cases. Serology is not useful because of the marked cross-reactivity of antibodies to *Blastomyces* with *Histoplasma*.

For treatment the drug of choice is amphotericin.

Invasive zygomycosis

Invasive zygomycosis (mucormycosis) is rare and is caused by several fungi, including *Mucor*, *Rhizopus* and *Absidia*. It occurs in ill patients. The hallmark of the disease is vascular invasion with marked haemorrhagic necrosis.

Rhinocerebral mucormycosis is the most common form. Nasal stuffiness, facial pain and oedema, and necrotic, black nasal turbinates are characteristic. It is rare and is mainly seen in diabetics with ketoacidosis. Other forms include pulmonary and disseminated infection (immunosuppressed), gastrointestinal infection (in malnutrition), and cutaneous involvement (in burns). Treatment is with amphotericin. This condition is invariably fatal if left untreated.

Subcutaneous infections

Sporotrichosis

Sporotrichosis is due to the saprophytic fungus *Sporothrix schenckii*, which is found worldwide. Infection usually follows cutaneous inoculation, at the site of which a reddish, non-tender, maculopapular lesion develops – referred to as 'plaque sporotrichosis'. Pulmonary involvement and disseminated disease rarely occur.

Treatment with saturated potassium iodide (10–12 mL daily orally for adults) is curative in the cutaneous form. Amphotericin or miconazole is required for systemic infection.

Subcutaneous zygomycosis

Subcutaneous zygomycosis, a disease seen in children in Africa and Indonesia, is caused by several filamentous fungi of the *Basidiobolus* genus. The disease usually remains confined to the subcutaneous tissues and muscle fascia. It presents as a brawny, woody infiltration involving the limbs, neck and trunk. Less commonly, the pharyngeal and orbital regions may be affected.

Treatment is with saturated potassium iodide solution given orally.

Chromomycosis

Chromomycosis (chromoblastomycosis) is caused by fungi of the genus *Philalophora* and *Cladosporium carrionii*, and Fonsecara and is found mainly in tropical and subtropical countries. It presents initially as a small papule, usually at the site of a previous injury. This persists for several months before ulcerating. The lesion later becomes warty and encrusted and gradually spreads. Satellite lesions may be present. Itching is frequent. The drug of choice is flucytosine in combination with amphotericin in small doses. Cryosurgery is used to remove local lesions.

Mycetoma (Madura foot) (see also p. 39)

Mycetoma may be due to subcutaneous infection with fungi (e.g. *Eumycates spp.*) or to *Actinomyces*. Infection results in local swelling which may discharge through sinuses. Bone involvement may follow.

Treatment is with ketoconazole or antibacterials for *Actinomyces*.

Pneumocystis carinii infection

(see also pp. 115 and 798)

Genetic analysis has shown this organism to be homologous with fungi. It exists as a trophozoite which is probably motile and reproduces by binary fission. After invasion the trophozoite wall thickens and forms a cyst. On maturation further division takes place to yield eight merozoites which after cell wall rupture develops into trophozoites. Infection probably occurs in infancy but in otherwise healthy infants it remains undetected. It is usually cleared from the lungs. *P. carinii* disease in adults is associated with immunodeficiency states, particularly AIDS, and is discussed on p. 115.

Superficial infections

Dermatophytosis

Dermatophytoses are chronic fungal infections of keratinous structures such as the skin, hair or nails. *Trichophyton, Microsporum* and *Epidermophyton candida* can also infect keratinous structures.

Malassezia infection

Malassezia spp. are found on the scalp and greasy skin and are responsible for seborrhoeic dermatitis, pityriasis versicolor (hypo- or hyperpigmented rash on trunk) and *Malassezia* folliculitis (itchy rash on back). Treatment is with topical antifungals (e.g. terbinafine) or with oral agents if infection is extensive.

FURTHER READING

Walsh TJ, Hiemenz JW, Anaissie E (1996) Recent progress and current problems in treatment of invasive fungal infections in neutropenic patients. *Infectious Diseases Clinics of North America* **10**: 365-400

Protozoal infections in blood and tissues

Leishmaniasis

Leishmaniasis is caused by the protozoa *Leishmania* transmitted by the sandfly. In humans the disease is usually visceral or cutaneous. The disease varies according to the geographical areas to which different *Leishmania* species are restricted and the host response. The geographical distribution is shown in Fig 1.37.

The life-cycle of the parasite involves two stages:

- The *amastigote* (Leishman–Donovan body) occurs in vertebrate hosts such as humans, dogs or rodents. The parasites infect macrophages and reticuloendothelial cells and multiply until the cells rupture, releasing the organisms into the circulation. When the female sandfly (*Phlebotomus* or *Lutzomyia*) bites an infected host, it draws blood containing the amastigotes.
- In the sandfly the parasites develop into the infective *promastigotes*, which move to the salivary glands in about 10 days. The cycle is completed by the sandfly biting another vertebrate.

The presentation in humans is dependent on the patient's cellular immunity as well as the parasite species.

- In the *kala-azar syndrome* there is little or no immune response and the reticuloendothelial system is laden with amastigote-laden macrophages. In subjects with an increased immune response, hepatic and lymph node granulomas are found, and either there are no clinical symptoms or a localized lesion is seen.
- *Inapparent infection* is common in endemic areas and is recognized by the high incidence of leishmanin-positive skin tests. There is usually no previous history of skin ulceration or systemic disease. Infection is eradicated by the immune system and the subject is left with permanent immunity to that species of *Leishmania*.

Three clinical entities caused by *Leishmania* have been described: visceral, cutaneous and mucocutaneous.

Visceral leishmaniasis

- *Visceral leishmaniasis (kala-azar)* is caused by *L. donovani* and occurs in Asia, the Mediterranean, South America and Africa. Dogs, foxes, jackals and wild

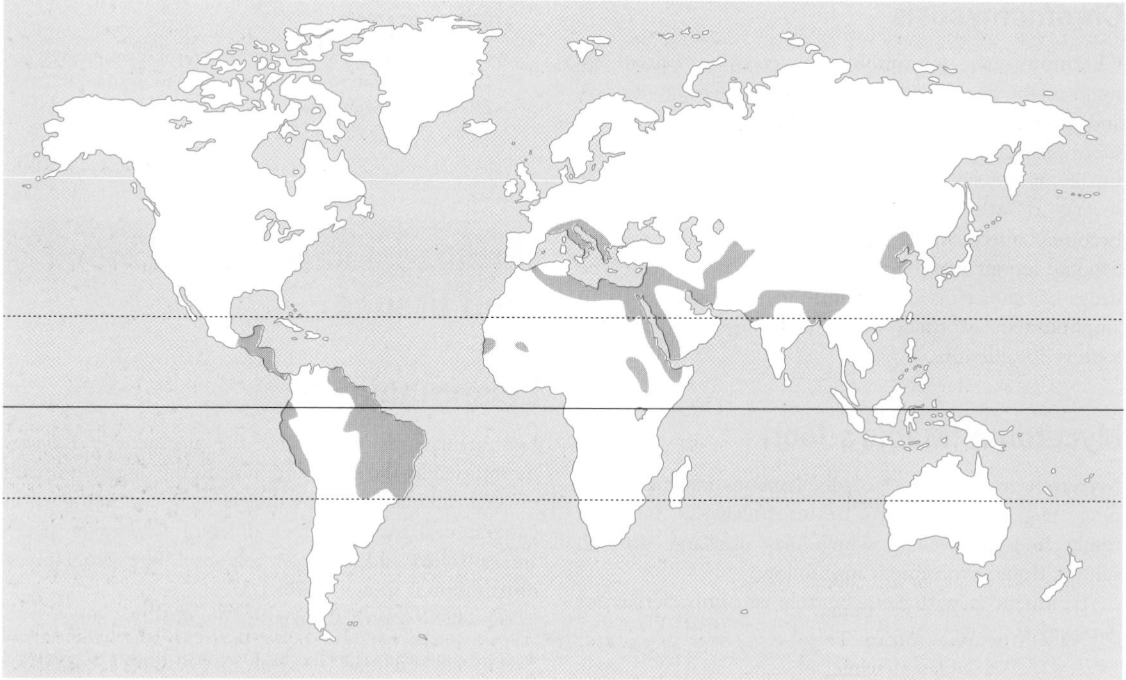

Fig 1.37
Leishmaniasis – geographical distribution

rodents can be reservoirs, but in India humans are the only known reservoir. Only 5–10% of those infected go on to develop visceral leishmaniasis. The incidence is increasing in immunocompromised patients, such as those with AIDS. Primary skin lesions are only rarely found at the site of the sandfly bite.

CLINICAL FEATURES

Visceral leishmaniasis usually affects young people. The incubation period may be months or years. The onset is abrupt or insidious. The patient feels remarkably well despite many symptoms and signs. Fever occurs and may exhibit a characteristic biphasic pattern. Cough is frequent and diarrhoea may occur. The skin is dry and rough and with time becomes pigmented. Splenic enlargement may be massive and hypersplenism is chiefly responsible for the pancytopenia seen. Epistaxis may occur as a result of thrombocytopenia. Hepatomegaly is less prominent than the splenomegaly. In *African kala-azar*, warty skin eruptions and lymphadenopathy also occur. If left untreated, death occurs within three years in the majority of patients and is due to pulmonary or gastrointestinal superinfection, to which these patients are predisposed.

Infantile kala-azar

This is seen chiefly in the Mediterranean region and is a disease of children below the age of five years.

Post kala-azar dermal leishmaniasis (PKDL)

PKDL occurs 1–2 years after successful treatment for visceral leishmaniasis in a small proportion of patients in India and less often in Africa. It is characterized by macular, erythematous lesions and pale pink nodules on the face.

INVESTIGATIONS FOR DIAGNOSIS

- **Full blood count** for normochromic normocytic, anaemia – Hb below 7 g dL^{-1} in 50% of patients. Neutropenia and thrombocytopenia also occur.
- **Hypoalbuminaemia** and **hyperglobulinaemia**.
- **Characteristic Leishman–Donovan bodies** may be demonstrated in buffy coat preparations of blood or in bone-marrow smears or lymph node, liver or spleen aspirates.
- **Culture**. The organism can be cultured in the Nicolle–Novy–McNeal culture medium.
- **Antibodies** may be detected by ELISA which is >95% specific and sensitive.

An intradermal leishmanin skin test (a test of delayed hypersensitivity) is of no value in diagnosis since it is negative early in the course of the disease.

TREATMENT

Pentavalent antimony compounds are the drugs of choice (e.g. sodium stibogluconate). The antimony dose is 20 mg kg^{-1} daily i.v. or i.m. for 21 days or longer in patients with AIDS. Antibiotics are given for intercurrent pulmonary infections. Blood transfusions are rarely required.

Intravenous amphotericin or pentamidine (up to four courses of 3 mg kg^{-1} daily for 10 days) may be required for patients whose initial response to therapy is poor. Liposomal amphotericin B is very effective but expensive. Pentamidine is ineffective in the treatment of PKDL.

PROGNOSIS

Response to therapy varies. African kala-azar is relatively resistant to treatment and the duration of therapy is necessarily longer. Clinical relapses occur in approximately 2% and requires prolonged treatment.

Cutaneous leishmaniasis

Following the sandfly bite, *Leishmania* multiply in the macrophages of the skin. The local response depends on the *Leishmania* species, the size of the inoculum, and the host immune response. Single or multiple painless nodules occur on exposed areas within one week to three months following the bite. These enlarge and ulcerate with a characteristic erythematous raised border. An overlying crust may develop. The lesions heal slowly over months or years, sometimes leaving a disfiguring scar. Different clinical patterns are described as follows.

In the Old World

L. major and *L. tropica* are found in Russia and Eastern Europe, the Middle East, around the Mediterranean and sub-Sahara and West Africa. The reservoir for *L. major* is infected desert rodents, while *L. tropica* has an urban distribution with dogs and humans as reservoirs. *L. aethiopica* is found in the highlands of Ethiopia and Kenya and the animal reservoir is often the hyrax. The vectors are usually the phlebotomus sandfly.

The lesions described above heal spontaneously with scarring but this may take years. 'Leishmaniasis recidivans', which is characterized by features resembling lupus vulgaris, describes the lesions seen many years after the healing of the primary lesions; it is rare.

In the New World

L. mexicana is found in Mexico, Guatemala, Brazil, Venezuela and Panama. The condition runs a benign course with spontaneous healing within six months. However, infection of the pinna (*chiclero's ear*) results in gross destruction of the external ear. A lesion at this site may persist for over 20 years.

L. amazonensis causes *diffuse cutaneous leishmaniasis*. This is rare and is characterized by diffuse infiltration of the skin by Leishman–Donovan bodies. Visceral lesions are absent. Clinically this chronic condition resembles lepromatous leprosy, although it does not involve the nasal septum.

L. peruviana occurs in cooler climates in the Andes. It produces single or multiple ulcers, (uta) which usually heal spontaneously.

INVESTIGATIONS FOR DIAGNOSIS

- **Giemsa's stain** on a split skin smear will demonstrate *Leishmania* in 80% of cases
- **Culture** followed by smear, isoenzyme or DNA studies if available.
- **Leishmanin skin test** is positive in over 90% of cases, although it is negative in diffuse cutaneous leishmaniasis.

Serology is unhelpful.

TREATMENT

Small lesions usually require no treatment. Large lesions or those in cosmetically important sites are treated either:

- locally by surgery, curetage, cryotherapy or hyperthermia (40–42°C), or
- systemically with pentavalent antimony compounds or azole drugs.

Treatment is less successful than for visceral leishmaniasis as antimonials are poorly concentrated in the skin. *L. aethiopica* is not sensitive to antimonials.

Mucocutaneous leishmaniasis

This is caused by *L. braziliensis* and is found in Brazil, Ecuador, Bolivia, Uruguay and northern Argentina. Initially painful, itchy nodules appear on the lower limbs, and then ulcerate. Lymphangitis is usual. Healing occurs spontaneously in six months.

In up to 40% of patients, secondary lesions develop several years later at mucocutaneous junctions such as the nasopharynx. There is evidence of nasal obstruction, ulceration, septal perforation and destruction of the nasal cartilages (Espundia).

Diagnosis can be difficult as few *Leishmania* are present. A deep punch biopsy is required. The Leishman test is positive and serum antibodies are often present.

Treatment is with systemic antimonial compounds but relapses are common. Amphotericin is sometimes used. Death usually occurs from secondary bacterial infection.

PREVENTION

In endemic areas control of vectors plays an important part. Spraying with an effective insecticide should be carried out at regular intervals. There should also be an attempt to decrease the reservoir of infection by destroying infected animals and treating infected humans early. All these methods are difficult to achieve. Travellers should wear long-sleeved clothes, use insect repellants, and sleep under impregnated fine-mesh nets.

Trypanosomiasis

African trypanosomiasis

African trypanosomiasis (sleeping sickness) follows the bite of the tsetse fly and is caused by *Trypanosoma brucei*. *T. brucei* is found in West and Central Africa between latitudes 20°N and 20°S (Fig 1.38).

- *Gambian sleeping sickness* is found mainly in West Africa, but also in southern Sudan and Uganda. Gambian sleeping sickness is caused by *T. b. gambiense* and transmitted to humans by the tsetse fly species *Glossina palpalis* and *G. tachinoides*. Humans are the only important reservoirs although domestic and wild animals may carry

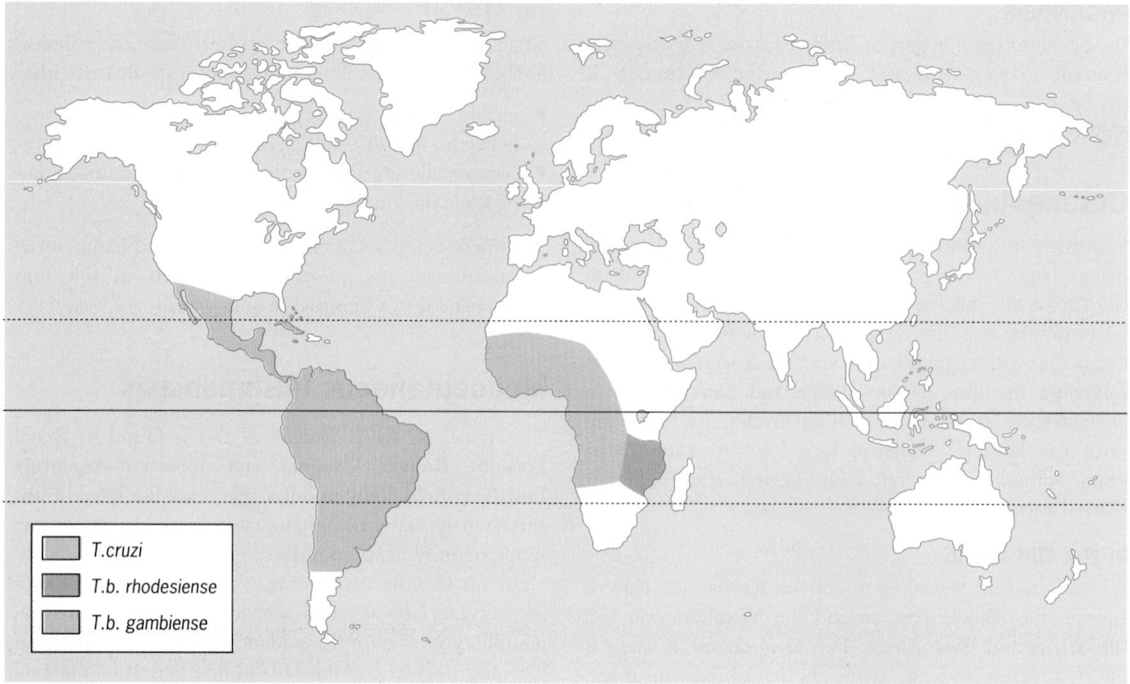

Fig 1.38
Trypanosomiasis – geographical distribution

the infection. Transmission occurs most frequently at river banks where the flies lie under trees.

- *Rhodesian sleeping sickness* is found from Ethiopia in the north to Botswana in the south. *T. b. rhodesiense*, the causative agent of Rhodesian sleeping sickness, is a zoonosis and is transmitted by *G. morsitans*, *G. swynnertoni*, *G. pallidipes*, and *G. palpalis*. Antelopes and other wild animals as well as domestic animals are reservoirs.

Tsetse flies bite in the daylight and both male and female flies can be infected. Following the bite, metacyclic forms (the infective forms of trypomastigotes) are deposited into the subcutaneous tissue, where a marked perivascular reaction occurs. Lymphatics are then invaded, followed by spread to the lymph nodes. Invasion of the bloodstream occurs in 2–3 weeks, at which time the organisms reach all parts of the body, especially the CNS. In the CNS they elicit a marked perivascular mononuclear infiltration that results in leptomeningitis or encephalomyelitis.

CLINICAL FEATURES

A tender nodule appears at the site of the bite. This is referred to as a 'trypanosoma chancre' and is seen more commonly in Rhodesian sleeping sickness and in Caucasians. Tachycardia and persistent headache are common. Spontaneous healing of the chancre occurs at about three weeks and this is followed by haematogenous dissemination.

The lymph glands are discrete, non-tender and have a peculiar rubbery consistency. Splenomegaly and hepatomegaly may also occur. After a variable period of time, there is evidence of CNS involvement and features of a chronic meningo-encephalomyelitis with behavioural changes. The patient loses interest in the surroundings, becomes apathetic, has mask-like facies, and a tendency to fall asleep during the day and inability to sleep at night. The eyelids tend to droop, there is facial puffiness, the lower lips are swollen and hang loosely and the patient's attention span decreases. Later, tremor of the hands, areas of hyperaesthesia, especially over the ulnar nerve (Kerandel's sign), choreiform movements, seizures and finally coma develop. Myocarditis, hepatitis, petechiae and pleural effusions may occur, particularly in Rhodesian sleeping sickness.

Gambian sleeping sickness is a chronic illness with symptom-free periods, while Rhodesian sleeping sickness is an acute, more severe form, and death usually occurs within one year, often from myocarditis. Features of CNS involvement are therefore less prominent than in the Rhodesian form (see Table 1.37).

Unusual manifestations

An erythematous, patchy, annular rash that fades in a week may be seen in the early stages of infection in Caucasians. Facial oedema, paraesthesiae, periosteitis, especially of the tibia resulting in hyperaesthesia, iridocyclitis and choroiditis may occur. Endocrine dysfunction may develop, manifesting as amenorrhoea or impotence.

INVESTIGATIONS FOR DIAGNOSIS

- **Trypomastigotes** may be demonstrated in the peripheral blood or lymph node aspirates. If the organism is not easily demonstrated, concentration techniques are required.

Table 1.37
Comparison between Gambian and Rhodesian sleeping sickness

	Gambian	Rhodesian
Causative agent	*Trypanosoma brucei gambiense*	*Trypanosoma brucei rhodesiense*
Main insect vector	*Glossina palpalis*	*Glossina morsitans*
Reservoir	Humans (pigs, goats, cattle, ? dogs)	Wild animals (antelopes and hogs), cattle and humans
Geographical distribution	West Africa (Gambia to Congo), Central Africa, scattered areas in East Africa	East Africa
Clinical features:		
Duration	Chronic	Acute
Severity	Mild	Severe
Trypanosoma chancre	Uncommon	Common
Fever	Insidious and low grade	Acute and with large variations
Lymphadenopathy	Prominent, especially posterior cervical group (Winterbottom's sign)	Less prominent
Hepatosplenomegaly	Present	Present
CNS abnormalities	Marked	Less marked
Other organs	Uncommon	Common
Chemoprophylaxis	Effective	Less effective

- **Serology** is required. An indirect immunofluorescent antibody test, ELISA and card agglutination tests for trypanosomiasis (CATT) are valuable for screening.
- **CSF examination** is essential. Increased lymphocytes and raised protein levels are present. IgM is elevated.

TREATMENT

Therapy is usually effective if commenced *before CNS symptoms develop*.

Before CNS involvement

Suramin, a polysulphated compound, is given intravenously. Initially 0.1 g is given as a test dose to exclude an idiosyncratic reaction, followed by 1.0 g i.v. on the first, third, seventh, fourteenth and twenty-first days. If proteinuria or haematuria develop, therapy should be discontinued. Pentamidine 3–4 mg kg^{-1} intramuscularly on alternate days for 10 injections is an effective alternative. Rapid intravenous injection of pentamidine results in hypotension.

Although suramin and pentamidine have been found to be effective and should be used initially to control the fever, they do not cross the blood–brain barrier. It is believed that relapse or failure to respond to therapy will occur when CNS involvement occurs early in the disease.

After CNS involvement. Drugs that penetrate the blood–brain barrier are recommended as part of the initial treatment of trypanosomiasis. Melarsoprol, a trivalent arsenic, is used most widely for this purpose. Three to four consecutive injections of 2.0–3.6 mg kg^{-1} (up to a maximum of 250 mg per injection) are given intravenously. The course is usually repeated after an interval of two weeks. Major side-effects include an acute encephalitis-like condition and skin rashes. Jarisch–Herxheimer-type reactions can be reduced by clearing the parasites from the blood with suramin initially.

Oral nitrofurazone 10 mg kg^{-1} in divided doses thrice daily for 10 days has also been found to be useful in cerebral trypanosomiasis. Peripheral neuropathy and haemolytic anaemia may be troublesome side-effects in patients with glucose-6-phosphate dehydrogenase deficiency.

Difluoromethylornithine is also used for Gambian sleeping sickness.

PREVENTION AND CONTROL

Elimination of the vector – the tsetse fly – by insecticide traps or by making environmental conditions unsuitable for its inhabitation would effectively eradicate trypanosomiasis. Both these approaches require formidable mobilization of manpower and money. Insect repellents, as well as protective, light-coloured clothing and insecticide-impregnated sleeping nets, should be used when visiting endemic areas.

A single intramuscular prophylactic injection of pentamidine 4 mg kg^{-1} (up to a maximum dose of 300 mg) gives effective protection against Gambian sleeping sickness, but is less effective against Rhodesian sleeping sickness.

African trypanosomiasis in children

In children the early manifestations and CNS symptoms overlap. Lymphadenopathy and neurological abnormalities may occur together. Seizures and choreiform movements are not uncommon. Treatment is as for the adult form.

American trypanosomiasis (Chagas' disease)

This is a zoonotic disease caused by *T. cruzi* that is transmitted by various reduviid insects. The principal vectors are *Triatoma infestans* and *Rhodnius prolixus* (Latin

America) and *Panstrongylus megistus* (Brazil). Once infected, these insects remain infective for at least two years. Domestic and wild animals are important reservoirs. Humans are infected usually at night when the insect feeds and infected faeces are rubbed into a skin abrasion or mucosal surface such as the conjunctiva. Less commonly the infection may spread via blood transfusions or transplacentally.

Chagas' disease is confined to South and Central America, but occasional cases have also been reported from southern Texas.

CLINICAL FEATURES

The incubation period is 1–2 weeks. Two clinically distinct presentations are recognized.

Acute Chagas' disease

Acute Chagas' disease predominantly affects children. In 50% of cases an erythematous, indurated papule (chagoma) develops at the site of the bite, and is associated with regional lymphadenopathy. This resolves spontaneously. If the portal of entry is the conjunctiva, unilateral periorbital and palpebral oedema (Romana's sign), conjunctivitis and preauricular lymphadenopathy develop. Systemic findings such as fever, a transient morbilliform or urticarial rash, a peculiar gelatinous oedema of the face and trunk, tender lymphadenopathy and hepatosplenomegaly may be present. Death occurs in a small proportion of patients owing to myocarditis or meningo-encephalitis. More commonly the patient recovers completely in a few weeks.

Chronic Chagas' disease

Chronic Chagas' disease occurs after a latent period of many years. It is due to an autoimmune reaction mediated by cytotoxic T cells and antibodies against the endocardium, vascular tissue and striated muscle, together with myenteric plexus damage by amastigotes. The heart is invariably involved. The patient may complain of chest pain, dyspnoea or syncope. Cardiac abnormalities and arrhythmias are usual. Signs of right-sided cardiac failure may be present. Thromboembolic phenomena may occur.

With gastrointestinal involvement, megaoesophagus leading to dysphagia and aspiration pneumonia, and megacolon giving constipation and progressive abdominal distension, occur. Dilatation of the biliary tree and of the bronchi have also been documented.

INVESTIGATIONS FOR DIAGNOSIS

In acute Chagas' disease, trypomastigotes may be demonstrated in peripheral blood. If parasites are not demonstrated in the blood, xenodiagnosis may be used: a parasite-free laboratory-reared vector feeds on a patient (or the patient's blood) suspected to have the disease and 2–3 weeks later the intestinal contents of the vector are examined for parasites.

In chronic Chagas' disease, complement fixation (Machado–Guerreiro reaction), indirect fluorescent antibody or haemagglutination tests may be used. Radiological assessment of gastrointestinal abnormalities is helpful.

TREATMENT

Nifurtimox has been widely used in acute disease but is no longer produced. Benzimidazole 7.5 mg kg^{-1} for 60 days is now the drug of choice for all patients with acute or early chronic disease. Over 80% of patients with the acute form of the disease and slightly more with the chronic form are cured of the infection.

PREVENTION AND CONTROL

No vaccine or chemoprophylactic agent is available. Prevention therefore involves a 'vertical' attack phase when all houses in a district are treated with a modern pyrethroid such as deltamethrin, cyfluthrin or lambda-cyhalothrin followed by 'horizontal' vigilance where householders report the findings of any bug. Blood donors must be screened.

Toxoplasmosis

Toxoplasmosis is caused by *Toxoplasma gondii*, an intracellular protozoon, which requires for completion of its life-cycle the definitive host, the cat, and an intermediate host such as a human. Infection of humans occurs either by ingestion of foodstuffs contaminated by infected cat faeces or lamb or pork contaminated with *T. gondii* cysts or transplacentally (when the mother has an acute infection). The prevalence of toxoplasma antibodies varies from 30% (UK) to 90% in different countries

CLINICAL FEATURES

Five major clinical forms of toxoplasmosis are recognized.

- *Asymptomatic lymphadenopathy* is the most common mode of presentation.
- *Lymphadenopathy* usually involves the cervical lymph nodes and is associated with a febrile illness. This may be clinically indistinguishable from infectious mononucleosis but the Paul–Bunnell test is negative.
- *Neurological abnormalities* include neck stiffness and headache, associated with sore throat and maculopapular rashes. The CSF is under pressure and the level of protein is elevated.
- An *acute febrile illness* occurs, with a maculopapular rash, hepatosplenomegaly and reactive lymphocytes in the peripheral blood. Uveitis, chorioretinitis, myocarditis and hepatitis may occur.
- In *congenital toxoplasmosis* the symptoms and signs are indicative of CNS involvement. The characteristic 'syndrome of Savin', which comprises internal hydrocephalus, chorioretinitis, convulsions and cerebral calcification, may be seen. Tremors,

nystagmus, micro-ophthalmia and pneumonitis are also present. The prognosis is usually poor, the survivors generally exhibiting mental retardation, epilepsy and spastic paraplegia.

The immunocompromised host presents with features of both the acute febrile and neurological forms and is due to reactivation of previously acquired infection.

INVESTIGATIONS FOR DIAGNOSIS

Serological tests are the mainstay of diagnosis of acquired infection. The Sabin–Feldman dye test, a measure of IgG antibodies, has been widely used. Antibodies can also be detected by indirect fluorescence or indirect haemagglutination. Raised antibody levels are common in the general population and only a rising antibody titre is highly suggestive of toxoplasmosis. The IgM-immunofluorescent antibody (IgM-IFA) test is particularly useful for detecting acute infection since titres rise early and fall rapidly.

T. gondii can be isolated by injecting bone marrow, body fluids or CSF into mice, examining the peritoneal fluid 6–10 days later for the organism. The organism can also be cultured in tissue culture cell lines and *T. gondii* DNA can be detected by PCR. Patients with eye involvement, those with immunosuppression and those with severe disease need treatment.

TREATMENT

Most patients require no therapy as the disease is mild. Pyrimethamine (25–50 mg thrice-daily) and sulphadiazine (4–5 g daily) are used in combination for severe disease since they are synergistic. Folinic acid (15 mg twice-weekly) should also be given. Therapy should be continued for at least one month. Since pyrimethamine is teratogenic, spiramycin is a useful alternative during pregnancy. Steroids are probably useful in ocular toxoplasmosis.

PREVENTION

Domestic cats that kill mice and birds are the chief source of infection and care should be taken in handling their faeces. Good basic hygiene in the house and garden should be observed.

Babesiosis

This is a tick-borne disease, found chiefly in North America and Europe, and is occasionally transmitted to humans, especially those who are immunocompromised following splenectomy. The causative organisms are the plasmodium-like *Babesia microti* (rodents) and *B. divergens* (cattle). The incubation period averages 10 days.

CLINICAL FEATURES

In patients with normal splenic function, the symptoms are mild and usually comprise fever, nausea, myalgia, chills, vomiting and abdominal pain. Hepatosplenomegaly and mild to moderate haemolytic anaemia may also be present. In splenectomized individuals, systemic symptoms are more pronounced and haemolysis is associated with haemoglobinuria, jaundice and renal failure. Examination of a peripheral blood smear may reveal the characteristic plasmodium-like organisms.

TREATMENT

The treatment of choice is a combination of quinine 650 mg and clindamycin 600 mg orally thrice-daily for seven days. This reduces the fever and parasitaemia but is not curative. Combination of pentamidine and co-trimoxazole have been used partially successfully in *B. divergens* infection.

Malaria

Malaria currently affects 250 million people and has a mortality rate of 1%.

Endemic and epidemic malaria are found in all countries between latitudes 30°S and 40°N (Fig 1.39). Malaria is primarily a disease of hot, humid countries at altitudes less than 2200 m above mean sea level, where conditions are ideal for prolific breeding of the mosquito vector, *Anopheles*. It is endemic in India, in parts of Africa and parts of South and Central America. Malaria may also be transmitted by the importation of infected mosquitoes by air, so-called 'airport malaria'.

In humans, malaria is caused by four species of *Plasmodium*: *P. vivax*, *P. ovale*, *P. falciparum* and *P. malariae*. The four species are distinguishable from each other on examination of peripheral blood smears.

P. ovale has been reported predominantly from East and West Africa. *P. vivax* is the major species in temperate zones, whereas in the tropics all forms of malaria are seen. With present-day ease and speed of travel, sporadic cases of malaria are being increasingly recognized. Unfortunately, the initial impact of the WHO eradication programme lost its impetus in several countries in the early 1970s and malaria has once more become a major cause of morbidity and mortality in tropical and subtropical countries. In addition, the emergence of drug (chloroquine) and insecticide (DDT) resistance is a major problem.

Humans, the intermediate hosts, are infected following the bite of an infected female *Anopheles* mosquito, the definitive host. The parasite can also be transmitted by blood transfusion, transplacentally, and, increasingly, between drug addicts who use improperly cleaned syringes.

The introduction of sporozoites, the infective form of the parasite, through the skin by the *Anopheles* mosquito heralds the commencement of the human cycle (Fig 1.40). The following stages occur.

Pre-erythrocytic schizogony

During this phase clinical symptoms are absent and humans are not infective. Those sporozoites that are not removed by the body's defence mechanisms undergo

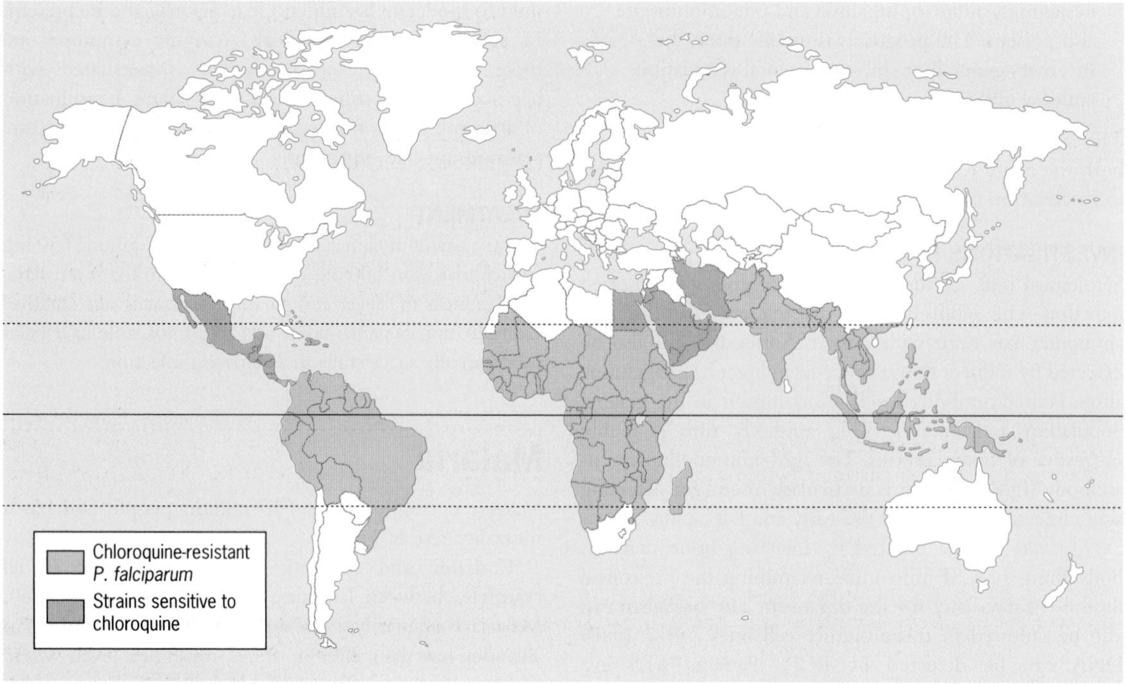

Fig 1.39
Malaria – geographical distribution

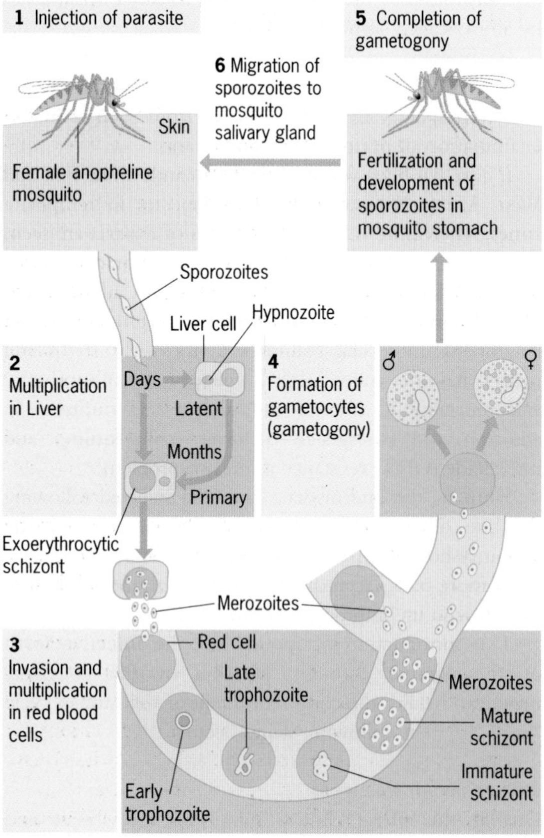

Fig 1.40
A schematic life-cycle of *Plasmodium vivax*

development within the liver. A variable number of days later, merozoites are liberated (primary attack) from the liver. Other sporozoites (*P. vivax* and probably *P. ovale*) remain in a latent form in the liver as hypnozoites.

Erythrocytic schizogony

This is the phase when red blood cells (RBCs) become infected by the released merozoites. In the RBCs they pass through several stages of development, namely trophozoites, schizonts and finally merozoites again. These asexual parasitic forms are found in peripheral blood about 12 days after inoculation of the sporozoites in *P. vivax* infection and after nine days in *P. falciparum* infection.

The different *Plasmodium* species differ in their ability to invade RBCs. *P. falciparum* is capable of invading all RBCs, especially young RBCs. It therefore has the potential to produce the most severe form of malaria. *P. vivax* and *P. ovale* preferentially invade reticulocytes and young RBCs, whereas *P. malariae* invades senescent RBCs.

Each cycle in the RBCs terminates with rupture of the cell and release of merozoites into the circulation. This occurs every 48 hours in *P. falciparum* infection, every 48–72 hours in *P. vivax* and *P. ovale* infection, and approximately every 72 hours in *P. malariae*.

Gametogony

The erythrocytic phase may continue for a considerable period of time before the stage of gametogony occurs. In this stage a few merozoites develop into the sexual form of the parasites known as gametocytes. Of these only the mature forms are found in peripheral blood. At this stage the patient is infective.

Exoerythrocytic schizogony

This fourth stage, which occurs in the liver, is found only with *P. vivax*, probably *P. ovale* and possibly *P. malariae* infections. It does not occur with *P. falciparum* infection and is believed to be responsible for the relapses in *P. vivax* and *P. ovale* infections. The parasites in this phase are referred to as hypnozoites.

When an *Anopheles* mosquito ingests human blood containing gametocytes it marks the commencement of the sexual cycle in the mosquito. The external incubation period is 7–20 days.

PATHOGENESIS

The severity of malaria can be explained partly on the magnitude of the parasitaemia, with *P. falciparum* causing severe disease as it can invade RBCs of any age.

Immunity may be natural or acquired. Natural immunity is present in individuals of West African extraction who are blood group Duffy-negative (FyFy) and therefore lack the specific receptor on the RBC surface to which the merozoites attach. They cannot develop *P. vivax* malaria. The presence of haemoglobin S, glucose-6-phosphate dehydrogenase deficiency, thalassaemia and pyruvate kinase deficiency also offer resistance against *P. falciparum*. The presence of abnormal haemoglobins or altered RBC metabolism retards *P. falciparum* maturation and reduces the severity of the disease. Certain HLA antigens have been shown to be protective against *P. falciparum* in Gambian children.

The spleen plays an important role in natural immunity, since splenectomized individuals are highly susceptible to the malarial parasite.

Infants are protected by the transfer of maternal IgG antibodies across the placenta.

Partial immunity may be acquired following an attack of malaria, and is attributed to macrophage stimulation by T cells.

Tumour necrosis factor α (TNF-α) blood levels correlate with the severity of the disease but a cause-and-effect relationship has not been shown. Certain polymorphisms of ICAM-1 predispose those individuals to develop cerebral malaria.

CLINICAL FEATURES

The incubation period varies, being:

- 10–14 days in *P. vivax*, *P. ovale* and *P. falciparum*
- 18 days to six weeks in *P. malariae* infection.

Although individual variations in clinical presentation are noted, febrile paroxysms, anaemia, splenomegaly and hepatomegaly are usually present. Malarial febrile paroxysms typically have three stages:

- The '*cold stage*' is characterized by marked vasoconstriction and lasts from 30 minutes to one hour. The patient feels intensely cold and uncomfortable. There is marked shivering. The temperature rises rapidly, often to as high as 41°C.
- The '*hot stage*' abruptly follows and lasts for 2–6 hours. The patient feels intensely hot and uncomfortable. Delirium may be present.
- The '*sweating stage*' then occurs, during which the bedclothes are drenched. The patient feels fatigued and exhausted but otherwise well and often sleeps. The fever is due to schizont rupture and the release of pyrogens.

Herpes labialis frequently occurs in established malaria. Anaemia is usually present and is largely a result of haemolysis.

P. vivax and *P. ovale* disease

The fever occurs every other day when established. These species of *Plasmodium* give rise to a clinically mild infection. The presence of an exoerythrocytic stage in the liver is responsible for relapses and makes eradication of the organisms difficult.

P. malariae disease

This is usually a mild disease with a fever, but tends to run a more chronic course. The nephrotic syndrome can complicate this type of malaria and may be fatal between the ages of four and five years. Because of its chronicity, the patient develops a sallow complexion, marked muscle wasting, mild icterus and massive splenomegaly. Growth retardation may occur in children.

P. falciparum disease

This is the most severe form of malaria (pernicious malaria), with high levels of parasitaemia. Infected RBCs develop peculiar knob-like surface projections that facilitate adhesion of these RBCs to the endothelium of blood vessels (sequestration) via, for example, ICAM-1. The consequent vascular occlusion causes severe anoxic organ damage, chiefly in the kidneys, liver, brain and gastrointestinal tract. Sequestration means that the mature trophozoites and schizonts are not seen in the peripheral blood and thus evade destruction by the spleen. The prodrome tends to be severe. The fever follows no particular pattern. Splenomegaly tends to occur late and the characteristic cold, hot and sweating stages are not prominent. Severe falciparum malaria when more than 2% of RBCs are parasitized shows the clinical consequences shown in Information box 1.4. Impaired conciousness and respiratory distress identify children at high risk of death.

Cerebral malaria. Cerebral malaria is characterized by a marked elevation in body temperature, a rapid deterioration in consciousness, convulsions, coma and death. Individuals with a genetic variant in the promoter region of the TNF gene (termed the TNF Z allele) have an increased risk of developing cerebral malaria.

Blackwater fever. Blackwater fever – so called because of the production of dark brown-black urine owing to intravascular haemolysis – is seen only in falciparum malaria.

Information

CNS Cerebral malaria (coma, convulsion) **Renal** Haemoglobinuria (blackwater fever) Oliguria Uraemia (acute tubular necrosis) **Blood** Severe anaemia (haemolysis and dyserythropoiesis) Disseminated intravascular coagulation (DIC – haemorrhage)	**Respiratory** Acute respiratory distress syndrome **Metabolic** Hypoglycaemia (particularly in children) Metabolic acidosis **Gastrointestinal/liver** Diarrhoea Jaundice Splenic rupture **Other** Shock – hypotensive Hyperpyrexia

Information box 1.4 Some features of severe falciparum malaria

It can be precipitated by very small amounts of quinine in quinine-sensitive cases. This is a rapidly progressive illness characterized by the abrupt onset of fever, marked haemolysis, haemoglobinuria, hyperbilirubinaemia, vomiting, circulatory collapse and acute renal failure. Malarial parasites cannot usually be detected in peripheral blood smears after the onset of intravascular haemolysis.

Tropical splenomegaly syndrome

Tropical splenomegaly syndrome is seen in areas where malaria is hyperendemic. It is uncommon before 10 years of age. Characteristic features are anaemia, massive splenomegaly, marked elevation in serum IgM levels, and IgM aggregates (detected by immunofluorescence) in Kupffer cells in the liver. The splenomegaly responds to antimalarial therapy. However, malarial parasites are not detected in the spleen or peripheral blood smears.

PREVALENCE

The following indices are used to measure the prevalence of malaria:

- *Spleen rate* is defined as the percentage of children between two and 10 years of age with splenomegaly. It is used as a measure of the endemicity of malaria in a community.
- *Infant parasite rate* is defined as the percentage of infants below one year of age in whom malarial parasites are demonstrable in peripheral blood smears. It is regarded as the most sensitive index of transmission of malaria to a locality.

DIAGNOSIS

A history of travel and awareness of the possible diagnosis is vital and should be considered in any febrile patient. The parasite can be demonstrated in either thin or thick peripheral blood smears stained with Giemsa, Wright or Leishman stains. The blood film should indicate the *Plasmodium* species and the percentage of red blood cells infected. Two to three blood smears taken each day for three or four days and found to be negative are necessary before a patient is declared malaria-free.

Serological methods are not widely used but include indirect immunofluorescence, indirect haemagglutination and gel diffusion techniques. ELISA for antigen detection and probes for parasite DNA are currently being evaluated.

TREATMENT

General

Analgesics and antipyretics such as aspirin and paracetamol are given as necessary. However, paracetamol has no antipyretic benefit over mechanical antipyresis and prolongs the time taken to clear the parasite, possibly by reducing production of TNF and oxygen radicals. Intravenous fluids may be required to combat dehydration and shock.

Treatment of an acute attack

The 4-aminoquinolines are the drugs of choice. Chloroquine-sensitive malaria is treated with chloroquine 600 mg of the base followed by 300 mg in six hours and then 300 mg twice-daily for two days.

In most parts of the world, *P. falciparum* is resistant to chloroquine and is therefore treated with quinine sulphate 600 mg of salt thrice-daily for seven days, followed by a single dose of pyrimethamine 75 mg and sulfadoxine 1.5 g (i.e. three tablets of Fansidar). Tetracycline (250 mg four times daily for seven days) is used for Fansidar-resistant cases.

Mefloquine is a synthesized quinolone which is useful in chloroquine-resistant and some quinine-resistant cases; again resistance to this is developing. Halofantrine, an amino alcohol, is another drug for resistant cases. Halofantrine prolongs the QT_c interval and is contraindicated in pre-existing heart disease and when there is a family history of heart disease.

Artemisin and its derivatives are highly effective agents isolated from the chinese medicinal herb *Artemisia annua*. They are effective against chloroquine-resistant malaria and their use is generally restricted to severe, complicated infection.

Drug side-effects. These drugs are potentially toxic. Haemolytic anaemia, drug fever and tinnitus may occur with quinine. Chloroquine may cause vomiting, abdominal pain, agranulocytosis or convulsions. Mefloquine can produce severe neuropyschiatric side-effects which may persist for several days owing to the drug's long half-life.

Eradication

- *P. vivax*, *P. malariae* and *P. ovale*. Primaquine, an 8-aminoquinoline, is essential for eliminating the exoerythrocytic cycle and effecting a radical cure.

A course of one of the 4-aminoquinolines should therefore be followed by primaquine 15 mg daily for 14 days. Primaquine can cause severe haemolysis in G6PD-deficient patients and therefore the G6PD status should be checked prior to therapy. In pregnancy, radical cure is postponed and chloroquine 600 mg weekly is given.

- *P. falciparum* requires no additional therapy as there is no exo-erythrocyte stage.

Treatment of severe malaria

Severe malaria (more than 1% of RBCs infected) or any of the pernicious forms of falciparum malaria constitutes a medical emergency. *Quinine*, given by a slow intravenous infusion, is the drug of choice – quinine dihydrochloride 20 mg kg^{-1} intravenously over four hours, followed by 10 mg kg^{-1} infused over four hours at eight–hourly intervals until the patient is able to tolerate oral therapy.

Ill patients require full intensive care. Anaemia should be treated by blood transfusion, convulsions controlled with diazepam, hypoglycaemia (which is made worse by quinine therapy as this releases insulin) should be monitored and the fluid balance carefully evaluated as pulmonary oedema is common. Exchange transfusion is required with heavy infestation (>10%). The parasites disappear with adequate treatment in 3–5 days.

Artemisin is an alternative agent which can be given orally or by intramuscular injection.

PREVENTION AND CONTROL

Owing to changing patterns of resistance, advice about chemoprophylaxis should be sought prior to leaving for a malaria-endemic area. Chemoprophylaxis is essential for those visiting endemic areas. This is generally chloroquine 300 mg once a week in areas where there is no chloroquine resistance, but where there is resistance it should be combined with proguanil 200 mg daily. In Oceania, dapsone/pyrimethamine (Maloprim) one tablet (100 mg and 125 mg respectively) as well as 300 mg each week should be given. Mefloquine 250 mg weekly (adults) is an alternative where falciparum malaria is highly resistant to chloroquine (sub-Saharan Africa, South America and South East Asia) for periods of up to six months. Doxycycline has also been used successfully in South East Asia. Prophylaxis should be continued for six weeks after leaving a high-risk area. Travellers should be warned that malaria can occur after return to the UK even if seemingly appropriate prophylaxis has been taken.

On the basis of the WHO Expert Committee report on malaria in 1979, the following preventive measures have been suggested. Measures to be applied to the community include prevention of man–vector contact, destruction of adult mosquitoes and mosquito larvae, and active elimination of human infection by presumptive treatment (i.e. treatment of all fevers in endemic areas with antimalarials) and radical treatment. Measures to be applied to individuals include use of mosquito repellents, impregnated bed nets, protective clothing, chemoprophylaxis and chemotherapy where indicated.

FURTHER READING

Kwiatkowski D, Marsh K (1997) Vaccine development and trials. *Lancet* **350**: 1696-1703.

Olliaro PL, Bryceson ADM (1993) Practical progress and new drugs for changing patterns of leishmaniasis. *Parasitology Today* **9**: 323-328.

Pasvol G (ed) (1995) Malaria: *Baillière's Clinical Infectious Diseases* **2**: no 3.

Protozoal infections in intestines and genitalia

Human intestinal protozoal infections are found worldwide, particularly in the developing countries (Table 1.38). Intestinal protozoa are being increasingly recognized as a cause of diarrhoea in patients with AIDS.

Amoebiasis

The most important human disease due to amoebae is amoebiasis, which is caused by *Entamoeba histolytica*. This intestinal pathogen can be differentiated from other enteric amoebae such as *Entamoeba hartmani*, *Entamoeba coli* and *Endolimax nana*, since *E. histolytica* is the only amoeba found in the intestine that phagocytoses RBCs. It occurs

Table 1.38
Human intestinal protozoa

Sarcodina (amoebae)	
Pathogenic	*Entamoeba histolytica*
Non-pathogenic	*Entamoeba dispar*
Non-pathogenic (usually)	*Entamoeba moshkovkii*
	Entamoeba chattoni
	Entamoeba coli
	Endolimax nana
	Iodamoeba butchlii
	Dientamoeba fraginalis
Mastigophora (flagellates)	
Pathogenic	*Giardia intestinalis*
Non-pathogenic	*Trichomonas hominis*
	Chilomastic mesnili
	Enbadomonas intestinalis
	Enteromonas hominis
Cillophora (cillates)	*Balantidium coli*
Coccidia	*Cryptosporidium parvum*
	Isospora belli
	Sarcocystis spp.
	Cyclospora cayetanensis
Microspora	*Enterocytozoon bienensi*
	Encephalitazoon intestinalis

worldwide, although much higher incidence rates are found in the tropics and subtropics. It can be found in active male homosexuals who carry the pathogen (usually strains of low virulence) and between whom it is spread by sexual contact.

LIFE-CYCLE AND PATHOGENESIS

The organism exists both as a motile trophozoite and as a cyst that can survive outside the body. Cysts are transmitted chiefly by ingestion of contaminated food or water or spread directly by person-to-person contact. Trophozoites emerge from the cyst in the small intestine and then pass on to the colon, where they multiply (Fig 1.41).

Many individuals can carry the pathogen without obvious evidence of clinical disease (asymptomatic cyst passers). However, under certain conditions, *E. histolytica* trophozoites invade the colonic epithelium, probably with the aid of their own cytotoxins and proteolytic enzymes. The parasites continue to multiply and finally frank ulceration of the mucosa occurs. If penetration continues, trophozoites may enter the portal vein, via which they reach the liver and cause hepatitis and intrahepatic abscesses. This invasive form of the disease is particularly serious and unless treated promptly is often fatal.

CLINICAL FEATURES

The incubation period is highly variable and may be as short as a few days or as long as several months or even a year. The presenting features may be gradual, severe or fulminating.

- *Gradual-onset colitis* presents with mild intermittent diarrhoea and abdominal discomfort, usually progressing to bloody diarrhoea with mucus. Systemic manifestations such as headache, nausea and anorexia are often present.

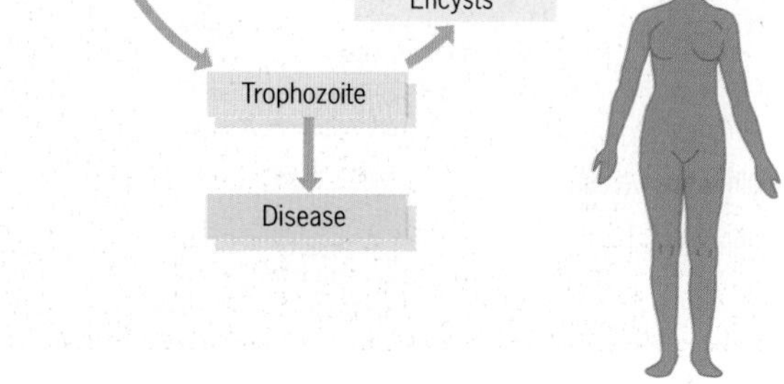

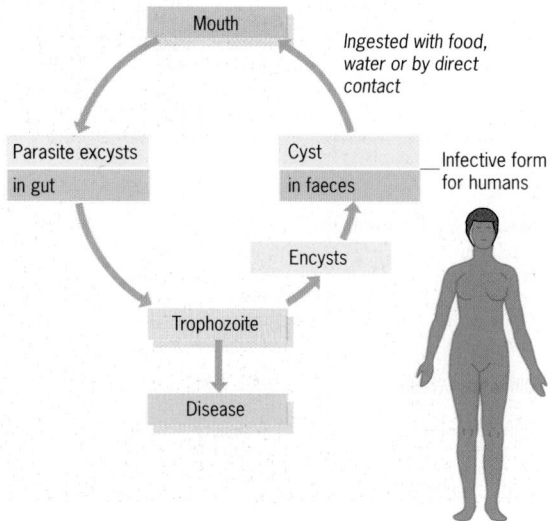

Fig 1.41
A schematic life-cycle of intestinal protozoa

- *Severe acute (amoebic) dysentery* closely resembles that due to *Shigella* (bacillary dysentery).
- Patients with a *fulminating amoebic colitis* appear less unwell than those with bacillary dysentery. Fever is low-grade or absent, and dehydration is unusual.

COMPLICATIONS

Complications are unusual, but include:

- progression of fulminant colitis to toxic dilatation of the colon with perforation and peritonitis
- chronic infection leading to stricture formation
- severe haemorrhage
- amoeboma (i.e. a mass of fibrotic granulation tissue)
- amoebic liver abscess.

Amoebomas, which develop most commonly in the caecum or rectosigmoid region, occur in 10% of patients and are sometimes mistaken for carcinoma. They may bleed, cause obstruction or intussuscept.

Amoebic liver abscesses often develop in the absence of a recent episode of colitis. Tender hepatomegaly, a high swinging fever and profound malaise are characteristic, although early in the course of the disease both symptoms and signs may be minimal. The clinical features are described in more detail on p. 331.

DIAGNOSIS

Serodiagnosis

The amoebic fluorescent antibody test is positive in at least 90% of patients with liver abscess and in 75% with active colitis. Seropositivity is low in asymptomatic cyst passers.

Colonic disease

Direct examination of colonic exudate obtained at sigmoidoscopy or of freshly passed stool as a saline-wet mount is the most rapid and least expensive way of confirming amoebic infection. *E. histolytica* trophozoites must be distinguished from non-pathogenic amoebae and from polymorphonuclear leucocytes, with which they are sometimes confused. Cysts may also be present in the stool. Sigmoidoscopy and barium enema examination may show colonic ulceration but are rarely diagnostic.

Liver disease

Liver abscess should be suspected if the serum alkaline phosphatase is elevated, even when clinical signs are absent. Hepatic ultrasound scan should confirm the presence of an abscess, which may be either single or multiple. Pus from an amoebic abscess has a classic 'anchovy sauce' appearance and may contain trophozoites.

TREATMENT

Metronidazole 800 mg thrice-daily for five days is given in amoebic colitis and a more prolonged course for 10–14 days in liver abscess or other extraintestinal spread.

An alternative drug is the other nitroimidazole derivative, tinidazole. Dehydroemetine is used when nitroimidazoles fail (rarely). Diloxanide furoate is a luminal amoebicide and may be a helpful adjunct in clearing cysts. Quinfamide is also used and is more readily available.

Large, tense abscesses in the liver may require percutaneous drainage, using an ultrasound scan to localize accurately the abscess and to position the drainage needle.

CONTROL AND PREVENTION

This disease will be difficult to eradicate because of the substantial human reservoir of asymptomatic cases. There is no immediate hope of vaccine development, particularly as the same individual may experience several episodes of amoebic infection, indicating that only partial protective immunity develops after exposure to the pathogen. Improved standards of personal hygiene and water quality are important. Cysts are destroyed by boiling water for at least 10 minutes, but the effects of chlorination are variable.

Balantidiasis

Balantidium coli is the only ciliate that produces clinically significant infection in humans. It is found throughout the tropics, particularly in Central and South America, Iran, Papua New Guinea and the Philippines. It is usually carried by pigs and infection is most common in those communities that live in close association with swine. Its life-cycle is identical to that of *E. histolytica*.

B. coli produces a dysenteric illness owing to invasion of the distal ileal and colonic mucosa. The colitis may be acute and fulminant and if untreated may be fatal. Trophozoites rather than cysts are found in the stool. Treatment is with tetracycline, ampicillin or metronidazole.

Giardiasis

Giardia intestinalis (lamblia) is a flagellate (Fig 1.42) that is found worldwide. It causes small-intestinal disease, with diarrhoea and malabsorption. Prevalence is high throughout the tropics. It is an important cause of traveller's diarrhoea worldwide, usually occurring on return from travel. In certain parts of Europe, Russia, and in some rural and mountainous areas of North America, large water-borne epidemics have been reported. Person-to-person spread is common in day nurseries and residential institutions and between male homosexuals. Like *E. histolytica*, the organism exists both as a trophozoite and a cyst, the latter being the form in which the protozoon is transmitted.

The organism colonizes and multiplies within the small intestine and may remain there without causing detriment to the host. Severe malabsorption may occur and is thought to be related to morphological damage to the small intestine; changes in villous architecture vary from mild partial villous atrophy to (rarely) subtotal villous atrophy. The mechanism by which *Giardia* causes alteration in mucosal architecture and produces diarrhoea and intestinal malabsorption is unknown. There is evidence that the morphological damage may be immune mediated. Bacterial overgrowth has also been found in association with giardiasis and may contribute to fat malabsorption.

CLINICAL FEATURES

Many individuals excreting *Giardia* cysts have no symptoms and are therefore carriers. Others develop symptoms within 1–2 weeks of ingesting cysts. These include diarrhoea, often watery in the early stage of the illness, nausea, anorexia, abdominal discomfort and distension. Stools may then become paler, with the characteristic features of steatorrhoea. If the illness is prolonged, weight loss ensues, which, even in previously healthy adults, can be marked. Chronic giardiasis can result in growth retardation in children.

DIAGNOSIS AND TREATMENT

Both cysts and trophozoites can be found in the stool, but negative stool examination does not exclude the diagnosis since the parasite may be excreted at irregular intervals. The parasite can also be seen in duodenal aspirates and in histological sections of jejunal mucosa. Raised specific anti-*Giardia* IgG and, in acute infections, IgM antibodies are found.

Metronidazole 2 g as a single dose on three successive days will cure the majority of infections, although sometimes a second or third course is necessary. Preventive measures are similar to those outlined above for *E. histolytica*. Alternative drugs include mepacrine and albendazole.

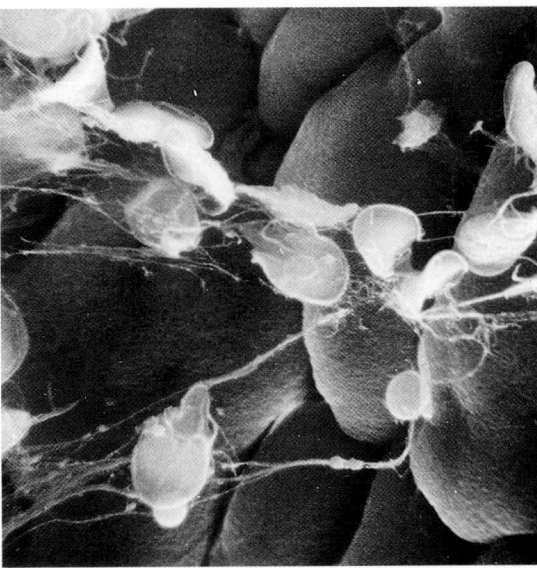

Fig 1.42
Giardia intestinalis. Courtesy of Dr A. Phillips, Department of Electron Microscopy, Royal Free Hospital, London

Cryptosporidium parvum

This organism is found worldwide, cattle being a major natural reservoir. It has also been demonstrated in drinking water supplies. It produces a devastating diarrhoeal illness in patients with immunodeficiency, particularly those with AIDS. It is a recognized cause of gastroenteritis, particularly in children.

The parasite is able to reproduce both sexually and asexually and has a life-cycle in the intestine very similar to that of *Plasmodium*. The disease is spread by oocysts excreted in the faeces.

CLINICAL FEATURES

In healthy individuals cryptosporidiosis is a self-limiting illness lasting for 7–10 days. Acute watery diarrhoea is associated with fever and general malaise, but otherwise the disease follows a benign course. In the immunocompromised patient diarrhoea is severe (see p. 84).

DIAGNOSIS AND TREATMENT

The parasite can be detected in intestinal biopsies but is now most commonly found in faeces (as oocysts) using concentration techniques and a modified Ziehl–Nielsen stain.

As yet there is no effective antimicrobial treatment for this infection. AZT can reduce diarrhoea temporarily in AIDS, as can paromomycin, although the agent does not affect the cryptospiridiosis itself. Good hygiene, especially hand washing, prevents spread of the organism.

Other diseases

Blastocystis hominis infection

B. hominis is a strictly anaerobic protozoan pathogen that inhabits the colon. For decades its pathogenicity for humans was questioned, but there is increasing evidence that it may cause diarrhoea. It is sensitive to metronidazole.

Cyclospora cayetanensis infection

Cyanobacterium-like bodies were detected in the stools of travellers returning from Nepal with diarrhoea, and although this coccidian parasite has not been detected within enterocytes, it is thought to cause diarrhoea. It has been named *Cyclospora cayetanensis*. Treatment is with co-trimoxazole for 7–10 days.

Microsporidiosis

This is now a common cause of diarrhoea in patients with HIV/AIDS. Spores can be detected with high accuracy in the stools. Albendazole is effective in eradication of *Encephalitazoon intestinalis* and can suppress *E.bienensi*.

Trichomoniasis

Trichomonas vaginalis is a flagellate that causes vaginitis and urethritis (see p. 105).

FURTHER READING

Farthing MJG, Cevallos AM, Kelly MP (1995) Intestinal protozoa. In: Cook GA (ed) Manson's tropical disease, 7th edn. WB Saunders, London, pp 1255-1298.

Kelsall BL, Ravidin JI (1994) Amebiasis. *Progress in Clinical Parasitology* **4**: 27-54.

Nematode (roundworm) infections

Filariasis

Several nematodes belonging to the superfamily Filarioidea are responsible for filariasis (Table 1.39). The adult worms are thread-like. The females are larger than the males. The viviparous females give birth to larvae known as microfilariae. The microfilariae of various species can be differentiated from each other easily by the presence or absence of a sheath and the pattern of nuclear distribution in the tail. These nematodes require two hosts to complete their life-cycle.

Bancroftian and Malayan (lymphatic) filariasis

Wuchereria bancrofti is found mainly in the tropics and subtropics – in northern Australia, the Pacific Islands, West and Central Africa, South America and India. *Brugia malayi* infection is less widespread than Bancroftian filariasis and is found in India, southern China, Malaysia, Indonesia and Borneo (Fig 1.43).

Humans are the definitive hosts and mosquitoes of various types are the intermediate hosts. Humans are the only known reservoirs of Bancroftian filariasis, whereas, in addition to humans, animals such as cats are reservoirs of Malayan filariasis. *Culex fatigans*, which bites at night, is the main vector of Bancroftian filariasis. *Aedes* and *Anopheles* spp. have also been implicated. The major vector for Malayan filariasis is *Mansonia annulifera* and the anophelus mosquito. *Brugla timori* is transmitted by *Anopheles barbirostris*.

Following the bite of an infected mosquito, the larvae penetrate the skin, enter the lymphatics and are carried to the regional lymph nodes. Here they grow and mature for up to 18 months. After fertilization the microfilariae produced are carried from the lymphatics into the blood; here they do not produce any symptoms or signs. Adult worms produce lymphangitis, which is believed to be a hypersensitivity reaction. The lymphangitis is followed by fibrosis, a granulomatous reaction and later irreversible lymphatic blockade. Secondary bacterial infection may add considerably to the inflammatory response and resultant fibrosis.

Table 1.39
Habitat, vectors and major clinical manifestations of some nematodes of the superfamily Filarioidea

Organism	Habitat of adult worms in humans	Vector	Clinical manifestations
Wuchereria bancrofti	Lymphatics, lymph nodes	*Culex, Aedes, Anopheles*	Fever, lymphangitis, elephantiasis of limbs, breasts and scrotum
Brugia malayi	Lymphatics	*Mansonia* *Anopheles*	Fever, lymphangitis, elephantiasis (scrotal involvement is uncommon)
Loa loa	Subcutaneous tissue, subconjunctiva	*Chrysops*	'Calabar swellings', urticaria
Onchocerca volvulus	Subcutaneous tissue	*Simulium*	Subcutaneous nodules, elephantiasis, ocular lesions
Dipetalonema	Body cavities	*Culicoides*	Occasionally dermatitis

CLINICAL FEATURES

These are variable and depend on the age of first exposure and immunity, the duration of exposure and the sex of the infected person. In endemic areas many infected people are asymptomatic despite having circulating filarial antigens; these people are immune or are hyporesponsive. Others may demonstrate an inappropriate immune response and produce clinical features – particularly if infected for the first time in adult life. Prolonged repeated exposure is necessary for chronic filariasis and females have lower rates of the disease.

Acute presentation

Following an incubation period that averages 10–12 months, the patient presents with fever in the range 39–41°C accompanied by lymphangitis, both of which usually subside in 3–5 days. Lymphangitis typically involves the lymphatics of the lower or upper limbs or of the abdomen. Involvement of the lymphatics of the epididymis, testis and spermatic cord occurs almost exclusively in Bancroftian filariasis. The involved superficial lymphatics appear as red streaks on the skin, and are tender and cord-like. The inflammation may subside either with treatment or spontaneously but there is a tendency for recurrences.

Chronic presentation

This occurs following prolonged exposure but not all patients give a history of acute attacks. Many are amicrofiliaraemic. The progressive lymph vessel obstruction leads to lymphoedema and elephantiasis. Many sites may be affected, but lower limb and scrotal oedema occur frequently. Longstanding obstruction produces thick, rough skin, which occasionally ulcerates. Less frequently chyluria, chylous ascites and pleural effusions occur. The obstructive phase may be punctuated by episodes of acute lymphangitis.

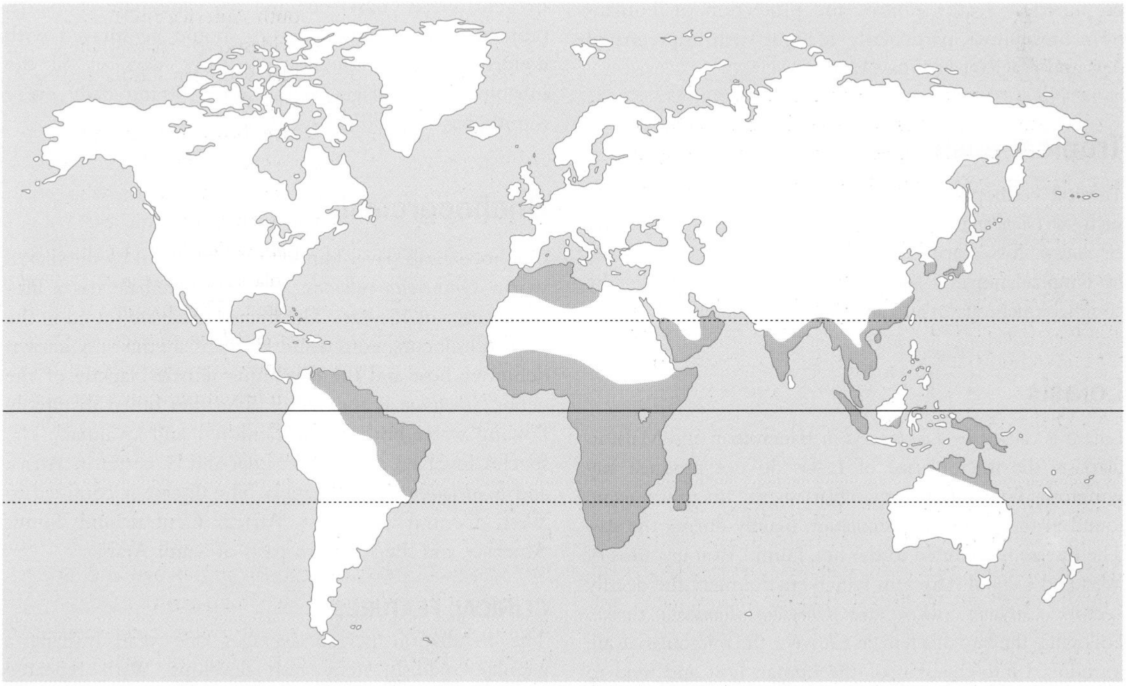

Fig 1.43
Filariasis – geographical distribution

Nonfilarial elephantiasis is seen in areas where silicates in soil are absorbed through the skin and damage the lymphatics.

DIAGNOSIS

The clinical presentation is characteristic. Eosinophilia and the presence of microfilariae in thin or thick peripheral blood smears is diagnostic. Since *W. bancrofti* and *B. malayi* are released into the peripheral circulation at night – coinciding with the time of the mosquito bite – blood for examination should be taken between 9 p.m. and 1 a.m. Serological tests are available but are not highly specific; they are particularly useful in tropical eosinophilia (see below).

TREATMENT

Diethylcarbamazine (DEC) 6–8 mg kg^{-1} daily in single or divided doses for 14 days has been the recommended treatment.

Associated bacterial infections should be treated appropriately. Reconstructive surgery plays an important role in removing unsightly tissue.

PREVENTION AND CONTROL

Mass chemotherapy with DEC (often added to table salt) has been effective in decreasing the *microfilariae rate* (the percentage of individuals who have microfilariae in a unit volume of their blood in a given population) and the *microfilariae density* (the number of microfilariae per unit volume of blood in individual patients). Annual single-dose community-wide treatment with DEC and ivermectin has been shown to be effective in reducing the rate and density of infection. Primary prophylaxis should be aimed at vector control and protection of humans from mosquitoes, particularly at night with impregnated nets and repellant creams and sprays.

Tropical eosinophilia

Tropical eosinophilia has been attributed to microfilariae such as *Dirofilaria* and more recently to *W. bancrofti* and *B. malayi*. Two forms are recognized, one characterized by lymphadenopathy and splenomegaly, and the other by cough, bronchospasm and an asthma-like picture.

Loiasis

Loiasis is caused by *Loa loa*. As in Bancroftian and Malayan filariasis, the microfilariae of *L. loa* do not produce any symptoms. Unlike Bancroftian filariasis, the microfilariae are found in the peripheral circulation mainly during the day. The disease is confined to the hot, humid, swampy areas of West and Central Africa, in which environment the deerfly vectors *Chrysops silacea* and *Chrysops dimidiata* thrive. Following the bite of a female *Chrysops*, the microfilariae are introduced into the skin of the human host and tend to migrate in the subcutaneous tissues. They have a predilection for subconjunctival and periorbital tissues.

CLINICAL FEATURES

The main feature of loiasis is *Calabar swellings*, which are painless, localized, transient, hot, soft-tissue swellings, often near joints. They persist for periods varying from a few hours to several weeks. They occur more commonly during the hotter months and may be preceded by numbness and tingling. They are produced by toxin released from the adult worm.

Urticaria, pruritus, lymphoedema, arthritis and chorioretinitis may occur.

A picture resembling meningo-encephalitis that occurs only during treatment is thought to be an allergic reaction.

DIAGNOSIS

The worm can be seen in subcutaneous tissues or crossing the conjunctivae. The characteristic microfilariae may be demonstrable in peripheral blood smears. Marked eosinophilia is present. Serological tests such as the complement-fixation test are also useful.

TREATMENT

DEC 2–6 mg kg^{-1} in gradually increasing dosage is effective against both adult worms and microfilariae, although multiple courses may be necessary. Treatment should be continued for 2–3 weeks. Side-effects of treatment (caused by death of parasites) are fever, headache, urticaria and encephalopathy; steroids may be necessary to counter these effects. Asymptomatic patients are often best left untreated because of these side-effects.

PREVENTION AND CONTROL

Prevention is best effected by adequate personal protection. In addition, houses should be sprayed with dieldrin. Mass treatment over three days of all the inhabitants of villages, with DEC 400 mg daily every month, has reduced the incidence of this disease.

Onchocerciasis

Onchocerciasis (river blindness) is produced by the filarial worm *Onchocerca volvulus*. The gravid female has a life-expectancy of 15 years. The microfilariae are found in the skin and subcutaneous tissue. Humans are the only known definitive host and the day-biting female blackfly of the genus *Simulium* is the vector. The flies breed in rapidly flowing water both in the rainforest and savannah. The species involved are *S. damnosum* and *S. neavei* in Africa and *S. metallicum* in Venezuela. The disease is confined to West, Central and East Africa, Central and South America, and the southern parts of Saudi Arabia.

CLINICAL FEATURES

The incubation period averages one year. Initially a papular, reddish, itchy rash develops. With repeated infections, characteristic subcutaneous nodules of various sizes appear. Usually they number fewer than 10 and are unevenly distributed over the body. In chronic disease, lichenification, xeroderma, pseudoichthyosis and atrophy of the skin occur. The nodules may be associated with the development of genital elephantiasis, hydrocele and the so-called 'hanging groin', in which large folds of wrinkled and thickened skin develop in the groin.

Ocular lesions represent the most serious manifestation of this disease and in some communities 40% of people are blind by 50 years of age. Eye disease is most common in the savannah. Initially the patient complains of lacrimation, photophobia and a foreign-body sensation in the eye. Conjunctivitis, iridocyclitis, chorioretinitis, secondary glaucoma and optic atrophy may occur. The eye lesions have been attributed to toxin production by the microfilariae and adult worms, mechanical irritation and hypersensitivity.

DIAGNOSIS

This is established by demonstrating microfilariae in snips of bloodless tissue obtained from the nodules and kept in saline for 30–60 minutes before microscopic examination. The organism may also be identified in the anterior chamber of the eye by slit-lamp examination. Serological tests are not helpful in the indigenous population as the positivity rate is high. Eosinophilia occurs. If no microfilariae are found, 50 mg DEC should be given to the patient; an acute itching rash within 24 hours suggests infection (Mazzotti test).

TREATMENT

Ivermectin, a broad-spectrum antiparasitic drug, is very effective. A single dose of 150 mg kg^{-1} orally produces a prolonged reduction in microfilarial levels. Therapy every 6–12 months must be given in endemic areas as ivermectin is not curative and re-infection occurs.

PREVENTION AND CONTROL

Prevention and control depends partly on personal protection to avoid bites and attempts at destroying the vector. Eradication of blackfly is expensive, and so mass treatment with ivermectin (Mectizan, currently provided free by the manufacturer, Merck, Sharp & Dohme Ltd) once a year is being used in endemic areas with good success. In areas where *Loa loa* is endemic, ivermectin therapy should be monitored carefully as serious encephalopathy can occur when the two conditions coexist.

Dracunculiasis

Dracunculiasis (Guinea worm infection) results from infection with *Dracunculus medinensis*. It is found sporadically throughout the tropics but is common in certain parts of India, Central, East and West Africa, Pakistan, the Middle East, parts of South America and the eastern regions of the former USSR.

Humans are the definitive host and are infected by ingestion of water containing infected *Cyclops*. The larvae are liberated in the human stomach by the action of acid. These penetrate the intestinal wall, where the male dies after fertilizing the female. The gravid female then wanders in connective tissue for several months before emerging through the skin. On reaching the skin, the parasite elicits an allergic reaction with blister formation and later protrusion of the worm associated with the discharge of motile larvae. The larvae are then taken up by *Cyclops*, which once again are infective to humans.

CLINICAL FEATURES

A generalized reaction can occur that is associated with nausea, vomiting, generalized urticaria and diarrhoea. These symptoms abate with rupture of the blister. Secondary bacterial infection, especially with streptococci, is common and results in cellulitis and abscess formation. In Nigeria, tetanus is a frequent complication. If attempts at extraction of the worm result in damage to it, intense cellulitis may occur. Arthritis, synovitis, ankylosis of joints and epididymitis are rare sequelae.

DIAGNOSIS

Keeping the appropriate part of the body immersed in water may induce the worm to wriggle out. Fluorescent antibody tests are useful. Radiography may reveal the presence of the worm.

TREATMENT

Gradual physical extraction of the worm by winding it carefully around a stick is the treatment of choice. It may take several days before the entire worm is extruded. Niridazole and thiabendazole are of questionable value in facilitating worm extrusion.

PREVENTION AND CONTROL

Prevention of this parasitosis is easily effected by chemically treating infected sources of water. It is likely that Guinea worm infection will be totally eradicated within the next few years.

Animal nematodes

Toxocariasis

Toxocariasis (visceral larva migrans) occurs worldwide and is caused by *Toxocara canis* or *T. cati*. The adult worm is found in the intestine of dogs and occasionally cats. The infective ova are passed in animal faeces and may be accidentally ingested by humans. The liberated larvae penetrate the intestinal wall and reach the liver and lung via the circulation. Epidemiologically, puppies who acquire worms tranplacentally are the most important natural hosts.

The infection is most commonly seen in children 1–4 years of age. Several viscera may be involved and the clinical manifestations are dependent on the organ involved and the intensity and frequency of infection. Anorexia, abdominal pain and fever and hepatomegaly occur. Urticaria and dermatitis may occur. With pulmonary involvement the presentation is that of bronchial asthma with cough and wheeze. Chest radiographs may reveal transient pulmonary infiltrates. Splenomegaly and hepatomegaly occur. Rarely involvement of the myocardium and CNS results in death. Eye involvement (ocular larva migrans) produces a posterior chorioretinitis or an intraretinal granuloma; the latter resembles a retinoblastoma-like picture. Other organs are usually spared.

Prevention of the condition can be achieved by controlling infection in dogs by regular deworming.

DIAGNOSIS AND TREATMENT

The presence of marked eosinophilia, anaemia and elevated plasma IgG, IgM and IgE is suggestive. Specific diagnosis is by detection of specific antibodies by ELISA.

Treatment is difficult to evaluate in view of the mild nature of the illness and the tendency for spontaneous cure. Albendazole 400 mg for one week has emerged as the most satisfactory therapy.

Cutaneous larva migrans

Cutaneous larva migrans (creeping eruption) is a disease of the hot, humid areas of tropical and subtropical countries. It is caused by the dog and cat hookworms *Ancylostoma braziliense* and *A. caninum* and, occasionally, the human parasites *A. duodenale*, *Necator americanus* and *Strongyloides stercoralis*. The adult forms of these worms are found in the intestine of the host. The filariform larva emerges from the ova passed in the faeces and penetrates intact human skin. An itchy papule develops at the site of larval entry. Two to three days later a markedly itchy, erythematous, serpiginous skin lesion develops. This is due to the larva, which migrates at approximately 1 cm per day. The skin over the lesion may vesiculate. Healing occurs by crusting. Although the lesions are more frequent on the lower limbs, any part of the body may be affected. Secondary bacterial infection may result in a mistaken diagnosis of pyoderma. The only systemic manifestations are transient pulmonary infiltrates and occasional breathlessness. Eosinophilia is seen.

TREATMENT

Thiabendazole applied locally as a 10% solution or given systemically (25 mg kg^{-1} for five days) is effective. Ivermectin is also effective.

Anisakiasis

Anisakiasis (herring worm disease) is caused by the larval stage of several species of *Anisakis*, and possibly of the related nematode *Phocanema*, which are found in abundance in herring, dolphins, whales and other large sea mammals. The disease is prevalent in Japan and northern Europe, where raw herring and other raw fish are considered a delicacy. In Japan the illness is characterized by an acute gastric syndrome that presents as epigastric pain, nausea and vomiting. Upper gastrointestinal endoscopy may reveal the presence of larvae in the gastric mucosa. In contrast, in Europe the small intestine is predominantly involved and the patient presents with colicky, generalized abdominal pain and fever. Eosinophilia is unusual.

Trichinosis

This is caused by the intestinal nematode *Trichinella spiralis*. The larval form is found in rats, hares, pigs, dogs, cats and bears. Although cases of trichinosis have been reported from all parts of the world, it is found predominantly in the USA and Europe. It is uncommon in India. Transmission to humans occurs when improperly cooked meats, contaminated with infective larvae, are eaten.

CLINICAL FEATURES

Most infections are asymptomatic. Vomiting, diarrhoea, abdominal pain and headache occur 24–72 hours after ingestion of contaminated meat. The severity of the clinical manifestations depends on the number of infecting larvae.

The larvae mature into the adult form in the intestine, where they reproduce and discharge larvae into the circulation. When these larvae migrate into the bloodstream and striated muscles (a stage that lasts 10–21 days), periorbital oedema, conjunctivitis, photophobia, fever with chills, and muscle pain and spasm occur. An urticarial rash, diarrhoea, dyspnoea and pleurisy may also occur. Myocardial and CNS involvement is unusual and, if it occurs, may result in death. In the next stage of development, larvae encyst in striated muscle. During encystment, symptoms gradually subside, although weakness, muscle pain and cramps may persist for several months.

DIAGNOSIS AND TREATMENT

A firm diagnosis can be made on the clinical presentation, marked eosinophilia, and positive serology using ELISA. A biopsy of the deltoid or gastrocnemius muscle three weeks after the onset of illness will demonstrate larvae, but with good serology this is not needed.

Analgesics, sedatives and bedrest are the mainstays of treatment. Steroids are indicated only in the presence of myocarditis, CNS involvement or marked allergic phenomena. Thiabendazole 25 mg kg^{-1} twice daily for seven days is effective against intestinal worms and larvae, but not if muscle invasion has occurred.

Intestinal nematode infection (Table 1.40 and Fig 1.44)

Some adult nematodes live within the intestinal lumen. The disease is spread to humans either by the ingestion of

Table 1.40
Intestinal nematode (roundworm) infections

Organism	Site	Clinical manifestations
Strongyloides stercoralis	Small intestine	Malabsorption
Hookworm: *Ancylostoma duodenale* and *Necator americanus*	Small intestine	Iron-deficiency anaemia
Capillaria philippinensis	Small intestine	Malabsorption
Ascaris lumbricoides (roundworm)	Small intestine	?Undernutrition, intestinal obstruction
Trichuris trichiura (whipworm)	Large intestine	Usually nil, colitis, rectal prolapse
Enterobius vermicularis (threadworm)	Large intestine	Usually nil, pruritis ani

infective eggs, as occurs with *Ascaris lumbricoides* (roundworm), *Trichuris trichiura* (whipworm) and *Enterobius vermicularis* (threadworm), or alternatively by percutaneous spread of filariform larvae that penetrate the skin (hookworm and *Strongyloides*).

Ascaris deviates from the simplified life-cycle shown in Fig 1.44 in that it invades the duodenum and enters the venous system, via which it reaches the lungs. The worm is eventually expectorated and swallowed, entering the intestine where it completes its maturation. *Strongyloides* is the only nematode that is able to complete its life-cycle in humans; its rhabditiform larvae, which hatch in the intestine, are able to reinfect the host by penetrating the intestinal wall and entering the venous system.

Strongyloidiasis

Strongyloides stercoralis is found worldwide but is particularly common in warm, wet regions such as parts of Central America and South East Asia. Infection can persist for decades and is still being discovered in war veterans, particularly prisoners of war who worked on the Burma–Thailand railway and veterans from Vietnam. Adult worms inhabit the crypts of the small intestine, causing little damage, but in heavy infection worms are embedded in the mucosa, and cause an inflammatory response with mucosal injury. The worms are passed in the stools and autoinfection is common.

CLINICAL FEATURES

After penetration of the skin by the filariform larvae, a local reaction occurs characterized by itching, erythema, oedema and urticaria. This subsides within two days. A week later, migration of the adolescent worms causes irritation of the upper airways, producing cough and occasionally more severe respiratory symptoms. After about three weeks, intestinal colonization occurs, often leading to abdominal discomfort, intermittent diarrhoea and constipation. These symptoms can be mild and may pass unnoticed. However, in some individuals, heavy infection may lead to persistent diarrhoea, nausea, anorexia and evidence of intestinal malabsorption, notably steatorrhoea. Hypoalbuminaemia and weight loss also occur. Disseminated strongyloidiasis is a very serious and often fatal condition and has been described in patients receiving corticosteroid or other immunosuppressive therapy or in those who are immunocompromised for other reasons.

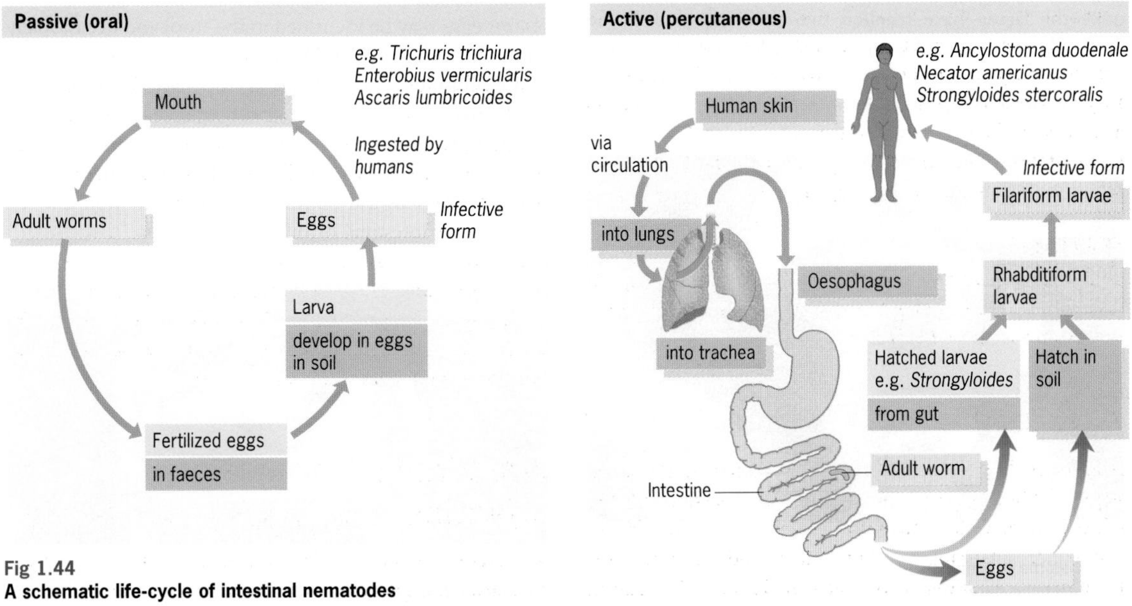

Fig 1.44
A schematic life-cycle of intestinal nematodes

DIAGNOSIS AND TREATMENT

Motile rhabditiform larvae can be detected in fresh stool or in duodenal aspirate. Eosinophilia is common. In heavy infection, anaemia and biochemical evidence of malabsorption are found.

Treatment consists of thiabendazole 25 mg kg^{-1} twice-daily for three days. Therapy should be given for at least five days (often longer) in the hyperinfected patient with disseminated disease. Albendazole 400 mg kg^{-1} for three days is also effective. Repeated therapy may be required. The mortality is high in the hyperinfected group owing to an accompanying Gram-negative septicaemia and treatment should include intravenous broad-spectrum antibiotics. *S. stercoralis* is also sensitive to ivermectin.

Hookworm infection

Hookworm is seen worldwide and affects approximately 25% of the world's population. *Ancylostoma duodenale* is found in Europe, the Middle East and North Africa, whereas *Necator americanus* is found in the western hemisphere, sub-Saharan Africa, South East Asia, the Far East and tropical America.

Adult worms inhabit the small intestine and attach firmly to the intestinal mucosa by their teeth or by 'cutting plates' in their large buccal capsule. Blood loss is approximately 0.2 mL daily in *A. duodenale* infection (five- to ten-fold less with *N. americanus*); in heavy infection it has been estimated that up to 100 mL of blood is lost daily.

CLINICAL FEATURES

Local irritation at the site of larval entry in the skin is known as 'ground itch', but this rapidly disappears to be followed some two weeks later by mild and transitory pulmonary symptoms. Most patients are asymptomatic once the larvae have reached the small intestine. Some patients experience ulcer-like symptoms and those with heavy chronic infection eventually develop symptoms and signs of anaemia. Hookworm infection is the commonest cause of iron deficiency anaemia worldwide. *A. braziliensis* (dog hookworm) causes characteristic patterns of subcutaneous infection in children (Fig 1.45).

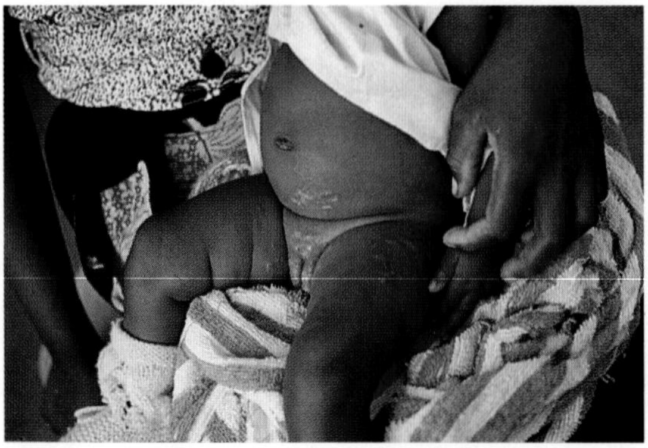

Fig 1.45
***Ancylostoma braziliensis* (dog hookworm) causes this characteristic cutaneous lesion**

DIAGNOSIS AND TREATMENT

Hookworm ova appear in the stool, the number of eggs present giving a guide to the severity of the infection. Early in the infection, eosinophilia may be found in the peripheral blood. This is followed later by the appearance of iron deficiency anaemia.

Mebendazole 100 mg twice-daily for three days is effective in both types of hookworm, although the infection may not be cleared with a single course of treatment. Iron therapy is given if necessary.

Ascaris lumbricoides (roundworm) infection

A. lumbricoides is a large worm (Fig 1.46) that is found worldwide but is particularly common in poor rural communities where there is heavy faecal contamination of the immediate environment. Infection may be entirely asymptomatic, although heavy infections are associated with nausea, vomiting, abdominal discomfort and anorexia. Worms may obstruct the small intestine, the most common site being at the ileocaecal valve. Worms occasionally invade the appendix, causing acute appendicitis, or the bile duct, resulting in biliary obstruction and suppurative cholangitis. Larvae in the lung may produce pulmonary eosinophila.

The nutritional impact of *Ascaris* infection in children is controversial, although it is very likely that heavy infection in malnourished children compounds the situation, largely by competition for host nutrients.

DIAGNOSIS AND TREATMENT

Ascaris eggs may be identified in the stool and occasionally adult worms emerge from the mouth or the anus.

Levamisole 120–150 mg as a single dose is now considered to be the drug of choice. Mebendazole 100 mg twice-daily for three days or a single dose of piperazine 100 mg kg^{-1} or pyrantel pamoate 10 mg kg^{-1} are effective. Surgical or endoscopic intervention may be required for intestinal or biliary obstruction.

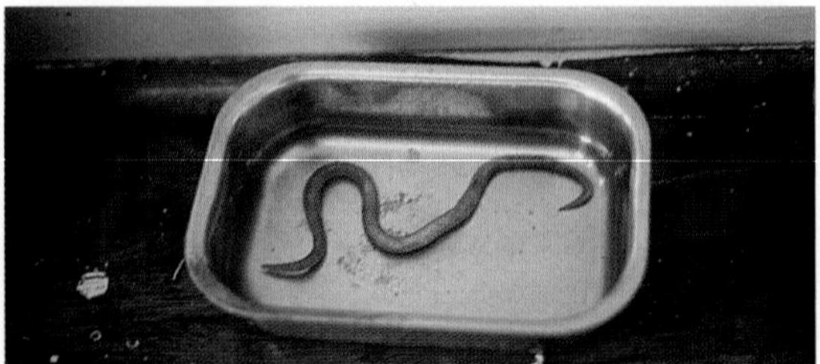

Fig 1.46
***Ascaris lumbricoides*, approximately 20 cm long**

Trichuris trichiura (whipworm) infection

T. trichiura is a common parasite and is found worldwide particularly in some tropical regions with a high rainfall (e.g. South East Asia). Prevalence varies from 1% to 90%, being highest in poor communities with inadequate sanitation. Adult worms are most commonly found in the distal ileum and caecum, although in heavy infection no part of the colon is spared. The adult worm embeds its cephalic region into the intestinal mucosa, leaving the distal tail free within the lumen. Such invasion damages the intestinal mucosa and in heavy infection overt colonic and rectal ulceration may result, leading to significant blood and protein loss.

CLINICAL FEATURES

Most infections are asymptomatic and haematological or biochemical deficits do not occur provided nutritional intake is adequate. Heavy infection is associated with diarrhoea with blood and mucus, often associated with abdominal discomfort, tenesmus, anorexia and weight loss. Involvement of the appendix can cause appendicitis, and rectal prolapse has been reported in children.

DIAGNOSIS AND TREATMENT

Stool examination confirms the presence of typical barrel-shaped eggs. Proctosigmoidoscopy may reveal adult worms firmly attached to the rectal mucosa.

Mebendazole 100 mg twice-daily for three days or a single dose of pyrantel pamoate 10 mg kg^{-1} are effective therapies.

Enterobius vermicularis (threadworm) infection

This parasite occurs worldwide but is more prevalent in temperate and cold climates. Children are most commonly infected, but it may affect whole families, inhabitants of residential institutions, and any group of people living in overcrowded circumstances. Adult worms reside largely in the colon, the female migrating to the anus to deposit embryonated eggs on the perianal and perineal areas. Superficial damage to the colonic mucosa occurs during heavy infection and secondary bacterial infection of these lesions may rarely result in submucosal abscesses.

CLINICAL FEATURES

Intense pruritus ani is usually the only symptom of threadworm infection. This is usually nocturnal and related to egg-laying in the perianal region by the female worms. Scratching results in dissemination of eggs and autoinfection. Infection has little significance while the parasite remains within the intestinal lumen, although on occasions migration occurs to the peritoneum and the viscera may be involved.

DIAGNOSIS AND TREATMENT

Diagnosis is best achieved by applying a piece of clear adhesive tape to the perianal region; this tape may then be examined microscopically for the presence of adherent eggs. Adult worms may be observed leaving the anus by the child's parents.

A single dose of mebendazole 100 mg followed by a second dose two weeks later is usually effective. Alternatives include pyrantel pamoate or piperazine. Family members should also be treated.

FURTHER READING

Burnham S (1998) Onchocerciasis. *Lancet* **351**: 1341-1346.

Reports of WHO Expert Committee on Filariasis (1992) 1-17; on Onchocerciasis (1995) 1-103. WHO; Geneva.

Trematode (fluke) infections (Table 1.41)

Blood infections

Schistosomiasis (bilharzia)

Three major species of schistosomes produce human disease. These have marked differences in geographical distribution (Fig 1.47). Prevalence is dependent on the presence of a susceptible intermediate snail host and faecal contamination of water supplies. The size of snail populations varies with the season and availability of freshwater breeding grounds. An increase in the world prevalence of schistosomiasis is partly due to dam construction and irrigation programmes. In *S. japonicum* or *S. mansoni*, animals such as pigs, water buffalo and cattle as well as humans can act as hosts, and this makes eradication programmes more difficult.

Table 1.41
Trematode (fluke) infection

Organism	Location	Major disease site(s)
Schistosoma mansoni	Mesenteric veins	Liver, colon
Schistosoma japonicum	Mesenteric veins	Liver, colon, small intestine
Schistosoma haematobium	Pelvic veins, vesical plexus	Bladder, distal colon, rectum
Fasciola hepatica	Bile ducts	Bile ducts, liver
Clonorchis sinensis	Bile ducts	Bile ducts, liver
Fasciolopsis buski	Small intestine	Small intestine
Paragonimus westermani	Lung	Lung

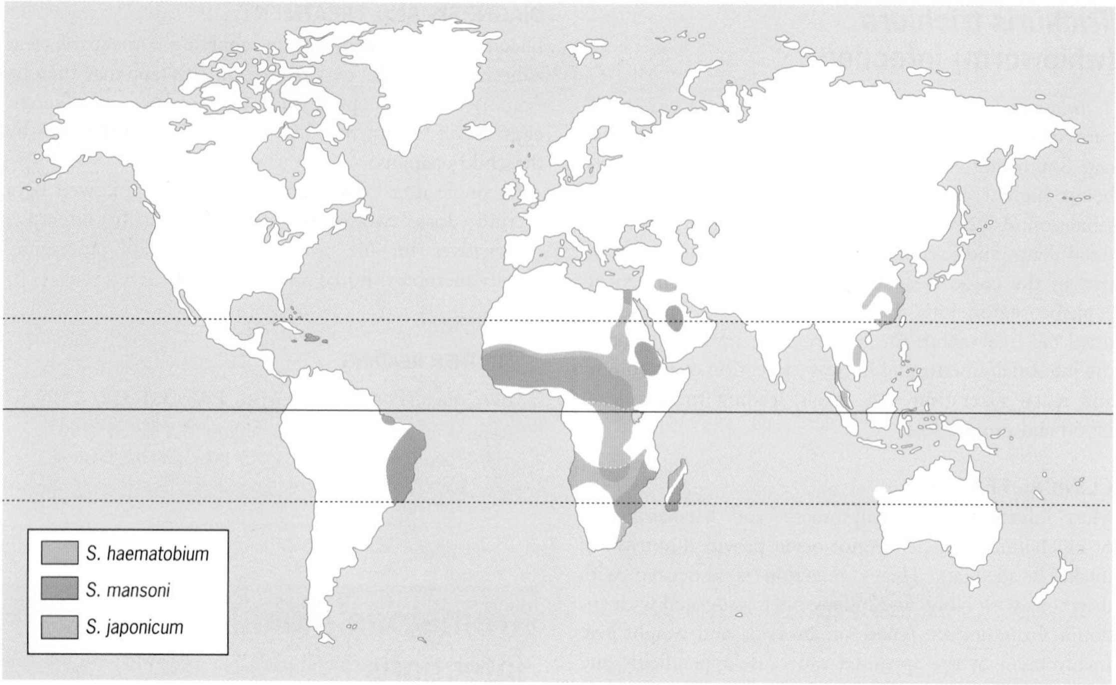

Fig 1.47
Schistosomiasis – geographical distribution

LIFE-CYCLE AND PATHOGENESIS

Human infection occurs after penetration of the skin or mucous membranes by cercariae, the infective form of the parasite that is liberated into fresh water by the specific intermediate snail host (Fig 1.48). Cercariae penetrate unbroken skin and migrate as schistosomules via the venous circulation through the lungs and then to the liver, where the adult worms mature. Eventually pairs of male and female worms migrate from the liver upstream along the portal vein to the mesenteric venules, until the calibre of the vessels halts their progress. They remain in this location for many years copulating continuously and producing enormous numbers of eggs. To complete the life-cycle, eggs must leave the body, either by penetrating the intestinal wall (*S. mansoni* and *S. japonicum*) or the bladder wall (*S. haematobium*) and returning to the environment via faeces or urine, respectively. The larvae (miracidia) develop inside the eggs but do not hatch until they arrive in fresh water, when they search actively for the specific snail host to invade. Once inside the snail, multiplication occurs – a single miracidium produces up to 100 000 cercariae, released at the rate of 5000 per day.

Eggs retained in host tissues, particularly the liver, urinary bladder and intestine, are responsible for the clinical manifestations of schistosomiasis. Egg antigens initiate both immediate and delayed-type hypersensitivity reactions with granuloma formation. Humoral substances such as lymphokines, macrophage migration inhibitory factor and fibroblast stimulating factors are found at the site of these granulomas and presumably support the cellular inflammatory response. Healing eventually occurs by fibrosis.

CLINICAL FEATURES

The peak of infection is between the ages of five and 15 years. Older individuals are less susceptible owing to reduction in exposure and development of immunity.

The first clinical sign of an *acute infection* is a local inflammatory response at the site of the invading cercariae known as 'swimmer's itch'. Within a week or more there is a generalized allergic response characterized by fever, urticaria, eosinophilia, myalgia and malaise. Nausea, vomiting and profuse diarrhoea are common, as are respiratory symptoms, particularly cough. Clinical findings at this time include generalized lymphadenopathy, hepatosplenomegaly and signs of patchy pneumonia. In Asia the acute disease is called Katayama fever. It is most pronounced in infection with *S. japonicum* and *S. mansoni*. Following acute infection in adults by *S. mansoni* and *S. haematobium*, a radiculitis and/or transverse myelitis can occur.

Chronic schistosomiasis varies in its clinical presentation depending on the type of schistosome involved.

Schistosoma mansoni and *japonicum*

S. mansoni is found predominantly in Africa, South America and the West Indies, whereas *S. japonicum* is common in China and other specific sites in South East Asia.

S. mansoni predominantly affects the colon, where the presence of ova produces macroscopic lesions such as mucosal granularity, erythema and superficial ulceration. However, a particularly severe form of colonic disease is seen in Egyptians, with gross ulceration and polyp formation, particularly in the rectosigmoid; extensive

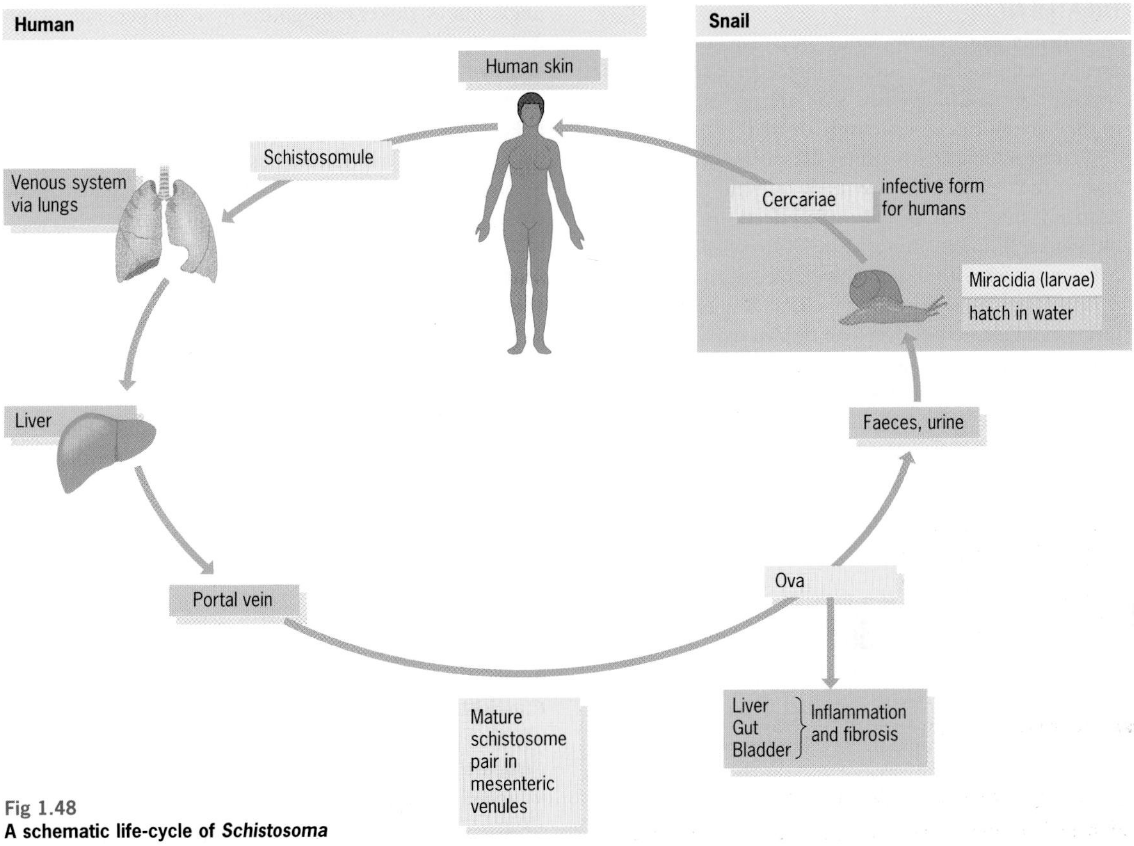

Fig 1.48
A schematic life-cycle of *Schistosoma*

polyposis results in significant blood and protein loss from the colon. Progressive fibrosis in the intestinal wall leads to rigidity and stricture formation, although intestinal obstruction is rare. A localized granulomatous reaction in the intestine (pseudotumour or bilharzioma) may be mistaken for a colonic cancer.

The development of granulomatous hepatitis, followed by progressive periportal fibrosis and portal hypertension, is signified by marked hepatosplenomegaly, often associated with oesophageal varices. In advanced cases death is due to the complications of portal hypertension, as hepatocellular function remains remarkably good.

S. japonicum affects the small intestine and proximal colon in addition to causing fibrotic liver disease. *S. japonicum* produces larger numbers of eggs than *S. mansoni*, which accounts for the more extensive pattern of disease and the frequency of ectopic deposition of ova, particularly in the lungs, spinal cord and brain. The latter may result in fits or hemiplegia.

Epithelial dysplasia in the colon has been reported in patients with chronic *S. japonicum* colitis, and it is now clear that this condition has premalignant potential in endemic areas.

Schistosoma haematobium

This is a mainly urinary tract schistosome found predominantly in Egypt, East Africa and the Middle East. Chronic inflammation is found in the bladder, ureters and urethra, causing urinary frequency, dysuria and haematuria. Chronic infection leads to obstructive uropathy, chronic pyelonephritis and renal failure, and contraction of the bladder. Epidemiological studies confirm an association between bladder carcinoma and this infection. The internal genitalia may be involved and rectal inflammation and ulceration may be found in up to 70% of patients.

DIAGNOSIS

In endemic areas a confident diagnosis can often be obtained on clinical grounds. Confirmation is achieved by detecting the characteristic eggs in the stools, the urine or in a rectal biopsy. Different species of *Schistosoma* can be distinguished not only by the clinical pattern but also by egg morphology.

A plain abdominal radiograph may reveal intramural calcification in the wall of the bladder or the colon. Barium contrast studies of the colon show spiculating mucosal ulceration, polyposis, strictures, and possibly a mass lesion that could either be a bilharzioma or, in the case of *S. japonicum* infection, a carcinoma.

Intravenous urography or ultrasound may confirm an obstructive uropathy and demonstrate bladder contraction. The liver can also be examined by ultrasound examination.

Immunodiagnostic tests are available, the most sensitive of which detect antibodies against a gut-associated polysaccharide antigen by either ELISA or indirect immunofluorescence.

TREATMENT

In endemic and hyperendemic areas, curative therapy is usually inappropriate, since reinfection occurs rapidly, whereas infected individuals who are no longer exposed to the parasite can be effectively treated.

Praziquantel is active against all species of schistosome and is the drug of choice as it is well tolerated and relatively free from serious side-effects. A single dose (40 mg kg^{-1}) cures more than 90% of patients with *S. haematobium*, with slightly lower rates against *S. mansoni*. *S. japonicum* is best treated with a total dose of 60 mg kg^{-1} given in divided doses over one or two days.

Oxamniquine is active against *S. mansoni* and metriphonate against *S. haematobium*.

Colonscopic polypectomy can control the number of colonic polyps, but surgery may be required to relieve obstructive uropathy and for inflammatory masses in the CNS.

PREVENTION

Personal protection for the traveller is to avoid infected water. If there has been contact, vigorous washing is recommended. Any individual returning from endemic areas must be carefully screened even if asymptomatic.

General control is difficult but depends on the provision of good sanitation, which is largely an economic problem. Community-based mass chemotherapy in endemic areas has been tried but is expensive and results in treating individuals who are not infected. Selective chemotherapy may be the better alternative in high-risk groups, such as children. Efforts to control the snail vector have been largely unsuccessful.

Liver and biliary tract infections

Fascioliasis

Fasciola hepatica infects sheep, goats and cattle, in which it produces liver disease, and is only accidentally transmitted to humans via consumption of wild watercress or other plants grown on the grazing land of infected animals. The disease is found worldwide, including the UK. Animals excrete eggs in their faeces, from which ciliated miracidia emerge. These enter the freshwater snail (the intermediate host) in which larval development takes place. Eventually cercaria are released and these encyst on aquatic or surface vegetation.

After ingestion by a mammalian host, the parasites excyst, migrate through the intestinal wall and penetrate the liver capsule after traversing the peritoneal cavity. Immature flukes reach the bile duct by passing through liver parenchyma and after maturation begin to produce eggs. Adult flukes remain within the biliary tract for many years.

CLINICAL FEATURES

Early symptoms of intermittent fever, malaise, weight loss, right upper quadrant pain and urticaria relate to migration of flukes through the liver and generally occur 2–3 months after infection. This migration can be detected on CT or MRI.

A second phase of the illness relates to the presence of flukes in the biliary tract, where they can cause obstruction with jaundice and cholangitis, although infection may remain asymptomatic. Flukes have been found in many ectopic sites, including lung, brain and skin.

DIAGNOSIS AND TREATMENT

Eosinophilia is common in the early phase of the illness and is often associated with liver biochemical abnormalities and a positive ELISA. Ova are not found in the stool until the second phase of the illness when the mature flukes are established in the biliary tract. However, in up to 30% of cases, stools remain negative; the diagnosis can then be confirmed either by identifying ova in duodenal aspirate or by serological tests.

Treatment is with triclabendazole 10 mg kg^{-1} as a single dose, but repeated doses may be required.

Clonorchiasis

Clonorchis sinensis is a common fluke of the dog, cat and pig that affects millions of animals in the Far East, particularly Indo-China, Japan, Korea, Hong Kong and Vietnam. A related fluke, Opisthorchis felineus, also affects foxes and is found predominantly in India, the Philippines, Korea and Japan, and *O. viverrini* is an important human infection in Thailand. The life-cycles of both these flukes are similar to that of *F. hepatica*, except that freshwater fish become infected by the cercaria and thereby function as a second intermediate host. Human infection occurs by ingestion of infected raw fish.

CLINICAL FEATURES

Infected individuals may remain symptom-free, although prolonged exposure with heavy infection results in recurrent cholestatic jaundice, suppurative cholangitis, liver abscess and cholangiocarcinoma.

DIAGNOSIS AND TREATMENT

The diagnosis is made on microscopic examination of faeces or duodenal aspirate.

Praziquantel 25 mg kg^{-1} thrice-daily for two days is highly effective.

Intestinal infections

Fasciolopsiasis

Fasciolopsis buski causes intestinal infection in humans and pigs. There are two intermediate hosts – freshwater snails and water plants. Human infection is initiated by oral contact with contaminated water plants. These large flukes, which are several centimetres in length, are common in China, Vietnam, Thailand and Taiwan.

Mucosal ulceration and inflammation are apparent at the site of attachment in the intestine; abscess formation, haemorrhage and occasionally bowel obstruction may result. The symptoms are usually non-specific. Heavy infection in children may simulate or precipitate protein-energy malnutrition. Anaemia and eosinophilia are common.

DIAGNOSIS AND TREATMENT

The diagnosis may be simple if the patient is vomiting or passing flukes per rectum, but may be confirmed by identifying ova in the stools.

Praziquantel as a single dose 15 mg kg^{-1} is very effective.

FURTHER READING

Cook GC (ed) (1996) Manson's tropical diseases, 20th edn. WB Saunders, Philadelphia.

Cestode (tapeworm) infections

Tapeworms belong to the subclass Cestoda. These are flat worms measuring a few millimetres (*Echinococcus granulosus*) to several metres (*Taenia saginata*) in length. Structurally they consist of a head that is adorned with suckers and hooks (*Taenia solium*) or suckers alone (*T. saginata*). The head is attached via a short slender neck to several segments or proglottids that form a chain-like structure or strobila. The terminal proglottide is the most mature. The entire worm is covered with a continuous elastic cuticle. Tapeworms are devoid of a gastrointestinal tract or vascular system; nutrients are absorbed directly through the cuticle. They are hermaphrodites and cross-fertilization between proglottids is frequent.

Adults live in the intestinal tract of vertebrates, whereas the larvae (oncospheres) exist in the tissues of vertebrates and invertebrates. Infection is transmitted to humans by ingestion of meats infected with larval forms. Four tapeworms commonly infect humans: *T. saginata*, *T. solium*, *Diphyllobothrium latum* and *Hymenolepsis nana*.

Taenia saginata (beef tapeworm) infection

T. saginata measures up to 10 m in length, inhabits the upper jejunum, and is prevalent in humans in all beef-eating countries. The majority of patients are asymptomatic. Symptoms are mild, with vague epigastric and abdominal pain, and occasional diarrhoea and vomiting. Weight loss is unusual. Rarely, appendicitis and pancreatitis due to obstruction of the appendix and pancreatic ducts, respectively, by the adult worms may occur. The most common symptom is the presence of proglottids in the faeces, bed or underclothing.

DIAGNOSIS AND TREATMENT

The presence of proglottids, which are visible macroscopically, or the eggs, which are seen microscopically, in the faeces or perianal region is diagnostic. A higher positive yield is obtained by examining perianal clear adhesive tape swabs for ova, in which case the scolex (the head) or proglottids are required to establish the species.

Niclosamide 2 g as a single chewed dose is effective. Praziquantel 10 mg kg^{-1} as a single dose is effective but is not available on the UK market.

PREVENTION

Prevention is easily effected by careful inspection of beef for cysticerci (encysted larval forms). Refrigeration of beef at 0°C for five days or cooking it at 57°C for a few minutes destroys the cysticerci.

Taenia solium infection and cysticercosis

T. solium (the pork tapeworm) measures up to 6 m in length. It has a worldwide distribution but is seen most frequently in eastern Europe, South East Asia and Africa. In the adult form it lives in the human upper jejunum. The clinical features are similar to those caused by *T. saginata*.

Treatment is similar to that for *T. saginata*. However, because release of ova can occur during treatment and, theoretically, could be carried back into the stomach, releasing the intermediate larval stage, treatment for *T. solium* should be followed by a saline purge.

Human cysticercosis (Fig 1.49)

Cysticercosis occurs after autoinfection or heteroinfection by eggs of *T. solium* and invasion of tissues by the intermediate larval form – cysticercus cellulosae. Cysticercosis is most commonly seen in parts of Asia, Africa and South America. Cysticerci may develop in any tissue in the body. Most commonly, however, three clinical forms are recognized:

- *Cerebral cysticercosis* may present as various forms of epilepsy, as a space-occupying lesion, or as focal neurological deficits including hemiplegia and behavioural changes.
- *Ocular cysticercosis* may present as retinitis, uveitis, conjunctivitis or choroidal atrophy. Blindness may ensue.
- *Subcutaneous cysticercosis* presents as small, pea-sized, hard nodules in the subcutaneous tissue.

The diagnosis is established by biopsy of a subcutaneous nodule and demonstrating the characteristic translucent membrane. Radiography may demonstrate calcified

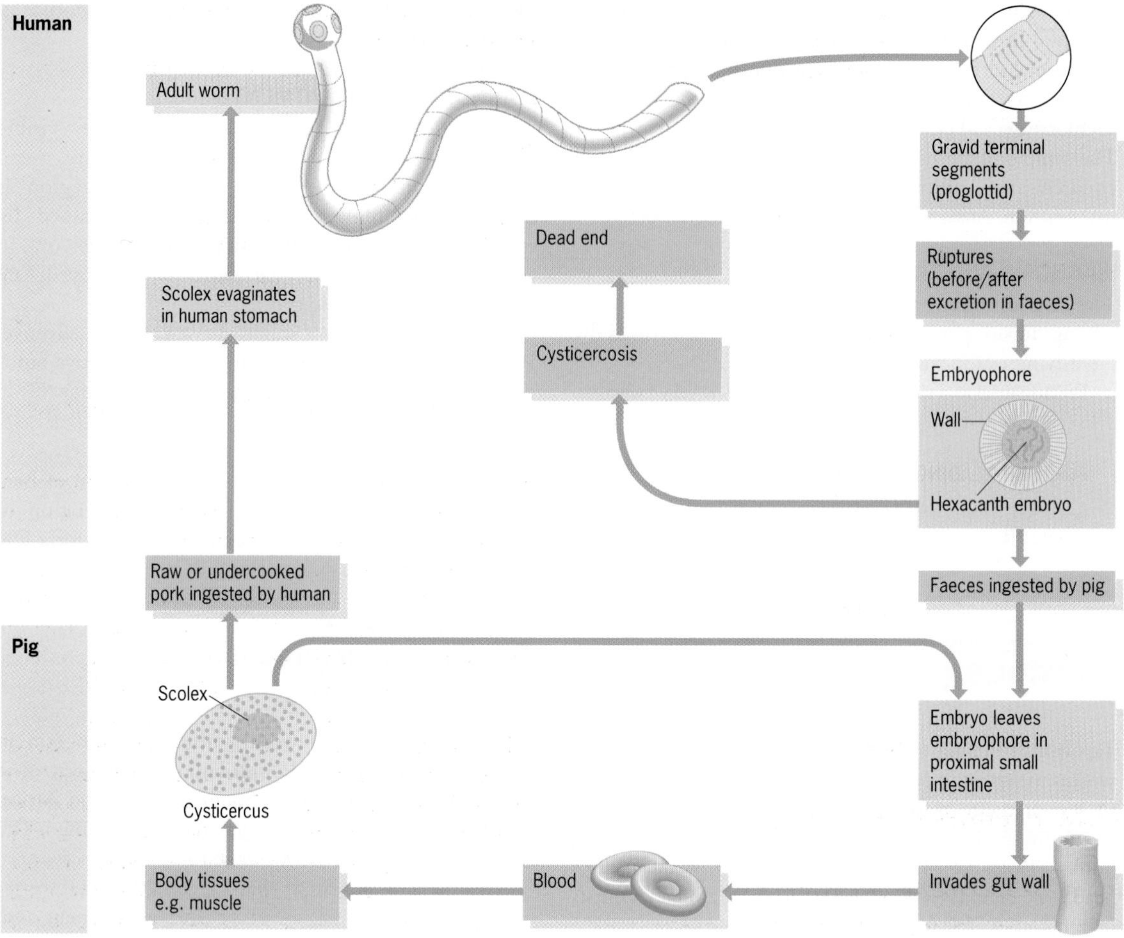

Fig 1.49
A schematic life-cycle of *Taenia solium*

degenerating cysticerci. CT brain scan should be performed when subcutaneous cysticercosis has been diagnosed. Indirect haemagglutination tests are useful.

Treatment involves surgical excision of the cysticerci if possible. Praziquantel is the drug of choice for cysticercosis; steroids are given during therapy to avoid reactions. Anti-epileptic drugs are usually necessary for cerebral cysticercosis.

Diphyllobothrium latum infection

Diphyllobothriasis is particularly prevalent in Scandinavian countries, the Baltic region, Japan and the lake region of Switzerland. Infection in humans, the definitive host, results from ingestion of fish that contain the infected plerocercoid form. The adult tapeworm measures several metres in length. The proglottids differ from those of *Taenia* in that they are more wide than long. The adult worm usually attaches itself to the jejunum.

The clinical features are usually mild and consist of vague abdominal discomfort, anorexia, nausea and vomiting. Megaloblastic anaemia, due to competitive utilization of ingested vitamin B_{12} by the parasite, may occur in a small percentage of patients. Rarely, intestinal obstruction occurs.

Treatment is similar to that described for *T. saginata*.

Hydatid disease

Hydatid disease occurs when humans ingest the hexacanth embryos of the dog tapeworm *Echinococcus granulosus* or of *E. multilocularis*.

Human infection with *E. granulosus* frequently occurs in early childhood by direct contact with infected dogs, or by eating uncooked, improperly washed vegetables contaminated with infected canine faeces. In the duodenum the hexacanth embryos hatch, penetrate the intestinal wall, enter the portal system and are then carried to the liver. Further dissemination of embryos to the lung and to almost every organ in the body may occur, where they form hydatid cysts (Fig 1.50).

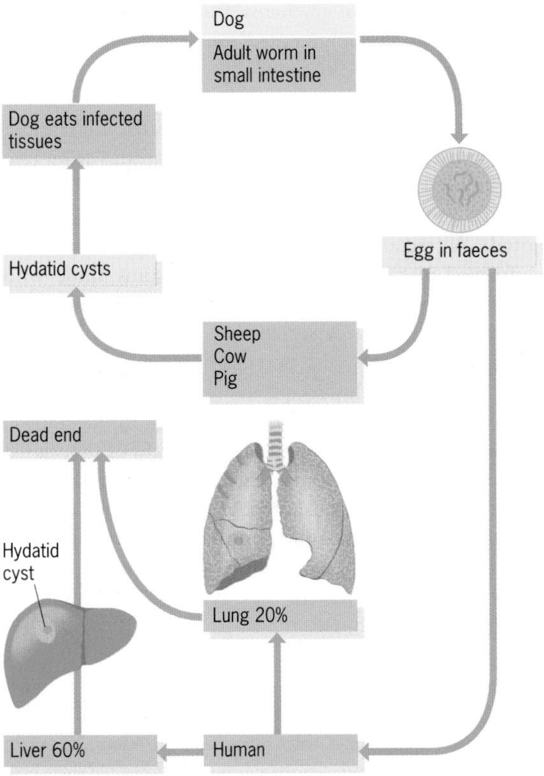

Fig 1.50
A schematic life-cycle of *Echinococcus granulosus*

The disease is seen in all parts of the world particularly in those countries where sheep and cattle-raising constitutes an important means of livelihood. It is rare in the UK but is seen in the Middle East, North and East Africa, Australia and Argentina. These animals perpetuate the life-cycle of the parasite.

Symptoms largely depend upon the site of the unilocular hydatid cyst. The liver is the most common site for cyst formation (60%), followed by the lung (20%), kidneys (3%) and brain (1%). In the liver the majority of cysts are situated in the right lobe. The symptoms are those of a slowly growing benign tumour. Pressure on the bile ducts may cause jaundice. Rupture into the abdominal cavity, pleural cavity or biliary tree may occur. In the latter instance, intermittent jaundice, abdominal pain and fever associated with eosinophilia result. A cyst rupturing into a bronchus may result in its expectoration and spontaneous cure, but if secondary infection supervenes a chronic pulmonary abscess will form. Haemoptysis, dyspnoea and chest pain may lead to a mistaken diagnosis of malignancy. Focal seizures may occur if cysts are present in the brain. Renal involvement produces lumbar pain and haematuria. Calcification of the cyst occurs in about 40% of cases.

The alveolar hydatid cyst caused by *E. multilocularis* results from its larval stage. *E. multilocularis* is seen in parts of Canada, Russia and Alaska. Foxes and small rodents constitute the intermediate hosts; humans are accidental hosts. The majority of the lesions are in the liver and metastases may occur.

The diagnosis and treatment of hydatid liver disease are described on p. 332.

FURTHER READING

Ammann RW, Eckert J (1996) Cestodes: echinococcus. *Gastroenterology Clinics of North America* **25**: 655-689.

Sexually transmitted diseases

Sexually transmitted diseases (STDs) remain epidemic in all societies and the range of pathogens that are known to be spread by sex continues to increase.

Over the past twenty years there has been a marked increase in the incidence of STDs in the UK (as in the rest of the world) with 671 000 new cases seen in genitourinary medicine (GUM) clinics in the UK in 1993. People aged from 15 to 30 years are the most likely to acquire STDs. Changes in incidence reflect earlier sexual maturity and age at first intercourse. Widespread use of oral contraceptives has reduced the use of barrier methods of contraception. Increased travelling both within and between countries, recreational drug use, alcohol and more frequent partner change are also implicated. Multiple infections frequently coexist, some of which may be asymptomatic and facilitate spread.

Changes in the patterns of infection have been seen in the UK over the last 50 years. The incidence of syphilis has declined since the widespread introduction of penicillin into medical practice. A high incidence of gonorrhoea during the 1970s has been followed by a sharp decline from the mid 1980s when the emergence of human immunodeficiency virus (HIV) produced substantial behavioural change. Nevertheless, viral conditions, particularly herpes simplex virus (HSV) and human papillomavirus, as well as nonspecific genital infection including *Chlamydia*, have all increased substantially. The recognition of AIDS and HIV has heightened awareness of STDs. Many people attend GUM clinics to seek information, advice and checks of their sexual health, but have no active STD.

Approach to the patient

Patients presenting with possible STDs are frequently anxious, embarassed and concerned about confidentiality. Staff must be alert to these issues and respond sensitively. The clinical setting must ensure privacy and reinforce confidentiality.

HISTORY

The history of the presenting complaint frequently focuses on genital symptoms, the three most common being vaginal discharge (Table 1.42), urethral discharge (Table 1.43), and genital ulceration (Table 1.44). Details should be obtained of any associated fever, pain, itch, malodour, genital swelling, skin rash, joint pains and eye symptoms. All patients should be asked about dysuria, haematuria and loin pain. A full general medical, family and drug history, particularly of any recent antibacterial or antiviral treatment, allergies and use of oral contraceptives, must be obtained. In women, menstrual, contraception and obstetric history should be obtained. Any past or current history of drug misuse should be explored.

A detailed sexual history should be taken and include the number and types of sexual contacts (genital/genital, oral/genital, anal/genital, oral/anal) with dates, partner's sex, whether regular or casual partner, use of condoms and other forms of contraception, previous history of STDs including dates and treatment received, HIV testing and results and hepatitis B vaccination status.

Enquires should be made concerning travel abroad to areas where antibiotic resistance is known or where particular pathogens are endemic.

EXAMINATION

General examination must include the mouth, throat, skin and lymph nodes in all patients. Signs of HIV infection are covered on p. 108. The inguinal, genital and perianal areas should be examined with a good light source. The groins should be palpated for lymphadenopathy and hernias. The pubic hair must be examined for nits and lice. The external genitalia must be examined for signs of erythema, fissures, ulcers, chancres, pigmented or hypopigmented areas and condylomata. Signs of trauma may be seen.

In men, the penile skin should be examined and the foreskin retracted to look for balanitis, ulceration, condylomata or tumours. The urethral meatus is located and the presence of discharge noted. Scrotal contents are palpated and the consistency of the testes and epididymis noted. A rectal examination/proctoscopy should be performed in patients with rectal symptoms, those who practise anoreceptive intercourse and patients with prostatic symptoms. A search for rectal condylomata is indicated in patients with perianal lesions.

In women, Bartholin's glands must be identified and examined. The cervix should be inspected for ulceration, discharge, bleeding and ectopy and the walls of the vagina for condylomata. A bimanual pelvic examination is performed to elicit adnexal tenderness or masses, cervical tenderness, and to assess the position, size and mobility of the uterus. Rectal examination and proctoscopy are performed if the patient has symptoms or practises anoreceptive intercourse.

INVESTIGATIONS

Although the history and examination will guide investigation, it must be remembered that multiple infections may coexist, some being asymptomatic. Full screening is indicated in any patient who may have been in contact with an STD.

In men

- Urethral smears for Gram staining
- Urethral swabs for gonococcal culture and Chlamydia testing
- Two-glass urine test and urinalysis
- Rectal swabs for Gram staining and culture
- Throat swab for culture
- Blood for syphilis serology.

Table 1.42
Causes of vaginal discharge

Infective	Non-infective
Candida albicans	Cervical polyps
Trichomonas vaginalis	Neoplasms
Bacterial vaginosis	Retained products (e.g. tampons)
Neisseria gonorrhoeae	Chemical irritation
Chlamydia trachomatis	
Herpes simplex	

Table 1.43
Causes of urethral discharge

Infective	Non-infective
Neisseria gonorrhoeae	Physical or chemical trauma
Chlamydia trachomatis	Nonspecific (aetiology unknown)
Ureaplasma urealyticum	
Mycoplasma spp.	
Trichomonas vaginalis	
Herpes simplex	
Urethral warts	
Urinary tract infection (rare)	
Treponema pallidum	

Table 1.44
Causes of genital ulceration

Infective	Non-infective
Syphilis	Behçet's syndrome
Primary chancre	Stevens–Johnson syndrome
Secondary mucous patches	Carcinoma
Tertiary gumma	Trauma
Chancroid	
Lymphogranuloma venereum	
Granuloma inguinale	
Herpes simplex	
Primary	
Recurrent	
Herpes zoster	

In women

- Smears from the lateral vaginal wall for Gram staining
- Vaginal swab for culture of *Candida* and *Trichomonas*
- A wet preparation is made from the posterior fornix for Trichomonas and for the potassium hydroxide test for bacterial vaginosis
- The pH of vaginal secretions using narrow-range indicator paper
- Endocervical smears and swabs for Gram staining, gonococcal culture and Chlamydia tests
- Urethral smears and swabs for Gram staining and gonococcal culture
- Rectal and throat swabs, if indicated
- Urinalysis
- Cervical cytology
- Blood syphilis serology.

Additional investigations when appropriate

- Blood for hepatitis B and C serology, HIV antibody testing (with full counselling)
- Swabs for HSV and *Haemophilus ducreyi* from clinically suspicious lesions in special media
- Smears and swabs from the subpreputial area in men with balanoposthitis (inflammation of glans penis and prepuce)
- Scrapings from lesions suspicious of early syphilis for immediate dark-ground microscopy
- Pregnancy testing
- Stools for *Giardia*, *Shigella* or *Salmonella* from homosexual men.

TREATMENT, PREVENTION AND CONTROL

The treatment of specific conditions is considered in the appropriate section. Many GUM clinics keep basic stocks of medication and dispense directly to the patient.

Tracing the sexual partners of patients is crucial in controlling spread of STDs. The aims are to prevent the spread of infection within the community and to ensure that people with asymptomatic infection are properly treated. Interviewing people about their sexual partners requires considerable tact and sensitivity and specialist health advisors are available in GUM clinics.

Prevention starts with education and information. People begin sexual activity at ever younger ages and education programmes need to include school pupils as well as young adults. Education of health professionals is also crucial. Appropriate and accessible services must be well advertised. The risks of acquiring an STD may be reduced by avoiding multiple partners, correct and consistent use of condoms and avoiding sex with people who have symptoms of infection. For those who change their sexual partners frequently regular check-ups (approximately three-monthly) are advisable. Once people develop symptoms they should be encouraged to seek medical advice as soon as possible to reduce complications and spread to others.

Clinical syndromes

HIV and AIDS

These are discussed in the section starting on p. 107.

Gonorrhoea

The incidence of gonorrhoea (GC) in developing countries has fallen dramatically since the early 1970s but in Asia and Africa it still remains high. In 1990 the WHO estimated 35 million cases worldwide, second to *Chlamydia trachomatis* amongst STDs. The causative organism, *Neisseria gonorrhoeae* (gonococcus), is a Gram-negative intracellular diplococcus which infects epithelium particularly of the urogenital tract, rectum, pharynx and conjunctivae. Humans are the only host and the organism is spread by intimate physical contact. It is very intolerant to drying and although occasional reports of spread by fomites exist this route of infection is extremely rare.

CLINICAL FEATURES

Forty per cent of women and some men are asymptomatic. The incubation period is 2–14 days with most symptoms occurring between days 2 and 5. In men the most common syndrome is one of anterior urethritis causing dysuria and/or urethral discharge. Complications include ascending infection involving the epididymis, testes or prostate leading to acute or chronic infection. In homosexual men rectal infection may produce proctitis with pain, discharge and itch.

In women the primary site of infection is usually the endocervical canal. Symptoms consist of a vaginal discharge, dysuria and intermenstrual bleeding. Complications include ascending infection leading to salpingitis with associated pelvic pain and fever. In rare cases a perihepatitis may develop (Fitzhugh–Curtis syndrome). Bartholin's abscesses may develop. On a global basis GC is one of the most common causes of female infertility. Rectal infection, due to local spread, may occur in women and is usually asymptomatic, as is pharyngeal infection. Conjunctival infection is seen in neonates born to infected mothers and is one cause of ophthalmia neonatorum.

Disseminated GC leads to arthritis (usually monoarticular or pauciarticular) (see p. 486) and a characteristic purplish macular rash in association with fever and malaise. It is more common in women.

DIAGNOSIS

The organism is identified from infected areas by Gram stain and culture on special media. Blood culture and synovial fluid investigations should be performed in cases of disseminated GC. Coexisting pathogens such as *Chlamydia*, *Trichomonas* and syphilis must be sought.

TREATMENT

The gonococcus is sensitive to a wide range of antimicrobial agents but an increase in antibiotic resistance has been seen over the past two decades. Therapy initiated in the clinic on the basis of Gram-stained slides prior to culture results is influenced by travel history or details known from contacts.

In the UK it is still reasonable to give single-dose amoxycillin 3 g with probenecid 1 g in uncomplicated cases. Spectinomycin 2 g i.m. or ciprofloxacin 250 mg are used in penicillin-resistant or allergic cases. Longer courses of antibiotics are required for complicated infections. Patients must be followed up to ensure that the organism has been eradicated and all sexual contacts should be examined and treated as necessary.

Chlamydia infection

Chlamydia trachomatis (see p. 49) is an obligate intracellular bacterial parasite which cannot be grown on artificial culture media. Cell culture systems are not universally available and indirect diagnostic methods are being perfected. The organism has a worldwide distribution and silent infection is common. In men 30–40% of non-gonococcal and post-gonococcal urethritis is due to *Chlamydia*. It is frequently found in association with other pathogens: 20% of men and 40% of women with gonorrhoea have been found to have coexisting chlamydial infections.

CLINICAL FEATURES

In men *Chlamydia* gives rise to an anterior urethritis with dysuria and discharge; infection is often asymptomatic and detected by contact tracing. Ascending infection leads to epididymitis. Rectal infection leading to proctitis may occur in men practising anoreceptive intercourse. In *women* the most common site of infection is the endocervix where it may go unnoticed; ascending infection causes acute salpingitis. In women subfertility may be the first problem encountered. Reiter's syndrome (see p. 482) has been related to infection with *C. trachomatis*. Neonatal infection, acquired from the birth canal, can result in mucopurulent conjunctivitis and pneumonia.

INVESTIGATIONS FOR DIAGNOSIS

- **Antigen detection systems** – direct fluorescent antibody or enzyme. In view of the intracellular nature of the organism, care must be taken to obtain adequate specimens and it is essential that cells are collected. Wooden swabs may interfere with assay techniques. Special transport media are required.
- **Serum antibodies** – high or rising titres (IgM > 1:8 for acute; high IgG for chronic).
- **Cell culture** systems are still considered the definitive method of diagnosis but are costly and not suitable for routine use.

TREATMENT

Tetracyclines or macrolide antibiotics are most commonly used to treat *Chlamydia*. Oxytetracycline 500 mg six-hourly or doxycycline 100 mg 12-hourly for seven days are effective. Tetracyclines are contraindicated in pregnancy, and erythromycin 500 mg six-hourly for 7–14 days is used. Contacts must be traced and treated.

Urethritis

Urethritis is usually characterized in men by a discharge from the urethra, dysuria and varying degrees of discomfort within the penis. In 10–15% of cases there may be no symptoms. A wide array of aetiologies can give rise to the clinical picture, but may be divided into two broad bands: gonococcal or non-gonococcal urethritis (NGU). NGU occurring shortly after infection with gonorrhoea is known as postgonococcal urethritis (PGU). Gonococcal urethritis and chlamydial urethritis (a major cause of NGU) are discussed above.

In *Chlamydia*-negative NGU, *Ureaplasma urealyticum* is the next most frequent organism. *Bacteroides* spp. and *Mycoplasma* are responsible for a minority of cases. HSV can cause urethritis in about 30% of cases of primary infection, considerably fewer in recurrent episodes. Other causes include syphilitic chancres and warts within the urethra. Non-sexually transmitted NGU may be due to urinary tract infections, prostatic infection, foreign bodies and strictures.

CLINICAL FEATURES

The urethral discharge is often mucoid and worse in the mornings. It may be noted as crusting at the meatus or stains on underwear. Dysuria is common but not universal. Discomfort or itch within the penis may be present. The incubation period is 1–5 weeks with a mean of 2–3 weeks. The importance of asymptomatic urethritis must be recognized as a major reservoir of infection. Associated features of conjunctivitis and/or arthritis may occur, particularly in HLA B27-positive individuals.

DIAGNOSIS

Smears should be taken from the urethra when the patient has not voided urine for at least four hours and should be Gram stained and examined under a high-power (×1000) oil immersion lens. The presence of five or more polymorphonucleocytes per high power field is diagnostic. Men who are symptomatic but have no objective evidence of urethritis should be re-examined and tested after holding urine overnight. Cultures for gonorrhoea must be taken together with swabs for *Chlamydia* testing.

TREATMENT

Therapy is with tetracyclines initially, using either oxytetracycline 500 mg six-hourly or doxycycline 100 mg 12-hourly for seven days. Sexual intercourse should be avoided. The vast majority of patients will show partial or total response. For those left with objective evidence of urethritis, erythromycin 500 mg six-hourly for 1–2 weeks should be prescribed. Sexual partners must be traced and treated; *C. trachomatis* can be isolated from the cervix in 50–60% of the female partners of men with gonorrhoea or NGU, many of whom are asymptomatic. This causes long-term morbidity in such women, acts as a reservoir of infection for the community, and may lead to reinfection in the index case if not treated.

Recurrent/persistent NGU

This is a common and difficult clinical problem. The usual time for patients to re-present is 2–3 weeks following treatment. Tests for *Chlamydia* and *Ureaplasma* are usually negative. It is necessary to document objective evidence of urethritis, check compliance and establish any possible contact with untreated sexual partners. Investigations should include wet preparation and culture of a urethral smear for *Trichomonas vaginalis* and fungi. Cultures should be taken for HSV. A mid-stream urine sample should be examined and cultured. A further two weeks' treatment with erythromycin may be given and any specific additional infection treated appropriately. If symptoms are mild and all partners have been treated, patients should be reassured and further antibiotic therapy avoided. In cases of frequent recurrence and/or florid unresponsive urethritis, the prostate should be investigated and urethroscopy or cystoscopy performed to investigate possible strictures, periurethral fistulae or foreign bodies.

Lymphogranuloma venereum (LGV)

Chlamydia trachomatis types 1, 2 and 3 (see p. 49) is responsible for this sexually transmitted infection. It is endemic in the tropics, with the highest incidences in Africa, India and South East Asia.

CLINICAL FEATURES

The primary lesion is a painless ulcerating papule on the genitalia occurring 7–21 days following exposure. It frequently is unnoticed. A few days after this heals, regional lymphadenopathy develops. The lymph nodes are painful and fixed and the overlying skin develops a dusky erythematous appearance. Finally, nodes may become fluctuant (buboes) and can rupture. Acute LGV also presents as proctitis with perirectal abscesses, the appearances sometimes resembling anorectal Crohn's disease.

INVESTIGATIONS FOR DIAGNOSIS

The diagnosis is made on the basis of:

- the characteristic clinical picture
- isolation of an LGV strain of *C. trachomatis* (only possible in specialized laboratories)
- immunofluorescence using specific monoclonal antibodies for identifying organisms in pus from a bubo
- a rising titre in a complement-fixation test.

The intradermal Frei test is nonspecific and unreliable. Great care must be taken to exclude syphilis and genital herpes.

TREATMENT

Early treatment with doxycycline 100 mg four times daily for at least two weeks is generally necessary. Chronic infection may result in extensive scarring and abscess and sinus formation. Surgical drainage may be required. Sexual partners should also be treated.

Table 1.45
Classification and clinical features of syphilis

	Clinical features
Acquired	
Early stages	
Primary	Hard chancre Painless, regional lymphadenopathy
Secondary	*General*: Fever, malaise, arthralgia, sore throat and generalized lymphadenopathy *Skin*: Red/brown maculopapular non-itchy, sometimes scaly rash; condylomata lata *Mucous membranes*: Mucous patches, 'snail-track' ulcers in oropharynx and on genitalia
Late stages	
Tertiary	*Late benign*: Gummas (bone and viscera) *Cardiovascular*: Aortitis and aortic regurgitation *Neurosyphilis*: Meningovascular involvement, general paralysis of the insane (GPI) and tabes dorsalis
Congenital	
Early stages	Stillbirth or failure to thrive 'Snuffles' (nasal infection with discharge) Skin and mucous membrane lesions as in secondary syphilis
Late stages	'*Stigmata*': Hutchinson's teeth, 'sabre' tibia and abnormalities of long bones Keratitis, uveitis, facial gummas and CNS disease

Syphilis

The causative organism, *Treponema pallidum* (TP), is a motile spirochaete that is generally acquired by close sexual contact. The organism enters the new host through breaches in squamous or columnar epithelium. Primary infection of non-genital sites may occasionally occur but is rare. Syphilis is a chronic systemic disease which can be quiescent or show protean manifestations. It can also be transmitted transplacentally from mother to fetus.

Both congenital and acquired syphilis have early and late stages, each of which has classic clinical features (Table 1.45).

Primary

Between 10 and 90 days (mean 21 days) after exposure to the pathogen a papule develops at the site of inoculation. This ulcerates to become a painless, firm chancre. There is usually painless regional lymphadenopathy in association. The primary lesion may go unnoticed especially if it is on the cervix or within the rectum. Healing occurs spontaneously within 2–3 weeks.

Secondary

Between four and ten weeks after the appearance of the primary lesion constitutional symptoms with fever, sore throat, malaise and arthralgia appear. Any organ may be affected – leading, for example, to hepatitis, nephritis, arthritis and meningitis. In a minority of cases the primary chancre may still be present and should be sought.

Signs include:

- generalized lymphadenopathy (50%)
- generalized skin rashes involving the whole body including the palms and soles but excluding the face (75%) – the rash, which rarely itches, may take many different forms, ranging from pink macules, through coppery papules, to frank pustules
- condylomata lata – warty, plaque-like lesions found in the perianal area and other moist body sites
- superficial confluent ulceration of mucosal surfaces – found in the mouth and on the genitalia, described as 'snail track ulcers'
- acute neurological signs in less than 10% of cases (e.g. aseptic meningitis).

Latent

Without treatment, symptoms and signs abate over 3–12 weeks, but in up to 20% of individuals may recur during a period known as early latency, a two-year period in the UK (one year in USA). Late latency is based on reactive syphilis serology with no clinical manifestations for at least two years. This can continue for many years before the late stages of syphilis become apparent.

Tertiary

Late benign syphilis, so called because of its response to therapy rather than its clinical manifestations, generally involves the skin and the bones. The characteristic lesion, the gumma (granulomatous, sometimes ulcerating, lesions), can occur anywhere in the skin, frequently at sites of trauma. Gummas are commonly found in the skull, tibia, fibula and clavicle, although any bone may be involved. Visceral gummas occur mainly in the liver (hepar lobatum) and the testes.

Cardiovascular and neurosyphilis are discussed on p. 741 and p. 1074.

Table 1.46
Syphilis serology

Stage of infection	Results		
	FTA-abs	TPHA	VDRL
Very early primary	–	–	–
Early primary	+	–	–
Primary	+	±	+
Secondary or latent	+	+	+
Late latent	+	+	–
Treated	+	+	–
Biological false-positive	–	–	+

FTA-abs, fluorescent *Treponema* antibodies absorbed; TPHA, *Treponema pallidum* haemagglutination assay; VDRL, Veneral Disease Research Laboratory.

Congenital syphilis

Congenital syphilis usually becomes apparent between the second and sixth week after birth, early signs being nasal discharge, skin and mucous membrane lesions, and failure to thrive. Signs of late syphilis generally do not appear until after two years of age and take the form of 'stigmata' relating to early damage to developing structures, particularly teeth and long bones. Other late manifestations parallel those of adult tertiary syphilis.

INVESTIGATIONS FOR DIAGNOSIS

Treponema pallidum is not amenable to *in vitro* culture – the most sensitive and specific method is identification by dark-ground microscopy. Organisms may be found in variable numbers, from primary chancres and the mucous patches of secondary lesions. Individuals with either primary or secondary disease are highly infectious.

Serological tests used in diagnosis are either treponemal-specific or nonspecific. Three main tests are used routinely (Table 1.46):

- The VDRL (Venereal Disease Research Laboratory) is a nonspecific but useful screening test, becoming positive within 3–4 weeks of the primary infection. It generally becomes negative by six months after treatment. It is a quantifiable test which can be used to monitor treatment efficacy and is helpful in assessing disease activity. The VDRL may also become negative in untreated patients (50% of patients with late-stage syphilis). False-positive results may occur in other conditions – particularly: infectious mononucleosis, hepatitis, *Mycoplasma* infections, some protozoal infections, cirrhosis, malignancy, autoimmune disease and chronic infections.
- *T. pallidum* haemagglutination assay (TPHA) and fluorescent treponema antibodies absorbed (FTA-abs) test are both highly specific for treponemal disease but will not differentiate between syphilis and other treponemal infection such as yaws.
- The FTA-abs test is positive in more than 90% of patients with primary infection and in all patients with latent and late syphilis. It remains positive for life, even after treatment.

All serological investigations may be negative in early primary syphilis. The diagnosis will then hinge on positive dark-ground microscopy and treatment should not be delayed if serological tests are negative in such situations.

In certain cases, examination of the CSF for evidence of neurosyphilis and a chest X-ray to determine the extent of cardiovascular disease will be indicated.

TREATMENT

Early syphilis (primary or secondary) should be treated with long-acting procaine benzylpenicillin 3 ml daily by intramuscular injection for 10 days. When compliance is in doubt, a single injection of benzathine penicillin 2.4 g will maintain adequate levels of drug for approximately two weeks, although it may not cross the blood–brain barrier. For late-stage syphilis, particularly when there is cardiovascular or neurological involvement, the treatment course should be extended to four weeks. For patients sensitive to penicillin, either tetracycline or erythromycin is given. Tetracycline is contraindicated in pregnancy.

The *Jarisch–Herxheimer reaction*, which is due to release of TNF-α when large numbers of organisms are killed by antibiotics, is seen in 50% of patients with primary syphilis and up to 90% of patients with secondary syphilis. It occurs about eight hours after the first injection and usually consists of mild fever, malaise and headache lasting several hours. In cardiovascular or neurosyphilis the reaction, although rare, may be severe and exacerbate the clinical manifestations. Prednisolone given for 24 hours prior to therapy ameliorates the reaction. Penicillin should not be withheld because of the Jarisch–Herxheimer reaction; since it is not a dose-related phenomenon, there is no value in giving a smaller dose.

The prognosis depends on the stage at which the infection is treated. Early and early latent syphilis have an excellent outlook but once extensive tissue damage has occurred in the later stages the damage will not be reversed although the process may be halted. Symptoms in cardiovascular and neurosyphilis may therefore persist.

All patients treated for syphilis must be followed up at about three-monthly intervals for the first two years following treatment. Serological markers should be followed and a fall in titre of the VDRL of at least four-fold is consistent with adequate treatment. The sexual partners of all patients with early syphilis must be contacted and screened. Babies born to mothers who have been treated for syphilis in pregnancy may be retreated at birth.

Chancroid

Chancroid or soft chancre is an acute STD caused by *Haemophilus ducreyi*. It is common in tropical areas of the world and is endemic in parts of Africa and Asia. Epidemiological studies in Africa have shown an association between genital ulcer disease, frequently chancroid, and the acquisition of HIV infection. A new urgency to control chancroid has resulted from these observations.

CLINICAL FEATURES

The incubation period is 4–7 days. An initial erythematous papular lesion forms which then breaks down into an ulcer. Several ulcers merge to form giant serpiginous lesions. Ulcers appear most commonly on the prepuce and frenulum in men and can erode through tissues. In women the most commonly affected site is the vaginal entrance and the perineum. The lesions in women sometimes go unnoticed.

At the same time inguinal lymphadenopathy develops (usually unilateral) and can progress to form large buboes which suppurate.

DIAGNOSIS AND TREATMENT

Chancroid must be differentiated from other genital ulcer diseases (see Table 1.44). Isolation of *H. ducreyi* in specialized culture media is definitive but difficult. Swabs should be taken from the ulcer and material aspirated from the local lymph nodes for culture.

Clinically significant plasmid-mediated antibiotic resistance to *H. ducreyi* is developing. Single-dose regimens now include azithromycin 1 g orally, ciprofloxacin 500 mg orally or spectinomycin 2 g i.m. Multiple-dose regimens are needed in patients with HIV (e.g. erythromycin 500 mg four times daily for seven days, and ciprofloxacin 500 mg twice-daily for three days). All sexual partners should be seen and treated.

Granuloma inguinale

Granuloma inguinale is the least common of all STDs in North America and Europe, but is endemic in the tropics and subtropics, particularly the Caribbean, South East Asia and South India. Infection is caused by *Calymmatobacterium granulomatis*, a short, encapsulated Gram-negative bacillus. The infection was also known as Donovanosis, the organism originally being known as Donovan's body. Although sexual contact appears to be the most important mode of transmission, the infection rates are low, even between sexual partners of many years' standing.

CLINICAL FEATURES

In the vast majority of patients, the characteristic, heaped-up ulcerating lesion with prolific red granulation tissue appears on the external genitalia, perianal skin or the inguinal region within 1–4 weeks of exposure. However, almost any cutaneous or mucous membrane site can be involved, including the mouth and anorectal regions. Extension of the primary infection from the external genitalia to the inguinal regions produces the characteristic lesion, the 'pseudo-bubo'.

DIAGNOSIS AND TREATMENT

The clinical appearance usually strongly suggests the diagnosis but *C. granulomatis* (Donovan bodies) may be identified intracellularly in scrapings or biopsies of an ulcer. Culture or serological methods of diagnosis are not available.

Antibiotic treatment should be given for at least 10–14 days. Tetracycline 500 mg four times daily, streptomycin 1 g i.m. twice-daily or ampicillin 500 mg four times daily are the three most commonly used drugs. Alternatives include erythromycin and chloramphenicol.

Herpes simplex (p. 51)

Genital herpes is one of the most common STDs worldwide - in 1990 in the UK 20 000 new cases were seen in GUM clinics. Transmission occurs during close contact with a person who is shedding virus. Most genital herpes is due to type II. Genital contact with oral lesions caused by HSV-1 can also produce genital infection.

Susceptible mucous membranes include the genital tract, rectum, mouth and oropharynx. The virus has the ability to establish latency in the dorsal root ganglia by ascending peripheral sensory nerves from the area of inoculation. It is this ability which allows for recurrent attacks.

CLINICAL FEATURES

Asymptomatic infection has been reported but is rare. Primary genital herpes is usually accompanied by systemic symptoms of varying severity including fever, myalgia and headache. Multiple painful shallow ulcers develop which may coalesce. Tender inguinal lymphadenopathy is usual. Over a period of 10–14 days the lesions develop crusts and dry. In women with vulval lesions the cervix is almost always involved. Rectal infection may lead to a florid proctitis. Neurological complications can include aseptic meningitis and/or involvement of the sacral autonomic plexus leading to retention of urine.

Recurrent attacks may be expected in a significant proportion of people following the initial episode. Precipitating factors vary amongst individuals as does the frequency of recurrence. Recurrent attacks are usually less severe. A symptom prodrome is present in some people prior to the appearance of lesions. Systemic symptoms are rare in recurrent attacks.

The clinical manifestations in immunosuppressed patients (including those with HIV) may be more severe and recurrences occur with greater frequency. Systemic spread has been documented (see p. 115).

DIAGNOSIS

Although the history and examination can be highly suggestive of HSV infection, a firm diagnosis can be made only on the basis of isolation of virus from lesions. Swabs should be taken and placed in viral transport medium. Virus is most easily isolated from new lesions.

MANAGEMENT

Primary

Saltwater bathing or sitting in a warm bath is soothing and may allow the patient to pass urine with some degree of comfort. Oral acyclovir (200 mg five times daily initially for five days) is useful if patients are seen whilst lesions are still moist. Famciclovir and valaciclovir are also being used. If lesions are already crusting, acyclovir will do little to change the clinical course. Secondary bacterial infection may occasionally be present and should be treated. Rest, analgesia and antipyretics should be advised. In rare instances patients may need to be admitted to hospital and acyclovir given intravenously, particularly if HSV encephalitis is suspected.

Recurrence

Recurrent attacks tend to be much less severe and can be managed with simple measures such as saltwater bathing. Psychological morbidity may be associated with recurrent genital herpes and frequent recurrences impose strains on relationships; patients need considerable support. Long-term suppressive acyclovir therapy is given in patients with frequent recurrences. An initial course of 200 mg three to four times daily for six months usually reduces the frequency of attacks although there may still be some breakthrough.

HSV in pregnancy

If HSV is acquired for the first time during pregnancy, transplacental infection of the fetus may occur. For women with previous infection or primary infection at the time of labour concern focuses on the baby acquiring HSV from the birth canal. The risk is very low in recurrent attacks but rather greater in a primary episode. Obstetric opinion is divided, but if the woman has an attack around the time of labour Caesarian section may be performed. Acyclovir is not licensed for use in pregnancy but studies are still being carried out to evaluate its use in the last few weeks of pregnancy in women with recurrent HSV.

PREVENTION AND CONTROL

Patients must be advised that they are infectious when lesions are present; sexual intercourse should be avoided during this time or during prodromal stages. Condoms may not be effective as lesions may occur outside the areas covered. Sexual partners should be examined and may need information on avoiding infection.

Warts

Anogenital warts are amongst the most common sexually acquired infections with ever growing numbers of people seeking treatment. The causative agent is human papillomavirus (HPV) especially types 6 and 11. HPV is acquired by direct sexual contact with a person with either clinical or subclinical infection. Neonates may acquire HPV from an infected birth canal which may result either in anogenital warts or in laryngeal papillomas. The incubation period may range from two weeks to eight months or even longer.

CLINICAL FEATURES

Warts develop around the external genitalia in women, usually starting at the fourchette and involve the perianal region. The vagina may be infected. Flat warts may develop on the cervix and are not be easily visible on routine examination. Such lesions may have an association with cervical intraepithelial neoplasia and may be diagnosed on cervical cytology or at colposcopy. In men the penile shaft and subpreputial space are the most common sites although warts involve the urethra and meatus. Perianal lesions are more common in men who practise anoreceptive intercourse but can be found in any patient. The rectum may become involved. Warts become more florid during pregnancy or in immunosuppressed patients.

DIAGNOSIS

The diagnosis is essentially clinical. It is important to differentiate condylomata lata of secondary syphilis. Unusual lesions should be biopsied if the diagnosis is in doubt. Up to 30% of patients have coexisting infections with other STDs and a full screen is important.

TREATMENT

Local agents include podophyllin extract 10–25%, podophyllotoxin and trichloroacetic acid. In extensive or recalcitrant infection, cryotherapy, electrocautery or laser ablation is indicated. Podophyllin is contraindicated in pregnancy.

Sexual contacts should be examined and treated if necessary. In view of the difficulties of diagnosing subclinical HPV, condoms should be used for up to eight months after treatment. Because of the association of HPV with cervical intraepithelial neoplasia, women with warts and female partners of men with warts are advised to have cervical cytology carried out annually. Colposcopy should be performed in all women with vaginal and cervical warts.

Hepatitis B

This is discussed in Chapter 5. Sexual contacts should be screened and given vaccine if they are not immune (see p. 306).

Trichomoniasis

Trichomonas vaginalis (TV) is a flagellated protozoon which is predominantly sexually transmitted. It is able to attach to squamous epithelium and can infect the vagina and urethra.

Infected women may, unusually, be asymptomatic. Commonly the major complaints are of vaginal discharge which may be offensive and of local irritation.

Examination often reveals a frothy yellowish vaginal discharge and erythematous vaginal walls. The cervix may have multiple small haemorrhagic areas which lead to the description 'strawberry cervix'.

In men the infection is usually asymptomatic but may be a cause of NGU.

DIAGNOSIS AND TREATMENT

Phase-contrast microscopy of a drop of vaginal discharge shows TV swimming with a characteristic motion. Many polymorphonuclear leucocytes are also seen. Culture techniques are good and confirm the diagnosis.

Metronidazole 400 mg twice-daily for seven days is the treatment of choice. There is some evidence of metronidazole resistance and nimorazole is effective in these cases. Topical therapy with clotrimazole is effective, but if extravaginal infection exists this may not be eradicated and vaginal infection reoccurs. It is important that male partners be followed up, especially as they are likely to be asymptomatic.

Candidiasis

Vulvovaginal infection with *Candida albicans* is extremely common. The organism is also responsible for balanitis in men. *Candida* may be isolated from the vagina in a high proportion of women of childbearing age, many of whom will have no symptoms.

The role of *Candida* as pathogen or commensal is difficult to disentangle and it may be changes in host environment which allow the organism to produce pathological effects. Predisposing factors include pregnancy, the oral contraceptive pill, diabetes and broad-spectrum antibiotics. Immunosuppression can produce more florid infection.

CLINICAL FEATURES

In women, pruritus vulvae is the dominant symptom. Vaginal discharge is present in varying degree. Many women have only one or occasional isolated episodes but in a minority of patients the symptoms may be recurrent or chronic. Examination reveals erythema and swelling of the vulva with broken skin in severe cases. The vagina may contain adherent curdy discharge. Men may have a florid balanoposthitis. More commonly, self-limiting burning penile irritation immediately after sexual intercourse with an infected partner is described. Diabetes must be excluded in men with balanoposthitis.

DIAGNOSIS

Microscopic examination of a smear from the vaginal wall reveals the presence of spores and mycelia. Culture of swabs should be undertaken but may be positive in women with no symptoms. It is important to exclude *Trichomonas* and bacterial vaginosis in women with itch and discharge.

TREATMENT

Topical. Pessaries or creams containing one of the imidazole antifungals such as clotrimazole used intravaginally are usually effective. Nystatin is also useful.

Oral. The triazole drugs such as fluconazole 150 mg as a single dose or itraconazole 200 mg twice in one day may be used systemically in circumstances where topical therapy has failed or is inappropriate. Successful treatment to prevent recurrent attacks is difficult, but low-dose ketoconazole 100 mg per day for six months has been used.

The evidence for sexual transmission of *Candida* is slight and there is no evidence that treatment of male partners reduces recurrences in women.

Bacterial vaginosis

Bacterial vaginosis (BV) or nonspecific vaginosis is a disorder characterized by an offensive vaginal discharge. The aetiology and pathogenesis are unclear but the normal lactobacilli of the vagina are replaced by a mixed flora of *Gardnerella vaginalis*, anaerobes including *Bacteroides*, and *Mycoplasma hominis*. Amines and their breakdown products from the abnormal vaginal flora are thought to be responsible for the characteristic odour associated with the condition. As vaginal inflammation is not part of the syndrome the term vaginosis is used rather than vaginitis. It is not clear to what extent BV is a sexually transmitted condition.

CLINICAL FEATURES

Vaginal discharge and odour are the most common complaints although a proportion of women are asymptomatic. A homogeneous, greyish white, adherent discharge is present in the vagina, the pH of which is raised (greater than 5). Associated complications are ill-defined but may include chorioamnionitis and an increased incidence of premature labour in pregnant women. Whether BV disposes non-pregnant women to upper genital tract infection is unclear.

DIAGNOSIS

Different authors have differing criteria for making the diagnosis of BV. In general it is accepted that three of the following should be present for the diagnosis to be made:

- characteristic vaginal discharge
- the amine test: raised vaginal pH using narrow range indicator paper (>4.7)
- a fishy odour on mixing a drop of discharge with 10% potassium hydroxide
- the presence of clue cells on microscopic examination of the vaginal fluid.

Clue cells are squamous epithelial cells from the vagina which have bacteria adherent to their surface giving a granular appearance to the cell. A Gram stain gives a typical mixed reaction.

Additional laboratory tests include cultures for *G. vaginalis*, but this is nonspecific as the organism can be recovered in over 50% of women who do not meet the clinical diagnostic criteria for BV. Metabolic byproducts of the altered vaginal flora may be detected using gas or thin-layer chromatography.

TREATMENT

Metronidazole given orally in doses of 800–1200 mg daily for 5–7 days is usually recommended. A single dose of 2 g metronidazole is less effective. Topical 2% clindamycin cream 5 g intravaginally is effective.

Recurrence is high, with some studies giving a rate of 80% within nine months of completing metronidazole therapy. There is debate over the treatment of asymptomatic women who fulfil the diagnostic criteria for BV. The diagnosis should be fully discussed and treatment offered if the woman wishes. Until the relevance of BV to other pelvic infections is elucidated the routine treatment of all women with BV is not to be recommended. There is no convincing evidence that simultaneous treatment of the male partner influences the rate of recurrence of BV and routine treatment of male partners is not indicated.

Infestations (see also p. 1158)

Pediculosis pubis

The pubic louse (*Phthirius pubis*) is a blood-sucking insect which attaches tightly to the pubic hair. It is relatively host-specific and is transferred only by close bodily contact. Eggs (nits) are laid at hair bases and hatch within a week. Although infestation may be asymptomatic the most common complaint is of itch.

DIAGNOSIS

Lice may be seen on the skin at the base of pubic hairs. They may resemble small scabs or freckles but if they are picked up with forceps and placed on a microscope slide will move and walk away. Nits are usually closely adherent to hairs. Both are highly characteristic under the low-power microscope.

As with all sexually transmitted infections the patient must be screened for coexisting pathogens.

TREATMENT

It is important that both lice and eggs be killed. This is achieved with 1% benzene hexachloride or 0.5% malathion. The preparation should be applied to all areas of the body from the neck down and washed off after 24 hours. In a few cases a further application after one week may be necessary. For severe infestations, antipruritics may be indicated for the first 48 hours. All sexual partners should be seen and screened.

Scabies

This is discussed on p. 1158.

FURTHER READING

Adler M (1995) *The ABC of Sexually Transmitted Diseases*, 3rd edn. London: BMA Publications.

Sobel JD (1997) Vaginitis. *New England Journal of Medicine* **337**: 1896–1903.

HIV and AIDS

EPIDEMIOLOGY

The acquired immune deficiency syndrome (AIDS) was first described as a clinical entity in 1981 and HIV was identified as the causative organism in 1983. In December 1997 the World Health Organization (WHO) estimated that 29 million adults and 1.5 million children were already infected, and worldwide up to 16 000 new infections occur daily. Patterns of spread have varied greatly within different regions influenced by social, behavioural, cultural and political factors. WHO long-term projections estimate a cumulative total of over 40 million infections by the year 2000.

HIV infection is predominantly concentrated in developing countries in people in early adult life. Despite the fact that HIV can be isolated from a wide range of body fluids and tissues, the majority of infections are transmitted via semen, cervical secretions and blood. The character of the epidemic in different regions of the world has been influenced by the relative frequency of each of the routes of transmission.

Sexual intercourse (vaginal and anal)

Worldwide, heterosexual intercourse accounts for the vast majority of infections, and coexistent STDs, especially those causing genital ulceration, enhance transmission. Passage of HIV appears to be more efficient from men to women, and to the passive partner in anal intercourse, than vice versa.

Homosexual transmission still accounts for the majority of infections seen in the UK but there is now an increasing rate of heterosexual transmission in developed countries (particularly in urban populations). Up to 18% of the infections in Europe are thought to be heterosexually acquired. In central and sub-Saharan Africa the epidemic has always been heterosexual and more than half the infected adults in these regions are women. South East Asia and the Indian subcontinent are still in the early phases of a possible explosive epidemic, driven by promiscuous heterosexual intercourse and a high incidence of other sexually transmitted diseases.

Mother to child (parentally, perinatally, breastfeeding)

Vertical transmission is the most common route of HIV infection in children. As more women in their reproductive years are infected the numbers of babies acquiring HIV will increase. European studies suggest that 15% of babies born to HIV-infected mothers are likely to be themselves infected although rates of up to 40% have been reported from Africa and USA. Factors associated with increased vertical transmission include advanced disease in the mother, prolonged and premature rupture of membranes, and chorioamnionitis. Transmission can occur *in utero* and also, possibly, during the passage of the baby down the birth canal. Breastfeeding has been shown to increase the risk of vertical transmission by up to 20%. Vertical transmission can be reduced by the use of zidovudine (see below), and the numbers of infected children have fallen in areas where zidovudine is used.

Contaminated blood, blood products and organ donations

Screening of blood and blood products was introduced in 1985 in Europe and North America. Prior to this HIV infection was associated with the use of clotting factors (for haemophilia) and with blood transfusions. In some developing countries where blood is not screened or treated, and in areas where the rate of new HIV infections is very high, transfusion-associated transmission remains significant.

Contaminated needles (intravenous drug misuse, injections, needlestick injuries)

The practice of sharing needles and syringes for intravenous drug use continues to be a major route for transmission of HIV in both developed countries and parts of South East Asia and Latin America. In some areas successful education and needle exchange schemes have reduced the rate of transmission by this route. Iatrogenic transmission from needles and syringes used in developing countries is reported. Healthcare workers have a risk of approximately 0.3% following a single needlestick injury with known HIV infected blood.

There is no evidence that HIV is spread by social or household contact nor by blood-sucking insects such as mosquitoes and bed bugs.

THE VIRUS

HIV belongs to the lentivirus group of the retrovirus family. There are at least two types, HIV-1 and HIV-2. HIV-2 is almost entirely confined to West Africa although there is evidence of some spread to the Indian subcontinent. It is associated with an AIDS-type illness. The structure of the virus is shown in Fig 1.51.

Retroviruses are characterized by the possession of the enzyme reverse transcriptase, which allows viral RNA to be transcribed into DNA, and thence incorporated into the host cell genome. Reverse transcription is a highly error-prone process with a significant rate of misincorporation of bases. This, combined with a high rate of viral turnover, leads to considerable genetic variation and a diversity of viral subtypes or clades. On the basis of DNA sequencing, HIV-1 is divided into two subtypes:

- *Group M (major) subtypes*. There are at least ten, which are denoted A–J. There is a predominance of subtype B in Europe, North America and Australia, but areas of central and sub-Saharan Africa have multiple M subtypes.

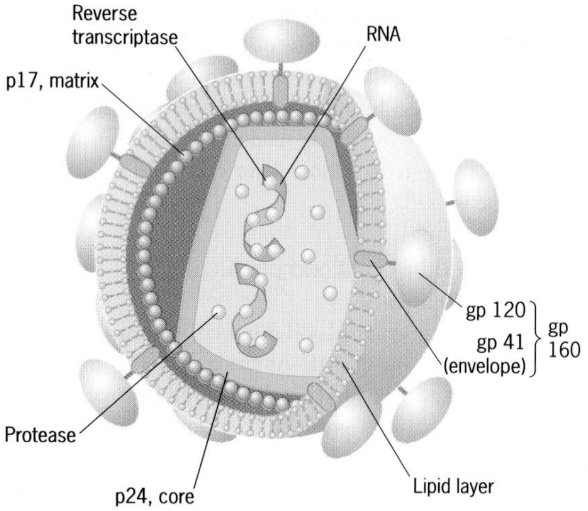

Fig 1.51
The structure of HIV

- *Group O (outlier) subtypes*. This is highly divergent from group M and is confined to small numbers centred around the Cameroons.

PATHOGENESIS

The interrelationship between HIV and the host immune system is the basis of the pathogenesis of HIV disease. The host cellular receptor that is recognized by HIV surface glycoprotein is the CD4 molecule which defines the cell populations that are susceptible to infection (Fig 1.52). The interaction between CD4 and HIV surface glycoprotein together with recently identified chemokine co-receptors is responsible for HIV entry into cells. Mutations in the chemokine gene (CCR5) may partly explain the lack of entry of HIV into cells and therefore resistance to this infection. The process of syncytium formation which is a cytopathic effect of HIV infection is mediated by CD4 receptors and HIV surface glycoprotein interactions.

Studies of viral turnover in HIV-infected individuals have demonstrated a virus half-life in the circulation of about six hours. To maintain observed levels of plasma viraemia, 10^8–10^9 virus particles need to be released and cleared daily. Virus production by infected cells lasts for about two days and is probably limited by the death of the cell owing to direct HIV effects, linking HIV replication to the process of CD4 destruction and depletion. Recent studies suggest that immunopathogenesis is a result of defective T-cell homeostasis in HIV infection. The progressive and severe depletion of CD4 helper lymphocytes has profound repercussions for the functioning of the immune system (see p. 180). Cell mediated immunodeficiency which is the major consequence leaves the host open to infections with intracellular pathogens, whilst the coexisting antibody abnormalities predispose to infections with capsulated bacteria. HIV also has a direct effect on certain tissues, notably the nervous system.

DIAGNOSIS AND NATURAL HISTORY (Fig 1.53)

HIV infection is diagnosed either by the detection of virus-specific antibodies (anti-HIV) or by direct identification of viral material.

Detection of IgG antibody to envelope components (gp120 and its subunits). This is the most commonly used marker of infection. The routine tests used for screening are based on ELISA techniques which may be confirmed with western blot assays. Up to three months may elapse from initial infection to antibody detection (serological latency, or window period). These antibodies to HIV have no protective function and persist for life. As with all IgG antibodies, anti-HIV will cross the placenta. All babies born to HIV-infected women will thus have the antibody at birth. In this situation, anti-HIV antibody is not a reliable marker of active infection and in uninfected babies will be gradually lost over the first 18 months of life.

Other than in exceptional circumstances, HIV antibody testing should be carried out only after full discussion of the implications with the patient and with the patient's express consent.

IgG antibody to p24 (anti-p24). This can be detected from the earliest weeks of infection and through the asymptomatic phase. It is frequently lost as disease progresses.

Antigen assays. Nucleic acid-based assays are available which amplify and test for components of the HIV genome. All are based on HIV-1 subtype B material, and there are potential inaccuracies with other subtypes, especially group O variants. These assays are used to aid diagnosis of HIV in the babies of HIV-infected mothers, or in situations where serological tests may be inadequate such as subtyping HIV variants for medicolegal reasons. (see the discussion of viral load monitoring, p. 119).

Viral p24 antigen (p24ag). This is detectable shortly after infection but has usually disappeared by 8–10 weeks after exposure. It can be a useful marker in individuals who have been infected recently but have not had time to mount an antibody response. It may reappear at low levels intermittently during the period of clinical latency and in some people as infection progresses. Its use as a surrogate marker of viral activity has been superseded by HIV RNA assays in many areas (see p. 119).

Isolation of virus in culture. This is a specialized technique available in some laboratories to aid diagnosis and as a research tool.

Clinical features of HIV infection

The spectrum of illnesses associated with HIV infection is broad and is the result of both direct HIV effects and the associated immune dysfunction. Several classification systems exist, the most widely used being the 1993 Centres for Disease Control (CDC) classification

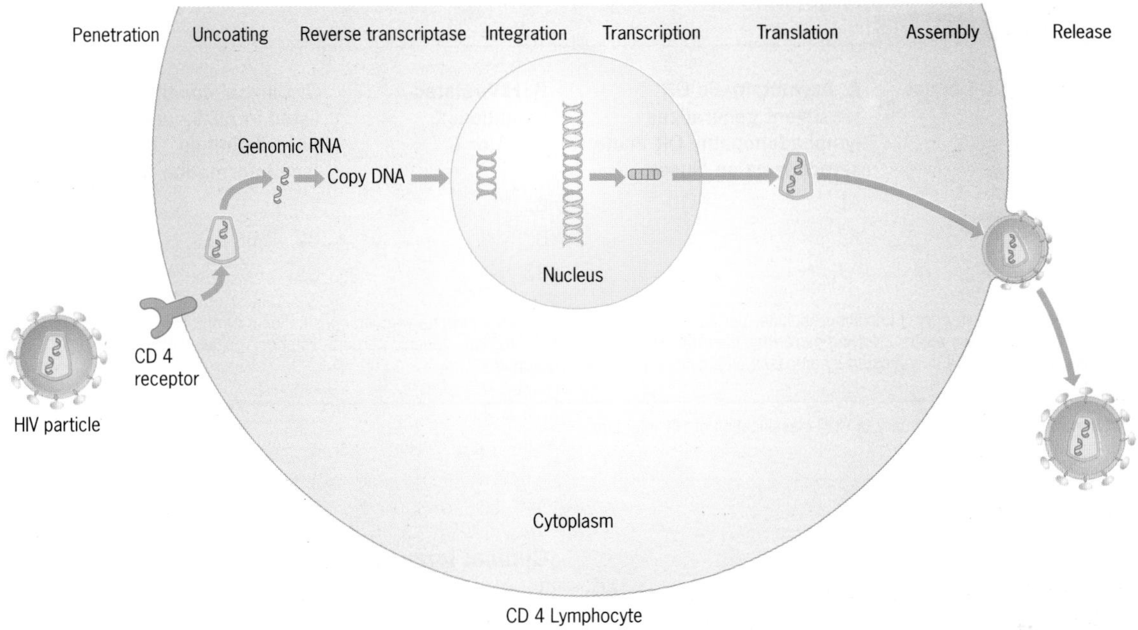

Fig 1.52
HIV entry and replication in CD4 T lymphocytes. The virus replicates by making a DNA copy (provirus) of its diploid RNA (using reverse transcriptase) which then becomes inserted into the host cell chromosomal DNA. This then provides RNA genomes for a progeny of new viruses

(Information box 1.5). This classification depends to a large extent on definitive diagnoses of infection, which makes it more difficult to use in those areas of the world without sophisticated laboratory support. As immunosuppression progresses the patient is susceptible to an increasing range of opportunistic infections and tumours, certain of which meet the criteria for the diagnosis of AIDS (Information box 1.6).

Since 1993 the definition of AIDS has differed between the USA and Europe. The USA definition includes individuals with CD4 counts below 200 in addition to the clinical classification based on the presence of specific indicator diagnoses shown in Information box 1.6. In Europe the definition remains based on the diagnosis of specific clinical conditions with no inclusion of CD4 lymphocyte counts.

Incubation

The 2–4 weeks immediately following infection are usually silent both clinically and serologically.

Seroconversion/primary illness

The majority of HIV seroconversions are also clinically silent. In a proportion, a self-limiting nonspecific illness occurs 6–8 weeks after exposure. Symptoms may include fever, arthralgia, myalgia, lethargy, lymphadenopathy, sore throat, mucosal ulcers and occasionally a transient faint pink maculopapular rash. Neurological symptoms are common, including headache, photophobia, myelopathy, neuropathy and in rare cases encephalopathy. The illness lasts up to three weeks and recovery is usually complete.

Laboratory abnormalities include lymphopenia with atypical reactive lymphocytes noted on blood film, thrombocytopenia and raised liver enzymes. CD4 lymphocytes may be markedly depleted and the CD4:CD8 ratio reversed. Antibodies to HIV may be absent during this early stage of infection although the level of circulating viral RNA is high and p24 core protein may be detectable. There is evidence to suggest that patients experiencing a seroconversion illness may have a more rapidly progressive course of infection.

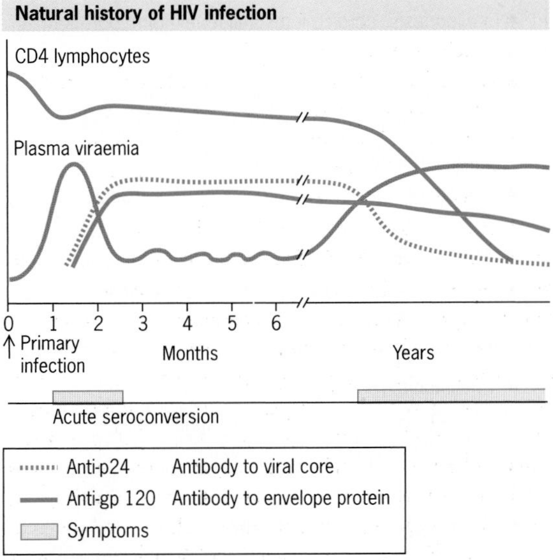

Fig 1.53
Natural history of HIV infection

Information

Absolute CD4 count (mm^{-3})	A: Asymptomatic OR persistent generalized lymphadenopathy OR acute seroconversion illness	B: HIV-related conditions*, not A or C	C: Clinical conditions listed in AIDS surveillance case definition (see Information box 1.6)
>500	A1	B1	C1
200–499	A2	B2	C2
<200	A3	B3	C3

* Examples of category B conditions include: bacillary angiomatosis, candidiasis (oropharyngeal), constitutional symptoms, oral hairy leucoplakia, herpes zoster involving more than one dermatome, idiopathic thrombocytopenic purpura, listeriosis, pelvic inflammatory disease especially if complicated by tubo-ovarian abscess, peripheral neuropathy.

Information box 1.5 Summary of CDC classification of HIV infection

Information

- Candidiasis of bronchi, trachea or lungs
- Candidiasis, oesophageal
- Cervical carcinoma, invasive
- Coccidioidomycocis, disseminated or extrapulmonary
- Cryptococcosis, extrapulmonary
- Cryptosporidiosis, chronic intestinal (one-month duration)
- Cytomegalovirus (CMV) disease (other than liver, spleen or nodes)
- CMV retinitis (with loss of vision)
- Encephalopathy, HIV-related
- Herpes simplex, chronic ulcers (one-month duration); or bronchitis, pneumonitis or oesophagitis
- Histoplasmosis, disseminated or extrapulmonary
- Isosporiasis, chronic intestinal (one-month duration)
- Kaposi's sarcoma
- Lymphoma, Burkitt's (or equivalent term)
- Lymphoma, immunoblastic (or equivalent term)
- Lymphoma, primary, of brain
- *Mycobacterium avium* complex or *M. kansasii*, disseminated or extrapulmonary
- *Mycobacterium tuberculosis*, any site
- *Mycobacterium*, other species or unidentified species, disseminated or extrapulmonary
- *Pneumocystis carinii* pneumonia
- Pneumonia, recurrent
- Progressive multifocal leukoencephalopathy
- *Salmonella* septicaemia, recurrent
- Toxoplasmosis of brain
- Wasting syndrome, due to HIV

Information box 1.6 AIDS defining conditions

Clinical latency

The majority of people with HIV infection are asymptomatic for a substantial but variable length of time. However, the virus continues to replicate and the person is infectious. Studies suggest a median time of 10 years from infection to development of AIDS, although some patients progress much more rapidly and others have remained symptom-free for up to 15 years. Older age is associated with more rapid progression, and the influence of putative protective genetic factors is under scrutiny. Gender and pregnancy *per se* do not appear to influence the rate of progression, although women may fare less well for a variety of reasons. It is still too soon to know whether all those with asymptomatic infection progress to AIDS.

A subgroup of patients with asymptomatic infection have persistent generalized lymphadenopathy (PGL), defined as lymphadenopathy (>1 cm) at two or more extrainguinal sites for more than three months in the absence of causes other than HIV infection. The nodes are usually symmetrical, firm, mobile and non-tender. There may be associated splenomegaly. The architecture of the nodes shows hyperplasia of the follicles and proliferation of the capillary endothelium. Biopsy is rarely indicated. Similar disease progression has been noted in asymptomatic patients with or without PGL. Nodes may disappear with disease progression.

Symptomatic HIV infection

As HIV infection progresses the CD4 count falls, the viral load rises and the patient develops an array of symptoms and signs. The clinical picture is the result of direct HIV effects and of the associated immunosuppression.

In an individual patient the clinical consequences of HIV-related immune dysfunction will depend on at least three factors:

- *The microbial exposure of the patient throughout life.* Many clinical episodes represent reactivation of previously acquired infection which has been latent. Geographical factors are important in determining the microbial repertoire of an individual patient. Those organisms requiring intact cell-mediated immunity for their control are most likely to cause clinical problems.

- *The pathogenicity of organisms encountered.* High-grade pathogens such as *Mycobacterium tuberculosis*, *Candida* and the herpes viruses are clinically relevant even when immunosuppression is mild, and will thus occur earlier in the course of the disease. Less virulent organisms occur at later stages of immunodeficiency.
- *The degree of immunosuppression of the host.* When patients are severely immunocompromised (CD4 count < $100/mm^3$) disseminated infections with organisms of very low virulence such as *M. avium intracellulare* and *Cryptosporidium* are able to establish themselves. These infections are very resistant to treatment, mainly because there is no functioning immune response to clear organisms. This hierarchy of infection allows for appropriate intervention with prophylactic drugs.

Effects of HIV infection

Neurological disease

The nervous system is a target for HIV infection quite independent of the immunosuppressive effects of the virus. Clinical neurological involvement is more common as HIV advances, but infection of nervous tissue occurs at an early stage. The clinical consequences include *AIDS dementia complex* (ADC) and *distal sensory polyneuropathy.* The pathogenesis is thought to be due both to the release of neurotoxic products by HIV itself and to cytokine abnormalities secondary to immune dysregulation.

ADC has varying degrees of severity, ranging from mild memory impairment and poor concentration through to severe cognitive deficit, personality change and psychomotor slowing. Changes in affect are common and depressive or psychotic features may be present. The spinal cord may show vacuolar myelopathy histologically. In severe cases brain CT scan shows atrophic change of varying degrees. MRI changes consist of white matter lesions of increased density on T2 weighted sections. EEG may show nonspecific changes consistent with encephalopathy. The CSF is usually normal, although the protein and neopterin concentrations may be raised. Patients with mild neurological dysfunction may be unduly sensitive to the effects of other insults such as fever, metabolic disturbance or psychotropic medication, any of which may lead to a marked deterioration in cognitive functioning.

A degree of sensory polyneuropathy is seen frequently in HIV infection, most commonly in the legs and feet although hands may be affected in advanced disease. In its most severe form it causes intense pain, usually in the feet, which may disrupt sleep, impair mobility and generally reduce the quality of life.

Autonomic neuropathy may also occur with postural hypotension and diarrhoea. Autonomic nerve damage is found in the small bowel.

Drugs. Zidovudine has a beneficial effect on HIV neurological disease, with startling improvement in cognitive function in many patients with ADC. It may also have a neuroprotective role. Other antiretrovirals have not yet been found to be as efficacious in this area but studies are continuing.

Zalcitabine, didanosine and stavudine produce a similar neuropathy as a major toxic side-effect and must be used with caution (if at all) in patients with HIV neuropathy.

Eye disease

Eye pathology is a regular finding in HIV infection, usually in the later stages. The most serious is cytomegalovirus retinitis (see p. 114) which is sight-threatening. Retinal cotton wool spots due to HIV *per se* are rarely troublesome but they may be confused with CMV retinitis. There are reports of anterior uveitis presenting as acute red eye associated with rifabutin therapy for mycobacterial infections in HIV. Steroids used topically are usually effective but modification of the dose of rifabutin is required to prevent relapse. Pneumocystis, toxoplasmosis, syphilis and lymphoma can all affect the retina and the eye may be the site of first presentation.

Mucocutaneous manifestations (see Table 1.48)

The skin is a common site for HIV-related pathology as the function of dendritic and Langerhans' cells, both target cells for HIV, is disrupted. Delayed-type hypersensitivity (p. 183), a good indicator of cell-mediated immunity, is frequently reduced or absent even before clinical signs of immunosuppression appear. Pruritus is a common complaint at all stages of HIV. Generalized dry, itchy, flaky skin is typical and the hair may become thin and dry. An intensely pruritic papular eruption favouring the extremities may be found, particularly in patients from sub-Saharan Africa. Eosinophilic folliculitis presents with urticarial lesions particularly on the face, arms and legs.

Drug reactions with cutaneous manifestations are extremely frequent, with rashes developing notably to sulphur-containing drugs amongst others. Recurrent aphthous ulceration which is severe and may be slow to heal is common and may impair the patient's ability to eat. Biopsy may be indicated to exclude other causes of ulceration. Topical steroids are useful and resistant cases may respond to thalidomide.

In addition to the above the skin is a common site of opportunistic infections (see below).

Haematological complications

Anaemia, neutropenia and thrombocytopenia are all common in advanced HIV infection.

- Anaemia of chronic HIV infection is usually mild, normochromic and normocytic.
- Neutropenia is common and usually mild.

- Isolated thrombocytopenia may occur early in infection and be the only manifestation of HIV for some time. Platelet counts are often moderately reduced but may fall dramatically (10–20 × 10^9/L) producing easy bleeding and bruising. Circulating antiplatelet antibodies lead to peripheral destruction. Megakaryocytes are increased in the bone marrow but their function may be impaired. Zidovudine therapy usually produces a rise in platelet count. Thrombocytopenic patients undergoing dental, medical or surgical procedures may need therapy with human immunoglobulin which gives a transient rise in platelet count, or be given platelet transfusion.

Underlying opportunistic infection or malignancies are frequently associated with pancytopenia, in particular *Mycobacterium avium intracellulare*, disseminated cytomegalovirus and lymphoma. Myelotoxic drugs commonly used in HIV management include zidovudine (megaloblastic anemia, red cell aplasia, neutropenia), ganciclovir (neutropenia), systemic chemotherapy (pancytopenia) and cotrimoxazole.

Gastrointestinal effects

Weight loss and diarrhoea are extremely common in HIV-infected patients. Wasting is a common feature of advanced HIV infection which although attributed to direct HIV effects on metabolism, is usually a consequence of other systemic infections producing anorexia. There is a small increase in resting energy expenditure in all stages of HIV, but weight and lean body mass usually remain normal during the period of clinical latency when the patient is eating normally.

HIV enteropathy is a term that has been used to describe a syndrome of diarrhoea, malabsorption and weight loss for which no other pathology has been found. HIV infection of the lymphocytes (in the lamina propria) which are distributed throughout both the large and small bowel, with disturbance of cytokine production, may be responsible. Villous atrophy is a common histological finding. Small bowel permeability is increased even in asymptomatic HIV-infected patients.

Hypochlorhydria is reported in patients with advanced HIV disease and may have consequences for drug absorption and bacterial overgrowth in the gut.

Rectal lymphoid tissue cells are the targets for HIV infection during penetrative anal sex and may be a reservoir for infection to spread through the body.

Renal complications

HIV-associated nephropathy (HIVAN) (see p. 538), although rare, can cause significant renal impairment particularly in more advanced disease. It is most frequently seen in black male patients and appears to be exacerbated by heroin use.

Nephrotic syndrome subsequent to focal glomerulosclerosis is the usual pathology which may be a consequence of HIV cytopathic effects on renal tubular epithelium. The course is usually relentlessly progressive and dialysis may be required.

Many nephrotoxic drugs are used in the management of HIV-associated pathology, particularly foscarnet, amphotericin B, pentamidine, sulphadiazine and indinavir.

Respiratory complications

The upper airway and lungs serve as a physical barrier to airborne pathogens and any damage will decrease the efficiency of protection, leading to an increase in upper and lower respiratory tract infections. The sinus mucosa may function abnormally in HIV infection and is frequently the site of chronic inflammation. Superadded bacterial infection is common. Response to antibacterial and topical steroids is usual but some patients require surgical intervention. A similar process is seen in the middle ear which can lead to chronic otitis media requiring grommets.

Lymphoid interstitial pneumonitis (LIP) is well described in paediatric HIV infection but is uncommon in adults. There is lymphocytic and plasma cell infiltration of the alveolar tissue which is seen on lung biopsy. The patient presents with dyspnoea, and a dry cough which may be confused with pneumocystis infection (see p. 798). Reticular nodular shadowing is seen on chest X-ray. Therapy with steroids may produce clinical and histological benefit in some patients.

Endocrine complications

Various endocrine abnormalities have been reported, including reduced levels of testosterone and abnormal adrenal function. The latter may assume clinical significance in more advanced disease when intercurrent infection superimposed upon borderline adrenal function may precipitate clear adrenal insufficiency requiring replacement doses of cortico- and mineralo-corticoid. CMV is also implicated in adrenal-deficient states.

Cardiac complications

Cardiomyopathy associated with HIV may lead to congestive cardiac failure. Lymphocytic or necrotic myocarditis have been described. Ventricular biopsy should be performed to ensure other treatable causes of myocarditis are excluded. Antiretrovirals, particularly zidovudine, may be helpful.

Conditions due to immunodeficiency (Table 1.47)

Immunodeficiency allows the development of opportunistic infections. These are diseases caused by organisms that are not usually considered pathogenic, unusual presentations of known pathogens, and the occurrence of tumours that may have an oncogenic viral aetiology. The process of diagnosis in an immunosuppressed patient may be complicated by a lack of typical signs as the inflammatory response is impaired. Examples are lack of neck stiffness in cryptococcal meningitis or minimal clinical findings in early *Pneumocystis carinii* pneumonia (PCP). Multiple pathogens may coexist. Indirect serological tests are frequently unreliable. These factors mean that in many instances material must be obtained from the appropriate site for examination and culture in order to make a diagnosis.

Opportunistic pathogens associated with HIV

Protozoal infections

Toxoplasmosis (see p. 76)

Toxoplasma gondii most commonly causes encephalitis and cerebral abscess in the context of AIDS, usually as a result of reactivation of previously acquired infection. The incidence depends on the rate of seropositivity to toxoplasmosis in the particular population. Particularly high levels are found in France where up to 90% of the adult population is seropositive. About 50% of the adult UK population is toxoplasmosis seropositive. Approximately 45% of AIDS patients who have antibodies to *T. gondii* may develop cerebral toxoplasmosis.

The clinical presentation is of focal neurological features, convulsions, fever, headache and possible confusion. Examination reveals focal neurological signs in more than 50% of cases. Eye involvement with chorioretinitis may also be present. In most but not all cases toxoplasmosis serology is positive. Typical CT scan of the brain shows multiple ring enhancing lesions. A single lesion on CT may be found to be one of several on MRI. A solitary lesion on MRI, however, mitigates against toxoplasmosis.

The definitive method of diagnosis is brain biopsy, but in most cases an empirical trial of anti-toxoplasmosis therapy is instituted and if this leads to radiological improvement within three weeks this is considered diagnostic. The differential diagnosis includes cerebral lymphoma, tuberculoma or focal cryptococcal infection.

Treatment is with pyrimethamine for at least six weeks (loading dose 200 mg, then 50 mg daily) combined with sulphadiazine and folinic acid. Clindamycin and pyrimethamine may be used in patients allergic to sulphonamide. Anticonvulsants should be given. Lifelong maintenance is required to prevent relapse. There is some evidence to suggest that co-trimoxazole as PCP prophylaxis has some ability to reduce the incidence of toxoplasmosis.

Table 1.47
Major HIV-associated pathogens

Protozoa	Bacteria
Toxoplasma gondii	*Salmonella* spp.
Cryptosporidium parvum	*Mycobacterium tuberculosis*
Microsporidia spp.	*Mycobacterium avium intracellulare*
Leishmania donovani	*Streptococcus pneumoniae*
Isospora belli	*Staphylococcus aureus*
Viruses	*Haemophilus influenzae*
Cytomegalovirus	*Moraxella catarrhalis*
Herpes simplex	*Rhodococcus equi*
Varicella zoster	*Bartonella quintana*
Human papilloma virus	*Nocardia*
Papovavirus	
Fungi and yeasts	
Pneumocystis carinii	
Cryptococcus neoformans	
Candida spp.	
Dermatophytes (Tricophytum, *Tinea* spp.)	
Aspergillus fumigatus.	
Histoplasma capsulatum	
Coccidioides immitis	

Cryptosporidiosis (see p. 84)

Cryptosporidium parvum can cause a self-limiting acute diarrhoea in an immunocompetent individual. In HIV infection it can cause severe and progressive watery diarrhoea which may be associated with anorexia, abdominal pain, nausea and vomiting. Cysts attach to the epithelium of the small bowel wall causing secretion of fluid into the gut lumen and leading to failure of fluid absorption. It is associated with sclerosing cholangitis (see p. 343). The cysts may be seen on stool specimen microscopy using Kinyoun acid-fast stain. The organism is readily identified on small bowel biopsy specimens.

Treatment is largely supportive as there are no effective antimicrobial agents available other than a non-absorbable aminogylycoside, paromamycin, which may have a limited effect on diarrhoea.

Microsporidiosis (see p. 84)

Enterocytozoon bieneusi and *Septata intestinalis* are associated with diarrhoeal illness in HIV infection. Spores can be detected in stools using a trichrome or fluorescent stain that attaches to the chitin of the spore surface. Albendazole eradicates the infection with amelioration of symptoms.

Leishmaniasis (see p. 71)

This is a cause of illness in immunosuppressed HIV-infected individuals who have been in endemic areas, which include South America, tropical Africa and much of the Mediterranean. Symptoms are frequently nonspecific with fever, malaise, diarrhoea and weight loss. Splenomegaly, anaemia and thrombocytopenia are significant findings. Amastigotes may be seen on bone marrow biopsy or from splenic aspirates. Serological tests exist for *Leishmania* but they are not reliable in this setting.

Treatment is based on sodium stibgluconate (pentavalent antimony) but in HIV infection the response may be better to liposomal amphotericin. Relapse is common unless long-term secondary prophylaxis is given.

Viral infections

Cytomegalovirus (see p. 53)

CMV is a cause of considerable morbidity in HIV-infected individuals, especially in the later stages of disease. The major problems encountered are retinitis, colitis, oesophageal ulceration, encephalitis and pneumonitis. CMV infection is associated with an arteritis which may be the major pathogenic mechanism. Polyradiculopathy and adrenalitis may also be caused by CMV.

CMV retinitis

This tends to occur once the CD4 count is below 100 and is found in up to 30% of AIDS cases. It is the most common cause of eye disease and blindness. Although usually unilateral to begin with, the infection frequently progresses to involve both eyes. Presenting features depend on the area of retina involved (loss of vision being most common with macular involvement) and include floaters, loss of visual acuity, field loss and scotomata, orbital pain and headache.

Examination of the fundus (Fig. 1.54) reveals haemorrhages and exudates which follow the vasculature of the retina (so called 'pizza pie' appearances). The features are highly characteristic and the diagnosis is made clinically. Retinal detachment and papillitis may occasionally occur. If untreated, retinitis spreads within the eye, destroying the retina wihin its path. Routine fundoscopy should be carried out on all HIV-infected patients to look for evidence of early infection. Any patient with symptoms of visual disturbance should have a thorough examination with pupils dilated, and if no evident pathology is seen a specialist ophthalmological opinion should be sought.

Treatment for CMV should be started as soon as possible with either ganciclovir (10 mg kg^{-1} daily) or foscarnet (60 mg kg^{-1} eight-hourly) given intravenously. The decision about which drug to use is based on the overall condition of the patient and concurrent medication, because a major side-effect of ganciclovir is myelosupression and foscarnet is

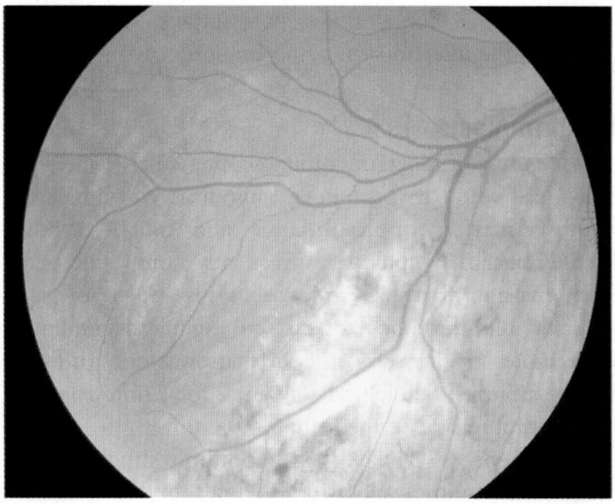

Fig 1.54
Untreated CMV retinitis

nephrotoxic. Treatment doses should be continued for at least three weeks or until the retinitis is quiescent. These agents halt disease but do not eradicate it and damaged retinal tissue does not regenerate. Reactivation is common and with each attack further retina is destroyed and vision lost, which may eventually lead to blindness in one or both eyes. Maintenance therapy with either ganciclovir or foscarnet self-administered intravenously requires long-term vascular access through either a Hickman line or subcutaneous reservoir device. This is not without hazards, especially of line sepsis, and may cause psychological distress. Recently an oral form of ganciclovir has been developed which has some long-term benefit when used as maintenance therapy, thus avoiding lines and their complications for some time. It is not suitable for all patients and has a lower efficacy than intravenous ganciclovir. Ganciclovir can be given directly into the vitreous cavity but regular injections are required. A new sustained-release implant of ganciclovir has been developed which is surgically implanted into the affected eye. These 'topical' therapies will only protect the eye and will not offer any systemic protection against CMV elsewhere in the body. A new compound, cidofovir, has recently become available for use in refractory cases. It has renal toxicity.

CMV colitis

The usual presenting features include abdominal pain, often generalized or left iliac, diarrhoea which may be bloody, generalized abdominal tenderness with rebound in some cases, and a low-grade fever. Loops of dilated large bowel may be seen on abdominal X-ray. Sigmoidoscopy shows a friable or ulcerated mucosa which should be biopsied.

The diagnosis is made on the histological appearances with characteristic 'owls eye' cytoplasmic inclusion bodies (see Fig. 1.31).

Treatment with either intravenous ganciclovir or foscarnet for three weeks improves symptoms and the histological changes are reversed. However, relapse is common once therapy is stopped. The issue of long-term maintenance therapy in this situation is controversial since, unlike CMV retinitis, repeated attacks of colitis do not necessarily have significant long-term sequelae of the sort associated with retinitis. Given the complications associated with maintenance anti-CMV therapy there may be no overall benefit.

Other sites along the gastrointestinal tract also be prone to CMV infection. Solitary ulceration of the oesophagus, usually in the lower third, causes painful dysphagia. CMV can also cause hepatitis.

CMV neurological conditions

CMV polyradiculopathy usually affects the lumbosacral roots, leading to paraparesis and sphincter disturbance. The CSF has an increase in white cells which surprisingly are almost all neutrophils. Although progression may be arrested by anti-CMV medication, functional recovery may not occur. The encephalopathy of CMV has similarities to that caused by HIV but tends to respond poorly to therapy.

Herpesviruses (see p. 51 and p. 103)

Herpes simplex infection occurs with greater frequency and severity, presenting in an ulcerative rather than vesical form in profoundly immunosuppressed individuals. Genital, oral and occasionally disseminated infection may be seen. Viral shedding may be prolonged in comparison with immunocompetent patients.

Varicella zoster can occur at any stage of HIV but tends to be more aggressive and longer-lasting in the more immunosuppressed patient. Multidermatomal zoster may occur.

Herpes virus 8 (HHV-8) is associated with Kaposi's sarcoma (see p. 118).

Therapy with acyclovir is usually effective but frequent recurrences may need suppressive therapy. Acyclovir-resistant strains (usually due to thymidine kinase deficient mutants) in HIV-infected patients have become more common. Such strains may respond to foscarnet.

Epstein–Barr virus (see p. 54)

Oral hairy leucoplakia due to this is a sign of immunosuppression first noted in HIV but now also recognized in other conditions. It appears intermittently on the lateral borders of the tongue or the buccal mucosa as a pale ridged lesion. Although usually asymptomatic, patients may find it unsightly and occasionally painful. The virus can be identified histologically and on electronmicroscopy. There is a variable response to acyclovir.

Human papilloma virus (see p. 55)

HPV produces genital, plantar and occasionally oral warts which may be slow to respond to therapy and recur repeatedly. HPV is associated with the more rapid development of cervical and anal intra-epithelial neoplasia which in time may progress to squamous cell carcinoma of the cervix or rectum in HIV-infected individuals.

Papovavirus (see p. 55)

Progressive multifocal leukencephalopathy (PML) is caused by JC virus, a member of the papovavirus family which infects oligodendrocytes. This leads to demyelination particularly within the white matter of the brain. The features are of progressive neurological and/or intellectual impairment, often including hemiparesis or aphasia. The course is usually inexorably progressive but a stuttering course may be seen.

Radiologically the lesions are usually multiple and confined to the white matter. They do not enhance with contrast and do not produce a mass effect. MRI (Fig. 1.55) is more sensitive than CT and reveals enhanced signal on T2 weighted images of the lesions. Definitive diagnosis is made on histological and viral examination of brain tissue obtained at biopsy.

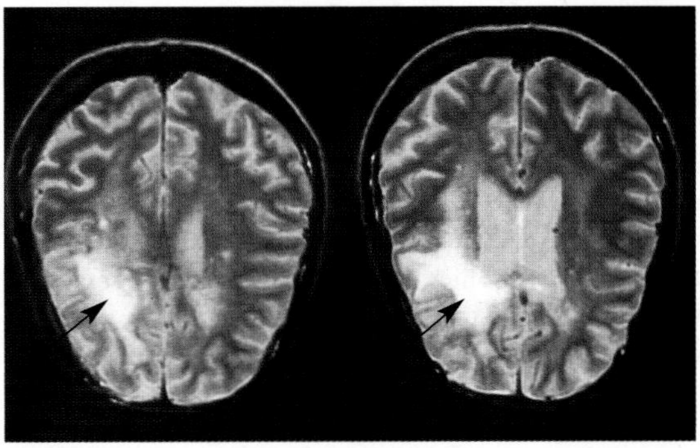

Fig 1.55
MRI scan showing progressive multifocal leukoencephalopathy

There is no specific therapy, although attempts to enhance the immune system with antiretrovirals may have a role. The prognosis is very poor with many patients dying within a few months of diagnosis.

Fungal infections

Pneumocystis carinii (see p. 798)

This organism most commonly causes pneumonia (PCP) but can cause disseminated infection. It is not usually seen until patients are severely immunocompromised with a CD4 count below 200. The infection remains common although the use of primary prophylaxis in patients with CD4 < 200 has reduced the incidence. The organism damages alveolar epithelium which impedes gas exchanges and reduces lung compliance.

The onset is often insidious over a period of weeks, with a prolonged period of increasing shortness of breath (usually on exertion), non-productive cough, fever and malaise. Clinical examination reveals tachypnoea, tachycardia, cyanosis and signs of hypoxia. Fine crackles are heard on auscultation, although in mild cases there may be no auscultatory abnormality. In early infection the chest X-ray is normal but the typical appearances are of bilateral perihilar interstitial infiltrates which can progress to confluent alveolar shadows throughout the lungs. High-resolution CT scans of the chest demonstrate a characteristic ground-glass appearance even when there is little to see on the chest X-ray. The patient is usually hypoxic and desaturates on exercise. Definitive diagnosis rests on demonstrating the organisms in the lungs via bronchoalveolar lavage. As the organism cannot be cultured *in vitro* it must be directly observed either with silver staining or immunofluorescent techniques.

Treatment should be instituted as early as possible. First-line therapy is with intravenous co-trimoxazole (100 mg kg^{-1} per day sulphamethoxazole and 20 mg kg^{-1} per day trimethoprim in divided doses) for 21 days. Up to 40% of patients receiving this regimen will develop some adverse drug reaction, including typical allergic rash. If the patient is sensitive to co-trimoxazole, intravenous pentamidine (4 mg kg^{-1} per day) or dapsone and trimethoprim are given for the same duration. Atovaquone or a combination of clindamycin and primaquine is also used. In severe cases (P_aO_2 less than 9.5 kPa), systemic corticosteroids have been shown to reduce mortality and should be added. Continuous positive airways pressure (CPAP) or mechanical ventilation (see p. 851) may be required if the patient remains severely hypoxic or becomes too tired. Pneumothorax not uncommonly complicates the clinical course and is very difficult to manage in an already severely hypoxic patient.

Long-term secondary prophylaxis is required to prevent relapse, the usual regimen being co-trimoxazole 960 mg thrice-weekly. Patients sensitive to sulphonamide are given either dapsone and pyrimethamine or nebulized pentamidine. The latter only protects the lungs and does not penetrate the upper lobes particularly efficiently; hence if relapses occur on this regimen they may be either atypical or may be extrapulmonary.

Cryptococcus (see p. 69)

The most common presentation of *Cryptococcus* in the context of HIV is meningitis, although pulmonary and disseminated infections can also occur. The organism, *C. neoformans*, is widely distributed – often in bird droppings – and is usually acquired by inhalation. The onset may be insidious with nonspecific fever, nausea and headache. As the infection progresses the consciousness level is impaired and changes in affect are noted. Fits or focal neurological presentations are uncommon. Neck stiffness and photophobia may be absent as these signs depend on the inflammatory response of the host, which in this setting is abnormal.

The diagnosis is made on examination of the CSF (a CT scan must be carried out before lumbar puncture to exclude space-occupying pathology). Indian ink staining shows the organisms directly and CSF cryptococcal antigen is positive at variable titre. It is unusual for the cryptococcal antigen to become negative after treatment, although the levels should fall substantially. Cryptococci can be cultured from CSF and/or blood.

Signs associated with a poor prognosis include a high organism count in the CSF, a low white cell count in the CSF, and an impaired consciousness level at presentation.

Initial treatment is usually with intravenous amphotericin B (0.7 mg kg^{-1} per day), although intravenous fluxonazole (400 mg daily) is useful in some circumstances. Once the patient is making a sustained recovery therapy may be changed to oral fluconazole if the organism is shown to be fully sensitive.

The mortality from a first episode of cryptococcal meningitis is up to 20%. Relapse is very common, possibly from a prostatic reservoir in men, and lifelong secondary prophylaxis is required.

Candida (see p. 67)

Mucosal infection with *Candida* is very common in HIV-infected patients. Oral *Candida* is one of the most common conditions. *C. albicans* is the usual form, although *C. krusei* and *C. glabrata* occur and have therapeutic implications. Pseudomembranous candidiasis consisting of creamy plaques in the mouth and pharynx is the best recognized. Erythematous *Candida* is more subtle and appears as reddened areas on the hard palate or as atypical areas on the tongue which may be overlooked. Angular cheilitis can occur in association with either form or more rarely alone. Vulvovaginal *Candida* is often problematic.

Oesophageal *Candida* infection (see p. 231) produces dysphagia with retrosternal discomfort or may present as 'heartburn' or other peptic symptoms. Barium swallow or endoscopy shows multiple areas of ulceration throughout the length of the oesophagus. Fluconazole or itraconazole are the agents of choice. With prolonged exposure to these agents in HIV-infected patients, azole-resistant *C. albicans* is becoming an increasingly common phenomenon. Switching azoles may produce a response in this setting. Symptom relief may require intravenous amphotericin. Disseminated *Candida* is uncommon in the context of HIV infection. *C. krusei* may colonize patients who have been treated with fluoconazole as it is fluconazole-resistant. Amphotericin is useful in the treatment of this infection, which makes it important to attempt to type *Candida* from clinically azole-resistant patients.

Superficial dermatophyte infections

These are common. Nail infection with *Tricophyton rubrum* causes onychomycocis (see p. 1157 and Table 1.48).

Aspergillus (see p. 811)

Infection with *Aspergillus fumigatus*, although still unusual, is becoming increasingly common in advanced HIV disease. *Aspergillus* is controlled by functioning neutrophils, and patients with longstanding neutropenia

Table 1.48 Some mucocutaneous manifestations of HIV infection (see also chapter 20)

Skin	**Mucous membranes**
Dry skin and scalp	Candidiasis
Onychomycosis	oral
Seborrhoeic dermatitis	vulvovaginal
Tinea	Hairy oral leucoplakia
cruris	Aphthous ulcers
pedis	Herpes simplex
Pityriasis	genital
versicolor	oral
rosea	labial
Folliculitis	Periodontal disease
Acne	Warts
Molluscum contagiosum	oral
Warts	genital
Herpes zoster	
multidermatomal	
disseminated	
Papular pruritic eruption	
Scabies	
Ichthyosis	
Kaposi's sarcoma	

(often due to chemotherapy), those on ganciclovir therapy for CMV and myelotoxic antiretrovirals, are prone to this infection. Spores are airborne and ubiquitous. Following inhalation, lung infection proceeds to haematogenous spread to other organs. Sinus infection may occur.

The prognosis is very poor, with amphotericin B being the mainstay of therapy. Itraconazole is also effective. It is almost impossible to deal effectively with *Aspergillus* unless the neutrophil count can be sustained, and neutropenic patients should be supported with granulocyte colony stimulating factors.

Histoplasmosis (see p. 68)

This infection is a well-recognized complication of HIV in the USA where it is endemic in soil. The most common manifestation is with pneumonia which may be confused with *Pneumocystis carinii* in its presentation (see above).

Bacterial infections

Bacterial infection in HIV is common and frequently disseminated. Cell-mediated immune responses control infection; intracellular bacteria, e.g. *Mycobacterium* and *Salmonella,* are the prime examples. The abnormalities of B cell function associated with HIV lead to infections with encapsulated bacteria as reduced production of IgG_2 cannot protect against the polysaccharide coat of such organisms. These functional abnormalities may be present well before there is a significant decline in CD4 numbers and so bacterial sepsis may be seen at early stages of HIV infection. *Streptococcus pneumoniae, Haemophilus influenzae* and *Moraxella catarrhalis* are examples. Bacterial infection is often disseminated and, although usually amenable to standard antibiotic therapy, may reoccur. Long-term prophylaxis is required if recurrent infection is frequent.

Skin conditions such as folliculitis, abscesses and cellulitis are common and are usually caused by *Staphylococcus aureus*. Periodontal disease, which may be necrotizing, causes pain and damage to the gums. It is more common in smokers, but no specific causative agent has been identified. Therapy is with local debridement and systemic antibiotics.

Salmonella (non-typhoidal) (see p. 34) are frequent pathogens in HIV infection. *Salmonella* are able to survive within macrophages, this being a major factor in their pathogenicity. Organisms are usually acquired orally and frequently result in disseminated infection. Gastro-intestinal disturbance may be disproportionate to the degree of dissemination, and once the pathogen is in the blood stream any organ may be infected. *Salmonella* osteomyelitis and cystitis have been reported. Diagnosis is from blood and stool cultures.

Response to standard antibiotic therapy, depending on laboratory sensitivities, is usually good. Recurrent infection is, however, common and long-term prophylaxis may be required.

Education on food hygiene should be provided.

Mycobacteria

Mycobacterium tuberculosis (see p. 801)

TB can cause disease when there is only minimal immunosuppression and thus often appears early in the course of infection. In many countries where HIV is spreading and TB is endemic there has been a substantial increase in the incidence of tuberculosis. HIV-related TB frequently represents reactivation of latent TB, but there is also clear evidence of newly acquired infection and nosocomial spread in HIV-infected populations.

The pattern of disease differs with immuno-suppression. Patients with relatively well-preserved CD4 counts have a clinical picture similar to that seen in HIV-negative patients with pulmonary infection. In more advanced HIV disease atypical pulmonary presentations without cavitation and prominent hilar lymphadenopathy, or extrapulmonary TB affecting lymph nodes, bone marrow or liver occur. Bacteraemia may be present.

The diagnosis depends on demonstrating the organisms in appropriate tissue specimens. The response to tuberculin testing is blunted in HIV-positive individuals and is unreliable. Sputum microscopy may be negative even in pulmonary infection and culture techniques are the best diagnostic tool.

M. tuberculosis infection usually responds well to standard treatment regimens, although the duration of therapy may be extended especially in extrapulmonary infection. Multidrug resistance is becoming a problem, particularly in the USA where it is becoming a nosocomial danger. Isolated cases from HIV units in the UK have recently been reported. Compliance with antituberculous therapy needs to be emphasized. Treatment of TB in the HIV-infected individual is not curative and long-term isoniazid prophylaxis may be given. In patients from TB endemic areas, primary prophylaxis may prevent emergence of infection.

Mycobacterium avium intracellulare

Atypical mycobacteria, particularly *M. avium intracellulare* (MAI), generally appear only in the later stages of HIV infection when patients are profoundly immunosuppressed. It is a saprophytic organism of low pathogenicity that is ubiquitous in soil and water. Entry may be via the gastrointestinal tract or lungs with dissemination via infected macrophages.

The major clinical features are fevers, malaise, weight loss, anorexia and sweats. Dissemination to the bone marrow causes anaemia. Gastrointestinal symptoms may be prominent with diarrhoea and malabsorption. At this stage of disease patients frequently have other concurrent infections, so differentiating MAI is difficult on clinical grounds. Direct examination and culture of blood, lymph node, bone marrow or liver give the diagnosis most reliably.

MAI is typically resistant to standard antituberculous therapies, although ethambutol may be useful. Newer drugs such as rifabutin in combination with clarithromycin or azithromycin have shown promise in reducing the burden of organisms and in ameliorating symptoms. A common combination is ethambutol, rifabutin and clarithromycin. Addition of amikacin may produce a good symptomatic response in patients failing on other regimens. Primary prophylaxis with rifabutin or azithromycin may delay the appearance of MAI, but no corresponding increase in survival has been shown.

Infections due to other organisms

Strongyloides (see p. 89), a nematode found in tropical areas, may produce a hyperinfection syndrome in HIV-infected patients. Larvae are produced which invade through the bowel wall and migrate to the lung and occasionally to the brain. Albendazole or ivermectin may be used to control infection. Gram-negative septicaemia can develop (see p. 838).

Scabies (see p. 1158) may be much more severe in HIV infection. It may be widely disseminated over the body and appear as atypical, crusted papular lesions known as 'Norwegian scabies' from which mites are readily demonstrated. Superadded staphylococcal infection may occur. Treatment with conventional agents such as lindane may fail, and ivermectin has been used to good effect in some patients.

Neoplasms

The mortality and morbidity associated with neoplasia in HIV is substantial, with Kaposi's sarcoma and non-Hodgkin's lymphoma being the most significant tumours.

Kaposi's sarcoma (see p. 1185)

Kaposi's sarcoma (KS) in association with HIV (epidemic KS) behaves more aggressively than that associated with HIV-negative populations (endemic KS). The tumour is most common in homosexual men and others who have acquired HIV sexually, particularly from a partner who has KS, implicating a sexually transmitted cofactor in the pathogenesis. Human herpes virus 8 (HHV-8) has been implicated in pathogenesis. Polymerase chain reaction (PCR) evidence of HHV-8 infection in HIV-infected subjects has a high predictive value for the subsequent development of KS.

KS skin lesions are characteristically pigmented, well-circumscribed and occur in multiple sites. It is a multicentric tumour consisting of spindle cells and vascular endothelial cells which together form slit-like spaces in which red blood cells become trapped. This process is responsible for the characteristic purple hue of the tumour. In addition to the skin lesions, KS affects lymphatics and lymph nodes, the lung and gastrointestinal tract, giving rise to a wide range of symptoms and signs. Most patients with visceral involvement also have skin or

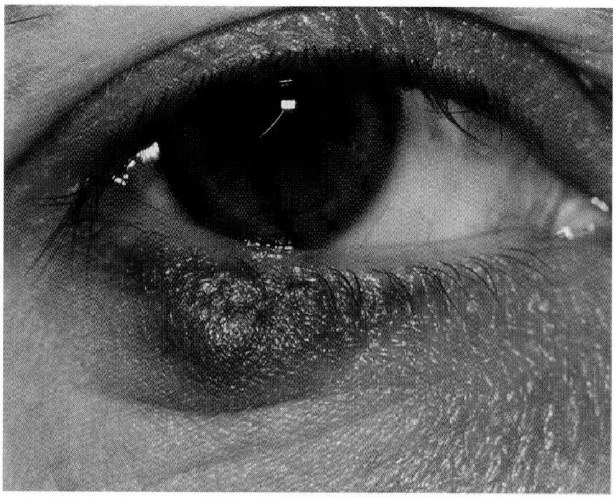

Fig 1.56
Kaposi's sarcoma of the eyelid

mucous membrane lesions. Visceral KS carries a worse prognosis than that confined to the skin. Kaposi's sarcoma is seen around the eye (Fig. 1.56), particularly in the conjunctivae, which can lead to periorbital oedema.

Treatment with local radiotherapy gives good results in skin lesions and is helpful in lymph node disease. For patients with aggressive disease, systemic chemotherapy is indicated using combinations of vincristine and bleomycin or the newer liposomal preparations of doxorubicin. Response is often very good although of uncertain duration. Antiretroviral medication and interferon-α are also effective.

Lymphoma

A significant proportion of patients with HIV will at some stage develop lymphoma, mostly of the non-Hodgkin's, large B cell type. These are frequently extranodal, often affecting the brain, lung and gastrointestinal tract. Many of these tumours are strongly associated with Epstein–Barr virus (EBV), with evidence of expression of latent gene nuclear antigens such as EBNA 1–6, some of which are involved in the immortalization of B cells and drive a neoplastic pathway.

HIV-associated lymphomas are frequently very aggressive. Patients often present with systemic 'B' syndromes and progress rapidly despite chemotherapy. Primary cerebral lymphoma is variably responsive to radiotherapy but overall carries a poor prognosis. Lymphomas occurring early in the course of HIV infection tend to respond better to therapy and carry a better prognosis, occasionally going into complete remission.

Squamous cell carcinoma

Squamous cell carcinoma, especially of the cervix and anus, is associated with HIV. Human papilloma virus may have a role in the pathogenesis of these malignancies. Women with HIV infection should have yearly cervical cytology for detection of premalignant change.

Practical

Haematology
Full blood count, differential count and film
Erythrocyte sedimentation rate

Biochemistry
Serum, liver and renal function tests

Immunology
Lymphocyte subsets
Serum neopterin
Serum β_2 microglobulin

Virology
HIV antibody (confirmatory)
HIV viral load (p24 antigen/antibody if unavailable)
Hepatitis serology (A, B and C)
Cytomegalovirus antibody

Microbiology
Toxoplasmosis serology
Syphilis serology
Cryptococcal antigen
Screen for other sexually transmitted diseases

Other
Baseline chest X- ray
Lung function tests
Cervical cytology

Practical box 1.1 Baseline investigations in HIV infection

Investigations and monitoring

INITIAL ASSESSMENT

A full history should be taken, followed by examination. Baseline investigations will depend on the clinical setting, but those for an asymptomatic person in the UK are shown in Practical box 1.1.

Monitoring the progression of disease

Patients are regularly monitored to assess the progression of the infection. Clinical examination will identify signs of immunosuppression (such as hairy oral leucoplakia) and detect early evidence of major opportunistic events. Decisions about appropriate intervention can be made.

Immunological monitoring

CD4 lymphocytes. The absolute CD4 count and the percentage of total lymphocytes that this represents falls as HIV progresses. These figures bear a relationship to the risk of the occurrence of HIV-related pathology, with patients with counts below 200 cells at greatest risk. The currently available routine assays measure numbers of circulating CD4 lymphoctyes but are unable to assess cellular function which may be abnormal even when numbers are relatively well preserved. Factors other than HIV (e.g. smoking, exercise, intercurrent infections and diurnal variation) also affect CD4 numbers and results must be interpreted with caution. CD4 counts are performed at approximately three-monthly intervals unless values are approaching critical levels for intervention, in which case they are performed more frequently.

β_2 microglobulin and neopterin. β_2 microglobulin is a protein marker of lymphocyte activation, and neopterin is produced by activated macrophages. Both rise as HIV progresses. However, there is considerable overlap between clinical stages of infection, making them unreliable markers.

Virological monitoring

Viral load (HIV RNA)

The replication of HIV continues at a high rate throughout the course of infection, with many billion new virus particles being produced daily. The rate of viral clearance is relatively constant in any individual and thus the level of viraemia is a reflection of the rate of virus replication. This has both prognostic and therapeutic value.

The commonly used term 'viral load' has been coined to encompass viraemia and HIV RNA levels. Three assays are in current use:

- branched-chain DNA (bDNA)
- reverse transcription polymerase chain reaction (RT-PCR)
- nucleic acid sequence-based amplification (NASBA).

Results are given in copies of viral RNA per millilitre of plasma, or converted to a logarithmic scale. Methodological differences mean that the three assay techniques are not interchangeable, but there is good correlation. Some assays may be less reliable at estimating non-B subtypes of HIV, but the most sensitive test is able to detect as few as 20 copies of viral RNA per millilitre. If the HIV RNA level in plasma is below the sensitivity of the assay, the viral load is described as below the limits of detection. Transient increases in viral load are seen following immunizations (e.g. for influenza and *Pneumococcus*) or during episodes of acute intercurrent infection (e.g. tuberculosis); for meaningful information to be obtained, viral load measurements should not be carried out within a month of these events.

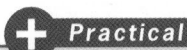

By about six months after seroconversion to HIV, the viral set point for an individual is established and there is a correlation between HIV RNA levels and long-term prognosis, independent of the CD4 count. Those patients with a viral load consistently greater than 10 000 copies per millilitre have a 10 times higher risk of progression to AIDS over the ensuing five years than those consistently below 10 000/mL. Although a correlation exists between viral load and CD4 cell numbers, the viral load appears to be the best predictor of the long-term prognosis, whilst the CD4 count will give warning of the risks of immediate or shorter term problems.

HIV RNA is a useful marker of treatment efficacy, with levels falling in response to the introduction of effective antiretroviral medication (see below). Both duration and magnitude of virus suppression are pointers to clinical outcome. None of the currently available therapies seem able to suppress viral replication indefinitely, and rising viral load to pretreatment values indicates drug failure.

Various guidelines exist for viral load monitoring in clinical practice. Baseline measurements are followed by repeat estimations at intervals of 3–4 months, ideally in conjunction with CD4 counts to allow both pieces of evidence to be used together in decision-making. Following initiation of antiretroviral therapy or changes in therapy, effects on viral load should be seen by four weeks, reaching a maximum at 10–12 weeks, when repeat viral load testing should be carried out.

Phenotype determination

Two phenotypes of HIV, syncytium-inducing (SI) and non-syncytium-inducing (NSI), exist and appear to correlate with disease progression. This is a specialized technique that is currently available only as a research tool.

Genotype determination

Clear genotypic variation exists within HIV and there are increasing numbers of well-identified point mutations associated with antiretroviral drugs. The genotype may in the future be used to guide antiretroviral use, although this is not currently a feasible routine practice.

Management of the HIV-infected patient

Despite the introduction of new antiretroviral agents there is still no cure for HIV and AIDS, so the patient must live with a chronic, progressive, infectious and unpredictable condition. The aims of management in HIV infection are to maintain physical and mental health, to avoid transmission of the virus, and to provide appropriate palliative support as needed. The complexity of HIV infection means that it is best managed via a multidisciplinary team approach. Confidentiality must be strictly observed and care taken over establishing who is aware of the patient's diagnosis and who is excluded from that knowledge. Psychological support is needed not only for the patient but also for family, friends and carers. Dietary assessment and advice should be freely accessible.

Clear advice on reducing the risk of HIV transmission must be provided and future sexual practices discussed. Information must be available to allow people to make informed choices about childbearing. The implications for existing family members should be considered. General health promotion advice on smoking, drug misuse and exercise is necessary.

Table 1.49
Antiretroviral agents

Nucleoside-analogue reverse-transcriptase inhibitors (NRTI)	Protease inhibitors	Non-nucleoside reverse-transcriptase inhibitors (NNRTI)
Zidovudine (AZT)	Saquinavir	Nevirapine
Didanosine (DDI)	Indinavir	Delavirdine*
Zalcitabine (DDC)	Ritonavir	DMP 266*
Stavudine (D4T)	Vx-478*	
Lamivudine (3TC)	Nelfinavir*	
	Abacavir*	

*Currently not licensed in Europe.

Antiretroviral drugs

Substantial progress has been made in the development and uses of antiretroviral drug regimens. The principal aim of antiretroviral drug therapy is to suppress viral replication to as low a level as possible for as long as possible. In doing so, continuing damage to the immune system can be checked and disease progression delayed. Opportunities for spontaneous mutations in the viral genetic material which occur only when there is active replication are reduced, and the potential for emergence of drug-resistant strains is lessened. Evidence from controlled trials has shown clear clinical benefits of antiretrovirals used in combination compared with their use as monotherapy, with concomitant marked decline in plasma HIV RNA levels. However, none of the current combinations eradicate HIV, and plasma RNA levels rise when therapy is stopped. Combinations of drugs might be expected to be more efficient at delaying the emergence of resistant strains than the use of single agents.

The drugs available for the treatment of HIV infection have increased in number and complexity. Various events in the HIV life-cycle have been identified as potential targets for antiretroviral therapy. Inhibitors of HIV reverse transcriptase and of HIV protease are so far the most developed (Table 1.49), although the integrase inhibitors are being developed.

Nucleoside-analogue reverse-transcriptase inhibitors (NRTIs)

NRTIs inhibit reverse transcriptase and also act as a DNA chain terminator.

Zidovudine (AZT) is well-absorbed with a high bioavailability and penetrates the blood–brain barrier. Adverse effects include nausea, abdominal discomfort, headache and insomnia, but these frequently resolve after several weeks of therapy. The major toxicity is bone marrow suppression leading to anaemia and neutropenia. Megaloblastic change is usual in patients taking the drug. Myopathy may be seen after extended usage. Dose regimens range from 500 to 1000 mg orally daily in divided doses. An intravenous preparation exists for use in specific circumstances such as during labour (see below).

Didanosine (DDI) is a nucleoside analogue of inosine which has a potent anti-HIV effect. It is unstable in acid and so is formulated with a buffer which is taken on an empty stomach twice-daily. Side-effects include nausea, diarrhoea, pancreatitis and polyneuropathy. The standard dose is 200 mg twice-daily. Work is in progress to evaluate the efficacy of 400 mg once daily.

Zalcitabine (DDC), an analogue of cytidine, has a similar activity profile to didanosine although it is acid-stable. The main toxicities are a polyneuropathy and aphthous ulceration of the mouth. The usual dose is 0.75 mg thrice-daily.

Lamivudine, a synthetic dideoxynucleoside analogue, has potent activity against HIV-1 and HIV-2, acting as chain terminator of reverse transcriptase. It also inhibits hepatitis B DNA replication. It is well absorbed, with a bioavailability of 85%. Side-effects are not common, but nausea, headache, rashes and polyneuropathy have been noted. Marrow suppression leading to neutropenia and thrombocytopenia occurs. The dose is 150 mg twice daily, without restriction on food.

Stavudine (D4T) is a thymidine nucleoside analogue exhibiting good anti-HIV activity with a high bioavailability and good penetration of the central nervous system. The major toxicity is polyneuropathy, although some people tolerate reintroduction of the drug at reduced dosage. This may limit combination with other antiretrovirals with overlapping toxicities. There is a theoretical interaction with zidovudine, which competes for phosphorylation pathways to the active triphosphate form. The usual dose is 40 mg twice-daily (30 mg for persons less than 60 kg).

Non-nucleoside reverse-transcriptase inhibitors (NNRTIs)

NNRTIs bind to and inhibit the reverse transcriptase of HIV-1 but are ineffective against HIV-2. The major drugs in this category are *nevirapine* and *delavridine*

Nevirapine has a high bioavailability, a long half-life and wide tissue distribution which includes the central nervous system. Metabolism is via the liver and dependent on cytochrome CYP3A, which has drug interaction implications especially with saquinavir (see below) and ketoconazole. Nevirapine induces its own metabolism and dosing needs to be escalated over the first month of treatment, starting at 200 mg once-daily for two weeks increasing to 200 mg twice-daily thereafter. Nevirapine must be used as part of a powerful combination with other antiretrovirals as resistant strains of HIV emerge within weeks if it is given as monotherapy. Major toxicities are rash and elevation of liver enzymes.

Protease inhibitors

The protease inhibitors act competitively on the HIV aspartyl protease enzyme which is involved in the production of functional viral proteins and enzymes. In consequence, viral maturation is impaired and immature dysfunctional viral particles are produced. Most of the protease inhibitors are active at very low concentrations and *in vitro* are found to have synergy with reverse-transcriptase inhibitors. There appears to be no activity against human aspartyl proteases (e.g. renin), although there are clinically significant interactions with the cytochrome P450 system.

Resistance and cross-resistance are considerations in the use of protease inhibitors. *Ritonavir* and *saquinavir* seem to have different resistance patterns, but mutations leading to ritonavir resistance also appear to reduce the sensitivity of the virus to *indinavir*, and vice versa.

Saquinavir was the first protease inhibitor developed for clinical use. Despite a very potent anti-HIV effect *in vitro*, poor absorbtion (4%) results in very low bioavailability. The drug is at least 98% protein-bound. The current recommended dose is 600 mg three times daily. A new soft gel formulation of saquinavir (1.2 g three times daily with food) is now available and has increased bioavailability. Side-effects include diarrhoea, abdominal pain and nausea.

Ritonavir is a potent protease inhibitor of HIV-1 with bioavailability of about 60%. The efficacy against HIV-2 may be less. It also inhibits human CYP3A and CYP2D6, the two enzymes by which the drug itself is metabolized. The consequences clinically are of potentially serious drug interactions. Ritonavir will reduce the rate of metabolism of drugs using these pathways, and any drugs which themselves induce CYP3A will increase the metabolism of ritonavir. Contraindicated drugs are, *inter alia*, alprazolam, amiodarone, astemizole, cisapride, dextropropoxyphene, diazepam, flecanide, midazolam, pethidine, pimozide, piroxicam, rifabutin and terfenidine. Metabolism of the recreational drug ecstasy may be slowed with potentially catastrophic consequences.

There is evidence that ritonavir may inhibit the metabolism of other proteinase inhibitors, and co-administration of ritonavir and saquinavir has been shown to increase the levels of the latter.

Side-effects associated with starting ritonavir include nausea, diarrhoea and vomiting, although these can be reduced by escalating the dose over the initial few weeks of treatment. Paraesthesia in the hands, feet and around the mouth have been described. The dose is 600 mg twice-daily with food. Capsules need to be stored in a refrigerator.

Indinavir is an increasingly used potent protease inhibitor. The dose is 800 mg thrice-daily, taken two hours after food or with a fat-free snack to ensure optimum absorption. The major toxicity is nephrolithiasis and so adequate hydration must be maintained. Isolated hyperbilirubinaemia has been reported.

Nelfinavir is another of the new proteases which appears to be promising in terms of cross-resistance patterns and efficacy.

Antiretroviral drug therapy in practice

Starting therapy

Although clear clinical benefit has been demonstrated with the use of antiretroviral drugs in advanced HIV disease, the evidence for the introduction of medication at earlier stages of infection is less clear-cut. So far there are no randomized trial data on the use of combination therapy specifically addressing this question. The scientific rationale for early intervention – the 'hit early and hit hard' philosophy – is based on the rapid viral turnover that has been demonstrated throughout all stages of infection, and the view that the earlier and more thoroughly viral replication is suppressed the less likely the immune system is to be damaged and the virus develop resistance. However, it must be remembered that HIV has a long period of clinical latency despite continuing viral activity. None of the current therapeutic regimens is likely to be able to eradicate the virus from an individual, and there is a lack of data on the long-term effectiveness and toxicity of antiretrovirals. Strategic planning in antiretroviral use is becoming increasingly important.

Various national guidelines and treatment frameworks exist (e.g. PACT framework, BHIVA guidelines). In general, a combination of clinical assessment and laboratory marker data, including viral load and CD4 counts, will influence therapeutic decision-making. In the UK, indications to consider initiation of antiretroviral therapy in an adult patient wishing to be treated are any of the following:

- symptomatic HIV disease
- CD4 count < 350
- very rapidly falling CD4 count
- high viral load (> log 4).

Special situations (seroconversion, children, pregnancy, post-exposure prophylaxis) in which antiretrovirals may be used are described on p. 123.

Choice of drugs

The drug regimen used for starting therapy must be individualized to suit the particular patient needs. Factors to be considered include:

- the stage of HIV disease
- clinical trial data, with appropriate extrapolation
- other medical history, e.g. renal stones (*indinavir*)
- drug characterization with regard to efficacy/synergy
- side-effect profile and toxicity considerations
- potential for interactions with other medications
- ease of compliance
- the source of HIV infection
- CNS penetration
- resistance patterns of the individual drugs and the potential to limit future therapeutic manoeuvres via cross-resistance
- the preferences of the patient.

Treatment is initiated with at least two or three drugs depending on the particular circumstances of the individual. Two NRTIs in combination, with or without a proteinase inhibitor or NNRTI, is the foundation of most therapeutic strategies. Proven initial NRTI combinations include zidovudine/didanosine, zidovudine/zalcitabine, and zidovudine/lamivudine. The first two combinations have been successful in large-scale clinical trials, while zidovudine/lamivudine gives similar changes in viral load and CD4 count.

Initiation of therapy with two NRTIs plus a potent protease inhibitor produces a more substantial and longer-lasting reduction in viral load in a greater proportion of patients than that obtained with two NRTIs alone. Two NRTIs plus nevirapine have also been shown to be efficacious. However, the potential for adverse reactions and drug interactions is greater with more drugs, compliance may be more difficult, and drug options for future use may be reduced by this strategy. For these reasons it is not yet clear which approach is best.

The choice of which protease to include in initial therapy is governed by the clinical effectiveness, ease of compliance and the resistance and cross-resistance patterns of the drug. Given that long-term patient compliance is essential to gain the most enduring viral suppression and to impede the emergence of drug resistance, it is crucial that patients be fully involved in therapeutic decision-making throughout and be treated with drug regimens that are manageable as part of their day-to-day lives.

Changing therapy

Changes in antiretroviral therapy may be made if the original combination is felt to be failing in some respect. Reasons for treatment failure include the emergence of resistant viral strains or poor patient compliance. Intolerance or adverse drug reactions may occur. New clinical events that imply progression of HIV disease, a falling CD4 count, a rise in viral load towards pre-treatment values are all reasons to review therapy. The emergence of new data in this rapidly changing field may lead to therapeutic changes.

If the patient is stable but a change needs to be made then one or more drugs may be altered. If, however, the patient is deteriorating clinically, virologically or immunologically then two or more drug changes should be made, either additions or substitutions. The compounds chosen at this stage must take account both of past drug exposure which might be expected to have engendered viral resistance, and future therapeutic options which ideally should not be compromised.

Stopping therapy

Stopping antiretroviral drugs may be the proper course of action in a number of circumstances. Examples of this are cumulative toxicity, or potential drug interactions with medications needed to deal with another more pressing problem. Poor quality of life and the view of the patient on the matter must be considered.

Specific therapeutic situations

Acute seroconversion

Antiretroviral therapy in patients presenting with an acute seroconversion illness is controversial. Preliminary evidence shows that the viral load can be reduced substantially by aggressive therapy at this stage, although it rises when treatment is withdrawn. The longer-term clinical sequelae are not yet known. If treatment is contemplated in this situation an aggressive approach is likely to be most appropriate, although the risk of limiting future options must be assessed.

Pregnancy

Management of HIV-infected pregnant women requires close collaboration between obstetric, medical and paediatric teams. Antiretroviral therapy may be initiated for maternal indications depending on clinical, immunological and virological assessment. Although zidovudine is the only drug licensed for use in pregnancy, current US guidelines suggest combination therapy should be used.

A further indication for the use of antiretroviral agents in pregnancy is to reduce the risk of transmission of HIV to the fetus. Data from a randomized placebo-controlled clinical trial of zidovudine in pregnancy (ACTG 076) showed a 67.5% reduction in vertical transmission with use of the drug. However, the timing of maternofetal transmission is unclear, and the long-term toxicity of zidovudine on the infant is unknown. Given a vertical transmission rate of 15% without intervention, 85% of babies who are uninfected will be exposed to zidovudine.

Treatment of the mother with zidovudine monotherapy is at variance with the data on combination therapy for adults as described above. This may have longer-term implications for the course of the mother's HIV infection, particularly with regard to the possible emergence of zidovudine-resistant virus. On the other hand, early data suggest that since the availability of zidovudine prophylaxis in pregnancy the numbers of HIV-infected children born to HIV-positive mothers has fallen substantially.

Pregnant HIV-infected women should be made aware of all these facts and treatment decisions made in this knowledge. Those electing to take the drug should be given zidovudine orally in a dose of 100 mg five times daily from the second trimester. During labour, intravenous zidovudine should be given at a dose of 2 mg kg^{-1} for the first hour, reducing to 1 mg kg^{-1} per hour thereafter until delivery. The neonate should be given zidovudine syrup at a dose of 2 mg kg^{-1} for the first six weeks of life.

Children

The management of HIV infection in children should be carried out by pediatricians with specialized knowledge of current practice. Many of the drugs available for adult use do not have paediatric licences.

Post-exposure prophylaxis

The use of zidovudine following needlestick injuries or other parenteral exposure with known HIV-infected material has been shown to reduce but not remove the risk of seroconversion in healthcare workers. Expert advice should be sought promptly.

Treatment will depend upon a number of factors, including the clinical status and antiretroviral history of the source patient, the severity of the exposure, and the medical needs of the recipient. The combination of zidovudine and lamivudine with or without indinavir, taken for 4–6 weeks, is the recommendation of the UK Expert Advisory Group on AIDS (EAGA) if prophylaxis is elected.

Prevention and control

The development of an effective vaccine against HIV is being pursued and progress is being made.

Changing behaviour is therefore the main tool available for prevention of infection. This is notoriously difficult, especially in areas that carry as many taboos as HIV and AIDS. Education programmes providing factual knowledge and strategies to avoid infection are fundamental to the process. The use of condoms has been shown to reduce the spread of HIV infection in discordant couples and their use has been strongly promoted.

Control of other STDs is also crucial, particularly in view of their role in enhancing HIV transmission. Some STD control programmes in Africa are beginning to bear fruit with a reduction in STDs and a consequent fall in HIV transmission rates. Access to clean needles and syringes to prevent sharing amongst drug users is important, as are programmes to reduce drug use.

Screening of blood products has reduced iatrogenic infection in developed countries but is expensive and not globally available. The need for blood transfusions in developing countries could be reduced by improved control of conditions such as malaria and hookworm which lead to chronic anaemia.

Partner notification schemes are developing but are sensitive and controversial. Availability and accessibility of confidential HIV testing is important and provides an opportunity for individual health education and risk reduction to be discussed.

FURTHER READING

Adler M (1997) *The ABC of AIDS*, 4th edn. London: BMA Publications.

British HIV Association (1997) Guidelines for antiretroviral treatment of HIV seropositive individuals *Lancet* **349**: 1086-1092.

Flexner C (1998) HIV protease inhibitors. *New England Journal of Medicine* **338**: 1281-1292.

Sexually transmitted diseases (1998) *Lancet* **351** Suppl III.

GENERAL READING

Mandell GL, Bennett JE, Dolin R (eds) (1995) Mandell, Douglas and Bennett's Principles and Practice of Infectious Diseases, 4th edn. Churchill Livingstone, Edinburgh.

Lambert HP, O'Grady F, Finch P, Greenwood D (1996) Antibiotic and Chemotherapy, 7th edn. Churchill Livingstone, Edinburgh.

Halstead SB (1992) Arboviruses of the Pacific and Southeast Asia, In: Feigin RD, Cherry JD (eds) Textbook of Pediatric Infectious Diseases, 3rd edn. Vol II. WB Saunders, Philadelphia, pp. 1468-1488

Tropical Medicine (1997) Supplement to *Lancet* **349**: 1-32

Cell and molecular biology, genetic disorders and immunology

2

The cell: structure and function

Most cells within the human body are specialized to perform certain specific functions (for example, absorptive cells). However, all cells have certain common structures or *organelles* which are essential for their function (Fig 2.1). Each cell is a compact unit, but it can 'talk' to an adjacent cell via specific channels. Within a cell, there is a constant flow of traffic between the organelles.

The cell membrane

The cell membrane consists of a bilayer of non-polar and amphipathic lipid molecules. It is a dynamic fluid compartment and acts as a barrier for water and hydrophilic solutes.

The major lipids in the membrane are phospholipids such as phosphatidylcholine and phosphatidylethanolamine and cholesterol. The phospholipids are amphipathic molecules with the phosphate portion being relatively soluble in water (polar or hydrophilic) while the fatty acid tails are insoluble (non-polar or hydrophobic).

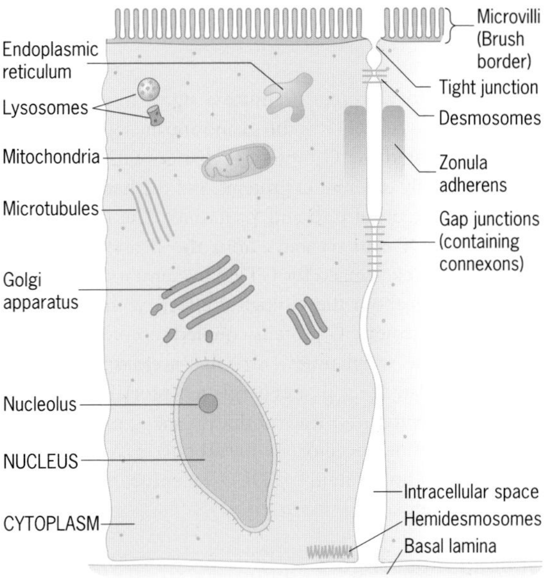

Fig 2.1
Ultrastructure of the cell. This is an intestinal cell showing the cellular constituents and connections with an adjacent cell

The hydrophilic ends of the molecules are exposed to the outside of the cells whilst the hydrophobic ends are in the lipid interior of the cell.

Proteins are found either within the membrane or attached to the exterior or interior surface. Some proteins are *structural* while others are functional, acting as *pumps* (e.g. the sodium pump which actively transports sodium out of the cell). Other proteins act as carriers, transporting solutes (e.g. glucose) into a cell. *Ion channels* are also made up of proteins involved in transport of electrolytes across the membrane (see Fig 2.20). The exterior proteins act as *receptors* (see p. 896), and immunoglobulins are also found in the cell membrane. Finally, *enzymes* (e.g. alkaline phosphatase) are part of the membrane structure.

Receptors

Specific receptor molecules that are present on the outer surface of the membrane of target cells interact with physiological ligands, such as lipoproteins, immunoglobulins, peptide hormones, and neurotransmitters; these are *first messengers*. The activated receptor then interacts with an enzyme system within the cell that produces *second messengers*, such as cyclic adenosine monophosphate (cAMP), inositol triphosphate (IP_3) and diacylglycerol (DAG). These in turn trigger a chain of intracellular reactions that eventually leads to the usual response of the cell to its physiological ligand (see Fig 16.1 on p. 897).

The number of receptors on a cell membrane increases and decreases in response to stimuli. Thus, for example, if a neurotransmitter or hormone (first messenger) is present in excess, the number of active receptors decreases (down-regulation); if there is a deficiency the number of receptors increases (up-regulation).

When activated, these receptors initiate the release of the second messengers via GTP-binding proteins (G protein).

G proteins

These regulatory proteins translate a signal to a biological event within a cell. GTP is the guanosine analogue of ATP. When stimulated the G protein exchanges GDP for GTP. There are many different G proteins, and the heterotrimeric ones are made up of α, β and γ subunits. The α subunit is bound to GDP and separates from the β and γ subunits when GDP is exchanged for GTP. This separation of the α subunit brings about the biological effects within the cell. These heterotrimeric G protein-coupled receptors span the cell membrane seven times (*serpentine receptors*) and many have been isolated (e.g. β_2 adrenergic receptor). Defective or damaged receptors can lead to disease states; examples are the acetylcholine receptor in myasthenia gravis, and the low-density lipoprotein (LDL) receptor in familial hypercholesterolaemia.

Second messengers

These can alter the function of the cell in the short term in many ways. For example, they can trigger exocytosis, alter enzyme function or induce transcription of many genes. They do this by activating protein kinases which catalyse the phosphorylation of, for example, tyrosine or serine residues in proteins (see p. 345).

Differential domains

Certain areas of the cell membrane are structurally different; for example, the low-density lipoprotein (LDL) receptor lies in an evagination or 'pit'. This pit is coated with heavy and light chains of clathrin (see Fig 17.1 on p. 960). These coated pits become detached and form coated vesicles (endocytosis). Another example is the absorptive cell which has a characteristic brush border with microvilli containing enzymes for digestion.

Cell-to-cell recognition and communication (see also p. 129)

At certain points the cell membrane is joined to its neighbouring cell and intercellular channels allow diffusion of ions or small molecules (Fig 2.2).

Cytoplasm

The cytoplasm contains many specialized organelles that serve different functions. These include *storage* of substances (e.g. glycogen and lipids), the *synthesis* of essential substances (e.g. amino acids, fatty acids, monosaccharides), the *metabolism* of these substances, and *protein synthesis* and

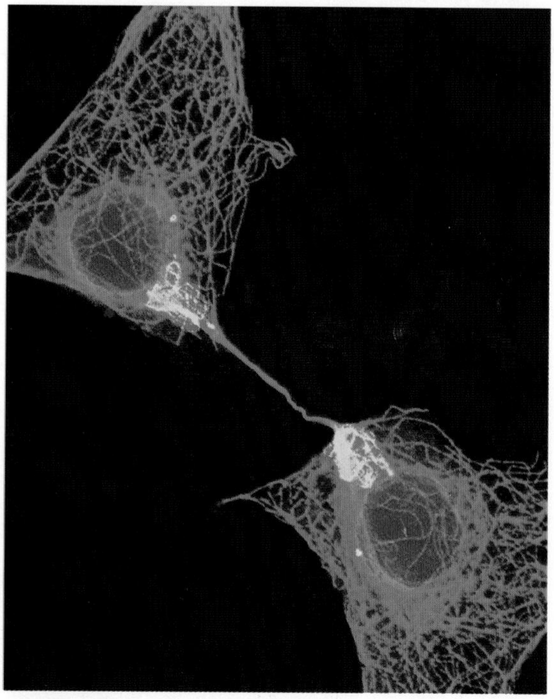

Fig 2.2
Immunofluorescence of dividing fibroblasts. Microtubules are shown in green, Golgi apparatus in yellow and the nuclei in blue. (Reproduced with permission of Dr Philip Huie, Stanford University, from *Biotechniques* July/August 1995)

translation. Microtubules are cylindrical structures formed from the protein tubulin; they help to maintain the structure of the cells and form channels for communication between the subcellular organelles.

Endoplasmic reticulum

This is a network of tubules throughout the cytoplasm from the nucleus to the cell membrane. It is divided into:

- the nuclear *membrane* surrounding the nucleus and controlling traffic in and out of the nucleus
- the *rough endoplasmic reticulum* (RER), which is lined by ribosomes that synthesize proteins
- the *smooth endoplasmic reticulum* (SER), consisting of tubules and vesicles containing microsomes.

Endoplasmic reticulum is involved in the processing of secretory proteins. Some contain enzyme systems (e.g. mixed-function oxygenases, including cytochrome P450) that hydroxylate hydrophobic compounds, making them more soluble and therefore easier to metabolize (e.g. vitamin D) or eliminate (e.g. drugs).

The Golgi apparatus

This consists of channels or vesicles. Functions include modification and packaging of secretory proteins, transport of lysosomal enzymes to lysosomes, and storage. The Golgi apparatus acts as a focal point for the complex intracellular traffic that takes place between all of the subcellular components.

Mitochondria

These consist of double membranes with an extensively infolded inner membrane, forming cristae. There are several hundred per cell. They contain enzymes responsible for oxidative phosphorylation, the citric acid cycle, the electron-transport chain and ATP synthesis. ATP is the principal source of energy in man. Mitochondria contain their own DNA, and teleologically they were autonomous micro-organisms that became incorporated into the eukarytic cell. Proteins of the oncogene family *Bcl*-2 are found in the outer membrane of the mitochondria where they inhibit or facilitate apoptosis (see p. 153).

Lysosomes

These contain digestive enzymes, mostly acid hydrolases, capable of digesting many constituents of cells and tissues. The substrates can enter the lysosome directly or via the Golgi apparatus. Lysosomes are involved in:

- the killing and digesting of infective agents by polymorphs and macrophages
- removal of unwanted cells during embryonic development
- disposal of excess secretory products in glandular cells
- osteoclastic remodelling of bone by secreted enzymes.

Lysosomal proteolysis is not quantitatively important in the normal turnover of most cellular proteins. Most are degraded by a multienzymatic process that requires ATP. The proteins are repeatedly linked to a small protein co-factor, ubiquitin, via their lysine residues. These ubiquitin conjugated proteins which contain five or more ubiquitin molecules are rapidly degraded by a large proteolytic complex, the 26S proteasome. This ubiquitin–proteasome pathway is capable of selectively degrading most cell proteins.

The cytoskeleton

This consists of a complex network of structural elements which determine the shape of the cell, its ability to move and to respond to external stimuli. The major components are microtubules, intermediate filaments and microfilaments.

- *Microtubules*. These are made up of two protein subunits α and β tubulin (50 kDa) and are continuously changing length. They form a 'highway' for motor proteins to move up and down the cell. Thus if an organelle is attached to a motor protein it can rapidly travel through the cytoplasm. There are two motor microtubule-associated proteins (MAP) – dynein and kinesin – allowing antegrade and retrograde movement. Dynein is also responsible for the beating of cilia. During interphase the microtubules are rearranged by the microtubule organizing centre (MTOC), which consists of centrosomes containing tubulin and provides a structure on which the daughter chromosomes can separate. Another protein involved in the binding of organelles to microtubules is the cytoplasmic linker protein (CLIP). The intracellular position of the Golgi apparatus also involves microtubules. Drugs that disrupt the microtubule assembly (e.g. colchicine and vinblastine) affect the positioning and morphology of the organelles (Golgi apparatus and mitochondria). The anticancer drug paclitaxel causes cell death by binding to microtubules and stabilizing them so much that organelles cannot move, and thus mitotic spindles cannot form.
- *Intermediate filaments*. These form a network around the nucleus and extend to the periphery of the cell. They make cell-to-cell contacts with the adjacent cells via desmosomes. Their function is uncertain but they may have a structural role.
- *Microfilaments*. Muscle cells contain a highly ordered structure of actin (a globular protein, 42–44 kDa) and myosin filaments which form the contractile system. These filaments are also present throughout the non-muscle cells as truncated myosins (e.g. myosin 1), in the cytosol (forming a contractile actomyosin gel), and beneath the plasma membrane. Cell movement is mediated by the ancorage of actin filaments to the plasma membrane and these filaments control the organization and shape of the cell.

Actin-binding proteins (e.g. fimbria) modulate the behaviour of microfilaments and their effects are often calcium-dependent. Control of the actin cytoskeleton may be partly controlled by small *ras*-like GTP-binding proteins.

Intracellular calcium and calcium-binding proteins

Calcium within the cell plays a major role in signalling. Most of the calcium is bound by the endoplasmic reticulum and by the other organelles. Calcium enters the cell by voltage-gated Ca^{2+} channels (activated by depolarization) and ligand-gated channels (activated by hormones and neurotransmitters). Ca^{2+}-H^{+}-ATPase pumps calcium ions out of the cell in exchange for hydrogen ions. Second messengers frequently act by increasing cytoplasmic calcium concentration.

There are many calcium-binding proteins, such as troponin (involved in contraction of skeletal muscle), calmodulin and calbindin. Calmodulin, by binding Ca^{2+}, activates many calmodulin-dependent kinases, such as myosin light-chain kinase (which phosphorylates myosin), phosphorylase kinase (activates phosphorylation), and calcineurin (which inactivates calcium channels). Calmodulin kinases are also involved with synaptic function, activating T cells, and can be inhibited by immunosuppressants. Calbindin binds and transports calcium ions across membranes.

The nucleus

A nucleus is present in all eukaryotic cells that divide. It contains the cell's genome, consisting of DNA and all the apparatus for replication and transcription into RNA (see p. 131). When the cell is not dividing, the nuclear envelope – consisting of an outer and an inner membrane – separates it from the cytoplasm. The outer membrane is continuous with the endoplasmic reticulum.

A *nucleolus* (rich in RNA) is present in most nuclei, and nucleoli are the site of synthesis for ribosomes. There are two types of cell division – meiosis and mitosis. In *meiosis*, which occurs only in germ cells, the chromosome complement is halved (haploid) and, at fertilization, the union of two cells restores the full complement of 46 chromosomes. *Mitosis* occurs in dividing cells after fertilization, and results in two identical daughter cells. It is only during cell division that chromosomes (see p. 139) become visible.

The cell cycle (Fig 2.3)

Regulation of the cell cycle is complex. Cells in the quiescent G0 phase (G, gap) of the cycle are stimulated by the receptor-mediated actions of growth factors (e.g. EGF, epithelial growth factor; PDGF, platelet-derived growth factor; IGF, insulin growth factor) via intracellular second messengers. Stimuli are transmitted to the nucleus (see below) where they activate transcription factors and lead to the initiation of DNA synthesis, followed by mitosis and cell division. Cell cycling is modified by the cyclin family of proteins which activate (by phosphorylation via kinases) proteins involved in DNA replication. Thus from G0 the cell moves on to G1 (gap 1) when the chromosomes are prepared for replication. This is followed by the synthetic (S) phase, when the 46 chromosomes are duplicated into chromatids, followed by another gap phase (G2) which eventually leads to mitosis (M).

Cytokines (e.g. interferon) bind to receptors on target cells, causing the formation of protein complexes that are transferred to the nucleus. These receptors are part of a signalling complex (the JAK-STAT pathway) made up of JANUS kinases (JAK) and signal transducers and activators of transcription (STATs).

Binding of interferon brings the JANUS kinases close to each other. They, the receptor chain and the STATs are activated by phosphorylation. The STAT dimer is transferred to the nucleus where it binds to regulatory DNA elements, thereby activating the genes that encode for the protein mediators produced by interferon stimulation.

Intercellular connections

There are two types of junction between cells, tight junctions and gap junctions (see Fig 2.1).

Tight junctions

These (zonula occludens) hold cells together. They are at the apical margins of epithelial cells (e.g. intestinal and renal cells) and form a barrier to the movement of ions and solutes across the epithelium, although they can be variably 'leaky' to certain solutes. The zonula adherens is continuous on the basal side of cells, it contains cadherins, and is the major site of the attachment of intracellular microfilaments. Intermediate filaments attach to desmosomes, which are apposed areas of thickened membranes of two adjacent cells.

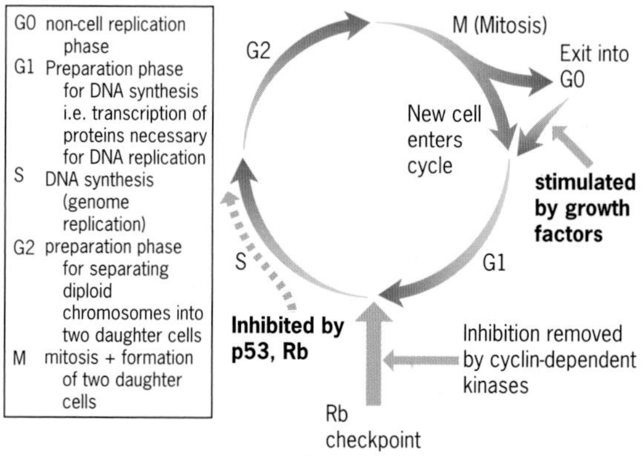

Fig 2.3
The cell cycle. Cells are stimulated to leave non-cycle G0 to enter G1 phase by growth factors. During G1, transcription of the DNA synthesis molecules occurs. Rb is a 'checkpoint' (inhibition molecule) between G1 and S phases and must be removed for the cycle to continue. This is achieved by the action of the cyclin-dependent kinase produced during G1. During the S phase any DNA defects will be detected and *p53* will halt the cycle (see p. 152). Following DNA synthesis (S phase) cells enter G2, a preparation phase for cell division. Mitosis takes place in the M phase. The new daughter cells can now either enter G0 and differentiate into specialized cells, or re-enter the cell cycle

Hemidesmosomes attach cells to the basal lamina and are also connected to intermediate filaments. Trans-membrane integrins link the extracellular matrix to microfilaments at focal areas where cells also attach to their basal laminae.

Gap junctions

These allow substances to pass directly between cells without entering the extracellular fluids. Protein channels (connexons) are lined up between two adjacent cells and allow the passage of solutes up to molecular weight 1000 kDa (e.g. amino acids and sugars), as well as ions, chemical messengers and other factors. The diameter of these channels is regulated by intracellular Ca^{2+}, pH and voltage. Connexons are made up of six subunits surrounding a channel and its isoforms in tissues are encased by different genes. Mutant connexons can cause disorders, such as the X-linked form of Charcot–Marie–Tooth disease (p. 1096).

Cell adhesion molecules (see also p. 167)

Cells are attached to the basal membrane and to each other by cell adhesion molecules (CAMS). There are four types:

- *integrins* that bind to receptors
- *adhesion molecules* of the IgG super-family of immunoglobulins, which bind to other molecules
- *cadherins*, which are calcium-dependent molecules that mediate cell-to-cell adhesion
- *selectins*, which have lectin-like domains that bind to carbohydrates.

Many of these cell adhesion molecules bind to laminins, which are molecules found in the extracellular matrix (see Fig 20.26).

FURTHER READING

Mitch WE, Goldberg AL (1996) The role of the ubiquitin-proteasome pathway. *New England Journal of Medicine* **335**: 1897–1905.

Cohen N (ed) (1991) Cell structure, function and metabolism. Hodder and Stoughton, Open University Press, UK.

Molecular biology and genetic disorders

Over 200 genetic disorders have been identified, and the role of molecular biology in the diagnosis of monogenic disease is clear cut. The interaction of 'at risk' genes in multifactorial diseases has also increased the role of genetics in rheumatology, cancer, schizophrenia and many other more common human afflictions. The future promise of direct gene therapy makes the understanding of the principles and the basic tools of molecular genetics essential.

A glossary of terms commonly used in genetics is given in Information box 2.1.

DNA structure and function

Genetic information is stored in the form of double-stranded deoxyribonucleic acid (DNA). Each strand of DNA is made up of a deoxyribose–phosphate backbone and a series of purine (adenine (A) and guanine (G)) and pyrimidine (thymine (T) and cytosine (C)) bases of the nucleic acid. For practical purposes the length of DNA is generally measured in numbers of base-pairs (bp).

The monomeric unit in DNA (and in RNA) is the nucleotide, which is a base joined to a sugar–phosphate unit (Fig 2.4(a)). The two strands of DNA are held together by hydrogen bonds between the bases. There are only four possible pairs of nucleotides – TA, AT, GC and CG (Fig 2.4(b)). The two strands twist to form a double helix with major and minor grooves, and the large stretches of helical DNA are coiled around histone proteins to form nucleosomes and further condensed into the chromosomes that are seen at metaphase (Figs 2.4(c) and (d)).

Genes

A gene is a portion of DNA that contains the codes for a polypeptide sequence. Three adjacent nucleotides (a *codon*) code for a particular amino acid, such as AGA for arginine, and TTC for phenylalanine. There are only 20 common amino acids, but 64 possible codon combinations that make up the genetic code. This means that some amino acids are encoded for by more than one triplet; other codons are used as signals for 'initiating' or 'terminating' polypeptide-chain synthesis, while others read as 'nonsense' and no amino acid is produced.

Genes consist of lengths of DNA that contain sufficient nucleotide triplets to code for the appropriate number of amino acids in the polypeptide chains of a particular protein. Genes vary greatly in size: most extend over 20–40 kbp, but a few, such as the gene for the muscle protein dystrophin, can extend over millions of base-pairs.

In bacteria the coding sequences are continuous, but in higher organisms these coding sequences (exons) are interrupted by intervening sequences that are non-coding (introns) at various positions (see Fig 2.5). Some genes code for RNA molecules which will not be further translated into proteins. The genes code for functional ribosomal RNA (rRNA) and transfer RNA (tRNA), which play vital roles in polypeptide synthesis.

Information

Acrocentric. Term used to describe a chromosome in which the centromere lies close to one end, producing one long and one short arm

Allele (allelomorph). Alternative form of a gene occupying the same locus on a particular chromosome

Aneuploid. Any chromosomal number that is not the exact multiple of the normal haploid number

Autosome. Any chromosome that is not a sex chromosome or mitochondrial chromosome; there are 22 pairs of autosomes in humans

Bacteriophage. A bacterial virus; these are modified and used as vectors for DNA cloning

cDNA. DNA synthesized from an mRNA template by the enzyme reverse transcriptase

Centromere. The point at which two chromatids of a chromosome are joined, and also where the spindle fibres become attached during mitosis and meiosis

Character (trait). An observable phenotypic feature of an individual

Chromatid. One of the two strands, held together by the centromere, that make up the chromosome as seen during cell division

Chromatin. Genomic DNA coiled and supercoiled in association with histone proteins

Chromosomal aberration. An abnormality in the number or structure of a chromosome

Chromosome. A thread-like body containing DNA and protein, situated in the nucleus, and carrying genetic information

Clone. Cells having the same genetic constitution and derived from a single cell by repeated mitoses

Codon. Three adjacent nucleotides in a nucleic acid that code for one amino acid

Concordance. The occurrence of the same trait in both members of a pair of twins

Deletion. Loss of a part of a chromosome

Diploid. The number of chromosomes found in somatic cells, i.e. two sets

DNA ligase. The enzyme that joins two DNA ends together

DNA polymerase. The enzyme that replicates DNA

Dominant. Term used to describe a trait expressed in individuals who are heterozygous for a particular gene

Episomal DNA. Gene carrying DNA found outside the main genome; i.e. bacterial plasmids and mitochondrial DNA

Eukaryote. Organisms whose genome is bound by a nuclear membrane

Euchromatin. Regions of chromosome which are not tightly coiled and therefore accessible for gene expression

Exon. A segment of a gene that is represented in the final spliced mRNA product

Expressivity. The degree to which the effect of a gene is expressed

Gene. Part of a DNA molecule that directs the synthesis of a specific polypeptide chain

Gene pool. The total genetic information contained in all the genes in a breeding population at a given time

Genetic marker. A genetically controlled phenotypic feature used in inheritance studies

Genetics. The science of heredity and variation

Genome. The total amount of genetic material in the cell

Genotype. The genetic constitution of an individual

Haploid. The number of chromosomes found in germ cells, i.e. one set

Heterochromatin. Condensed chromatin where supercoiling prevents expression of the encoded genes

Heterozygote. An individual possessing two different alleles at the corresponding loci on a pair of homologous chromosomes

Histones. Nuclear proteins which hold genomic DNA in coils and supercoils

Homozygote. An individual possessing identical alleles at the corresponding loci on a pair of homologous chromosomes

Hybridization. The pairing of complementary DNA or RNA strands to give DNA–DNA or DNA–RNA strands; for example, it is used to search for particular DNA fragments after Southern blotting

Intron. A segment of a gene not represented in the final mRNA product because it has been removed through splicing together of exons on each side of it

Karyotype. The number, size and shape of the chromosomes in a cell

Linkage. The co-segregation of two unrelated DNA sequences which are physically close together on the chromosome

Linkage disequilibrium. The association of particular alleles at two linked loci more frequently than expected by chance

Locus. The site of a gene on a chromosome

Metacentric. Term used to describe a chromosome in which the centromere lies in the middle

Monosomy. A state in which one chromosome of a pair is missing

Mosaics. Patients with two different cell lines in their constitution

Non-disjunction. Failure of a chromosome pair to separate during cell division, resulting in both chromosomes passing to the same daughter cell

Information box 2.1 Glossary of terms in molecular biology

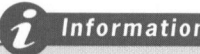

Information

Nucleotide. The basic unit of nucleic acids, which is made up of a pyrimidine or purine base, a pentose sugar and a phosphate group

Oncogenes. Normal genes which when altered in their structure or expression contribute to the abnormal growth of cancer cells

Penetrance. The proportion of individuals with a particular genotype who also have the corresponding phenotype; full penetrance occurs when a dominant trait is always seen in an individual with one such allele, or when a recessive trait is seen in all individuals possessing two such alleles

Phenotype. The appearance of an individual, resulting from the effects of both environment and genes

Plasmid. A simple circular DNA molecule derived from bacteria which can be modified and used as a vector for DNA cloning

Ploidy. Term that describes the number of chromosome sets, namely 23 = haploid (1 set), 46 = diploid (2 sets)

Polymerase chain-reaction (PCR). Technique for rapid analysis of DNA; oligonucleotide primers corresponding to each end of DNA of interest are synthesized and amplified in genomic DNA using DNA polymerase

Positional cloning (or reverse genetics). Methodology used to isolate genes whose protein products are not known but whose existence can be inferred from the disease phenotype

Prokaryote. Organisms whose genome is not bound by a nuclear membrane

Pulsed-field gel electrophoresis. Technique for separation of large fragments of DNA

Recessive. Term used to describe a trait expressed in individuals who are homozygous for a particular gene but not seen in the heterozygote

Restriction fragment length polymorphisms (RFLPs). When variations in non-coding DNA sequences affect restriction enzyme cleavage sites, DNA fragments of different sizes (RFLPs) will result from enzyme digestion

RNA polymerase. The enzyme that synthesizes RNA, based on a DNA template

Sex linkage. Genes carried on the sex chromosomes

'Somy'. Term referring to the number of copies of an individual chromosome per cell, e.g. 'trisomy' = three copies

Splicing. Removing the introns from an unprocessed RNA molecule

Synteny. Term used to describe genes on the same chromosome

Transcription. The process by which an RNA molecule is synthesized from a DNA template

Translation. The process by which genetic information from mRNA is 'translated' into protein synthesis

Translocation. The transfer of a piece of one chromosome to another non-homologous chromosome

Trisomy. Representation of a chromosome three times rather than twice, giving a total of 47 chromosomes

tRNA. Transfer RNA, a molecule which carries a single amino acid (depending on its anticodon) and which brings the amino acid to the ribosome

Vector. A DNA molecule used to carry DNA regions of interest

Information box 2.1 (*cont.*) Glossary of terms in molecular biology

Transcription and translation (Fig 2.5)

The conversion of genetic information to polypeptides and proteins relies on the transcription of sequences of bases in DNA to RNA molecules. These messenger (m) RNAs are found mainly in the nucleolus and the cytoplasm, and are polymers of nucleotides containing a ribose–phosphate unit attached to a base. The bases are adenine, guanine, cytosine and uracil (U) (which replaces the thymine found in DNA). RNA is a single-stranded molecule but it can hybridize with a complementary sequence of single-stranded DNA (ssDNA). Genetic information is carried from the nucleus to the cytoplasm by mRNA, which in turn acts as a template for protein synthesis.

Each base in the mRNA molecule is lined up opposite to the corresponding base in the DNA: C to G, G to C, U to A and A to T. A gene is always read in the 5′–3′ orientation and at 5′ promoter sites which specifically bind the enzyme RNA polymerase and so indicate where transcription is to commence. Eukaryotic genes have two AT-rich promoter sites. The first, the TATA box, is located about 25 bp upstream of (or before) the transcription start site, while the second, the CAAT box, is 75 bp upstream of the start site. The initial or primary mRNA is a complete copy of one strand of DNA and therefore contains both introns and exons. While still in the nucleus the mRNA undergoes post-transcriptional modification whereby the 5′ and 3′ ends are protected by the addition of an inverted guanidine nucleotide (CAP) and a chain of adenine nucleotides (PolyA) (see Fig 2.5). In higher organisms the primary transcript mRNA is further processed inside the nucleus whereby the introns are spliced out. Splicing is achieved by small nuclear RNA in association with specific proteins. Furthermore, alternative splicing is possible whereby an entire exon can be omitted. Thus more than one protein can be coded from the same gene.

The processed mRNA then migrates out of the nucleus into the cytoplasm. Polysomes (groups of ribosomes)

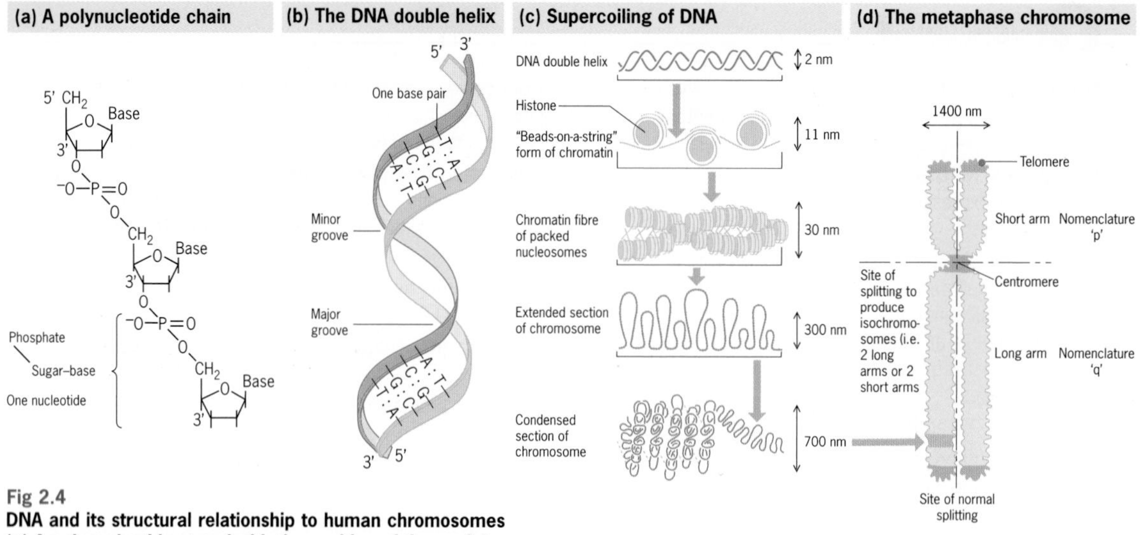

Fig 2.4
DNA and its structural relationship to human chromosomes
(a) A polynucleotide strand with the position of the nucleic bases indicated. Individual nucleotides form a polymer linked via the deoxyribose sugars. The 5′ carbon of the heterocyclic sugar structure links to the 3′ carbon of the next via a phosphate molecule forming the sugar–phosphate backbone of the nucleic acid. The 5′–3′ linkage gives an orientation to a sequence of DNA
(b) Double-stranded DNA. The two strands of DNA are held together by hydrogen bonds between the bases. As T always pairs with A, and G with C, there are only four possible pairs of nucleotides – TA, AT, GC and CG. The orientation of the complementary single strands of DNA (ssDNA) is always opposite; i.e. one will be 5′–3′ whilst the partner will be 3′–5′. CG base-pairs form three hydrogen bonds whilst the AT bonds form only two. Thus, CG bonds are stronger than AT bonds, which affects the biophysical nature of different sequences of DNA. In a random sequence of DNA with equal proportions of CG and AT base-pairs, complementary strands form a helical 3D structure. This helix will have major and minor grooves and a complete turn of the helix will contain 12 base-pairs. These grooves are structurally important as DNA-binding proteins predominantly interact with the major grooves. DNA sequences rich in repetitive CG base-pairs distort the helical shape whereby the minor grooves become more equal in size to the major grooves, giving a Z-like structure. These CG-rich regions are sites were DNA-binding proteins are likely to bind.
(c) Supercoiling of DNA. In humans, and other higher organisms, the large stretches of helical DNA are coiled to form nucleosomes and further condensed into the chromosomes that can be seen at metaphase. DNA is first packaged by winding around nuclear proteins – histones – every 180 bp. This can then be coiled and supercoiled to compact nucleosomes and eventually visible chromosomes.
(d) At the end of the metaphase DNA replication will result in a twin chromosome joined at the centromere. This picture shows the chromosome, its relationship to supercoiling, and the position of structural regions: centromeres, telomeres and sites where the double chromosome can split
Nomenclature of chromosomes. This is the assigned number or X or Y plus short arm (p) or long arm (q). The region or subregion is defined by the transverse light and dark bands observed when staining with Giemsa (hence G-banding) or quinacrine and numbered from the centromere outwards
Chromosome constitution = chromosome number + sex chromosomes + abnormality; e.g.
46XX = normal female
47XX+21 = Down's syndrome (trisomy 21)
46XYt (2;19) (p21;p12) = male with a normal number of chromosomes but a translocation between chromosome 2 and 19 with breakages at short-arm bands 21 and 12 of the respective chromosomes.

become attached to the mRNA; the ribosomes consist of subunits composed of small RNA molecules (rRNA) and proteins. The rRNA components are key to the binding and translation of the genetic code. Held by the ribosomes, triplets of adjacent bases on the mRNA called codons are exposed and recognized by complementary sequences, or anti-codons, in transfer RNA (tRNA) molecules. Each tRNA molecule carries an amino acid that is specific to the anti-codon. As the ribosome passes along the mRNA in the 5′–3′ direction, amino acids are transferred from tRNA molecules and sequentially linked by the ribosome in the order dictated by the order of codons. The ribosome, in effect, moves along the mRNA like a 'zipper', linking the assembled amino acids to form a polypeptide chain. The first 20 or more nucleotides are recognition and regulatory sequences and are untranslated but necessary for translation and possibly earlier transcription. Translation begins when the triplet AUG (methionine) is encountered. All proteins start with methionine but this is often lost as the leading sequence of amino acids of the native peptides are removed during protein folding and post-translational modification into a mature protein. Similarly the Poly A tail is not translated (3′ untranslated region) and is proceeded by a stop codon, UAA, UAG or UGA.

The control of gene expression

Gene expression can be controlled at many points in the steps between the translation of DNA to proteins. Proteins and RNA molecules are in a constant state of turnover; as soon as they are produced, processes for their destruction are at work. For many genes transcriptional control is the most important point of regulation. Deleterious, even oncogenic, changes to a cell's biology

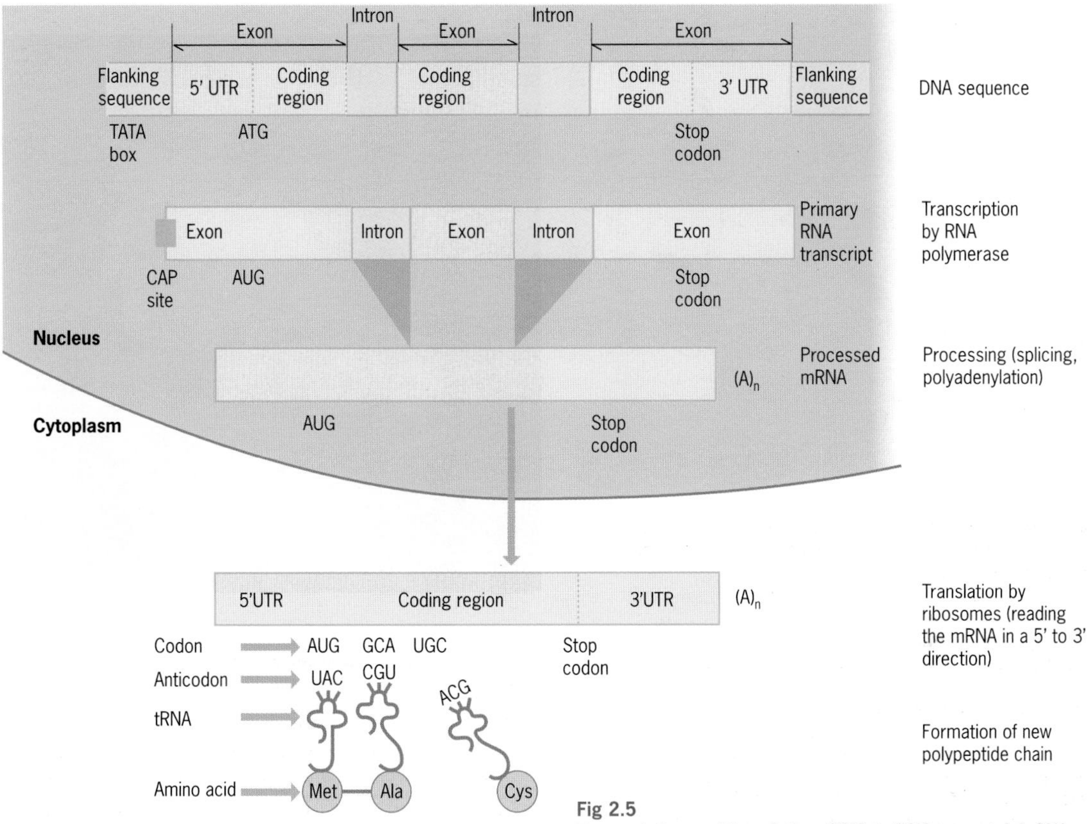

Fig 2.5
Transcription and translation (DNA to RNA to protein). RNA polymerase creates an RNA copy of the gene sequence. This primary transcript is processed: capping of the 5′ free end of the mRNA precursor involves the addition of an inverted guanine residue to the 5′ terminal which is subsequently methylated forming a 7-methylguanosine residue. (The corresponding position on the gene is thus called the CAP site.) The 3′ end of an mRNA defined by the sequence AAUAAA acts as a cleavage signal for an endonuclease which cleaves the growing transcript about 20 bp downstream from the signal. The 3′ end is further processed by a Poly A polymerase which adds about 250 adenosine residues to the 3′ end, forming a Poly A tail (polyadenylation). Without these additions the mRNA sequence will be rapidly degraded 5′–3′ but the inverted cap nucleotide prevents nuclease attachment. The activity of specific 5′ mRNA nucleases to remove the cap is further regulated by the Poly A tail which must first be removed by other degradation enzymes. Splicing out of the introns then produces the mature mRNA (prokaryote genes do not contain introns). This then moves out of the nucleus via nuclear pores and aligns on endoplasmic reticulum. Ribosomal subunits assemble on the mRNA moving along 5′ to 3′. With the transport of amino acids to their active sites by specific tRNAs, the complex translates the code producing the peptide sequence. Once formed the peptide is released into the cytoplasmic reticulum for post-translational modification into a mature protein

may arise through no fault in the expression of a particular gene. Apparent over-expression may be due to non-breakdown of mRNA or protein product.

Transcriptional control

Gene transcription (DNA to mRNA) is not a spontaneous event and is possible only as a result of the interaction of a number of DNA-binding proteins with genomic DNA.

Regulation of a gene's expression must first start with the opening up of the double helix of DNA in the correct region of the chromosome. In order to do this a class of protein molecules which recognize the outside of the DNA helix have evolved (see Fig 2.7 on p. 135).

These DNA-binding proteins preferentially interact with the major groove of the DNA double helix (see Fig 2.4(b)). The base-pair composition of the DNA sequence can change the geometry of a DNA helix to facilitate the fit of a DNA-binding protein with its target region: CG-rich areas form the Z-structure DNA helix (Fig 2.4(b)); sequences such as AAAANNN cause a slight bend, and if this is repeated every 10 nucleotides it produces pronounced curves. DNA-binding proteins that recognize these distorted helices result either in the opening up of the helix so that the gene may be transcribed, or in the prevention of the helix being opened.

Structural classes of DNA-binding proteins

There are four basic classes of DNA-binding protein, classified according to their structural motifs (Fig 2.6):

- *helix–turn–helix* (HTH)
- *zinc finger*
- *leucine zipper*
- *helix–loop–helix* (HLH).

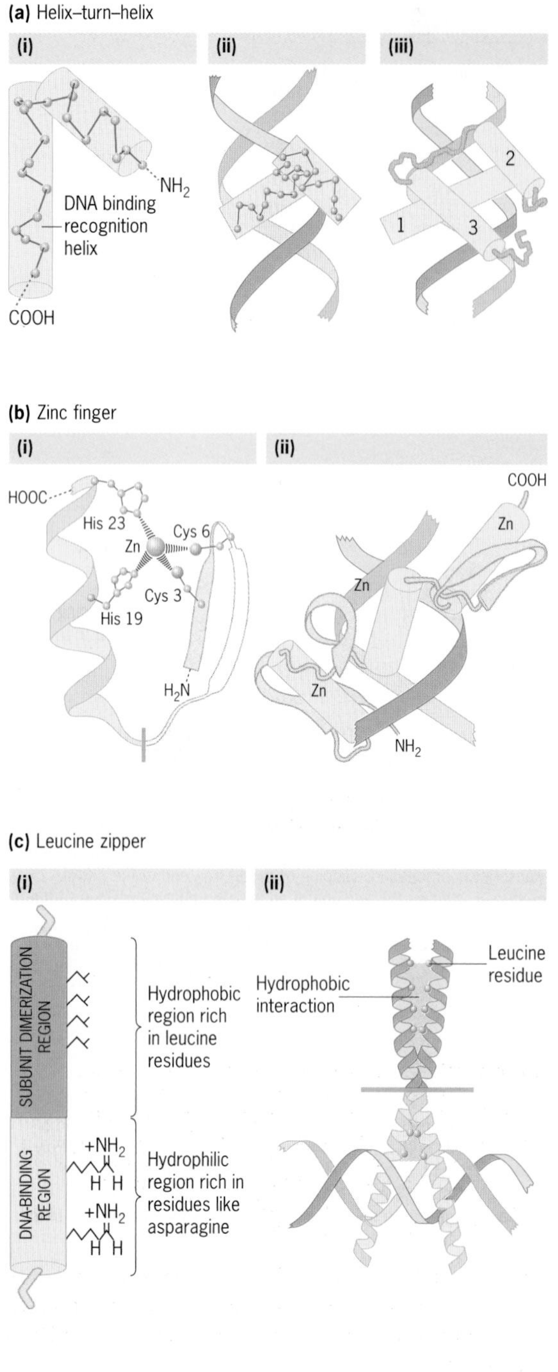

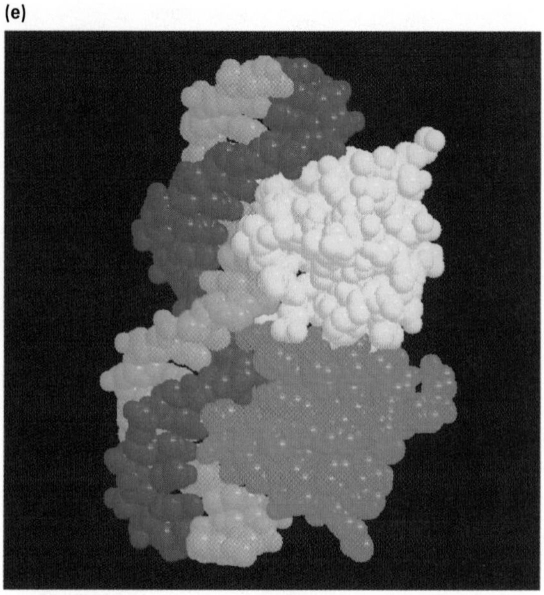

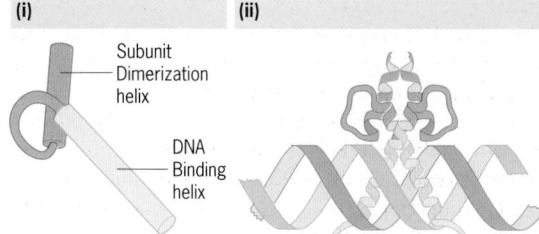

Fig 2.6

The four classes of DNA-binding proteins

(a) Helix–turn–helix (HTH) motifs. The simplest and most common, it consists of a helix connected by a fixed angle to a second helix. This represents the 'core' motif of HTH DNA-binding proteins but considerable modifications occur **(i)**. Like all DNA-binding proteins they interact as dimers, binding at exactly one turn of the double helix (3.4 nm or 12 bp) apart **(ii)**. The Homeodomain HLH DNA-binding proteins are a special class of HTH proteins. Discovered in the 1980s during investigation of the gene controlling Drosophila development, they contain an almost identical stretch of 60 amino acids. They have a third helix which holds the DNA-binding region in a fixed orientation. Indeed, all homeodomain proteins appear to have specific conserved amino acid positions and residues which interact with DNA. Furthermore, random orientation extension chains at the N-terminal can interact with the minor groove **(iii)**

(b) Zinc finger motifs, characterized by the incorporation of zinc, in some form, into the protein's quartenary structure. The term originated from the structural model of a Xenopus lavis protein which uses a zinc ion to hold a loop in a 'finger' shape by cross-linking two histidine residues with two cysteine residues. The Cys–Cys–His–His family of zinc finger DNA regulator proteins typically consists of an anti-parallel sheet forming a tight tertiary association with its own helix by zinc interaction with Cys and His residues within each of the two secondary structures. Several clusters of zinc fingers are found together and form a repeating structure which can interact with repetitive sequences in DNA **(ii)**

(c) Leucine zipper motif, consisting of a long α-helix which has many hydrophobic leucine residues at one end, responsible for dimer formation, whilst the opposite hydrophilic ends interact with DNA across the major groove of the double helix **(i)**. The quaternary structure of the leucine zippers need not be homodimeric, and indeed heterodimers are extremely common **(ii)**. Thus multiple sequences may be recognized by two or three DNA leucine zipper proteins depending on the type of dimer formed

(d) Helix–loop–helix (HLH) motifs. These consist of a DNA binding α-helix joined to a protein dimerization secondary α-helix via a loop (i). These combine leucine zipper properties with those of helix motif DNA-binding proteins. A helix interacting with DNA is linked via a loop to a large second helix which non-covalently binds to a similar HLH protein. Homo- and heterodimers can form, but the loop gives flexibility in the orientation of the given DNA-binding α-helix domain **(ii)**

(e) A crystallography-generated image of a bacterial HLH DNA-binding protein interacting with DNA as a dimer (green and yellow chains) binding into the major grooves of the DNA double helix (light blue and dark blue chains) exactly one turn (12 bp) apart

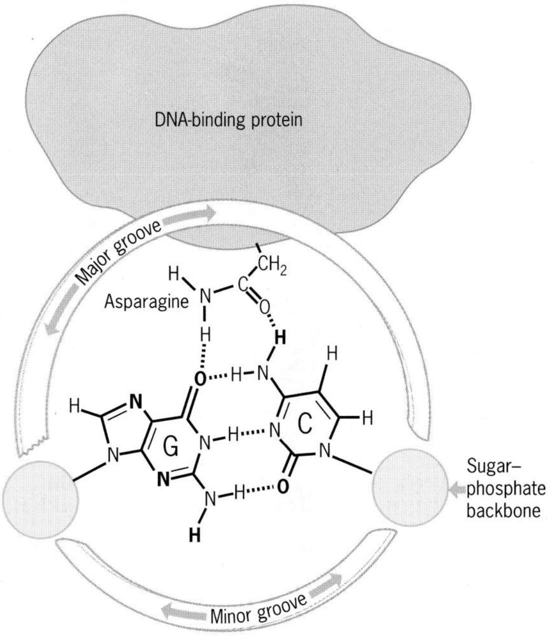

Fig 2.7
Recognition sites for DNA binding proteins. A cross-section through a DNA double helix, showing the base-pairing between cytidine and guanidine nucleic acids. Emboldened atom symbols show constituent atomic residues of the major and minor grooves available to form hydrogen pairing with DNA-binding proteins. The relative position of a DNA-binding protein molecule in cross-section above the major groove is shown, as is the interaction of an asparagine amino acid residue with DNA recognition sites of the C–G pairing

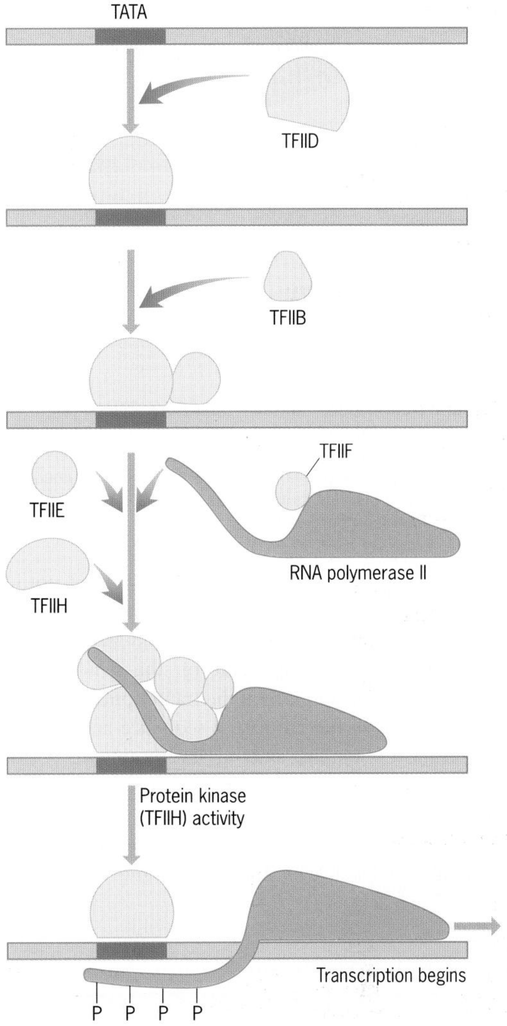

Fig 2.8
The general transcription factors – promoters. Promoters of gene transcription are initiated by the binding of the transcription factor (TF) IID protein to the recognition sequence TATA. Other transcription factors then bind to the TFIID (TFIIB, TFIIE, TFIIH and TFIIF) along with the RNA polymerase II protein. Once assembled the RNA polymerase II molecule is activated by phosphorylation and is able to proceed to transcribe the DNA gene into RNA
(Modified from Aberts *et al.* (1994))

Control regions and proteins

DNA-binding proteins act as regulators of gene expression in three different ways. They are the promoters, the operators and the enhancers.

The primary gene expression regulators are the *promoters*. The RNA polymerases bind to a promoter region normally adjacent to the transcribed sequence of DNA. In prokaryotes these are single DNA-binding proteins, but in eukaryotes active transcription is possible only when a number of DNA-binding and associated proteins come together and interact. Known as 'general transcription factors', these proteins are thought to assemble at promoter sites used by the enzyme RNA polymerase II (Pol II) which are characterized by the TATA sequence (Fig 2.8). Following the sequence of events shown in Fig 2.8, activated Pol II begins transcription of the genetic code.

Other DNA regulator proteins operate in close proximity to the site of promoter binding. These are called *operator proteins/regions* and act either as repressors by binding to DNA sequences within the promoter site (Fig 2.9(a)), or as positive regulators facilitating RNA polymerase binding (Fig 2.9(b)).

The third class of regulator proteins operates as *enhancer* sequences a considerable distance from the site of transcription initiation. Binding of regulator proteins to enhancer regions up-regulates the expression of a gene up to several kilobases from the promoter site. This turns out to be a distance favourable for DNA to loop back on itself without straining the backbone bonds of the DNA double helix.

The GAL4 enhancer of yeast physically aids the binding of transcription factors to the TATA region of the promoter, and thus acts like a catalyst for general transcription factor assembly, and consequently also the rate of RNA polymerase activity (Fig 2.10). In mammals, it is frequently a region termed the 'cyclic AMP response element' (CRE) that acts in this manner. Increasing intracellular cAMP levels cause activation and release of CRE binding protein (CREB). This binds to the CRE sequence and enhances the transcription rate.

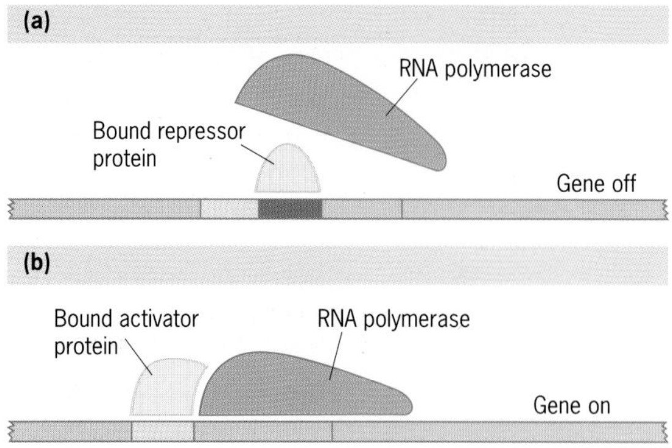

Fig 2.9
The general transcription factors – operators. DNA-binding proteins/region can **(a)** bind to recognition sequences which lie within the binding region of the RNA polymerase and therefore prevent gene transcription, or **(b)** bind to regions adjacent to the RNA polymerase assembly point and facilitate its binding/assembly and promote gene transcription (Modified from Aberts *et al.* (1994))

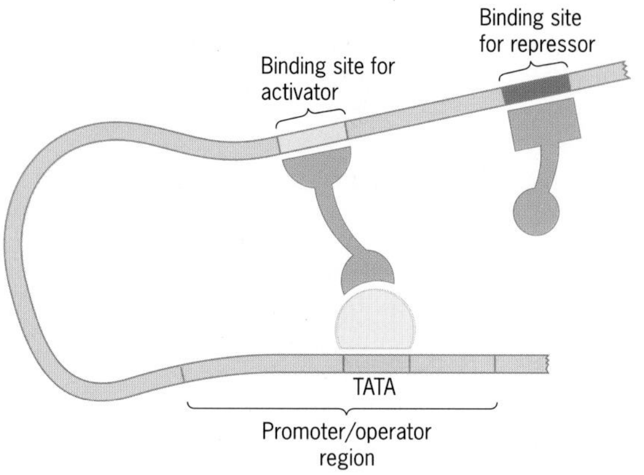

Fig 2.10
The general transcription factors – enhancers. DNA-binding proteins/regions. These are usually at least 500 bp away from the promoter region of gene transcription. The DNA loops back on itself, and the DNA-binding protein is brought into close proximity to the target gene. This can either facilitate the assembly of factors such as the general factors of transcription and hence enhance gene expression, or hinder such assembly (Modified from Aberts *et al.* (1994)

These relatively remote regulatory regions need not just enhance gene expression but may also repress transcription. Indeed, loops can be formed from regulatory regions downstream as well as upstream of the gene's coding sequence. Repressors can inhibit the transcription of a given gene by binding to the regulatory sequence and blocking positive regulators, binding and thus inactivating the positive regulator, or by interfering with the promoter protein assembly. Multiple regulatory regions and DNA-binding proteins can surround a given gene and precisely control its expression at a basal level and in response to a cellular stimulus (Table 2.1).

The reason for chromosomes and introns

Human genetics differs from that of bacteria in structural components of the genetic code and in the way DNA is packaged. The fact that humans have chromosomes and introns effects how much DNA we require to code for all our proteins in an unusual way. We have far more DNA than protein coding genes, whereas simple bacteria appear to have a much more economic DNA to gene ratio. Simple organisms like bacteria that have circular genomes which are not contained within a membrane bound organelle, the nucleus, are termed 'prokaryotes'. Higher *eukaryotic* organisms have their linear genomic packages, chromosomes, separated from the general cytoplasm by the nuclear envelope. In eukaryotes, genomic DNA is associated with nuclear proteins called *histones*.

Coiling around histones requires regions of DNA devoted specifically to the purpose of packaging and not coding for a protein (see Fig 2.4(c)). Most of human DNA is highly repetitive or *satellite* DNA consisting of long arrays of tandem repeats. These regions tend to be supercoiled around histones in condensed regions termed *heterochromatin*, even when the cell is not undergoing division. In contrast, most other DNA regions – in particular, those coding for proteins – are relatively uncondensed during interphase and constitute the *euchromatin*. This remaining DNA is either moderately repetitive (50–100 × 10^3), accounting for about 1% of the total, or codes for unique genes and gene families, some 50–100 × 10^3, occupying some 2% of the genome.

Thus the reason for chromosomes is that supercoiling around histones gives tighter control of specific gene expression. Introns enable the production of alternative proteins for one gene, e.g. parathyroid-like proteins for the parathyroid hormone (PTH) gene.

FURTHER READING

Aberts B, Bray D, Lewis J, Raff M, Roberts K, Watson JD (1994) *Molecular Biology of the Cell*, 3rd edn. New York: Garland Publishing.

Table 2.1
Examples of DNA-binding proteins causing human pathology

Class of DNA-binding protein	Examples
Helix–turn–helix	CREB (cAMP Response Element Binding Protein)
Zinc finger	Steroid and thyroid hormone receptors Retinoic acid and vitamin D receptors *Bcl-6* oncogene product (large-cell lymphoma) *WT-1* oncogene product (Wilms' tumour) GATA-1 erythrocyte differentiation and Hb expression factor
Leucine zippers	*cJun* cell replication oncogene *cFos* cell replication oncogene
Helix–loop–helix	*Myc* oncogene *Mad* oncogene *Max* oncogene

Tools for molecular biology

Preparation of genomic DNA

The first step in studying the DNA of an individual involves preparation of genomic DNA. This is a simple procedure in which any cellular tissue including blood (the nucleated cells are isolated from the erythrocytes) can be used. The cells are lysed in order to open their cell and nuclear membranes, releasing chromosomal DNA. Following digestion of all cellular protein by the addition of proteolytic enzymes, the genomic DNA is isolated by chemical extraction with phenol. DNA is stable and can be stored frozen for years.

Restriction enzymes and gel electrophoresis

Genomic DNA can be cut into a number of fragments by enzymes called 'restriction enzymes', which are obtained from bacteria. Restriction enzymes recognize specific DNA sequences and cut double-stranded DNA at these sites. For example, the enzyme EcoRI will cut DNA wherever it reads the sequence GAATTC, and so human genomic DNA is cut into hundreds of thousands of fragments. Whenever the genomic DNA from an individual is cut with EcoRI, the same 'restriction fragments' are produced.

As DNA is a negatively charged molecule, the genomic DNA that has been digested with a restriction enzyme can be separated according to its size and charge, by electrophoresing the DNA through a gel matrix. The DNA sample is loaded at one end of the gel, a voltage is applied across the gel, and the DNA migrates towards the positive anode. The small fragments move more quickly than the large fragments, and so the DNA fragments separate out. Fragment size can be determined by running fragments of known size on the same gel.

Pulsed-field gel electrophoresis (PFGE) can be used to separate very long pieces of DNA (hundreds of kilobases) which have been cut by restriction enzymes that cut at rare sites in the genome. In this technique, DNA molecules are subjected to two perpendicular electric fields that are switched on alternately. The DNA molecules are separated on the basis of molecular size, and this technique can be used for long-range mapping of the genome to detect major deletions and rearrangements.

Southern blotting and DNA probes

This technique allows the visualization of individual DNA fragments (Fig 2.11).

A DNA probe is used to indicate where the fragment of interest lies. DNA probes are useful because a fundamental property of DNA is that when two strands are separated, for example by heating, they will always reassociate and stick together again because of their complementary base sequences. Therefore the presence or position of a particular gene can be identified using a gene 'probe' consisting of DNA with a base sequence that is complementary to that of the sequence of interest. A DNA probe is thus a piece of single-stranded DNA that can be labelled with a radioactive isotope (usually ^{32}P) or a fluorescent signal. The probe is added to a hybridization solution into which the membrane with the DNA is also placed. The single-stranded probe will locate and bind to its complementary sequence on the blot and can be identified by autoradiography or fluorescence.

A similar technique for blotting RNA fragments (which are not cut by restriction enzymes, but which are blotted as full-length mRNAs) on to membranes is called *Northern blotting* and one for blotting proteins is called *Western blotting.*

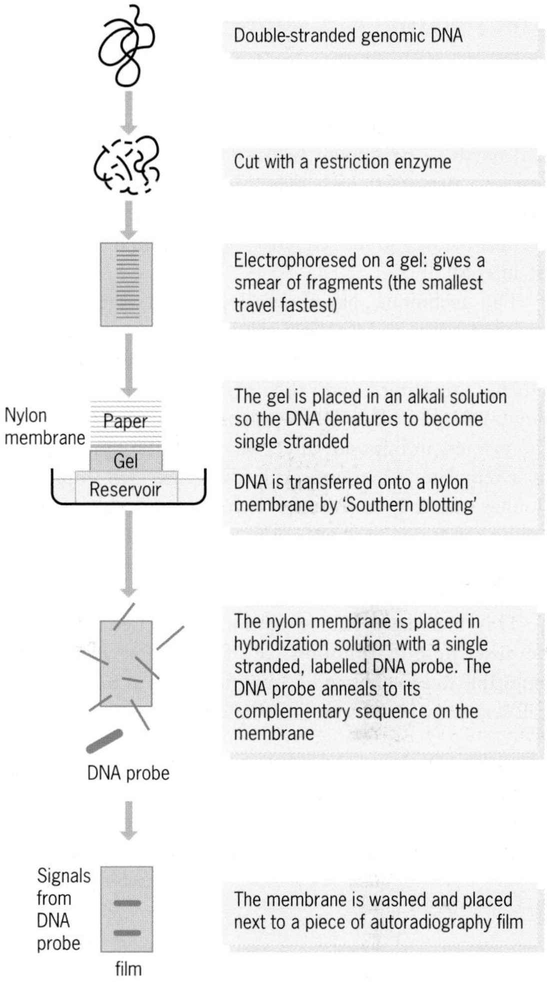

Fig 2.11
Southern blotting and DNA probes

The polymerase chain-reaction (PCR)

Minute amounts of DNA can be amplified over a million times within a few hours using this *in vitro* technique (Fig 2.12). The exact DNA sequence to be amplified needs to be known because the DNA is amplified between two short (generally 17–25 bp) single-stranded DNA fragments ('oligonucleotide primers') which are complementary to the sequences at each end of the DNA of interest.

The technique has three steps. First, the double-stranded genomic DNA is denatured by heat into single-stranded DNA. The reaction is then cooled to favour DNA annealing, and the primers bind to their target DNA. Finally, a DNA polymerase is used to extend the primers in opposite directions using the target DNA as a template. After one cycle there are two copies of double-stranded DNA, after two cycles there are four copies, and this number rises exponentially with the number of cycles. Typically a polymerase chain-reaction is set for 25–30 cycles, allowing millions of amplifications.

This technique has revolutionized genetic research because minute amounts of DNA not previously amenable to analysis can be amplified, such as from buccal cell scrapings, blood spots, or single embryonic cells.

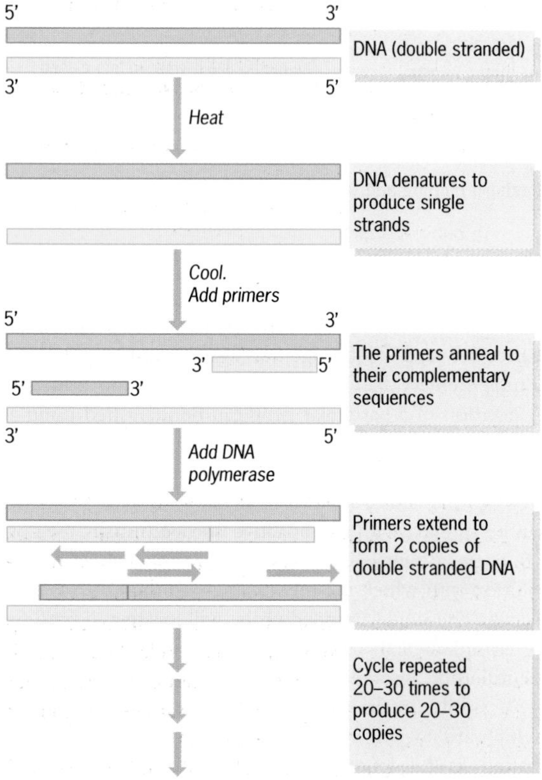

Fig 2.12
Polymerase chain reaction

DNA cloning

A particular DNA fragment of interest can be isolated and inserted into the genome of simple self-replicating organisms or organelles such as viruses and plasmids. When used for this purpose they are referred to as *vectors*. Replication by the million of the vector results in multiple copies or clones of the inserted sequence. Thus, after removal from the host vector, cloned gene sequences can be prepared in large quantities independently of other sequences.

Vectors include: bacteriophage viruses; plasmids, which are self-replicating episomal circular DNA molecules found in bacteria which carry antibody resistance genes; and 'yeast artificial chromosomes' (YACs), which are derived from centromeric and telomeric DNA sequences found in yeast. Each vector takes an optimum size of cloned DNA insert. Typically, viruses can accommodate only small sequences up to a maximum of a kilobase, larger fragments of 2–10 kilobases can be inserted into a plasmid, and sequences of several hundred kilobases can be inserted into a YAC. Each have their relative merits – viruses being very efficient, but the vectors which take large clones being considerably less so. A hybrid between a plasmid and a bacteriophage (called a *cosmid*) has been constructed artificially. This has the ability to clone reasonably large sequences as plasmids within a host bacteria. However, cosmids trick bacteriophages into packaging them into a viral body, and this viral body is then able to infect the target bacteria, giving efficient transfection rates.

The DNA fragment of interest is inserted into the vector DNA sequence using an enzyme called a *ligase*. This takes place *in vitro*. The next step, cloning, creates many copies of the 'recombinant DNA molecule' and takes place *in vivo* when the plasmid or other vector is placed back into the bacterial (or yeast) host. Bacteria that have successfully taken up the recombinant plasmid can be selected if the plasmid also carries an antibiotic resistance gene (so bacteria without the plasmid die in the presence of antibiotic) (Fig 2.13).

The DNA fragment of interest to be cloned may be a restriction fragment. Alternatively it could be DNA (cDNA) which has been copied from an mRNA sequence. mRNA provides the template from which a viral enzyme called *reverse transcriptase* (RT) can synthesize a complementary single-stranded DNA copy (cDNA). A DNA polymerase may then be used to produce a double-stranded copy by PCR. A cDNA molecule contains all the sequences necessary for a functional gene, but unlike genomic DNA it lacks introns.

DNA libraries

These are pools of isolated and cloned DNA sequences that form a permanent resource for further experiments. Two types of library are used:

- *Genomic libraries* are prepared from genomic DNA that has been digested with restriction enzymes, ligated into a vector and each individual clone passed into a bacterial (plasmid, bacteriophage, cosmid) or yeast (YAC) host. A genomic library usually contains almost every sequence in the genome.

- *cDNA libraries* are prepared from the total mRNA of a tissue, which is copied into cDNA by reverse transcriptase. The cDNA is ligated into a vector and passed into a host as above. A cDNA library should contain sequences derived from all the mRNAs expressed in that tissue type.

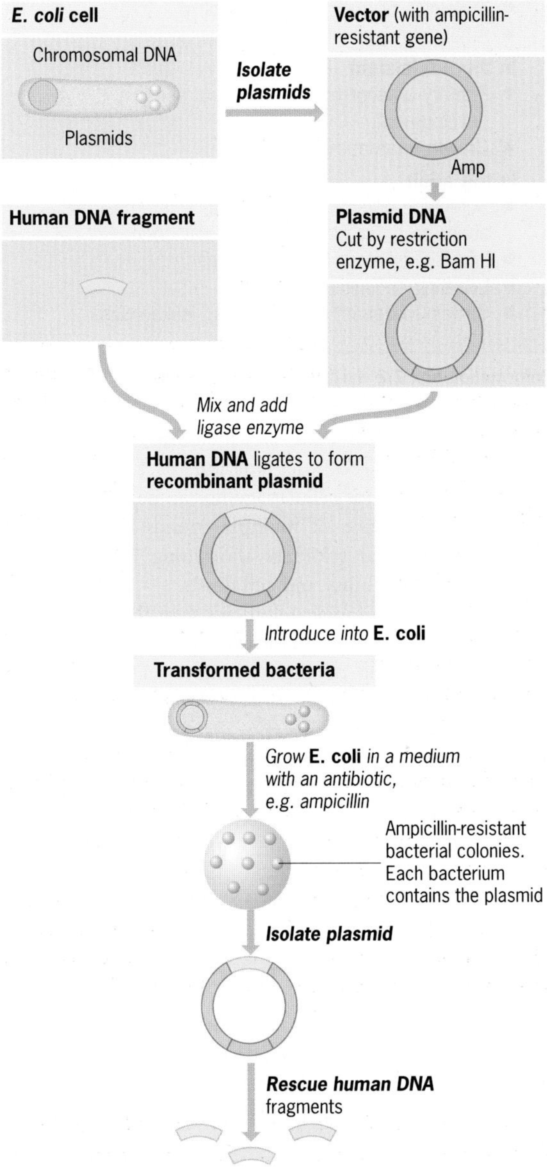

Fig 2.13
DNA cloning. Recombinant DNA technique, showing incorporation of foreign DNA into a plasmid. The ampicillin-resistant genes can be used to distinguish transformed *Escherichia coli* cells

DNA sequencing

A chemical process known as dideoxy-sequencing allows the identification of the exact nucleotide sequence of a piece of DNA. The DNA of interest is single-stranded and an oligonucleotide primer is annealed adjacent to the region of interest. This primer acts as the starting point for a DNA polymerase to build a new DNA chain that is complementary to the sequence under investigation.

The reaction is carried out in four tubes to each of which a mixture of nucleotides is added, one of which is radioactive. To each tube one dideoxytriphosphate of either adenine, guanine, cytosine or thymine is also added at a low level. These are incorporated into the growing chain and stop enzymatic synthesis (because they lack the necessary 3′-hydroxyl group). As the dideoxynucleotides are present at a low concentration, not all the chains in a reaction tube will incorporate a dideoxynucleotide in the same place, so the tubes contain sequences of different lengths but which all terminate with a particular dideoxynucleotide. These fragments are electrophoresed in four columns and a sequence of DNA is deduced by autoradiography.

Sequencing machines work by using fluorescent labels on the four nucleotides. By laser scanning a gel these machines can rapidly sequence a stretch of DNA.

FURTHER READING

Brown TA (1990) *Gene Cloning: An Introduction*, 2nd edn. London: Chapman & Hall.

Maniatis T, Fritsch EF, Sambrook J (1989) *Molecular Cloning: A Laboratory Manual*, 2nd edn. New York: Cold Spring Harbour.

Papavassilioy AG (1995) Transcription factors. *New England Journal of Medicine* **332**: 45–47.

Smith CA, Wood EJ (1991) *Molecular Biology and Biotechnology*. London: Chapman & Hall.

The biology of chromosomes

Human chromosomes

The nucleus of each diploid cell contains 6×10^9 bp of DNA in long molecules called *chromosomes*. Chromosomes are massive structures containing one linear molecule of DNA that is wound around histone proteins into small units called *nucleosomes*, and these are further wound to make up the structure of the chromosome itself. Diploid human cells have 46 chromosomes, 23 inherited from each parent; thus there are 23 'homologous' pairs of chromosomes (22 pairs of 'autosomes' and two 'sex chromosomes').

The sex chromosomes, called X and Y, are not homologous but are different in size and shape. Males have an X and a Y chromosome, females have two

X chromosomes. (Primary male sexual characteristics are determined by the *SRY* gene – sex determining region, Y chromosome.)

The chromosomes can be classified according to their size and shape, the largest being chromosome 1. The constriction in the chromosome is the *centromere*, which can be in the middle of the chromosome (metacentric) or at one extreme end (acrocentric). The centromere divides the chromosome into a short arm and a long arm, which are referred to as the *p arm* and the *q arm* respectively (see Fig 2.4(d)). In addition, chromosomes can be stained when they are in the metaphase stage of the cell cycle and are very condensed. The stain gives a different pattern of light and dark bands that is diagnostic for each chromosome. Each band is given a number, and gene mapping techniques allow genes to be positioned within a band within an arm of a chromosome. For example, the *CFTR* gene (in which a defect gives rise to cystic fibrosis) maps to 7q21, that is on chromosome 7 in the long arm in band 21.

During cell division (mitosis), each chromosome divides into two so that each daughter nucleus has the same number of chromosomes as its parent cell. During gametogenesis, however, the number of chromosomes is halved by meiosis, so that after conception the number of chromosomes remains the same and is not doubled. In the female, each ovum contains one or other X chromosome but, in the male, the sperm bears either an X or a Y chromosome.

Chromosomes can only be seen easily in actively dividing cells. Typically, lymphocytes from the peripheral blood are stimulated to divide and are processed to allow the chromosomes to be examined. Cells from other tissues can also be used – for example amniotic fluid, placental cells from chorionic villus sampling, bone marrow and skin (Information box 2.2).

Information

Chromosome studies may be indicated in the following circumstances.

Antenatal
- Pregnancies in women over 35 years
- Positive maternal serum screening test for trisomy 21
- Ultrasound markers of chromosomal abnormalities
- Severe fetal growth retardation
- Sexing of fetus in X-linked disorders

In the neonate
- Congenital malformations
- Suspicion of trisomy or monosomy
- Ambiguous genitalia

In the adolescent
- Primary amenorrhoea or failure of pubertal development
- Growth retardation

In the adult
- Screening parents of a child with a chromosomal abnormality for further genetic counselling
- Infertility or recurrent miscarriages
- Learning difficulties
- Certain malignant disorders (e.g. leukaemias)

Information box 2.2 Indications for chromosomal analysis

The X chromosome and inactivation

Although female chromosomes are XX, females do not have two doses of X-linked genes (compared with just one dose for a male XY), because of the phenomenon of X inactivation or *Lyonization* (after its discoverer, Dr Mary Lyon). In this process, one of the two X chromosomes in the cells of females becomes transcriptionally inactive, so the cell has only one dose of the X-linked genes. Inactivation is random and can affect either X chromosome.

Telomeres and immortality

The ends of chromosomes, telomeres (see Fig 2.4(d)), do not contain genes but many repeats of a hexameric sequence TTAGGG. Replication of linear chromosomes starts at coding sites (origins of replication) within the main body of chromosomes and not at the two extreme ends. The extreme ends are therefore susceptible to single-stranded DNA degradation back to double-stranded DNA. Thus cellular ageing can be measured as a genetic consequence of multiple rounds of replication with consequential telomere shortening. This leads to chromosome instability and cell death.

Stem cells have longer telomeres than their terminally differentiated daughters. However, germ cells replicate without shortening of their telomeres. This is because they express an enzyme called *telomerase* which protects against telomere shortening by acting as a template primer at the extreme ends of the chromosomes. Not surprisingly, increased telomerase activity is found in tumour cells and may contribute to their immortality. Conversely, cells from patients with progeria (premature aging syndrome) have extremely short telomeres.

The mitochondrial chromosome

In addition to the 23 pairs of chromosomes in the nucleus of every diploid cell, the mitochondria in the cytoplasm of the cell also have their own chromosomes. The mitochondrial chromosome is a circular DNA molecule of approximately 16 500 bp, and every base-pair makes up part of the coding sequence. These genes principally encode proteins or RNA molecules involved in mitochondrial function. These proteins are components of the mitochondrial respiratory chain involved in oxidative phosphorylation. Every cell contains several hundred mitochondria, and therefore several hundred mitochondrial chromosomes. All mito-chondria are inherited from the mother as sperm contains no (or very few) mitochondria.

FURTHER READING

Haber DA (1995) Telomeres, cancer, and immortality. *New England Journal of Medicine* **332**: 955–956.

Human genetic disorders

The spectrum of inherited or congenital genetic disorders can be classified as the chromosomal disorders, including mitochondrial chromosome disorders, the Mendelian and sex-linked single-gene disorders, a variety of non-Mendelian disorders, and the multifactorial and polygenic disorders (Table 2.2 and Information box 2.3). All are a result of a mutation in the genetic code. This may be a change of a single base-pair of a gene, resulting in functional change in the product protein (e.g. thalassaemia) or gross rearrangement of the gene within a genome (e.g. Down's syndrome). These mutations can be *congenital* (inherited at birth) or *somatic* (arising during a person's life). The latter are responsible for the collective disease known as cancer, and the principles underlying Mendelian inheritance act in a similar manner to dominant and recessive traits. Both gross chromosomal and point mutations occur in somatic genetic disease.

Chromosomal disorders

Chromosomal abnormalities are much more common than generally appreciated. Over half of spontaneous abortions have chromosomal abnormalities, compared with only 4–6 abnormalities per 1000 live births. Specific chromosomal abnormalities can lead to well-recognized and severe clinical syndromes, although autosomal aneuploidy (a differing from the normal diploid number) is usually more severe than the sex-chromosome aneuploidies. Abnormalities may occur in either the number or the structure of the chromosomes.

Table 2.2
Prevalence of genetic disease

Type	Estimated prevalence per 1000 population
Single-gene disorders	
Autosomal dominant	2–10
Autosomal recessive	2
X-linked recessive	1–2
Chromosomal abnormalities	6–7
Common disorders with a genetic component	7–10
Congenital malformation	20
Total	38–51

From Kingston H (1989) Clinical genetic services. *British Medical Journal* **298**: 306–307

Abnormal chromosome numbers

If a chromosome or chromatids fail to separate ('non-disjunction') either in meiosis or mitosis, one daughter cell will receive two copies of that chromosome and one daughter cell will receive no copies of the chromosome. If this non-disjunction occurs during meiosis it can lead to an ovum or sperm having either (i) an extra chromosome, so resulting in a fetus that is 'trisomic' and has three instead of two copies of the chromosome; or (ii) no chromosome, so the fetus is 'monosomic' and has one instead of two copies of the chromosome. Non-disjunction can occur with autosomes or sex chromosomes. However, only individuals with trisomy 13, 18 and 21 survive to birth, and most children with trisomy 13 and trisomy 18 die in early childhood. Trisomy 21 (Down's syndrome) is observed with a frequency of 1 in 700 live births regardless of geography or ethnic background. This should be reduced with widespread screening (p. 140). Full autosomal monosomies are extremely rare and very deleterious. Sex-chromosome trisomies (e.g. Klinefelter's syndrome, XXY) are relatively common. The sex-chromosome monosomy in which the

i **Information**

Mendelian
- Inherited or new mutation
- Mutant allele or pair of mutant alleles at single locus
- Clear pattern of inheritance (autosomal or sex-linked) dominant or recessive
- High risk to relatives

Chromosomal
- Loss, gain or abnormal rearrangement of one or more of 46 chromosomes in diploid cell
- No clear pattern of inheritance
- Low risk to relatives

Multifactorial
- Common
- Interaction between genes and environmental factors
- Low risk to relatives

Mitochondrial
- Due to mutations in mitochondrial genome
- Transmitted through maternal line
- Different pattern of inheritance from Mendelian disorders

Somatic cell
- Mutations in somatic cells
- Somatic event is not inherited
- Often give rise to tumours

Information box 2.3 Genetic disorders

individual has an X chromosome only and no second X or Y chromosome is known as Turner's syndrome and is estimated to occur in 1 in 2500 live-born girls (Table 2.3).

Occasionally, non-disjunction can occur during mitosis shortly after two gametes have fused. It will then result in the formation of two cell lines, each with a different chromosome complement. This occurs more often with the sex chromosome, and results in a 'mosaic' individual.

Very rarely the entire chromosome set will be present in more than two copies, so the individual may be triploid rather than diploid and have a chromosome number of 69. Triploidy and tetraploidy (four sets) result in spontaneous abortion.

Abnormal chromosome structures

As well as abnormal numbers of chromosomes, chromosomes can have abnormal structures, and the disruption to the DNA and gene sequences may give rise to a genetic disease.

- *Deletions*. Deletions of a portion of a chromosome may give rise to a disease syndrome if two copies of the genes in the deleted region are necessary, and the individual will not be normal with just the one copy remaining on the non-deleted homologous chromosome. Many deletion syndromes have been well described. For example, Prader–Willi syndrome (p. 207) is the result of cytogenetic events resulting in deletion of part of the long arm of chromosome 15, Aniridia–Wilms is characterized by deletion of part of the short arm of chromosome 11, and microdeletions in the long arm of chromosome 22 give rise to the DiGeorge syndrome.
- *Duplications*. Duplications occur when a portion of the chromosome is present on the chromosome in two copies, so the genes in that chromosome portion are present in an extra dose. A form of the neuropathy Charcot–Marie–Tooth disease (p. 1096) is due to a small duplication of a region of chromosome 17.
- *Inversion*. Inversions involve an end-to-end reversal of a segment within a chromosome; e.g. abcdefgh becomes abcfedgh.

Table 2.3
Examples of chromosomal disorders in live births

Abnormal chromosome disorders	
Autosomal disorders	
Trisomy 21 (Down's syndrome)	1 in 650
Trisomy 18 (Edward's syndrome)	1 in 3000
Trisomy 13 (Patau's syndrome)	1 in 5000
Sex-chromosome disorders	
47, XXY (Klinefelter's syndrome)	1 in 1000 males
47, XYY	1 in 800 males
47, XXX	1 in 1000 females
45, X (Turner's syndrome)	1 in 2500 females
Abnormal chromosome structures	
Balanced translocations	1 in 500
Unbalanced translocations	1 in 2000

- *Translocations*. Translocations occur when two chromosome regions join together, when they would not normally. Chromosome translocations in somatic cells may be associated with tumourigenesis (see p. 151).

Translocations can be very complex, involving more than two chromosomes, but most are simple and fall into one of two categories.

Reciprocal translocations occur when any two non-homologous chromosomes break simultaneously and rejoin, swapping ends. In this case the cell still has 46 chromosomes but two of them are rearranged. Someone with a balanced translocation is likely to be normal (unless a translocation breakpoint interrupts a gene); but at meiosis, when the chromosomes separate into different daughter cells, the translocated chromosomes will enter the gametes and any resulting fetus may inherit one abnormal chromosome and have an unbalanced translocation, with physical manifestations.

Robertsonian translocations occur when two acrocentric chromosomes join and the short arm is lost, leaving only 45 chromosomes. This translocation is balanced as no genetic material is lost and the individual is healthy. However, any offspring have a risk of inheriting an unbalanced arrangement. This risk depends on which acrocentric chromosome is involved. Clinically important is the 14/21 Robertsonian translocation. A woman with this karyotype has a 1 in 8 risk of delivering a baby with Down's syndrome (a male carrier has a 1 in 50 risk). However, they have a 50% risk of producing a carrier like themselves, hence the importance of genetic family studies. Relatives should be alerted about the risk of a Down's offspring and should have their chromosomes checked.

Table 2.4 shows some of the syndromes resulting from chromosomal abnormalities.

Mitochondrial chromosome disorders

The mitochondrial chromosome (p. 140) carries its genetic information in a very compact form; for example there are no introns in the genes. Therefore any mutation has a high chance of having an effect. However, as every cell contains hundreds of mitochondria, a single altered mitochondrial genome will not be noticed. As mitochondria divide there is a statistical likelihood that there will be more mutated mitochondria, and at some point this will give rise to a mitochondrial disease.

Most mitochondrial diseases are myopathies and neuropathies with a maternal pattern of inheritance. Many syndromes have been described, including myoclonic epilepsy with ragged red fibres (MERRF) and mitochondrial encephalomyopathy, lactic acidosis and stroke-like episodes (MELAS) (see p. 1104). Leber's optic atrophy, with late-onset bilateral loss of central vision and cardiac arrhythmias, is an example of a mitochondrial disease caused by a point mutation in one gene.

Table 2.4
Chromosomal abnormalities: examples of a few syndromes

Syndrome	Chromosome karyotype	Incidence and risks	Clinical features	Mortality
Autosomal abnormalities				
Trisomy 21 (Down's syndrome)	47, +21 (95%) Mosaicism Translocation 5%	1:650 (Risk with 20–29 year old mother 1:1000; >45 year old mother 1:30)	Flat face, slanting eyes, epicanthic folds, small ears, simian crease, short stubby fingers, hypotonia, variable learning difficulties, congenital heart disease (up to 50%)	High in first year, but some survive to adulthood
Trisomy 13 (Patau's syndrome)	47, +13	1:5000	Low-set ears, cleft lip and palate, polydactyly, micro-ophthalmia, learning difficulties	Rarely survive for more than a few weeks
Trisomy 18 (Edwards' syndrome)	47, +18	1:3000	Low-set ears, micrognathia, rocker-bottom feet, mental retardation	Rarely survive for more than a few weeks
Sex-chromosome abnormalities				
Fragile X syndrome	46, XX, fra (X) 46, XY, fra (X)	1:2000	Most common inherited cause of learning difficulties predominantly in males Macro-orchidism	
Female				
Turner's syndrome	45, XO	1:2500	Infantilism, primary amenorrhoea, short stature, webbed neck, cubitis valgus, normal IQ	
Triple X syndrome	47, XXX	1:1000	No distinctive somatic features, learning difficulties	
Others	48, XXXX 49, XXXXX	Rare	Amenorrhoea, infertility, learning difficulties	
Male				
Klinefelter's syndrome	47, XXY (or XXYY)	1:1000 (more in sons of older mothers)	Decreased crown–pubis:pubis–heel ratio, eunuchoid, testicular atrophy, infertility, gynaecomastia, learning difficulties (20%; related to number of X chromosomes)	
Double Y syndrome	47, XYY	1:800	Tall, fertile, minor mental and psychiatric illness, high incidence in tall criminals	
Others	48, XXXY 49, XXXXY		Learning difficulties, testicular atrophy	

Analysis of chromosome disorders

The analysis of gross chromosomal disorders has traditionally involved the culture of isolated cells in the presence of toxins such as colchicine. These toxins arrest the cell cycle at mitosis and, following staining, the chromosomes with their characteristic banding can be seen. A highly trained cytogeneticist can then identify each chromosome pair and any abnormalities (Fig 2.14).

New molecular biology techniques have made things simpler: YAC-cloned probes are available and cover large genetic regions of individual chromosomes. These probes can be labelled with fluorescently tagged nucleotides and used in *in situ hybridization* of the nucleus of isolated tissue from patients. These tagged probes allow rapid and relatively unskilled identification of metaphase chromosomes, and allow the identification of chromosomes dispersed within the nucleus (Fig 2.15). Furthermore, tagging two chromosome regions with different fluorescent tags allows easy identification of chromosomal translocations (Fig 2.15).

Gene defects

Mendelian and sex-linked single-gene disorders are the result of mutations in a protein coding sequence. These mutations can have various effects on the expression of the gene, as explained below, but all cause a dysfunction of the protein product.

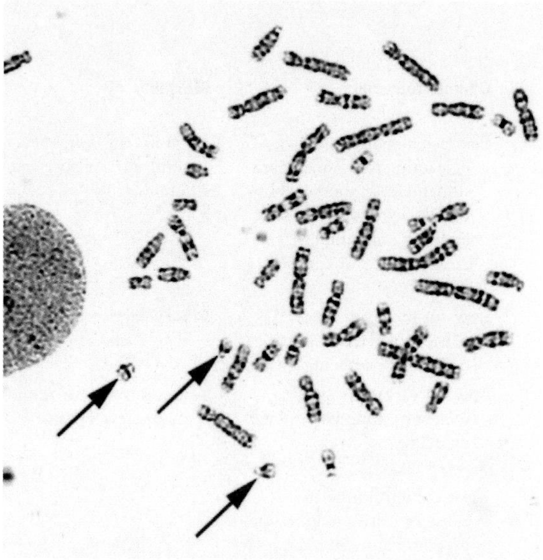

Fig 2.14
Karyotyping. G-banded spread of metaphase chromosomes, showing trisomy 21 (arrowed) Down's syndrome
Courtesy of D Lillington, Medical Oncology Unit, St Bartholomew's Hospital

Mutations

Although DNA replication is a very accurate process, occasionally mistakes occur to produce changes or mutations. These changes can also occur owing to other factors such as radiation, ultraviolet light or chemicals. Mutations in gene sequences or in the sequences which regulate gene expression (transcription and translation) may alter the amino acid sequence in the protein encoded by that gene. In some cases protein function will be maintained; in other cases it will change or cease, perhaps producing a clinical disorder. Many different types of mutation occur.

Point mutation

This is the simplest type of change and involves the substitution of one nucleotide for another, so changing the codon in a coding sequence. For example, the triplet AAA, which codes for lysine, may be mutated to AGA, which codes for arginine. Whether a substitution produces a clinical disorder depends on whether it changes a critical part of the protein molecule produced. Fortunately, many substitutions have no effect on the function or stability of the proteins produced as several codons code for the same amino acid. However, some mutations may have a severe effect; for example, in sickle cell disease a mutation within the globin gene changes one codon from GAG to GTG, so that instead of glutamic acid, valine is incorporated into the polypeptide chain, which radically alters its properties.

Insertion or deletion

Insertion or deletion of one or more bases is a more serious change, as it results in the alteration of the rest of the following sequence to give a frame-shift mutation. For example, if the original code was

TAA GGA GAG TTT

and an extra nucleotide (A) is inserted, the sequence becomes

TAA AGG AGA GTT T

Alternatively, if the third nucleotide (A) is deleted, the sequence becomes

TAG GAG AGT TT

In both cases different amino acids are incorporated into the polypeptide chain. This type of change is responsible for some forms of thalassaemia (p. 375).

Insertions and deletions can involve many hundreds of base-pairs of DNA. For example, some large deletions in the dystrophin gene remove coding sequences and this results in Duchenne's muscular dystrophy. Insertion/deletion (ID) polymorphism in the angiotensin converting enzyme (ACE) gene has been shown to result in the genotypes II, ID and DD. The deletion is of a 287 bp repeat sequence and DD is associated with higher concentrations of circulating ACE and possibly cardiac disease (see p. 687).

Splicing mutations

If the DNA sequences which direct the splicing of introns from mRNA are mutated, then abnormal splicing may occur. In this case the processed mRNA which is translated into protein by the ribosomes may carry intron sequences, so altering which amino acids are incorporated into the polypeptide chain.

Termination mutations

Normal polypeptide chain termination occurs when the ribosomes processing the mRNA reach one of the chain termination or 'stop' codons (see above). Mutations involving these codons will result in either late or premature termination. For example, Haemoglobin Constant Spring is a haemoglobin variant where instead of the 'stop' sequence, a single base change allows the insertion of an extra amino acid (see p. 377).

Single-gene disease

Monogenetic disorders involving single genes can be inherited as dominant, recessive or sex-linked characteristics. Inheritance occurs according to simple Mendelian laws, making predictions of disease in offspring and therefore genetic counselling more straightforward.

(a)

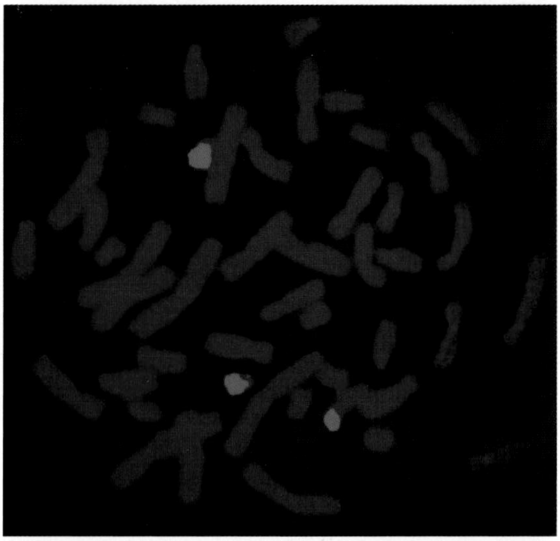

(b)

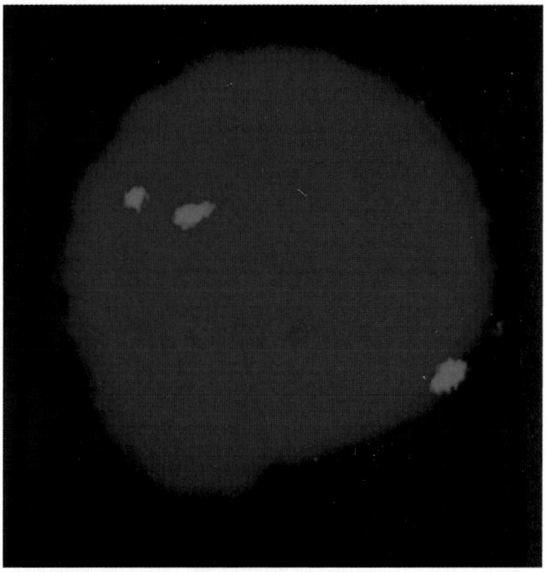

(c)

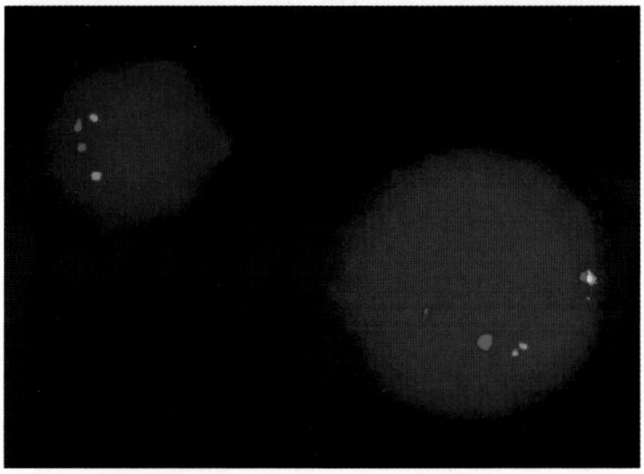

Fig 2.15
Fluorescence in situ hybridization (FISH).
Trisomy 21 chromosomes **(a)** painted red in the metaphase of chromosomes and **(b)** as an anaphase cell nucleus. **(c)** Two coloured FISH using a red paint for the ABL gene on chromosome 9 and a green paint for the BCR gene on chromosome 22 in the anaphase cell nucleus. Where a translocation has occurred the two genes become juxtaposed on the Philadelphia chromosome and a hybrid yellow florescence can be seen only in the affected cell nucleus on the right of **(c)**.
Courtesy of D Lillington, Medical Oncology Unit, St. Bartholomew's Hospital

Autosomal dominant disorders (Fig 2.16(a) and Table 2.5)

Each diploid cell contains two copies of all the autosomes. An autosomal dominant disorder occurs when one of the two copies has a mutation and the protein produced by the normal form of the gene cannot compensate. In this case a *heterozygote* individual who has two different forms (or *alleles*) of the same gene will manifest the disease.

The offspring of heterozygotes have a 50% chance of inheriting the chromosome carrying the disease allele, and therefore also of having the disease. However, estimation of risk to offspring for counselling families can be difficult because of three factors:

- These disorders have a great variability in their manifestation. 'Incomplete penetrance' may occur if patients have a dominant disorder but it does not manifest itself clinically in them. This gives the appearance of the gene having 'skipped' a generation.
- Dominant traits are extremely variable in severity (variable expression) and a mildly affected parent may have a severely affected child.

Table 2.5
Examples of autosomal dominant disorders

Achondroplasia	Hereditary elliptocytosis
Acute intermittent porphyria	Hereditary haemorrhagic telangiectasia
Adult polycystic disease	Hereditary spherocytosis
Alzheimer's disease (familial)	Huntington's chorea
α_1-Antitrypsin deficiency	Marfan's syndrome
C_1 esterase inhibitor deficiency	Dystrophia myotonica
Crigler–Najjar syndrome type II	Neurofibromatosis
Epidermolysis bullosa (some forms)	Osteogenesis imperfecta (some forms)
Familial adenomatous polyposis	Peutz–Jegher's syndrome
Familial hypercholesterolaemia	Rotor syndrome
Facio-scapulohumeral dystrophy	Tuberose sclerosis
	Von Willebrand's disease

- New cases in a previously unaffected family may be the result of a new mutation. If it is a mutation, the risk of a further affected child is negligible. Most cases of achondroplasia are due to new mutations.

The overall incidence of autosomal dominant disorders is 7 per 1000 live births.

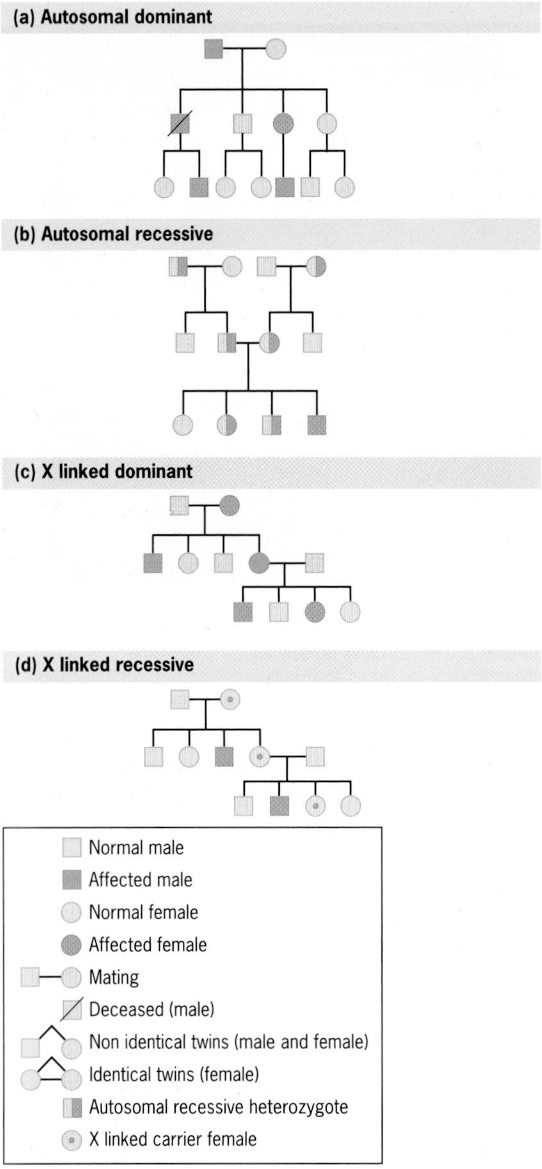

Fig 2.16
Modes of inheritance of simple gene disorders, with a key to the standard pedigree symbols

Table 2.6
Examples of autosomal recessive disorders

Albinism (oculocutaneous)	Hereditary haemochromatosis
Ataxia telangiectasia	Homocystinuria
Crigler–Najjar syndrome type I	Hurler's syndrome (mucopolysaccharidosis)
Cystic fibrosis	Infantile polycystic kidney disease
Deafness (some forms)	Laurence–Moon–Biedl syndrome
Dubin–Johnson syndrome	Phenylketonuria
Epidermolysis bullosa (some forms)	Sickle cell disease
Fanconi syndrome	Tay–Sachs disease
Friedreich's ataxia	β-Thalassaemia
Galactosaemia	Wilson's disease
Gaucher's disease	
Glycogen storage disease	

Autosomal recessive disorders (Fig 2.16(b) and Table 2.6)

These disorders manifest themselves only when an individual is homozygous for the disease allele; i.e. both chromosomes carry the mutated gene. In this case the parents are generally unaffected healthy carriers (heterozygous for the disease allele). There is usually no family history, although the defective gene is passed from generation to generation. The offspring of an affected person will be healthy heterozygotes unless the other parent is also a carrier. If carriers marry, the offspring have a 1 in 4 chance of being homozygous and affected, a 1 in 2 chance of being a carrier, and a 1 in 4 chance of being genetically normal. Consanguinity increases the risk of two carriers having a child who has a 25% chance of being affected. The clinical features of autosomal recessive disorders are usually severe; patients often present in the first few years of life and have a high mortality.

Many inborn errors of metabolism are recessive diseases. The most common recessive disease in the UK is cystic fibrosis (see p. 157 and p. 783). The overall incidence of autosomal recessive disorders is about 2.5 per 1000 live births in the UK. World-wide, diseases such as thalassaemia and sickle cell disease are very common; the frequency of these diseases may be as high as 20 per 1000 births in some populations. Prenatal diagnosis for recessive disorders may be possible by analysing the DNA of the fetus for mutations known in the parents.

Table 2.7 lists some autosomal dominant and autosomal recessive genetic diseases with their chromosomal localization. Some diseases show a racial or geographical prevalence. Thalassaemia (see p. 375) is seen mainly in Greeks, South East Asians and Italians, porphyria variegata occurs more frequently in the South African white population, and Tay–Sachs (p. 1001) disease particularly occurs in Ashkenazi Jews.

Sex-linked disorders

(Figs 2.16(c) and (d) and Table 2.8)

Genes carried on the X chromosome are said to be X-linked and can be dominant or recessive in the same way as autosomal genes. As females have two X chromosomes they will be unaffected carriers of X-linked recessive diseases. However, since males have just one X chromosome, any deleterious mutation in an X-linked gene will manifest itself because no second copy of the gene is present.

X-linked dominant disorders

These are rare. Vitamin D-resistant rickets is the best-known example. Females who are heterozygous for the mutant gene and males who have one copy of the mutant

Table 2.7
Examples of single-gene disorders and their chromosomal locations

Disorder	Chromosome
Autosomal dominant disorders	
Familial adenomatous polyposis	5
Hypertrophic cardiomyopathy	14
Neurofibromatosis type I	17
Familial hypercholesterolaemia	19
Malignant hyperpyrexia	19
Amyotrophic lateral sclerosis	21
Autosomal recessive disorders	
Haemochromatosis	6
Cystic fibrosis	7
Friedreich's ataxia	9
β-Thalassaemia	11
Sickle cell disease	11
Phenylketonuria	12
α-Thalassaemia	
Triplet repeat expansion disorders	
Huntington's disease (autosomal dominant)	4
Myotonic dystrophy (autosomal dominant)	19

Table 2.8
Examples of X-linked disorders

Recessive
Albinism (ocular)
Becker's muscular dystrophy
Christmas disease
Colour blindness
Duchenne muscular dystrophy
Fabry's disease
Fragile X syndrome
Glucose-6-phosphate dehydrogenase deficiency
Haemophilia A
Hunter's syndrome (mucopolysaccharidosis)
Lesch–Nyhan syndrome
Menkes syndrome
Mental retardation (with or without fragile site)
Nephrogenic diabetes insipidus
Red–green colour blindness
Wiskott–Aldrich syndrome

Dominant
Vitamin D-resistant rickets (X-linked hypophosphataemia)

gene on their single X chromosome will manifest the disease. Half the male or female offspring of an affected mother and all the female offspring of an affected man will have the disease. Affected males tend to have the disease more severely than the heterozygous female.

X-linked recessive disorders

These disorders present in males and present only in (usually rare) homozygous females. X-linked recessive diseases are transmitted by healthy female carriers or affected males if they survive to reproduce. An example of an X-linked recessive disorder is haemophilia A (see p. 404), which is caused by a mutation in the X-linked gene for the essential clotting factor, factor VIII. It has recently been shown that in 50% of cases there is an intrachromosomal rearrangement (inversion) of the tip of the long arm of the X chromosome (one break point being within intron 22 of the factor VIII gene).

Of the offspring from a carrier female and a normal male:

- *50% of the girls will be carriers* as they inherit a mutant allele from their mother and the normal allele from their father; the other 50% of the girls inherit two normal alleles and are themselves normal
- *50% of the boys will have haemophilia* as they inherit the mutant allele from their mother (and the Y chromosome from their father); the other 50% of the boys will be normal as they inherit the normal allele from their mother (and the Y chromosome from their father).

The male offspring of a male with haemophilia and a normal female will not have the disease as they do not inherit his X chromosome. However, all the female offspring will be carriers as they all inherit his X chromosome.

Y-linked genes

Genes carried on the Y chromosome are said to be Y-linked and only males can be affected. However, there are no known examples of Y-linked single-gene disorders which are transmitted.

Sex-limited inheritance

Occasionally a gene can be carried on an autosome but manifests itself only in one sex. For example, frontal baldness is an autosomal dominant disorder in males but behaves as a recessive disorder in females.

Other single-gene disorders

These are disorders which may be due to mutations in single genes but which do not manifest as simple monogenic disorders. They can arise from a variety of mechanisms, including the following.

Triplet repeat mutations

In the gene responsible for myotonic dystrophy (p. 1103), the mutated allele was found to have an expanded 3′ UTR region in which three nucleotides, GCT, were repeated up to about 35 times. In families with myotonic dystrophy, people with the late-onset form of the disease had 20–40 copies of the repeat, but their children and grandchildren who presented with the disease from birth had vast increases in the number of repeats, up to 2000 copies. It is thought that some mechanism during meiosis causes this 'triplet repeat expansion' so that the offspring inherit an increased number of triplets. The number of triplets affects mRNA and protein function. See also p. 155 for the phenomenon of 'anticipation'.

Imprinting

It is known that normal humans need a diploid number of chromosomes, 46. However the maternal and paternal contributions are different and, in some way which is not yet clear, the fetus can distinguish between the chromosomes inherited from the mother and the chromosomes inherited from the father, although both give 23 chromosomes. In some way the chromosomes are 'imprinted' so that the maternal and paternal contributions are different. Imprinting is relevant to human genetic disease because different phenotypes may result depending on whether the mutant chromosome is maternally or paternally inherited. A deletion of part of the long arm of chromosome 15 (15q11–q13) will give rise to the Prader–Willi syndrome (PWS) if it is paternally inherited. A deletion of a similar region of the chromosome gives rise to Angelman syndrome (AS) if it is maternally inherited. Two different genes seem to be involved in PWS and AS as the necdin gene (found mainly in the brain and hypothalamus) is deleted in PWS but not in AS.

FURTHER READING

Brock DJH (1993) *Molecular Genetics for the Clinician*. Cambridge: Cambridge University Press.

Conner JM, Ferguson-Smith MA (1991) *Essential Medical Genetics*, 3rd edn. Oxford: Blackwell Scientific.

Gelehrter TD, Collins FS (1990) *The Principles of Medical Genetics*. Baltimore: Williams and Wilkins.

Saenger P (1996) Turner's syndrome. *New England Journal of Medicine* **335**: 1749–1754.

Weatherall DJ (1991) *The New Genetics in Clinical Practice*, 3rd edn. Oxford: Oxford University Press.

Complex traits: multifactorial and polygenic inheritance

Characteristics resulting from a combination of genetic and environmental factors are said to be *multifactorial*; those involving multiple genes can also be said to be *polygenic*.

Measurements of most biological traits (e.g. height) show a variation between individuals in a population and a unimodal, symmetrical (Gaussian) frequency distribution curve can be drawn. This variability is due to variation in genetic factors and environmental factors. Environmental factors may play an important part in determining some characteristics, such as weight, whilst other characteristics such as height may be largely genetically determined. This genetic component is thought to be due to the additive effects of a number of alleles at a number of loci, many of which can be individually identified using molecular biological techniques, for example studying identical twins in different environments.

One such condition that has been studied is congenital pyloric stenosis. This is most common in boys but if it occurs in girls the latter have a larger number of affected relatives. This difference suggests that a larger number of the relevant genes are required to produce the disease in girls than in boys. Most of the important human diseases, such as heart disease, diabetes and common mental disorders, are multifactorial traits (Table 2.9).

Table 2.9
Examples of disorders that may have a polygenic inheritance

Disorder	Frequency (%)	Heritability (%)[a]
Hypertension	5	62
Asthma	4	80
Schizophrenia	1	85
Congenital heart disease	0.5	35
Neural tube defects	0.5	60
Pyloric stenosis	0.3	75
Ankylosing spondylitis	0.2	70
Cleft palate	0.1	76

[a] Percentage of the total variation of a trait which can be attributed to genetic factors.

Analysis of mutations and genetic disease

Tracking a disease gene

Of the estimated 3400 inherited genetic disorders, only a very small number have been characterized in terms of their biochemistry and genetics. Their clinical phenotype may have been described extensively but the identity of the culpable gene is still unknown. However, it is not necessary to identify the gene because two genes that are situated close together on a chromosome are nearly always co-inherited. Only on rare occasions do they segregate during meiosis when the two chromosomes of a diploid pair cross over and exchange parts (recombination) – even then the crossover point must be between the two genes. The closer the genes, the less chance of a segregating crossover such that two genes that are one million base-pairs apart will only have a 1% chance of being separated by recombination. This might be an enormous distance in molecular terms, but for clinical genetic analysis this is acceptable for diagnosis. If a known gene or non-coding repetitive DNA sequence is within this one million base-pairs of the disease gene it will act as the *tag* or *marker* probe for the disease.

The large amount of non-coding DNA between genes, like all DNA, accumulates random base-pair changes throughout many generations. If these changes occur within genes, then they cause inherited disorders. The rate of mutation in some genes is quite low as there is a strong genetic selection against variants, but this is not true of non-coding DNA where a base-pair change has no deleterious effect. The frequency of change can approach 1 in 100 base-pairs. These changes occur randomly throughout the non-coding DNA, as do restriction enzyme sites. Sometimes a base-pair change will create or destroy a particular restriction site. Generally two members of a chromosome pair (*homologues*) will have broadly the same restriction patterns at any one point (Fig 2.17). However, owing to a random base-pair change, one chromosome will show a different restriction pattern for one enzyme (BamHI in Fig 2.17) compared with its homologue. These differences in restriction pattern are inherited, and are known as *polymorphisms*. Because they are observable as differences in length of particular restriction fragments they are known as *restriction fragment length polymorphisms* (RFLPs).

The inheritance of RFLPs

The blue area in Fig 2.17 shows a cloned area of DNA from two chromosomes. If this is used as a probe, it will detect any restriction fragment that contains an identical piece of DNA sequence, and thus it can be used to detect the BamHI polymorphism shown. A person with these two chromosomes will be heterozygous for the BamHI polymorphism, as the two chromosomes are different. The person will produce gametes that have only one of these chromosomes: 50% of the cells will have one type, 50% the other. If the mate of this person is also heterozygous for the same polymorphism, he or she will produce gametes that are 50% of one type and 50% the other. At fertilization there is a random chance that any one gamete will fuse with any gamete from the other parent, and thus four types of progeny will be produced. Two will be heterozygous for the polymorphism (Fig 2.18), one will be homozygous for the large BamHI fragment, the other will be homozygous for the small BamHI fragment.

If the chromosome carrying the BamHI polymorphism has a closely linked gene that when defective causes an inherited disorder, then by studying the family pedigree, the inheritance of both the disorder and the RFLP can be monitored. Generally, inherited disorders are caused by recessive genes. Both parents can therefore be carriers without being affected. If both parents come from families that have affected relatives, or they themselves have produced affected children, then they may wish to know if any subsequent children will also be sufferers. Suppose that the small BamHI fragment of the polymorphism is on the same chromosome as the defective gene, the large fragment being on the same chromosome as the normal allele. This can be checked by showing that any sufferers of the condition must be homozygous for the defective gene and thereby homozygous for the small BamHI fragment. To determine if any subsequent children are likely sufferers, DNA from a chorionic villi or amniocentesis sample can be digested with BamHI and electrophoresed on an agarose gel. It can then be probed with a cloned fragment using a Southern blot.

DNA can be amplified from very small tissue samples using PCR. If a polymorphism is reasonably well characterized, PCR across the RFLP will yield a suitable fragment to test for its prescence. Other markers used to trace disease genes are simple sequence repeats. More common and more polymorphic (i.e. having greater variability) than RFLPs, these are short di-, tri-, tetra- or penta-nucleotide repeats (such as $(CA)_n$) which are present throughout the genome and have highly variable lengths. By designing primers to the sequence either side of one of these repeats, the repeat can be amplified by PCR. The amplified product is electrophoresed on a gel and different sized products are produced from different people. If the mutant gene is close by, then a particular size repeat in that region will always segregate with the disease allele.

The likelihood of recombination between the marker under study and the disease allele must be taken into account. This measure of likelihood is known as the '*lod score*' (the logarithm of the odds) and is a measure of the statistical significance of the observed co-segregation of

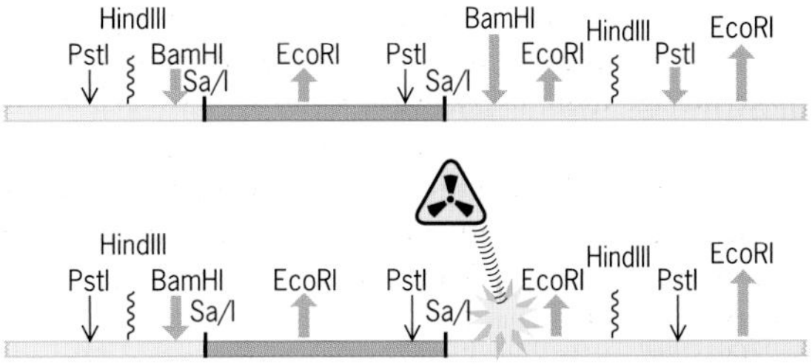

Fig 2.17
Restriction fragment length polymorphism. Diagrammatic representation of two allelic sections of DNA from a chromosome pair. The restriction site map of the two is identical except for a BamHI sequence which has been mutated by environmental radiation resulting in a restriction fragment length polymorphism (RFLP). The blue area represents a cloned sequence which acts as a marker probe or tag for the polymorphism

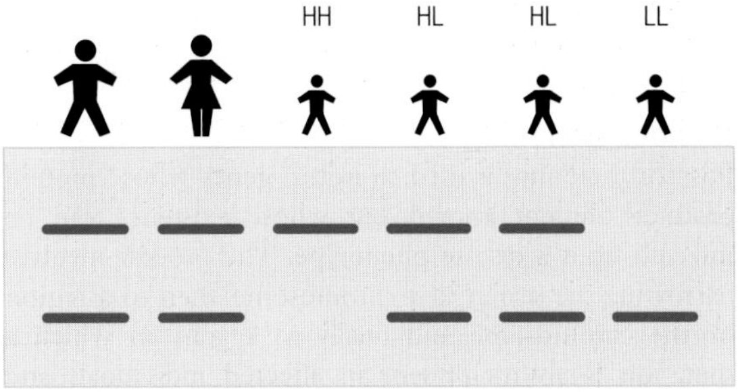

Fig 2.18
RFLP and disease tracking. Diagrammatic representation of the effect of the RFLP on a Southern blot of DNA extracted and digested with the BamHI restriction enzyme from a family whose parents were heterozygous for the polymorphism. The bands represent the hybridization of labelled marker probed sequence shown in Fig 2.17. Where the mutation had occurred the DNA would not have been cut and would therefore be heavier (H) and move down the gel slower than where the restriction site was still present (L). If the polymorphism which gives the small (L) fragment is on the same chromosome carrying the defective gene, a fetus homozygous for the large fragment (HH) will not be a sufferer and will be free of the disease. Fetuses that are heterozygous for the polymorphism will not be affected by the disease, but they will be carriers. Only if the fetus is homozygous for the small fragment (LL) will it be affected by the disease

the marker and the disease gene, compared with what would be expected by chance alone. Positive lod scores make linkage more likely, negative lod scores make it less likely. By convention a lod score of +3 is taken to be definite evidence of linkage because this indicates 1000 to 1 odds that the co-segregation of the DNA marker and the disease did not occur by chance alone.

Linkage analysis has provided many breakthroughs in mapping the positions of genes that cause genetic diseases, such as the gene for cystic fibrosis which was found to be tightly linked to a marker on chromosome 7, or the gene for Friedreich's ataxia which is tightly linked to a marker on chromosome 9.

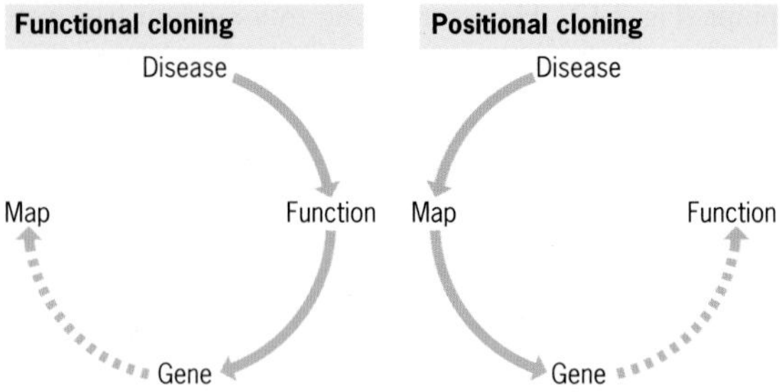

Fig 2.19
Diagrammatic representation of the two approaches to gene cloning

Gene hunting

Two approaches to the identification of a disease gene are possible – functional or positional cloning (Fig 2.19).

Functional cloning

Functional cloning requires a working knowledge of the biochemistry of the disease such that the defective protein/enzyme has previously been characterized in some way. Extracted mRNA from tissue expressing the disease gene (from both normal and affected individuals) is cloned into a vector. The clones are engineered such that the gene product is expressed by the host organism (i.e. bacteria) which may then be screened by antibodies or functional (enzyme–substrate) assay for those clones producing the desired gene product. The selected clones are isolated, propagated and the insert sequenced. The isolated cDNA insert can then be used as a probe to identify the location of the gene on a chromosome by *in situ* hybridization and to identify the genomic sequence from genome libraries.

As already stated, the biochemistry of most genetic disease is unknown and positional cloning is required.

Positional cloning

Positional cloning is used to isolate genes whose protein products are not known, but whose existence can be inferred from a disease phenotype. The process involves narrowing the search to a chromosome, then to a region of the chromosome, and finally to a gene in which a mutation is always present in affected individuals and absent in normal individuals.

The first step in the analysis is to study the pattern of inheritance. This may provide valuable clues about whether a single gene is affected, and whether this gene is likely to be autosomal or on the sex chromosomes or the mitochondrial chromosome. Gross chromosome analysis can be useful and geneticists look for chromosomal aberrations (for example deletions) which are present at an unusually high frequency in individuals affected with the disease, compared with the normal population.

If there are no further clues, often the next stage in locating the gene that is mutated in the disease is to look for genetic markers as described earlier. Once polymorphic markers from across the genome have been tested, it should be possible by linkage analysis to see if any segregate with the disease allele in a family. If the position of the polymorphic marker is known, then the affected gene is likely to be close by and is therefore mapped to a region of the genome (i.e. a specific band on a chromosome arm).

Isolating the gene

Once linkage analysis has established which chromosome and which region of the chromosome contains the disease gene, the next step is to identify the gene. The region of DNA which contains the gene may span several million base-pairs, and a variety of techniques exist for cloning cDNAs and gene sequences from such regions. Genes which have been cloned and are very tightly linked to a genetic disease may be 'candidate genes' for that disease, and researchers have to show that a mutation in the gene is likely to give rise to the disease.

However, most are unknown and markers which span the disease gene's physical location on the chromosome are traced through the affected families' genetic samples. These markers define the target interval of genetic code – often several million base-pairs – within which the disease gene lies. Essentially the whole target interval is cloned and partially or entirely sequenced by 'chromosome walking' or searching cDNA libraries for uncharacterized sequences which hybridize to regions of the target interval. Sequencing approaches require searching for motif sequences, such as areas rich in repetitive cytosine and guanidine base pairs, which are characteristic of a gene. Further, criteria for candidacy is that the gene is expressed in the affected tissues. It is unlikely that a gene giving rise to a liver disease might give the instructions for making protein purely in neuronal tissue. Probably the most important criterion is to find a mutation in the gene in affected and not unaffected individuals. When candidate genes have been identified, they are cloned and expressed in order to establish the function of the protein product.

The genetic basis of cancer

Cancers are genetic diseases and involve changes to the normal function of cellular genes. However, multiple genes interact during oncogenesis and an almost stepwise progression of defects leads from an overproliferation of a particular cell to the breakdown of control mechanisms such as apoptosis (programmed cell death). This would be triggered if a cell were to attempt to survive in an organ other than its tissue of origin. For the vast majority of cancer cases (especially those in older people) we believe that the multiple genetic changes which occur are somatic. However, it is clear that susceptibility to the development of a particular form of cancer can be inherited. Indeed for some rare cancers a dominant single-gene defect can give rise to an almost Mendelian trend. In some other cancers (e.g. forms of breast cancer) the mode of inheritance is much more complex. In these cases close relatives may have an increased susceptibility to cancer (Table 2.10), and the genetics are clearly those of a multifactorial trait.

- Cancer tissues are clonal, and tumours arise from changes in only one cell which then proliferates in the body.
- The genes that are primarily damaged by the genetic changes which lead to cancer fall into two categories: oncogenes and tumour suppressor genes.
- Oncogenesis is a multistep process in that a number of mutations or alterations to key genes are required before a malignant phenotype is expressed.
- Once mutations have begun to cause unchecked clonal expansion of the primary tumour cells, further mutations occur within the subsequent generations of daughter cells that give rise to clones which are invasive and/or form metastases.

Oncogenes (see p. 418)

The genes coding for proteins which are either growth factors, growth factor receptors, secondary messengers or even DNA-binding proteins would act as promoters of abnormal cell growth if mutated. This concept was verified when viruses were found to carry genes which, when integrated into the host cell, promoted oncogenesis. These were originally termed viral or 'v-oncogenes', and later their normal cellular counterparts, c-oncogenes, were found. Thus, oncogenes encode proteins that are known to participate in the regulation of normal cellular proliferation (Table 2.11).

Activation of oncogenes

Non-activated oncogenes which are functioning normally have been referred to as 'proto-oncogenes'. Their transformation to oncogenes can occur by three routes.

Mutation

Carcinogens such as those found in cigarette smoke, ionizing radiation and ultraviolet light can cause point mutations in genomic DNA. By chance some of these point mutations will occur in regions of the oncogene which lead to activation of that gene. Not all bases in an oncogene cause cancer if mutated, but some (e.g. those in the coding region) do.

Chromosomal translocation

If during cell division an error occurs and two chromosomes translocate, so that a portion swaps over, the translocation breakpoint may occur in the middle of two genes. If this happens then the end of one gene is translocated on to the beginning of another gene, giving rise to a 'fusion gene'. Therefore sequences of one part of

Table 2.10
Inherited cancer syndromes

Syndrome	Chromosome localization	Tumour suppressor gene	Neoplasms
Familial adenomatous polyposis	5q21	*APC*	Colon
Familial non-polyposis colon cancer	2	*MLH1* or *MSH2*	Colon
Wilms' tumour	11p13p15	*WT-1*	Kidney
Retinoblastoma	13q14.1	*RB-1*	Retina
Li-Fraumeni syndrome	17p13.1	*p53*	Breast adrenal cortex, sarcomas, leukaemia, brain tumours
Neurofibromatosis type I	17q11	*NF 1*	Neural tumours
Neurofibromatosis type II	22q	*NF 2*	Central Schwannomas and meningiomas
Von Hippel–Lindau disease	3p25	*VHL*	Haemangioblastoma and renal cell carcinoma
Multiple endocrine neoplasia (MEN 2a)	10p11–q11	*Ret*	Thyroid C cells Adrenal medulla

Table 2.11
Well-known examples of oncogenes (see also Table 7.3)

Name	Chromosomal location	Function if known
SIS	22q13.1	Secreted tissue specific growth factor
INT-2	11q13	Secreted tissue specific growth factor
FMS	5q34	Colony stimulating factor receptor
Erb-A	17q11–q12	Thyroid hormone receptor
Erb-B	7p13–p12	Epidermal growth factor receptor
Abl	9q34	Non-receptor tyrosine kinase/ signal transduction molecule
Src	20q12–q13	Non-receptor tyrosine kinase/ signal transduction molecule
H-ras	11p14.1	Inner membrane bound signal transduction protein
K-ras	12p12.1	Inner membrane bound signal transduction protein
Myc	8q24	Gene expression regulatory protein
Jun	1p32–p31	Gene expression regulatory protein
Fos	14q24.3	Gene expression regulatory protein

the fusion gene are inappropriately expressed because they are under the control of the other part of the gene.

An example of such a fusion gene occurs in chronic myeloid leukaemia (CML). In patients with CML a translocated chromosome (the Philadelphia chromosome; see p. 426) is seen in the leukaemic cells. This chromosome arises from a translocation between chromosomes 9 and 22 in which they exchange a portion of their long arms. Consequently the *ABL* gene on chromosome 9 becomes joined to the *BCR* gene on chromosome 22. The resulting fusion protein is thought to cause the changes which lead to CML. Similarly in Burkitt's lymphoma a translocation causes the regulatory segment of the *myc* oncogene to be replaced by a regulatory segment of an unrelated immunoglobulin.

Viral stimulation

When viral RNA is transcribed by reverse transcriptase into viral cDNA and in turn is spliced into the cellular DNA, the viral DNA may integrate within an oncogene and activate it. Alternatively the virus may pick up cellular oncogene DNA and incorporate it into its own viral genome. Subsequent infection of another host cell might result in expression of this viral oncogene. For example, the Rous sarcoma virus of chickens was found to induce cancer because it carried the *ras* oncogene.

After the initial activation event other changes occur within the DNA. A striking example of this is amplification of gene sequences, which can affect the *myc* gene for example. Instead of the normal two copies of a gene, multiple copies of the gene appear either within the chromosomes (these can be seen on stained chromosomes as homogeneously staining regions) or as extra-chromosomal particles (double minutes). N-*myc* sequences are amplified in neuroblastomas as are N-*myc* or L-*myc* in some lung small-cell carcinomas.

Tumour suppressor genes

A series of genes, originally termed 'tumour supressor genes', were discovered which restrict undue cell proliferation (in contrast to oncogenes), and which induce the repair or self-destruction (apoptosis) of cells containing damaged DNA. Therefore mutations in these genes which disable their function lead to uncontrolled cell growth in cells with active oncogenes. An example is the germline mutations in genes found in non-polyposis colorectal cancer which are responsible for repairing DNA mismatches (p. 274).

The first tumour suppressor gene to be described was the *Rb* gene. Mutations in *Rb* lead to retinoblastoma which occurs in 1 in 20 000 young children and can be sporadic or familial. In the familial variety, the first mutation is inherited and by chance a second somatic mutation occurs with the formation of a tumour. In the sporadic variety, by chance both mutations occur in both the *RB* genes in a single cell.

Since the finding of *Rb*, other tumour suppressor genes have been described, including the gene *p53*. Mutations in *p53* have been found in almost all human tumours, including sporadic colorectal carcinomas, carcinomas of breast and lung, brain tumours, osteosarcomas and leukaemias. The protein, encoded by *p53*, is a cellular 53 kDa nuclear phosphoprotein that plays a role in DNA repair and synthesis, in the control of the cell cycle and cell differentiation and programmed cell death – apoptosis. *p53* is a DNA-binding protein which activates many gene expression pathways but it is normally only short-lived. In many tumours, mutations that disable *p53* function also prevent its cellular catabolism. Although in some cancers there is a loss of *p53* from both chromosomes, in most cancers (particularly colorectal carcinomas; see Fig 4.34) such long-lived mutant *p53* alleles can disrupt the normal alleles' protein. As a DNA-binding protein, *p53* is likely to act as a dimer. Thus, a mutation in a single copy of the gene can promote tumour formation because a heterodimer of mutated and normal *p53* subunits would still be dysfunctional.

How tumour suppressor genes work

Tumour suppressor gene products are intimately involved in control of the cell cycle (see Fig 2.3). Progression through the cell cycle is controlled by many molecular gateways which are opened or blocked by the *cyclin* group of proteins that are specifically expressed at various stages of the cycle. The *RB* and *p53* proteins are important in the control of the cell cycle and interact specifically within many cyclin proteins. The latter are affected by INK 4α acting on p16 proteins. The general principle is that being held at one of these gateways will ultimately lead to programmed cell death. *p53* is a DNA-binding protein which induces the expression of other genes and is a major player in the induction of cell death. Its own expression is induced by broken DNA. The induction of *p53* by damage initially causes the expression of DNA repair enzymes. If DNA repair is too slow or cannot be effected, then other proteins that are induced by *p53* will effect programmed cell death.

One gateway event which has been largely elucidated is that between the G1 and the S phase of the cell cycle. The transcription factor dimer E2F-DP1 causes progression from the G1 to the S phase. However, the *RB* protein binds to this transcription factor, preventing its induction of DNA synthesis. Other, cyclin D-related molecules inactivate the *RB* protein thus allowing DNA synthesis to proceed. This period of rapid DNA synthesis is susceptible to mutation events and will propagate a pre-existing DNA mistake. Damaged DNA-induced *p53* expression rapidly results in the expression of a variety of closely related (and possibly tissue-specific) proteins WAF-1/p21, p16, p27. These inhibit the inactivation of *RB* by cyclin D-related molecules. As a result *RB*, the normal gate which stops the cell cycle, binds to the E2F-DP1 transcription factor complex, halting S phase DNA synthesis. If the DNA damage is not repaired apoptosis ensues.

Viral inactivation of tumour suppressors

The suppression of normal tumour suppressor gene function can be achieved by disabling the normal protein once it has been transcribed, rather than by mutating the gene. Viruses have developed their own genes which produce proteins to do precisely this. The main targets of these proteins are *RB* and *p53* to which they bind and thus disable. The best understood are the adenovirus E1A and human papilloma virus (HPV) E7 gene products which bind *RB*, whilst the adenovirus E1B and HPV E6 gene products bind *p53*. The SV40 virus large T antigen binds both *RB* and *p53*.

Cancer aetiology: inheritance or environment?

It is clear that a mutation causing the dysfunction of a single oncogene or tumour supressor gene is not sufficient to induce unregulated clonal expansion. The *Knudson multi-hit hypothesis* elegantly unites the genetics of familial and sporadic tumour development: an inherited mutation in one gene allele may be insufficient to cause a tumour but will cause a significant susceptibility to the development of a particular cancer. Subsequent lifetime exposure to environmental carcinogens (viral, chemical, radiation), along with simple mistakes during cell division, may deregulate the normal allele. Other mutations which accumulate in a similar manner then lead to tumour development. Research has clearly shown that germline mutations in particular genes, such as *p53* and *RB*, have a much stronger influence on the chance of subsequent tumour development than others.

Apoptosis (programmed cell death)

Necrotic cell death is where some external factor (e.g. hypoxia, chemical toxins) damages the cell's physiology and results in the disintegration of the cell. Characteristically there is an influx of water and ions, after which cellular organelles swell and rupture. Cell lysis induces acute inflammatory responses *in vivo* owing to the release of lysosomal enzymes into the extracellular environment. In *apoptosis, physiological cell death* occurs owing to the deliberate activation of constituent genes whose function is to cause their own demise. Apoptotic cell death has characteristic morphological features:

- chromatin aggregation, with nuclear and cytoplasmic condensation into distinct membrane bound-vesicles which are termed apoptotic bodies
- organelles remain intact
- cell 'blebs' (which are intact membrane vesicles)
- there is no inflammatory response
- cellular 'blebs' and remains are phagocytosed by adjacent cells and macrophages.

This process requires energy (ATP), and several Ca^{2+} and Mg^{2+}-dependent nuclease systems are activated which specifically cleave nuclear DNA at the inter-histone residues.

Recently an endonuclease has, at last, been found that destroys DNA following apoptosis. This involves the enzyme CASPASE (cysteine-containing aspartase-specific protease) which activates the CAD (caspase-activated DNase)/ICAD (inhibitor of CAD) system which can destroy DNA.

The genetics of apoptosis

Programmed cell death has been principally studied in the nematode *Caenorhabditis elegans*. The genes identified as responsible for the process are termed *ced* (cell death defective). Of particular interest are those termed *ced-3*, *ced-4* and *ced-9* since the first two need to be active for apoptosis to occur and the last protects cells from undergoing apoptosis if triggered. In mammals, at least 10 homologues to *ced-3* have been found. The first of these to be discovered was the protease *interleukin 1β-converting enzyme* – ICE (now called caspace-1).

Subsequently several classes of homologous proteins have been discovered (e.g. caspace 2–10 proteases). The genes for these cysteine proteases are initially transcribed to produce inactive precursors which are constitutively expressed in most cells. Thus they are always present, ready to be immediately activated. The mammalian homologue of *ced-9* is the known oncogene *Bcl-2*. The expression of the *Bcl-2* protein is protective against apoptosis and heightens the threshold to which a cell will respond to a signal to undergo apoptosis. Thus, over-expression of *Bcl-2* is an important component of oncogenesis for some tumours and proliferative states (e.g. polycythaemia vera). There are several homologues of *Bcl-2* termed *Bax*, *Bcl-x* and *Mcl*. *Bcl-2* forms a dimer when acting as an inhibitor of apoptosis. However, its dimeric partner can be any of the proteins arising from the homologous genes. This disrupts *Bcl-2*'s function to varying degrees, and *Bax–Bax* homodimers are in fact enhancers of apoptosis. Thus the ratio of pro-apoptotic to anti-apoptotic proteins is important for the survival of a cell.

FURTHER READING

Duke RC, Ojcius DM, Young JD-E (1996) Cell suicide in health and disease. *Scientific American* December: 48–56.

Krontiris TG (1995) Oncogenes. *New England Journal of Medicine* **333**: 303–306.

Macdonald F, Ford CHJ (1997) Molecular Biology of Cancer. Oxford: BIOS Science Publishers.

Wyllie AH (ed) (1997) Apoptosis: an overview. *British Medical Bulletin* **53**: 451–465.

Population genetics

The genetic constitution of a population depends on many factors. The Hardy–Weinberg equilibrium is a concept, based on a mathematical equation, that describes the outcome of random mating within populations. It states that 'in the absence of mutation, non-random mating, selection and genetic drift, the genetic constitution of the population remains the same from one generation to the next'.

This genetic principle has clinical significance in terms of the number of abnormal genes in the total gene pool of a population. The Hardy–Weinberg equation states that

$$p^2 + 2pq + q^2 = 1$$

where p is the frequency of the normal gene in the population, q is the frequency of the abnormal gene, p^2 is the frequency of the normal homozygote, q^2 is the frequency of the affected abnormal homozygote, $2pq$ is the carrier frequency, and $p + q = 1$.

Example. The equation can be used, for example, to find the frequency of heterozygous carriers in cystic fibrosis. The incidence of cystic fibrosis is 1 in 2000 live births. Thus $q^2 = 1/2000$, and therefore $q = 1/44$. Since $p = 1 - q$, then $p = 43/44$. The carrier frequency is represented by $2pq$, which in this case is 1/22. Thus 1 in 22 individuals in the whole population is a heterozygous carrier for cystic fibrosis.

Clinical genetics and genetic counselling

Genetic disorders pose considerable health and economic problems because often there is no effective therapy. In any pregnancy the risk of a serious developmental abnormality is approximately 1 in 30 pregnancies; approximately 15% of paediatric inpatients have a multifactorial disorder with a predominantly genetic element.

People with a history of a congenital abnormality in a member of their family often seek advice as to why it happened and about the risks of producing further abnormal offspring. Interviews must be conducted with great sensitivity and psychological insight, as parents may feel a sense of guilt and blame themselves for the abnormality in their child.

Genetic counselling should have the following aims:

- *A full and careful history should be taken.* The pregnancy history, drug and alcohol ingestion during pregnancy and maternal illnesses (e.g. diabetes) should be detailed.
- *Establishing an accurate diagnosis.* Examination of the child may help in diagnosing a genetically abnormal child with characteristic features (e.g. trisomy 21) or whether a genetically normal fetus was damaged *in utero*.
- *Drawing a family tree is essential.* Questions should be asked about abortions, stillbirths, deaths, marriages, consanguinity and medical history of family members. Diagnoses may need verification from other hospital reports.
- *Estimating the risk of a future pregnancy being affected or carrying a disorder.* Estimation of risk should be based on the pattern of inheritance. Mendelian disorders (see earlier) carry a high risk; chromosomal abnormalities carry a low risk. Empirical risks may be obtained from population or family studies.
- *Information.* On prognosis and management.
- *Continued support and follow-up.* Explanation of the implications for other siblings and family members.
- *Genetic screening.* This includes prenatal diagnosis if requested, carrier detection and data storage in genetic registers.

Genetic counselling should be non-directive, with the couple making their own decisions on the basis of an accurate presentation of the facts and risks in a way they can understand.

Carrier detection

This is offered in autosomal recessive disorders for conditions that are relatively common such as thalassaemia (Asian and Mediterranean populations), cystic fibrosis (Caucasian populations), sickle cell disease (African origin) and Tay–Sachs disease (Ashkenazi Jews). Families segregating the severe form of haemophilia A can now have more accurate genetic counselling to detect the inversion of the X chromosome (flip-tip inversion) using Southern blotting.

Genetic anticipation

An unusual phenomenon observed by geneticists studying myotonic dystrophy and Huntington's chorea in the early 1900s was termed 'anticipation'. Successive generations of patients with these genetic diseases presented earlier and with progressively worse symptoms; in the case of myotonic dystrophy the disease could be traced back to an ancestor with the mildest of symptoms such as cataracts.

It has only recently been shown that this was due to a previously unknown phenomenom of unstable mutations occurring within the disease gene. Trinucleotide repeats such as CTG (myotonic dystrophy) and CAG (Huntington's chorea) expand within the disease gene with each generation, and somatic expansion with cellular replication is also observed. This novel type of genetic mutation can occur within the translated region or untranslated (and presumably regulatory) regions of the target genes. This genetic distinction has been used to subclassify a number of genetic diseases which have now been shown to be caused by trinucleotide repeat expansion and display phenotypic 'anticipation' (Table 2.12).

Table 2.12 The location of the trinucleotide repeat in 'anticipation' genetic diseases[a]

Trinucleotide repeat (untranslated)
Myotonic dystrophy (19q13)
Fragile X (Xq28)
Friedreich's ataxia (9q13–21)
Trinucleotide repeat (translated)
Huntington's chorea (4p16)
Spinobulbar muscular atrophy – SBMA (Xq21)
Spinocerebellar ataxia 1 and 2 – SCA1/2 (6p21)
Machado–Joseph ataxia – SCA-3 (14p32)
Dento–Rubro–Pallido–Luysian atrophy – DRPLA (12p12)

[a] The chromosomal locations of the genes are given in in parentheses.

Prenatal diagnosis (Information box 2.4)

For families at risk of genetic disease, an intrauterine diagnosis is important – either to reassure parents if the fetus is unaffected, or to allow termination of the pregnancy if requested. Prenatal diagnosis might be carried out if there is a high genetic risk of a severe disorder and if no treatment is available for the particular disorder.

High-resolution ultrasonography has replaced amniocentesis in some centres for the diagnosis of neural tube defects. However, for diagnosing gene defects in which it is necessary to study fetal DNA, amniocentesis (sampling of fluid under ultrasound control from the amniotic sac) gives access to fetal cells. Chorionic villus sampling (CVS), transcervical or transabdominal under ultrasound guidance, can be performed at an earlier time (from 10 weeks' gestation), which has the advantage of earlier and easier termination if requested. However, there is a 1% increase in the rate of spontaneous abortion following these procedures, and limb bud deformations have been associated with CVS when performed before 9.5 weeks' gestation. With embryos produced by *in vitro* fertilization, DNA analysis of one or two embryonic cells at the 8–16 cell stage can be undertaken and if normal the embryo is implanted.

Screening for fetal aneuploidies

Maternal serum is widely used in the second trimester (15–22 weeks) for screening for neural tube defects and aneuploid fetuses. High levels of maternal serum fetoprotein are associated with neural tube defects and some other fetal abnormalities. Altered levels of maternal serum α-fetoprotein, unconjugated oestriol and human chorionic gonadotrophin (hCG) are associated with aneuploid pregnancies, in particular trisomy 21 (Down's syndrome). Various other oncofetal antigens have been investigated, but hCG – and in particular the free β-subunit – is the single most important.

The measurement of these markers is corrected for gestation ages as a multiple of the median (MoM) value for the appropriate week of gestation. Individual samples are compared with the distribution of MoMs found for the individual analyte of those with normal and affected pregnancies. Summing the odds of the MoM value (found corresponding to either an aneuploid or normal pregnancy for each marker), combined with maternal age, gives a risk value of the mother carrying an affected fetus. Currently a risk of 1/250 is taken as high risk and the mother is then recommended to undergo amniocentesis. Second-trimester serum screening can detect 60–70% of Down's pregnancies. The sole measurement of the urinary metabolite of hCG, beta-core, is reported to detect as many Down's cases as do current serum biochemical tests, and this may prove much cheaper and easier. First-trimester maternal serum screening for

Information

	Risk and gestation for performing test	Comments
Prenatal diagnosis		
Ultrasound	1st trimester	Increased nuchal translucency for major chromosomal abnormalities (e.g. trisomies and Turner's[a])
	2nd trimester	Structural abnormalities (e.g. neural tube defects, congenital heart defects, chromosomal markers such as abnormal digits)
Amniocentesis	Risk < 1% From 14 weeks	Chromosomal analysis Measurement of α-fetoprotein (AFP) or acetylcholine esterase Biochemical analysis Widely available
Chorionic villus sampling	Risk 1–2% From 10 weeks	Chromosomal and DNA analysis Biochemical analysis Highly specialized
Cordocentesis	Risk 1–2% From 19 weeks	Fetal blood sampling for chromosomal and DNA analysis Highly specialized
Maternal blood screening	***Test***	***Abnormality in fetus***
2nd trimester	α-Fetoprotein (high)	Neural tube defects
	Triple test: α-Fetoprotein (low) Unconjugated oestradiol (low) Human chorionic gonadotrophin (high)	Trisomy 21

[a] Sensitivity for trisomy 21 = 85%; for trisomy 13 = 90%; for trisomy 18 = 90%.

Information box 2.4 Methods available for prenatal diagnosis and screening

trisomy 21 using pregnancy-associated plasma protein-A (PAP-A from the syncytial trophoblast) is under evaluation. Ultrasound detection of a thickened oedematous flap of skin at the base of the neck – *nuchal translucency* – is reported to detect as many as 80% of Down's fetuses during the first trimester. However, highly skilled ultrasonographers are required for this level of scan measurement.

The following points must be borne in mind when considering a prenatal screening test for aneuploidies:

- The most common congenital chromosomal aneuploidy in which the afflicted individual lives into old age is Down's syndrome – trisomy 21
- Most Down's individuals have an IQ of between 20 and 80; 61% will require surgery for congenital heart, gastrointestinal and ophthalmic defects; there is a strong association with the development of acute childhood leukaemia; and 60–70% will develop Alzheimer-like neuronal degeneration after the age of 40 years.
- The risk of having a Down's child increases with maternal age, such that at age 35 the risk is 1 in 380.
- Although women over 35 are at higher risk, they account for only 7% of pregnancies. In fact, 70–80% of all Down's children are born to women under this age.
- Karyotyping is the only definitive test, but cannot be offered to all as it is expensive and time-consuming and requires skilled technicians.
- Fetal tissue sampling is associated with a 1% risk of spontaneous termination.
- Screening aims to select a high-risk group, irrespective of maternal age, to be offered a diagnostic procedure; it does not provide a diagnosis itself.
- Of paramount importance is the ability of screening to give parents a more informed choice.

FURTHER READING

Harper PS (1996) New genes for old diseases: the molecular basis of myotonic dystrophy and Huntington's disease. *Journal of the Royal College of Physicians of London* **30**: 221–231.

Stranc LC *et al.* (1997) CVS and amniocentesis in prenatal. *Lancet* **349**: 711–714.

Wald *et al.* (1992) Screening for Down's. *British Medical Journal* **305**: 391–394.

Applications of molecular genetics

The use of molecular biological techniques in genetics is having a massive impact on the investigation, diagnosis, treatment and control of genetic disorders.

The avoidance and control of genetic disease

Some genetic disorders, such as phenylketonuria or haemophilia, can be managed by diet or replacement therapy, but most have no effective treatment. By understanding what causes genetic damage, potential mutagens such as radiation, environmental chemicals, viruses or drugs (e.g. thalidomide) can be avoided.

Gene therapy

There are many technical problems to overcome in gene therapy, particularly in finding delivery systems to introduce DNA into a mammalian cell. Very careful control and supervision of gene manipulation will be necessary because of its potential hazards and the ethical issues.

Treatment of congenital genetic disease

Conventional therapy consists of controlling rather than curing the genetic defect. In some conditions, gene product replacement may ameliorate the symptoms; examples are the production of insulin (from recombinant DNA) for the treatment of diabetes, and factor VIII replacement in haemophilia A. Current research suggests that for many defects 'gene therapy' may be an option in the future.

Gene therapy entails placing a normal copy of a gene into the cells of a patient who has a defective copy of the gene. For example, it might be possible to remove bone marrow cells from a patient with thalassaemia, culture the cells *in vitro*, and introduce a functional normal human globin gene; then re-introduce the cells with normal globin into the patient's bone marrow. This type of experiment involves somatic tissue only, so altered DNA would not be inherited by the offspring of a person who has undergone gene therapy. To alter germline cells in a human conceptus is banned as it is considered to promote eugenic medical technology.

Current experiments are concentrated on recessive disorders, such as cystic fibrosis where the disease is due to the absence of a normal gene product. In these cases it is sufficient to introduce one functional normal allele of the relevant gene in order to overcome the genetic deficiency. However, in dominant disorders the pathogenic potential of the mutant allele is normally expressed in the presence of a normal allele. This requires gene correction, whereby the mutant sequence is replaced by an equivalent sequence from a normal allele, or the mutant allele is inactivated. Such procedures are more difficult and, therefore, attempts have concentrated on recessive disorders focusing on gene insertion into somatic cells. Technically this is still a daunting challenge.

The two major problems in this type of gene therapy are:

- the introduction of the functional gene sequence into target cells
- the expression and permanent integration of the transfected gene into the host cell genome.

Success is based largely on probability. *In vitro* cells can be simply transfected by swamping them with the gene sequence (complete with transcription regulating sequences) and much of the DNA will be absorbed by pinocytosis. Alternatively, altered viral vectors can be used to infect the target cells. Once inside the cell the gene has to be expressed and also incorporated into the host genome if it is to be passed on to subsequent generations of daughter cells.

The latter is a particularly difficult issue to address. It is relatively easy to demonstrate transient expression of DNA transfected into a cell, but genomic integration has many problems. Retroviruses are potential vectors which will overcome the problem of integration as they insert their genome into that of the host, specifically targeting dividing cells. However, such integration is random and may interrupt important genes, and only a 7 kbp gene can be inserted into the virus owing to physical limitation. Adenoviruses target non-dividing cells and form an episomal genome which is self-regulating and expressed. However, again, only a 7 kbp gene can be inserted. Large genes can be absorbed into a cell if they are packaged into a lipid bilayer. Lipid bilayer analogues and liposomes have been developed as delivery systems for genes, cytotoxins and enzymes.

The biological nature of the genetic disease is also important. If the defect is in a specific organ in which a local paracrine interaction is disrupted, we are unlikely to be able to specifically target the stem cells of that tissue/organ.

Suitable diseases for current gene therapy experiments include cystic fibrosis, adenosine deaminase deficiency, and familial hypercholesterolaemia.

Cystic fibrosis (see also p. 783)

The gene responsible for cystic fibrosis was first localized to chromosome 7 by linkage analysis. The cystic fibrosis transmembrane regulator gene (*CFTR*) was then isolated by chromosome-mediated gene transfer, chromosome walking and jumping. The *CFTR* gene spans about 250 kbp and contains 27 exons. The DNA sequence analysis predicts a polypeptide sequence of 1480 amino acids. The *CFTR* gene also encodes a simple chloride ion channel within the *CFTR* (Fig 2.20). In most patients there is a single mutation with a 3 bp deletion in exon 10 resulting in the removal of a codon specifying phenylalanine. There are also over 100 different minor mutations of the *CFTR* gene with most mapping to the ATP-binding domains. This has led to the improved diagnosis of cystic fibrosis as well as new strategies for conventional drug-based therapies.

Gene therapy experiments are under way that take two different routes to putting a normal version of the *CFTR* gene into the lung epithelial cells of a patient who is homozygous for a defect in this gene. One route entails placing the *CFTR* gene in an adenovirus vector, and infecting the epithelial cells of the patient with the virus. Infection causes the *CFTR* gene to be taken into the cell where it may start functioning normally. A second route entails placing the DNA for the *CFTR* gene into a liposome. Liposomes are then conveyed to the lung using an aerosol spray, and the fatty surface of the liposome fuses with the cell membrane to deliver the *CFTR* DNA into the cell, where again the gene should function normally. Ultimately this type of gene therapy should give cystic fibrosis patients a normal life without the need for drugs and intensive physiotherapy.

Adenosine deaminase (*ADA*) deficiency

Gene therapy for this rare immunodeficiency disease entails introducing a normal human *ADA* gene into the patient's lymphocytes to reconstitute the function of the cellular and humoral immune system in severe combined immunodeficiency (SCID). Currently it is being tried using lymphocytes for short-term therapy, but for longer-term treatment bone marrow transplantation would be the definitive approach (see p. 436).

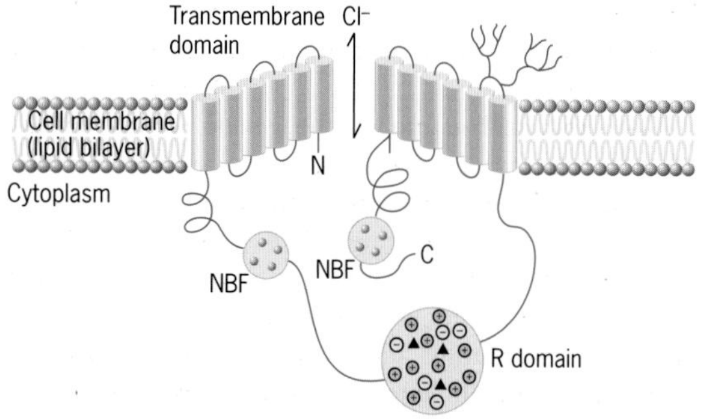

Fig 2.20
Model of cystic fibrosis transmembrane conductor regulator (*CFTR*). This is an integral membrane glycoprotein, consisting of two repeated elements. The cylindrical structures represent six membrane-spanning helices in each half of the molecule. The nucleotide-binding folds (NBFs) are in the cytoplasm, and the dots in these hatched areas represent the means of entry by the nucleotide. The regulatory (R) domain links the two halves and contains charged individual amino acids and protein kinase phosphorylation sites (black triangles). N and C are the N and C terminals. The branched structure on the right half represents potential glycosylation sites. The chloride channel is shown

Familial hypercholesterolaemia

This disorder is a result of a defective low-density lipoprotein (LDL) receptor gene. In therapy, a receptor gene is inserted into hepatocytes, removed by liver biopsy from the patient. Gene-corrected hepatocytes are then re-injected into the portal circulation of the patient. These cells migrate back to the liver where they are re-incorporated and should start to produce LDL receptor protein, which would dramatically lower the patient's cholesterol level.

Muscle-cell-mediated gene therapy

Much of the problem associated with gene therapy of chronic genetic disease is how long the transfected cells will survive. Isolated myoblasts transfected with a retrovirus have been shown to function and live for the lifetime of mouse models (two years). The myoblasts fuse with the patient's muscle fibres and express the transfected protein. The long life of the muscle fibres and their rich blood supply make them an ideal site for treatment of diseases in which functional serum-born factors are missing (e.g. human growth hormone, coagulation factors and erythropoietin).

Obviously, myoblast transfection would appear to be the best option for the treatment of Duchenne's muscular dystrophy. However, the Duchenne's gene is far too large to fit into any current viral vector, and re-implanted myoblasts do not colonize muscles fibres distant from the site of injection.

Treatment of somatic disease

Gene therapy which requires only a transient expression of the transfected genetic material circumvents the problems currently plaguing gene therapy of inherited disorders. This may also prove to be the front-line of gene therapy.

Vascular disease

The ideal therapy in heart disease would be neovascularization to increase blood flow and the repair of cardiac tissue after a myocardial infarction. In fact, any vascular disease might require regeneration or new blood vessel growth. Temporary expression of angiogenic factors at the site of a blockage would induce new blood vessels. Alternatively, local temporary expression of clot-disintegrating enzymes such as streptokinase and lipases may repair damaged and diseased arteries. It is quite possible to deliver liposomes loaded with DNA or, in fact, directly inject DNA plasmids into the tissue and the protein will be expressed by the cells which take it up. Only 1–3% will do so, but this is sufficient for the local effect required and it is a transient expression. This gives a controllable gene therapy.

Neuronal disease

Neurotrophic factors can be transiently expressed as described above for vascular diseases. The local expression of neurotrophins is essential for nerve cell regeneration and maintenance. It is possible to extend the expression period of the neurotrophin by injecting transfected myocytes into the damaged area. They will fuse with any adjacent muscle tissue to give a prolonged expression of the factor gene.

Cancer

Cancer is a genetic disease and many genes are deregulated. *p53* is particularly important as a tumour suppressor gene; the reintroduction and overexpression of a functional *p53* in tumours is being investigated with some success. Since *p53* will induce apoptosis in cells with damaged genetic material, the transient expression of high levels in a tumour cell with *p53* pathway defects should induce its own (apoptotic) demise. Since this is only likely to occur in rapidly dividing cells, this is a perfect target for cancer gene therapy. Transient expression induced by repeat exposure to vectors such as retroviruses, liposomes and naked DNA plasmids is all relatively straightforward. Initial trials using aerosols of these vectors in patients with lung cancer has so far been encouraging.

Tumour growth depends on the development of new blood vessels (angiogenesis), and inhibitors of this process are also being used in trials.

Creating and using animal models

There is a need for model systems in which to test gene therapies prior to use in patients. To some extent gene 'knock-out' experiments in mice are providing new animal models of disease. In these experiments the normal gene of interest in a mouse is targeted using recombinant DNA techniques so that gene function is impaired, in analogy to the situation in the particular gene of a human patient. However, mice and humans are different and it will not be possible to mimic some human genetic diseases in mice.

Transgenic mice are created when exogenous DNA carrying a gene of interest is injected into a mouse egg. If this egg is fertilized then all the cells of the resulting animal will carry the extra gene sequences. Transgenic mice have also been used as animal models of human diseases in which new therapies may be tested.

Other animal models have paved the way for gene therapy techniques. For example, some of the first experiments in the transfer of globin genes (which will be useful for gene therapy for sickle cell disease and thalassaemia) have taken place in mice. These include transplanting normal donor cells with normal genes into lethally irradiated mice, which results in engraftment of the donor cells.

The human genome project (HGP)

An international effort to sequence the entire human genome, all 3×10^9 bp on the 24 different chromosomes, was officially launched in 1986. An initial aim was to construct genetic and physical maps of the chromosomes: 40 three-generation families were studied for microsatellite and restriction enzyme (RFLP) polymorphisms. Some 70 000 polymorphisms were characterized and physically assigned to chromosomal band locations. These landmarks in the genome are used as reference points in the subsequent genome mapping project. However, as already described, these polymorphisms are the first step in positional cloning of a disease gene and are used as genetic markers if they co-segregate with the disease. Up to the beginning of 1997 some 1–2% of the genome had been sequenced, but with the current exponential rise in sequencing automation the projected completion date of 2005 should easily be achieved. Having the complete sequence of the genome will make it much easier to identify candidate genes in genetic disorders, and will be a great aid to genetic research.

As only 2% of the genome codes for actual proteins, it has been suggested that we should only sequence cDNA, which would be cheaper and much quicker. However, many genetic disorders are the result of deregulation of expression and it is the control elements surrounding the coding that are deregulated. Thus complete sequencing will eventually give rise to an understanding of how genes are packaged as euchromatin or heterochromatin.

The human proteome project

A more direct route to understanding genetic and somatic disease is by studying the protein expression characteristics of normal and diseased cells – the *proteome*. This relies on the separation of proteins expressed by a given tissue by molecular size and charge on a simple two-dimensional display and is achieved by using 2D gel electrophoresis. The pattern of dots corresponds to the different proteins expressed. With the improvement in technology the patterns are reproducible and can be stored as electronic images. Non-, over- and under-expression of a given protein can be detected by a corresponding change on the proteome 2D electrophoresis image. Furthermore, post-translational modifications of the protein show up as a change in either size or charge on the proteome picture. This cannot be detected by genome analysis. Looking for such changes has already lead to the discovery of new protein markers for the diagnosis of Creutzfeldt–Jakob disease, multiple sclerosis, schizophrenia, Parkinson's disease (spinal fluid protein) and Alzheimer's disease (blood and brain proteins). Though still in its infancy, the proteome approach may prove more useful to medical advances than the genome project.

Ethical considerations

Ethical considerations must be taken into account in any discussion of clinical genetics. For example, prenatal diagnosis with the option of termination may be unacceptable on moral or religious grounds. With diseases for which there is no cure and currently no treatment (e.g. Huntington's), genetic tests can predict accurately which family members will be affected; however, many people would rather not know this information. One very serious outcome of the new genetic information is that disease susceptibility may be predictable, for example in Alzheimer's disease, so the medical insurance companies can decline to give policies for individuals at high risk.

Society has not yet decided who should have access to an individual's genetic information and to what extent privacy should be preserved.

FURTHER READING

Blau HM, Springer ML (1995) Gene therapy: a novel form of drug delivery. *New England Journal of Medicine* **333**: 1204–1207.

Blau HM, Springer ML (1995) Muscle-mediated gene therapy. *New England Journal of Medicine* **333**: 1554–1556.

McDonnell WM, Askari FK (1996) DNA vaccines. *New England Journal of Medicine* **334**: 42–46.

Weatherall DJ (1996) *Basic Molecular and Cell Biology*, 3rd edn. London: BMJ Publishing.

SECTION BIBLIOGRAPHY

Brock DJH (1993) *Molecular Genetics for the Clinician.* Cambridge: Cambridge University Press.

Conner JM, Ferguson-Smith MA (1991) *Essential Medical Genetics*, 3rd edn. Oxford: Blackwell Scientific.

McKusick VA (1994) Mendelian Inheritance in Man, 11th edn. London: Johns Hopkins Press.

Weatherall DJ (1991) *The New Genetics in Clinical Practice*, 3rd edn. Oxford: Oxford University Press

The immune system in health and disease

The immune system is made up of a complex network of lymphoid organs, cells, humoral factors and soluble cellular messengers or cytokines, which enable us to recognize 'self' from 'non-self' or altered self, and thereby confer protection against disease. The most common clinical problems are:

- *overactivity* of the immune response, leading to allergic and autoimmune disease
- *underactivity*, resulting in immunodeficiency.

The immune system, by recognizing 'foreign' tissue, may also act as a barrier to effective organ or bone marrow transplants unless suppressed.

This section of the chapter first covers the basic structure and function of the immune system in order to help an understanding of the disorders associated with its dysfunction.

The immune system in health

Innate immunity

Innate immunity consists of the rapidly acting 'front-line' host defence mechanisms and includes both physical or chemical barriers as well as elements of the immune system (Table 2.13).

Certain factors, many common in clinical practice, reduce the effectiveness of this protection:

- breach of physical barriers (e.g. trauma, burns, eczema)
- loss of chemical barriers (e.g. drugs which inhibit gastric acid secretion)
- suppression of the cough reflex (e.g. by opiates, neurological disease)
- failure of respiratory mucus clearance:
  (a) ciliary paralysis (e.g. smoking, primary ciliary dyskinesis syndromes)
  (b) increased mucus production (e.g. asthma)
  (c) abnormally viscid secretions (e.g. cystic fibrosis)
- failure of the washing mechanism (e.g. urinary stasis in prostatic hypertrophy)
- loss of colonization resistance (e.g. during broad-spectrum antibiotic use).

In these situations, pathogenic organisms may gain access and cause disease, despite a normal immune system.

Innate immunity also comprises elements of the immune system that can mount a nonspecific, 'immediate' response. These are directly activated by infectious agents,

Table 2.13
Innate immunity: host defence mechanisms

Physical or chemical barriers Skin and mucous membranes Gastic acid, lysozyme, lactoferrin, nitric oxide in secretions	**Colonization resistance** Presence in skin and gut of normal flora preventing colonization by pathogenic organisms
Mechanical removal Sneezing, coughing Secretions and urine (washing) Ciliary escalator of respiratory mucosa	**Nonspecific immune system** Phagocytes Natural killer cells Complement Interferons

Table 2.14
Origins and biological functions of cytokines

Cytokine	Source	Mode of Action
IL-1	Macrophages/monocytes	Immune activation: induces an inflamatory response
IL-2	Primarily T cells	Activates T (and NK) cells and supports their growth Formerly called *T cell growth factor*
IL-3	T cells	Primarily promotes growth of haematopoietic cells
IL-4	T cells	Lymphocyte growth factor; involved in IgE responses
IL-5	T cells	Promotes growth of B cells and eosinophils
IL-6	Fibroblasts	Promotes B cell growth and antibody production
IL-7	Stromal cells	Lymphocyte growth factor important in the development of immature cells
IL-8	Primarily macrophages	Chemoattractant
IL-10	CD4 cells, activated monocytes	Inhibits the production of IFN-γ, IL-1, IL-6, TNF-α and antigen presentation
IL-12	Monocyte/macrophages	Augments TH1 responses and induces IFN-γ
IL-13	Activated T cells	Stimulates B cells
G-CSF	Primarily monocytes	Promotes growth of myeloid cells
M-CSF	Primarily monocytes	Promotes growth of macrophages
GM-CSF	Primarily T cells	Promotes growth of mono-myelocytic cells
IFN-α	Leucocytes	Immune activation and modulation
IFN-β	Fibroblasts	Immune activation and modulation
IFN-γ	T cells and NK cells	Immune activation and modulation
TNF-α	Macrophages	Stimulates generalized immune activation as well as tumour necrosis; formerly known as *cachectin*
TNF-β	T cells	Stimulates immune activation and generalized vascular effects; formerly known as *lymphotoxin*
TGF-β	Platelets	Immunoinhibitory but stimulates connective tissue growth and collagen formation

G-CSF, granulocyte colony stimulating factor; GM-CSF, granulocyte-macrophage colony stimulating factor; IFN, interferon; IL, interleukin; M-CSF, monocyte colony stimulating factor; TGF, transforming growth factor; TNF, tumour necrosis factor.

tissue damage or tumours and provide the first line of defence. This has the advantage of speed, but because it lacks specificity it may cause excessive host tissue damage. The main components are summarized in Table 2.13 and considered in detail below. Despite the separate categorization, it must be remembered that there is considerable interaction between the innate and specific immune responses (Fig 2.21).

Phagocytes

The *neutrophil* (polymorphonuclear, or PMN cell) is a highly specialized microbicidal (microbe killing) phagocyte. The human body contains over 10^{11} cells per kilogram, most of which are in the bone marrow. These cells are released in large numbers during acute infection, and new cells are produced by the action of granulocyte and granulocyte-macrophage colony stimulating factors (G-CSF and GM-CSF; Table 2.14) on progenitor cells. This response causes the characteristic neutrophil leukocytosis observed in the peripheral blood of patients with infectious or inflammatory disease. The raised white cell count can be useful in diagnosis and monitoring of patients. However, it must be remembered that in premature infants, or others with poorly functioning bone marrow, '*storage pool exhaustion*' occurs and results in paradoxical neutropenia during severe infections.

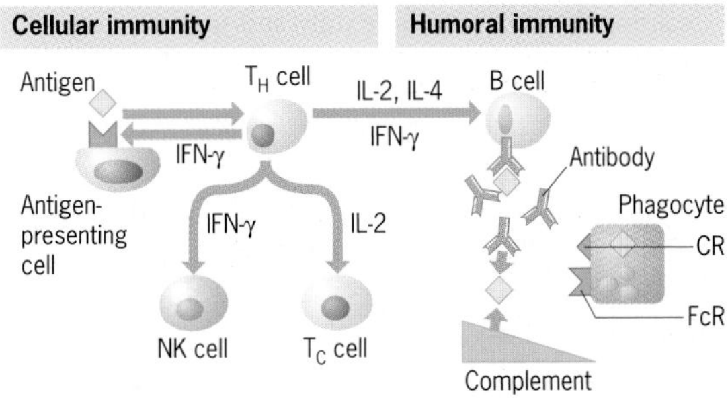

Fig 2.21
Components of the immune response. Antigen is presented to T-helper cells (T_H cells) by an antigen-presenting cell. T_H cells secrete lymphokines, which activate cytotoxic T cells (T_C cells) that are involved in antiviral activity. The lymphokines also activate NK cells, which are involved in tumour surveillance. B cells are activated when the antigen binds to the surface immunoglobulins in the presence of lymphokines. This leads to secretion of antibodies. Antibody and complement coat the antigen (opsonize), leading to phagocytosis by phagocytes via binding to the complement receptor (CR) and *Fc* receptor (FcR). NK = natural killer cell

Mechanisms of neutrophil function

Recruitment and role in inflammation (Fig 2.22)

The recruitment of cells such as phagocytes and lymphocytes to tissue sites is vital to host defence and occurs as a result of interactions between cell adhesion molecules (CAMs) on the inflammatory cells and tissues. Examples are the adhesion molecule members of the immunoglobulin superfamily, as well as integrins, selectins and cadherins (calcium-dependent adherins). Surface adhesion molecules associate with cytoplasmic proteins and the cytoskeleton to cause cytoskeletal reorganization, such as formation of pseudopodia, migration and spreading. Ligation of adhesion molecules may also cause signal transduction, leading to activation of other receptors and affecting cellular proliferation, altered gene expression and cell survival.

The initiation of recruitment of neutrophils to sites of tissue damage is usually by the local release of powerful chemoattractants (chemicals which attract phagocytes) produced by invading organisms or factors released by damaged tissues. The main chemoattractants *in vivo* are the complement activation products C5a and C3a (see p. 164) and the macrophage-derived cytokine-leukotriene B4. Chemoattractants induce the migration of neutrophils by three mechanisms:

- Up-regulation of the adhesion molecules L-selectin and integrins (leukocyte function antigen LFA-1) on neutrophils (Table 2.15) increases the 'stickiness' of the phagocyte.
- Increase in E-selectin and ICAM-1 (intercellular adhesion molecule type 1) on the blood vessel endothelial cells causes these cells also to become 'sticky'. The result is that selectin expression causes the previously circulating neutrophil to be tethered or 'marginate' and roll along the endothelium slowly. This slowing allows the much stronger reaction between the integrins LFA-1 and ICAM-1 to occur, causing the cells to adhere fully and stop moving.

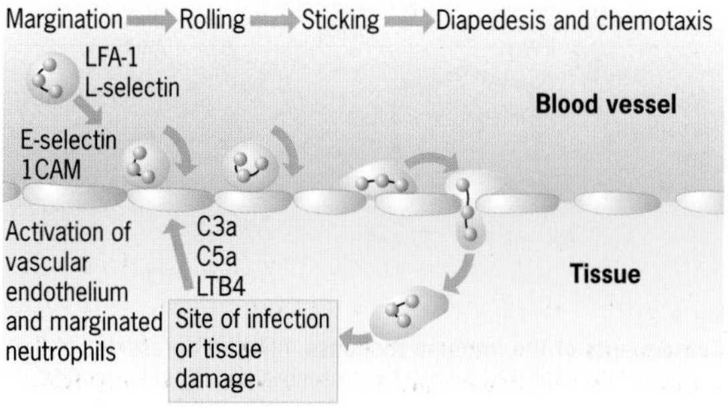

Fig 2.22
Neutrophil migration
Release of C3a, C5a and LTB4 by damaged or infected tissue causes upregulation of adhesion molecules on the vascular endothelium and neutrophils. This causes neutrophils to stick to the endothelium and eventually migrate to the site of damage by chemotaxis. LFA-1, Leucocyte function antigen; ICAM-1, Intracellular adhesion molecule type I

- The final mechanism used by chemoattractants, including C3a, C5a and chemokines (see Table 2.16) is to stimulate neutrophil chemotaxis (movement towards the stimulus along a concentration gradient). The cells pass between endothelial cells into the tissues by the formation of foot-like processes that push through the intercellular spaces; this is called *diapedesis*. The exodus of neutrophils leads to the inflammatory response, and if cells are present in large numbers causes the formation of pus, the characteristic yellow colour being due to the peroxidase enzymes within the cells. Patients with congenital deficiencies of adhesion molecules or those on systemic corticosteroids who have acquired adhesion-molecule defects (steroids reduce ICAM-1 expression on endothelial cells) cannot target their neutrophils to sites of infection and suffer with recurrent infections.

Similar mechanisms of cell recruitment and trafficking control, by the use of adhesion molecules, are being described for lymphocytes and other cells within the immune system. For example, L-selectin on leucocytes facilitates 'homing' of lymphocytes to lymph nodes.

Phagocytosis and intracellular killing

Once the polymorphonuclear cells have been recruited, *phagocytosis* (ingestion) and intracellular killing of microbes or the clearing of cellular debris begins. Phagocytosis occurs by the formation of pseudopodia (projections of cytoplasmic membrane) around the organism or particle to be ingested. Owing to the fluidity of the cell membrane, the tips eventually fuse to form a membrane-bound vesicle called a *phagosome*. This fuses with the neutrophil cytoplasmic granules (Table 2.17) to form a *phago-lysosome*. Within this localized environment killing occurs, the remainder of the cytoplasm being protected.

There are two major mechanisms:

- *O_2-dependent response* or 'respiratory burst', in which there is production of reactive oxygen metabolites, such as hydrogen peroxide, hydroxyl radicals and singlet oxygen, via the reduction of oxygen by an NADPH oxidase present in the phagocyte cytoplasm. Most of the current knowledge was derived from the study of patients with chronic granulomatous disease who cannot activate this enzyme system. This condition is discussed in detail later in the section on immunodeficiency (see p. 178).
- *O_2-independent response*, owing to the toxic action of preformed cationic proteins and enzymes contained within the neutrophil cytoplasmic granules.

Opsonization

Ingestion and killing of organisms is much more effective if the particle is first coated or opsonized ('made ready to eat') with specific antibody and complement. This is because neutrophils have receptors both for the *Fc* portion of antibody molecules (FcR) and complement components

Table 2.15
Adhesion molecules

Adhesion molecule	Tissue distribution	Ligand
Immunoglobulin superfamily		
ICAM-1	Endothelial cells, monocytes, T and B cells, dendritic cells, keratinocytes, chondrocytes, epithelial cells	LFA-1
ICAM-2	Endothelial cells, monocytes, dendritic cells, subpopulations of lymphocytes	LFA-1
ICAM-3	Lymphocytes	LFA-1, Mac-1
VCAM-1	Endothelial cells, kidney epithelium, macrophages, dendritic cells, myoblasts, bone marrow fibroblasts	VLA-4
PECAM-1	Platelets, T cells, endothelial cells, monocytes, granulocytes	?
MAdCAM-1	Endothelial venules in mucosal lymph nodes	$\alpha 4\beta 7$ integrin and L-selectin
Selectin family		
E-selectin/ELAM-1	Endothelial cells	?
L-selectin	Lymphocytes, neutrophils, monocytes	CD34
P-selectin	Megakaryocytes, platelets and endothelial cells	?
Integrin family		
VLA subfamily		
VLA-1 to VLA-4	Endothelial cells, resting T cells, monocytes, platelets and epithelial cells	Various molecules including laminin, fibronectin, collagen and VCAM1
VLA-5 (fibronectin receptor)	Endothelial cells, monocytes and platelets	Laminin
VLA-6 (laminin receptor)	Endothelial cells, monocytes and platelets	Laminin
$\beta 1\alpha 7$	Endothelial cells, ?	Laminin
$\beta 1\alpha 8$	Endothelial cells, ?	?
$\beta 1\alpha$	Platelets and megakaryocytes	Fibronectin
$\beta 2$	Widely distributed	Collagen, laminin, vitronectin
Leucam subfamily		
LFA-1	Leucocytes	ICAMs-1 to 3
Mac-1	Endothelial cells, ?	ICAM-1, fibrinogen, C3bi
Cytoadhesin subfamily		
Vitronectin receptor	Platelets and megakaryocytes	Vitronectin, fibrinogen, laminin, fibronectin, von Willebrand factor, thrombospondin
$\beta 4\alpha 6$	Endothelial cells, thymocytes and platelets	Laminin
$\beta 5\alpha$	Platelets and megakaryocytes, ?	Vitronectin, fibronectin
$\beta 6\alpha$	Platelets and megakaryocytes, ?	Fibronectin
$\beta 7\alpha 4$/LPAM-1	Endothelial cells, thymocytes, monocytes	Fibronectin, Vcam-1
$\beta 8\alpha$	Platelets and megakaryocytes, ?	?

E-selectin or ELAM, endothelial leucocyte adhesion molecule; ICAM, intercellular adhesion molecule; LPAM, lymphocyte Peyer's patch adhesion molecule; MAdCAM-1, mucosal addressin; PECAM, platelet/endothelial cell adhesion molecule; VCAM vascular cell adhesion molecule; VLA, very late antigen; LFA, leucocyte function antigen.

(CR), which bind strongly to the coated particle. Binding of the receptors not only increases the force of adhesion between particle and phagocyte, but also causes transduction of intracellular signals which further activate the cell and promote phagocytic and killing activity. The role of antibody in this situation demonstrates the interaction of the innate (neutrophil) and specific (antibody) immune responses.

It should be noted that neutrophils are mainly active against *extracellular infections*, particularly bacteria and fungi. *They have no means of recognizing intracellular organisms* such as viruses, mycobacteria, protozoa, and some fungi, which are destroyed mainly by lymphocyte–macrophage responses.

Eosinophils (see p. 397)

These cells comprise up to 5% of white blood cells in healthy individuals and appear to be used selectively for fighting parasitic (particularly nematode) infections. Eosinophils also participate in immediate hypersensitivity (allergic) reactions (see p. 182). In allergic inflammatory disorders chemokines such as MCP and eotaxin bind to the CCR receptor in the eosinophils, inducing cell migration and activation. They have low-affinity surface receptors for antibodies of the IgE class (see p. 170). Unlike neutrophils, they do not appear to be phagocytic,

Table 2.16
Chemokines and associated functions

Chemokine	Class[a]	Site of production	Biological activity
MCP-1	-CC-	Monocytes, macrophages, fibroblasts, keratinocytes	Attracts monocytes and memory T cells to inflammatory sites
MIP-1α	-CC-	Macrophages	Attracts monocytes and T cells
MIP-1β	-CC-	Monocytes, macrophages, endothelial cells, T and B cells	Attracts monocytes and CD8+ T cells
Eotaxin	-CC-	Macrophages, activated leucocytes, endothelial cells	Attracts eosinophils, basophils
RANTES	-CC-	Platelets and T cells	Attracts monocytes, T cells and eosinophils
IL-8	-CXC-	Macrophages	Attracts neutrophils, naive T cells

[a] Refers to a double cysteine amino acid structure (-CC-) within the cytokine; in some cases this is interspersed with another amino acid (-CXC-).
MCP, macrophage chemoattractant protein; MIP, macrophage inflammatory protein; RANTES, regulated on activation, normal T-cell expressed and secreted.

but they contain many large granules, which are cytotoxic when released on to the surface of organisms. These granular structures have been characterized as follows.

Major basic protein (MBP)
This is the major protein component of eosinophil granules and directly damages helminths, producing ballooning and detachment of the tegumental membrane.

Eosinophil cationic protein (ECP)
This is present in the matrix of eosinophil granules and its deposition has been seen in the kidneys of patients with renal disease, certain types of myocardial infarction, and allergic gastroenteritis. It is highly toxic to parasites, being eight to ten times more active than MBP, producing complete fragmentation and disruption of the organisms. ECP is a potent neurotoxin.

Eosinophil-derived neurotoxin
This is released from the matrix of eosinophil granules and can damage myelinated neurones in experimental animals.

Eosinophil peroxidase
This is localized in the granule matrix of the eosinophil. In combination with a halide and hydrogen peroxide it can kill bacteria, helminths and tumour cells. It inactivates leukotrienes C4 and D4 and causes mast cell degranulation.

Basophils and mast cells (p. 397)

Mast cells consist of at least two distinct populations, which are distinguished by their enzyme content. The *T mast cells* contain trypsin alone and were formerly termed 'mucosal mast cells' owing to their location near mucosal surfaces. The *TC mast cells* contain both trypsin and chymotrypsin and were formerly described as 'connective tissue mast cells', owing to their location.

Basophils and the morphologically similar mast cells make up only a very small proportion of the granulocytic white blood cell population. Basophils are involved in inflammation, possibly attracted by chemokines which bind to surface receptors CCR2 and CCR3. The cytoplasmic granules of basophils and mast cells contain histamine and other vasoactive amines. These cells also bear high-affinity IgE *Fc* receptors and participate in immediate hypersensitivity reactions, which is described in more detail in the section on allergic disease (see p. 182).

Complement

Complement is involved in the eradication of organisms and immune complexes, as well as in inflammation and immunoregulation. The complement system comprises a series of at least 20 serum glycoproteins that are activated in a cascade sequence, consisting of proenzymes that undergo sequential proteolytic cleavage, in a mechanism similar to the coagulation pathway. The nomenclature of the complement proteins is complex. For those that are cleaved during activation, the smaller fragment is given the 'a' designation and, being soluble, is released; the larger 'b' fragment is usually deposited on the surface of the activating cell. Further fragmentation of the larger 'b' fragment may occur to 'c', 'd', 'e', for example. The numbering of the components relates to the order in which they were discovered, not the sequence of activation.

Two main pathways of C′ activation exist, termed the *classical* and *alternative pathways* (Fig 2.23). They are triggered by different factors, but converge in the activation of the same central component – C3 (by the formation of either a 'classical' or 'alternative' pathway C3 convertase). Activated C3 leads into a final common pathway sequence with the eventual assembly of components C5, C6, C7, C8 and finally C9 which forms the *membrane attack complex* (MAC). This is a 'doughnut-like' transmembrane channel which leads to cell destruction by osmotic lysis.

Activation of the classical pathway

Activation of the classical pathway is dependent on calcium and magnesium. It is initiated by activation of C1 through the binding of C1q (a subcomponent of the whole C1qrs molecule) by:

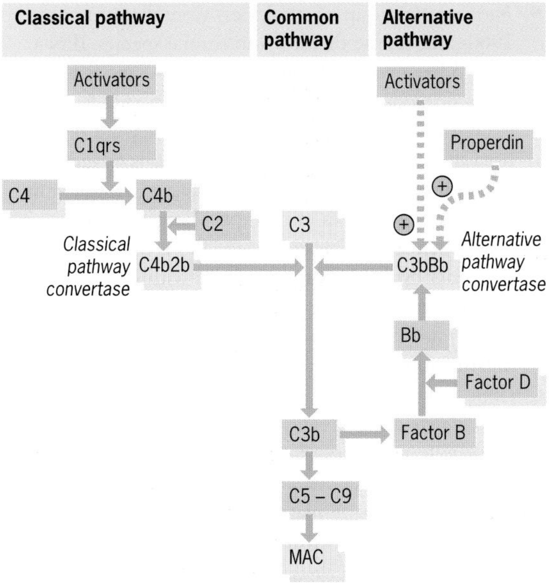

Fig 2.23
Complement activation pathways
In the **classical pathway**, activated C1 causes cleavage of C4 to C4a (a soluble factor which is released) and C4b, which in turn cleaves C2 to C2a (soluble and released) and C2b. C2b combines with C4b to become C4b2b (classical pathway convertase)
In the **alternative pathway** convertase is formed by the combination of C3b with the cleavage product of factor B (Bb). This is catalysed by factor D, and the convertase is stabilized by properdin and alternative pathway activators (see text)
The **final common pathway** leads through C3 to the formation of membrane attack complex (MAC) and lysis of the cell

- antigen–antibody immune complexes
- IgM alone
- mannan binding protein.

Activation of C1 in turn activates C4 and C2 and thence C3. Usually the classical pathway does not turn over as C1 is kept in an inactive form by the presence of C1 esterase inhibitor. In the condition of hereditary angio-oedema (see p. 1168), the inhibitor is lacking and patients have recurrent attacks of angio-oedema owing to uncontrolled activation of the classical pathway and resultant tissue inflammation.

Activation of the alternative pathway

Activation and control of this pathway is more complex. The main components are factor B, factor D and properdin as well as C3b. In the presence of factor D, factor B is cleaved (to Bb) and combines with C3b to form the alternative pathway C3 convertase, C3bBb. This convertase is stabilized by properdin. The alternative pathway is continually turning over at a low rate. This turnover is markedly accelerated by substances which provide a 'protected' site for the C3bBb convertase. These 'activators' function by enhancing the binding of properdin and preventing degradation of the C3bBb complex.

Activators of the alternative pathway include:

- yeast cell walls
- IgA
- endotoxin (found in Gram-negative bacterial cell walls)
- C3 nephritic factor (an autoantibody that stabilizes the convertase) which is found in some patients with membrano-proliferative glomerulonephritis.

Table 2.17 Neutrophil granule proteins (there are two types distinguished by staining characteristics)

Primary granule (azurophilic)
Defensins
Lysozyme
Elastase
Bactericidal/permeability-increasing factor
Cathepsin G
Myeloperoxidase
Acid glycolases
Collagenase
Secondary granule (specific)
Lysozyme
Lactoferrin
Collagenase
Cytochrome B
Vitamin B_{12}-binding protein

Regulation of complement activation

Complement activation does not occur in the fluid phase, but is localized on the surface of the organism, cell or immune complex that triggered the reaction. In addition to the activation sequences described, there are regulatory proteins (factors H and I) that suppress the activation. This is essential, as many of the by-products of complement activation are potent mediators of inflammation, and would cause extensive tissue damage if not controlled.

Actions of complement

The following are the most important effects of complement activation:

- *Recruitment of cells and proteins* to inflammatory sites, by the potent chemoattractant activity of the pro-inflammatory soluble products C5a and C3a. These factors also cause an increase in vascular permeability (sometimes called anaphylatoxins, as overproduction causes the vascular leak syndrome and anaphylaxis).
- *Destruction of pathogens and tumour cells* by the lytic process described above and by opsonizing them for phagocytosis.
- *Removal of immune complexes* by opsonization, solubilization (alternative pathway) and prevention of precipitation (classical pathway). Patients who have congenital complement deficiencies of C1, C2 or C4 are highly susceptible to immune complex diseases such as systemic lupus erythematosus.
- *Immunomodulation* of B-cell responses to specific antigen through binding to complement receptors on the B-cell surface.

Table 2.18
Acute phase proteins

Pentraxins – C-reactive protein, serum amyloid P protein
Complement components
Fibrinogen
Haptoglobulin
Caeruloplasmin
α-1-antitrypsin
Mannan binding protein

Other cells or factors active in nonspecific immunity

Natural killer (NK) cells

NK cells have the morphology of lymphocytes but do not bear the markers for T or B cells. They appear to have nonspecific antiviral and antitumour activity, recognizing particular proteins and causing lysis of cells with which they react. They are described in more detail on p. 171.

Acute-phase proteins

Acute-phase reactants are proteins that are synthesized in response to infection, necrosis, tumours or other inflammatory events (Table 2.18). Although of secondary importance in host defence, fibronectin has some opsonic activity. The measurement of C-reactive protein in the serum is used to monitor disease activity, and serum amyloid P protein may be helpful in the diagnosis or monitoring of secondary amyloidosis.

Heat-shock proteins (HSP)

Heat-shock proteins are a family of highly conserved proteins which act as immunodominant antigens in many infections. They act as molecular chaperones, housekeeping proteins within cells, preserving the cell's protein structure. They are similar in configuration to antigens found on certain micro-organisms and may induce autoimmunity through molecular mimicry.

Cytokines

Much of the immune system's ability to communicate between its different compartments is achieved through the use of soluble messenger molecules called *cytokines*, a generic term meaning 'made by any cell', such as lymphokines (produced by lymphocytes) or interleukins (made by other white cells). Once the cytokine reaches its destination cell it then induces a biological effect, which will of course vary according to the cytokine and the cell involved; but typically these molecules will signal certain cell populations to activate, divide or home in on a particular site in the body. Many cytokines have been isolated, cloned and characterized by the use of recombinant DNA technology. The origins and biological functions of the major cytokines are summarized in Table 2.14.

A number of cytokines are involved in innate immunity. Some are now being used in clinical practice.

- *Interferons* (a group of cytokines) were discovered in the 1960s and can be divided into several species. IFN-α and -β have potent general antiviral activity as well as immunomodulation function (increasing HLA class I expression and antigen presentation); they are being used in the treatment of chronic hepatitis B and C infections as well as showing an effect in reducing the frequency of relapses in multiple sclerosis. IFN-γ is a potent activator of macrophages and is used to improve the phagocyte function of patients with chronic granulomatous disease (see p. 178).
- *Tumour necrosis factor* (TNFα) plays a key role in inflammation, and antibodies to this molecule may have clinical effect in the control of rheumatoid arthritis.
- *Granulocyte-colony stimulating factor* (G-CSF) and *granulocyte/macrophage CSF*, substances that cause bone marrow cells to divide and mature, have found application in bone marrow transplantation and in the treatment of neutropenia.

Interleukins (IL), are cytokines involved in signalling between white cells (p. 171). IL-1 is a pro-inflammatory molecule produced mainly by monocytes/macrophages, IL-2 has a key role in the activation of T cells, IL-4 increases IgE production by B cells and is involved in allergy, and IL-6 activates the acute-phase response and stimulates T-lymphocytes.

Chemokines are low-molecular-weight cytokines (Table 2.16), which are primarily associated with chemoattractant function. They are secreted at sites of infection and inflammation, and they induce cell migration and activation by binding to specific G-protein-coupled cell surface receptors on target cells. They control the movement of leucocytes, and their dramatic increase at the site of inflammation results in an upsurge of leucocytes. They also have a role in a number of diseases (e.g. asthma, rheumatoid arthritis, atherosclerosis).

Nuclear factor-κB (NFκB) is a pivotal transcription factor in chronic inflammatory diseases. It is a heterodimer of two proteins (*p65* and *p50*) and is found in the cytoplasm bound to an inhibitor (IKB), which prevents it from entering the nucleus. It is released from IKB on stimulation of the cell, and passes into the nucleus where it binds to specific sequences in the promoter regions of target genes. It is stimulated by, for example, cytokines, protein C activators and viruses, and itself regulates various proteins (e.g. pro-inflammatory cytokines, chemokines, adhesion molecules, inflammatory enzymes and receptors).

Specific immunity

Specific or 'adaptive' immunity is the hallmark of the immune system of higher animals and is provided by T- and B-lymphocytes. It is characterized by antigen specificity, the generation of memory and for a heightened response on subsequent antigen exposure. The ability to respond specifically to many millions of different antigens is achieved by an unusual mechanism of multiple rearrangements of germline DNA in the T- and B-lymphocytes. The altered DNA encodes for proteins with hyper-variable regions and creates the specific antigen-binding T-cell receptors (TCR) and antibody molecules. This genetic diversity allows the production, for example, of over 10^8 different antibodies, enough to cover the spectrum of antigens encountered by humans.

FURTHER READING

Barnes PJ, Karin M (1997) Nuclear factor-κB. *New England Journal of Medicine* **336**: 1066–1071.

Bevilacqua MP (1993) Endothelial-leukocyte adhesion molecules. *Annual Review of Immunology* **11**: 767–804.

Luster AD (1998) Chemokines. *New England Journal of Medicine* **338**: 436–445.

Tomlinson S (1993) Complement defence mechanisms. *Current Opinion in Immunology* **5**: 83–89.

Cells of the immune system

Circulating leucocytes can be subdivided into several groups, characterized on morphology, cell surface markers and biological function. There are two families of molecular structure on the cell surface, called *clusters of differentiation* (Table 2.19) and *adhesion molecules*. There is an overlap between these two families and certain adhesion molecules have also been assigned CD numbers.

The biological function of many of the CD molecules is known, and knowledge of their presence is very useful in identifying specific leucocyte subpopulations.

Adhesion molecules facilitate many biological activities, particularly those involved in cell–cell recognition. Their functions include cellular activation, cytokine release, capture and 'rolling' of leucocytes along the endothelial cell lining of blood vessels, and extravasation (Fig 2.22).

Lymphocytes

Lymphocytes are spherical cells, approximately 10 μm diameter, with a prominent nucleus of densely packed nuclear chromatin (Fig 2.24(a)).

B cells

These cells produce *antibody* and comprise approximately 25% of the lymphocyte population. Once a B cell has been

Table 2.19
Major CD antigens and their cellular distribution[a]

Cluster designation	Tissue distribution	Function
CD1	Cortical thymocytes	
CD2	All T cells and NK cells	Ligand for CD58; pair (e.g. between T cell and antigen-presenting cell)
CD3	Found on all mature T cells. Intimately associated with the T cell receptor	Signal transduction following antigen presentation
CD4	T-helper/inducer lymphocytes Comprise 2/3 circulating T cells	Ligand for class II MHC molecules associated with processed antigen fragments
CD5	T cells; also B cells	Ligand for CD72
CD8	Cytotoxic/suppressor T cells	Ligand for class I MHC molecules associated with processed antigen fragments
CD11a	Lymphocytes (especially memory T cells), granulocytes, monocytes and macrophages	Part of adhesion molecule LFA-1
CD14	Macrophages	Receptor for bacterial lipopolysaccharide
CD16	Natural killer cells and macrophages	CD16 is a low-affinity *Fc* receptor involved in signal transduction
CD19	All mature B cells	Signal transduction
CD20	All mature B cells	Involved in cell activation; may be a calcium channel
CD21	Mature B cells, follicular dendritic cells, pharyngeal and cervical epithelial cells	Complement C3d receptor
CD28	Activated T cells and some B cells	Activation of naive T cells
CD45	All cells of a haematopoietic origin; also called leucocyte common antigen	Two isoforms, RO and RA RO is associated with memory. Functions by cell signalling through the T cell receptor
CD56	NK cell marker	Mediates cell adhesion
CD72	All mature B cells	Ligand for CD5; involved in signalling
CD80/86	Antigen-presenting cells	Co-stimulatory ligands for CD28

[a]This list is far from exhaustive and has been confined to CD types most commonly encountered in a clinical immunology setting.

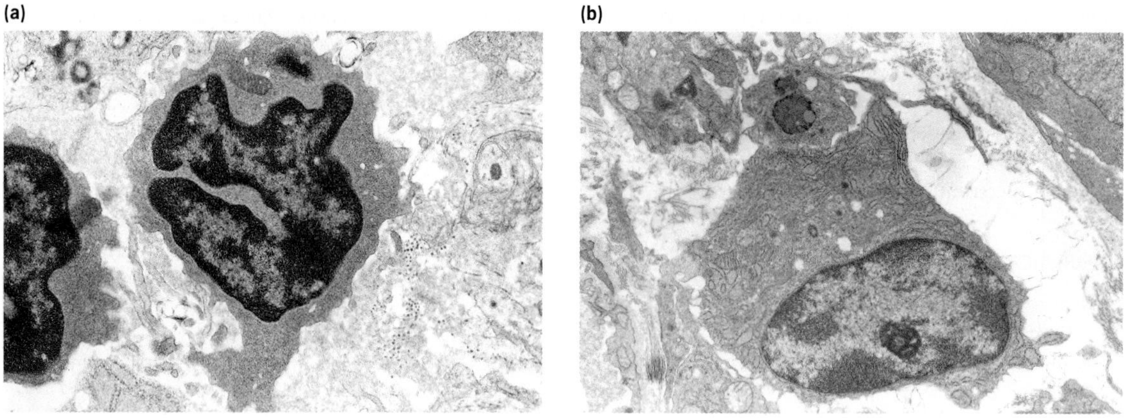

Fig 2.24
(a) Electron micrograph of a T lymphocyte showing a prominent nucleus containing nuclear chromatin
(b) Electron micrograph of a plasma cell derived from a B cell containing large amounts of endoplasmic recticulum Courtesy of Dr G McPhail

exposed to a specific antigen (which it recognizes through immunoglobulin molecules located in the cell membrane), and in the presence of cytokines (interleukins 1–6 and B-cell growth factors), it is activated and divides. Following this expansion step, B lymphocytes differentiate to become plasma cells which produce large amounts of antibody.

Morphologically, plasma cells are distinguished by a cytoplasm containing large amounts of endoplasmic reticulum (Fig 2.24(b)). The plasma cell has a relatively short half-life and is 'terminally differentiated'; i.e. after it has fulfilled its antibody-producing function it dies. Following the death of these cells, the expanded B cell population shrinks back to its original size, although some remain as *memory cells*. As well as surface immunoglobulin, B lymphocytes can be distinguished by the presence of the CD19 and CD20 molecules.

Antibody molecules (immunoglobulins)

Antibodies are glycoproteins (Fig 2.25). They consist of two heavy chains (each with four 'domains') and two light chains (termed either κ or λ polypeptides, each with two domains). This leads to the formation of a molecule having two 'arms' with antigen-binding sites and a single stem which bears the *Fc* portion which is not antigen-specific and attaches to cellular immunoglobulin receptors (FcR). Details of the major regions of immunoglobulins are as follows.

Variable 'V' domains. These have great variation in amino acid sequence between immunoglobulins, and have short segments of hypervariable regions. Antigen binding occurs in the area where the loops bearing the hypervariable regions of the light and heavy chains come together in space, called the *Fab* (fragment antigen binding) region. The shape of the binding site determines the 'goodness of fit' or affinity/avidity of any particular antibody for an antigen.

Idiotypes. These are markers found in the hypervariable region and are associated with the antigen-binding site. The idiotype is antigenic and can be defined by serological techniques.

Constant (C) domains. These are domains in which the amino acid sequences are relatively conserved. The *Fc* (Fragment crystalline) is formed from the constant domains. This is the part that binds to cell surface immunoglobulin receptors or causes complement fixation, and hence controls the effects of the antibody molecule after it has bound its antigen.

The hinge region. This gives flexibility to the antibody molecule, allowing ease of binding to antigen and cell surface receptors.

The type of heavy chain determines the antibody *isotypes* or class (i.e. IgG, A, M, D or E). *Allotypes* are a result of different allelic forms of κ and λ light chains, and heavy chains. These are inherited as autosomal co-dominants, and have various disease associations.

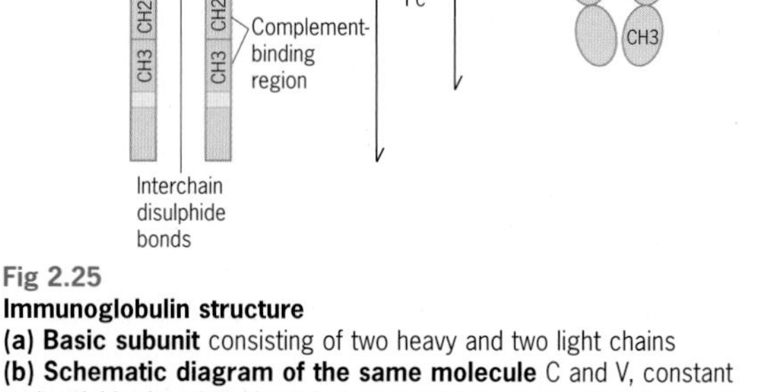

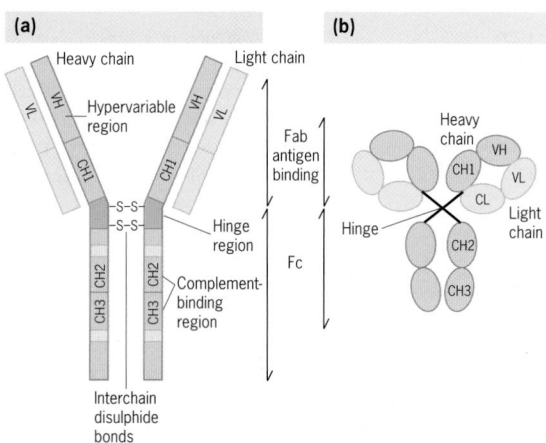

Fig 2.25
Immunoglobulin structure
(a) Basic subunit consisting of two heavy and two light chains
(b) Schematic diagram of the same molecule C and V, constant and variable domains; H and L, heavy and light chains; Fab, fragment antigen binding; Fc, fragment crystalline

Genetics of antibody production

Rearrangement of the germline DNA occurs within developing B cells, leading to production of antibodies with many different antigen-binding sites or *clonal diversity* (Fig 2.26). In the B-cell immunoglobulin gene there are three parts, called the variable (V), diversity (D) and joining (J) regions (Fig 2.27). In the germline stage these are separated, but need to be spliced together as the cell matures to form the final genetic sequence from which protein will be transcribed to form the antibody molecule.

It is during this splicing that much of the variability occurs. Firstly, there is a multiplicity of all these regions within the DNA (V = 25–100 genes, D = 10 genes and J = 5–6 genes). Any one of these multiple genes can join any one other (called *combinational freedom*) to form the final VDJ region. Secondly, splicing of the genes together is frequently inaccurate and 'frame-shift' in base-pairs leads to misreading and production of the 'wrong' amino acid (this is called *junctional diversity*). Thirdly, somatic mutation in the genes may occur during cell division.

Once the VDJ region is spliced it combines successively to the IgM, IgD, IgG, IgA, and IgE constant genes to cause progressive switching in the isotype of the antibody with subsequent antigen challenges. However, as the *Fab* gene is not further altered the same antigen-binding region is maintained. Thus a mature but naive B cell, that has rearranged its VDJ gene, will initially make an IgM response on antigen stimulation as this is the first to be translocated. The primary immune response is therefore always of the IgM isotype; IgG and other isotype responses develop later and require additional T-cell help. However, once the 'switch' from IgM to another isotype has occurred, memory B cells remain in the body for many years. These react rapidly to any re-challenge with the same antigen, and the characteristic IgG production of the secondary response occurs.

Immunoglobulin isotypes and their functions

The main biological features of the human antibodies are summarized in Table 2.20. Different classes of antibody tend to predominate at different sites. The major functions of antibody are:

- elimination of infective organisms by:
  - (a) binding to prevent adhesion and invasion of organisms (e.g. preventing the entry of poliovirus and other enteroviruses)
  - (b) opsonization of particles for phagocytosis
  - (c) lysis (in combination with complement)
- antitoxin activity (e.g. in prevention of tetanus)
- sensitization of cells for antibody-dependent cell cytotoxicity (ADCC)
- immune regulation, acting as the antigen receptor on B cells and presenting the antigen to helper T cells.

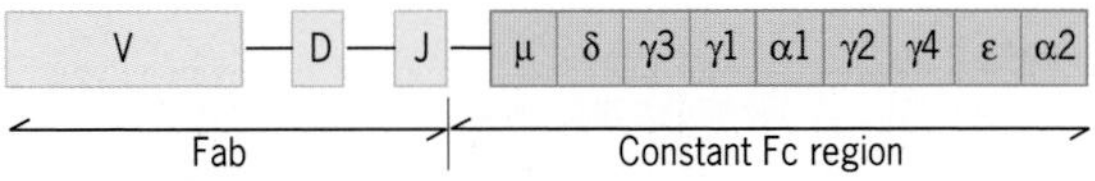

Fig 2.26
Genes on the Fab and Fc regions of an immunoglobulin. The chain is made up of a 'V' variable gene which is translocated to the 'J' joining chain. The VJ segment is then spliced to the (C) constant gene. Heavy chains have an additional D (diversity) segment which forms the VDJ segment that bears the antigen-binding site determinants

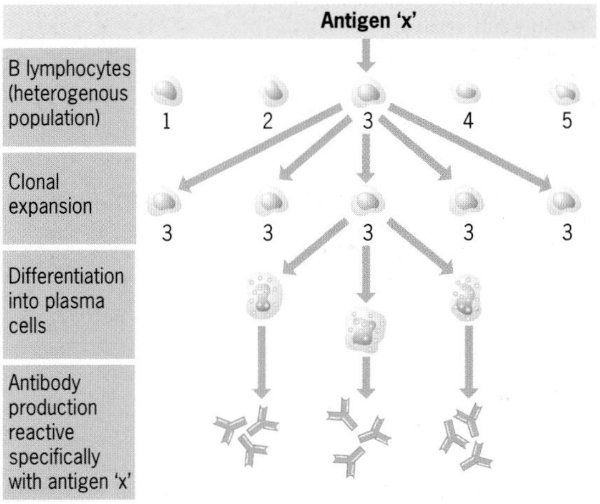

Fig 2.27
Clonal expansion of the B cell population in response to a specific antigenic stimulus

IgM

This antibody is confined mainly to the intravascular pool. It is a large pentameric molecule, the single IgM molecules being bound together by the joining 'J' chain. It is the major antibody of the primary immune response. It does not cross the placenta, and is not normally produced in the child until after birth. Therefore, if present in the newborn infant, antigen-specific IgM is a good marker for intrauterine infection.

IgG

This is the most abundant immunoglobulin in serum, present as a monomer. IgG is the antibody of secondary response, and has high antigen affinity. It is the only antibody to cross the placenta in significant quantities. There are four subclasses: IgG_1, IgG_2, IgG_3 and IgG_4. IgG_1 and IgG_3 are produced mainly in response to protein antigens, such as tetanus toxin and many viruses. These subclasses are good opsonins, binding *Fc* receptors on neutrophils, and activating complement. IgG_2 and IgG_4 are produced in response to polysaccharide antigen (e.g. the capsule of bacteria such as *Pneumococcus* and *Haemophilus influenzae*) and are the major opsonins for such organisms. IgG appears to be the most important antibody in resistance to infection as patients who are lacking in IgG suffer with recurrent, even life-threatening bacterial infections. Those with isolated IgA or IgM deficiency have much less severe problems.

Table 2.20
Characteristics of the immunoglobulins

	IgG	IgM	IgA	IgE	IgD
	Dominant class of antibody	**Produced first in immune response**	**Found in mucous membrane secretions**	**Responsible for symptoms of allergy; used in defence against nematode parasites**	**Found almost solely on lymphocyte membrane**
Heavy chain	γ	μ	α	ε	δ
Mean adult serum levels (mg mL^{-1}):	IgG (total) = 12 G_1 = 6.5 G_2 = 2.5 G_3 = 0.7 G_4 = 0.3	1.5	IgA_1 = 1.5 IgA_2 = 0.2	0.0002	0.03
Half-life (days)	21	10	6	2	3
Complement fixation					
Classical	++	+++	–	–	–
Alternative	–	–	+	–	–
Binding to mast cells	–	–	–	+	–
Crosses placenta	+	–	–	–	–

IgA

This is mainly the antibody of secretions, being present in the respiratory, gastrointestinal and urinary tracts. There are two subclasses, IgA_1 and IgA_2, but their functions appear to be similar. IgA is mainly monomeric in the serum, but dimeric in secretions, the two molecules being complexed by a joining (J) chain. The mechanism for transport from serum to mucosal surface is well established for the gut. IgA in serum binds to a poly *Fc* receptor for IgA and IgM on the basal surface of enterocytes and hepatocytes. Transcellular transport delivers the immunoglobulin to the luminal surface where it is secreted still bound to the receptor, which is termed the *secretory component* (SC). For IgA responses, localized antigen exposure gives rise to generalized mucosal immunity, which is of importance in vaccination. This is because after encountering antigen, IgA precursor B cells in the mucosal lymphoid follicles journey to regional lymph nodes. After clonal expansion the cells return to the systemic circulation via the thoracic duct and circulate to settle widely in the mucosal associated lymphoid tissue (MALT; see p. 249), not just the area where antigen exposure occurred.

IgD

Serum levels are very low and its function at this site is uncertain. IgD is present on the surface of B lymphocytes, and may have an immunoregulatory role. Levels are high in conditions with B-cell activation such as systemic lupus erythematosus (SLE), AIDS and Hodgkin's disease.

IgE

IgE is a monomer that is normally present in very low levels in serum, as most is membrane-bound to the high-affinity receptors on mast cells and basophils. Its main physiological role is its antinematode activity, but its most common clinical relevance is in the pathogenesis of type 1 hypersensitivity (atopic or allergic) disease.

T cells

T cells are characterized by the possession of the CD3 surface molecule and the presence of a specific membrane antigen receptor called the T-cell receptor (TCR). T-lymphocytes have two principal functions, and are divided into helper/inducer cells and cytotoxic/ suppressor cells.

Helper/inducer cells

T-helper cells can be distinguished by the presence of the CD4 protein on their surface. These cells enhance certain immune responses. They receive antigen from specialized presenting cells and initiate or reinforce antibody production, natural killer cell and cytotoxic responses, mainly by the production of certain cytokines. CD4+ lymphocytes recognize antigen only when presented with MHC class II and therefore can only be activated by antigen-presenting cells that bear this molecule.

T-helper cells are categorized into two major subpopulations based on cytokine synthesis (Fig 2.28). Those of the T-helper 1 (Th1) class produce IL-2, IL-3 and γ-interferon. These cytokines will promote immune responses that are primarily cell-mediated or inflammatory. Lymphocytes of the T-helper 2 (Th2) category produce cytokines that favour antibody responses (i.e. IL-4, IL-5, IL-10). In particular these drive IgE responses and an overactive Th2 response may underlie predisposition to allergic diseases. Cells termed Th0 are CD4-positive T cells that have yet to differentiate. γ-Interferon acts in an autocrine way to increase differentiation to Th1, IL-4 to Th2.

Recently a third type of T-helper cell has been described. This population has been termed Th3 and is associated with immunosuppressive effects.

Cytotoxic/suppressor cells

Cytotoxic T cells have the ability to kill other cells by the induction of apoptosis (programmed cell death) or lysis by the production of perforins which punch holes in the membranes of cells. This kind of response is used in dealing with virus infections and cancer cells. The suppressor cell can down-regulate immune responses at an appropriate time. It may function by releasing soluble factors or messenger molecules which act on the B lymphocytes to reduce their output of antibodies. The cytotoxic/suppressor lymphocyte can be recognized by the presence of the CD8 cell surface molecule and its ability to recognize antigen only when presented with MHC class I molecules.

T-cell receptor complex

Antigen recognition at the T cell level is accomplished by a mechanism quite similar to that employed by immunoglobulin (and immunoglobulin genes), except that the receptor is not released as is the case for antibody, but forms a permanent part of the cell surface. Essentially a limited set of gene segments can recombine to encode a highly diverse set of receptor specificities. The T-cell antigen receptor is a structure on the surface of all thymus-derived lymphocytes. It comprises two transmembrane glycoprotein chains, termed α and β (although analogous structures named γ and δ can be found on some immature T cells). As with antibody, the polypetide chains have both a variable (V) and a constant (C) region of amino acid residues. In the β chain the variable region is encoded by V-, D- and J-like elements. The α chain is made up of V- and J-like elements. The whole molecule is arranged on the T-cell membrane as a complex with another structure known as CD3. The receptor also has a transmembrane tail. When an antigenic peptide is received by the receptor, a signal, manifesting as a series of enzyme phosphorylation reactions, is transmitted to the nucleus and the activated cell then responds accordingly, e.g. by releasing cytokines.

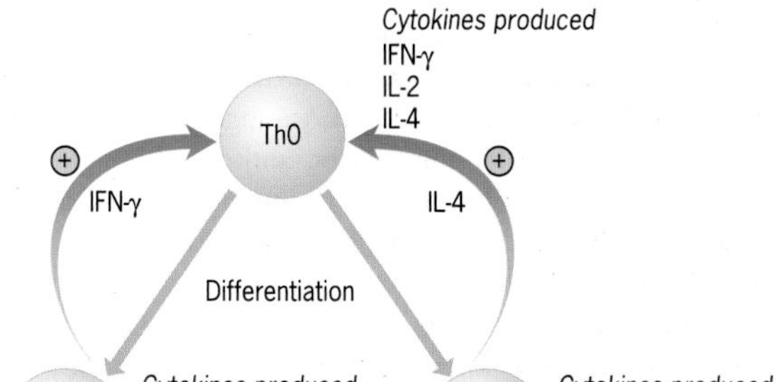

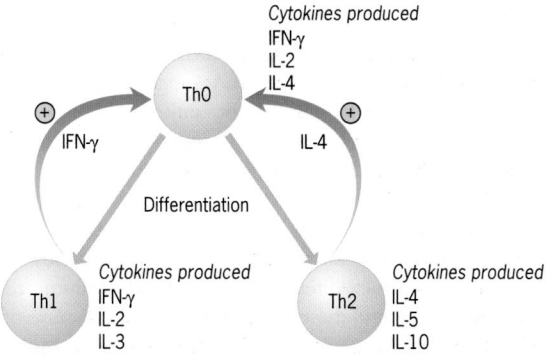

Fig 2.28
CD4 T cells: Th1 and Th2 sub-populations. $CD4^+$ T helper cells differentiate into either Th1or Th2 from Th0. The type of cell produced depends on the cytokine environment. The presence of IFN-γ leads to production of Th1 cells; IL-4 leads to Th2 predominance

Non-T non-B lymphocytes

Some lymphocytes do not have characteristics of T or B cells. Although they make up only a small proportion of cells, they may have an important role in immunity.

Natural killer cells

The role of natural killer (NK) cells is to eliminate tumour and virus-infected cells. This process is not antigen-specific. Many of the cells appear as large granular lymphocytes with an indented nucleus. The granules, which contain acid hydrolases including acid phosphatase, α-naphthyl acetate esterase and β-glucuronidase, are thought to be involved in the cytotoxic events. NK cells are non-phagocytic, and most are CD3, CD4 and surface immunoglobulin negative but carry the $CD56^+$ $CD2^+$ marker on their surface. They also contain chemokine receptors CCR2 and CCR5 which bind the chemokines MCP, MIP and RANTES. They also have the receptor CX_3 CR1 which binds fractalkine, a membrane-bound glycoprotein. The role of these chemokines in inflammation is currently being assessed.

Antibody-dependent cytotoxic cells (ADCC) and lymphokine-activated killer (LAK) cells

These are populations of lymphocytes that are not characterized by their surface molecules, but by function. ADCC bear *Fc* receptors on their surface, and recognize target cells coated with immunoglobulin. LAK cells are cytokine-stimulated lymphocytes. They may have a role in eradicating virus-infected and tumour cells.

FURTHER READING

Leder P (1982) The genetics of antibody diversity. *Scientific American* **246**: 72–83.

Allen JE, Maizels RM (1997) Th1–Th2: reliable paradigm or dangerous dogma? *Immunology Today* **18**: 387–392.

Organization of the lymphoid system

All lymphocytes originate from the bone marrow and are 'programmed' to carry out specific functions by certain lymphoid organs. T and B cells develop within the primary lymphoid tissues (thymus for T cells and bone marrow for B cells) and then circulate to the secondary lymphoid tissues (lymph nodes, spleen, tonsils and mucosa-associated lymphoid tissue).

Primary lymphoid tissues

Bone marrow

The bone marrow is the site of haemopoiesis in mature mammals. All blood cells are derived from a pluripotent stem cell (Fig 6.1). Stem cells are primitive cell types that have no specific function, divide rapidly and, under the influence of various cytokine signals, will differentiate into myeloid precursors (producing neutrophils, eosinophils and monocytes) or lymphoid cells. Pre-B lymphocytes remain here to mature, whereas cells destined to be T-lymphocytes home to the thymus for development.

The thymus

The thymus is formed in embryonic life from the third and fourth branchial pouches. Lymphocytes derived from the thymus are called T cells and comprise about 75% of the lymphoid population. In the passage through this organ, the immature T cells are converted into mature CD4+ (helper) or CD8+ (cytotoxic) cells by the influence of thymic epithelial hormones. Cells that are potentially reactive with the body's own tissues undergo clonal deletion here – 'negative selection'. A degree of recognition of self-MHC is important for later antigen responses, and cells that bind self-MHC are positively selected at this stage.

Secondary lymphoid tissues

Lymph nodes

These are sites of organized lymphoid tissue with B cells mainly in the outer cortex within follicles (which develop into germinal centres after antigen stimulation) and T cells in the paracortex. The lymph nodes also contain antigen-presenting cells (follicular dendritic cells within the B-dependent areas and interdigitating dendritic cells within the T-dependent areas). Afferent and efferent lymphatics carrying lymphocytes run to and from the nodes.

Tonsils

Tonsils function rather similarly to lymph nodes. They are located in the nasopharyngeal tract and are thus well placed to combat airborne antigens. B cells predominate.

MALT, GALT, BALT and SALT

Lymphoid tissue is frequently found distributed in mucosal surfaces in non-encapsulated patches. This is given the general term of *mucosa-associated lymphoid tissue* (MALT), or more specifically *gut-associated lymphoid tissue* (GALT, primarily Peyer's patches), *bronchus-associated lymphoid tissue* (BALT, found in the lobes of the lungs along the main bronchi) and *skin-associated lymphoid tissue* (SALT).

The spleen is another organ containing lymphoid tissue (see p. 390) which has both T- and B-dependent areas.

Immune recognition and cellular function

A unique feature of the immune response is its ability to react specifically and discriminate between 'self' and 'non-self' antigens. This process is facilitated by a recognition system called the *major histocompatibility complex* (MHC) which dictates the way antigen is processed, presented to T or B cells and recognized as foreign.

Human leucocyte antigens (HLA)

In humans the MHC is a cluster of genes located on the short arm of chromosome 6 (Fig 2.29). It encodes a series of molecules known as the *human leucocyte antigens* (HLAs). These structures (which can be defined as antigens because they can be recognized by cells of the immune system) were first seen to be important in transplantation reactions and would determine the acceptance of an organ or tissue graft between individuals. The system comprises several genetic loci – HLA-A, B, C, D, DR, DP and DQ. Each locus may be one of many polymorphic forms or alleles which number over 40 in the case of HLA-B. The combination or segregation of the A, B, C, D, DR, DP and DQ alleles in any one individual is called the *haplotype*. A list of some recognized HLA antigens associated with disease is presented in Table 2.21.

The HLA molecules are distributed throughout the body tissues, and it is through differences in this system that cells are classified as 'self' or 'non-self'. The possibility of two different individuals having the same combination of HLA molecules is very remote. It is this particular aspect of the immune system that presents problems for organ transplantation. Unless the HLA type of the donor and the recipient are virtually identical, the organ graft will be recognized as 'non-self' and rejected by the immune system of the host. Traditionally the process of tissue typing involves the identification of the set of HLA antigens in the tissues of a given individual using specific antisera, although the polymerase chain-reaction is now becoming the method of choice to determine HLA type at the molecular level.

Genetic linkage

The genes at a given locus are inherited co-dominantly, so that each individual expresses both alleles, one transmitted from the mother and the other from the father. Because of the close linkage between the loci, all the genes in the MHC tend to be inherited together. The term 'haplotype' is used to indicate the particular set of HLA genes an individual carries on each chromosome 6. 'Crossing over' can occur within the HLA region. However, certain alleles occur more

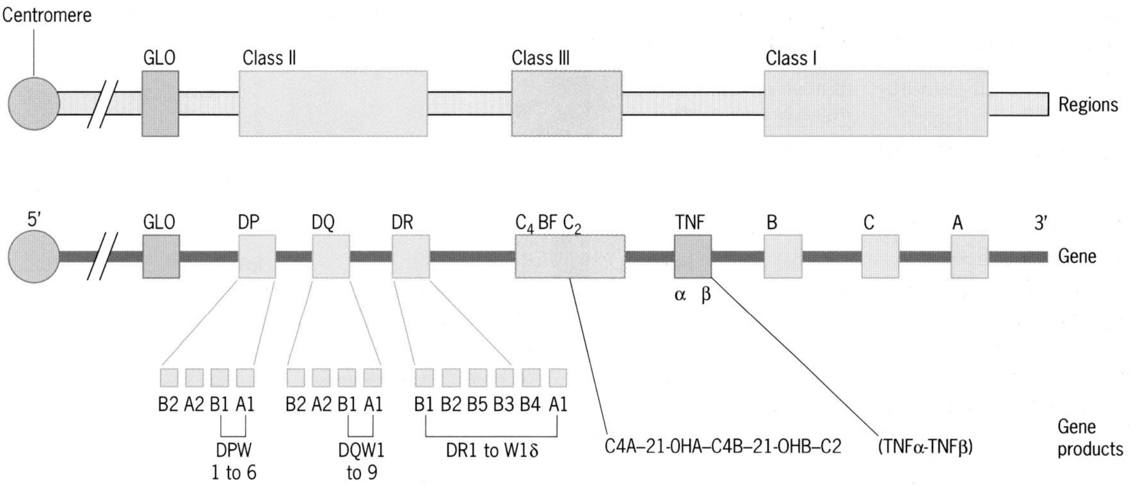

Fig 2.29
The major histocompatibility complex, showing the regions, genes and gene products on the short arm of chromosome 6
GLO, glyoxylase; TNF, tumour necrosis factor

frequently in the same haplotype than expected by chance, and this is known as *linkage disequilibrium*; for example, the haplotype A1 B8 occurs more frequently than would be expected from the individual gene frequencies of A1 or B8. There is a wide inter-racial variation in HLA antigens; for example, the HLA haplotype A1 B8 is found mainly in Caucasians, while the antigen B42 is seen only in Africans.

Products of the HLA genes

The HLA genes code for cell-surface glycoproteins that extend from the plasma membrane to the cytoplasm and are known as class I and class II molecules. These glycoproteins consist of two chains of unequal size (α and β chains), and are antigenic. The class III series of genes express complement.

Class I molecules (Fig 2.30)

Class I antigens are expressed on all cell types except erythrocytes and trophoblasts. Striated muscle cells and liver parenchymal cells are normally negative but become strongly positive in inflammatory reactions. HLA-A, -B and -C antigens can be distinguished serologically by the microlymphocytotoxic test. Lymphocytes from the peripheral blood are incubated with a range of antibodies of known specificity (obtained from parous women or immunized individuals) in the presence of complement and trypan blue dye (which penetrates and stains cells with a damaged cell membrane). If the antibody does not react with the antigen, the lymphocytes survive and exclude the dye; in a positive reaction the dye enters the dead cells, indicating the presence of the specific antigen on that cell.

Class II molecules (Fig 2.30)

Class II antigens are expressed on B cells, monocytes, dendritic cells and activated T cells. Inflammation causes aberrant class II expression in many other tissues. They are involved in presenting antigens to certain sub-populations of T cells.

Table 2.21
Diseases associated with HLA

A3, B14	Hereditary haemochromatosis
A28	Schizophrenia
B5	Behçet's syndrome Polycystic kidney disease Ulcerative colitis
B8	Tuberculoid leprosy (Asians)
B8, DR3	Autoimmune hepatitis Dermatitis herpetiformis Graves' disease Idiopathic membranous glomerulonephritis Myasthenia gravis (without thymoma) Addison's disease Sjögren's syndrome Systemic lupus erythematosus
B8, DR3, DR7, DQ2	Coeliac disease
B18	Hodgkin's disease
B27	Acute anterior uveitis Ankylosing spondylitis Psoriatic arthropathy Reiter's syndrome Juvenile arthritis
B47	Congenital adrenal hyperplasia
C6, B13, 17,	Psoriasis
DR7, DR2	Goodpasture's syndrome (anti-GBM) Multiple sclerosis Narcolepsy (100% association)
DR4	Rheumatoid arthritis Vitiligo
DR4, DR3 (B8, 15 [62] 18)	Diabetes mellitus (insulin-dependent)
DR5	Hashimoto's thyroiditis Systemic sclerosis
DR7	Minimal change disease (nephrotic)
MHC class III	C4A associated with SLE

GBM, glomerular basement membrane.

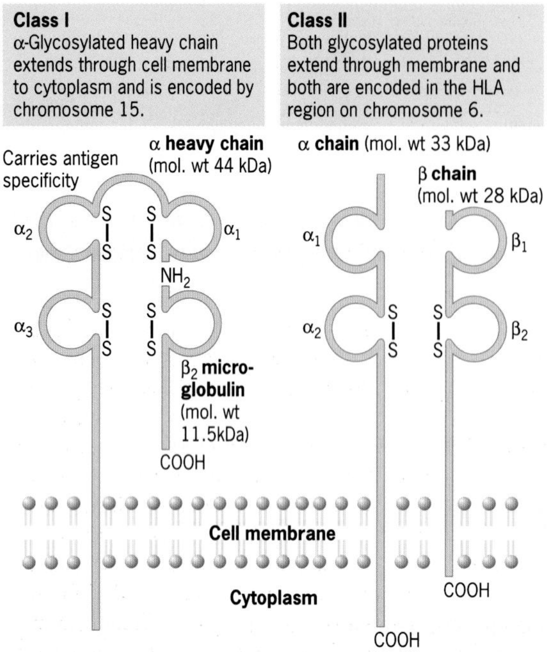

Fig 2.30
Histocompatibility antigens – classes I and II

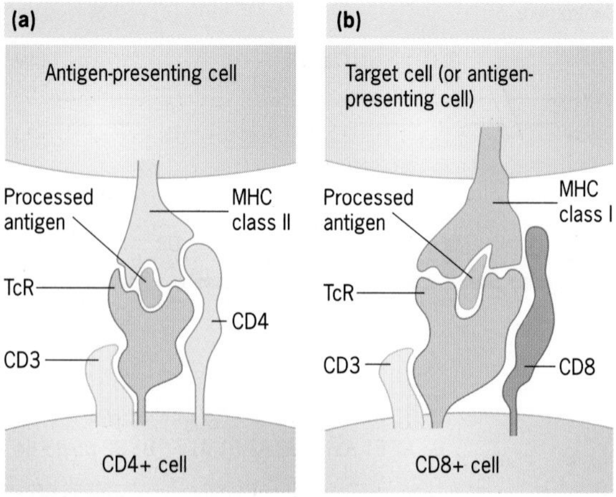

Fig 2.31
Antigen processing. The antigen is presented by an antigen-presenting cell (e.g. a macrophage). The T cells (CD4 (a) or CD8 (b)) recognize the antigen via the HLA glycoprotein.
TCR, T-cell receptor

HLA-D antigens are recognized by the mixed lymphocyte culture (MLC) technique, which requires a panel of different HLA-D homozygous standard typing cells. The homozygous typing cell (HTC) is treated with mitomycin or irradiation to prevent it dividing when it is cultured with the test responder lymphocytes. The latter will not proliferate (measured by incorporation of tritiated thymidine) if it possesses the same D antigen as the HTC, but it will proliferate if it lacks this antigen. The DR (D-related) antigens are very closely related to D antigens and are also detected on B cells (B cell alloantigens) using a cytotoxic antibody test. These serological and cellular techniques for HLA typing are largely being replaced by molecular typing by PCR for more accurate characterization.

Antigen presentation

Antigen fragments are presented to T cells in association with either class I or class II major histocompatibility complex (MHC) molecules. Antigens that are presented with class II molecules are recognized by CD4+ T-helper cells. Antigens that associate with class I molecules are presented to CD8+ T cells and a cytotoxic response results. This is because T cells recognize the combined shape of the antigen and the MHC molecule. The combination of T-cell receptor, MHC molecule and antigen fragment is known as the *trimolecular complex* (Fig 2.31). As there are differences in the three-dimensional shape of the MHC molecules owing to genetic variation, some antigens may be more effective than others in inducing immune responses because they present an optimum shape or conformation to the T cells. Immune responses that occur only with certain antigen-MHC combinations are called *MHC-restricted*.

Antigen presenting cells

Several cell types, sometimes termed *accessory cells*, facilitate the antigen-presenting process. These are characterized by surface expression of class II molecules and are therefore able to present processed antigen to CD4+ T-helper cells.

Macrophages and monocytes (mononuclear phagocytes)

These cells are distributed throughout the body, in the tissues (as macrophages) and in the blood (as monocytes). Macrophages are equipped with various features that make them particularly effective at removing foreign antigens, ready for presentation. They are phagocytic and have, on their surface, receptors that recognize the *Fc* region of antibody molecules as well as biologically active fragments of complement (*C3b*).

Follicular dendritic cells

Follicular dendritic cells are non-phagocytic and are located in the germinal centres of lymph nodes (follicles). They are surrounded by B lymphocytes to which they present antigen, usually complexed with antibody, on the surface of their dendrites. Their surfaces are rich in *Fc* and *C3b* receptors to facilitate antigen trapping.

Langerhans' cells and dendritic cells

Langerhans' cells are found primarily in the skin. The dendritic (or veiled) cell is present in the blood (and is different from the follicular dendritic cell described above). These cells are of macrophage/monocyte lineage.

Tolerance

Tolerance is a state in which the immune system fails to respond to a given antigen. This mechanism evolved from a need for the body to prevent its tissues being attacked by its own defence network. On occasions when tolerance fails or is incomplete, autoimmunity can result. T-cell tolerance develops in the thymus by the negative selection process described earlier (see p. 172), leading to clonal deletion of self-reactive cells by programmed cell death.

Peripheral tolerance

Self-reactive cells can occasionally escape the elimination process in the thymus and become part of the circulating pool of T cells. While these lymphocytes may become autoaggressive, there are several other forms of tolerance that occur outside the thymus. These mechanisms are rather complicated processes that exist to eliminate or inactivate (anergize) both self-reactive T and B lymphocytes. The so-called 'veto' effect can occur when self-peptides are presented to the autoreactive lymphocyte. Specialized cytotoxic T cells may kill the autoreactive cell if the self-peptide is presented in association with an MHC class I molecule. Self-reactive, antibody-producing B cells may be deleted in certain circumstances when they encounter an autoantigen. Alternatively it is thought that they may be regulated by anti-idiotypic antibodies which bind to the idiotype marker on the B cell in question.

Transplantation requirements

Tissue typing for organ grafting requires HLA typing for A, B, C and DR antigens. The match should be as close as possible, as this increases graft survival. Requirements for matching in bone marrow transplantation are much more stringent, as the rejection process can be either host-versus-graft or graft-versus-host.

HLA alleles and adverse drug reactions

There are associations between HLA antigens and adverse drug reactions. For example, HLA-DR4 is present in 75% of patients with systemic lupus erythematosus (SLE) due to hydralazine, compared with 25% of idiopathic SLE patients and slow acetylators who do not develop SLE on hydralazine. Autosomal genes also control the acetylator status, with the 'rapid' allele being dominant to the 'slow' allele. Homozygotes for the 'slow' allele have reduced levels of *N*-acetyltransferase in the liver. Acetylation is the controlling factor for the rate of drug metabolism. The percentage of rapid acetylators varies between ethnic populations – 50% in the West, 90% of Japanese, and 100% of Eskimos.

FURTHER READING

Knight SC, Stagg AJ (1993) Antigen-presenting cell types. *Current Opinion in Immunology* **5**: 374–382.

Lechler R (1994) *HLA and Disease*. London: Academic Press.

The immune system in concert

Following an antigenic stimulus, the components of the immune system co-operate to meet and eliminate the challenge. The foreign antigen is picked up by a cell of the monocyte/macrophage series and the antigen is degraded or processed and presented to both the B and T lymphocytes. T-helper cells are generated which enhance the antibody response made by B cells. Some of this augmentation is due to secreted lymphokines or cytokines from the T-helper population. It should be noted that cytotoxic T cells may be generated if foreign antigens, typically viruses, are presented directly to this cell population. Bacteria are most likely to be processed through the MHC class II pathway and thus generate, primarily, antibody responses. The B cells, once triggered, will differentiate into plasma cells producing specific antibody which binds to the antigen and further triggers the complement system. The complement system, in turn, recruits neutrophils which together eliminate the antigen, perhaps with additional help from lymphokine-activated macrophages.

Once the immune system has detected 'foreign antigens' it can communicate this information to other systems, particularly to the brain and neuroendocrine systems. For example, following infection, there is an increase in both pituitary and adrenal gland secretion. Fig 2.32 indicates the complex nature of these relationships.

Immunodeficiency

Unlike some diseases that are due to immunological abnormalities (e.g. rheumatoid arthritis, thyroid disease and allergy), which are common in clinical practice, immunodeficiency is relatively rare. However, the occurrence of certain infections in the context of specific immune defects can illuminate the physiological role of those parts of immune defence in the normal control of infection.

General principles

Infection is the result of microbial virulence on the one hand and host defence on the other. Pathogenic organisms have mechanisms of evading normal defence mechanisms. Organisms of low virulence can cause disease only if the host defence mechanisms that normally control them are defective.

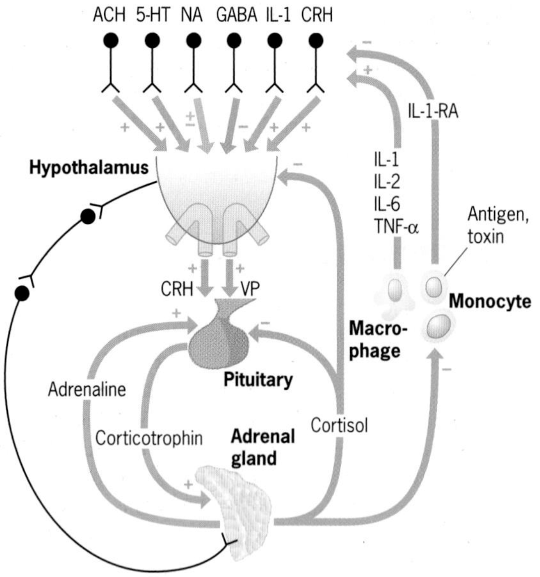

Fig 2.32
Interaction of the immune system with the hypothalamo–pituitary axis regulating adrenocortical secretion. In response to infection, activated T cells release cytokines which induce the hypothalamic release of corticotrophin-releasing hormone (CRH) and vasopressin (VP). This overrides the normal negative feedback relationship between corticotrophin and cortisol. Circulating cortisol also acts on peripheral immunocompetent cells to inhibit their activation and secretion of cytokines and other mediators of inflammation.
ACH, acetylcholine; NA, noradrenaline; TNF, tumour necrosis factor

Table 2.22
Immune defects and some opportunist organisms

Neutropenia and defective neutrophil function	Lytic complement pathway defects (C5–9)
Staphylococcus aureus *Staphylococcus epidermidis* *Escherichia coli* *Klebsiella pneumoniae* *Proteus mirabilis* *Pseudomonas aeruginosa* *Serratia marcescens* *Bacteroides* spp. *Aspergillus fumigatus* *Candida* spp. (systemic) *Mucor* spp.	Meningococcus Gonococcus (disseminated)
Opsonin defects (antibody/complement deficiency, splenectomy)	**Cell-mediated immunodeficiency**
Pneumococcus *Haemophilus influenzae* Meningococcus *Streptococcus* spp. (capsulated)	*Listeria monocytogenes* *Legionella pneumophilia* *Salmonella* spp. (non-typhi) *Nocardia asteroides* *Mycobacterium tuberculosis* Atypical mycobacteria, especially *M. avium-intracellulare* *Candida* spp. (mucocutaneous) *Cryptococcus neoformans* *Histoplasma capsulatum* *Pneumocystis carinii* *Toxoplasma gondii* Herpes simplex Herpes zoster Cytomegalovirus Epstein–Barr virus Measles virus Papovaviruses
Antibody deficiency only	
Campylobacter spp. *Mycoplasma* spp. *Ureaplasma* spp. Echovirus	

Opportunist infections

Organisms taking advantage of the opportunity of impaired host defence mechanisms are called *opportunists*. Different host defence defects cause increased susceptibility to different groups of organisms. Therefore, recognizing a pattern of infections can provide the best clinical clue to the type of underlying defence defect.

Patterns of opportunist infection

Examples of opportunist organisms in the setting of non-immunological defence defects include: staphylococci and pseudomonas in burns patients; *Haemophilus influenzae* and pneumococci in smokers; pseudomonas in cystic fibrosis patients; Gram-negative infections where there is urinary obstruction; staphylococcal and candidal infections with indwelling venous catheters and other foreign bodies; *Candida* and pathogenic *Escherichia coli* following elimination of gut flora after antibiotic therapy.

Table 2.22 shows the main infecting organisms for the principal classes of immunodeficiency. In broad terms, the following principles apply:

- *Neutrophil defects* lead to staphylococcal, Gram-negative enteric and systemic fungal infections, owing to difficulty in eradication of *extracellular* organisms.
- *Opsonic defects* due to antibody deficiencies, or defects of the main complement pathways, and splenectomy lead to infection with capsulated organisms. These cannot be eliminated by neutrophils alone, as the capsule prevents phagocytosis unless opsonized by either antibody or complement.
- *Defects of the lytic pathway of complement* cause susceptibility to disseminated infections with Gram-negative cocci (*Neisseria*).
- *Cell-mediated immune defects* affecting the cooperation between CD4 T cells and macrophages lead to susceptibility to infection with facultative intracellular pathogens (mycobacteria, *Salmonella*, *Listeria* and *Brucella* as well as some fungi and protozoa) and the herpes viruses and polyoma viruses.

Congenital immunodeficiencies

Congenital defects of specific metabolic or developmental disorders can lead to characteristic deficiencies and are rare. The main categories of immunodeficiency by host mechanism are as follows:

- reduced neutrophil number and function, with or without accompanying defects in the related phagocytes of the monocyte/macrophage lineage
- deficiencies of individual complement components
- B cell defects, causing various types of antibody deficiency

- T cell defects, impairing cell-mediated immunity
- combined T and B cell defects, which cause some of the most severe immunodeficiencies.

Table 2.23 shows the main types of immunodeficiency.

Acquired immunodeficiencies

Acquired immunodeficiencies are much more common but are often less precisely defined in terms of immunological mechanisms. They can in many cases be best understood against the background of the more specific defects. They include iatrogenic defects and immunosuppression.

Iatrogenic defects

These can result from malnutrition or deliberate immunosuppression, or from unwanted complications of certain therapies (e.g. splenectomy).

Immunosuppression

This can result from specific diseases that affect immune competence, such as tumours of the immune system and autoimmune disorders. Transient or progressive immunosuppression can be caused by certain infections. The most important of the latter is the acquired immunodeficiency syndrome (AIDS) resulting from HIV infection (see p. 107). Table 2.24 shows the mechanisms in the immunopathogenesis of HIV.

Table 2.23
Main types of immunodeficiency

Congenital	Acquired
Phagocytes	
Congenital neutropenia	Neutropenia due to myelosuppression
Cyclical neutropenia	
Leucocyte adhesion defects	Hypersplenism
Hyper-IgE syndrome	Autoimmune neutropenia
Shwachman's syndrome	
Chronic granulomatous disease	Corticosteroid therapy
Other intrinsic killing defects	Diabetes mellitus
Storage diseases	Hypophosphataemia
Chediak–Higashi syndrome	Myeloid leukaemias
	Influenza
Complement deficiency	
C3, Clq, I, H deficiencies	
C5, 6, 7, 8, 9, deficiencies	
Mannan-binding protein deficiency	
Complement-dependent opsonization defects	
Antibody deficiency (B cell defects)	
X-linked hypogammaglobulinaemia	Myeloma, lymphoma
Common variable immunodeficiency	Splenectomy
IgA ($\pm IgG_2$) deficiency	Congenital rubella
Specific antibody deficiencies	
T-cell deficiencies	
DiGeorge anomaly	Measles
IL-2 deficiency	Corticosteroid therapy
Signal transduction defect	Cyclosporin, tacrolimus
Combined immunodeficiencies	
Severe combined immunodeficiency:	AIDS
Adenosine deaminase deficiency	Protein-calorie malnutrition
Purine nucleoside phosphorylase deficiency	
Non-expression of MHC class II	
Reticular dysgenesis	
Wiskott–Aldrich syndrome	
Ataxia telangiectasia	
EBV-associated immunodeficiency	

Phagocyte deficiency

Neutropenia (see Table 6.19 on p. 397)

Congenital neutropenias are rare and, if severe, are often fatal at an early age. Most, however, are relatively benign and may even be incidental findings. They generally reflect defects of maturation and release of neutrophils from marrow. Staphylococcal skin infections are common manifestations. A particular variant is cyclical neutropenia with cycles of 3–5 weeks, but this disorder is typically benign.

Acquired neutropenia is most commonly due to myelosuppression by disease, such as the leukaemias or drug therapy. Myelosuppressive drugs are most often used in the treatment of tumours; deliberate immunosuppression is also used for prevention or treatment of graft rejection in transplantation and for treating severe autoimmune disease. A number of other drugs such as some antivirals are also immunosuppressive (e.g. zidovudine, ganciclovir), and some can cause neutropenia or agranulocytosis as an idiosyncratic side-effect (e.g. carbimazole). Neutropenia due to increased rate of destruction of neutrophils is seen in hypersplenism and in autoimmune neutropenia.

In adults, the risk of infection rises steeply once the neutrophil count falls below $0.5 \times 10^9/L$, regardless of the cause. The risk is less if the monocyte count is preserved, as these cells can serve as a backup phagocyte population. (In cyclical neutropenia, monocytes usually have cycles of opposite phase, which is probably why serious infections are uncommon.) Infections are typically disseminated, with septicaemia, fungaemia and deep abscess formation. Colonization of the gut with pathogens can readily lead to septicaemia. Local infections often affect the mouth, perianal area and sites of skin damage, including

Table 2.24
Mechanisms of CD4 loss/dysfunction in HIV infection

Direct cytopathic effects of HIV
Lysis of infected cells by HIV-specific cytotoxic T cells
Tc-mediated lysis of uninfected CD4+ T cells that have bound gp120 to the CD4 molecule
Immunosuppressive effects of soluble HIV proteins on uninfected cells, e.g. gp120 envelope protein leading to decreased proliferation
Molecular mimicry between gp120/160 and MHC class I-inducing autoimmune destruction
Signal transduction defects and induction of programmed cell death (apoptosis) by unknown mechanisms

indwelling vascular catheters, and these can readily lead to systemic infection. Pus, which largely comprises neutrophils, may be scanty and may appear serous.

If myelosuppressive therapy is being used, the dose should be reduced or the drug stopped. Neutropenic episodes can be reduced by the use of G-CSF or GM-CSF, which appear to reduce infective episodes and the duration of neutropenia. Antibiotic or antifungal prophylaxis are sometimes of value. Otherwise prompt antimicrobial therapy for febrile episodes during neutropenia is essential, using agents with broad cover for the common organisms encountered (see p. 8).

Defects in the function of neutrophils

Defects of neutrophil function (some of which also affect monocyte/macrophage function) interfere with migration into the tissues through vascular endothelium, locomotion in tissues, phagocytosis or intracellular killing (see Table 2.23).

Mucocutaneous sepsis in the mouth and perianal areas is common, and local infections often lead to chronic abscess formation in the tissues or draining lymph nodes. Granulomas may be seen, because of failure of neutrophils to degrade microbes effectively. Systemic spread is less common than with neutropenia. Congenital causes may first present with infection or delayed separation of the umbilical stump.

LEUKOCYTE ADHESION DEFECT

This is an autosomal recessive disorder caused by abnormal synthesis of the β-chain CD18 that is shared by the CD11a, b and c molecules to form leucocyte function antigen (LFA) LFA-1, the C3bi (inactivated C3b) receptor and the C3dg receptor (p150/95). There is impaired leucocyte tissue localization, locomotion and endocytosis. Bone marrow transplantation has been successful in a few cases.

HYPER-IGE SYNDROME

The syndrome is characterized by very high levels of IgE (much of it antistaphylococcal), impaired neutrophil locomotion and severe eczema, with frequent staphylococcal secondary infections and abscesses. Other immune defects may be seen causing a wider spectrum of pyogenic and fungal infections.

SHWACHMAN'S SYNDROME

This may resemble cystic fibrosis clinically, with exocrine pancreatic insufficiency and pyogenic infections, in which mild neutropenia is associated with a defect of neutrophil migration.

CHRONIC GRANULOMATOUS DISEASE (CGD)

This is the prototype congenital defect of neutrophil (and monocyte) killing.

PATHOGENESIS

In this disorder, the oxidative pathway of microbial killing is severely impaired, due either to a defective cytochrome b558 (X-linked CGD) or components of the associated NADPH oxidase (autosomal recessive CGD). Production of superoxide is abnormal, this being the first of a cascade of microbicidal oxygen radicals, including hydrogen peroxide, hypohalites, hydroxyl radicals and singlet oxygen. Impaired production of oxygen radicals can also affect the efficiency of non-oxidative killing.

CLINICAL FEATURES

Patients have chronic suppurative granulomas or abscesses affecting skin, lymph nodes and sometimes lung and liver, as well as osteomyelitis. They may present during early or late childhood years, depending on the severity of the defect. Most of the typical infections associated with neutrophil defects can be seen, particularly those that produce catalase, which inactivates any endogenous microbial peroxide that can kill organisms inside the phagocytic vacuole. Because macrophages are also affected, cell-mediated opportunist infections may also be seen such as atypical mycobacteria, *Nocardia* and salmonellae.

DIAGNOSIS AND TREATMENT

Diagnosis is made with the nitroblue tetrazolium (NBT) test, which uses a coloured dye reaction to assay the oxidative pathway. This can also be used to screen carriers.

Infections respond to appropriate antimicrobial therapy and surgical measures as needed; in some patients prophylaxis may be merited. Studies have shown that regular interferon-γ can reduce the frequency of infections, probably through enhanced monocyte/macrophage killing.

CHEDIAK–HIGASHI SYNDROME

This, an autosomal recessive disorder, is characterized by giant granules in myeloid cells and large granular lymphocytes; abnormal microbial killing is due to defective fusion with the phagosome in phagocytes; NK cell activity is similarly impaired. Similar fusion abnormalities in melanocytes causes partial oculocutaneous albinism, in addition to recurrent infections.

A wide variety of other rare disorders can impair microbial killing, including other inborn errors in microbicidal mechanisms, such as leucocyte G6PD deficiency (much less common than that affecting red cells) and myeloperoxidase deficiency. Various storage diseases, such as Gaucher's and glycogen storage diseases, impair the function of phagocytes, particularly macrophages, because of the accumulated material within them.

Acquired neutrophil function disorders

This defect is often caused by corticosteroid therapy, which also affects T cell-macrophage cooperation causing cell-mediated immunodeficiency. The main effect of corticosteroids on neutrophils is to impair leucocyte–endothelial adhesion. This reduces the marginated pool of leucocytes and impairs their attachment to endothelium at the site of tissue injury or infection. Corticosteroids thus prevent neutrophils reaching the tissues. The corollary of reduced margination is a rise in the neutrophil count; this can be deceptive if its significance is not appreciated.

The effect of corticosteroid therapy on neutrophil function is reflected by increased focal and systemic infections with staphylococci and Gram-negative bacteria. The effect is usually apparent above doses of 15 or 20 mg of prednisolone daily or equivalent, and can be reduced substantially (as can other side-effects) by alternate-day therapy.

An infective cause of acquired neutrophil dysfunction is *influenza*, which causes a specific transient impairment of phagosome–lysosome fusion. This is the main reason for the high risk of staphylococcal pneumonia in influenza epidemics.

Myeloid leukaemias can cause defective neutrophil function as well as effectively causing neutropenia of normal cells. Neutrophil and macrophage function can also be impaired in abnormal metabolic states such as uncontrolled diabetes mellitus and hypophosphataemia. The latter was seen during intravenous feeding of critically ill patients. Inhibitors of endogenous chemotactic factors for neutrophils may be seen in Hodgkin's disease and alcoholic cirrhosis, and are responsible for increased pyogenic infections in such patients.

Complement deficiencies

There are two major patterns of infection associated with complement deficiencies:

- *Deficiencies of C3, C1q or of Factors H or I* cause increased susceptibility to capsulated bacteria. These patients may also develop immune complex disorders and SLE-like disorders, as do patients with deficiencies of other classical pathway components of complement.
- *Deficiencies of the lytic complement pathway, C5-9*, causes susceptibility to disseminated neisserial infections, (meningococcaemia and gonococcaemia); the latter has also been seen in association with disorders of complement function.

These complement deficiencies are rare, but functional defects of complement deposition on microbial surfaces are common,. These are responsible for increased infections with haemophilus and pneumococcal infections, especially in the early childhood years before a sufficiently wide specific antibody repertoire is acquired. A common and well-defined opsonization defect is caused by Mannan binding protein deficiency. This protein is a member of the *collectin* family which is in the serum in the form of multimers of the basic 32 kDa peptide. It activates the classical complement C1 complex in the absence of other activating factors. Mutations in codons 52, 54 or 57 prevent the formation of the multimers, leading to intracellular degradation or defective function. The defect is present in up to 5% of Caucasian populations, but appears to be associated with recurrent viral and pyogenic infections in children.

The C3 depletion caused by C3nef, an autoantibody that stabilizes the alternative pathway convertase, and seen in association with partial lipodystrophy, may also increase the risk of pyogenic infection.

C1 esterase inhibitor deficiency (see p. 1168) is not associated with infection but with hereditary angio-oedema, with episodes of localized oedema in skin of limbs or face, and the mucosa of the larynx or gut. The latter can cause life-threatening respiratory obstruction or severe episodes of abdominal pain.

Antibody deficiencies

X-linked hypogammaglobulinaemia

There is a profound reduction in all immunoglobulin classes; B cells and plasma cells are reduced. The defect is in the differentiation of pre-B cells into B cells; T cells are normal. The specific gene defect has now been shown to be in the *btk* gene for a tyrosine kinase signal transducing molecule involved in the maturation of B cells; the gene is at a position Xq 21.2-22 on the long arm of the X chromosome. It typically presents with infections (e.g. meningitis, mycoplasmal infections) after the first 3–6 months of life, when the protection from passively transferred maternal antibody has largely been lost. Immunoglobulin replacement therapy is very successful and is generally given intravenously. Many patients treat themselves at home.

Common variable immunodeficiency (CVI)

This is a late-onset antibody deficiency, which may present in childhood or adult life. IgG levels are especially low. B cell numbers are usually normal; the defect appears to result from failure of their further differentiation. Some tests of T cell function may be abnormal, but few clinical manifestations of T cell immunodeficiency are documented. CVI is probably a heterogeneous group of disorders in its cellular and molecular origins, reflecting defective interactions between T and B cells, with arrested maturation of B cells.

CLINICAL FEATURES

The patients have similar infections to those with the X-linked variety. However, a particular feature is follicular hyperplasia of lymph nodes, which in the gut takes the form of nodular lymphoid hyperplasia, and there may be splenomegaly. CVI patients may develop autoimmune disease, and there is also an increased risk of lymphoreticular malignancy.

DIAGNOSIS AND TREATMENT

The finding of reduced immunoglobulin levels and normal B cell numbers indicates the diagnosis.

Most of the manifestations are satisfactorily prevented by regular immunoglobulin replacement therapy.

IgA deficiency

This is an extremely common disorder (affecting 1 in 600 of the UK population) but is often symptomless. Only a small proportion have an increased risk of pyogenic infection and many of these have another defect, such as IgG_2 subclass deficiency. Some have allergic disorders or a gluten-sensitive enteropathy, and autoimmune disorders may also occur.

Isolated IgG_2 subclass deficiency

This is a rare cause of increased infection with capsulated organisms, for which it is the main immunoglobulin subclass. Intravenous immunoglobulin replacement provides effective restoration.

A variety of other rare immunoglobulin deficiencies exist, including *hypogammaglobulinaemia with raised IgM*, in which there is a defect in isotype switching; the genetic basis has been shown to be due to the mutations in the gene for CD40 ligand, which is at Xq26 on the long arm of the X chromosome. Patients have recurrent bacterial infections and are susceptible to *Pneumocystis carinii* pneumonia. Other patients with increased bacterial infections have apparently normal levels of immunoglobulin but fail to produce specific antibodies to certain organisms (so-called *functional dysgammaglobulinaemia*).

Acquired hypogammaglobulinaemia

This is seen in the immune paresis of patients with myeloma and chronic lymphatic leukaemia or lymphoma. Infection with capsulated bacteria may be seen, especially in myeloma. Splenectomy causes impairment of defence against capsulated bacteria, especially pneumococcus, partly because T-independent antibody responses are largely made in the spleen and partly because of its role as part of the fixed reticuloendothelial system. Hyposplenism associated with severe sickle cell disease is responsible for the increased risk of infection in such patients. Pneumococcal vaccination (see p. 391) before elective splenectomy and the use of penicillin prophylaxis can largely eliminate risk of serious infection. Hypogammaglobulinaemia can be seen in congenital rubella.

Congenital T cell immunodeficiencies

DiGeorge anomaly

A defect of branchial arch development leads to abnormal thymic development. This is of varying severity and is associated with other branchial arch defects: dysmorphic facies, hypoparathyroidism and cardiac defects. Patients present with infections including mucocutaneous candidiasis and *Pneumocystis carinii* pneumonia, together with chronic diarrhoea, owing to a variety of pathogens. The absent thymus can be documented radiologically. CD3 T cells are variably reduced in number, but the CD4 subset is usually reduced and T-cell proliferative responses are impaired. Immunoglobulin production is typically normal. Thymic transplants and thymic hormone have been reported to have reconstituted some patients with severe disease, and bone marrow transplants have also had some success. The defect for this condition has been found on chromosome 22.

Other causes of cellular immunodeficiency

Various other rare congenital defects have been reported that predominantly affect T-cell responses, including:

- isolated CD4 lymphopenia
- IL-2/IL-2 receptor deficiency
- defects in signal transduction via the T-cell receptor (e.g. *Zap-70* deficiency)
- deficiency of the IFN-γ receptor.

Acquired T-cell defects

HIV infection

By far the most common immunodeficiency encountered in clinical practice is that due to infection with the human immunodeficiency virus (HIV), the cause of acquired immunodeficiency syndrome (AIDS).

PATHOGENESIS

The primary cellular receptor for HIV is the CD4 molecule, which defines the cells that are susceptible and includes the following cells within the immune system:

- CD4+ T lymphocytes (which are most affected)
- monocytes
- macrophages and other antigen-presenting cells
  (a) dendritic cells in the blood
  (b) Langerhans' cells of the skin
  (c) follicular dendritic cells of the lymph nodes, where much of the early infection and replication of HIV takes place.

Studies have shown that a second receptor is required for fusion/viral entry. This is CXCR4 in lymphocytes and CCR5 in cells of the monocyte/macrophage lineage. These are both chemokine receptors.

A number of pathogenic mechanisms have been described to account for the profound cellular immunodeficiency of HIV infection (see Table 2.24).

IMMUNOLOGICAL ABNORMALITIES

The central and most characteristic feature is the progressive and severe depletion of CD4+ 'helper' lymphocytes. These cells orchestrate the immune response, responding to antigen presented to them via antigen-presenting cells in the context of class II MHC. They proliferate and release cytokines, in particular IL-2, which leads to proliferation of other reactive T-cell clones, including cytotoxic T cells to eradicate viral infections, and interferon-γ, which activates B cells to antibody production, NK cells to cytotoxicity and macrophages to microbicidal activity against intracellular pathogens. Loss of this single cell type can therefore explain nearly all the immunological abnormalities of AIDS, as other cells' functioning is so dependent on it. In addition other cells are also affected, if not infected, by HIV. Antigen-presenting cells are directly and productively infected; B cells are polyclonally activated by the envelope proteins of HIV. For the presentation and management of HIV infection and AIDS, see p. 99.

Measles

Measles can cause a transient T-cell immunodeficiency, but it is rarely long-lasting enough for severe clinical problems to ensue.

Therapies causing T-cell defects

Immunosuppressive therapy

Immunosuppressive therapy with cytotoxic agents such as cyclophosphamide and azathioprine tends to cause predominant T-cell immunosuppression. Cyclosporin and tacrolimus are potent immunosuppressive agents which interfere with T-cell activation mechanisms at an intra-cellular level. Surprisingly, they are associated with only modest increases in infection, unless combined with corticosteroids or other agents. In such combinations, increased risk of Epstein–Barr virus (EBV)-associated lymphoma has been reported. Antilymphocyte immuno-globulin or monoclonal anti-CD3 antibody therapy also suppress T-cell responses transiently.

Corticosteroid therapy

This interferes with cell-mediated immunity, in particular T cell–macrophage cooperation. This is due to effects on T cell traffic and impairment of macrophage responses to cytokines, together with impaired antigen presentation. Mucocutaneous candidiasis, *Pneumocystis carinii* pneumonia, cytomegalovirus infection, mycobacterial infection, *Nocardia*, non-typhi *Salmonella* septicaemia and crypto-coccosis are some of the very many infections seen with prolonged high-dose steroid therapy.

Combined immunodeficiencies

These severe immunodeficiencies affect both B and T cell responses. These can stem from a variety of defective mechanisms in lymphocyte function, but tend to have rather similar clinical features, combining the opportunist infections of cell-mediated immunodeficiency with those of antibody deficiency.

Severe combined immunodeficiency (SCID)

This typically presents in the first weeks of life. Failure to thrive, absent lymphoid tissue, lymphopenia and hypogammaglobulinaemia with multiple severe infections are characteristic.

There are primary X-linked and autosomal recessive variants of SCID. The X-linked defect has been mapped to Xq13 which leads to mutations in the gamma chain common to the IL-2, IL-4, IL-7, IL-11 and IL-15 receptors, leading to failure to respond to these growth factors in T and B cells. Other causes include *adenosine deaminase (ADA) deficiency* (p. 158), in which a defective purine salvage enzyme that is expressed in all cells has a particular effect on lymphocytes owing to the accumulation of substrates and metabolites that interfere with lymphocyte function. An analogous disorder is seen in *purine nucleoside phosphorylase deficiency*. Non-expression of MHC class II, owing to a variety of defects in class II transactivating proteins and reticular dysgenesis, cause similar syndromes. Milder expressions of these defects exist, some presenting in later life, and are sometimes termed 'benign combined immunodeficiency' or *Nezeloff's syndrome.*

Even with supportive and antimicrobial therapy, most of these conditions have a very poor prognosis without recon-stitutive therapy. Immunoglobulin therapy is effective for the antibody deficiency, but the cell-mediated opportunists are the main determinant of outcome. Bone marrow transplant-ation is the definitive approach and has had significant success, especially if undertaken before extensive infection has set in. Attempts to restore the defective enzymes in *ADA* deficiency and gene therapy has had some success.

Other combined immune deficiencies

Wiskott–Aldrich syndrome

This is an X-linked defect (at Xp11–23 on the short arm) with associated eczema and thrombocytopenia. A mainly cell-mediated defect with falling immunoglobulins is seen, and autoimmune manifestations and lymphoreticular malignancy may develop.

Ataxia telangiectasia

In these patients a mutation prevents repair of DNA breaks, resulting in chromosomal instability. The gene responsible for a very rare variant (Nijmegen breakage syndrome, NBS) has just been cloned; it encodes the protein nibrin. Nibrin is probably an oncogene which interacts with the ataxia telangiectasia gene upstream from *p53*. *p53* is vital for the recognition of damaged DNA. Patients also have cell-mediated defects with low IgA and IgG_2, and lymphoid malignancy is again common.

EBV-associated immunodeficiency

Apparently normal, but genetically predisposed (usually X-linked) individuals develop overwhelming EBV infection, polyclonal EBV-driven lymphoproliferation, combined immunodeficiency, aplastic anaemia and lymphoid malignancy. EBV appears to act as a trigger for the expression of a hitherto silent immunodeficiency.

Protein–calorie malnutrition

Worldwide this is a very common cause of acquired combined immunodeficiency, with predominantly cell-mediated defects. Mechanisms are not fully established. Measles is a major cause of morbidity and mortality among children, and *Pneumocystis carinii* pneumonia is also a major pathogen; indeed, it was in this setting that *Pneumocystis* was first seen in the Warsaw ghetto.

The immunodeficiency of prematurity

An immune response is not essential for normal fetal development and growth, but is necessary for survival after birth. Premature infants of 28 weeks' gestation and under are now surviving and have several immunological deficiences and problems.

Antibody deficiency. IgM synthesis does not occur before 30 weeks' gestation, and IgG production does not occur until several weeks after birth. As active placental transfer of maternal antibody does not occur until the third trimester, babies born before 28 weeks have hypogammaglobulinaemia, and antibody levels continue to drop after birth owing to the loss of maternal IgG.

Other possible problems are:

- neutropenia and impaired chemotaxis
- invasion of foreign bodies, such as indwelling catheters and ventilator tubes
- antibiotic therapy, reducing colonization resistance.

FURTHER READING

Parkin JM, Morrow WJW (1993) Autoimmune mechanisms in HIV pathogenesis. In: Morrow WJW, Haigwood HL (eds) HIV: *Molecular Organization, Pathogenicity and Treatment*. Elsevier.

Nye KE, Parkin JM (1994) *HIV and AIDS*. Oxford: BIOS.

Rosen FS, Cooper MD, Wedgwood RJP (1995) The primary immunodeficiencies. *New England Journal of Medicine* **333**: 431–440.

Hypersensitivity diseases

Allergy or hypersensitivity was initially defined by Von Pirquet in 1906 as 'specifically changed reactivity of an host to an agent on a second or subsequent occasion'. This definition would apply to all specific immune responses, and allergy is now taken to mean a damaging reaction. Hypersensitivity reactions underlie a number of autoimmune and allergic conditions. The classification of these reactions is shown in Table 2.25. Immediate hypersensitivity (type I) and autoimmunity (types II and III) are discussed below.

Immediate hypersensitivity reaction

This is an allergic reaction produced within 5–10 minutes of exposure to a specific allergen. Type 1 reactivity is mediated by IgE, although later in the reaction other mechanisms of inflammation – including infiltration with eosinophils and lymphocytes – may contribute to the so-called 'late-phase response' which occurs at 4–6 hours. Low levels of allergens (e.g. house dust mite, pollens, animal danders or moulds) only elicit IgE reactions in certain genetically predisposed individuals, who are said to be *atopic*. Diseases due to type 1 reactivity include extrinsic asthma, atopic eczema, allergic rhinitis/conjunctivitis, food allergies, anaphylaxis and angio-oedema.

The diagnosis is made by a typical clinical history and examination in conjunction with either skin-prick testing (when a type 1 wheal and flare reaction is elicited by pricking the skin through a solution of the test antigens) or by measuring specific IgE in the serum.

Susceptibility to atopic disease

Hereditary predisposition. There is an inherited component: if one parent is atopic their child has a 25–40% chance of also being atopic; if both parents are affected the risk rises to 50–75%. This is compared to a background incidence in much of the developed world of around 15%. There is also an association with HLA-A1, B8, Dw3 and HLA-A3, Dw2. However, not all individuals who make IgE antibody to environ-mental allergens suffer with atopic disease, other factors play a part.

Allergen exposure. The individual must have been exposed to the allergen previously.

Age. Exposure in the first few years of life is more likely to induce atopic disease. In addition atopic disease tends to improve with age.

Intercurrent infections. Viral infections may induce atopic disease, potentially by damaging the respiratory mucosa and allowing greater allergen penetration and sensitization.

Table 2.25
Summary of hypersensitivity reactions

	I (immediate)	II (cytotoxic)	III (immune complex)	IV (delayed)	V (stimulating/ blocking)
Antigens	Pollens, moulds, mites, drugs, food and parasites	Cell surface or tissue bound	Exogenous (bacteria, fungi, parasites) Autoantigens	Cell/tissue bound	Cell surface receptors
Mediators	IgE and mast cells	IgG, IgM and complement	IgG, IgM, IgA and complement	T_D, T_C, activated macrophages and lymphokines	IgG
Diagnostic tests	Skin-prick tests: wheal and flare RAST	Coombs' test Indirect immuno-fluorescence (antibodies) Red cell agglutination Precipitating antibodies	Immune complexes	Skin test: erythema induration (e.g. tuberculin test)	Indirect immuno-fluorescence
Time taken for reaction to develop	5–10 min	6–36 hours	4–12 hours	48–72 hours	Variable
Histology	Oedema, vasodilatation, mast cell degranulation, eosinophils	Damage to target cells	Acute inflammatory reaction, neutrophils, vasculitis	Perivascular inflammation, mononuclear cells, fibrin Granulomas Caseation and necrosis in TB	Hypertrophy or normal
Diseases and conditions produced	Asthma (extrinsic) Eczema (atopic) urticaria Allergic rhinitis Anaphylaxis	Autoimmune haemolytic anaemia Transfusion reactions Haemolytic disease of newborn Goodpasture's syndrome Addisonian pernicious anaemia Myasthenia gravis	Autoimmune (e.g. SLE, glomerulo-nephritis, rheumatoid arthritis) Low-grade persistent infections (e.g. viral hepatitis) Disease caused by environmental antigens (e.g. farmer's lung)	Pulmonary TB Contact dermatitis Graft-versus-host disease Insect bites Leprosy	Neonatal hyper-thyroidism Graves' disease Myasthenia gravis
Treatment	Antigen avoidance Antihistamines Corticosteroids (usually topical) Sodium cromoglycate	Exchange transfusion Plasmapheresis Immuno-suppressives	Corticosteroids Immuno-suppressives Plasmapheresis	Immuno-suppressives Corticosteroids Removal of antigen	Treatment of individual disease

[a]Type V hypersensitivity may also be classified with type II reactions.
RAST, radioallergosorbent test; SLE, systemic lupus erythematosus; TB, tuberculosis; T_C, T cytotoxic; T_D, T delayed hypersensitivity.

Nonspecific irritants. Pollutants such as diesel emission particles (DEPs) increase bronchial reactivity and may also damage the mucosa.

Immunodeficiency. Patients with underlying immunodeficiency are more susceptible to atopic disease. This may be due to greater allergen exposure after damage to the respiratory or gut mucosa by infection, or to decreased T cell control of IgE regulation.

Mechanisms of allergic disease

The IgE response is mediated mainly by mast-cell degranulation. Both mast cells and basophils bear high-affinity receptors for IgE (FceRI). The low-affinity IgE receptor is called FceRII and is found on eosinophils, T and B lymphocytes and plays a part in the regulation of IgE production. FceRI on mast cells binds locally produced allergen-specific IgE. On subsequent allergen exposure, cross-linkage of the surface IgE molecules causes *degranulation* of the mast cell and release of pre-formed (granule-derived) and newly formed (membrane-derived) mediators. These initiate the allergic response through increasing vascular permeability (causing swelling of the tissue), inducing chemotaxis of neutrophils and eosinophils (inflammation) and increasing airway hyperactivity (bronchoconstriction) (Table 2.26).

Arachidonic acid metabolites (see Fig 12.32)

Arachidonic acid is generated in sensitized cells from membrane lipids following the binding of specific allergen. It is subsequently metabolized to produce prostaglandins (cyclooxygenase pathway), leukotrienes (lipoxygenase pathway) or platelet-activating factor (PAF acetylation), depending on which cell type is being activated. Leukotrienes and prostaglandins are together termed *eicosanoids*. The arachidonic acid metabolites involved in type 1 hypersensitivity reactions are PAF, leukotrienes (LT) B_4, C_4, D_4 and E_4, and prostaglandins (PG) D_2, E_2 and F_2. They have four main actions:

- *Inflammatory cell mucosal infiltration*. This is mediated by LTB_4 and PAF, which attract and activate neutrophils, eosinophils and monocytes/macrophages. LTB_4 is released by activated mast cells and macrophages and PAF is released by mast cells, neutrophils and eosinophils.
- *Bronchoconstriction*. This is mediated by several metabolites, including PAF, LTC_4, LTD_4, LTE_4, PGD_2 and PGF_2. LTC_4 and PGD_2 are the major arachidonic acid metabolites released by mast cells. The remaining eicosanoids are generated by human lung tissue and/or alveolar macrophages.
- Bronchial mucosal oedema is mediated by LTC_4, LTD_4 and PGE_2. PGE_2 is released from alveolar macrophages and human lung tissue.
- Mucus hypersecretion is mediated by LTC_4 and LTD_4.

Table 2.26
Mediators involved in the allergic response

Preformed mediators
Histamine and serotonin
Bronchoconstriction
Increased vascular permeability
Neutrophil and eosinophil chemotactic factors (NCF and ECF)
Induce inflammatory cell infiltration

Newly formed mediators (membrane-derived)
Leukotriene (LT) B_4
Chemoattractant +++
LTC_4, D_4, E_4 (slow-reacting substance of anaphylaxis, SRS-A)
Sustained bronchoconstriction and oedema
Prostaglandins and thromboxanes
Platelet activating factor (PAF)
Prolonged airway hyperactivity

This reaction is termed the *early phase response*. The *late phase reaction* comes 4–6 hours later and is characterized by inflammatory cell infiltrates with neutrophils, eosinophils and lymphocytes. It is likely that this reaction is important in asthma.

Regulation of IgE production

The regulation of IgE production appears to be controlled by functional subsets of helper T-lymphocytes termed Th1 and Th2, which develop after antigen stimulation from an undifferentiated population termed Th0 (p. 170).

Th1 cells produce the cytokines γ-interferon and interleukin-2 and suppress IgE production by B cells (see Fig 2.28). Th2 cells produce mainly IL-4 and IL-5. IL-4 is the switch factor for B cells to produce IgE. IL-5 attracts eosinophils. Thus Th2 cells drive an atopic response and Th1 cells suppress it. There appears to be a dysregulation towards a Th2 response in atopic individuals.

Autoimmunity

An autoimmune disease occurs when the immune system fails to recognize the body's own tissues as 'self' and mounts an attack on them. Disorders include rheumatoid arthritis, juvenile (insulin-dependent) diabetes, thyroiditis and multiple sclerosis. Illnesses are divided into those that affect just one organ (organ-specific) and those that affect many systems (organ nonspecific or multisystemic, Table 2.27). Autoimmune diseases are mostly of unknown

Table 2.27
Autoimmune diseases as classified by organ specificity

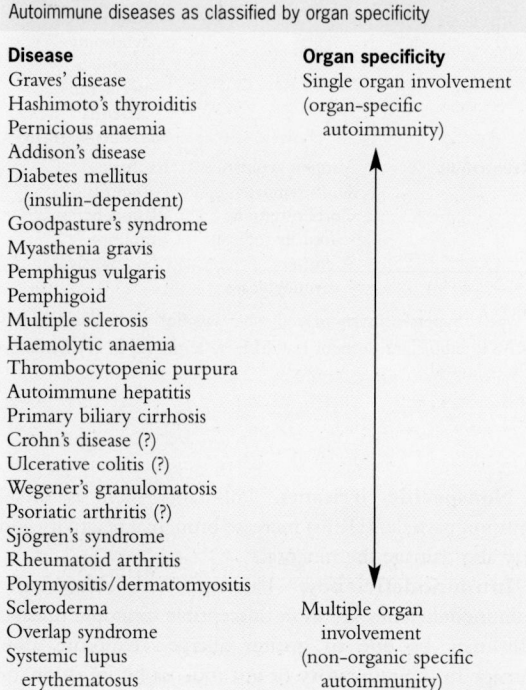

Disease	Organ specificity
Graves' disease	Single organ involvement (organ-specific autoimmunity) ↑
Hashimoto's thyroiditis	
Pernicious anaemia	
Addison's disease	
Diabetes mellitus (insulin-dependent)	
Goodpasture's syndrome	
Myasthenia gravis	
Pemphigus vulgaris	
Pemphigoid	
Multiple sclerosis	
Haemolytic anaemia	
Thrombocytopenic purpura	
Autoimmune hepatitis	
Primary biliary cirrhosis	
Crohn's disease (?)	
Ulcerative colitis (?)	
Wegener's granulomatosis	
Psoriatic arthritis (?)	
Sjögren's syndrome	
Rheumatoid arthritis	
Polymyositis/dermatomyositis	
Scleroderma	↓ Multiple organ involvement (non-organic specific autoimmunity)
Overlap syndrome	
Systemic lupus erythematosus	

Table 2.28
Factors influencing the pathogenicity of immune complexes

Size
Nature of the antigen
Class of antibodies
Subclass of antibodies
Affinity of antibodies
Complement-fixing ability
Ability of patient's complement to solubilize complex

aetiology although genetic, hormonal, microbiological and environmental factors are known to be implicated in their manifestation and severity.

IMMUNOPATHOLOGY

Formation of autoantibodies may be a normal physiological process. However, excessive production of such antibodies can be harmful. The way in which autoantibodies cause structural damage to the body's tissues are varied. Antibodies may react directly with a specific tissue, resulting in inflammation and tissue damage (e.g. antiglomerular basement membrane antibodies in Goodpasture's syndrome), or affect function directly (e.g. acetylcholine receptor antibodies in myasthenia gravis – type II hypersensitivity).

Alternatively, circulating immune complexes may be formed. Immune complexes are biologically active entities which in themselves have certain characteristics. These properties determine whether immune complexes become harmful and cause extensive tissue damage. Some of these features are detailed in Table 2.28. Inflammation or autoimmune conditions resulting from the formation of immune complexes are classified as *type III hypersensitivity reactions*. The complexes are often deposited in the kidney, skin, joint and nervous system. This results in complement activation, accumulation and activation of neutrophils with the release of proteolytic enzymes and further damage.

It should also be noted that mononuclear cells are also implicated in tissue destruction. Both CD4+ and CD8+ lymphocytes are observed routinely as infiltrates in inflammatory lesions. While there is little doubt these cells contribute to tissue destruction, their precise role in the pathological processes is uncertain. The complexity of the autoimmune diseases is quite formidable, largely because there is so much variation in the interplay of different factors that can influence the reactivity of the immune system to the body's tissues.

Immunological interventions

A number of products of the immune response can be produced in therapeutic volumes by purification from blood (immunoglobulins), cell culture (e.g. monoclonal antibodies, fibrobloast interferons) and molecular techniques (recombinant interferons, interleukin-2, colony stimulating factors, TNF). Some are still in trials. A summary of the current therapies is shown in Table 2.29.

Table 2.29
Immunological interventions

Intravenous immunoglobulin
Replacement (e.g. in hypogammaglobulinaemic states)
Fc-receptor blockade (e.g. in autoimmune cytopenias; idiopathic thrombocytopenia purpura)
Immunomodulation in autoimmune disease
Guillain–Barré syndrome
Chronic inflammatory demyelinating polyneuropathies
Lambert–Eaton myasthenic syndrome
Dermatomyositis
Interferons
Antiproliferative agents (e.g. hairy cell leukaemia; Kaposi's sarcoma; renal cell carcinoma)
Antiviral and immunomodulatory agents (e.g. chronic hepatitis B and C infection; multiple sclerosis)
Immunomodulation (e.g. γ-interferon in chronic granulomatous disease)
Colony stimulating factors
Granulocyte colony stimulating factor (GCSF) in neutropenia
Monoclonal antibodies
Immunosuppressives (e.g. anti-T-cell antibody to prevent graft-versus-host disease; anti-CD4 in treatment of rheumatoid arthritis)
Anti-inflammatory agents (e.g. anti-TNF in rheumatoid arthritis; leukotriene antagonist, e.g. montelukast sodium, in asthma)

FURTHER READING

Isenberg DA, Morrow NJW (1995) Friendly Fire. Oxford: OUP

Diagnostic tests in clinical immunology

The major investigations in the diagnosis and monitoring of disorders of the immune system are described below.

Autoantibodies

A characteristic feature of many autoimmune disorders is the presence of specific autoantibodies. These may be useful markers of disease activity, and in monitoring response to therapeutic interventions.

Indirect immunofluorescence (Fig 2.33)

This technique is used to detect organ-specific and tissue-specific antibodies, for example against thyroid, adrenal, smooth muscle, gastric parietal cell, mitochondrial, acetylcholine receptor, antinuclear, antineutrophil cytoplasm, or glomerular basement membrane. In these tests the tissue of interest is incubated with the patient's serum. Autoantibodies will bind to the tissue if present. Excess antibody is then washed off and a *developing* fluorescent antibody which binds to the *Fc* portion of the patient's autoantibody is then applied. By using a UV light microscope the specific autoantibodies can be detected.

Particle agglutination

This technique is used for the detection of rheumatoid factors (RF are antibodies to human immunoglobulin *Fc*), in the rheumatoid arthritis particle agglutination assay (RAPA), but can be used to detect many other antigens semi-quantitatively and can be a useful bedside test. In the RAPA particles are coated with rabbit or human immunoglobulin and the patient's serum added in doubling dilutions. If RF is present it will bind to the immunoglobulin and agglutinate the particles. The results are usually expressed as a titre of the highest serum dilution that gives a positive result.

Enzyme-linked immunosorbent test (ELISA)

ELISA is a commonly used technique for the detection of a wide range of proteins and autoantibodies. It is a useful technique as it is easily automated and therefore many samples can be processed. Wells of microtitre plates are coated with the antigen and the patient's serum applied. Any antibody present will bind to the antigen. A second layer of antihuman antibody conjugated with an enzyme (often alkaline phosphatase) is added, as a 'developing antibody'. A substrate that changes colour if the enzyme is present is added, and the colour intensity is measured spectrophotometrically. The intensity is proportional to the concentration of protein/antibody present. The test is quantitative as the intensity of the reaction of the patient's serum is compared with a standard curve plotted using a serum with known concentration of antibody/antigen.

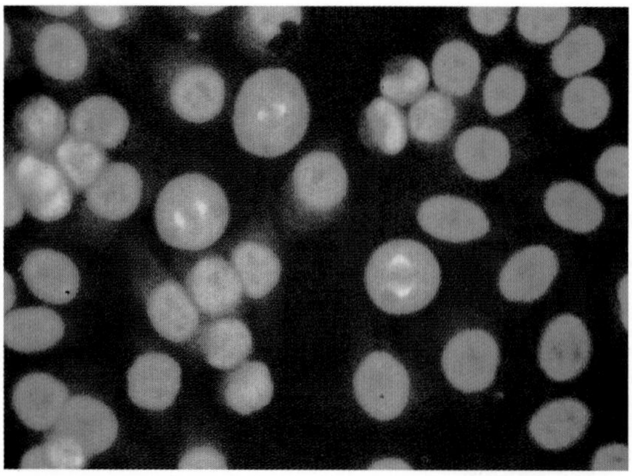

Fig 2.33
Antinuclear antibodies seen under indirect immunofluorescence

Cellular tests

The major immunodeficiencies involve abnormalities in the cells of the immune system: for example, T and B cells in SCID, DiGeorge syndrome, HIV infection, X-linked hypogammaglobulinaemia; and phagocytes in chronic granulomatous disease.

Lymphocyte subset phenotypes

Fluorescent-labelled monoclonal antibodies to the surface protein of interest are applied to the cells. The cells can then be analysed by a flow cytometer which 'lights up' cells bearing the fluorescent tag by a laser beam and counts each one. Commonly used antibodies are CD3 (all mature T lymphocytes), CD4 (CD4+ or 'helper' T cells), CD8 (CD8+ or 'suppressor' T cells), CD19 or CD20 (mature B cells).

Since the emergence of AIDS, T-cell subset counts have been done on many thousands of individuals, and it is clear that many factors outside of immunodeficiency affect the numbers:

- age (higher in infancy)
- exercise (increase)
- smoking (increase)
- diurnal variation
- pregnancy (decrease)
- splenectomy (increase).

Therefore, results have to be interpreted cautiously. Also, although HIV characteristically causes CD4-cell depletion, other conditions, such as tuberculosis and sarcoidosis, can cause similar findings.

Functional lymphocyte tests

In addition to the quantitative phenotypic studies above, functional tests of lymphocytes may also need to be performed. Peripheral blood lymphocytes are stimulated with:

- mitogens such as phytohaemagglutinin (activates T cells and B cells), concanavalin A (activates T cells), pokeweed mitogen (activates B cells)
- *recall antigens* such as purified protein derivative (PPD) and *Candida* to test memory responses.

The resulting proliferation is detected by the uptake of the radiolabelled thymidine into the DNA of the lymphocytes.

Neutrophil function tests

Tests of phagocytosis and intracellular killing/oxidative burst, random locomotion and chemotaxis are available in specialist centres, providing a useful screen for disorders such as chronic granulomatous disease.

CHAPTER BIBLIOGRAPHY

Brent LA (1997) *History of Transplantation Immunology*. London: Academic Press.

Chapel H, Haeney M (eds) (1993) *Essentials of Clinical Immunology*. Oxford, Blackwell Scientific.

Janeway C, Travers P (1997) *Immunobiology*, 3rd edn. London/New York: Current Science/Garland Publishing.

Life, death and the immune system. *Scientific American* 1993: 269.

Peakman M, Vergani D (1997) *Basic and Clinical Immunology*. Edinburgh: Churchill Livingstone.

Vogelstein B, Kinzler K (eds) (1998) The Genetic Basis of Human Cancer. New York: McGraw-Hill.

WORLD WIDE WEB ADDRESSES

Genome database
http://www.hgmp.mrc.ac.uk/gdb/gdbtop.html

UK Medical Research Council Human Gene Mapping Project Resource Centre
http://www.hgmp.mrc.ac.uk

Online Mendelian Inheritance in Man
http://www3.ncbi.nlm.nih.gov/omim/searchomim.html

Nutrition

3

In developing countries, lack of food and poor usage of the available food can result in protein–energy malnutrition (PEM); 50 million pre-school African children have PEM. In developed countries, excess food is available and the most common nutritional problem is obesity.

Diet and disease are interrelated in many ways. Excess energy intake, particularly when high in animal (saturated) fat content, is thought to be responsible for a number of diseases, including ischaemic heart disease and diabetes. A relationship between food intake and cancer has been found in many epidemiological studies; an excess of energy-rich foods (i.e. fat and sugar containing), often with physical inactivity, plays a role in the development of certain cancers, while diets high in vegetables and fruits reduce the risk of most epithelial cancers. Numerous carcinogens, either intentionally added to food (e.g. nitrates for preserving foods) or accidental contaminants (e.g. moulds producing aflatoxin and fungi), may also be involved in the development of cancer.

The proportion of processed foods eaten may affect the development of disease. A number of processed convenience foods have a high sugar and fat content and therefore predispose to dental caries and obesity respectively. They also have a low fibre content, and dietary fibre is possibly important in the prevention of a number of diseases (see p. 193). Some epidemiological data suggest that there are long-term effects of under-nutrition; low growth rates *in utero* being associated with high death rates from cardiovascular disease in adult life.

In 1991 the Department of Health published the dietary reference values for food and energy and nutrients for the UK. Values were based on all of the available information including data from the 1985 Food and Agriculture Organisation (FAO–WHO), United Nations University (UNU) expert committee, so that there is broad agreement on the reference values given. In the United Kingdom recommended daily amounts (RDAs) are no longer used, but have been replaced by the reference nutrient intake (RNI) to provide more help in interpreting dietary surveys.

The RNI is roughly equivalent to the previous RDA, and is sufficient or more than sufficient to meet the nutritional needs of 97% of healthy people in a population. Most people's daily requirements are less than this, and so an estimated average requirement (EAR) is also given, which will certainly be adequate for most. A lower reference nutrient intake (LRNI) which fails to meet the requirement of 97% of the population is also given. The RNI figures quoted in this chapter are for the age group 19–50 years.

FURTHER READING

Panel on Dietary Reference Values of the Committee on Medical Aspects of Food Policy (1991) *Dietary Reference for Food Energy and Nutrients for the United Kingdom* (Report 41DOH). London: HMSO.

Water and electrolyte balance

Water and electrolyte balance is dealt with fully in Chapter 10. About 1 L of water is required in the daily diet to balance insensible losses, but much more is usually drunk, the kidneys being able to excrete large quantities. The daily RNI for sodium is 70 mmol (1.6 g) but daily sodium intake varies in the range 90–440 mmol (2–10 g). These are needlessly high intakes which are thought by some to play a role in causing hypertension (see p. 730).

Dietary requirements

Energy

Food is necessary to provide the body with energy (Fig 3.1). The SI unit of energy is the joule (J), and 1 kJ = 0.239 kcal. The conversion factor of 4.2 kJ, equivalent to 1 kcal, is used in clinical nutrition.

Energy balance

Energy balance is the difference between energy intake and energy expenditure. Weight gain or loss is a simple, but accurate, way of indicating differences in energy balance.

Energy requirements

There are two approaches to assessing energy requirements:

- assessment of energy intake
- assessment of total energy expenditure.

Energy intake

This can be estimated from dietary surveys and in the past has been used to decide daily energy requirements. However, measurement of energy expenditure gives a more accurate assessment of requirements.

Energy expenditure

Daily energy expenditure (Fig 3.2) is the sum of:

- the basal metabolic rate (BMR)
- the thermic effect of food eaten
- occupational activities
- non-occupational activities.

Total energy expenditure can be measured using a double-labelled water technique. Water containing the stable isotopes ^2H and ^{18}O is given orally. As energy is expended carbon dioxide and water are produced. The difference between the rate of loss of the two isotopes is used to calculate the carbon dioxide production, which is then used to calculate energy expenditure. This can be done on urine samples over a three-week period with the subject ambulatory. The technique is accurate, but it is expensive and requires the availability of a mass spectrometer.

Basal metabolic rate

The BMR can be calculated by measuring oxygen consumption, but it is more usually taken from standardized tables (Table 3.1) that require knowledge of the subject's age, weight and sex. The resting metabolic rate (RMR) is 5–10% higher than the BMR and is also used.

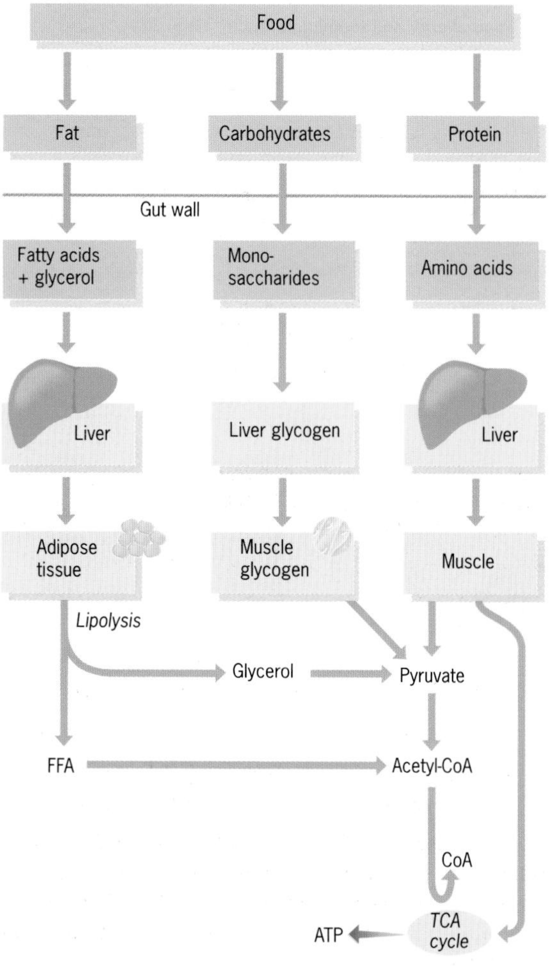

Fig 3.1
The production of energy from the main constituents of food. Alcohol produces up to 5% of total calories. 1 mol of glucose produces 36 mol of ATP. FFA, free fatty acids; ATP, adenosine triphosphate

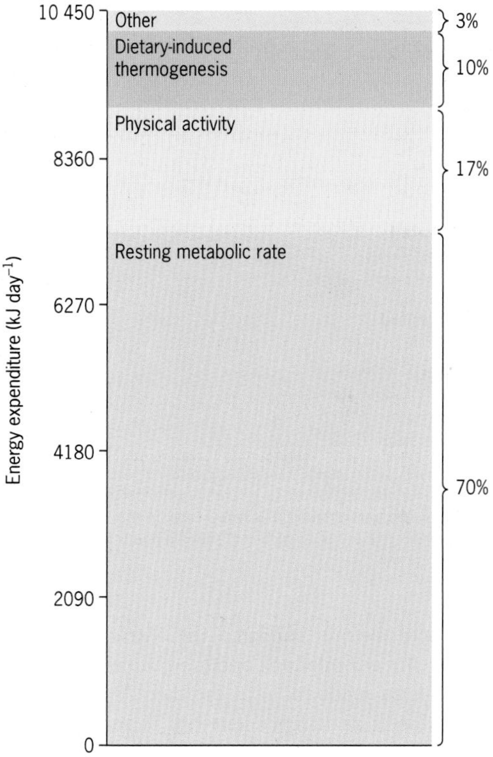

Fig 3.2
Daily energy expenditure in a sedentary adult

Physical activity
The physical activity ratio (PAR) is expressed as multiples of the BMR for both occupational and non-occupational activities of varying intensities (Table 3.2).

$$\textit{Total daily energy expenditure} = \text{BMR} \times [\text{Time in bed} + (\text{Time at work} \times \text{PAR}) + (\text{Non-occupational time} \times \text{PAR})].$$

Thus, for example, to determine the daily energy expenditure of a 55-year-old, 50 kg female doctor, with a BMRof 5240 kJ per day spending one-third of a day sleeping, working or engaged in non-occupational activities, the latter at a PAR of 2.1, the following calculation ensues:

$$(5240\ \text{kJ d}^{-1}) \times [0.3 + (0.3 \times 1.7) + (0.3 \times 2.10)] = 7550\ \text{kJ or } 1806\ \text{kcal/day}^{-1}$$

In the UK the estimated 'average' daily requirement is:

- for a 55-year-old female – 8100 kJ (1940 kcal)
- for a 55-year-old male – 10 600 kJ (2550 kcal).

This is made up of 50% carbohydrate, 35% fat, 15% protein plus or minus 5% alcohol. *In developing countries*, however, carbohydrate may be more than 75% of the total energy input, and fat less than 15% of the total energy input.

Energy requirements increase during the growing period, with pregnancy and lactation, and following infection or trauma.

Table 3.1
Equations for the prediction of basal metabolic rate (in MJ per day)

Age range (years)	Prediction equation (BMR =)	95% confidence limits
Men		
10–17	0.074 (wt)* + 2.754	± 0.88
18–29	0.063 (wt)* + 2.896	± 1.28
30–59	0.048 (wt)* + 3.653	± 1.40
60–74	0.0499 (wt)* + 2.930	N/A
75+	0.0350 (wt)* + 3.434	N/A
Women		
10–17	0.056 (wt)* + 2.898	± 0.94
18–29	0.062 (wt)* + 2.036	± 1.00
30–59	0.034 (wt)* + 3.538	± 0.94
60–74	0.0386 (wt)* + 2.875	N/A
75+	0.0410 (wt)* + 2.610	N/A

*Bodyweight (wt) in kilograms
Data reproduced with permission of Department of Health, 1991

Table 3.2 Physical activity ratio (PAR) for various activities (expressed as multiples of BMR)

	PAR
Occupational activity	
Professional/Housewife	1.7
Domestic helper/Sales person	2.7
Labourer	3.0
Non-occupational activity	
Reading/Eating	1.2
Household/Cooking	2.1
Gardening/Golf	3.7
Jogging/Swimming/Football	6.9

In the basal state, energy demands for resting muscle are 20% of the total energy required, abdominal viscera 50%, brain 20% and heart 10%. There is a 10-fold increase in muscle energy demands during exercise.

Energy stores

Energy is derived from various body stores. One-third of protein (e.g. in bone) is unavailable as an energy source, muscle being the main available protein source. Protein breakdown provides only 17 kJ (4 kcal) of energy per gram, whereas fat provides 37 kJ (9 kcal) of energy per gram. Adipose tissue is therefore an efficient way of storing energy and is the only major source of fuel available, apart from muscle protein, in the long-term fasting state. Carbohydrate provides 17 kJ (4 kcal) per gram; however, stores are small (Table 3.3), consisting of glycogen in the liver and a small amount of circulating glucose.

Bodyweight

Bodyweight depends on the energy balance. Intake depends not only on food availability but also on a number of complex interrelationships that include the stimulus of good food, the role of hunger, metabolic

Table 3.3
Normal composition of a 70 kg man

Constituent	kg	Percentage of bodyweight
Water	42	60
Fat	13	18
Protein	11	16
Carbohydrate	0.5	0.7
Minerals	3.5	5.2

changes (e.g. hypoglycaemia), and the pleasure and habit of eating. Some people are able to keep their bodyweight constant within a few kilograms for many years, but most gradually increase their weight owing to a small but continuous increase of intake over expenditure. A gain or loss of energy of 25–29 MJ (6000–7000 kcal) would respectively increase or decrease bodyweight by 1 kg.

Protein

In the UK the adult daily RNI for protein is 0.75 g kg^{-1}, with protein representing at least 10% of the total energy intake. Most affluent people eat more than this, consuming 80–100 g of protein per day. The total amount of nitrogen excreted in the urine represents the balance between protein breakdown and synthesis. In order to maintain nitrogen balance, at least 40–50 g of protein are needed. *The amount of protein required to maintain nitrogen balance* in a particular individual can be calculated from the amount of nitrogen excreted in the urine over 24 hours using the following equation:

Grams of protein required = Urinary nitrogen × 6.25
(most proteins contain about 16% of nitrogen).

In practice, urinary urea is more easily measured and forms 80–90% of the total urinary nitrogen.

Protein contains many amino acids, of which nine are indispensable (essential) amino acids. These amino acids cannot be synthesized and must be provided in the diet. The dispensable (non-essential) amino acids can be synthesized in the body, but some may still be needed in the diet unless adequate amounts of their precursors are available. Animal proteins, such as in milk, meat and eggs, are of high nutritional value as they contain all indispensable amino acids. Conversely, most proteins from vegetables are deficient in at least one indispensable amino acid.

In developing countries, adequate protein intake is achieved mainly from vegetable proteins. By combining foodstuffs with different low concentrations of indispensable amino acids (e.g. maize with legumes), protein intake can be adequate provided enough vegetables are available.

Adequate energy is required in addition to protein for the normal diet, otherwise protein will be directed towards oxidative pathways and eventually gluconeogenesis for energy. Alanine is the primary amino acid released from muscle; it is deaminated and converted into pyruvic acid before entering the citric acid cycle. Homocysteine is a sulphur-containing amino acid which is derived from methionine in the diet. A raised plasma concentration is an independent risk factor for vascular disease (see p. 687).

Table 3.4
The main fatty acids in foods

Saturated
Lauric C12:0
Myristic C14:0
Palmitic C16:0
Stearic C18:0

Monosaturated
Oleic C18:1 (n-9)
Elaidic C18:1 (n-9 *trans**)

Polyunsaturated
Linoleic C18:2 (n-6)
α-Linolenic C18:3 (n-3)
Arachidonic C20:4 (n-6)
Eicosapentaenoic C20:5 (n-3)
Docosahexaenoic C22:6 (n-3)

The number of carbon atoms is indicated before the colon; the number of double bonds after the colon. In parentheses the positions of the double bonds (designated either n as here or ω) are shown counted from the methyl end of the molecule. All double bonds are in the *cis* position except the *.

Fat

Dietary fat is chiefly in the form of triglycerides which are esters of glycerol and free fatty acids. Fatty acids vary in chain length and in saturation (Table 3.4). Unsaturated fatty acids are monounsaturated or polyunsaturated. The hydrogen molecules related to these double bonds can be in the *cis* or the *trans* position, most natural fatty acids in food being in the *cis* position (Information box 3.1).

The essential fatty acids (EFAs) are linoleic and α-linolenic acid, both of which are precursors of prostaglandins (see Fig 12.32). Eicosapentaenoic and docosahexaenoic are physiologically important, but can be made to a limited extent in the tissues from linoleic and linolenic and thus a dietary supply is not essential.

Information

Type of acid	Sources
Saturated fatty acids	Mainly animal fat
n-6 fatty acids	Vegetables oils and other plant foods
n-3 fatty acids	Vegetable foods, rapeseed oil, fish oils
trans fatty acids	Hydrogenated fat or oils, often in margarine

Information box 3.1 Dietary sources of fatty acids

Synthesis of triglycerides, sterols and phospholipids is very efficient, and even with low-fat diets subcutaneous fat stores can be normal.

Dietary fat provides 37 kJ (9 kcal) of energy per gram. A high fat intake has been implicated in the causation of:

- cardiovascular disease
- cancer (e.g. breast, colon and prostate)
- obesity
- non-insulin-dependent diabetes.

The data on causation are largely epidemiological and disputed by many. Nevertheless, it is often suggested that the consumption of saturated fatty acids should be reduced, accompanied by an increase in monounsaturated fatty acids (the 'Mediterranean diet') or polyunsaturated fatty acids. Any increase in polyunsaturated fats should not, however, exceed 10% of the total food energy, particularly as this requires a big dietary change.

Increased consumption of hydrogenated vegetable and fish oils in margarines has led to an increased *trans* fatty acid consumption and their intake should not, on present evidence, increase more than the current estimated average of 5 g per day or 2% of the dietary energy. The current recommendations for fat intake for the UK are as follows:

- Saturated fatty acids should provide approximately 10% of the dietary energy.
- *cis*-monounsaturated acids (mainly oleic acid) should continue to provide approximately 12% of the dietary energy.
- *cis*-polyunsaturated acids should provide 6% of dietary energy, and are derived from n-6 and n-3 polyunsaturated fatty acids
- Total fat intake should be no more than 35% of the total dietary energy, and restriction to 30% is desirable

Cholesterol is found in all animal products. Eggs are particularly rich in cholesterol, which is virtually absent from plants. The average daily intake in the UK is 300–500 mg. Cholesterol is also synthesized (see p. 289) and only very high or low dietary intakes will significantly affect blood levels.

Essential fatty acid deficiency

Essential fatty acid deficiency may accompany PEM, but it has been clearly defined as a clinical entity only in patients on long-term parenteral nutrition given glucose, protein and no fat. Alopecia, thrombocytopenia, anaemia and a dermatitis occur within weeks with an increased ratio of triene (n-9) to tetraene (n-6) in plasma fatty acids.

Carbohydrate

Carbohydrates are readily available in the diet, providing 17 kJ (4 kcal) per gram of energy.

Carbohydrate intake comprises the polysaccharide starch, the disaccharides (mainly sucrose) and monosaccharides (glucose and fructose). Carbohydrate is cheap compared with other foodstuffs; a great deal is therefore eaten, usually more than required.

Dietary fibre, which is largely *non-starch polysaccharide* (NSP), is often removed in the processing of food. This leaves highly refined carbohydrates such as sucrose which contribute to the development of dental caries and obesity. *Lignin* is included in dietary fibre, but it is not a polysaccharide. It is only a minor component of the human diet. The principal classes of NSP are:

- cellulose
- hemicelluloses
- pectins
- gums.

None of these is digested by gut enzymes. However, NSP is partly broken down in the gastrointestinal tract, mainly by colonic bacteria, producing gas and volatile fatty acids.

All plant food, when unprocessed, contains NSP, so that all unprocessed food eaten will increase the NSP content of the diet. *Bran*, the fibre from wheat, provides an easy way of adding additional fibre to the diet: it increases faecal bulk and is helpful in the treatment of constipation.

The average daily intake of NSP in the diet is 12 g. *NSP deficiency* is now accepted as an entity by many authorities in the UK. It is suggested that the total NSP be increased to 25–30 g daily. This could be achieved by increased consumption of bread, potatoes, fruit and vegetables, with a reduction in sugar intake in order not to increase total calories. Each extra gram of fibre daily adds approximately 5 g to the daily stool weight. A high intake of fruits and vegetables probably reduces the risk of cancer.

Pectins and gums have been added to food to slow down monosaccharide absorption, particularly in diabetes.

Health promotion

Many chronic diseases – particularly obesity, diabetes mellitus and cardiovascular disease – cause premature mortality and morbidity and are potentially preventable by dietary change.

Information box 3.2 suggests the composition of the 'ideal healthy diet'. The values given are based on the principle of:

- reducing total fat in the diet, particularly saturated fat
- increasing consumption of fish which contain n-3 (or ω-3) polyunsaturated fatty acids
- increasing intake of whole-grain cereals, green and orange vegetables and fruits, leading to an increase in fibre and antioxidants.

Reductions in dietary sodium and cholesterol have also been suggested. There would be no disadvantage in this, and most studies have suggested some benefit.

Olestra is a polymer of sucrose and six or more triglycerides. It is not absorbed and is therefore used particularly in savoury snack foods (where it has FDA

Information

Intake	Approximate amounts (%)	Helpful hints
Energy % derived from:		
Carbohydrates	40	Increase fruit, vegetables, beans, as well as bread and pasta
Protein	12	Decrease red meat
Sugar	10	
Total fat	30	Decrease meat, cheese and increase olive and other vegetable oils
Saturated fat	10	
Cholesterol (mg d^{-1})	<300	Decrease meat and eggs
NSP (g d^{-1})	30	Increase bran and cereal
Salt (g d^{-1})	6	Decrease prepared meats and do not add salt to food

NSP, non-starch polysaccharides

Information box 3.2 An 'Ideal' healthy diet

approval) as a 'fake fat'. It results in a reduced intake of fat and therefore a reduction in total calories. It has side-effects (mainly in the gut) and its use is being carefully monitored.

FURTHER READING

Calder PC (1997) n-3 polyunsaturated fatty acids and cytokine production in health and disease. *Annals of Nutrition and Metabolism* **41**:203–234

Connor WE, Connor SJ (1997) Should a ω-fat high-carbohydrate diet be recommended for everyone? for and against. *New England Journal of Medicine* **337**: 562–567

Willett WC, Sampson L (eds) (1997) Dietary assessment methods. *American Journal of Clinical Nutrition* **65** (Suppl 4)

Protein–energy malnutrition

In developed countries

Starvation is unusual in developed countries, although some degree of undernourishment is seen in very poor areas. Most nutritional problems occurring in the population at large are due to eating wrong combinations of foodstuffs, such as an excess of refined carbohydrate or a diet low in fresh vegetables.

Common causes of protein–energy malnutrition

Table 3.5 gives a list of conditions in which malnutrition is often seen. Surgical complications, with sepsis, are the most common cause in hospitals.

The majority of the weight loss, leading to malnutrition, *is due to poor intake secondary to the anorexia associated with the underlying condition.* Other possible factors are:

- increased catabolism in the septic patient
- tumour necrosis factor, or TNF, previously known as cachexia factor, in patients with cancer
- malabsorption in patients with gastrointestinal disease.

All of these contribute only a small amount to the weight loss.

Pathophysiology of starvation (Fig 3.3)

In the first 24 hours following low dietary intake, the body relies on the breakdown of hepatic glycogen to glucose for energy. Hepatic glycogen stores are small and therefore gluconeogenesis is soon necessary to maintain glucose levels. Gluconeogenesis takes place mainly from pyruvate, lactate, glycerol and amino acids, especially alanine and glutamine. The majority of protein breakdown takes place in muscle, with eventual loss of muscle bulk.

Lipolysis, the breakdown of the body's fat stores, also occurs. It is inhibited by insulin, but the level of this hormone falls off as starvation continues. The stored

Table 3.5
Common conditions associated with protein–energy malnutrition

Sepsis	Psychological: anorexia nervosa, depression
Trauma	Dementia
Surgery, particularly of GI tract with complications	Malignancy
GI disease, particularly involving the small bowel	Metabolic disease: renal failure
	Any very ill patient

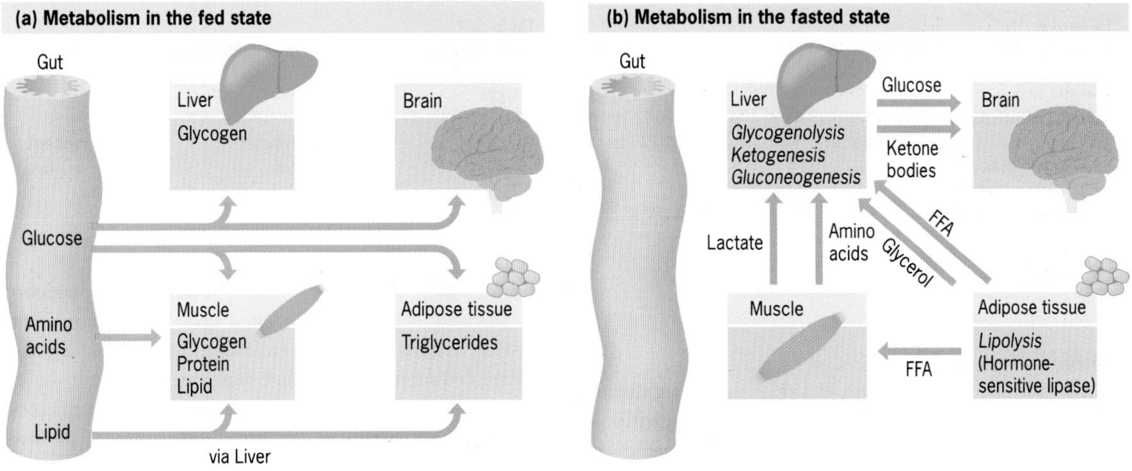

Fig 3.3
Metabolism in (a) the fed and (b) the fasted state. FFA, free fatty acids

triglyceride is hydrolysed by lipase to glycerol, which is used for gluconeogenesis, and also to non-esterified fatty acids that can be used directly as a fuel or oxidized in the liver to ketone bodies.

As starvation continues, *adaptive processes* take place lest the body's protein be completely utilized. There is a decrease in metabolic rate and total body energy expenditure. Central nervous metabolism changes from glucose as a substrate to ketone bodies, which now become the main source of energy for the brain. Gluconeogenesis in the liver decreases with a consequent reduction of protein breakdown in muscle, both of these processes being inhibited directly by ketone bodies. Most of the energy at this stage comes from adipose tissue, with some gluconeogenesis from amino acids, particularly glutamine, occurring in the kidney.

Following trauma or shock, adaptation does not take place and there is also a rise in glucocorticoid and catecholamine levels. Glucocorticoid and cytokines (see below) stimulate the ubiquitin–proteasome pathway (p. 127) in muscle which is responsible for accelerated proteolysis in muscle in many catabolic illnesses. Total energy requirements are often increased. These changes all result in continuing gluconeogenesis with massive muscle breakdown.

Regulation of metabolism

The unavailability of the various substrates in starvation produces dramatic changes in hormone levels, which are one of the main factors controlling intracellular metabolism.

- *In the fed state*, insulin/glucagon ratios are high. Insulin promotes synthesis of glycogen, protein and fat, and inhibits lipolysis and gluconeogenesis.
- *In the fasted state*, the insulin/glucagon ratios are low. Glucagon acts mainly on the liver and has no action on muscle. It increases glycogenolysis and gluconeogenesis, as well as increasing ketone body production from fatty acids. It also stimulates lipolysis in adipose tissue. Catecholamines have a similar action to glucagon but also affect muscle metabolism. These agents both act via cyclic adenosine monophosphate (cAMP) to stimulate lipolysis, producing free fatty acids that can then act as a major source of energy.

Cytokines, such as interleukin-1, interleukin-6 and tumour necrosis factor (TNF), have also been shown to play a role in regulating metabolism. TNF, which inhibits lipoprotein lipase, has been identified as the cachexia factor in patients with cancer. It is unclear how these cytokines interact with central feeding pathways to cause anorexia. However, in both animal models of cancer and inflammatory bowel disease, neuropeptide Y levels in the hypothalmus are inappropriately low so there is a reduced drive to feeding.

CLINICAL FEATURES

Patients are sometimes seen with loss of weight or malnutrition as the primary symptom (failure to thrive in children). Mostly, however, malnourishment is only seen as an accompaniment of some other disease process, such as malignancy. The major cause of the weight loss is failure to eat owing to anorexia. A careful history may indicate the cause of the weight loss but, if nothing obvious is found, hyperthyroidism must be considered. Anorexia nervosa commonly occurs in young adolescent females (see p. 1142).

Patients who have lost more than 10% of their bodyweight (unless dieting) suffer from malnutrition. Indicators of malnutrition are given in Table 3.6. The clinician can usually decide whether the patient is malnourished by the patient's general appearance. Retrospective dietary evaluation is not helpful, unfortunately, because of the degree of error in patients' recollection of their intake.

Severe malnutrition is seen mainly with advanced organic disease or after surgical procedures followed by complications. PEM leads to a depression of the immunological defence mechanism, resulting in a decreased resistance to infection (see p. 5).

Table 3.6
Hallmarks of protein–energy malnutrition

Weight loss	M + F > 10%
Triceps skinfold thickness*	M < 10 mm; F < 13 mm
Mid-arm muscle circumference*	M < 23 cm; F < 22 cm
Serum albumin	M + F < 35 g L^{-1}
Serum transferrin	M + F < 1.5 g L^{-1}
Lymphocyte count	M + F < 1.5 × 10^9 L^{-1}

*Values obtained in the UK.
M, male; F, female

TREATMENT (see also p. 210)

When malnutrition is obvious and the underlying disease cannot be corrected at once, some form of nutritional support is necessary. Nutrition should always be given enterally if the gastrointestinal tract is functioning adequately. This can most easily be done by encouraging the patient to eat more often and by giving a high-calorie supplement. If this is not possible, a liquefied diet may be given intragastrically via a fine-bore tube or by a percutaneous endoscopic gastrostomy (PEG). If both of these measures fail, parenteral nutrition is given.

In developing countries

In many areas of the world, people are on the verge of malnutrition. In addition, if events such as drought, war or changes in political climate occur, millions suffer from starvation. Although the basic condition of PEM is the same in all parts of the world from whatever cause, malnutrition resulting from long periods of near-total starvation produces unique clinical appearances in children virtually never seen in the West.

The term 'protein–energy malnutrition' covers the spectrum of clinical conditions seen in adults and children; one of a number of clinical classifications is shown in Table 3.7. The mild-to-moderate undernourished child is the most common. *Marasmus* is the childhood form of starvation. *Kwashiorkor* occurs typically in a young child displaced from breastfeeding by a new baby and fed a diet with a very low protein content, such as cassava.

This diet – which has sufficient energy but an inadequate amount of protein – results in a high plasma insulin and a low plasma cortisol. This hormonal pattern leads to an uptake of amino acids in the muscle (diverting these from the liver), leading to reduced albumin synthesis and, therefore, oedema (i.e. kwashiorkor). Conversely, when total energy is insufficient, there is an opposite hormonal pattern (i.e. low insulin and high cortisol). Amino acids are now released from the muscles, albumin is synthesized normally, and this results in marasmus rather than kwashiorkor. This classical hypothesis of protein deficiency with adequate carbohydrates as the aetiology of kwashiorkor is difficult to substantiate as most infants will have deficiency of total calorie intake as well as other unspecified nutrients. Alternatively, it has been suggested that kwashiorkor results from an imbalance of free radicals and their safe disposal, causing cell membrane damage and oedema.

Table 3.7
Wellcome classification of protein–energy malnutrition

Weight (% of standard for age)	Oedema present	Oedema absent
80–60	Kwashiorkor	Undernourished
< 60	Marasmic kwashiorkor	Marasmus

In addition to the above, infections such as measles, malaria and diarrhoea can affect the clinical picture, and children with one form of PEM may change to another form.

CLINICAL FEATURES

Adults

Starvation in adults leads to extreme loss of weight depending upon the severity and duration. They crave for food, are apathetic and complain of cold and weakness with a loss of subcutaneous fat and muscle wasting. Infections such as gastrointestinal or bronchopneumonia are common.

Children under the age of 5 years (Fig 3.4)

- *Marasmus* is the type of severe PEM seen most commonly. A child looks emaciated, there is obvious muscle wasting and loss of body fat. There is no oedema. The hair is thin and dry. The child is not so apathetic or anorexic as with kwashiorkor. Diarrhoea is frequently present and signs of infection must be looked for carefully.
- *Kwashiorkor* shows the child to be apathetic and lethargic with severe anorexia. There is generalized oedema with skin pigmentation and thickening. The hair is dry, sparse and may become reddish or yellow in colour. The abdomen is distended owing to hepatomegaly and/or ascites. The serum albumin is always low.

The undernourished child

Many children in developing countries are underweight, and subclinical PEM is often present if looked for carefully. Mild-to-moderate malnutrition is most easily detected in children by the mid upper-arm circumference (MUAC) which changes little in the normal child. An MUAC above 13.5 cm is normal, but MUAC < 12.5 cm indicates definite malnutrition.

Nutritional dwarfism is the term used to describe a child who appears normal until it is realized that he or she is short for age. Reduced linear growth occurs in response to undernutrition; dental development is less retarded so that the facial appearance is inappropriate for the age.

(a)

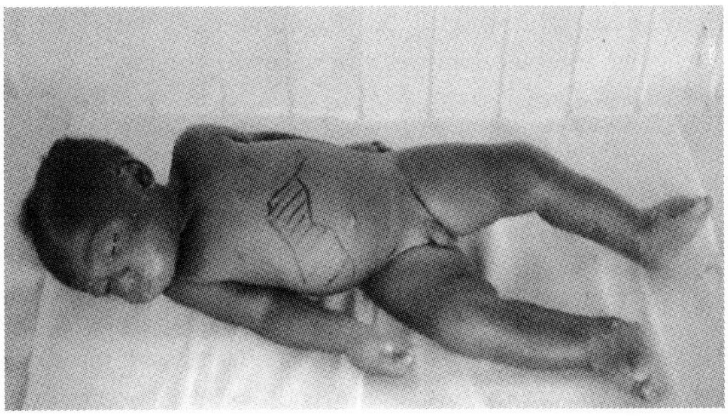

(b)

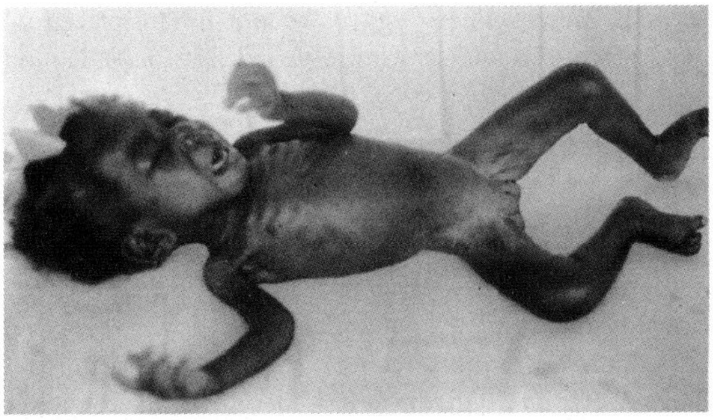

Fig 3.4
Malnourished children: (a) kwashiorkor and (b) marasmus.
Courtesy of Professor J Garrow

As with an adult, the undernourished child is very susceptible to respiratory and gastrointestinal infections, leading to an increased mortality in this group.

INVESTIGATION

It must be realized that this is not always practicable.

- **Blood tests**
  (a) Anaemia due to folate, iron and copper deficiency is often present, but the haematocrit may be high owing to dehydration.
  (b) Eosinophilia suggests parasitic infestation.
  (c) Electrolyte disturbances are common.
  (d) Malarial parasites should be looked for.
- **Stools** should be examined for parasitic infestations.
- **Chest X-ray** – tuberculosis is common and is easily missed if a chest X-ray is not performed.

TREATMENT

Treatment must involve the provision of protein and energy supplements and the control of infection.

Resuscitation

The severely ill child will require correction of fluid and electrolyte abnormalities, but intravenous therapy should be avoided if possible because of the danger of fluid overload.

Glucose electrolyte mixtures (such as the WHO formulation, p. 32) are sometimes necessary. Diarrhoea is often due to bacterial or protozoal overgrowth; metronidazole is very effective and is often given routinely. Parasites are also common and, as facilities for stool examination are usually not available, mebendazole 100 mg twice daily should be given for three days. In high-risk areas, antimalarial therapy is given.

Refeeding

This needs to be planned carefully. During the initial treatment of the acute situation, just enough energy and protein should be given to maintain a steady state. Large increases in energy lead to heart failure, circulatory collapse and death. A child requires approximately 450 kJ kg^{-1} (100 kcal kg^{-1}) daily, which is provided by 0.6 g kg^{-1} of protein. This is often given as milk with additional water, flour, maize or whatever is available locally. Sugar mixed with dried skimmed milk and small amounts of cotton-seed oil (DISCO) is frequently used. Attempts should be made to give the feeds as slowly and as often as possible, although anorexia is often a problem and can be exacerbated by excessive feeding. If necessary, fluids and food should be given by nasogastric tube. The child is then gradually weaned to liquids and then solids by mouth.

Hypothermia and hypoglycaemia occur in severely ill children, often with an accompanying infection, and need to be treated urgently. Because of the cold temperatures at night, blankets and sometimes additional heat are necessary.

Supplements of vitamins (A, D, B and C) should always be given, together with folic acid and iron. Many children are deficient in minerals such as zinc, copper and selenium, and supplements should be given if deficiency is suspected.

Rehabilitation

Gradually, as the child improves, more energy can be given, and during rehabilitation maximum weight gain is achieved in the shortest time by extra calories ('catch-up weight gain'). Children who have been severely ill need constant attention right through the convalescent period, as often home conditions are poor and feeds are refused.

Adults do not usually suffer such severe malnutrition, but the same principles of treatment should be followed.

PROGNOSIS

Children with extreme malnutrition have a mortality of over 50%. By careful management this can be reduced significantly to 1–2%, depending on the availability of facilities. Brain development takes place in the first years of life, a time when severe PEM frequently occurs. There is evidence that intellectual impairment and behavioural abnormalities occur in severely affected children. Physical growth is also impaired. Probably both of these effects can be alleviated if it is possible to maintain a high standard of living with a good diet and freedom from infection over a long period.

Information

- **G**rowth monitoring: The WHO has a simple growth chart that the mother keeps
- **O**ral rehydration, particularly for diarrhoea
- **B**reast feeding supplemented by food after 6 months
- **I**mmunization: against measles, tetanus, pertussis, diphtheria, polio and tuberculosis
- **F**amily planning

Information box 3.3 Prevention of protein–energy malnutrition – GOBIF (a WHO priority programme)

PREVENTION

Prevention of PEM depends not only on adequate nutrients being available but also on education of both governments and individuals of the importance of good nutrition and immunization (Information box 3.3). Short-term programmes are useful for acute shortages of food, but long-term programmes involving improved agriculture are equally important. Bad feeding practices and infections are more important than actual shortage of food in many areas of the world. However, good surveillance is necessary to avoid periods of famine.

Food supplements (and additional vitamins) should be given to 'at-risk' groups by adding high-energy food (e.g. milk powder, meat concentrates) to the diet. Pregnancy and lactation are times of high energy requirement and supplements have been shown to be beneficial.

FURTHER READING

Khanu MS, Ashworh A, Huttley SR (1994) Controlled trial of three approaches to the treatment of severe malnutrition. *Lancet* **334**: 1728–1732.

Schwarz MW, Seeley RT (1997) Neuro-endocrine responses to starvation and weight loss. *New England Journal of Medicine* **336**: 1802–1811.

Waterlow JC, (1992) Protein energy malnutrition. Edward Arnold, London.

Vitamins

Deficiencies due to inadequate intake associated with PEM (Table 3.8) are commonly seen in the developing countries. This is not, however, invariable. For example, vitamin A deficiency is never seen in Jamaica, but is common in PEM in Hyderabad. In the West, deficiency of vitamins is rare except in the specific groups shown in Table 3.9. The widespread use of vitamins as 'tonics' is unnecessary and should be discouraged. Toxicity from excess fat-soluble vitamins is occasionally seen.

Fat-soluble vitamins

Vitamin A

Vitamin A (retinol) is part of the family of retinoids which is present in food and the body as esters combined with long-chain fatty acids.

The richest food source is liver, but it is also found in milk, butter, cheese, egg yolks and fish oils. Retinol or carotene is added to margarine in the UK and other countries.

Beta-carotene is the main carotenoid found in green vegetables, carrots and other yellow and red fruits. Other carotenoids, lycopene and lutein, are probably of little quantitative importance as dietary precursors of vitamin A.

Beta-carotene is cleaved in the intestinal mucosa by carotene dioxygenase, yielding retinaldehyde which can be reduced to retinol. Between a quarter and a third of dietary vitamin A in the UK is derived from retinoids. Nutritionally, 6 μg of β-carotene is equivalent to 1 μg of preformed retinol; vitamin A activity in the diet is given as retinol equivalents.

Function

Retinol is stored in the liver and is transported in plasma bound to an α-globulin retinol binding protein (RBP). Vitamin A has several metabolic roles:

- Retinaldehyde in its *cis* form is found in the opsin proteins in the rods (rhodopsin) and cones (iodopsin) of the retina. Light causes retinaldehyde to change to its *trans* isomer, and this leads to changes in membrane potentials that are transmitted to the brain.
- Retinol and retinoic acid are involved in the control of cell proliferation and differentiation.
- Retinyl phosphate is a cofactor in the synthesis of most glycoproteins containing mannose.

Deficiency

Vitamin A deficiency and xerophthalmia (see below) is the major cause of blindness in young children despite intensive preventative programmes. The WHO estimates that between six and seven million new cases of xerophthalmia occur each year, with 20% of survivors being totally blind and 50–56% partially blind. South and East Asia, parts of Africa and Latin America as well as the Middle East are the most severely affected.

Xerophthalmia has been classified by the WHO (Table 3.10). Impaired adaptation followed by night blindness is the first effect. There is dryness and thickening of the conjunctiva and the cornea (xerophthalmia occurs as a result of keratinization). Bitot's

Table 3.8
Fat-soluble and water-soluble vitamins: reference nutrient intake (RNI) and lower reference nutrient intake (LRNI)

Vitamin	RNI/day (sufficient)	LRNI/day (insufficient)	Major clinical features of deficiency
Fat-soluble			
A (retinol)	700 μg	300 μg	Xerophthalmia, night blindness, keratomalacia, follicular hyperkeratosis
D (cholecalciferol)	No dietary intake required	10 μg (living indoors)	Rickets, osteomalacia
K	1 μg kg^{-1} bodyweight		Coagulation defects
E (α-tocopherol)	*		Neurological disorders, e.g. ataxia
Water-soluble			
B_1 (thiamin)	0.4 mg per 1000 kcal**	0.23 mg per 1000 kcal**	Beriberi, Wernicke–Korsakoff syndrome
B_2 (riboflavin)	1.3 mg	0.8 mg	Angular stomatitis
Niacin	6.6 mg per 1000 kcal	4.4 mg per 1000 kcal	Pellagra
B_6 (pyridoxine)	15 μg per g of dietary protein	11 μg per g of dietary protein	Polyneuropathy
B_{12} (cobalamin)	1.5 μg	1.0 μg	Megaloblastic anaemia, neurological disorders
Folate	200 μg	100 μg	Megaloblastic anaemia
C (ascorbic acid)	40 mg	10 mg	Scurvy

*No official RNI because amount varies depending upon polyunsaturated fatty acid content of diet
**Thiamin requirements are related to energy metabolism

spots – white plaques of keratinized epithelial cells – are found on the conjunctiva of young children with vitamin A deficiency. These spots can, however, be seen without vitamin A deficiency, possibly caused by exposure. Corneal softening, ulceration and dissolution (keratomalacia) eventually occur; superimposed infection is a frequent accompaniment and both lead to blindness.

Vitamin A in malnourished children

Vitamin A supplementation (usually with 200 000 i.u.) in groups of children with xerophthalmia showed a decrease in mortality. Several trials have now been undertaken in various parts of the world with varying results, but the consensus is that the benefit of supplements of vitamin A in reducing child mortality is highly significant and unlikely to be due to factors other than the supplements. This, however, is still controversial.

The evidence that vitamin A supplementation reduces diarrhoea and respiratory disease is also controversial with different results reported from various countries. Vitamin A may also reduce mortality from measles.

In PEM, retinol binding protein along with other proteins are reduced. This suggests vitamin A deficiency, although body stores are not necessarily reduced.

DIAGNOSIS

In parts of the world where the deficiency is common, diagnosis is made on the basis of the clinical features and deficiency should always be suspected if any degree of malnutrition is present. Blood levels of vitamin A will usually be low, but the best guide to the diagnosis is a response to replacement therapy.

Table 3.9
Some causes of vitamin deficiency in the West

Decreased intake
- Alcohol dependency: chiefly B vitamins (e.g. thiamin)
- Small bowel disease: chiefly folate, occasionally fat-soluble vitamins
- Vegans: vitamin D (if no exposure to sunlight), vitamin B_{12}
- Elderly with poor diet: chiefly vitamin D (if no exposure to sunlight), folate
- Anorexia from any cause: chiefly folate

Decreased absorption
- Ileal disease/resection: only vitamin B_{12}
- Liver and biliary tract disese: fat-soluble vitamins
- Intestinal bacterial overgrowth: vitamin B_{12}
- Oral antibiotics: vitamin K

Miscellaneous
- Long-term enteral or parenteral nutrition: usually vitamin supplements are given
- Renal disease: vitamin D
- Drug antagonists (e.g. methotrexate interfering with folate metabolism)

Table 3.10
Classification of xerophthalmia by ocular signs

Night blindness (XN)
Conjunctival xerosis (XIA)
Bitot's spot (X2)
Corneal xerosis (X2)
Corneal ulceration/keratomalacia < $\frac{1}{3}$ corneal surface (X3A)
Corneal ulceration/keratomlacia ≥ $\frac{1}{3}$ corneal surface (X3B)
Corneal scar (XS)
Xerophthalmic fundus (XF)

Reproduced with permission from WHO/Unicef/IVACG 1988

TREATMENT

Urgent treatment with retinol palmitate 30 mg orally should be given on two successive days. In the presence of vomiting and diarrhoea, 30 mg of vitamin A is given intramuscularly. Associated malnutrition must be treated and superadded bacterial infection should be treated with antibiotics. Referral for specialist ophthalmic treatment is necessary in severe cases.

PREVENTION

Most Western diets contain enough dairy products and green vegetables, but vitamin A is added to foodstuffs (e.g. margarine) in some countries. Vitamin A is not destroyed by cooking. Education of the population is important and people should be encouraged to grow their own vegetables. In particular, pregnant women and children should be encouraged to eat green vegetables. In some developing countries vitamin A supplements are given at the time the child attends for measles vaccination. Food fortification programmes are another approach.

Other effects of vitamin A

Possible beneficial effects

- *Protection against cancer.* In epidemiological studies, β-carotene (which acts as an antioxidant), and to a lesser extent vitamin A, have been shown to have a possible protective effect against certain cancers. Controlled trials using β-carotene supplements have, however, not confirmed this protective effect.
- *Reduction in cardiovascular events.* Epidemiological studies have shown an association between increased intake of antioxidant vitamins (β-carotene, vitamin E, vitamin C) and reduced morbidity and mortality from coronary artery disease. Recent randomized trials have so far shown no reduction with β-carotene supplementation.
- *Dermatological applications.* Retinoic acid and some synthetic retinoids are used in dermatology (p. 1170).

Possible adverse effects

- *High intakes of vitamin A.* Chronic ingestion of retinol can cause liver and bone damage, hair loss, double vision, vomiting, headaches and other abnormalities. Single doses of 300 mg in adults or 100 mg in children can be harmful.
- *Retinol is teratogenic.* The incidence of birth defects in infants is high with vitamin A intakes of more than 3 mg a day during pregnancy. In pregnancy, extra vitamin A or consumption of liver is not recommended in the UK. However, β-carotene is not toxic.

Vitamin D

See p. 504.

Vitamin K

Vitamin K is found as phylloquinone (vitamin K_1) in green leafy vegetables, dairy products, rape seed and soya bean oils. Intestinal bacteria can synthesize the other major form of vitamin K, menaquinone (vitamin K_2), in the terminal ileum and colon. Vitamin K is absorbed in a similar manner to other fat-soluble substances in the upper small gut. Some menaquinones must also be absorbed as this is the major form found in the human liver.

Function

Vitamin K is a cofactor necessary for the production not only of blood clotting factors (p. 406), but also for proteins necessary in the formation of bone (p. 502).

Vitamin K is a co-factor for the post-translational carboxylation of specific protein bound glutamate residues in γ-carboxyglutamate (Gla). Gla residues bind calcium ions to phospholipid templates, and this action on factors II, VII, IX and X, and on proteins C and S, is necessary for coagulation to take place.

Bone osteoblasts contain three vitamin K dependent proteins, osteocalcin, matrix Gla protein and protein S (p. 502) which have a role in bone matrix formation. Osteocalcin contains three Gla residues which bind tightly to the hydroxyapatite matrix depending on the degree of carboxylation; this leads to bone mineralization. There is, however, no convincing evidence that vitamin K deficiency or antagonism affects bone other than rapidly growing bone.

Vitamin K deficiency

Vitamin K deficiency results in inadequate synthesis of clotting factors (p. 406) which leads to an increase in the prothrombin time and haemorrhage. Deficiency occurs in the following circumstances.

The newborn

Deficiency occurs in the new born owing to:

- poor placental transfer of vitamin K
- little vitamin K in breast milk
- no hepatic stores of menaquinone (no intestinal bacteria in the neonate).

Deficiency leads to a haemorrhagic disease of the newborn which can be prevented by prophylactic vitamin K. However, in the UK there is no agreement on whether prophylactic therapy is necessary.

Cholestatic jaundice

When bile flow into the intestine is interrupted, malabsorption of vitamin K occurs as no bile salts are available to facilitate absorption and the prothrombin time increases. This can be corrected by giving 10 mg of phytomenadione intramuscularly. (Note that an increased prothrombin time due to liver disease does not respond to vitamin K injection, there being no shortage of vitamin K, just bad liver function.) In patients with chronic cholestasis (e.g. primary biliary cirrhosis) oral therapy using a water-soluble preparation Menadiol, sodium phosphate 10 mg daily is used.

Concomitant vitamin K antagonists
Oral anticoagulants antagonize vitamin K (p. 412). Antibacterial drugs also interfere with the bacterial synthesis of vitamin K.

Vitamin E

Vitamin E includes eight naturally occurring compounds divided into tocopherols and tocotrienoles. The most active compound and the most widely available in food is the natural isomer d- (or RRR) α-tocopherol which accounts for 90% of vitamin E in the human body. Vegetables and seed oils, including soya bean, saffron, sunflower, cereals and nuts, are the main sources. Animal products are poor sources of the vitamin.

Vitamin E is absorbed with fat, transported in the blood largely in low-density lipoproteins (LDL).

An individual's vitamin E requirement depends on the intake of polyunsaturated fatty acids (PUFAs). Since this varies widely, in the UK no daily requirement is given. The requirement stated in the USA is approximately 7–10 mg per day, but average diets contain much more than this. If PUFAs are taken in large amounts, more vitamin E is required.

Function

The biological activity of vitamin E results principally from its antioxidant properties. In biological membranes it contributes to membrane stability. It protects cellular structures against damage from a number of highly reactive oxygen species, including hydrogen peroxide, superoxide and other oxygen radicals. Vitamin E may also affect cell proliferation and growth.

Vitamin E deficiency

The first deficiency to be demonstrated was a haemolytic anaemia described in premature infants. Infant formulations now contain vitamin E.

Deficiency is seen only in children with abetalipoproteinaemia (p. 259). The severe neurological deficit (gross ataxia) can be prevented by vitamin E injection.

Plasma or serum levels of α-tocopherol can be measured and should be corrected for the level of plasma lipids by expressing the value as milligrams per milligram of plasma lipid.

Epidemiological data

Animals fed an atherogenic diet supplemented with α-tocopherol develop many fewer new atheromatous lesions than do those fed an atherogenic diet alone, and there may be regression of existing lesions.

There is also strong evidence for vitamin E intake and blood α-tocopherol levels as an independent risk factor for the development of *ischaemic heart disease* (IHD) in healthy, well-nourished individuals eating a Western diet. This has been shown in comparisons of different communities in the WHO 'MONICA' observational study. It may account for the 'Mediterranean paradox' of communities in Southern Europe – who eat a high-fat diet with a high prevalence of cigarette smoking – having an incidence of premature IHD just 10% of that of communities in Northern Europe, such as the Clyde Valley or Finland. This antioxidant hypothesis has been tested in one randomized controlled trial of 2002 individuals with advanced IHD, the Cambridge Heart Antioxidant Study (CHAOS). This demonstrated a beneficial effect of high doses of vitamin E (400 or 800 i.u. per day) on the subsequent risk of non-fatal myocardial infarction, which was reduced by 75%. There was no effect on mortality, which may have been due to a lack of 'statistical power' in the study. It is thus debatable whether vitamin E should be advocated as an accepted therapy for secondary prevention of IHD, although the evidence for it as an independent risk factor is strong.

Antioxidants may also have a role in the prevention of cancer, and vitamin E has also been shown to have some benefit in patients with Alzheimer's disease (p. 1114).

Water-soluble vitamins

Water-soluble vitamins are non-toxic and relatively cheap and can therefore be given in large amounts if a deficiency is possible. The daily requirements of water-soluble vitamins are given in Table 3.6.

Thiamin (vitamin B_1)

Thiamin consists of pyrimidine and thiazole rings. The alcohol side-chain is esterified with one, two or three phosphates (Fig 3.5).

Function

Thiamin diphosphate, often called thiamin pyrophosphate (TPP), is an essential co-factor, particularly in carbohydrate metabolism.

TPP is involved in the oxidative decarboxylation of acetyl CoA in mitochondria. In the Krebs cycle, TPP is the key enzyme for the decarboxylation of α-ketoglutarate to succinyl CoA. TPP is also the co-factor for transketolase, a key enzyme in the hexose monophosphate shunt.

Thiamin is found in many foodstuffs, including cereals, grains, beans, nuts, as well as pork and duck. It is often added to food (e.g. in cereals) in developed countries. The dietary requirement (see Table 3.8) depends on energy intake, more being required if the diet is high in carbohydrates.

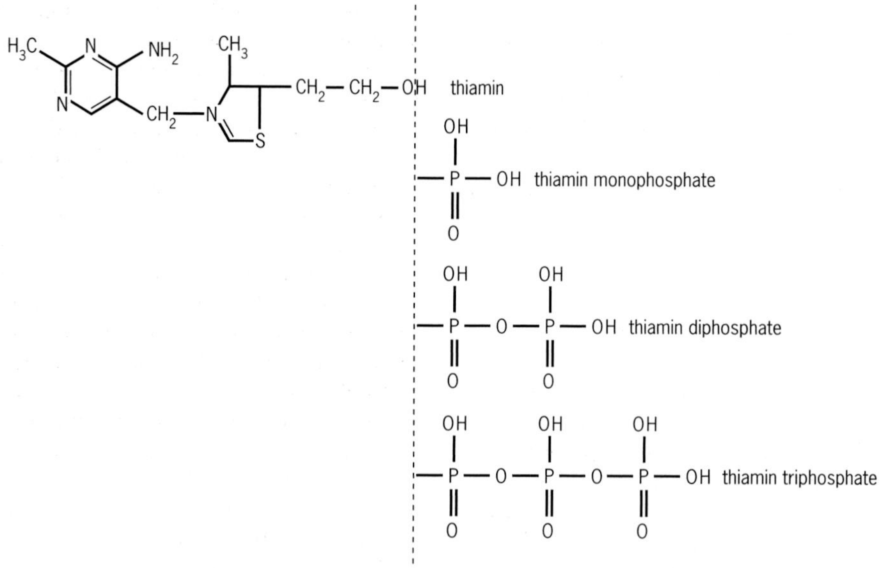

Fig 3.5
Thiamin

Following absorption, thiamin is found in all body tissues, the majority being in the liver. Body stores are small and signs of deficiency quickly develop with inadequate intake.

There is no evidence that a high oral intake is dangerous, but ataxia has been reported after high parentral therapy.

Thiamin deficiency

Thiamin deficiency is seen:

- as beriberi, where the only food consumed is polished rice
- in chronic alcohol-dependent patients who are consuming virtually no food at all
- rarely in starved patients (e.g. with carcinoma of the stomach), and in severe prolonged hyperemesis gravidarum, especially when treated by intravenous fluids alone.

Beriberi

This is now confined to the poorest areas of South East Asia. It can be prevented by eating undermilled or par-boiled rice, or by fortification of rice with thiamine. Probably the most important factor in the reduction of beriberi is the general increase in overall food consumption so that the staple diet is varied and contains legumes and pulses, which contain a large amount of thiamin. There are two main clinical types of beriberi, which, surprisingly, only rarely occur together.

Dry beriberi usually presents insidiously with a symmetrical polyneuropathy. The initial symptoms are heaviness and stiffness of the legs, followed by weakness, numbness, and pins and needles. The ankle jerk reflexes are lost and eventually all the signs of polyneuropathy that may involve the trunk and arms are found (p. 1093). Cerebral involvement occurs, producing the picture of the Wernicke–Korsakoff syndrome (p. 1095). In endemic areas, mild symptoms and signs may be present for years without unduly affecting the patient.

Wet beriberi causes oedema. Initially this is of the legs, but it can extend to involve the whole body, with ascites and pleural effusions. The peripheral oedema may mask the accompanying features of dry beriberi.

Thiamin deficiency impairs pyruvate dehydrogenase with accumulation of lactate and pyruvate, producing peripheral vasodilatation and eventually oedema. The heart muscle is also affected and heart failure occurs, causing a further increase in the oedema. Initially there are warm extremities, a full, fast, bounding pulse and a raised venous pressure ('high-output state'), but eventually heart failure advances and a poor cardiac output ensues. The electrocardiogram may show conduction defects.

Infantile beriberi occurs, usually acutely, in breast-fed babies at approximately 3 months of age. The mothers show no signs of thiamin deficiency but presumably their body stores must be virtually nil. The infant becomes anorexic, develops oedema and has some degree of aphonia. Tachycardia and tachypnoea develop and, unless treatment is instituted, death occurs quickly.

DIAGNOSIS

In endemic areas the diagnosis of beriberi should always be suspected and if in doubt treatment with thiamine should be instituted. A rapid disappearance of oedema after thiamine (50 mg i.m.) is diagnostic. Other causes of oedema must be considered (e.g. renal or liver disease), and the polyneuro-pathy is indistinguishable from that due to other causes. The diagnosis is confirmed by measurement of transketolase activity in red cells using fresh heparinized blood. This enzyme is dependent on TPP. The assay is performed with and without added TPP; an increase in activity of 25% with TPP indicates deficiency.

TREATMENT

Thiamine 50 mg i.m. is given for three days, followed by 25 mg of thiamine daily by mouth. The response in wet beriberi occurs in hours, giving dramatic improvement, but in dry beriberi improvement is often slow to occur. In most cases all the B vitamins are given because of multiple deficiency. Infantile beriberi is treated by giving thiamine to the mother, which is then passed on to the infant via the breast milk.

Thiamin deficiency in patients with alcohol dependence

In the West this is the only major group to suffer from thiamin deficiency. Rarely they develop wet beriberi, which must be distinguished from alcoholic cardiomyopathy. More usually, however, thiamin deficiency presents with polyneuropathy or with the Wernicke–Korsakoff syndrome. This syndrome, which consists of dementia, ataxia, varying ophthalmoplegia and nystagmus (see p. 1095), presents acutely and should be suspected in all heavy drinkers. If treated promptly it is reversible; if left it becomes irreversible. It is a major cause of dementia in the USA.

Urgent treatment with thiamine 50–100 mg i.m. or i.v. is given for three days, often combined with other B-complex vitamins. Thiamine must always be given before any intravenous glucose infusion.

Riboflavin

Riboflavin is widely distributed throughout all plant and animal cells. Good sources are dairy products, offal and leafy vegetables. Riboflavin is not destroyed appreciably by cooking, but is destroyed by sunlight. Riboflavin is a flavoprotein that is a co-factor for many oxidative reactions in the cell.

There is no definite deficiency, although many communities have low dietary intakes. Studies in volunteers taking a low riboflavin diet have produced:

- angular stomatitis or cheilosis (fissuring at the corners of the mouth)
- a red, inflamed tongue
- seborrhoeic dermatitis, particularly involving the face (around the nose) and the scrotum or vulva.

Conjunctivitis with vascularization of the cornea and opacity of the lens have also been described. It is probable, however, that many of the above features are due to multiple deficiencies rather than the riboflavin itself.

Riboflavin 5 mg daily can be tried for the above conditions, usually given as the vitamin B complex.

Niacin

This is the generic name for the two chemical forms, nicotinic acid and nicotinamide, the latter being found in the two pyridine nucleotides, nicotinamide adenine dinucleotide (NAD) and nicotinamide adenine dinucleotide phosphate (NADP). Both act as hydrogen acceptors in many oxidative reactions, and in their reduced forms (NADH and NADPH) act as hydrogen donors in reductive reactions. Many oxidative steps in the production of energy require NAD, and NADP is equally important in the hexose monophosphate shunt (p. 380) for the generation of NADPH, which is necessary for fatty-acid synthesis.

Niacin is found in many foodstuffs, including plants, meat (particularly offal) and fish. Niacin is lost by removing bran from cereals but is added to processed cereals and white bread in many countries.

Niacin can be synthesized in humans from tryptophan, 60 mg of tryptophan being converted to 1 mg of niacin (Fig 3.6). The amount of niacin in food is given as the 'niacin equivalent', which is equal to the amount of niacin plus one-sixtieth of the tryptophan content. Eggs and cheese contain tryptophan.

Kynureninase and kynurenine hydroxylase are both B_6 and riboflavin dependent and deficiency of these B vitamins can also produce pellagra.

Pellagra

This is rare and is found in people who eat virtually only maize, for example in parts of Africa. Maize contains niacin in the form of niacytin, which is biologically unavailable, and has a low content of tryptophan. In central America, pellagra has always been rare because maize (for the cooking of tortillas) is soaked overnight in calcium hydroxide which releases niacin. Many of the features of

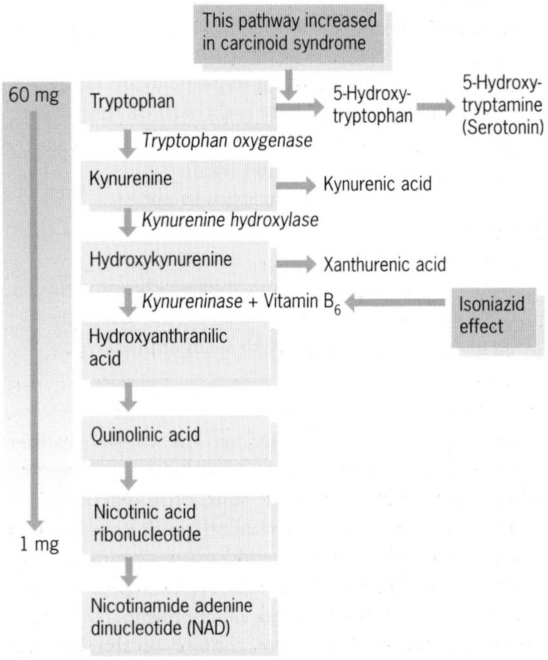

Fig 3.6
The oxidative pathway of tryptophan metabolism

pellagra can be explained purely by niacin deficiency; but some are probably due to multiple deficiencies, including deficiencies of proteins and of other vitamins.

CLINICAL FEATURES

The classical features are of dermatitis, diarrhoea and dementia. Although this is an easily remembered triad, not all are always present and the mental changes are not a true dementia.

- *Dermatitis.* In the areas of skin exposed to sunlight, initially there is redness followed by cracks with occasional ulceration. Chronic thickening, dryness and pigmentation develop. The lesions are always symmetrical and often affect the dorsal surfaces of the hands. The perianal skin and vulva are frequently involved. Casal's necklace or collar is the term given to the skin lesion around the neck, which is confined to this area by the clothes worn.
- *Diarrhoea.* This is often a feature but constipation is occasionally seen. Other gastrointestinal manifestations include a painful, red, raw tongue, glossitis and angular stomatitis. Recurring mouth infections occur.
- *Dementia.* This occurs in chronic disease. In milder cases there are symptoms of depression, apathy and sometimes thought disorders. Tremor and an encephalopathy frequently occur. Hallucinations and acute psychosis are seen with more severe cases.

Pellagra may also occur in the following circumstances:

- Isoniazid therapy can lead to a deficiency of vitamin B_6, which is needed for the synthesis of nicotinamide from tryptophan. Vitamin B_6 is now given concomitantly with isoniazid (Fig 3.5).
- In Hartnup's disease, a rare inborn error, in which basic amino acids including tryptophan are not absorbed by the gut. There is also loss of this amino acid in the urine.
- In generalized malabsorption (rare).
- Alcohol-dependent patients who do not eat.
- Very low protein diets given for renal disease or taken as a food fad.
- In the carcinoid syndrome and phaeochromocytomas, tryptophan metabolism is diverted away from the formation of nicotinamide to form amines.

DIAGNOSIS

In endemic areas this is based on the clinical features, remembering that other vitamin deficiencies can produce similar changes (e.g. angular stomatitis). Nicotinamide (approximately 300 mg daily by mouth) with a maintenance dose of 50 mg daily is given with dramatic improvement in the skin and diarrhoea. Mostly, however, vitamin B complex is given, as other deficiencies are often present.

An increase in the protein content of the diet and treatment of malnutrition and other vitamin deficiencies is essential.

Vitamin B_6

Vitamin B_6 exists as pyridoxine, pyridoxal and pyridoxamine, and is found widely in plant and animal foodstuffs. Pyridoxal phosphate is a co-factor in the metabolism of many amino acids. Dietary deficiency is extremely rare. Some drugs (e.g. isoniazid, hydralazine and penicillamine) interact with pyridoxal phosphate, producing B_6 deficiency. The polyneuropathy occurring after isoniazid usually responds to vitamin B_6. Sideroblastic anaemia occasionally responds to vitamin B_6 (see p. 363). A polyneuropathy has occurred after high doses (> 200 mg) given over many months. Vitamin B_6 is used for pre-menstrual tension: a daily dose of 10 mg should not be exceeded.

Biotin and pantothenic acid

Biotin is involved in a number of carboxylase reactions. It occurs in many foodstuffs and the dietary requirement is small. Deficiency is extremely rare and is confined to a few people who consume raw eggs, which contain an antagonist (avidin) to biotin. It causes a dermatitis that responds to biotin replacements.

Pantothenic acid is widely distributed in all foods and deficiency in humans has not been described.

Vitamin C

Ascorbic acid is a simple sugar and a powerful reducing agent, its main role being to control the redox potential within cells. It is involved in the hydroxylation of proline to hydroxyproline, which is necessary for the formation of collagen. The failure of this biochemical pathway in vitamin C deficiency accounts for virtually all of the clinical effects seen.

Humans, along with a few other animals (e.g. primates and the guinea-pig) are unusual in not being able to synthesize ascorbic acid from glucose.

Vitamin C is present in all fresh fruit and vegetables. Unfortunately, ascorbic acid is easily leached out of vegetables when they are placed in water and it is also oxidized to dehydro-ascorbic acid during cooking, exposure to copper or alkalis. Potatoes are a good source as many people eat a lot of them, but vitamin C is lost during storage.

It has been suggested that ascorbic acid in high dosage (1–2 g daily) will prevent the common cold. While there is some scientific support for this, clinical trials have shown no significant effect. Vitamin C supplements have also been advocated to prevent atherosclerosis and cancer, but again a clear benefit has not been demonstrated.

Vitamin C deficiency is seen mainly in infants fed boiled milk and in the elderly and single people who cannot be bothered to eat vegetables. In the UK it is also seen in Asians eating only rice and chapatis, and in food faddists.

Table 3.11
Clinical features of vitamin C deficiency

Keratosis of hair follicles with 'corkscrew' hair
Perifollicular haemorrhages
Swollen, spongy gums with bleeding and superadded infection, loosening of teeth
Spontaneous bruising
Spontaneous haemorrhage
Anaemia
Failure of wound healing

Scurvy

In adults the early symptoms may be nonspecific, with weakness and muscle pain. Other features are shown in Table 3.11. In infantile scurvy there is irritability, painful legs, anaemia and characteristic subperiosteal haemorrhages, particularly into the ends of long bones.

DIAGNOSIS

The anaemia is usually hypochromic but occasionally a normochromic or megaloblastic anaemia is seen. The type of anaemia depends on whether iron deficiency (owing to decreased absorption or loss due to haemorrhage) or folate deficiency (folate being largely found in green vegetables) is present.

Plasma ascorbic acid is very low in obvious deficiency and a vitamin C level of less than 11 μmol L^{-1} (10.2 mg per 100 mL) indicates vitamin C deficiency. The leucocyte–platelet layer (buffy coat) of centrifuged blood corresponds to vitamin C concentrations in other tissues. The normal level of leucocyte ascorbate is 1.1–2.8 pmol per 10^6 cells.

TREATMENT

Initially the patient is given 250 mg of ascorbic acid daily and encouraged to eat fresh fruit and vegetables. Subsequently, 40 mg daily will maintain a normal exchangeable body pool of about 900 mg (5.1 mmol).

PREVENTION

Orange juice should be given to bottle-fed infants. The intake of breast-fed infants depends on the mother's diet. In the elderly, eating adequate fruit and vegetables is the best way to avoid scurvy. Careful surveillance of the elderly, particularly those who live alone, is necessary. Ascorbic acid supplements should only be necessary occasionally.

Vitamin B_{12} and folate

These are dealt with on p. 364 and daily requirements are shown in Table 3.8. In many developed countries up to 15% of the population have a partial deficiency of 5,10-methylene-tetrahydrofolate reductase, a key folate-metabolizing enzyme. This is due to point mutation and is associated with an increase in neural tube defects and hyper-homocysteinaemia, which may lead to cardiovascular damage. In the USA folic acid fortification of enriched cereals at 1.4 mg per kg grain is being introduced, and other countries may also increase their daily folate requirements.

FURTHER READING

Gerster H (1997) Vitamin A. Functions, dietary requirements and safety in humans. *International Journal of Vitamin and Nutrition Research* **67**: 71–90.

Kusti LH, Folsom AR, Prineas RJ et al. (1996) Dietary antioxidants, vitamins and death from coronary disease in postmenopausal women. *New England Journal of Medicine* **334**: 1156–1162

Jones A (1995) [Series of review articles on vitamins A, D, E and K]. *Lancet* **345**.

Minerals

A number of minerals have been shown to be essential in animals and an increasing number of deficiency syndromes are becoming recognized in humans. Long-term total parenteral nutrition allowed trace-element deficiency to be studied in controlled conditions; now trace elements are always added to long-term parenteral nutrition regimens. It is highly probable (but difficult to study because of multiple deficiencies) that trace-element deficiency is also an important accompaniment of all PEM states. Sodium, potassium, magnesium and chloride are discussed in Chapter 10.

Iron (see also p. 360)

The daily RNI for men is 160 μmol (8.7 mg) and for women 260 μmol (14.8 mg). Iron deficiency is common worldwide, affecting both developing and developed countries. It is particularly prevalent in women of a reproductive age. Dietary iron overload is seen in the South African Bantu men who cook and brew in iron pots.

Copper

The daily RNI of copper is 1.2 mg (19 μmol). Shellfish, legumes, cereals and nuts are good dietary sources.

Deficiency

Menkes' kinky hair syndrome is a rare condition caused by malabsorption of copper. Infants with this sex-linked recessive abnormality develop growth failure, mental retardation, bone lesions and brittle hair. Anaemia and neutropenia also occur. This condition, which serves as a model for copper deficiency, supports the idea that some of the clinical features seen in PEM are due to copper deficiency. Breast and cows' milk are low in copper and supplementation is occasionally necessary when first treating PEM.

Copper toxicity

This occurs in Wilson's disease; see p. 326.

Zinc

The daily RNI of zinc is 9 mg (140 μmol) and it is widely available in food. Zinc is involved in many metabolic pathways, often acting as a co-enzyme; it is essential for the synthesis of RNA and DNA.

Deficiency

Acrodermatitis enteropathica is an inherited disorder caused by malabsorption of zinc. Infants develop growth retardation, severe diarrhoea, hair loss and associated *Candida* and bacterial infections. This condition provides a model for zinc deficiency. Zinc supplementation results in a complete cure. Deficiency probably also plays a role in PEM.

Zinc levels have been shown to be low in some patients with malabsorption or skin disease, and in patients with AIDS, but the exact role of zinc in these situations is disputed. Zinc has low toxicity, but high zinc levels from water stored in galvanized containers interfere with iron and copper metabolism. Wound healing is impaired with moderate zinc deficiency and is improved by zinc supplements.

Iodine

The daily RNI of iodine is 140 μg (1.1 μmol) and it is found in milk, meat and seafoods. It exists in foodstuffs as inorganic iodines which are efficiently absorbed. Iodine is a constituent of the thyroid hormones (p. 930).

Deficiency

Many mountainous areas throughout the world lack iodine in the soil, and so iodine deficiency which impairs brain development is a WHO priority. Endemic goitre occurs in remote areas where the daily intake is below 70 μg, and in those parts 1–5% of babies are born with cretinism. In these areas iodized oil should be given intramuscularly to all reproductive women every 3–5 years. In developed countries, salt is iodized and endemic goitre has disappeared.

Fluoride

In areas where the level of fluoride in drinking water is less than 1 p.p.m. (0.7–1.2 mg L^{-1}), dental caries is relatively more prevalent. Fluoridation of the water provides 1–2 mg daily, resulting in a reduction of about 50% of tooth decay in children. There is little fluoride in food except for seafish and tea, the latter providing 70% of the daily intake. Fluoride-containing toothpaste may add up to 2 mg a day.

Excessive fluoride intake in areas where the water fluoride level is above 3 mg L^{-1} can result in fluorosis, in which there is infiltration into the enamel of the teeth, producing pitting and discoloration.

Selenium

The daily RNI of selenium is 60 μg (0.8 μmol). Selenium is a component of several enzymes, including glutathione peroxidase and superoxide dimutase. These enzymes prevent oxidative and free radical damage to cells. Selenium works in conjunction with vitamin E. Selenium is also involved in the conversion of thyroxine to triiodothyronine.

Deficiency of selenium is rare except in areas of China where Keshan disease, a selenium-responsive cardiomyopathy, occurs. Toxicity has been described with very high intakes.

Calcium (see also p. 503)

The daily RNI of calcium is 700 mg (17.5 mmol). It is found in many foodstuffs, with two-thirds of the intake coming from milk and milk products, only 5% from vegetables. In the UK most flour is fortified. Calcium absorption from the gastrointestinal tract is vitamin D-dependent. Ninety-nine per cent of body calcium is in the skeleton.

Increased calcium is required in pregnancy and lactation, when dietary intake must be increased. Calcium deficiency is usually due to vitamin D deficiency.

Phosphate (see also p. 615)

The daily RNI of phosphate is the same as that of calcium, i.e. 17.5 mmol. Phosphates are present in all natural foods and dietary deficiency has not been described. Patients taking large amounts of aluminium hydroxide can, however, develop phosphate deficiency owing to binding in the gut lumen. It can also be seen in total parenteral nutrition. Symptoms include anorexia, weakness and osteoporosis.

Other trace elements

The possible significance of cadmium, chromium, cobalt, manganese, molybdenum, nickel and vanadium are shown in Table 3.12.

FURTHER READING

Bender DA, Bender AE (1997) Nutrition – a reference handbook. Oxford University Press, Oxford.

Table 3.12
Other trace elements (see text)

Element	Deficiency
Cadmium	?
Chromium	Glucose intolerance
Cobalt	Anaemia
Manganese	Growth retardation, skeletal abnormalities, glucose intolerance
Molybdenum	? Animals only
Nickel	? Animals only
Vanadium	? Nutritional oedema

Nutrition and ageing

Many animal studies have shown that life expectancy can be extended by restricting food intake. It is, however, not known whether the ageing process in humans can be altered by nutrition.

The ageing process

The process of ageing is not well understood. While wear and tear may play a role it is an insufficient explanation for the causation of ageing. A number of theories have been postulated.

- **Programmed ageing theory** suggests a predetermined, presumably genetic, age-related alteration in cellular function that leads to susceptibility to disease and death.
- **Genomic instability theory** suggests errors in genetic transcription and translation, resulting in impaired protein synthesis and deterioration in cell function as age increases.
- **Free radical theory** suggests that these highly reactive molecules are no longer metabolized rapidly; accumulation occurs, leading to irreversible cell damage.
- **Random genetic errors** have also been implicated; an accumulation of errors over time is said to result in impaired protein synthesis and a decrease in cellular function.

Several other mechanisms have been suggested, but it is still unclear whether one universal or several independent mechanisms are involved.

Nutritional requirements in the elderly

These are *qualitatively* similar to the requirements of younger adults, but as energy expenditure is less, there is a lower energy requirement. However, maintaining physical activity is required for the overall health of the elderly.

The daily energy requirement of 'elderly people' (aged 60 and above, irrespective of age) has been set to be approximately 1.5 × BMR. The BMR is reduced, owing to a fall in the fat-free mass, from an average of 60 kg to 50 kg in men and from 40 kg to 35 kg in women. The diet should contain the same *proportions* of nutrients, and essential nutrients are still required.

Nutritional deficits in the elderly may be due to many factors, such as dental problems, lack of cooking skills (particularly in widowers), depression and lack of motivation. Significant malnourishment in developed countries is usually secondary to social problems or disease. In the elderly who are institutionalized, vitamin D supplements may be required because often these people do not go into the sunlight.

Owing to the high prevalence of osteoporosis in elderly people, daily calcium intake should be 1–1.5 g.

FURTHER READING

American Journal of Clinical Nutrition (1997) Special issue on aging and nutrition. 66 (4)

Obesity

Obesity is almost invariable in the West, and almost all people develop some obesity as they get older. Obesity implies an excess storage of fat, and this can most easily be detected by looking at the undressed patient.

Most patients suffer from *simple obesity,* but in certain conditions obesity is an associated feature (Table 3.13). Even in the latter situation, the intake of calories must be exceeding expenditure. Hormonal imbalance is often incriminated in women (e.g. postmenopause or when taking contraceptive pills), but most weight gain in such cases is usually small and due to water retention.

Simple obesity

Not all obese people eat more than the average person, but all obviously eat more than they need.

Table 3.13
Conditions in which obesity is an associated feature

Genetic syndromes associated with hypogonadism (e.g. Prader–Willi syndrome, Laurence–Moon–Biedl syndrome)
Hypothyroidism
Cushing's syndrome
Stein–Leventhal syndrome
Drug-induced (e.g. corticosteroids)
Hypothalmic damage (e.g. due to trauma, tumour)

Suggested mechanisms

Genetic and environmental factors

These have always been difficult to separate when studying obesity. However, refeeding experiments in both monozygotic and dizygotic twins, reared together or apart, suggest that genetic influences account for 70% of the difference in body mass index (BMI) later in life, and that the childhood environment has little or no influence.

The refeeding experiments also showed that weight gain did not occur in all pairs of twins, suggesting that in some a facultative increase in thermogenesis occurred so that part of their extra dietary energy was expended inefficiently. Genetic factors have led to the discovery of a putative gene, firstly in the obese (*ob ob*), mouse and now in humans. The *ob* gene was shown to be expressed solely in both white and brown adipose tissue. The *ob* gene is found on chromsone 7 and produces a 16 kDa protein called leptin. In the *ob ob* mouse a mutation in the *ob* gene leads to production of a non-functioning protein. Administration of normal leptin to these obese mice reduces food intake and corrects the obesity.

In massively obese subjects, leptin mRNA in subcutaneous adipose tissue is 80% higher than in controls. Plasma levels of leptin are also very high, correlating with the BMI. Weight loss due to food restriction decreases plasma levels of leptin. In contrast to the *ob ob* mouse the leptin structure is normal and abnormalities in leptin are not the prime cause of human obesity.

Leptin secreted from fat cells could act as a feedback mechanism between the adipose tissue and the brain, acting as a 'lipostat' (adipostat), controlling fat stores by regulating hunger and satiety (see below).

Food intake

Many factors related to the home environment, such as finance and the availability of sweets and snacks, will affect food intake. Some patients eat more during periods of heavy exercise or during pregnancy and are unable to get back to their former eating habits. The increase in obesity in social class 5 can usually be related to the type of food consumed (i.e. food containing sugar and fat). Psychological factors and how food is presented may override complex biochemical interactions.

It has been shown that obese patients eat more than they admit to eating, and over the years a very small daily excess can lead to a large accumulation of fat. For example, a 44 kJ (10.5 kcal) excess would lead to a 10 kg weight gain over 20 years.

Control of appetite

This is complex and depends partly on external stimuli, such as the company, the type of food, the surroundings and the person's habitual behaviour.

Appetite is the desire to eat and this usually initiates food intake. Following a meal, satiation occurs. This depends on gastric and duodenal distension and the release of many substances peripherally and centrally.

Following a meal, cholecystokinin (CCK), bombesin and somatostatin are released from the small intestine and glucagon and insulin from the pancreas. All of these hormones have been implicated in the control of satiety. Centrally, the hypothalamus – particularly the paraventricular nucleus and the ventromedial wall – is thought to be the main satiety centre. Numerous neurotransmitters (e.g. CCK, opioids, serotonin, corticotrophin-releasing hormone and particularly neuropeptide Y) have a role in the central control of satiation.

A leptin receptor has been found in the ventromedial nucleus of the hypothalamus and it is possible that changes in this receptor impair the effect of leptin. This would lead to a decrease in the release of transmitters such as neuropeptide Y, so that appetite would not be suppressed, interfering with the feedback mechanism (Fig 3.7). Recent experimental evidence suggests that leptin inhibits release of neuropeptide Y which is known to be the most potent peptide to stimulate feeding. The leptin feedback is complex and many other genes are likely to be involved.

Energy expenditure

Obese patients tend to expend more energy during physical activity as they have a larger mass to move. On the other hand, many obese patients decrease their amount of physical activity. The energy expended on walking at 3 miles per hour is only 15.5 kJ min^{-1} (3.7 kcal min^{-1}) and therefore increasing exercise plays only a small part in losing weight. Nevertheless, because increased body fat develops insidiously over many years, any discrepancy in energy balance is important.

Thermogenesis

Brown adipose tissue in animals, when stimulated by cold or food, dissipates in the form of heat the energy derived from ingested food. This can be a major component of overall energy balance and it has been suggested that this may also apply to humans.

β_3-Adrenergic receptors are the principal receptors mediating catecholamine-stimulated lipolysis in brown and white fat tissue. After a meal or exposure to cold, relatively high concentrations of noradrenaline are released, stimulating the low-affinity receptors in brown adipose tissue. Low β_3-adrenergic receptor activity would decrease thermogenesis, and this can explain why most obese patients require a very low calorie intake to maintain any weight loss, and gain weight easily after only small calorie increases. Decreased function of the receptors in white adipose tissue could slow lipolysis, causing retention of lipid in fat cells. As β_3-receptors are more frequent in visceral adipose tissue, this would explain the regional distribution of fat in obese subjects.

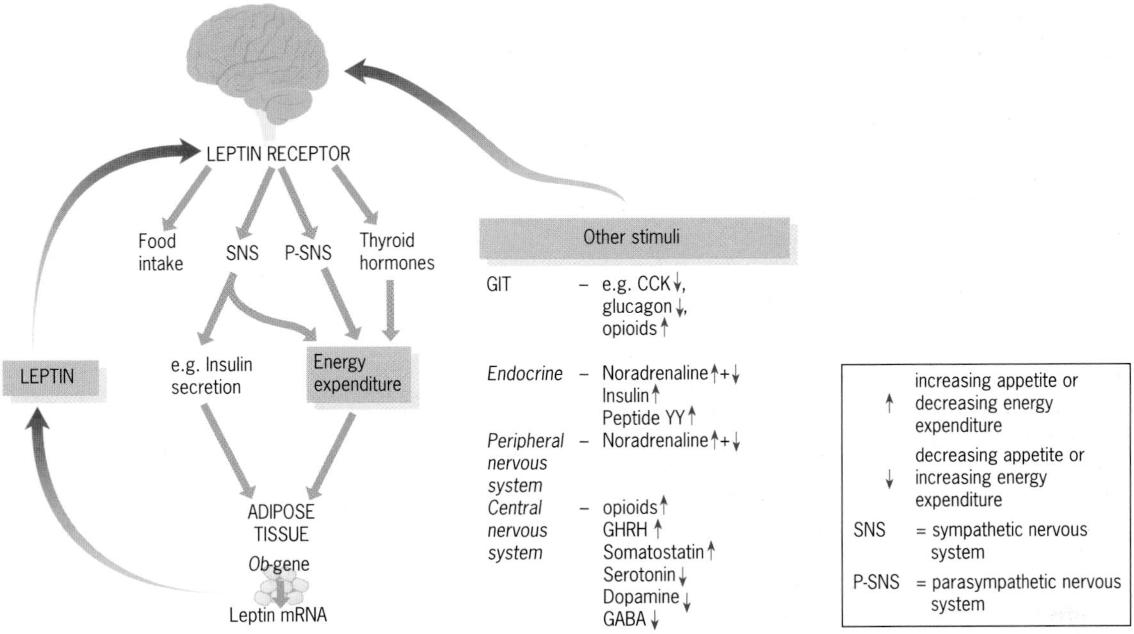

Fig 3.7
Shows the proposed feedback loop between peripheral adipose tissue and central feeding pathways.
Peripheral and central factors (listed under 'other stimuli') influence food intake; some may interact with leptin

Morbidity and mortality

Obese patients are at risk of early death, mainly from diabetes, coronary heart disease and cerebrovascular disease. The greater the obesity the higher the morbidity and mortality rates. For example, men who are 10% overweight have a 13% increased risk of death, while the increase in mortality for those 20% overweight is 25%. The rise is less in women and in men over 65 obesity is not an independent risk factor. Weight reduction reduces this mortality and therefore should be strongly encouraged.

CLINICAL FEATURES

Most patients recognize their own problems, although often they are unaware of the main foods that cause obesity. Many symptoms are related to psychological problems or social pressures, such as the woman who cannot find fashionable clothes to wear.

The degree of obesity can be assessed by comparison with tables of ideal weight for height (see Appendices), from the BMI (Information box 3.4), and by measuring skinfold thickness. The latter should be measured over the middle of the triceps muscle; normal values are 20 mm in a man and 30 mm in a woman. A central distribution of body fat (a waist/hip circumference ratio of >1.0 in men and >0.9 in women) is associated with a higher risk of morbidity and mortality than is a more peripheral distribution of body fat (waist/hip ratio <0.85 in men and <0.75 in women).

Table 3.14 shows the conditions and complications that are associated with obesity. The relationship between cardiovascular disease (hypertension or ischaemic heart disease), hyperlipidaemia, smoking, physical exercise and obesity is complex. Difficulties arise in interpreting mortality figures because of the number of factors involved. Many studies of obesity do not, for instance, differentiate between smokers and non-smokers or between the types of physical exercise taken. Many do not take into account the cuff-size artefact in the measurement of blood pressure (an artefact will occur if a large cuff is not used in patients with a large arm). Nevertheless, obesity almost certainly plays a part in all of these diseases and should be treated. The only exception is that stopping smoking, even if accompanied by weight gain, is more important than any of the other factors.

i Information

	Men	Women
Acceptable BMI range	20.1–25.0	18.7–23.8
Obesity	30+	28.6+

Information box 3.4 Body mass index values for men and women

Table 3.14
Conditions and complications associated with obesity

Psychological	Hypertension
Osteoarthritis of knees and hips	Breathlessness
Varicose veins	Ischaemic heart disease
Hiatus hernia	Stroke
Gallstones	Diabetes mellitus (NIDDM)
Postoperative problems	Hyperlipidaemia
Back strain	Menstrual abnormalities
Accident proneness	Increased morbidity and mortality

TREATMENT

Dietary control

This largely depends on a reduction in calorie intake. The most common diets allow a daily intake of approximately 4200 kJ (1000 kcal), although this may need to be nearer 6300 kJ (1500 kcal) for someone engaged in physical work. A diet that is too low in total calories will usually result in the patient cheating and keeping to the diet only for short periods. Patients must realize that prolonged dieting is necessary for large amounts of fat to be lost. Furthermore, a permanent change in eating habits is required to maintain the new low weight. It is relatively easy for most people to lose the first few kilograms, but long-term success in moderate obesity is poor, with an overall success rate of no more than 10%.

The aim of any dietary regimen is to lose approximately 1 kg per week. Weight loss will be greater initially owing to accompanying protein and glycogen breakdown and consequent water loss. After 3–4 weeks, incremental weight loss may be very small because only adipose tissue is broken down and there is no accompanying water loss.

Patients must understand the principles of energy intake and expenditure, and the best results are obtained in educated, well-motivated patients. Constant supervision by a doctor, by close relatives or through membership of a slimming club helps to encourage compliance.

An increase in exercise will increase energy expenditure and should be encouraged – provided there is no contra-indication – since weight control is usually not achieved without exercise. Weight cannot be lost by exercise alone, because even a 15-minute brisk daily walk will use less energy than is contained in a small slice of bread and butter. Regular exercise, however, will improve general health and often enables patients to control their diet.

The diet should contain adequate amounts of each nutrient. A diet of 4200 kJ (1000 kcal) per day should be made up of approximately 100 g of carbohydrate, 50 g of protein and 40 g of fat. The carbohydrate should be in the form of complex carbohydrates such as vegetables and fruit rather than simple sugars. Alcohol contains 29 kJ g^{-1} (7 kcal g^{-1}) and should be discouraged. It can be substituted for other foods in the diet, but it often reduces the willpower. With a varied diet, vitamins and minerals will be adequate and supplements are not necessary. A balanced diet, attractively presented, is of much greater value and safer than any of the slimming regimens often advertised in magazines.

Most obese people oscillate in weight; they often regain the lost weight, but many manage to lose weight again. This 'cycling' in bodyweight may play a role in the development of coronary artery disease.

Drug therapy

Drugs can be used in the short term (up to three months) as an adjunct to the dietary regimen, but they do not substitute for strict dieting. Fenfluramine, which acts through the serotinergic system in the brain, has frequent side effects. It has been associated with the development, albeit rarely, of primary pulmonary hypertension and valvular heart disease and, in the UK, along with dexfenfluramine, has now been withdrawn.

Surgical treatment

Operations that involve bypassing parts of the small intestine have fallen out of favour because of their side-effects and cannot be recommended. Jejunoileal bypass was the most common operation and involved the anastomosis of approximately 18 cm of jejunum to the terminal 18 cm of the ileum. Complications are chiefly those of intestinal resection (p. 257). A fatty liver often occurs and in a few patients cirrhosis is seen.

Three procedures are still performed in cases of severe morbid obesity:

- *Wiring the jaws to prevent eating*. This permits liquid feeds only. It can be used as a temporary measure but good dental hygiene is essential. Weight gain usually occurs after the wires have been removed, but this can be controlled by the use of a tight waist cord.
- *Gastric plication*. A small gastric pouch is created by stapling across the wall of the stomach. Good results have been claimed without the side-effects of bypass operations.
- *Gastric balloon*. A balloon is placed endoscopically inside the stomach and inflated. Its value has been over-exaggerated and complications include intestinal obstruction.

PREVENTION

Preventing obesity must always be the goal because most obese people find it difficult to maintain any weight loss they have managed to achieve. All health professionals must be aware of the dangers of obesity and encourage children, young as well as older adults, from gaining too much weight. A small gain each year over a long period produces an obese individual for whom treatment is difficult.

FURTHER READING

Rosenbaum M, Leibel RL, Hirsch J (1997) Medical progress: obesity. *New England Journal of Medicine* **337**: 396–407.

Scott J (1996) New chapter for the fat controller. *Nature* **379**: 113–114

Nutritional support in the hospital patient

Nutritional support is recognized as being necessary in many hospitalized patients. The pathophysiology and hallmarks of malnutrition have been described earlier (p. 195); here the forms of nutritional support that are available are discussed.

Principles

Some form of nutritional supplementation is required in those patients who cannot eat, should not eat, will not eat or cannot eat enough. It is necessary to provide nutritional support for:

- all severely malnourished patients on admission to hospital
- moderately malnourished patients who, because of their physical illness, are not expected to eat for 3–5 days
- normally nourished patients not expected to eat for 7–10 days.

Enteral rather than parenteral nutrition should always be used if the gastrointestinal tract is functioning normally.

Enteral nutrition (EN) (Practical box 3.1)

Feeds can be given by various routes:

- By *mouth*
- By *fine-bore nasogastric tube*
- *Percutaneous endoscopic gastrostomy* (PEG) is useful for patients who need enteral nutrition for a prolonged period (e.g. more than 30 days), such as with swallowing problems following a head injury or in elderly people after a stroke. A catheter is placed percutaneously into the stomach under endoscopic control.
- *With needle catheter jejunostomy*, a fine catheter is inserted into the jejunum at laparotomy and brought out through the abdominal wall.

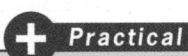

Practical

Procedure

- Insert fine-bore tube intranasally with wire stylet.
- Confirm position of tube in stomach by aspiration of gastric contents and auscultation of the epigastrium.
- Check by X-ray if aspiration or auscultation is unsuccessful.

Problems

No satisfactory way of keeping nasogastric tubes in place (up to 60% come out).

Main complications

- Regurgitation and aspiration into bronchus
- Blockage of the nasogastric tube
- Gastrointestinal side-effects, the most common being diarrhoea
- Metabolic complications including hyperglycaemia and hyperkalaemia, as well as low levels of potassium, magnesium, calcium and phosphate.

Practical box 3.1 Enteral feeding

Diet formulation (see Table 3.15)

A polymeric diet with whole-protein and fat can be used, except in patients with severely impaired gastrointestinal function who may require a predigested (i.e. elemental) diet. In these patients, the nitrogen source is purified low-molecular-weight peptides or amino acid mixtures, with sometimes the fat being given partly as medium-chain triglycerides.

MANAGEMENT

The aim of any regimen is to achieve a positive nitrogen balance, which can usually be obtained by giving 3–5 g of nitrogen in excess of output. Nitrogen loss can be calculated using the formula:

$$N_2 \text{ loss (g per 24 hours)} = \text{Urinary urea (mmol per 24 hours)} \times 0.028 + 2$$

(the 2 representing non-urinary nitrogen excretion).

Daily amounts of diet vary between 2 and 2.5 L and the full amount can be started immediately.

Hypercatabolic patients require a high supply of nitrogen (15 g daily) and often will not achieve positive nitrogen balance until the primary injury is resolved.

The success of enteral feeding depends on careful supervision of the patient with monitoring of weight, biochemistry and diet charts.

Total parenteral nutrition (TPN)

Peripheral parenteral nutrition

Specially formulated mixtures for peripheral use are available, with a low osmolality and containing lipid emulsions. Heparin and corticosteroids are added to the infusion and local application of glyceryl trinitrate patches reduces the occurrence of thrombophlebitis and prolongs catheter life. Initially, peripheral parenteral nutrition is preferred (each catheter will last for about 5 days), allowing time to consider the necessity for having to insert a central venous catheter.

Table 3.15 Standard enteric diet, providing 12 000 kJ per day (2000–3000 kcal)

Energy
Carbohydrate as glucose polymers (49–53% of total energy)
Fat as triglycerides (30–35% of total energy)

Nitrogen
Whole protein (6–7 g of nitrogen L^{-1})

Additional electrolytes, vitamins and trace elements

Features
Ratio of energy to nitrogen kJ:g = 620:1 (kcal:g = 150:1)
Osmolality = 285–300 mOsmol kg^{-1}

Parenteral nutrition via a central venous catheter (see Practical box 3.2)

A silicone catheter is placed into a central vein, usually using the infraclavicular approach to the subclavian vein. The skin-entry site should be dressed carefully and not disturbed unless there is a suggestion of catheter-related sepsis.

Complications of catheter placement include central vein thrombosis, pneumothorax and embolism, but the major problem is catheter-related sepsis. Organisms, mainly staphylococci, enter along the side of the catheter, leading to septicaemia. Sepsis can be prevented by careful and sterile placement of the catheter, by not removing the dressing over the catheter entry site, and by not giving other substances (e.g. blood products, antibiotics) via the central vein catheter.

Sepsis should be suspected if the patient develops fever and leucocytosis. In two-thirds of cases, organisms can be grown from the catheter tip. Treatment involves removal of the catheter and appropriate systemic antibiotics.

Nutrients

With TPN it is possible to provide sufficient nitrogen for protein synthesis and calories to meet energy requirements. Electrolytes, vitamins and trace elements are also necessary. All of these substances are infused simultaneously.

Nitrogen source

Synthetic L-amino acid solutions are used, which contain between 9 g L^{-1} and 17 g L^{-1} of nitrogen. Most patients require at least 14 g of nitrogen per day.

Energy source

This is mainly provided by glucose, with additional calories provided by a fat emulsion. Fat infusions provide a greater number of calories in a smaller volume than can be provided by carbohydrate. Fat infusions are not hypertonic and they also prevent essential fatty acid deficiency.

Table 3.16 Daily dietary electrolytes and trace elements required for long-term maintenance

Na^+	70–220 mmol	Fe^{3+}	70 μmol
K^+	60–120 mmol	Cu^{2+}	20 μmol
Mg^{2+}	5–20 mmol	Cl^-	70–220 μmol
Ca^{2+}	15–25 mmol	PO_4^{3-}	15–25 mmol
Zn^{2+}	50–100 μmol	F^-	50 μmol
Mn^{2+}	120 μmol	I^-	1 μmol

Essential fatty acid deficiency has been reported in long-term parenteral nutritional regimens without fat emulsions. It causes a scaly skin, hair loss and a delay in healing.

The calorie-to-nitrogen ratio (kcal:g) should be approximately 0.62 MJ per gram of protein (150:1).

Electrolytes and trace elements (see Table 3.16)

The electrolyte status should be monitored on a daily basis and electrolyte solutions given as appropriate. Water-soluble vitamins can be given daily but fat-soluble vitamins should be given weekly, as overdose can occur. A trace-metal solution is available for patients on long-term parenteral nutrition, but if the patient requires blood transfusions trace-metal supplements are not needed.

Administration and monitoring

Peripheral parenteral nutrition is administered via 3 L bags over 24 hours, with the constituents being premixed under sterile conditions by the pharmacy. Table 3.17 shows the composition which provides 9 g of nitrogen and 1700 non-protein calories in 24 hours.

For a central venous TPN regimen, most hospitals now use premixed 3 L bags. A standard parenteral nutrition regimen which provides 14 g of nitrogen and 2250 non-protein calories over 24 hours is given in Table 3.17.

Essential monitoring includes daily plasma electrolytes and weekly assessments of nutritional status (weight and skinfold thickness). Nitrogen balance should also be

Practical

This should be performed only by experienced clinicians under aseptic conditions in an operating theatre.

- The patient is placed supine with 5° of head-down tilt to avoid air embolism.
- The skin below the midpoint of the left clavicle is infiltrated with 1–2% lignocaine and a 1 cm skin incision is made.
- A 20-gauge needle on a syringe is inserted beneath the clavicle and first rib and angled towards the tip of finger held in the suprasternal notch.
- When blood is aspirated freely, the needle is used as a guide to insert the cannula through the skin incision and into the subclavian vein.
- The catheter is advanced so that its tip lies in the distal part of the superior vena cava.
- A skin tunnel is created under local anaesthetic using an introducer inserted through a point about 10 cm below and medial to the incision and passed upwards to the incision.
- The proximal end of the catheter (with hub removed) is passed backwards through the introducer to emerge 10 cm below the clavicle, where it is sutured to the chest wall.
- The original infraclavicular entry incision is now sutured.

Practical box 3.2 Central catheter placement for parenteral nutrition

Table 3.17
Examples of total parenteral nutrition regimens

Central: all mixed in 3 L bags and infused over 24 hours		
Nitrogen	L-Amino acids 14 g L^{-1}	1 L
Energy	Glucose 50%	0.5 L
	Glucose 20%	0.5 L
	plus	
	Lipid 10%	0.5 L
	as either Intralipid	Fractionated soya oil 100 g L^{-1}
	or Lipofundin	Soya oil 50 g, medium-chain triglycerides 50 g L^{-1}
	+ Electrolytes, water-soluble vitamins, fat-soluble vitamins, trace elements, heparin and insulin may be added if required. Nitrogen 14 g non-protein calories 9305 kJ (2250 kcal)	
Peripheral: all mixed in 3 L bags and infused over 24 hours		
Nitrogen	L-Amino acids 9 g L^{-1}	1 L
Energy	Glucose 20%	1 L
	Lipid 20%	0.5 L
	+ Trace elements, electrolytes, and water-soluble and fat-soluble vitamins. Heparin 1000 UL and hydrocortisone 100 mg. Insulin is added if required. Nitrogen 9 g non-protein calories 7206 kJ (1700 Kcal)	

measured on a weekly basis. Home parenteral nutrition is occasionally required for patients with virtually no small bowel.

Complications

- Catheter-related (see above)
- Metabolic (e.g. hyperglycaemia – insulin therapy is usually necessary)
- Electrolyte disturbances
- Hypercalcaemia
- Liver dysfunction.

FURTHER READING

Payne-James JJ, Grimble G, Silk D (1998) Artificial nutrition support in clinical practice. Greenwich Medical Media Ltd.

Sauba WW (1997) Nutritional support. *New England Journal of Medicine* **336**: 41–48.

Food allergy and food intolerance

Many people ascribe their various symptoms to food allergy or food sensitivity, and there are a number of clinics in the UK where such sufferers are seen and started on exclusion diets. The scientific evidence that food does harm in most instances is incomplete, but certainly some evidence supports the following disease 'entities':

- *Acute hypersensitivity*. Some patients develop acute reactions to a particular food; an example is urticaria, vomiting or diarrhoea after eating strawberries or shellfish. These reactions are presumably immunological hypersensitivity reactions mediated by IgE. This is usually not a clinical problem as the patients have already learned to avoid the suspected food.
- *Eczema and asthma*. Particularly in children, these have sometimes been treated successfully by removal of eggs from the diet, suggesting some form of food allergy.
- *Rhinitis and asthma*. These have been produced by foods such as milk and chocolate, mainly in atopic subjects, again suggesting a food allergy.
- *Chronic urticaria*. This has been treated successfully by an exclusion diet.
- *Migraine*. In some subjects this seems to follow the intake of foods such as chocolate, cheese and alcohol, suggesting a trigger mechanism, although probably not a true allergic phenomenon.

In addition, some people suffer a reaction due to:

- a constituent of food (e.g. the histamine in mackerel or canned food, or the tyramine in cheeses)
- chemical mediators released by food (e.g. histamine may be released by tomatoes or strawberries)
- toxic chemicals found in food (e.g. the food additive tartrazine)
- an enzyme deficiency (e.g. milk-induced diarrhoea in alactasia or fava-bean-induced haemolytic anaemia in glucose-6-phosphate dehydrogenase deficiency).

Many other additives and compounds with certain E numbers have been implicated as causing reactions, but here the evidence is less than complete.

There is little or no evidence to suggest that diseases such as arthritis, behaviour and affective disorders, irritable bowel syndrome and Crohn's disease are due to ingestion of a particular food.

Multiple vague symptoms such as tiredness or malaise are also not due to food allergy. Most of the patients in this group are suffering from a psychiatric disorder.

MANAGEMENT

- **A careful history** may help to delineate the causative agent, particularly when the effects are immediate.
- **Skin-prick testing** with allergen and measurement in the serum of antigen or antibodies have not correlated with symptoms and are usually misleading. 'Fringe' techniques such as hair analysis, although widely advertised, are valueless and possibly fraudulent.
- **Diagnostic exclusion diets** are sometimes used, but they are time-consuming. They can occasionally be of value in identifying a particular food causing problems.
- **Dietary challenge** consists of the food and the test being given sublingually or by inhalation in an attempt to reproduce the symptoms. Again this may be helpful in a few cases.

Most people who have acute reactions to food realize it and stop the food, and do not require medical attention. In the remainder of patients, a small minority seem to be helped by modifying their diet, but there is no good scientific evidence to support these exclusion diets.

FURTHER READING

Sampson HA (1997) Food allergies. In: Sleisenger and Fordtrans Gastrointestinal and Liver Disease. WB Saunders, Philadelphia

Information

- Alcohol dehydrogenase:

$$\underset{\text{(ethanol)}}{CH_3CH_2OH} + NAD^+ \xrightarrow{\text{(ADH)}\ CH_3CHO} \text{(acetaldehyde)} + NADH + H^+$$

- The liver microsomal enzyme oxidizing system (MEOS) including the specific p450 enzyme, p450 11E1, which is induced by ethanol.

$$CH_3CH_2OH + NADPH + H^+ + O_2 \xrightarrow{\text{MEOS}} CH_3CHO + NADP + 2H_2O$$

Information box 3.5 The main pathways of ethanol oxidization

Alcohol

Alcohol is a popular 'nutrient' consumed in large quantities all over the world. In many countries, alcohol consumption is becoming a major problem (see p. 1135).

Ethanol (ethyl alcohol) is oxidized, in the steps shown in Information box 3.5, to acetaldehyde. Acetaldehyde is then converted to acetate, mainly in the liver mitochondria. Acetate is released into the blood and oxidized by peripheral tissues to carbon dioxide, fatty acids and water.

Alcohol dehydrogenases are found in many tissues and it has been suggested that enzymes present in the gastric mucosa may contribute substantially to ethanol metabolism.

Ethanol itself produces 29.3 kJ g^{-1} (7 kcal g^{-1}), but many alcoholic drinks also contain sugar, which increases their calorific value. For example, one pint of beer provides 1045 kJ (250 kcal), so the heavy drinker will be unable to lose weight if he or she continues to drink.

Effects of excess alcohol consumption

Excess consumption of alcohol leads to two major problems, both of which can be present in the same patient:

- alcohol dependence syndrome (p. 1137)
- physical damage to various tissues.

Each unit of alcohol (defined as one half pint of normal beer, one single spirit, or one small glass of wine) contains 8 g of ethanol (Fig 3.8). All the *long-term* effects of excess alcohol consumption are due to excess ethanol, irrespective of the type of alcoholic beverage; i.e. beer and spirits are no different in their long-term effects. *Short-term* effects, such as hangovers, depend on additional substances, particularly other alcohols such as isoamyl alcohol, which are known as congeners. Brandy and bourbon contain the highest percentage of congeners.

The amount of alcohol that produces damage varies and not everyone who drinks heavily will suffer physical damage. For example, only 20% of people who drink heavily develop cirrhosis of the liver. The effect of alcohol on different organs of the body is not the same; in some patients the liver is affected, in others the brain or muscle. The differences may be genetically determined. Susceptibility to damage of different organs is variable and the figures in Information box 3.6 are given only as a guide. Heavy *persistent* drinkers for many years are at greater risk than heavy *sporadic* drinkers.

Liver disease

In general the effects of a given intake of alcohol seem to be worse in women. The following figures are for men and should be reduced by 50% for women:

- 160 g ethanol per day (20 single drinks) carries a high risk
- 80 g ethanol per day (10 single drinks) carries a medium risk
- 40 g ethanol per day (five single drinks) carries little risk.

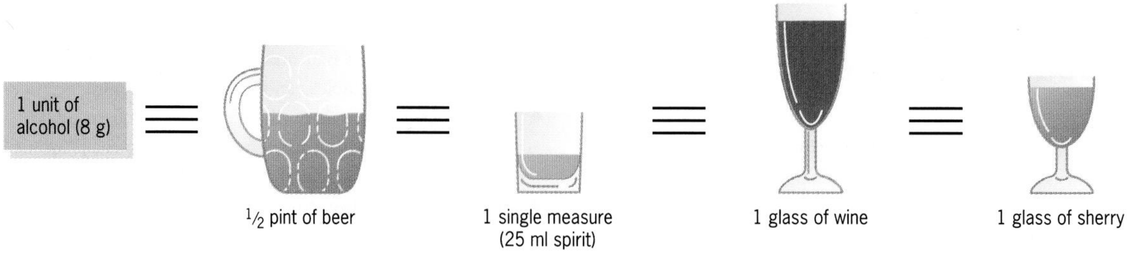

Fig 3.8
Measures of one unit of alcohol

Alcohol consumption in pregnancy

Women are advised not to drink alcohol at all during pregnancy because even small amounts of alcohol consumed can lead to 'small babies'. The fetal alcohol syndrome is characterized by mental retardation, dysmorphic features and growth impairment; it occurs in fetuses of alcohol-dependent women.

i Information

Daily maximum
3 units for men

2 units for women

To help achieve this
Use a standard measure.

Do not drink during the daytime.

Have alcohol-free days each week.

Remember
Health can be damaged without being 'drunk'.

Regular heavy intake is more harmful than occasional binges.

Do not drink to 'drown your problems'.

In the UK the drink-before-driving limit of alcohol in the blood is 800 mg L^{-1} (80 mg%).

One unit of alcohol is eliminated per hour, therefore spread drinking time.

Food decreases absorption and therefore results in a lower blood alcohol level.

4–5 units are sufficient to put the blood alcohol level over the legal driving limit in a 70 kg man (less in a lighter person.

Information box 3.6 Guide to sensible drinking of alcohol

Summary

A summary of the physical effects of alcohol is given in Table 3.18. Details of these diseases are discussed in the relevant chapters. The effects of alcohol withdrawal are discussed on p. 1138.

FURTHER READING

Lieber CS (1995) Medical disorders of alcoholism. *New England Journal of Medicine* **333**: 1058–1063.

Table 3.18
Physical effects of excess alcohol consumption

Central nervous system Epilepsy Wernicke–Korsakoff syndrome Polyneuropathy	**Respiratory system** Chest infections
Muscles Acute or chronic myopathy	**Gastrointestinal system** Acute gastritis Carcinoma of the oesophagus or large bowel Pancreatic disease Liver disease
Cardiovascular system Cardiomyopathy Beriberi heart disease Cardiac arrhythmias Hypertension	**Haemopoiesis** Macrocytosis (due to direct toxic effect on bone marrow or folate deficiency) Thrombocytopenia Leucopenia
Metabolism Hyperuricaemia (gout) Hyperlipidaemia Hypoglycaemia Obesity	**Bone** Osteoporosis Osteomalacia
Endocrine system Pseudo-Cushing's syndrome	

Gastroenterology

4

Gastrointestinal (GI) disease is a major cause of ill-health worldwide. In developing countries infection and malnutrition are common; for example, over a billion people are infested with roundworms and hookworms, and amoebiasis affects over 10% of the world's population. Poor hygiene and malnutrition allow the spread of infective organisms, and many infections could be prevented by improved sanitation and education.

In developed countries, much of the workload is due to non-organic disorders, which are also becoming a worldwide problem. In primary care and in outpatient clinics, patients with dyspepsia and the irritable bowel syndrome are very common. Nevertheless approximately 20% of all cancers occur in the gastrointestinal tract (Fig 4.1). In this chapter, the anatomy and physiology will be discussed in the relevant sections.

A brief summary of symptoms

Dysphagia

Dysphagia is difficulty in swallowing.

Heartburn

Heartburn is a retrosternal or epigastric burning sensation that spreads upwards to the throat. This is a common symptom of reflux and is often trivial.

Dyspepsia and indigestion

These are terms often used by lay people to describe any symptom (e.g. nausea, heartburn, acidity, pain or distension) that occurs as a result of eating or drinking.

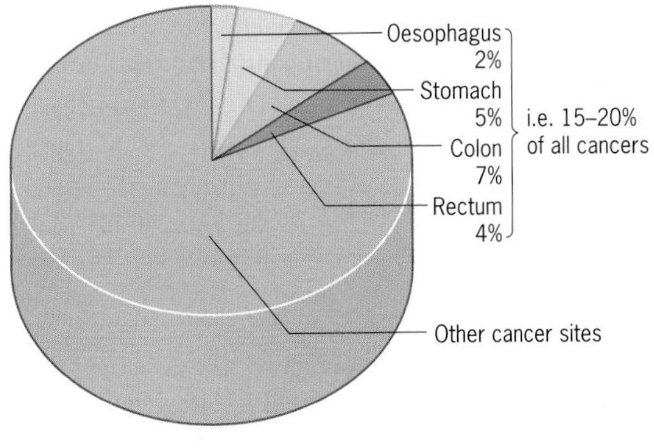

Fig 4.1
Incidence (approximate) of cancers at various sites of the gastrointestinal tract

They may also be used to describe an inability to digest food. Careful questioning is required to elicit the exact nature of the patient's complaint.

'Indigestion' is common; 80% of the general population will have had indigestion at some time.

Flatulence

Flatulence is the term used to describe excessive wind. It indicates belching, abdominal distension (see below) or the passage of flatus per rectum. Excessive belching is not usually associated with organic disease and is a common functional disorder. It is due to air swallowing (aerophagy), which many people do subconsciously. Some of the swallowed air is passed into the intestines, where most is absorbed. Intestinal bacterial breakdown of food, particularly high-fibre legumes, also produces a small amount of gas. Flatus consists of nitrogen, carbon dioxide, hydrogen and methane. On average, flatus is passed 10 to 20 times per day.

Halitosis

Halitosis (bad breath) can be due to poor oral hygiene. Anxious patients can complain of halitosis when it is often more imaginary than real. Very rarely, it can be due to oesophageal stasis (e.g. strictures), achalasia or pulmonary sepsis.

Hiccups

Hiccups are due to involuntary diaphragmatic contractions with closure of the glottis and are extremely common. Occasionally, patients present with persistent hiccups. This can be a result of diaphragmatic irritation (e.g. subphrenic abscess), or a metabolic cause (e.g. uraemia). Treatment for persistent hiccups may be effective with chlorpromazine 50 mg three times daily, or diazepam 5 mg three times daily. The cause should be treated, if known.

Vomiting

Vomiting is the forceful ejection of gastric contents through the mouth. There are three phases:

- nausea – a feeling of wanting to vomit often associated with autonomic effects including hypersalivation, pallor and sweating
- retching – a strong involuntary effort to vomit
- vomiting – the expulsion of gastric contents through the mouth.

The vomiting centres are located in the lateral reticular formation of the medulla and are stimulated by the chemoreceptor trigger zones (CTZs) in the floor of the fourth ventricle, and also by vagal afferents from the gut. The zones are directly stimulated by drugs, motion sickness and metabolic causes.

Many gastrointestinal conditions are associated with vomiting (Table 4.1), but nausea and vomiting without pain are frequently non-gastrointestinal in origin. Haematemesis is vomiting blood or coffee-grounds from the stomach. Large volumes of vomit suggest intestinal obstruction, and faeculent vomit suggests low intestinal obstruction from a gastrocolic fistula. Projectile vomiting is associated with pyloric stenosis.

Chronic nausea and vomiting with no other abdominal symptoms usually have psychological causes. Early-morning vomiting is seen in pregnancy, alcohol dependence and some metabolic disorders (e.g. uraemia).

Constipation

Constipation is difficult to define in terms of frequency of bowel action because there is considerable individual and geographical variation. Patients usually consider themselves constipated if their bowels are not opened on most days. The difficult passage of hard stools is also regarded as constipation, irrespective of stool frequency.

In the UK the normal daily stool weight is only 50–300 g. In developing countries with a high fibre intake, stool weight is 500 g or more with bowel actions two to three times per day.

Diarrhoea

Diarrhoea is extremely common, and a single episode is usually due to dietary indiscretion. A patient may define diarrhoea as either loose stools or an increased frequency. True diarrhoea implies the passing of increased amounts (> 300 g per 24 h) of loose stool. This is different from the frequent passage of small amounts of stool, which is not true diarrhoea and is seen commonly in functional bowel disease. The consistency of the stools is important; watery stools of large volume are always due to an organic cause. Bloody diarrhoea usually implies colonic disease.

Diarrhoea can be either acute or chronic. If it is acute, infective causes must be looked for.

Steatorrhoea

Steatorrhoea is the passage of pale, bulky offensive stools that contain fat, sometimes float in the lavatory pan and are difficult to flush away. These stools float because of the increased air content. Normally people with steatorrhoea complain of diarrhoea, but occasionally they may pass only one motion per day.

Table 4.1
Causes of vomiting

Any gastrointestinal disease	Drugs, e.g.
Acute infections, e.g.	digitalis toxicity
influenza	opiates
pertussis	cytotoxics
Central nervous disease, e.g.	Reflex, e.g.
raised intracranial pressure	severe pain: myocardial infarction
meningitis	Psychogenesis
vestibular disturbances	Pregnancy
migraine	Alcohol excess
Metabolic causes, e.g.	
uraemia	
diabetes: ketoacidosis or gastroparesis	
hypercalcaemia	

Abdominal pain

Pain is stimulated mainly by the stretching of smooth muscle or organ capsules. Severe acute abdominal pain can be due to a large number of gastrointestinal conditions, and normally presents as an emergency. An 'acute abdomen' can occasionally be due to referred pain from the chest, as in pneumonia, or to metabolic causes, such as diabetic ketoacidosis.

In patients with abdominal pain the following should be ascertained:

- the site, intensity, character, duration and frequency of the pain
- the aggravating and relieving factors
- associated symptoms, including non-gastrointestinal symptoms.

Localized abdominal pain with tenderness can very rarely arise from the abdominal wall itself. The cause is unknown, but may possibly be due to nerve entrapment; a local anaesthetic injection may help.

Upper abdominal pain

Epigastric pain is very common; it is often a dull ache, but sometimes sharp and severe. Its relationship to food intake should be ascertained. It is a common feature of peptic ulcer disease, but it can be caused by a variety of upper GI diseases.

Right hypochondrial pain is usually from the gallbladder or biliary tract. Hepatic congestion (e.g. in hepatitis) and sometimes peptic ulcer can present with pain in the right hypochondrium. Chronic, often persistent, pain in the right hypochondrium is a frequent symptom in healthy females suffering from functional bowel disease. This chronic pain is not due to gallbladder disease (p. 339).

Lower abdominal pain

Acute pain in the left iliac fossa is usually colonic in origin (e.g. acute diverticulitis). Pain over a long period is most commonly associated with functional bowel disease. In females, lower abdominal pain occurs in a number of gynaecological disorders and the differentiation from GI disease is often difficult.

Persistent pain in the right iliac fossa over a long period is not due to chronic appendicitis.

Proctalgia is a severe pain deep in the rectum that comes on suddenly but lasts only for a short time. It is not due to organic disease.

Abdominal distension

Abdominal distension or bloating is a common complaint often erroneously attributed to wind. In the absence of physical signs, the symptom is due to functional bowel disease.

Weight loss

This is due to anorexia (loss of appetite) and is a frequent accompaniment of all gastrointestinal disease. Anorexia is also common in systemic disease and may be seen in psychiatric disorders, particularly anorexia nervosa. Anorexia often accompanies carcinoma but it is a late symptom and not of diagnostic help. Weight loss with a normal or increased dietary intake occurs with hyperthyroidism. Malabsorption is never so severe as to cause weight loss without anorexia. Weight loss should be assessed objectively as patients often 'think' they have lost weight. Appetite is described on p. 208.

Rectal bleeding

Bright red blood on the toilet paper on wiping the anus is a common symptom of piles. There are many other causes (see Fig. 4.17).

Clinical examination

A general examination is performed, with particular emphasis on the examination of all lymph nodes and noting the presence of anaemia or jaundice. Detailed examination of the gastrointestinal tract starts with the mouth and tongue, before examining the abdomen.

Examination of the abdomen

Inspection

The organs found in a normal abdomen are shown in Fig 4.2, and Fig 4.3 shows a normal CT scan at the T12 level.

Abdominal distension, whether due to flatus, fat, fetus, fluid or faeces, must be looked for. Lordosis may give the appearance of a distended abdomen; it is a common feature of the 'abdominal distension' seen in functional bowel disease.

Palpation

The abdominal organs may be felt in some normal subjects (see Fig 4.2) but this is not common and such organs are usually only just palpable. A Reidel's lobe is an extension of the lateral portion of the right lobe of the liver and can occasionally be palpated.

Any palpable mass is carefully felt to decide which organs are involved and also to evaluate its size, shape and consistency and whether it moves with respiration.

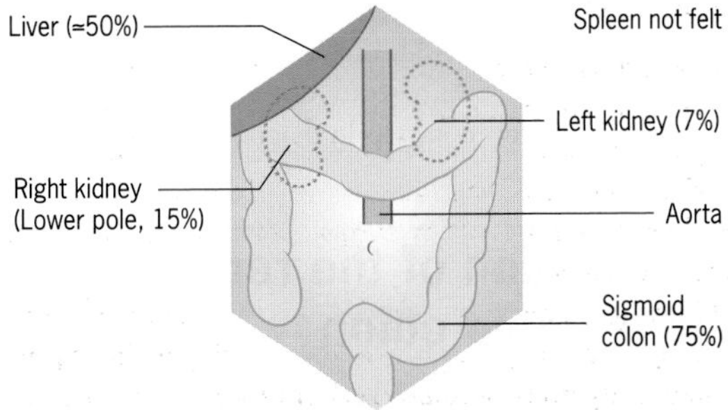

Fig 4.2
The organs sometimes palpable in thin subjects (%)

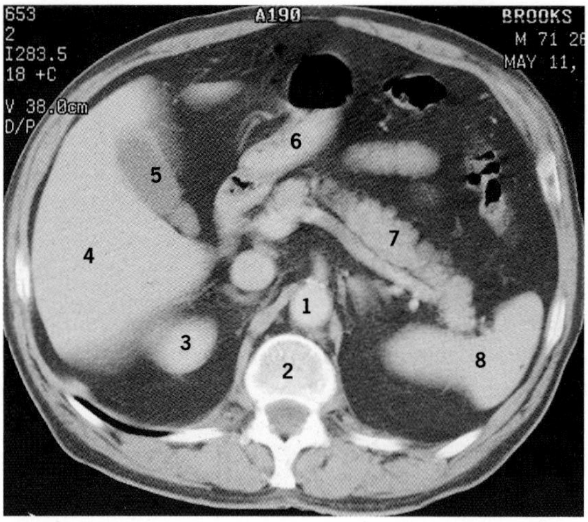

Fig 4.3
CT scan of the normal abdomen at the level of T12
1, aorta; 2, spine; 3, top of right kidney; 4, liver; 5, gallbladder; 6, stomach (containing air); 7, pancreas; 8, spleen

The hernial orifices should be examined if intestinal obstruction is suspected.

A succussion splash suggests gastric outlet obstruction if the patient has not drunk for 2–3 hours; the splash of fluid in the stomach can be heard with a stethoscope laid on the abdomen when the patient is moved.

Percussion

This is performed in the usual way to detect the area of dullness caused by the liver and spleen, and possibly bladder enlargement. The presence of fluid in the peritoneal cavity (i.e. ascites) is detected by shifting dullness. The percussion note changes from resonance to dullness when the patient is moved from one side to the other. It is a good physical sign if performed carefully, but 1–2 L of fluid must be present to elicit it. A fluid 'thrill' can be elicited, but is not always helpful. A large ovarian cyst can sometimes produce an enlarged abdomen, but the dullness is more centrally placed than in ascites.

Auscultation

Auscultation is not of great value in gastrointestinal disease, apart from in the evaluation of the acute abdomen (see p. 282). Abdominal bruits are often present in normal subjects, but these are not clinically significant. Intestinal sounds do not help in diagnosis.

Examination of the rectum and sigmoid colon

Digital examination of the rectum should be performed in all patients with a change in bowel habit and rectal bleeding (Practical box 4.1).

Practical

The patient should be positioned in the left lateral position with the hips flexed and the knees drawn up. The buttocks should be over the edge of the couch.

1 Explain what you are going to do.
2 Inspect the anus and perianal area for anal tags, external haemorrhoids, fissures or fistulae.
3 Insert lubricated gloved finger gently into anal canal.
4 Assess tone of anal musculature.
5 Rotate finger 360° in canal and feel:
the wall
(a) thickening or irregularity of the wall
(b) mass lesions, e.g. polyps, cancer
outside the wall
(a) prostate anteriorly in male patients
(b) cervix anteriorly in female patients
(c) any other lesions
inside the wall
stools – consistency
6 Withdraw finger and look at it for colour of stool. Is blood present?

Practical box 4.1 Rectal examination

Sigmoidoscopy (Practical box 4.2) should, in hospital, be part of the routine examination in all cases of diarrhoea and in patients with lower abdominal symptoms such as a change in bowel habit or bleeding.

Proctoscopy (Practical box 4.2) is performed in all patients with a history of bright red blood per rectum; the narrow sigmoidoscope does not distend the lumen and haemorrhoids can be missed.

Flexible-fibre sigmoidoscopy

The rigid sigmoidoscope allows inspection of only the lower 20–25 cm of the bowel, but a 70 cm flexible fibre-optic sigmoidoscope allows much more bowel to be visualized. It can be readily used in the outpatient department after minimal bowel preparation (a disposable enema). Seventy per cent of colonic neoplasms occur within the range of the flexible sigmoidoscope (see Fig 4.35a on p. 275).

Stool examination

This can be useful occasionally to confirm the patient's symptoms (e.g. passing of blood or steatorrhoea). The shape and size may be helpful (e.g. rabbity stools in the irritable bowel syndrome). Stool charts for recording volume and frequency of defecation are useful in inpatients to follow the progress of diarrhoea. Stool weights can be performed in outpatients to confirm true diarrhoea.

Practical

Sigmoidoscopy

- The technique is easy to learn, provides valuable information and is safe in competent hands.
- No bowel preparation is required.
- The technique is relatively painless. In the irritable bowel syndrome, the patient's pain is often reproduced by air insufflation.

1. Rectal examination is initially performed (Information box 4.1).
2. The sigmoidoscope is pointed towards the symphysis pubis and passed into the anus. The obturator is removed and the instrument passed under direct vision to the rectosigmoid junction and beyond if possible (using air insufflation).
3. The mucosa of the anus and rectum is inspected. The normal mucosa is shiny, superficial vessels can be seen and no contact bleeding should occur
4. Biopsies can be taken of any lesions that are seen or from apparently normal-looking mucosa which occasionally shows histological evidence of inflammation.

Proctoscopy

1. The proctoscope is passed into the anus directed towards the symphysis pubis and the obturator is removed.
2. The patient strains down as the proctoscope is removed.
3. Haemorrhoids are seen as purplish veins in the left lateral, right posterior or right anterior positions.
4. Fissures may also be seen.

Practical box 4.2 Sigmoidoscopy and proctoscopy

Investigations

Radiology and endoscopy are the principal investigations. These are usually preceded by routine haematology and biochemistry. The investigation of small bowel disease is discussed on p. 251.

Barium contrast studies

These are performed after an overnight fast. The radiologist should be given correct clinical information and directed to the particular area under suspicion. X-rays should be reviewed with the radiologist, if possible.

- **Barium swallow**. The oesophagus is visualized as barium is swallowed in the upright and prone positions. Motility abnormalities as well as anatomical lesions can then be observed. Reflux of barium from the stomach into the oesophagus is demonstrated with the patient tipped head down, but minimal reflux under these conditions may well have no clinical significance. Swallowing bread with the barium (to add bulk) is sometimes useful in a case of dysphagia.
- **Double-contrast barium meal**. This is performed to examine the stomach and duodenum. A small amount of barium is given together with effervescent granules or tablets to produce carbon dioxide so that a double contrast between air and barium is obtained. This technique has a high accuracy rate when performed carefully.
- **Small bowel follow-through**. This is used to examine the small bowel and ideally should be performed separately from a barium meal as a different technique is employed. Barium is swallowed and allowed to pass into the small intestine through the jejunum and into the ileum. This technique is the only way of demonstrating the gross anatomy of the small intestine. Views of the terminal ileum should be obtained with the use of a compression pad.
- **Small bowel enema (enteroclysis)**. A tube is passed through the duodenum and a large volume of dilute barium is introduced. This technique is only occasionally used and is useful for visualizing suspicious areas seen on the follow through, particularly strictures.
- **Barium enema**. Patients should be given a low-fibre diet for three days and be well prepared with laxatives and washouts so that the colon is empty. Barium and air are insufflated into the rectum via a retained catheter. A double contrast view is then obtained of the whole colon, often with views of the terminal ileum as well. Rectal examination and sigmoidoscopy usually precede this examination. The patient should be warned that this is an unpleasant examination.

Plain X-rays

Plain X-rays of the abdomen are chiefly used in the investigation of an acute abdomen (see p. 282). Areas of calcification can be seen in chronic pancreatitis (see p. 349). Routine abdominal X-rays are of little use in the management of most gastrointestinal disease.

Ultrasound, computed tomography (CT) and magnetic resonance imaging (MRI)

These techniques are used to define the intra-abdominal organs (e.g. liver, spleen, pancreas) but also to detect thickened bowel, masses, abscesses, fistulae or liver metastases.

- **Ultrasound**. This requires no radiation and is best for fluid-filled lesions. Mesenteric glands and thickened bowel can be visualized, but mucosal detail is not seen. In the acute abdomen it can be used to

diagnose acute cholangitis, aortic aneurysms or appendicitis. It has a complementary role to CT and is useful for follow-up and for draining collections.
- **Luminal ultrasonography**. A gastroscope incorporating an ultrasound probe is used to assess oesophageal and gastric wall thickening in cancer as well as other localized intraluminal lesions. In the duodenum, it is probably the most sensitive technique for the detection of small pancreatic tumours. An endorectal transducer is used to stage rectal carcinomas and also for the detection of anal fistulae and perianal absecess.
- **Computed tomography**. CT, particularly helical (spiral) CT, gives excellent anatomical definition. It can detect thickened bowel wall and gives good visualization of the mesentery, the retroperitoneal structures and the aorta. It can detect a perforated viscus, subdiaphragmatic abscesses, extraluminal abscesses in appendicitis and diverticulitis. It can assess the extent of Crohn's disease and can diagnose bowel obstruction. Contrast extravasated from the gut lumen can be detected, as can free air. CT-guided fine needle biopsies can be taken from tumours and lymph nodes. Cancer can be staged prior to surgery. Air insufflation into the colon followed by CT (air colonogram) gives a good definition of the colon (instead of using a barium enema).
- **Magnetic resonance imaging**. MRI has the advantage of using no ionizing radiation. It is particularly useful for abscesses around the anus, rectum and in the pelvis. It is currently used more in hepatobiliary and pancreatic disease (see p. 294).

Radioisotope imaging

Radionuclides are used to a varying degree depending on local enthusiasm and expertise. Indications are:

- to demonstrate oesophageal reflux using [^{99m}Tc] technetium–sulphur colloid
- to determine the rate of gastric emptying using [^{99m}Tc] technetium–sulphur colloid
- to demonstrate a Meckel's diverticulum using [^{99m}Tc] pertechnetate which has an affinity for gastric mucosa
- to show the extent of inflammation and the presence of any inflammatory collections in inflammatory bowel disease using ^{99m}Tc HMPAO (hexamethylpropylene amine oxime) labelled white cells.

Isotopes can also be used:

- to assess gastrointestinal loss of red cells by giving ^{51}Cr red cells and measuring radioactivity in the faeces or by labelling red cells with ^{99m}Tc and scanning the abdomen, e.g. Meckel's diverticulum
- to assess albumin loss in the stools in protein-losing enteropathy by giving $^{51}CrCl_3$ intravenously (p. 253)
- to assess bile salt malabsorption by whole-body scanning and counting the activity in the faeces following oral ^{75}Se-homochoyl taurine (SeHCAT)
- to detect bacterial overgrowth by measuring $^{14}CO_2$ in the breath following ^{14}C glycocholic acid orally (see Fig 4.23)
- to detect neuroendocrine tumours using radiolabelled octreotide and whole-body scanning
- to assess B_{12} malabsorption using $^{57}Co\text{-}B_{12}$ (see p. 367)

Endoscopy (Practical box 4.3)

Video endoscopes are replacing the old fibreoptic types. They have three chips (for blue, green and red light) mounted at the tip of the instrument. These send electronic signals which produce high-quality images on the monitor. Thus, they do not require the expensive fragile fibreoptic bundles. They are easier to use, and trainees and nurses can all view the progress of the endoscope on the screen. A permanent record can also be obtained.

The tip of the endoscope can be angulated in all directions. Channels are present in the endoscope for air insufflation, water injection, suction and for the passage of biopsy forceps or brushes for obtaining tissue. These latter channels can also be used for other therapeutic interventions (e.g. injection of varices).

- **Oesophagogastroduodenoscopy (OGD)**. This is often used as the investigation of choice for upper GI disorders by gastroenterologists because of easy access, the possibility of interventional therapy and obtaining mucosal biopsies. Contraindications include severe chronic obstructive pulmonary disease, a recent myocardial infarction, or instability of the atlanto-axial joints. The mortality for diagnostic endoscopy is 0.01%.
- **Colonoscopy**. This allows good visualization of the whole colon and terminal ileum. Biopsies can be obtained and polyps removed. The success rate for reaching the terminal ileum is approximately 80%. The mortality is 0.02% for diagnostic colonoscopy.
- **Enteroscopy**. The small bowel from the duodenum to the ileum can be visualized by enteroscopes. The indications for this technique are limited (mainly gastrointestinal blood loss), the instruments are expensive, and consequently they are used only in a few centres.

Barium studies and endoscopy are frequently complementary and the technique chosen often depends on local expertise and workload. Radiology is better than endoscopy for assessing motility disorders, extrinsic lesions and gastro-oesophageal reflux. Endoscopy is preferable in gastric ulcer disease (as biopsies can be obtained) and in the detection of oesophagitis. Colonoscopy is used in inflammatory bowel disease, for

Practical

Gastroscopy

1. The patient is fasted overnight and the procedure is carried out as an outpatient.
2. The throat is sprayed with lignocaine.
3. IV sedation is given for the very anxious patient or for additional procedures.
4. Oxygen saturation is monitored with a pulse oximeter.
5. Oxygen via nasal prongs is given to elderly patients.
6. The instrument is passed into the pharynx under direct vision, then down the oesophagus into the stomach and duodenum.
   (a) The forward-viewing instrument is used for visualization of the oesophagus, stomach and duodenal cap.
   (b) The side-viewing instrument is needed to visualize certain areas (e.g. the ampulla of Vater).
7. The patient must be 'nil by mouth' for approximately $1\frac{1}{2}$ hours following the procedure and may complain of a sore throat and abdominal discomfort.
8. Complications include local perforation and aspiration pneumonia.

Colonoscopy

1. Two days before the procedure, a low-residue diet is started.
2. One day before the procedure, clear fluids only are taken.
3. On the afternoon before the procedure, 71 mL extract of Senna with one pint of water is given.
4. Three hours later, one sachet of sodium picosulphate with one pint of water is given.
   An alternative preparation consists of giving large volumes of balanced electrolyte solution by mouth on the day of the test.
5. On the day of the procedure, one sachet of sodium picosulphate with one pint of water is given.
6. The instrument is passed under direct vision, and manoeuvred around to the caecum and into the terminal ileum. Sedation, with a benzodiazepine and pethidine, is required. Oxygen saturation is monitored with a pulse oximeter.
7. Observation is required of sedated patients for two hours following the procedure.
8. Complications include perforation or haemorrhage following a biopsy or polypectomy.

Practical box 4.3 Gastroscopy and colonoscopy

polyp follow-up, in the investigation of rectal bleeding, and for sick, immobile patients. Barium enema is usually performed for the investigation of change in bowel habit.

The mouth

The oral cavity extends from the lips to the pharynx and contains the tongue, teeth and gums. Its primary functions are mastication, swallowing and speech.

Problems in the mouth are extremely common and although they may be trivial, they can produce severe symptoms. Poor dental hygiene is often a factor.

Stomatitis is inflammation in the mouth from any cause, such as ill-fitting dentures. Angular stomatitis is inflammation of the corners of the mouth.

The burning mouth syndrome consists of a burning sensation in the context of a clinically normal oral mucosa. It occurs more commonly in middle-aged and elderly females. It is probably psychogenic in nature.

Oral ulceration

Recurrent ulceration

Recurrent aphthous ulceration of unknown aetiology is a common oral mucosa disorder affecting 20% of the population. It consists of recurrent bouts of one or more rounded, shallow, painful ulcers recurring at intervals of days to a few months. There are three main clinical types:

- *Minor aphthous ulcers* are the most common. They are less than 10 mm diameter, have a grey/white centre with a thin erythematous halo and heal within 14 days without scarring.
- *Major aphthous ulcers* are less common. They are larger (more than 20 mm diameter), often persist for weeks or months and heal with scarring. They present after puberty.
- *Herpetiform aphthous ulcers* are characterized by multiple (10–100), 2–3 mm diameter lesions. The term 'herpetiform' is purely descriptive and does not imply an infective aetiology.

Most patients with recurrent ulcers are otherwise well. Various nutritional deficiencies of iron, folic acid or vitamin B_{12} (with or without gastrointestinal disorders) are occasionally found.

There are no specific, effective therapies. Corticosteroids may lessen the duration and severity of the attacks. Chlorhexadine gluconate mouthwash, dapsone, colchicine, systemic steroids and azathioprine have all been tried.

Ulceration associated with systemic disorders

Oral ulceration is seen in gastrointestinal disorders, such as Crohn's disease, ulcerative colitis and coeliac disease in approximately 10–20% of cases. Other diseases associated with oral ulceration include lupus erythematosus (systemic and discoid), Behçet's disease, cyclic neutropenia (p. 177) and immunodeficiency disorders. In Reiter's disease, ulceration occurs in approximately 25–30% of patients.

Ulceration associated with dermatological disorders

These include erythema multiforme (e.g Stevens Johnson syndrome), lichen planus, pemphigus vulgaris, mucous membrane pemphigoid, 'epidermolysis bullosa' and dermatitis herpetiformis.

Ulceration associated with viral infection

Herpes simplex virus. Primary herpes simplex (usually type I but rarely type II) presents with fever and widespread confluent painful ulcers. After resolution, the virus remains latent and recurs as herpes labialis ('cold sores' – see p. 1155). Reactivation of persistent herpes simplex virus occurs secondary to a viral infection, fever, sunlight exposure or menstruation. There is a prodrome of lip burning or pricking sensation. Treatment with soluble tetracycline mouthwash three times daily gives pain relief. Oral systemic acyclovir shortens the course of the disease.

Coxsackie. Hand, foot and mouth disease due to coxsackie A virus produces small ulcers. Herpangina, due to a different coxsackie A, or rarely B, infection presents with an acute pharyngitis, cervical lymphadenopathy and pyrexia with multiple ulcers of the soft palate and pharyngeal mucosa.

Ulceration associated with bacterial infection

Syphilis and tuberculosis can rarely cause oral ulcerations and are seen mainly in developing countries.

Ulceration associated with drugs

Certain drugs can cause oral lichenoid eruptions. They include antimalarials, methyldopa, tolbutamide, penicillamine and gold salts.

Trauma

Traumatic ulcers may be due to ill-fitting dentures, toothbrushing or lacerations by sharp teeth.

Neoplastic lesions (squamous cell carcinoma)

Malignant tumours of the mouth account for 1% of all malignant tumours in the UK. The majority develop on the floor of the mouth or lateral borders of the tongue. Early tumours may be painless, but advanced tumours are easily recognizable as indurated aphthous ulcers with raised and rolled edges. Aetiological agents include tobacco, heavy alcohol consumption and the areca nut. Intra-oral lesions which undergo malignant transformation include leukoplakia, lichen planus, submucus fibrosis and erythroplakia (a red patch). The previous male predominance has declined. Treatment is by surgical excision and/or radiotherapy.

Oral white patches

White lesions may be transient or persistent. Transient white patches are either due to *Candida* infection or are very occasionally seen in systemic lupus erythematosis. Oral candidiasis in adults is seen in seriously ill or immunocompromised patients, or following therapy with broad-spectrum antibiotics or inhaled steroids. Local causes include mechanical, irritative or chemical trauma from drugs (e.g. aspirin).

Leukoplakia describes white patches for which no local cause can be found. It is associated with alcohol and (particularly) smoking, and is regarded as a premalignant condition. A biopsy should always be undertaken; histology shows alteration in the keratinization and dysplasia of the epithelium. Treatment with isotretinoin reduces disease progression. Oral lichen planus presents as white striae.

Oral pigmented lesions

Non-neoplastic lesions

Racial pigmentation is scattered and symmetrically distributed. Amalgam tattoo is the most common form of localized oral pigmentation and consists of blue-black macules involving the gingivae and results from the dental amalgam sequestering into the tissues. Diseases causing pigmentation include Peutz–Jegher's syndrome, Addison's disease and lichen planus. Heavy metals, such as lead, bismuth and mercury, and drugs (e.g. phenothiazines and antimalarials) all cause gingival pigmentation.

Neoplastic lesions

These include melanotic naevi on the hard palate and buccal mucosa. These are rarer in the mouth than on the skin. Malignant melanomas are rare, more common in males, and occur mainly on the upper jaw. The five year survival is only 5%.

The tongue

The tongue may be involved in a generalized stomatitis with similar lesions to those described above. *Glossitis* is a red, smooth, sore tongue seen in anaemia. It is also seen in infections due to *Candida* and in riboflavin and nicotinic acid deficiency.

A black hairy tongue is due to a proliferation of chromogenic micro-organisms causing brown staining of elongated filliform papillae. The causes are unknown, but heavy smoking and the use of antiseptic mouth washes have been indicated. A geographic tongue is an idiopathic condition occurring in 1–2% of the population and may be familial. There are erythematous areas surrounded by well-defined, slightly raised irregular margins. The lesions are usually painless and the patient should be reassured.

The gums

The gingivae consist of the mucus membranes covering the alveolar process of the mandible and the maxilla.

Chronic gingivitis is the most common cause of bleeding gums and is an inflammation following the accumulation of bacterial plaque. It resolves when the plaque is removed.

Acute (necrotizing) ulcerative gingivitis (Vincent's gingivitis) is characterized by the proliferation of spirochaete and fusi-form bacteria. Young male smokers with poor oral hygiene are predominantly affected. It responds to oral metro-nidazole 200 mg three times daily for three days, used with chlorhexadine gluconate mouthwash.

Desquamatous gingivitis is a clinical description of smooth, red atrophic gingivae caused by lichen planus or mucus membrane pemphigoid. The diagnosis is confirmed by biopsy.

Gingival swelling is due to fibrous hyperplasia or as a result of inflammatory changes. Fibrous gingival hyperplasia is a result of hereditary gingival fibromatosis or associated with drugs (e.g. phenytoin, cyclosporin, nifedipine). Inflammatory swellings are seen in pregnancy, gingivitis and scurvy. Swelling due to infiltration is seen in acute leukaemia and Wegener's granulomatosis.

The teeth

Streptococcus mutans is the main bacterial cause of dental caries in man. These bacteria are cariogenic only in the presence of dietary sugar. Dental caries can progress to pulpitis and pulp necrosis, and spreading infection can cause adentoalveolar abscesses. If there is soft tissue swelling, antibiotics (e.g. amoxycillin or metronidazole) should be prescribed prior to dental intervention. Erosion of the teeth can also result in exposure to acid (e.g. in bulimia nervosa – p. 1143) or, very occasionally, in patients with gastro-oesophageal reflux disease.

Oral manifestations of HIV infection

In the UK, 60% of HIV-infected patients have characteristic oral lesions. Lesions strongly associated with HIV infection include candidiasis (with erythema and/or white exudates), erythematous candidiasis, oral hairy leukoplakia, Kaposi's sarcoma, non-Hodgkin's lymphoma, necrotizing ulcerative gingivitis, and necrotizing ulcerative periodontitis.

Oral hairy leukoplakia is almost pathogonomic of HIV infection and may be an early sign. It is more common in HIV-infected homosexual men than in any other high-risk group. It is characterized by white vertical corrugations on the lateral borders of the tongue and immunostaining shows Epstein–Barr virus. Treatment is rarely necessary.

Kaposi's sarcoma presents as a red, purple or blue macule or nodule, most commonly on the palate. It is diagnostic of AIDs, but can occur at CD_4 lymphocyte counts of greater than 200 mm^3. The lesion has recently been associated with the herpes virus 8.

FURTHER READING

Lehner T (1996) The mouth and salivary glands. In: Weatherall DJ, Ledingham JG, Warrell DA (eds) Oxford Textbook of Medicine, 3rd edn. pp 1846-1865

The salivary glands

Ptyalism (excessive salivation)

Ptyalism occurs prior to vomiting, but may be secondary to other intra-oral pathology. It can be psychogenic.

Xerostomia (dry mouth)

This can result from:

- Sjögren's syndrome
- drugs (e.g. antiparkinsonian, antihistamines, lithium, monoamine oxidase inhibitors, tricyclic and related antidepressants, and clonidine)
- radiotherapy
- psychogenic causes
- dehydration, shock and renal failure.

The principles of management are to preserve what flow remains, stimulate flow and replace saliva (glycerine and lemon mouthwash and artificial saliva).

Sialadenitis

Acute sialadenitis is due to mumps (parotitis) or bacteria. Bacteria include *Staphylococcus aureus*, *Streptococcus pyogenes* and *Streptococcus pneumoniae*. There is an ascending infection, usually secondary to secretory failure. Pus can be expressed from the affected duct.

Salivary duct obstruction due to calculus

Obstruction to salivary flow is usually due to a calculus. There is a painful swelling of the submandibular gland after eating and stones can sometimes be felt in the floor of the mouth. Sialography and plain X-ray films will show the calculus. Removal of the obstruction gives complete relief.

Sarcoidosis (see also p. 806)

Sarcoidosis can involve the major salivary glands and forms part of Heerfordt's syndrome (parotitis, uveitis, low-grade fever). When combined with lacrimal gland enlargement it is known as the Mikulicz syndrome.

Neoplasms

Salivary gland neoplasms account for 3% of all tumours worldwide. The majority occur in the parotid gland. The pleomorphic adenoma is the most common and 15% of these undergo malignant transformation. Recurrence following surgical excision is common. Malignant tumours classically result in 7th cranial nerve lower motor neurone signs.

The pharynx and oesophagus

Structure and function

The oesophagus is a muscular tube, approximately 25 cm long, connecting the pharynx to the stomach. The muscle coat has two layers – an outer longitudinal layer and an inner circular layer of fibres. In the upper portion both muscle layers are striated. They gradually change to smooth muscle in the lower oesophagus, where they are continuous with the muscle layer of the stomach. The oesophagus is lined by stratified squamous epithelium, except near the gastro-oesophageal junction where columnar epithelium is found.

The oesophagus is separated from the pharynx by the *upper oesophageal sphincter*, which is normally closed by the continuous contraction of the cricopharyngeus muscle. The *lower oesophageal sphincter* (LOS) consists of an area of the distal end of the oesophagus that has a high resting tone and is largely responsible for the prevention of reflux. The reduction in tone and relaxation that occurs with swallowing is under the control of nervous (vagal) and hormonal mechanisms. The presynaptic neurotransmittter is acetyl choline. The postsynaptic neurotransmitter, which inhibits relaxation, is nitric oxide (NO), and vasoactive intestinal peptide (VIP) also contributes.

During swallowing, the bolus of food is moved from the mouth to the pharynx voluntarily. Immediately, the upper sphincter relaxes and food enters the oesophagus. A primary peristaltic wave starts in the pharynx at the onset of swallowing and sweeps down the whole oesophagus (Fig 4.4). Secondary peristalsis occurs locally in response to direct stimulation (e.g. distension by the bolus) and helps to clear food residue from the oesophagus. Non-peristaltic, non-propulsive tertiary waves are frequent in the elderly. The LOS relaxes when swallowing is initiated, before the arrival of the peristaltic wave.

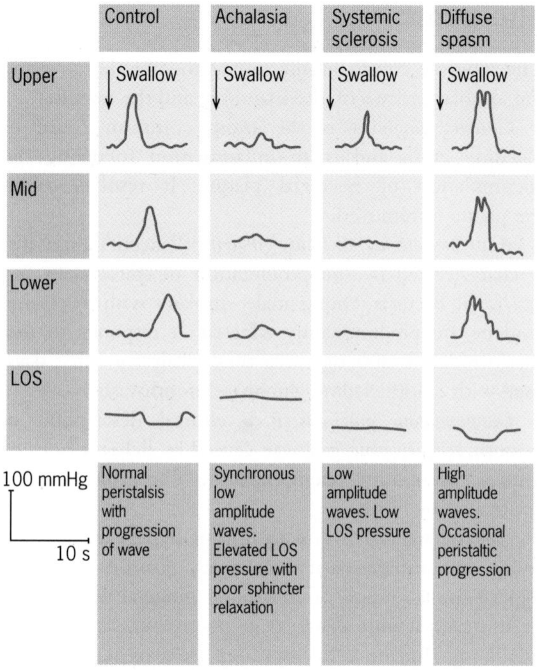

Fig 4.4
Oesophageal manometric patterns in normals and diseased states. LOS, lower oesophageal sphincter

SYMPTOMS OF OESOPHAGEAL DISORDERS

Major oesophageal symptoms are:

- dysphagia
- heartburn
- painful swallowing (odynophagia).

Dysphagia

This is either due to a local lesion or is part of a generalized disease. Patients will complain of something sticking in their throat or chest during swallowing or immediately afterwards. It is always a serious symptom and the cause must be found (Table 4.2); benign and malignant oesophageal strictures are the most common causes seen in hospital practice. *Globus hystericus* is the name given to apparent dysphagia – the sensation of a 'lump in the throat' in patients who do not have true dysphagia and can therefore swallow. It has no organic cause and the treatment is reassurance.

Heartburn

Heartburn is a common symptom of acid reflux. The pain can spread to the neck, across the chest, and can be difficult to distinguish from the pain of ischaemic heart disease. It can also occur at night when the patient lies flat or after bending or stooping. Hot drinks and alcohol often precipitate the pain.

Painful swallowing

Painful swallowing without real difficulty is a symptom of candidiasis and herpes simplex infection. Both these conditions are seen in AIDS patients. Ingestion of tablets such as bisphosphonates and potassium (slow release) will produce local ulceration if they lodge in the gullet when swallowed lying down and without water.

SIGNS OF OESOPHAGEAL DISORDERS

There are very few signs associated with oesophageal disease, the main one being of weight loss as a consequence of dysphagia.

INVESTIGATION OF OESOPHAGEAL DISORDERS

- **Barium swallow and meal**.
- **Oesophagoscopy**.
- **Manometry** is performed by passing a fluid-filled catheter through the nose into the oesophagus. Changes in pressure are transmitted up the fluid column and recorded. These studies are useful in motility disorders.
- **pH monitoring** – 24 hour monitoring using a pH-sensitive probe positioned in the lower oesophagus – is used for the identification of reflux episodes (pH < 4). Brief episodes can, however, occur in normal subjects.
- **Radioisotope studies** with technetium–sulphur colloid incorporated into food can also be used to study reflux. It is not widely used in the UK.
- **The Bernstein test** (alternate dilute acid and alkali infused into the oesophagus to reproduce the pain) is now seldom used. A positive test suggests oesophagitis, but there are many false negatives.

Hiatus hernia

This describes the 'herniation' of part of the stomach into the chest.

Table 4.2
Causes of dysphagia

Disease of mouth and tongue (e.g. tonsillitis)	Extrinsic pressure:
Neuromuscular disorders:	Mediastinal glands
Pharyngeal disorders	Goitre
Bulbar palsy (e.g. motor neurone disease)	Enlarged left atrium
Myasthenia gravis	Intrinsic lesion:
Oesophageal motility disorders:	Foreign body
Achalasia	Stricture
Scleroderma	benign – peptic, corrosive
Diffuse oesophageal spasm	malignant – carcinoma
Presbyoesophagus	Lower oesophageal rings
Diabetes mellitus	oesophageal web
Chagas' disease	pharyngeal pouch

In a *sliding hiatus hernia*, the gastro-oesophageal junction 'slides' through the hiatus so that it lies above the diaphragm. This type of hernia occurs in approximately 30% of people of 50 years of age and by itself is of no diagnostic significance. It does not produce symptoms on its own; symptoms occur because of the presence of associated reflux (see below).

A *para-oesophageal* or *rolling hernia* is when a small part of the fundus of the stomach rolls up through the hernia alongside the oesophagus. The sphincter remains below the diaphragm and remains competent. Occasionally a rolling para-oesophageal hernia will produce severe pain and require surgical treatment for gastric volvulus or strangulation.

Gastro-oesophageal reflux disease (GORD)

Gastro-oesophageal reflux occurs as a normal event, and the clinical features of GORD occur only when the antireflux mechanisms fail sufficiently to allow gastric contents to make prolonged contact with the lower oesophageal mucosa.

Antireflux mechanisms (Fig 4.5)

The most important mechanism is provided by the lower oesophageal sphincter (LOS) which is formed by the distal 4 cm of oesophageal smooth muscle. It rapidly regains its normal tone (following relaxation to allow a bolus to enter the stomach) and thereby prevents reflux. It is capable of increasing tone in response to rises in intra-abdominal and intragastric pressures.

Other antireflux measures involve the intra-abdominal segment of the oesophagus which acts as a flap valve, and the mucosal rosette formed by folds of the gastric mucosa also help to occlude the gastro-oesophageal junctional lumen. In addition, contraction of the crucal diaphragm exerts a 'pinchcock-like' action at the LOS.

The oesophagus is normally rapidly cleared of any reflux contents by secondary peristalsis.

PATHOGENESIS

The following mechanisms have been implicated:

- The resting LOS tone is low and LOS tone fails to increase when lying flat, as occurs in normal patients.
- The LOS tone fails to increase when intra-abdominal pressure is increased by tight clothing or pregnancy.
- There is reduced oesophageal mucosal resistance to acid.
- There is reduced oesophageal clearance of acid due to poor oesophageal peristalsis. The reduced acid clearance is exacerbated with a hiatus hernia owing to trapping of acid within the hernial sac.
- A large hiatus hernia can impair the 'pinchcock' mechanism of the diaphragm.

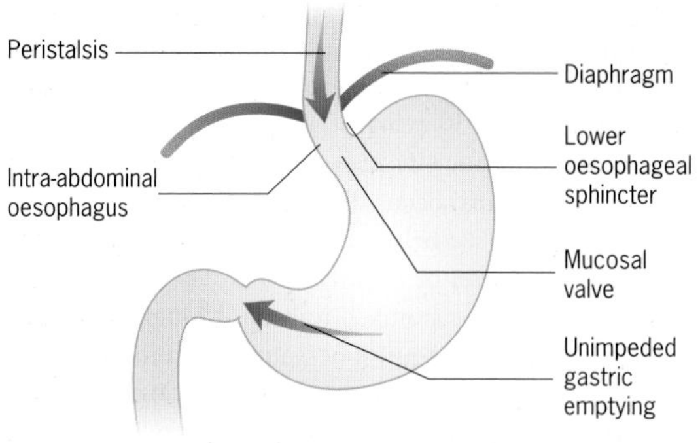

Fig 4.5
The main antireflux mechanisms

- Delayed gastric emptying occurs and thus may increase the chance of reflux.
- Prolonged episodes of gastro-oesophageal reflux occur at night and post-prandially.

Factors associated with increased gastro-oesophageal reflux are shown in Table 4.3. All or some of these features play a role in the individual patient and can occur whether or not a hiatus hernia is present. GORD can undoubtedly occur without a hiatus hernia.

CLINICAL FEATURES

Heartburn is the major feature of GORD. Pain is mainly due to direct stimulation of the hypersensitive oesophageal mucosa, but is also partly due to spasm of the distal oesophageal muscle. The burning is aggravated by bending, stooping or lying down and may be relieved by antacids. The patient may complain of pain on drinking hot liquids or alcohol. The correlation between heartburn and minor degrees of oesophagitis is poor. Some patients have mild oesophagitis, but severe heartburn; others have severe oesophagitis without symptoms and present with a haematemesis or an iron-deficiency anaemia from chronic blood loss. Regurgitation of food and acid into the mouth can occur, particularly when the patient is bending or lying flat. Aspiration into the lungs, producing pneumonia, is unusual without an accompanying stricture, but cough and nocturnal asthma from regurgitation and aspiration can occur. The differential diagnosis from angina can be difficult; 20% of cases admitted to a coronary care unit have GORD (Information box 4.1).

Table 4.3
Factors associated with increased gastro-oesophageal reflux

Pregnancy or obesity
Fat, chocolate, coffee or alcohol ingestion
Large meals
Cigarette smoking
Drugs – anticholinergic, calcium-channel blockers, nitrates
Systemic sclerosis
After treatment for achalasia
Hiatus hernia

DIAGNOSIS AND INVESTIGATIONS

GORD is a clinical diagnosis and many patients can be treated without investigation.

- **Oesophagoscopy** is used to show and confirm the presence of oesophagitis with a red friable mucosa and in more severe cases, linear ulceration. The mucosa can be normal in GORD. A biopsy can be taken in doubtful cases.
- **Barium swallow** is less sensitive than endoscopy in demonstrating oesophagitis. It may show a hiatus hernia (which by itself is of no diagnostic significance) with or without free reflux of barium.
- **Radiolabelled technetium** (see p. 227) can be used to demonstrate reflux.
- **24-hour intraluminal pH monitoring** (see p. 227) is the most accurate test available, there being a reasonable correlation between frequency of reflux and symptoms. It is often combined with manometry. The number of reflux episodes (below pH 4) occurring over 24 h is noted (Fig 4.6).

TREATMENT

Many patients (approximately 50%) can be treated successfully with simple antacids, loss of weight, and raising the head of the bed at night. Precipitating factors should be avoided with a reduction in alcohol consumption and cessation of smoking. These measures are simple to say, difficult to carry out, but are useful in mild cases.

Drugs

The chief antacids are magnesium trisilicate and aluminium hydroxide, but the former often causes diarrhoea whilst the latter causes constipation. Many antacids contain sodium

Information

Gastro-oesophageal reflux

Burning pain produced by bending, stooping or lying down
Pain seldom radiates to the arms
Pain precipitated by drinking hot liquids or alcohol
Relieved by antacids

Myocardial ischaemia

Gripping or crushing pain
Pain radiates into neck, shoulders and both arms
Pain produced by exercise
Accompanied by dyspnoea

Information box 4.1 Features of gastro-oesophageal reflux and myocardial ischaemia

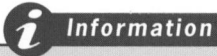

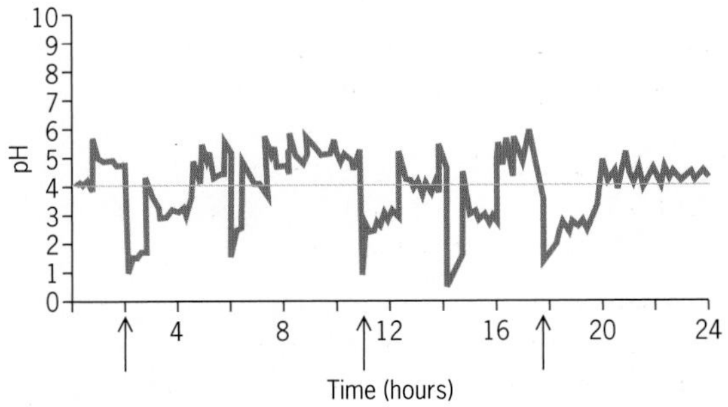

Fig 4.6
24-hour intraluminal pH monitoring. Five reflux episodes (pH < 4) occurred, but only three gave symptoms (arrows)

which may exacerbate fluid retention; aluminium hydroxide has less sodium than magnesium trisilicate.

Alginate-containing antacids (10 mL three times daily) are the most frequently prescribed agents for GORD. They form a gel or 'foam raft' with gastric contents and thereby reduce reflux.

H_2-receptor antagonists can be obtained over-the-counter and are frequently used (see p. 237).

Proton pump inhibitors (e.g. omeprazole, lansoprazole, pantoprazole) inhibit the gastric hydrogen–potassium ATPase (see Fig. 4.9). These produce almost complete reduction of gastric acid secretion and are the drugs of choice for all but mild cases. Patients with severe symptoms need prolonged treatment, often for years.

The *prokinetic agents* metoclopramide and cisapride can be used. Metoclopramide, a dopamine antagonist, is occasionally helpful as it enhances peristalsis and speeds gastric emptying. Cisapride is devoid of dopaminergic activity; it increases oesophageal peristalsis, increases LOS pressure and is of some value, particularly for maintenance therapy.

Eradication of *Helicobacter pylori* (see p. 237)

H. pylori is associated with hypersecretion of acid in some patients. In view of this, most experts recommend eradication therapy.

Surgery

Surgery should never be performed for a hiatus hernia alone. The properly selected case with severe reflux confirmed by pH manometry and oesophagitis responds well to surgery. Repair of the hernia and some sort of additional antireflux surgery (e.g. a modified Nissen fundoplication) is performed laparoscopically. Results show an improvement in symptoms in up to 80% of cases.

COMPLICATIONS

Peptic stricture usually occurs in patients over the age of 60. The symptoms are those of intermittent dysphagia over a long period. Treatment is by dilatation of the stricture and management of the reflux usually medically with a proton-pump inhibitor, but occasionally surgery is required.

Barrett's oesophagus was defined as more than 3 cm of specialized columnar epithelium was (intestinal type metaplasia) extending upwards into the lower oesophageal mucosa. However, short segments (<3 cm) of specialized columnar epithelium are found histologically even from normal-looking oesophagogastric junctions. It is due to longstanding acid reflux. It is seen in up to 20% of patients undergoing endoscopy for gastro-oesophageal reflux disease. It is most common in middle-aged men. Barrett's oesophagus (even short segment) is premalignant for adenocarcinoma (see p. 232). An indocarmine spray down the endoscope can detect intestinal metaplasia and possibly dysplasia. The dysplasia is patchy and biopsies from all four quadrants (every 2 cm) of the Barrett's segment must be performed. Surveillance – looking for severe dysplasia/cancer – is costly and subject to observer error; its value is disputed.

Motility disorders

Achalasia

Achalasia is a disease characterized by aperistalsis in the body of the oesophagus and failure of relaxation of the lower oesophageal sphincter on initiation of swallowing. In the majority of cases the aetiology is unknown (idiopathic). A similar clinical picture is seen in Chagas' disease (American trypanosomiasis – p. 75) where there is damage to the neural plexus of the gut.

PATHOGENESIS

Degenerative lesions are found in the vagus as well as a decrease in ganglionic cells in the myenteric nerve plexus of the oesophageal wall. Nitric oxide-containing neurones are affected more than the cholinergic nerves, and thus the relaxation of the sphincter is impaired in its absence. Recent studies suggest that two-thirds of patients have autoantibodies to a dopamine-carrying protein on the surface of the cells in the myenteric plexus.

CLINICAL FEATURES

The disease can present at any age but is rare in childhood. The incidence is about 1 per 100 000 per year. Patients usually have a long history of intermittent dysphagia for both liquids and solids. Regurgitation of food from the dilated oesophagus may be induced by the patient or may occur spontaneously, particularly at night, and aspiration pneumonia may result. Occasionally food gets stuck but patients often learn to overcome this by drinking large quantities, thereby increasing the head of pressure in the oesophagus and forcing the food through. Severe retrosternal chest pain occurs particularly in younger patients with vigorous non-peristaltic contraction of the oesophagus. The dysphagia in these patients can be mild and the pain misdiagnosed as cardiac in origin. Weight loss is usually not marked.

INVESTIGATIONS

- **Chest X-ray** may show a dilated oesophagus, with an occasional fluid level, behind the heart. The fundal gas shadow is not present.
- **Barium swallow** will show dilatation of the oesophagus, lack of peristalsis and often synchronous contractions. The lower end gradually narrows (beak deformity); this appearance is due to failure of the sphincter to relax (Fig 4.7a).
- **Oesophagoscopy** is necessary to exclude a carcinoma at the lower end of the oesophagus, as this can produce a similar X-ray appearance. When there is marked dilatation, extensive cleansing is necessary to remove food debris in order to obtain a clear view. In achalasia the oesophagoscope easily flops through the apparent narrowing without resistance.
- **Manometry** is used to measure oesophageal motility. It shows aperistalsis of the oesophagus as well as the failure of relaxation of the lower oesophageal sphincter (see Fig 4.4).

TREATMENT

The treatment of choice is endoscopic dilatation of the LOS using a pneumatic bag (passed under X-ray control). This weakens the sphincter and is successful in 80% of cases. Endoscopic injection of Botulinum toxin into the LOS has been used with variable success. If these measures fail, surgical division of the muscle at the lower end of the oesophagus (cardiomyotomy or Heller's operation) is performed laparoscopically. Reflux oesophagitis complicates all procedures and the aperistalsis of the oesophagus remains. In older patients, nifedipine (20 mg sublingually) can be tried initially.

COMPLICATIONS

There is a slight increase in the incidence of carcinoma of the oesophagus in both treated and untreated cases.

Systemic sclerosis (see also p. 490)

There is oesophageal involvement in 90% or more of patients with this disease. Diminished peristalsis, detected manometrically (see Fig 4.4) or by barium swallow, is due to replacement of the smooth muscle layers by fibrous tissue. The lower oesophageal sphincter pressure is also decreased, allowing reflux; mucosal damage occurs as a consequence. Strictures may develop. Initially there are no symptoms, but dysphagia and heartburn occur as the oesophagus becomes severely involved.

Similar motility abnormalities may be found in other connective-tissue disorders, particularly if Raynaud's phenomenon is present. Treatment is as for reflux (see p. 228) and stricture formation.

(a)

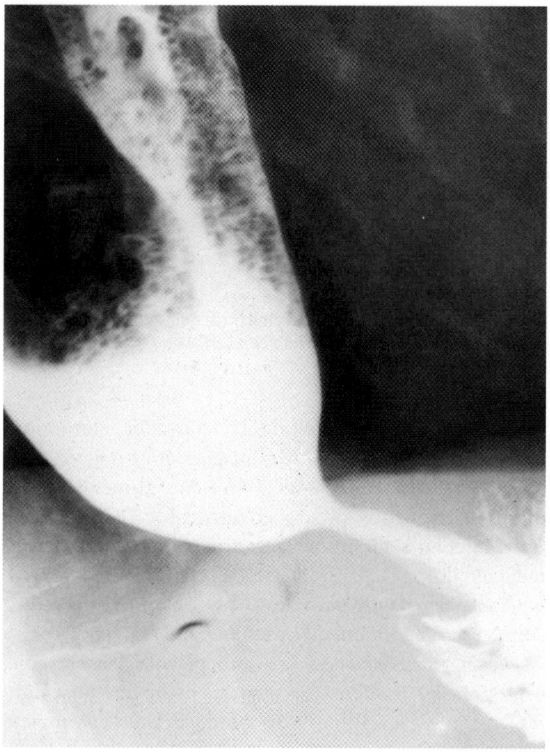

(b)

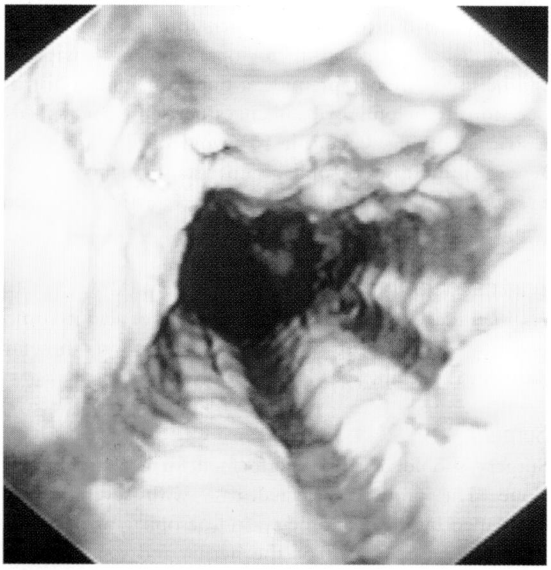

Fig 4.7
(a) Barium swallow, showing achalasia with atonic body of the oesophagus and a narrowed distal end. Note food residue in dilated oesophagus
(b) Endoscopic picture, showing Candida oesophagitis. Note the thick yellow exudate with underlying oesophagitis

Diffuse oesophageal spasm

This is a severe form of abnormal oesophageal motility that can sometimes produce retrosternal chest pain and dysphagia. It can accompany GORD. Swallowing is accompanied by bizarre and marked contractions of the oesophagus without progression of the waves (see Fig 4.4). On barium swallow the appearance may be that of a 'corkscrew'. However, asymptomatic changes in oesophageal motility are not infrequent, particularly in patients over the age of 60 years (presbyoesophagus). Care must therefore be taken that the symptoms, the manometry and X-ray findings of oesophageal spasm are not falsely correlated.

A variant of diffuse oesophageal spasm is the *'nutcracker' oseophagus*, which is characterized by finding very high-amplitude peristalsis (pressures >200 mmHg) within the oesophagus. Chest pain and dysphagia occur.

TREATMENT

True oesophageal spasm producing severe symptoms is rare and treatment is often unhelpful. Antispasmodics, nitrates, or calcium-channel blockers – such as sublingual nifedipine 10 mg three times daily – may be tried. Occasionally, balloon dilatation or even myotomy is necessary. When the spasm is associated with GORD, acid suppression is given.

Miscellaneous motility disorders

Abnormalities of motility that are mostly asymptomatic but occasionally produce dysphagia are found in the elderly, in diabetes mellitus, myotonica dystrophica and myasthenia gravis, as well as in any neurological disorder involving the brain stem.

Other oesophageal disorders

Oesophageal diverticulum

This is a pouch lined with epithelium that can produce dysphagia and regurgitation. It is usually asymptomatic and often detected accidentally on a barium swallow performed for other reasons. Diverticula can occur:

- immediately above the upper oesophageal sphincter (pharyngeal pouch) – if large, it may cause dysphagia as well as spillage of contents into the trachea
- near the middle of the oesophagus (traction diverticulum produced by extrinsic inflammation)
- just above the lower oesophageal sphincter (epiphrenic diverticulum).

Only when symptoms are severe should surgery be undertaken.

Rings and webs

A number of rings and webs have been described throughout the oesophagus.

Lower oesophageal or Schatzki ring

This is a narrowing of the lower end of the oesophagus due to a ridge of mucosa or a fibrous membrane. The ring may be asymptomatic, but it can very occasionally produce dysphagia after swallowing a large bolus of bread or meat. A barium swallow (with the oesophagus well distended with barium) often shows the narrowing; barium-coated bread will lodge at the narrowing. Treatment is with reassurance and dietary advice, but dilatation is occasionally necessary.

Upper oesophageal web

This is a constriction near the upper oesophageal sphincter in the post-cricoid region and appears radiologically as a web. The web may be asymptomatic or may produce dysphagia. In the Plummer–Vinson syndrome (Paterson–Brown–Kelly syndrome) this web is associated with iron-deficiency anaemia, glossitis and angular stomatitis. This rare syndrome affects mainly women and its aetiology is not understood. At oesophagoscopy the web may be difficult to see. Dilatation of the web is rarely necessary. Iron is given for the iron deficiency.

Benign oesophageal stricture

Peptic stricture secondary to reflux is the most common cause of benign strictures (for treatment, see p. 229). They also occur after the ingestion of corrosives, after radiotherapy, after sclerosis of varices, and following prolonged nasogastric intubation. All strictures give rise to dysphagia. They are usually treated by dilatation, but occasionally surgery is necessary.

Oesophageal infections

Infection is a cause of painful swallowing and is seen particularly in immunosuppressed debilitated patients and patients with AIDS. Infection can occur with:

- *Candida*
- herpes simplex
- cytomegalovirus.

It is occasionally difficult to distinguish between these either on barium swallow or oesophagoscopy, as only widespread ulceration is seen. In candidiasis the characteristic white plaques on top of friable mucosa are frequently found (Fig. 4.7b), but oral candidiasis is not always present. The diagnosis of *Candida* infection can be confirmed by examining a direct smear taken at endoscopy, but often infections are mixed and cultures and biopsies must be performed.

TREATMENT

Most patients on large doses of immunosuppressive agents are treated prophylactically with nystatin or amphotericin. Other antifungal or antiviral treatment is given appropriately (see Chapter 1).

The Mallory–Weiss syndrome

This is described on p. 245.

Oesophageal perforation or rupture

This can occur, with violent vomiting producing severe chest pain and collapse. It may follow alcohol ingestion and a chest X-ray shows a hydropneumothorax.

Oesophageal tumours

Benign tumours

These are rare, the most common being leiomyomas. They are usually discovered accidentally and they do not often produce symptoms.

Malignant tumours

Cancer of the oesophagus is the eighth most common cancer throughout the world. Approximately 40% occur in the middle third of the oesophagus and are squamous carcinomas. Adenocarcinomas (approx 45%) occur in the lower third of the oesophagus and at the cardia. Tumours of the upper third are rare (15%).

Kaposi's sarcoma is frequently found in the oesophagus as well as the mouth (see p. 225) and hypopharynx in patients with AIDS (see p. 118).

EPIDEMIOLOGY AND AETIOLOGICAL FACTORS

Squamous carcinoma

The incidence of carcinoma varies throughout the world, being high in China, parts of Africa and in the Caspian regions of Iran (where the incidence is the highest observed for any type of cancer anywhere in the world). In the UK it is 5–10 per 100 000 and represents 2.2% of all malignant disease. The variation in incidence throughout the world is greater than for any other carcinoma and is unusual in that sharp differences occur in regions very close to one another. Dietary and other environmental causes have been investigated and it is probable that different causative agents are involved in different parts of the world.

Carcinoma of the oesophagus is more common in men and there is an increased risk with heavy alcohol intake and heavy smoking. Monotonous diets, very high in cereals and *N*-nitroso compounds in preserved food, possibly increase the risk. Diets high in carotenoids and vitamin C (vegetables and fruit) possibly decrease the risk. Predisposing factors include the Plummer–Vinson syndrome, achalasia, coeliac disease and the familial condition of tylosis (an autosomal dominant condition with hyperkeratosis of palms and soles).

Adenocarcinoma

Eighty per cent of these tumours arise in the columnar-lined epithelium of the lower oesophagus (Barrett's oesophagus – p. 229). This columnarization results from longstanding reflux, although some patients will have no preceding symptoms. This premalignant lesion increases the chances of adenocarcinoma 30–40-fold. Extension of an adenocarcinoma of the gastric cardia can cause oesophageal obstruction; the incidence rate of this tumour is increasing.

CLINICAL FEATURES

Carcinoma of the oesophagus occurs mainly in those aged 60–70 years, although it is now occurring in younger age groups. Dysphagia is the most common single symptom and is progressive and unrelenting. Initially there is difficulty in swallowing solids, but eventually dysphagia for liquids also occurs. Benign strictures, on the other hand, initially produce intermittent dysphagia. Impaction of food causes pain, but more persistent pain implies infiltration.

The lesion is usually ulcerative, extending around the wall of the oesophagus to produce a stricture. Direct invasion of the surrounding structures occurs rather than widespread metastases, and at presentation 50% have regional lymph node involvement. Weight loss, due to the dysphagia as well as to anorexia, frequently occurs. The oesophageal obstruction eventually causes difficulty in swallowing saliva, and coughing and aspiration into the lungs is common.

Signs are often absent. Weight loss, anorexia and lymphadenopathy are occasionally found.

INVESTIGATIONS

- **Barium swallow** is often the initial investigation (Fig 4.8(a)), although many gastroenterologists like to go directly to oesophagoscopy which provides histological or cytological proof of the carcinoma; 90% of oesophageal carcinomas can be confirmed with this technique.
- **CT scan** of the thorax and abdomen will show the volume of the tumour and possible spread outside the oesophagus. It has been used to attempt to stage tumours prior to surgery, but results are disappointing.
- **Endoscopic ultrasound** (Fig 4.8(b)) has an accuracy rate of nearly 90% for assessing depth of tumour and infiltration and 80% for staging lymph node involvement.

TREATMENT

This depends on the age and fitness of the patient and the stage of the disease. Overall, the results are poor with a 10% five-year survival rate.

Surgery

Surgery provides the best chance of a cure and should be used only when screening (see above) has shown that the

(a)

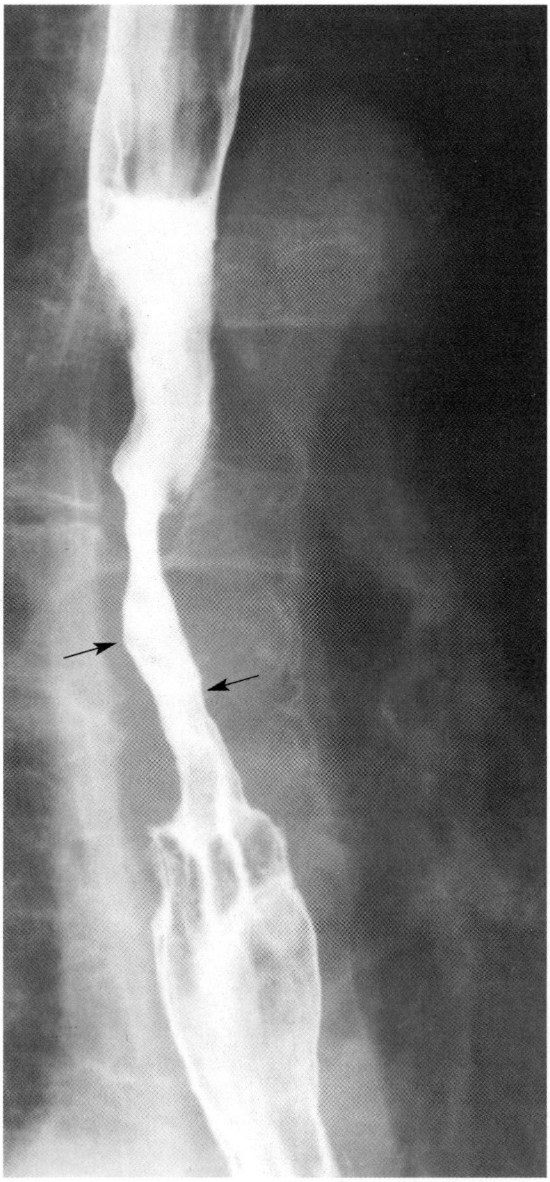

(b)

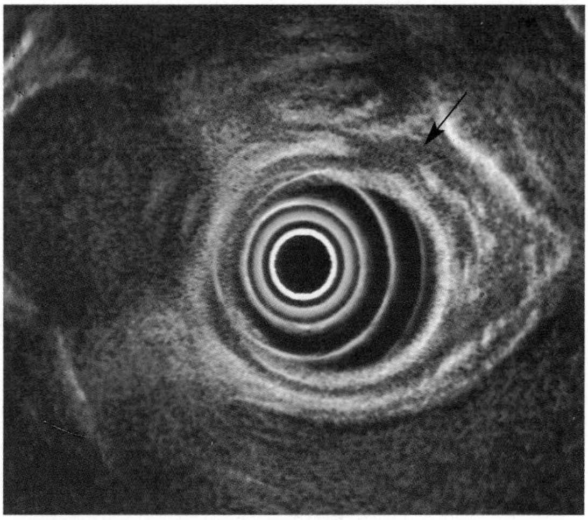

Fig 4.8
Carcinoma of the oesophagus
(a) Barium swallow, showing an irregular narrowed area (arrow) at the lower end of the oesophagus
(b) Endoscopic ultrasound. The central concentric circles are the probe. The arrow points to a break in the muscle layer and the soft tissue mass of the carcinoma

tumour has not infiltrated outside the oesophageal wall. Surgery in this group shows an 80% five-year survival rate if the postoperative pathology confirms the staging. Unfortunately, most patients present with advanced disease and surgery here is inappropriate.

Radiotherapy
This is used, with limited success, for squamous carcinoma of the upper and middle third of the oesophagus.

Chemotherapy
5FU, cisplatinum and combined chemoradiation are being used (see p. 44).

Palliative therapy
This is often the only realistic possibility. Repeated dilatation or dilatation of the stricture with the insertion of a plastic or expanding metal stent to keep the oesophageal lumen open can be performed via an endoscope. This allows liquids and soft foods to be eaten. Fizzy drinks are recommended to keep the tubes from blocking.

Tumours can be photocoagulated using a laser beam delivered through an endoscope, or necrosed using alcohol injections. This relieves the dysphagia, but repeated treatments are necessary. Photodynamic therapy is being tried to reduce the tumour bulk.

Nutritional support, as well as support for the patient and their family, is vital in this distressing condition.

FURTHER READING

Mittal RK, Balaban DH (1997) The esophago-gastric junction. *New England Journal of Medicine* **336**: 924–932.

Cameron AJ, Lombay CT, Pena M *et al.* (1995) Adenocarcinoma of the esophago gastric junction and Barrett's esophagus. *Gastroenterology* **108**: 1541-1546.

The stomach and duodenum

STRUCTURE
The stomach, which varies considerably in size, is divided into the upper portion (the fundus), the mid-region or body, and the antrum, which extends into the pyloric region.

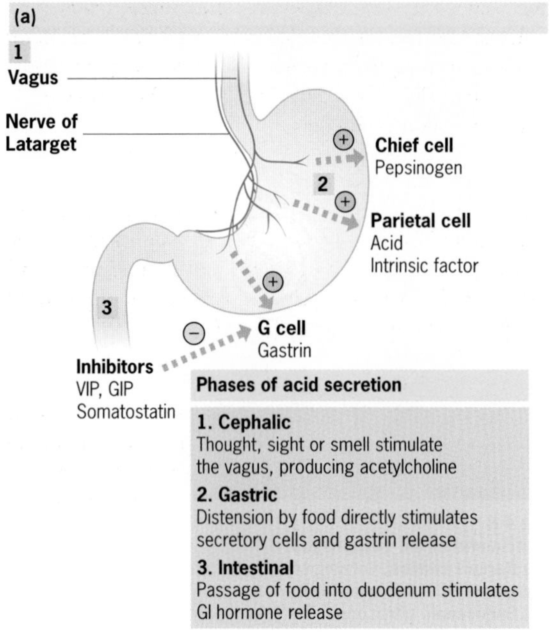

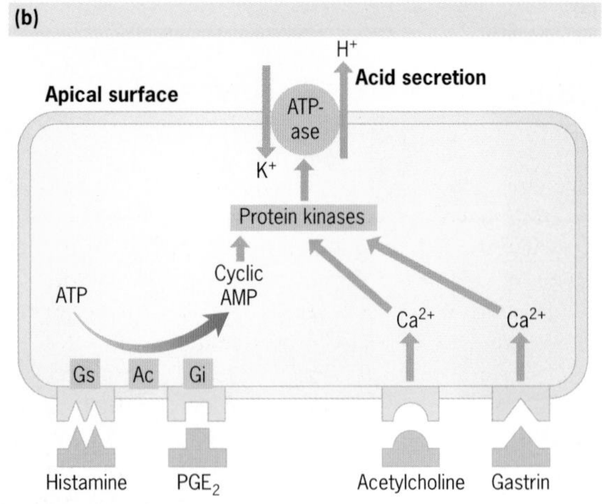

Fig 4.9
(a) Control of acid secretion
(b) Mechanisms involved in acid secretion. Gastrin and acetyl choline also act through enterochromaffin cells, stimulating histamine release. G_s, G_i, G proteins–inhibitory, stimulatory and inhibitory; Ac, adenyl cyclase; PGE_2, prostaglandin E_2

There are two sphincters, the gastro-oesophageal sphincter and the pyloric sphincter; the latter is largely made up of a thickening of the circular muscle layer. The muscle wall of the stomach has three layers – an outer longitudinal, an inner circular, and an innermost oblique layer of smooth muscle.

The duodenum has outer longitudinal and inner smooth muscle layers. It is C-shaped and the pancreas sits in the concavity. It terminates in the jejunum at the duodenojejunal flexure.

The mucosal lining of the stomach, particularly in the greater curvature, is thrown into thick folds or rugae. The upper two-thirds of the stomach contains parietal cells, which secrete hydrochloric acid, and chief cells, which secrete pepsinogen (which initiates proteolysis). The junction between the body and the antrum of the stomach can often be seen macroscopically, but can be confirmed by measuring surface pH. The antrum contains mucus-secreting and G cells, which secrete gastrin. There are two major forms of gastrin, G17 and G34, depending on the number of amino-acid residues. G17 is the major form found in the antrum. Mucus-secreting cells are present throughout the stomach and secrete mucus and bicarbonate which is trapped in the mucus gel. The mucus is made of glycoproteins called mucins. Somatostatin is also produced by specialized antral cells.

The mucosal barrier, made up of the surface membranes of mucosal cells and the mucus, protects the gastric epithelium from damage by, for example, alcohol, aspirin, NSAIDS, and bile salts. Prostaglandins stimulate mucus secretion and their synthesis is inhibited by aspirin and NSAIDS which inhibit cyclooxygenase (see Fig. 12.32).

The duodenal mucosa contains Brunner's glands, which secrete alkaline mucus. This, along with the pancreatic and biliary secretions, helps to neutralize the acid secretion from the stomach when it reaches the duodenum.

FUNCTION

The factors controlling *acid secretion* are shown in Fig 4.9. Secretion is under neural and hormonal control. Both stimulate acid secretion through the direct release of histamine on the parietal cell. Acetylcholine and gastrin also release histamine via the enterochromaffin cells. Somatostatin inhibits both histamine and gastrin release and therefore acid secretion.

Other major gastric functions are:

- acting as a reservoir for food
- for the emulsification of fat and mixing of gastric contents
- for the secretion of intrinsic factor
- for absorption (of only minimal importance).

Gastric emptying depends on many factors. There are osmoreceptors in the duodenal mucosa that control gastric emptying by local reflexes and the release of gut hormones. In particular, intraduodenal fat delays gastric emptying by negative feedback through duodenal receptors.

Gastritis

Acute gastritis, erosions and acute ulceration

In acute gastritis there is an acute inflammatory infiltrate in the superficial gastric mucosa predominantly with neutrophils. This is sometimes accompanied by mucosal erosions. Multiple small erosions, often with an oedematous mucosa, are described as *acute erosive gastritis*.

Acute gastric ulceration occurs in the same setting as erosions, but ulcers are larger and less superficial.

Gastritis can be commonly produced by drugs such as aspirin and other NSAIDS (Information box 4.2), and occasionally by infections (e.g. cytomegalovirus and herpes simplex), particularly in the immunocompromised. Aspirin and other NSAIDS deplete mucosal prostaglandins by inhibiting the cyclooxygenase (COX) pathway, which leads to mucosal damage. Cyclooxygenase occurs in two forms: COX I, the constituitive enzyme, and COX II, the inducible form which is produced by cytokine stimulation in areas of inflammation. NSAIDS more specific for COX II are currently being developed (e.g. etodolac), as these drugs would have less effect on the COX I enzyme in the gastric mucosa.

Alcohol in high concentration damages the gastric mucosal barrier and is associated with acute gastric mucosal lesions and upper GI bleeding.

Information

- NSAIDs cause gastroduodenal erosions and ulcers (10–25% of patients on long-term NSAIDs).
- NSAIDs increase the incidence of complications in patients with both DUs and GUs (20 000 hospitalizations per year in USA).
- Rectal administration does not prevent upper GI adverse effects.
- Concurrent therapy with proton pump inhibitors or misoprostol may be used to prevent peptic ulcers.
- In patients with a long history of peptic ulcer disease, *Helicobacter pylori* should be looked for and eradicated prior to long-term NSAID therapy.
- An enteropathy and colitis can occur, producing diarrhoea.
- All NSAIDs, including aspirin, have been implicated in GI problems to varying degrees.
- H_2 receptor against (H_2RA) may be effective in preventing DUs.
- In patients who need to continue NSAIDs, H_2RAs, PPIs (proton pump inhibitors) or misoprostol can be used to heal the ulcer.

Information box 4.2 Non-steroidal anti-inflammatory drugs (NSAIDs) and the GI tract

Acute ulcers are also seen after severe stress (stress ulcers) and secondary to burns (Curling ulcers), trauma, shock, renal or liver disease. The underlying mechanism for these ulcers is unknown but may be related to an alteration in mucosal flow.

CLINICAL FEATURES

The correlation between the pathological changes and symptoms is poor, but some patients with acute gastritis may suffer from indigestion and vomiting, usually shortlived. Gastrointestinal haemorrhage can occur (see p. 244) usually from NSAIDS.

DIAGNOSIS AND TREATMENT

In many patients symptoms settle without diagnosis, but endoscopy is necessary in patients with a GI haemorrhage to confirm the presence of acute ulcers or erosions.

No specific therapy is required apart from removal of the offending cause, if possible.

Chronic gastritis

Chronic active gastritis consists of an infiltration of the lamina propria with lymphocytes and plasma cells. This can lead to the development of atrophic changes in the mucosa, including loss of parietal and chief cells, and subsequent intestinal metaplasia.

- *Helicobacter pylori* (*H. pylori*) is the chief cause of chronic active gastritis affecting the antrum and body of the stomach.
- Autoimmune gastritis affects the fundus and body of the stomach (pangastritis) and is the cause of pernicious anaemia. Auto-antibodies to gastric parietal cells and intrinsic factors are found in the serum (pernicious anaemia – p. 366).
- Chronic ingestion of NSAIDS or aspirin produces gastritis.
- Biliary reflux possibly produces gastritis.

CLINICAL FEATURES

A consistent relationship between upper gut symptoms and histological chronic gastritis has not been established. There may be a subset of patients in whom the gastritis accounts for the symptoms. Most chronic gastritis is asymptomatic and requires no treatment.

Helicobacter pylori and the upper gastrointestinal tract

H. pylori is a spiral-shaped Gram-positive urease-producing bacterium (Fig 4.10). Its complete genomic sequence is now known and available to all on the World Wide Web. It is found predominantly in the gastric antrum and in areas of gastric metaplasia in the duodenum. *H pylori* is found in greatest numbers under the mucus layers in gastric pits in close apposition to gastric epithelial cells.

(a) (b)

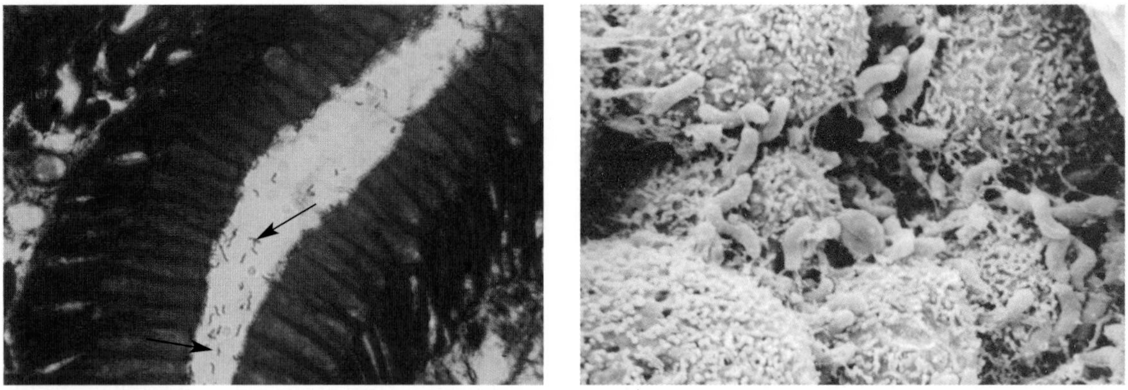

Fig 4.10
Helicobacter pylori.
(a) Organisms (arrows) are shown on the gastric mucosa (cresyl fast violet (modified Giemsa) stain) Courtesy of Dr Alan Phillips, Department of Paediatric Gastroenterology, Royal Free Hospital **(b) Scanning electron microscopy,** showing the spiral-shaped bacterium

EPIDEMIOLOGY

The exact mode of transmission is unclear, but intrafamilial clustering suggests person-to-person spread, either oral-oral or faeco-oral. Childhood acquisition of *H. pylori* is prevalent in developing countries and its presence is also associated with lower socioeconomic status worldwide. Between one and two-thirds of the Western populations have this infection and the prevalence is high in the older population – presumably acquired in their childhood.

MECHANISM OF ACTION

The possible pathogenetic factors of *H. pylori* infection result in:

- an increase in fasting and meal-stimulated gastrin release
- a decrease in somatostatin (D cells) in the antrum
- an increase in pepsinogen I secretion
- an alteration in the mucus protective layer
- cytotoxin release.

H. pylori causes tissue damage by releasing toxins – Vac A (vacuolating toxin) and Cag A (cytotoxin-associated protein). Type I *H. pylori* strains release both these toxins whilst type II are non-cytotoxic, Vac A negative and Cag A negative.

CLINICOPATHOLOGICAL FEATURES

Initially, *H. pylori* infection produces acute gastritis which rapidly becomes chronic active gastritis, and in some, peptic ulcer disease may develop. Some strains of *H. pylori* (Cag A positive strains) may be particularly associated with gastroduodenal disease. The fact that up to two-thirds of the population are *H. pylori* positive and only 10–15% of the general population develop a duodenal ulcer in their lifetime, is partly explained by the different infecting strains as well as host and environmental factors. In addition, *H. pylori* positive healthy volunteers have a decreased sensitivity to gastrin whereas duodenal ulcer patients hypersecrete acid in response to gastrin.

Longstanding chronic gastritis leads to atrophy and intestinal metaplasia which can lead to gastric cancer (see Fig 4.13), implicating *H. pylori* as a causative factor. Thus the earlier the *H. pylori* is acquired, the greater the risk of atrophy and metaplasia.

Over 90% of patients with gastric B cell lymphomas (mucosal-associated lymphoid tissue – MALT lymphoma) have *H. pylori*. Recently it has been shown that *H. pylori* gastritis contains the clonal B cell that eventually gives rise to the MALT lymphoma. Low-grade tumours have been shown to regress with *H. pylori* eradication. This association with malignancy has led to the view that all patients with *H. pylori* infection should have eradication therapy.

H. pylori is present in a greater proportion of patients with non-ulcer dyspepsia, than in asymptomatic controls. The relationship with symptoms is poor, and its significance unclear.

DIAGNOSIS

Non-invasive methods

- **Urea breath test with ^{13}C or ^{14}C** (see p. 253, but using urea as the substrate). This is a quick and easy way of detecting the presence of *H. pylori* and is used as a screening test. ^{13}C urea avoids using a radioisotope, but the measurement of $^{13}CO_2$ in the breath requires a mass spectrometer which is expensive and not available in every hospital. The breath test is also used to demonstrate eradication of the organism following treatment.
- **Serological tests** detect IgG antibodies and are reasonably sensitive and specific. They are used in the diagnosis and in epidemiological studies. IgG titres may take up to one year to fall by 50% after eradication therapy and therefore are not useful for confirming eradication. Antibodies can also be found in the saliva, but tests are currently not as sensitive or specific as serology.

Invasive (endoscopy)

- **Rapid urease test**. Gastric biopsies are added to a urea solution containing phenol red. If *H. pylori* is present, the urease enzyme splits the urea to release ammonia which raises the pH of the solution and causes a rapid colour change. Gel kits are available commercially.
- **Culture**. Biopsies obtained can be cultured on special medium and sensitivities to antibiotics can be ascertained, if necessary.
- **Histology**. *H. pylori* can be detected histologically on routine (Giemsa) stained sections of gastric mucosa obtained at endoscopy.

ERADICATION THERAPY

If *H. pylori* infection is demonstrated, with or without peptic ulceration, eradication therapy should be given.

In patients with peptic ulcer disease, eradication of the organism leads to a 'cure' with a very low recurrence of ulceration unless re-infection occurs. This is, however, uncommon (1%) in developed countries, although high (50%–60%) in developing countries, where compliance may be poor.

There are several regimens for eradication, but all regimens must take into account the following factors:

- the necessity of good compliance with the chosen treatment regimen
- the high incidence of antibiotic resistance to metronidazole (25%+)
- the increased side effects of treatment with oral metronidazole
- bismuth chelate is unpleasant to take, even as tablets.

Currently favoured *regimens* use proton-pump inhibitor (PPI)-based triple therapy (rather than bismuth) along with two antibiotics for one week. For example:

- omeprazole (PPI) 20 mg twice daily + metronidazole 400 mg twice daily and clarithromycin 250 mg twice daily
- omeprazole 20 mg twice daily + metronidazole 400 mg twice daily and amoxycillin 1 g twice daily.

Resistance to amoxycillin has not yet been demonstrated. Clarithromycin can be substituted for metronidazole if resistance to the latter is suspected in the second regimen.

Tripotassium dicitratobismuthate (bismuth chelate) binds to the ulcer crater and stimulates prostaglandin secretion. It is effective against *H. pylori* and is used in some eradication therapies with two antibiotics. It blackens the tongue and stools.

In some regimens, H_2-receptor antagonists are included instead of a PPI (e.g. ranitidine 150 mg twice daily).

Ménétrièr's disease

Ménétrièr's disease is a rare condition in which there is thickening and enlargement of the gastric mucosal folds. Histologically there is hyperplasia of the mucin-producing cells with glandular proliferation and loss of the parietal and chief cells. Hypochlorhydia is usually present.

The patient may complain of epigastric pain and occasionally peripheral oedema may occur due to hypoalbuminaemia resulting from protein loss through the gastric mucosa. It is possibly premalignant.

Recent evidence suggests that many of these patients have *H. pylori* and that they improve with eradication therapy.

Management of dyspepsia in the community

Dyspepsia (or indigestion) is very common in the general population. Over-the-counter antacids and H_2-receptor antagonists are available and are widely used.

In young people (<45 years) with dyspepsia, significant gastrointestinal pathology is very uncommon. Investigation with endoscopy is therefore not necessary. Their *H. pylori* status can be assessed serologically and, if positive, eradication therapy instituted. Further investigation should be reserved for those who remain symptomatic and for those whose *H. pylori* test is negative.

Older people (>45 years) with persistent dyspepsia, who have had *H. pylori* eradication therapy, and all patients with 'alarm symptoms' such as dysphagia, weight loss or gastrointestinal bleeding, must be investigated with endoscopy to exclude significant organic disease.

THERAPIES

Antacids are described on p. 228.

H_2-receptor antagonists have molecular structures that fit the H_2-receptors on the parietal cells. They can produce up to 80% reduction in nocturnal acid production. They are useful in the mangement of dyspepsia and are part of some *H. pylori* eradication regimens. There is little difference between the several H_2-receptor antagonists available, but some have side effects and cross-react with other medication, such as warfarin.

Peptic ulcer disease

This is mainly due to *Helicobacter pylori* infection; most peptic ulcers occur in the stomach or proximal duodenum. The other main cause of peptic ulceration is NSAIDs. Peptic ulcers can also occur in the oesophagus (with oesophageal reflux), in the jejunum due to the Zollinger–Ellison syndrome, after a gastroenterostomy at the anastamotic (stomach) site, or in a Meckel's diverticulum which contains ectopic gastric mucosa.

EPIDEMIOLOGY

Duodenal ulcers (DUs) are very common and are two to three times more common than gastric ulcers (GUs). Approximately 15% of the population will suffer from a DU. Ulcer rates are declinig rapidly for younger men and increasing for older individuals, particularly women. Both DUs and GUs are common in the elderly. There is a considerable geographical variation; for example, DUs are more common in northern England and Scotland than in other parts of the UK.

AETIOLOGY

The traditional theory that peptic ulcers are due to an imbalance between acid and pepsin against the mucosal defences (mucus, bicarbonate, prostaglandins) is probably one of several aetiological factors, many of which are influenced by infection with *H. pylori*. DU patients with *H. pylori* infection secrete more acid after stimulation by gastrin and have more parietal cells in the stomach than healthy people with *H. pylori* infection.

Non-steroidal anti-inflammatory drugs cause gastric ulceration, but the evidence for producing chronic duodenal ulceration is not so convincing. Peptic ulcers are also said to be increased in certain diseases (hyperparathyroidism, as calcium stimulates acid secretion; cirrhosis; chronic obstructive pulmonary disease) but this may be due to false correlations.

Genetic susceptibility may play a role. Peptic ulceration is more common in patients who have blood group O and are non-secretors of blood group substances in the saliva.

PATHOLOGY

Gastric ulcers are found in any part of the stomach, but are most commonly seen on the lesser curve. Most duodenal ulcers are found in the duodenal cap; the surrounding mucosa appears inflamed, haemorrhagic or friable (duodenitis).

Histologically, there is a break in the superficial epithelial cells penetrating down to the muscularis mucosa at the site of the ulcer; there is a fibrous base and an increase in inflammatory cells. *H. pylori* may be found scattered on the surface of the gastric mucosa or in the ectopic gastric mucosa in the duodenum. There is an associated chronic active gastritis.

CLINICAL FEATURES

The characteristic feature is epigastric pain. It has been shown that if a patient points to the epigastrium as the site of the pain this has a high discriminatory value for diagnosis. The relationship of the pain to food is variable and on the whole not helpful in the diagnosis. The pain of duodenal ulceration classically occurs at night (as well as during the day) and is worse when the patient is hungry. Both gastric and dudoenal ulcers are helped by antacids.

Nausea may accompany the pain; vomiting is infrequent but often relieves the pain. Heartburn occurs owing to acid regurgitation. Anorexia and weight loss may occur, particularly with gastric ulcers. If the patient complains of persistent and severe pain, complications such as penetration into other organs should be considered. Back pain suggests a penetrating posterior duodenal ulcer. Severe ulceration can occasionally be symptomless as 50% of patients who have died from the complications of peptic ulceration were unaware of the diagnosis prior to the final event. Patients can present for the first time with either a haematemesis or melaena or a perforation.

Untreated, the symptoms of a duodenal ulcer are periodic with spontaneous relapses and remissions. The natural history is for the disease to remit over many years with the onset of gastritis with atrophy and a decrease in acid secretion. Fifty per cent of patients with gastric ulceration will have a recurrence within two years if untreated.

INVESTIGATION AND MANAGEMENT

If peptic ulcer disease is suspected, serology or a breath test is performed to confirm *H. pylori* status before the commencement of eradication therapy. Further investigation is required only in patients with persistent dyspepsia following successful eradication therapy (checked with a breath test) or in symptomatic patients who are *H. pylori* negative.

- **Endoscopy – for the exclusion of GORD or cancer**. All gastric ulcers (Fig 4.11) should be biopsied.
- **Barium meal** (double contrast) is less commonly used than endoscopy in this situation. A gastric ulcer and a duodenal ulcer are shown in Fig 4.12.
- **Acid secretion measurement** is not helpful in peptic ulcer disease. It may be measured in the Zollinger–Ellison syndrome, but a serum gastrin is more useful.

TREATMENT

Peptic ulcers associated with *H. pylori*

Successful eradication of *H. pylori* (see p. 237) results in healing rates of 90% and prevents recurrence of the ulcer. Anti-secretory treatment (PPI or H_2-receptor

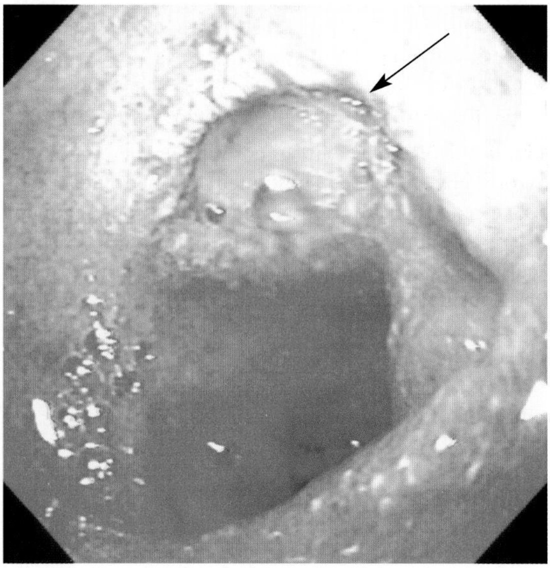

Fig 4.11
Endoscopic picture of a benign gastric ulcer

(a) (b)

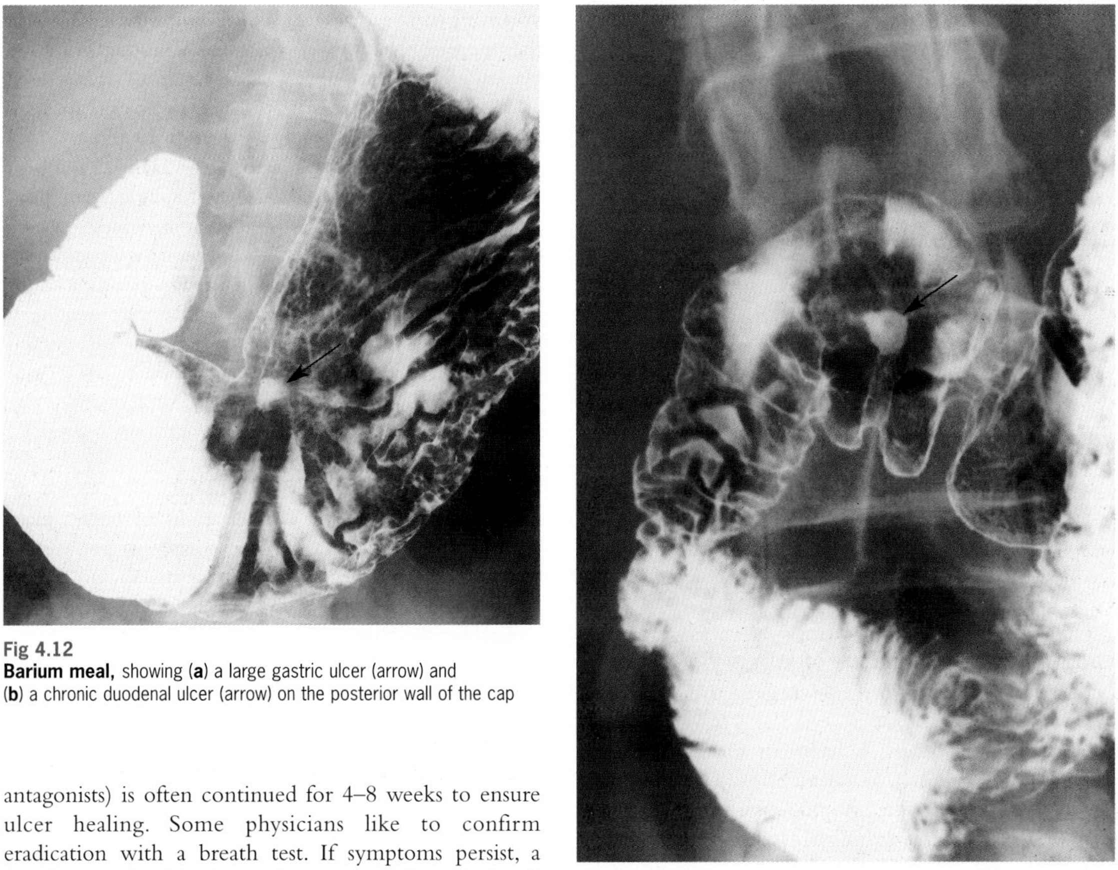

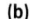

Fig 4.12
Barium meal, showing (**a**) a large gastric ulcer (arrow) and (**b**) a chronic duodenal ulcer (arrow) on the posterior wall of the cap

antagonists) is often continued for 4–8 weeks to ensure ulcer healing. Some physicians like to confirm eradication with a breath test. If symptoms persist, a breath test should always be performed and if still positive, a further course of eradication therapy with different antibiotics is given (p. 237).

Ulcers not associated with *H. pylori*

These are mainly due to NSAID ingestion. Treatment involves acid suppression and discontinuation of NSAIDs if possible. This may be difficult in those with severe arthritis, and proton-pump inhibitors, H_2-receptor antagonists or misoprostol may be used concurrently with NSAIDs.

- *Proton-pump inhibitors* (PPIs) include omeprazole 20 mg daily, lansoprazole 30 mg daily, or pantoprazole 40 mg daily. Recent evidence shows higher healing rates (80%) than with H_2-receptor antagonists and better patient tolerance than with misoprostol.
- *H_2-receptor antagonists* include cimetidine 800 mg, ranitidine 300 mg, famotidine 40 mg and nizatidine 300 mg, all daily.
- Misoprostol is a synthetic analogue of prostaglandin E1 and inhibits gastric acid secretion. It is mainly used as a cytoprotective agent against NSAID-associated gastric ulcers, particularly in the elderly. Prophylaxis is 200 mg, two to four times per day. The main side-effects are diarrhoea and abdominal pain.

Miscellaneous

Stopping smoking should be strongly encouraged as smoking slows healing. Special diets, together with the avoidance of coffee, alcohol or acid substances, are not required.

The effectiveness of treatment should be assessed symptomatically. There is no need for follow-up endoscopy for duodenal ulcers. Patients with gastric ulcers should be re-endoscoped at six weeks to exclude a malignant tumour. If the patient fails to respond, the diagnosis should be reviewed. Duodenal ulcers are common and care must be taken not to falsely attribute abdominal symptoms to the finding of an ulcer.

SURGICAL MANAGEMENT

Since the introduction of H_2-receptor antagonists in the 1970s and now the importance of *H. pylori*, surgery for peptic ulceration is rarely necessary and is used only for the complications:

- recurrent uncontrolled haemorrhage when the bleeding vessel is ligated
- perforation which is oversown.

For both of these conditions no other procedure, such as a gastrectomy or vagotomy, is required.

Two types of operation were performed:

- *Partial gastrectomy*. The principle for this was to remove the antral area that secretes gastrin, since this in turn stimulated acid production. In Billroth I partial gastrec-tomy, the lower part of the stomach was removed and the stomach remnant connected to the duodenum; in Billroth II (Polya gastrectomy), the stomach remnant was connected to the first loop of jejunum (a gastroenterostomy) and the duodenum closed.
- *Vagotomy*:
  (a) Truncal vagotomy plus gastroenterostomy/pyloroplasty
  (b) Selective vagotomy (preserving the hepatic and coeliac branch of the vagus) plus gastroenterostomy/pyloroplasty.
  (c) Highly selective vagotomy or proximal gastric vagotomy, in which only the nerves supplying the parietal cells were transected, and therefore no drainage was required. With this type of operation there was little diarrhoea but the recurrence rate was still 5–10%.

Long-term complications of surgery

Long-term complications of surgery are still seen occasionally.

A recurrent ulcer. A recurrent ulcer, which can occur in the stomach, duodenum or jejunum, often occurs at the stoma. The symptoms are similar to those seen in the unoperated stomach, with pain invariably being present, although patients may present with haemorrhage. Because of the deformity of the stomach, investigation by endoscopy is preferred to X-ray examination. Treatment is with acid suppression and eradication of *H. pylori*, if present. Consideration should be given to the possibility of the Zollinger–Ellison syndrome (see p. 352).

Dumping. This is the term used to describe a number of upper abdominal symptoms (e.g. nausea and distension associated with sweating, faintness and palpitations) that occur in patients following gastrectomy or gastro-enterostomy. It is due to 'dumping' of food into the jejunum, which is followed by rapid fluid dilution of the high osmotic load. A number of patients had mild symptoms of dumping but learned to cope with them. It was rare for it to be a clinical problem and, if it was, the symptoms had a functional element. Treatment was with reassurance and symptomatic therapy. Further operations were rarely needed.

Diarrhoea. This was chiefly seen after vagotomy. Urgency or recurrent severe episodes occurred in 1% and could be a major problem. Treatment consists of antidiarrhoeals such as codeine phosphate but is not entirely satisfactory. Cholestyramine – a resin that binds bile salts – helps in some cases. Very occasionally the diarrhoea or steatorrhoea can be due to bacterial overgrowth in the blind loop of a Polya gastrectomy (see p. 256).

Vomiting (afferent loop syndrome/bilious vomiting). The incidence of vomiting decreased with the more conservative operations. Vomiting occurred because food was trapped as a result of the altered anatomy. Treatment is symptomatic, except on the rare occasions when reconstructive surgery is required.

Nutritional complications. Anaemia is most commonly due to iron deficiency resulting from poor absorption. Treatment is with oral iron, which may be needed long-term. Megaloblastic anaemia is uncommon, but can be due to either folate deficiency (poor intake) or B_{12} deficiency (long-term gastritis with atrophy resulting in intrinsic factor deficiency). Osteomalacia is an uncommon late complication (see p. 510). Patients often fail to gain weight owing to anorexia after gastric surgery and a few suffer from severe protein-energy malnutrition as a result.

COMPLICATIONS OF PEPTIC ULCER

In all patients with any complications of peptic ulcer disease, *H. pylori* eradication is necessary (if positive). If the patient has been given eradication therapy previously a further course of eradication therapy is necessary, preferably following a positive breath test.

Haemorrhage

This is discussed on p. 243.

Perforation (Information box 4.3; see also p. 283)

The frequency of perforation of peptic ulceration is decreasing; this is partly attributable to better medical therapy. Duodenal ulcers perforate more commonly than gastric ulcers, usually into the peritoneal cavity; perforation into the lesser sac may occur.

Management of perforation. Detailed management is described on p. 283. Surgery is performed to close the perforation and drain the abdomen. Conservative management using nasogastric suction, intravenous fluids and antibiotics is occasionally used in elderly and very sick patients.

Information

Look for:

- other acute gastrointestinal conditions (e.g. cholecystitis, pancreatitis – check serum amylase)
- non-GI conditions (e.g. myocardial infarction)
- silent perforations in the elderly or patients on steroids.

Remember:

- There is harm in leaving an undiagnosed perforation.
- Avoid laparotomy if pancreatitis is diagnosed.

Information box 4.3 Perforation of peptic ulcer

Pyloric stenosis or obstruction

This is more accurately called *gastric outflow obstruction*, as the obstruction may be prepyloric or in the duodenum. The obstruction occurs either because of an active ulcer with surrounding oedema or because the healing of an ulcer has been followed by scarring. The obstruction can also be due to a gastric malignancy or external compression from a pancreatic carcinoma.

The main symptom of this condition is vomiting, usually without pain as the characteristic ulcer pain has abated owing to healing.

Vomiting is projectile and huge in volume, and the vomitus contains particles of yesterday's food. On examination of the abdomen the patient may have a succussion splash.

Severe or persistent vomiting causes loss of acid from the stomach and a metabolic alkalosis occurs (see p. 623).

The diagnosis is made by barium meal examination (less commonly by endoscopy) but can be suspected when large quantities of fluid are removed by gastric intubation in the fasting state. Fluid and electrolyte replacement is necessary, together with the regular removal of gastric contents via a nasogastric tube. In some patients with oedema rather than scarring, the symptoms will settle with this conservative management. However, most patients require surgery. Postoperative gastric stasis can be a problem, particularly if a vagotomy has been performed, even when accompanied by drainage.

Gastric tumours

Benign tumours

The most common benign tumour is a leiomyoma. This tumour is usually discovered by chance but it can occasionally ulcerate and produce haematemesis. Treatment is surgical removal.

Gastric polyps are uncommon and again are found usually by chance. They produce no symptoms. The most common are regenerative or hyperplastic polyps, which are often multiple and require no treatment. Rarely adenomatous polyps are found and endoscopic removal is recommended because of possible malignant potential. Most gastric cancers appear not to arise from pre-existing adenomas (in contrast to colonic carcinomas).

Malignant tumours

Carcinoma of the stomach (see Fig 4.1) is one of the most common malignant tumours of the GI tract and is the sixth most common fatal cancer in the UK. The frequency varies throughout the world, being high in Japan and Chile and relatively low in the USA.

In the UK, 15 per 100 000 males are affected per year. Although the overall world-wide incidence of gastric carcinoma appears to be falling, even in Japan, proximal gastric cancers are increasing in the West. The incidence increases with age, being rare under the age of 30 years, and more men than women are affected.

EPIDEMIOLOGY AND PATHOGENESIS

There is a strong link between *H. pylori* infection and gastric cancer. *H. pylori* infection results in chronic gastritis which eventually leads to gastritis with atrophy and intestinal metaplasia – a premalignant pathological change (Fig 4.13). Much of the earlier epidemiological data (i.e. the increase of cancer in lower socioeconomic groups) can be explained by the intrafamilial spread of *H. pylori*.

Dietary factors may still be important as both initiators and promoters may have separate roles in carcinogenesis. Diets high in salt probably increase the risk. Dietary nitrates can be converted into nitrosamines by bacteria at neutral pH, and nitrosamines are known to be carcinogenic in animals. Nitrosamines are also present in the stomach of patients with achlorhydria who have an increased cancer risk. Consumption of diets high in vegetables and fruits, and low in salt, protect against cancer. Smoking is also associated with an increased incidence of stomach cancer.

Genes underlying the inherited susceptibility to gastric cancer have not yet been identified, but certain patterns are emerging as seen in colonic cancer. There is a higher incidence of gastric cancer in blood group A patients.

Benign gastric ulcers have not been shown to develop into gastric cancer. It can, however, be difficult to differentiate a benign ulcer from a malignant ulcer, as even malignant ulcers can partially heal on medical treatment. For these reasons it was originally thought that gastric ulcers could become malignant.

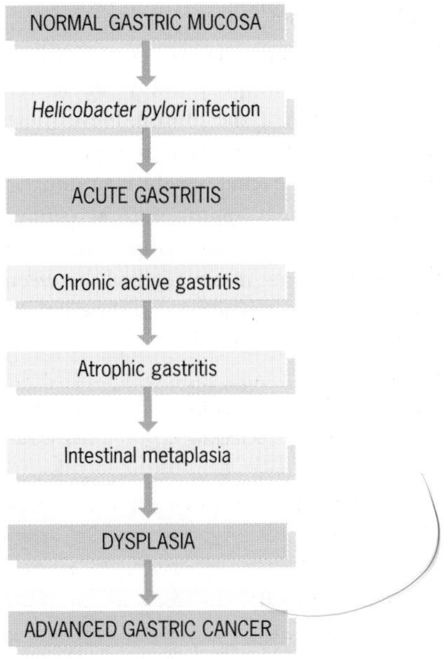

Fig 4.13
Flow diagram showing the development of gastric cancer associated with *H. pylori* infection

Pernicious anaemia carries a small increased risk of developing gastric carcinoma. Gastritis with atrophy present in the body and fundus of the stomach of these patients may be a precancerous lesion.

There is an increased risk of gastric cancer after a partial gastrectomy (*post-operative stomach*) whether performed for a gastric or a duodenal ulcer. This may be a reflection of *H. pylori* causing the original ulceration.

SCREENING

Gastric cancer has an appalling prognosis despite treatment, and earlier diagnosis has been advocated in an attempt to improve this. Unfortunately, earlier diagnosis does not necessarily mean longer survival. The patient is merely operated on at an earlier date and, although the survival may appear longer, death will still occur at the same time from the point of genesis of the cancer (called lead time bias) (Fig 4.14).

With lead time bias a greater number of slowly growing tumours are detected when screening asymptomatic individuals. In Japan, mass screening with mobile X-ray units has increased the proportion of early gastric cancers diagnosed. Early gastric cancer is defined as a carcinoma that is confined to the mucosa or submucosa. It is associated with five-year survival rates of approximately 90%. In a large series of patients with gastric cancer from the UK, only 0.7% were identified as having early gastric cancer and therefore screening would not be warranted.

An effective screening procedure should:

- be cheap
- be acceptable to all social groups so that they attend for examination
- have a good discriminatory index from benign lesions
- result in an improvement in prognosis.

Unless all these criteria are fulfilled, screening is unwarranted except possibly in individuals with an increased risk for the disease. Nevertheless, even in this high-risk group, screening asymptomatic subjects is not justified as the overall benefit is minimal.

An alternative approach to screening asymptomatic patients is to investigate symptomatic patients as quickly as possible. The mean interval between the onset of symptoms and attendance at hospital is approximately

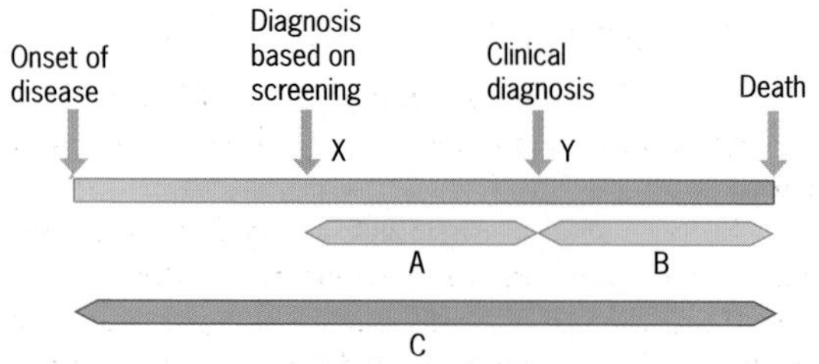

Fig 4.14
Lead time bias. Earlier diagnosis, at X, made by screening tests before the clinical diagnosis, at Y, suggests an increased survival time of A + B compared with B. The actual survival time (C) remains unchanged

6–9 months. However, dyspepsia is very common in the general population without any gastric lesions and it would obviously be impracticable for every dyspeptic member of the general population to consult a physician. Even if they did, most primary physicians would think it unjustified to arrange a complicated series of investigations on the first visit.

Thus, the detection of early gastric cancer in symptomatic patients is not a feasible proposition at present in the UK.

PATHOLOGY

Most gastric cancers occur in the antrum and are almost invariably adenocarcinomas. The common type is 'intestinal' and the tumours are polypoid or ulcerating lesions with heaped-up, rolled edges. Intestinal metaplasia is often seen in the surrounding mucosa, often with *H. pylori*. The diffuse type is composed of scattered or small clusters of cells, often with extensive submucosal spread which may result in the picture of 'linitis plastica', where the stomach appears rigid on X-ray.

CLINICAL FEATURES

Symptoms

The most common symptom is epigastric pain, which is indistinguishable from the pain of peptic ulcer disease, both being relieved by food and antacids. The pain can vary in intensity, but may be constant and severe. Most patients with carcinoma of the stomach have advanced disease at the time of presentation, and also have nausea, anorexia and weight loss. Vomiting is frequent and can be severe if the tumour is near the pylorus. Dysphagia can occur with tumours involving the fundus. Gross haematemesis is unusual, but anaemia from occult blood loss is frequent.

Patients can present with metastases causing abdominal swelling due to ascites or jaundice due to liver involvement. Metastases also occur in bone, brain and lung, producing appropriate symptoms.

Signs

Nearly 50% of patients have a palpable epigastric mass with abdominal tenderness. Often weight loss is the only feature. A palpable lymph node is sometimes found in the supraclavicular fossa (Virchow's node) and signs of metastases are present in up to one-third of patients. Carcinoma of the stomach is the cancer most frequently associated with dermatomyositis (p. 492) and acanthosis nigricans.

INVESTIGATIONS

- **Routine full blood count and liver biochemistry**.
- **Barium meal**. A good-quality double-contrast barium meal has a diagnostic accuracy of up to 90%. The carcinoma is usually seen as a filling defect or an

irregular ulcer with rolled edges. With a diffuse (linitis plastica) infiltrating type, the X-ray may show a rigid stomach.

- **Gastroscopy** (Fig 4.15). Gastroscopy is usually performed as the primary procedure and has the advantage that biopsies can be performed for histological assessment and to exclude lymphoma. Positive biopsies can be obtained in almost all cases of obvious carcinoma, but a negative biopsy does not necessarily rule out the diagnosis. For this reason, 8–10 biopsies should be taken from around the ulcer margin and its base. Superficial brushings for cytology will further improve the diagnostic rate.
- **CT and ultrasound**. CT can demonstrate gastric wall thickening, but has limited vlaue in determining tumour invasion into adjacent tissues. Ultrasound can demonstrate masses and wall thickening. Liver secondaries can be detected. Endoscopic ultrasound can demonstrate the penetration of the cancer through the gastric wall and extension into lymph nodes. It complements CT and ultrasound.

TREATMENT

The five-year survival rate of patients operated on for early gastric cancer (EGC) in Japan is 90%, but outside Japan EGC is rare. Surgery remains the best form of treatment if the patient is operable. Better preoperative staging has reduced the numbers undergoing operation and has improved the overall five-year survival rates to around 30%. Five-year survival rates in curative operations are as high as 50%. Despite these improved figures, the overall survival rate for a patient with gastric carcinoma has not dramatically improved, with a 10% five-year survival.

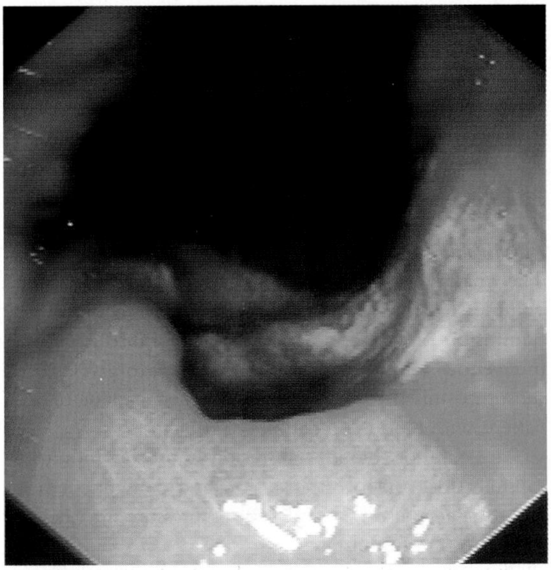

Fig 4.15
Carcinoma of the stomach. Endoscopic picture showing a large irregular ulcer with rolled edges

Treatment with chemotherapy (see p. 441) is often given for unresectable lesions. Survival may be prolonged by a few months and better results are being obtained with a combination of cytotoxic agents. Adjuvant chemotherapy following apparently curative surgery has not been clinically successful.

Palliative care with relief of pain and counselling is essential, as described on p. 442.

Primary lymphoma

Lymphoma of the stomach can account for 10% of all gastric malignancies in the developed world. It is a non-Hodgkin's lymphoma of the B-cell type. Gastric lymphomas in mucosal-associated lymphoid tissue (MALT) are caused by *Helicobacter pylori* (p. 236). The clinical presentation is the same as with gastric carcinoma. Lymphomas due to *H. pylori* can be treated successfully by eradication therapy. Otherwise, treatment is surgical with postoperative radiotherapy and chemotherapy. Prognosis is good, with a 75% five-year survival depending on the type of lymphoma.

FURTHER READING

Blaser MJ (ed) (1998) *Helicobacter pylori* infection, atrophic gastritis and gastric cancer. *Alimentary Pharmacology and Therapeutics* **12**: Suppl 1.

Blok N (1997) Carcinoma of the stomach. *Quarterly Journal of Medicine* **90**: 735.

Dent J, Talley NJ (eds) (1997) Heartburn and dyspepsia. *Alimentary Pharmacology and Therapeutics* **11**: Suppl 2.

Hawkey CJ et al (1998) Omeprazole compared with misoprostol for ulcers associated with NSAIDS. *New England Journal of Medicine* **338**: 727–734.

Laine L (ed) (1997) Management of *H. pylori* infection. *Alimentary Pharmacology and Therapeutics* **11**: Suppl 1.

Acute and chronic gastrointestinal bleeding

This section should be read in conjunction with the descriptions of the specific conditions mentioned.

Acute upper gastrointestinal bleeding

Haematemesis is the vomiting of blood. Melaena is the passage of black tarry stools; the black colour is due to altered blood – 50 mL or more is required to produce this. Melaena can occur with bleeding from any lesion from areas proximal to and including the caecum. Following a massive bleed from the upper GI tract, unaltered blood (owing to rapid transit) can appear per rectum, but this is rare. The colour of the blood appearing per rectum is dependent not only on the site of bleeding but also on the time of transit in the gut.

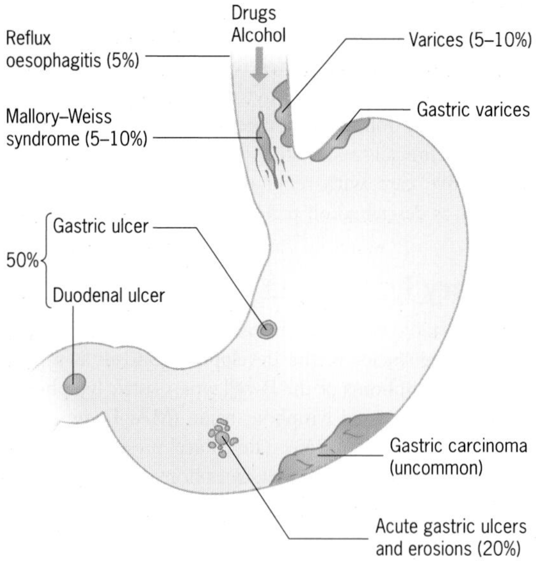

Other uncommon causes
Hereditary telangiectasia (Osler–Weber–Rendu syndrome)
Pseudoxanthoma elasticum
Blood dyscrasias
Dieulafoy gastric vascular abnormality
Portal gastropathy

Fig 4.16
Causes of upper gastrointestinal haemorrhage. The approximate frequency is also given

AETIOLOGY

Chronic peptic ulceration still accounts for approximately half of all cases of upper GI haemorrhage. This and other causes are shown in Fig 4.16. The relative incidences of these causes vary depending on the patient population.

Drugs. Aspirin and other non-steroidal anti-inflammatory drugs can undoubtedly produce gastric lesions. These agents are also responsible for GI haemorrhage from both duodenal and gastric ulcers, particularly in the elderly. Corticosteroids in the usual therapeutic doses probably have no influence on GI haemorrhage.

CLINICAL APPROACH TO THE PATIENT

All cases with a recent (i.e. within 48 hours) significant gastrointestinal bleed should be sent to hospital. In many, no immediate treatment is required as often there has been only a small amount of blood loss and the patient's cardiovascular system can compensate for this. Approximately 85% of patients stop bleeding spontaneously within 48 hours. The cause of the haemorrhage may be obvious from the history, such as a long history of indigestion or, more significantly, previous haemorrhage from an ulcer. A history of aspirin or non-steroidal anti-inflammatory drug ingestion suggests acute ulceration.

The following are factors that will affect the management:

- age (see below)
- the amount of blood lost, which may give some guide to the severity
- continuing visible blood loss
- signs of chronic liver disease on examination
- presence of the classical clinical features of shock (pallor, cold nose, tachycardia and low blood pressure – see Emergency box 4.1).

! Emergency

- History and examination.
- Monitor the pulse and blood pressure half-hourly.
- Take blood for haemoglobin, urea, electrolytes, grouping and cross-matching.
- Establish intravenous access – central line if brisk bleed.
- Give blood transfusion/colloid if necessary.
  Indications for blood transfusion are:
  (a) SHOCK (pallor, cold nose, systolic BP below 100 mmHg, pulse >100 bpm)
  (b) haemoglobin <10 g dL^{-1} in patients with recent or active bleeding.
- Urgent endoscopy.
- Continue to monitor pulse and BP.
- RE-endoscope for continued bleeding/hypovolaemia.
- Surgery.

Emergency box 4.1 Management of acute gastrointestinal bleeding

With liver disease the bleeding is often severe and recurrent if it is from varices. Splenomegaly suggests portal hypertension but its absence does not rule out oesophageal varices. Liver failure can develop.

With shock, remember that the peripheral arterial constriction that occurs may keep the blood pressure falsely high.

IMMEDIATE MANAGEMENT

Urgent resuscitation is required in patients with large bleeds and the clinical signs of shock. Details of the management of shock are given in Fig 13.17. Many hospitals have multidisciplinary specialist teams with agreed protocols and these should be followed carefully.

Blood volume

The major principle is to rapidly restore the blood volume to normal. This can be best achieved by transfusion of whole blood via one or more large-bore intravenous cannulae. It may be necessary to give a blood substitute initially to a severely shocked patient or to a patient with blood compatibility problems.

The rate of blood transfusion must be monitored carefully to avoid overtransfusion and consequent heart failure. The pulse rate and venous pressure are the best guides to transfusion rates.

Anaemia does not develop immediately as haemodilution has not taken place, and therefore the haemoglobin level is a poor indicator of the need to transfuse. If the level is low (less than 10 g dL^{-1}) and the patient has either bled recently or is actively bleeding, transfusion may be necessary. In most patients the bleeding stops, albeit temporarily, so that further assessment can be made.

Endoscopy

Endoscopy should be performed as soon as practically possible, but urgently in patients with shock, suspected liver disease or with continued bleeding. Endoscopy can detect the cause of the haemorrhage in 80% or more of cases, but in some no definite lesion is found. In patients with a peptic ulcer, if the stigmata of a recent bleed are seen (i.e. a spurting artery, active oozing, fresh or organized blood clot or black spots) the patient is more likely to re-bleed.

At endoscopy:

- varices should be injected – see p. 319 for management of varices
- all bleeding ulcers should be either injected with adrenalin and a sclerosant or the vessel coagulated either with a heater probe or with laser therapy.

These methods reduce the incidence of re-bleeding, although they do not significantly improve mortality.

Drug therapy

There is little evidence that H_2-receptor antagonists or proton-pump inhibitors affect the mortality rate of GI haemorrhage, but they are usually given to patients with ulcers because of their longer term benefits. Octreotide (which reduces the splanchnic blood flow as well as acid secretion) can be given as an infusion if the bleeding is difficult to stop, although a meta-analysis of clinical trials has shown no clear benefit.

Important factors in reassessment

- Age is clearly significant. Below the age of 60 years mortality from GI bleeding is small, but above the age of 80 the mortality is greater than 20%.
- Patients with recurrent haemorrhage have an increased mortality.
- Most re-bleeds (approximately 25% of all cases) occur within 48 hours.
- Melaena is usually less hazardous than haematemesis.

Uncontrolled or repeat bleeding

Endoscopy should be repeated to assess the bleeding site and to treat, if possible. Surgery is necessary only if bleeding is persistent and/or uncontrollable.

Discharge policy

The patient's age, diagnosis on endoscopy, co-morbidity and the presence or absence of shock should be taken into consideration. In general, patients under the age of 60 years, as well as older patients who are dynamically stable and have no stigmata of recent haemorrhage on endoscopy, can be discharged from hospital within 24 hours. All shocked patients need careful observation.

Specific conditions

Chronic peptic ulcer. Eradication of *H. pylori* is started as soon as possible (see p. 237). A proton-pump inhibitor is continued for four weeks to ensure healing. If necessary to control haemorrhage, surgery with ligation of the bleeding vessel is performed, but no other surgical procedure is undertaken.

Gastric carcinoma. Most patients do not have large bleeds with this condition but surgery may be performed for the lesion itself.

Oesophageal varices. These are discussed on p. 318.

Mallory–Weiss tear. This is a linear mucosal tear occurring at the oesophagogastric junction and produced by a sudden increase in intra-abdominal pressure. It often occurs after a bout of coughing or retching and is classically seen after an alcohol binge. There may, however, be no antecedent history of retching. The haemorrhage may be large but most patients stop spontaneously and can be discharged from the hospital within 24 hours. Rarely, surgery with over-sewing of the tear will be required.

PROGNOSIS

The mortality from gastrointestinal haemorrhage has not changed from 5–10% over the years, despite many changes in management, partly owing to more patients being elderly. Early endoscopy has not so far reduced the mortality, although bleeding episodes are reduced.

Acute lower gastrointestinal bleeding

Massive bleeding from the lower GI tract is rare. On the other hand, small bleeds from haemorrhoids occur very commonly. Massive bleeding is usually due to diverticular disease or ischaemic colitis and may require urgent resuscitation. Surgery is rarely required as bleeding usually stops spontaneously. The causes of lower gastrointestinal bleeding are shown in Fig 4.17.

MANAGEMENT

The patient may need to be resuscitated. Then a diagnosis is made using the following investigations as appropriate:

- rectal examination (e.g. carcinoma)
- proctoscopy (e.g. haemorrhoids)
- sigmoidoscopy (e.g. inflammatory bowel disease)
- colonoscopy – for any mucosal lesion and removal of polyps
- angiography – vascular abnormality (e.g. angiodysplasia).

Individual lesions are treated as appropriate.

Chronic gastrointestinal bleeding

Patients with chronic bleeding usually present with iron-deficiency anaemia (see Chapter 6).

Chronic blood loss producing anaemia in all men and all women after the menopause is always due to bleeding from the gastrointestinal tract. Occult blood tests are therefore not necessary (Information box 4.4).

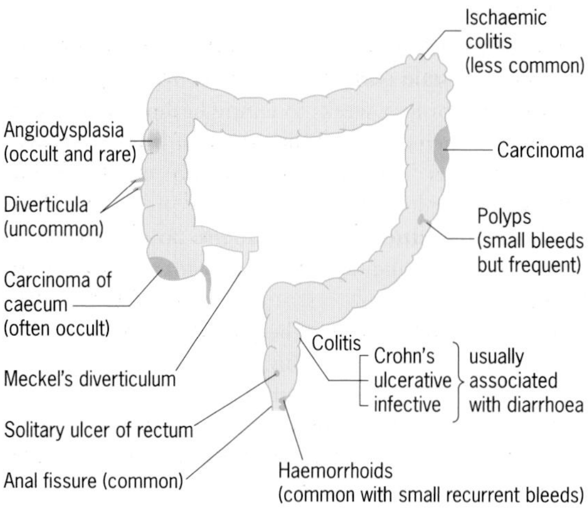

Fig 4.17
Causes of lower gastrointestinal bleeding. The sites shown are illustrative – many of the lesions can be seen in other parts of the colon

Information

This is frequently performed *unnecessarily*. It is *only* of value in:

- premenopausal women – if a history of menorrhagia is uncertain and the cause of iron deficiency is unclear
- mass population screening for large bowel malignancy.

Advantages: cheap and easy to perform.

Disadvantages: high false-positive rate, leading to unnecessary investigations.

Information box 4.4 Measurement of faecal occult blood

DIAGNOSIS

Chronic blood loss can occur with any lesion of the gastrointestinal tract that produces acute bleeding (see Figs. 4.16 and 4.17). In addition, a Meckel's diverticulum and carcinoma of the caecum may present with an iron-deficiency anaemia. It should be remembered that, world-wide, hookworm is the most common cause of chronic gastrointestinal blood loss.

Careful history and examination may indicate the most likely site of the bleeding, but if no clue is available it is usual to investigate both the upper and lower gastrointestinal tract endoscopically at the same session ('top and tail').

For practical reasons an upper gastrointestinal endoscopy is performed first as this takes minutes only, followed by colonoscopy when any lesion can be removed or biopsied. A barium enema is performed only if colonoscopy is unavailable.

A small bowel follow-through is the next investigation, but the diagnostic yield is very low.

Following negative investigations, an angiography may show the site of bleeding, particularly when acute bleeding is occurring. Occasionally intravenous technetium-labelled colloid may be used to demonstrate the bleeding site in a Meckel's diverticulum. Endoscopes to visualize the whole of the small bowel (enteroscopy) are available at specialist centres.

TREATMENT

The cause of the bleeding should be treated, if found. Oral iron is given to treat anaemia (see p. 362).

FURTHER READING

Langman MJS, Weil J, Wainwright P *et al.* (1994) Risk of bleeding peptic ulcer associated with individual non-steroidal anti-inflammatory drugs. *Lancet* **343**: 1075–1078

Rockall TA, Logan RFA, Devlin HB, Northfield TC (1995) Incidence of and mortality from upper gastrointestinal haemorrhage in the UK. *British Medical Journal* **311**: 222–226.

Rockall TA *et al.* (1996) National audit for acute upper gastrointestinal haemorrhage. *Lancet* **347**: 1138–1140.

The small intestine

STRUCTURE

The small intestine extends from the duodenum to the ileum. Its surface area is enormously increased by mucosal folds. In addition, the mucosa has numerous finger-like projections called villi and the surface area is further increased by microvilli (Fig 4.18). Each villus consists of a core containing blood vessels, lacteals (lymphatics) and cells (e.g. plasma cells and lymphocytes), and is covered by epithelial columnar cells that are absorptive. The crypts of Lieberkühn open into the lumen between the villi.

The epithelial cells are formed at the bottom of these crypts and migrate to the tops of the villi, from where they are shed. This process takes 3–4 days. On its luminal side the epithelial cell has a brush border of microvilli that is covered by the glycocalyx. The lamina propria contains plasma cells, lymphocytes, macrophages, eosinophils and mast cells. Scattered throughout the gut are peptide-secreting cells.

Most of the *blood supply* to the small intestine is via branches of the superior mesenteric artery. The terminal branches are end arteries – there are no local anastomotic connections.

Histochemically there are three types of *nerves* in the gut:

- cholinergic parasympathetic (with muscarinic or nicotinic receptors)
- adrenergic sympathetic (with both α and β receptors)
- non-cholinergic non-adrenergic.

For the latter the transmitters are thought to be either cyclic nucleotides and ATP (the purinergic system) or intestinal hormones (e.g. VIP – the peptidergic hypothesis) or nitric oxide.

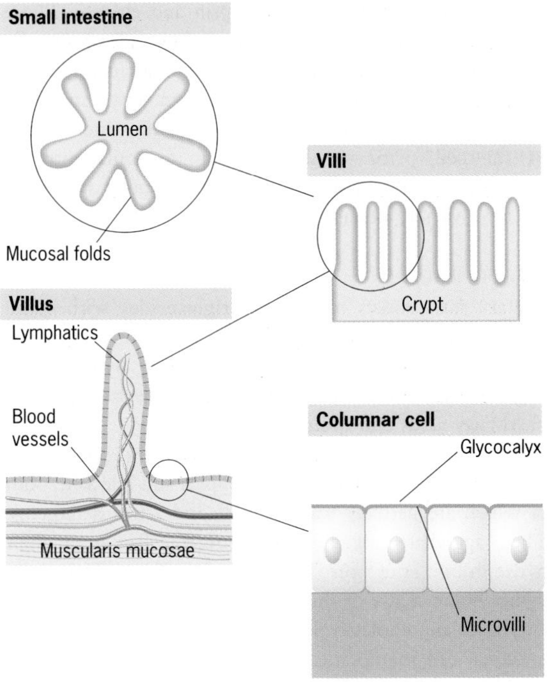

Fig 4.18
Structure of the small intestine

FUNCTIONS (Table 4.4)

The epithelial cells form a physical barrier permeable to ions, small molecules and macromolecules. The small intestine is concerned with the digestion and absorption of nutrients, salt and water. Digestive enzymes (e.g. proteases, disaccharidases) are produced by intestinal cells; some of these enzymes are membrane-bound whilst others (e.g. lipases produced by the pancreas) are associated with the glycocalyx. Nutrients can be absorbed throughout the small intestine with the exception of vitamin B_{12} and bile salts, which have specific receptors in the terminal ileum.

General principles of absorption

Simple diffusion

This process requires no energy and takes place if there is a concentration gradient from the intestinal lumen (high concentration) to the bloodstream (low concentration).

Table 4.4
Functions of the small intestine

Digestion and absorption
Continuous cell renewal and cell death
Defence against antigen entry
Structural
Immunological – innate (see p. 160); e.g. antimicrobial peptides, trefoil peptides
Immunological – acquired
Neuro-endocrine peptide production
Motor function – transit of nutrients

Active transport

This requires energy and can work against a concentration gradient. A carrier protein is required and the process is sodium-dependent. For example, glucose enters the enterocyte on the luminal side via a sodium-dependent carrier molecule (sodium/glucose cotransporter I, SGLTI) and leaves on the serosal side via a sodium-independent carrier (Glut 2) that is found in the basolateral membrane. An Na^+ gradient is maintained across the membrane by an energy-dependent sodium pump (Na^+–K^+-ATPase) that keeps the intracellular sodium concentration low (Fig 4.19).

Facilitated diffusion

This is an energy-independent carrier-mediated transport system that allows a faster absorption rate than simple diffusion (e.g. fructose absorption).

Absorption in the small intestine

Carbohydrate

Dietary carbohydrate consists mainly of starch with some sucrose and a small amount of lactose. Starch is a polysaccharide made up of numerous glucose units. Its hydrolysis begins in the mouth by salivary amylase. The

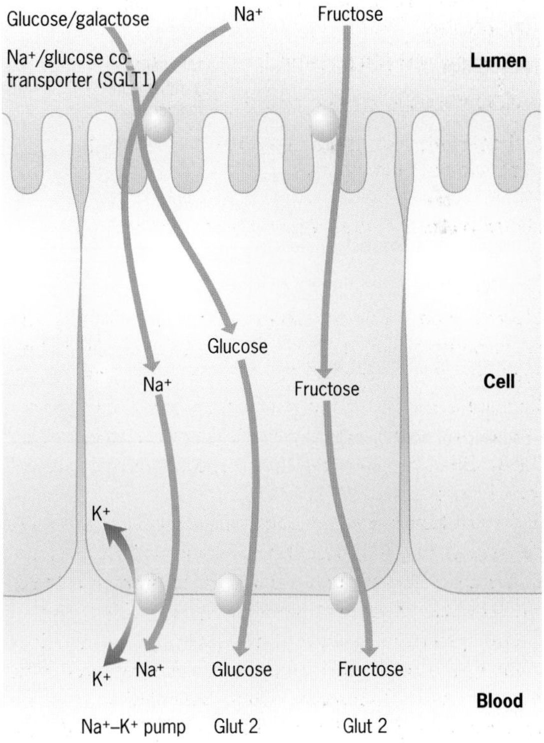

Fig 4.19
Solute (glucose, galactose, fructose) transport across the apical membrane, showing glucose/galactose sodium-linked transport. Galactose is transported by the same mechanism as glucose. Fructose is transported across the apical and basolateral membrane down the concentration gradient. The sodium–potassium ATPase pump is located in the basolateral membrane

Starch —Amylase→ { α-limit dextrins (5+ glucose units); maltotriose (3 glucose units); maltose (2 glucose units) }

majority of hydrolysis takes place in the upper intestinal lumen by pancreatic amylase. This hydrolysis is limited by the fact that amylases have no specificity for some glucose–glucose branching links.
These breakdown products, together with sucrose and lactose, are hydrolysed on the brush border membrane by their appropriate oligo- and disaccharidases to form the monosaccharides glucose, galactose and fructose. These monosaccharides are transported into the cells (Fig 4.19).

Protein

Dietary and endogenous proteins (desquamated cells, intestinal secretions) are mainly digested by pancreatic enzymes prior to absorption. These proteolytic enzymes are secreted as proenzymes and transformed to active enzymes in the lumen. The presence of protein in the lumen stimulates the release of enterokinase, which activates trypsinogen to trypsin, and this in turn activates the other proenzymes, chymotrypsin and elastase. These enzymes break down protein into oligopeptides. Some di- and tripeptides are absorbed intact by a carrier-mediated process, while the remainder are broken down into free amino acids by peptidases on the microvillus membranes of the cell, prior to absorption in a similar way to disaccharides. These amino acids are transported into the cell by a variety of carrier systems.

Fat (Fig 4.20)

Dietary fat consists mainly of triglycerides with some cholesterol and fat-soluble vitamins. Emulsification of fat occurs in the stomach and is followed by hydrolysis of triglycerides in the duodenum by pancreatic lipase to yield fatty acids and monoglycerides.

Bile enters the duodenum following gallbladder contraction. Bile contains phospholipids and bile salts, both of which are partially water-soluble and act as detergents. They aggregate together to form micelles with their hydrophilic ends on the outside. Trapped in the hydrophobic centre of this micelles are the monoglycerides, fatty acids and cholesterol; these are then transported to the intestinal cell membrane. At the cell membrane the lipid contents of the micelles are absorbed, while the bile salts remain in the lumen. Inside the cell the monoglycerides and

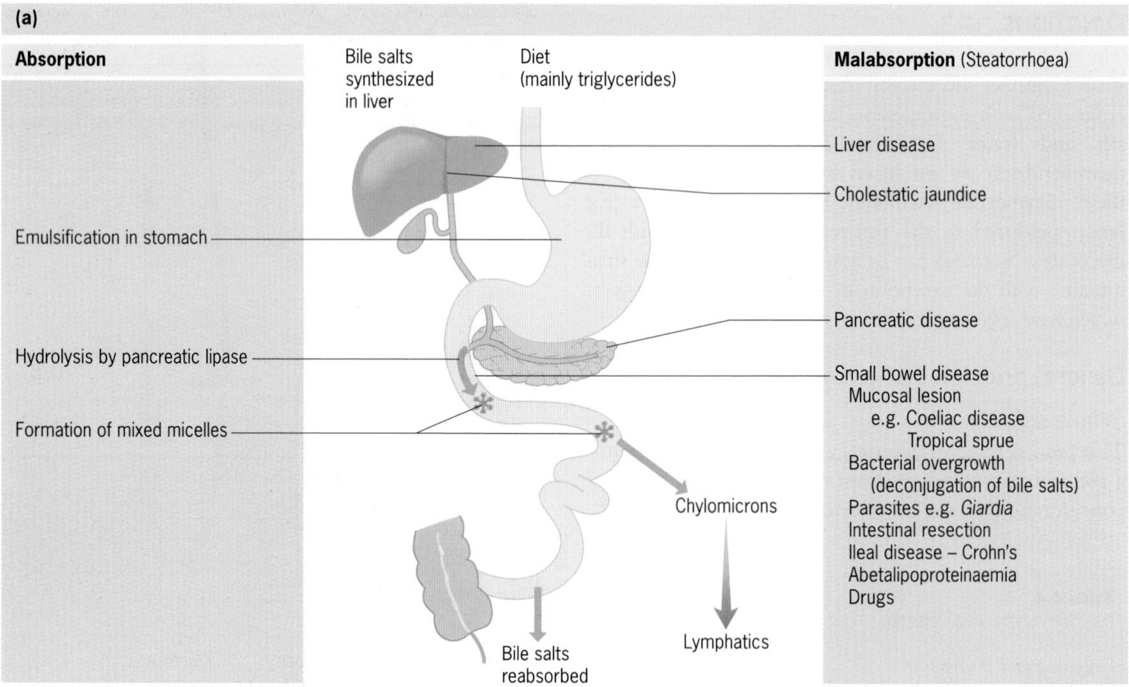

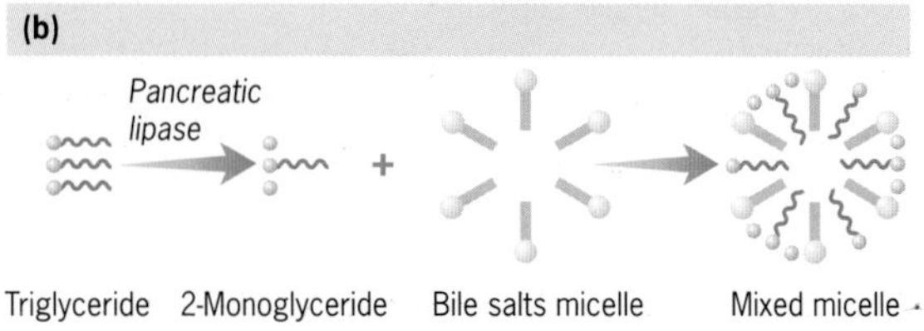

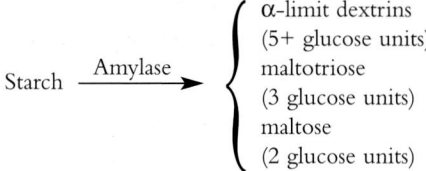

Fig 4.20
(a) The pathophysiology of fat absorption
(b) Diagram showing the formation of mixed micelles

fatty acids are re-esterified to triglycerides. The triglycerides and other fat-soluble molecules (e.g. cholesterol, phospholipids) are then incorporated into chylomicrons to be transported into the lymph.

Medium-chain triglycerides (which contain fatty acids of chain length 6–12) as well as a small amount of long-chain fatty acids are transported via the portal vein.

Bile salts are not absorbed in the jejunum, so that the intraluminal concentration in the upper gut is high. They pass down the intestine to be absorbed in the terminal ileum and are transported back to the liver. This enterohepatic circulation prevents excess loss of bile salts (see p. 290).

The pathophysiology of fat absorption is shown in Fig 4.20. Interference with absorption can occur at all stages, as indicated, giving rise to steatorrhoea.

Water and electrolytes

A large amount of water and electrolytes, partly dietary, but mainly from intestinal secretions, are absorbed coupled with monosaccharides and amino acids in the upper jejunum. Some water and electrolytes are absorbed in the ileum and right side of the colon, where active sodium transport occurs but this is not coupled to solute absorption. Intestinal secretion also takes place and abnormalities of this mechanism cause secretory diarrhoea (see p. 276).

Water-soluble vitamins, essential metals and trace elements

These all have to be absorbed in the small intestine. It must be remembered that vitamin B_{12} (see p. 365) is the only substance other than bile salts that is specifically absorbed in the terminal ileum alone, and malabsorption of both these substances will always occur following ileal resection.

Calcium absorption

Calcium absorption is discussed on p. 503.

Iron absorption

Iron absorption is discussed on p. 360.

Defence against antigens (see also p. 172)

The mucosa contains scattered lymphoid cells as well as lymphoid aggregates (e.g. the tonsils and Peyer's patches) to form the gut-associated lymphoid tissue (GALT) (Fig 4.21).

The normal mucosal immune system protects the host from micro-organisms and dietary proteins. Protective defence can be either innate or adaptive. *Innate* or natural immunity is provided in the gut by, for example, the mucus layer overlying epithelial cells, phagocytic cells, and enzymes (e.g. lysozyme which has antibacterial properties against Gram-positive organisms); also, the acid secreted by the stomach gives relative sterility to the small bowel. Recently, a novel form of innate immunity due to antimicrobial peptides has been described in animals. These peptides (defensins, magainins and cecropins) act in the lumen and at the mucosal surface and have potent activity against both Gram-negative and Gram-positive bacteria.

Adaptive immunity is provided by specific responses generated by the immune system. Antigenic priming of the GALT can give rise to specific secretory immunity, not only in the gut, but also in other mucosal-associated lymphoid tissue (MALT) (e.g. respiratory tract, lacrimal, salivary and

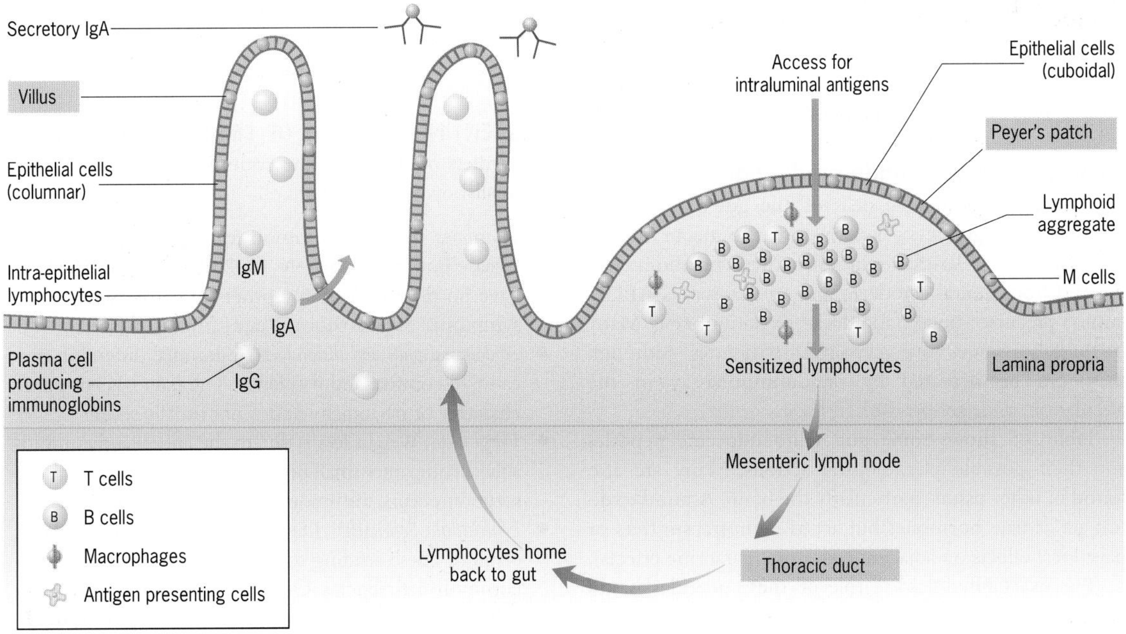

Fig 4.21
Small intestinal mucosa with a Peyer's patch, showing the gut-associated lymphid tissue (GALT)

mammary glands). This is because of the migration of specifically primed T and B cells from the GALT via the local mesenteric lymph nodes, and the thoracic duct and peripheral circulation back to the lamina propria (of gut or other mucosal tissue) where they become immunoglobulin (Ig)-producing plasma cells.

Local mucosal immunity is provided by the secretory immunoglobulin (sIg) system. There are approximately 10^{10} Ig-producing immunocytes (plasma cells and plasmoblasts) per metre of human small bowel, of which 70–90% are IgA immunocytes. Dimeric and polymeric IgA (pIgA) and IgM, containing a disulphide-linked polypeptide called 'J' (or 'joining') chain, are transported through the glandular epithelium via the transmembrane pIg receptor called 'secretory component' (SC) into the gut lumen. These antibodies are the first-line defence antigens in the lumen and may take part in the immunological homeostasis within the mucosa (e.g. dampening T-cell mediated hypersensitivity responses against harmless absorbed luminal antigens). SC expression can be up-regulated by lymphokines (e.g. IFNγ and TNFα) secreted by activated T-cells and macrophages respectively, thus promoting the transport of IgA and IgM into the lumen.

A specialized epithelial cell above the Peyer's patches, called the 'M' or 'membrane' cell, lacks SC and HLA-DR expression; these cells allow non-selective inward transport of luminal antigens. Antigens may also be taken up by other epithelial cells (expressing HLA-DR) on a genetically restricted basis and may subsequently be presented directly by antigen-presenting cells (macrophages) to primed (memory) T lymphocytes.

Intra-epithelial lymphocytes (IELs) are mainly T cells with a predominance of T8 (CD8+) cells, whereas the lamina prop-ria contains mainly T4 (CD4+) subsets. Most human IELs express the T cell receptor α/β (TCRα/β) which, along with considerable CD45RO expression, suggest that they are traditional memory T cells. Few cells express TCRγ/δ.

Neuroendocrine peptide production

The hormone-producing cells of the gut are scattered diffusely throughout its length and also occur in the pancreas. The cells that synthesize these hormones are derived from neural ectoderm and are known as APUD (amine precursor uptake and decarboxylation) cells. Many of these hormones have very similar structures. Although they can be detected by radioimmunoassay in the circulation, their action is often local.

Table 4.5 shows some gut neuroendocrine peptides and their possible physiological actions. Many are also found in other tissues, particularly the brain. A number do not act as true hormones but act as neurotransmitters or have local effects on adjacent cells only (paracrine effects).

The exact physiological role of these peptides is still being evaluated. Their importance clinically is that they may be secreted in excess, particularly in endocrine tumours of the pancreas (see p. 352).

Trefoil peptides

These are a family of small proteins each consisting of a three-loop structure. They help to protect the lining of the gastrointestinal tract by stabilizing the mucus in normal conditions and by up-regulating and stimulating the repair process (e.g. epithelial restitution) in acute injury. Intestinal trefoil factor (ITF) is produced predominantly by goblet cells of the small and large intestine, whereas spasmolytic polypeptide (SP) and p52 are produced in the stomach. All three trefoil peptides can also be secreted ectopically in the cells around damaged areas (e.g. in inflammatory bowel disease and peptic ulceration).

Gut motility

The contractile patterns of small intestinal muscles are primarily determined by integrated neural circuits within the gut wall – the enteric nervous system. The CNS and gut hormones also have a modulatory role on motility. During fasting, a distally migrating sequence of motor events termed the migrating motor complexes (MMC) occurs in a cyclical fashion. The MMC consists of a period of motor quiescence (phase I) followed by a period of irregular contractile activity (phase II), culminating in a short (5–10 minutes) burst of regular phasic contractions (phase III). Each MMC cycle lasts for approximately 90 minutes. In the duodenum, phase III is associated with increased gastric, pancreatic and biliary secretions. The role of the MMC is unclear, but the strong phase III contractions propel secretions, residual food and desquamated cells towards the colon, acting as an 'intestinal housekeeper'.

After a meal, the MMC pattern is disrupted and replaced by irregular contractions. This seemingly chaotic-fed pattern lasts typically for 2–5 hours, depending on the size and nutrient content of the meal. The irregular contractions of the fed pattern have a mixing function, moving intraluminal contents to and fro, aiding the digestive process.

PRESENTING FEATURES OF SMALL BOWEL DISEASE

Regardless of the cause, the common presenting features of small-bowel disease are:

- *Diarrhoea.* This is a common feature of small bowel disease but approximately 10–20% of patients will have no diarrhoea or any other gastrointestinal symptoms. Steatorrhoea is occasionally present.
- *Abdominal pain and discomfort.* Abdominal distension can cause discomfort and flatulence. The pain has no specific character or periodicity and is not usually severe.
- *Weight loss.* Weight loss is due to the anorexia that invariably accompanies small bowel disease. Although malabsorption occurs, the amount is small relative to intake.
- *Nutritional deficiencies.* Deficiencies of iron, B_{12}, folate or all of these, leading to anaemia, are the only common deficiencies. Occasionally malabsorption of other vitamins or minerals occurs, causing bruising (vitamin K deficiency), tetany (calcium deficiency), osteomalacia (vitamin D deficiency), or stomatitis, sore

Table 4.5
Gastrointestinal hormones

Hormone	Physiological action	Main gut localization
Peptides with similar structure		
Cholecystokinin(CCK)	Stimulates gallbladder contraction and colonic motility Pancreatic secretion (minor role) Role in satiety	Duodenum and jejunum Enteric nerves
Gastrin	Stimulates acid secretion Stimulates growth of gut mucosa	Gastric antrum, duodenum
Secretin and related peptides (all possess structural homology with secretin)		
Secretin	Pancreatic bicarbonate secretion	Duodenum and jejunum
Vasoactive intestinal polypeptide (VIP)	Intestinal secretion Splanchnic vasodilation	Enteric nerves
Peptide–histidine methionine	As for VIP	Enteric nerves
Glucose-dependent insulinotropic peptide (GIP)	Facilitates insulin release by islets ? Inhibits acid secretion	Duodenum
Enteroglucagon	? Inhibits acid secretion ? Contributes to glucagon effects on pancreas	Ileum
Glucagon-like peptide-1 (GLP-1)	Increases insulin secretion	Ileum – pancreas
Growth hormone releasing factor (GHRF)	Unclear	Small gut
Other		
Pancreatic polypeptide	? Inhibitor of pancreatic and biliary secretion	Pancreas
Peptide YY	Inhibition of pancreatic exocrine secretion	Ileum and colon
Neuropeptide Y	Regulation of intestinal blood flow	Enteric nerves
Motilin	Increases gastric emptying and small bowel contraction	Whole gut
Bombesin	Stimulates pancreatic exocrine secretion and gastric acid secretion	Whole gut and pancreas
Somatostatin	Inhibits secretion and action of most hormones	Stomach and pancreas
Galanin	Inhibits insulin secretion	Enteric nerves
Pancreastatin	Inhibits pancreatin exocrine and endocrine secretion	Pancreas
Substance P	? Unclear	Enteric nerves
Calcitonin gene-related peptide	? Unclear	Enteric nerves
Neurotensin	? Unclear	Ileum

tongue and aphthous ulceration (multiple vitamin deficiencies). Ankle oedema may be seen and is partly nutritional and partly due to intestinal loss of albumin.

PHYSICAL SIGNS OF SMALL BOWEL DISEASE

These are few and nonspecific. If present they are associated with anaemia and the nutritional deficiencies described above.

Abdominal examination is often normal, but sometimes distension and, rarely, hepatomegaly or an abdominal mass are found. In the severely ill patient, gross malnutrition with muscle wasting is seen. A neuropathy, not always due to B_{12} deficiency, can be present.

INVESTIGATION OF SMALL BOWEL DISEASE (Fig 4.22)

Blood tests

- **Full blood count and film**. Anaemia can be microcytic (low mean corpuscular volume – MCV) or macrocytic (high MCV). The blood film may also show other abnormal cells (e.g. Howell–Jolly bodies which are seen in splenic atrophy associated with coeliac disease).
- *If the MCV is low*, serum iron and total iron-binding capacity or serum ferritin are performed.
- *If the MCV is high*, serum B_{12}, serum and red cell folate are performed. However, with mixed deficiencies, the MCV may be normal. The red cell folate is a good indicater of the presence of small bowel disease. It is frequently low in both coeliac disease and Crohn's disease which are the two most common causes of small bowel disease in developed countries.
- **Serum albumin** gives some indication of the nutritional status.
- **Low serum calcium and raised alkaline phosphatase**. These may indicate the presence of osteomalacia.
- **Autoantibodies**. Measurement in the serum of antireticulin and/or endomysial antibodies are a useful adjunct for the diagnosis of coeliac disease.

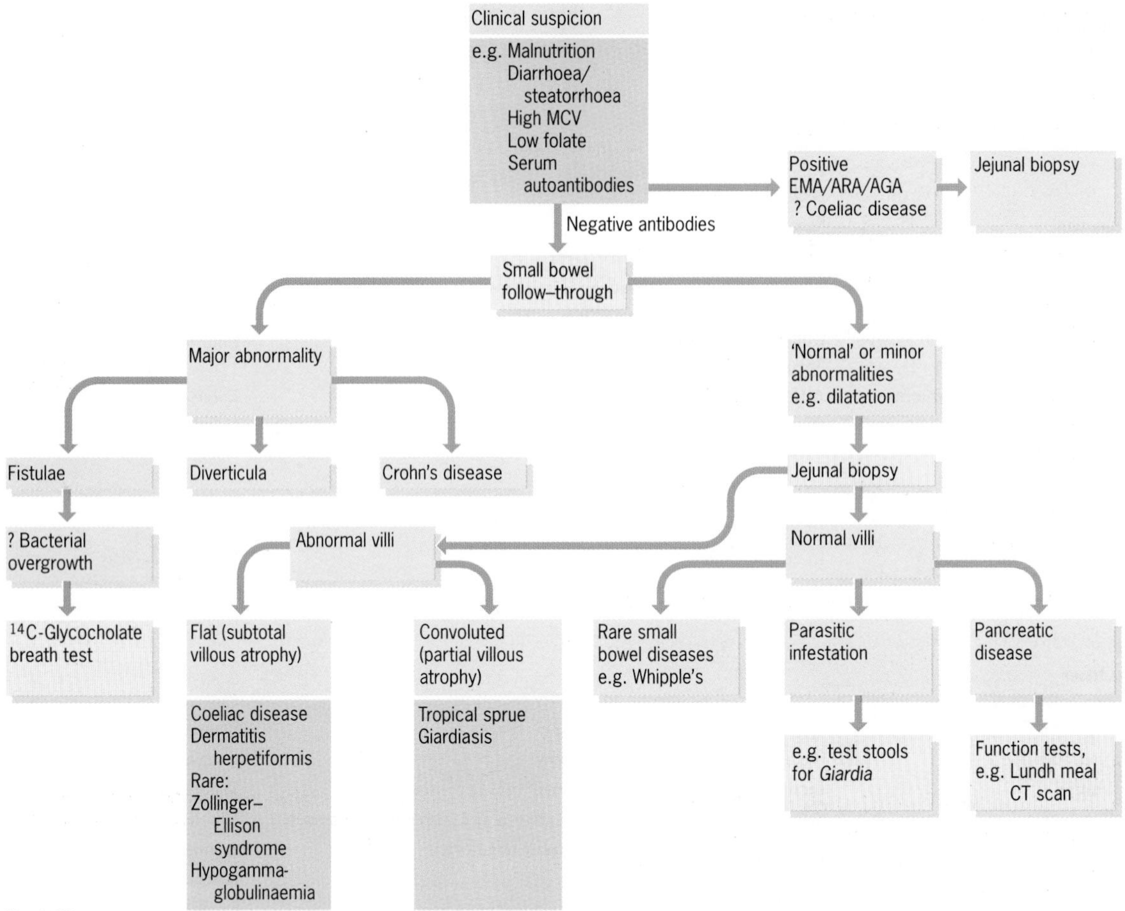

Fig 4.22
Flow diagram for investigation of patients with suspected small bowel disease. EMA, endomysial antibody; ARA, antireticulin antibody; AGA, antigliadin antibody

Small bowel anatomy

The macroscopic and microscopic appearances of the small bowel are studied unless the diagnosis has already been made (e.g. the presence of endomysial antibodies in coeliac disease).

- **Small bowel follow-through** (see p. 221). This detects gross anatomical defects such as diverticula, strictures and Crohn's disease. Dilatation of the folds and a changed fold pattern may suggest malabsorption but, as these are not specific findings, the diagnosis should not be based on these alone. Gross dilatation is seen in pseudo-obstruction.
- **Jejunal biopsy**. This is used to assess the microanatomy of the small bowel. Biopsies are usually obtained via an endoscope passed into the duodenum using large forceps. Alternatively, specimens can be obtained by swallowing a Crosby–Kugler capsule. With either technique, an adequate piece of tissue, well-orientated, is necessary for correct evaluation initially under a dissecting microscope. The histological appearances are described in the sections on individual diseases.

A smear of the jejunal juice or a mucosal impression can also be made and is helpful in the diagnosis of *Giardia intestinalis* (see p. 83).

Tests of absorption

These are required only in complicated cases.

- **Fat malabsorption**. The confirmation of the presence of steatorrhoea is only occasionally necessary. The fat content of stools is measured using a three-day collection of faeces with the patient on a diet containing 100 g of fat daily. Normal faecal fat excretion is less than 17 mmol (6 g) per day. To avoid faecal collections, fat absorption can also be measured using breath analysis. Following oral administration of a radiolabelled fat load, the amount of $^{14}CO_2$ in the expired breath gives an indication of the amount of fat malabsorption. Comparison between a labelled triglyceride (^{14}C triolein) and a labelled fatty acid (tritiated oleic acid) is used to diagnose pancreatic disease, when fatty-acid absorption will be normal.
- **D-Xylose tolerance test**. Xylose is a sugar which is absorbed from the proximal small intestine. The

urinary xylose excretion and the blood xylose level following an oral dose reflect its absorption. This test tends to produce many false-positives and should not be used in adults.

- **Lactose tolerance test**. This involves the oral ingestion of 50 g of lactose and the measurement of blood glucose. The test is of little use in adults as lactose intolerance is not a clinical problem since these patients avoid milk by choice. There is a high incidence of lactase deficiency in many parts of the world (e.g. the Mediterranean countries, and parts of Africa and Asia). It should be remembered that a glass of milk contains only approximately 11 g of lactose. A glucose tolerance test should not be performed, as it is influenced by many factors other than absorption.
- **Schilling test**. This is performed to look for vitamin B_{12} malabsorption. It is described in detail on p. 367. In gastrointestinal disease it is used to detect:
  (a) pernicious anaemia
  (b) ileal disease (when oral vitamin B_{12} given with intrinsic factor will show malabsorption)
  (c) bacterial overgrowth (measurement of vitamin B_{12} plus intrinsic factor absorption is repeated after antibiotics).

Other tests

- **^{14}C-glycocholic acid breath test** (Fig 4.23). This is performed to look for bacterial overgrowth (see below). The patient is given ^{14}C-labelled bile salts by mouth. Bacteria deconjugate the bile salts, releasing [^{14}C]-glycine, which is metabolized and appears in the breath as $^{14}CO_2$. This radioactivity in the breath can easily be measured. An early rise indicates either bacterial overgrowth in the upper small intestine or rapid transit to the colon where, of course, bacteria are normally present.
- **Hydrogen breath test**. This is frequently used as a screening test to detect bacterial overgrowth. Oral lactulose or glucose is metabolized by bacteria with the production of hydrogen. An early rise in the breath hydrogen will indicate bacterial breakdown in the small intestine. Rapid transit of the lactulose to the large intestine will also produce a rise in breath hydrogen. As bacteria are present in the oral cavity, the mouth should be rinsed out with an antiseptic mouthwash prior to the test being performed. This test is simple to perform and it does not involve radioisotopes. However, interpretation is often difficult.
- **Direct intubation**. Aspiration of intestinal juices is another method by which bacterial contamination can be detected, but is now seldom used. Bacterial counts are performed on aerobic and anaerobic cultures. Chromatography of bile salts can also be performed on the aspirate to detect evidence of deconjugation by bacteria.

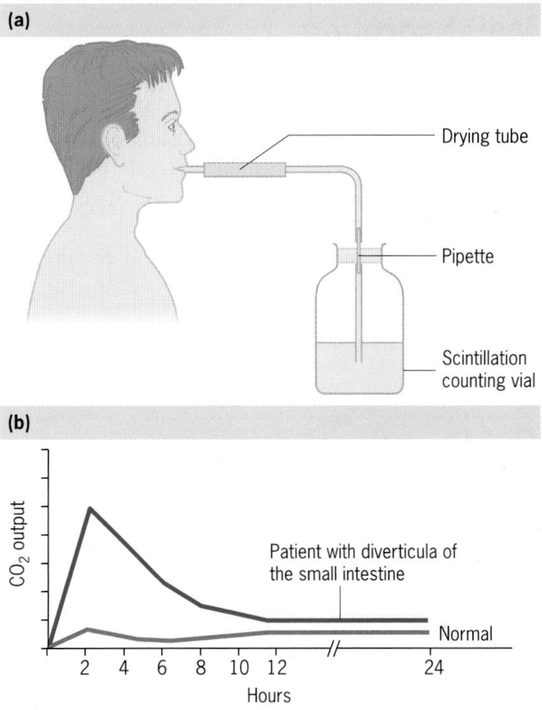

Fig 4.23
The ^{14}C-glycocholic acid breath test
(a) Apparatus
(b) The amount of $^{14}CO_2$ expired in the breath after an oral dose of ^{14}C-glycocholic acid in a normal subject and in a patient with diverticula of the small intestine

- **Pancreatic tests** (see p. 345). These are used in the differential diagnosis of steatorrhoea.
- **Other blood tests**. Serum immunoglobulins are measured to exclude immune deficiencies. Hormones (e.g. vasoactive intestinal peptide – VIP) are measured in high-volume secretory diarrhoea.
- **Test for protein-losing enteropathy**. Intravenous radioactive chromium chloride ($^{51}CrCl_3$) is used to label circulating albumin. In excess gastrointestinal protein loss, the faeces will contain radioactivity. This test is rarely required unless a low serum albumin is a major clinical feature.
- **Bile salt loss**. This can be demonstrated by giving oral 75-selena homotaurocholate (SeHCAT – a synthetic taurine conjugate) and measuring the retention of the bile acid by whole-body counting at seven days.
- **Intestinal permeability tests**. These tests can be used for the detection of small bowel disease but are not in general use. They are based on the fact that the abnormal intestinal mucosa is permeable to large molecules such as lactulose and cellobiose. An oral load of these sugars is given and the sugars are then measured in the urine. A radiolabelled sodium-EDTA solution has been used in a similar way and is said to be a more accurate investigation.

Malabsorption

In many small bowel diseases, malabsorption of specific substances occurs, but these deficiencies do not dominate the clinical picture. An example is Crohn's disease, in which malabsorption of vitamin B_{12} can be demonstrated, but this is not usually a problem and diarrhoea and general ill-health are the major features.

Steatorrhoea – malabsorption of fat – is discussed on p. 248.

The major disorders of the small intestine that cause malabsorption are shown in Table 4.6.

Table 4.6
Disorders of the small intestine causing malabsorption

Coeliac disease
Dermatitis herpetiformis
Tropical sprue
Bacterial overgrowth
Intestinal resection
Whipple's disease
Radiation enteritis
Parasite infestation (e.g. *Giardia intestinalis*)

Coeliac disease (gluten-sensitive enteropathy)

Coeliac disease is a condition in which there is an abnormal jejunal mucosa that improves morphologically when the patient is treated with a gluten-free diet and relapses when gluten is reintroduced. Gluten is contained in the cereals wheat, rye and barley. Oats are probably not harmful.

Dermatitis herpetiformis is a skin disorder that is associated with a gluten-sensitive enteropathy (see below).

INCIDENCE

Coeliac disease is common in Europe, with an incidence in the UK of approximately 1 in 1500. In Ireland, however, this is 1 in 300. It occurs throughout the world, but is rare in the black African.

There is an increased incidence of coeliac disease within families but the exact mode of inheritance is unknown; 10–15% of first-degree relatives will have the condition, although it may be asymptomatic. The haplotype HLA-A1, B8, DR3, DR7, DQ2 (DQA ° 0501, DQB1 ° 0201) is seen in coeliac disease. Over 90% of patients will have DQ2, compared with 20–30% of the general population. However, the fact that not all patients have this haplotype, and that as many as 30% of identical twins are discordant for the condition, suggests an additional factor, e.g. environmental.

AETIOLOGY

Gluten is a high-molecular-weight, heterogeneous compound that can be fractionated to produce α, β, γ, ω-gliadin peptides. α-Gliadin is injurious to the small intestinal mucosa although there is some disagreement about the toxicity of other peptides. The exact mechanism of how the damage is produced is still not understood. There are many immunological abnormalities that revert to normal on treatment. An immunogenetic mechanism may be possible in view of the increased incidence of the particular HLA haplotype. An environmental factor, such as a viral infection, may play a role. There is a sequence homology between gliadin and adenovirus 12 but this virus has not been substantiated as being an actiological factor.

PATHOLOGY

The mucosa of the proximal small bowel is predominantly affected, the mucosal damage decreasing in severity towards the ileum as the gluten is digested into smaller non-toxic fragments.

Under the dissecting microscope there is an absence of villi, making the mucosal surface flat. Histological examination shows that the crypts are elongated, with chronic inflammatory cells in the lamina propria (Fig 4.24). The lesion is described as *subtotal villus atrophy*, although true atrophy of the mucosa is not present because the crypt hyperplasia compensates for villus atrophy and the total mucosal thickness is normal. A partial villus atrophy can also be found.

The surface cells become cuboidal. There is an increase in the number of intra-epithelial lymphocytes which show an increased expression of the γ/δ T-cell receptor, instead of the α/β receptor, and this is specific to coeliac disease. In the lamina propria there is an increase in lymphocytes and plasma cells.

CLINICAL FEATURES

Coeliac disease can present at any age. In infancy it appears after weaning on to gluten-containing foods. The peak incidence in adults is in the third and fourth decades, with a female preponderance. The symptoms are very variable and often nonspecific with tiredness and malaise. Common GI symptoms include diarrhoea or steatorrhoea, abdominal discomfort or pain and weight loss.

Mouth ulcers and angular stomatitis are frequent and can be intermittent. Rare complications include tetany, osteomalacia, or gross malnutrition with peripheral oedema. Neurological symptoms such as paraesthesia, muscle weakness or a polyneuropathy can occur.

There is an increased incidence of atopy and autoimmune disease, including thyroid disease and insulin-dependent diabetes. Other associated diseases include inflammatory bowel disease, chronic liver disease, and fibrosing allergic alveolitis.

Physical signs are usually few and nonspecific and are related to anaemia and malnutrition.

INVESTIGATIONS

- **Endomysial antibodies** (IgA). These antibodies have a high sensitivity and specificity for the diagnosis of untreated coeliac disease. They are now the investigation of first choice. This immunofluorescent test is performed on monkey oesophagus or umbilical cord tissue and the antigen is a transglutamase. In the presence of a typical clinical picture and the presence of these antibodies, a confirmatory jejunal biopsy may not always be required.

- **Anti-reticulin antibodies** are also very sensitive but not so specific as they are seen in other gastrointesinal conditions (e.g. Crohn's disease).
- **Jejunal biopsy**. The mucosal appearance (Fig. 4.24) of a jejunal biopsy specimen is diagnostic. Other causes of a flat mucosa in adults are rare and are shown in Fig 4.22. At endoscopy, a dye can be injected on to the duodenal mucosa to accentuate the smoothness of the mucosa (positive dye test) before the biopsy is taken.
- **Haematology**. A mild or moderate anaemia is present in 50% of cases. Folate deficiency is almost invariably present in coeliac disease, giving rise in most instances to a high MCV. B_{12} deficiency is rare but iron deficiency due to malabsorption of iron and increased loss of desquamated cells is common. A blood film may therefore show microcytes and macrocytes as well as hypersegmented polymorphonuclear leucocytes and Howell–Jolly bodies (due to splenic atrophy).
- **Absorption tests** are often abnormal (see p. 252) but are seldom performed.
- **Small bowel follow-through** may show dilatation of the small bowel with a change in fold pattern. Folds become thicker and in the severer forms total effacement is seen.
- *In the severely ill patient*, other biochemical abnormalities are seen (e.g. hypoalbuminaemia).

TREATMENT AND MANAGEMENT

A gluten-free diet usually produces a rapid clinical and morphological improvement. Replacement haematinics are given initially to replace body stores. The usual cause for failure to respond to the diet is poor compliance. A gluten challenge – i.e. reintroduction of gluten with evidence of jejunal morphological change – confirms the diagnosis, but is only performed if the diagnosis is equivocal. A transient gluten intolerance has been described in early childhood.

Despite advice, many patients do not keep to a strict diet but nevertheless maintain good health. The long-term effects of this low gluten intake are uncertain. Osteoporosis is seen even in the treated case.

COMPLICATIONS

A few patients do not improve on a strict diet (unresponsive 'coeliac disease'). Often no cause for this is found, but intestinal lymphoma, ulcerative jejunitis or carcinoma are sometimes responsible. The incidence of small intestinal

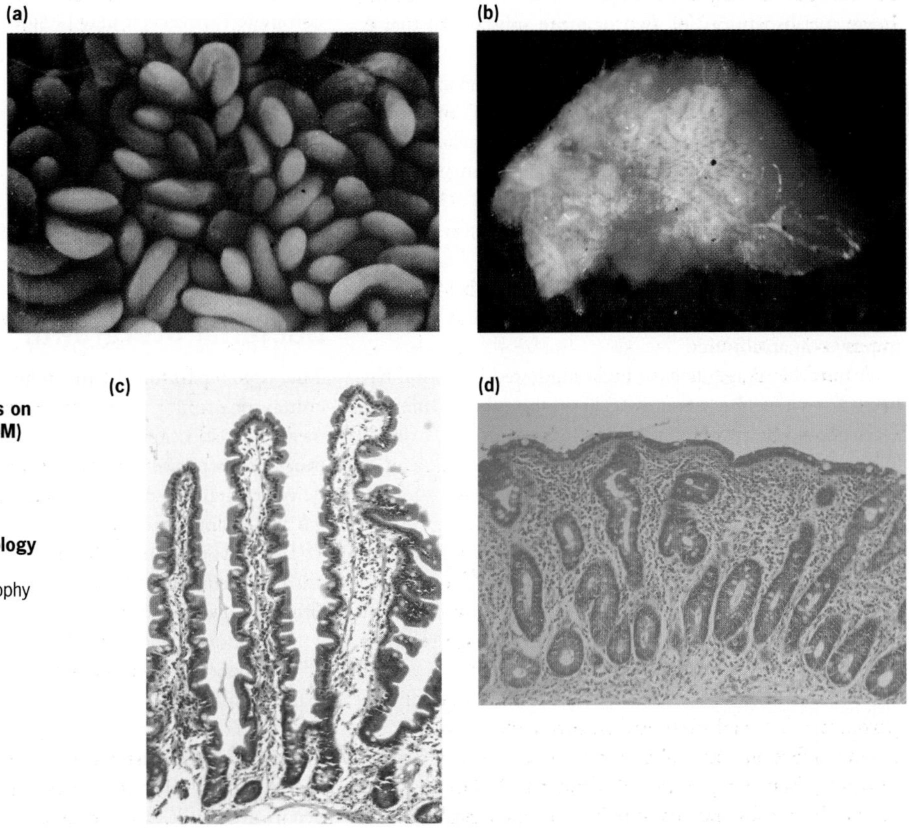

Fig 4.24
Small bowel appearances on dissecting microscopy (DM) and histology
(a) Normal mucosa DM
(b) Coeliac disease DM – flattened mucosa
(c) Normal mucosal histology
(d) Coeliac disease – showing subtotal villous atrophy

T-cell lymphoma (see p. 260) is increased in coeliac disease. Carcinoma of the small bowel and oesophagus as well as extra-gastrointestinal cancers are also seen. Table 4.7 shows the incidence of malignancy compared with the incidence in other GI disorders. Malignancy seems to be unrelated to the duration of the disease but the incidence may be reduced by a gluten-free diet.

Dermatitis herpetiformis (see also p. 1180)

This is an uncommon blistering subepidermal eruption of the skin associated with a gluten-sensitive enteropathy. Rarely there may be gross malabsorption, but usually the jejunal morphological abnormalities are not as severe as in coeliac disease. The inheritance and immunological abnormalities are the same as for coeliac disease. The skin condition responds to dapsone but both the gut and the skin will improve on a gluten-free diet.

Tropical sprue

This is a condition presenting with malabsorption that occurs in residents or visitors to a tropical area where the disease is endemic.

Malabsorption of a mild degree, sometimes following an enteric infection, is quite common and is usually asymptomatic. This is sometimes called tropical malabsorption. The term *tropical sprue* is reserved for severe malabsorption (of two or more substances) that is usually accompanied by diarrhoea and malnutrition. Tropical sprue is endemic in most of Asia, some Caribbean islands, Puerto Rico and parts of South America. Epidemics occur, lasting up to two years, and in some areas repeated epidemics occur at varying intervals of up to ten years.

AETIOLOGY

The aetiology is unknown, but is likely to be infective because the disease occurs in epidemics and patients improve on antibiotics.

A number of agents have been suggested but none has been shown to be unequivocally responsible. Different agents could be involved in different parts of the world.

Table 4.7 Incidence of malignancy in various GI disorders compared to familiar adenomatous polyposis

Disorders	%
Familial adenomatous polyposis	100
Barrett's oesophagus	15
Chronic ulcerative colitis	13
Coeliac disease	13
Pernicious anaemia	< 5
Postgastrectomy stomach	< 5

CLINICAL FEATURES

These vary in intensity and consist of diarrhoea, anorexia, abdominal distension and weight loss. The onset is sometimes acute and occurs either a few days or many years after being in the tropics. Epidemics can break out in villages, affecting thousands of people at the same time. The onset can also be insidious, with chronic diarrhoea and evidence of nutritional deficiency.

The clinical features of tropical sprue vary in different parts of the world, particularly as different criteria are used for diagnosis.

DIAGNOSIS

Acute infective causes of diarrhoea must be excluded (see p. 277), particularly *Giardia*, which can produce a syndrome very similar to tropical sprue.

Malabsorption should be demonstrated, particularly of fat and B_{12}.

The jejunal mucosa is abnormal, showing some villus atrophy (partial villus atrophy). In most cases the lesion is less severe than that found in coeliac disease, although it affects the whole small bowel. Mild changes can be seen in asymptomatic individuals in the tropics, so jejunal mucosal changes must be interpreted carefully.

TREATMENT AND PROGNOSIS

Many patients improve when they leave the sprue area and take folic acid (5 mg daily). Most patients also require an antibiotic (usually tetracycline 1 g daily) to ensure a complete recovery; it may be necessary to give this for up to six months.

The severely ill patient requires resuscitation with fluids and electrolytes for dehydration; any nutritional deficiencies should be corrected. Vitamin B_{12} (1000 μg) is also given to all acute cases.

The prognosis is excellent. Mortality is usually associated with water and electrolyte depletion, particularly in epidemics.

Bacterial overgrowth

The upper part of the small intestine is almost sterile, containing only a few organisms derived from the mouth. Gastric acid kills most organisms and intestinal motility keeps the jejunum empty. The normal terminal ileum contains faecal-type organisms, mainly *Escherichia coli* and anaerobes.

Bacterial overgrowth is normally only found associated with a structural abnormality of the small intestine, although it can occur occasionally in the elderly.

Aspiration of the upper jejunum will reveal the presence of *E. coli* and/or *Bacteroides*, both in concentrations greater than 10^6/mL as part of a mixed flora. These bacteria are capable of deconjugating and dehydroxylating bile salts, so that unconjugated and dehydroxylated bile salts can be detected in aspirates by chromatography. Steatorrhoea (see p. 248) occurs as a result of conjugated bile salt deficiency.

The bacteria are able to metabolize B_{12} and interfere with its binding to intrinsic factor, thereby leading to B_{12} deficiency; this can be demonstrated using the Schilling test (p. 367). Conversely some bacteria produce folic acid.

Bacterial overgrowth has only minimal effects on other substances absorbed from the small intestine. The clinical features are chiefly diarrhoea and steatorrhoea. The vitamin B_{12} deficiency is not so severe as to produce a neurological deficit.

Although bacterial overgrowth may be responsible for the presenting symptoms, it must be remembered that many of the symptoms may be due to the underlying small bowel pathology.

TREATMENT

If possible, the underlying lesion should be corrected (e.g. a stricture should be resected). With multiple diverticula, grossly dilated bowel, or in Crohn's disease, this may not be possible and rotating courses of antibiotics are necessary, such as metronidazole and tetracycline, or ciprofloxacin.

Intestinal resection (Fig 4.25)

Intestinal resection is usually well tolerated, but massive resection is followed by the short-gut syndrome. The effects of resection depend on the extent and the areas involved. Because the gut is long, a 30–50% resection can usually be tolerated without undue problems.

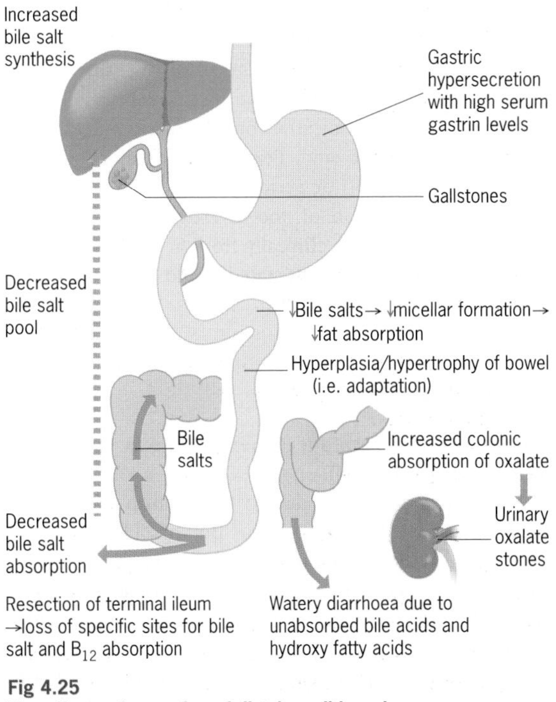

Fig 4.25
The effects of resection of distal small bowel

Ileal resection

The ileum has specific receptors for the absorption of bile salts and vitamin B_{12}, so that relatively small resections will lead to malabsorption of these substances. Removal of the ileocaecal valve increases the incidence of diarrhoea. The following occur in ileal resection:

- Bile salts and fatty acids enter the colon and interfere with water and electrolyte absorption, causing diarrhoea.
- Increased bile salt synthesis can compensate for loss of approximately one-third of the bile salts in the faeces. Greater loss than this results in decreased micellar formation and steatorrhoea, and lithogenic bile and gallstone formation.
- Increased oxalate absorption is caused by the presence of bile salts in the colon. This gives rise to renal oxalate stones.
- There is a low serum B_{12} and macrocytosis.

Investigations include a small bowel follow-through, measurement of B_{12}, bile salt and occasionally fat absorption (see p. 248). Many patients require B_{12} replacement and some need a low-fat diet if there is steatorrhoea. If diarrhoea is a problem, cholestyramine or aluminium hydroxide mixture, to bind bile salts, sometimes helps.

Jejunal resection

The ileum can take over the jejunal absorptive function. Jejunal resection may lead to gastric hypersecretion with high gastrin levels; the exact mechanism of this is unclear. Intestinal adaptation takes place, with an increase in the absorption per unit length of bowel.

Massive resection (short-gut syndrome)

This occurs following resection in Crohn's disease, mesenteric occlusion or trauma. Severe symptoms occur when there is less than 90–100 cm of small bowel remaining. Diarrhoea with severe loss of water and electrolytes occurs together with malnutrition. Parenteral nutrition (sometimes long-term) is necessary. With intestinal adaptation most will eventually recover, although they continue to have diarrhoea and little functional reserve should another GI problem occur.

Whipple's disease

This is a rare disease usually affecting males. It presents with steatorrhoea and abdominal pain along with systemic symptoms of fever and weight loss. Peripheral lymphadenopathy, arthritis and involvement of the heart, lung and brain may occur. Histologically, the villi are stunted and contain diagnostic periodic acid–Schiff (PAS)-positive macrophages. On electron microscopy, bacilli can be seen 'within' the macrophages. The organism has been identified by the polymerase chain reaction; it is similar to actinomycetes and has been given the name

Tropheryma whippeii. A dramatic improvement occurs with antibiotic therapy, which should include an antibiotic that crosses the blood–brain barrier (e.g. chloramphenicol).

Radiation enteritis

Radiation of more than 50 Gy will damage the intestine. The ileum and rectum are the areas most often involved, as pelvic irradiation is the common cause. There may be diarrhoea and abdominal pain at the time of the irradiation. These symptoms usually improve within six weeks after completion of therapy. Chronic radiation enteritis is diagnosed if symptoms persist for three months or more. The prevalence is more than 15%. Many patients suffer from an increased bowel frequency.

Radiation enteritis produces muscle fibre atrophy, ulcerative changes due to ischaemia, and obstruction due to strictures produced by radiation-induced fibrosis. The symptoms are often that of obstruction, which is usually partial but eventually may be complete. Malabsorption due to mucosal damage as well as bacterial overgrowth in dilated segments can occur. Treatment is symptomatic although often unsuccessful in chronic enteritis. Surgery should be avoided if at all possible, being reserved for life-threatening situations such as complete obstruction or occasionally perforation.

Radiation damage to the rectum produces a radiation proctitis with diarrhoea, with or without blood and tenesmus. Treatment is symptomatic; local steroids sometimes help.

Parasite infestation

Giardia intestinalis (see p. 83) not only produces diarrhoea but can produce malabsorption with steatorrhoea. Minor changes are seen in the jejunal mucosa and the organism can be found in the jejunal fluid or mucosa.

Cryptosporidiosis (see p. 84) can also produce malabsorption.

Patients with HIV infection are particularly prone to parasitic infestation (see Table 4.18).

Other causes of malabsorption

- Drugs that bind bile salts (e.g. cholestyramine) and some antibiotics (e.g. neomycin) produce steatorrhoea.
- Diarrhoea, rarely with steatorrhoea, occurs in thyrotoxicosis owing to increased gastric emptying and increased motility. Steatorrhoea occurs in the Zollinger–Ellison syndrome (see p. 352).
- Intestinal lymphangiectasia produces diarrhoea and rarely steatorrhoea.
- Lymphoma that has infiltrated the small bowel mucosa causes malabsoption.
- In some patients with diabetes mellitus, diarrhoea, malabsorption and steatorrhoea occur, sometimes due to bacterial overgrowth from stasis.
- Hypogammaglobulinaemia, which is seen in a number of conditions including lymphoid nodular hyperplasia, causes steatorrhoea owing either to an abnormal jejunal mucosa or to secondary infestation with *Giardia intestinalis*.

Miscellaneous intestinal diseases

Protein-losing enteropathy

Protein-losing enteropathy is seen in many gastrointestinal and systemic conditions. Increased protein loss across an abnormal mucosa causes hypoalbuminaemia. Causes include inflammatory or ulcerative lesions (e.g. Crohn's disease), tumours, Ménétrièr's disease, coeliac disease and lymphatic disorders (e.g. lymphangiectasia). Usually it forms a minor part of the generalized disorder, but occasionally hepatic synthesis of albumin cannot compensate for the hypoalbuminaemia, and the peripheral oedema produced may dominate the clinical picture. The investigations are described on p. 253 and treatment is that of the underlying disorder.

Meckel's diverticulum

This is the most common congenital abnormality of the GI tract, affecting 2–3% of the population. The diverticulum projects from the wall of the ileum approximately 60 cm from the ileocaecal valve. It is usually symptomless, but 50% contain gastric mucosa that secretes hydrochloric acid. Peptic ulcers can occur and may bleed (see p. 244) or perforate.

Acute inflammation of the diverticulum also occurs and is indistinguishable clinically from acute appendicitis. Obstruction from an associated band rarely occurs. Treatment is surgical removal.

Tuberculosis

Tuberculosis (TB) can affect the intestine as well as the peritoneum (see p. 284).

Intestinal tuberculosis is due to reactivation of primary disease caused by *M. tuberculosis*. Bovine TB occurs in areas where milk is unpasteurized and is very rare in the UK. The ileocaecal area is most commonly affected, but the colon, and rarely other parts of the gastrointestinal tract, can be involved too.

Tuberculosis is being seen more frequently in patients with HIV infection.

CLINICAL FEATURES

These are chiefly diarrhoea and abdominal pain with generalized systemic manifestations, including anorexia and weight loss. Intestinal obstruction may develop.

On examination, a mass may be palpable and 50% have X-ray evidence of pulmonary tuberculosis; this is an important aid to the diagnosis.

DIAGNOSIS

In the West, TB must be differentiated from Crohn's disease and should always be considered as a possible diagnosis in Asian immigrants. A caecal carcinoma can present with similar symptoms. An ultrasound of the abdomen may show mesenteric thickening and lymph node enlargement. Histological verification and culture of tissue is highly desirable, but it is not always possible to obtain bacteriological confirmation and treatment should be started if there is a high degree of suspicion. Specimens can be obtained by colonoscopy but laparotomy is required in some cases.

TREATMENT

Drug treatment is similar to that for pulmonary TB – rifampicin, isoniazid and pyrazinamide (see p. 804) – but treatment should last one year.

Amyloid (see also p. 1002)

In systemic amyloidosis there is usually a diffuse involvement that may affect any part of the GI tract. Occasionally amyloid deposits occur as polypoid lesions. The symptoms depend on the site of involvement; amyloidosis in the small intestine gives rise to diarrhoea.

Connective-tissue disorders

Systemic sclerosis (see p. 487) most commonly affects the oesophagus (p. 230), although the small bowel and colon are often found to be involved if the appropriate radiological studies are performed. Frequently there are no symptoms of this involvement, but diarrhoea and steatorrhoea can occur. This is usually due to bacterial overgrowth of the small bowel as a result of reduced motility, dilatation and the presence of diverticula.

In *rheumatoid arthritis* (p. 470) and systemic lupus erythematosus (p. 487), gastrointestinal symptoms may occur, but rarely predominate.

Chronic intestinal ischaemia

This is due to atheromatous occlusion or cholesterol emboli to the mesenteric vessels, particularly in the elderly. Such an occlusion does not always produce clinical effects because of the collateral circulation. The characteristic symptom is abdominal pain occurring after food. This may be followed by acute mesenteric vascular occlusion. Loud bruits may be heard but, as these are heard in normal subjects, they are of doubtful significance. The diagnosis is made using angiography.

The term 'coeliac axis compression syndrome' has been used in young patients with chronic abdominal pain, bruits and minor angiographic changes. Despite its plausible title, it is not an organic syndrome. Its suggested existence results from the false correlation of pain and bruits.

Eosinophilic gastroenteritis

This is a condition of unknown aetiology in which there may be eosinophilic infiltration and oedema of any part of the gastrointestinal mucosa. It usually involves the gastric antrum and proximal small intestine either as a localized lesion (eosinophilic granuloma) or diffusely with sheets of eosinophils seen in the serosal and submucosal layers. An association with asthma, eczema and urticaria has been described.

The condition may occur at any age, but mainly in the third decade. Males are affected twice as often as females. The clinical presentation depends on the site of involvement. Abdominal pain, nausea and vomiting occur. An increased number of eosinophils in the blood is present in only 20% of patients. Radiology or endoscopy will demonstrate the lesion. Steroids are used for the widespread infiltration, particularly if peripheral eosinophilia is present.

In some adults the condition appears to be allergic (allergic gastroenteritis) and is associated with peripheral eosinophilia and high levels of blood and tissue IgE.

Intestinal lymphangiectasia

Dilatation of the lymphatics may be primary or secondary to lymphatic obstruction, such as that occurring in malignancy or constrictive pericarditis. In the rare primary form it may be detected incidentally as dilated lacteals on a jejunal biopsy or it can produce steatorrhoea of varying degrees. Hypoproteinaemia with ankle oedema is the other main feature. Serum immunoglobulin levels are reduced with low circulating lymphocytes. Treatment is with a low-fat diet.

Abetalipoproteinaemia

In this rare condition, there is failure of apo B100 synthesis in the liver and apo B48 in the intestinal cell, so that chylomicrons are not formed. This leads to fat accumulation in the intestinal cells, giving a characteristic histological appearance of the jejunal mucosa. Clinical features include acanthocytosis (spiky red cells due to membrane abnormalities), a form of retinitis pigmentosa, and mental and neurological abnormalities. The latter can be prevented by vitamin E injections.

GI problems in patients with HIV infection

See Table 4.18.

Tumours of the small intestine

The small intestine is relatively resistant to the development of neoplasia and only 3–6% of all GI tumours and fewer than 1% of all malignant lesions occur here. The reasons for the rarity of tumours is unknown. Explanations include the fluidity and relative sterility of small bowel contents and the rapid transit time, reducing the time of exposure to potential carcinogens. It is also possible that the high population of lymphoid tissue and secretion of IgA in the small intestine protects against malignancy.

Benign tumours

Adenomas, leiomyomas or lipomas are rarely found and are usually asymptomatic and picked up incidentally. In familial adenomatous polyposis the upper gut, particularly the duodenum, is affected in one-third of patients. Peutz–Jeghers syndrome consists of mucocutaneous pigmentation (circumoral, hands and feet) and gastrointestinal polyps and has a Mendelian dominant inheritance. The brown buccal pigment is characteristic of this condition. The polyps, which are hamartomas, can occur anywhere in the GI tract but are most frequent in the small bowel. They may bleed or cause intussusception. They virtually never become malignant. Treatment is by individual polypectomy. Multiple polypectomies may have to be performed, but bowel resection should be avoided.

Malignant tumours

Adenocarcinoma of the small intestine is rare and found most frequently in the duodenum (in the periampullary region) and in the jejunum. It is the most common malignancy of the small intestine accounting for up to 50% of primary tumours. *Lymphomas* are most frequently found in the ileum. These are of the non-Hodgkin's type and must be distinguished from peripheral or nodal lymphoma involving the gut secondarily.

In developed countries, the most common type of lymphoma is the B-cell type arising from MALT (see p. 172). These lymphomas tend to be annular or polypoid masses in the distal or terminal ileum, whilst most T-cell lymphomas are ulcerated plaques or strictures in the proximal small bowel.

A tumour similar to Burkitt's lymphoma also occurs and commonly affects the terminal ileum of the children in North Africa and the Middle East.

Carcinoid tumours form the next major group with lymphoma and muscle tumours making up the remainder.

PREDISPOSING FACTORS

Coeliac disease

There is an increased incidence of lymphoma of the T-cell type and adenocarcinoma of the small bowel in coeliac disease (see Table 4.7), as well as an unexplained increase in all malignancies both in the GI tract and elsewhere. The reason for the local development of malignancy is unknown. It is now accepted that coeliac disease is a pre-malignant condition, but there is no association with a poor response to a gluten-free diet or to the chronicity of symptoms. There is some evidence that treatment of coeliac disease with a gluten-free diet protects against the development of either lymphoma or carcinoma.

Crohn's disease

There is a small increase in the incidence of adenocarcinoma of the small bowel in Crohn's disease.

Immunoproliferative small intestinal disease (IPSID)

IPSID is a B-cell lymphocyte disorder in which there is proliferation of plasma cells in the lamina propria of the upper small bowel. These cells produce truncated monoclonal heavy chains, but lack associated light chains. The α heavy chains are found in the gut mucosa on immunofluorescence and these can also be detected in the serum. IPSID occurs usually in countries surrounding the Mediterranean, but it has also been found in other developing countries in South America and the Far East. IPSID predominantly affects people in lower socioeconomic groups in areas with poor hygiene and a high incidence of bacterial and parasitic infection of the gut. IPSID presents itself as a malabsorptive syndrome associated with diffuse lymphoid infiltration of the small bowel and neighbouring lymph nodes. This then progresses in some cases to a lymphoma. Recently the condition has been documented in the developed world.

CLINICAL FEATURES

Patients present with abdominal pain, diarrhoea, anorexia, weight loss and symptoms of anaemia.

There may be a palpable mass and a small bowel follow-through will detect most lesions. Ultrasound and CT will show bowel wall thickening and the involvement of lymph nodes which is common with lymphoma.

TREATMENT

Adenocarcinoma Most patients are treated surgically with a segmental resection. The overall 5-year survival rate is 20–35%; this varies with the histological grade and the presence or absence of lymph nodes. Radiotherapy and chemotherapy are used in addition.

IPSID If there is no evidence of lymphoma, antibiotics, e.g. tetracycline, should be tried initially. In the presence of lymphoma combination chemotherapy is used; in one series the 3–5-year survival was 58%.

Lymphoma Most patients require surgery and radiotherapy with chemotherapy for more extensive disease. The prognosis varies with the type.

The five-year survival rate for T-cell lymphomas is 25%, but is better for B-cell lymphomas, varying from 50% to 75%, depending on the grade of lymphoma.

Carcinoid tumours

These originate from the enterochromaffin cells (APUD cells) of the intestine. They make up 10% of all small bowel neoplasms, the most common sites being in the appendix, terminal ileum and the rectum. It is often difficult to be certain histologically whether a particular tumour is benign or malignant. Clinically most carcinoid tumours are asymptomatic until metastases are present. Ten per cent of carcinoid tumours in the appendix present as acute appendicitis, the inflammation being secondary to obstruction. Surgery is sometimes necessary for localized tumours.

Carcinoid syndrome occurs in only 5% of patients with carcinoid tumours and only when there are liver metastases. Patients complain of spontaneous or induced bluish-red flushing, predominantly on the face and neck. This can lead to permanent changes with telangiectasis. Gastrointestinal symptoms consist of abdominal pain and recurrent watery diarrhoea. Cardiac abnormalities are found in 50% of patients and consist of pulmonary stenosis or tricuspid incompetence. Examination of the abdomen reveals hepatomegaly.

There are *biochemical abnormalities*. The tumours secrete a variety of biologically active amines and peptides, including serotonin (5-hydroxytryptamine; 5HT), bradykinin, histamine and tachykinins as well as prostaglandins.

The diarrhoea and cardiac complications are probably caused by 5HT itself, but the cutaneous flushing is thought to be produced by one of the kinins, such as bradykinin, which is known to cause vasodilatation, bronchospasm and increased intestinal motility.

DIAGNOSIS AND TREATMENT

Ultrasound examination confirms the presence of liver secondary deposits, and the major metabolite of 5HT, 5-hydroxyindoleacetic acid (5HIAA), is found in high concentration in the urine.

Octreotide is an octapeptide somatostatin analogue that has been shown to inhibit the release of many gut hormones. It alleviates the flushing and diarrhoea and can control a carcinoid crisis. It is given subcutaneously in doses up to 200 μg three times daily.

Octreotide sometimes inhibits tumour growth and, since its introduction, other therapy is usually unnecessary. Interferon and other chemotherapeutic regimens occasionally reduce tumour growth, but have not been shown to increase survival. Most patients survive for 5–10 years after diagnosis.

FURTHER READING

Johnson LR (1994) *Physiology of the Gastrointestinal Tract*. New York: Raven Press.

Mäki M, Collin P (1997) Coeliac disease. *Lancet* **349**: 1755–1759.

Inflammatory bowel disease

Two major forms of *nonspecific* inflammatory bowel disease are recognized: Crohn's disease (CD), which can affect any part of the GI tract, and ulcerative colitis (UC), which affects only the large bowel.

There is overlap between these two conditions in their clinical features, and histological and radiological abnormalities; in 10% of cases of colitis a definitive diagnosis of either ulcerative colitis or Crohn's disease is not possible. Currently, it is necessary to distinguish between these two conditions because of certain differences in their managment. However, it is possible that these conditions represent two aspects of the same disease.

EPIDEMIOLOGY

The incidence of Crohn's disease is rising. It varies from country to country but is approximately 5–8 per 100 000 annually, with a prevalence of 50–60 per 100 000. The incidence of ulcerative colitis is stable at 6–15 per 100 000 annually, with a prevalence of 80–120 per 100 000.

Both conditions have a world-wide distribution but are more common in the West. The incidence is lower in the non-white races. Jews are more prone to inflammatory bowel disease than non-Jews, and the Ashkenazi Jews have a higher risk than the Sephardic Jews.

AETIOPATHOGENESIS

The aetiology is unknown, but the racial differences and geographical clusterings suggest both genetic and environmental causes.

- *Familial*. Both conditions are more common amongst relatives of patients than in the general population. There is a high rate of disease concordance in monozygotic twins in Crohn's disease.
- *Genetic*. There are no HLA markers but HLA-B27 is increased in patients with inflammatory bowel disease and ankylosing spondylitis.
- *Diet*. There is little evidence to support a dietary factor, although a high sugar intake has been found in patients with Crohn's disease.
- *Smoking*. Patients with CD are more likely to be tobacco smokers, but conversely there is an increased risk of UC amongst non-smokers or ex-smokers.
- *Infective agent*. In CD the most attractive hypothesis is that of a transmissible agent. However, no bacterium, virus or parasite has been definitely identified.

(a) *Measles virus* – A higher than expected rate of Crohn's disease in children born during measles epidemics suggested a role for this virus and this also implicated the measles vaccination. In one study, measles-specific DNA fragments were found in Crohn's tissue, but this has not been corroborated.

(b) *Mycobacterium* – In cattle and sheep, Johne's disease, which is a chronic inflammatory disorder of the distal ileum, is caused by *M. paratuberculosis*. Isolation of mycobacterium from Crohn's tissue has been inconsistent and current evidence is against this being an aetiological agent.

- *Multifocal gastrointestinal infarction* due to granulomatous angiitis has been suggested as a primary event in CD.
- *Inducible nitric oxide synthase* (iNOS) is expressed after activation by bacterial endotoxins or certain pro-inflammatory cytokines. This intramucosal enzyme produces large amounts of nitric oxide intraluminally in an acute attack of colitis. It has antimicrobial properties but could also damage host cells.

Additionally, many *immunological abnormalities* have been described in inflammatory bowel disease. It is unclear whether they are the primary or secondary event in the pathogenesis. A suggested mechanism is that a specific or generalized luminal antigen can cause stimulation of immune (antigen-specific) or inflammatory (antigen-nonspecific) responses. It is possible that these responses are abnormal or exaggerated in inflammatory bowel disease. Activation of T lymphocytes, tissue macrophages, eosinophils, mast cells, neutrophils and fibroblasts produce a wide variety of cytokines (e.g. interleukin IL-1, IL-6, TNF), chemokines (e.g. eotaxin, macrophage inflammatory protein (MIP), monocyte chemoattractant protein (MCP, IL-8), eicosanoids (e.g. prostaglandins, thromboxane, LTB4), cell adhesion markers (e.g. E-selectins and endothelial cell leucocyte adhesion molecule (ELAM)) and free oxygen radicals, all of which can lead to tissue damage. The serum antineutrophil cytoplasmic antibody (ANCA) is increased in ulcerative colitis, but not in Crohn's; the significance of this is unknown.

PATHOLOGY

Crohn's disease is a chronic inflammatory condition that may affect any part of the GI tract from the mouth to the anus but has a particular tendency to affect the terminal ileum and ascending colon (ileocolonic disease). The disease can involve one small area of the gut such as the terminal ileum, or multiple areas with relatively normal bowel in between ('skip lesions'). It may also involve the whole of the colon (total colitis) sometimes without bowel involvement.

Ulcerative colitis can affect the rectum alone (proctitis), can extend proximally to involve the sigmoid and descending colon ('left-sided colitis'), or may involve the whole colon ('total colitis'). In a few of these patients there is also inflammation of the distal terminal ileum ('backwash ileitis').

Macroscopic changes

In *Crohn's disease* the involved small bowel is usually thickened and narrowed. There are deep ulcers and fissures in the mucosa, producing a cobblestone appearance. Fistulae and abscesses may be seen in the colon. An early feature is aphthoid ulceration, usually seen at colonoscopy (see Fig 4.26); later, larger and deeper ulcers appear in a patchy distribution, again producing a cobblestone appearance.

(a) (b)

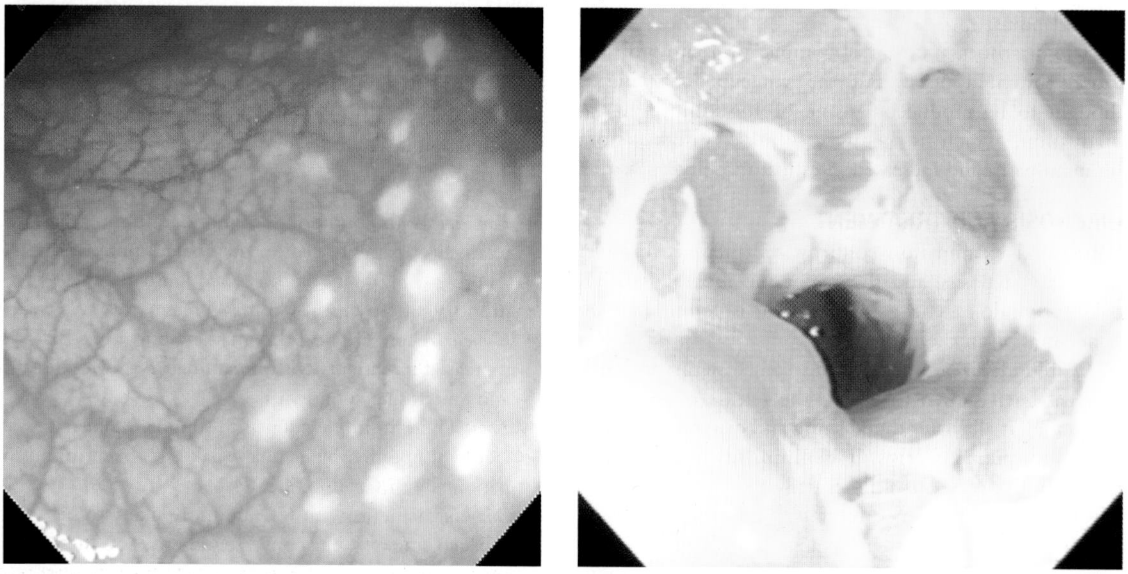

Fig 4.26
Crohn's disease: Colonoscopic appearances of
(a) Aphthoid ulcers typical of Crohn's disease
(b) Cobblestone appearance

In *ulcerative colitis* the mucosa looks reddened, inflamed and bleeds easily. In severe disease there is extensive ulceration, with the adjacent mucosa appearing as inflammatory polyps.

In fulminant colonic disease of either type, most of the mucosa is lost, leaving a few islands of oedematous mucosa (mucosal islands) and toxic dilatation occurs. On healing, the mucosa can return to normal, although there is usually some residual glandular distortion.

Microscopic changes

In *Crohn's disease* the inflammation extends through all layers (transmural) of the bowel, whereas in ulcerative colitis a superficial inflammation is seen. In Crohn's disease there is an increase in chronic inflammatory cells and lymphoid hyperplasia, and in 50–60% of patients granulomas are present. These granulomas are non-caseating epithelioid cells aggregates with Langhan's giant cells.

In *ulcerative colitis* the mucosa shows a chronic inflammatory cell infiltrate in the lamina propria. Crypt abscesses and goblet cell depletion are also seen.

The differentiation between these two diseases is made not only on the basis of clinical and radiological data but also on the histological differences seen in the rectal and colonic mucosa obtained by biopsy (Table 4.8).

CLINICAL FEATURES

Crohn's disease

This can present at any age; it is uncommon before the age of 10 years and has a peak incidence at between 20 and 40 years. A late peak affecting mainly the colon has been reported in women aged over 60 years. Both sexes are equally affected.

The major symptoms are of diarrhoea, abdominal pain and weight loss. Constitutional symptoms of malaise, lethargy, anorexia, nausea, vomiting and low-grade fever may be present. Despite the recurrent nature of this condition, many patients remain well and have an almost normal lifestyle. However, patients with extensive disease may have frequent recurrences necessitating multiple hospital admissions.

The clinical features are very variable and depend partly on the region of the bowel that is affected. The disease may present insidiously or acutely. The abdominal pain may be colicky, suggesting obstruction but it usually has no special characteristics and sometimes in colonic disease only minimal discomfort is present. Diarrhoea is present in 80% of all cases and in colonic disease it usually contains blood, making it difficult to differentiate from ulcerative colitis. Steatorrhoea can be present in small bowel disease. Some patients (15%) present with only anorexia, weight loss and general ill-health, with an absence of any other GI symptoms.

Crohn's disease may present as an emergency with acute right iliac fossa pain mimicking appendicitis. If laparotomy is undertaken, an oedematous, reddened terminal ileum is found. There are other causes of an acute ileitis (e.g. infections such as *Yersinia*). Crohn's disease is the cause of approximately 10% of acute ileitis.

The presentation of Crohn's colitis may be similar to that seen in UC (see below).

Examination

Physical signs are few, apart from loss of weight and general ill-health. Aphthous ulceration of the mouth is often seen. Abdominal examination is often normal, although tenderness and a right iliac fossa mass are occasionally found. This mass is due either to inflamed loops of bowel that are matted together or to an abscess. A careful examination of the anus should always be made to look for oedematous anal tags, fissures or perianal abscesses. These abnormalities are particularly common (80%) in colonic involvement.

Other extra-gastrointestinal features of inflammatory bowel disease should be looked for, such as erythema nodosum, arthritis, or iritis (see below).

Sigmoidoscopy should always be performed in a patient with Crohn's disease. With small bowel involvement the rectum may appear normal, but a biopsy must be taken as nonspecific histological changes may sometimes be found in the mucosa. Even with extensive colonic Crohn's disease the rectum may be spared and be relatively normal, but patchy involvement with an oedematous haemorrhagic mucosa can be present.

Ulcerative colitis

This also occurs at any age, but most frequently between 20 and 40 years with women affected more than men.

The major symptom in ulcerative colitis is diarrhoea with blood and mucus, sometimes accompanied by lower abdominal discomfort. General features include malaise, lethargy and anorexia. Aphthous ulceration in the mouth is seen. The disease can be mild, moderate or severe, and in most patients runs a course of remissions and exacerbations. Ten per cent of patients have persistent chronic symptoms, while some patients may have only a single attack.

When the disease is confined to the rectum, blood mixed with the stool, urgency and tenesmus are common. There are normally very few constitutional symptoms, but patients are nevertheless greatly inconvenienced by the frequency of defaecation.

Table 4.8 Histological differences between Crohn's disease and ulcerative colitis

	Crohn's disease	**Ulcerative colitis**
Inflammation	Deep (transmural) Patchy	Mucosal Continuous
Granulomas	++	Rare
Goblet cells	Present	Depleted
Crypt abscesses	+	++

In an acute attack patients have bloody diarrhoea, passing 10–20 liquid stools per day. Diarrhoea also occurs at night, with urgency and incontinence that is severely disabling for the patient. Occasionally blood and mucus alone are passed.

The definition of a severe attack is given in Table 4.9. The patient may be very ill and needs careful monitoring in hospital with prompt treatment to avoid the development of complications, such as septicaemia, toxic dilatation and perforation.

Examination

In general there are no specific signs in ulcerative colitis. The abdomen may be slightly distended or tender to palpation. The anus is usually normal. Rectal examination will show the presence of blood. Sigmoidoscopy is always abnormal and shows an inflamed, bleeding, friable mucosa. A biopsy should be taken for histological diagnosis.

Extra-gastrointestinal manifestations

These occur with both diseases and some are related to the intestinal disease activity (Table 4.10). Patients with Crohn's colitis have more extra-gastrointestinal complications than those with small bowel lesions alone.

INVESTIGATIONS

Blood tests

Anaemia is common and is usually the normocytic, normochromic anaemia of chronic disease. Deficiency of iron and/or folate also occurs. Despite terminal ileal involvement in Crohn's disease, megaloblastic anaemia due to B_{12} deficiency is unusual, although the B_{12} level can be low. There is often a raised ESR and CRP and a raised white cell count. Hypoalbuminaemia is present in severe disease. Liver biochemistry may be abnormal. Blood cultures are required if septicaemia is suspected.

Stool cultures

These should always be performed on presentation if diarrhoea is present.

Imaging for Crohn's disease

A small bowel follow-through is usually performed first unless the disease is predominantly Crohn's colitis (see below).

A small bowel follow-through shows an asymmetrical alteration in the mucosal pattern with deep ulceration and areas of narrowing (string sign) largely confined to the ileum (Fig 4.27). Skip lesions with normal bowel between are also seen.

Table 4.9
Definition of a severe attack of ulcerative colitis

Stool frequency	>6 stools per day with blood
Fever	>37.5°C
Tachycardia	>90 per minute
ESR	>30 mm per hour
Anaemia	Haemoglobin <10 g dL^{-1}
Albumin	<30 g L^{-1}

Table 4.10
Extra-gastrointestinal manifestations of inflammatory bowel disease (as percentage of cases)

	Crohn's disease	Ulcerative colitis
Eyes		
Uveitis Episcleritis Conjunctivitis	3–10	5–8
Joints		
Monoarticular arthritis	14	10–15
Ankylosing spondylitis	2–6	1–2
Sacroiliitis[c]	<15	12–15
Skin		
Erythema nodosum	5–10	2
Pyoderma gangrenosum	1	1–2
Liver[a,b] and biliary tree	5–6	3
Fatty change	Common	Common
Sclerosing cholangitis	<1%	3–10%
Chronic hepatitis	Uncommon 2–3	Uncommon
Cirrhosis	Uncommon 2–3	Uncommon
Cholangiocarcinoma	Related to sclerosing cholangitis	
Kidney[a]		
Stones	30	–
Gallbladder[a]		
Stones	30	5 (as in normal population)

[a]These manifestations are not related to disease activity.
[b]Biochemical abnormalities are common, but clinically overt disease is uncommon.
[c]Usually asymptomatic.

Barium enema has been superseded by colonoscopy, for colonic disease (see below). Early changes on barium enema consist of aphthous ulceration. This involvement is again usually patchy with deep ulceration developing later.

CT scanning (particularly spiral) is helpful in delineating abscesses, masses, thickened bowel wall and mesentery, or other extraluminal problems in Crohn's disease.

Ultrasound is useful if there is a mass. It is also used for follow-up.

Imaging for ulcerative colitis

A plain X-ray of the abdomen is performed in cases of severe colitis to look for colonic dilatation. The extent of the disease can be judged by the air distribution in the colon.

An instant, unprepared barium enema is where barium is run into the rectum without pressure and a single film taken. This is a good investigation to show the extent of the disease.

The prepared barium enema has been superseded by colonoscopy. If performed, there may be ulceration (Fig 4.28).

Early changes include scattered aphthoid ulceration, with oedema and deep ulceration in later stages. Rectal sparing can occur, although this is unusual in UC. Biopsies can also be taken from the terminal ileum.

In longstanding disease, the colon is shortened and narrowed. The disease is usually continuous.

Colonoscopy

In *Crohn's disease*, colonoscopy is performed if colonic involvement is suspected when biopsies of the whole colon can be taken.

In *ulcerative colitis*, colonoscopy shows the exact extent of the disease. Again, biopsies from the whole colon and ileum can be taken to differentiate between Crohn's and UC. The mucosa is oedematous, friable and bleeds, and the involvement is continuous. In patients with symptoms of proctitis, a flexible sigmoidoscopy will show the extent of the disease.

Small bowel function tests (see also p. 251)

When Crohn's disease involves the small bowel, other tests may be necessary (e.g. a breath test for bacterial overgrowth or a test for vitamin B_{12} absorption).

ACTIVITY OF DISEASE

A rough estimate of the activity can be made on the clinical picture and laboratory tests of ESR, serum albumin and acute-phase protein (e.g. CRP or orosomucoids). In some centres, scans to localize areas of inflammation are performed using radiolabelled leucocytes injected intravenously; these may help in localizing abscesses (see p. 7).

DIFFERENTIAL DIAGNOSIS

Crohn's disease has to be considered in the differential diagnosis of all chronic diarrhoeas, malabsorption and malnutrition. It is also a differential diagnosis of small

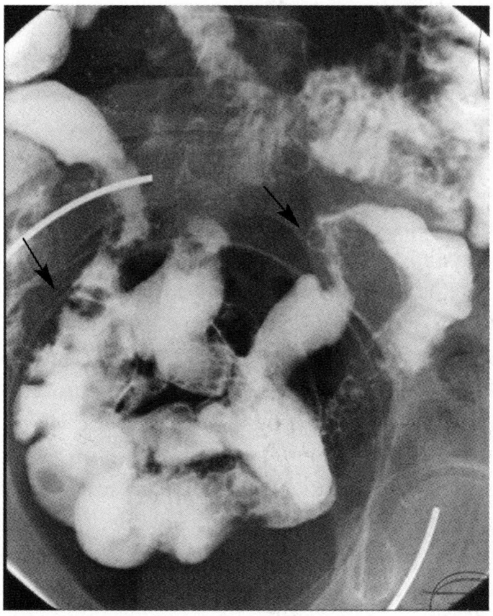

Fig 4.27
Small bowel follow-through in Crohn's disease, showing narrowing and ulceration of the terminal ileum (arrow) and a further stricture in the ileum

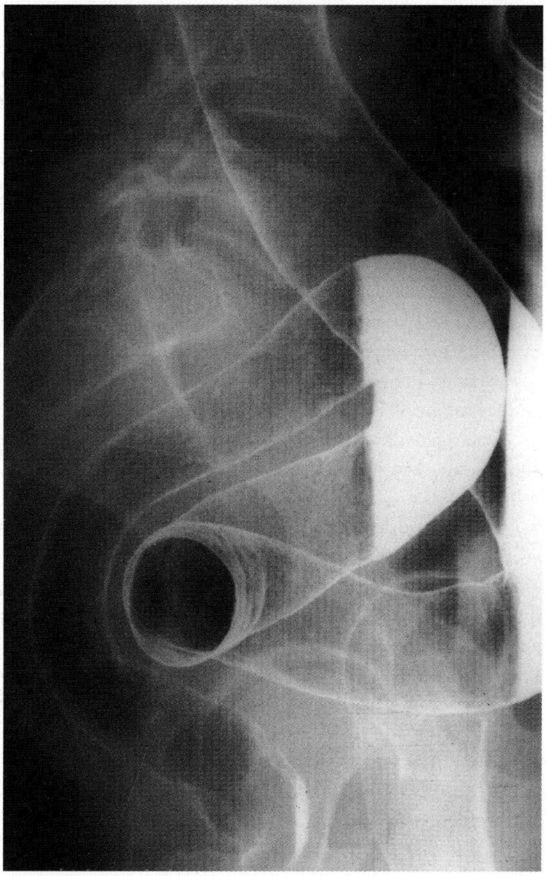

Fig 4.28
Double-contrast barium enema showing ulcerative colitis Note the fine ulceration of the muscosa

stature in children (see p. 927). A small bowel follow-through usually differentiates it from other forms of small bowel disease.

Ileocaecal tuberculosis is common in Asia and Africa and in Asian immigrants in the UK. Acute ileitis due to *Yersinia* can be distinguished serologically. Lymphomas occasionally cause a major diagnostic difficulty.

Colitis, both ulcerative and Crohn's, must be differentiated from amoebic and ischaemic colitis as well as infective causes of diarrhoea. The latter are becoming more common in homosexuals and should be suspected if multiple or unusual organisms are found. A rare cause of colitis is *Behçet's disease*, which also gives orogenital ulceration.

In a few patients the mucosal appearance on colonoscopy and sigmoidoscopy is macroscopically normal and the inflammation is only detected histologically. This '*microscopic colitis*' presents with chronic diarrhoea and is treated as a nonspecific colitis. *Collagenous colitis* also presents as chronic diarrhoea; there is a thick subepithelial deposit of collagen in the macroscopically normal colonic mucosa. Both of these conditions are probably variants of ulcerative colitis and are treated in a similar fashion. Response to treatment is variable.

Neutropenic enterocolitis is due to infection with *Clostridium septicum* and occurs in patients with severe neutropenia.

MEDICAL MANAGEMENT OF CROHN'S DISEASE

Some patients require only symptomatic treatment. Diarrhoea can be controlled with agents such as loperamide 2–4 mg three times daily, codeine phosphate 30–60 mg three times daily, or diphenoxylate with atropine 1–2 tablets four times daily. Patients with more severe disease require specific medical therapy and acute attacks often require admission to hospital. Medical therapy relies mainly on anti-inflammatory and immunosuppressive drugs. The mechanism of action of these drugs in inflammatory bowel disease is unknown and treatment is largely empirical.

Anaemia will improve as the patient gets better, but appropriate haematinics may be required (e.g. ferrous sulphate 400 mg daily, or folic acid 5 mg daily).

Acute (moderate/severe) attacks require oral corticosteroids 30–60 mg daily, and any dehydration and electrolyte loss should be corrected with intravenous fluids. On this regimen patients usually improve quickly and the steroid dosage can then be reduced. Azathioprine (2 mg kg^{-1} daily) is an immunosuppressive agent that has been shown to be helpful in maintaining the steroid-induced remission. It is often started in an acute attack as it takes a few weeks to be effective. 6-Mercaptopurine (6MP), its metabolite, is used in some centres. Many other anti-inflammatory and immunosuppressive drugs (e.g. cyclosporin) have been tried with variable success. Mesalazine or sulphasalazine (see below) is used in patients with colonic involvement who can also be given rectal steroids (see below). Metronidazole (800 mg three times daily) and cotrimoxazole (two tablets twice daily) are useful in severe perianal disease, possibly owing to their antibacterial action.

Budesonide, a corticosteroid analogue with low systemic activity due to its rapid hepatic conversion, is useful in mild attacks at a dose of 9 mg per day for eight weeks. It is less effective than prednisolone in more severe attacks.

Elemental diets (see p. 211) can induce remissions, particularly in small bowel disease. They improve nutrition, allow the bowel to 'rest' and reduce antigen load to the bowel, but their precise mode of action is unclear. Unfortunately, the diets are unpalatable and expensive, and many patients relapse on restarting a normal diet. The treatment is useful in some patients, particularly children, who refuse steroids or who have marked side-effects.

Remission. Some patients can come off all therapy. Others require a small dose of steroids and/or long-term azathioprine. Because of the relapses and remissions seen in the majority of patients with Crohn's disease, all new therapy must be carefully evaluated. Good evidence-based medicine requires at least one large randomized controlled trial.

SURGICAL MANAGEMENT OF CROHN'S DISEASE

Approximately 80% of patients will require an operation at some time during the course of their disease. Nevertheless, surgery should be avoided if possible and only minimal resections undertaken, as recurrence (15% per year) is almost inevitable. The indications for surgery are:

- failure of medical therapy, with acute or chronic symptoms producing ill-health
- complications (e.g. toxic dilatation, obstruction, perforation, abscesses, enterocutaneous fistula)
- failure to grow in children.

In patients with small bowel disease, strictures can be widened (stricturoplasty), whereas in others resection and end-to-end anastomosis is necessary. The surgery of colonic disease is discussed below.

MEDICAL MANAGEMENT OF ULCERATIVE COLITIS

Severe attacks require careful management in hospital as the mortality of this condition is still high. All patients with ulcerative colitis are treated with a 5-aminosalicylic acid (5-ASA or mesalamine) compound. Sulphasalazine consists of a 5-aminosalicylic acid (5-ASA) attached to sulphapyridine as a carrier. This combination is broken down in the colon by bacteria to release the active agent, 5-ASA. Sulphasalazine is started at a dose of 3–4 g daily, reducing to a maintenance dose of 2 g daily. In mild cases it may induce a remission. Its main role, however, is to reduce the number of relapses when taken long-term. Sulphasalazine may induce nausea and has some reversible side-effects, including haemolytic anaemia, skin rashes and infertility in men. These are produced by the sulphapyridine and preparations of slow-release mesalamine without sulphapyridine have been developed and are superseding sulphasalazine for new patients. Mesalazine consists of mesalamine itself in a delay-release tablet that dissolves at pH 7 or greater. A dose of 400–1200 mg three times daily is used.

Olsalazine consists of two molecules of 5-ASA linked by an azo bond which separates in the large bowel and is also used.

Balsalazide is a prodrug in which 5-ASA is linked via a diazo bond to 4-aminobenzoyl-β-alanine (4-ABA), an inert and biologically inactive carrier molecule. A dose of 6.75 g daily has been shown to be effective in colitis and is better tolerated than mesalazine.

Mild attacks and proctitis can be treated with local rectal steroids in the form of enemas (prednisolone-21 phosphate 20 mg) or a 10% hydrocortisone foam. Mesalamine retention enemas are also useful.

Moderate attacks are treated with oral prednisolone 30–40 mg daily. Patients with their first attack or those who do not respond quickly should be admitted to hospital.

Severe attacks (see also toxic dilatation for management) should be treated with high-dose corticosteroids in the form of prednisolone 60 mg or hydrocortisone 100 mg i.v. 6-hourly. In addition, dehydration and electrolyte disturbances should be corrected by intravenous therapy. Accompanying septicaemia, which is usually due to Gram-negative bacteria, should be treated with antibiotics.

Azathioprine 2 mg kg^{-1} has been shown to induce a remission (see Crohn's treatment above) in some patients who have not responded to steroid therapy.

Cyclosporin given intravenously has also been shown in some studies to induce a remission, and probably should be tried before advocating colectomy. Surgical treatment is necessary if there is then no improvement.

Remission. All patients are maintained on a 5-ASA compound for many years.

SURGICAL MANAGEMENT OF UC (AND CROHN'S COLITIS)

In UC the disease is confined to the colon and therefore colectomy is curative. The main indication for surgery is usually a severe attack which does not respond to medical therapy. A prophylactic colectomy is sometimes performed in patients who have a high cancer risk.

Protocolectomy with an ileostomy is the standard operation, in which the colon and rectum are removed and the ileum is brought out through an opening in the right iliac fossa and attached to the skin. The patient wears an ileostomy bag, which is stuck on to the skin over the ileostomy spout. The bag needs to be emptied once or twice daily, so this is compatible with a near-normal lifestyle. Stoma-care therapists are readily available with help and advice.

Problems associated with ileostomies include:

- mechanical problems
- dehydration, particularly in hot climates
- psychosexual problems
- infertility in men
- recurrence of Crohn's disease.

In ulcerative colitis, but *not* in Crohn's disease, *colectomy with an ileorectal or ileoanal anastomosis* is used to avoid ileostomy.

Ileorectal anastomoses leave a diseased rectum *in situ* and frequent diarrhoea still occurs. With an ileoanal anastomosis (Fig 4.29), a pouch of ileum is formed that acts as a reservoir and the patient is continent with only a few bowel motions per day. The ileoanal operation is being increasingly used, but inflammation of the pouch ('pouchitis') can be a problem. It is not used for Crohn's disease because of the high recurrence rate.

COMPLICATIONS

These are similar in both conditions, but vary in frequency. Crohn's disease, with its transmural inflammation, has a higher incidence of fistulae, fissures and abscess formation.

Perforation

This is a rare but serious complication that occurs in association with toxic megacolon in both diseases. In Crohn's disease local perforations occur, usually of the terminal ileum, forming walled-off abscesses, and occasionally small bowel perforation gives rise to peritonitis.

Haemorrhage

Massive haemorrhage is rare.

Toxic dilatation

Toxic dilatation may occur during an acute severe attack of colitis. This is more common in UC than in CD. The diagnosis should be suspected in a patient with a severe episode (see above) who develops abdominal distension. A plain abdominal X-ray (Fig 4.30) will show a dilated thin-walled colon with a diameter greater than 5 cm that is gas-filled and contains mucosal islands. Treatment is as for a severe attack of colitis plus daily abdominal X-rays and measurements of abdominal girth. If the patient does not

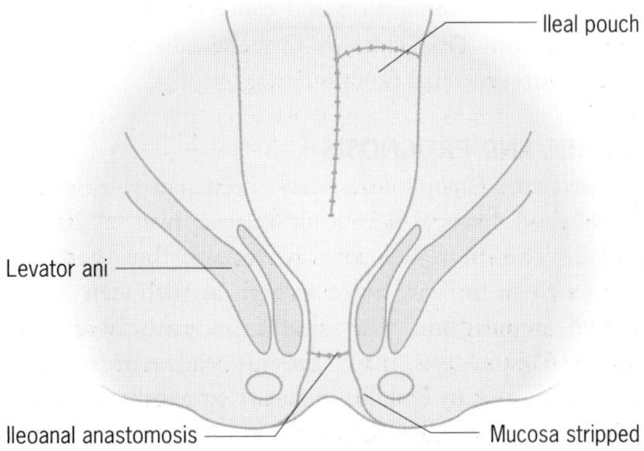

Fig 4.29
An ileoanal pouch for ulcerative colitis

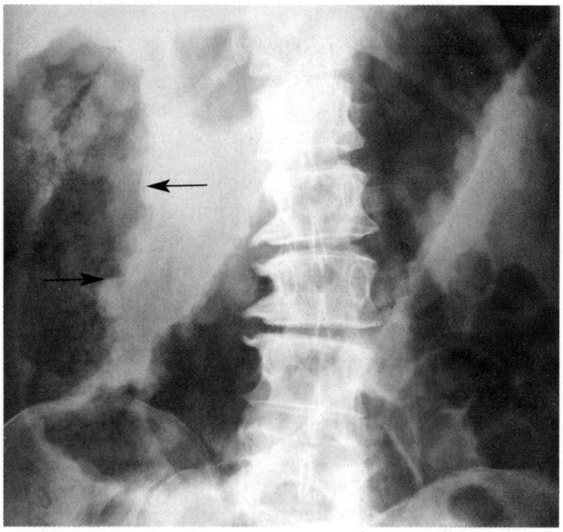

Fig 4.30
Plain abdominal X-ray, showing toxic dilatation in ulcerative colitis. The arrows indicate mucosal islands

settle in 48 hours with high-dose corticosteroids, emergency surgery should be performed. When mucosal islands are present, the risk of perforation is high, as is the mortality, and many favour immediate surgery without medical therapy.

Carcinoma

The incidence is increased in both conditions (3–5%). In Crohn's disease the incidence of carcinoma is only marginally increased and does not influence management. In ulcerative colitis the risk of carcinoma of the colon in a patient who has had total colitis for more than 10 years is greater than it is for the general population. It was suggested that regular sigmoidoscopy and colonoscopy with biopsies might detect early premalignant changes, but this is not recommended as repeated studies, not surprisingly, have shown no benefit.

Cholangiocarcinoma is also found in increased frequency.

Amyloid

This is a rare complication and can affect the bowel or other organs. The kidneys may be affected with a deterioration of renal function.

COURSE AND PROGNOSIS

Patients with *Crohn's disease* have recurrent relapses and virtually all have a significant relapse over a 20-year period. The mortality rate is variable but generally appears to be at least twice as high as that seen in the normal population. Most deaths are associated with surgery. Despite this, many patients lead a normal life. Crohn's disease in childhood causes growth retardation. Self-help groups provide patient information, and a number of booklets that are invaluable for health staff and patients with inflammatory bowel disease.

The course and prognosis of *ulcerative colitis* is variable. In proctitis it is very good; only 10% of these cases go on to develop more extensive disease. On the other hand, severe fulminant disease still carries a 15–25% mortality. The mortality is reduced if the acute attack is treated promptly and surgery is performed if no improvement occurs in the first 2–3 days. Overall, because many cases are mild, the mortality of this disease is not much greater than the mortality rates for the general population, in contrast to Crohn's disease.

There is no particular risk to mother or child during *pregnancy* in either form of inflammatory bowel disease.

FURTHER READING

Hyde GM, Jewell DP (1997) Management of severe ulcerative colitis. *Alimentary Pharmacology and Therapeutics* **11**: 419-425.

Satsangi J, Parkes M, Jewell DP, Bell JL (1998) Genetics of inflammatory bowel disease. *Clinical Science* **94**: 473-478

Sheath SG, Lamont JT (1998) Toxic megacolon. *Lancet* **351**: 509–513.

The colon and rectum

STRUCTURE

The large intestine starts at the caecum, on the posterior medial wall of which is the appendix. The colon is made up of ascending, transverse, descending and sigmoid parts, which join the rectum at the rectosigmoid junction.

The muscle wall consists of an inner circular layer and an outer longitudinal layer. The outer layer is incomplete, coming together to form the taenia coli, which produce the haustral pattern seen in the normal colon.

The mucosa of the colon is lined with epithelial cells with crypts but no villi, so that the surface is flat. The mucosa is full of goblet cells. A variety of cells, mainly lymphocytes and macrophages, are found in the lamina propria.

Table 4.11 Input and output of water and electrolytes in the gastrointestinal tract over 24 hours

	Water (mL)	Sodium (mmol)	Potassium (mmol)
Input			
Diet	1500	150	80
GI secretions	7500	1000	40
Totals	9000	1150	120
Output			
Faeces	150	5	12
Ileostomy (adapted)	500–1500	60–120	4

The blood supply to the colon is from the superior and inferior mesenteric vessels. Generally there are good anastomotic channels, but the caecum and splenic flexure are areas where ischaemia can occur.

The rectum is about 12 cm long. Its interior is divided by three crescentic circular muscles producing shelf-like folds. These are the rectal valves and can be seen at sigmoidoscopy. The anal canal has an internal and an external sphincter.

PHYSIOLOGY

The main role of the colon is the absorption of water and electrolytes (Table 4.11). Approximately 2 L of fluid passes the ileocaecal valve each day. The absorption of fluid and electrolytes takes place mainly in the right side of the colon, and only about 150 mL is passed in the faeces.

The role of the rectum and anus in defaecation is complex. The rectum is usually empty and collapsed; the entry of faeces from the colon produces relaxation of the internal sphincter and the puborectalis muscle. This decreases the acute angle between the rectum and the anal canal. When the rectum contains approximately 100 mL of faeces the urge to defecate is experienced. The rectum is emptied by relaxation of the external anal sphincter (under voluntary control) and an increase in intra-abdominal pressure.

Diverticular disease

Diverticula are frequently found in the colon and occur in 50% of patients over the age of 50 years. They are most frequent in the sigmoid, but can be present over the whole colon.

The term *diverticulosis* indicates the presence of diverticula; *diverticulitis* implies that these diverticula are inflamed. It is perhaps better to use the more general term *diverticular disease*, as it is often difficult to be sure whether the diverticula are inflamed. The precise mechanism of diverticula formation is not known. There is thickening of the muscle layer and, because of high intraluminal pressures, pouches of mucosa extrude through the muscular wall through weakened areas near blood vessels to form diverticula. Diverticular disease seems to be related to the low-fibre diet eaten in the West.

Diverticulitis occurs when faeces obstruct the neck of the diverticulum causing stagnation and allowing bacteria to multiply and produce inflammation. This can then lead to bowel perforation (peridiverticulitis), abscess formation, fistulae into adjacent organs, or even generalized peritonitis.

(a)

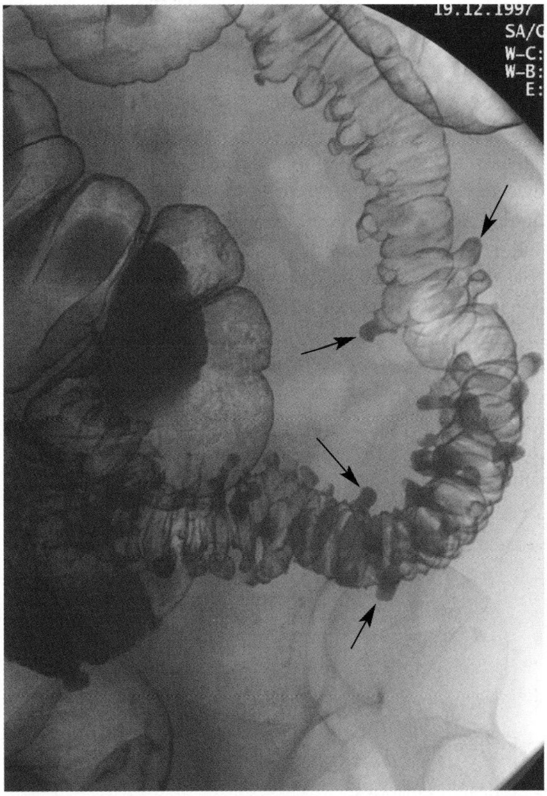

(b)

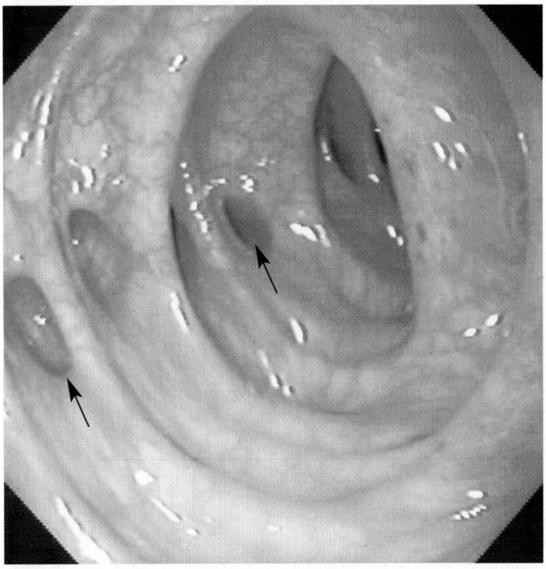

Fig 4.31
(a) Double-contrast enema, showing diverticular disease (the diverticula are arrowed). The barium is black on these films
(b) Diverticula seen on colonoscopy (arrows)

CLINICAL FEATURES AND MANAGEMENT

Diverticular disease is asymptomatic in 90% and is usually discovered incidentally on a barium enema examination (Fig 4.31). No treatment is required.

Intermittent left iliac fossa pain and alternating constipation and diarrhoea are often attributed to diverticular disease, but as these symptoms are very similar to those seen in the irritable bowel syndrome, it is debatable whether they are due to diverticular disease. In practice, both conditions are treated symptomatically with a high-fibre diet, antispasmodic drugs (e.g. mebeverine 135 mg three times daily) and agents to regulate the bowel. A barium enema is often performed to exclude colonic carcinoma.

Diverticular disease can produce rectal bleeding, which is sometimes massive, particularly from right-sided diverticula. In most cases the bleeding stops and the cause of the bleeding can be established by X-ray, colonoscopy and sometimes angiography. In rare cases emergency colectomy is necessary. It is unwise to ascribe an iron-deficiency anaemia to a bleeding diverticulum unless all other causes (e.g. piles or carcinoma) have been excluded.

Acute diverticulitis almost always affects diverticula in the sigmoid colon. It presents with severe pain in the left iliac fossa, often accompanied by fever and constipation. These symptoms and signs are similar to appendicitis but on the left side. On examination the patient is often febrile with a tachycardia. Abdominal examination shows tenderness, guarding and rigidity on the left side of the abdomen. A palpable tender mass is sometimes felt in the left iliac fossa.

The *complications* of acute diverticulitis can be:

- perforation, leading to generalized peritonitis (see p. 283)
- fistula formation into the bladder, causing dysuria or pneumaturia, or into the vagina, causing discharge
- intestinal obstruction (see p. 283), usually after repeated episodes.

INVESTIGATIONS

- **Blood tests**. A polymorphonuclear leucocytosis is often present. The ESR is raised.
- **Spiral CT** of the lower abdomen (Fig 4.32) will show colonic wall thickening, diverticulae and often pericolic collections and abscesses. There is usually a streaky increased density extending into the immediate pericolic fat with thickening of the pelvic fascial planes. These findings are diagnostic of acute diverticular disease and differ from malignant disease.
- **Ultrasound** examination is often more readily available and is cheaper. It can demonstrate thickening bowel and large pericolic collections, but is less sensitive than CT.

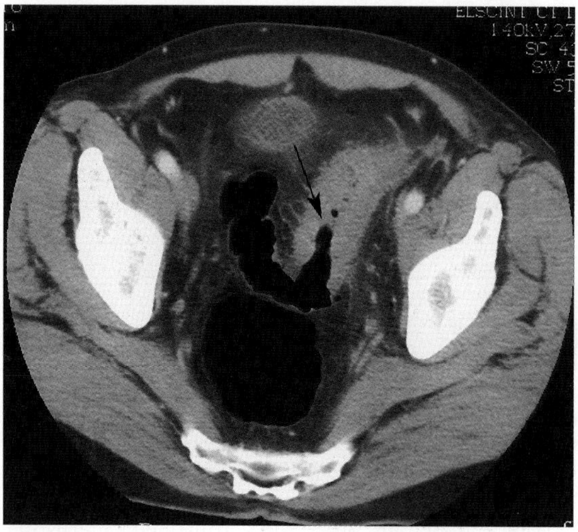

Fig 4.32
Spiral CT of lower abdomen, showing acute diverticulitis (arrow). The bowel wall is thickened and there is loss of clarity of the pericolic fat. A narrow segment of bowel is seen to the left of the diseased segment

TREATMENT

Acute attacks can be treated on an outpatient basis using a cephalosporin and metronidazole. Patients who are more ill will require admission for bowel rest, intravenous fluids and antibiotic therapy (e.g. gentamicin, or a cephalosporin) and metronidazole. Most attacks settle on this regimen, but a few require emergency surgery, with resection of the diseased segment and the formation of a defunctioning colostomy which is later reversed.

Acute episodes do not necessarily recur and elective surgery (laparoscopically if possible) is reserved mainly for patients with intestinal obstruction or fistulae.

Constipation (see also p. 218)

Constipation is such a major problem in the general population that it need not be considered a disease. Most people simply require reassurance and dietary advice. Constipation is common in the elderly, possibly owing to immobility and a poor diet. Constipation in young women is common, and in some, slow transit through the colon has been identified as the cause, whilst some women after childbirth have pelvic floor abnormalities preventing defaecation. A list of the causes of constipation is given in Table 4.12. Most have simple constipation, often due to a low fibre intake. Drugs are a common cause and may need to be stopped. A rectal examination should always be performed. Longstanding constipation does not require investigation, but a change in bowel habit in the middle-aged or elderly merits a barium enema examination.

TREATMENT

Laxatives should be avoided if at all possible and patients encouraged to take a high-fibre diet. Glycerol suppositories, which can be used by the patient, are often

Table 4.12
Causes of constipation

Simple
Intestinal obstruction
Colonic disease (e.g. carcinoma)
Painful anal conditions
Drugs (e.g. opiates, aluminium antacids, antidepressants, codeine, iron)
Hypothyroidism, hypercalcaemia
Depression
Immobility
Hirschsprung's disease (very occasionally seen in adults)

Table 4.13
Laxatives and enemas

	Mechanism of action
Bulking agents	Increased faecal mass due to fibre and water
Dietary fibre	
Bran	
Ispaghula husks	
Sterculia	
Methylcellulose	
Stimulant laxatives	Stimulate intestinal secretion
Anthraquinones (e.g. senna, sodium picosulphate)	
Dioctyl sodium sulphosuccinate	
Danthron[a]	
Bisacodyl	
Osmotic laxatives	Osmotic effect
Magnesium (sulphate or hydroxide)	
Lactulose	
Suppositories	
Bisacodyl	
Glycerol	
Enemas	
Phosphate	
Sodium citrate	

[a]For elderly or for opiate-induced constipation in terminally ill.

useful. The types of laxatives available are shown in Table 4.13. Bulking agents should be tried first. Stimulant laxatives often cause cramp and their long-term use should be avoided as they cause an atonic non-functioning colon. Magnesium sulphate is useful in very severe constipation.

Megacolon

The term 'megacolon' is used to describe a number of congenital and acquired conditions in which the colon is dilated. In many instances it is secondary to chronic constipation and in some parts of the world Chagas' disease is a common cause.

All young patients with megacolon should have Hirschsprung's disease excluded. In this disease, which presents in the first years of life, an aganglionic segment of the rectum gives rise to constipation and subacute obstruction. Occasionally Hirschsprung's disease affecting only a short segment of the rectum can be missed in childhood. A preliminary rectal biopsy is performed and stained with special stains for ganglion cells in the submucosal plexus. In doubtful cases a full thickness biopsy, under anaesthesia, should be obtained. A frozen section is stained for acetyl cholinesterase, which is elevated in Hirschsprung's disease. Pressure studies show failure of relaxation of the internal sphincter, which is diagnostic of Hirschsprung's disease. This disease can be successfully treated surgically.

Treatment of megacolon is similar to simple constipation, but saline washouts and manual removal of faeces are sometimes required.

Pneumatosis cystoides intestinalis

This is a rare condition in which multiple gas-filled cysts are found in the submucosa of the intestine, chiefly the colon. The cause is unknown, but many cases are associated with chronic bronchitis and some with peptic ulceration. Patients are usually asymptomatic, but abdominal pain and diarrhoea do occur and occasionally the cysts rupture to produce a pneumoperitoneum. This condition is diagnosed on X-ray of the abdomen, barium enema or at sigmoidoscopy when cysts are seen.

Treatment is often unnecessary but continuous oxygen therapy will help to disperse the largely nitrogen-containing cysts. Metronidazole may help.

Ischaemic disease of the colon (ischaemic colitis)

This commonly presents in the older age group (over 50 years) with sudden onset of abdominal pain and the passage of bright red blood with or without diarrhoea. There may be signs of shock and there is sometimes evidence of other cardiovascular disease. This condition has also been described in young women taking the contraceptive pill.

On examination, the abdomen is distended and tender. Sigmoidoscopy is normal apart from the presence of blood. Investigations include an abdominal X-ray to exclude perforation. Thumb-printing – a characteristic sign for ischaemic disease – can be seen on a barium enema performed when the patient is well; strictures can also be seen.

The differential diagnosis is of other causes of acute colitis, but these can usually be excluded on the basis of the normal sigmoidoscopic findings in ischaemic colitis.

TREATMENT

Most patients with this condition settle on symptomatic treatment. A few develop gangrene and perforation and require urgent surgery. Some develop strictures.

Anorectal conditions

These important conditions largely present to surgeons. The major conditions presenting initially to the physicians include the following.

Pruritus ani

Pruritus ani, or an itchy bottom, is common and often no cause is found. Treatment consists of good personal hygiene and keeping the area dry. Secondary causes include any local anal lesions such as haemorrhoids, infestation (e.g. with threadworm – *Enterobius vermicularis*), or fungal infection (e.g. candidiasis). The latter condition often occurs secondary to the use of hydrocortisone creams, which should be avoided.

Haemorrhoids

Haemorrhoids usually produce rectal bleeding and pruritus ani. Patients may notice red blood on their toilet paper. They are the most common cause of rectal bleeding (see Fig 4.17) and require no treatment if minor. Diagnosis is made on proctoscopy.

Anal fissures

Anal fissures cause painful defaecation and minor rectal bleeding and can often be seen in the anal margin on inspection. Treatment is by application of a local anaesthetic gel. Dilatation is not required.

Faecal incontinence

The physiology of defaecation is described on p. 269. The common causes of faecal incontinence are shown in Table 4.14. In younger patients, neurological disorders and trauma during childbirth are more common causes. It is a major problem in the elderly, infirm or demented patient. It is often secondary to faecal loading and impaction. The patient should be carefully examined and investiged as appropriate. Treatment is that of the underlying problem but is often unsatisfactory.

Table 4.14
Aetiology of faecal incontinence

Faecal impaction with overflow diarrhoea	Neurological disorders Spinal trauma (level S2–S4) Spina bifida Multiple sclerosis
Anorectal disease Rectal prolapse Anal stricture Haemorrhoidectomy Anal dilatation Rectal carcinoma	Senile dementia
Post-childbirth Damage to pelvic floor innervation during parturition	Congenital abnormalities of anus/rectum e.g. surgery for imperforate anus
	Impalement injuries
	Diabetes mellitus (with autonomic involvement)

Faecal impaction

This occurs in the elderly with constipation. It can lead to overflow incontinence. It usually requires manual removal of faeces, and care to prevent recurrences (see constipation).

Solitary rectal ulcer

These ulcers occur in young adults and produce bowel irregularity and rectal bleeding with the passage of mucus. Most cases are due to excess straining at stool with prolapse of the rectal mucosa (descending perineal syndrome).

Rectal examination is usually normal but sigmoidoscopy reveals redness or an ulcer approximately 10 cm from the anal margin on the anterior rectal wall. It often has an appearance not unlike that of a carcinoma.

Histology is diagnostic. There are nonspecific inflammatory changes with bands of smooth muscle extending into the lamina propria.

Treatment is unsatisfactory and many cases run an indolent chronic course with continuation of symptoms. Local steroids may help and surgical excision should be avoided. Patients should be advised to stop straining on defaecation.

Rectal prolapse

In this common condition affecting children and elderly women the rectal mucosa prolapses through the anus owing to excessive straining. Initially prolapse occurs only during defaecation causing mucous discharge and bleeding from the engorged mucosa. Later ulceration, mucosal discharge and faecal incontinence can occur. Surgical treatment is required in complete prolapse.

REFERENCE

Ferzoco LB, Raptopovias V, Silen W (1998) Acute diverticulitis. *New England Journal of Medicine* **338**: 1521-1526.

Colonic tumours

Colon polyps and polyposis syndromes (Table 4.15)

A polyp is an elevation above the mucosal surface. The majority of colorectal polyps are adenomas with malignant potential. Polyps range in size from a few millimetres to 10 cm diameter. They may be single or multiple and in the polyposis syndromes hundreds may be found.

In adults, 2–5 mm polyps in the rectum are often found, and 90% of these will be of the innocent metaplastic type. Larger polyps in the rectum and 70–80% of all polyps in the colon are adenomas, and 5% (20% of those 2 cm or greater in diameter) will contain invasive carcinoma at discovery. Most polyps are asymptomatic and found by chance when patients are investigated for pain, altered bowel habit, bleeding haemorrhoids or some other cause.

Non-neoplastic polyps

Hamartomatous polyps are commonly large and stalked and are either juvenile or Peutz–Jeghers in type. Other non-neoplastic polyps are less common and are shown in Table 4.15.

Juvenile polyps (occurring in children and teenagers) are confined mainly to the colon and histologically show mucus-retention cysts. They are inherited as an autosomal dominant and are a cause of bleeding and intussusception, often in the first year of life. In juvenile polyposis (more

Table 4.15
Classification of colorectal polyps

Type	Solitary	Multiple polyposis syndrome
Hamartomas	Peutz–Jeghers polyps Juvenile polyps	Peutz–Jeghers syndrome Juvenile polyposis Cronkhite–Canada syndrome
Inflammatory	Inflammatory polyps e.g. Ulcerative colitis Crohn's colitis Schistosomiasis	Inflammatory polyposis
Neoplastic	Adenomas – tubular, tubulovillous, villous	Familial adenomatous polyposis
Miscellaneous	Metaplastic (hyperplastic) polyps Lymphoid polyps	Benign lymphoid polyposis

than 10 colonic polyps) there is an increased risk of colonic cancer and surveillance and removal of polyps must be undertaken.

Peutz–Jeghers polyps are usually multiple and histologically have characteristic fibromuscular fronds radiating between disorganized mucosal crypts. They can occur in the large intestine, producing chronic anaemia.

In the Cronkhite–Canada syndrome, polyps similar to Peutz–Jegher are associated with ectodermal abnormalities such as alopecia, nail dystrophy and skin hyperpigmentation.

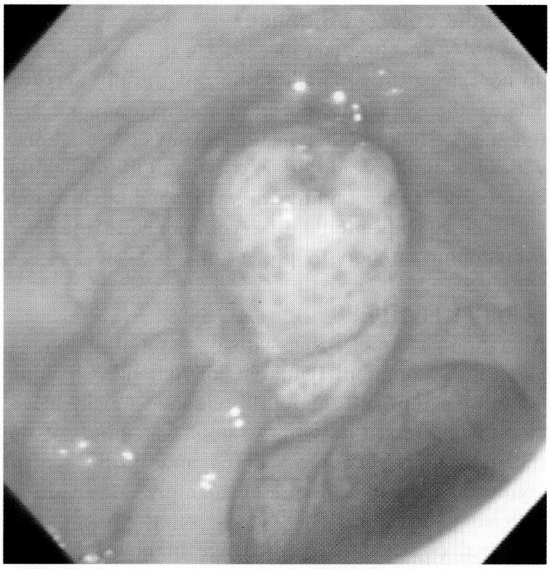

Fig 4.33
Colonoscopic appearance of a large peduncular polyp

Neoplastic polyps

Adenomas occur in about 10% of the population in the West but are rare elsewhere in the world. Genetic and environmental factors have been implicated but no definite aetiological factors have been identified (see below).

Polyps rarely produce symptoms and most are diagnosed on X-ray or on colonoscopy performed for other reasons. Large polyps (Fig 4.33) may bleed intermittently and cause anaemia. Large sessile villous adenomas of the rectum can present with profuse diarrhoea and hypokalaemia.

The frequency with which invasive carcinoma occurs in adenomas increases with the size of the polyp and most colonic carcinomas originate as adenomas. Once a polyp has been found on X-ray or endoscopy it is usually removed endoscopically. Further polyps may develop (30–50% probability) and continuous surveillance in patients under 75 years of age is necessary. An initial colonoscopy examination is made at three years, with 3–5 yearly colonoscopies thereafter.

Familial adenomatous polyposis (FAP) is inherited as an autosomal dominant trait. Linkage studies in families have shown that the gene involved (*apc*) is on the long arm of chromosome 5 (between q21 and q22).

In FAP, multiple polyps are found throughout the GI tract, the colon and duodenum being particularly involved. Constant endoscopic surveillance is necessary as all patients with eventually develop cancer if followed long enough. An attempt should be made to remove all colonic polyps, but this is often impossible and therefore, in this high-risk group and in any relative found to have polyps (relatives must be screened after 12 years of age), a colectomy with an ileorectal anastomosis is performed with long-term surveillance of the rectal stump. The NSAID sulindac has been shown to decrease the number and size of polyps in FAP.

Congenital hypertrophy of the retinal pigment epithelium (CHRPE) can be seen in two-thirds of FAP patients and is useful for screening in young patients.

Gardner's syndrome is a variant of this condition in which, in addition to adenomatosis, there are mesodermal tumours (e.g. dermoid tumours, osteomas of the skull) and pigmented occular fundal lesions.

Colorectal carcinoma

Adenocarcinoma of the large bowel is the second most common tumour in the UK with a lifetime incidence of about 1 in 27 (both male and females). The incidence increases with age, the average age at diagnosis being 60–65 years. The disease is rare in Africa and Asia and this difference is thought to be largely environmental rather than racial. There is a correlation between the consumption of meat and animal fat and colonic cancer. Western diets are low in fibre and the resulting intestinal stasis increases the time for which any potential carcinogen is in contact with the bowel wall. Case control and colort studies suggest that the risk of developing adenoma and carcinoma is substantially reduced among aspirin and NSAID users.

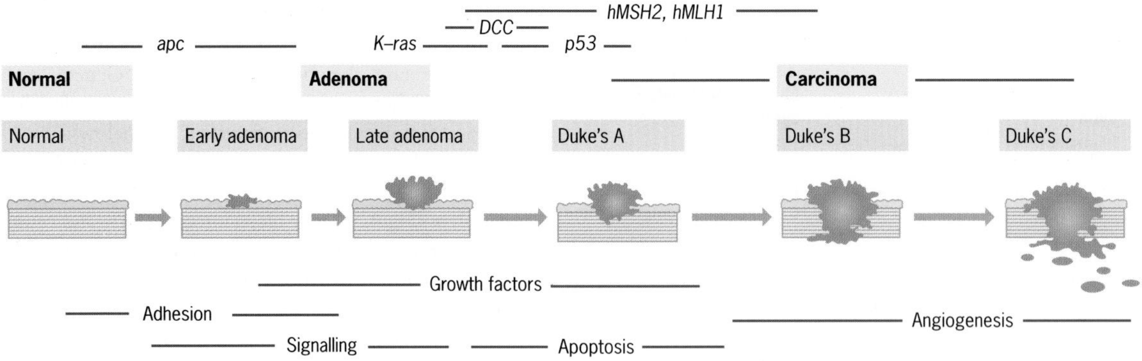

Fig 4.34
Genetic model for colorectal tumourigenesis, showing the progression from adenoma to carcinoma. The stages are shown at which mutations occur in the genes *apc* (adenomatous polyposis coli), *K-ras*, *hMSH2*, and *hMLH1*. From Bodmer W (1997) *Journal of the Royal College of Physicians of London* **31**, with permission

The bacterial flora in the colon are also affected by different diets, particularly in amount of fibre present, and it is speculated is that certain bacteria convert bile acids to potential carcinogens.

Ulcerative colitis (see p. 268) and familial adenomatous polyposis are predisposing factors.

GENETICS

Most colorectal cancers develop as a result of a stepwise progression from normal mucosa to adenomatous polyp to invasive cancer. This progression is associated with accumulating mutations in a number of growth-regulating genes (Fig 4.34). Genetic changes include the activation of dominantly acting proto-oncogenes, many of which have a physiological role in the regulation of normal cell division and differentiation. Mutations within these genes result in inappropriate stimulation signals, and the K-*ras* and c-*myc* genes are mutated in up to 50% and 70% of colorectal cancers respectively. Conversely, tumour suppressor genes inhibit cellular proliferation and tumorigenesis, and inactivation of these genes leads to excess tumour growth. Mutation of the *apc* gene, located on the long arm of chromosome 5, is responsible for the FAP syndrome, but is also found in 60% of sporadic colon cancers. Other tumour suppressor genes associated with colorectal cancer include the *p53*, *DCC* (deleted in colonic cancer) and *Nm23* genes. About 15% of sporadic colorectal cancers are also associated with microsatellite instability, but it appears that the accumulation of mutations is more important in cancer progression rather than the particular order in which they occur.

Cancer families

The risk of developing colorectal cancer is closely related to a positive family history. There is a 1.7 times increased lifetime risk of developing colorectal cancer if one first-degree relative is affected, but rises progressively with the number of affected family members. At the upper end of the risk spectrum is the hereditary non-polyposis colon cancer (HNPCC) syndrome accounting for 5–10% of colorectal cancers. HNPCC results from a dominantly inherited DNA mismatch repair gene mutation, on chromosomes 2, 3 or 7, which results in defective repair of mismatched bases during cell replication. Mutations in two mismatch repair genes, *MSH2* and *MSH1*, account for most cases. This leads to widespread genomic instability and manifests itself as microsatellite instability in the tumours of affected family members. HNPCC patients tend to develop right-sided cancers at an early age. Some (type II patients) also have an increased risk of upper gastrointestinal, gynaecological and urinary tract cancers whilst others are colon-specific (type I patients). The average age of cancer diagnosis in HNPCC patients is 45 years, and colonoscopic surveillance beginning at 23–35 years is necessary to detect and remove polyps from affected patients.

Sporadic colorectal cancer

About 90% of colorectal cancers occur in individuals who do not have a strong family history of this disease. Over half of these tumours occur in the rectosigmoid area (Fig 4.35). The tumour, which is usually a polypoid mass with ulceration, spreads by direct infiltration through the bowel wall. It then invades lymphatics and blood vessels with subsequent spread, most commonly to the liver. Synchronous tumours are present in 2% of cases.

CLINICAL FEATURES

Alteration in bowel habit, with or without abdominal pain, is a common symptom of left-sided colonic lesions. Rectum and sigmoid carcinomas usually bleed, blood being mixed in with the stool. Carcinoma of the caecum may become large and still remain asymptomatic. It can present simply as an iron-deficiency anaemia. The elderly often present with intestinal obstruction. Any change in bowel habit or bleeding per rectum must be investigated, particularly in the older age group.

Clinical examination is usually unhelpful, but a mass may be palpable. With liver metastases, hepatomegaly is found. Digital examination of the rectum is essential and sigmoidoscopy should be performed in all cases. Fibre-optic sigmoidoscopy can be performed on an outpatient basis after a single enema and increases 3–4 times the extent of the colon seen covering the area of the highest risk of carcinoma (Fig 4.35).

INVESTIGATIONS

- **Blood count and routine biochemistry** are performed.
- **Double-contrast barium enema** is still the usual investigation initially, but good preparation to ensure that the colon is free of faeces is essential.
- **Colonoscopy** is used for confirmation of doubtful lesions and to obtain specimens for histological examination.
- **Occult blood tests** have been used for mass screening but are of no value in hospital practice.
- **Abdominal and rectal ultrasound** is performed prior to surgery, for evaluation of tumour size and local and secondary spread.
- **CT** is useful for evaluating hepatic metastases.

TREATMENT

The primary tumour can be removed surgically in over 90% of cases. The specific procedure will depend on the tumour site, but resection and end-to-end anastomosis is performed if possible. Long-term survival is 40% overall, but depends upon the extent of the primary tumour and the presence of metastatic disease (Table 4.16). Adjuvant chemotherapy increases survival in patients with stage C colon cancer and, when combined with radiotherapy, increases survival for those with stage C rectal cancer. Chemotherapy is of little benefit for patients with stage A or B cancer, but is sometimes used when metastases are present; 5-fluorouracil and raltitrexed are the agents most commonly used.

Table 4.16
Modified Duke's classification of colorectal carcinoma

- Stage A – cancer confined to the bowel wall
- Stage B – cancer extending beyond the bowel wall, but without mestatases
- Stage C – cancer involving lymph nodes
- Stage D – cancer with distant metastases or with residual disease following surgery.

Tumour stage	Percentage of cases	Five-year cancer-related survival (%)
A	10	90–100
B	35	65–75
C	30	30–40
D	25	<5

(a)

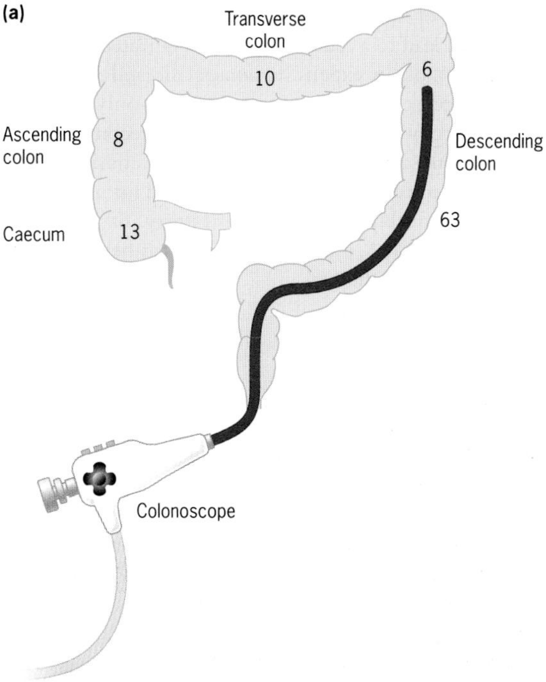

(b)

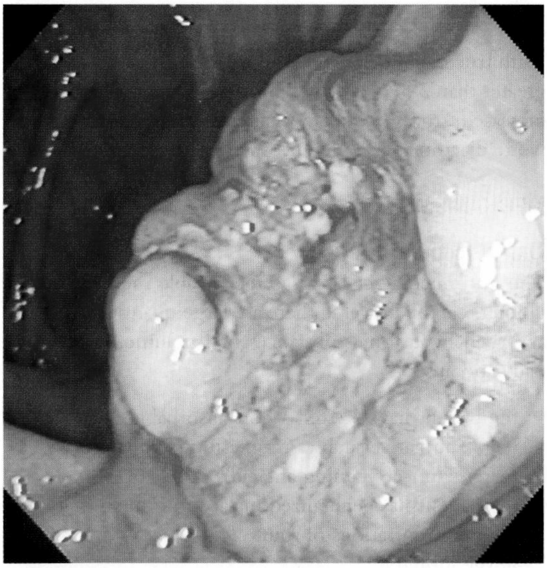

Fig 4.35
(a) Distribution of colorectal cancer (%). The flexible sigmoidoscope can reach 60–70 cm up the colon; approximately 70% of cancers occur in this area
(b) Colonoscopic appearance of a carcinoma in the ascending colon – a large irregular ulcer

PREVENTION AND SCREENING

Health-care agencies advocate a low-fat high-fibre diet in the prevention of sporadic colorectal cancer, while endoscopic screening with polyp removal is established for patients with FAP and HNPCC. A case for average-risk population screening has also been made, based upon the results of faecal occult blood (FOB) testing. FOB testing can lead to a reduction in cancer-related mortality of 15–33%, but is expensive, nonspecific and insensitive for the presence of cancer. A once-only flexible sigmoidoscopy at 55 years has also been recommended. Total colonoscopy is too expensive to consider as a population screening tool, but may be used for individuals with a reasonably strong family history of colorectal cancer. In the USA, universal screening has been adopted but not, so far, in the UK.

FURTHER READING

Bodmer W (1997) The somatic evolution of cancer. *Journal of the Royal College of Physicians* **31**: 82–89.

Lynch HT et al (1993) Genetics, natural history, tumour spectrum and pathology of hereditary non-polyposis colorectal cancer. *Gastroenterology* **104**: 1535–1549.

Winawer SJ (1997) Colorectal cancer screening: clinical guidelines and rationale. *Gastroenterology* **112**: 594–642.

Diarrhoea

With true diarrhoea there is an increase in stool weight to greater than 300 g per day. This is usually accompanied by increased stool frequency. Patients often interpret the word 'diarrhoea' in different ways (see p. 218).

MECHANISMS

Osmotic diarrhoea

The gut mucosa acts as a semipermeable membrane and fluid enters the bowel if there are large quantities of non-absorbed hypertonic substances in the lumen. This may occur because:

- the patient has ingested a non-absorbable substance (e.g. a purgative such as magnesium sulphate or magnesium-containing antacid)
- the patient has generalized malabsorption so that high concentrations of solute (e.g. glucose) remain in the lumen
- the patient has a specific absorptive defect (e.g. disaccharidase deficiency or glucose-galactose malabsorption).

The volume of diarrhoea produced by these mechanisms is reduced by the absorption of fluid by the ileum and colon. The diarrhoea stops when the patient stops eating or the malabsorptive substance is discontinued.

Secretory diarrhoea

In this disorder there is both active intestinal secretion of fluid and electrolytes as well as decreased absorption. The mechanism of intestinal secretion is shown in Fig 4.36a.

Common causes of secretory diarrhoea are:

- enterotoxins (e.g. cholera, *E. coli* – thermolabile or thermostable toxin)
- hormones (e.g. vasoactive intestinal peptide in the Verner–Morrison syndrome (p. 352)
- bile salts (in the colon) following ileal resection
- fatty acids (in the colon) following ileal resection
- some laxatives (e.g. dioctyl sodium sulphosuccinate).

With secretory diarrhoea, the stool volumes may be very high. Food does not affect the diarrhoea and it therefore continues during fasting.

Inflammatory diarrhoea (mucosal destruction)

Diarrhoea occurs because of damage to the intestinal mucosal cell so that there is a loss of fluid and blood. In addition, there is defective absorption of fluid and electrolytes. Common causes are infective conditions (e.g. dysentery due to *Shigella*), and inflammatory conditions (e.g. ulcerative colitis, see Fig 4.36b).

Abnormal motility

Diabetic, post-vagotomy and hyperthyroid diarrhoea are all due to abnormal motility of the upper gut. In many of these cases the volume and weight of the stool is not all that high, but frequency of defecation occurs; this therefore is not true diarrhoea.

Causes of diarrhoea are shown in Table 4.17. It should be noted that the irritable bowel syndrome, and diverticular disease and faecal impaction with overflow in the elderly, are not mentioned as they do not cause 'true' diarrhoea, even though the patients may complain of diarrhoea. World-wide, infection and infestation are a major problem and these are discussed under the causative organisms in Chapter 1.

Table 4.17
Causes of diarrhoea

Acute	Chronic
Dietary indiscretion	Inflammatory bowel disease
Infective Food poisoning, see p. 33 Viral gastroenteritis, see p. 58	Parasitic/fungal infections Malabsorption Gut resection
Traveller's diarrhoea, see p. 34; e.g. *E. coli* *Giardia intestinalis* *Shigella* *Entamoeba histolytica*	Drugs Colonic neoplasia Endocrine Pancreatic tumours (e.g. gastrinoma) Medullary carcinoma of the thyroid Thyrotoxicosis Diabetic neuropathy
	Faecal impaction – in the elderly

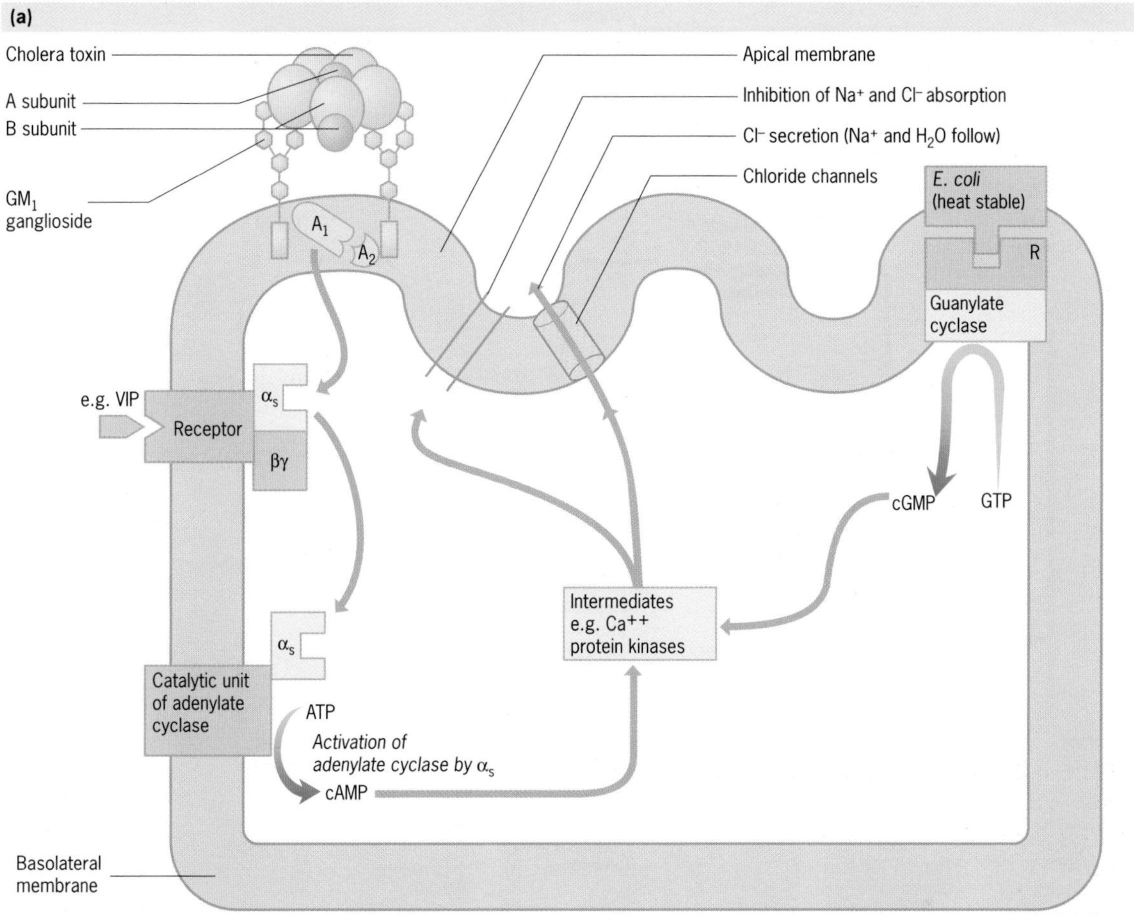

Fig 4.36
Mechanisms of diarrhoea
(a) Small intestinal cell. Cholera toxin binds to its receptor (monosialoganglioside GM$_1$) via its B subunits. The enzymatically active A_1 subunit activates G_s protein shown as its three subunits γ, β and α_s. α_s dissociates from G_s protein and activates the catalytic unit of adenylate cyclase on the basolateral membrane. The resulting increase in cAMP activates intermediates (e.g. protein kinases and Ca^{2+}), which act on the apical microvillous membrane to cause Cl$^-$ secretion and inhibition of Na$^+$ and Cl$^-$ absorption. Heat-labile *E. coli* shares the same receptor as cholera toxin. Heat-stable *E. coli* (ST) binds to its receptor protein R and this complex activates guanylate cyclase which produces the same effect. The ST receptor is specific for the intestine. In both mechanisms, stimulation occurs without invasion

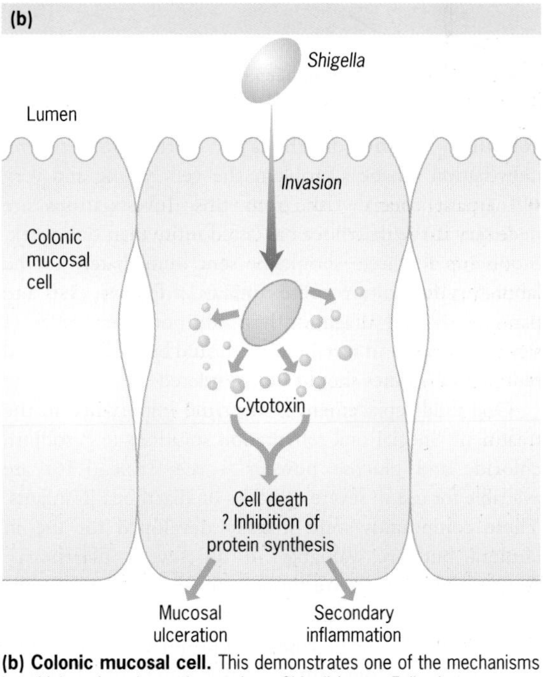

(b) Colonic mucosal cell. This demonstrates one of the mechanisms by which an invasive pathogen (e.g. *Shigella*) acts. Following penetration, the pathogens generate cytotoxins which lead to mucosal ulceration and cell death

Acute diarrhoea

(excluding cholera, discussed on p. 34)

Diarrhoea of sudden onset is very common, often short-lived and requires no investigation or treatment. This type of diarrhoea is seen after dietary indiscretions, but diarrhoea due to viral agents also lasts 24–48 hours (see p. 58). The causes of other infective diarrhoeas are shown on p. 276. Traveller's diarrhoea, which affects people travelling outside their own countries, particularly to developing countries, usually lasts 2–5 days; it is discussed on p. 34. Clinical features associated with the acute diarrhoeas include fever, abdominal pain and

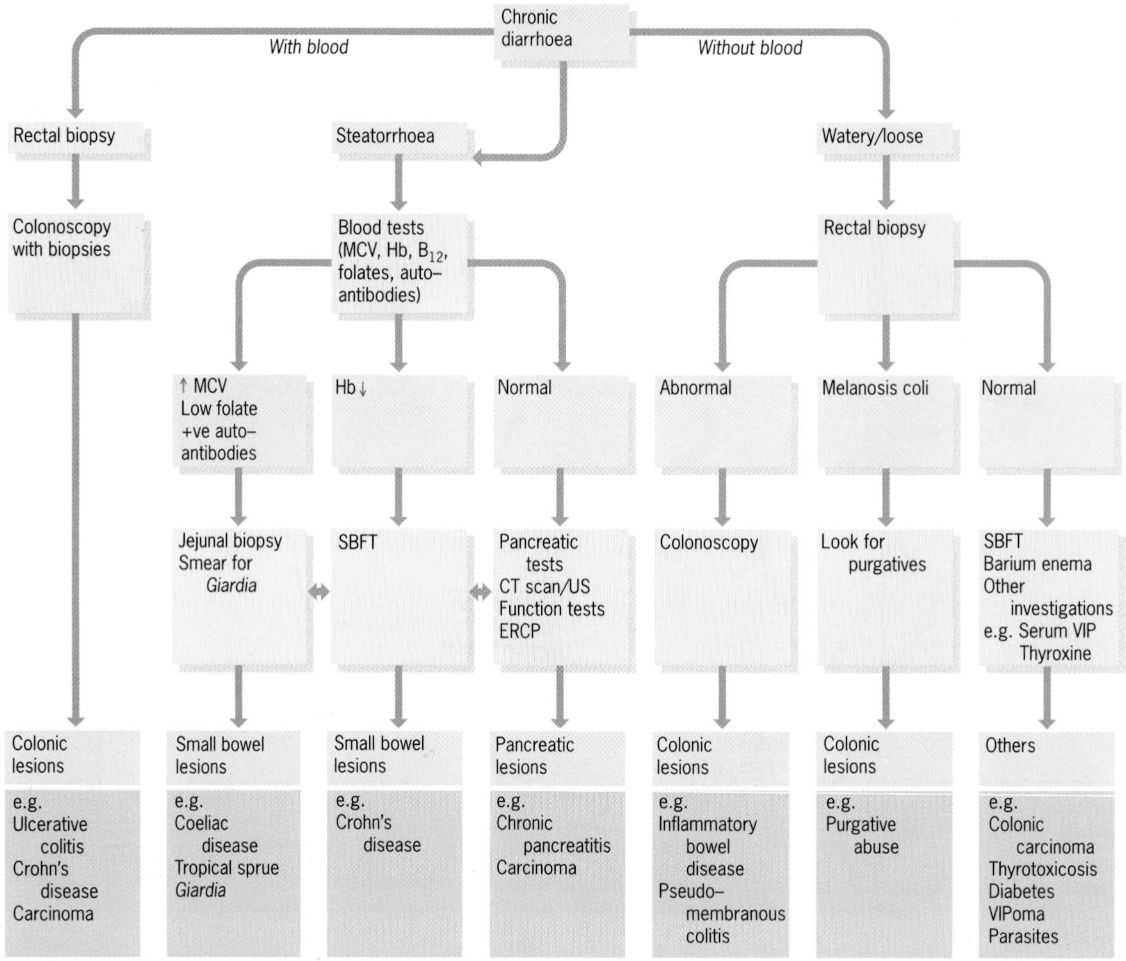

Fig 4.37
Flow diagram for the investigation of chronic diarrhoea. NB: All patients should have had stool cultures. SBFT, small bowel follow-through; VIP, vasoactive intestinal polypeptide; ERCP, endoscopic retrograde cholangiopancreatography

vomiting. If the diarrhoea is particularly severe, dehydration can be a problem; the very young and very old are at special risk from this. Investigations are necessary if the diarrhoea has lasted more than one week. Stools (up to three) should be sent immediately to the laboratory for culture and examination for ova, cysts and parasites. If the diagnosis has still not been made, a sigmoidoscopy and rectal biopsy should be performed and radiological studies should be considered.

Oral fluid replacement is of prime importance in the treatment. Special oral rehydration solutions (e.g. sodium chloride and glucose powder – see Table 1.16) are available for use in severe episodes of diarrhoea in infants. These compounds were initially developed for use in cholera but are valuable in all severe diarrhoeas. Antidiarrhoeal drugs are thought to impair the clearance of any pathogen from the bowel but may be necessary for short-term relief (e.g. codeine phosphate 30 mg four times daily, or loperamide 2 mg three times daily). Antibiotics are sometimes given (see p. 34), depending on the organism.

Chronic diarrhoea

This always needs investigation. All patients should have a sigmoidoscopy and rectal biopsy. The flow diagram in Fig 4.37 is illustrative; whether the large or the small bowel is investigated first will depend on the clinical story of, for example, bloody diarrhoea or steatorrhoea. The investigations and treatment are described in detail under the individual diseases.

Purgative abuse

This is most commonly seen in females who surreptitiously take high-dose purgatives and are often extensively investigated for chronic diarrhoea. The diarrhoea is usually of high volume (1 L daily). Sigmoidoscopy may show a pigmented mucosa, a condition known as *melanosis coli*. Histologically the rectal biopsy shows pigment-laden macrophages in patients taking an anthraquinone purgative (e.g. Senokot). Melanosis coli is also seen in people regularly taking purgatives in normal doses.

Table 4.18
GI problems in patients with AIDS

Site	Symptoms	Problems
Mouth/oesophagus	Dysphagia Retrosternal discomfort Oral ulceration	Candidiasis Herpes simplex virus (HSV) Cytomegalovirus (CMV)
Small bowel/colon	Chronic diarrhoea Steathorrhoea Weight loss	Parasites: Amoebae *Giardia intestinalis* *Cryptosporidium* *Isospora belli* Microsporidia *Cyclospora cayetanensis* Viruses: CMV/HSV, adenovirus Bacteria: *Salmonella* *Campylobacter* *Mycobacterium avum intracellulare* Non-infective enteropathy – cause unknown
Rectum/colon	Bloody diarrhoea	Bacterial infection (e.g. *Shigella*)
Any	Weight loss Diarrhoea	Neoplasia Kaposi's sarcoma Lymphoma Squamous carcinoma Infection – disseminated, e.g. *Mycobacterium avium intracellulare*

Phenolphthalein laxatives can be detected by pouring an alkali (e.g. sodium hydroxide) on the stools, which then turn pink; a magnesium-containing purgative will give a high faecal magnesium content. Anthraquinones can be measured in the urine. A barium enema shows loss of haustral pattern and there may be mild abnormalities of absorption tests and a low serum potassium.

Management is difficult as the patient often denies purgative ingestion. If the diagnosis is suspected, a locker or bed search (while the patient is out of the ward) is occasionally necessary. If the diagnosis is confirmed, the patient needs psychiatric help.

Antibiotic-associated diarrhoea (pseudomembranous colitis – see p. 27)

Pseudomembranous colitis may develop following the use of any antibiotic. Diarrhoea occurs in the first few days after taking the antibiotic or even up to six weeks after stopping the drug. The causative agent is *Clostridium difficile*.

Diarrhoea in patients with HIV infection

Chronic diarrhoea is a common symptom in HIV infection, but HIV's role in the pathogenesis of diarrhoea is unclear. *Cryptosporidium* (see p. 84) is the pathogen most commonly isolated. *Isospora belli* and microsporidia have also been found. An enteropathy has been described. The cause of the diarrhoea is often not found and treatment is symptomatic.

Table 4.18 shows the conditions affecting the gastrointestinal tract in patients with AIDS.

Functional bowel disease

Functional bowel disease is the general term used to embrace two syndromes, *non-ulcer dyspepsia* and the *irritable bowel syndrome*. These conditions are extremely common world-wide, making up to 60–80% of patients seen in a gastroenterology clinic. The two conditions overlap, with some symptoms being common to both. Table 4.19 give some gastrointestinal symptoms that are suggestive of psychosomatic disorders.

Table 4.19
Chronic GI symptoms suggestive of psychosomatic disorders

Nausea alone
Vomiting alone
Bad breath (halitosis)
Belching
Abdominal bloating
Chronic right hypochondrial pain
Left iliac fossa pain
Frequent bowel actions in the morning

Information

	Functional dyspepsia	Peptic ulceration
Site of pain	Diffuse 'all over'. Fits no recognized pattern	Epigastric Points with one finger
Frequency of pain	Daily for long periods	Episodic
Food/meals	Pain unaffected Lasts all day	Exacerbate or help pain
Antacids	No help	Help pain
Nocturnal pain waking patient	Rare	Common
Vomiting	No effect	Reduces pain

Information box 4.5 Clinical clues

Non-ulcer dyspepsia

This characterizes a heterogenous group of patients whose symptoms are mainly stress-related. Patients complain of indigestion, wind, nausea, early satiety or heartburn (dyspepsia) when no ulcer is found. It can be difficult on the history to differentiate it from the symptoms of peptic ulceration, but typically patients with ulcers have nocturnal pain and also respond to antacids (Information box 4.5).

Barium studies or endoscopy are often performed to exclude ulceration, but are best avoided in patients under 35 years, as no abnormality is found in the majority (80%).

Chronic antral gastritis due to *Helicobacter pylori* is found more frequently than in asymptomatic controls, but the relationship of this finding with symptoms is unclear.

Treatment is by reassurance. Antacids and H_2-receptor antagonists are probably of little benefit apart from the placebo effect. Cisapride 10 mg three times daily, or metoclopramide 10 mg three times daily, sometimes help, particularly in patients with fullness and early satiety, some of whom have been shown to have slow gastric emptying. Patients who are found to have *H. pylori* infection should have eradication therapy (see p. 237).

The irritable bowel syndrome

CLINICAL FEATURES

The pain is classically situated in the left iliac fossa and is usually relieved by defaecation or the passage of wind. The patient may complain of constipation or diarrhoea with the passage of frequent small volume stools and a feeling of incomplete emptying of the rectum. Stools may be ribbon-like or rabbity in appearance. True watery diarrhoea suggests organic disease. The pain, however, can be very variable and occur in any part of the abdomen and the bowel habit may be normal.

Abdominal distension and bloating are extremely common and, if present, strongly suggest the diagnosis of the irritable bowel. Women are more frequently affected than men, and often the symptoms occur at the time of menstruation. The length of history is usually long with frequent recurrent episodes and long symptom-free intervals. The patient may give a history of recurrent episodes of abdominal pain as a child and there is an increase of childhood or sexual abuse in some series. Mild episodes of pain occur frequently (approximately 40%) in the normal population and are often disregarded. The reason why some patients attend doctors is unclear, but it is sometimes related to psychological and social factors. The patient with the irritable bowel syndrome looks well despite frequent episodes of pain, some of which can be very acute and require hospital admission to rule out an acute abdominal condition.

Information

- *Beware of false correlations.* Diverticular disease is common in the elderly and because diverticular disease is seen on the barium enema it must not be assumed to be the cause of the pain. Hiatus hernias are also common findings and are also often asymptomatic.
- *Gynaecological problems must be excluded.* On the other hand, it must not be assumed that all lower abdominal pain in women is due to some gynaecological problem. Many unnecessary operations are carried out as a consequence.
- *Recurrent pain in the right iliac fossa* is not due to chronic appendicitis, but to the irritable bowel syndrome.
- *Recurrent pain in the right hypochondrium* is usually not due to gallbladder disease, but to the irritable bowel syndrome.
- *Abdominal bruits are common* and abdominal pain should not be ascribed to an ischaemic bowel on this basis alone.

Information box 4.6 Traps for the unwary

PATHOPHYSIOLOGY

Motility abnormalities have been found in the irritable bowel syndrome, but these abnormal findings have not been consistent and do not always correlate with episodes of pain.

Psychological factors are important and most patients find the symptoms are exacerbated by stress. Some patients are depressed, and this fact may be missed unless looked for carefully.

EXAMINATION AND DIAGNOSIS

Examination reveals no abnormality. Rectal examination and sigmoidoscopy should be performed. Although sigmoidoscopy shows a normal mucosa, air insufflation may reproduce the pain.

INVESTIGATION

The amount of investigation varies in individual patients. A young girl with pain in the left iliac fossa exacerbated by stress will require no investigation. Conversely, an elderly person who has developed pain or diarrhoea for the first time must be investigated, with a full radiological assessment, before the diagnosis of functional bowel disease is made.

Information box 4.6 gives tips towards avoiding an incorrect diagnosis.

MANAGEMENT

In many patients symptoms are not severe and are clearly stress-related. These patients often require nothing but a discussion of their lifestyle and reassurance. Over-investigation and drug therapy should be avoided.

- Patients must be reassured of the benign nature of the condition. Cancer phobia must be dispelled. Patients are encouraged to learn to cope with their symptoms, as they tend to be recurrent.
- A high-fibre diet or even a change in diet help some patients.
- Antispasmodics (e.g. mebeverine) are given.
- A small group of patients who are often hospital attenders have severe symptoms and treatment here is difficult. Many are depressed and improve with antidepressant therapy. Other therapies, such as biofeedback and hypnotherapy, have been tried.

The acute abdomen

This section deals with acute abdominal conditions that cause the patient to be hospitalized within a few hours of the onset of their pain. It is important to make the diagnosis as quickly as possible to reduce morbidity and mortality. Although a specific diagnosis should be attempted, the immediate problem in management is to decide whether an 'acute abdomen' exists and whether surgery is required.

HISTORY

This should include previous operations, any gynaecological problems, and whether any concurrent medical condition is present.

Pain

The onset, site, type and subsequent course of the pain should be determined as accurately as possible. In general, the pain of an acute abdomen can either be constant (usually due to inflammation) or a colic due to a blocked 'tube'. The inflammatory nature of a *constant* pain will be supported by a temperature, tachycardia and/or a raised white cell count. If these are normal, then other causes (e.g. musculoskeletal, aortic aneurysm) or rare causes (e.g. porphyria) should be considered. A *colic* can be due to an obstruction of the gut, biliary system, urogenital system or the uterus. These will probably initially require conservative management along with analgesics. If the colic becomes a constant pain, then inflammation of the organ may have supervened (e.g. strangulated hernia, ascending cholangitis or salpingitis).

A *sudden onset of pain* suggests:

- a perforation (e.g. of a duodenal ulcer)
- a rupture (e.g. of an aneurysm)
- torsion (e.g. of an ovarian cyst)
- acute pancreatitis.

Back pain suggests:

- pancreatitis
- rupture of an aortic aneurysm
- renal tract disease.

Inflammatory conditions (e.g. appendicitis) produce a more gradual onset of pain. With peritonitis (see below) the pain is continuous and may be made worse by movement.

Vomiting

Vomiting may accompany any acute abdominal pain, but if persistent, it suggests an obstructive lesion of the gut. The character of the vomit should be asked – does it contain blood, bile or small bowel contents?

Other symptoms

Any change in bowel habit or of urinary frequency should be documented and, in females, a gynaecological history taken.

PHYSICAL EXAMINATION

The general condition of the person should be noted. Does the patient look ill? Is he or she shocked? Large volumes of fluid may be lost from the vascular compartment into the peritoneal cavity or into the lumen of the bowel giving rise to hypovolaemia, i.e. a pale cold skin, a weak rapid pulse and hypotension.

The abdomen

- **Inspection**. Look for the presence of scars, distension or masses.

- **Palpation**. The abdomen should be examined gently for sites of tenderness and the presence or absence of guarding. Guarding is involuntary spasm of the abdominal wall and it indicates peritonitis. This can be localized to one area or it may be generalized, involving the whole abdomen.
- **Bowel sounds**. Increased high-pitch tinkling bowel sounds indicate fluid obstruction; this occurs because of fluid movement within the large dilated bowel lumen. Absent bowel sounds suggest peritoneal involvement. In an obstructed patient, absent bowel sounds suggest strangulation or ischaemia or ileus. It is essential that the hernial orifices be examined if intestinal obstruction is suspected.

Pelvic and rectal examination

Pelvic examination can be very helpful, particularly in diagnosing gynaecological causes of an acute abdomen (e.g. a ruptured ectopic pregnancy). Rectal examination is less helpful as localized tenderness may be due to any cause; it may show blood on the finger stall.

Other observations

- **Mouth**. The tongue is furred in some cases and a fetor is present.
- **Temperature**. Fever is more common in acute inflammatory processes.
- **Urine**. Examine for:
  (a) blood – suggests urinary tract infection or renal colic
  (b) glucose and ketones – ketoacidosis can present with acute pain
  (c) protein and white cells – to exclude acute pyelonephritis).
- Think of other conditions, such as:
  (a) diabetes mellitus (ketoacidosis)
  (b) pneumonia (referred pain)
  (c) myocardial infarction (referred pain)
  (d) lead poisoning
  (e) irritable bowel syndrome (this can produce acute severe pain)
  (f) renal colic
  (g) porphyria (a rare cause of abdominal pain).

INVESTIGATIONS

- **Blood count**. A raised white cell count occurs in inflammatory conditions.
- **Serum amylase**. High levels (more than five times normal) indicate acute pancreatitis. Raised levels below this can occur in any acute abdomen and should not be considered diagnostic of pancreatitis.
- **Serum electrolytes**. These are not particularly helpful for diagnosis, but useful for general evaluation of the patient.
- **Pregnancy**. A urine dipstix is used with women of child-bearing age.
- **X-rays**. A CXR is useful to detect air under the diaphragm owing to a perforation or dilated loops of bowel or fluid levels suggestive of obstruction (supine abdominal X-ray).
- **Ultrasound**. This is useful in the diagnosis of acute cholangitis and aortic aneurysm, and in expert hands is reliable in the diagnosis of acute appendicitis. Gynaecological and other pelvic causes of pain can also be detected.
- **CT scan**. Spiral CT is an accurate investigation (where available) in most acute emergencies. It is becoming more widely used and reduces unnecessary laparotomies for cases of suspected appendicitis.
- **Laparoscopy**. This has gained increasing importance as a diagnostic tool proir to proceding with surgery, particularly in men and women over the age of 50 years. In addition, therapeutic manoeuvres, such as appendicectomy, can be performed.

Acute appendicitis

This is the most common surgical emergency. It affects all age groups, but is rare in the very young and the very old. Appendicitis should always be considered in the differential diagnosis if the appendix has not been removed.

Acute appendicitis mostly occurs when the lumen of the appendix becomes obstructed with a faecolith; however, in some cases there is only generalized acute inflammation. If the appendix is not removed at this stage, gangrene occurs with perforation, leading to a localized abscess or to generalized peritonitis.

CLINICAL FEATURES AND MANAGEMENT

Most patients present with abdominal pain; in many it starts vaguely in the centre of the abdomen, becoming localized to the right iliac fossa in the first few hours. Nausea, vomiting and occasional diarrhoea can occur. Because of the mobile position of the appendix, symptoms and signs are variable.

Examination of the abdomen reveals tenderness in the right iliac fossa, with guarding due to the localized peritonitis. There may be a tender mass in the right iliac fossa. Laboratory tests are unhelpful, except that the white cell count may be raised. An ultrasound is accurate for the detection of an inflamed appendix and will also indicate an appendix mass or other localized lesion. CT is being used more frequently. It is highly sensitive and specific, and reduces the incidence of removing the 'normal' appendix.

DIFFERENTIAL DIAGNOSIS

All abdominal conditions must be considered:

- nonspecific mesenteric lymphadenitis – may mimic appendicitis
- acute terminal ileitis (see p. 263) – due to Crohn's disease; *Yersinia* infection also gives similar symptoms and signs
- acute salpingitis – should be considered in women; there is usually a vaginal discharge and on vaginal examination, adnexal tenderness is found

- inflamed Meckel's diverticulum
- functional bowel disease.

It should be noted that 45% of women aged 15–45 years who have had an appendicectomy have a normal appendix removed.

TREATMENT

The appendix is removed by open surgery or laparoscopically. If an appendix mass is present, the patient is treated conservatively with intravenous fluids and antibiotics. The pain subsides over a few days and the mass usually disappears over a few weeks. Interval appendicectomy is recommended at a later date to prevent further acute episodes.

Acute peritonitis

Localized peritonitis

There is virtually always some degree of localized peritonitis with all acute inflammatory conditions of the GI tract (e.g. acute appendicitis, acute cholecystitis). Pain and tenderness are largely features of this localized peritonitis. The treatment is for the underlying disease.

Generalized peritonitis

This is a serious condition resulting from irritation of the peritoneum owing to infection (e.g. perforated appendix), or from chemical irritation due to leakage of intestinal contents (e.g. perforated ulcer). In the latter case, superadded infection gradually occurs; *E. coli* and *Bacteroides* are the most common organisms.

The peritoneal cavity becomes acutely inflamed with production of an inflammatory exudate that spreads throughout the peritoneum leading to intestinal dilatation and paralytic ileus.

CLINICAL FEATURES AND MANAGEMENT

In perforation, the onset is sudden with acute severe abdominal pain, followed by general collapse and shock. The patient may improve temporarily, only to become worse later as generalized toxaemia occurs.

When the peritonitis is secondary to inflammatory disease, the onset is less rapid with the initial features being those of the underlying disease.

Investigations should always include an erect chest X-ray to detect free air under the diaphragm, and a serum amylase to diagnose acute pancreatitis which is treated conservatively. Imaging with ultrasound and/or CT is being increasingly used for diagnosis.

Peritonitis is always treated surgically after adequate resuscitation with the re-establishment of a good urinary output. This includes insertion of a nasogastric tube, intravenous fluids and antibiotics. Surgery has a twofold objective:

- peritoneal lavage of the abdominal cavity
- specific treatment of the underlying condition.

Table 4.20
Some causes of intestinal obstruction

Small bowel obstruction	Large bowel obstruction
Adhesions	Carcinoma of the colon
Herniae	Volvulus
Crohn's disease	Diverticular disease

COMPLICATIONS

Any delay in treatment of peritonitis produces more profound toxaemia and septicaemia. In addition, local abscess formation occurs and should be suspected if the patient continues to remain unwell postoperatively with a swinging fever, high white cell count and continuing pain. Abscesses are commonly pelvic or subphrenic. Both are now localized chiefly by ultrasound examination. Treatment is with drainage and antibiotics.

Intestinal obstruction

Most intestinal obstruction is due to a mechanical block. Sometimes the bowel does not function, leading to a paralytic ileus. This occurs temporarily after most abdominal operations and with peritonitis. Some causes of intestinal obstruction are shown in Table 4.20.

Obstruction of the bowel leads to bowel distension above the block, with increased secretion of fluid into the distended bowel. Bacterial contamination occurs in the distended stagnant bowel. In strangulation the blood supply is impeded, leading to gangrene, perforation and peritonitis unless urgent treatment of the condition is undertaken.

CLINICAL FEATURES

The patient complains of abdominal colic, vomiting and constipation without passage of wind. In upper gut obstruction the vomiting is profuse but in lower gut obstruction it may be absent.

Examination of the abdomen reveals distension with increased bowel sounds. Marked tenderness suggests strangulation and urgent surgery is necessary. Examination of the hernial orifices and rectum must be performed. X-ray of the abdomen reveals distended loops of bowel proximal to the obstruction. Fluid levels are seen in small bowel obstruction on an erect film. In large bowel obstruction, the caecum and ascending colon are distended. An instant water-soluble barium enema without air insufflation may help to demonstrate the site of the obstruction.

MANAGEMENT

Initial management is by resuscitation with intravenous fluids (mainly isotonic saline with potassium) and decompression. The majority will settle on conservative management, but an increasing temperature, raised pulse rate, increasing pain and a rising white cell count require exploratory laparotomy.

Laparotomy with removal of the obstruction is necessary in most cases of small bowel obstruction. If the bowel is gangrenous owing to strangulation, gut resection will be required. A few patients (e.g. those with Crohn's disease) may have recurrent episodes of incomplete intestinal obstruction that can be managed conservatively.

In large bowel obstruction, if surgery is necessary, primary resection with or without primary anastomosis should be performed. In critically ill patients, a defunctioning colostomy may be the only alternative.

Volvulus of the sigmoid colon can be managed by the passage of a flexible sigmoidoscope or a rectal tube to unkink the bowel, but recurrent volvulus may require sigmoid resection.

A pseudo-obstruction is occasionally seen in diabetics owing to an autoimmune neuropathy, and in patients taking certain drugs (e.g. antidepressants) and those on continuous morphine pumps. Very rarely the clinical features of obstruction are produced by a condition in which the nerve plexuses of the bowel are damaged (intestinal pseudo-obstruction). This condition is managed conservatively.

Intestinal vascular emergencies

These are uncommon, but are usually seen in elderly patients with cardiac arrthyrmias. Artery occlusion can occur from either an embolus or thrombosis in an arteriosclerotic artery leading to ischaemia and bowel necrosis.

Patients present with sudden severe abdominal pain and vomiting, but often with a paucity of physical signs. The abdomen is usually tender and bowel sounds may be absent.

Large bowel ischaemia is treated conservatively. Small bowel ischaemia invariably requires surgery, but the outcome will depend on the site of occlusion. A limited resection has a reasonable prognosis, but extensive gangrene of the bowel is invariably fatal.

Mesenteric venous thrombosis occurs mainly in patients who have circulatory failure and can lead to gut necrosis. Often the patient is extremely ill from the underlying condition and requires intensive care and a GTN intravenous infusion. If there is no response, an exploratory laparotomy is performed.

FURTHER READING

McColl I (1998) More precision in diagnosing appendicitis [Editorial]. *New England Journal of Medicine* **338**: 190-191.

The peritoneum

The peritoneal cavity is a closed sac lined by mesothelial cells. The peritoneal mesothelial cells produce surfactant that acts as a lubricant within the peritoneal cavity. The cavity contains less than 100 mL of serous fluid containing less than 30 g L^{-1} of protein.

Table 4.21
Diseases of the peritoneum

Infective (bacterial) peritonitis	Neoplasia
Secondary to gut disease; e.g. appendicitis, perforation of any organ	Secondary deposits (e.g. from ovary, stomach)
Chronic peritoneal dialysis	Primary mesothelioma
Spontaneous, usually in ascites with liver disease	**Vasculitis**
Tuberculosis	Connective tissue disease

The mesothelial cells lining the diaphragm have gaps that allow communication between the peritoneum and the diphragmatic lymphatics. Approximately one-third of fluid drains through these lymphatics, the remainder through the parietal peritoneum. These mechanisms allow particulate matter to be removed rapidly from the peritoneal cavity.

Complement activation is an early defence mechanism followed rapidly by up-regulation of the peritoneal mesothelial cells and migration of polymorphonuclear neutrophils and macrophages into the peritoneum.

Mast cells release potent mediators of inflammation and interact with T cells to generate an immune response.

The peritoneal-associated lymphoid tissue includes the omental milky spots, the lymphocytes within the peritoneal cavity and the draining lymph nodes. B cells with a unique CD^{5+} are common. This defence system plays an important role in localizing peritoneal infection. Some conditions that can affect the peritoneum are shown in Table 4.21.

Peritonitis can be acute or chronic, as seen in tuberculosis. Most cases of infective peritonitis are secondary to gastrointestinal diseases, but it occurs occasionally without intra-abdominal sepsis in ascites due to liver disease. Very rarely, fungal and parasitic infections can also cause primary peritonitis (e.g. amoebiasis, candidiasis). Peritonitis is discussed further on p. 283.

The peritoneum can be involved by *secondary malignant deposits*, and the most common cause of ascites in a young to middle-aged woman is an ovarian carcinoma.

A *subphrenic abscess* is usually secondary to infection in the abdomen and is characterized by fever, malaise, pain in the right or left hypochondrium and shoulder-tip pain. An erect chest X-ray shows gas under the diaphragm, impaired movement of the diaphragm on screening, and a pleural effusion. Ultrasound is usually diagnostic.

Ascites is associated with all diseases of the peritoneum. The fluid that collects is an exudate with a high protein content. It is also seen in liver disease. The mechanism, causes and investigation of ascites are discussed on p. 320.

Tuberculous peritonitis (see also p. 258)

This is due to reactivation of a tuberculous focus in the abdomen, often a lymph node. It is common in developing countries and is seen in the UK in debilitated patients, alcohol-dependent patients and in certain racial groups (e.g. Asians). Usually the onset is insidious, with fever, anorexia and weight loss. Abdominal pain is common, accompanied by ascites (75%) or an abdominal mass caused by an inflamed mesentery.

Diagnosis is made by examination of the peritoneal fluid, if present, which shows an increase in lymphocyte count; occasionally tubercle bacilli are seen on staining. Culture of the fluid should be performed. Ultrasound shows mesenteric thickening and enlargement of lymph nodes. At laparoscopy the peritoneum is seen to be studded with tubercles that can be biopsied and sent for culture and histology. Treatment is with conventional chemotherapy for 18 months to two years.

Retroperitoneal fibrosis (periaortitis)

This is a rare condition in which there is a marked fibrosis over the posterior abdominal wall and retroperitoneum. The aetiology is usually unknown but it has been associated with the drug methysergide and occasionally with the carcinoid syndrome. The disease usually presents in middle age with malaise, fever, and loss of weight. There is often anaemia and a raised ESR – a CT scan is diagnostic (see Fig. 9.35). The major complication is urinary tract obstruction from ureteric involvement, which may require surgery.

FURTHER READING

Hall JC et al (1998) The pathobiology of peritonitis. *Gastroenterology* **114**: 185–196.

CHAPTER BIBLIOGRAPHY

Guide to the Internet (1998) *Lancet* **351** (Suppl 1): 1–17.

Sleisenger and Fordtran's Gastrointestinal and Liver Disease, 6th edn (1997) Philadelphia: WB Saunders.

5

Liver, biliary tract and pancreatic diseases

In the West, alcohol is the major cause of liver disease, whilst elsewhere the hepatitis B virus is still a significant factor. The longer term clinical consequences of hepatitis C have been recognized, and a new virus – hepatitis G – has been identified. Health education and the improvement of social conditions should help to stop the spread of viral infections, as should widespread vaccination against hepatitis A and B.

Imaging techniques now enable the liver and biliary tree to be visualized with precision, resulting in earlier diagnosis. Therapeutic endoscopy, and laparoscopic and minimally invasive surgery, avoid the necessity of major surgery, particularly for biliary tract disease. Finally, liver transplantation is now established for the treatment of acute and chronic liver disease.

The liver

Structure of the liver and biliary system

The liver

The liver is the largest internal organ in the body and is situated in the right hypochondrium. Functionally, it is divided into right and left lobes by the middle hepatic vein. The right lobe is larger and contains the caudate and quadrate lobes. The liver is further subdivided into a total of eight sectors (Fig 5.1) by divisions of the right, middle and left hepatic veins. Each sector receives its own portal pedicle, permitting individual sector resection at surgery.

The blood supply to the liver constitutes 25% of the resting cardiac output and is via two main vessels:

- The *hepatic artery*, which is a branch of the coeliac axis, supplies 25% of the total blood flow. Autoregulation of blood flow by the hepatic artery ensures a constant total liver blood flow.
- The *portal vein* drains most of the gastrointestinal tract and the spleen. It supplies 75% of the blood flow. The normal portal pressure is 5–8 mmHg; flow increases after meals.

Both vessels enter the liver via the hilum (porta hepatis). The blood from these vessels is distributed to the sectors and passes into the sinusoids via the portal tracts.

Blood leaves the sinusoids, entering branches of the hepatic vein which join into three main branches before entering the inferior vena cava.

The caudate lobe is an autonomous segment as it receives an independent blood supply from the portal vein and hepatic artery, and its hepatic vein drains directly into the inferior vena cava.

Lymph, formed mainly in the perisinusoidal space, is collected in lymphatics which are present in the portal tracts. These small lymphatics enter larger vessels which eventually drain into the hepatic ducts.

The functional unit of the liver is the acinus. This consists of parenchyma supplied by the smallest portal tracts containing portal vein radicles, hepatic arterioles and bile ductules (Fig 5.2). The hepatocytes near this triad (zone 1) are well supplied with oxygenated blood and are more resistant to damage than the cells nearer the terminal hepatic (central) veins (zone 3).

The sinusoids lack a basement membrane and are loosely surrounded by specialist fenestrated endothelial cells and Kupffer's cells (phagocytic cells). Sinusoids are separated by plates of liver cells (hepatocytes). The subendothelial space that lies between the sinusoids and hepatocytes is the space of Disse which contains a matrix of basement membrane constituents and stellate cells.

Stellate cells (previously called 'fat storage cells' or Ito cells) store retinoids and contain the intermediate filament, desmin. They are contractile and probably regulate sinusoidal blood flow. Endothelin and nitric oxide play an important role in modulating stellate cell contractility. Stellate cells, after activation, produce collagen types I, III and IV (see p. 517).

The biliary system

Bile canaliculi form a network between the hepatocytes. These join to form thin bile ductules near the portal tract, which in turn enter the bile ducts in the portal tracts. These then combine to form the right and left hepatic ducts that leave each liver lobe. The hepatic ducts join at the porta hepatis to form the common hepatic duct. The cystic duct connects the gallbladder to the lower end of the common hepatic duct. The gallbladder lies under the right lobe of the liver and stores and concentrates hepatic bile; it has a capacity of approximately 50 mL. The common bile duct is formed by the combination of the cystic and hepatic ducts and is approximately 8 mm in diameter, narrowing at its distal end to pass into the duodenum. The common bile duct and pancreatic duct open into the second part of the duodenum through a common channel at the ampulla of Vater. The lower end of the common bile duct contains the muscular sphincter of Oddi, which contracts rhythmically and prevents bile from entering the duodenum in the fasting state.

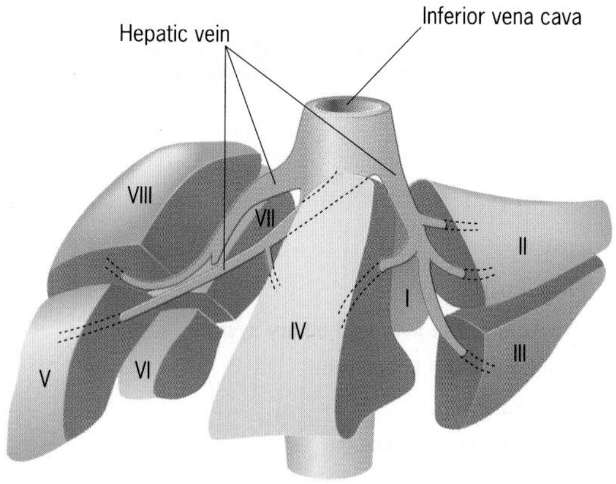

Fig 5.1
Segmental anatomy of the liver showing the eight hepatic segments.
I = caudate lobe, II–IV the left hemiliver, V–VIII the right hemiliver.
Modified from Bismuth H (1982) *World Journal of Surgery* with permission

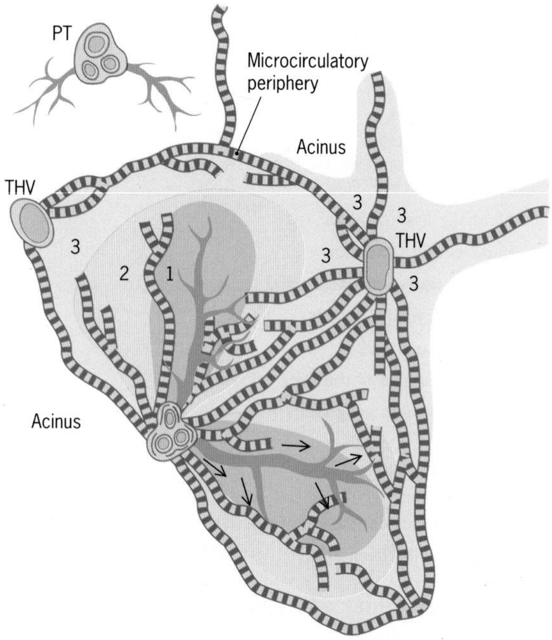

Fig 5.2
Diagram of an acinus.
Zones 1, 2 and 3 represent areas supplied by blood, with zone 1 being best oxygenated. Zone 3 is supplied by blood remote from afferent vessels and is in the microcirculatory periphery of the acinus. The perivascular areas (star shaped) is formed by the most peripheral parts of zone 3 of several adjacent acini and is the least well oxygenated. THV, terminal hepatic venule; PT, portal triad.
From Sherlock S, Dooley J (1997) with permission

FURTHER READING

Sherlock S, Dooley J (1997) *Anatomy and Function in Diseases of the Liver and Biliary System*, 10th edn. Oxford: Blackwell Science.

Functions of the liver

Protein metabolism (see also p. 192)

Synthesis

The liver is the principal site of synthesis of all circulating proteins apart from γ-globulins, which are produced in the reticuloendothelial system. The liver receives amino acids from the intestine and muscles and, by controlling the rate of gluconeogenesis and transamination, regulates levels in the plasma. Plasma contains 60–80 g L^{-1} of protein, mainly in the form of albumin, globulin and fibrinogen.

Albumin has a half-life of 16–24 days and 10–12 g are synthesized daily. Its main functions are first to maintain the intravascular oncotic (colloid osmotic) pressure, and second to transport water-insoluble substances such as bilirubin, hormones, fatty acids and drugs. Reduced synthesis of albumin over prolonged periods produces hypoalbuminaemia and is seen in chronic liver disease and malnutrition. Hypoalbuminaemia is also found in hypercatabolic states (e.g. trauma with sepsis), and in diseases where there is an excessive loss (e.g. nephrotic syndrome, protein-losing enteropathy).

Transport or carrier proteins such as transferrin and caeruloplasmin, acute phase and other proteins (e.g. α_1-antitrypsin and α-fetoprotein) are also produced in the liver.

The liver also synthesizes all coagulation factors (apart from factor VIII) – that is, fibrinogen, prothrombin, factors V, VII, IX, X and XIII (see Chapter 6), and components of the complement system.

Degradation (nitrogen excretion)

Amino acids are degraded by transamination and oxidative deamination to produce ammonia, which is then converted to urea and excreted by the kidneys. This is a major pathway for the elimination of nitrogenous waste. Failure of this process occurs in severe liver disease.

Carbohydrate metabolism

Glucose homeostasis and the maintenance of the blood sugar is an important function of the liver. It stores approximately 80 g of glycogen. In the immediate fasting state, blood glucose is maintained either by glucose released from the breakdown of glycogen (glycogenolysis) or by newly synthesized glucose (gluconeogenesis). Sources for gluconeogenesis are lactate, pyruvate, amino acids from muscles (mainly alanine and glutamine) and glycerol from lipolysis of fat stores. In prolonged starvation, ketone bodies and fatty acids are used as alternative sources of fuel and the body tissues adapt to a lower glucose requirement (see Chapter 3).

Lipid metabolism

Fats are insoluble in water and are transported in the plasma as protein–lipid complexes (lipoproteins). These are discussed in detail on p. 989.

The liver has a major role in the metabolism of lipoproteins. It synthesizes very-low-density lipoproteins (VLDLs) and high-density lipoproteins (HDLs). HDLs are the substrate for lecithin–cholesterol acyltransferase (LCAT), which catalyses the conversion of free cholesterol to cholesterol ester (see below). Hepatic lipase removes triglyceride from intermediate-density lipoproteins (IDLs) to produce low-density lipoproteins (LDLs) which are degraded by the liver after uptake by specific cell-surface receptors (see Fig 17.19).

Triglycerides are mainly of dietary origin but are also formed in the liver from circulating free fatty acids (FFAs) and glycerol and incorporated into VLDLs. Oxidation or *de novo* synthesis of FFA occurs in the liver, depending on the availability of dietary fat.

Cholesterol may be of dietary origin but most is synthesized from acetyl-CoA mainly in the liver, intestine, adrenal cortex and skin. It occurs either as free cholesterol or is esterified with fatty acids; this reaction is catalysed by LCAT. This enzyme is reduced in severe liver disease, increasing the ratio of free cholesterol to ester, which alters membrane structures. One result of this is the red cell abnormalities (e.g. target cells) seen in chronic liver disease. Phospholipids (e.g. lecithin) are synthesized in the liver.

The complex interrelationships between protein, carbohydrate and fat metabolism are shown in Fig 5.3.

Formation of bile

Bile secretion

Bile consists of water, electrolytes, bile acids, cholesterol, phospholipids and conjugated bilirubin. Two processes are involved in bile secretion across the canalicular membrane of the hepatocyte – a *bile salt-dependent* and a *bile salt-independent process* – each contributing about 230 mL per day. The remainder of the bile (about 150 mL daily) is produced by the epithelial cells of the bile ductules.

Bile formation requires firstly the uptake of bile acids and other organic and inorganic ions across the basolateral (sinusoidal) membranes by multiple transport proteins. This process is driven by Na^+–K^+-ATPase in the basolateral membrane. Intracellular transport across the hepatocyte is partly through microtubules and partly by cytosol transport proteins. The canalicular membrane contains additional transporters, mainly ATPase-dependent, which carry molecules into the biliary canaliculi against a concentration gradient. The canalicular multispecific organic anion transporter (cMOAT) mediates transport of a broad range of compounds including bilirubin diglucuronide.

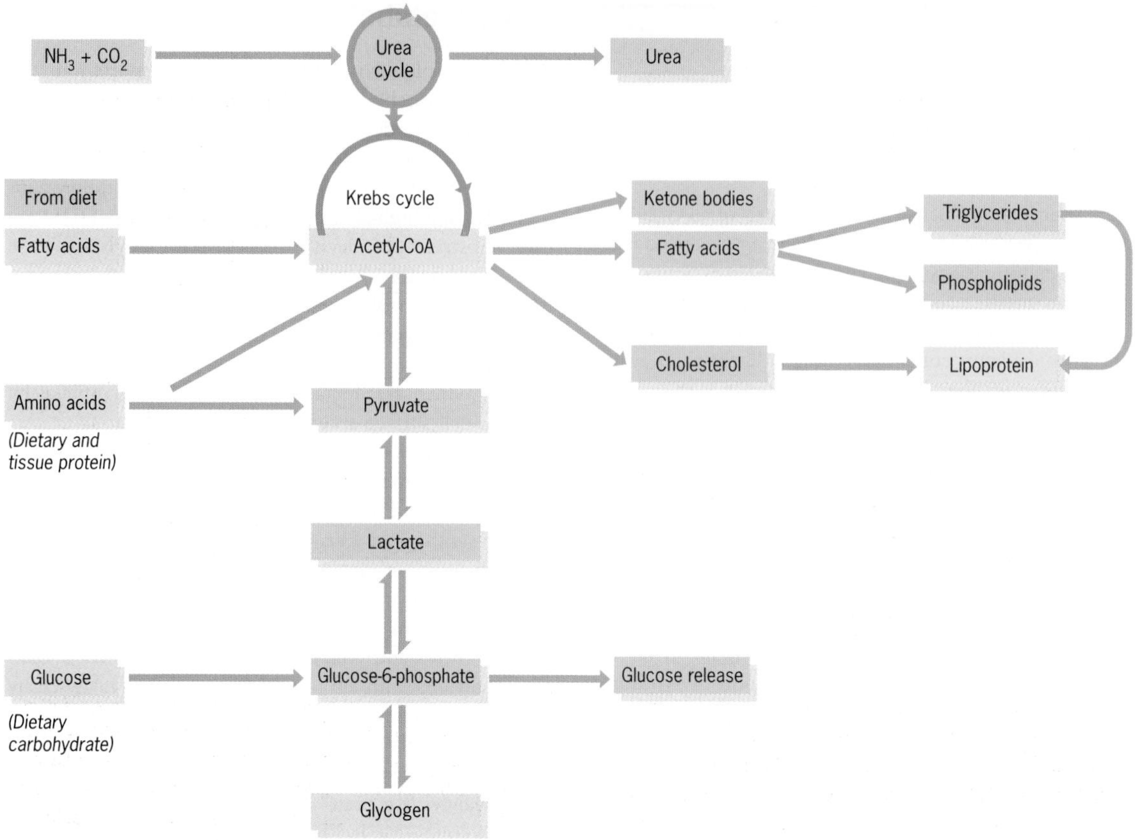

Fig 5.3
Interrelationships of protein, carbohydrate and lipid metabolism in the liver

Na^+ and water follow the passage of bile salts into the biliary canaliculus by diffusion across the tight junction between hepatocytes (a bile salt-dependent process). In the bile salt-independent process water flow is due to other osmotically active solutes such as glutathione and bicarbonate.

Secretion of a bicarbonate-rich solution is stimulated mainly by secretin and is inhibited by somatostatin. In this process several membrane proteins are involved, including the Cl^-/HCO_3^- exchanger and the cystic fibrosis transmembrane conductance regulator which controls Cl^- secretion, as well as water channels (aquaporins) in cholangiocyte membranes.

The average total bile flow is approximately 600 mL per day. In the fasted state half of the bile flows directly into the duodenum and half is diverted into the gallbladder. The mucosa of the gallbladder absorbs 80–90% of the water and electrolytes, but is impermeable to bile acids and cholesterol. Following a meal, cholecystokinin is secreted by the duodenal mucosa and stimulates contraction of the gallbladder and relaxation of the sphincter of Oddi, so that bile enters the duodenum. An adequate bile flow is dependent on bile salts being returned to the liver by the enterohepatic circulation.

Bile acid metabolism

Bile acids are synthesized in hepatocytes from cholesterol. The rate-limiting step in their production is that catalysed by cholesterol-7α-hydroxylase. They are excreted into the bile and then pass into the duodenum. The two primary bile acids – cholic acid and chenodeoxycholic acid (Fig 5.4) – are conjugated with glycine or taurine (in a ratio of 3:1 in humans) and this process increases their solubility. Intestinal bacteria convert these acids into secondary bile acids, deoxycholic and lithocholic acid. Fig 5.5 shows the enterohepatic circulation of bile acids.

Bile acids act as detergents; their main function is lipid solubilization. Bile acid molecules contain both a hydrophilic and a hydrophobic end. In aqueous solutions they aggregate to form micelles, with their hydrophobic (lipid-soluble) ends in the centre. Micelles are expanded by cholesterol and phospholipids (mainly lecithin), forming mixed micelles.

Bilirubin metabolism

Bilirubin is produced mainly from the breakdown of mature red cells in the Kupffer cells of the liver and in the reticuloendothelial system; 15% of bilirubin comes from the catabolism of other haem-containing proteins, such as myoglobin, cytochromes and catalases.

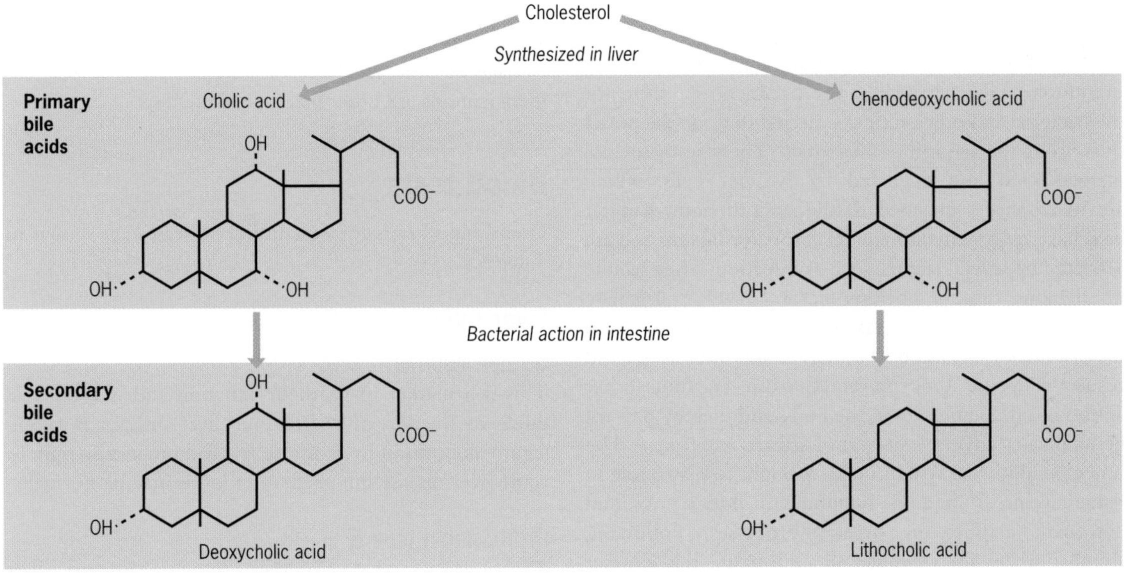

Fig 5.4
Primary and secondary bile acids.
All bile acids are normally conjugated with glycine or taurine

Normally, 250–300 mg of bilirubin are produced daily. The iron and globin are removed from the haem and are reused. Biliverdin is formed from the haem and this is reduced to form bilirubin. The bilirubin produced is unconjugated and water-insoluble, and is transported to the liver attached to albumin. Bilirubin dissociates from albumin and is taken up by the hepatic cell membrane and transported to the endoplasmic reticulum by cytoplasmic proteins, where it is conjugated with glucuronic acid and excreted into bile. The microsomal enzyme, uridine diphosphoglucurosyl transferase, catalyses the formation of bilirubin monoglucuronide and then diglucuronide. This conjugated bilirubin is water-soluble and is actively secreted into the bile canaliculi and excreted into the intestine within the bile (Fig 5.5). It is not absorbed from the small intestine because of its large molecular size. In the terminal ileum, bacterial enzymes hydrolyse the molecule, releasing free bilirubin, which is then reduced to urobilinogen. Some of this is excreted in the stools as stercobilinogen. The remainder is absorbed by the terminal ileum, passes to the liver via the enterohepatic circulation, and is re-excreted into the bile. Urobilinogen bound to albumin enters the circulation and is excreted in the urine via the kidneys. When hepatic excretion of conjugated bilirubin is impaired, a small amount of conjugated bilirubin is found strongly bound to serum albumin. It is not excreted by the kidneys and accounts for the continuing hyperbilirubinaemia for a short time after cholestasis has resolved.

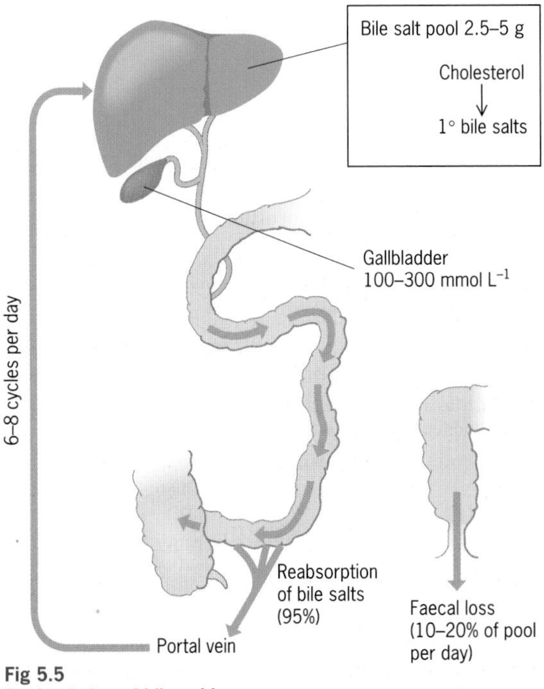

Fig 5.5
Recirculation of bile acids.
The bile salt pool is relatively small and the entire pool recycles 6–8 times via the enterohepatic circulation. Up to 40 g are excreted daily into the bile and the synthesis of new bile acids only compensates for faecal loss

Hormone and drug inactivation

The liver catabolizes hormones such as insulin, glucagon, oestrogens, growth hormone, glucocorticoids and parathyroid hormone. It is also the prime target organ for many hormones (e.g. insulin). It is the most important site for the metabolism of drugs (see p. 335) and alcohol (see p. 328). Fat-soluble drugs are converted to water-soluble substances that facilitate their excretion in the bile or urine.

Immunological function

The reticuloendothelial system of the liver contains many immunologically active cells. The liver acts as a 'sieve' for the bacterial and other antigens carried to it via the portal tract from the gastrointestinal tract. These antigens are phagocytosed and degraded by Kupffer cells, which are macrophages attached to the endothelium. Kupffer cells have specific membrane receptors for ligands and are activated by several factors, such as infection. They secrete interleukins, tumour necrosis factor (TNF), collagenase and lysosomal hydrolases. Antigens are degraded without the production of antibody as there is very little lymphoid tissue. They are thus prevented from reaching other antibody-producing sites in the body and thereby prevent generalized adverse immunological reactions. The reticuloendothelial system is also thought to play a role in tissue repair, T and B lymphocyte interaction, and cytotoxic activity in disease processes. Following stimulation by, for example, an endotoxin, the Kupffer cells release IL-6, IL-8 and TNF-α and play a key role in producing parenchymal damage. These cytokines stimulate the sinusoidal cells, stellate cells and killer cells to release proinflammatory cytokines. The stimulated hepatocytes themselves express adhesion molecules and release IL-8, which is a potent neutrophil chemoattractant. These exogenous leukocytes again release more cytokines – all damaging the function of the hepatocyte including hepatocellular bile formation which leads to cholestasis. Cytokines also stimulate hepatic apoptosis.

Investigations

Investigative tests can be divided into:

- **Blood tests**
  - (a) Liver 'function' tests:
    - (i) serum albumin
    - (ii) prothrombin time
  - (b) Liver biochemistry:
    - (i) serum aspartate and alanine aminotransferases – reflecting hepatocellular damage
    - (ii) serum alkaline phosphatase, γ-glutamyl transpeptidase – reflecting cholestasis
    - (iii) total protein
  - (c) Viral markers
  - (d) Additional blood investigations; haematological, biochemical and immunological.
- **Urine tests** – for bilirubin and urobilinogen.
- **Imaging techniques** – to define gross anatomy.
- **Liver biopsy** – for histology.

Most routine 'liver function tests' sent to the laboratory will be processed by an automated multichannel analyser to produce serum levels of bilirubin, aminotransferases, alkaline phosphatase, γ-glutamyl transpeptidase (γ-GT) and total proteins. These routine tests are markers of liver damage, but not actual tests of 'function' *per se*. Subsequent investigations are often based on these tests.

Blood tests

Useful blood tests for certain liver diseases are shown in Table 5.1.

Liver function tests

Serum albumin

This is a marker of synthetic function and is a valuable guide to the severity of chronic liver disease. A falling serum albumin in liver disease is a bad prognostic sign. In acute liver disease initial albumin levels may be normal.

Prothrombin time (PT)

This is also a marker of synthetic function. Because of its short half-life, it is a sensitive indicator of both acute and chronic liver disease. Vitamin K deficiency should be excluded as the cause of a prolonged PT by giving an intravenous bolus (10 mg) of vitamin K. Vitamin K deficiency commonly occurs in biliary obstruction, as the low intestinal concentration of bile salts results in poor absorption of vitamin K.

Prothrombin times vary in different laboratories depending upon the thromboplastin used in the assay. The International Normalized Ratio (INR) is therefore used in the UK (see p. 412).

Liver biochemistry

Bilirubin

In the serum, bilirubin is normally almost all unconjugated. In liver disease, increased serum bilirubin is usually accompanied by other abnormalities in liver biochemistry.

Table 5.1
Useful blood tests for certain liver diseases

Test	Disease
Antimitochondrial antibody	Primary biliary cirrhosis
Antinuclear, smooth muscle (actin), liver/kidney microsomal antibody	Autoimmune hepatitis
Raised serum immunoglobulins:	
IgG	Autoimmune hepatitis
IgM	Primary biliary cirrhosis
Viral markers (IgG and IgM)	Hepatitis A, B, C, D and others
α-Fetoprotein	Hepatocellular carcinoma
Serum iron, transferrin saturation, serum ferritin	Hereditary haemochromatosis
Serum and urinary copper, serum caeruloplasmin	Wilson's disease
α_1-Antitrypsin	Cirrhosis (± emphysema)
Antinuclear cytoplasmic antibodies	Sclerosing cholangitis

Determination of whether the bilirubin is conjugated or unconjugated is only necessary in congenital disorders of bilirubin metabolism (see below) or to exclude haemolysis.

Aminotransferases

These enzymes (often referred to as transaminases) are present in hepatocytes and leak into the blood with liver cell damage. Two enzymes are measured:

- *Aspartate aminotransferase* (AST), which was previously known as serum glutamic oxaloacetic transaminase (SGOT), is a mitochondrial enzyme and is also present in heart, muscle, kidney and brain. High levels are seen in hepatic necrosis, myocardial infarction, muscle injury and congestive cardiac failure.
- *Alanine aminotransferase* (ALT), which was previously known as serum glutamic pyruvic transaminase (SGPT), is a cytosol enzyme, more specific to the liver so that a rise only occurs with liver disease.

Alkaline phosphatase (ALP)

This is present in the canalicular and sinusoidal membranes of the liver, but is also present in many other tissues, such as bone, intestine and placenta. If necessary, its origin can be determined by electrophoretic separation of isoenzymes or bone-specific monoclonal antibodies. Alternatively, if there is also an abnormality of, for example, the γ-GT, the ALP can be presumed to come from the liver.

Serum ALP is raised in cholestasis from any cause, whether intrahepatic or extrahepatic disease. The synthesis of ALP is increased and this is released into the blood. In cholestatic jaundice, levels may be 4–6 times the normal limit. Raised levels may also occur in conditions with infiltration of the liver (e.g. metastases) and in cirrhosis, frequently in the absence of jaundice. The highest serum levels due to liver disease (>1000 IU L^{-1}) are seen with hepatic metastases and primary biliary cirrhosis.

γ-Glutamyl transpeptidase

This is a microsomal enzyme that is present in many tissues as well as the liver. Its activity can be induced by such drugs as phenytoin and by alcohol. If the ALP is normal, a raised serum γ-GT is a good guide to alcohol intake and can be used as a screening test (see p. 1137). Mild elevation of the γ-GT is common even with a small alcohol consumption and does not necessarily indicate liver disease if the other liver biochemical tests are normal. In cholestasis the γ-GT rises in parallel with the ALP as it has a similar pathway of excretion. This is also true of the 5-nucleotidase, another microsomal enzyme that can be measured in blood.

Total proteins

This measurement, in itself, is of little value. Serum albumin is discussed above. The globulin fraction consists of many proteins that can be separated on electrophoresis. A raised globulin fraction, seen in liver disease, is usually due to increased circulating immunoglobulins (see below).

Viral markers

Viruses are a major cause of liver disease. Virological studies have a key role in diagnosis (see p. 303); markers are available for most common viruses that cause hepatitis.

Additional blood investigations

Haematological

A full blood count is always performed. Anaemia may be present. The red cells are often macrocytic and can have abnormal shapes – target cells and spur cells – owing to membrane abnormalities. Vitamin B_{12} levels are normal or high, while folate levels are often low owing to poor dietary intake. Other changes are caused by the following:

- Bleeding produces a hypochromic, microcytic picture.
- Alcohol causes macrocytosis, sometimes with leucopenia and thrombocytopenia.
- Hypersplenism results in pancytopenia.
- Cholestasis can often produce abnormal-shaped cells and also deficiency of vitamin K.
- Haemolysis accompanies acute liver failure and jaundice.
- Aplastic anaemia is present in up to 2% of patients with acute viral hepatitis.
- A raised serum ferritin with transferrin saturation (>60%) is seen in hereditary haemochromatosis.

Biochemical

- *α_1-Antitrypsin.* A deficiency of this enzyme can produce cirrhosis.
- *α-Fetoprotein.* This is normally produced by the fetal liver. Its reappearance in increasing and high concentrations in the adult indicates hepatocellular carcinoma. Increased concentrations in pregnancy in the blood and amniotic fluid suggest neural-tube defects of the fetus. Blood levels are also slightly raised in patients with hepatitis, chronic liver disease and also in teratomas.
- *Serum and urinary copper and serum caeruloplasmin* – for Wilson's disease (see p. 326).

Immunological tests

There are no specific antibodies to the liver itself that are measured routinely.

Serum immunoglobulins

Increased γ-globulins are thought to be due to reduced phagocytosis by sinusoidal and Kupffer cells of the antigens absorbed from the gut. These antigens then stimulate antibody production in the spleen, lymph nodes and lymphoid and plasma cell infiltrate in the portal tracts. In primary biliary cirrhosis, the predominant serum immunoglobulin that is raised is IgM, while in autoimmune hepatitis it is IgG.

Serum autoantibodies

- *Antimitochondrial antibody* (AMA) is found in the serum in over 95% of patients with primary biliary cirrhosis (p. 324). Many different AMA subtypes have been described, depending on their antigen specificity. AMA is demonstrated by an immunofluorescent technique and is neither organ- nor species-specific. Some subtypes are occasionally found in autoimmune hepatitis and other autoimmune diseases.
- *Nucleic, smooth muscle (actin), liver/kidney microsomal antibodies* can be found in the serum in high titre in patients with autoimmune hepatitis. These antibodies can be found in the serum in other autoimmune conditions and other liver diseases.
- *Antinuclear cytoplasmic antibodies* (ANCA) are present in primary sclerosing cholangitis.

Bromsulphthalein (BSP) clearance test

This is now very rarely performed. The liver normally clears BSP from the blood. The level of BSP in the blood after an intravenous injection of BSP is a sensitive guide to hepatocellular damage. A second recirculation peak occurs in the congenital hyperbilirubinaemia of the Dubin–Johnson syndrome. Anaphylactic reactions may occur.

Urine tests

Dipstick tests are available for bilirubin and urobilinogen. Bilirubinuria is due to the presence of conjugated (soluble) bilirubin. It is found in the jaundiced patient with hepatobiliary disease; its absence implies that the jaundice is due to increased unconjugated bilirubin. Urobilinogen in the urine is, in practice, of little value but suggests haemolysis or hepatic dysfunction of any cause.

Imaging techniques

Ultrasound examination

This is a non-invasive, safe and relatively cheap technique. It involves the analysis of the reflected ultrasound beam detected by a probe moved across the abdomen. The normal liver appears as a relatively homogeneous structure. The gallbladder, common bile duct, pancreas, portal vein and other structures in the abdomen can be visualized. Abdominal ultrasound is useful in:

- a jaundiced patient (p. 299)
- hepatomegaly/splenomegaly
- the detection of gallstones (Fig 5.6)
- focal liver disease – lesions >1 cm
- general parenchymal liver disease
- assessing portal and hepatic vein patency
- lymph node enlargement.

Other abdominal masses can be delineated and biopsies can be obtained under ultrasonic control. Doppler ultrasound can show the direction of blood flow in the portal and hepatic veins.

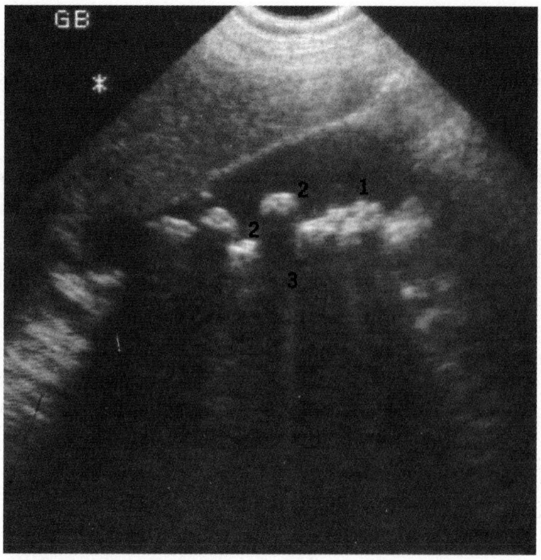

Fig 5.6
Gall bladder ultrasound with multiple echogenic gallstones causing well defined acoustic shadowing
1, gallbladder; 2, gallstones; 3, echogenic shadow

Computed tomography (CT) examination

This is useful in all hepatobiliary problems and is complementary to ultrasound. Pancreatic disease, enlargement of regional lymph nodes, and lesions in the porta hepatis can be visualized. Abnormalities of size, shape and density as well as focal lesions of the liver can be detected. CT can detect calcification not seen on plain X-rays. It is not as useful as ultrasound for biliary tract disease but has advantages in obese subjects.

Spiral CT involves rapid acquisition of a volume of data during or immediately after i.v. contrast injection. Data can thus be acquired in both arterial and portal venous phases of enhancement, enabling more precise characterization of a lesion and its vascular supply (Fig 5.7). Retrospective analysis of data allows multiple overlapping slices to be obtained with no increase in the radiation dose. Multi-planar and 3-dimensional reconstruction in the arterial phase can create a CT angiogram, often making formal invasive angiography unnecessary. As with ultrasound, biopsies can be taken under CT control.

Magnetic resonance imaging (MRI)

(see also p. 1038)

MRI produces cross-sectional images in any plane within the body. Diffuse liver disease alters the T1 and T2 characteristics and MRI is now probably the most sensitive investigation of focal liver disease, although not widely used because of limited availability.

Magnetic resonance cholangiopancreatography (MRCP)

This technique involves the manipulation of a volume of data acquired by MRI. A heavily T2 weighted sequence enhances visualization of the 'water-filled' bile ducts and

(a) (b) (c)

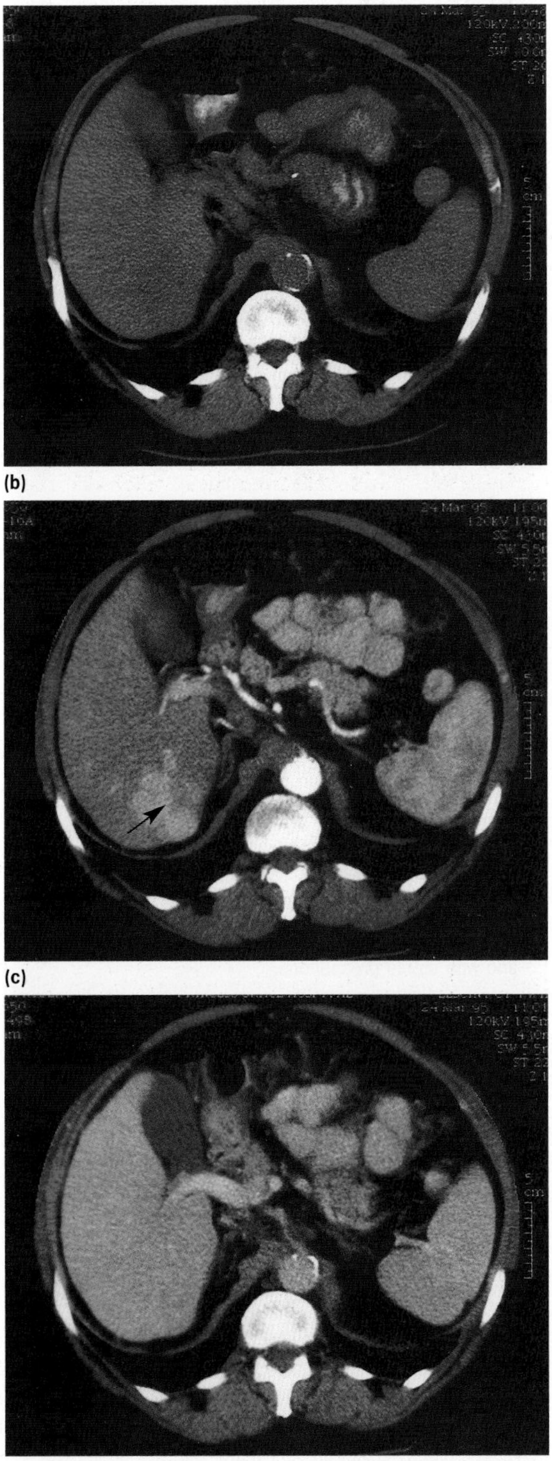

Fig 5.7
Use of contrast-enhanced spiral CT. Unenhanced **(a)**, arterial phase (note high density contrast in the aorta) **(b)**, and portal venous phase **(c)** scan through the right lobe of the liver.

There is an irregular mass (arrow) in the posterior aspect of the right lobe of the liver which is only well seen on the early arterial phase enhanced scan (b).

pancreatic ducts to produce high-quality images of ductal anatomy. The impact of this non-invasive technique is being evaluated.

Plain X-rays of the abdomen

These are rarely requested but may show:

- gallstones –10% contain enough calcium to be seen
- air in the biliary tree owing to its recent instrumentation, surgery or to a fistula between the intestine and the gallbladder
- pancreatic calcification
- rarely, calcification of the gallbladder (porcelain gallbladder).

Cholecystogram

This has been almost universally replaced by ultrasound, but may be useful in certain circumstances. Oral iopanoic acid is absorbed from the gut, conjugated in the liver, secreted in bile and concentrated in the gallbladder, which opacifies homogeneously. A fatty meal is given to make the gallbladder contract. The dye is excreted by the liver via the same mechanism as bilirubin, so that non-visualization will occur in the jaundiced patient and in the patient with liver disease.

Intravenous cholangiography

This has been replaced by ultrasound, MRCP and endoscopic retrograde cholangiopancreatography (see below).

Radionuclide imaging – scintiscanning

In a technetium-99m (^{99m}Tc) colloid scan, the colloid is injected intravenously to be taken up by the reticuloendothelial cells of the liver and spleen. In chronic liver disease there is poor intake in the liver and most of the colloid is taken up in the spleen and bone marrow. Ultrasound has largely replaced this technique.

In a ^{99m}Tc-Iodida scan, technetium-labelled iododiethyl IDA is taken up by the hepatocytes and excreted rapidly into the biliary system. Its main uses are in the diagnosis of:

- acute cholecystitis
- jaundice due to either biliary atresia or hepatitis in the neonatal period.

Endoscopy

Upper GI endoscopy

This is used for the diagnosis and treatment of varices, for the detection of portal hypertensive gastropathy, and for associated lesions such as peptic ulcers.

Endoscopic ultrasound (EUS)

In this technique, a small high-frequency ultrasound probe is mounted on the tip of an endoscope and placed by direct vision into the duodenum. The close proximity of the probe to the pancreas and biliary tree permits high-resolution ultrasound imaging. It allows accurate staging of small, potentially operable, pancreatic tumours and offers a less-invasive method for bile duct imaging. It has a reported high accuracy in detection of small neuro-endocrine tumours of the pancreas. EUS-guided fine-needle aspiration of tumours provides cytological/histological confirmation of malignancy.

Endoscopic retrograde cholangiopancreatography (ERCP)

This technique is used to outline the biliary and pancreatic ducts. It involves the passage of an endoscope into the second part of the duodenum and cannulation of the ampulla. Contrast is injected into both systems and the patient is screened radiologically. Contrast medium with a low iodine content of 1.5 mg mL^{-1} is used for the common bile duct so that gallstones are not obscured; a higher iodine content of 2.8 mg mL^{-1} is used for the pancreatic duct. In addition, other diagnostic and therapeutic procedures can be carried out:

- Common bile duct stones can be removed after a diathermy cut to the sphincter has been performed to facilitate their withdrawal (p. 340). *Sphincterotomy* has a complication rate of 8–12%: acute pancreatitis in 5% of cases; severe haemorrhage in 2%, with an overall mortality of 0.5–1%. Endoscopic balloon dilatation, where the opening of the bile duct is enlarged by inflating a balloon, is now being used as it preserves biliary sphincter function and appears safer.
- The biliary system can be drained by passing a tube (stent) through an obstruction.

The complication rate in *diagnostic* ERCP is 2–3%. A raised serum amylase is often seen and pancreatitis is the most common complication. Cholangitis is also seen, and broad-spectrum antibiotics (e.g. 1 g of cefotaxime i.v. 8-hourly) should be given prophylactically to all patients with suspected biliary obstruction.

Percutaneous transhepatic cholangiography (PTC)

Under a local anaesthetic, a fine flexible needle is passed into the liver. Contrast is injected slowly until a biliary radicle is identified and then further contrast is injected to outline the whole of the biliary tree. In patients with dilated ducts the success rate is near 100%. ERCP is the preferred first investigation because therapy (e.g. stone removal) can be undertaken at the same time.

In difficult cases the two techniques are sometimes combined, PTC showing the biliary anatomy above the obstruction, with ERCP showing the more distal anatomy. If an obstruction in the bile ducts is seen, a bypass stent can sometimes be inserted, draining either externally or, for long-term use, internally. Contraindications are as for liver biopsy (see below). The main complications are bleeding and cholangitis with septicaemia, and prophylactic antibiotics should be given as for ERCP.

Angiography

This is performed by selective catheterization of the coeliac axis and hepatic artery. It was used for detecting the abnormal vasculature of hepatic tumours, but spiral CT has taken over. The portal vein can be demonstrated with increased definition using subtraction techniques, and splenoportography (by direct splenic puncture) is rarely performed. In digital vascular imaging (DVI), contrast given intravenously or intra-arterially can be detected in the portal system using computerized subtraction analysis. Hepatic venous cannulation also allows an indirect measurement of portal pressure to be made, although this has seldom been shown to be of any diagnostic or therapeutic value.

Liver biopsy (see Practical box 5.1)

Histological examination of the liver is valuable in the differential diagnosis of diffuse or localized parenchymal disease. Liver biopsy can be performed on a day-case or overnight-stay basis. The indications and contraindications are shown in Table 5.2. The mortality rate is less than 0.02% when performed by experienced operators.

Liver biopsy guided by ultrasound or CT is often performed routinely, particularly when specific lesions need to be biopsied. Laparoscopy with guided liver biopsy is performed through a small incision in the abdominal wall under local anaesthesia (general anaesthesia is preferred in

Practical

This should be performed only by experienced doctors and with sterile precautions.

- The patient's coagulation status (prothrombin time, platelets) is checked.
- The patient's blood group is checked and serum saved for cross-matching.
- The patient lies on his back at the edge of the bed.
- The liver margins are delineated using percussion.
- Local anaesthetic is injected at the point of maximum dullness in the mid-axillary line through the intercostal space during expiration. Anaesthetic (1% lignocaine, approximately 5 mL) should be injected down to the liver capsule.
- A tiny cut is made in the skin with a scalpel blade.
- A special needle (Menghini, Trucut or Surecut) is used to obtain the liver biopsy whilst the patient holds his breath in expiration.
- The biopsy is laid on filter paper and placed in 10% formalin. If a culture of the biopsy is required it should be placed in a sterile pot.
- The patient should be observed, with pulse and blood pressure measurements taken regularly for 6 h.

Practical box 5.1 Needle biopsy of the liver

Table 5.2
Indications and contraindications for liver biopsy

Indications	
Liver disease	
Unexplained hepatomegaly	
Some cases of jaundice	
Persistently abnormal liver biochemistry	
Occasionally in acute hepatitis	
Chronic hepatitis	
Cirrhosis	
Drug-related liver disease	
Infiltrations	
Tumours: primary or secondary	
Infections (e.g. tuberculosis)	
Storage disease (e.g. glycogen storage)	
Screening relatives of patients with certain diseases (e.g. hereditary haemochromatosis)	
Pyrexia of unknown origin	
Usual contraindications to percutaneous needle biopsy	
Uncooperative patient	
Prolonged prothrombin time (by more than 3 s)	
Platelets $< 80 \times 10^9$/L	
Ascites	
Extrahepatic cholestasis	
Renal transplant	

some centres). A transjugular approach is used when liver histology is essential for management but coagulation abnormalities prevent the percutaneous approach.

Most complications of liver biopsy occur within 24 hours (usually in the first two hours). They are often minor and include abdominal or shoulder pain which settles with analgesics. Minor intraperitoneal bleeding is common, but this settles spontaneously. Rare complications include major intraperitoneal bleeding, pleurisy and perihepatitis, biliary peritonitis, haemobilia and transient septicaemia. Haemobilia produces biliary colic, jaundice and melaena within three days of the biopsy.

FURTHER READING

Saini S (1997) Imaging of the hepatobiliary tract. *New England Journal of Medicine* **336**: 1889–1894.

Symptoms of liver disease

Acute liver disease

This may be asymptomatic and anicteric. Symptomatic disease, which is often viral, produces generalized symptoms of malaise, anorexia and fever. Jaundice may appear as the illness progresses.

Chronic liver disease

Patients may be asymptomatic or complain of nonspecific symptoms. Specific symptoms include:

- right hypochondrial pain due to liver distension
- abdominal distension due to ascites
- ankle swelling due to fluid retention
- haematemesis and melaena from gastrointestinal haemorrhage
- pruritus due to cholestasis – this is often an early symptom of primary biliary cirrhosis
- breast swelling (gynaecomastia), loss of libido and amenorrhoea due to endocrine dysfunction
- confusion and drowsiness due to neuropsychiatric complications (portosystemic encephalopathy).

Signs of liver disease

Acute liver disease

There may be few signs apart from jaundice and an enlarged liver. Jaundice is a yellow coloration of the skin and mucous membranes and is best seen in the conjunctivae. In the cholestatic phase of the illness, pale stools and dark urine are present. Spider naevi and liver palms usually indicate chronic disease but they can occur in severe acute disease.

Chronic liver disease

The physical signs are shown in Fig 5.8. However, it is possible for the physical examination to be normal in patients with advanced chronic liver disease.

The skin

The chest and upper body may show spider naevi. These are telangiectases that consist of a central arteriole with radiating small vessels. They are found in the distribution of the superior vena cava (i.e. above the nipple line). They are also found in pregnancy. In haemochromatosis the skin may have a slate-grey appearance.

The hands may show palmar erythema, which is a nonspecific change indicative of a hyperdynamic circulation; it is also seen in pregnancy, thyrotoxicosis or rheumatoid arthritis. Clubbing occasionally occurs, and a Dupuytren's contracture is often seen in alcoholic cirrhosis.

Xanthomas (cholesterol deposits) are seen in the palmar creases or above the eyes in primary biliary cirrhosis.

The abdomen

Initial hepatomegaly will be followed by a small liver in well-established cirrhosis. Splenomegaly is seen with portal hypertension.

The endocrine system

Gynaecomastia (occasionally unilateral) and testicular atrophy may be found in males. The cause of gynaecomastia is complex, but it is probably related to altered oestrogen metabolism or to treatment with spironolactone.

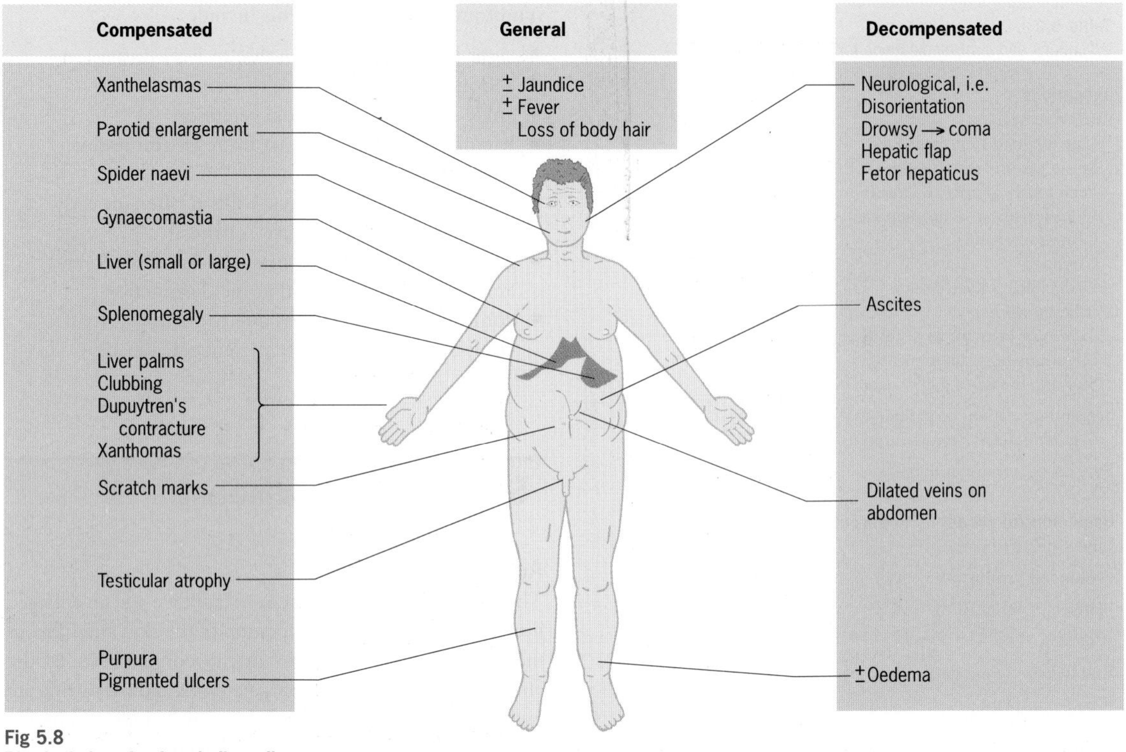

Fig 5.8
Physical signs in chronic liver disease

In decompensated cirrhosis, additional signs that can be seen are:

- jaundice
- ascites with or without peripheral oedema
- evidence of portosystemic encephalopathy (PSE) (p. 322), including drowsiness, stupor, fetor hepaticus and a flapping tremor of the outstretched hands
- collateral veins and veins around the umbilicus (caput medusae – very rare).

Jaundice

Jaundice (icterus) is detectable when the serum bilirubin is greater than 30–60 μmol L^{-1} (3 mg dL^{-1}). The usual division of jaundice into prehepatic, hepatocellular and obstructive (cholestatic) is an oversimplification as in hepatocellular jaundice there is invariably cholestasis and the clinical problem is whether the cholestasis is intrahepatic or extrahepatic. Jaundice will therefore be considered under the following headings:

- haemolytic jaundice – increased bilirubin load for the liver cells
- congenital hyperbilirubinaemias – defects in conjugation
- cholestatic jaundice, including hepatocellular (parenchymal) liver disease and large duct obstruction.

Haemolytic jaundice

The increased breakdown of red cells (see p. 371) leads to an increase in production of bilirubin. The resulting jaundice is usually mild (serum bilirubin of 68–102 μmol L^{-1} or 4–6 mg dL^{-1}) as normal liver function can easily handle the increased bilirubin derived from excess haemolysis. Unconjugated bilirubin is not water-soluble and therefore will not pass into the urine; hence the term 'acholuric jaundice'. Urinary urobilinogen is increased.

The causes of haemolytic jaundice are those of haemolytic anaemia (p. 373). The clinical features depend on the cause; anaemia, jaundice, splenomegaly, gallstones and leg ulcers may be seen.

Investigations show features of haemolysis (p. 372). The level of unconjugated bilirubin is raised but the serum ALP, transferases and albumin are normal. Serum haptoglobulins are low. The differential diagnosis is from other forms of jaundice.

Congenital hyperbilirubinaemias (non-haemolytic)

Unconjugated

Gilbert's syndrome

This is the most common familial hyperbilirubinaemia and affects 2–7% of the population. It is asymptomatic and is usually detected as an incidental finding of a slightly raised bilirubin (17–102 μmol L^{-1} or 1–6 mg dL^{-1}) on a routine check. No signs of liver disease are seen. There is a family history of jaundice in 5–15% of patients. Many abnormalities of bilirubin handling have been demonstrated. Most patients have reduced levels of UDP-glucuronosyl transferase activity, the enzyme that conjugates bilirubin with glucuronic acid. Recent evidence has shown mutations in the gene encoding this enzyme with an expanded nucleotide repeat in the upstream promoter element. This abnormality appears to be necessary for the syndrome, but is not in itself sufficient for the phenotypic expression of the syndrome.

The major importance of establishing this diagnosis is to inform the patient that this is not a serious disease and to prevent unnecessary investigation in the future. Investigations show only a raised unconjugated bilirubin, which rises on fasting and during a mild illness. The reticulocyte count is normal, and no treatment is necessary.

Crigler–Najjar syndrome

This is very rare. Only patients with type II (autosomal dominant) with a decrease rather than absence (type I – autosomal recessive) of UDP-glucuronosyl transferase can survive into adult life. Mutations of the gene for UDP-glucuronosyl transferase has been demonstrated in the coding region. Liver histology is normal. Transplantation is the only effective treatment.

Conjugated

In the *Dubin–Johnson* (autosomal recessive) and *Rotor* (possibly autosomal dominant) syndromes, there are defects in bilirubin handling in the liver. The prognosis is good in both. In the Dubin–Johnson syndrome a mutation in the cMOAT (p. 289) transporter gene has recently been described. The liver is black owing to melanin deposition.

Cholestatic jaundice

This can be divided into extrahepatic and intrahepatic cholestasis. The causes are shown in Fig 5.9.

- Extrahepatic cholestasis is due to large duct obstruction of bile flow at any point in the biliary tract distal to the bile canaliculi.
- Intrahepatic cholestasis occurs owing to failure of bile secretion. A number of cellular mechanisms in cholestasis have been described in animal models, including inhibition of the Na^+–K^+-ATPase in the basal lateral membranes, decreased fluidity of the sinusoidal plasma membrane, disruption of the microfilaments responsible for canalicular tone, and damage to the tight junctions. In addition, inflammatory change in ductular cells interfere with bile flow.

Clinically in both types there is jaundice with pale stools and dark urine, and the serum bilirubin is conjugated. However, intrahepatic and extrahepatic cholestatic jaundice must be differentiated as their clinical management is entirely different.

DIFFERENTIAL DIAGNOSIS OF JAUNDICE

A careful history may give a clue to the diagnosis. Patients should be asked a series of questions, keeping in mind that certain causes of jaundice are more likely in particular categories of people.

For example, a young person is more likely to have hepatitis, so questions should be asked about drug and alcohol use, and sexual behaviour. An elderly person with gross weight loss is more likely to have a carcinoma. All patients may complain of malaise. Abdominal pain occurs in patients with biliary obstruction by gallstones and, sometimes with an enlarged liver there is pain resulting from distension of the capsule.

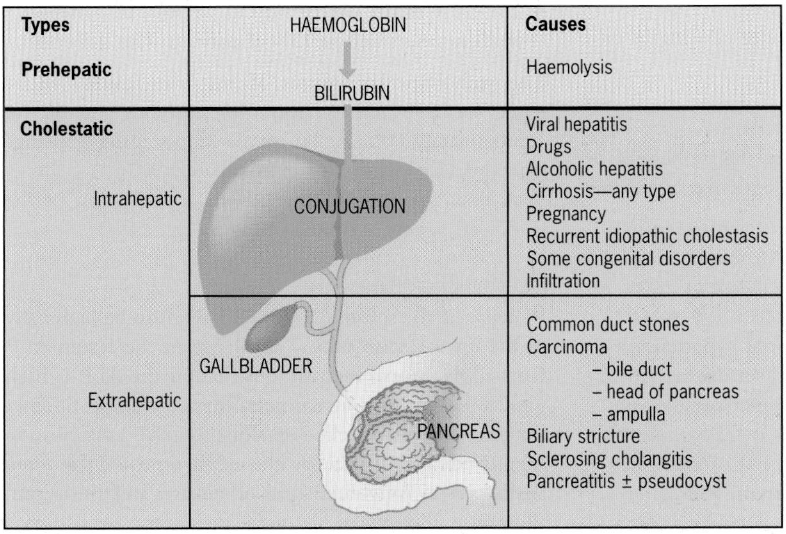
Types
HAEMOGLOBIN
Causes
Prehepatic
BILIRUBIN
Haemolysis
Cholestatic
Intrahepatic
CONJUGATION
Viral hepatitis
Drugs
Alcoholic hepatitis
Cirrhosis—any type
Pregnancy
Recurrent idiopathic cholestasis
Some congenital disorders
Infiltration
Extrahepatic
GALLBLADDER
PANCREAS
Common duct stones
Carcinoma
- bile duct
- head of pancreas
- ampulla
Biliary stricture
Sclerosing cholangitis
Pancreatitis ± pseudocyst

Fig 5.9
Causes of jaundice

Questions should be appropriate to the particular situation, and the following aspects of the history should be covered.

- .*Country of origin*. The incidence of hepatitis B virus (HBV) infection is increased in many parts of the world (p. 305).
- *Duration of illness*. A history of jaundice with prolonged weight loss in an older patient suggests malignancy. A short history, particularly with a prodromal illness of malaise, suggests a hepatitis.
- *Recent outbreak of jaundice*. An outbreak in the community suggests hepatitis A virus (HAV).
- *Recent consumption of shellfish*. This suggest HAV.
- *Intravenous drug abuse*, or recent injections or tattoos. These all increase the chance of HBV and hepatitis C virus (HCV) infection.
- *Male homosexuality*. This increases the chance of HBV infection.
- *Female prostitution*. This increases the chance of HBV infection.
- *Blood transfusion or infusion of pooled blood products*. Increased risk of HBV and HCV. In developed countries all donors are screened for HBV and HCV.
- *Alcohol consumption*. A careful history of drinking habits should be taken, although many patients often understate the actual amount they drink.
- *Drugs taken* (particularly in the previous 2–3 months). Many drugs cause jaundice (see p. 335).
- *Travel*. Certain areas have an increased risk of HAV infection.
- *Recent anaesthetics*. Halothane, for example, may cause jaundice.
- *Family history*. Patients with, for example, Gilbert's disease may have family members who get recurrent jaundice.
- *Recent surgery* on the biliary tract or for carcinoma.
- *Environment*. People engaged in recreational activities in rural areas, as well as farm and sewage workers, are at risk for leptospirosis.
- *Fevers or rigors*. These are suggestive of cholangitis or possibly a liver abscess.

CLINICAL FEATURES

The signs of acute and chronic liver disease should be looked for (p. 298). Certain additional signs may be helpful:

- **Hepatomegaly**. A smooth tender liver is seen in hepatitis and with extrahepatic obstruction, but a knobbly irregular liver suggests metastases. Causes of hepatomegaly are shown in Table 5.3.
- **Splenomegaly**. This indicates portal hypertension in patients when signs of chronic liver disease are present. The spleen can also be 'tipped' occasionally in viral hepatitis.
- **Ascites**. This is found in cirrhosis but can also be due to carcinoma (particularly ovarian) and many other causes (see Table 5.14).

Table 5.3
Causes of hepatomegaly

Apparent Low-lying diaphragm Reidel's lobe	**Haematological** Leukaemias Lymphoma Myeloproliferative disorders Thalassaemia
Cirrhosis (early)	
Inflammation Hepatitis Schistosomiasis Abscesses (pyogenic or amoebic)	**Tumours: primary and secondary carcinoma**
	Venous congestion Heart failure Hepatic vein occlusion
Cysts Hydatid Polycystic	**Biliary obstruction (particularly extrahepatic)**
Metabolic Fatty liver Amyloid Glycogen storage disease	

A palpable gallbladder can suggest a carcinoma of the pancreas obstructing the bile duct. Generalized lymphadenopathy suggests a lymphoma.

INVESTIGATIONS

Jaundice is not itself a diagnosis and the cause should always be sought. The two most useful tests are the viral markers for HAV, HBV and HCV (in high-risk groups), plus an ultrasound examination. Liver biochemistry confirms the jaundice and may help in the diagnosis.

An ultrasound examination should always be performed to exclude an extrahepatic obstruction, unless the patient is young and the diagnosis of viral hepatitis is suspected. Ultrasound will demonstrate:

- the size of the bile ducts, which are dilated in extrahepatic obstruction (Fig 5.10)
- the level of the obstruction
- the cause of the obstruction in virtually all patients with tumours and in 75% of patients with gallstones.

The pathological diagnosis of any mass lesion can be made by fine-needle aspiration cytology (sensitivity approximately 60%) or by needle biopsy using a spring-loaded device (sensitivity approximately 90%).

A flow diagram for the general investigation of the jaundiced patient is shown in Fig 5.11.

Liver biochemistry

In hepatitis, the serum AST or ALT tends to be high early in the disease with only a small rise in the serum ALP. Conversely, in extrahepatic obstruction the ALP is high with a smaller rise in aminotransferases. These findings cannot, however, be relied on alone to make a diagnosis in an individual case. The prothrombin time (PT) is often prolonged in longstanding liver disease, and the serum albumin is also low.

(a) (b)

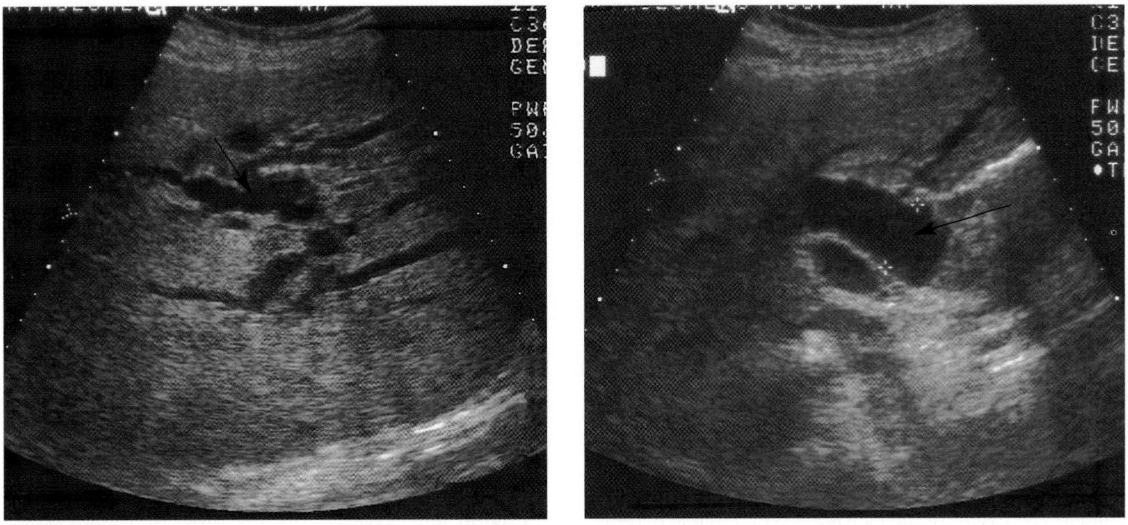

Fig 5.10
Liver ultrasound showing (a) dilated intrahepatic bile ducts (arrow). **(b) Common bile duct** (arrow).
The normal bile duct measures 6 mm at the porta hepatis

Haematological tests

These are helpful in a case of haemolytic jaundice (p. 298). A raised white cell count may indicate infection (e.g. cholangitis). A leucopenia often occurs in viral hepatitis, while abnormal mononuclear cells suggest infectious mononucleosis and a Monospot test should be performed.

Other blood tests

These include tests to exclude unusual causes of liver disease (e.g. cytomegalovirus antibodies), autoimmune antibodies (e.g. antimitochondrial antibodies, AMA) for the diagnosis of primary biliary cirrhosis, and α-fetoprotein for a hepatocellular carcinoma.

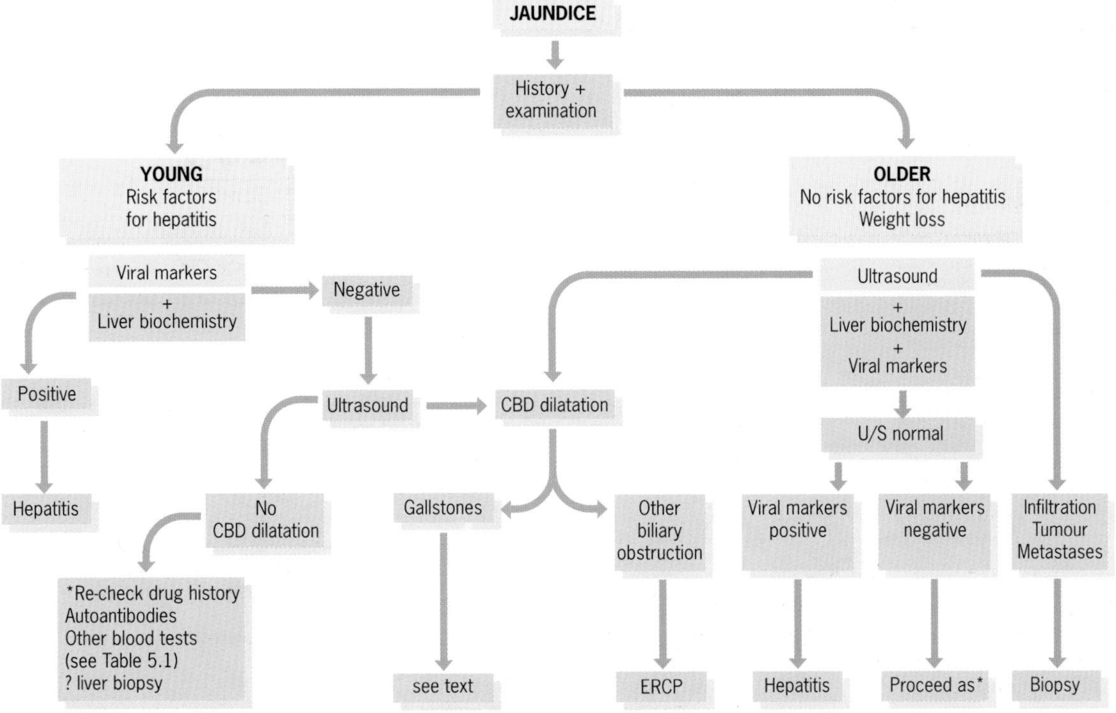

Fig 5.11
Approach to patient with jaundice.
ERCP, endoscopic retrograde cholangiopancreatography; CBD, common bile duct.

Acute hepatitis

Acute parenchymal liver damage can be caused by many agents (Fig 5.12). If there is widespread damage of hepatocytes, the normal liver architecture may collapse. The extent of hepatocellular damage may be extremely variable.

PATHOLOGY

Although some histological features are suggestive of the aetiological factor, most of the changes are essentially similar whatever the cause. Hepatocytes show degenerative changes (swelling, cytoplasmic granularity, vacuolation), undergo necrosis (becoming shrunken, eosinophilic Councilman bodies) and are rapidly removed. The distribution of these changes varies somewhat with the aetiological agent, but necrosis is usually maximal in zone 3. The extent of the damage is very variable between individuals affected by the same agent: at one end of the spectrum, single and small groups of hepatocytes die (spotty or focal necrosis), while at the other end there is multiacinar necrosis involving a substantial part of the liver (massive hepatic necrosis) resulting in fulminant hepatic failure. Between these extremes there is limited confluent necrosis with collapse of the reticulin framework resulting in linking (bridging) between the central veins, the central veins and portal tracts, and between the portal tracts. The extent of the inflammatory infiltrate is also variable, but portal tracts and lobules are infiltrated mainly by lymphocytes. Other variable features include cholestasis in zone 3 and fatty change, the latter being prominent in hepatitis that is due to alcohol or certain drugs.

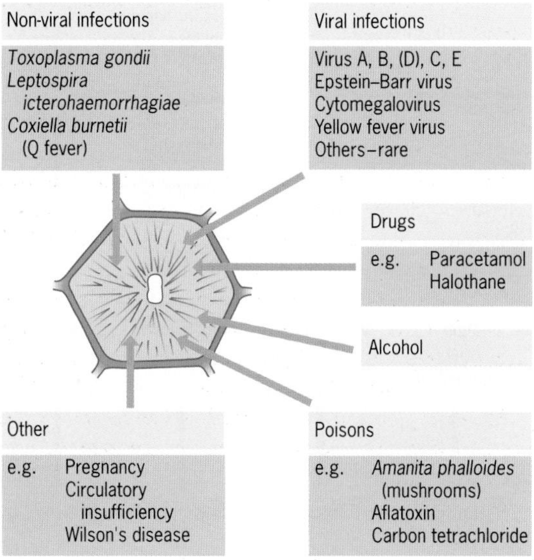

Fig 5.12
Some causes of acute parenchymal damage

MANAGEMENT

This is discussed below under the individual aetiological factors.

Viral hepatitis

The differing features of the common forms of viral hepatitis are summarized in Table 5.4.

Hepatitis A

Hepatitis A virus (HAV)

HAV is a picornavirus, having the structure shown in Fig 5.13. It has a single serotype as only one epitope is immunodominant. It replicates in the liver, is excreted in bile and is then excreted in the faeces of infected persons for about two weeks before the onset of clinical illness and for up to seven days after. The disease is maximally infectious just before the onset of jaundice. HAV particles can be demonstrated in the faeces by electron microscopy.

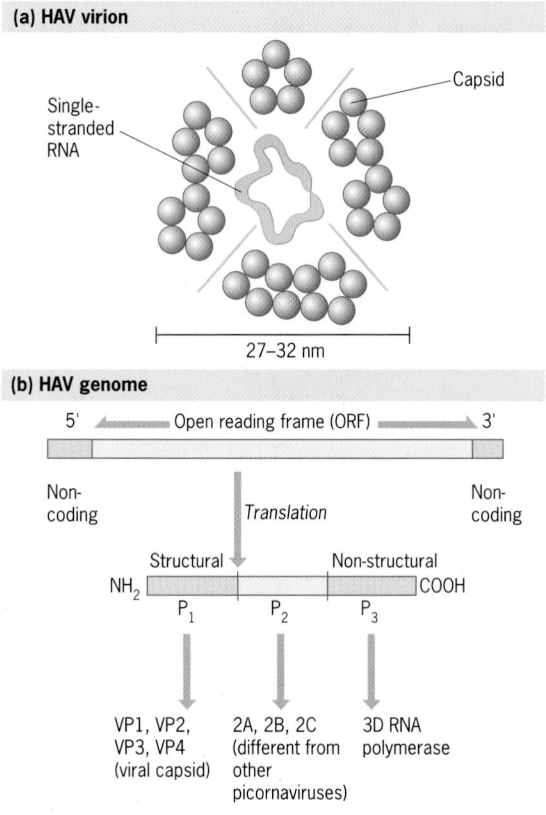

Fig 5.13
(a) The hepatitis A (HAV) virion consists of four polypeptides (VP1–VP4) which form a tight protein shell, or capsid, containing the RNA. The major antigenic component is associated with VP1.
(b) Arrangement of HAV genome.

Table 5.4
Some features of hepatitis viruses

	A	B	D	C	E
Virus	RNA 27 nm	DNA 42 nm	RNA 36 nm(with HBsAg coat)	RNA 30–60 nm	RNA 27 nm
	Picorna	Hepadna	Unclassified	Flavi	Calici
Spread					
Faecal	Yes	No	No	No	Yes
Blood	Rare	Yes	Yes	Yes	No
Vertical	No	Yes	Rare	Rare	No
Saliva	Yes	Yes	Yes	? No	?
Sexual	Rare	Yes	Yes (rare)	Rare	No
Incubation	Short (2–3 weeks)	Long (1–5 months)	Long	Intermediate	Short
Age	Young	Any	Any	Any	Any
Carrier state	No	Yes	Yes	?	No
Chronic liver disease	No	Yes	Yes	Yes	No
Liver cancer	No	Yes	Rare	Yes	No
Mortality (acute)	<0.5%	<1%		<1%	1–2% (pregnant women 10–20%)
Immunization:					
Passive	Normal immunoglobulin serum i.m. (0.04–0.06 mL kg^{-1})	Hepatitis B immunoglobin (HBIg)	–	–	–
Active	Vaccine	Vaccine	HBV vaccine	–	–

EPIDEMIOLOGY

Hepatitis A is the most common type of viral hepatitis occuring worldwide, often in epidemics. The disease is commonly seen in the autumn and affects children and young adults. Spread of infection is mainly by the faecal–oral route and arises from the ingestion of contaminated food or water (e.g. shellfish). Overcrowding and poor sanitation facilitate spread. There is no carrier state. In the UK it is a notifiable disease.

CLINICAL FEATURES

The viraemia causes the patient to feel unwell with nonspecific symptoms that include nausea, anorexia and a distaste for cigarettes. Many recover at this stage and remain anicteric.

After one or two weeks some patients become jaundiced and symptoms often improve. As the jaundice deepens, the urine becomes dark and the stools pale owing to intrahepatic cholestasis. The liver is moderately enlarged and the spleen is palpable in about 10% of patients. Occasionally, tender lymphadenopathy is seen, with a transient rash in some cases. Thereafter the jaundice lessens and in the majority of cases the illness is over within 3–6 weeks. Extrahepatic complications are rare but include arthritis, vasculitis, myocarditis and renal failure. Relapses occasionally occur, with the return of jaundice. Rarely the disease may be very severe with fulminant hepatitis, liver coma and death. The typical sequence of events after HAV exposure is shown in Fig 5.14.

INVESTIGATIONS

Liver biochemistry

In the prodromal stage the serum bilirubin is usually normal. However, there is bilirubinuria and increased urinary urobilinogen. A raised serum AST or ALT, which can sometimes be very high, precedes the jaundice.

In the icteric stage the serum bilirubin reflects the level of jaundice. Serum AST reaches a maximum 1–2 days after the appearance of jaundice, and may rise above 500 IU L^{-1}. Serum ALP is usually less than 300 IU L^{-1}.

After the jaundice has subsided, the aminotransferases may remain elevated for some weeks and occasionally for up to six months.

Haematological tests

There is leucopenia with a relative lymphocytosis. Very rarely there is a Coombs'-positive haemolytic anaemia or

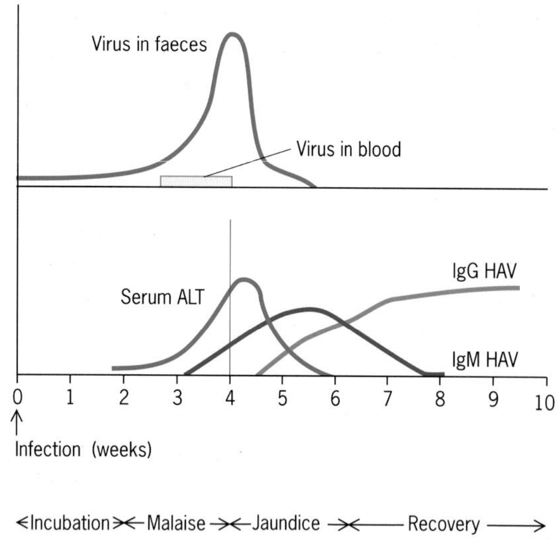

Fig 5.14
HAV – sequence of events after exposure

an associated aplastic anaemia. The prothrombin time (PT) is prolonged in severe cases. The erythrocyte sedimentation rate (ESR) is raised.

Viral markers: antibodies to HAV

IgG antibodies are common in the general population over the age of 50 years, but an anti-HAV IgM means an acute infection. In areas of high prevalence most children have antibodies by the age of 3 years following asymptomatic infection.

Other tests

Further tests are not necessary in the presence of an IgM antibody.

DIFFERENTIAL DIAGNOSIS

Clinically the differential diagnosis is from all other causes of jaundice – but in particular from other types of viral and drug-induced hepatitis.

COURSE AND PROGNOSIS

The prognosis is excellent, with most patients making a complete recovery. The mortality in young adults is 0.1% but it increases with age. Death is due to fulminant hepatic necrosis. During convalescence, 5–15% of patients may have relapse of the hepatitis but this settles spontaneously. Occasionally a more severe jaundice with cholestasis will run a prolonged course of 7–20 weeks and is called 'cholestatic viral hepatitis'.

There is no reason to stop alcohol consumption other than for the few weeks when the patient is ill. Patients may complain of debility for several months following resolution of the symptoms and biochemical parameters. This is known as the post-hepatitis syndrome; it is a functional illness. Treatment is by reassurance. HAV never progresses to chronic liver disease.

TREATMENT

There is no specific treatment, and rest and dietary measures are unhelpful. Corticosteroids have no benefit. Admission to hospital is not usually necessary.

PREVENTION AND PROPHYLAXIS

Control of hepatitis depends on good hygiene. The virus is resistant to chlorination but is killed by boiling water for 10 minutes.

Active immunization

A formaldehyde inactivated vaccine is available commercially. This is used for people travelling frequently to endemic areas, patients with chronic liver disease, people with haemophilia, and workers in frequent contact with hepatitis cases (e.g. in residential institutions for patients with learning difficulties). Community outbreaks can be interrupted by vaccination. A single dose produces antibodies that persist for at least one year when a booster is given. Immunity then can last for up to ten years.

Passive immunization

Normal human immunoglobulin (0.04–0.06 mL kg^{-1} i.m.) gives protection for 3–4 months and is useful for persons who are occasionally at risk.

Hepatitis B

Hepatitis B virus (HBV)

The complete infective virion or Dane particle is a 42 nm particle comprising an inner core or nucleocapsid (27 nm) surrounded by an outer envelope of surface protein (HBsAg). This surface coat is produced in excess by the infected hepatocytes and can exist separately from the whole virion in serum and body fluid as 22 nm particles or 22 nm tubules.

HBsAg contains a major 'a' antigenic determinant as well as several subtypes: 'd', 'y', 'w' and 'r'. Combinations of these subdeterminants (e.g. adr, adw, ayw and ayr) are used in epidemiology for studying geographical patterns of infection.

The core or nucleocapsid is formed of core protein (HBcAg) containing incompletely double-stranded circular DNA and the DNA polymerase/reverse transcriptase. One strand is almost a complete circle and contains overlapping genes that encode both structural proteins (pre S, surface (s), core(c)) and replicative proteins (polymerase and X). The other strand is variable in length (Fig 5.15).

HBeAg is a protein formed via specific self-cleavage of the precore/core gene product which is secreted separately by the cell.

Pre S_1 and pre S_2 regions are involved in attachment to the specific HBV receptor on the hepatocyte. After penetration, the virus core is transported to the nucleus without processing with transcription of HBV into mRNA taking place.

Translation into HBV proteins (Table 5.5) as well as replication of the genome takes place in the endoplasmic

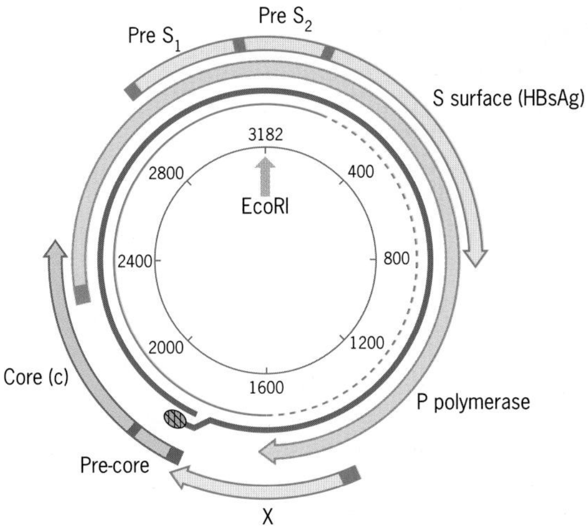

Fig 5.15
Hepatitis B virus (HBV) genome. The viral DNA is partially double stranded (red incomplete circle and blue circle). The long strand (blue) encodes seven proteins from four overlapping reading frames (S, surface (Pre S_1, Pre S_2, S), C, core (Pre C, C) P, polymerase (P) and X gene (X). EcoRI restriction enzyme binding site is included as a reference point (see Table 5.5)

Table 5.5
HBV proteins

HBV protein	Clinical significance
Core	Protein of core particle; kinase activity (role in replication?)
Pre-core (HBeAg)	Pre-core/core cleaves to HBeAg; good marker of active replication and role in inducing immunotolerance
Surface (HBsAg)	Envelope protein of HBV; basis of current vaccine
Pre-S_2	HBV binding and entry into hepatocytes
Pre-S_1	HBV binding and entry into hepatocytes
Polymerase	Viral replication
X protein	Trans-activation

reticulum; they are then packaged together and exported from the cell. During the period of replication, the viral genome may integrate into the chromosomal DNA of the hepatocyte.

The HBV is not directly cytopathic and the liver damage produced is by the cellular immune response of the host. Specific failure of T cells to recognize HBV antigens leads to viral persistence.

Hepatitis B mutants

Mutations occur in the various reading frames of the HBV genome (see Fig 5.15). These mutants can emerge in chronic HBV carriers or can be acquired by infection. Patients have HBsAg and HBV DNA but not the e antigen itself: anti-HBe may or may not be present. The amino acid sequence of the e antigen protein is almost identical to that of the core antigen which is involved in viral replication. Separate messenger RNAs have not been described for the two antigens, but HBeAg is initiated several nucleotides upstream of HBcAg. A guanosine (G) to adenosine (A) mutation in the precore region of the genome creates a stop codon (TAG) that prevents the production of HBeAg, but the synthesis of HBcAg is unaffected. Mutants have also been seen following interferon therapy and in patients with fulminant and fatal hepatitis. Their existence means that serological markers such as the HBeAg are less useful in detecting infectivity and HBV DNA must be measured.

EPIDEMIOLOGY

The hepatitis B virus is present worldwide and has infected more than 2000 million people. There are an estimated 300 million carriers. The UK and the USA have a low carrier rate (0.5%), but it rises to 10–15% in parts of Africa, the Middle and the Far East.

Spread of this virus is either by the intravenous route (e.g. by transfusion of infected blood or blood products, or by contaminated needles used by drug addicts, tattooists or acupuncturists), or by close personal contact, such as during sexual intercourse, particularly in male homosexuals. The virus can be found in semen and saliva. Vertical transmission from mother to child during parturition or soon after birth is the most important means of transmission worldwide. The role of insect vectors is controversial; there is no evidence that HBV replicates in these insects but the virus has been detected in mosquitoes and bed bugs.

CLINICAL FEATURES

The sequence of events following acute HBV infection are shown in Fig 5.16. In many cases, however, the infection is subclinical. The clinical picture is the same as that found in HAV infection, although the illness may be more severe. In addition, a serum sickness-like immunological syndrome may be seen. This consists of rashes (e.g. urticaria or a maculopapular rash) and polyarthritis affecting small joints occurring in up to 25% of cases in the prodromal period. Fever is usual. Extrahepatic immune complex-mediated conditions such as an arteritis or glomerulonephritis are occasionally seen.

INVESTIGATIONS

These are generally the same as for hepatitis A.

Specific tests

The markers for HBV are shown in Table 5.6. HBsAg is looked for initially; if it is found, a full viral profile is then performed. In acute infection, HBsAg may be cleared rapidly and in such cases IgM anti-core antibodies are helpful. However, in any other situation anti-core antibodies will always accompany surface antigen positivity, and is therefore of little help. HBV DNA is the most sensitive index of viral replication and is found without e antigen in hepatitis due to mutants.

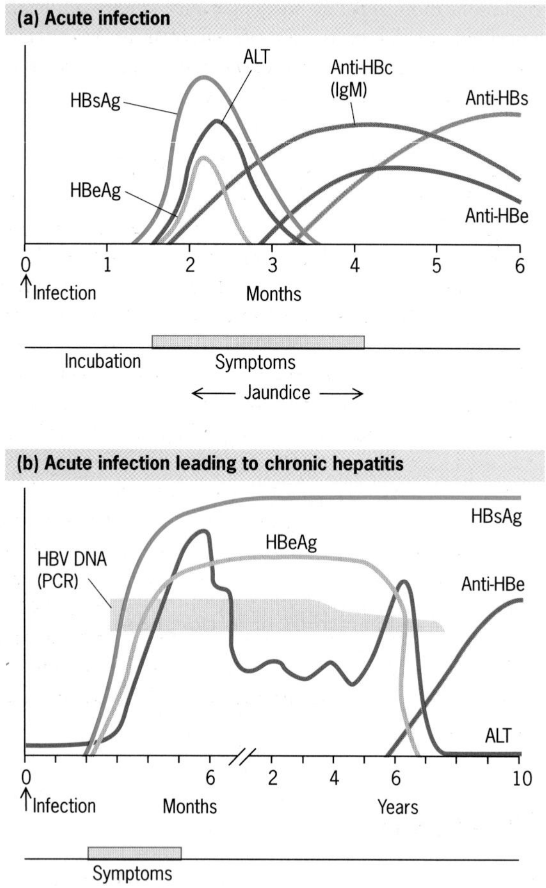

Fig 5.16
Time course of the events and serological changes seen following infection with hepatitis B virus.

(a) Acute infection

Antigens

HBsAg appears in the blood from about 6 weeks to 3 months after an acute infection and then disappears.

HBeAg rises early and usually declines rapidly.

Antibodies

Anti-HBs appears late and indicates immunity.

Anti-HBc is the first antibody to appear and high titres of IgM anti-HBc suggest an acute and continuing viral replication. It persists for many months. IgM anti-HBc may be the only serological indicator of recent HBV infection in a period when HBsAg has disappeared and anti-HBs is not detectable in the serum.

Anti-HBe appears after the anti-HBc and its appearance relates to a decreased infectivity, i.e. a low risk.

(b) Acute infection leading to chronic hepatitis B

HBsAg persists and indicates a chronic infection (or carrier state).

HBeAg persists and correlates with increased severity and infectivity and the development of chronic liver disease. When anti-HBe develops (seroconversion) the Ag disappears and there is a rise in ALT.
HBV DNA suggests continual viral replication

Table 5.6
Significance of viral markers in hepatitis B

Antigens	
HBsAg	Acute or chronic infection
HBeAg	Acute hepatitis B Persistence implies: continued infectious state development of chronicity increased severity of disease
HBV DNA	Implies viral replication Found in serum and liver
Antibodies	
Anti-HBs	Immunity to HBV; previous exposure
Anti-HBe	Seroconversion
Anti-HBc	
IgM	Acute hepatitis B (high titre) Chronic hepatitis B (low titre)
IgG	Past exposure to hepatitis B (HBsAg-negative)

COURSE

The majority of patients recover completely, fulminant hepatitis occurring in up to 1%. Some patients go on to develop chronic hepatitis and hepatocellular carcinoma (p. 333) or become asymptomatic carriers (Fig 5.17). The outcome depends upon several factors, including the virulence of the virus and the immunocompetence and age of the patient. Genetic factors have been identified. The class II allele DRB1°1302 protects against persistent HBV infection, while abnormalities in mannose binding protein (p. 179) may alter host defence to HBV.

TREATMENT

There is no specific treatment apart from symptomatic therapy.

PREVENTION AND PROPHYLAXIS

Prevention depends on avoiding risk factors, such as shared needles, multiple male homosexual partners, and prostitutes. Infectivity is highest in those with the e antigen and HBV DNA in their blood. These patients should be counselled about their infection. In developing countries, blood and blood products are still a hazard. Standard safety precautions in laboratories and hospitals must be enforced strictly to avoid accidental needle punctures and contact with infected body fluids.

Passive and active immunization

Vaccination should be given to:

- all healthcare personnel in the UK
- members of emergency and rescue teams
- morticians and embalmers
- children in high-risk areas
- people with haemophilia
- patients in some psychiatric units
- long-term travellers

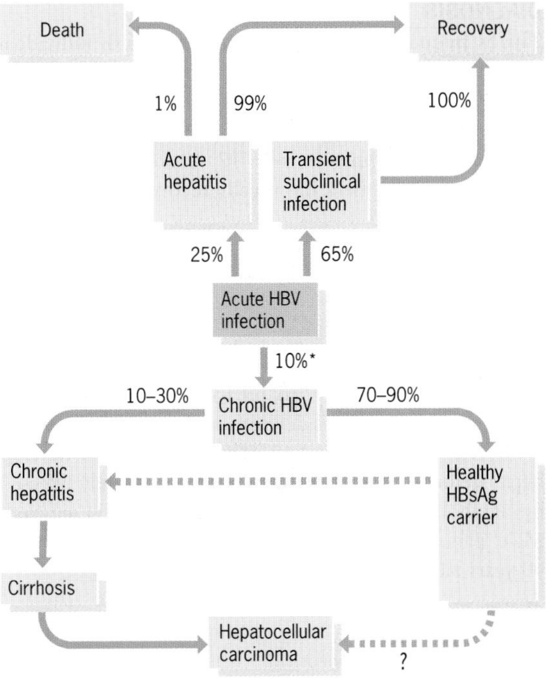

Fig 5.17
Clinical course of hepatitis B infection.
*, percentage variable worldwide

- homosexual and bisexual men and prostitutes
- intravenous drug abusers.

Combined prophylaxis (i.e. vaccination and immunoglobulin) should be given to:

- staff with accidental needlestick injury
- all newborn babies of HBsAg-positive mothers
- regular sexual partners of HBsAg-positive patients, who have been found to be HBV-negative.

To adults give 500 IU of specific hepatitis B immunoglobulin (HBIG) (200 IU to newborns) and the vaccine i.m. at another site.

Active immunization

This is with a recombinant yeast vaccine produced by insertion of a plasmid containing the gene of HBsAg into a yeast.

Dosage regimen. Three injections (at 0, 1 and 6 months) are given into the deltoid muscle; this gives short-term protection in over 90% of patients. People who are over 50 years of age or clinically ill and/or immunocompromised (including those with HIV infection or AIDS) have a poor antibody response; more frequent and larger doses are required. Antibody levels should be measured at 7–9 months after the initial dose in all at-risk groups. Antibody levels fall steadily after vaccination and booster doses may be required after approximately 3–5 years. It is not cost-effective to check antibody levels prior to active immunization. There are few side-effects from the vaccine; soreness at the site of injection may occur, with very occasionally a fever, rash or a 'flu-like' illness.

Chronic asymptomatic carriers of HBV

Following an acute HBV infection which may be subclinical, approximately 5–10% of patients will not clear the virus and most will become carriers of HbsAg. This occurs more readily with neonatal or childhood infection than when HBV is acquired in adult life. There is a vast geographical variation in the incidence of carriers. In the UK, carriers are usually discovered incidentally on blood tests, such as when they are screened for donating blood for transfusion or when attending genital medicine clinics. Carriers have HBsAg in their serum and are HBeAg-negative, Hbe antibody-positive with no HBV DNA in the serum. They have no evidence of active liver disease and are not highly infective. Most remain HBsAg positive, but do not develop active liver disease; there is an annual spontaneous clearance rate of HBsAg of 1–2%.

Asymptomatic people who have the e antigen and HBV DNA in the serum can progress to active liver disease and are best considered as having occult liver disease rather than being true carriers.

Hepatitis D

This is caused by the hepatitis D virus (HDV or delta virus). It is an incomplete RNA particle enclosed in a shell of HBsAg. It is unable to replicate on its own but is activated by the presence of HBV. It is particularly seen in intravenous drug abusers but can affect all-risk groups for HBV infection. Active HBV synthesis is reduced by delta infection and patients are usually negative for HBeAg and HBV DNA. Hepatitis D viral infection can occur either as a co-infection with HBV or as a super-infection in an HBsAg-positive patient.

Co-infection of HDV and HBV is clinically indistinguishable from an acute icteric HBV infection, but a biphasic rise of serum aminotransferases may be seen. *Diagnosis* is confirmed by finding serum IgM anti-δ in the presence of IgM anti-HBc. IgM anti-δ appears at one week and disappears by 5–6 weeks (occasionally 12 weeks) when serum IgG anti-δ is seen. The infection may be transient but the clinical course is variable.

Super-infection results in an acute flare-up of previously quiescent chronic HBV infection. A rise in serum AST or ALT may be the only indication of infection. *Diagnosis* is by finding serum IgM anti-δ at the same time as IgG HBc; patients are usually negative for IgM anti-HBc.

Fulminant hepatitis can follow both types of infection but is more common after co-infection. HDV RNA in the serum and liver can be measured and is found in acute and chronic HDV infection.

Hepatitis C

Hepatitis C virus (HCV)

HCV is a single-stranded RNA virus of the Flaviviridae family. The RNA genome is approximately 10 Kb in length, encoding a polyprotein product consisting of a structural (capsid and envelope) and non-structural viral proteins (Fig 5.18). Comparisons of subgenomic regions, such as E1, NS4 or NS5, have allowed variants to be classified into at least six genotypes. Variability is distributed throughout the genome with the non-structural gene of different genotypes showing only 65–70% nucleotide sequence similarity. Genotypes 1a or 1b account for 70–80% of cases in the USA and Europe. Antigens from the nucleocapsid regions have been used to develop enzyme-linked immunosorbent assays (ELISA). The current assay, ELISA-3, incorporates antigens NS3, NS4 and NS5 regions.

EPIDEMIOLOGY

HCV was identified in 1988 and was found to be responsible for 70–90% of post-transfusion hepatitis in all countries where blood was tested for HBV markers. The prevalence rate of infection in healthy blood donors is about 0.02% in northern Europe, 6% in Africa and with rates as high as 19% in Egypt. The virus is transmitted by blood and blood products and it is postulated that 80% of people with haemophilia in the UK may have been infected. The incidence in intravenous drug abusers is high, up to 90%. The low rate of HCV infection in high-risk groups, such as homosexuals, prostitutes and attendees at STD clinics, suggests a limited role for sexual transmission. Vertical transmission from mother to child can occur. Other routes of community-acquired infection (e.g. close contact) are unlikely. In 20% of cases the exact mode of transmission is unknown.

CLINICAL FEATURES

Most infections are asyptomatic with about 10% of patients having a mild 'flu-like illness with jaundice and a rise in serum aminotransferases. Most patients will not be diagnosed until they present, years later, with evidence of chronic liver disease. Extrahepatic manifestations are seen, including arthritis, agranulocytosis and aplastic anaemia, as well as diffuse neurological problems.

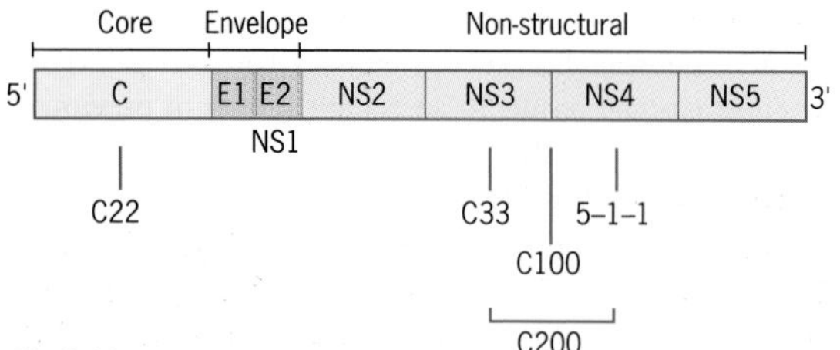

Fig 5.18
Hepatitis C virus.
Diagram showing a single-stranded RNA virus with viral proteins.
C = core, NS = non-structural, E = envelope

DIAGNOSIS

This is frequently by exclusion in a high-risk individual with negative markers for HAV, HBV and other viruses. A drug cause should be excluded if possible. HCV RNA can be detected one or two weeks after infection. HCV antibodies take approximately 12 weeks to develop by which time the patient has usually recovered.

TREATMENT

Interferon has been used in some acute cases with some success.

COURSE

At least 50% of patients go on to develop chronic liver disease (p. 312). Cirrhosis develops in about 20–30% within 5–30 years, and of these patients about 15% will develop hepatocellular carcinoma. The course is adversely affected by alcohol consumption which should be discouraged. Male patients and patients acquiring the infection over 40 years have a more rapid development of fibrosis.

Hepatitis E

Hepatitis E virus (HEV) is an RNA virus (Calicivirus) which causes a hepatitis clinically very similar to hepatitis A. It is enterally transmitted, usually by contaminated water. Epidemics have been seen in many developing countries. It has a mortality from fulminant hepatic failure of 1–2% which rises to 20% in pregnant women. There is no carrier state and it does not progress to chronic liver disease. An ELISA for IgG and IgM anti-HEV is available for diagnosis, although this ELISA is not always reliable. HEV RNA can be detected in the serum or stools by PCR (polymerase chain reaction). Prevention and control depend on good sanitation and hygiene.

Non-A–E hepatitis

The GB hepatitis agent was isolated from a surgeon (GB) with hepatitis in 1967 and propagated in the Tamarin. The agent GB has subsequently been found to be two normal RNA viruses of the Flaviviridae family – hepatitis GB virus A (HGBV-A) and hepatitis GB virus B (HGBV-B).

Another closely related virus was then isolated from patients with non-A non-B hepatitis called hepatitis GB virus C (HGBV-C). This is a single-stranded RNA virus that structurally also belongs to the Flaviviridae family. It resembles HCV, but its nucleotide structure is too dissimilar to be classified as a genotype of HCV.

Later, *HGV* was cloned from a patient with community-acquired chronic hepatitis whose plasma transmitted hepatitis to Tamarins. HGV and HGBV-C are more than 95% homologous and it is now accepted that they are the same virus. This agent, now known as HGV, is parenterally transmitted and is found in intravenous drug-users, haemophiliacs and dialysis patients. It is also found in 1–2% of voluntary blood donors in the USA, more prevalent than the HCV virus. It has been found in 15% of people in West Africa.

Seventy-five per cent of patients found to have HGV following transfusion do not have any biochemical evidence of liver disease. Any rise in serum aminotransferases after acquiring HGV has been small and can sometimes be explained by co-infection with another virus, such as HCV.

There is, at the moment, no definite evidence that HGV causes either acute or chronic hepatitis.

A few cases of hepatitis still occur with no obvious aetiological agents involved. When a viral aetiology is suspected, it is best classified as hepatitis non-A–E. The letter F was used for a possible virus, but this has not been substantiated.

Table 5.7
Causes of fulminant hepatic failure

Viruses A, B, (D), E **Other viruses** **Drugs** (examples) Analgesics (e.g. paracetamol) Monoamine oxidase inhibitors (e.g. imipramine) Anaesthetics (e.g. halothane) Anti-tuberculosis (e.g. isoniazid) Antiepileptic (e.g. valproate) 'Social' drugs (e.g. 'Ecstasy')	**Toxins** *Amanita* poisoning Halohydrocarbons **Miscellaneous** Wilson's disease Pregnancy Reye's syndrome

Fulminant hepatic failure (FHF)

This is defined as severe hepatic failure in which encephalopathy develops in under two weeks in a patient with a previously normal liver (occasionally in some patients with previous liver damage; e.g. δ virus superinfection in a previous carrier of HBsAg). Cases that evolve at a slower pace (2–12 weeks) are called subacute or subfulminant hepatic failure. FHF is a rare but often life-threatening syndrome that is due to acute hepatitis from any cause (Table 5.7). The causes vary throughout the world; the majority are due to viral hepatitis, but paracetamol overdose is commonly implicated in the UK (50% of cases). HCV appears to cause FHF very rarely.

Histologically there is multiacinar necrosis involving a substantial part of the liver. Severe fatty change is seen in pregnancy (p. 332), Reye's syndrome (p. 335), or following tetracycline administration intravenously.

CLINICAL FEATURES

Examination shows a jaundiced patient with a small liver and signs of hepatic encephalopathy. The mental state varies from slight drowsiness, confusion and disorientation (grades I and II) to unresponsive coma (grade IV) with convulsions. Fetor hepaticus is common, but ascites and splenomegaly are rare. Fever, vomiting, hypotension and hypoglycaemia occur. Neurological examination shows spasticity and extension of the arms and legs; plantar responses remain flexor until late. Cerebral oedema is found in 80% of patients and its consequences of intracranial hypertension and brain herniation are the most common causes of death. Other complications include bacterial infections, gastrointestinal bleeding, respiratory arrest, renal failure (hepatorenal syndrome and acute tubular necrosis) and pancreatitis.

INVESTIGATIONS

There is hyperbilirubinaemia, high serum aminotransferases and low levels of coagulation factors, including prothrombin and factor V. Aminotransferases are not useful indicators of the course of the disease as they tend to fall along with the albumin with progressive liver damage. An EEG is sometimes helpful in grading the encephalopathy. An isotope scan may show no uptake in the liver. Ultrasound will show liver size and any evidence of underlying liver pathology.

TREATMENT

There is no specific treatment, but patients should be managed in a specialized unit. Supportive therapy as for hepatic encephalopathy is necessary (see p. 332). When signs of raised intracranial pressure (which is measured directly) are present, 20% mannitol (1 g kg^{-1} bodyweight) should be infused intravenously; this dose may need to be repeated. Dexamethasone is of no value. Hypoglycaemia, hypokalaemia and hypocalcaemia should be anticipated and corrected with 10% dextrose infusion (checked by 2-hourly Dextrostix testing), potassium and calcium. Coagulopathy is managed with intravenous vitamin K, platelets, blood or fresh frozen plasma. Haemorrhage may be a problem and patients are given H_2-receptor antagonists to prevent gastrointestinal bleeding. Infection should be treated with suitable antibiotics, and renal and respiratory failure treated as appropriate. Flumazenil, a benzodiazepine receptor antagonist, may give a transient improvement in encephalopathy.

Liver transplantation has been a major advance for patients with FHF. It is difficult to judge the timing or the necessity for transplantation, but various transplant centres have developed guidelines depending on prognosis (see below).

COURSE AND PROGNOSIS

In mild cases (grades I and II encephalopathy with drowsiness and confusion), two-thirds of the patients will survive. The outcome of severe cases (grades III and IV encephalopathy with stupor or deep coma) is related to the aetiology. In special units, 70% of patients with paracetamol overdosage and grade IV coma survive, as do

30–40% of patients with HAV or HBV hepatitis. In patients with drug reactions and viral hepatitis, poor prognostic variables include aetiology (non-A–E or drugs), age (<10 years and >40 years), time interval from onset of jaundice to encephalopathy (more than 7 days – subfulminant), a serum bilirubin >300 μmol L^{-1} and a prothrombin time over 50 s. In addition, for paracetamol overdose an arterial pH <7.3, a serum creatinine >300 μmol L^{-1}, a PT >100 s with grade III–IV encephalopathy indicates a very poor prognosis and should be considered for transplantation.

Acute hepatitis due to other viruses

Infectious mononucleosis (see also p. 54)

This is due to the Epstein–Barr (EB) virus. Mild jaundice associated with minor abnormalities of liver biochemistry is extremely common, but 'clinical' hepatitis is rare. Hepatic histological changes occur within five days of onset; the sinusoids and portal tracts are infiltrated with large mononuclear cells but the liver architecture is preserved. A Paul–Bunnell or Monospot test is usually positive, and atypical lymphocytes are present in the peripheral blood. Treatment is of the symptoms.

Cytomegalovirus (CMV) (see also p. 53)

This can cause acute hepatitis, particularly in a patient with a poor immune response. The virus may be isolated from the urine. The liver biopsy shows intranuclear inclusions and giant cells.

Yellow fever (see also p. 60)

This viral infection is carried by the mosquito *Aedes aegypti* and can cause acute hepatic necrosis. There is no specific treatment.

Herpes simplex (see also p. 51)

Very occasionally the herpes simplex virus causes a generalized acute infection, particularly in the immunosuppressed patient. Liver biopsy shows extensive necrosis. Acyclovir is used for treatment.

Other infectious agents

Abnormal liver biochemistry is frequently found in a number of acute infections. The abnormalities are usually mild and have no clinical significance.

Toxoplasmosis (see also p. 76)

This produces a clinical picture similar to that of infectious mononucleosis, with abnormal liver biochemistry, but the Paul–Bunnell test is negative.

FURTHER READING

Dusheiko G (ed) (1996) Review in depth: hepatitis *A to Z. European Journal of Gastroenterology and Hepatology* **8**: 287–288.

Lau YNJ, Wright TL (1993) Molecular virology and pathogenesis of hepatitis B. *Lancet* **342**: 1335–1340.

Lee WM (1997) Hepatitis B virus infection. *New England Journal of Medicine* **337**: 1733–1745

Mas AJ, Rodés J (1997) Fulminant hepatitic failure. *Lancet* **349**: 1081–1085.

Chronic hepatitis

Clinically this is defined as any hepatitis lasting for six months or longer. Chronic hepatitis is best classified according to the aetiology (Table 5.8):

- due to viral disease
- due to autoimmune disease
- drug-induced
- unknown cause.

Terms such as 'chronic persistent' or 'chronic active' hepatitis are now used less commonly.

Chronic viral hepatitis is the principal cause of chronic liver disease, cirrhosis and hepatocellular carcinoma in the world.

PATHOLOGY

Chronic inflammatory cell infiltrates comprising lymphocytes, plasma cells and sometimes lymphoid follicles are usually present in the portal tracts. The amount of inflammation varies from mild to severe. In addition, there may be:

- periportal or periseptal interface hepatitis (the term 'interface hepatitis' is preferred to 'piecemeal necrosis' because the damage is due to apoptosis rather than necrosis)
- lobular change, focal lytic necrosis, apoptosis and focal inflammation

Table 5.8
Causes of chronic hepatitis

Viral	**Hereditary**
Hepatitis B ± delta virus Hepatitis C	α_1-antitrypsin deficiency Wilson's disease
Autoimmune	**Others**
Drugs (e.g. methyldopa, oxyphenisatin (withdrawn in UK), isoniazid, ketoconazole, nitrofurantoin)	Inflammatory bowel disease – ulcerative colitis Alcohol (rarely)

- confluent necrosis
- fibrosis which may be mild, bridging (across portal tracts) or severe
- cirrhosis.

The overall severity of the hepatitis is judged by the degree of the necrosis and inflammation and the severity of the fibrosis or cirrhosis.

Chronic hepatitis due to viral disease

Two main viruses (HBV and HCV) that cause chronic hepatitis (CH) can produce similar clinical features, biochemical abnormalities and histological characteristics, although some features are more suggestive of one virus than the other being involved.

Chronic hepatitis B infection

This is common in developing countries where vertical transmission still frequently occurs. In the UK it is mainly confined to high-risk groups (see p. 300) and immigrants from developing countries. The outcome of HBV infection is shown in Fig 5.17.

PATHOGENESIS

Cytotoxic T cells recognize the viral antigen via HLA class I molecules on the infected hepatocyte; this mechanism may be defective in patients leading to viral persistence. Viral persistence in patients with a very poor cell mediated response leads to a healthy carrier state. A better response, however, results in continuing hepatocellular damage with the development of CH.

Chronic HBV infection goes through a replicative and an integrated phase. In the former there is active viral replication with hepatic inflammation and the patient is highly infectious with HBeAg and HBV DNA positivity. At some stage the viral genome becomes integrated into the host DNA and the viral genes are then transcribed along with those of the host. At this stage, the level of HBV DNA in the serum is low and the patient is HBeAg-negative and HBe antibody-positive. The aminotransferases are now normal or only slightly elevated and liver histology shows little inflammation, often with cirrhosis. Hepatocellular carcinoma (HCC) develops in patients with this late-stage disease, but the mechanism is still unclear. Integration of the viral DNA with the host-cell chromosomal DNA does appear to have an important role in carcinogenesis. Recent evidence implicates inactivation of the p53-induced apoptosis by protein X (Table 5.5), allowing accumulation of abnormal cells and, eventually, carcinogenesis.

CLINICAL FEATURES AND INVESTIGATIONS

Chronic hepatitis occurs mainly in men and it is often not preceded by an acute attack. The condition may be asymptomatic or may present as a mild, slowly progressive hepatitis; 50% present with established chronic liver disease. Clinical relapses occur, sometimes associated with seroconversion (see below).

Investigations show a moderate rise in aminotransferases and a slightly raised ALP. The serum bilirubin is often normal. HBsAg and HBV DNA are found in the serum, usually with HBe antigen, unless a mutant virus is involved (see p. 305).

Histologically, there is a full spectrum of changes from near normal with only a few lymphocytes and interface hepatitis to a full-blown cirrhosis. HBsAg may be seen as a 'ground-glass' appearance in the cytoplasm on haematoxylin and eosin staining, and this can be confirmed on orcein staining or more specifically with immunohistochemical staining. HBcAg can also be demonstrated in hepatocytes by appropriate immunohistochemical staining.

TREATMENT

Patients with HBsAg, HBeAg and HBV DNA in the serum with abnormal serum aminotransferases and chronic hepatitis on liver biopsy should be treated. Patients with normal aminotransferases and those with decompensated liver disease should not be treated (see below).

The main aim of treatment is the disappearance of the HbeAg and HBV DNA from the serum with consequent reduction in inflammatory necrosis of the hepatocyte. This seroconversion occurs spontaneously at a rate of 10–15% per year, and this varies in different countries.

In patients in whom HBeAg disappears, remission is usually sustained. The patient remains a carrier with HbsAg present, although many will eventually become HBsAg-negative.

Antiviral agents

α-Interferon is the best agent available. It is given in a dose of 5M units daily or 10M units three times weekly for 4–6 months. Drug treatment, which often causes transient elevation in aminotransferases, is sometimes accompanied by systemic symptoms. Treatment should be continued.

Side effects of treatment are many, with an acute 'flu-like illness occurring 6–8 hours after the first injection. This usually disappears after subsequent injections, but malaise, headaches, myalgia, depression, diarrhoea, reversible hair loss and bone marrow depression commonly occur. The platelet count should be monitored. These drug reactions occur in up to 30% of patients, and the dose may have to be lowered; in 10% the treatment has to be discontinued. Severe reactions occur infrequently, and include infection, severe depression, cardiac and renal failure.

Overall, the response rate with disappearance of HBeAg is 25–40%. The success rate depends on factors shown in Table 5.9.

Those with chronic hepatitis with no HBeAg (i.e. a mutant HBV – see p. 305) generally do not respond, neither do patients with concominant HIV infection. Patients with decompensated liver disease often have severe side-effects and should not be treated with this drug.

New antiviral therapies

Famciclovir and lamivudine have activity against HBV *in vitro* and *in vivo*. They can be given orally and are well-tolerated. Longer courses of therapy are currently being given with hopeful results.

PROGNOSIS

The progression is slow and remission may occur. Established cirrhosis is associated with a poor prognosis. Primary liver cell carcinoma is a frequent association and is one of the most common carcinomas in HBV endemic areas such as the Far East.

Chronic hepatitis C infection

(see also p. 308)

Patients with chronic hepatitis C infection are usually asymptomatic, the disease being discovered only following a routine biochemical test when mild elevations in the aminotransferases (usually ALT) are noticed. The elevation in ALT may be minimal and fluctuating, and probably 50% of patients have a normal ALT – the disease being detected by checking HCV antibodies (e.g. in blood donors).

Despite this, severe chronic hepatitis and even cirrhosis can be present with only minimal elevation in aminotransferases. A few patients present with the symptoms and signs found in cirrhosis.

Table 5.9 Factors predictive of a sustained response to α-interferon in patients with chronic hepatitis

	Chronic hepatitis B	Chronic hepatitis C
Duration of disease	Short	Short
Liver biochemistry	High serum aminotransferase concentrations	
Histology	Active liver disease with fibrosis	Absence of cirrhosis or minimal amounts of hepatic fibrosis
Viral levels	Low HBV DNA levels Wild-type (HBeAg-positive) virus	Low HCV RNA levels Genotype 2 or 3 or absence of a high degree of genetic heterogenicity
Other	Absence of immunosuppression	Low hepatic iron stores Young age

Modified from Hoofnagle and Di Bisceglie (1997)

DIAGNOSIS

This is made by finding HCV antibody in the serum. Third-generation ELISA-3 tests are most widely used, but should be confirmed using a specific recombinant immunoblast assay (RIBA). HCV RNA should be assayed using either a PCR or branched-chain DNA signal amplification; both methods allow quantitation of the amount of HCV RNA present. The viraemia is usually of low grade and variable.

The HCV genotype should be characterized, if possible, in patients who are to be given treatment (see below).

Liver biopsy is indicated if active treatment is being considered. The changes on liver biopsy are highly variable. Sometimes only minimal inflammation is detected, but in most cases the features of CH are present, as previously described (p. 310). Lymphoid follicles are often present in the portal tracts and fatty change is frequently seen.

TREATMENT

Treatment is appropriate for patients with chronic hepatitis on liver histology who have HCV RNA in their serum and who have raised serum aminotransferases for more than six months. The presence of cirrhosis is not a contraindication. Patients with decompensated cirrhosis should be considered for transplantation. The aim of treatment is to eliminate the HCV RNA from the serum in order to:

- stop the progression of active liver disease
- prevent the development of hepatocellular carcinoma.

Antiviral agents

α-Interferon is still the best drug available. It is given as a dose of 3M units thrice-weekly for 12 months. Side-effects (p. 307) are less than for the treatment of HBV infection because of the lower dose.

Monitoring results. The effects of treatment are monitored by measurement of the aminotransferases with measurement of the HCV RNA at three months. If the aminotransferases remain abnormal and HCV RNA is present in the serum at three months, treatment is stopped because a response to further treatment is then unlikely.

After six months of therapy, 40–50% of patients will have normal aminotransferases. About a half of these, however, will relapse after treatment with a sustained response in the remainder of 15–25%. Because of this, the current recommended therapy is for 12 months. Best results are obtained in the patients with the predictive factors shown in Table 5.9. Long-term follow-up shows that the good response is continued in most and some may be cured of their infection.

Patients with normal aminotransferases do not have a good response and treatment is not currently recommended.

New therapies

Ribavirin in combination with interferon has shown a higher rate of long-term response (40–77%).

Chronic D hepatitis

This is a relatively infrequent chronic hepatitis, but spontaneous resolution is rare. Between 60% and 70% of patients will develop cirrhosis eventually. In 15% the disease is rapidly progressive with development of cirrhosis in only a few years. The diagnosis is made by finding antibodies against the δ virus in a patient with chronic liver disease and who is HBsAg-positive. It can be confirmed by finding HDV in the liver or HDV RNA in the serum by reverse transcription–polymerase reaction.

Treatment is with α-interferon, usually at the high dose of 10M thrice-weekly for 12 months. Between 15% and 25% of patients will show disappearance of HBsAg from the serum.

Autoimmune hepatitis

This condition occurs most frequently in women. There is an association with other autoimmune diseases (e.g. pernicious anaemia, thyroiditis and Coombs'-positive haemolytic anaemia), and 60% of cases are associated with HLA class I B8, and HLA class II DR3 and DR52a loci.

PATHOGENESIS

The cause is unknown. It is proposed, in a genetically predisposed person, that an environmental agent causes an autoimmune process to develop against liver antigens, producing a progressive necroinflammatory process which results in fibrosis and cirrhosis. *In vitro* observations have shown that there is a defect of suppressor (regulatory) T cells which may be primary or secondary. However, no clear mechanism causing the inflammation has been found.

CLINICAL FEATURES

Patients may be asymptomatic, the disease being discovered by abnormalities in liver biochemistry or because of signs of chronic liver disease on routine examination. Twenty-five per cent of patients present as an acute hepatitis with jaundice and very high aminotransferases.

Examination can show hepatosplenomegaly, cutaneous striae, acne, hirsuities, bruises and, sometimes, ascites. An ill patient can also have features of an autoimmune disease with a fever, migratory polyarthritis, glomerulonephritis, pleurisy, pulmonary infiltration or fibrosing alveolitis.

INVESTIGATIONS

Liver biochemistry

The serum aminotransferases are high, with lesser elevations in the ALP and bilirubin. The serum γ-globulins are high, frequently twice normal.

Haematology

A mild normochromic normocytic anaemia with thrombocytopenia and leukopenia is present, even before portal hypertension and splenomegaly. The prothrombin time is often high.

Autoantibodies

Two types of autoimmune hepatitis have been recognized:

- Type I with antibodies: (a) antinuclear, (b) anti-smooth muscle (or actin), or (c) occasionally antimitochondrial.
- Type II with antibodies: (a) anti-liver/kidney microsomal (anti-LKM1) or (b) anti-liver cytosol.

Type II occurs most frequently in girls and young women.

Liver biopsy

This shows the changes of CH described previously. The amount of interface hepatitis is variable, but tends to be high in untreated patients. Lymphoid follicles are less often seen than in hepatitis C. Approximately one-third of patients have cirrhosis at presentation.

TREATMENT

Prednisolone 30 mg is given daily for two weeks, followed by a maintenance dose of 10–15 mg daily, along with azathioprine 1–2 mg kg^{-1} daily.

COURSE AND PROGNOSIS

Steroid and azathioprine therapy induce remission in 80% of cases. The length of treatment is unclear. Those with initial cirrhosis are more likely to relapse following treatment withdrawal and require indefinite therapy. Liver transplantation is performed if treatment fails, although the disease may recur.

Drug-induced chronic hepatitis

Many drugs can cause a CH which clinically bears many similarities to autoimmune hepatitis (see Table 5.8). Patients are often female, present with jaundice and hepatomegaly, have raised serum transaminases and globulin levels, and LE cells and anti-LKM1 antibodies may be detected. Improvement follows drug withdrawal but exacerbations can occur with drug reintroduction.

Chronic alcoholic liver disease can occasionally have the histological appearances more like a chronic hepatitis.

Chronic hepatitis of unknown cause

As more and more people are having routine blood tests, mild elevations in the serum aminotransferases are found. Many of these patients have no symptoms and no evidence of liver disease clinically. All known aetiological agents should be excluded (see above), as well as tests to exclude primary biliary cirrhosis, primary sclerosing cholangitis, Wilson's disease, haemochromatosis and α_1-antitrypsin deficiency.

Liver biopsy should be performed if the elevation in the aminotransferases continues for over a year, confirming the presence of chronic hepatitis.

The prognosis is unknown, but appears to be very good.

FURTHER READING

Hoofnagle JH, Di Bisceglie AM (1997) The treatment of chronic viral hepatitis. *New England Journal of Medicine* **336**: 347–356.

Ishak K, Baptista A, Bianchi L *et al.* (1995) Histological grading and staging of chronic hepatitis. *Journal of Hepatology* **22**: 696–699.

Krawitt EL (1996) Autoimmune hepatitis. *New England Journal of Medicine* **334**: 897–903.

Cirrhosis

Cirrhosis results from the necrosis of liver cells followed by fibrosis and nodule formation. The liver architecture is diffusely abnormal and this interferes with liver blood flow and function. This derangement produces the clinical features of portal hypertension and impaired liver cell function.

AETIOLOGY

The causes of cirrhosis are shown in Table 5.10. Alcohol is now the most common cause in the West, but viral infection is the most common cause worldwide. With the identification of HCV, idiopathic (cryptogenic) cirrhosis is diagnosed less commonly. Young patients with cirrhosis must be investigated carefully as the cause may be treatable (e.g. Wilson's disease).

PATHOGENESIS

Chronic injury to the liver results in inflammation, necrosis and, eventually, fibrosis (Fig 5.19). Fibrosis is initiated by activation of the stellate cells (see p. 288). Kupffer cells seem to have a role in their activation, but hepatocytes and other cells are probably involved.

In the early stage of activation the stellate cells become swollen and lose retinoids with up-regulation of receptors for proliferative and fibrogenic cytokines, such as platelet-derived growth factor (PDGF), and possibly transforming growth factor β_1 (TGFβ_1). TGFβ_1 is the most potent fibrinogenic mediator identified so far.

Table 5.10
Causes of cirrhosis

Common	Others
Alcohol	Biliary cirrhosis
Hepatitis B ± D	Primary
Hepatitis C	Secondary
? other viruses	Autoimmune hepatitis
	Hereditary haemochromatosis
	Hepatic venous congestion
	Budd–Chiari syndrome
	Wilson's disease
	Drugs (e.g. methotrexate)
	α_1-Antitrypsin deficiency
	Cystic fibrosis
	Intestinal bypass operations for obesity
	Galactosaemia
	Glycogen storage disease
	Veno-occlusive disease
	Idiopathic (cryptogenic)

In the space of Disse, the normal matrix is replaced by collagens, predominantly types 1 and 3, and fibronectin. Subendothelial fibrosis leads to loss of the endothelial fenestrations (ports), and this impairs liver function.

PATHOLOGY

The characteristic features of cirrhosis are regenerating nodules separated by fibrous septa and loss of the normal lobular architecture within the nodules (Fig 5.20a). Two types of cirrhosis have been described which give clues to the underlying cause:

- *Micronodular cirrhosis*. Regenerating nodules are usually less than 3 mm in size and the liver is involved uniformly. This type is often caused by ongoing alcohol damage or biliary tract disease.
- *Macronodular cirrhosis*. The nodules are of variable size and normal acini may be seen within the larger nodules. This type is often seen following previous hepatitis, such as HBV infection.

A mixed picture with small and large nodules is sometimes seen.

Symptoms and signs are described on p. 300.

INVESTIGATIONS

These are performed to assess the severity and type of liver disease.

Severity

- **Liver function**. Serum albumin is the best indicator of liver function: the outlook is poor with a level below 25 g L^{-1}. The prothrombin time is prolonged commensurate with the severity of the liver disease.
- **Liver biochemistry**. This can be normal depending on the severity of cirrhosis. In most cases there is at least a slight elevation in the serum ALP and serum aminotransferases. In decompensated cirrhosis all biochemistry is deranged.

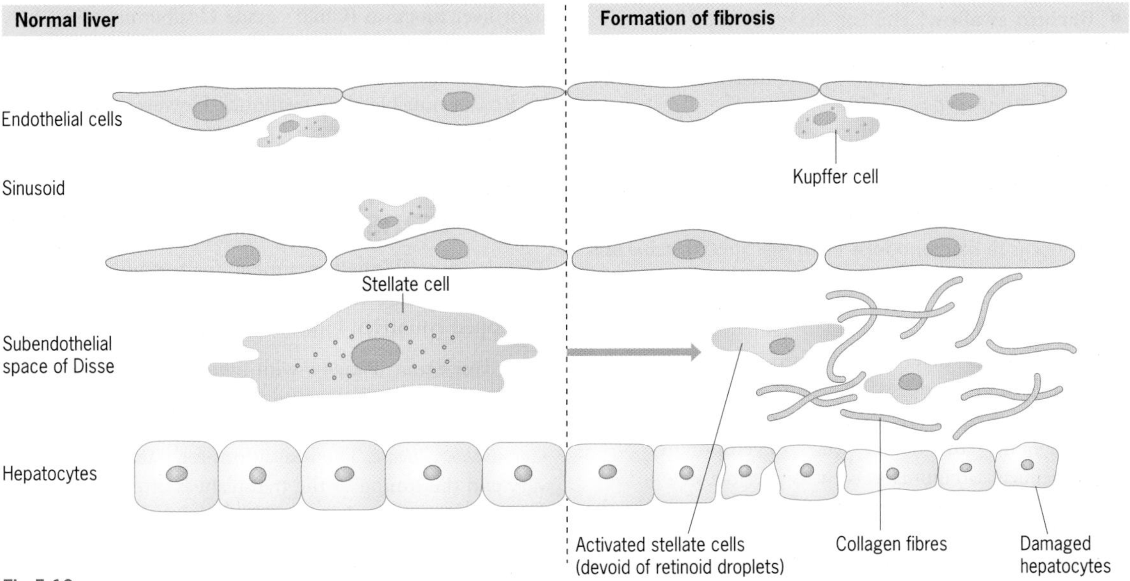

Fig 5.19
Pathogenesis of fibrosis. Activation of the stellate cell is followed by proliferation of fibroblasts and the deposition of collagen

- **Serum electrolytes**. A low sodium indicates severe liver disease because of dilution secondary to a defect in free water clearance or to excess diuretic therapy.

In addition, serum α-fetoprotein is a useful screening test for a hepatocellular carcinoma.

Type

This can be determined by:

- viral markers
- serum autoantibodies
- serum immunoglobulins
- miscellaneous measures.

Among the miscellaneous measures, serum copper (p. 327) and serum α_1-antitrypsin (p. 327) should always be done in young cirrhotics. Serum iron, total iron binding capacity (TIBC) and ferritin should be measured to exclude hereditary haemochromatosis; genetic markers are also available.

Imaging

- **Ultrasound examination**. This can demonstrate changes in size and shape of the liver. Fatty change and fibrosis produce a diffuse increased echogenicity. In established cirrhosis there may be marginal nodularity of the liver surface and distortion of the arterial vascular architecture. The patency of the portal and hepatic veins can be evaluated. It is useful in detecting hepatocellular carcinoma.
- **CT scan** (see p. 294). Fig 5.20b shows hepatosplenomegaly and dilated collaterals seen in chronic liver disease. Arterially phased contrast-enhanced scans are useful in the detection of hepatocellular carcinoma.

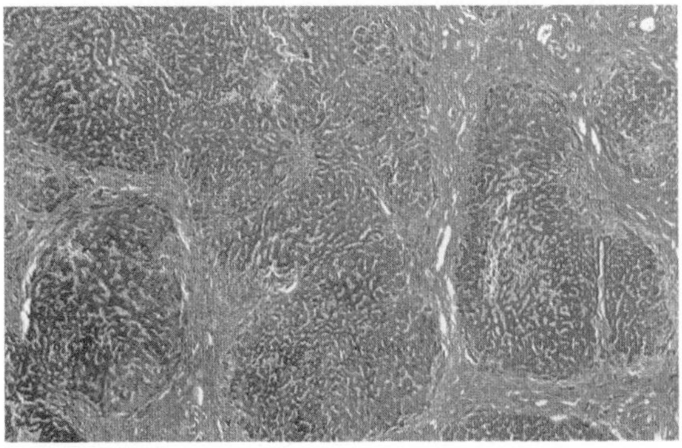

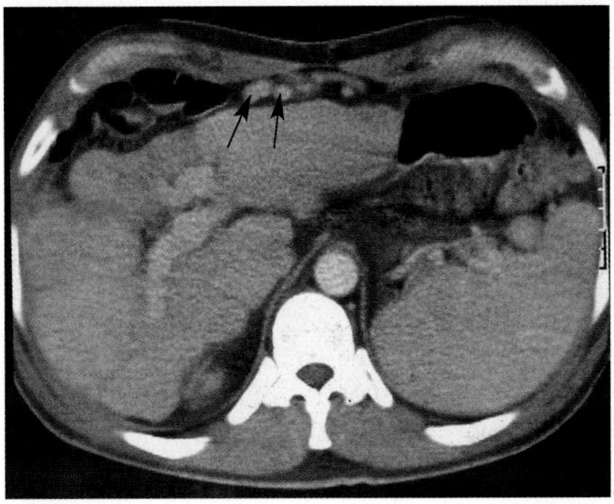

Fig 5.20
(a) Pathology of cirrhosis. Histological appearance showing nodules of liver tissue of varying size surrounded by fibrosis
(b) CT scan showing an irregular lobulated liver. There is splenomegaly and enlargement of collateral vessels beneath the anterior abdominal wall (arrows) as a result of portal hypertension.

- **Barium swallow**. This can detect varices.
- **Scintiscanning**. This is occasionally helpful
- **Endoscopy**. is performed for the detection and treatment of varices.

Liver biopsy

This is necessary to confirm the severity and type of liver disease. The core of liver often fragments and sampling errors occur in macronodular cirrhosis. Special stains may be required for iron and copper.

MANAGEMENT

Management is that of the complications seen in decompensated cirrhosis. Patients should have six-monthly ultrasound and serum α-fetoprotein measurements to detect the development of a hepatocellular carcinoma as early as possible (see p. 333).

There is no treatment that will arrest or reverse the cirrhotic changes. Progression may be halted by correcting the underlying cause (see below). Patients with compensated cirrhosis should lead a normal life and no particular diet is helpful. Alcohol should be avoided, although if the cirrhosis is not due to alcohol, small amounts are probably not harmful.

COURSE AND PROGNOSIS

This is extremely variable, depending on many factors, including the aetiology and the presence of complications. Poor prognostic indicators are given in Table 5.11. Development of any complication usually worsens the prognosis. In general, the five-year survival rate is approximately 50%, but this also varies depending on the aetiology and the stage at which the diagnosis is made.

There are a number of prognostic classifications based on modifications of Child's grading (A, B and C). This is based on the presence of jaundice, ascites, encephalopathy and the level of serum albumin. Patients with good liver function (Child's grade A) do better than patients with poor liver function (Child's grade C: albumin <30 g L^{-1}, bilirubin >50 μmol L^{-1}, and ascites).

Surgical procedures carry an overall operative mortality of 30% in non-bleeding cirrhotics. However, the range is from 10% in Child's grade A to 76% in grade C.

Table 5.11
Poor prognostic indicators in cirrhosis

Blood tests
Low albumin (< 25 g L^{-1})
Low serum sodium (< 120 mmol L^{-1})
Prolonged prothrombin time/INR

Clinical
Persistent jaundice
Failure of response to therapy
Ascites
Haemorrhage from varices, particularly with poor liver function
Neuropsychiatric complications developing with progressive liver failure
Small liver
Persistent hypotension
Aetiology
(e.g. alcoholic cirrhosis, if the patient continues drinking)

INR, International Normalized Ratio

Liver transplantation

This is an established treatment for a number of liver diseases. Shortage of donors is a major problem in all developed countries. Indications include the following:

Acute liver disease. Patients with fulminant hepatic failure of any cause, including acute viral hepatitis (p. 303), may be considered.

Chronic liver disease. The indications for transplantation vary and the timing of the transplant is often difficult. All patients with end-stage (Child's grade C) cirrhosis should be considered.

- *Primary biliary cirrhosis*. Patients with this disease should be transplanted when their serum bilirubin rises above 100 μmol L^{-1}.
- *Chronic hepatitis B*. Following transplantation, recurrence of the hepatitis occurs in 60–70% of cases and cirrhosis develops, in some, in 2–3 years. Recurrence of HBV infection can be reduced to 30% by hepatitis B immunoglobulin prophylaxis. Interferon therapy and other antiviral drugs (see p. 311) also reduce recurrence.
- *Chronic hepatitis C*. In end-stage disease the prognosis of the graft is good, despite HCV RNA being found in the grafted liver, indicating reinfection.
- *Autoimmune hepatitis*. These are patients who have failed to respond to medical treatment or have major side-effects of corticosteroid therapy.
- *Alcoholic liver disease*. Well-motivated patients who have stopped drinking can be offered a transplant.
- *Primary metabolic disorders*. Examples are Wilson's disease and α_1-antitrypsin deficiency.
- Other conditions, such as sclerosing cholangitis.

CONTRAINDICATIONS

Absolute contraindications include active sepsis outside the hepatobiliary tree, metastatic malignancy, HIV infection, and if the patient is not psychologically committed.

Relative contraindications are mainly anatomical considerations that would make surgery more difficult, such as portal vein thrombosis, previous portocaval shunts or complex surgery. With exceptions, patients aged 65 years or over are not transplanted. In hepatocellular carcinoma the recurrence rate is high and transplantation is not recommended.

SURGICAL PROCEDURE

Pretransplant workup includes confirmation of the diagnosis, ultrasound and CT scanning, radiological demonstration of the hepatic arterial and biliary tree.

Because of the ethical and financial implications of this operation, psychiatric counselling and regular psychosocial support are vital.

The donor should be ABO-compatible, but not necessarily HLA-compatible. He or she should ideally be under 50 years of age and have no evidence of sepsis, malignancy, HIV or HBV infection. The liver is cooled and stored on ice; its preservation time is then 11–20 hours. The recipient operation takes approximately 8 hours and requires a large blood transfusion.

The operative mortality is low. Most postoperative deaths occur in the first three months. Sepsis, haemorrhage, metabolic acidosis and hyperkalaemia occur. Opportunistic infections (see p. 176) are still a problem owing to immunosuppression. Various immunosuppressive agents have been used, but cyclosporin and corticosteroids are the most common. Tacrolimus, a macrolide immunosuppressant, has a more powerful effect than cyclosporin in inhibiting interleukin-2. A pretransplant serum creatinine above 160 μmol L^{-1} (2 mg dL^{-1}) is the best predictor of post-transplant death.

REJECTION

Rejection can be early (reversible) or late (irreversible). Acute or cellular rejection is usually seen 5–10 days post-transplant; the patient feels ill with a pyrexia and tender hepatomegaly. Histologically, there is portal inflammation, bile duct damage and endothelialitis of the liver. This type of rejection responds to immunosuppressive therapy.

Irreversible chronic ductopenic rejection is seen 6 weeks to 9 months post-transplant, with disappearing bile ducts (vanishing bile duct syndrome, VBDS) and an arteriopathy with narrowing and occlusion of the arteries. Ductopenic rejection is not reversed by immunosuppression and requires retransplantation. Graft-versus-host disease is extremely rare.

PROGNOSIS

Elective liver transplantation in low-risk patients now has a 90% one-year survival. Five-year survivals are as high as 70–85% largely owing to the introduction of cyclosporin and tacrolimus. Patients require lifelong immunosuppression, although the doses can be reduced over time without significant problems.

Complications and effects of cirrhosis

These are shown in Table 5.12.

Table 5.12
Complications and effects of cirrhosis

Portal hypertension and gastrointestinal haemorrhage
Ascites
Portosystemic encephalopathy
Renal failure
Hepatocellular carcinoma

Portal hypertension

The portal vein is formed by the union of the superior mesenteric and splenic veins. The pressure within it is normally 5–8 mmHg with only a small gradient across the liver to the hepatic vein in which blood is returned to the heart via the inferior vena cava. Portal hypertension can be classified according to the site of obstruction:

- *prehepatic* – due to blockage of the portal vein before the liver
- *intrahepatic* – due to distortion of the liver architecture, which can be presinusoidal (e.g. in schistosomiasis) or postsinusoidal (e.g. in cirrhosis)
- *posthepatic* - due to venous blockage outside the liver (rare).

As portal pressure rises above 10–12 mmHg, the compliant venous system dilates and collaterals occur with the systemic venous system. The main sites of the collaterals are at the gastro-oesophageal junction, the rectum, the left renal vein, the diaphragm, the retroperitoneum and the anterior abdominal wall via the umbilical vein.

The collaterals at the gastro-oesophageal junction (varices) are superficial in position and tend to rupture. Portosystemic anastomoses at other sites seldom give rise to symptoms. Rectal varices are found frequently (30%) if carefully looked for and can be differentiated from haemorrhoids, which are lower in the anal canal.

PATHOPHYSIOLOGY

Portal vascular resistance is increased in chronic liver disease. During liver injury, stellate cells are activated (see p. 315) and transform into myofibroblasts. In these cells there is *de novo* expression of the specific smooth muscle protein α-actin. Under the influence of mediators, such as endothelin, nitric oxide or prostaglandins, the contraction of these activated cells contributes to abnormal blood flow patterns and increased resistance to blood flow. This increased resistance leads to portal hypertension and opening of portosystemic anastomoses in both precirrhotic and cirrhotic livers. Patients with cirrhosis have a hyperdynamic circulation. This is thought to be due to the release of mediators, such as nitric oxide and glucagon, which leads to peripheral and splanchnic vasodilatation. This effect is followed by plasma volume expansion due to sodium retention (see the discussion on ascites, p. 320), and this has a significant effect in maintaining portal hypertension.

CAUSES (see Table 5.13)

The most common cause is cirrhosis. Other causes include the following.

Table 5.13
Causes of portal hypertension

Prehepatic / Intrahepatic	Posthepatic
Prehepatic	**Posthepatic**
Portal vein thrombosis	Budd–Chiari syndrome
	Veno-occlusive disease
Intrahepatic	Right heart failure (rare)
Cirrhosis	Constrictive pericarditis
Hepatitis (alcoholic)	
Idiopathic non-cirrhotic portal hypertension (subtle liver disease)	
Schistosomiasis	
Partial nodular transformation	
Congenital hepatic fibrosis	
Myelosclerosis (extramedullary haemopoiesis)	
Granulomata	

Prehepatic causes

Extrahepatic blockage is due to portal vein thrombosis. The cause is often unidentified, but some cases are due to portal vein occlusion secondary to congenital portal venous abnormalities or neonatal sepsis of the umbilical vein. Patients usually present with bleeding, often at a young age. They have normal liver function and, because of this, their prognosis following bleeding is excellent. The portal vein blockage can be identified by ultrasound or Doppler imaging. A splenectomy should never be performed, as it may be possible to perform a splenorenal shunt in adult life. Treatment is usually with repeated sclerotherapy.

Intrahepatic causes

Although cirrhosis is the most common intrahepatic cause of portal hypertension, there are other causes:

- *Non-cirrhotic portal hypertension or subtle-change liver disease.* Patients present with portal hypertension and variceal bleeding but without cirrhosis. Histologically, the liver shows mild portal tract fibrosis. The aetiology is unknown, but arsenic, vinyl chloride and other toxic agents have been implicated. A similar disease is found frequently in India. The liver lesion does not progress and the prognosis is therefore good.
- *Schistosomiasis* with extensive pipe-stem fibrosis is a common cause worldwide, but is confined to endemic areas.
- Other causes include congenital hepatic fibrosis, nodular regenerative hyperplasia, and partial nodular transformation. The last two conditions are rare. They share the common features of hyperplastic liver cell growth in the form of nodules, but in contrast to cirrhosis, fibrosis is typically absent. A wedge liver biopsy is usually required to establish the diagnosis.

Posthepatic causes

Prolonged severe heart failure with tricuspid incompetence and constrictive pericarditis can both lead to portal hypertension. The Budd–Chiari syndrome is described on p. 329.

CLINICAL FEATURES

Patients with portal hypertension are often asymptomatic and the only clinical evidence of portal hypertension is splenomegaly. Clinical features of chronic liver disease are usually present (see p. 298). Presenting features may include:

- haematemesis or melaena from rupture of gastro-oesophageal varices
- ascites
- encephalopathy.

Variceal haemorrhage

Approximately 70% of patients with cirrhosis will develop gastro-oesophageal varices, but only one-third of these will bleed from them. Bleeding is likely to occur with large varices, high pressure (>12 mmHg) and in severe liver disease.

MANAGEMENT

The management can be divided into the active bleeding episode, the prevention of rebleeding, and prophylactic measures to prevent the first haemorrhage. Despite all the therapeutic techniques available, the prognosis depends on the severity of the underlying liver disease, with an overall mortality from variceal haemorrhage of 30% – reaching 50% in Child's grade C.

Initial management of acute variceal bleeding

(Fig 5.21)

See also the discussion of the general management of gastrointestinal haemorrhage on p. 244.

Resuscitation

- Assess the general condition of the patient – pulse and blood pressure.
- Insert an intravenous line and obtain blood for grouping and crossmatching, haemoglobin, PT, urea, electrolytes and liver biochemistry.
- Restore blood volume with plasma expanders or, if possible, blood transfusion. These measures are discussed in more detail in the treatment of shock (p. 843). Prompt correction of hypovolaemia is necessary in patients with cirrhosis as their baroreceptor reflexes are diminished.

Urgent endoscopy

Endoscopy should be performed to confirm the diagnosis of varices (Fig 5.22) and to exclude bleeding from other sites (e.g. gastric ulceration), which are sometimes the source of haemorrhage in these patients. *Portal hypertensive*

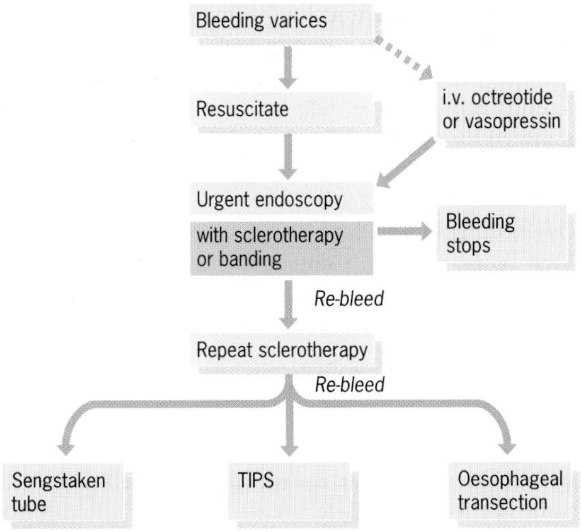

Fig 5.21
Management of gastrointestinal haemorrhage due to oesophageal varices.
TIPS, transjugular intrahepatic portocaval shunt.

(or congestive) gastropathy is the term used for chronic gastric congestion, punctate erythema and gastric erosions and is a source of bleeding. Varices may or may not be present. Propranolol (see below) is the best treatment for this.

Injection sclerotherapy or variceal banding

The varices should be injected with a sclerosing agent that may arrest bleeding by producing vessel thrombosis. A needle is passed down the biopsy channel of the endoscope and a sclerosing agent is injected into the varices. Alternatively, the varices can be banded by mounting a band on the tip of the endoscope, sucking the varix just into the end of the scope and dislodging the band over the varix using a trip-wire mechanism.

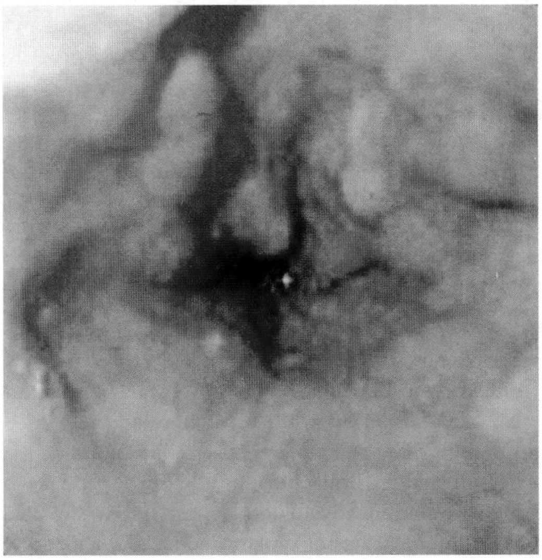

Fig 5.22
Endoscopic picture of oesophageal varices

Acute variceal sclerotherapy and banding are the treatment of choice; this arrests bleeding in 80% of cases and reduces early rebleeding. Between 15% and 20% of bleeding comes from gastric varices and here results of sclerotherapy are poor.

Other measures available

Vasoconstrictor therapy

The main use of this is for emergency control of bleeding either whilst waiting for endoscopy and sclerotherapy or – if the latter has failed – to control the bleeding. The aim of vasoconstrictor agents is to restrict portal inflow by splanchnic arterial constriction.

- *Octreotide*. This drug (a somatostatin analogue – 50 μg bolus followed by an infusion of 50 μg per hour for 48 hours) will produce splanchnic vasoconstriction without significant systemic vascular effect or complications. Octreotide is safe, as effective as balloon tamponade, and is often used while awaiting sclerotherapy.
- *Vasopressin*. An infusion of 25 units per hour should be administered by a central venous catheter (if possible) to avoid the risks of local leakage and necrosis. Vasopressin should not be given to patients with ischaemic heart disease. The addition of nitrates either by the intravenous, sublingual or patch route has been shown to enhance the efficacy of vasopressin and to reduce its complications. The patient will complain of abdominal colic, will defaecate and have facial pallor owing to the generalized vasoconstriction. Terlipressin (2 mg bolus 6-hourly) is longer acting than vasopressin and is an alternative.

Balloon tamponade

This procedure is used mainly to control bleeding if sclerotherapy has failed or is unavailable, or if vasoconstrictor therapy has failed or is contraindicated. The tube should be left in place for up to 12 hours and removed in the endoscopy room prior to sclerotherapy. The usual tube is a Sengstaken–Blakemore. The tube is passed into the stomach and the gastric balloon is inflated with air and pulled back. It should be positioned in close apposition to the gastro-oesophageal junction to prevent the cephalad variceal blood flow to the bleeding point. The oesophageal balloon should be inflated only if bleeding is not controlled by the gastric balloon alone.

This technique is successful in up to 90% of patients and is very useful in the first few hours of haemorrhaging. However, it has serious complications such as aspiration pneumonia, oesophageal rupture and mucosal ulceration, which lead to a 5% mortality. The procedure is very unpleasant for the patient.

Additional management of acute episode

- *Measures to prevent encephalopathy*. Portosystemic encephalopathy (PSE) can be precipitated by a large bleed (since blood contains protein). The management is described on p. 322.
- *Nursing*. Patients require high-dependency/intensive-care nursing. They should have nil by mouth until bleeding has stopped.
- *Sucralfate*. 1 g four times daily is given to reduce oesophageal ulceration following sclerotherapy.

Management of an acute rebleed

Fifty per cent of patients rebleed within 10 days. The source of the rebleed should be established by endoscopy. It is sometimes due to an ulcer produced by previous sclerotherapy and this is difficult to manage. Management starts with:

- repeat sclerotherapy – once only to control rebleeding (further sclerotherapy is not advisable)
- octreotide infusion for 3–5 days.

Transjugular intrahepatic portocaval shunt (TIPS)

In this technique, a guidewire is passed from the jugular vein into the liver and an expandable metal shunt is forced over it into the liver substance to form a channel between the systemic and portal venous systems. It reduces the hepatic sinusoidal and portal vein pressure by creating a side-to-side shunt, but without the risks of general anaesthesia and major surgery. TIPS is used in cases where the bleeding cannot be stopped after two sessions of sclerotherapy 24 hours apart. It is useful in the short term, but recurrent portal hypertension owing to stent stenosis can occur within two years.

Emergency surgery

This is used when other measures fail or if TIPS is not available and, particularly, if the bleeding is from gastric fundal varices. Oesophageal transection and ligation of the feeding vessels to the bleeding varices is the most common surgical technique. Acute portosystemic shunt surgery (see below) is infrequently performed in the UK.

Prevention of recurrent variceal bleeding

Following an episode of variceal bleeding, the risk of recurrence is 60–80% over a two-year period with an approximate mortality of 20% per episode. These facts justify the use of measures to prevent rebleeding.

Long-term injection sclerotherapy or banding

The use of repeated courses of injection sclerotherapy or banding at weekly intervals leads to the obliteration of the varices by fibrous tissue. This markedly reduces rebleeding, most occurring before the varices have been fully obliterated. Between 30% and 40% of varices return per year, so that follow-up endoscopy with ablation should be performed.

Although a reduction in bleeding episodes occurs, the effect on survival is controversial and probably small. Complications include oesophageal ulceration, mediastinitis and strictures, which occur in about 10% with repeated sclerotherapy. Banding has fewer complications, particularly in stricture formation.

β-Adrenoreceptor blockade

Oral propranolol in a dose sufficient to reduce resting pulse rate by 25% has been shown to decrease portal pressure. Portal inflow is reduced by two mechanisms: by a decrease in cardiac output (β_1), and by the blockade of β_2 vasodilator fibres on the splanchnic arteries, leaving an unopposed vasoconstrictor effect. This has been shown to decrease the frequency of rebleeding in patients with well-compensated liver disease, and some studies show it to be as effective as sclerotherapy.

Surgical procedures

Portosystemic shunting is associated with an extremely low risk of rebleeding, but the diversion of portal blood away from the liver produces significant *encephalopathy*. Operative mortality is low in patients with Child's grade A (0–5%) but encephalopathy still occurs. Child's grade C has a very poor prognosis. The 'shunts' performed now are usually an end-to-side portocaval anastomosis or a selective distal splenorenal shunt (Warren shunt), which maintains hepatic blood flow via the superior mesenteric vein. Oesophageal transection does not produce encephalopathy, but rebleeding eventually occurs and it is only used acutely. Liver transplantation (p. 316) should always be considered.

Prophylactic measures

Patients with cirrhosis and varices, who have not bled, should be prescribed non-selective β-blockers (e.g. propranolol). This reduces the chances of variceal haemorrhage, may increase survival and is cost-effective.

Ascites

Ascites is the presence of fluid within the peritoneal cavity and is a common complication of cirrhosis of the liver. The pathogenesis of the development of ascites in liver disease is controversial, but is probably secondary to renal sodium and water retention. Several factors are involved.

- *Sodium and water retention* occur as a result of peripheral arterial vasodilatation and consequent reduction in the effective blood volume. Nitric oxide has been postulated as the putative vasodilator, although other substances (e.g. atrial natriuretic peptide and prostaglandins) may be involved. The reduction in effective blood volume activates various neurohumoral pressor systems such as the sympathetic nervous system and the renin–angiotensin system, thus promoting salt and water retention.

- *Portal hypertension* exerts a local hydrostatic pressure and leads to increased hepatic and splanchnic production of lymph and transudation of fluid into the peritoneal cavity.
- *Low serum albumin* (a consequence of poor synthetic liver function) may further contribute by a reduction in plasma oncotic pressure.

In patients with ascites, urine sodium excretion rarely exceeds 5 mmol in 24 hours. Loss of sodium from extrarenal sites accounts for approximately 30 mmol in 24 hours. The normal daily dietary sodium intake may vary between 120 and 200 mmol, resulting in a positive sodium balance of approximately 90–170 mmol in 24 hours (equivalent to 600–1300 mL of fluid retained).

CLINICAL FEATURES

The abdominal swelling associated with ascites may accumulate over many weeks or as rapidly as a few days. Precipitating factors include a high sodium diet or the development of a hepatocellular carcinoma. Mild generalized abdominal pain and discomfort are common but, if more severe, should raise the suspicion of spontaneous bacterial peritonitis (see below). Respiratory distress may accompany tense ascites.

The presence of fluid is confirmed by the demonstration of shifting dullness. Many patients will also have peripheral oedema. A pleural effusion (usually on the right side) may infrequently be found and is believed to arise from the passage of ascitic fluid through congenital defects in the diaphragm.

INVESTIGATIONS

A diagnostic aspiration of 10–20 mL of fluid should be obtained and the following performed:

- **Cell count**. A neutrophil count above 250 cells mm^{-3} is indicative of an underlying (usually spontaneous) bacterial peritonitis.
- **Gram stain and culture** – for bacteria and acid-fast bacilli.
- **Protein**. The ascitic protein level enables a division into transudative and exudative ascites. For this division the serum albumin must be used as a reference point. An ascitic protein of 11 g L^{-1} or more below the serum albumin level suggests a transudate. The level of ascitic protein provides an indirect estimate of opsonization capacity, and thereby the risk of developing spontaneous bacterial peritonitis. Patients at most risk are those with ascitic protein levels below 10 g L^{-1}.
- **Cytology** – for malignant cells.
- **Amylase** – to exclude pancreatic ascites.

The differential diagnosis of ascites is listed in Table 5.14.

Table 5.14
Causes of ascites divided according to the type of ascitic fluid

Straw-coloured	Chylous
Malignancy (most common cause)	Obstruction of main lymphatic duct (e.g. by carcinoma) – chylomicrons are present
Cirrhosis	
Infective	**Haemorrhagic**
Tuberculosis	Malignancy
Following intra-abdominal perforation - any bacteria may be found (e.g. *E. coli*)	Ruptured ectopic pregnancy
Spontaneous in cirrhotics	Abdominal trauma
Hepatic vein obstruction (Budd–Chiari syndrome) – protein level high in fluid	Acute pancreatitis
Chronic pancreatitis	
Congestive cardiac failure	
Constrictive pericarditis	
Meigs' syndrome (ovarian tumour)	
Hypoproteinaemia, (e.g. nephrotic syndrome)	

MANAGEMENT

The aim is to both reduce sodium intake and increase renal excretion of sodium – and by doing so produce a net reabsorption of fluid from the ascites back into the circulating volume. The maximum rate at which ascites can be mobilized is 500–700 mL in 24 hours (see below). The management is as follows:

- Check serum electrolytes and creatinine at the start and every other day; weigh and measure urinary output daily.
- Bed rest alone will lead to a diuresis in a small proportion of people by improving renal perfusion, but in practice is not helpful.
- By dietary sodium restriction it is possible to reduce sodium intake to 22 mmol in 24 hours and still maintain an adequate protein and calorie intake. Many patients find this difficult and a 40 mmol diet is frequently an adequate compromise.
- Fluid restriction is probably not necessary unless the serum sodium is under 128 mmol L^{-1} (see below).
- The diuretic of first choice is the aldosterone antagonist spironolactone, 200 mg daily. Chronic administration produces gynaecomastia; amiloride, 10–15 mg daily, is then substituted.

The aim of diuretic therapy should be to produce a net loss of fluid approaching 700 mL in 24 hours (0.700 kg weight loss or 1.5 kg if peripheral oedema is present). Although 60% of patients respond with this regimen, diuresis is often poor and the spironolactone can be increased to 500 mg daily. A loop diuretic, such as frusemide 80 mg or bumetanide 1 mg daily, may be added if response is poor. These loop diuretics have several potential disadvantages, including hyponatraemia, hypokalaemia and volume depletion.

Ascitic fluid is mobilized more slowly than interstitial fluid and diuretics should be given with great care in those without peripheral oedema.

Diuretics should be temporarily discontinued if a rise in serum creatinine level (to approximately 160 μmol L^{-1})

occurs, representing overdiuresis and hypovolaemia. Hyponatraemia occurring during therapy almost always represents haemodilution secondary to a failure to clear free water (usually a marker of reduced renal perfusion) and should be treated by stopping the diuretics if the sodium level falls below approximately 128 mmol L^{-1} as well as introducing water restriction. Diuretics should also be stopped if there is hypokalaemia or precoma.

Paracentesis

This is used to relieve symptomatic tense ascites. It is also used as a means of rapid therapy in patients with ascites and peripheral oedema, thus avoiding prolonged hospital stay. The main danger of this approach is the production of hypovolaemia as the ascites reaccumulates at the expense of the circulating volume. In patients with normal renal function and in the absence of hyponatraemia, this has largely been overcome by the administration of albumin (6 g per litre of ascitic fluid removed) or a plasma expander to maintain the plasma volume – e.g. dextran-70 (8 g per litre of ascitic fluid removed) or gelatin infusion (125 mL of a 3.5–4% solution per litre removed). In practice, up to 20 L can be removed over 4–6 hours. This should always be followed by the plasma expander given over half an hour, three hours after the paracentesis. This procedure should not be performed in end-stage cirrhosis or if the patient has renal failure.

Shunts

The introduction of peritoneo-venous shunt – a catheter from the peritoneal cavity (subcutaneously) to the internal jugular vein, incorporating a one-way valve – allows passage of the ascites directly into the circulation. This is occasionally useful in patients with resistant ascites but the tube often blocks.

A transjugular intrahepatic portocaval shunt (TIPS) is useful occasionally for resistant ascites.

Spontaneous bacterial peritonitis

This condition represents one of the more serious complications of ascites and occurs in approximately 8% of cirrhotics with ascites. The infecting organisms are believed to gain access to the peritoneum by haematogenous spread. The most frequently incriminated bacteria are *Escherichia coli*, *Klebsiella* and enterococci. The condition should be suspected in any patient with ascites with evidence of clinical deterioration. Features such as pain and pyrexia are frequently absent. Diagnostic aspiration should always be performed in patients with ascites (see above). The raised neutrophil count in the ascites is alone sufficient evidence to start treatment immediately. A third-generation cephalosporin, such as cefotaxime or ceftazidime, is used and may be modified on the basis of culture results.

The prognosis is grave and depends on the severity of the liver disease. It has a 50% mortality and recurs in 70% of patients within a year. It is an indication for liver transplantation.

Portosystemic encephalopathy

The term 'portosystemic encephalopathy' (PSE) refers to a chronic neuropsychiatric syndrome secondary to chronic liver disease. This condition occurs with cirrhosis, but a similar acute encephalopathy can occur in acute FHF (see p. 309). PSE is seen in patients with portal hypertension that is due to spontaneous 'shunting', or in patients following a portosystemic shunt procedure, e.g. TIPS. Encephalopathy is potentially reversible.

PATHOGENESIS

The mechanism is unknown but several factors are thought to play a part. In cirrhosis, the blood bypasses the liver via the collaterals and the 'toxic' metabolites pass directly to the brain to produce the encephalopathy.

Many 'toxic' substances have been suggested as the causative factor, including ammonia, free fatty acids, mercaptans and accumulation of false neurotransmitters (octopamine) or activation of the γ-aminobutyric acid (GABA) inhibitory neurotransmitter system. Increased blood levels of aromatic amino acids (tyrosine and phenylalanine) and reduced branched-chain amino acids (valine, leucine and isoleucine) also occur. Nevertheless, ammonia seems to have a major role, and ammonia-induced alteration of brain neurotransmitter balance – especially at the astrocyte–neurone interface – is currently the leading concept of the causation. Ammonia is produced by the breakdown of protein by intestinal bacteria, and a high blood ammonia is seen in most patients. The factors that can precipitate PSE are shown in Table 5.15.

CLINICAL FEATURES

An acute onset often has a precipitating factor (Table 5.15). The patient becomes increasingly drowsy and comatose.

Chronically, there is a disorder of personality, mood and intellect, with a reversal of normal sleep rhythm. These changes may be fluctuating and a history from a relative must be obtained. The patient is irritable, confused, disorientated and has slow slurred speech. General features

Table 5.15
Factors precipitating portosystemic encephalopathy

High dietary protein
Gastrointestinal haemorrhage
Constipation
Infection, including spontaneous bacterial peritonitis
Fluid and electrolyte disturbance due to:
diuretic therapy
paracentesis
Drugs (e.g. any CNS depressant)
Portosystemic shunt operations, TIPS
Any surgical procedure
Progressive liver damage
Development of hepatocellular carcinoma

TIPS, transjugular intrahepatic portocaval shunt

include nausea, vomiting and weakness. Convulsions and coma occur as the encephalopathy becomes more marked. Hyperventilation and pyrexia are seen.

Signs include:

- fetor hepaticus (a sweet smell to the breath)
- a coarse flapping tremor seen when the hands are outstretched and the wrists hyperextended (asterixis)
- constructional apraxia, with the patient being unable to write or draw, for example, a five-pointed star).
- decreased mental function, which can be assessed by using the serial-sevens test (see p. 1109). A trail-making test (the ability to join numbers and letters with a pen within a certain time – a standard psychological test for brain dysfunction) is prolonged and is a useful bedside test to assess encephalopathy.

Diagnosis is clinical. Routine liver biochemistry merely confirms the presence of liver disease, not the presence of encephalopathy.

Additional investigations.

- Electroencephalogram (EEG) shows a decrease in the frequency of the normal α-waves (8–13 Hz) to δ-waves of 1.5–3 Hz. These changes occur before coma supervenes.
- Visual evoked responses (see p. 1041) also detect subclinical encephalopathy.
- Arterial blood ammonia is occasionally useful in the differential diagnosis of the cause of the coma and to follow the course of the PSE, but is not readily available.

MANAGEMENT

Management consists of restricting protein intake and sterilizing the bowel.

Immediate management

- Identify and remove the possible precipitating cause, such as drugs with cerebral depressant properties.
- Give purgation and enemas to empty the bowels of nitrogenous substances. Lactulose (10–30 mL thrice daily) is an osmotic purgative that reduces the colonic pH and limits ammonia absorption. Lactilol (β-galactoside sorbitol 30 g daily) is metabolized by colonic bacteria and is comparable in efficacy to lactulose. Hypernatraemia can result from water loss.
- Institute a protein-free diet, with adequate calories, given if necessary via a fine-bore nasogastric tube.
- Give antibiotics. One gram of oral neomycin 6-hourly can be used if lactulose fails. Neomycin can also be used in retention enemas. It is mainly unabsorbed, but in the long term it can produce deafness. Metronidazole (200 mg four times daily) is also effective in the acute situation.
- Stop or reduce diuretic therapy.
- Correct any electrolyte imbalance.
- Give intravenous fluids as necessary (beware of too much sodium).
- Treat any infection.
- Flumazenil, a benzodiazepine receptor antagonist, can induce a transient improvement.

Long term management

- Increase protein in the diet to the limit of tolerance (20–50 g) as the encephalopathy improves.
- Give lactulose 10–30 mL thrice daily to avoid constipation.
- Avoid precipitating factors such as narcotic drugs, which depress cerebral function, and over-diuresis producing electrolyte imbalance.

COURSE AND PROGNOSIS

Acute encephalopathy, often seen after FHF, has a very poor prognosis as the disease itself has a high mortality. In cirrhosis, chronic PSE is very variable and the prognosis is that of the underlying liver disease.

Renal failure (hepatorenal syndrome)

The hepatorenal syndrome occurs typically in a patient with advanced cirrhosis with jaundice and ascites. The urine output is low with a low urinary sodium concentration, a maintained capacity to concentrate urine (i.e. tubular function is intact) and an almost normal renal histology. The renal failure here is described as 'functional'. It is sometimes precipitated by overvigorous diuretic therapy, diarrhoea or paracentesis, but often no precipitating factor is found. Advanced cases may progress beyond the 'functional' stage to produce an acute tubular necrosis.

The mechanism is similar to that producing ascites. The initiating factor is thought to be extreme peripheral vasodilation possibly due to nitric oxide, leading to an extreme decrease in the effective blood volume and hypotension. This activates the homeostatic mechanisms, causing a rise in plasma renin, aldosterone, noradrenaline and vasopressin, leading to vasoconstriction of the renal vasculature. There is an increased preglomerular vascular resistance causing the blood flow to be directed away from the renal cortex. This leads to a reduced glomerular filtration rate and plasma renin remains high. Salt and water retention occur with reabsorption of sodium from the renal tubules.

A number of other mediators have been incriminated in the pathogenesis of the hepatorenal syndrome, in particular the eicosanoids. This has been supported by the precipitation of the syndrome by inhibitors of prostaglandin synthetase such as non-steroidal anti-inflammatory agents.

Diuretic therapy should be stopped and intravascular hypovolaemia corrected. TIPS has been used as a short-term measure with improvement, but the overall prognosis is poor. Liver transplantation is the best option with long-term survival similar in patients to those without renal failure.

Primary hepatocellular carcinoma

This is discussed on p. 333.

Types of cirrhosis

Alcoholic cirrhosis

This is discussed in the section on alcoholic liver disease (p. 328).

Primary biliary cirrhosis

Primary biliary cirrhosis (PBC) is a chronic disorder in which there is a progressive destruction of bile ducts, eventually leading to cirrhosis. Ninety per cent of those affected are women in the age range 40–50 years. It used to be rare but is now being diagnosed more frequently in its milder forms. The prevalence is approximately 7.5 per 100 000, with a marked increase in first-degree relatives. PBC has been called 'chronic non-suppurative destructive cholangitis'; this term is more descriptive of the early lesion and emphasizes that true cirrhosis occurs only in the later stages of the disease.

AETIOLOGY

The aetiology is unknown, but immunological mechanisms may play a part. Serum antimitochondrial antibodies are found in almost all patients with PBC, and of the mitochondrial proteins involved, the antigen M2 is specific to PBC. The finding of M4 and M8 antigens in patients with M2 may be associated with more progressive disease.

Five M2 specific antigens have been further defined using immunoblot techniques, of which the E2 component of the pyruvate dehydrogenase complex (PDC) is the major M2 autoantigen. The five antigens are a 72 kDa E2 subunit (PDC.E2), the 52 kDa protein X, the 50 kDa branched-chain 2-oxo-acid dehydrogenase complex (BCOADC.E2), the 48 kDa 2-oxo-glutarate dehydrogenase complex (OGDC.E2), and the 41 kDa E1 α-subunit of PDC.

The presence of AMA in high titre is unrelated to the clinical or histological picture and its role in pathogenesis is unclear.

It seems likely that an environmental factor acts on a genetically predisposed host. *E. coli* and other enterobacteria have been proposed as the triggering infective agent.

Although damage to bile ducts is a feature, antibodies to bile ductules are not specific to PBC. Biliary epithelium from patients with PBC expresses aberrant class II HLAs, but it is not known whether this expression is the cause or result of the inflammatory response. Cell-mediated immunity is impaired (demonstrated both *in vitro* and by skin testing), suggesting that sensitized T lymphocytes might be involved in producing damage. There may be a defect in immunoregulation, or a decrease in T suppressor cells which may allow cytotoxic T cells to produce damage to the bile ducts. There is also evidence to suggest that lymphokine secretion and cell activation by T lymphocytes is impaired at the site of tissue destruction. There is an increased synthesis of IgM, thought to be due to a failure of the switch from IgM to IgG antibody synthesis.

CLINICAL FEATURES

Asymptomatic patients are discovered on routine examination or screening to have hepatomegaly, a raised serum alkaline phosphatase or autoantibodies.

Pruritus is often the earliest symptom, preceding jaundice by a few years. When jaundice appears, hepatomegaly is usually found. In the later stages, patients are jaundiced with severe pruritus. Pigmented xanthelasma on eyelids or other deposits of cholesterol in the creases of the hands may be seen. Hepatosplenomegaly is present.

ASSOCIATIONS

Autoimmune disorders (e.g. Sjögren's syndrome, scleroderma, rheumatoid arthritis) occur with increased frequency. Keratoconjunctivitis sicca (dry eyes and mouth) is seen in 70% of cases. Renal tubular acidosis and membranous glomerulonephritis may occur.

INVESTIGATIONS

- **Mitochondrial antibodies** - measured routinely by ELISA (in titres >1:160) – are present in over 95% of patients. M2 antibody is specific. Other nonspecific antibodies (e.g. antinuclear factor and smooth muscle) may also be present.
- **High serum alkaline phosphatase** is often the only abnormality in the liver biochemistry.
- **Serum cholesterol** is raised.
- **Serum IgM** may be very high.
- **Ultrasound** can show a diffuse alteration in liver architecture.
- **Liver biopsy** shows characteristic histological features of a portal tract infiltrate mainly of lymphocytes and plasma cells; approximately 40% have granulomas. Most of the early changes are in zone 1. Later, there is damage to and loss of small bile ducts with ductular proliferation. Portal tract fibrosis and, eventually, cirrhosis is seen.

Hepatic granulomas are not specific and are also seen in sarcoidosis, tuberculosis, schistosomiasis, drug reactions (e.g. phenylbutazone), brucellosis, parasitic infestation (e.g. strongyloidiasis) and other conditions.

DIFFERENTIAL DIAGNOSIS

The classical picture presents little difficulty with diagnosis (high serum alkaline phosphatase and the presence of AMA); this can be confirmed by the characteristic features on liver biopsy. There is a group of patients with the histological changes of PBC, but the serology of autoimmune hepatitis (i.e. positive antinuclear and smooth muscle antibodies but negative AMA). This has been given the name of *autoimmune cholangitis* and responds to steroids and azathioprine.

In the jaundiced patient, extrahepatic biliary obstruction should be excluded by ultrasound and, if there is doubt about the diagnosis, ERCP (or MRCP) should be performed to make sure that the bile ducts are normal.

TREATMENT

Ursodeoxycholate (10–15 mg kg L^{-1}) is of benefit in some patients with improvement in serum liver enzymes and pruritus, and should be given to all patients. The results from all trials have shown a modest reduction in time to death or transplant. Corticosteroids and other immunosuppressive drugs have shown no clear benefit and are not now used.

Malabsorption of fat-soluble vitamins (A, D and K) occurs and supplementation is required when deficiency is detected and in the jaundiced patient prophylactically. Calcium is required for osteoporosis. Hyperlipidaemia should be treated (see p. 994).

Pruritus is difficult to control, but cholestyramine, one 4 g sachet three times daily, can be helpful, although it is unpalatable. Rifampicin and naloxone hydrochloride (an opioid antagonist) have been shown to be of benefit in trials.

The lack of effective medical therapy has made PBC a major indication for orthotopic liver transplantation (p. 316).

COMPLICATIONS

The complications are those of cirrhosis. In addition, osteoporosis, osteomalacia and a polyneuropathy can also occur.

COURSE AND PROGNOSIS

This is very variable. Asymptomatic patients and those presenting with pruritus will survive for more than 20 years. Symptomatic patients with jaundice have a more rapidly progressive course and die of liver failure or bleeding varices in approximately 5 years. Liver transplantation should therefore be offered when the serum bilirubin reaches 100 μmol L^{-1}. Transplantation has a five-year survival of at least 70%.

Secondary biliary cirrhosis

Cirrhosis can result from prolonged (for months) large duct biliary obstruction. Causes include bile duct strictures, gallstones and sclerosing cholangitis. An ultrasound examination, followed by ERCP or PTC, is performed to outline the ducts and any remedial cause is dealt with.

Hereditary haemochromatosis

Hereditary haemochromatosis (HH) is an inherited disease characterized by excess iron deposition in various organs leading to eventual fibrosis and functional organ failure.

PREVALENCE AND AETIOLOGY

HH is transmitted by an autosomal recessive gene with a prevalence in caucasians of homozygotes (affected) of 1 in 400 and a heterozygote (carrier) frequency of 1 in 10. It is the most common single gene disorder in caucasians. It is associated with HLA-A3 (72% versus 28% of the general population); in addition HLA-B14 is increased in France and HLA-B7 in Australia.

HH has been shown to be due to a mutation in a gene initially designated HLA-H – now HFE – on the short arm of chromosome 6.

Between 83% and 90% of patients with overt HH are homozygous for the Cys 282 Tyr mutation. A second mutation (His 63 Asp; C 187G) occurs in about 25% of the population and is in complete linkage disequilibrium with Cys 282 Tyr.

Dietary intakes of iron and chelating agents (ascorbic acid) are probably also important. Iron overload may be present in alcoholics, but alcohol excess *per se* does not cause HH. There is a history of excess alcohol intake in 25% of patients.

Mechanism of damage. This is still unclear. The HFE gene may be involved in regulating the expression of other gene products including the recently described divalent-cation transporter (DCTI) which may be a mediator in intestinal iron absorption. Iron is taken up by the mucosal cells inappropriately, exceeding the binding capacity of transferrin; excess iron is then taken up by the liver and other tissues gradually over a long period. It seems likely that it is the iron itself that precipitates fibrosis.

PATHOLOGY

In symptomatic patients the total body iron content is 20–40 g, compared with 3–4 g in a normal person. The iron content is particularly increased in the liver and pancreas (50–100 times normal) but is also increased in all other organs (e.g. the endocrine glands, heart and skin). Gonadal function is impaired despite a low testicular iron content.

In established cases the liver shows extensive iron deposition and fibrosis. Early in the disease, iron is deposited in the periportal hepatocytes (in pericanalicular lysosomes). Later it is distributed widely throughout all acinar zones, biliary duct epithelium, Kupffer cells and connective tissue. Cirrhosis is a late feature.

CLINICAL FEATURES

The course of the disease depends on a number of factors, including sex, dietary iron intake, presence of associated hepatotoxins (especially alcohol) and genotype. Overt clinical manifestations occur more frequently in men; the reduced incidence in women is probably explained by physiological blood loss and a smaller dietary intake of iron. Most affected individuals present in the fifth decade. The classic triad of bronze skin pigmentation (due to melanin deposition), hepatomegaly and diabetes mellitus is only present in cases of gross iron overload.

Hypogonadism secondary to pituitary dysfunction is the most common endocrine feature. Deficiency of other pituitary hormones is also found, but symptomatic endocrine deficiencies, such as loss of libido, are very rare. Cardiac manifestations, particularly heart failure and arrhythmias, are common, especially in younger patients. Calcium pyrophosphate is deposited asymmetrically in both large and small joints (chondrocalcinosis) leading to an arthropathy. The exact relationship of chondrocalcinosis to iron deposition is uncertain.

COMPLICATIONS

Thirty per cent of patients with cirrhosis will develop primary hepatocellular carcinoma (HCC). HCC has only rarely been described in non-cirrhotic patients in whom the excess iron stores have been removed. This has important implications for early diagnosis.

INVESTIGATIONS

Homozygotes

- **Serum iron** is elevated (>30 μmol L^{-1}), with a reduction in the TIBC and complete or almost complete transferrin saturation (>60%).
- **Serum ferritin** is elevated (usually >500 μg L^{-1} or 240 nmol L^{-1}).
- **Liver biochemistry** is often normal, even with established cirrhosis.

Heterozygotes

Heterozygotes may have normal biochemical tests or modest increases in serum iron transferrin saturation (>50%) or serum ferritin (usually >400 μg L^{-1}).

Liver biopsy

This can define the extent of tissue damage, assess tissue iron, and the hepatic iron concentration can be measured (>180 μmol g^{-1} dry weight of liver indicates haemochromatosis).

Mild degrees of parenchymal iron deposition in patients with alcoholic cirrhosis can often cause confusion with true homozygous HH. It is highly likely that many of this former group are heterozygotes for the haemochromatosis gene.

Magnetic resonance imaging

MRI shows dramatic reduction in the signal intensity of the liver and pancreas owing to the paramagnetic affect of ferritin and haemosiderin which profoundly shortens both the T1 and T2 relaxation times. In secondary iron overload (haemosiderosis) which involves the reticuloendothelial cells, the pancreas is spared – enabling distinction between these two conditions.

TREATMENT AND MANAGEMENT

Venesection

Venesection prolongs life and may reverse tissue damage; the risk of malignancy still remains if cirrhosis is present. All patients should have excess iron removed as rapidly as possible. This is achieved using venesection of 500 mL performed twice-weekly for up to two years; i.e. 160 units × 250 mg of iron per unit, which equals 40 g removed. During venesection, serum iron and ferritin and the mean corpuscular volume (MCV) should be monitored. These fall only when available iron is depleted. Three or four venesections per year are required to prevent reaccumulation of iron. Serum ferritin should remain within the normal range. Liver biopsy is useful to ensure removal of iron and to assess progress of hepatic disease.

Manifestations of the disease usually improve or disappear, except for diabetes, testicular atrophy and chondrocalcinosis. The requirements for insulin often diminish in diabetic patients. Testosterone replacement is often helpful.

Chelation therapy

In the rare patient who cannot tolerate venesection (because of severe cardiac disease or anaemia), chelation therapy with desferrioxamine either intermittently or continuously by infusion has been successful in removing iron.

SCREENING

In all cases of HH, all first-degree family members must be screened to detect early and asymptomatic disease. Serum ferritin is an excellent test with only occasional false-positives in hepatocellular necrosis and rare false-negatives in some family studies. Genetic markers are now available for diagnosis.

In the general population, the serum iron and transferrin saturation are the best and cheapest tests available.

Wilson's disease (hepatolenticular degeneration)

Dietary copper is normally absorbed from the stomach and upper small intestine. It is transported to the liver loosely bound to albumin. Here it is incorporated into caeruloplasmin, a glycoprotein synthesized in the liver, and secreted into the blood. Copper is normally excreted in the bile.

Wilson's disease is a very rare inborn error of copper metabolism that results in copper deposition in various organs, including the liver, the basal ganglia of the brain and the cornea. It is potentially treatable and all young patients with liver disease must be screened for this condition.

AETIOLOGY

It is an autosomal recessive disorder with a molecular defect within a copper-transporting ATPase encoded by a gene (designated ATP7B) located on chromosome 13. Over 60 mutations have been identified, the most frequent being His1070Gly found in approximately 50% of cases in the USA and Europe. It occurs worldwide, particularly in countries where consanguinity is common. The basic problem is a failure of biliary excretion of copper. There is a low serum caeruloplasmin in over 80% of patients owing to poor synthesis, but the precise mechanism for the failure of copper excretion is not known.

PATHOLOGY

The liver histology is not diagnostic and varies from that of chronic hepatitis to macronodular cirrhosis. Stains for copper show a periportal distribution but this can be unreliable (see below). The basal ganglia are damaged and show cavitation, the kidneys show tubular degeneration, and erosions are seen in bones.

CLINICAL FEATURES

Children usually present with hepatic problems, whereas young adults have more neurological problems, such as tremor, dysarthria, involuntary movements and eventually dementia. The liver disease varies from episodes of acute hepatitis, especially in children, which can go on to fulminant hepatic failure to chronic hepatitis or cirrhosis.

Typical signs are of chronic liver disease with neurological signs of basal ganglia involvement (p. 1065). A specific sign is the Kayser–Fleischer ring, which is due to copper deposition in Descemet's membrane in the cornea. It appears as a greenish brown pigment at the corneoscleral junction just within the cornea. Identification of this ring frequently requires slit-lamp examination. It may be absent in young children.

INVESTIGATIONS

- **Serum copper and caeruloplasmin** are usually reduced but can be normal.
- **Urinary copper** is usually increased (100–1000 μg in 24 hours; normal levels <40 μg in 24 hours).
- **Liver biopsy**. The diagnosis depends on the measurement of the amount of copper in the liver, although high levels of copper are also found in the liver in chronic cholestasis. Measurement of ^{64}Cu incorporation into the liver may be helpful.
- **Haemolysis and anaemia** may be present.

TREATMENT

Lifetime treatment with penicillamine, 1–2 g daily, is effective in chelating copper. If treatment is started early, clinical and biochemical improvement can occur. Urine copper levels should be monitored and the drug dose adjusted. Serious side-effects of the drug occur in 10% and include skin rashes, leucopenia and renal damage. All siblings and children of patients should be screened and treatment given even in the asymptomatic if there is evidence of copper accumulation.

PROGNOSIS

Early diagnosis and effective treatment have improved the outlook. Neurological damage is, however, permanent. Fulminant hepatic failure or decompensated cirrhosis should be treated by liver transplantation.

α_1-Antitrypsin deficiency (see also p. 776)

A deficiency of α_1-antitrypsin (α_1AT) is sometimes associated with liver disease and pulmonary emphysema (particularly in smokers). α_1AT is a glycoprotein, part of a family of *ser*ine *p*rotease *in*hibitors, or serpin, superfamily. α_1AT is inherited as an autosomal dominant and 1 in 10 northern Europeans carry a deficiency gene.

The protein is a 394-amino acid 52 kDa acute phase protein that is synthesized in the liver and comprises 90% of the serum α_1-globulin seen on electrophoresis. Its main role is to inhibit the proteolytic enzyme, neutrophil elastase.

The gene is located on chromosome 14. The genetic variants of α_1AT are characterized by their electrophoretic mobilities as medium (M), slow (S) or very slow (Z). The normal genotype is protease inhibitor MM (PiMM), the homozygote for Z is PiZZ, and the heterozygotes are PiMZ and PiSZ. S and Z variants are due to a single amino acid replacement of glutamic acid at positions 264 and 342 of the polypeptide, respectively. This results in decreased synthesis and secretion of the protein by the liver as protein–protein interactions occur between the reactive centre loop of one molecule and the β-pleated sheet of a second (loop sheet polymerization).

How this causes liver disease is uncertain. The failure of secretion of the abnormal protein leads to an accumulation in the liver which leads to plasma levels of antitrypsin in the S variant being 60% of that normally found in the M allele, with the Z variant being 10% of the normal levels.

CLINICAL FEATURES

The majority of patients with clinical disease are homozygotes with a PiZZ phenotype. Some may present in childhood and a few require transplantation. Approximately 10–15% of adult patients will develop cirrhosis, usually over the age of 50 years, and 75% will have respiratory problems. Approximately 5% of patients die of their liver disease. Heterozygotes (e.g. PiSZ or PiMZ) may develop liver disease, but the risk is small.

INVESTIGATIONS

- **Serum α_1-antritrypsin** is low, at 10% of the normal level in the PiZZ phenotypes.

Liver biopsy

Periodic acid–Schiff (PAS)-positive, diastase-resistant globules are seen in periportal hepatocytes. These can be shown to be α_1AT using specific antiserum. Fibrosis and cirrhosis can be present.

TREATMENT

There is no treatment apart from dealing with the complications of liver disease. Patients with hepatic decompensation should be considered for liver transplantation. Patients should be advised to stop smoking (see p. 777).

FURTHER READING

Abbasoglu O *et al.* (1997) Ten years of liver transplantation. *Transplantation* **64**: 1801-1807.

Arroyo V, Gines P, Gerbes AL *et al* (1996) Definition and diagnostic criteria of refractory ascites and hepatorenal syndrome in cirrhosis. *Hepatology* **23**: 164–175.

Jazwnska EG, Powell LW (1997) Haemochromatosis and 'HLA-H' definite. *Hepatology* **25**: 495–496.

Lomas DA (1996) New insights into the structural basis of α_1-antitrypsin deficiency. *Quarterly Journal of Medicine* **89**: 807–812.

Major ME, Feinstone SM (1997) The molecular biology of hepatitis C. *Hepatology* **25**: 1527–1538.

Moore K (1997) The hepatorenal syndrome. *Clinical Science* **92**: 433–443.

O'Donoghue J, Williams R (1996) Primary biliary cirrhosis. *Quarterly Journal of Medicine* **89**: 5–13.

Rees CJ, Hiubon M, Record CO (1997) Therapeutic modalities in portal hypertension. *European Journal of Gastroenterology and Hepatology* **9**: 9–11.

Riordan SM, Williams R (1997) Current concepts: treatment of hepatic encephalopathy. *New England Journal of Medicine* **337**: 473–479.

Scott L, Friedman MD (1993) The cellular basis of hepatic fibrosis. *New England Journal of Medicine* **328**: 1828–1836.

Rockey D (1997) The cellular pathogenesis of portal hypertension: stellate cell contractility, endothelin, and nitric oxide. *Hepatology* **25**: 2–5.

Alcoholic liver disease

This section gives the pathology and clinical features of alcoholic liver disease. The amounts needed to produce liver damage, alcohol metabolism, and other clinical effects of alcohol are described on p. 214.

Ethanol is metabolized in the liver by two pathways (see p. 214), resulting in an increase in the NADH/NAD ratio. The altered redox potential results in increased hepatic fatty acid synthesis with decreased fatty acid oxidation, both events leading to hepatic accumulation of fatty acid that is then esterified to glycerides.

The changes in oxidation–reduction also impair carbohydrate and protein metabolism and are the cause of the centrilobular necrosis of the hepatic acinus typical of alcohol damage.

Acetaldehyde is formed by the oxidation of ethanol and its effect on hepatic proteins may well be an important factor in producing liver cell damage. The exact mechanism of alcoholic hepatitis and cirrhosis is unknown, but since only 10–20% of people who drink heavily will suffer from cirrhosis, a genetic predisposition is proposed. Immunological mechanisms have also been proposed.

Alcohol can enhance the effects of toxic metabolites of drugs (e.g. paracetamol) on the liver, as it induces microsomal metabolism via the microsomal ethanol oxidizing system (MEOS) (p. 214).

PATHOLOGY

Alcohol can produce a wide spectrum of liver disease from fatty change to hepatitis and cirrhosis.

Fatty change

The metabolism of alcohol invariably produces fat in the liver, mainly in zone 3. This is minimal with small amounts of alcohol, but with larger amounts the cells become swollen with fat (steatosis) giving, eventually, a Swiss-cheese effect on haematoxylin and eosin stain. Steatosis can also be seen in obesity, diabetes, starvation and occasionally in chronic illness. There is no liver cell damage and therefore in general this is not precirrhotic. The fat disappears on stopping alcohol.

In some cases collagen is laid down around the central hepatic veins (perivenular fibrosis) and this can sometimes progress to cirrhosis without a preceding hepatitis. Alcohol directly affects stellate cells, transforming them into collagen-producing myofibroblast cells. Cirrhosis might then develop if there is an imbalance between degradation and production of collagen.

Alcoholic hepatitis

In addition to fatty change there is infiltration by polymorphonuclear leucocytes and hepatocyte necrosis mainly in zone 3. Dense cytoplasmic inclusions called Mallory bodies are sometimes seen in hepatocytes and giant mitochondria are also a feature. Mallory bodies are suggestive of, but not specific for, alcoholic damage as they can be found in other liver disease, such as Wilson's disease and PBC. If alcohol consumption continues, alcoholic hepatitis may progress to cirrhosis.

Alcoholic cirrhosis

This is classically of the micronodular type, but a mixed pattern may also be seen accompanying fatty change and evidence of pre-existing alcoholic hepatitis may be present.

CLINICAL FEATURES

Fatty liver

There are often no symptoms or signs. Vague abdominal symptoms of nausea, vomiting and diarrhoea are due to the more general effects of alcohol on the gastrointestinal tract. Hepatomegaly, sometimes huge, can occur together with other features of chronic liver disease.

Alcoholic hepatitis

The clinical features vary in degree:

- The patient may be well, with few symptoms, the hepatitis only being apparent on the liver biopsy in addition to fatty change.

- Mild to moderate symptoms of ill-health, occasionally with mild jaundice, may occur. Signs include all the features of chronic liver disease. Liver biochemistry is deranged and the diagnosis is made on liver histology.
- In the severe case, usually superimposed on patients with alcoholic cirrhosis, the patient is ill, with jaundice and ascites. Abdominal pain is frequently present, with a high fever associated with the liver necrosis. On examination there is deep jaundice, hepatomegaly, sometimes splenomegaly, and ascites with ankle oedema. The signs of chronic liver disease are also present.

Alcoholic cirrhosis

This represents the final stage of liver disease from alcohol abuse. Nevertheless, patients can be very well with few symptoms. On examination, there are usually signs of chronic liver disease. The diagnosis is confirmed by liver biopsy.

Usually the patient presents with one of the complications of cirrhosis. In many cases there are features of alcohol dependency (see p. 1137) as well as evidence of involvement of other systems, such as polyneuropathy.

INVESTIGATIONS

Fatty liver

An elevated MCV often indicates heavy drinking. Liver biochemistry shows mild abnormalities with elevation of both serum aminotransferase enzymes. The γ-GT level is a sensitive test for determining whether the patient is taking alcohol. With severe fatty infiltration, marked changes in all liver biochemical parameters can occur. Ultrasound or CT will demonstrate fatty infiltration, as will liver histology.

Alcoholic hepatitis

Investigations show a leucocytosis with markedly deranged liver biochemistry with elevated:

- serum bilirubin
- serum AST and ALT
- serum alkaline phosphatase
- prothrombin time (PT).

A low serum albumin may also be found. Rarely, hyperlipidaemia with haemolysis (Zieve's syndrome) may occur.

The prolonged PT makes liver biopsy impossible in the severe form. In these severe cases the mortality is at least 50%, and with a PT twice the normal, progressive encephalopathy and renal failure, the mortality approaches 90%.

Alcoholic cirrhosis

Investigations are as for cirrhosis in general.

MANAGEMENT AND PROGNOSIS

General management

Patients should be advised to stop drinking. Delirium tremens (a withdrawal symptom) may be treated with diazepam or chlormethiazole. Bedrest with a diet high in protein and vitamin supplements is given. Dietary protein may have to be limited because of encephalopathy. Follow-up of patients with alcoholic liver disease shows, however, that – apart from highly motivated groups – most patients continue to drink alcohol.

Fatty liver

In all but the mildest cases the patient is advised to stop drinking alcohol; the fat will disappear and the liver biochemistry usually returns to normal. Small amounts of alcohol can be drunk subsequently as long as patients are aware of the problems and can control their consumption.

Alcoholic hepatitis

In severe cases the patient is confined to bed. Treatment for encephalopathy and ascites is commenced. Patients should be fed preferably via a fine-bore nasogastric tube or sometimes intravenously. Nitrogen solutions enriched with branched-chain amino acids (e.g. leucine, isoleucine and valine) may be helpful. Vitamins B and C should be given by injection. Corticosteroids are often given, but controlled trials have shown them to be of little benefit.

Patients are advised to stop drinking for life, as this is undoubtedly a precirrhotic condition. The prognosis is variable and, despite abstinence, the liver disease is progressive in many patients. Conversely, a few patients continue to drink heavily without developing cirrhosis.

Alcoholic cirrhosis

The management of cirrhosis is described on p. 316. Again, all patients are advised to stop drinking for life. Abstinence from alcohol results in an improvement in prognosis, with a five-year survival of 90%, but with continued drinking this falls to 60%. With advanced disease (i.e. jaundice, ascites and haematemesis) the five-year survival rate falls to 35%, with most of the deaths occurring in the first year. Liver transplantation is being used widely in some countries with good survival figures. Patients must demonstrate their ability to abstain from alcohol.

HCC is a complication in men in approximately 10–15% of cases.

FURTHER READING

Lieber C (1995) Medical disorders of alcoholism. *New England Journal of Medicine* **133**: 1058–1065.

Budd–Chiari syndrome

In this condition there is obstruction to the venous outflow of the liver owing to occlusion of the hepatic vein. In one-third of patients the cause is unknown, but specific causes include hypercoagulability states, such as polycythaemia vera, taking the contraceptive pill, or leukaemia. Other causes include occlusion of the hepatic vein owing to posterior abdominal wall sarcomas, renal or adrenal tumours, HCC, hepatic infections (e.g. hydatid cyst), congenital venous webs, radiotherapy, or trauma to the liver.

The acute form presents with abdominal pain, nausea, vomiting, tender hepatomegaly and ascites. The liver histology shows centrilobular congestion with hepatocyte atrophy. In the chronic form there is enlargement of the liver (particularly the caudate lobe), mild jaundice, ascites, a negative hepatojugular reflex, and splenomegaly with portal hypertension.

INVESTIGATIONS

Investigations show a high protein content in the ascitic fluid and characteristic liver histology. Ultrasound, CT or MRI will demonstrate hepatic vein occlusion with diffuse abnormal parenchyma on contrast-enhancement which spares the caudate lobe because of its independent blood supply and venous drainage. There may be compression of the inferior vena cava. Pulsed Doppler sonography or a colour Doppler are useful as they show abnormalities in the direction of flow in the hepatic vein. Investigations to identify a cause are also performed, such as blood tests and coagulation studies.

DIFFERENTIAL DIAGNOSIS

A similar clinical picture can be produced by inferior vena caval obstruction, right-sided cardiac failure or constrictive pericarditis, and appropriate investigations should be performed.

TREATMENT

Ascites should be treated as well as any underlying cause (e.g. polycythaemia). Congenital webs should be resected surgically. A side-to-side portocaval or splenorenal anastomosis may decompress the congested liver, with considerable improvement in the clinical state of the patient. A peritoneal–jugular LeVeen shunt for resistant ascites is occasionally useful. Liver transplantation is the treatment of choice.

PROGNOSIS

The prognosis depends on the aetiology, but some patients can survive for several years.

Veno-occlusive disease

This is due to injury of the hepatic veins and presents clinically like the Budd–Chiari syndrome. It was originally described in Jamaica, where the ingestion of the toxic pyrrolizidine alkaloids in bush tea (made from plants of the genera *Senecio*, *Heliotropium* and *Crotolaria*) caused damage to the hepatic veins. It can be seen in other parts of the world. It is also seen as a complication of chemotherapy and total body irradiation before allogeneic bone marrow transplantation. The development of veno-occlusive disease after transplantation carries a high mortality. Treatment is supportive with control of ascites and hepatocellular failure.

Fibropolycystic diseases

These diseases are usually inherited and lead to the presence of cysts or fibrosis in the liver, kidney and occasionally the pancreas, and other organs.

Polycystic disease of the liver

In adults

This is inherited as an autosomal dominant and usually presents in middle age with abdominal swelling or right hypochondrial discomfort. It can also be detected by ultrasound scanning or may only be discovered at autopsy. There may or may not be hepatomegaly and bilateral irregular palpable polycystic kidneys. The cysts are of variable size and consist of thin-walled cavities containing clear fluid or altered blood. Liver function is normal and complications such as oesophageal varices are very rare. The prognosis is excellent and is often dependent on whether the kidneys are involved.

In children

Childhood polycystic disease is inherited in a different way from the adult type. It is an autosomal recessive condition presenting in the first few months of life. Renal involvement is common, with cystic changes in the renal tubules.

Congenital hepatic fibrosis

In this rare condition the liver architecture is normal but there are broad collagenous fibrous bands extending from the portal tracts. It is often inherited as an autosomal recessive condition but can also occur sporadically. It usually presents in childhood with hepatosplenomegaly, and portal hypertension is common. It may present later in life and can be misdiagnosed as cirrhosis. A wedge biopsy of the liver may be required to confirm the diagnosis. The outlook is good and the condition should be distinguished from cirrhosis. Patients who bleed do well after variceal sclerotherapy or a portocaval anastomosis because of their good liver function.

Congenital intrahepatic biliary dilatation (Caroli's disease)

In this rare, non-familial disease there are saccular dilatations of the intrahepatic or extrahepatic ducts. It can present at any age (although usually in childhood) with fever, abdominal pain and recurrent attacks of cholangitis with Gram-negative septicaemia. Jaundice and portal hypertension are absent. Diagnosis is by ultrasound, PTC, ERCP or MRCP.

Solitary non-parasitic cysts

These are rare and probably a variant of polycystic disease.

Liver abscess

Pyogenic abscess

These abscesses are uncommon, but may be single or multiple. The most common cause used to be a portal pyaemia from intra-abdominal sepsis (e.g. appendicitis or perforations), but now in many cases the aetiology is not known. Biliary sepsis, particularly in the elderly, is a common cause. Other causes include trauma, bacteraemia and direct extension from, for example, a perinephric abscess.

The organism found most commonly is *E. coli*. Other organisms include *Streptococcus faecalis*, *Proteus vulgaris* and *Staphylococcus aureus*. *Streptococcus milleri* and anaerobic organisms such as *Bacteroides* are also seen. Often the infection is mixed. Failure to culture an organism may be due to previous antibiotic therapy or inadequate anaerobic culture.

CLINICAL FEATURES

Some patients are not acutely ill and present with malaise lasting several days or even months. Others can present with fever, rigors, anorexia, vomiting, weight loss and abdominal pain. In these patients a Gram-negative septicaemia with shock can occur. On examination there may be little to find. Alternatively, the patient may be toxic, febrile and jaundiced. In such patients, the liver is tender and enlarged and there may be signs of a pleural effusion or a pleural rub in the right lower chest.

INVESTIGATIONS

Patients are often investigated as a 'pyrexia of unknown origin' (PUO) and in the mild chronic case most investigations will be normal. Often the only clue to the diagnosis is a raised serum alkaline phosphatase.

- **Serum bilirubin** is raised in 25% of cases.
- **Normochromic normocytic anaemia** may occur, usually accompanied by a polymorphonuclear leucocytosis.
- **Serum alkaline phosphatase and ESR** are often raised.
- **Serum B_{12}** is very high, as vitamin B_{12} is stored in and subsequently released from the liver.
- **Blood cultures** are positive in only 30% of cases.

Imaging

Ultrasound is useful for detecting abscesses. A CT scan may be of value in complex and multiple lesions. A chest X-ray will show elevation of the right hemidiaphragm with a pleural effusion in the severe case.

MANAGEMENT

Aspiration of the abscess should be attempted under ultrasound control. Antibiotics should initially cover Gram-positive, Gram-negative and anaerobic organisms until the causative organism is identified.

Further drainage via a large-bore needle under ultrasound control or surgically should almost always be performed if a localized abscess is found. The underlying cause must also be treated.

PROGNOSIS

The overall mortality depends on the nature of the underlying pathology and has been reduced to approximately 16% with needle aspiration and antibiotics. A unilocular abscess in the right lobe has a better prognosis. Scattered multiple abscesses have a very high mortality, with only one in five patients surviving.

Amoebic abscess (see also p. 81)

This condition occurs worldwide and must be considered in patients travelling from endemic areas. *Entamoeba histolytica* (p. 182) can be carried from the bowel to the liver in the portal venous system. Portal inflammation results, with the development of multiple microabscesses and eventually single or multiple large abscesses.

Clinically the onset is usually gradual but may be sudden. There is fever, anorexia, weight loss and malaise. There is often no history of dysentery. On examination the patient looks ill and has tender hepatomegaly and signs of an effusion or consolidation in the base of the right side of the chest. Jaundice is unusual.

INVESTIGATIONS

These are as for pyogenic abscess, plus:

- **Serological tests for amoeba** (e.g. haemagglutination inhibition, amoebic complement-fixation test, ELISA). These are always positive, particularly if there are bowel symptoms, and remain positive after a clinical cure and therefore do not indicate current disease. A repeat negative test, however, is good evidence against an amoebic abscess.
- **Diagnostic aspiration of fluid** looking like anchovy sauce.

TREATMENT

Metronidazole 800 mg thrice daily is given for 10 days. Aspiration is used in patients failing to respond, in multiple and large abscesses, and in those with abscesses in the left lobe of the liver.

COMPLICATIONS

Complications include rupture, secondary infection and septicaemia.

Other infections of the liver

Schistosomiasis (see also p. 91)

Schistosoma mansoni and *S. japonicum* affect the liver, but *S. haematobium* rarely does so. During their life-cycle the ova reach the liver via the venous system and obstruct the portal branches, producing granulomas, fibrosis and inflammation but not cirrhosis.

Clinically there is hepatosplenomegaly and presinusoidal portal hypertension, which is particularly severe with *S. mansoni*.

Investigations show a raised serum alkaline phosphatase, and ova can be found in the stools (centrifuged deposits) and in rectal and liver biopsies. Skin tests and other immunological tests often have false results and may also be positive because of past infection.

Treatment is with praziquantel, but fibrosis still remains with a potential risk of portal hypertension.

Hydatid disease (see also p. 96)

Cysts caused by *Echinococcus granulosus* are single or multiple. They usually occur in the lower part of the right lower lobe. The cyst has three layers: an outside layer derived from the host, an intermediate laminated layer, and an inner germinal layer that buds off brood capsules to form daughter cysts.

Clinically there may be no symptoms or a dull ache and swelling in the right hypochondrium. Investigations show a peripheral eosinophilia in 30% of cases and usually a positive hydatid complement-fixation test or haemaglutination (85%). Plain abdominal X-ray may show calcification of the outer coat of the cyst. Ultrasound and CT scan demonstrate cysts and may show diagnostic daughter cysts within the parent cyst (Fig 5.23)

Fine-needle aspiration under ultrasound control with chemotherapeutic cover is now used therapeutically. Surgery can be performed with removal of the cyst intact if possible after first sterilizing the cyst with formalin or alcohol. Medical treatment (e.g. with albendazole, which penetrates into large cysts) can result in reduction of cyst size. Chronic calcified cysts can be left.

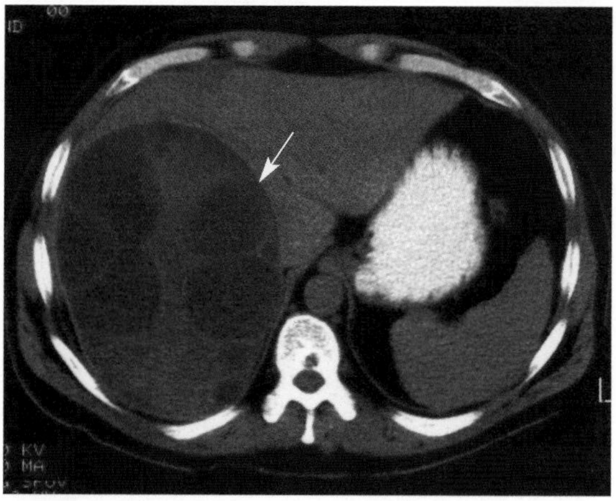

Fig 5.23
CT scan of liver showing a large hydatid cyst (arrow) with 'daughter' cysts lying within it

Complications include rupture, secondary infection and involvement of other organs. The *prognosis* without any complications is good, although there is always the risk of rupture. *Preventative measures* are important, including deworming of pet dogs and prevention of pets from eating infected carcasses where possible.

Acquired immunodeficiency syndrome (see also p. 107)

The liver is often involved but rarely causes significant morbidity or mortality. HIV itself is probably not the cause of the liver abnormalities. The following are seen:

- pre-existing/coincidental viral hepatitis (HBV, HCV, HDV)
- neoplasia: Kaposi's sarcoma and non-Hodgkin's lymphoma
- opportunistic infection (e.g. *Mycobacterium tuberculosis*, *Myco. avium intracellulare*, *Cryptococcus*, *Candida albicans*, toxoplasmosis
- drug hepatotoxicity
- sclerosing cholangitis (see p. 343).

Clinical hepatomegaly is common (60% of patients).

Liver disease in pregnancy

Liver function is not impaired in pregnancy. Any liver disease from whatever cause can occur incidentally and coincide with pregnancy. For example, viral hepatitis accounts for 40% of all cases of jaundice during pregnancy. Pregnancy does not necessarily exacerbate established liver disease, but it is uncommon for women with advanced liver disease to conceive.

The following changes take place:

- Plasma and blood volumes increase during pregnancy but the hepatic blood flow remains constant.
- The proportion of cardiac output delivered to the liver therefore falls from 35% to 29% in late pregnancy; drug metabolism can thus be affected.
- The size of the liver remains constant.
- Liver biochemistry remains unchanged apart from a rise in serum alkaline phosphatase from the placenta (up to three to four times) and a decrease in total protein owing to increased plasma volume.
- Triglycerides and cholesterol levels rise, and caeruloplasmin, transferrin, α_1-antitrypsin and fibrinogen levels are elevated owing to increased hepatic synthesis.

There are a number of liver diseases that complicate pregnancy.

Hyperemesis gravidarum

Pathological vomiting during pregnancy can be associated with liver dysfunction and jaundice. This is never severe and resolves when vomiting subsides.

Intrahepatic cholestasis of pregnancy

This condition of unknown aetiology presents usually with pruritus alone in the third trimester. It has a familial tendency and there is a higher prevalence in Scandinavia, Chile and Bolivia.

Liver biochemistry shows a cholestatic picture with high serum ALP (up to four times normal) and raised aminotransferases which occasionally can be very high. The serum bilirubin is slightly raised with jaundice in 60% of cases. Liver biopsy is not indicated but would show centrilobular cholestasis.

Treatment is symptomatic with cholestyramine in high doses (up to 24 g daily) for the pruritus. *Prognosis* is usually excellent and the condition resolves after delivery. Recurrent cholestasis may occur during subsequent pregnancies or with the ingestion of oestrogen-containing oral contraceptive pills.

Pre-eclampsia and eclampsia

Pre-eclampsia is characterized by hypertension, proteinuria and oedema occurring in the second or third trimester. Eclampsia is marked by seizures or coma in addition. Hepatic complications include subcapsular haematoma and infarction, and occasionally fulminant hepatic failure. The HELLP syndrome – a combination of *h*aemolysis, *e*levated *l*iver enzymes and a *l*ow *p*latelet count – can occur in association with severe pre-eclampsia. In the HELLP syndrome, there is epigastric pain, nausea and vomiting, with jaundice in 5% of patients. Delivery is the best treatment for eclampsia.

Acute fatty liver of pregnancy

This is a rare, serious condition of unknown aetiology. There is an association between acute fatty liver and long-chain 3-hydroxylacyl-CoA-dihydroxyl (LCHAD) deficiency. The mechanism is unclear, but abnormal fatty acid metabolites produced by the heterozygous fetus enter the circulation and overcome maternal hepatic mitochondrial oxidation systems. It presents in the last trimester with symptoms of fulminant hepatitis – jaundice, vomiting, abdominal pain, possibly haematemesis and coma.

Investigations show hepatocellular damage, hyperuricaemia and possibly DIC. CT scanning shows a low density of the liver owing to the high fat content. It can sometimes be difficult to differentiate from the HELLP syndrome. Liver biopsy is contraindicated but histology shows fine droplets of fat (microvesicles) in the liver cells with little necrosis.

Immediate delivery of the child may save both baby and mother. Early diagnosis and treatment has reduced the mortality to less than 20%. T*reatment* is as for acute liver failure.

FURTHER READING

Koux TA, Olans LB (1996) Liver disease in pregnancy. *New England Journal of Medicine* **335**: 569–576.

Liver tumours

The most common liver tumour is a secondary (metastatic) tumour (Fig 5.24), particularly from the gastrointestinal tract, breast or bronchus. Clinical features are variable but usually include hepatomegaly. Ultrasound is the primary investigation, with CT or MRI used when available; MRI is comparable to CT at detecting metastases. Primary liver tumours may be benign or malignant, but the most common are malignant.

Malignant tumours

Hepatocellular carcinoma (HCC)

Hepatocellular carcinoma (HCC) is one of the ten most common cancers worldwide, although it is uncommon in the West.

(a) (b)

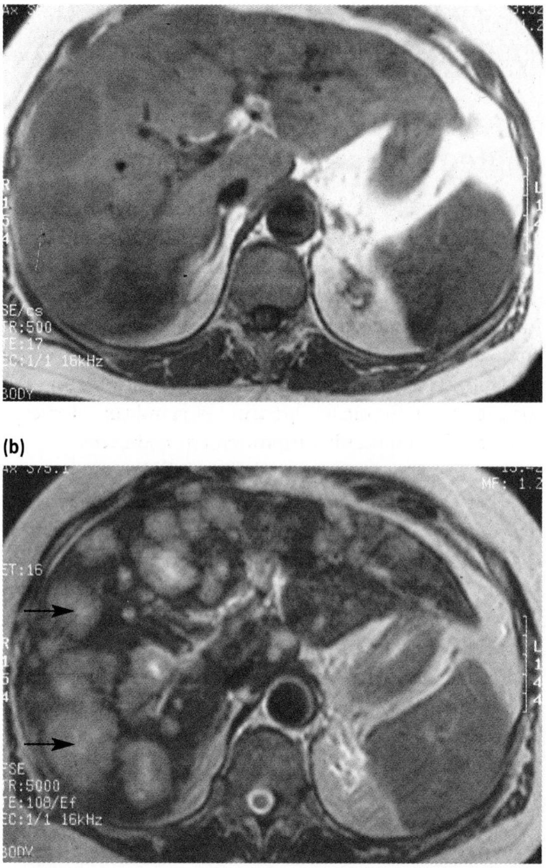

Fig 5.24
Liver MRI. T1(a) and T2(b) weighted sequences showing multiple liver metastases. Structures of fluid density have high signal on T2 images. Note the central tumour necrosis in (b) (arrows).

AETIOLOGY

Carriers of HBV and HCV have an extremely high risk of developing HCC. In areas where HBV is prevalent, 90% of patients with this cancer are positive for hepatitis B. Cirrhosis is present in over 80% of these patients. The development of HCC is related to the integration of viral DNA into the genome of the host hepatocyte (see p. 304). Primary liver cancer is also associated with other forms of cirrhosis, such as alcoholic cirrhosis and haemochromatosis. Males are affected more than females; this may account for the high incidence seen in haemochromatosis and low incidence in PBC. Other suggested aetiological factors are aflatoxin (a metabolite of a fungus found in groundnuts) and androgenic steroids, and there is an association with the contraceptive pill.

PATHOLOGY

The tumour is either single or occurs as multiple nodules throughout the liver. Histologically it consists of cells resembling hepatocytes. It can metastasize via the hepatic or portal veins to the lymph nodes, bones and lungs.

CLINICAL FEATURES

HCC usually presents below the age of 50 years. The clinical features include weight loss, anorexia, fever, an ache in the right hypochondrium, and ascites. The rapid development of these features in a cirrhotic patient is suggestive of HCC. On examination, an enlarged, irregular, tender liver may be felt.

INVESTIGATIONS

Serum α-fetoprotein is raised. Ultrasound scans show large filling defects in 90% of cases. A liver biopsy, particularly under ultrasonic guidance, is performed for diagnosis.

TREATMENT AND PROGNOSIS

Surgical resection is occasionally possible. Small tumours in patients with cirrhosis do not always prevent transplantation. Chemotherapy and radiotherapy are unhelpful.

Survival, except in very selected groups, is seldom more than six months.

PREVENTION

Persistant HBV infection usually acquired after perinatal infection is a high risk factor for HCC in many parts of the world. Widespread vaccination against HBV is being used and this has already shown a reduction in the annual incidence of HCC.

Cholangiocarcinoma

Cholangiocarcinomas can be extrahepatic (see p. 344) or intrahepatic. Intrahepatic adenocarcinomas arising from the bile ducts account for approximately 10% of primary tumours. They are not associated with cirrhosis or hepatitis B. In the Far East they may be associated with infestation with *Clonorchis sinensis* or *Opisthorchis viverrini*. The clinical features are similar to primary HCC except that jaundice is frequent with hilar tumours.

Treatment is unsuccessful and patients usually die within six months.

Benign tumours

The most common benign tumour is a haemangioma. It is usually small and single but can be multiple and large. They are usually found incidentally on ultrasound, CT or MRI and have characteristic appearances. They require no treatment.

Hepatic adenomas are associated with oral contraceptives. They can present with abdominal pain or intraperitoneal bleeding. Resection is only required for symptomatic patients.

FURTHER READING

Bruix J (1997) Treatment of hepatocellular carcinoma. *Hepatology* **25**: 259–262.

Miscellaneous conditions of the liver

Hepatic mitochondrial injury syndromes

These syndromes – in which there is mitochondrial damage with inhibition of β-oxidation of fatty acids – can be categorized as follows:

- *Genetic*, with abnormalities which include medium-chain acyl-coenzyme A dehydrogenase deficiency leads to microsteatosis.
- *Toxins* leading to liver failure include aflatoxin and cerulide (produced by *Bacillus cereus*) which causes food poisoning (see p. 33).
- *Drugs* (e.g. i.v. tetracycline, valproic acid and zidovudine) can produce a fatal microsteatosis.
- *Idiopathic*, the best known being fatty liver of pregnancy (p. 333) and *Reye's syndrome*. This condition, due to inhibition of β-oxidation and uncoupling of oxidative phosphorylation in mitochondria, leads in children to an acute encephalopathy and diffuse microvesicular fatty infiltration of the liver. Aspirin ingestion and viral infections have been implicated as precipitating agents. Mortality is about 50%, usually due to cerebral oedema.

Benign recurrent intrahepatic cholestasis

This condition often presents in children and consists of bouts of cholestatic jaundice with pruritus. Jaundice may last for weeks or months. There is no treatment; cholestyramine 12 g daily may help relieve the itching.

Idiopathic adult ductopenia

This unexplained condition is characterized by pruritus and cholestatic jaundice. Histology of the liver shows a decrease in intrahepatic bile ducts in at least 50% of the portal tract, together with the features of cholestasis and marked fibrosis or cirrhosis. In most the disease is progressive and the only treatment is liver transplantation.

Indian childhood cirrhosis

This condition of children is seen in the Indian subcontinent. The cause is unknown. Eventually there is development of a micronodular cirrhosis with excess copper in the liver.

Hepatic porphyrias

These are dealt with on p. 1003.

Cystic fibrosis (see also p. 784)

This disease affects mainly the lung and pancreas, but patients can develop fatty liver, cholestasis and cirrhosis. The aetiology of the liver involvement is unclear.

Drugs and the liver

Drug metabolism

The liver is the major site of drug metabolism. Drugs are converted from fat-soluble to water-soluble substances that can be excreted in the urine or bile. This metabolism of drugs is mediated by a group of mixed-function enzymes, including the cytochrome P450 system of haem-proteins and cytochrome C-reductase, located on the smooth endoplasmic reticulum of the liver cell. It takes place in two stages:

- *Phase I metabolism* involves oxidation or demethylation of the drug, mediated by cytochrome P450 and cytochrome C-reductase.
- *Phase II metabolism* involves the conjugation of the derivatives produced in phase I with glucuronide or sulphate. These conjugates, which are now water-soluble, are excreted in the urine and bile as they cannot be reabsorbed by renal tubular or bile ductular cells.

Glutathione binds to a number of potential harmful compounds via glutathione S-transferase. This is central to detoxification of a number of compounds, such as paracetamol.

Factors affecting drug metabolism

The microsomal enzyme system. The speed of metabolism of drugs is dependent on the microsomal enzyme system. Certain drugs (e.g. phenytoin, barbiturates and alcohol) can themselves increase the activity of these enzymes such as cytochrome P450 – that is, they cause 'enzyme induction' – and are known as 'inducing agents'. Therapy with any of these drugs will produce increased metabolism of the drug and consequently a reduction in its effectiveness. Equally, if two drugs are metabolized by the same microsomal enzymes, metabolism of both drugs will be reduced, prolonging their actions. Genetically determined subtypes of cytochrome P450 have different activities and this may explain some adverse reactions to drugs.

Route of administration. Many drugs are partially inactivated on passage through the liver (the first-pass effect). If this is pronounced, drugs taken orally are inactive.

Liver blood flow. The rate of removal of the drug from the liver is influenced by the liver blood flow.

Competitive inhibition. Some drugs compete with bilirubin at various stages:

- uptake by the liver (e.g. rifampicin)
- conjugation (e.g. novobiocin)
- excretion into the bile canaliculus (e.g. oral contraceptives).

Drug hepatotoxicity

Many drugs impair liver function and drugs should always be considered as a cause when mildly abnormal liver tests are found. Damage to the liver by drugs is usually classified as being either predictable (or dose-related) or non-predictable (not dose-related) (see p. 862). This classification should not be used rigidly, as there is considerable overlap and many mechanisms may be involved in the production of damage.

Biochemical pathways

When a small amount of hepatotoxic drug whose effect is dose-dependent (e.g. paracetamol) is ingested, a large proportion of it undergoes conjugation with glucuronide and sulphate, whilst the remainder is metabolized by microsomal enzymes to produce toxic derivatives that are immediately detoxified by conjugation with glutathione. If larger doses are ingested, the former pathway becomes saturated and the toxic derivative is produced at a faster rate. Once the hepatic glutathione is depleted, large amounts of the toxic metabolite accumulate and produce damage.

The 'predictability' of drugs to produce damage can, however, be affected by metabolic events preceding their ingestion. For example, chronic alcohol abusers may become more susceptible to liver damage because of the enzyme-inducing effects of alcohol, or ill or starving patients may become susceptible because of the depletion of hepatic glutathione produced by starvation. Many other factors such as environmental or genetic effects may be involved in determining the 'susceptibility' of certain patients to certain drugs.

Immunological mechanisms

These can be involved in the production of hepatic cell damage by certain drugs. The toxic metabolite produced by the microsomal enzymes may bind to the liver cell protein, thereby altering its antigenicity. The production of antibody against this will lead to immunologically mediated damage. An example of this mechanism is halothane-induced hepatic necrosis, which requires prior sensitization of the patient to halothane, although direct toxicity may also play a part.

Other pointers for the involvement of immunological mechanisms are the development of skin rashes, fever and arthralgia (serum-sickness syndrome) following ingestion of certain drugs. Eosinophilia and circulating immune complexes and antibodies may occasionally be detected.

Hepatic damage

The type of damage produced by various drugs is shown in Table 5.16. The diagnosis of these conditions is usually by exclusion of other causes. Most reactions occur within three months of starting the drug. Monitoring liver biochemistry in patients on long-term treatment, such as antituberculosis therapy, is advisable. If a drug is suspected of causing hepatic damage it should be stopped immediately. Liver biopsy is of limited help in confirming the diagnosis, but occasionally hepatic eosinophilia or granulomas may be seen. Diagnostic challenge with subtherapeutic doses of the drug is sometimes required after the liver biochemistry has returned to normal, to confirm the diagnosis.

Individual drugs

Paracetamol

In high doses paracetamol produces liver cell necrosis (see above). The toxic metabolite binds irreversibly to liver cell membranes. Overdosage is discussed on p. 875.

Halothane

This commonly used anaesthetic agent rarely produces a hepatitis in patients having repeated exposures. The mechanism is thought to be a hypersensitivity reaction. An unexplained fever occurs approximately 10 days after the second or subsequent halothane anaesthetic and is followed by jaundice, typically with a hepatitic picture. Most patients recover spontaneously but there is a high mortality in severe cases. There are no chronic sequelae.

Steroids

Cholestasis is caused by natural and synthetic oestrogens as well as methyltestosterone. These agents interfere with canalicular biliary flow and cause a pure cholestasis. Cholestasis is rare with the contraceptive pill because of the low dosage used. However, the contraceptive pill is associated with an increased incidence of gallstones, hepatic adenomas (rarely HCCs), the Budd–Chiari syndrome and *peliosis hepatis*. The latter condition, which also occurs with anabolic steroids, consists of dilatation of the hepatic sinusoids to form blood-filled lakes.

Table 5.16
Some drugs causing types of liver damage

Types of liver damage	Drugs
Zone 3 necrosis	Carbon tetrachloride *Amanita* mushrooms Paracetamol Salicylates Piroxicam Cocaine
Zone 1 necrosis	Ferrous sulphate
Microvesicular fat	Sodium valproate Tetracyclines
'Alcoholic' hepatitis (phospholipidosis)	Perhexiline maleate Amiodarone Synthetic oestrogens Nifedipine
Fibrosis	Methotrexate Other cytotoxic agents Arsenic Vitamin A Retinoids
Heparlobatum	Combination chemotherapy for metastatic breast cancer
Vascular	
Sinusoidal dilatation	Contraceptive drugs Anabolic steroids Azathioprine
Pelioses hepatis	Oral contraceptives Anabolic steroids e.g. Danazol Azathioprine
Veno occlusive	Pyrrolizidine alkaloids (*Senecio* in bush tea) Cytotoxics – cyclophosphamide, azathioprine
Acute hepatitis	Isoniazid Rifampicin Methyldopa Atenolol Enalapril Verapamil Ketoconazole Cytotoxic drugs Clonazepam Disulfiram Niacin Halothane
Chronic hepatitis	Methyldopa Nitrofurantoin Fenofibrate Isoniazid
General hypersensitivity	Sulphonamides e.g. Sulphasalazine, Cotrimoxazole, Fansidar Penicillins e.g. Flucloxacillin, Ampicillin, Amoxacillin, Co-amoxiclav NSAIDs e.g. Salicylates, Diclofenac Allopurinol Anti-thyroid e.g. Propylthiouracil, Carbimazole Quinine e.g. Quinidine Diltiazem Anticonvulsants e.g. Phenytoin
Canalicular cholestasis	Sex hormones Cyclosporin A
Hepato-canalicular cholestasis	Chlorpromazine Haloperidol Erythromycin Cimetidine/ranitidine Nitrofurantoin Imipramine Azathioprine Oral hypoglycaemics Dextropropoxyphene
Ductular cholestasis	Benoxyprofen
Biliary sludge	Ceftriaxone
Sclerosing cholangitis	Hepatic arterial infusion of 5-fluorouracil Thiabendazole into hydatid cysts
Hepatic tumours	Pills with high hormone content (adenomas)
Hepatocellular carcinoma	Contraceptive pill Danazol

NSAID, non-steroidal anti-inflammatory drugs

Phenothiazines

Phenothiazines (e.g. chlorpromazine) can produce a cholestatic picture owing to a hypersensitivity reaction. It occurs in 1% of patients, usually within four weeks of starting the drug. Typically it is associated with a fever and eosinophilia. Recovery occurs on stopping the drug.

Antituberculous chemotherapy

Isoniazid produces elevated aminotransferases in 10–20% of patients. Hepatic necrosis with jaundice occurs in a smaller percentage. The hepatotoxicity of isoniazid appears to be related to acetylator status, as the damage is due to the metabolites.

Rifampicin produces a hepatitis, usually within three weeks of starting the drug, particularly in patients on high doses.

Pyrazinamide produces abnormal liver biochemical tests and, rarely, liver cell necrosis.

Drug prescribing for patients with liver disease

The metabolism of drugs is impaired in severe liver disease (with jaundice and ascites) as the removal of many drugs depends on liver blood flow and the integrity of the hepatocyte. In general, therefore, the effect of drugs is prolonged by liver disease and also by cholestasis. This is further accentuated by portosystemic shunting, which diminishes the first-pass extraction of drugs. With hypoproteinaemia there is decreased protein binding of some drugs, and bilirubin competes with many drugs for the binding sites on serum albumin. In patients with portosystemic encephalopathy, care must be taken in prescribing drugs with a central depressant action.

FURTHER READING

Lee WM (1995) Drug-induced hepatotoxicity. *New England Journal of Medicine* **333**: 1118–1127.

The gallbladder and biliary system

The main cause of disease of the gallbladder and biliary tract is gallstones. The structure, formation and function of bile is discussed on pp. 288 and 289.

Gallstones

Prevalence of gallstones

Gallstones are present in 10–20% of the population in the West, but the exact prevalence is unknown. There is a geographical variation. Gallstones are rare in the Far East and Africa and very common in native North Americans and in Chile and Sweden. They occur twice as frequently in young women than in men but this difference decreases with increasing age.

Types of gallstones

Gallstones can be divided into those composed of cholesterol and those composed of bile pigment. Cholesterol stones, which account for 80% of all gallstones in the West, contain more than 70% cholesterol, often with some bile pigment and calcium (mixed stones). Pure cholesterol stones are often solitary.

Cholesterol gallstones

Cholesterol is derived partly from dietary sources. In addition, it is synthesized, chiefly in the liver, but also in the small intestine, skin and adrenals. The rate-limiting step in cholesterol synthesis is β-hydroxy-β-methyl-glutaryl-CoA (HMG-CoA) reductase, which catalyses the first step – i.e. the conversion of acetate to mevalonate. The cholesterol formed is co-secreted with phospholipids into the biliary caniliculus as unilamellar vesicles.

Cholesterol stones develop only in bile that has an excess of cholesterol relative to bile salts and phospholipids (supersaturated bile). This could occur because of excess of cholesterol or because of a decrease in bile salts. There is a reduced bile salt pool in some patients with cholesterol gallstones and the pool circulates more frequently. This may account for the reduction in the rate-limiting cholesterol-7α-hydroxylase found in some patients (feedback inhibition).

Diminished bile salt synthesis is not the only cause of supersaturated bile; there appears to be an increase in HMG-CoA reductase with an increase in cholesterol secretion into bile in some patients.

In supersaturated bile the bile acids solubilize phospholipids from the unilamellar vesicles more than cholesterol. This results in unstable vesicles which are more prone to aggregate, fuse and form multilamellar vesicles. It is from these vesicles that cholesterol crystals nucleate. Factors other than cholesterol saturation are required to form gallstones, as supersaturated bile is found in normal subjects during an overnight fast. The rate of cholesterol crystallization and gallbladder motor dysfunction also play a role. Glycoproteins in bile promote nucleation of cholesterol crystals, leading to stone formation, but why this occurs only in bile from patients with gallstones is unclear. It may depend on the presence or absence of solubilizing factors. The role of infection is unknown. Definite risk factors for gallstones are shown in Table 5.17.

Bile pigment stones

Black pigment stones contain calcium salts of bilirubin, phosphate and carbonate in addition to bilirubin polymers and mucin glycoproteins. The biliary lipids are normal. These stones form in the gallbladder and are seen in patients with chronic haemolysis (e.g. hereditary spherocytosis and sickle cell disease) where there is an increase in bilirubin, and in cirrhosis. In other situations the pathogenesis is unclear.

Brown pigment stones have layers of cholesterol, calcium salts of fatty acids (mainly palmitate) and calcium bilirubinate. They form in the common bile duct when there is bile stasis and infected bile and are due to precipitation of deconjugated bilirubin with calcium.

Table 5.17
Risk factors for cholesterol gallstones

Increasing age	Drugs (e.g. contraceptive pill)
Sex (F > M)	Ileal disease or resection
Multiparity	Diabetes
Obesity	Acromegaly treated with octreotide
Rapid weight loss	Liver cirrhosis
Diet (e.g. high in animal fat)	

They are also found with strictures, sclerosing cholangitis and Caroli's syndrome (p. 331). In the Far East these stones are associated with parasitic infestation of the biliary tract.

Clinical presentation of gallstones

(Fig 5.25)

The majority of gallstones (approximately 80%) remain in the gallbladder and are asymptomatic.

A gallstone may impact in the neck of the gallbladder or in the cystic duct, giving biliary pain or acute cholecystitis.

Finally, gallstones may pass into the common bile duct, giving rise to biliary obstruction that produces severe biliary pain and sometimes cholestatic jaundice. Bacterial infection can occur and produce cholangitis.

Biliary pain occurs in the epigastrium and right hypochondrium and is not colicky. Biliary 'colic' therefore is a misnomer.

Rarely a gallstone may perforate through the wall of an inflamed gallbladder into the intestine, producing a fistula.

Gallstones do not give rise to any other symptom complex, and the idea that they produce indigestion, chronic right hypochondrial pain or intolerance to fatty food is based on a false correlation. Gallstones and upper abdominal symptoms are both common, so great care must be taken to establish that the two are truly related. Fair, fat, fertile females of 40 years of age have the same chance of having gallstones as the rest of the general population (10–20%). Thus, if they are investigated regardless of symptoms, gallstones will obviously be seen frequently by chance alone.

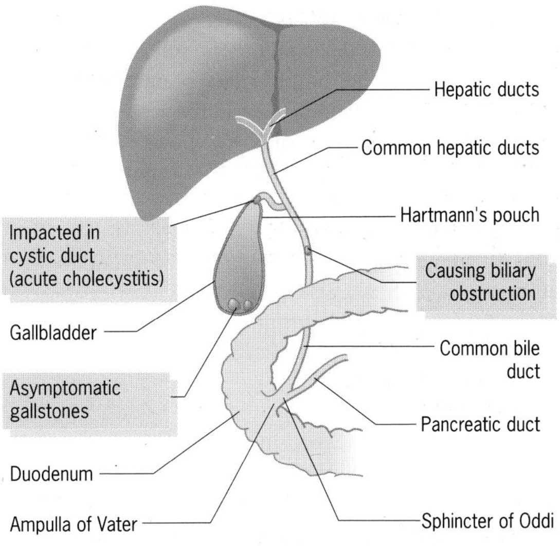

Fig 5.25
Clinical presentation of gallstones

Asymptomatic (silent) gallstones

Gallstones may be discovered accidentally when a patient is being investigated for some other reason. They require no treatment since the natural history is for them to remain asymptomatic, with only approximately 18% of patients having symptoms over a 15-year period.

Acute cholecystitis

PATHOPHYSIOLOGY

In over 90% of cases the gallbladder contains gallstones. Initially there is obstruction to the neck of the gallbladder or the cystic duct by an impacted stone, leading to distension and inflammation. The inflammation is usually sterile, but within 24 hours gut organisms can be cultured from the gallbladder. Occasionally the inflammation may be mild and quickly subsides, sometimes leaving a gallbladder distended by mucus (mucocele). In this situation the patient may only have slight abdominal pain with a palpable gallbladder.

More commonly, however, the inflammation is more severe, involving the whole wall and giving rise to localized peritonitis and acute pain. Occasionally the gallbladder can become distended by pus (an empyema) and rarely an acute gangrenous cholecystitis occurs with perforation and a more generalized peritonitis.

CLINICAL FEATURES

The disease can occur at any age. The main symptoms are severe pain in the epigastrium and right hypochondrium. The pain is continuous, increasing in intensity over 24 hours. It can radiate to the back and shoulder. It may be accompanied by nausea and vomiting. Mild jaundice occurs in 20% of cases owing to accompanying common duct stones or to surrounding oedema occluding the common hepatic duct.

The patient is usually ill with a fever and shallow respirations. Right hypochondrial tenderness is present, being worse on inspiration (Murphy's sign). There is guarding and rebound tenderness.

INVESTIGATIONS

- **Blood count**. A moderate leucocytosis is found.
- **Biochemistry**. The serum bilirubin, alkaline phosphatase and aminotransferases may be slightly raised.
- **Ultrasound** examination (Fig 5.26). The detection of gallstones *alone* is insufficient for a diagnosis of acute cholecystitis. Additional criteria are:
  (a) sonographic Murphy's sign (focal tenderness directly over the visualized gallbladder)
  (b) gallbladder wall thickening – not specific for acute disease
  (c) distension of gallbladder
  (d) the presence of biliary sludge
  (e) pericholecystic fluid.

- **Iodida scintiscan**. This shows blockage of the cystic duct with the bile duct, but not the gallbladder, being visualized. There are, however, false positives and ultrasound is more commonly used in the acute situation.
- **X-ray**. A plain abdominal X-ray shows gallstones in 10% of cases, but this is not useful diagnostically.

DIFFERENTIAL DIAGNOSIS

The differential diagnosis includes other abdominal emergencies, such as a perforated peptic ulcer, retrocaecal appendicitis or acute pancreatitis. Right basal pneumonia and myocardial infarction must also be considered.

MANAGEMENT

The majority of patients improve with conservative management consisting of bedrest, nil-by-mouth and intravenous fluids, with the addition of an antibiotic, usually amoxycillin or a cephalosporin. In all but the mild cases, pain relief with an opiate is required.

In the absence of vomiting, the patient can soon tolerate oral fluids and nasogastric aspiration is not often required. Signs of complications such as an empyema, generalized peritonitis or gangrene of the gallbladder (which causes increasing pain and fever) require urgent repeat ultrasound for assessment. Immediate surgery is usually required.

Cholecystectomy (see below) within days of the acute attack has been advocated for all patients who are not an anaesthetic risk. A firm diagnosis can usually be made using an Iodida scintiscan or ultrasound. Alternatively, cholecystectomy can be performed 2–3 months later. However, early surgery means only one hospital visit and no possibility of a recurrent attack while waiting for surgery to be performed. It does not increase operative morbidity or mortality and is, therefore, the recommended treatment.

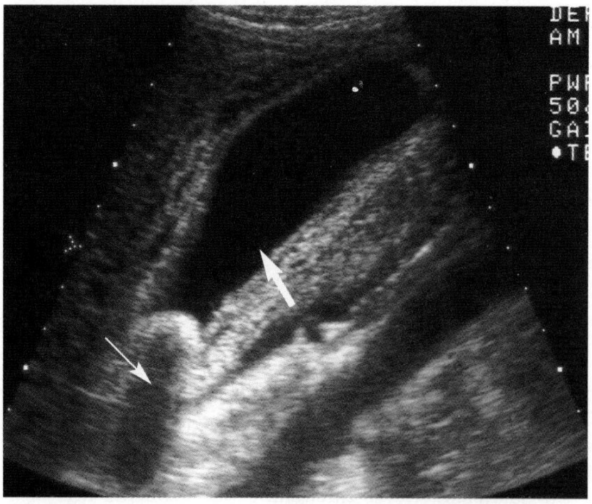

Fig 5.26
Ultrasound scan in a patient with acute cholecystitis.
There is a stone (casting an acoustic shadow – thin arrow) impacted in the gallbladder neck, with a distended gallbladder (thick arrow) and thickening and oedema of the gallbladder wall.

Chronic cholecystitis

There are no symptoms or signs that can conclusively be shown to be due to chronic cholecystitis. Symptoms attributed to this condition are vague, such as indigestion, upper abdominal discomfort or distension. There is no doubt that gallbladders studied histologically can show signs of chronic inflammation, and occasionally a small, shrunken gallbladder is found either radiologically or on ultrasound examination. However, these findings can be seen in asymptomatic people and therefore this clinical diagnosis should not be made. Most patients with chronic right hypochondrial pain suffer from functional bowel disease.

Common bile duct stones

These may be asymptomatic or they may present with any one or all of the triad of abdominal pain, jaundice and fever. The pain is usually severe and situated in the epigastrium and right hypochondrium. The pain may be accompanied by vomiting. The pain usually lasts for a few hours and then clears up, only to return days, weeks or even months later. Between attacks the patient is well.

The jaundice is variable in degree, depending on the amount of obstruction. The urine is dark and the stools are pale. High fevers and rigors indicate cholangitis.

The liver is enlarged if the obstruction lasts for more than a few hours. Prolonged biliary obstruction or repeated attacks lead to secondary biliary cirrhosis, but this is now rare.

INVESTIGATIONS

- **Blood count**. A leucocytosis is present.
- **Blood cultures**. These may grow an intestinal organism (*E. coli*, *Strep. faecalis*).
- **Biochemistry**. This may show a cholestatic picture (see p. 300) with a raised conjugated bilirubin and alkaline phosphatase in the serum and relatively normal serum aminotransferases.
- **Prothrombin time**. This may become elevated over a few weeks owing to poor vitamin K absorption.
- **Ultrasound examination**. This reveals a dilated common bile duct (see Fig 5.10) sometimes with a visible stone. Stones in the common bile duct are detected in only about 75% of cases. Endoscopic ultrasound is a more accurate method of detecting a stone. Stones in the gallbladder suggest, but do not prove, that gallstones are the cause of the dilatation.
- **X-ray**. A plain abdominal X-ray may reveal gallstones.
- **ERCP**. This is performed to confirm the diagnosis (Fig 5.27) and to remove the stones (see below).
- **Magnetic resonance cholangiopancreatography** (MRCP; see p. 294) is being used to detect common bile duct stones (Fig 5.28).

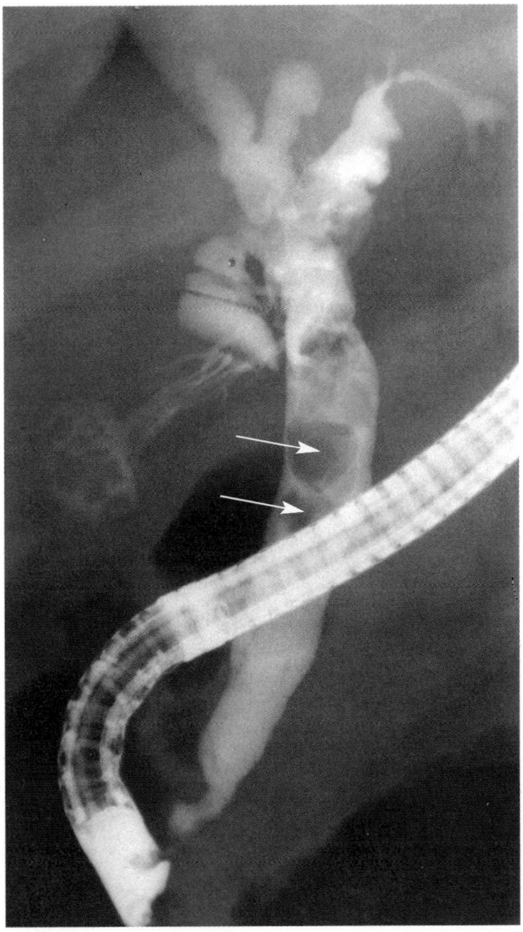

Fig 5.27
ERCP showing a dilated common bile duct containing multiple stones (arrowed)

DIFFERENTIAL DIAGNOSIS

The differential diagnosis includes all causes of jaundice and other causes of upper abdominal pain.

MANAGEMENT

The acute episode is usually allowed to settle and the serum bilirubin falls to normal levels. During this stage the patient only requires pain relief but occasionally antibiotics are necessary.

The serum ALP falls more slowly than the serum bilirubin, and if the patient is seen some time after an acute attack, elevation of this enzyme may be the only evidence of biliary tract disease.

Further management of common duct stones is discussed below.

Acute cholangitis

Acute cholangitis is due to bacterial infection of the bile ducts and is always secondary to bile duct abnormalities. The common causes are common duct stones, biliary

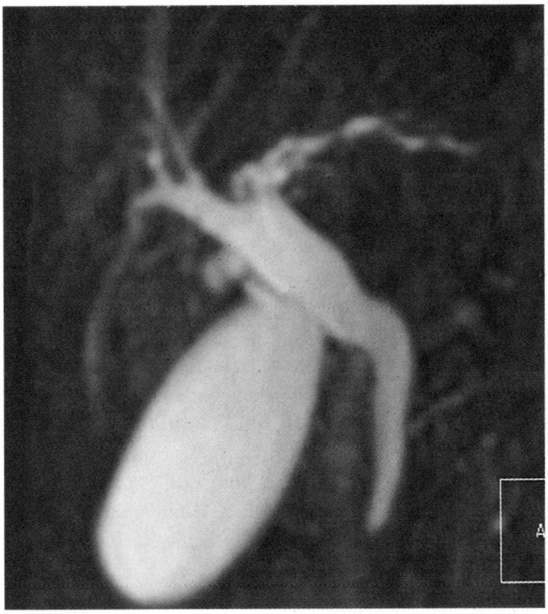

Fig 5.28
MRCP (magnetic resonance cholangio-pancreatography).
The image is constructed from a heavily T2-weighted sequence which accentuates fluid-filled structures. The gallbladder, bile ducts and pancreatic ducts are outlined.

strictures, neoplasms, or following ERCP in the presence of large duct obstruction.

Symptoms are fever, often with a rigor, upper abdominal pain and jaundice. All three symptoms are present in 70% of cases. Older patients can present with collapse and Gram-negative septicaemia. *Specific signs* may be minimal but tenderness over the liver occurs.

When all three symptoms are present the diagnosis is not difficult, but the patient can present with only a fever and an accompanying leucocytosis. Blood cultures are often positive (usually for *E. coli*) and a severe Gram-negative septicaemia can occur.

Treatment is with 6-hourly intravenous amoxycillin 1 g, along with intravenous gentamicin 2–5 mg kg^{-1} daily in divided doses for severe cases. Ceftazidime is also used.

Suppurative cholangitis can occur as a *complication*. The fever continues and shock develops despite adequate antibiotics. Urgent decompression of the duct should be performed, usually endoscopically with placement of a nasobiliary drain. The subsequent treatment of the obstruction is either endoscopic or surgical (see below).

Management of gallstones

Stones in the gallbladder

Cholecystectomy

A cholecystectomy is the treatment of choice for virtually all patients with gallbladder stones and symptoms. In developed countries, the earlier surgical method using a

Kocher incision has been largely superseded by the following minimally invasive techniques. Only patients who refuse surgery should be considered for alternative therapy (see below).

Laparoscopic cholecystectomy

Laparoscopic cholecystectomy is thought by many to be the operation of choice. The abdominal cavity is insufflated with carbon dioxide under a general anaesthetic and the laparoscope and operating channels are inserted at the umbilicus and through three other small incisions. The gallbladder is dissected from its bed on the liver and removed whole after the cystic duct and vessels have been clipped and haemostasis achieved with electrocautery or laser. The mortality is less than 0.1% and the patients can leave hospital in 24–48 hours. Complications are low and include wound sepsis, bile duct injury (0.5%) and retained gallstones in the common bile duct. Patients can return to full activity in approximately one week.

Mini laparotomy

Some surgeons prefer this approach to laparoscopic surgery. The surgical incision is small so that the length of stay in hospital and return to full activity is similar to that of laparoscopic surgery.

Post-cholecystectomy syndrome

Some patients continue to complain of right hypochondrial pain, flatulence, indigestion and intolerance to fatty foods after cholecystectomy, despite a normal radiological appearance of the biliary tree. In the vast majority of these patients the original diagnosis was incorrect and the patient was suffering from functional bowel disease, the gallstones being an incidental finding. The occurrence of severe pain with jaundice or abnormal liver biochemistry suggests a retained stone in the common duct and this can usually be confirmed by ultrasound.

Pain has been attributed to dysfunction of the sphincter of Oddi, but, even with manometry, this is difficult to substantiate, and sphincterotomy is not usually justified.

Gallstone dissolution or disruption

Cholesterol gallstones can be dissolved by the bile acids chenodeoxycholic acid and ursodeoxycholic acid, which increase cholesterol solubility in bile. They dissolve only radiolucent stones in a functioning gallbladder and not calcified stones. Only about 10% of patients are therefore suitable for this therapy.

Gallstone dissolution takes anything from 6 months to 2 years and when the treatment is stopped 50% of the gallstones recur. Chenodeoxycholate also produces diarrhoea.

Shock-wave treatment of gallstones can be carried out using ultrasound-guided lithotripters that do not require a general anaesthetic or waterbath.

Minimally invasive surgery has made the above techniques redundant except in a very few cases where an anaesthetic is contraindicated.

Stones in the common bile duct

These are found in approximately 15% of patients undergoing cholecystectomy, whose bile ducts are visualized at surgery.

Unfortunately, techniques for detecting stones preoperatively are not foolproof. Predictors of common duct stones are:

- clinical history (see above)
- abnormal liver biochemistry
- stones seen in the common bile duct on ultrasound or CT scan
- endoscopic ultrasound showing stones (best predictive value, but not always available).

Patients likely to have CBD stones from the above criteria should have their common bile ducts visualized directly. Many surgeons prefer this to be done endoscopically (ERCP) preoperatively, with removal of any stone found. This entails a sphincterotomy (p. 296) which has risks, and it is also an expensive procedure to add to the cost of subsequent surgery. Following sphincterotomy, stones can be removed using a Dormia basket and the duct swept with a balloon to ensure all stones have been removed. This can be confirmed by further cholangiography.

Endoscopic removal is appropriate in all older patients since subsequent cholecystectomy is not indicated in this group, the chance of further complications – even with stones in the gallbladder after CBD stone removal – being only 5–15%.

In patients who require cholecystectomy, laparoscopic common bile duct exploration should be performed at the same time. Fluoroscopic cholangiography is first performed and then a choledochoscope is passed through the cystic duct into the common bile duct. Up to 90% of stones can be removed. Retained stones after surgery are removed endoscopically.

In the persistently jaundiced patient, often with cholangitis, stones in the common duct are almost always removed endoscopically prior to cholecystectomy. The patient is usually offered cholecystectomy at a later date. Large stones cannot always be removed and an endoprosthesis is inserted into the common bile duct around the stone to allow biliary drainage. These large stones occasionally need to be crushed with mechanical lithotripsy or fragmented by extracorporeal shock-wave lithotripsy prior to removal.

Complications of gallstones

- Pancreatitis (p. 346).
- Gallstone ileus and biliary enteric fistula.
- Gallstones can occasionally erode through the wall of the gallbladder into the intestine. They can cause obstruction, mainly in the terminal ileum but occasionally in the duodenum.
- Carcinoma of the gallbladder may be causally related.

FURTHER READING

Hunter JG (1997) Advanced laparoscopic surgery. *American Journal of Surgery* **173**: 14–18.

Tait N, Little JM (1995) The treatment of gallstones. *British Medical Journal* **311**: 99-105

Miscellaneous conditions of the biliary tract

Primary sclerosing cholangitis

Primary sclerosing cholangitis (PSC) results from inflammation and fibrosis of the intrahepatic and extrahepatic bile ducts, leading to multiple areas of narrowing throughout the biliary system. The cause is unknown but immunological mechanisms have been implicated. HLA associations have been reported with HLA-B8, DR3, DR2 and HLA-DR52a. With DR4 there is a tendency for rapid disease progression. Seventy per cent of patients are men with the average age at presentation being 39 years. Smoking is associated with a decrease in the development of PSC.

Seventy-five per cent of patients have inflammatory bowel disease (usually ulcerative colitis), but this may be asymptomatic. Patients with AIDS can develop sclerosing cholangitis. The cause here is unclear but infection particularly with *Cryptosporidium parvum* is a probable aetiological factor.

CLINICAL FEATURES AND MANAGEMENT

The majority (60%) have no symptoms initially and the diagnosis is suggested by a raised serum ALP, but a negative mitochondrial antibody; 80% have myeloperoxidase ANCA antibodies. Symptoms that may fluctuate are pruritus, jaundice and occasionally abdominal pain. Cirrhosis and portal hypertension can develop. Liver biopsy shows a fibrous obliterating cholangitis with eventual loss of interlobular and adjacent septal bile ducts. The classical finding is the onion-skin lesion with dense connective tissue surrounding a necrotic, often obliterated, bile duct. An ERCP will show the multiple strictures.

Treatment is unsatisfactory. The mean survival time from diagnosis to death or liver transplantation in symptomatic patients is 12 years, while 75% of asymptomatic patients are alive at 15 years. Although most die of chronic liver disease both hepatocellular and cholangiocarcinomas occur. Steroids, azathioprine, methotrexate and ursodeoxycholate are of unproven value but seem to help some patients. When associated with ulcerative colitis, colectomy does not affect the progress of the condition. Obvious extrahepatic biliary strictures can sometimes be dilated or stented at endoscopy with short-term improvement in symptoms and biochemistry. Liver transplantation should be considered in those with advanced disease; there is now a 90% survival at 5 years.

Non-calculous cholecystitis

Occasionally cholecystitis occurs in patients with diabetes mellitus, polyarteritis nodosa and systemic infections.

Cholesterolosis of the gallbladder

In this condition, deposits of cholesterol are seen in the mucosal wall, producing a fine yellow pattern on a red background (strawberry gallbladder). Cholesterol stones may or may not be present. The relationship to symptoms is unclear.

Adenomyomatosis of the gallbladder

This may be found as an incidental finding on a cholecystogram and consists of thickening of the mucosal and muscle layers with the presence of Rokitansky–Aschoff sinuses, often associated with small gallstones. It does not usually produce symptoms.

Choledochal cyst

This is a congenital cystic dilatation of the extrahepatic ducts producing jaundice and abdominal pain. Fifty per cent of the patients do not present until early adult life. Treatment is surgical.

Haemobilia

Haemobilia can occur as a result of hepatic trauma, sometimes from a tumour, and rarely after liver biopsy. Blood enters the biliary tree and produces either cholestatic jaundice or gastrointestinal bleeding.

FURTHER READING

Lee YM, Kaplan MM (1995) Medical progress: primary sclerosing cholangitis. *New England Journal of Medicine* **322**: 924–933.

Tumours of the biliary tract

Gallbladder polyps

Polyps are found in 4% of patients referred for ultrasonography. These polyps are a mixture of true adenomatous polyps, inflammatory polyps and epithelium-covered aggregates of lipid-laden macrophages, also called 'cholesterol polyps'. Two questions arise: do these lesions cause symptoms, and can adenomatous polyps become malignant?

Both of these questions are unanswered. Current advice suggests cholecystectomy in patients with large polyps (>10 mm), or a wait-and-watch policy for smaller polyps.

Primary carcinoma of the gallbladder

This adenocarcinoma represents under 1% of all cancers. It occurs chiefly in those over 70 years of age and is most common in females. Gallstones are usually present but a definite relationship is uncertain. The presenting features are of jaundice and occasionally right hypochondrial pain. A mass may be palpable in the right hypochondrium. The diagnosis is often made at operation and cholecystectomy is performed if possible. Few patients survive one year.

Cholangiocarcinoma (see also p. 334)

This sometimes affects the extrahepatic biliary tree, giving rise to jaundice. Surgery, if possible, is the only effective treatment. Alternatively, a stent or tube can be passed through the obstruction during PTC or ERCP to relieve the obstruction. The prognosis is poor.

Malignant tumours of the ampulla

These present with a cholestatic jaundice which may occasionally be intermittent. They may ulcerate and produce gastrointestinal haemorrhage. The diagnosis is usually made at ERCP. Carcinoma of the ampulla can sometimes be resected, with a five-year survival rate of 40% (compare this with pancreatic carcinoma, p. 350).

The pancreas

Structure

The pancreas extends retroperitoneally across the posterior abdominal wall from the second part of the duodenum to the spleen. The head is encircled by the duodenum; the body, which forms the main bulk of the organ, ends in a tail that lies in contact with the spleen. The pancreas consists of exocrine and endocrine cells, the former making up 98% of the human pancreas. The pancreatic acinar cells are grouped into lobules, forming the ductal system which eventually joins into the main pancreatic duct. The main pancreatic duct has many tributary ductules and gradually tapers towards the tail of the pancreas. The main pancreatic duct usually joins the common bile duct to enter the duodenum as a single duct at the ampulla of Vater. Pancreas divisum is an anatomical variant in which a small proportion of the pancreas drains through an accessory duct into the duodenum.

Function

Pancreatic acini synthesize digestive enzymes which are stored in secretory granules and released by exocytosis in response to stimulation by several hormones (Fig 5.29).

Neurohormonal control of exocrine pancreas

Pancreatic exocrine function is regulated by both neural and hormonal mediators.

Cholecystokinin (CCK) is secreted by I cells in the gut mucosa in response to nutrients, particularly fat, protein and amino acids. CCK then acts by cholinergic pathways

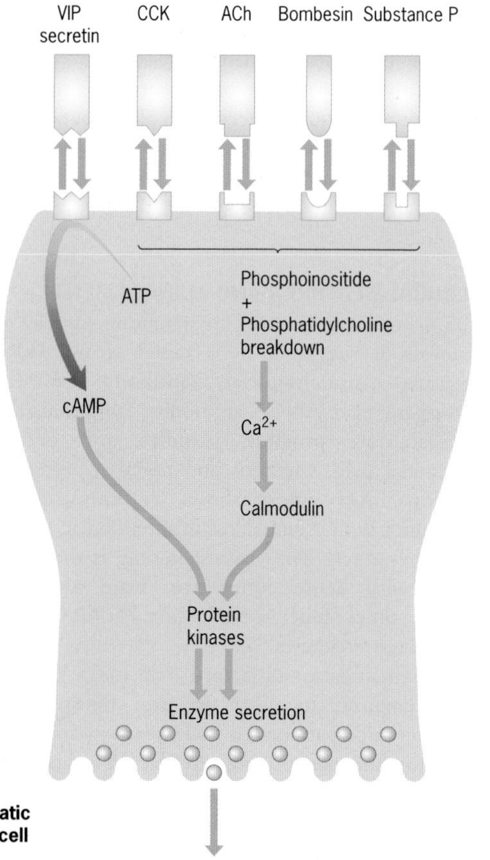

Fig 5.29
Diagram showing stimulus–secretion coupling of pancreatic cell protein secretion.
VIP = vasoactive intestinal polypeptide; CCK = cholecystokinin; ACh = acetylcholine.

to stimulate pancreatic secretion of enzymes and bicarbonate. The enzymes produced are amylase, lipase, colipase, phospholipase and proteases (trypsinogen and chymotrypsinogen). These proteases are activated in the duodenum by enterokinase. Pancreatic polypeptide (PP) also acts via the vagus to inhibit pancreatic secretion.

Secretin is released by duodenal acidification and also acts through cholinergic pathways to stimulate pancreatic secretion of bicarbonate-rich fluid. The vagal cholinergic pathway interacts with specific receptors on the acinar cell.

Cholecystokinin, acetylcholine and gastrin-releasing peptide all act on the pancreatic acinar cell through specific high-affinity interaction with guanine nucleotide-binding protein (G protein) coupled receptors. This is initiated by coupling to a member of the G_q family leading to activation of a phosphoinositide-specific phospholipase C. This enzyme hydrolyses phosphatidylinositides to yield inositol phosphates which stimulate Ca^{++} release (see Fig 5.29).

Secretin and VIP (vasoactive intestinal peptides) act via receptors that are coupled to a different G protein (G_s) to stimulate adenylate cyclase. These two cascades are interdependent. The increase in intracellular free Ca^{++} that results is the key step leading to release of intracellular stores of digestive enzymes following fusion of the granule membrane with the apical plasma membrane.

The endocrine pancreas

This consists of hormone-producing cells arranged in nests or islets – the islets of Langerhans. They do not connect directly to the duct system. There are four main types of islet cell and these have different secretory granules in their cytoplasm:

- β-cells, which are the most common cells, produce insulin
- α-cells produce glucagon
- D cells produce somatostatin
- PP cells produce pancreatic polypeptide (PP).

A number of other hormones (e.g. bombesin, neuropeptide Y and galanin) are present in pancreatic neurones and probably act as neurotransmitters.

Investigations (Table 5.18)

Exocrine function

The choice of individual tests is made on the clinical situation.

Serum amylase

This is useful in acute disease but is of no value in chronic disease.

Serum lipase

This is also raised in acute pancreatitis.

Table 5.18 Investigations available for the assessment of pancreatic disease

Exocrine	**Visualization of the pancreas**
Serum amylase/lipase	Abdominal X-ray - to detect calcification
Duodenal enzymes after:	Ultrasound – to demonstrate size, presence of calcification, tumours
Hormone stimulation with CCK and secretin	CT scan – useful for all pancreatic disease
Food stimulation (Lundh meal)	MRI and MRCP
PABA test	ERCP - to examine the ductular system
Fat excretion	Angiography - to detect tumours
Faecal fat (see p. 252)	Somatostatin receptor scintography – to detect neuro-endocrine tumours
Breath tests	Barium meal - to show an abnormal duodenal loop (seldom used)
Endocrine	Endoscopic ultrasound – good for small tumours
Serum level of peptides (examples)	
Insulin	
Glucagon	
Pancreatic polypeptide (PP)	
Gastrin	
Vasoactive intestinal polypeptide (VIP)	
Glucose tolerance test measuring glucose and insulin	

Measurement of duodenal enzymes

These tests have been largely superseded by imaging techniques. Direct measurement, either after hormone stimulation or after food, is only sometimes helpful in the diagnosis of chronic pancreatitis because of the large reserve in enzyme capacity. A tube is passed into the duodenum and pancreatic secretions are collected after stimulation. Stimulation with secretin or CCK causes a rise in bicarbonate and enzyme (e.g. trypsin) levels, which are low with chronic disease. The differential diagnosis between pancreatic tumour and pancreatitis is difficult.

The Lundh test is performed in a similar fashion, the stimulation being produced by a meal. Measurement of intraluminal trypsin and lipase is undertaken. These are low in chronic pancreatitis. The Lundh meal test is particularly useful in the investigation of steatorrhoea (p. 248).

PABA test

N-Benzoyl-L-tyrosyl *p*-aminobenzoic acid is a synthetic peptide hydrolysed by pancreatic chymotrypsin to release free PABA, which is absorbed, metabolized and excreted in the urine. Reduction in absorption of free PABA occurs (after an oral load of the peptide) in pancreatic insufficiency, and the test is highly specific in expert hands, although not widely utilized.

Tests for fat malabsorbtion

Faecal fat estimation is occasionally performed to demonstrate steatorrhoea.

A *breath test* can also be used; here the amount of $^{14}CO_2$ in expired air is measured following oral ingestion of a labelled fatty acid compared with that after a labelled triglyceride (e.g. [^{14}C]oleic acid compared with

[^{14}C]triolein). Impaired triglyceride absorption with normal fatty acid absorption indicates that pancreatic disease is the cause of the steatorrhoea.

Endocrine function

Assessment of endocrine function is useful only if a hormone-secreting tumour is suspected and the serum measurements are often diagnostic. Plasma PP is raised with all endocrine tumours.

Visualization of the pancreas

Imaging of the pancreas is becoming increasingly more accurate using newer techniques.

- *Conventional ultrasound* is still widely used; it is inexpensive and easy to perform. It is used to detect gallstones in acute pancreatitis, and to detect pancreatic and peripancreatic fluid collections, although CT is better (see below).
- *Endoscopic ultrasound* is probably the best technique for detecting small pancreatic tumours and for detecting small stones in the common bile duct in pancreatitis.
- *Laparoscopic ultrasound* and intravascular ultrasound are being used.
- *Helical CT*, with dynamic enhancement, enables the pancreas to be completely imaged within one 30-second breath hold and is extremely useful in all forms of pancreatic disease.
- *MRI* has the advantage over CT in that it does not involve ionizing radiation, but prolonged scan times are required. It is equally sensitive to CT.
- *Magnetic resonance cholangio-pancreatography (MRCP)* is being used and may challenge diagnostic ERCP as the best way of outlining the biliary tree.
- *Arteriography* with selective catheterization is less frequently used.

A combination of two or three tests is often necessary and none of the investigations is completely diagnostic. Fine-needle aspiration of any abnormality discovered can be performed under ultrasound or CT scan control. The presence of malignant cells in the aspirate indicates tumour but, of course, a negative sample does not exclude malignancy.

Pancreatitis

Classification

The classification of pancreatitis is difficult owing to the inability to separate acute and chronic pancreatitis clearly.

By definition, acute pancreatitis may occur as isolated or as recurrent attacks. The gland is normal before the attack and can return to normal after resolution of the attack. In chronic pancreatitis there is continuing inflammation, irreversible structural changes and eventual permanent loss of exocrine and endocrine pancreatic function. The causes of pancreatitis are shown in Table 5.19.

Acute pancreatitis

This is an acute inflammatory process of the pancreas which may subsequently involve peripancreatic tissue.

PATHOGENESIS

The exact mechanism by which pancreatic necrosis occurs is unclear. Associated gallstones are found mainly in the gallbladder and only occasionally in the common bile duct. Reflux of bile up the pancreatic duct associated with occlusion of the ampulla may play a role in the pathogenesis. Autodigestion of the pancreas by proteolytic enzymes (particularly trypsin and phospholipase A) released in the pancreas rather than in the intestinal lumen may also be involved in the pathogenesis. Active enzymes could digest cell membranes, leading to proteolysis, oedema, vascular damage and necrosis.

The mildest and most common (75%) form of pancreatitis is characterized by interstitial oedema with an inflammatory exudate and some fat necrosis (oedematous pancreatitis), while in the severe form there is extensive pancreatic and peripancreatic necrosis, and haemorrhage.

CLINICAL FEATURES

These vary depending on the severity of the attack. In all patients the principal symptom is abdominal pain that is usually localized to the epigastrium or upper abdomen. It may radiate to the back between the scapulae. The pain will vary from mild discomfort to excruciating pain in severe cases. Rarely, acute pancreatitis can occur in the absence of pain. Nausea and vomiting accompany the pain in most cases.

In severe acute pancreatitis there is often associated organ failure and/or development of a local complication, such as necrosis abscess or pseudocyst.

Table 5.19
Causes of pancreatitis

Acute	Chronic
Gallstones	Alcohol (> 85%)
Alcohol	Idiopathic
Infections (e.g. mumps, coxsackie B)	Tropical (nutritional)
Pancreatic tumours	Hereditary
Drugs (e.g. azathioprine, oestrogens, corticosteroids)	Trauma
Iatrogenic (e.g. post-surgical, ERCP)	Hypercalcaemia
Hyperlipidaemias	
Miscellaneous	
Trauma	
Scorpion bite	
Cardiac surgery	
Idiopathic	

Physical examination may reveal tenderness, guarding and rigidity of the abdomen, with varying degrees of shock depending on the severity of the attack. Rarely, body wall ecchymoses occur – e.g. umbilical (Cullen's sign) or in the flanks (Grey Turner's sign). The remaining clinical features depend on the local and systemic complications that occur (Table 5.20).

Local pancreatic complications can occasionally occur with mild attacks of pancreatitis, but systemic complications occur only with severe attacks.

INVESTIGATIONS AND DIAGNOSIS

The clinical manifestations are so varied that pancreatitis must be considered in the differential diagnosis of all causes of upper abdominal pain. Most patients present as an acute abdomen and differentiation from an acute perforated ulcer is the most difficult, as both may give rise to abdominal rigidity.

Serum amylase

The diagnosis of acute pancreatitis depends on the serum amylase or lipase. A raised serum amylase level can be seen in other acute abdominal emergencies such as acute cholecystitis and perforated peptic ulcer; but if the serum amylase level is five times greater than normal, acute pancreatitis is very likely. However, the serum amylase cannot be relied upon entirely and must be evaluated in conjunction with the history and physical signs. A plain abdominal X-ray may show ileus initially limited to the loop of bowel (sentinel loop) or calcification in acute on chronic pancreatitis.

Other investigations

- **Ultrasound** is used to detect gallstones in the biliary tree. It may also demonstrate pancreatic swelling, necrosis and the presence or absence of peripancreatic fluid collections. In severe pancreatitis the pancreas is often obscured by gas.
- **Contrast-enhanced dynamic CT scanning** (Fig 5.30) is the most valuable technique. It can detect swelling of the pancreas and the presence of pancreatic necrosis, peripancreatic fluid collections or diffuse inflammatory changes in the retroperitoneum. The demonstration of gallstones may indicate the aetiology.
- **MRI** is increasingly being used and can discriminate between fluid and solid inflammatory masses.
- **Peritoneal aspiration and lavage**, with estimation of amylase in the peritoneal fluid obtained, is useful in difficult cases.

If there is doubt about the diagnosis, exploratory laparotomy must be performed in all but mild cases to exclude a potentially fatal but treatable non-pancreatic lesion. Factors indicating the severity, which is assessed chiefly on blood investigations, are given in Table 5.21. APACHE II score (see p. 859) is also used to grade severity.

Biliary pancreatitis (also see below) is very likely if the serum bilirubin is raised and a stone is found in the common bile duct on ultrasound. Many patients, however, have no direct evidence of a biliary cause for the pancreatitis. An ERCP is sometimes performed – see below.

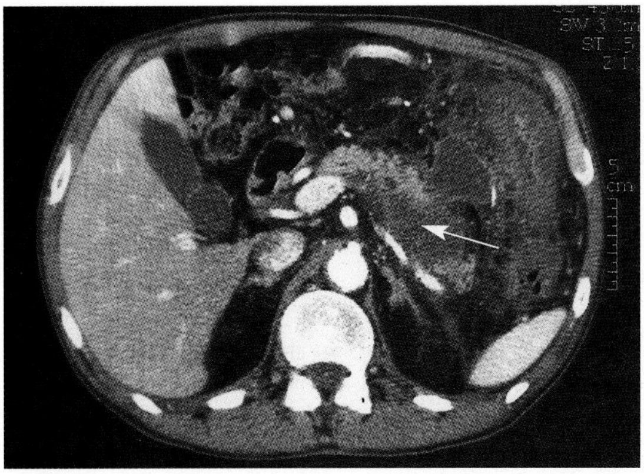

Fig 5.30
CT scan in patient with acute pancreatitis showing necrosis of the pancreatic parenchyma (arrow) and a fluid collection extending outside the gland with inflammatory thickening of the colon

Table 5.20
Complications of acute pancreatitis

Pancreatic	Systemic
Acute fluid collection	Metabolic
Necrosis	Malnutrition
Pseudocyst	Hypocalcaemia
Abscess	Hypoglycaemia
Ascites	Haematological
	Disseminated intravascular coagulation
Intestinal	Portal vein thrombosis
Paralytic ileus	Renal
GI haemorrhage	Acute renal failure
	Cardiovascular
Hepatobiliary	Circulatory failure (shock)
Jaundice	Respiratory
Obstruction of CBD	Hypoxic acute respiratory failure
Portal vein thrombosis	

Table 5.21 Factors during the first 48 hours that indicate severe pancreatitis and a poor prognosis

Age	> 55 years
WBC	$> 15 \times 10^9/L$
Blood glucose	> 10 mmol L^{-1}
Serum urea	> 16 mmol L^{-1}
Serum albumin	< 30 g L^{-1}
Serum aminotransferase	> 200 U L^{-1}
Serum calcium	< 2 mmol L^{-1}
Serum LDH	> 600 U L^{-1}
$P_{a}O_2$	< 8.0 kPa (60 mmHg)

LDH, lactate dehydrogenase

TREATMENT

Mild cases usually respond quickly to nil-by-mouth and nasogastric suction to reduce vomiting and abdominal distension. Water and electrolyte replacement and analgesia with an opiate (other than morphine) are also required.

Severe pancreatitis involves similar measures to those above. Intravenous nutrition is often required because of the length of time that feeding is stopped.

Local complications require treatment (see below), while patients in shock and/or respiratory failure require intensive care.

Specific therapy, such as peritoneal lavage and protease inhibitor therapy, have not been shown to affect overall mortality, but may be of value in high-risk patients.

A recent study using the platelet activating factor antagonist (Lexipafant) showed a reduction in complications and overall mortality when given within 48 hours of onset.

Biliary pancreatitis. In patients who have cholangitis or progressive jaundice with mild or severe biliary pancreatitis, an ERCP will be necessary for stone removal usually within 24–72 hours after the onset of symptoms.

In patients with no direct evidence of biliary pancreatitis (see above), but in which a biliary cause is suspected, ERCP is often advocated, but the evidence that this is beneficial is controversial.

LOCAL COMPLICATIONS

- *Acute fluid collection*. This occurs in the peripancreatic region early in the disease in 30–50% of patients and can be seen on ultrasound or CT. Diffuse retroperitoneal inflammatory change may accompany the collections. Approximately 50% regress spontaneously.
- *Pancreatic necrosis*. This is an area of non-viable pancreatic parenchyma, often associated with peripancreatic fat necrosis. It is diagnosed by dynamic contrast CT. Infected pancreatic necrosis carries a bad prognosis without surgical drainage and antibiotic therapy, usually with intravenous cefuroxime.
- *Pseudocysts* (see also p. 349). These evolve from acute fluid collections four weeks or more after the start of the acute attack. Pseudocysts contain enzyme-rich fluid and may be intra- or peripancreatic. Pseudocysts are lined by granulation tissue, whereas true cysts would be lined by epithelium. Large collections persisting for weeks or those suspected of secondary infection can be aspirated under ultrasonic control or be removed surgically.
- *Pancreatic abscesses*. These are circumscribed intra-abdominal collections of pus, usually near the pancreas, containing little or no pancreatic necrosis. They arise as a consequence of the acute pancreatitis usually some weeks after the attack has started. These abscesses can often be treated by percutaneous drainage (compare necrosis above).
- *Pancreatic ascites*. This is more commonly associated with chronic pancreatitis and has a high amylase content. In acute pancreatitis, ascites indicates a poor prognosis.

PROGNOSIS

The mortality rate varies from 1% in mild cases to 50% in severe cases. With multiple complications and the presence of all the bad prognostic signs, the mortality is nearer 100%. The patients who recover may have recurrent attacks, depending on the aetiology and whether accompanying gallstones are dealt with.

Chronic pancreatitis

This is defined as a continuing inflammatory disease of the pancreas characterized by irreversible morphological change and typically causing pain and/or permanent impairment of function. Acute pancreatitis (e.g. from gallstones) does not usually lead to chronic pancreatitis.

PATHOGENESIS

The earliest change appears to be deposition of protein plugs within pancreatic ducts. These then lead to ductular dilatation followed by acinar atrophy. There is some accompanying cellular infiltration but this is variable. Extensive fibrous tissue is deposited near the pancreatic ducts. Eventually only a few acinar and islet cells remain, with widely dilated pancreatic ducts. Intraluminal calcification of the protein plugs occurs, leading to stone formation. The role of lithostatine – a protein secreted by acinar cells in the causation of stones – remains controversial.

In chronic pancreatitis caused by alcohol the patient may give a history of bouts of abdominal pain suggesting recurrent episodes of acute inflammation. Many other patients have no previous history and it is likely that chronic pancreatitis results from a chronic insiduous process.

TYPES

Chronic calcifying pancreatitis. This is the most common form in developed countries and is usually caused by alcohol. Alcohol consumption is usually above 150 g per day over a long period (more than 10 years). A high-protein diet, sometimes with a high fat content, may potentiate the effect of alcohol.

Tropical pancreatitis. These patients are usually young, of either sex, primarily from a region where there is protein and fat malnutrition. Pancreatic insufficiency, diabetes mellitus and recurrent attacks of pain occur. The cause is unclear.

Hereditary pancreatitis. This is a rare condition where there is the lack of a protein stabilizer, permitting the formation of calcifying plugs. The defect is caused by a mutation in the cationic trypsinogen gene.

Obstructive pancreatitis. In this condition there is obstruction of the main pancreatic duct owing to a scar, stricture or tumour. The lesions are uniformly distributed with a paucity of intraductal plugs; calculi are unusual. The pancreatitis may regress if the obstruction can be cleared.

CLINICAL FEATURES

The major symptom is abdominal pain situated mainly in the epigastrium and upper abdomen and radiating to the back. The pain can be severe; in some cases it is comparable to that occurring in acute pancreatitis.

Continuing episodes of pain may occur; sometimes these are mild and of brief duration. In other cases there may be chronic pain interspersed with acute episodes (relapsing pancreatitis). The relationship to alcohol is variable; nevertheless, some acute episodes seem to be precipitated by heavy alcohol consumption. The abdominal pain is accompanied by severe weight loss that is due to anorexia.

Steatorrhoea occurs when the secretion of pancreatic lipase is reduced by 90%. It occurs in about half the patients. The steatorrhoea is often severe and the patient may notice drops of oil in the lavatory pan. The development of diabetes is more common. Both diabetes and steatorrhoea occur more commonly with calcified pancreatitis.

Less common presentations include biliary obstruction with jaundice and occasionally cholangitis. Obstruction of the splenic vein can lead to portal hypertension.

INVESTIGATIONS

These include assessment of some of the endocrine and exocrine functions as outlined earlier, as well as visualization of the pancreas (see p. 346). The serum amylase is of little value in chronic pancreatitis but may be raised during an acute episode of pain. Early cases are difficult to diagnose and a combination of all tests is often required.

Endoscopic ultrasound can detect early changes in both ducts and the parenchyma, as well as cysts (<20 mm) and tiny calcifications and is very specific for the diagnosis. It complements ERCP which outlines the duct system well and is more readily available. With severe chronic pancreatitis, there is pancreatic duct dilatation with stenotic areas often associated with pancreatic duct stones.

Conventional ultrasound is not very sensitive, particularly in early cases. *CT scan*, however, shows evidence of focal enlargement or atrophy, as well as abnormalities in duct size and calcification in most cases (Fig 5.31). *MRCP* is beginning to rival ERCP in some centres.

For patients presenting with steatorrhoea, a *Lundh test* can be performed to estimate exocrine function (see p. 345). However, if pancreatic imaging is diagnostic this is seldom performed.

DIFFERENTIAL DIAGNOSIS

Carcinoma of the pancreas must be suspected, particularly when the history is short. Very occasionally laparotomy may be necessary to distinguish between these two conditions.

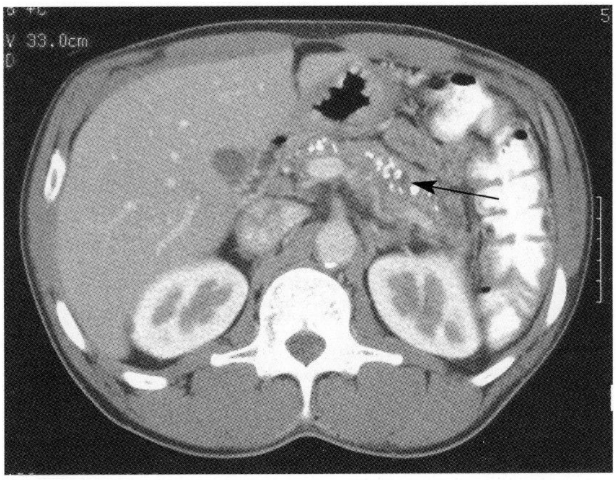

Fig 5.31
Contrast-enhanced CT scan demonstrating multiple calcific densities (arrow) along the line of the main pancreatic duct in a patient with chronic pancreatitis

TREATMENT

In alcoholic pancreatitis the patient should stop drinking alcohol. The pain needs to be controlled, often with narcotics. There is a frequent problem of addiction. Surgery is used for the treatment of intractable pain, pancreatic resection combined with drainage of an obstructed pancreatic duct into the small bowel being required. The use of surgery is controversial; good results are obtained only in a small number of cases, usually those who stop drinking.

Steatorrhoea is treated with a low-fat diet, pancreatic supplements (e.g. pancreatin 2–4 g with each meal), with occasionally cimetidine 400 mg twice-daily. Diabetes mellitus is treated with diet, oral hypoglycaemic agents and/or insulin as appropriate. The insulin requirement is greater than in idiopathic diabetes, and patients may experience frequent or severe hypoglycaemia. This may be because pancreatic glucagon is not being produced.

COMPLICATIONS

The most common complication is a *pancreatic pseudocyst*. These are found very frequently if careful ultrasound examinations are performed. Small cysts require no treatment. Large cysts can give rise to increased pain, nausea and vomiting 3–4 weeks after the onset of the most recent attack of pain. A smooth, tender mass may be palpable and the cyst can usually be easily identified using ultrasound. Surgical treatment has been used for most large pseudocysts, but a more conservative approach is preferable, with aspiration and close follow-up using ultrasound examination. Internal drainage into the stomach may be achieved by endoscopy, ideally with initial localization of the optimal drainage site by endoscopic ultrasound.

Pancreatic ascites occurs, usually in alcoholic pancreatitis, when there is a communication between the pancreatic duct and the peritoneal cavity. The amylase content of the ascitic fluid is high.

A good prognosis depends on complete abstention from alcohol.

FURTHER READING

Baillie J (1997) Treatment of acute biliary pancreatitis. *New England Journal of Medicine* **336**: 286–287.

Baron TH, Morgan DE (1997) The diagnosis and management of fluid collections associated with pancreatitis. *American Journal of Medicine* **102**: 555–563.

Bradley EL (1993) A clinically based classification for acute pancreatitis. *Archives of Surgery* **128**: 586–590.

Imrie CW (1997) Acute pancreatitis: review in depth. *European Journal of Gastroenterology and Hepatology* **9**: 103–144.

Steer MS, Waxman I, Freedman S (1995) Chronic pancreatitis. *New England Journal of Medicine* **332**: 1482–1490.

Cystic fibrosis (see also p. 157)

This is the most common cause of pancreatic disease in childhood. It is inherited as an autosomal recessive condition and a specific gene mutation ΔF508 is present in 70% of cases. The resultant protein defect produces an abnormality in the regulation of a cAMP-regulated Cl^- channel in the epithelial cell membrane. This cystic fibrosis gene product has been named cystic fibrosis transmembrane conductance regulator (CFTR) (see Fig 2.20). The resultant defective chloride transport in all exocrine glands produces thick viscoid dehydrated secretions which cause cystic dilatation of the ducts with eventual fibrosis. Increased numbers of patients are now surviving into adult life because of improved therapy.

CLINICAL FEATURES

These are described on p. 784.

DIAGNOSTIC TESTS

- **Sweat testing** (see p. 784) of symptomatic people and siblings of patients with cystic fibrosis – identifies 77% by two years of age and 95% by the age of 12 years.
- **Immunoreactive trypsin assay** of dried blood (in infants).
- **Genetic studies** (see p. 157)
- **Pancreatic function tests** (see p. 345).

TREATMENT

Treatment is required for pancreatic insufficiency and respiratory problems (see p. 784). Steatorrhoea is treated with pancreatic supplements. High-dose pancreatin-containing trypsin and lipase can be given in microsphere-containing capsules which deliver high doses of enzyme to the duodenum. Fibrosing colonopathy with stricture formation have been reported in young children on these high-dose pancreatic enzyme supplements. Current recommendation is that the daily dose of lipase should remain below 10 000 units kg^{-1}. H_2 antagonists are not usually required with these preparations, and the fat content of the diet can be kept normal. Optimal nutrition has been recognized as improving prognosis, and a high calorie intake (150% of recommended daily allowance) with vitamin supplements should be given.

Carcinoma of the pancreas

The incidence of pancreatic carcinoma has remained steady over the last 20 years. The incidence in the West is estimated at 9 cases per 100 000. This tumour is now the fifth most common cause of cancer death in the UK and USA. The incidence increases with age and most patients are over 60 years of age. Males are affected more than females. There are no definite aetiological factors, but the high incidence has been attributed to smoking, and diets containing substantial amounts of red meat and cholesterol. Alcohol and coffee probably do not affect the risk. Diets high in of fruit and vegetables are probably protective, possibly owing to their high fibre and vitamin C content. Environmental factors include occupational exposure to petroleum products, napthalanine and benzidine.

About 90% of pancreatic tumours are adenocarcinomas and arise from the duct epithelium. Neuroendocrine (see p. 352) and acinar cell carcinomas make up most of the remainder.

In 70% of cases the tumour is in the head of the pancreas. The tumour spreads locally to involve all adjacent organs, including the duodenum, peritoneum and some spread to the liver and spleen.

K-*Ras* mutations have been demonstrated in most pancreatic tumours studied, with high levels of *p53* gene expression in about 60% of tumours.

CLINICAL FEATURES

Symptoms

Carcinoma of the head of the pancreas or the ampulla of Vater. This presents with painless jaundice owing to obstruction of the common duct. However, most patients will have pain at some time in the course of their disease. Anorexia and weight loss also occur.

Carcinoma of the body or tail of the pancreas. This presents with abdominal pain, anorexia and weight loss. The pain is often a dull, boring pain that radiates through to the back. It may be relieved by sitting forward. Jaundice is rare. Diabetes occurs in about 15% of cases owing to insulin resistance. This is thought to be caused by islet amyloid polypeptide, a hormonal factor secreted from pancreatic cells. There is an increased incidence of thrombophlebitis.

Signs

In carcinoma of the head of the pancreas, examination will reveal jaundice with the dilated gallbladder sometimes being palpable (Courvoisier's sign). A dilated gallbladder is not found with gallstone disease because of the accompanying chronic inflammation of the gallbladder.

A palpable mass can be felt in 20% of patients, with hepatomegaly being present in most cases eventually.

INVESTIGATIONS AND DIAGNOSIS

Haematological or biochemical tests (including blood glucose) are not helpful. Tumour markers (e.g. CEA and carbohydrate antigen (CA 19.9 and CA 242) are used, but may give false positives and false negatives and their use should be discouraged.

The diagnosis is usually made by ultrasound (Fig 5.32) or thin-section, spiral contrast-enhanced CT scan. Tumours are usually advanced at diagnosis and imaging will demonstrate evidence of local spread as well as distal metastases so that surgery is not performed unnecessarily. Fine-needle aspirate or Tru-cut biopsy is used to confirm the diagnosis histologically in patients who are inoperable. Duodenoscopy with ERCP can detect tumours at the head of the pancreas or of the ampulla. Endoscopic ultrasound is valuable both in the detection and staging of small, potentially operable lesions. MRI is particularly good at determining vascular invasion.

(a)

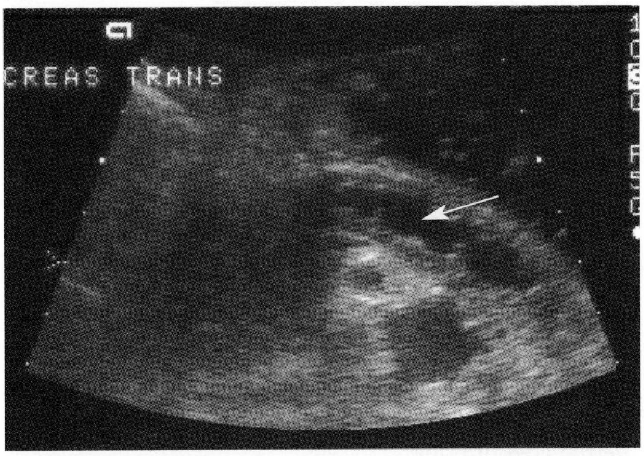

(b)

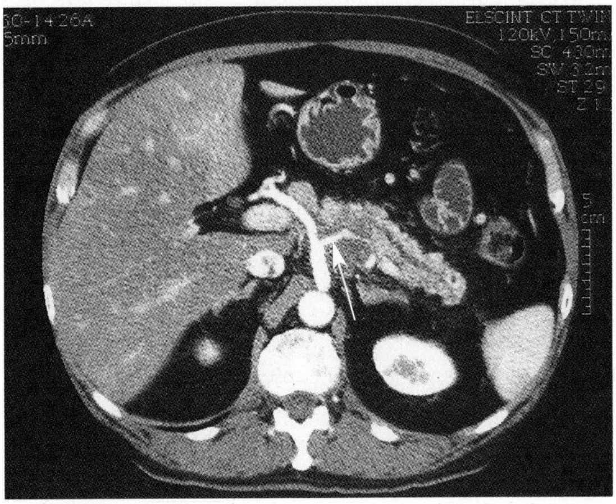

Fig 5.32
(a) Ultrasound of the pancreas showing a tumour in the pancreatic head, with dilation of the main pancreatic duct (arrow). (b) Cancer of the body of the pancreas. There is retroperitoneal tumour extension enclosing the branches of the coeliac axis (arrow). Early retroperitoneal spread makes most pancreatic cancers inoperable.

DIFFERENTIAL DIAGNOSIS

The differential diagnosis includes all causes of painless jaundice and persistent upper abdominal pain in the elderly.

MANAGEMENT

The five-year survival rate is miserably low at 2%, with most patients surviving less than one year from diagnosis. Pancreatic-duodenectomy performed for a cure has a five-year survival of 10–20%. Unfortunately, this survival benefit is only seen with small tumours (<3 cm) without evidence of tumour spread, this occurring in only a small proportion of cases (<10%). The operative mortality is about 5% with morbidity of 30–40% so that pancreatic-duodenectomy is attempted only in a few patients in whom all investigations indicate a small tumour.

Palliation

Jaundice from carcinoma of the head of the pancreas is usually relieved by a bypass procedure. This is performed endoscopically with the placement of a stent through the narrowed area of the common bile duct to allow drainage. An expandable metal stent is sometimes used which remains patent for longer. Patients frequently feel better after this procedure and quality of life is improved.

Surgical bypass where the common bile duct is anastomosed to the jejunum is reserved for cases where the tumour has obstructed the duodenum. Chemotherapy and radiotherapy have had little success in decreasing mortality. Ampullary tumours have a better prognosis than pancreatic carcinomas, and every attempt should be made to diagnose these rare lesions, as if a resection is possible, long-term survival is approximately 40% in 5 years.

Pain and symptoms of anxiety and depression are an important part of management. Analgesia with long-acting oral morphines should be used liberally (see p. 442). Addiction is not a problem in these terminally ill patients. Palliative care teams play an important role in this distressing condition.

FURTHER READING

Cello JP (1997) Carcinoma of the pancreas. In: Sleisenger and Fordtran's Gastrointestinal and Liver Disease. WB Saunders, Philadelphia, pp 863-870

Neuro-endocrine tumours

These tumours arise mainly in the pancreas from APUD (amine precursor uptake and decarboxylation) cells and are sometimes called 'apudomas'.

Pancreatic endocrine tumours can occur in association with other endocrine tumours, particularly parathyroid adenoma and pituitary adenoma, as part of multiple endocrine neoplasias (see p. 956). Neuro-endocrine tumours predominantly secrete one hormone that produces its clinical effect, but other hormones are often synthesized and can be detected either in the blood or in the resected tumour.

Most neuro-endocrine tumours express large numbers of somatostatin receptors. Intravenous injection of ^{111}In-labelled octreotide is therefore taken up readily by these tumours, and this has become the first investigation of choice for patients suspected of having a neuro-endocrine tumour. The test is also useful in detecting metastases.

Gastrinoma (Zollinger–Ellison syndrome)

These tumours mainly arise from G cells in the pancreas and secrete large amounts of gastrin. This stimulates maximal gastric acid secretion, so that the main clinical problem is peptic ulceration. Peptic ulcers occur in the usual areas of the stomach and duodenum and in the jejunum. The ulcers are often large and deep and sometimes multiple. Haemorrhage and perforation can occur.

Diarrhoea resulting from the low pH in the upper intestine is also a common feature. Jejunal mucosal abnormalities are also seen. A high serum gastrin confirms the diagnosis. Acid studies show high acid output. The tumour may be demonstrated by isotope scans, ultrasound, CT or local venous sampling for gastrin. Treatment is with a proton pump inhibitor. Octreotide is also used, usually while the diagnosis is being made. Surgery is reserved for removal of the primary tumour only. These tumours are malignant and although they grow slowly the patients die of malignancy rather than gastrointestinal problems if the primary cannot be removed.

Other endocrine tumours

Islet cell tumours

These are described on p. 987.

Vipomas

These rare pancreatic tumours produce severe intestinal secretion and watery diarrhoea leading to dehydration. Vasoactive intestinal polypeptide (VIP) is a neurotransmitter that stimulates adenyl cyclase to produce intestinal secretion. Plasma concentrations of VIP are very high and are diagnostic. Levels of PP hormone are also raised. The role of peptide histidine isoleucine (PHI), levels of which are also raised in this condition, is uncertain but this hormone may be involved in secretion.

Corticosteroids help to reduce the stool volume, but octreotide is the most effective agent. An attempt should be made to localize the tumour and, if possible, it should be resected.

Glucagonomas

These are α-cell tumours of the pancreas that produce pancreatic glucagon. The patients have a unique, characteristic necrolytic migratory erythematous rash, as well as cheilosis, diarrhoea, diabetes mellitus and a normochromic normocytic anaemia, venous thrombosis, weight loss and neuropsychiatric symptoms. The diagnosis is made by measuring pancreatic glucagon in the serum. Most patients have metastatic disease at presentation; nevertheless, debulking surgery and medical therapy are effective for long-term palliation.

A tumour originating in the right kidney has been described that produces marked hypertrophy of the villi in the jejunum and produces enteroglucagon (enteroglucagonoma).

Somatostatinomas

These have also been described. They produce diabetes, steatorrhoea and weight loss.

FURTHER READING

Modilin IM, Tang LH (1997) Approaches to the diagnosis of gut neuro-endocrine tumours. *Gastroenterology* **112**: 583–590.

GENERAL FURTHER READING

Current Opinions in Gastroenterology. Philadelphia: Rapid Science Publishers (gives useful updates with extensive references).

Sherlock S, Dooley J (1997) *Diseases of the Liver and Biliary System*, 10th edn. Oxford: Blackwell Scientific.

Sleisenger and Fordtran's Gastrointestinal and Liver Disease (1997) 6th edn. WB Saunders, Philadelphia.

Haematological disease

6

Introduction and general aspects

Blood consists of:

- red cells
- white cells
- platelets
- plasma, in which the above elements are suspended.

Plasma is the liquid component of blood, which contains soluble fibrinogen. Serum is what remains after the formation of the fibrin clot.

The formation of blood cells (haemopoiesis)

Blood islands are formed in the yolk sac in the third week of gestation, and produce primitive blood cells which migrate to the liver and spleen. These organs are the chief sites of haemopoiesis from 6 weeks to 7 months, when the bone marrow becomes the main source of blood cells. The bone marrow is the only source of blood cells during normal childhood and adult life.

At birth, haemopoiesis is present in the marrow of nearly every bone. As the child grows the marrow cavity is gradually replaced by fat so that haemopoiesis in the adult becomes confined to the central skeleton and the proximal ends of the long bones. Only if the demand for blood cells increases and persists do the areas of red marrow extend once again. Pathological processes interfering with normal haemopoiesis may result in resumption of haemopoietic activity in the liver and spleen, which is referred to as *extramedullary haemopoiesis*.

All peripheral blood cells are derived from pluripotential stem cells by a number of *differentiation* steps (Fig 6.1). Stem cells probably resemble small lymphocytes, although their exact appearance remains unknown. However, their presence can be shown by bone marrow culture techniques, involving the detection of *colony-forming units* (CFUs) in agar culture medium. The earliest detectable CFU is CFU-S (spleen); this gives rise to CFU-GEMM, which produces CFU 'committed' to the production of:

- granulocytes (G)
- erythroid cells (E)
- monocytes (M)
- megakaryocytes (Meg).

Stem cells also produce lymphoid cells.

Stem cells have the capability for *self-renewal*, as well as differentiation. Normal haemopoiesis is dependent on the presence of haemopoietic growth factors and occurs in close association with bone marrow stromal cells.

About 1–3% of bone marrow cells express the CD34 antigen, and this population contains virtually all the myeloid and lymphoid precursor cells. CD34-positive cells are heterogeneous, and the most primitive cells may be further characterized by the presence or absence of other cell markers. The ability to purify stem cells on the basis of cell markers could lead to important refinements in clinical haemopoietic cell transplantation.

Haemopoietic growth factors

Haemopoietic growth factors are glycoproteins which regulate the differentiation and proliferation of haemopoietic progenitor cells and the function of mature blood cells. They act on receptors expressed on haemopoietic cells at

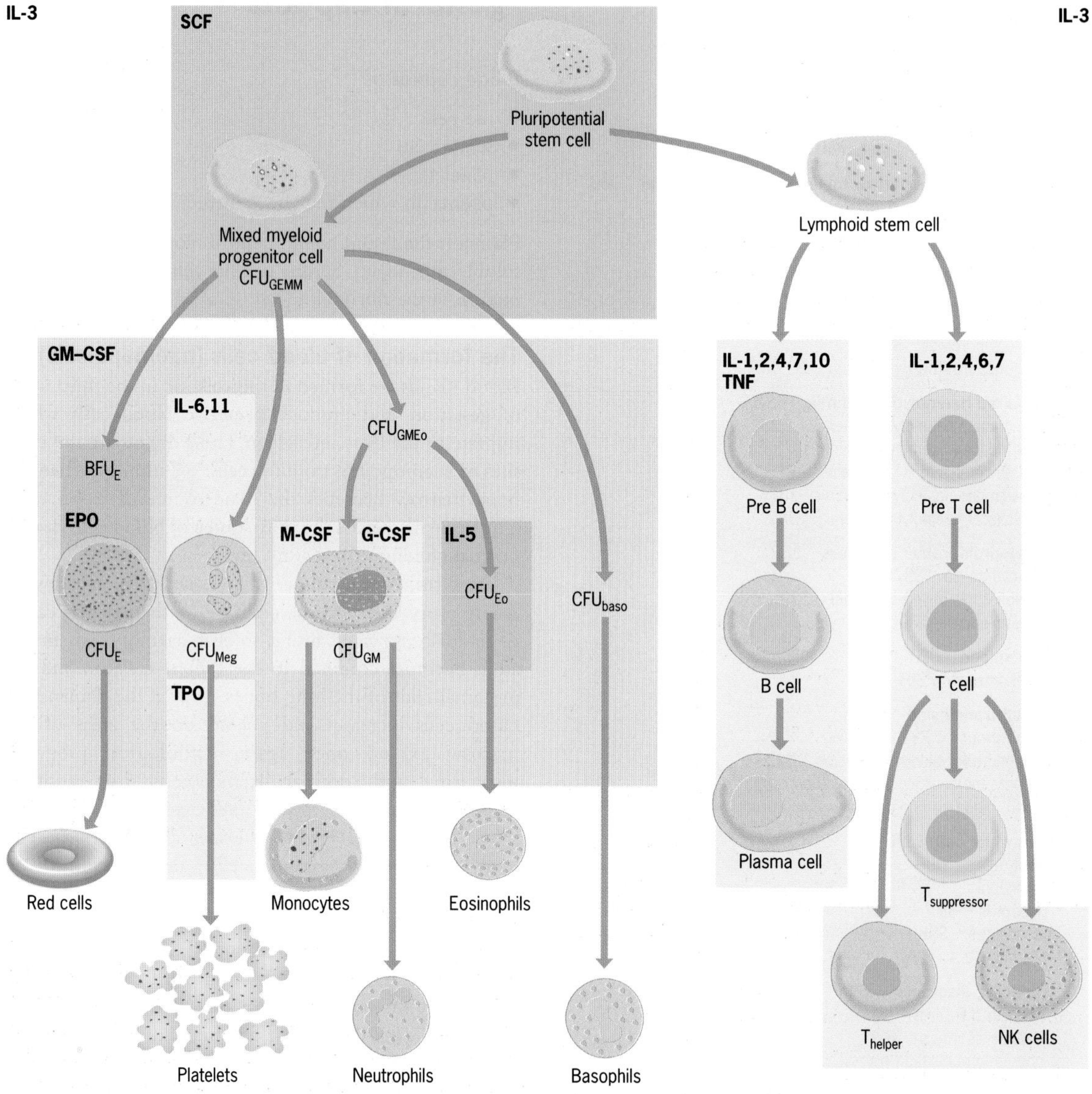

Fig 6.1
Role of growth factors in normal haemopoiesis. Multiple growth factors act on stem cells and early progenitor cells.
BFU, burst-forming unit
CFU, colony-forming unit
CSF, colony-stimulating factor
E, erythroid
Eo, eosinophil
EPO, erythropoietin
G, granulocyte
GEMM, mixed granulocyte, erythoid, monocyte, megakaryocyte
GM, granulocyte, monocyte
IL, interleukin
M, monocyte
Meg, megakaryocyte
SCF, stem cell (Steel) factor
TNF, tumour necrosis factor
TPO, Thrombopoietin

various stages of development to maintain the haemopoietic progenitor cells and to stimulate increased production of one or more cell lines in response to stresses such as blood loss and infection (Fig 6.1).

The pluripotential stem cells are under the influence of a number of haemopoietic growth factors including interleukin-3 (IL-3), IL-6, IL-11 and stem cell factor (SCF, Steel factor). Colony stimulating factors (CSFs, the prefix indicating the cell type, see Fig 6.1), as well as interleukins and erythropoietin (EPO) regulate the lineage committed progenitor cells. Thrombopoietin (which, like erythropoietin, is produced in the kidneys and the liver) along with IL-6 and IL-11 control platelet production. In addition to these factors stimulating haemopoiesis, other factors inhibit the process and include tumour necrosis factor (TNF) and transforming growth factor-β (TGF-β). Many of the growth factors are produced by activated T cells, monocytes, and bone marrow stromal cells such as fibroblasts, endothelial cells and macrophages; these cells are also involved in inflammatory responses.

Many growth factors have been produced by recombinant DNA techniques and are being used clinically. Examples include G-CSF which is used to accelerate haemopoietic recovery after chemotherapy and haemopoietic cell transplantation, and erythropoietin which is used to treat anaemia in patients with chronic renal failure. Thrombopoietin is undergoing clinical trials in patients treated for malignant disease to reduce the need for platelet transfusions after intensive chemotherapy.

Peripheral blood

Automated cell counters are used to measure the level of haemoglobin (Hb) and the number and size of red cells, white cells and platelets (Table 6.1). Other indices can be derived from these values. The mean corpuscular volume (MCV) of red cells is the most useful of the indices and is used to classify anaemia (see p. 358).

The white cell count (WCC) gives the total number of circulating leucocytes and many automated cell counters produce differential counts as well.

Normally, less than 2% of the red cells are *reticulocytes*. The reticulocyte count gives a guide to the erythroid activity in the bone marrow. An increased count is seen with haemorrhage or haemolysis, and during the response to treatment with a specific haematinic. A low count in the presence of anaemia indicates an inappropriate response by the bone marrow and may be seen in bone marrow failure (from whatever cause) or where there is a deficiency of a haematinic.

A carefully evaluated *blood film* is still an essential adjunct to the above, as definitive abnormalities of cells can be seen, and some examples are shown in Fig 6.8.

Table 6.1
Normal values for peripheral blood

	Male	Female
Hb (g dL^{-1})	13–18	11.5–15.5
PCV (haematocrit; L/L)	0.42–0.53	0.36–0.45
RCC (10^{12}/L)	4.5–6.0	3.9–5.
MCV (fl)	80–96	
MCH (pg)	27–33	
MCHC (g dL^{-1})	32–35	
WCC (10^9/L)	4.0–11.0	
Platelets (10^9/L)	150–400	
ESR (mm h^{-1})	< 20	
Reticulocytes (%)	0.5–2.5	

ESR, erythrocyte sedimentation rate, Hb, haemoglobin, MCH, mean corpuscular haemoglobin, MCHC, mean corpuscular haemoglobin concentration, MCV, mean corpuscular volume of red cells, PCV, packed cell volume, RCC, red cell count, WCC, white cell count.

Erythrocyte sedimentation rate (ESR)

This is the rate of fall of red cells in a column of blood and is a measure of the acute phase response. The pathological process may be immunological, infective, ischaemic, malignant or traumatic. A raised ESR reflects an increase in the plasma concentration of large proteins, such as fibrinogen and immunoglobulins. The proteins cause rouleaux formation, when cells clump together like a stack of coins, and therefore fall more rapidly. The ESR increases with age, and is higher in females than males. It is low in polycythaemia vera, owing to the high red cell concentration, and increased in patients with severe anaemia.

Plasma viscosity

Plasma viscosity measurement is used instead of the ESR in many laboratories. As with the ESR, the level is dependent on the concentration of large molecules such as fibrinogen and immunoglobulins. There is no difference between levels found in males and females, and viscosity increases only slightly in the elderly. It is not affected by the level of Hb and the result may be obtained within 15 minutes.

C-reactive protein

C-reactive protein is one of the proteins produced in the acute phase response. It is synthesized exclusively in the liver and rises within 6 hours of an acute event. It rises with temperature (possibly triggered by IL-1) and in inflammatory conditions and after trauma. It follows the clinical state of the patient much more rapidly than does the ESR and is unaffected by the level of Hb, but it is less helpful than the ESR or plasma viscosity in monitoring chronic inflammatory diseases. Its measurement is easy and quick to perform using an immunoassay that can be automated. Sophisticated equipment is required and it is more expensive than the ESR, particularly when assayed in small numbers.

The red cell

Erythropoiesis

Red cell precursors pass through several stages in the bone marrow. The earliest morphologically recognizable cells are *pronormoblasts*. Smaller *normoblasts* result from cell divisions and precursors at each stage progressively contain less RNA and more Hb in the cytoplasm. The nucleus becomes more condensed and is eventually lost from the late normoblast in the bone marrow, when the cell becomes a *reticulocyte*.

Reticulocytes contain residual ribosomal RNA and are still able to synthesize Hb. They remain in the marrow for about 1–2 days and are released into the circulation, where they lose their RNA and become mature red cells (or erythrocytes) after another 1–2 days. Mature red cells are non-nucleated biconcave discs.

Nucleated red cells (normoblasts) are not normally present in peripheral blood, but are present if there is extramedullary haemopoiesis and in some marrow disorders (see leucoeryothroblastic anaemia, p. 397).

About 10% of erythroblasts die in the bone marrow even during normal erythropoiesis. Such *ineffective erythropoiesis* is substantially increased in some anaemias such as thalassaemia major and megaloblastic anaemia.

Erythropoiesis is controlled by the hormone *erythropoietin*. The gene for erythropoietin on chromosome 7 codes for a heavily glycosylated polypeptide of 165 amino acids. Erythropoietin has a molecular weight of 30 400 and is produced in the peritubular cells in the kidneys (90%) and in the liver (10%). Its production is regulated mainly by tissue oxygen tension. Production is increased if there is hypoxia from whatever cause – for example, anaemia or cardiac or pulmonary disease. Erythropoietin stimulates an increase in the proportion of bone marrow precursor cells committed to erythropoiesis, and CFU-E are stimulated to proliferate and differentiate. Increased 'inappropriate' production of erythropoietin is also seen in patients with renal disease and neoplasms in other sites resulting in polycythaemia (see Table 6.15).

Other requirements for normal erythropoiesis

- Iron for Hb synthesis
- Vitamin B_{12} and folate for normal DNA synthesis
- Other vitamins – B_6 (pyridoxine), thiamin, riboflavin, and vitamins C and E
- Trace metals such as cobalt
- Hormones – androgens and thyroxine.

Haemoglobin synthesis

Haemoglobin performs the main functions of red cells – carrying O_2 to the tissues and returning CO_2 from the tissues to the lungs.

Each normal adult Hb molecule (Hb A) has a molecular weight of 68 000 and consists of two α and two β polypeptide chains ($\alpha_2\beta_2$) which have 141 and 146 amino acids respectively. Hb A comprises about 97% of the Hb in adults. Two other types, Hb A_2 ($\alpha_2\delta_2$) and Hb F ($\alpha_2\gamma_2$), are found in adults in small amounts (1.5–3.2% and <1%, respectively).

Haemoglobin synthesis occurs in the mitochondria of the developing red cell (Fig 6.2). The major rate-limiting step is the conversion of glycine and succinic acid to δ-aminolaevulinic acid (ALA) by ALA synthetase. Vitamin B_6 is a coenzyme for this reaction which is inhibited by haem and stimulated by erythro-poietin. Two molecules of δ-ALA condense to form a pyrrole ring (porphobilinogen). These rings are then grouped in fours to produce protoporphyrins. Finally, iron is inserted to form haem. Haem is then inserted into the globin chains to form Hb. The structure of Hb is shown in Fig 6.3.

Haemoglobin function

The biconcave shape of red cells provides a large surface area for the uptake and release of oxygen and carbon dioxide. Haemoglobin becomes saturated with oxygen in the pulmonary capillaries where the partial pressure of oxygen is high and Hb has a high affinity for oxygen. Oxygen is released in the tissues where the partial pressure of oxygen is low and Hb has a low affinity for oxygen.

The four haem units in Hb molecules successively take up oxygen in the lungs. The binding of oxygen to each haem unit becomes stronger in turn because of a

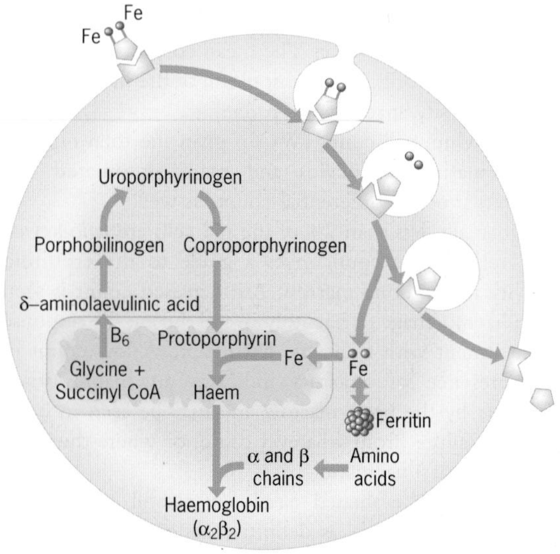

Fig 6.2
Haemoglobin synthesis. Transferrin attaches to a surface receptor on developing red cells. Iron is released and transported to the mitochondria, where it combines with protoporphyrin to form haemoglobin. Haem combines with α and β chains (formed on ribosomes) to make haemoglobin

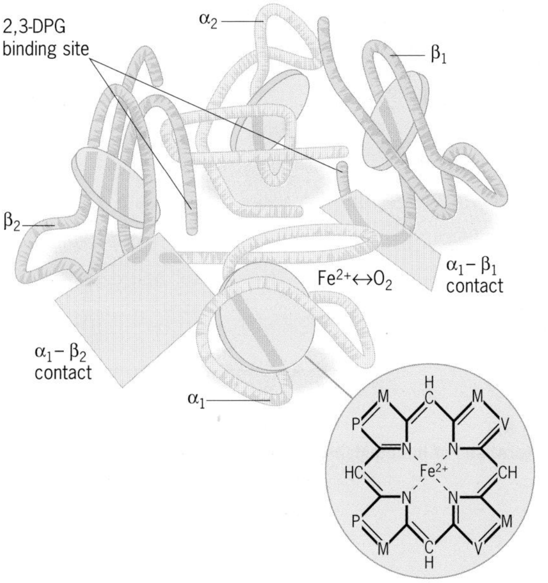

Fig 6.3
Model of the haemoglobin molecule showing α (pink) and β (blue) chains. 2,3-DPG binds in the centre of the molecule and stabilizes the deoxygenated form by cross-linking the β chains (also see Fig 6.4). M, methyl; P, propionic acid; V, vinyl. From Schrier SL (1988) *Scientific American* **10**, with permission

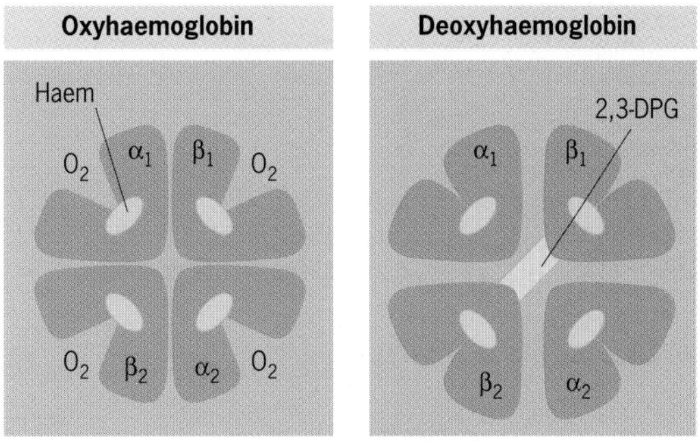

Fig 6.4
Oxygenated and deoxygenated haemoglobin molecule. The haemoglobin molecule is predominantly stabilized by α–β chain bonds rather than α–α and β–β chain bonds. The structure of the molecule changes during O_2 uptake and release. When O_2 is released, the β chains rotate on the $\alpha_1\beta_2$ and $\alpha_2\beta_1$ contacts, allowing the entry of 2,3-DPG which causes a lower affinity of haemoglobin for O_2 and improved delivery of O_2 to the tissues. From Hoffbrand AV, Pettit JE (1993) *Essential Haematology*, 3rd edn. Oxford: Blackwell Scientific Publications, with permission

conformational change in the Hb molecule allowing it to acquire more oxygen until it becomes saturated. The reverse occurs in the tissues, loss of oxygen becoming more difficult as Hb becomes desaturated. 2,3-diphosphoglycerate (2,3-DPG), an intermediate in red cell glycolysis (see Fig 6.22), influences this process by binding preferentially to deoxyhaemoglobin, stabilizing it, and thus making oxygen more readily available to the tissues (Fig 6.4). During hypoxia, such as during acclimatization to altitude, 2,3-DPG levels increase as a compensatory mechanism before erythropoietin produces an increase in level of Hb.

Haemoglobin is efficient for oxygen transport largely because the steepest part of the oxygen dissociation curve occurs at the partial pressures of oxygen which occur in the tissues. The *oxygen affinity* of Hb is expressed as the P_{50}, which is the partial pressure of oxygen at which 50% saturation occurs. When oxygen affinity increases, the oxygen dissociation curve shifts to the left and the P_{50} falls, and vice versa (Fig 13.5).

The oxygen dissociation curve is influenced by 2,3-DPG, the pH, the concentration of carbon dioxide in the red cell, and the structure of Hb. High concentrations of 2,3-DPG or carbon dioxide, a low pH and certain haemoglobins such as sickle Hb (Hb S), shift the curve to the right, thus decreasing oxygen affinity. A shift in the curve to the left occurs with some rare abnormal haemoglobins where erythrocytosis may result from the increased oxygen affinity and decreased release of oxygen to the tissues, and also with Hb F which is unable to bind 2,3-DPG. The resulting high oxygen affinity of Hb F means that it carries more oxygen at a given partial pressure than does Hb A, and the combination of high oxygen affinity with low blood pH ensures adequate oxygenation of fetal tissues.

A summary of normal red cell production and destruction is given in Fig 6.5.

FURTHER READING

Haynes AP, Hunter AE, Russell NH (1996) The clinical use of haemopoietic growth factors. In: Brenner MK, Hoffbrand AV (eds) *Recent Advances in Haematology*, 8th edn. Edinburgh: Churchill Livingstone.

Hoelzer D (1997) Hematopoietic growth factors: not whether, but when and where. *New England Journal of Medicine* **336**: 1822–1824.

Levin J (1997) Thrombopoietin: clinically realized? *New England Journal of Medicine* **336**: 434–436.

Lowe GDO (1994) Should plasma viscosity replace the ESR? *British Journal of Haematology* **86**: 6–11.

Scott MA, Gordon MY (1995) In search of the haemopoietic stem cell. *British Journal of Haematology* **90**: 738–743.

Anaemia

Anaemia is present when there is a decrease in the level of haemoglobin in the blood below the reference level for the age and sex of the individual (Table 6.1). Alterations in the level of Hb may occur as a result of changes in the plasma volume, as shown in Fig 6.6. A reduction in the plasma volume will lead to a spuriously high Hb – this is seen with dehydration and in the clinical condition of

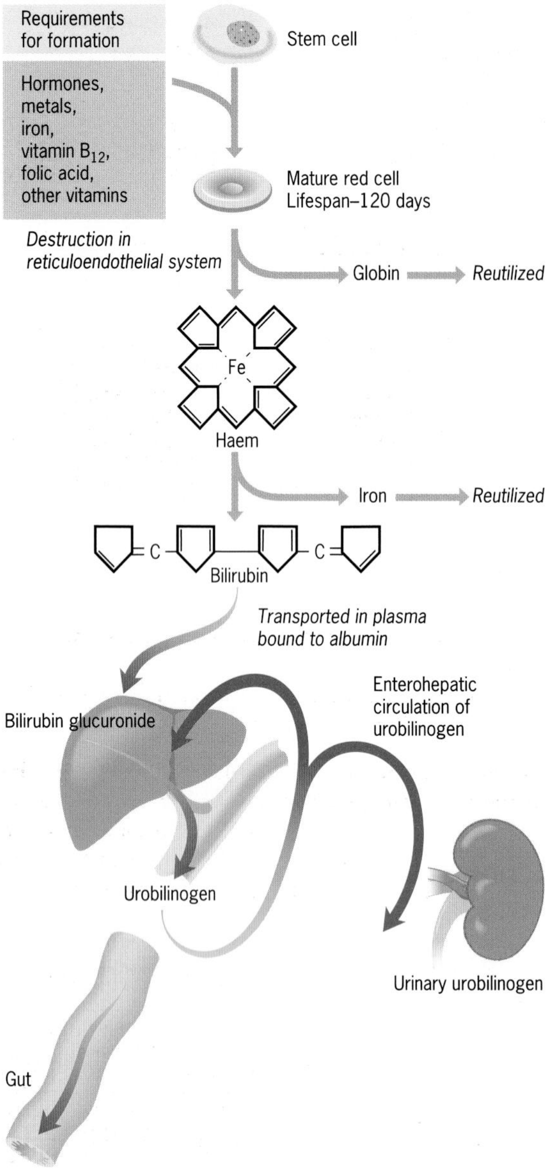

Fig 6.5
Red cell production and breakdown

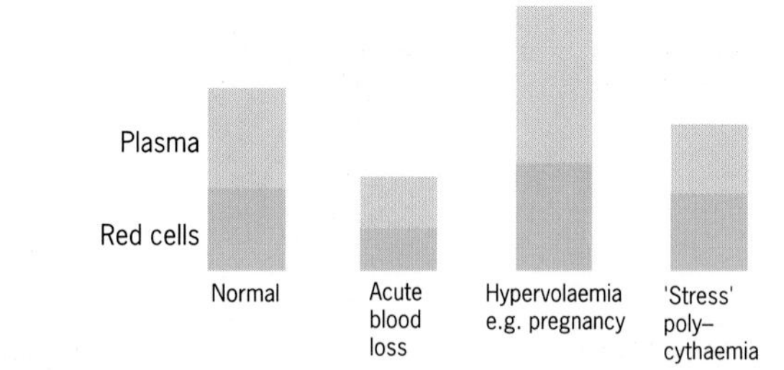

	Normal	Acute blood loss	Hypervolaemia e.g. pregnancy	'Stress' poly–cythaemia
Hb level	N	N	↓	↑
Red cell volume	N	↓	↑	N
Plasma volume	N	↓	↑↑	↓

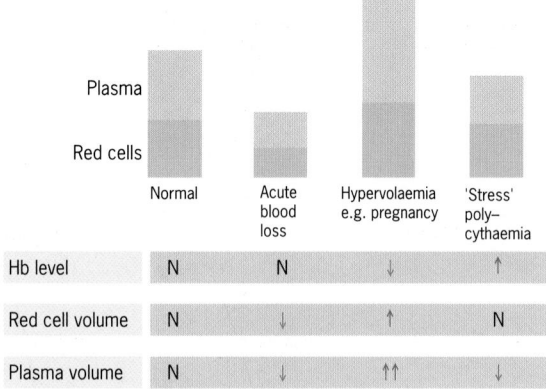

Fig 6.6
Alterations of haemoglobin in relation to plasma

stress polycythaemia (see p. 389). A raised plasma volume produces a spurious anaemia, even when combined with a small increase in red cell volume as occurs in pregnancy. After a major bleed, anaemia may not be apparent for several days until the plasma volume returns to normal.

The various types of anaemia, classified in terms of the red cell indices, particularly the MCV, are shown in Fig 6.7. There are three major types:

- hypochromic microcytic with a low MCV
- normochromic normocytic with a normal MCV
- macrocytic with a high MCV.

CLINICAL FEATURES

Patients with anaemia may be asymptomatic. A slowly falling level of Hb allows for haemodynamic compensation and enhancement of the oxygen-carrying capacity of the blood. A rise in 2,3-DPG causes a shift of the oxygen dissociation curve to the right, so that oxygen is more readily given up to the tissues. Where blood loss is rapid, more severe symptoms will occur, particularly in elderly people.

Symptoms (all nonspecific)

- Fatigue
- Headaches
- Faintness
  (the above three are all very common in the general population)
- Breathlessness
- Angina of effort
- Intermittent claudication
- Palpitations.

Signs

- Pallor
- Tachycardia
- Systolic flow murmur
- Cardiac failure
- Rarely papilloedema and retinal haemorrhages after an acute bleed (can be accompanied by blindness).

Specific signs of the different types of anaemia will be discussed in the appropriate sections. Examples include:

- koilonychia – spoon-shaped nails seen in iron deficiency anaemia
- jaundice – found in haemolytic anaemia
- bone deformities – found in thalassaemia major
- leg ulcers – occur in association with sickle cell disease.

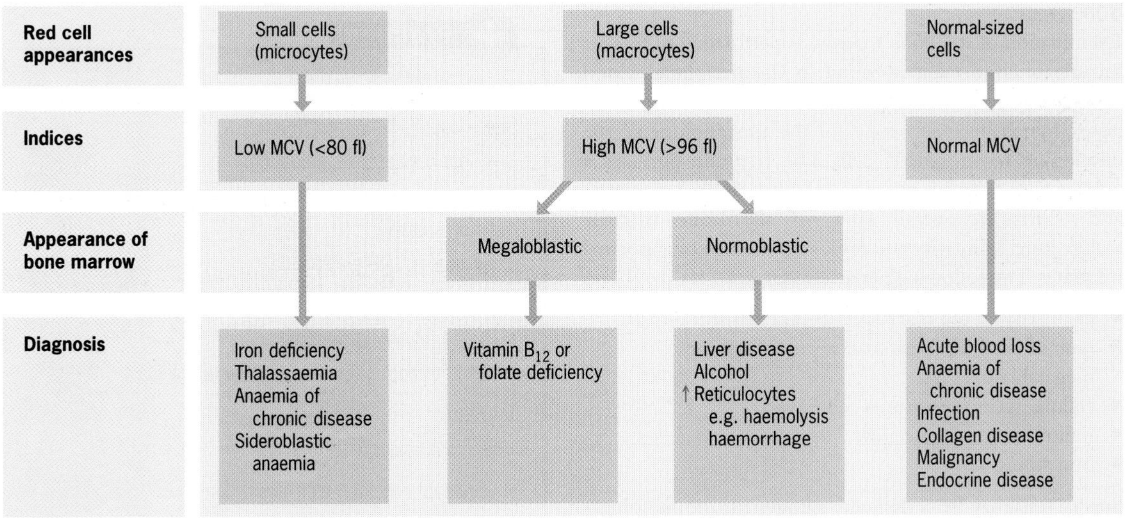

Fig 6.7
Classification of anaemia

It must be emphasized that *anaemia is not a diagnosis*, and a cause must be found.

INVESTIGATIONS

Peripheral blood

A low haemoglobin should always be considered in relation to:

- the white blood cell (WBC) count
- the platelet count
- the reticulocyte count (as this indicates marrow activity)
- the blood film, as abnormal red cell morphology (see Fig 6.8) may indicate the diagnosis.

Where two populations of red cells are seen, the blood film is said to be *dimorphic*. This may, for example, be seen in patients with 'double deficiencies' (e.g. combined iron and folate deficiency in coeliac disease), or following treatment of anaemic patients with the appropriate haematinic.

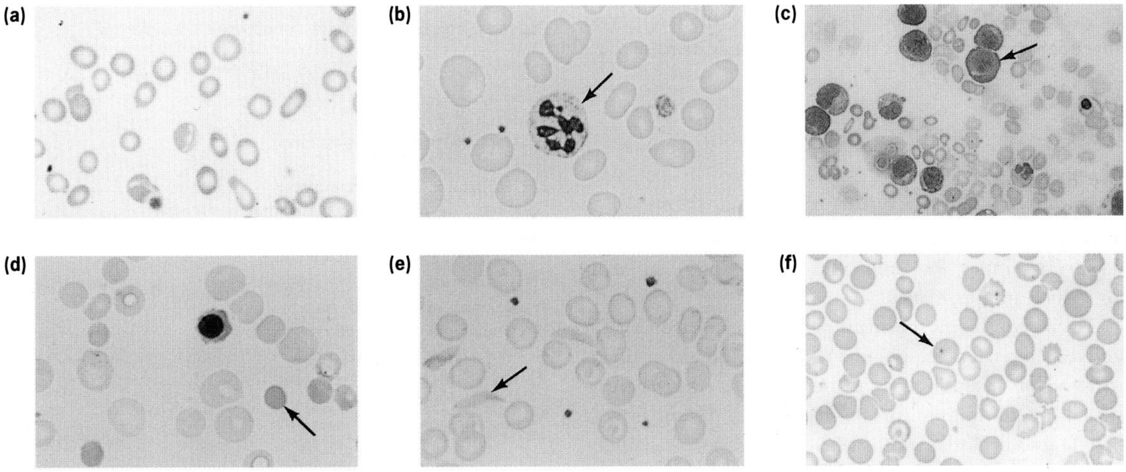

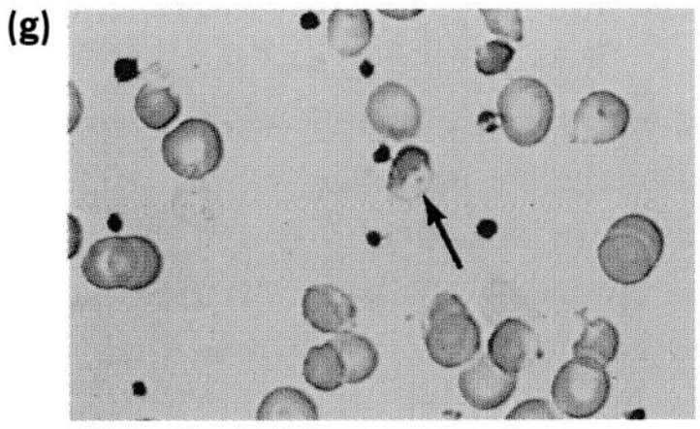

Fig 6.8
Shapes of cells.
(a) Hypochromic microcytic cells
(b) Macrocytes and a hypersegmented neutrophil (arrowed)
(c) Megaloblasts (arrowed) in the bone marrow
(d) Spherocytes (arrowed), reticulocytes, polychromasias and a nucleated erythroblast
(e) Sickle cells (arrowed) and target cells
(f) Postsplenectomy film with Howell–Jolly bodies (arrowed), target cells and irregularly contracted cells
(g) 'Blister' cells (arrowed) in G6PD deficiency

Bone marrow

Examination of the bone marrow is performed to further investigate abnormalities found in the peripheral blood (Practical box 6.1). Aspiration provides a film which can be examined by microscopy for the morphology of the developing haemopoietic cells. The trephine provides a core of bone which is processed as a histological specimen and allows an overall view of the bone marrow architecture, cellularity and presence/absence of abnormal infiltrates. The following are assessed:

- cellularity of the marrow
- type of erythropoiesis (e.g. normoblastic or megaloblastic)
- cellularity of the various cell lines
- infiltration of the marrow
- iron stores.

Special tests may be performed: cytogenetic, immunological, cytochemical markers, biochemical analyses (e.g. deoxyuridine suppression test), microbiological culture.

Practical

Aspiration

Site – usually iliac crest

Give local anaesthetic injection

Use special bone marrow needle (e.g. Salah)

Aspirate marrow

Make smear with glass slide

Stain with:

- Romanowsky technique
- Perls' reaction (acid ferrocyanide) for iron.

Trephine

Indications include:

- 'Dry tap' obtained with aspiration
- Better assessment of cellularity, e.g. aplastic anaemia
- Better assessment of presence of infiltration or fibrosis.

Technique

Site – usually posterior iliac crest

Give local anaesthetic injection

Use special needle (e.g. Jamshidi – longer and wider than for aspiration)

Obtain core of bone

Fix in formalin; decalcify – this takes a few days

Stain with:

- Haematoxylin and eosin
- Reticulin stain.

Practical box 6.1 Techniques for obtaining bone marrow

Microcytic anaemia

Iron deficiency is the most common cause of anaemia in the world. This is because of the body's limited ability to absorb iron and the frequent increased loss of iron owing to haemorrhage. The other causes of a microcytic hypochromic anaemia are anaemia of chronic disease, sideroblastic anaemia, and thalassaemia. In thalassaemia (described on p. 375) there is a defect in globin synthesis, in contrast to the other three causes of microcytic anaemia where the defect is in the synthesis of haem.

Table 6.2
Factors influencing iron absorption

Haem iron is absorbed better than non-haem iron
Ferrous iron is absorbed better than ferric iron
Gastric acidity helps to keep iron in the ferrous state and soluble in the upper gut
Formation of insoluble complexes with phytate or phosphate decreases iron absorption
Iron absorption is increased with low iron stores and increased erythropoietic activity, e.g. bleeding, haemolysis, high altitude
There is a decreased absorption in iron overload, except in hereditary haemochromatosis, where it is increased

Iron

Dietary intake

The average daily diet in the UK contains 15–20 mg of iron, although normally only 10% of this is absorbed. Absorption may be increased to 20–30% in iron deficiency and pregnancy.

Haem iron forms the main part of dietary iron and is derived from haemoglobin and myoglobin in red or organ meats. Non-haem iron is mainly derived from cereals which are commonly fortified with iron. Haem iron is better absorbed than non-haem iron whose availability is more affected by other dietary constituents.

Absorption

This takes place in the duodenum and jejunum. The absorption of iron is a complex process; some of the factors influencing it are shown in Table 6.2. Haem iron is partly broken down to non-haem iron, but some haem iron is absorbed intact into mucosal cells. Absorption is favoured by factors such as the acidity of the stomach keeping the iron soluble and in the ferrous rather than the ferric form.

The iron content of the body is kept within narrow limits and its loss and intake are normally finely balanced. The precise mechanisms by which iron is absorbed and transported across the epithelial cell are uncertain, but its absorption appears to be closely related to the total iron stores of the body. The body is unable to excrete iron once it has been absorbed. Iron overload may occur owing to excessive absorption of iron (haemochromatosis, see p. 325).

Iron absorption seems to be controlled by mucosal cells in the small intestine, possibly at both the stages of uptake of iron into the cells and transfer of iron into the portal blood (see below). Excess iron in mucosal cells is joined to apoferritin to form ferritin. Ferritin is lost into the gut lumen when the mucosal cells are shed. In iron deficiency, more iron enters the cells and a greater proportion of the intracellular iron is transported to the portal vein. In iron overload, less iron enters the cells and a greater proportion is shed into the gut lumen.

Transport in the blood

The normal serum iron level is about 11–30 μmol L^{-1}; there is a diurnal rhythm with higher levels in the morning. Iron is transported in the plasma bound to transferrin, a β-globulin that is synthesized in the liver. Each transferrin molecule binds two atoms of ferric iron and is normally one-third saturated. Most of the iron bound to transferrin comes from macrophages in the reticuloendothelial system and not from iron absorbed by the intestine. Transferrin-bound iron becomes attached by specific receptors to erythroblasts and reticulocytes in the marrow and the iron is removed (see Fig 6.2).

In an average adult male, 20 mg of iron, chiefly obtained from red cell breakdown in the macrophages of the reticuloendothelial system, is incorporated into Hb every day.

Iron stores

About two-thirds of the total body iron is in the circulation as haemoglobin (2.5–3 g in a normal adult man). Iron is stored in reticuloendothelial cells, hepatocytes and skeletal muscle cells (500–1500 mg). About two-thirds of this is stored as ferritin and one-third as haemosiderin in normal individuals. Small amounts of iron are also found in plasma (about 4 mg bound to transferrin), with some in myoglobin and enzymes.

Ferritin is a water-soluble complex of iron and protein. It is more easily mobilized than haemosiderin for Hb formation. It is present in small amounts in plasma.

Haemosiderin is an insoluble iron–protein complex found in macrophages in the bone marrow, liver and spleen. Unlike ferritin, it is visible by light microscopy in tissue sections and bone marrow films after staining by Perls' reaction.

Cellular iron homeostasis

This depends on the storage protein ferritin and the entry of iron into the cell via the transferrin receptor. The regulation appears to be dependent on the 'iron responsive element-binding protein' (IRE-BP encoded on chromosome 9) in the cytosol which undergoes a reversible change depending on iron availability. If iron levels are high, IRE-BP binds to the 5′ sequence in ferritin mRNA, allowing translation to take place thereby increasing ferritin synthesis and thus iron storage. At the same time transferrin receptors are downregulated because its mRNA is degraded.

Requirements

Each day 0.5–1.0 mg of iron is lost in the faeces, urine and sweat. Menstruating women lose 40 mL of blood per month, an average of about 0.7 mg of iron per day. Blood loss through menstruation in excess of 100 mL will usually result in iron deficiency as increased iron absorption from the gut cannot compensate for such losses of iron. The demand for iron also increases during growth (about 0.6 mg per day) and pregnancy (1–2 mg per day).

In the normal adult the iron content of the body remains relatively fixed. Increases in the body iron content (haemochromatosis) are classified into:

- hereditary haemochromatosis (p. 325)
- secondary haemochromatosis (transfusion siderosis; see p. 376).

The latter is due to iron overload in conditions where repeated transfusion is the only therapy.

Iron deficiency

Iron deficiency anaemia develops when there is inadequate iron for haemoglobin synthesis. A normal level of Hb is maintained for as long as possible after the iron stores are depleted; *latent iron deficiency* is said to be present during this period.

CAUSES

- Blood loss
- Increased demands such as growth and pregnancy
- Decreased absorption (e.g. postgastrectomy)
- Poor intake.

Most iron deficiency is due to *blood loss*, usually from the uterus or gastrointestinal tract. Premenopausal women are always in a state of precarious iron balance owing to menstruation. Iron deficiency affects more than a quarter of the world's population, but isolated nutritional iron deficiency is rare in developed countries. The most common cause of iron deficiency worldwide is blood loss from the gastrointestinal tract resulting from hookworm infestation. The poor quality of the diet, predominantly containing vegetables, also contributes to the high prevalence of iron deficiency in developing countries.

CLINICAL FEATURES

The symptoms of anaemia are described on p. 358. Other clinical features occur as a result of tissue iron deficiency. These are mainly epithelial changes induced by the effect of inadequate iron in the cells:

- brittle nails
- spoon-shaped nails (koilonychia)

- atrophy of the papillae of the tongue
- angular stomatitis
- brittle hair
- a syndrome of dysphagia and glossitis (Plummer–Vinson or Paterson–Brown–Kelly syndrome, see p. 231).

The diagnosis of iron deficiency anaemia relies on a good clinical history with questions about dietary intake, regular self-medication with non-steroidal anti-inflammatory drugs (which may give rise to gastrointestinal bleeding), and the presence of blood in the faeces (which may be a sign of haemorrhoids or carcinoma of the lower bowel). In women, a careful enquiry about the duration of periods, the occurrence of clots and the number of sanitary towels or tampons (normal 3–5/day) used should be made.

INVESTIGATIONS

Blood count and film

A characteristic blood film is shown in Fig 6.8. The red cells are microcytic (MCV < 80 fl) and hypochromic (MCH < 27 pg). There is *poikilocytosis* (variation in shape) and *anisocytosis* (variation in size). Target cells are seen.

Serum ferritin

The level of serum ferritin reflects the amount of stored iron, probably more accurately than the serum iron and iron-binding capacity, which are less frequently used to assess iron status now. The normal values for serum ferritin are 30–300 μg L^{-1} (11.6–144 nmol L^{-1}) in males and 15–200 μg L^{-1} (5.8–96 nmol L^{-1}) in females.

Serum iron and iron-binding capacity

The changes in serum iron and iron-binding capacity in iron deficiency compared with normal are included in Fig 6.9; the serum iron falls and the total iron-binding capacity (TIBC) rises compared with normal. Iron deficiency is regularly present when the *transferrin saturation* (i.e. serum iron divided by TIBC) falls below 19%.

Serum-soluble transferrin receptor

This immunoassay is now available, and when combined with serum ferritin compares well with results from bone marrow aspiration at estimating iron stores.

Bone marrow

Erythroid hyperplasia with ragged normoblasts are seen in the marrow in iron deficiency. Staining using Perls' reaction (acid ferrocyanide) does not show the characteristic Prussian-blue granules of stainable iron in the bone marrow fragments or in the erythroblasts.

Examination of the bone marrow is not essential for the diagnosis of iron deficiency but it may be helpful in the investigation of complicated cases of anaemia.

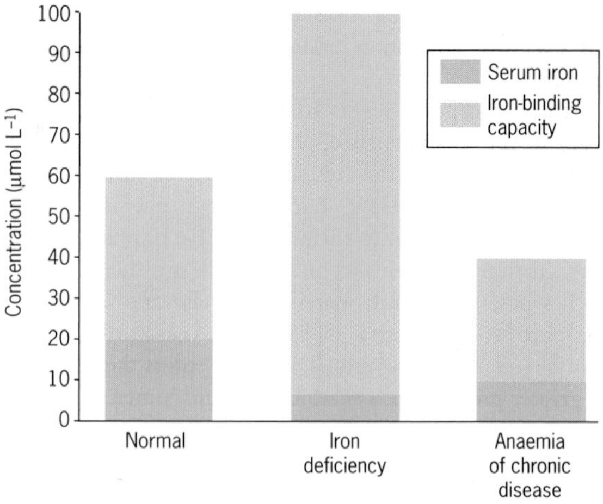

Fig 6.9
Serum iron and total iron-binding capacity in normal subjects, iron deficiency anaemia and anaemia of chronic disease

Other investigations

These will be indicated by the clinical history and examination. Investigations of the gastrointestinal tract are often required (see p. 246).

DIFFERENTIAL DIAGNOSIS

The presence of anaemia with microcytosis and hypochromia does not necessarily indicate iron deficiency. The most common other causes are thalassaemia, sideroblastic anaemia and anaemia of chronic disease, and in these disorders the iron stores are normal or increased. The differential diagnosis of microcytic anaemia is shown in Table 6.3.

TREATMENT

The correct management of iron deficiency is to find and treat the underlying cause, and to give iron to correct the anaemia and replace iron stores. The response to iron therapy can be monitored using the reticulocyte count and Hb level with an expected rise in haemoglobin of 1 g per week.

Oral iron is all that is required in most cases. The best preparation is ferrous sulphate (600 mg daily, 120 mg ferrous iron) which is absorbed best when the patient is fasting. If the patient has side-effects such as nausea, diarrhoea or constipation, taking the tablets with food or reducing the dose using a preparation with less iron such as ferrous gluconate (600 mg daily, only 70 mg ferrous iron) is all that is usually required to reduce the symptoms. The use of expensive iron compounds, particularly the slow-release ones which release iron beyond its main sites of absorption, is unnecessary.

In developing countries, distribution of iron tablets is the main approach for the alleviation of iron deficiency. However, iron supplementation programmes have been ineffective, probably mainly because of poor compliance.

Table 6.3
Microcytic anaemia: the differential diagnosis

	Iron deficiency	Anaemia of chronic disease	Thalassaemia trait (α or β)	Sideroblastic anaemia
MCV	Reduced	Low normal or normal	Very low for degree of anaemia	Low in inherited type but often raised in acquired type
Serum iron	Reduced	Reduced	Normal	Raised
Serum TIBC	Raised	Reduced	Normal	Normal
Serum ferritin	Reduced	Normal or raised	Normal	Raised
Iron in marrow	Absent	Present	Present	Present
Iron in erythroblasts	Absent	Absent or reduced	Present	Ring forms

TIBC, total iron binding capacity.

Oral iron should be given for long enough to correct the Hb level and to replenish the iron stores. This can take six months. Failure of response to oral iron may be due to:

- lack of compliance
- continuing haemorrhage
- severe malabsorption
- another cause for the anaemia.

These possibilities should be considered before parenteral iron is used. However, parenteral iron is required by occasional patients, including those who have general intolerance of oral preparations even at low dose, those with severe malabsorption, and those who have chronic gastrointestinal diseases such as ulcerative colitis or Crohn's disease. Iron stores are replaced much faster with parenteral iron than with oral iron, but the haematological response is no quicker. Parenteral iron can be given as repeated deep intramuscular injections of iron-sorbitol. No preparations of iron are currently available for intravenous use in the UK.

Anaemia of chronic disease

One of the most common types of anaemia, particularly in hospital patients, is the anaemia of chronic disease, occurring in patients with chronic infections such as infective endocarditis and tuberculosis and osteomyelitis in developing countries, chronic inflammatory diseases such as rheumatoid arthritis, systemic lupus erythematosus (SLE) and polymyalgia rheumatica, and in patients with malignant disease. There is decreased release of iron from the bone marrow to developing erythroblasts, an inadequate erythropoietin response to the anaemia, and decreased red cell survival. The exact mechanisms responsible for these effects are not clear, but they seem to be mediated by inflammatory cytokines such as IL-1, tumour necrosis factor and interferons.

The serum iron is low and the TIBC is also low (Fig 6.9). Serum ferritin is normal or raised because of the inflammatory process. There is stainable iron present in the bone marrow and, therefore, patients do not respond to iron therapy. However, iron is not seen in the developing erythroblasts. Treatment is, in general, that of the underlying disorder. However, trials are being carried out with recombinant erythropoietin in rheumatoid arthritis with some success, and also in inflammatory bowel disease, where treatment in combination with oral iron produced an increase of more than 1 g dL^{-1} in more than 80% of patients after 12 weeks' therapy.

Sideroblastic anaemia

Sideroblastic anaemias are inherited or acquired disorders characterized by a refractory anaemia, a variable number of hypochromic cells in the peripheral blood, and excess iron and *ring sideroblasts* in the bone marrow. The presence of ring sideroblasts is the diagnostic feature of sideroblastic anaemia; there is disordered accumulation of iron in the mitochondria of erythroblasts owing to disordered haem synthesis. A ring of iron granules is formed around the nucleus that can be seen with Perls' reaction. The blood film is often dimorphic; ineffective haem synthesis is responsible for the microcytic hypochromic cells. Sideroblastic anaemias can be classified as shown in Table 6.4. A structural defect in δ-aminolaevulinic acid (ALA) synthetase, the pyridoxine-dependent enzyme responsible for the merger of glycine and succinic acid as the first step in haem synthesis, has been identified in one form of inherited sideroblastic anaemia. Primary acquired sideroblastic anaemia is one of the myelodysplastic syndromes (see p. 390).

TREATMENT

Some patients respond when drugs or alcohol are withdrawn if these are the causative agents. In occasional cases, there is a response to pyridoxine. Treatment with folic acid may be required to treat accompanying folate deficiency.

Table 6.4
Classification of sideroblastic anaemia

Inherited	
X-linked disease – transmitted by females	
Acquired	
Primary (one of the myelodysplastic syndromes, see p. 390)	
Secondary	
Other types of myelodysplasia	
Myeloproliferative disorders	
Myeloid leukaemia	
Drugs, e.g. isoniazid	
Alcohol	
Lead	
Other disorders, e.g. rheumatoid arthritis, carcinoma, megaloblastic and haemolytic anaemias, malabsorption	

Lead poisoning

The causes, clinical features and treatment are discussed on p. 880. The characteristic haematological features include:

- *sideroblastic anaemia*, due to inhibition by lead of several enzymes involved in haem synthesis, including ALA synthetase
- *haemolysis*, which is usually mild, resulting from damage to the red cell membrane
- *punctate basophilia* (or basophilic stippling: the blood film shows red cells with small, round, blue particles), due to aggregates of RNA in red cells owing to inhibition by lead of pyrimidine-5-nucleotidase, which normally disperses residual RNA to produce a diffuse blue staining seen in reticulocytes on blood films (*polychromasia*).

Normocytic anaemia

Normocytic, normochromic anaemia is seen in anaemia of chronic disease, in some endocrine disorders (e.g. hypopituitarism, hypothyroidism and hypoadrenalism) and in some haematological disorders (e.g. aplastic anaemia and some haemolytic anaemias) (see Fig 6.7). In addition, this type of anaemia is seen acutely following blood loss.

Macrocytic anaemias

These can be divided into *megaloblastic* and *non-megaloblastic* types, depending on bone marrow findings.

Megaloblastic anaemia

Megaloblastic anaemia is characterized by the presence in the bone marrow of erythroblasts with delayed nuclear maturation because of defective DNA synthesis (*megaloblasts*). Megaloblasts are large and have large immature nuclei. The nuclear chromatin is more finely dispersed than normal and has an open stippled appearance (see Fig 6.8). A characteristic abnormality of white cells, *giant metamyelocytes*, is frequently seen in megaloblastic anaemia. These cells are about twice the size of normal cells and often have twisted nuclei. Megaloblastic changes occur in:

- vitamin B_{12} deficiency or abnormal vitamin B_{12} metabolism
- folic acid deficiency or abnormal folate metabolism
- other defects of DNA synthesis, such as congenital enzyme deficiencies in DNA synthesis (e.g. orotic aciduria), or resulting from therapy with drugs interfering with DNA synthesis (e.g. hydroxyurea, azathioprine, azidothymidine – AZT)
- myelodysplasia due to dyserythropoiesis.

Haematological values

Anaemia may be present. The MCV is characteristically >96 fl unless there is a coexisting cause of microcytosis. The peripheral blood film shows macrocytes with *hypersegmented polymorphs* with six or more lobes in the nucleus (see Fig 6.8). If severe, there may be leucopenia and thrombocytopenia.

Biochemical basis of megaloblastic anaemia

The key biochemical problem common to both vitamin B_{12} and folate deficiency is a block in DNA synthesis owing to an inability to methylate deoxyuridine monophosphate to deoxythymidine monophosphate, which is then used to build DNA (Fig 6.10). The methyl group is supplied by the folate coenzyme, methylene tetrahydrofolate polyglutamate. Deficiency of folate reduces the supply of this coenzyme; deficiency of vitamin B_{12} also reduces its supply by slowing the demethylation of methyl tetrahydrofolate and preventing cells receiving tetrahydrofolate for synthesis of methylene tetrahydrofolate.

Other congenital and acquired forms of megaloblastic anaemia are due to interference with purine or pyrimidine synthesis causing an inhibition in DNA synthesis.

Deoxyuridine suppression test

This is a useful method for rapidly determining the nature and severity of the vitamin B_{12} or folate deficiency in severe or complex cases of megaloblastic anaemia.

Tritiated thymidine is added to the patient's bone marrow *in vitro*. In a normoblastic marrow, the thymidine requirement is supplied by the methylation of deoxyuridine and this 'suppresses' the requirement for preformed tritiated thymidine to less than 5%. In a megaloblastic marrow, however, much more tritiated thymidine is used (5–50%). If the addition of B_{12} corrects the abnormality, it suggests that B_{12} is the cause of the deficiency. The addition of folate corrects the abnormality in both vitamin B_{12} and folate deficiency.

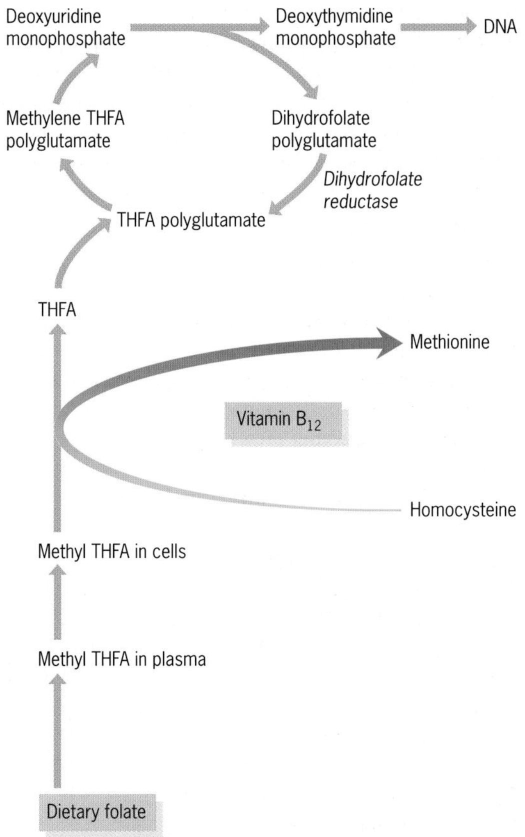

Fig 6.10
Biochemical basis of megaloblastic anaemia. The metabolic relationship between vitamin B_{12} and folate and their role in DNA synthesis. THFA, tetrahydrofolic acid

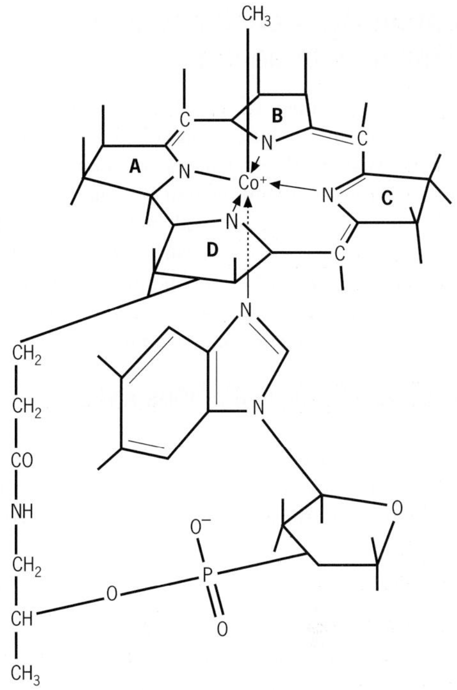

Fig 6.11
Methylcobalamin structure. This is the main form of vitamin B_{12} in the plasma

Vitamin B_{12}

Vitamin B_{12} is synthesized by certain micro-organisms, and humans are ultimately dependent on animal sources. It is found in meat, fish, eggs and milk, but not in plants. Vitamin B_{12} is not usually destroyed by cooking. The average daily diet contains 5–30 μg of vitamin B_{12}, of which 2–3 μg is absorbed. The average adult stores some 2–3 mg, mainly in the liver, and it may take two years or more after absorptive failure before B_{12} deficiency develops, as the daily losses are small (1–2 μg).

Structure and function

Cobalamins consist of a planar group with a central cobalt atom (corrin ring) and a nucleotide set at right-angles (Fig 6.11). Vitamin B_{12} was first crystallized as cyanocobalamin, but the main natural cobalamins have deoxyadenosyl-, methyl- and hydroxocobalamin groups attached to the cobalt atom.

Methylcobalamin is a coenzyme for the methylation of homocysteine to methionine by methyltetrahydrofolate, as described above (see Fig 6.10).

Deoxyadenosylcobalamin is a coenzyme for the conversion of methylmalonyl CoA to succinyl CoA. Measurement of methylmalonic acid in urine was used as a test for vitamin B_{12} deficiency but it is no longer carried out routinely.

Absorption and transport

Vitamin B_{12} is liberated from protein complexes in food by gastric enzymes and then binds to two vitamin B_{12}-binding proteins, intrinsic factor and 'R' binder derived from saliva. Vitamin B_{12} bound to 'R' binder is released by pancreatic enzymes and also becomes bound to intrinsic factor.

Intrinsic factor is a glycoprotein with a molecular weight of over 44 000. It is secreted by gastric parietal cells along with H^+ ions. It combines with vitamin B_{12} and carries it to specific receptors on the surface of the mucosa of the ileum. Vitamin B_{12} enters the ileal cells and intrinsic factor remains in the lumen. Vitamin B_{12} is transported from the enterocytes to the bone marrow and other tissues by the glycoprotein *transcobalamin II* (TC II). Although TC II is the essential carrier protein for vitamin B_{12}, the amount of B_{12} on TC II is low; it has a rapid clearance and is able to deliver cobalamin to all cells of the body. Vitamin B_{12} in plasma is mainly bound to *transcobalamin I* (TC I) (70–90%), but its functional role is unknown.

Vitamin B_{12} deficiency and pernicious anaemia

There are a number of causes of B_{12} deficiency and abnormal B_{12} metabolism (Table 6.5). The most common cause of vitamin B_{12} deficiency in adults is *pernicious anaemia*. Malabsorption of vitamin B_{12} due to pancreatitis, coeliac disease or treatment with metformin is mild and does not usually result in significant vitamin B_{12} deficiency.

Pernicious anaemia (PA) is a condition in which there is atrophy of the gastric mucosa with consequent failure of intrinsic factor production and vitamin B_{12} malabsorption.

PATHOGENESIS OF PERNICIOUS ANAEMIA

This disease is common in the elderly, with 1 in 8000 of the population aged over 60 years being affected in the UK. It can be seen in all races, but is particularly common in fair-haired and blue-eyed people. It is more common in females than males.

There is an association with other autoimmune diseases, particularly thyroid disease, Addison's disease and vitiligo. Approximately one-half of all patients with PA have thyroid antibodies. There is a higher incidence of gastric carcinoma in males with PA than in the general population; females have a normal life expectancy with replacement therapy.

Parietal cell antibodies are present in the serum in 90% of patients with PA – and also in many older patients with gastric atrophy. Conversely, intrinsic factor antibodies, although found in only 50% of patients with PA, are specific for this diagnosis. Two types of intrinsic factor antibodies are found: a *blocking* antibody, which inhibits binding of intrinsic factor to B_{12}, and a *precipitating* antibody, which inhibits the binding of the B_{12}-intrinsic factor complex to its receptor site in the ileum.

B_{12} deficiency may rarely occur in children from a congenital deficiency or abnormality of intrinsic factor, or as a result of early onset of the adult autoimmune type.

Table 6.5 Vitamin B_{12} deficiency and abnormal B_{12} metabolism: other causes (see text)

Low dietary intake	**Abnormal metabolism**
Vegans	Congenital transcobalamin II deficiency
Impaired absorption	Nitrous oxide (inactivates B_{12})
Stomach	
Pernicious anaemia	
Gastrectomy	
Congenital deficiency of intrinsic factor	
Small bowel	
Ileal disease or resection	
Bacterial overgrowth	
Tropical sprue	
Fish tapeworm (*Diphyllobothrium latum*)	

PATHOLOGY

Atrophic gastritis (see p. 235) is present with plasma cell and lymphoid infiltration. There is achlorhydria and absent secretion of intrinsic factor. The histological abnormality can be improved by corticosteroid therapy, which supports an autoimmune basis for the disease.

CLINICAL FEATURES

The onset of PA is insidious, with progressively increasing symptoms of anaemia. Patients are sometimes said to have a lemon-yellow colour owing to a combination of pallor and mild jaundice caused by excess breakdown of haemoglobin due to ineffective erythropoiesis in the bone marrow. A red sore tongue (glossitis) and angular stomatitis are sometimes present.

The neurological changes are of greatest importance because if left untreated they can be irreversible. The neurological abnormalities occur only with very low levels of serum B_{12} (less than 60 ng L^{-1}) and occasionally occur in patients who are not clinically anaemic. The classical neurological features are those of a polyneuropathy progressively involving the peripheral nerves and the posterior and eventually the lateral columns of the spinal cord (subacute combined degeneration). Patients present with symmetrical paraesthesia in the fingers and toes, early loss of vibration sense and proprioception, and progressive weakness and ataxia. Paraplegia may result. Dementia and optic atrophy also occur from vitamin B_{12} deficiency.

INVESTIGATIONS

- **Haematological findings** show the features of a megaloblastic anaemia as described on p. 364.
- **Bone marrow** shows the typical features of megaloblastic erythropoiesis (see Fig 6.8).
- **Serum bilirubin** may be raised as a result of ineffective erythropoiesis. Normally a minor fraction of serum bilirubin results from premature breakdown of newly formed red cells in the bone marrow. In many megaloblastic anaemias, where the destruction of developing red cells is much increased, the serum bilirubin can be increased.
- **Serum vitamin B_{12}** is usually well below the normal level of 160 ng L^{-1}. Serum vitamin B_{12} can be assayed using radioisotope dilution or immunological assays. Microbiological assays were often used in the past, but have largely been abandoned in favour of less labour-intensive assays.
- **Serum folate level** is normal or high, and the red cell folate is normal or reduced owing to inhibition of normal folate synthesis.

Absorption tests

The absorption of B_{12} can be measured using the *Schilling* test (Practical box 6.2). This test may give a falsely low result if there is an incomplete 24 hour collection of urine or if renal function is impaired. An alternative to the Schilling test is *whole-body counting* where a radioactive dose of B_{12} is given orally and the total body activity is measured. The level of radioactivity is counted no less than 7 days later to measure how much vitamin B_{12} has been retained. A normal result is retention of 50% or more of the 1 μg dose of radioactive B_{12}.

Gastrointestinal investigations

In PA there is marked gastric atrophy with achlorhydria. Intubation studies can be performed to confirm this but are rarely carried out in routine practice. Endoscopy or barium meal examination of the stomach is performed only if gastric symptoms are present.

DIFFERENTIAL DIAGNOSIS

Vitamin B_{12} deficiency must be differentiated from other causes of megaloblastic anaemia, principally folate deficiency, but usually this is quite clear from the blood level of these two vitamins.

Pernicious anaemia must be distinguished from other causes of vitamin B_{12} deficiency (see Table 6.5). Any disease involving the terminal ileum or bacterial overgrowth in the small bowel can produce vitamin B_{12} deficiency (see p. 256). Gastrectomy can lead, in the long term, to vitamin B_{12} deficiency. Vegans are strict vegetarians and eat no meat or animal products. A careful dietary history should be obtained.

Folic acid

Folic acid monoglutamate is not present in nature but is the parent compound of folates, which are polyglutamates (extraglutamic acid residues).

Practical

Part 1

- Give 1 μg $^{58}Co\text{-}B_{12}$ orally to fasting patient
- Give 1000 μg B_{12} (non-radioactive) by intramuscular injection to saturate B_{12}-binding proteins and to flush out $^{58}Co\text{-}B_{12}$
- Collect urine for 24 hours
- Normal subjects excrete more than 10% of the radioactive dose.

Part 2

Repeat part 1 with oral intrinsic factor capsules

Result

- If excretion now normal, diagnosis is pernicious anaemia or gastrectomy
- If excretion is still abnormal, lesion is in the terminal ileum or there is bacterial overgrowth.
- Vitamin B_{12} malabsorption due to bacterial overgrowth may be corrected by antibiotic therapy

Practical box 6.2 Schilling test

Folates are present in food as polyglutamates in the reduced dihydrofolate or tetrahydrofolate forms (Fig 6.12), with methyl (CH_3), formyl (CHO) or methylene (CH_2) groups attached to the pteridine part of the molecule. Polyglutamates are broken down to monoglutamates in the upper gastrointestinal tract, and during the absorptive process these are converted to methyltetrahydrofolate monoglutamate which is the main form in the serum. Vitamin B_{12} converts methyltetrahydrofolate to tetrahydrofolate, which is the substrate for the synthesis of folate polyglutamates in cells. These intracellular folates are the active forms of folate and act as coenzymes in the transfer of single carbon units in amino acid metabolism and DNA synthesis (see Fig 6.10).

Dietary intake

Folate is found in green vegetables such as spinach and broccoli, and offal, such as liver and kidney. Cooking causes a loss of 60–90% of the folate. The minimal daily requirement is about 100 μg.

Folate deficiency

The causes of folate deficiency are shown in Table 6.6. The main cause is poor intake which may occur alone or in combination with excessive utilization or malabsorption. The body's reserves of folate, unlike vitamin B_{12}, are low. On a deficient diet, folate deficiency develops over the course of about four months, but folate deficiency may develop rapidly in patients who have both a poor intake and excess utilization of folate (e.g. patients in intensive care units).

CLINICAL FEATURES

Patients with folate deficiency may be asymptomatic but may present with symptoms of anaemia or of the underlying cause. Glossitis can occur. Unlike with B_{12} deficiency, neuropathy does not occur.

INVESTIGATIONS

The haematological findings are those of a megaloblastic anaemia as discussed on p. 364.

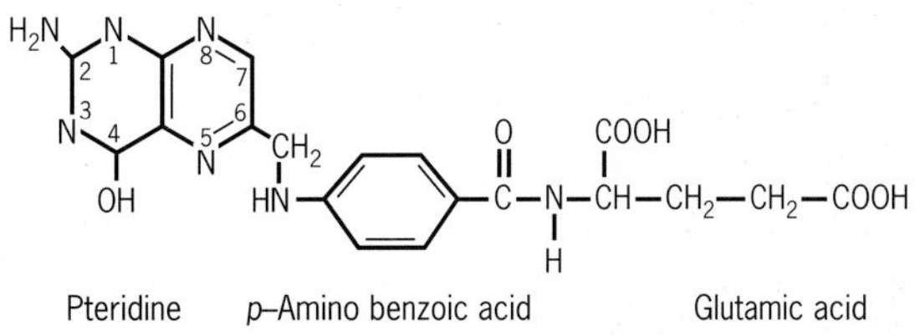

Fig 6.12
Folic acid structure. This is formed from three building blocks as shown. Tetrahydrofolate has additional hydrogen atoms at positions 5, 6, 7 and 8

Table 6.6
Causes of folate deficiency

Nutritional (major cause)	**Pathological**
Poor intake	Haematological disease with excess red cell production, e.g. haemolysis
Old age	Malignant disease with increased cell turnover
Poor social conditions	Inflammatory disease
Starvation	Metabolic disease, e.g. homocystinuria
Alcohol excess (also causes impaired utilization)	Haemodialysis or peritoneal dialysis
Poor intake due to anorexia	**Malabsorption**
Gastrointestinal disease, e.g. partial gastrectomy, coeliac disease, Crohn's disease	Occurs in small bowel disease, but the effect is minor compared with that of anorexia
Cancer	**Antifolate drugs**
Excess utilization	Anticonvulsants
Physiological	Phenytoin
Pregnancy	Primidone
Lactation	Methotrexate
Prematurity	Pyrimethamine
	Trimethoprim

Blood measurements

Serum and red cell folate are assayed by radioisotope dilution or immunological methods. Microbiological methods were used in the past, but had the disadvantage that antibiotic therapy could lead to falsely low results. Normal levels of serum folate are 4–18 $\mu g\ L^{-1}$ (5–63 $nmol\ L^{-1}$). The amount of folate in the red cells is a better measure of tissue folate; the normal range is 160–640 $\mu g\ mL^{-1}$.

Further investigations

In many cases of folate deficiency the cause is not obvious from the clinical picture or dietary history. Occult gastrointestinal disease should then be suspected and appropriate investigations, such as jejunal biopsy, should be performed (p. 252).

Treatment and prevention of megaloblastic anaemia

Treatment depends on the type of deficiency. Blood transfusion is not indicated in chronic anaemia; indeed, it is dangerous to transfuse elderly patients, as heart failure may be precipitated. Folic acid may produce a haematological response in vitamin B_{12} deficiency but may aggravate the neuropathy. Large doses of folic acid alone should not be used to treat megaloblastic anaemia unless the serum vitamin B_{12} level is known to be normal.

TREATMENT OF VITAMIN B_{12} DEFICIENCY

Hydroxocobalamin 1000 μg can be given intramuscularly to a total of 5–6 mg over the course of three weeks; 1000 μg is then necessary every three months for the rest of the patient's life. Clinical improvement may occur within 48 hours and a reticulocytosis can be seen some 2–3 days after starting therapy, peaking at 5–7 days. Improvement of the polyneuropathy may occur over 6–12 months, but longstanding spinal cord damage is irreversible. Hypokalaemia can occur and, if severe, supplements should be given. Iron deficiency often develops in the first few weeks of therapy. Hyperuricaemia occurs but clinical gout is uncommon. In patients who have had a total gastrectomy or an ileal resection, vitamin B_{12} should be monitored; if low levels occur, prophylactic vitamin B_{12} injections should be given.

TREATMENT OF FOLATE DEFICIENCY

Folate deficiency can be corrected by giving 5 mg of folic acid daily; the same haematological response occurs as seen after treatment of vitamin B_{12} deficiency.

Prophylactic folic acid (400 μg daily) is recommended for all women planning a pregnancy. Many authorities also recommend prophylactic administration of folate throughout pregnancy. Whether this can be achieved by increased consumption of foods with a high folate content or whether women should take folate supplements is being debated at present. The US Food and Drugs Administration has introduced a requirement for the fortification with folic acid of grain products such as bread, flour and rice.

Women who have had a child with a neural tube defect should have 5 mg folic acid before and during a subsequent pregnancy.

Prophylactic folic acid is also given in chronic haematological disorders where there is rapid cell turnover. A dose of 5 mg each week is probably sufficient.

Macrocytosis without megaloblastic changes

A raised MCV with macrocytosis on the peripheral blood film can occur with a normoblastic rather than a megaloblastic bone marrow.

A common *physiological* cause of macrocytosis is pregnancy, and a newborn may also suffer.

Common *pathological* causes are:

- alcohol excess
- liver disease
- reticulocytosis
- hypothyroidism
- some haematological disorders (e.g. aplastic anaemia, sideroblastic anaemia, pure red cell aplasia

- drugs (e.g. cytotoxics – azathioprine)
- spurious (agglutinated red cells measured on red cell counters)
- cold agglutinins due to autoagglutination of red cells (see p. 383) (the MCV decreases to normal with warming of the sample to 37°C).

In all these conditions, normal levels of vitamin B_{12} and folate will be found. The exact mechanisms in each case are uncertain, but in some there is increased lipid deposition in the red cell membrane.

An increased number of reticulocytes leads to a raised MCV because they are large cells.

Alcohol is a frequent cause of a raised MCV in an otherwise normal individual. A megaloblastic anaemia can also occur in people who abuse alcohol; this is due to a toxic effect of alcohol on erythropoiesis or to dietary folate deficiency.

Table 6.7
Causes of aplastic anaemia

Primary
Congenital, e.g. Fanconi's anaemia
Idiopathic acquired (50% of cases)

Secondary
Chemicals, e.g. benzene
Drugs
  chemotherapeutic
  idiosyncratic
Insecticides
Ionizing radiation
Infections:
  viral, e.g. hepatitis, measles, HIV, Parvo
  other, e.g. tuberculosis
Pregnancy
Paroxysmal nocturnal haemoglobinuria

FURTHER READING

Chanarin I, Metz J (1997) Diagnosis of cobalamin deficiency: the old and the new. *British Journal of Haematology* **97**: 695–700.

Wickramsinghe SN (1997) Folate and vitamin B_{12} deficiency and supplementation. *Prescribers Journal* **37**: 88–95.

Toh BH, vanDriel IR, Gleeson PA (1997) Pernicious anaemia. *New England Journal of Medicine* **337**: 1441–1448

Anaemia due to marrow failure (aplastic anaemia)

Aplastic anaemia is defined as pancytopenia with hypocellularity (aplasia) of the bone marrow. It is an uncommon but serious condition that may be inherited but is more commonly acquired.

Aplastic anaemia is due to a reduction in the number of pluripotential stem cells (see Fig 6.1) together with a fault in those remaining or an immune reaction against them so that they are unable to repopulate the bone marrow. Failure of one cell line may occur, resulting in isolated deficiencies such as the absence of red cell precursors in pure red cell aplasia. Evolution to myelodysplasia, paroxysmal nocturnal haemoglobinuria (PNH) or acute myeloblastic leukaemia occurs in some cases, probably due to the emergence of an abnormal clone of haemopoietic cells.

CAUSES

A list of causes of aplasia is given in Table 6.7. Immune mechanisms are probably responsible for most cases of idiopathic acquired aplastic anaemia and play a part in at least the persistence of many secondary cases. Activated cytotoxic T cells in blood and bone marrow are responsible for the bone marrow failure.

Many drugs may cause marrow aplasia, including cytotoxic drugs such as busulphan and doxorubicin, which are expected to cause transient aplasia as a consequence of their therapeutic use. However, some individuals develop aplasia due to sensitivity to non-cytotoxic drugs such as chloramphenicol, gold, carbimazole, chlorpromazine, phenytoin, tolbutamide, non-steroidal anti-inflammatory agents, and many others which have been reported to cause occasional cases of aplasia.

Congenital aplastic anaemias are rare. *Fanconi's anaemia* is inherited as an autosomal recessive and is associated with skeletal, renal and central nervous system abnormalities. It usually presents between the ages of 5 and 10 years.

CLINICAL FEATURES

The clinical manifestations of marrow failure are anaemia, bleeding and infection. Physical findings include ecchymoses, bleeding gums and epistaxis. Mouth infections are common. Lymphadenopathy and hepatosplenomegaly are rare in aplastic anaemia.

INVESTIGATIONS

The laboratory diagnosis is made on the basis of:

- pancytopenia
- the virtual absence of reticulocytes
- a hypocellular or aplastic bone marrow with increased fat spaces (Fig 6.13).

DIFFERENTIAL DIAGNOSIS

This is from other causes of pancytopenia (Table 6.8). A bone marrow trephine is essential for assessment of the bone marrow cellularity.

TREATMENT AND PROGNOSIS

The main danger is infection and stringent measures should be undertaken to avoid this (see also p. 423). Any suspicion of infection in a severely neutropenic patient

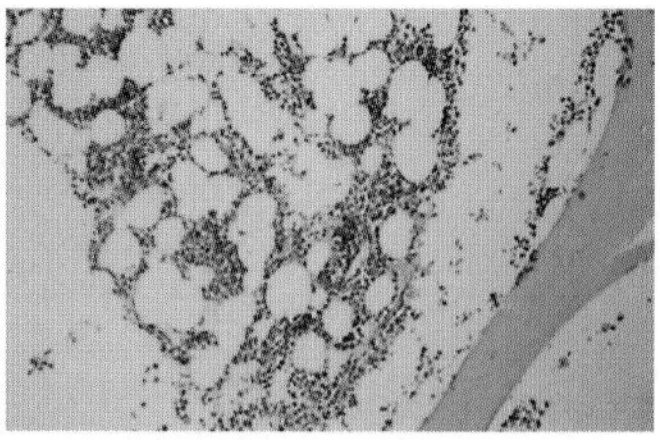

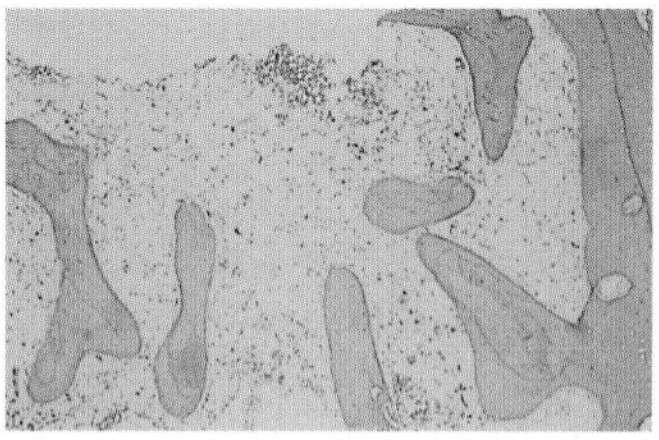

Fig 6.13
Bone marrow trephine biopsies in low power view. (a) Normal cellularity; **(b)** hypocellularity in aplastic anaemia

should lead to immediate institution of broad-spectrum parenteral antibiotics. Supportive care including transfusions of red cells and platelets should be given as necessary. Leucocyte-depleted red cells and platelets should be given to prevent HLA alloimmunization to minimize the risk of rejection of a bone marrow transplant and to prevent febrile transfusion reactions (see p. 395). The cause of the aplastic anaemia must be eliminated if possible.

The course of aplastic anaemia can be variable, ranging from a rapid spontaneous remission to a persistent increasingly severe pancytopenia, which may lead to death through haemorrhage or infection. The most reliable determinants for the prognosis are the number of neutrophils, reticulocytes, platelets, and the cellularity of the bone marrow.

A bad prognosis (i.e. severe aplastic anaemia) is associated with the presence of two of the following three features:

- neutrophil count $< 0.5 \times 10^9/L$
- platelet count of $< 20 \times 10^9/L$
- reticulocyte count of $< 40 \times 10^9/L$.

In *severe aplastic anaemia*, there is a very poor outcome without treatment. Bone marrow transplantation is the treatment of choice for patients under 20 years of age who have an HLA-identical sibling donor (Fig 6.14). Older patients up to the age of 45 years may also be treated by transplantation if an HLA-identical sibling is available, although immunosuppression produces similar long-term survival. Transplantation versus immuno-suppression is a contentious issue in the 20–45 age range. Some centres recommend transplantation, and others recommend immunosuppression as an initial trial and transplantation if there is no response. Patients over the age of 45 are not eligible for bone marrow transplantation whether an HLA-identical donor is available or not, because of the high risk of graft-versus-host disease as a complication of bone marrow transplantation.

With matched transplants, the 3 year survival rate is up to 90%, but about 70% of patients with aplastic anaemia eligible for bone marrow transplantation do not have an HLA-identical sibling. The results of bone marrow transplantation using unrelated donors or mismatched family donors are improving, but this is best restricted to very young patients (<6 years) failing to respond to immunosuppressive therapy.

Immunosuppressive therapy is used for those patients outlined above and for patients over the age of 45 years; antilymphocyte globulin (ALG) and cyclosporin are used alone or in combination. ALG alone produces a haematological recovery in 50–60% of cases and this is increased to 80% in patients also receiving cyclosporin.

Levels of haemopoietic growth factors (see Fig 6.1) are normal or increased in most patients with aplastic anemia, and are ineffective as primary treatment. They may be useful in promoting haemopoietic recovery after transplantation, and in chronically pancytopenic patients refractory to conventional therapy.

Androgens (e.g. oxymethalone) are sometimes useful in patients not responding to immunosuppression and in patients with moderately severe aplastic anaemia.

Steroids have little activity in severe aplastic anaemia but are used for serum sickness due to ALG. They are also used to treat children with *congenital pure red cell aplasia* (Diamond–Blackfan syndrome). *Adult pure red cell aplasia* is associated with a thymoma in 30% of cases and thymectomy may induce a remission. It may also be associated with autoimmune disease or may be idiopathic. Steroids and cyclosporin are effective treatment in some cases.

Table 6.8
Causes of pancytopenia

Aplastic anaemia (see Table 6.7)
Drugs
Megaloblastic anaemia
Bone marrow infiltration or replacement
Hodgkin's and non-Hodgkin's lymphoma
Acute leukaemia
Myeloma
Secondary carcinoma
Myelofibrosis
Hypersplenism
Systemic lupus erythematosus
Disseminated tuberculosis
Paroxysmal nocturnal haemoglobinuria
Overwhelming sepsis

FURTHER READING

Young NS (1995) Aplastic anaemia. *Lancet* **346**: 228–232.

Young NS, Maciejewski J (1997) The pathophysiology of acquired aplastic anaemia. *New England Journal of Medicine* **336**: 1365–1372.

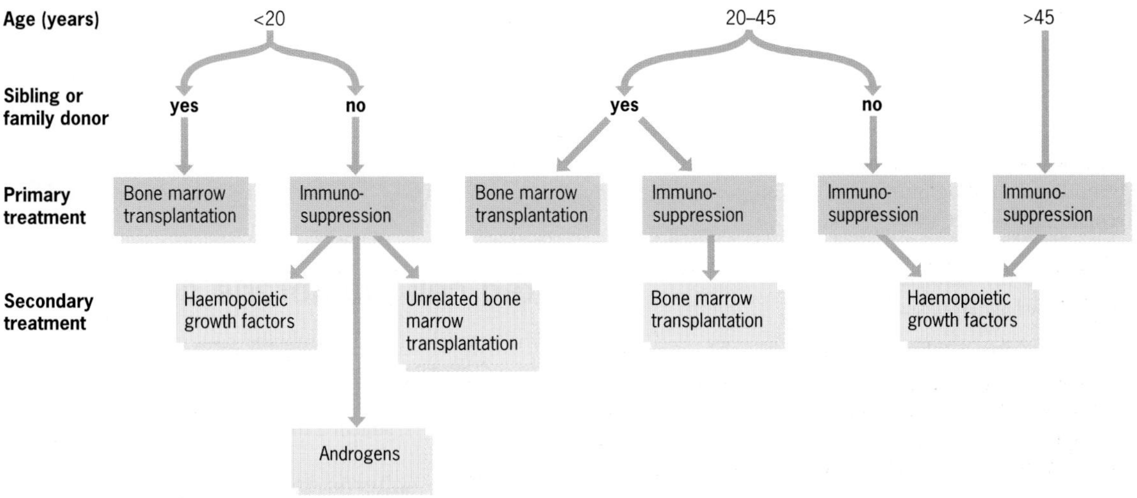

Fig 6.14
Treatment of severe acquired aplastic anaemia. Modified from Young NS (1995) *Lancet* **346**: 228–232, with permission

Haemolytic anaemias: an introduction

Haemolytic anaemias are caused by increased destruction of red cells. The red cell normally survives about 120 days, but in haemolytic anaemias the red cell survival times are considerably shortened (Fig 6.15).

There is no definite explanation why red cells are removed from the circulation at the end of their life-span. Breakdown of normal red cells occurs in the macrophages of the bone marrow, liver and spleen (see Fig 6.5).

Consequences of haemolysis

Shortening of red cell survival does not always cause anaemia as there is a compensatory increase in red cell production by the bone marrow. If the red cell loss can be contained within the marrow's capacity for increased output, then a haemolytic state can exist without anaemia (*compensated haemolytic disease*). The bone marrow can increase its output by six to eight times by increasing the proportion of cells committed to erythropoiesis (*erythroid hyperplasia*) and by expanding the volume of active marrow. In addition, immature red cells (*reticulocytes*) are released prematurely. These cells are larger than mature cells and stain light blue on a peripheral blood film (the description of the appearance of the blood film is *polychromasia*). They may be counted accurately as a percentage of all red cells on a blood film using a supravital stain for residual RNA (e.g. new methylene blue).

Sites of haemolysis

Extravascular haemolysis

In most haemolytic conditions red cell destruction is extravascular. The red cells are removed from the circulation by macrophages in the reticuloendothelial system, particularly the spleen.

Intravascular haemolysis

When red cells are rapidly destroyed within the circulation, haemoglobin is liberated (Fig 6.16). This is initially bound to *plasma haptoglobins* but these soon become saturated.

Excess free plasma Hb is filtered by the renal glomerulus and enters the urine, although small amounts are reabsorbed by the renal tubules. In the renal tubular cell, Hb is broken down and becomes deposited in the cells as *haemosiderin*. This can be detected in the spun sediment of urine using Perls' reaction. Some of the free plasma Hb is oxidized to *methaemoglobin*, which dissociates into *ferrihaem* and globin. *Plasma haemopexin* binds

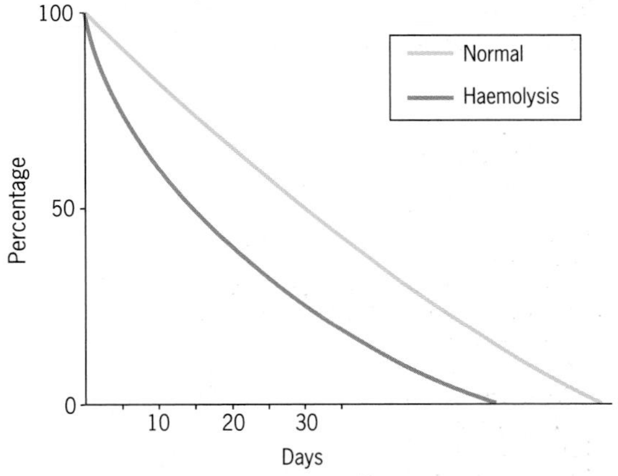

Fig 6.15
Survival curves of normal red cells and cells affected by haemolysis, using labelling of red cells with ^{51}Cr. The half-life of normal cells is about 30 days and is reduced to less than 15 days in patients with haemolytic anaemia

ferrihaem; but if its binding capacity is exceeded, ferrihaem becomes attached to albumin, forming *methaemalbumin*. On spectrophotometry of the plasma, methaemalbumin forms a characteristic band; this is the basis of *Schumm's test*.

The *liver* plays an important role in removing Hb bound to haptoglobin and haemopexin and any remaining free Hb.

Evidence for haemolysis

Increased red cell breakdown leads to:

- elevated serum bilirubin (unconjugated)
- excess urinary urobilinogen (resulting from bilirubin breakdown in the intestine, Fig 6.5)
- reduced plasma haptoglobin
- raised serum lactic dehydrogenase (LDH).

Increased red cell production leads to:

- reticulocytosis
- erythroid hyperplasia of the bone marrow.

There may be evidence of abnormal red cells in some haemolytic anaemias:

- spherocytes (see Fig 6.8)
- sickle cells (see Fig 6.8)
- red cell fragments.

Demonstration of shortened red cell life-span

Red cell survival studies using ^{51}Cr-labelled red cells are useful in complicated cases, and for quantitation of the severity of haemolysis. The dominant site of red cell destruction can be shown with external body counting over the liver and spleen.

Intravascular haemolysis

This is suggested by raised levels of plasma Hb, haemosiderinuria, very low or absent haptoglobins, and the presence of methaemalbumin (positive Schumm's test).

Various laboratory studies will be necessary to determine the exact type of haemolytic anaemia present. The causes of haemolytic anaemias are shown in Table 6.9.

Inherited haemolytic anaemia

Red cell membrane defects

The normal red cell membrane consists of a lipid bilayer crossed by integral proteins with an underlying lattice of proteins (or cytoskeleton), including spectrin, actin, ankyrin and protein 4.1, attached to integral proteins (Fig 6.17).

Hereditary spherocytosis (HS)

HS is the most common inherited haemolytic anaemia in northern Europeans, affecting 1 in 5000. It is inherited in an autosomal dominant manner, but in 25% of patients neither parent is affected and it is presumed that HS has occurred by spontaneous mutation. HS is due to a defect in the red cell membrane, resulting in the cells losing part of the cell membrane as they pass through the spleen, possibly because the lipid bilayer is inadequately supported by the cytoskeleton. The surface-to-volume ratio decreases, and the cells become spherocytic. Spherocytes are more rigid and less deformable than normal red cells. They are unable to pass through the splenic microcirculation and they die.

Several defects in the cell membrane have been identified in HS. The best characterized is a deficiency in the structural protein spectrin, but quantitative defects in other membrane proteins have been identified (Fig 16.17). The abnormal red cell membrane in HS is associated functionally with an increased permeability to sodium, and this requires an increased rate of active transport of sodium out of the cells which is dependent on ATP produced by glycolysis.

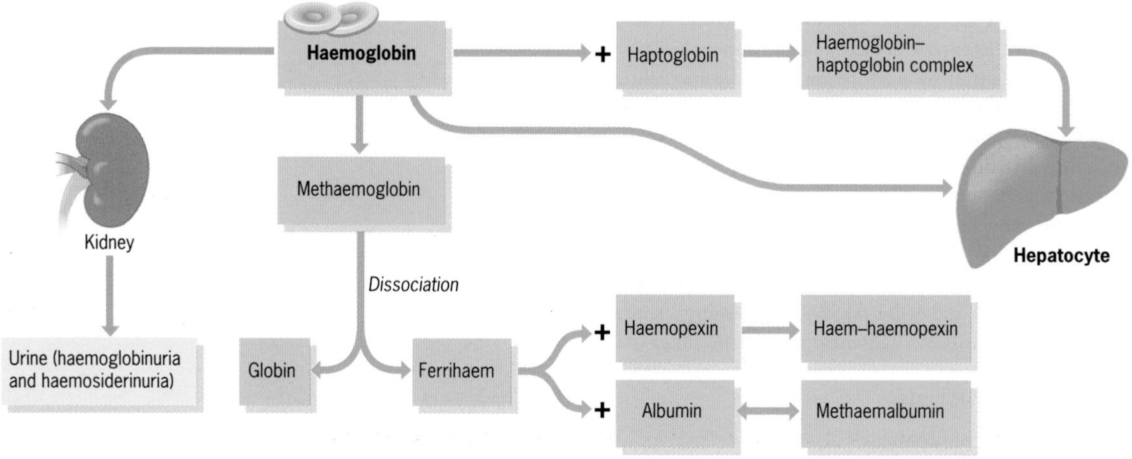

Fig 6.16
The fate of haemoglobin in the plasma

Table 6.9
Causes of haemolytic anaemia

Inherited	Non-immune
Red cell membrane defect Hereditary spherocytosis Hereditary elliptocytosis **Haemoglobin abnormalities** Thalassaemia Sickle cell disease **Metabolic defects** Glucose-6-phosphate dehydrogenase deficiency Pyruvate kinase deficiency	Acquired membrane defects Paroxysmal nocturnal haemoglobinuria Mechanical Microangiopathic haemolytic anaemia Valve prosthesis March haemoglobinuria Secondary to systemic disease: Renal and liver failure **Miscellaneous** Infections, e.g. malaria, *Clostridium welchii* Drugs and chemicals causing damage to the red cell membrane or oxidative haemolysis Hypersplenism Burns
Acquired **Immune** Autoimmune (see Table 6.14) Warm Cold Alloimmune Haemolytic transfusion reactions Haemolytic disease of the newborn After allogeneic bone marrow or organ transplantation Drug-induced	

CLINICAL FEATURES

The condition may present with jaundice at birth. However, the onset of jaundice can sometimes be delayed for many years and some patients may go through life with no symptoms and are detected only during family studies. The patient may eventually develop anaemia, splenomegaly and ulcers on the leg. As in many haemolytic anaemias, the course of the disease may be interrupted by aplastic, haemolytic and megaloblastic crises. Aplastic anaemia usually occurs after infections, particularly with parvovirus, whereas megaloblastic anaemia is the result of folate depletion owing to the hyperactivity of the bone marrow. Chronic haemolysis leads to the formation of pigment gallstones (see p. 338).

INVESTIGATIONS

- **Anaemia**. This is usually mild, but occasionally can be severe.
- **Blood film**. This shows spherocytes and reticulocytes.
- **Haemolysis** is evident (e.g. the serum bilirubin and urinary urobilinogen will be raised).
- **Osmotic fragility**. When red cells are placed in solutions of increasing hypotonicity, they take in water, swell, and eventually lyse. Spherocytes tolerate hypotonic solutions less well than do normal biconcave red cells. Osmotic fragility tests are infrequently carried out in routine practice, but may be useful to confirm a suspicion of spherocytosis on a blood film.
- **Direct antiglobulin (Coombs') test** is negative in spherocytosis, virtually ruling out autoimmune haemolytic anaemia where spherocytes are also commonly present.

TREATMENT

The spleen, which is the site of cell destruction, should be removed in all but the mildest cases. The decision about splenectomy in symptomless patients is difficult, but a raised bilirubin and especially the presence of gallstones should encourage splenectomy.

It is best to postpone splenectomy until after childhood, as sudden overwhelming fatal infections, usually due to encapsulated organisms such as pneumococci, may

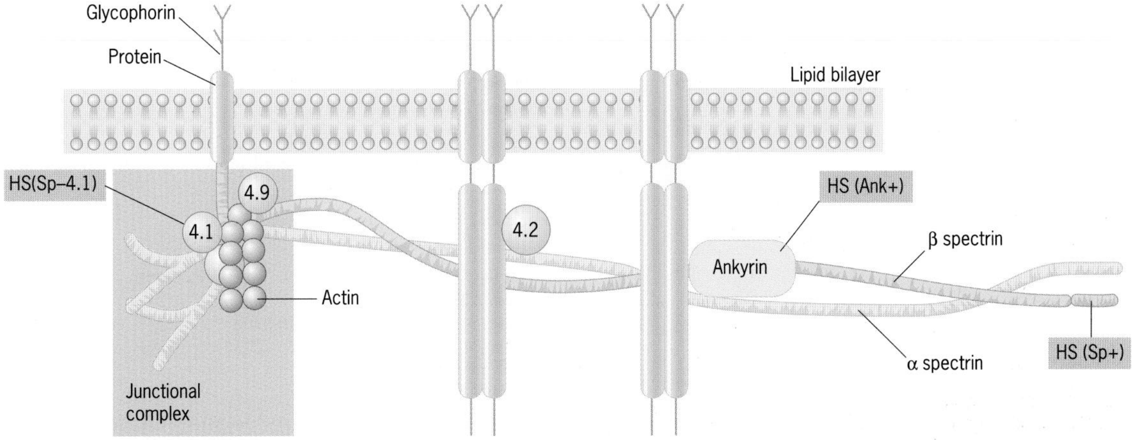

Fig 6.17
Red cell membrane showing the sites of the principal defects in hereditory spherocytosis (HS).
HS (Ank+), ankyrin deficiency
HS (Sp+), spectrin deficiency
HS (Sp-4.1) abnormal spectrin/protein 4.1 binding

occur (see p. 391). Splenectomy should be preceded by pneumococcal and Hib immunization and followed by lifelong penicillin prophylaxis (see p. 9).

Following splenectomy, the spherocytosis is reduced and the Hb level usually returns to normal as the red cells are no longer destroyed.

Folate deficiency often occurs in chronic haemolysis with rapid cell turnover. Folate levels should be monitored, or folic acid can be given prophylactically.

Hereditary elliptocytosis

This disorder of the red cell membrane is inherited in an autosomal dominant manner and has a prevalence of 1 in 2500 in Caucasians. The red cells are elliptical owing to spectrin and other protein abnormalities. Clinically it is a similar condition to HS but milder. Only a minority of patients have anaemia and only occasional patients require splenectomy.

Hereditary stomatocytosis

Stomatocytes are red cells in which the pale central area appears slit-like. Their presence in large numbers may occur in a hereditary haemolytic anaemia associated with a membrane defect, but excess alcohol intake is also a common cause.

Haemoglobin abnormalities

Normal haemoglobin

Normal adult Hb (Hb A) has two polypeptide globin chains, the α and β chains (Table 6.10), which have 141 and 146 amino acids, respectively. These are folded so that haem molecules can be held within the fold and are yet able to combine reversibly with oxygen.

In early embryonic life, haemoglobins Gower 1, Gower 2 and Portland predominate (Fig 6.18). Later, fetal haemoglobin (Hb F), which has two α and two γ chains, is produced. There is increasing synthesis of β chains from 13 weeks of gestation and at term there is 80% Hb F and 20% Hb A. The switch from Hb F to Hb A occurs after birth when the genes for γ chain production are further suppressed and there is rapid increase in the synthesis of β chains. The exact mechanism responsible for the switch remains unknown. There is little Hb F produced (normally less than 1%) from six months after birth. The β chain is synthesized just before birth and Hb A_2 ($\alpha_2\delta_2$) remains at a level of about 2% throughout adult life.

Globin chains are synthesized in the same way as any protein (see Chapter 2). Four globin chain genes are required to control α-chain production (Fig 6.18). Two are present on each haploid genome (genes derived from one parent). These are situated close together on

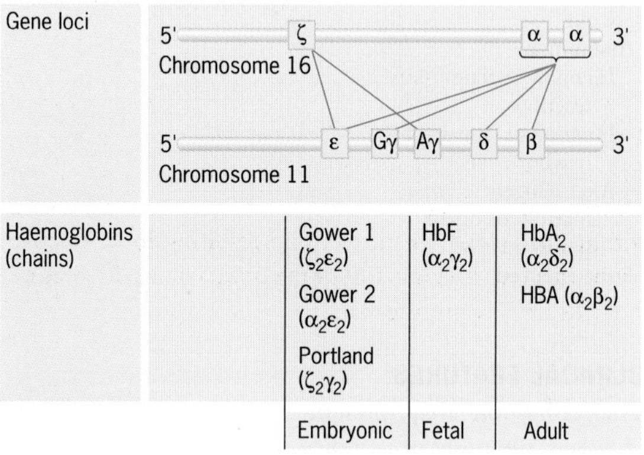

Fig 6.18
Loci of genes on chromosomes 16 and 11 and the combination of various chains to produce different haemoglobins

Table 6.10
Some types of haemoglobin

	Haemoglobin	Structure	Comment
Normal	A	$\alpha_2\beta_2$	Comprises 92% of adult haemoglobin
	A_{1c}	$\alpha_2\beta_2$ (β-NH glucose)	Comprises 5% of adult haemoglobin Glycosylated haemoglobin is increased in patients with uncontrolled diabetes
	A_2	$\alpha_2\delta_2$	Comprises 2% of adult haemoglobin Elevated in β-thalassaemia
	F	$\alpha_2\gamma_2$	Normal haemoglobin in fetus from 3rd to 9th month Increased in β-thalassaemia Comprises <1% of haemoglobin in adult
Abnormal chain production	H	β_4	Found in α-thalassaemia Biologically useless
	Barts	γ_4	Comprises 100% of haemoglobin in homozygous α-thalassaemia Biologically useless
Abnormal chain structure	S	$\alpha_2\beta_2$	Substitution of valine for glutamic acid in position 6 of β chain
	C	$\alpha_2\beta_2$	Substitution of lysine for glutamic acid in position 6 of β chain

chromosome 16. The genes controlling the production of ε, γ, δ and β chains are close together on chromosome 11. The globin genes are arranged on chromosomes 16 and 11 in the order in which they are expressed.

Abnormal haemoglobins

Abnormalities occur in:

- globin chain production (e.g. thalassaemia)
- structure of the globin chain (e.g. sickle cell disease)
- combined defects of globin chain production and structure, e.g. sickle cell β-thalassaemia.

Genetic defects in haemoglobin are the most common of all genetic disorders.

The thalassaemias

The thalassaemias (Greek *thalassa* = sea) are anaemias originally found in people living on the shores of the Mediterranean but which are now known to affect people throughout the world (Fig 6.19).

Normally there is balanced (1:1) production of α and β chains. The defective synthesis of globin genes in thalassaemia leads to 'imbalanced' globin chain production, leading to precipitation of globin chains within the red cell precursors and resulting in ineffective erythropoiesis. Precipitation of globin chains in mature red cells leads to haemolysis.

β-Thalassaemia

In homozygous β-thalassaemia, either *no* normal β chains are produced (β^0), or β-chain production is very reduced (β^+). There is an excess of α chains which precipitate in erythroblasts and red cells causing ineffective erythropoiesis and haemolysis. The excess α chains combine with whatever β, δ and γ chains are produced, resulting in increased quantities of Hb A_2 and Hb F and, at best, small amounts of Hb A. In heterozygous β-thalassaemia there is usually symptomless microcytosis with or without mild anaemia. Table 6.11 shows the findings in the homozygote and heterozygote for the common types of β-thalassaemia.

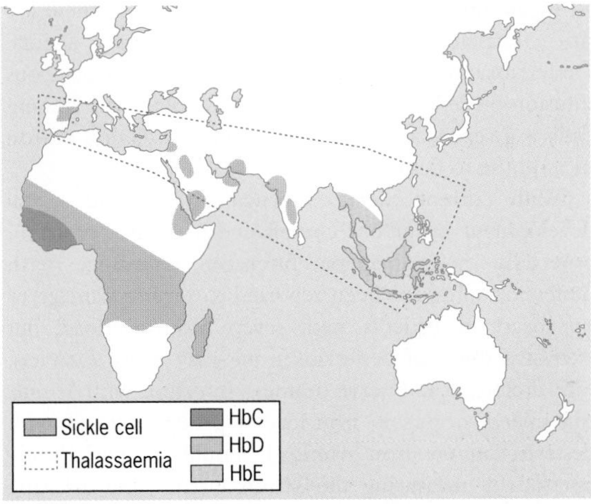

Fig 6.19
Major haemoglobin abnormalities: geographical distribution

Molecular genetics

The molecular errors accounting for over 100 genetic defects leading to β-thalassaemia genes have been characterized. Unlike α-thalassaemia, the defects are mainly point mutations rather than gene deletions. The mutations result in defects in transcription, RNA splicing and modification, translation via frame shifts and nonsense codons producing highly unstable β-globin which cannot be utilized.

Clinical syndromes

Clinically, β-thalassaemia can be divided into the following:

- *thalassaemia minor* (or *trait*), the symptomless heterozygous carrier state
- *thalassaemia intermedia*, with moderate anaemia, rarely requiring transfusions
- *thalassaemia major*, with severe anaemia requiring regular transfusions.

Thalassaemia minor (trait)

This common carrier state is asymptomatic. Anaemia is mild or absent. The red cells are hypochromic and microcytic with a low MCV and MCH, and it may be confused with iron deficiency. However, the two are easily

Table 6.11
Thalassaemia findings in β-, δβ- and γδβ-thalassaemias

Type of thalassaemia	Findings in homozgote	Findings in heterozygote
β^+	Thalassaemia major Hb A + F + A_2	Thalassaemia minor Hb A_2 raised
β^0	Thalassaemia major Hb F + A_2	Thalassaemia minor Hb A_2 raised
δβ	Thalassaemia intermedia Hb F only	Thalassaemia minor Hb F 5–15% Hb A_2 normal
δβ(Lepore)	Thalassaemia major or intermedia Hb F and Lepore	Thalassaemia minor Hb Lepore 5–15% Hb A_2 normal
γδβ	Not viable	Neonatal haemolysis Thalassaemia minor in adults with normal Hb F and A_2

Adapted with permission from Weatherall DJ (1996) Disorders of the synthesis or function of haemoglobin. In Weatherall DJ, Ledingham JGG, Warrell DA (eds), *Oxford Textbook of Medicine*. Oxford: Oxford University Press.

distinguished as in thalassaemia trait the serum ferritin and the iron stores are normal (see Table 6.3). Hb electrophoresis usually shows a raised Hb A_2 and often a raised Hb F (Fig 6.20). Iron should not be given to these patients unless they develop coincidental iron deficiency.

Thalassaemia intermedia

Thalassaemia intermedia includes patients who are symptomatic with moderate anaemia (Hb 7–10 g dL^{-1}) and who do not require regular transfusions. That is, it is more severe than in β-thalassaemia trait but milder than in transfusion-dependent thalassaemia major.

Thalassaemia intermedia may be due to a combination of homozygous mild β^+- and α-thalassaemia, where there is reduced α chain precipitation and less ineffective erythropoiesis and haemolysis. The inheritance of hereditary persistence of Hb F with homozygous β-thalassaemia also results in a milder clinical picture than unmodified β-thalassaemia major because the excess α chains are partially removed by the increased production of γ chains.

Patients may have splenomegaly and bone deformities. Recurrent leg ulcers, gallstones and infections are also seen.

Thalassaemia major (Cooley's anaemia)

Children affected by severe β-thalassaemia present during the first year of life with:

- failure to thrive and recurrent bacterial infections
- severe anaemia from 3–6 months when the switch from γ- to β-chain production should normally occur
- extramedullary haemopoiesis that soon leads to hepatosplenomegaly and bone expansion, giving rise to the classical thalassaemic facies (Fig 6.21a)

Skull X-rays in these children show the characteristic 'hair on end' appearance of bony trabeculation as a result of

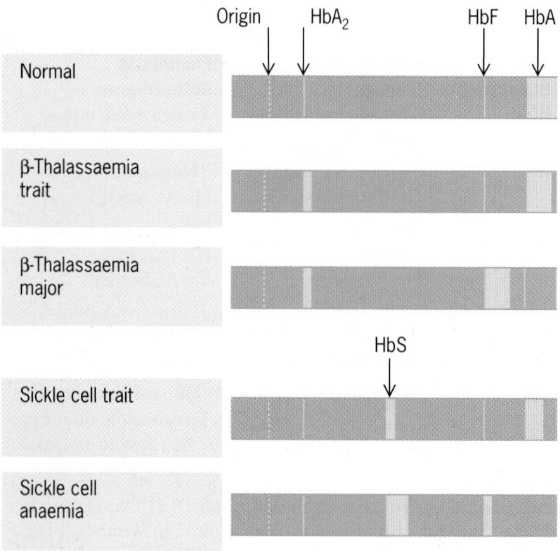

Fig 6.20
Patterns of haemoglobin electrophoresis

expansion of the bone marrow into cortical bone (Fig 6.21b). The expansion of the bone marrow is also shown in an X-ray of the hand (Fig 6.21c).

INVESTIGATIONS

- **Blood count** shows a moderate to severe anaemia with reduced MCV and MCH. The reticulocyte count is raised and nucleated red cells are present in the peripheral blood. The WCC and the number of platelets are normal unless hypersplenism is present.
- **Blood film** shows a hypochromic and predominantly microcytic picture. Postsplenectomy features will be present after splenectomy has been carried out (see Fig 6.8).
- **Saturated iron-binding capacity and high serum ferritin levels** are caused by multiple blood transfusions.
- **Hb electrophoresis** shows an increase in Hb F, markedly reduced or absent Hb A, and Hb A_2 is normal or slightly increased (see Fig 6.20).

MANAGEMENT

The aims of treatment are to suppress ineffective erythropoiesis, prevent bony deformities and allow normal activity and development. Long-term folic acid supplements are required, and regular transfusions should be given to keep the Hb above 10 g dL^{-1}. Blood transfusions may be required every 4–6 weeks. Febrile transfusion reactions can be prevented by the use of leucocyte-depleted blood (p. 395). If transfusion requirements increase, splenectomy should be considered although this is usually delayed until after the age of 6 years because of the risk of infection. Prophylaxis against infection is required for patients undergoing splenectomy (see p. 391).

Iron overload caused by repeated transfusions (*transfusion haemosiderosis*) may lead to damage to the endocrine glands, liver, pancreas and the myocardium by the time patients reach adolescence. The iron-chelating agent of choice remains desferrioxamine, although it has to be administered parenterally. Unfortunately, there are no satisfactory oral iron-chelating agents. Desferrioxamine is given as an overnight subcutaneous infusion on 5–7 nights each week. Ascorbic acid 200 mg daily is given, as it increases the urinary excretion of iron in response to desferrioxamine.

With current therapy, normal growth and sexual development occur but compliance may be a problem, especially in teenagers. Intensive treatment with desferrioxamine has been reported to reverse damage to the heart in patients with severe iron overload, but excessive doses of desferrioxamine may cause cataracts, retinal damage and nerve deafness. Infection with *Yersinia enterocolitica* occurs in iron-loaded patients treated with desferrioxamine. Iron overload should be periodically assessed by measuring the serum ferritin and assessing damage to organs, particularly the heart, liver and endocrine glands.

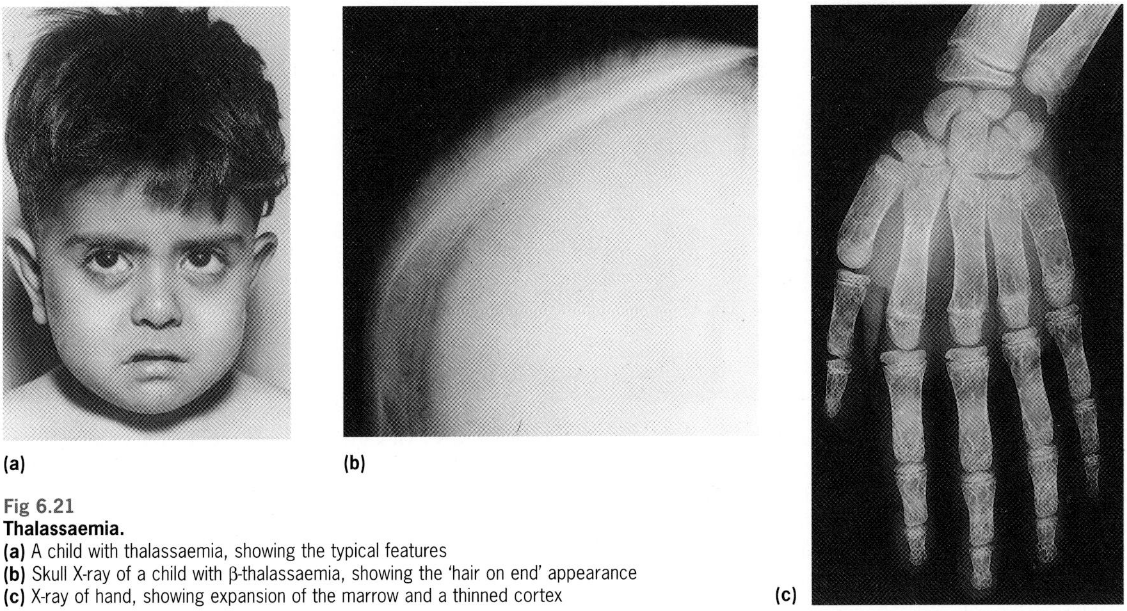

Fig 6.21
Thalassaemia.
(a) A child with thalassaemia, showing the typical features
(b) Skull X-ray of a child with β-thalassaemia, showing the 'hair on end' appearance
(c) X-ray of hand, showing expansion of the marrow and a thinned cortex

Bone marrow transplantation has been used in young patients with HLA-matched siblings. It has been successful in cases in good clinical condition with a mortality of less than 5%, but there is a high mortality (>50%) in patients in poor condition with iron overload and liver dysfunction.

Prenatal diagnosis and gene therapy are discussed on p. 156.

δβ-Thalassaemias, Hb Lepore and hereditary persistence of fetal haemoglobin (HPFH) (see Table 6.11)

These variants are due to deletions of the α- and β-globin genes and produce a milder form of thalassaemia than homozygous β^0-thalassaemia because the reduced β-chain production is partially compensated by increased γ-chain synthesis.

α-Thalassaemia

Molecular genetics

In contrast to β-thalassaemia, α-thalassaemia is caused by gene deletions. The gene for α chains is duplicated on both chromosomes 16; i.e. there are four genes. Deletion of one α-chain gene (α^+) or both α-chain genes (α^0) on each chromosome 16 may occur (Table 6.12). The former is the most common of these abnormalities.

If all four genes are absent (deletion of both genes on both chromosomes) there is no α-chain synthesis and only Hb Barts (γ_4) is present. Hb Barts cannot carry oxygen and is incompatible with life (Tables 6.10 and 6.12). Infants are either stillborn at 28–40 weeks or die very shortly after birth. They are pale, oedematous and have enormous livers and spleens – a condition called *hydrops fetalis*.

If three genes are deleted, there is moderate anaemia (Hb 7–10 g dL^{-1}) and splenomegaly (*Hb H disease*). The patients are not usually transfusion-dependent. Hb A, Hb Barts and Hb H (β_4) are present. Hb A_2 is normal or reduced.

If two genes are deleted (*α-thalassaemia trait*) there is microcytosis with or without mild anaemia. Hb H bodies may be seen on staining a blood film with brilliant cresyl blue. With one gene deletion the blood picture is usually normal.

Globin chain synthesis studies for the detection of a reduced ratio of α to β chains may be necessary for the definitive diagnosis of α-thalassaemia trait.

Less commonly, α-thalassaemia may result from genetic defects other than deletions, for example mutations in the stop codon producing an α chain with many extra amino acids (Hb Constant Spring).

Sickle syndromes

The most important structural abnormality of the Hb chain is sickle cell haemoglobin (Hb S). Hb S results from a single-base mutation of adenine to thymine which produces a substitution of valine for glutamine at the sixth codon of the β-globin chain. In the homozygous state (*sickle cell anaemia*) both genes are abnormal (Hb SS), whereas in the heterozygous state (*sickle cell trait*, Hb AS) only one chromosome carries the gene. As the synthesis of Hb F is normal, the disease usually does not manifest itself until the Hb F decreases to adult levels at about 6 months of age.

The disease occurs mainly in Africans (25% carry the gene) but is also found in India, the Middle East, and southern Europe (see Fig 6.19).

Table 6.12
The α-thalassaemias

Gene deletion			Haemoglobin type	Clinical picture
4 genes	α^0	– – / – –	Hb Barts (γ_4)	Hydrops fetalis
3 genes	α^0	– – / – α	Hb H (β_4)	Moderate anaemia Splenomegaly
2 genes	α^0	– – / α α or – α / – α	Some Hb H bodies Hb A	Mild anaemia α-Thalassaemia trait
1 gene	α^+	– α / α α	'Normal'	α-Thalassaemia trait

PATHOGENESIS

Deoxygenated Hb S molecules are insoluble and polymerize. The flexibility of the cells is decreased and they become rigid and take up their characteristic sickle appearance (see Fig 6.8). This process is initially reversible but, with repeated sickling, the cells eventually lose their membrane flexibility and remain in the sickle form. Sickling can produce:

- a shortened red cell survival
- impaired passage of cells through the microcirculation leading to obstruction of small vessels and tissue infarction.

Sickling is *precipitated* by infection, dehydration, cold, acidosis or hypoxia. In many cases the cause is unknown, but adhesion proteins on activated endothelial cells may play a role, particularly in vaso-occlusion. Hb S releases its oxygen to the tissues more easily than does normal Hb (see Fig 13.5), and patients therefore feel well despite being anaemic except during crises or complications.

Sickle cell anaemia

Symptoms vary from a mild asymptomatic disorder to a severe haemolytic anaemia and recurrent severe painful crises. The condition may present in childhood with anaemia and mild jaundice. The hand-and-foot syndrome due to infarcts of small bones is quite common in children and may result in digits of varying lengths.

In the older patient, vaso-occlusive problems occur owing to sickling in the small vessels of any organ, mimicking many medical and surgical emergencies.

Typical infarctive sickle crises include:

- bone pain (most common)
- chest – pleuritic pain
- cerebral – hemiparesis, fits
- kidney – papillary necrosis causing haematuria, renal tubular defect resulting in lack of concentration of the urine
- spleen – painful infarcts
- penis – priapism
- liver – pain with abnormal biochemistry.

Attacks of pain with low-grade fever last from a few hours to a few days. In a given patient the degree of anaemia is usually stable, and during a crisis Hb does not fall unless there is one or more of the following:

- *Aplasia* – due to decreased erythropoiesis, associated with viral infections, particularly parvovirus.
- *Acute sequestration* – the liver and spleen become engorged with sickle cells.
- *Haemolysis* – due to drugs, acute infection or associated G6PD deficiency.

Long-term problems

- *Susceptibility to infections*, particularly to *Streptococcus pneumoniae*, which can cause a fatal meningitis or pneumonia. Osteomyelitis can occur in necrotic bone, often due to *Salmonella.*
- *Chronic leg ulcers*, due to ischaemia.
- *Gallstones*: pigment stones from persistent haemolysis.
- *Aseptic necrosis of bone*, particularly of the femoral heads.
- *Blindness,* due to retinal detachment and/or proliferative retinopathy.
- *Chronic renal disease.*

INVESTIGATIONS

- **Blood count**: the level of Hb is in the range 6–8 g dL^{-1} with a high reticulocyte count (10–20%).
- **Blood films** can show features of hyposplenism (see Fig 6.8).
- **Sickling** of red cells on a blood film can be induced in the presence of sodium metabisulphite.
- **Sickle solubility test**: a mixture of Hb S in a reducing solution such as sodium dithionite gives a turbid appearance due to precipitation of Hb S, whereas normal Hb gives a clear solution. A number of commercial kits such as *Sickledex* are available for this rapid screening for the presence of Hb S, for example before surgery in appropriate ethnic groups.
- **Hb electrophoresis** (see Fig 6.20) is always needed to confirm the diagnosis. There is no Hb A, 80–95% Hb SS, and 2–20% Hb F.
- **The parents** of the affected child will show features of sickle cell trait.

MANAGEMENT

The 'steady state' anaemia requires no treatment. Precipitating factors (see above) should be avoided or treated quickly. Acute attacks require supportive therapy with intravenous fluids, oxygen, antibiotics and adequate analgesia. Prophylaxis is given to prevent pneumococcal infection (see p. 391). Folic acid is given to pregnant women and those with severe haemolysis.

Regular transfusions are given only if there is severe anaemia or if patients are having frequent crises in order to suppress the production of Hb S. Before elective operations and during pregnancy, repeated transfusions may be used to reduce the proportion of circulating Hb S to less than 20% to prevent sickling. Exchange transfusions may be necessary in patients with severe or recurrent crises, or before emergency surgery. Transfusion and splenectomy may be life-saving for young children with splenic sequestration.

Research is being carried out to find a way to increase production of Hb F, because its presence inhibits sickling. Hydroxyurea increases Hb F production by an unknown mechanism and reduces the frequency of painful crises, but there is a variable response and blood counts need to be checked every two weeks to detect myelotoxicity. The results of haemopoietic cell transplantation for patients with HLA-identical siblings and severe disease are improving, and gene therapy may be possible in the future.

PROGNOSIS

Some patients with Hb SS die in the first few years of life from either infection or episodes of sequestration. However, there is marked individual variation in the severity of the disease and some patients have a relatively normal life-span with few complications.

Sickle cell trait

These individuals have no symptoms unless extreme circumstances cause anoxia, such as flying in non-pressurized aircraft or problems with anaesthesia. Anaesthesia should always be carried out with care to avoid hypoxia. Sickle cell trait protects against *Plasmodium falciparum* malaria (see p. 79). Typically there is 60% Hb A and 40% Hb S. The blood count and film are normal. The diagnosis is made by a positive sickle test or by Hb electrophoresis (see Fig 6.20).

Other structural globin chain defects

There are many Hb variants (e.g. Hb C, D), many of which are not associated with clinical manifestations.

Hb C disease may be associated with Hb S (*Hb SC disease*). The clinical course is similar to that with Hb SS, but there is an increased likelihood of thrombosis, and in particular this may lead to life-threatening episodes of thrombosis in pregnancy, and retinopathy.

Combined defects of globin chain production and structure

Abnormalities of Hb structure (e.g. Hb S, C) can occur in combination with thalassaemia. The combination of β-thalassaemia trait and sickle cell trait (sickle cell β-thalassaemia) resembles sickle cell anaemia (Hb SS) clinically. Hb E is the most common Hb variant in South East Asia. Homozygous Hb E causes a mild microcytic anaemia, but the combination of Hb E and β-thalassaemia produces the clinical and haematological features of β-thalassaemia major.

PRENATAL DIAGNOSIS OF SEVERE HAEMOGLOBIN ABNORMALITIES

Of the offspring of parents who both have either β-thalassaemia or sickle cell trait, 25% will have β-thalassaemia major or sickle cell anaemia, respectively. Recognition of these heterozygous states in parents and family counselling provides a basis for antenatal diagnosis.

If a pregnant woman is found to have a haemoglobin defect, her partner should be tested. Antenatal diagnosis is offered if both are affected as there is a risk of a severe fetal Hb defect, particularly β-thalassaemia major. Fetal DNA analysis can be carried out using amniotic fluid, chorionic villus or fetal blood samples. Abortion is offered if the fetus is found to be affected. Chorionic villus biopsy has the advantage that it can be carried out in the first trimester, thus avoiding the need for second trimester abortions.

GENE THERAPY

The ultimate corrective therapy for severe Hb abnormalities would be gene therapy. This might involve inserting normal Hb genes into the patient's haemopoietic cells *in vitro* and then transplanting these cells back into the patient after ablative treatment had been given to remove the abnormal bone marrow. However, numerous problems remain to be overcome before gene therapy for Hb defects becomes a practical option.

Metabolic disorders of the red cell

Red cell metabolism

The mature red cell has no nucleus, mitochondria or ribosomes and is therefore unable to synthesize proteins. Red cells have only limited enzyme systems but they are of major importance in maintaining the viability and function of the cells. In particular, energy is required in the form of ATP for the maintenance of the flexibility of the membrane and the biconcave shape of the cells to allow passage through small vessels, and for regulation of the sodium and potassium pumps to ensure osmotic equilibrium. In addition, it is essential that Hb be maintained in the reduced state.

The enzyme systems responsible for producing energy and reducing power are (Fig 6.22):

- the glycolytic (Embden–Meyerhof) pathway, in which glucose is metabolized to pyruvate and lactic acid with production of ATP
- the hexose monophosphate (pentosephosphate) pathway, which provides reducing power for the red cell in the form of NADPH.

About 90% of glucose is metabolized by the former and 10% by the latter. The importance of the hexose monophosphate shunt is that it maintains glutathione (GSH) in a reduced state. Glutathione is important in combating oxidative stress to the red cell, and failure of this mechanism may result in:

- *rigidity* due to cross-linking of spectrin, which decreases membrane flexibility (see Fig 6.17) and causes 'leakiness' of the red cell membrane
- *oxidation of the Hb molecule*, producing methaemoglobin and precipitation of globin chains as Heinz bodies localized on the inside of the membrane; these bodies are removed from circulating red cells by the spleen.

2,3-DPG is formed from a side-arm of the glycolytic pathway (see Fig 6.22). It binds to the central part of the Hb tetramer, fixing it in the low-affinity state (see Fig 6.4). A decreased affinity with a shift in the oxygen dissociation curve to the right enables more oxygen to be delivered to the tissues (see Fig 13.5).

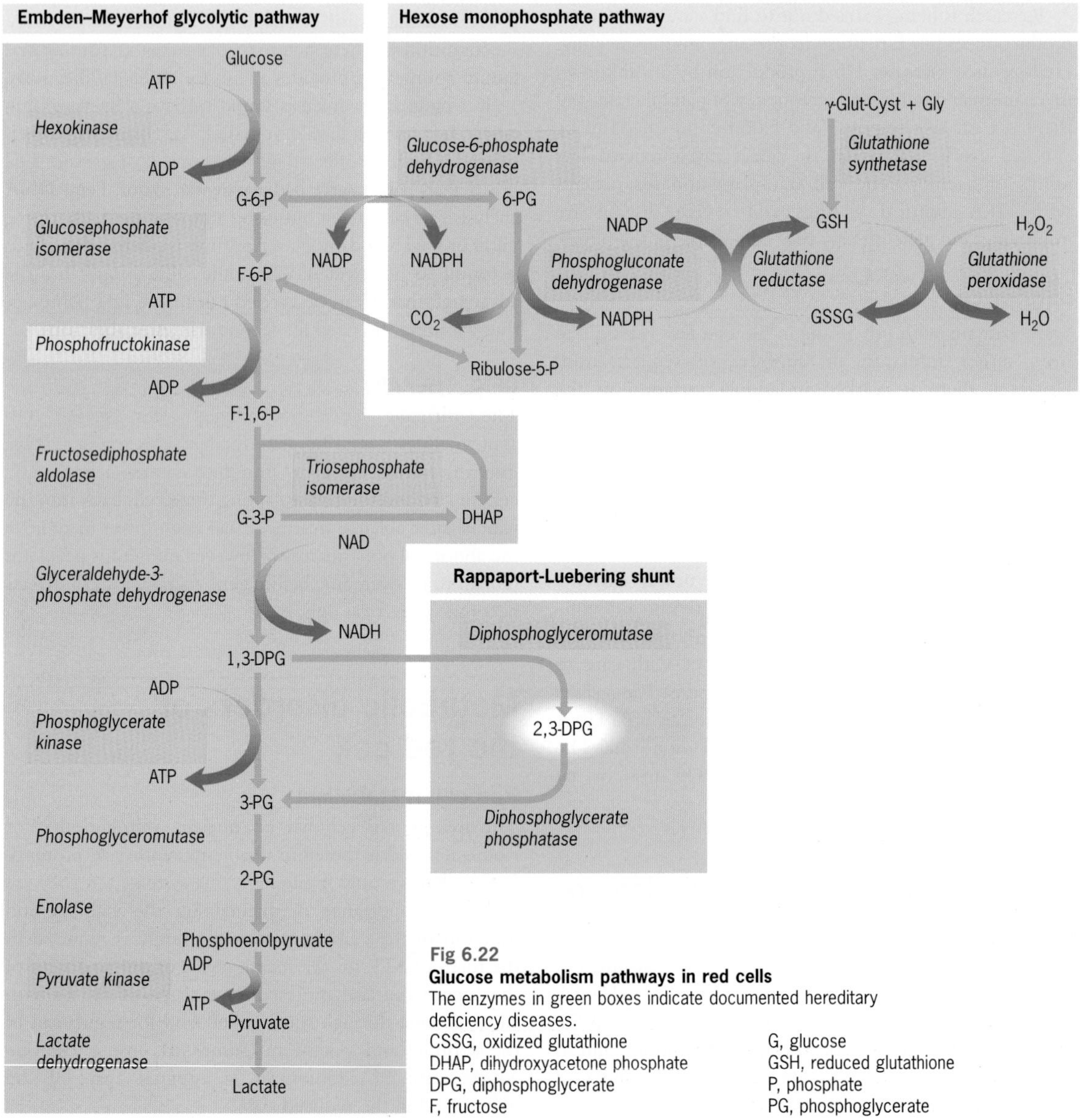

Fig 6.22
Glucose metabolism pathways in red cells
The enzymes in green boxes indicate documented hereditary deficiency diseases.

CSSG, oxidized glutathione
DHAP, dihydroxyacetone phosphate
DPG, diphosphoglycerate
F, fructose
G, glucose
GSH, reduced glutathione
P, phosphate
PG, phosphoglycerate

In addition to the G6PD and pyruvate kinase deficiencies described below, there are a number of rare enzyme deficiencies that need specialist investigation.

Glucose-6-phosphate dehydrogenase (G6PD) deficiency

The enzyme G6PD holds a vital position in the hexose monophosphate shunt (see Fig 6.22) oxidizing glucose-6-phosphate to 6-phosphogluconate with the reduction of NADP to NADPH. The reaction is particularly important in red cells where it is the only source of NADPH which is used via glutathione to protect the red cell from oxidative damage. G6PD deficiency is a common condition that presents with a haemolytic anaemia and affects millions of people throughout the world, particularly in Africa, around the Mediterranean, the Middle East and South East Asia.

The gene for G6PD is sex-linked, being carried on the X chromosome. The deficiency therefore affects males. It is carried by females, who show half the normal levels of the enzyme and can be affected in the neonatal period or after exposure to oxidant drugs. Imbalanced Lyonization (see p. 140) can exaggerate the response if there is a large excess of G6PD-deficient cells in a heterozygote. Heterozygotes have some protection against *Plasmodium falciparum*.

There are over 400 structural types of G6PD, and mutations are mostly single amino acid substitutions. The most common types with *normal* activity are called type B^+, which is present in almost all Caucasians and about 70% of Blacks, and type A^+, which is present in about 20% of Blacks. There are many variants with *reduced* activity but only two are common. In the African, or A^- type, the degree of deficiency is mild and more marked in older cells. Haemolysis is self-limiting as the young red cells newly produced by the bone marrow have nearly normal enzyme activity. However, in the Mediterranean type, both young and old red cells have very low enzyme activity. After an oxidant shock the Hb level may fall precipitously; death may follow unless the condition is recognized and the patient is transfused urgently.

Clinical syndromes

- Acute drug-induced haemolysis (Table 6.13).
- Favism (ingestion of fava beans).
- Chronic haemolytic anaemia.
- Neonatal jaundice.
- Infections and acute illnesses will also precipitate haemolysis in patients with G6PD deficiency.

The clinical features are due to rapid intravascular haemolysis with symptoms of anaemia, jaundice and haemoglobinuria.

INVESTIGATIONS

- **Blood count** is normal between attacks.
- **During an attack** the blood film may show irregularly contracted cells, bite cells (cells with an indentation of the membrane), blister cells (cells in which the Hb appears to have become partially detached from the cell membrane; see Fig 6.8), Heinz bodies (best seen on films stained with methyl violet) and reticulocytosis.
- **Haemolysis** is evident (see p. 372).
- **G6PD deficiency** can be detected using several screening tests, such as demonstration of the decreased ability of G6PD-deficient cells to reduce dyes. The level of the enzyme may also be directly assayed.

TREATMENT

- Any offending drugs should be stopped.
- Underlying infection should be treated.
- Blood transfusion may be life-saving.
- Splenectomy is not usually helpful.

Pyruvate kinase deficiency

This is the most common defect of red cell metabolism after G6PD deficiency, affecting thousands rather than millions of people. The site of the defect is shown in Fig 6.22. There is reduced production of ATP causing rigid red cells. Homozygotes have haemolytic anaemia and splenomegaly. It is inherited as an autosomal recessive.

INVESTIGATIONS

- **Anaemia** of variable severity is present (Hb 5–10 g dL^{-1}). The oxygen dissociation curve is shifted to the right as a result of the rise in intracellular 2,3-DPG (Fig 13.5), and this reduces the severity of symptoms due to anaemia.
- **Blood film** shows distorted ('prickle') cells and a reticulocytosis.
- **Pyruvate kinase activity** is low (affected homozygotes have levels of 5–20%).

Table 6.13
Drugs causing haemolysis in glucose-6-phosphate deficiency

Analgesics, such as:	**Antibacterials**, such as:
Aspirin	Most sulphonamides
Phenacetin (withdrawn in the UK)	Dapsone
Acetanilide	Nitrofurantoin
	Nitrofurazone
	Furazolidone
Antimalarials, such as:	Chloramphenicol
Primaquine	Ciprofloxacin
Pyrimethamine	
Quinine	**Miscellaneous drugs**, such as:
Chloroquine	Vitamin K
Pamaquine	Probenecid
	Nalidixic acid
	Quinidine
	Dimercaprol
	Phenylhydrazine
	p-Aminosalicylic acid

TREATMENT
Blood transfusions may be necessary during infections and pregnancy. Splenectomy may improve the clinical condition and is usually advised for patients requiring frequent transfusions.

FURTHER READING
Bunn HF (1997) Pathogenesis and treatment of sickle cell disease. *New England Journal of Medicine* **337**: 762–769.

Mason PJ (1996) New insights into G6PD deficiency. *British Journal of Haematology* **94**: 585–591.

Serjeant GR (1997) Sickle cell disease. *Lancet* **350**: 725–730.

Weatherall DJ (1997) The thalassaemias. *British Medical Journal* **314**: 1675–1678.

Acquired haemolytic anaemia

These anaemias may be divided into those due to immune, non-immune, or other causes (see Table 6.9).

Immune destruction of red cells
Immune destruction of red cells can be caused by:

- autoantibodies
- drug-induced antibodies
- alloantibodies.

Non-immune destruction of red cells
Non-immune destruction of red cells may be due to:

- acquired membrane defects (e.g. paroxysmal nocturnal haemoglobinuria – see p. 386)
- mechanical factors (e.g. prosthetic heart valves, or microangiopathic haemolytic anaemia – see p. 387).

It may also be secondary to systemic disease (e.g. renal and liver disease).

Miscellaneous causes
- Various *toxic substances* can disrupt the red cell membrane and cause haemolysis (e.g. arsenic, and products of *Clostridium welchii*).
- *Malaria* frequently causes anaemia owing to a combination of a reduction in red cell survival and reduced production of red cells.
- *Hypersplenism* (p. 391) results in a reduced red cell survival, which may also contribute to the anaemia seen in malaria.
- *Extensive burns* result in denaturation of red cell membrane proteins and reduced red cell survival.
- *Some drugs* (e.g. dapsone, sulphasalazine) cause oxidative haemolysis with Heinz bodies in normal subjects.
- *Some chemicals* (e.g. weed killers such as sodium chlorate) may cause severe oxidative haemolysis leading to acute renal failure.

Autoimmune haemolytic anaemias

Autoimmune haemolytic anaemias (AIHA) are acquired disorders resulting from increased red cell destruction due to red cell autoantibodies. These anaemias are characterized by the presence of a positive direct antiglobulin (Coombs') test, which detects the autoantibody on the surface of the patient's red cells (Fig 6.23).

AIHA is divided into 'warm' and 'cold' types, depending on whether the antibody attaches better to the red cells at body temperature (37°C) or at lower temperatures. The major features and the causes of these two forms of AIHA are shown in Table 6.14. In warm AIHA, IgG antibodies predominate and the direct antiglobulin test is positive with IgG alone, IgG and complement, or complement only. In cold AIHA, the antibodies are usually IgM. They easily elute off red cells, leaving complement which is detected as C3d.

Immune destruction of red cells
IgM or IgG red cell antibodies which fully activate the complement cascade cause lysis of red cells in the circulation (*intravascular haemolysis*).

IgG antibodies frequently do not activate complement and the coated red cells undergo *extravascular haemolysis* (Fig 6.24). They are either completely phagocytosed in the spleen through an interaction with Fc receptors on macrophages, or they lose part of the cell membrane through partial phagocytosis and circulate as spherocytes until they too become sequestered in the spleen. Some IgG antibodies partially activate complement, leading to deposition of C3b on the red cell surface, and this may enhance phagocytosis as macrophages also have receptors for C3b.

Non-complement-binding IgM antibodies are rare and have little or no effect on red cell survival. IgM antibodies which partially rather than fully activate complement cause adherence of red cells to C3b receptors on macrophages, particularly in the liver, although this is an ineffective mechanism of haemolysis. Most of the red cells are released from the macrophages when C3b is cleaved to C3d and then circulate with C3d on their surface.

'Warm' autoimmune haemolytic anaemias

CLINICAL FEATURES
These anaemias may occur at all ages and in both sexes, although they are most frequent in middle-aged females. They can present as a short episode of anaemia and

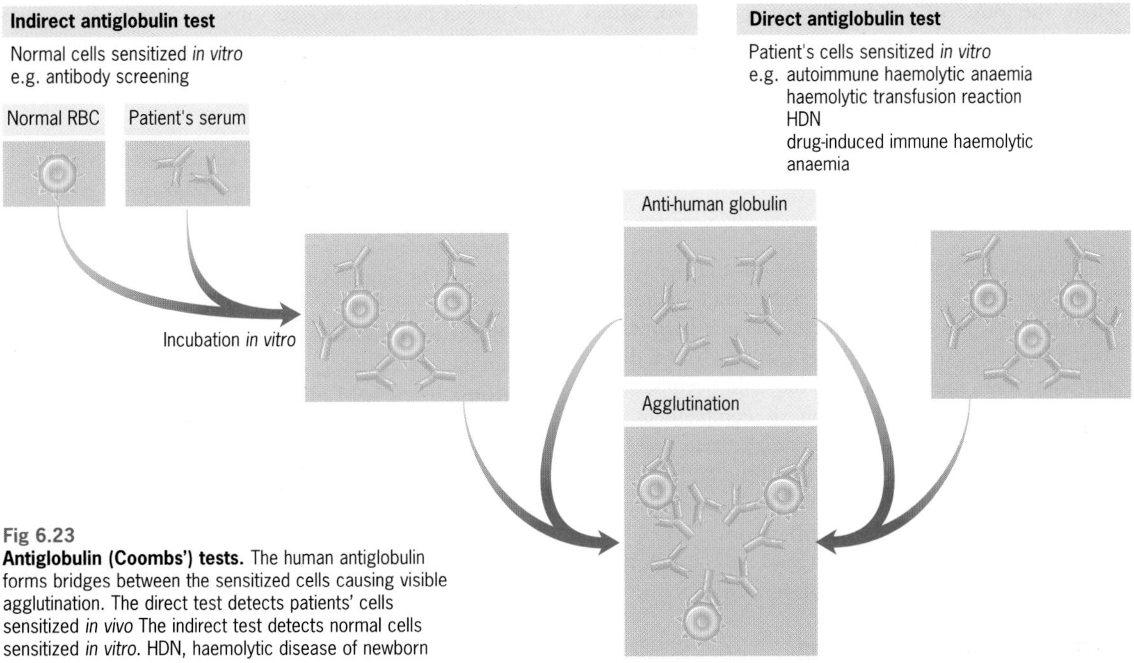

Fig 6.23
Antiglobulin (Coombs') tests. The human antiglobulin forms bridges between the sensitized cells causing visible agglutination. The direct test detects patients' cells sensitized *in vivo* The indirect test detects normal cells sensitized *in vitro*. HDN, haemolytic disease of newborn

jaundice but they often remit and relapse and may progress to an intermittent chronic pattern. The spleen is often palpable. Infections or folate deficiency may provoke a profound fall in the haemoglobin level.

In more than 30% of cases, the cause remains unknown. These anaemias may be associated with lymphoid malignancies or diseases such as rheumatoid arthritis and SLE or drugs (Table 6.14).

INVESTIGATIONS

- **Haemolytic anaemia** is evident (see p. 372).
- **Spherocytosis** is present as a result of red cell damage.
- **Direct antiglobulin test** is positive, with either IgG alone (67%), IgG and complement (20%), or complement alone (13%) being found on the surface of the red cells.
- **Autoantibodies** may have specificity for the Rh blood group system (e.g. for the e antigen).
- **Autoimmune thrombocytopenia** and/or **neutropenia** may also be present (Evans' syndrome).

TREATMENT AND PROGNOSIS

Corticosteroids (e.g. prednisolone in doses of 40–60 mg daily for adults) are effective in inducing a remission in about 80% of patients. Steroids reduce both production of the red cell autoantibody and destruction of antibody-coated cells. Splenectomy may be necessary if there is no response to steroids or if the remission is not maintained

Table 6.14
Causes and major features of autoimmune haemolytic anaemias

	Warm	**Cold**
Temperature at which antibody attaches best to red cells	37°C	Lower than 37°C
Type of antibody	IgG	IgM
Direct Coombs' test	Strongly positive	Positive
Causes of primary conditions	Idiopathic	Idiopathic
Causes of secondary condition	Autoimmune disorders, e.g. systemic lupus erythematosus Lymphomas Chronic lymphatic leukaemia Hodgkin's disease Carcinomas Drugs, e.g. methyldopa	Infections, e.g. infectious mononucleosis, *Mycoplasma pneumoniae* other viral infections (rare) Lymphomas Paroxysmal cold haemoglobinuria (IgG)

when the dose of prednisolone is reduced. Other immunosuppressive drugs, such as azathioprine and cyclophosphamide, may be effective in patients who fail to respond to steroids and splenectomy.

'Cold' autoimmune haemolytic anaemias

This is due to antibodies, usually of the IgM type. Normally, low titres of these IgM cold agglutinins reacting at 4°C are present in serum and are harmless. At low temperatures these antibodies can attach to red cells and cause their agglutination in the cold peripheries of the body. In addition, activation of complement may cause intravascular haemolysis when the cells return to the higher temperatures in the core of the body.

After certain infections (such as *Mycoplasma*, cytomegalovirus (CMV), Epstein–Barr virus (EBV)) there is increased synthesis of *polyclonal* cold agglutinins producing a mild to moderate transient haemolysis.

Chronic cold haemagglutinin disease (CHAD)

This usually occurs in the elderly with a gradual onset of haemolytic anaemia owing to the production of *monoclonal* IgM cold agglutinins. After exposure to cold the patient develops an acrocyanosis similar to Raynaud's (see p. 741) as a result of red cell autoagglutination.

INVESTIGATIONS

- **Red cells** agglutinate in the cold or at room temperature. Agglutination is sometimes seen in the sample tube after cooling but is more easily seen on the peripheral blood film made at room temperature. The agglutination is reversible after warming the sample. The agglutination may cause a spurious increase in the MCV (see p. 369).
- **Direct antiglobulin test** is positive with complement alone.
- **Monoclonal IgM antibodies** with specificity for the Ii blood group system, usually for the I antigen but occasionally for the i antigen.

TREATMENT

The underlying cause should be treated, if possible. Patients should avoid exposure to cold. Treatment with steroids, alkylating agents and splenectomy is usually ineffective.

Paroxysmal cold haemoglobinuria (PCH)

This is a rare condition associated with common childhood infections, such as measles, mumps and chickenpox, but was originally described in association

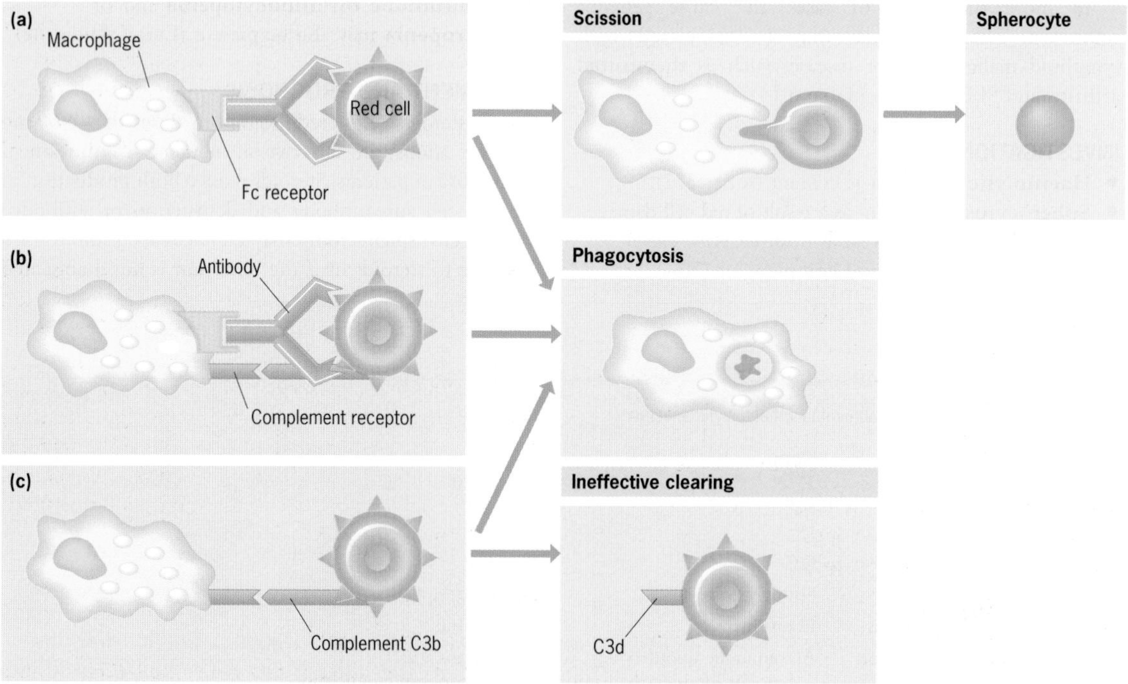

Fig 6.24
Extravascular haemolysis is due to interaction of antibody-coated cells with cells in the reticuloendothelial system, predominantly in the spleen.
(a) Spherocytosis results from partial phagocytosis
(b) Complete phagocytosis may occur and this is enhanced if there is complement as well as antibody on the cell surface
(c) Cells coated with complement only are ineffectively removed and circulate with C3d or C3b on their surface

with syphilis. Intravascular haemolysis is associated with polyclonal IgG complement-fixing antibodies. These antibodies are *biphasic*, reacting with red cells in the cold in the peripheral circulation, with lysis occurring due to complement activation when the cells return to the central circulation. The antibodies have specificity for the P red cell antigen. The lytic reaction is demonstrated *in vitro* by incubating the patient's red cells and serum at 4°C and then warming the mixture to 37°C (*Donath–Landsteiner test*). Haemolysis is self-limiting but supportive transfusions of warmed blood may be necessary.

Drug-induced haemolytic anaemia

Drugs have been classically thought to cause immune haemolytic anaemia by the following mechanisms.

- **Immune complex**. Drug–antibody immune complexes form and become attached to red cells, activating complement and resulting in cell destruction (e.g. quinine).
- **Membrane adsorption**. An antigenic drug-red cell complex is formed. Production of IgG antibodies results in cell destruction (e.g. penicillin).
- **Autoantibody**. The drug induces the production of a red cell autoantibody (e.g. methyldopa).

However, the mechanisms involved in drug-induced haemolytic anaemia may be simpler than indicated above. The interaction between a drug and red cell membrane may produce a composite antigenic structure (or *neo-antigen*), provoking two types of antibodies:

- *Drug-dependent antibodies*, which bind to both the drug and the cell membrane but not to either separately. Clinically there is usually severe complement-mediated intravascular haemolysis, which resolves quickly after withdrawal of the drug.
- *Drug-independent antibodies*, which are induced by a subtle alteration of the red cell membrane. Such antibodies react with red cells *in vitro* in the absence of the drug and are indistinguishable from 'true' autoantibodies. There is extravascular haemolysis and the clinical course tends to be more protracted.

This concept for drug-induced immune haemolytic anaemia probably also applies to drug-induced thrombocytopenia and neutropenia.

Alloimmune haemolytic anaemia

Antibodies produced in one individual react with the red cells of another. This situation occurs in haemolytic disease of the newborn, haemolytic transfusion reactions (see p. 393) and after allogeneic bone marrow, renal, liver or cardiac transplantation when donor lymphocytes transferred in the allograft may produce red cell antibodies against the recipient and cause haemolytic anaemia.

Haemolytic disease of the newborn (HDN)

HDN is due to fetomaternal incompatibility for red cell antigens. Maternal alloantibodies against fetal red cell antigens pass from the maternal circulation via the placenta into the fetus, where they destroy the fetal red cells. Only IgG antibodies are capable of transplacental passage from mother to fetus.

The most common type of HDN is that due to ABO incompatibility, where the mother is usually group O and the fetus group A.

HDN due to ABO incompatibility is usually mild and exchange transfusion is rarely needed. HDN due to RhD incompatibility has become much less common following the introduction of anti-D prophylaxis (see below). HDN may be caused by antibodies against antigens in many blood group systems (e.g. other Rh antigens such as c and E, and Kell, Duffy and Kidd – see p. 392).

Sensitization occurs as a result of passage of fetal red cells into the maternal circulation (which most readily occurs at the time of delivery), so that first pregnancies are rarely affected. However, sensitization may occur at other times, for example after a miscarriage, ectopic pregnancy or blood transfusion, or due to episodes during pregnancy which cause transplacental bleeding such as amniocentesis, chorionic villus sampling and threatened miscarriage.

CLINICAL FEATURES

These vary from a mild haemolytic anaemia of the newborn to intrauterine death from 18 weeks' gestation with the characteristic appearance of *hydrops fetalis* (hepatosplenomegaly, oedema and cardiac failure).

Kernicterus occurs owing to severe jaundice in the neonatal period, where the unconjugated (lipid-soluble) bilirubin exceeds 250 mmol L^{-1} and bile pigment deposition occurs in the basal ganglia. This can result in permanent brain damage, choreoathetosis, and spasticity. In mild cases it may cause deafness.

INVESTIGATIONS

Routine antenatal serology

All mothers should have their ABO and RhD groups determined and their serum tested for atypical antibodies after attending the antenatal booking clinic. Tests for red cell antibodies should be repeated at 26 and 34 weeks' gestation.

If an antibody is detected, its blood group specificity should be determined and the mother should be retested at least monthly. A rising antibody titre of IgG antibodies or a history of HDN in a previous pregnancy is an indication for referral to a specialist unit to determine the need for amniocentesis (to assess the level of bilirubin in the amniotic fluid) or fetal blood sampling to determine the severity of HDN and to guide further management.

At the birth of an affected infant

A sample of cord blood is obtained. This shows:

- anaemia with a high reticulocyte count
- a positive direct antiglobulin test
- a raised serum bilirubin.

TREATMENT

Management of the baby

In mild cases, phototherapy may be used to convert bilirubin to water-soluble biliverdin. Biliverdin can be excreted by the kidneys and this therefore reduces the chance of kernicterus.

In more severely affected cases, exchange transfusion may be necessary to replace the infant's red cells and to remove bilirubin. Indications for exchange transfusion include:

- a cord Hb of <14 g dL^{-1}
- a cord bilirubin of >60 $\mu mol\ L^{-1}$
- a later bilirubin of >300 $\mu mol\ L^{-1}$
- a rapidly rising bilirubin level.

Further exchange transfusions may be necessary to remove the unconjugated bilirubin.

The blood used for exchange transfusions should be ABO-compatible with the mother and infant, lack the antigen against which the maternal antibody is directed, be fresh (no more than 5 days from the day of collection), and leucocyte-depleted to prevent transmission of cytomegalovirus which is leucocyte-associated.

A fetus severely affected before 33 weeks' gestation may need intrauterine blood transfusions carried out in a special unit.

Prevention of RhD immunization in the mother

Anti-D should be given after delivery when all of the following are present:

- the mother is RhD negative
- the fetus is RhD positive
- there is no maternal anti-D detectable in the mother's serum; i.e. the mother is not already immunized.

The dose is 500 i.u. of IgG anti-D intramuscularly within 48 hours of delivery. The *Kleihauer test* is used to assess the number of fetal cells in the maternal circulation. A blood film prepared from maternal blood is treated with acid, which elutes Hb A. Hb F is resistant to this treatment and can be seen when the film is stained with eosin. If large numbers of fetal red cells are present in the maternal circulation, a higher dose of anti-D is necessary.

It may be necessary to give prophylaxis to RhD-negative women at other times when sensitization may occur, for example after an ectopic pregnancy, threatened miscarriage or amniocentesis. The dose of anti-D is 250 i.u. before 20 weeks' gestation and 500 i.u. after 20 weeks.

Of previously non-immunized RhD-negative women carrying RhD-positive fetuses, 1–2% are immunized by the time of delivery. *Antenatal prophylaxis* with administration of anti-D to RhD-negative women at 28 and 34 weeks' gestation has been shown to reduce the incidence of immunization in some studies. Antenatal prophylaxis is already used in some centres, and it has recently been recommended that all RhD-negative women should be given antenatal anti-D in the UK. Monoclonal anti-D could in principle replace polyclonal anti-D which is collected from RhD-negative women immunized in pregnancy and deliberately immunized RhD-negative males, but it is likely to be some years before trials have been completed and it is available in sufficient quantity.

Non-immune haemolytic anaemia

Paroxysmal nocturnal haemoglobinuria (PNH)

This is a rare acquired red cell defect in which a clone of red cells is particularly sensitive to destruction by activated complement. These cells are continually haemolysed intravascularly. Platelets and granulocytes are also affected and there may be thrombocytopenia and neutropenia.

The underlying defect is an inability of PNH cells to make glycosyl-phosphatidylinositol (GPI) which anchors surface proteins such as delay accelerating factor (DAF) and membrane inhibitor of reactive lysis (MIRL) to cell membranes. DAF and MIRL and other proteins are involved in complement degradation, and in their absence the haemolytic action of complement is not regulated. The molecular basis of PNH has been found to be mutations in the *pig*-A (phosphatidyl inositol glycan complementation group A) gene responsible for synthesis of the GPI anchor.

CLINICAL FEATURES

Patients present with haemolysis which may be precipitated by infection, iron therapy or surgery. Characteristically only the urine voided at night and in the morning on waking is dark in colour, although the reason for this phenomenon is not clear. In severe cases all urine samples are dark. Urinary iron loss may be sufficient to cause iron deficiency.

Some patients present insidiously with signs of anaemia and recurrent abdominal pains.

Venous thrombotic episodes are very common, and unusual and severe thromboses may occur, for example in hepatic (Budd–Chiari syndrome), mesenteric or cerebral veins.

INVESTIGATIONS

- **Intravascular haemolysis** is evident (see p. 372).
- **Ham's test**. Cells from a patient with PNH lyse more readily in acidified serum than do normal cells.
- **Bone marrow** is sometimes hypoplastic despite haemolysis.

TREATMENT AND PROGNOSIS

There is no specific treatment for PNH. It is a chronic disorder requiring supportive measures such as blood transfusions, which are necessary for patients with severe anaemia. Leucocyte-depleted blood should be used in order to prevent transfusion reactions resulting in complement activation and acceleration of the haemolysis.

Long-term anticoagulation may be necessary for patients with recurrent thrombotic episodes. Bone marrow transplantation has been successfully carried out in a small number of patients, but only patients under the age of 50 years with an HLA-identical sibling are eligible.

The course of PNH is variable. PNH may transform into aplastic anaemia or acute leukaemia, but it may remain stable for many years and the PNH clone may even disappear, which must be taken into account if considering potentially dangerous treatments such as bone marrow transplantation. The median survival is 10–15 years.

The gene that is defective in PNH is known, and so gene therapy will perhaps be possible in the future.

Mechanical haemolytic anaemia

Red cells may be injured by physical trauma in the circulation. Direct injury may cause immediate cell lysis or may be followed by resealing of the cell membrane with the formation of distorted red cells or 'fragments'. These cells may circulate for a short period before being destroyed prematurely in the reticuloendothelial system.

The causes of mechanical haemolytic anaemia include:

- damaged artificial heart valves
- March haemoglobinuria, where there is damage to red cells in the feet associated with prolonged marching or running
- microangiopathic haemolytic anaemia (MAHA), where fragmentation of red cells occurs in an abnormal microcirculation caused by malignant hypertension, eclampsia, haemolytic uraemic syndrome, thrombotic thrombocytopenic purpura, vasculitis, or disseminated intravascular coagulation.

FURTHER READING

Hillmen P, Lewis SM, Bessler M, Luzzatto L, Dacie JV (1995) Natural history of paroxysmal nocturnal haemoglobinuria. *New England Journal of Medicine* **333**: 1253–1258.

Rosse WF (1997) Paroxysmal nocturnal haemoglobinuria. *Medicine* **76**: 63–93.

Myeloproliferative disorders

In these disorders there is uncontrolled clonal proliferation of one or more of the cell lines in the bone marrow, namely erythroid, myeloid and megakaryocyte lines. Myeloproliferative disorders include *polycythaemia vera* (PV), *essential thrombocythaemia* (ET), *myelofibrosis* and *chronic myeloid leukaemia* (CML). These disorders are grouped together as there can be transition from one disease to another; for example PV can lead to myelofibrosis. They may also transform to acute myeloblastic leukaemia. The *non-leukaemic myeloproliferative disorders* (PV, ET and myelofibrosis) will be discussed in this section. Chronic myeloid leukaemia is described on p. 430.

Polycythaemia

Polycythaemia (or erythrocytosis) is defined as an increase in haemoglobin, PCV and red cell count. PCV is a more reliable indicator of polycythaemia than is Hb, which may be disproportionately low in iron deficiency. Polycythaemia can be divided into *absolute erythrocytosis* where there is a true increase in red cell volume, or relative erythrocytosis where the red cell volume is normal but there is a decrease in the plasma volume (see Fig 6.6).

Absolute erythrocytosis is due to primary polycythaemia (PV) or secondary polycythaemia. Secondary polycythaemia is due to either an *appropriate* increase in red cells in response to anoxia, or to an *inappropriate* increase associated with tumours, such as a renal carcinoma. The causes of polycythaemia are given in Table 6.15.

Primary polycythaemia: polycythaemia vera

PV is a clonal stem cell disorder in which there is an alteration in the pluripotent progenitor cell leading to excessive proliferation of erythroid, myeloid and megakaryocytic progenitor cells. This is due to a failure of apoptosis as a result of deregulation of the Bcl-x_L gene, which is known to oppose programmed cell death (p. 153).

Table 6.15
Causes of polycythaemia

Primary Polycythaemia vera **Secondary** **Due to an appropriate increase in erythropoietin:** High altitude Lung disease Cardiovascular disease (right-to-left shunt) Heavy smoking Increased affinity of haemoglobin, e.g. familial polycythaemia	**Due to an inappropriate increase in erythropoietin:** Renal disease, renal cell carcinoma, Wilms' tumour Hepatocellular carcinoma Adrenal tumours Cerebellar haemangioblastoma Massive uterine fibroma **Relative** Stress or spurious polycythaemia Dehydration Burns

CLINICAL FEATURES

The onset is insidious. It usually presents in patients aged over 60 years with tiredness, depression, vertigo, tinnitus and visual disturbance. It should be noted that these symptoms are also common in the normal population over the age of 60 and consequently PV is easily missed. These features, together with hypertension, angina, intermittent claudication and a tendency to bleed, are suggestive evidence for PV.

Severe itching after a hot bath or when the patient is warm is common. Gout due to increased cell turnover may be a feature, and peptic ulceration occurs in a minority of patients. Thrombosis and haemorrhage are the major complications of PV.

The patient is usually plethoric and has a deep dusky cyanosis. Injection of the conjunctivae is commonly seen. The spleen is palpable in 70% and is useful in distinguishing PV from secondary causes. The liver is enlarged in 50% of patients.

INVESTIGATIONS

- **Hb and PCV** are increased. The WCC is raised in about 70% of cases of PV and the platelet count is elevated in about 50%.
- **Bone marrow** shows erythroid hyperplasia and increased numbers of megakaryocytes.
- **Red cell volume** measured using ^{51}Cr-labelled red cells is increased (>36 mL kg^{-1} in males and 32 mL kg^{-1} in females).
- **Plasma volume** shows normal or increased values (normal range is 45 ± 5 mL kg^{-1}).
- **Serum uric acid** levels may be raised.
- **Leucocyte alkaline phosphatase** (LAP) score is usually high.
- **Serum vitamin B_{12} and vitamin B_{12}-binding protein** (TC I) levels may be high, although these are not routinely measured.

DIFFERENTIAL DIAGNOSIS

An increase in the red cell volume should be established. Raised WBC and platelet counts with splenomegaly makes a diagnosis of PV very likely. The principal secondary causes can often be excluded by the history and examination, but a renal ultrasound, an arterial Po_2 and carboxyhaemoglobin levels are usually performed.

The *serum erythropoietin* level is not diagnostic but may be helpful in distinguishing PV from secondary polycythaemia. In PV the level is low or normal, whereas in secondary polycythaemia the level may be raised, as expected, but also can be normal.

COURSE AND MANAGEMENT

Treatment is designed to maintain a normal blood count and to prevent the complications of the disease, particularly thromboses and haemorrhage. Treatment is aimed at keeping the PCV below 0.45 L/L and the platelet count below 400×10^9/L. There are three types of treatment:

- **Venesection.** This will successfully relieve many of the symptoms of PV. Iron deficiency limits erythropoiesis. Venesection is often used as the sole treatment and other therapy is reserved to control the thrombocytosis.
- **Chemotherapy**. Continuous or intermittent treatment with hydroxyurea is used frequently because of the ease of controlling thrombocytosis and general safety in comparison to the alkylating agents such as busulphan which carry an increased risk of acute leukaemia. Low-dose intermittent busulphan may be more convenient for elderly people, and this must be weighed against the potential risk of long-term complications.
- **Radioactive ^{32}P**. One dose may give control for up to 18 months, but the administration of ^{32}P carries an increased risk of transformation to acute leukaemia. ^{32}P is confined to the over-70 years age group.

Allopurinol is given to block uric acid production. The pruritus is lessened by avoiding very hot baths. H_1-receptor antagonists have largely proved unsuccessful in relieving distressing pruritus, but H_2-receptor antagonists such as cimetidine are occasionally effective.

It should be noted that patients with uncontrolled PV have a high operative risk; 75% of patients have severe haemorrhage following surgery and 30% of these patients die. Polycythaemia should be controlled before surgery. In an emergency, reduction of the haematocrit by venesection and appropriate fluid replacement must be carried out.

PROGNOSIS

PV develops into myelofibrosis in 30% of cases and into acute myeloblastic leukaemia in 5% as part of the natural history of the disease.

Secondary polycythaemias

The causes of these are shown in Table 6.15. The treatment is that of the precipitating factor; for example, renal or posterior fossa tumours need to be resected. Heavy smoking can produce as much as 10% carboxyhaemoglobin and this can produce polycythaemia because of a reduction in the oxygen-carrying capacity of the blood. Complications are similar to those seen in PV, including thrombosis, haemorrhage and cardiac failure, but the complications due to myeloproliferative disease such as progression to myelofibrosis or acute leukaemia do not develop. Venesection may be symptomatically helpful in the hypoxic patient, particularly if the PCV is above 0.55 L/L.

'Relative' or 'stress' polycythaemia (Gaisböck's syndrome)

This condition was originally thought to be stress-induced. The red cell volume is normal but, as the result of a decreased plasma volume, there is a *relative* polycythaemia. 'Stress' polycythaemia is more common than PV and occurs in middle-aged men, particularly in smokers who are obese and hypertensive. The condition may present with cardiovascular problems such as myocardial or cerebral ischaemia. For this reason, it may be justifiable to venesect the patient. Smoking should be stopped.

Essential thrombocythaemia (ET)

ET is closely related to PV. The platelet count is usually $>1000 \times 10^9$/L. It presents with bruising, bleeding and cerebrovascular symptoms. Initially splenic hypertrophy may be seen but, as the condition progresses, recurrent thromboses owing to the increased number of platelets reduce the size of the spleen and it may atrophy.

ET should be distinguished from *secondary thrombocytosis* that is seen in haemorrhage, connective tissue disorders, malignancy, after splenectomy and in other myeloproliferative disorders.

Treatment is with hydroxyurea or busulphan to control the platelet count at less than 400×10^9/L. α-Interferon is also effective but it is expensive and is administered by subcutaneous injection. ET may eventually transform into PV, myelofibrosis or acute leukaemia, but the disease may not progress for many years.

Myelofibrosis (myelosclerosis)

The terms myelosclerosis and myelofibrosis are interchangeable. There is clonal proliferation of stem cells and myeloid metaplasia in the liver, spleen and other organs. There is increased fibrosis in the bone marrow caused by hyperplasia of abnormal megakaryocytes which release fibroblast-stimulating factors such as platelet-derived growth factor. In about 25% of cases there is a preceding history of PV.

CLINICAL FEATURES

The disease presents insidiously with lethargy, weakness and weight loss. Patients often complain of a 'fullness' in the upper abdomen due to splenomegaly. Severe pain related to respiration may indicate perisplenitis secondary to splenic infarction, and bone pain and attacks of gout can complicate the illness. Bruising and bleeding occur due to thrombocytopenia or abnormal platelet function. Other physical signs include anaemia, fever and massive splenomegaly (for other causes see p. 391).

INVESTIGATIONS

- **Anaemia** with leucoerythroblastic features is present (p. 397). Poikilocytes and red cells with characteristic tear-drop forms are seen. The WBC count may be over 100×10^9/L, and the differential WBC count may be very similar to that seen in CML; later leucopenia may develop.
- **The platelet count** may be very high but, in later stages, thrombocytopenia occurs.
- **Bone marrow aspiration** is often unsuccessful and this gives a clue to the presence of the condition. A bone marrow trephine is necessary to show the markedly increased fibrosis. Increased numbers of megakaryocytes may be seen.
- **The Philadelphia chromosome** is absent; this helps to distinguish myelofibrosis from most cases of CML.
- **The LAP score** is normal or high.
- **A high serum urate** is present.
- **Low serum folate** levels may occur owing to the increased haemopoietic activity.

DIFFERENTIAL DIAGNOSIS

The major diagnostic difficulty is the differentiation of myelofibrosis from CML as in both conditions there may be marked splenomegaly and a raised WBC count with many granulocyte precursors seen in the peripheral blood. The main distinguishing features are the appearance of the bone marrow and the absence of the Philadelphia chromosome in myelofibrosis.

Fibrosis of the marrow, often with a leucoerythroblastic anaemia, can occur secondarily to leukaemia or lymphoma, tuberculosis or malignant infiltration with metastatic carcinoma, or to irradiation.

TREATMENT

This consists of general supportive measures such as blood transfusion, folic acid, analgesics and allopurinol. Drugs such as hydroxyurea and busulphan are used to reduce metabolic activity and high WBC count and platelet levels; hydroxyurea is the most common drug used. Chemotherapy and radiotherapy are used to reduce splenic size. If the spleen becomes very large and painful, and transfusion requirements are high, it may be advisable to perform splenectomy. Splenectomy may also result in relief of severe thrombocytopenia.

PROGNOSIS

Patients may survive for 10 years or more; median survival is three years. Death may occur in 10–20% of cases from transformation to acute myeloblastic leukaemia. The most common causes of death are cardiovascular disease, infection and gastrointestinal bleeding.

Myelodysplasia

Myelodysplasia (MDS) describes a group of acquired bone marrow disorders that are due to a defect in stem cells. They are characterized by increasing bone marrow failure with quantitative and qualitative abnormalities of all three myeloid cell lines (red cells, granulocyte/monocytes and platelets). The natural history of MDS is variable, but there is a high morbidity and mortality owing to bone marrow failure, and transformation into acute myeloblastic leukaemia occurs in about 30% of cases. There are a number of different types of MDS:

- refractory anaemia (RA)
- refractory anaemia with ringed sideroblasts (>15% ringed sideroblasts – RARS)
- refractory anaemia with an excess of blasts (blasts 5–20% – RAEB)
- refractory anaemia with an excess of blasts in transformation (blasts 20–30%) (RAEB-T)
- chronic myelomonocytic leukaemia (CMML).

CLINICAL AND LABORATORY FEATURES

MDS occurs mainly in the elderly and presents with symptoms of anaemia, infection or bleeding due to pancytopenia. Serial blood counts show evidence of increasing bone marrow failure with anaemia, neutropenia, monocytosis and thrombocyopenia, either alone or in combination. In CMML, monocytes are $> 1 \times 10^9$/L and the WBC count may be $>100 \times 10^9$/L.

The bone marrow usually shows increased cellularity despite the pancytopenia. Dyserythropoiesis is present, and granulocyte precursors and megakaryocytes also have abnormal morphology. Ring sideroblasts are present in all types. In RAEB and RAEB-T, the number of blasts in the bone marrow is increased, and the prognosis is worse than in those types with a normal number of blast cells (<5%).

MANAGEMENT

Patients with <5% blasts in the bone marrow are usually managed conservatively with red cell and platelet transfusions and antibiotics for infections, as they are needed. Haemopoietic growth fators (e.g. erythropoietin, G-CSF) may be useful in some patients.

Patients with >5% blasts have a less favourable prognosis, and a number of treatment options are available:

- **Supportive care only** is suitable for elderly patients with other medical problems.
- **'Gentle' chemotherapy** (low-dose or single-agent) may be useful in patients with high WBC counts.
- **Intensive chemotherapy** schedules used for acute myeloblastic leukaemia (see p. 426) may be tried in patients under the age of 60, but the remission rate is less, and prolonged pancytopenia may occur owing to poor haemopoietic regeneration because of the defect in stem cells.
- **Bone marrow transplantation** offers the hope of cure in the small proportion of MDS patients who are under the age of 50 and who have an HLA-identical sibling or an unrelated HLA-matched donor.

FURTHER READING

Provan D (1997) Myelodysplastic syndromes. *Prescriber's Journal* **37**: 17–23.

Schwartz RC (1998) Polycythaemia vera – chance, death and mutability. *New England Journal of Medicine* **338**: 613–615.

The spleen

The spleen is the largest lymphoid organ in the body and is situated in the left hypochondrium. There are two anatomical components:

- the red pulp, consisting of sinuses lined by endothelial macrophages and cords (spaces)
- the white pulp, which has a structure similar to lymphoid follicles.

Blood enters via the splenic artery and is delivered to the red and white pulp. During the flow the blood is 'skimmed', with leucocytes and plasma preferentially passing to white pulp. Some red cells pass rapidly through into the venous system while others are held up in the red pulp.

Functions

Sequestration and phagocytosis. Normal red cells, which are flexible, pass through the red pulp into the venous system without difficulty. Old or abnormal cells are damaged by the hypoxia, low glucose and low pH found in the sinuses of the red pulp and are therefore removed by phagocytosis along with other circulating foreign matter. Howell–Jolly and Heinz bodies and sideroblastic granules have their particles removed by 'pitting' and are then returned to the circulation. IgG-coated red cells are removed through their Fc receptors by macrophages.

Extramedullary haemopoiesis. Pluripotential stem cells are present in the spleen and proliferate during severe haematological stress, such as in haemolytic anaemia or thalassaemia major.

Immunological function. About 25% of the body's T lymphocytes and 15% of B lymphocytes are present in the spleen. The spleen shares the function of production of antibodies with other lymphoid tissues.

Blood pooling. Up to one-third of the platelets are sequestrated in the spleen and can be rapidly mobilized. Enlarged spleens pool a significant percentage (up to 40%) of the red cell mass.

Splenomegaly

CAUSES

A clinically palpable spleen can have many causes.

- *Infection*:
  (a) acute – e.g. septic shock, infective endocarditis, typhoid, infectious mononucleosis
  (b) chronic – e.g. tuberculosis and brucellosis
  (c) parasitic – e.g. malaria, kala-azar and schistosomiasis.
- *Inflammation*: rheumatoid arthritis, sarcoidosis, SLE.
- *Haematological*: haemolytic anaemia, haemoglobinopathies and the leukaemias, lymphomas and myeloproliferative disorders.
- *Portal hypertension*: liver disease.
- *Miscellaneous*: storage diseases, amyloid, primary and secondary neoplasias, tropical splenomegaly.

Massive splenomegaly

Massive splenomegaly is seen in myelofibrosis, chronic myeloid leukaemia, chronic malaria, kala-azar or, rarely, Gaucher's disease. *Investigation* is that of the primary disorder. The spleen can be visualized by ultrasound or CT scanning. Splenic function can be assessed with isotope scanning.

Hypersplenism

This can result from splenomegaly due to any cause. It is commonly seen with splenomegaly due to haematological disorders, portal hypertension, rheumatoid arthritis (Felty's syndrome) and lymphoma. Hypersplenism produces:

- pancytopenia
- haemolysis due to sequestration and destruction of red cells in the spleen
- increased plasma volume.

Treatment is often dependent on the underlying cause, but splenectomy is sometimes required for severe anaemia or thrombocytopenia.

Splenectomy

Splenectomy is performed mainly for:

- trauma
- autoimmune thrombocytopenic purpura (p. 402)
- haemolytic anaemias (p. 372)
- hypersplenism.

Problems after splenectomy

An immediate problem is an increased platelet count (usually 600–1000 × 10^9/L) for 2–3 weeks. Thromboembolic phenomena may occur. In the longer term there is an increased risk of overwhelming infections, particularly pneumococcal infections.

Prophylaxis against infection after splenectomy or splenic dysfunction

All patients should be educated about the risk of infection and the importance of early recognition and treatment. They should be given an information leaflet and should carry a card to alert health professionals to their risk of overwhelming infection.

Pneumococcal immunization should be given 2–3 weeks before splenectomy. It is effective if the types of pneumonia are reflected in the polysaccharides contained in the serum. The vaccination may need to be repeated in 5–10 years. The currently available polyvalent vaccine contains purified capsular polysaccharide from the 23 most prevalent serotypes. *Haemophilus* influenzae type B vaccine should be given to those who have not previously been immunized. Meningococcal immunization is not routinely recommended, except for travellers to areas where there is an increased risk of group A infection. Long-term prophylactic penicillin (e.g. penicillin V 500 mg 12 hourly) is recommended.

Postsplenectomy haematological features

- *Thrombocytosis* persists in about 30% of cases.
- *The WBC count* is usually normal but there may be a mild lymphocytosis and monocytosis.
- *Abnormalities in red cell morphology* are the most prominent changes and include Howell–Jolly bodies, Pappenheimer bodies (contain sideroblastic granules), target cells and irregular contracted red cells (see Fig 6.8). Pitted red cells can be counted.

Splenic atrophy

This is seen in sickle cell disease due to infarction. It is also seen in coeliac disease, in dermatitis herpetiformis, and occasionally in ulcerative colitis and essential thrombocythaemia. Postsplenectomy haematological features are seen.

FURTHER READING

British Committee for Standards in Haematology (1996) Guidelines for the prevention and treatment of infection in patients with an absent or dysfunctional spleen. *British Medical Journal* **312**: 430–434.

Blood transfusion

The cells and proteins in the blood express antigens which are controlled by polymorphic genes; that is, a specific antigen may be present in some individuals but not in others. A blood transfusion may immunize the recipient against donor antigens that the recipient lacks (*alloimmunization*), and repeated transfusions increase the risk of the occurrence of alloimmunization. Similarly, the transplacental passage of fetal blood cells during pregnancy may alloimmunize the mother against fetal antigens inherited from the father. Antibodies stimulated by blood transfusion or pregnancy, such as Rhesus antibodies, are termed *immune* antibodies and are usually IgG, in contrast to *naturally occurring* antibodies, such as ABO antibodies, which are made in response to environmental antigens present in food and bacteria and which are usually IgM.

Blood groups

The blood groups are determined by antigens on the surface of red cells; more than 400 blood groups have been found. The ABO and Rh systems are the two most important blood groups, but incompatibilities involving many other blood groups (e.g. Kell, Duffy, Kidd) may cause haemolytic transfusion reactions and/or haemolytic disease of the newborn (HDN).

ABO system

This blood group system involves naturally occurring IgM anti-A and anti-B antibodies which are capable of producing rapid and severe intravascular haemolysis of incompatible red cells.

The ABO system is under the control of a pair of allelic genes, *H* and *h*, and also three allelic genes, *A*, *B* and *O*, producing the genotypes and phenotypes shown in Table 6.16. The A, B and H antigens are very similar in structure; differences in the terminal sugars determine their specificity. The *H* gene codes for enzyme H, which attaches fructose to the basic glycoprotein backbone to form H substance, which is the precursor for A and B antigens.

The *A* and *B* genes control specific enzymes responsible for the addition to H substance of *N*-acetylgalactosamine for Group A and D-galactose for Group B. The *O* gene is amorphic and does not transform H substance and therefore O is not antigenic. The A, B and H antigens are present on most body cells. These antigens are also found in soluble form in tissue fluids such as saliva and gastric juice in the 80% of the population who possess *secretor* genes.

Table 6.16
The ABO system: antigens and antibodies

Phenotype	Genotype	Antigens	Antibodies	Frequency UK (%)
O	OO	None	Anti-A and anti-B	44
A	AA or AO	A	Anti-B	45
B	BB or BO	B	Anti-A	8
AB	AB	A and B	None	3

Rh system

There is a high frequency of development of IgG RhD antibodies in RhD-negative individuals after exposure to RhD-positive red cells. The antibodies formed are of major importance in causing HDN and haemolytic transfusion reactions.

This system is coded by allelic genes, *C* and *c*, *E* and *e*, *D* and no *D*, which is signified as *d*; they are inherited as triplets on each chromosome, one from each pair of genes (i.e. *CDE/cde*). The presence of the d antigen has not been demonstrated and the presence or absence of the D antigen determines whether an individual is characterized as RhD positive or negative.

Procedure for blood transfusion

The safety of blood transfusion depends on meticulous attention to detail at each stage leading to and during the transfusion. Avoidance of simple errors involving patient and blood sample identification at the time of collection of the sample for crossmatching and at the time of transfusion would avoid most serious haemolytic transfusion reactions, almost all of which involve the ABO system. Over 50% of fatalities associated with blood transfusion are due to immediate haemolytic transfusion reactions; the remainder are mainly due to post-transfusion hepatitis in developing countries.

Pretransfusion compatibility testing

Blood grouping

The ABO and RhD groups of the patient are determined.

Antibody screening

The patient's serum is screened for atypical antibodies that may cause a significant reduction in the survival of the transfused red cells. The patient's serum is tested against red cells from at least two group O donors, expressing a wide range of red cell antigens, for detection of IgM red cell alloantibodies (using a direct agglutination test of cells suspended in saline) and IgG antibodies (using an indirect antiglobulin test, see p. 383). If there is a positive result, the blood group specificity of the antibody should be determined using a comprehensive panel of typed red cells.

Selection of donor blood and crossmatching

Donor blood of the same ABO and RhD group as the patient is selected.

Crossmatching procedures

Patients *without* atypical red cell antibodies. The full crossmatch involves testing the patient's serum against the donor red cells suspended in saline in a direct agglutination test, and also using an indirect antiglobulin test. In some hospitals this has been shortened to an *immediate spin crossmatch* where the patient's serum is briefly incubated with the donor red cells, followed by centrifugation and examination for agglutination; this rapid crossmatch is an acceptable method of excluding ABO incompatibility in patients known to have a negative antibody screen.

Patients *with* atypical red cell antibodies. Donor blood should be selected that lacks the relevant red cell antigen(s), as well as being the same ABO and RhD group as the patient. A full crossmatch should always be carried out.

Hospital guidelines and new procedures. Many hospitals have guidelines for the ordering of blood for elective surgery (*maximum surgical blood ordering schedules*). These are aimed at unnecessary crossmatching and reducing the amount of blood that eventually becomes outdated. Many operations in which blood is required only occasionally for unexpectedly high blood loss can be classified as 'group and save serum'; this means that, where the antibody screen is negative, blood is not reserved in advance but can be made available quickly if necessary. If a patient has atypical antibodies, compatible blood should always be reserved in advance.

Several new systems for blood grouping, antibody screening and crossmatching have become available to hospital transfusion laboratories. They do not depend on agglutination of red cells in suspension, but rather on the differential passage of agglutinated and unagglutinated red cells through a column of dextran gel matrix (e.g. DiaMed, and Ortho Biovue systems), or on the capture of antibodies by red cells immobilized on the surface of a microplate well (e.g. Capture-R solid phase system). These new systems are easy to use, but are costly.

Complications of blood transfusion (see Table 6.17)

Immunological complications

Alloimmunization

Blood transfusion carries a risk of alloimmunization to the many 'foreign' antigens present on red cells, leucocytes, platelets and plasma proteins. Alloimmunization may also occur during pregnancy – to fetal antigens inherited from the father and not shared by the mother.

Alloimmunization does not usually cause clinical problems with the first transfusion but these may occur with subsequent transfusions. There may also be important delayed consequences of alloimmunization, such as HDN and rejection of tissue transplants.

Incompatibility

This may result in poor survival of transfused cells, such as red cells and platelets, and also in the harmful effects of antigen–antibody reaction.

Haemolytic transfusion reactions

Immediate reaction

This is the most serious complication of blood transfusion and is usually due to ABO incompatibility. There is complement activation by the antigen–antibody reaction, usually caused by IgM antibodies, leading to rigors, lumbar pain, dyspnoea, hypotension, haemoglobinuria and renal failure. The initial symptoms may occur a few minutes after starting the transfusion. Activation of coagulation may also occur and bleeding due to disseminated intravascular coagulation (DIC) is a bad prognostic sign. Emergency treatment may be needed to maintain the blood pressure and renal function.

DIAGNOSIS

This is confirmed by finding evidence of *haemolysis* (e.g. haemoglobinuria), and *incompatibility* between donor

Table 6.17
Complications of blood transfusion

Immunological	Non-immunological
Alloimmunization	Transmission of infection
Incompatibility	Hepatitis
Red cells	HIV
Immediate haemolytic transfusion reactions	Other viruses – CMV, EBV, HTLV-1
Delayed haemolytic transfusion reactions	Parasites – malaria, trypanosomiasis, toxoplasmosis
Leucocyte and platelets	Syphilis
Non-haemolytic (febrile) transfusion reactions	Transfusion of blood contaminated with bacteria
Post-transfusion purpura	Circulatory failure due to volume overload
Poor survival of transfused platelets and granulocytes	Iron overload due to multiple transfusions (see p. 376)
Graft-versus-host disease	Massive transfusion of stored blood may cause bleeding and electrolyte changes (see p. 844)
Plasma proteins	Physical damage due to freezing or heating
Urticarial and anaphylactic reactions	Thrombophlebitis
	Air embolism

and recipient. All documentation should be checked to detect errors such as:

- failure to check the identity of the patient when taking the sample for compatibility testing (i.e. sample from the wrong patient)
- mislabelling the blood sample with the wrong patient's name
- simple labelling or handling errors in the laboratory
- failure to perform proper identity checks before the blood is transfused (i.e. blood transfused to the wrong patient).

The serious consequences of such failures emphasize the need for meticulous checks at all stages in the procedure of blood transfusion.

INVESTIGATIONS

To confirm where the error occurred, blood grouping should be carried out on:

- the patient's original sample (used for the compatibility testing)
- a new sample taken from the patient after the reaction
- the donor units.

At the first suspicion of any serious transfusion reaction, the transfusion should always be stopped and the donor units returned to the blood transfusion laboratory with a new blood sample from the patient to exclude a haemolytic transfusion reaction.

Delayed reaction

This may occur in patients alloimmunized by previous transfusions or pregnancies. The antibody level is too low to be detected by pretransfusion compatibility testing, but a secondary immune response occurs after transfusion, resulting in destruction of the transfused cells, usually by IgG antibodies.

Haemolysis is usually extravascular as the antibodies are IgG, and the patient may develop anaemia and jaundice about a week after the transfusion, although most are clinically silent. The blood film shows spherocytosis and reticulocytosis. The direct antiglobulin test is positive and detection of the antibody is usually straightforward.

Non-haemolytic (febrile) transfusion reactions

Febrile reactions are a common complication of blood transfusion in patients who have previously been transfused or pregnant. The usual cause is the presence of leucocyte antibodies in the recipient acting against transfused leucocytes, leading to release of pyrogens. Typical signs are flushing and tachycardia, fever (>38°C), chills and rigors. Aspirin may be used to reduce the fever, although it should not be used in patients with thrombocytopenia. Febrile reactions may be prevented after further transfusions by the use of leucocyte-depleted blood.

Potent leucocyte antibodies in the plasma of donors, who are usually multiparous women, may cause severe pulmonary reactions (called *transfusion-related acute lung injury* or TRALI) characterized by dyspnoea, fever, cough, and shadowing in the perihilar and lower lung fields on the chest X-ray.

Urticaria and anaphylaxis

Urticarial reactions are often attributed to plasma protein incompatibility but, in most cases, they are unexplained. They are common but rarely severe; stopping or slowing the transfusion and administration of chlorpheniramine 10 mg i.v. are usually sufficient treatment.

Anaphylactic reactions (see p. 862) occasionally occur; severe reactions are seen in patients lacking IgA who produce anti-IgA that reacts with IgA in the transfused blood. The transfusion should be stopped and adrenaline 0.5 mg i.m. and chlorpheniramine 10 mg i.v. should be given immediately; endotracheal intubation may be required. Patients who have had severe urticarial or anaphylactic reactions should receive either washed red cells, autologous blood, or blood from IgA-deficient donors for patients with IgA deficiency.

Non-immunological complications

Transmission of infection

The incidence of post-transfusion hepatitis was estimated to be about 1% in the UK before testing for antibodies against hepatitis C virus (HCV) was introduced in 1991. As most cases were the result of non-A, non-B hepatitis due to HCV, the incidence of post-transfusion hepatitis has decreased. Each donation has been tested for HBsAg for many years. The incidence of transmission of HBV and HCV is about 1 in 200 000 units transfused for each virus. Other viruses which may cause post-transfusion hepatitis include CMV and EBV, and there are likely to be other as yet unidentified viruses.

In the UK the incidence of transmission of HIV by blood transfusion is extremely low – probably under 1 in 3 million units transfused. Prevention is based on self-exclusion of donors in 'high-risk' groups and testing each donation for anti-HIV.

Testing for anti-HTLV-1 (see p. 65) is currently being considered in the UK. Only about 1 in 20 000 donors are seropositive, and there is a low risk of developing disease after infection because of the long incubation period.

There is an increased risk of viral transmission from coagulation factor concentrates prepared from large pools of plasma. However, these are now subjected to measures for inactivating viruses – such as treatment with heat, solvents and detergents. The problem of viral transmission is still a major issue in the developing world.

Transfusion-transmitted syphilis is now very rare in the UK. Spirochaetes do not survive for more than 72 hours in blood stored at 4°C, and each donation is tested using the *Treponema pallidum* haemagglutination assay (TPHA).

Autologous transfusion

An alternative to using blood from volunteer donors is to use the patient's own blood. Interest in autologous transfusion was stimulated mainly by concern about transmission of infection, especially HIV, by blood transfusion. There are three types of autologous transfusion:

- *Predeposit.* The patient donates 2–5 units of blood at approximately weekly intervals before elective surgery.
- *Preoperative haemodilution.* One or two units of blood are removed from the patient immediately before surgery and retransfused to replace operative losses.
- *Blood salvage.* Blood lost during or after surgery may be collected and retransfused. Several techniques of varying levels of sophistication are available. The operative site must be free of bacteria, bowel contents and tumour cells.

There has been little demand for autologous transfusion in the UK as blood is generally perceived as being 'safe'. In addition, there are considerable costs in setting up a hospital-based predeposit autologous transfusion service, which would benefit only a minority of patients. In developing countries, however, autologous blood and blood from relatives is increasingly being used.

Blood, blood components and blood products

Most blood collected from donors is processed as follows.

- **Blood components**, such as red cell and platelet concentrates, fresh frozen plasma (FFP) and cryoprecipitate, are prepared from a single donation of blood by simple separation methods such as centrifugation and are transfused without further processing.
- **Blood products**, such as coagulation factor concentrates and albumin and immunoglobulin solutions, are prepared by complex processes using the plasma from many donors as the starting material.

In most circumstances it is preferable to transfuse only the blood component or product required by the patient (*component therapy*) rather than use whole blood. This is the most effective way of using donor blood, which is a scarce resource, and reduces the risk of complications from transfusion of unnecessary components of the blood.

Whole blood

The average volume of blood withdrawn is 470 mL (recently increased to this level from 450 mL), taken into 63 mL of anticoagulant. Blood stored at 4°C has a 'shelf-life' of 5 weeks when at least 70% of the transfused red cells should survive normally. Whole blood is rarely used even for acute blood loss; packed cells or red cell concentrates plus crystalloid or colloid solutions are acceptable alternatives.

Packed red cells

Some 200–250 mL of plasma are removed from whole blood to be frozen as FFP or to be further processed.

Red cell concentrates

Virtually all the plasma is removed and is replaced by about 100 mL of an *optimal additive solution*, such as SAG-M which contains sodium chloride, adenine, glucose and mannitol. The PCV is about 0.65 L/L, but the viscosity is low as there are no plasma proteins in the additive solution, and this allows fast administration if necessary.

Buffy coat-depleted red cell concentrates

These are prepared by removal of the buffy coat, which contains most of the leucocytes and platelets. They are useful in preventing febrile reactions in patients with a previous history of reactions and in those likely to receive multiple transfusions, e.g. patients with haematological diseases.

Leucocyte-depleted red cell concentrates

These are usually prepared by filtration. They are used to prevent alloimmunization to leucocyte antigens, e.g. in aplastic anaemia patients who are potential recipients of allogeneic bone marrow transplants.

Washed red cell concentrates

These are preparations of red cells suspended in saline, produced by cell separators to remove all but traces of plasma proteins. They are used in patients who have had severe recurrent urticarial or anaphylactic reactions.

Platelet concentrates

These are prepared either from whole blood by centrifugation or by plateletpheresis of single donors using cell separators. They may be stored for up to 5 days at 22°C. They are used to treat bleeding in patients with severe thrombocytopenia, and prophylactically to prevent bleeding in patients with bone marrow failure.

Granulocyte concentrates

These are prepared from single donors using cell separators. They are used for patients with severe neutropenia with definite evidence of bacterial infection where antibiotic therapy has failed. Today they are rarely used.

Fresh frozen plasma

FFP is prepared by freezing the plasma from 1 unit of blood at –30°C within 6 hours of donation. The volume is approximately 200 mL. FFP contains all the coagulation factors present in fresh plasma and is used mostly for replacement of coagulation factors in acquired coagulation factor deficiencies.

Cryoprecipitate

This is obtained by allowing the frozen plasma from a single donation to thaw at 4–8°C and removing the supernatant. The volume is about 20 mL and it is stored at –18°C. It contains factor VIII:C, von Willebrand factor (vWF) and fibrinogen. It is no longer used for the treatment of haemophilia A and von Willebrand's disease because of the greater risk of virus transmission compared with virus-inactivated coagulation factor concentrates.

Factor VIII and IX concentrates

These are freeze-dried preparations of specific coagulation factors prepared from large pools of plasma. They are used for treating patients with haemophilia and von Willebrand's disease, where recombinant factors are unavailable.

High-purity products are prepared using purification procedures involving chromatography columns and either monoclonal antibodies or ion exchanges. *Intermediate-purity* products are prepared by conventional fractionation methods. Solvents, detergents and heat treatment are used for viral inactivation. High-purity products should be used in preference to the intermediate-purity products (although their cost is higher), because of their greater safety and because they possibly cause less immunosuppression in HIV-seropositive patients with haemophilia. Recombinant factor VIII (see p. 405) is another alternative, but is even more costly than high-purity products.

Albumin

There are two preparations:

- *Human albumin solution 4.5%*, previously called plasma protein fraction (PPF), contains 45 g L^{-1} albumin and 160 mmol L^{-1} sodium. It is available in 50, 100, 250 and 500 mL bottles.
- *Human albumin solution 20%*, previously called 'salt-poor' albumin, contains approximately 200 g L^{-1} albumin and 130 mmol L^{-1} sodium and is available in 50 and 100 mL bottles.

Human albumin solutions are generally considered to be inappropriate fluids for acute volume replacement or for the treatment of shock because they are no more effective in these situations than synthetic colloid solutions such as polygelatins (Gelofucin) or hydroxyethyl starch (Haemaccel). However, albumin solutions are indicated for treatment of acute severe hypoalbuminaemia and as the replacement fluid for plasma exchange. The 20% albumin solution is particularly useful for patients with nephrotic syndrome or liver disease who are fluid overloaded and resistant to diuretics. Albumin solutions should not be used to treat patients with malnutrition or chronic renal or liver disease.

Normal immunoglobulin

This is prepared from normal plasma. It is used in patients with hypogammaglobulinaemia, to prevent infections, and in patients with immune thrombocytopenia.

Specific immunoglobulins

These are obtained from donors with high titres of antibodies. Many preparations are available, such as anti-D, anti-hepatitis B, and anti-varicella zoster.

The white cell

(see also Chapter 2)

The five types of leucocytes found in peripheral blood are neutrophils, eosinophils and basophils (which are all called *granulocytes*) and lymphocytes and monocytes. The development of these cells is shown in Fig 6.1.

Neutrophils

The earliest morphologically identifiable precursors of neutrophils in the bone marrow are *myeloblasts*, which are large cells constituting up to 3.5% of the nucleated cells in the marrow. The nucleus is large and contains 2–5 nucleoli. The cytoplasm is scanty and contains no granules. *Promyelocytes* are similar to myeloblasts but have some primary cytoplasmic granules containing enzymes such as myeloperoxidase. *Myelocytes* are smaller cells without nucleoli but with more abundant cytoplasm and both primary and secondary granules. Indentation of the nucleus marks the change from myelocyte to *metamyelocyte*. The mature *neutrophil* is a smaller cell with a nucleus with 2–5 lobes with predominantly secondary granules in the cytoplasm which contain lysozyme, collagenase and lactoferrin.

Peripheral blood neutrophils are equally distributed into a circulating pool and a marginating pool lying along the endothelium of blood vessels. In contrast to the prolonged maturation time of about 10 days for neutrophils in the bone marrow, their half-life in the peripheral blood is extremely short, only 6–8 hours. In response to stimuli (e.g. infection, corticosteroid therapy) neutrophils are released into the circulating pool from both the marginating pool and the marrow. Immature white cells are released from the marrow when a rapid response (within hours) occurs in acute infection (described as a 'shift to the left' on a blood film).

Function

The prime function of neutrophils is to ingest and kill bacteria, fungi and damaged cells. Neutrophils are attracted to sites of infection or inflammation by chemotaxins. Recognition of foreign or dead material is aided by coating of particles with immunoglobulin and complement (*opsonization*) as neutrophils have Fc and C3b receptors (see p. 162). The material is ingested into vacuoles where it is subjected to enzymic destruction, which is either oxygen-dependent with the generation of hydrogen peroxide (myeloperoxidase) or oxygen-independent (lysosomal enzymes and lactoferrin).

Neutrophil leucocytosis

A rise in the number of circulating neutrophils to $>10 \times 10^9/L$ occurs in bacterial infections or as a result of tissue damage. This may also be seen in pregnancy, during exercise and after corticosteroid administration (Table 6.18). With any tissue necrosis there is a release of various soluble factors, causing a leucocytosis. Interleukin-1 is also released in tissue necrosis and causes a pyrexia. The pyrexia and leucocytosis accompanying a myocardial infarction are a good example of this and may be wrongly attributed to infection.

A *leukaemoid reaction* (an overproduction of white cells, with many immature cells) may occur in severe infections, tuberculosis, malignant infiltration of the bone marrow and occasionally after haemorrhage or haemolysis.

In *leucoerythroblastic anaemia*, nucleated red cells and white cell precursors are found in the peripheral blood. Causes include marrow infiltration with metastatic carcinoma, myelofibrosis, osteopetrosis, myeloma, lymphoma, and occasionally severe haemolytic or megaloblastic anaemia.

Neutropenia and agranulocytosis

Neutropenia is defined as a circulatory neutrophil count below $1.5 \times 10^9/L$. A virtual absence of neutrophils is called *agranulocytosis*. The causes are given in Table 6.19. Neutropenia caused by viruses is probably the most common type. Chemotherapy and radiotherapy predictably produce neutropenia; many other drugs have been known to produce an idiosyncratic cytopenia and a drug cause should always be considered.

CLINICAL FEATURES

Infections may be frequent, often serious, and are more likely as the neutrophil count falls. A characteristic glazed mucositis occurs in the mouth, and ulceration is common.

INVESTIGATION

The blood film shows marked neutropenia. The appearance of the bone marrow will indicate whether the neutropenia is due to depressed production or increased destruction of neutrophils. Neutrophil antibody studies may be performed if an immune mechanism is suspected.

TREATMENT

Antibiotics should be given as necessary to patients with acute severe neutropenia (see p. 423).

If the neutropenia seems likely to have been caused by a drug, all current drug therapy should be stopped. Recovery of the neutrophil count usually occurs after about 10 days. G-CSF (see p. 355) is used to decrease the period of neutropenia after chemotherapy and haemopoietic transplantation. It is also used successfully in the treatment of chronic neutropenia.

Steroids and high-dose intravenous immunoglobulin are used to treat patients with severe autoimmune neutropenia and recurrent infections, and G-CSF has produced responses in some cases.

Eosinophils

Eosinophils are slightly larger than neutrophils and are characterized by a nucleus with usually two lobes and large cytoplasmic granules that stain deeply red. The eosinophil seems to play some part in allergic responses (p. 163) and in the defence against infections with helminths and protozoa.

Eosinophilia is said to occur when the number of eosinophils is $>0.4 \times 10^9/L$ in the peripheral blood. It is associated with a wide variety of disorders. The causes of eosinophilia are listed in Table 6.20.

Basophils

The nucleus of basophils is similar to neutrophils but the cytoplasm is filled with large black granules. The granules contain histamine, heparin and enzymes such as myeloperoxidase. The physiological role of the basophil is not known. Binding of IgE causes the cells to degranulate and release histamine and other contents involved in acute hypersensitivity reactions.

Table 6.18
Neutrophil leucocytosis

Bacterial infections
Tissue necrosis, e.g. myocardial infarction, trauma
Inflammation, e.g. gout, rheumatoid arthritis
Drugs, e.g. corticosteroids, lithium
Haematological
Myeloproliferative disease
Leukaemoid reaction
Leucoerythroblastic anaemia
Physiological, e.g. pregnancy, exercise
Malignant disease, e.g. bronchial, breast, gastric
Metabolic, e.g. renal failure, acidosis

Table 6.19
Causes of neutropenia

Congenital (Kostmann's syndrome)
Racial (neutropenia is common in Black races)
Viral infection
Severe bacterial infection, e.g. typhoid
Felty's syndrome
Autoimmune neutropenia
Pancytopenia from any cause, including drug-induced marrow aplasia (see p. 390)
Cyclic (genetic defect with neutropenia every 2–3 weeks)

Table 6.20
Causes of eosinophilia

Parasitic infestations, such as: Ascaris Hookworm Strongyloides	**Pulmonary disorders,** such as: Bronchial asthma Tropical pulmonary eosinophilia Allergic bronchopulmonary aspergillosis Churg–Strauss syndrome
Allergic disorders, such as: Hayfever (allergic rhinitis) Other hypersensitivity reactions, including drug reactions	**Malignant disorders,** such as: Hodgkin's disease Carcinoma Eosinophilic leukaemia
Skin disorders, such as: Urticaria Pemphigus Eczema	**Miscellaneous,** such as: Hypereosinophilic syndrome Sarcoidosis Hypoadrenalism Eosinophilic gastroenteritis

Basophils are usually few in number ($<1 \times 10^9$/L) but are significantly increased in myeloproliferative disorders.

Monocytes

Monocytes are slightly larger than neutrophils. The nucleus has a variable shape and may be round, indented or lobulated. The cytoplasm contains fewer granules than neutrophils. Monocytes are precursors of tissue macrophages and spend only a few hours in the blood but can continue to proliferate in the tissues for many years.

A monocytosis ($>0.8 \times 10^9$/L) may be seen in chronic bacterial infections such as tuberculosis or infective endocarditis, chronic neutropenia and patients with myelodysplasia, particularly chronic myelomonocytic leukaemia.

Lymphocytes

Lymphocytes form nearly half the circulating white cells. They descend from pluripotential stem cells. Circulating lymphocytes are small cells, a little larger than red cells, with a dark-staining central nucleus. There are two main types: the thymus-dependent or T lymphocytes, which are concerned with cellular immunity and form about 80% of the circulating lymphocytes, and the 'bursa dependent' or B lymphocytes, which are concerned with humoral immunity (see p. 167).

Lymphocytosis (lymphocyte count $>5 \times 10^9$/L) occurs in response to viral infections, particularly EBV, CMV and HIV, and chronic infections such as tuberculosis and toxoplasmosis. It also occurs in chronic lymphocytic leukaemia and in some lymphomas.

Bleeding disorders

The integrity of the circulation is maintained by blood flowing through intact vessels lined by endothelial cells. Injury to the vessel wall exposes collagen and together with tissue injury sets in motion a series of events leading to haemostasis.

Haemostasis

Haemostasis is a complex process depending on interactions between the vessel wall, platelets and coagulation factors (Fig 6.25).

Vessel wall

An immediate reflex vasoconstriction of the injured vessel and adjacent vessels results in a transient reduction of blood flow to the affected area. Damage to the endothelium of the vessel results in activation of platelets and coagulation; release of serotonin and thromboxane A_2 (TXA_2) from activated platelets contributes to the vasoconstriction.

Platelets

Platelet adhesion to collagen is dependent on platelet membrane receptors, glycoprotein Ia (GPIa), which binds directly to collagen, and glycoprotein Ib (GPIb), which binds to von Willebrand factor (vWF) in the plasma, and vWF in turn adheres to collagen. Following adhesion, platelets undergo a shape change from a disc to a sphere, spread along the subendothelium and *release* the contents of their cytoplasmic granules, i.e. the dense bodies (containing ADP and serotonin) and the α-granules (containing platelet-derived growth factor, platelet factor 4, β-thromboglobulin, fibrinogen, vWF and other factors).

The release of ADP leads to a conformational change in the fibrinogen receptor, the glycoprotein IIb–IIIa complex (GPIIb–IIIa), on the surfaces of adherent platelets, allowing it to bind to fibrinogen (see also Fig 6.33). Fibrinogen then binds platelets into activated aggregates (*platelet aggregation*) and further platelet release occurs. A self-perpetuating cycle of events is set up leading to formation of a platelet plug at the site of the injury.

Further platelet membrane receptors are exposed during aggregation, providing a surface for the interaction of coagulation factors; this platelet activity is referred to as platelet factor 3 (PF-3). The presence of thrombin encourages *fusion of platelets*, and fibrin formation reinforces the stability of the platelet plug.

Central to normal platelet function is platelet prostaglandin synthesis, which is induced by platelet activation and leads to the formation of TXA_2 in platelets (Fig 6.26). TXA_2 is a powerful vasoconstrictor and also lowers cyclic AMP levels and initiates the platelet release reaction.

Prostacyclin (PGI_2) is synthesized in vascular endothelial cells and opposes the actions of TXA_2. It produces vasodilatation and increases the level of cyclic AMP, preventing platelet aggregation on the normal vessel wall as well as limiting the extent of the initial platelet plug after injury.

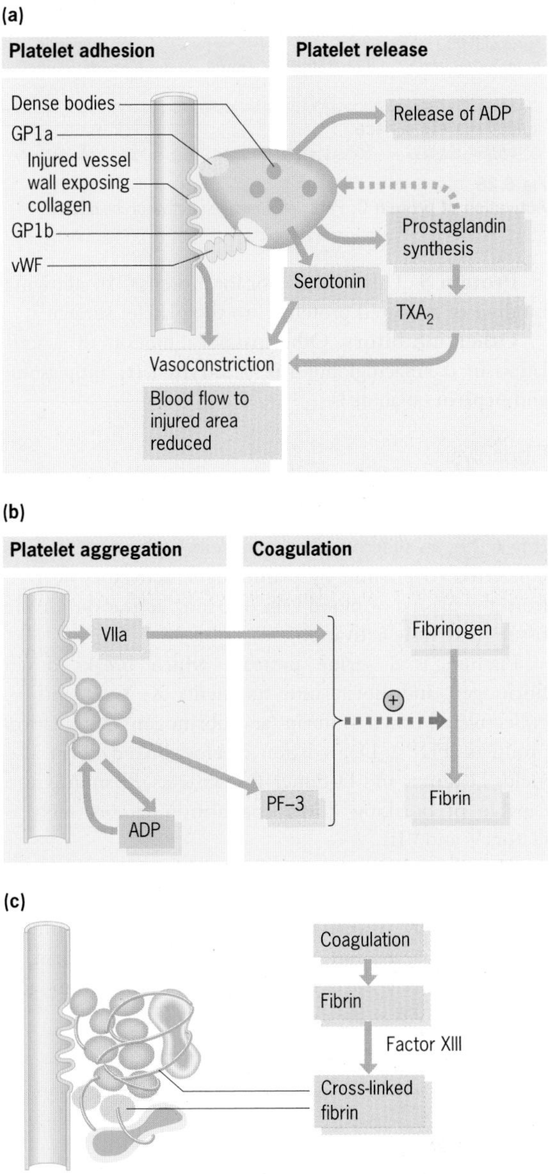

Fig 6.25
Formation of the haemostatic plug: sequential interactions between the vessel wall, platelets and coagulation factors.
(a) Contact of platelets with collagen, either via the platelet receptor GPIb and factor vWF in plasma, or directly via GPIa, activates platelet prostaglandin synthesis which stimulates release of ADP from the dense bodies. Vasoconstriction of the vessel occurs as a reflex and by release of serotonin and thromboxin A_2 (TXA_2) from platelets
(b) Release of ADP from platelets induces platelet aggregation and formation of the platelet plug. The coagulation pathway is stimulated leading to formation of fibrin
(c) Fibrin strands are cross-linked by factor XIII and stabilize the haemostatic plug by binding platelets and red cells

Coagulation and fibrinolysis

The coagulation cascade involves a series of enzymatic reactions leading to the conversion of soluble plasma fibrinogen to fibrin clot (Fig 6.27). Roman numerals are used for most of the factors, but I, II and III are referred to as fibrinogen, prothrombin and tissue factor respectively; VI is redundant. The active forms are denoted by 'a'.

The coagulation factors are primarily synthesized in the liver and are either enzyme precursors (factors XII, XI, X, IX and thrombin) or cofactors (V and VIII), except for fibrinogen, which is degraded to form fibrin. The enzymes apart from factor XIII are serine proteases and hydrolyse peptide bonds.

Coagulation pathway

This cascade was divided into 'extrinsic' and 'intrinsic' pathways, but that is an over-simplification. Coagulation is initiated by tissue factor, which is expressed on the surface of perivascular endothelial cells, coming into contact with plasma after an injury. The complex of activated factor VII and tissue factor (TF:VIIa) does activate factor X but its main role *in vivo* is to activate factor IX (Fig 6.27).

Factor XII was thought to be activated by 'contact' with the injured surface and then to initiate a series of reactions beginning with activation of factor XI and leading to activation of factor X. However, recent evidence suggests that the principal haemostatic mechanism *in vivo* is through factor VIIa complexes and that the factor XI pathway is relatively unimportant.

It is thought that factor IX is activated by a complex of tissue factor and factor VII. Activated factor IX together with factor VIII and calcium ions activate factor X. Factor XI is activated *in vivo* by thrombin and only makes an important contribution after major trauma.

Activated factor X induces the conversion of prothrombin to thrombin. Thrombin hydrolyses the peptide bonds of fibrinogen, releasing fibrinopeptides A and B, and allowing polymerization between fibrinogen molecules to form fibrin. At the same time thrombin, in the presence of calcium ions, activates factor XIII, which

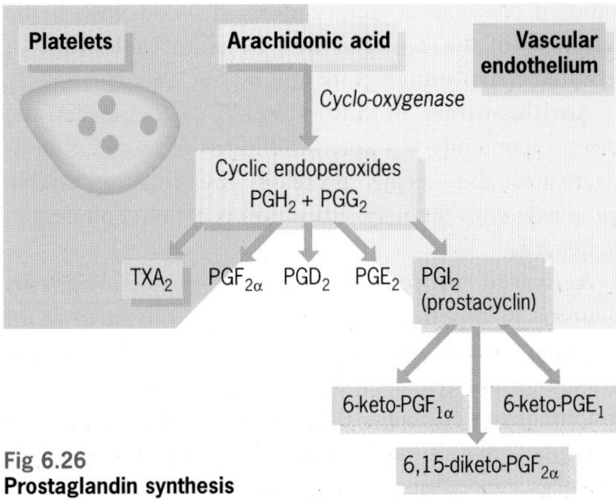

Fig 6.26
Prostaglandin synthesis

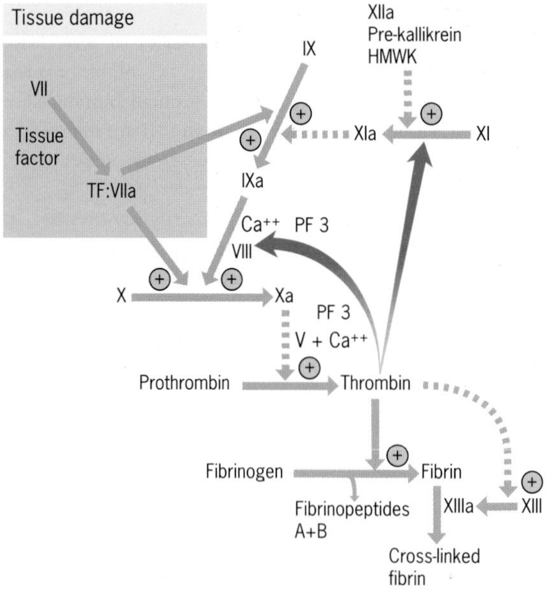

Fig 6.27
Coagulation cascade. The pathway *in vivo* begins with activation of factor IX by factor VIIa. The factor XII and pre-kallikrein reactions are probably only relevant *in vitro*. Factor XI is activated by thrombin *in vivo*. HMWK, high-molecular-weight kininogen

stabilizes the fibrin clot by cross-linking adjacent fibrin molecules. The presence of thrombin helps in the activation of factors XI, V, VIII and XIII.

Factor VIII consists of a molecule with coagulant activity (VIII:C) associated with von Willebrand factor whose function is to stabilize factor VIII:C and to promote platelet–endothelial interactions. VIII:C is a single-chain protein with a molecular weight of about 350 000. vWF is a glycoprotein with a molecular weight of about 200 000 which readily forms multimers in the circulation with molecular weights of up to 20×10^6. The high-molecular-weight multimeric forms of vWF are the most effective in promoting platelet function.

Limitation of coagulation

Coagulation is limited to the site of injury by removal of activated coagulation factors by rapid blood flow at the periphery of the damaged area, by plasma inhibitors of activated coagulation factors, and by fibrinolysis.

Antithrombin. Antithrombin (AT), a member of the serpin superfamily, is a potent inhibitor of coagulation. It inactivates the serine proteases by forming stable complexes with them, and its action is greatly potentiated by heparin.

Activated protein C. This is generated from its vitamin K-dependent precursor by the action of thrombin; thrombin activation of protein C is enhanced when thrombin is bound to thrombomodulin, which is an endothelial cell receptor (Fig 6.28). Activated protein C destroys factor V and factor VIII, reducing further thrombin generation.

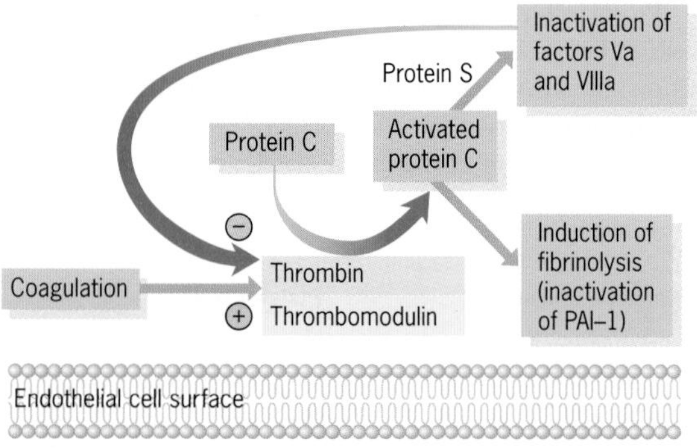

Fig 6.28
Activation of protein C. PAI-1, plasminogen activator inhibitor 1

Protein S. This is a cofactor for protein C by allowing binding of activated protein C to the platelet surface.

Other inhibitors. Other natural inhibitors of coagulation are α_2-macroglobulin, α_1-antitrypsin, α_1-antiplasmin and heparin cofactor II.

Fibrinolysis

Fibrinolysis, which helps to restore vessel patency, also occurs in response to vascular damage. In this system (Fig 6.29), an inactive plasma protein – plasminogen – is converted to plasmin by plasminogen activators derived from the plasma or blood cells (intrinsic activation) or the tissues (extrinsic activation).

Plasmin is a serine protease which breaks down fibrinogen and fibrin into fragments X, Y, D and E, collectively known as fibrin (and fibrinogen) degradation products (FDPs). Degradation of cross-linked fibrin also yields D-dimer and D-dimer-E fragments. Plasmin is also capable of breaking down coagulation factors such as factors V and VIII.

The fibrinolytic system is activated by the presence of fibrin. Plasminogen is specifically adsorbed to fibrin and fibrinogen by lysine-binding sites. However, little plasminogen activation occurs in the absence of fibrin, as fibrin also has a specific binding site for plasminogen activators, whereas fibrinogen does not (Fig 6.30).

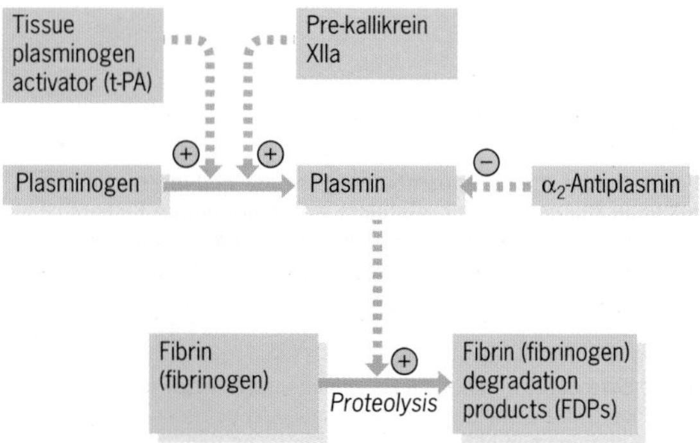

Fig 6.29
Fibrinolytic system

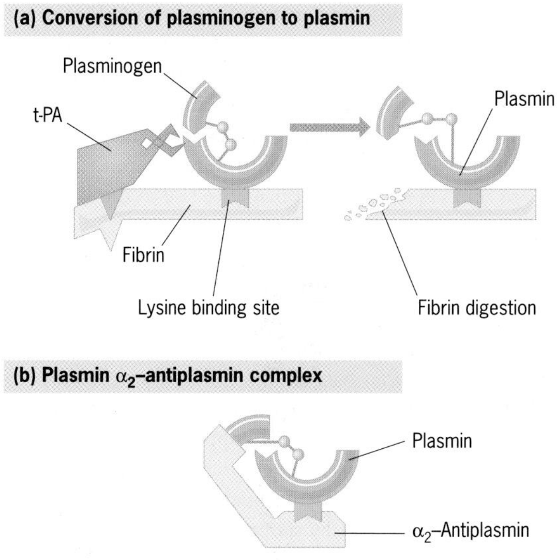

Fig 6.30
Fibrinolysis.
(a) The conversion of plasminogen to plasmin by plasminogen activator (t-PA) occurs most efficiently on the surface of fibrin which has binding sites for both plasminogen and t-PA
(b) Free plasmin in the blood is rapidly inactivated by α_2-antiplasmin. Plasmin generated on the fibrin surface is partially protected from inactivation. The lysine-binding sites on plasminogen are important for the interaction between plasmin(ogen) and fibrin and between plasmin and α_2-antiplasmin

The most important plasminogen activator is tissue-type plasminogen activator (t-PA); vascular endothelium is the major source of t-PA in plasma. Its release is stimulated by thrombin. Another plasminogen activator is urokinase, synthesized in the kidney and released into the urogenital tract. Intrinsic plasminogen activators such as factor XII and pre-kallikrein are of minor physiological importance.

t-PA is inactivated by plasminogen activator inhibitor-1 (PAI-1). Activated protein C inactivates PAI-1 and therefore induces fibrinolysis (Fig 6.28). Inactivators of plasmin (such as α_2-antiplasmin) are also present in the plasma and contribute to the regulation of fibrinolysis (Fig 6.30).

Investigation of bleeding disorders

Although the precise diagnosis of a bleeding disorder may depend on laboratory tests, much information may be obtained from the history and physical examination, which should aim to determine the following:

- **Is there a generalized haemostatic defect?** Supportive evidence for this includes bleeding from multiple sites, spontaneous bleeding, and bleeding into the skin.
- **Is the defect inherited or acquired?** A family history of a bleeding disorder should be sought. Severe inherited defects usually become apparent in infancy, while mild inherited defects may only come to attention later in life, for example with excessive bleeding after surgery, childbirth, dental extractions or trauma.
- **Is the bleeding suggestive of a vascular/platelet defect or a coagulation defect?**

Vascular/platelet bleeding is characterized by easy bruising and spontaneous bleeding from small vessels. The bleeding is mainly into the skin. The term *purpura* includes both *petechiae*, which are small skin haemorrhages varying from pinpoint size to a few millimetres in diameter and which do not blanch on pressure, and *ecchymoses*, which are larger areas of bleeding into the skin and from mucous membranes, often from the nose and mouth.

Coagulation disorders are typically associated with haemarthroses and muscle haematomas, and bleeding after injury or surgery.

LABORATORY INVESTIGATIONS

- **Blood count and film** show the number and morphology of platelets and any blood disorder such as leukaemia.
- **Bleeding time** measures platelet plug formation *in vivo*. It is determined by applying a sphygmomanometer cuff to the arm and inflating it to 40 mmHg. Two 1 mm deep, 1 cm long incisions are made in the forearm with a template. Each wound is blotted every 30 s and the time taken for bleeding to stop is recorded, normally between 3 and 10 minutes. Prolonged bleeding times are found in patients with platelet function defects and there is a progressive prolongation with platelet counts less than 80×10^9/L. The bleeding time should not be performed at low platelet counts.
- **Coagulation tests** are performed using blood collected into citrate, which neutralizes calcium ions and prevents clotting.

The *prothrombin time* (PT) (also see p. 412) is measured by adding tissue thromboplastin in the form of animal brain extract and calcium to the patient's plasma. The normal PT is 16–18 s, and it is prolonged with abnormalities of factors VII, X, V or II, liver disease, or if the patient is on warfarin (see Fig 6.27).

The *partial thromboplastin time with kaolin* (PTTK) is also known as the APTT (activated PTT). It is performed by adding a surface activator, kaolin, phospholipid (as platelet substitute) and calcium to the patient's plasma. The normal PTTK is 30–50 s depending on the exact methodology, and it is prolonged with deficiencies or inhibitors to one or more of the following factors: XII, XI, IX, VIII, X, V, II or I (but not factor VII) (see Fig 6.27).

The *thrombin time* (TT) is performed by adding thrombin to the patient's plasma. The normal TT is about 12 s, and it is prolonged with fibrinogen deficiency, dysfibrinogenaemia (normal level of fibrinogen but abnormal function) or inhibitors such as heparin or FDPs.

Correction tests can be used to differentiate prolonged times in the PT, PTTK and TT due to various coagulation factor deficiencies and inhibitors of coagulation. Prolonged PT, PTTK or TT due to coagulation factor deficiencies are corrected by addition of normal plasma to the patient's plasma; no correction of an abnormal result after the addition of normal plasma is suggestive of the presence of an inhibitor of coagulation.

Factor assays are used to confirm coagulation defects, especially where a single inherited disorder is suspected.

Special tests of coagulation will often be required to confirm the precise haemostatic defect. Such tests include estimation of fibrinogen and FDPs, platelet function tests such as platelet aggregation and tests of the fibrinolytic pathway which include the euglobulin clot lysis time (ELT) and assays of plasminogen, t-PA and PAI-1. The ELT involves precipitation by acidification of the euglobulin fraction of plasma which contains fibrinogen, plasminogen and plasminogen activators. The euglobulin is clotted with thrombin and the time taken for lysis of the fibrin clot is a measure of fibrinolytic activity; the normal range is 60–270 minutes.

Vascular disorders

The vascular disorders (Table 6.21), sometimes previously classified as non-thrombocytopenic purpuras, are characterized by easy bruising and bleeding into the skin. Bleeding from mucous membranes sometimes occurs but the bleeding is rarely severe. Laboratory investigations including the bleeding time are normal. The vascular disorders include the following.

Hereditary haemorrhagic telangiectasia is a rare disorder with autosomal dominant inheritance. Dilatation of capillaries and small arterioles produces characteristic small red spots that blanch on pressure in the skin and mucous membranes, particularly the nose and gastrointestinal tract. Recurrent epistaxis and chronic gastrointestinal bleeding are the major problems and may cause chronic iron deficiency anaemia.

Easy bruising syndrome is a benign disorder occurring in otherwise healthy women. It is characterized by bruises on the arms, legs and trunk with minor trauma, possibly due to skin vessel fragility. It may give rise to the suspicion of a serious bleeding disorder.

Senile purpura and purpura due to steroids are both due to atrophy of the vascular supporting tissue.

Purpura due to infections is mainly caused by damage to the vascular endothelium.

Henoch–Schönlein purpura (p. 535) occurs mainly in children. It is a type III hypersensitivity reaction that is often preceded by an acute upper respiratory tract infection. Purpura is mainly seen on the legs and buttocks. Abdominal pain, arthritis, haematuria and nephritis also occur. Recovery is usually spontaneous, but some patients develop renal failure.

Episodes of inexplicable bleeding or bruising may represent abuse, either self-inflicted or caused by others. These various forms of artificial or *factitious purpura* are expressions of severe emotional or psychiatric disturbances.

Table 6.21
Vascular disorders

Congenital	**Allergic**
Hereditary haemorrhagic telangiectasia (Osler–Weber–Rendu disease)	Henoch–Schönlein purpura
Connective tissue disorders (Ehlers–Danlos syndrome, osteogenesis imperfecta, pseudoxanthoma elasticum, Marfan's syndrome)	Autoimmune disorders (SLE, rheumatoid arthritis)
	Drugs
	Steroids
	Sulphonamides
Acquired	**Others**
Severe infections:	Senile purpura
Septicaemia	Easy bruising syndrome
Meningococcal infections	Scurvy
Measles	Factitious purpura
Typhoid	

Platelet disorders

Bleeding due to thrombocytopenia or abnormal platelet function is characterized by purpura and bleeding from mucous membranes. Bleeding is uncommon with platelet counts above 50×10^9/L, and severe spontaneous bleeding is unusual with platelet counts above 20×10^9/L.

Thrombocytopenia

This is caused by reduced platelet production in the bone marrow or excessive peripheral destruction of platelets (Table 6.22). A bone marrow aspirate to assess whether the numbers of megakaryocytes are reduced or normal/increased is an essential part of the investigation.

Autoimmune (idiopathic) thrombocytopenic purpura (AITP)

Thrombocytopenia is due to immune destruction of platelets. The sensitized platelets are removed by the reticuloendothelial system. There are two distinct clinical syndromes.

Acute AITP

Acute AITP is usually seen in children, often following a viral infection. It has been suggested that the thrombocytopenia is due to the deposition of immune complexes on platelets, but the acute development of platelet autoantibodies is probably responsible for the shortened platelet survival.

Table 6.22
Causes of thrombocytopenia

Impaired production	Excessive destruction
Generalized bone marrow failure	**Immune**
Leukaemia	Autoimmune idiopathic thrombocytopenic purpura
Aplastic anaemia	Secondary immune thrombocytopenia (SLE, chronic lymphatic leukaemia, viral infections, drugs)
Megaloblastic anaemia	Alloimmune neonatal thrombocytopenia
Myeloma	Post-transfusion purpura
Myelofibrosis	**Coagulation**
Marrow infiltration by solid tumours	Disseminated intravascular coagulation
Selective reduction in megakaryocytes	Thrombotic thrombocytopenic purpura
Drugs, e.g. co-trimoxazole	Haemolytic uraemic syndrome (see p. 541)
Chemicals	**Sequestration**
Viral infection	Hypersplenism
	Dilutional loss
	Massive transfusion of stored blood

Chronic AITP

Chronic AITP is characteristically seen in adult women. It is usually idiopathic but may occur in association with other autoimmune disorders such as SLE, thyroid disease and autoimmune haemolytic anaemia (Evans' syndrome), in patients with chronic lymphocytic leukaemia and solid tumours, and after viral infections with viruses such as HIV. Platelet autoantibodies are detected in about 60–70% of patients, and are presumed to be present, although not detectable, in the remaining patients; the antibodies often have specificity for platelet membrane glycoproteins IIb/IIIa and/or Ib/IX.

CLINICAL FEATURES

Major haemorrhage is rare and is seen only in patients with severe thrombocytopenia. Easy bruising, purpura, epistaxis and menorrhagia are common. Physical examination is normal except for evidence of bleeding. Splenomegaly is rare.

INVESTIGATION

The only blood count abnormality is thrombocytopenia. Normal or increased numbers of megakaryocytes are found in the bone marrow, which is otherwise normal. The detection of platelet autoantibodies is not essential for confirmation of the diagnosis, which often depends on exclusion of other causes of excessive destruction of platelets.

TREATMENT

Acute AITP in children usually remits spontaneously. Treatment in the acute phase with steroids or high-dose intravenous immunoglobulin is required only when the platelet count is $<20 \times 10^9$/L and there is bleeding.

Chronic AITP. Spontaneous remissions are rare.

The main aims of treatment are to reduce the production of platelet autoantibodies and the removal of antibody-coated platelets. Initial treatment is with prednisolone, 40–60 mg daily in adults, with cautious reduction of the dose after remission has occurred.

Twenty per cent of patients have a complete response and require no further treatment; 60% have a partial response, and half of these have little bleeding associated with mild or moderate thrombocytopenia (platelet count $30–100 \times 10^9$/L). They may require small doses of steroids, such as prednisolone 5–15 mg daily, or no further treatment. The other half of the partial responders eventually relapse and require splenectomy, as do the 20% of patients who failed to respond to steroids at all.

There is a 90% response rate to splenectomy, although about 30% of responders eventually relapse. Some of these refractory patients may respond to immunosuppressive drugs such as azathioprine, cyclophosphamide or vincristine or to danazol, which is a non-virilizing androgen. Splenectomy should be avoided in young children because of the subsequent risk of severe pneumococcal infection (see p. 391).

Intravenous infusion of high-dose immunoglobulin produces a rapid rise in the platelet count due to blockade of Fc receptors on macrophages in the spleen. The increase in platelet count is usually transient but may be useful in patients with acute haemorrhage and in preparing patients with chronic AITP for surgery.

Transfused platelets survive no longer than the patient's own platelets but may sometimes be beneficial in patients with life-threatening bleeding, when emergency splenectomy may be justified.

Other immune thrombocytopenias

Drugs cause immune thrombocytopenia by the same mechanisms as described for drug-induced immune haemolytic anaemia (p. 382). The same drugs may be responsible for immune haemolytic anaemia, thrombo-cytopenia or neutropenia in different patients. It is not known what determines the target cell in each case.

Fetomaternal alloimmune thrombocytopenia is due to fetomaternal incompatibility for platelet-specific antigens, usually for HPA-1a (human platelet alloantigen, previously called Pl^{A1}), and is the platelet equivalent of HDN. The mother is HPA-1a-negative and produces antibodies which destroy the HPA-1a-positive fetal platelets.

Thrombocytopenia is self-limiting after delivery, but platelet transfusions may be required initially to prevent or treat bleeding associated with severe thrombocytopenia; platelets may be prepared from HPA-1a-negative volunteers or the mother herself. Severe bleeding such as intracranial haemorrhage may also occur *in utero*. Antenatal treatment of the mother – with platelet transfusions given directly to the fetus by ultrasound-guided needling of the umbilical vessels – has been effective in preventing haemorrhage in severely affected cases.

Post-transfusion purpura (PTP) is rare, occurring 2–12 days after a blood transfusion. PTP is associated with a platelet-specific alloantibody, usually anti-HPA-1a in a HPA-1a-negative individual. PTP almost invariably occurs in females who have been previously immunized by pregnancy or blood transfusion. The cause of the destruction of the patient's own platelets is not well understood, but they may be destroyed as 'bystanders' during the acute immune response to HPA-1a. PTP is self-limiting, but high-dose intravenous immunoglobulin may limit the period of thrombocytopenia.

Platelet function disorders

These are usually associated with excessive bruising and bleeding and, in some of the acquired forms, with thrombosis. The platelet count is normal or increased and the bleeding time is prolonged. The rare inherited defects of platelet function require more detailed investigations such as platelet aggregation studies and factor VIII:C and vWF assays, if von Willebrand's disease is suspected.

Inherited types of platelet dysfunction

- *Glanzmann's thrombasthenia* – lack of the platelet membrane glycoprotein IIb/IIIa complex resulting in defective fibrinogen binding
- *Bernard–Soulier syndrome* – lack of platelet membrane glycoprotein Ib/IX, the binding site for factor vWF
- *Storage pool disease* – lack of platelet granules causing poor platelet aggregation.

Aquired types of platelet dysfunction

- Myeloproliferative disorders
- Uraemia and liver disease
- Paraproteinaemias
- Drug-induced, such as by aspirin or dipyridamole.

If there is serious bleeding or if the patient is about to undergo surgery, drugs with antiplatelet activity should be withdrawn and any underlying condition should be corrected if possible. In patients with renal failure, the haematocrit should be increased to greater than 0.30 L/L and the use of desmopressin (DDAVP) may be helpful. Platelet transfusions may be required if these measures are unsuccessful.

Inherited coagulation disorders

Coagulation disorders may be *inherited* or *acquired*. The inherited disorders are uncommon and usually involve deficiency of one factor only. The acquired disorders occur more frequently and almost always involve several coagulation factors; they are considered in the next subsection.

In inherited coagulation disorders, deficiences of all factors have been described. Those leading to abnormal bleeding are rare, apart from haemophilia A (factor VIII deficiency), haemophilia B (factor IX deficiency) and von Willebrand's disease.

Haemophilia A

In haemophilia A, the level of factor VIII:C is reduced but the level of factor vWF is normal (see Fig 6.31). The prevalence of haemophilia A is about 1 in 5000 of the male population. It is inherited as an X-linked disorder. If a female carrier has a son, he has a 50% chance of having haemophilia, and a daughter has a 50% chance of being a carrier. All daughters of haemophiliacs are carriers and the sons are normal.

The human factor VIII gene is enormous, constituting about 0.1% of the X chromosome, encompassing 186 kilobases of DNA. Various genetic defects have been found, including deletions, duplications, frameshift mutations and insertions. In approximately 50% of families with severe disease, the defect is an inversion. There is a high mutation rate, with one-third of cases being apparently sporadic with no family history of haemophilia.

CLINICAL AND LABORATORY FEATURES

The clinical features depend on the level of factor VIII:C.

- *Levels of less than 1%* are associated with frequent spontaneous bleeding from early life. Haemarthroses are common and may lead to joint deformity and crippling if adequate treatment is not given. Bleeds into muscles are also common, and intramuscular injections should be avoided.
- *Levels of less than 5%* are associated with severe bleeding following injury and occasional spontaneous episodes.
- *Levels above 5%* produce mild disease, usually with bleeding only after injury or surgery. It should be noted that patients with mild haemophilia can still bleed badly once haemostasis has failed. Diagnosis in this group is often delayed until quite late in life.

The most frequent cause of death in patients with severe haemophilia used to be cerebral haemorrhage, but is now AIDS. HIV was transmitted to many patients by coagulation factor concentrates between 1979 and 1985.

The main laboratory features of haemophilia A are shown in Table 6.23. The abnormal findings are a prolonged PTTK and a reduced level of factor VIII:C. The PT, bleeding time and vWF level are normal.

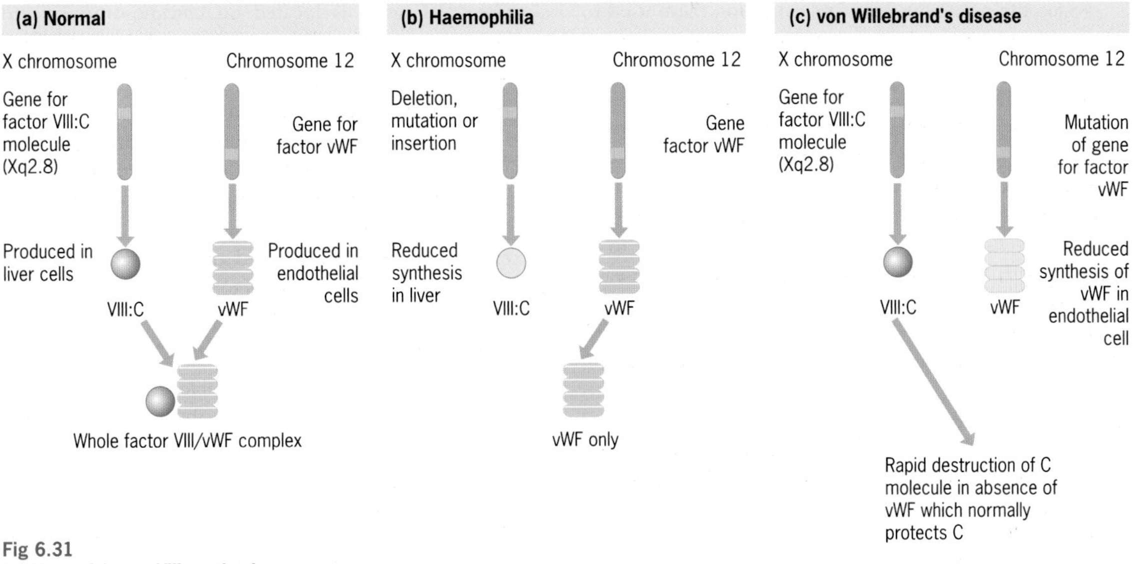

Fig 6.31
(a) Normal factor VIII synthesis
(b) Haemophilia A showing defective synthesis of factor VIIIc
(c) von Willebrand's disease showing reduced synthesis of vWF

TREATMENT

Bleeding is treated by administration of factor VIII concentrate by intravenous infusion.

- *Minor bleeding:* the factor VIII:C level should be raised to 20–30%.
- *Severe bleeding:* the factor VIII:C should be raised to at least 50%.
- *Major surgery:* the factor VIII:C should be raised to 100% preoperatively and maintained above 50% until healing has occurred.

Factor VIII has a half-life of 12 hours and therefore must be administered at least twice daily to maintain the required therapeutic level. Factor VIII concentrate is freeze-dried and may be stored in domestic refrigerators at 4°C. This allows it to be administered by the patient immediately after bleeding has started, reducing the likelihood of chronic damage to joints and the need for inpatient care.

Recombinant factor VIII concentrate is now well established as the treatment of choice for people with haemophilia, but economic constraints have resulted in many previously treated patients still being offered treatment with plasma-derived concentrates.

The majority of severely affected patients are now given prophylaxis three times per week from early childhood in an attempt to prevent permanent joint damage.

Synthetic vasopressin (DDAVP) – intravenous, subcutaneous or intranasal – produces a rise in factor VIII:C proportional to the initial level of factor VIII. It avoids the complications associated with blood products and is useful for treating bleeding episodes in mild haemophiliacs and as prophylaxis before minor surgery.

People with haemophilia should be registered at comprehensive care centres (CCC), which take responsibility for their full medical care, including social and psychological support. Each person with haemophilia carries a special medical card giving details of the defect and treatment.

COMPLICATIONS

Ten per cent of people with haemophilia have antibodies to factor VIII:C. These inhibitors develop most commonly in severely affected patients with no detectable VIII:C. Management of such patients may be very difficult, and even extremely high doses of factor VIII may not produce a rise in the plasma level of factor VIII:C. Purified porcine factor VIII may not cross-react with the patient's antibody. Some factor IX concentrates contain activated factors, which may 'bypass' the inhibitor and stop the bleeding. Recombinant factor VIIa also has this bypassing potential and shows great promise as an agent for treating patients with inhibitors. There is a growing interest in immune tolerance induction, especially in the management of recently developed inhibitors. Similar strategies, including immunosuppression and immunoabsorption, have been described.

Table 6.23 Blood changes in haemophilia A, von Willebrand's disease and vitamin K deficiency

	Haemophilia A	von Willebrand's disease	Vitamin K deficiency
Bleeding time	Normal	$\uparrow$	Normal
PT	Normal	Normal	$\uparrow$
PTTK	$\uparrow^{+}$	$\uparrow\pm$	$\uparrow$
VIII:C	$\downarrow^{++}$	$\downarrow$	Normal
vWF	Normal	$\downarrow$	Normal

Following numerous blood transfusions, there used to be a high risk of acquiring transfusion-transmitted infections, particularly hepatitis B and C, and HIV. The risk has been virtually eliminated in developed countries by excluding high-risk blood donors, testing all donations for HBsAg, HCV and HIV antibodies, and by including steps to inactivate viruses during the preparation of plasma-derived concentrate.

Hepatitis A and B vaccination is offered routinely to all patients with haemophilia and von Willebrand's disease. The clinical consequences of haemophilia patients infected with HIV are similar to other HIV-infected patients (see p. 111), except that Kaposi's sarcoma is rare. A number of patients with hepatitis C will progress to develop chronic liver disease and cirrhosis (see p. 312).

The use of recombinant factor VIII eliminates any residual risk of transfusion-transmitted infection, and it is safe and effective; but there is a similar incidence of inhibitor development as with plasma-derived factor VIII.

Carrier detection and antenatal diagnosis

Determination of carrier status in females depends on detailed information from the family history and results of coagulation factor assays. Female carriers usually have a factor VIII level of about 50% of normal, but the exact value is very variable, partly because of Lyonization. Owing to this process early in embryonic life (that is, random inactivation of one chromosome – see p. 140), some carriers have very low levels of factor VIII while others will have normal levels. Carriers could be diagnosed with reasonable confidence if the level of factor VIII:C was 50% or less of that expected from the level of factor vWF, but often no clear-cut answer was provided by this method. Carrier detection can be carried out using molecular genetic testing either by direct detection of mutations within the factor VIII gene or by indirect detection of the abnormal gene using DNA polymorphisms within or adjacent to the factor VIII gene as markers of the abnormal gene.

Antenatal diagnosis may be carried out by molecular analysis of fetal tissue obtained by chorionic villus biopsy at 9–11 weeks' gestation.

Haemophilia B (Christmas disease)

Haemophilia B is caused by a deficiency of factor IX. The inheritance and clinical features are identical to haemophilia A, but the incidence is only about 1 in 30 000 males. It is treated with factor IX concentrates.

von Willebrand's disease (vWD)

In vWD, there is defective platelet function as well as factor VIII:C deficiency and both are due to a deficiency or abnormality of vWF (see Fig 6.31). vWF plays a role in platelet adhesion to damaged subendothelium as well as stabilizing factor VIII:C in plasma (see p. 400).

The vWF gene is located on chromosome 12 and numerous mutations of the gene have been identified. vWD has been classified into three types:

- *Type 1* is characterized by a mild reduction in vWF and is inherited as an autosomal dominant.
- *Type 2* is due to a decrease in the proportion of high-molecular-weight multimers, and it too is inherited as an autosomal dominant.
- *Type 3* is recessively inherited and patients have barely detectable levels of factor VIII:vWF (and therefore factor VIII:C). Their parents are often phenotypically normal.

The *clinical features* of vWD are variable. Type 1 and type 2 patients usually have mild clinical features. Bleeding follows minor trauma or surgery and epistaxis and menorrhagia often occur. Haemarthroses are rare. Type 3 patients have more severe bleeding but rarely experience the joint and muscle bleeds seen in haemophilia A.

Characteristic *laboratory findings* are shown in Table 6.23. These also include defective platelet aggregation with ristocetin.

Treatment depends on the severity of the condition and may be similar to that of mild haemophilia, including the use of DDAVP for minor surgery. Intermediate purity factor VIII or von Willebrand factor concentrates should be used to treat bleeding or to cover surgery in patients with vWD who require replacement therapy. Cryoprecipitate should be avoided because of the greater risk of transfusion-transmitted infection.

Acquired coagulation disorders

Vitamin K deficiency (see also p. 200)

Vitamin K is necessary for the γ-carboxylation of glutamic acid residues on factors II, VII, IX and X and on proteins C and S. Without it, these factors cannot bind calcium and form complexes with PF-3 to carry out their normal functions.

Deficiency of vitamin K may be due to:

- *inadequate stores*, as in haemorrhagic disease of the newborn and protein-energy malnutrition (see p. 200)
- *malabsorption of vitamin K*, a fat-soluble vitamin, which occurs in cholestatic jaundice due to the lack of intraluminal bile salts
- *oral anticoagulant drugs*, which are vitamin K antagonists.

The PT and PTTK are prolonged (see Table 6.23) and there may be bruising, haematuria and gastrointestinal or cerebral bleeding. Minor bleeding is treated with phytomenadione (vitamin K_1) 10 mg intravenously. Some correction of the PT is usual within 6 hours but it may not return to normal for two days.

Newborn babies have low levels of vitamin K, and this may cause minor bleeding in the first week of life (*classical haemorrhagic disease of the newborn*). Vitamin K deficiency may also cause *late haemorrhagic disease of the newborn* which occurs 2–26 weeks after birth and may result in severe bleeding such as intracranial haemorrhage. Most infants with these syndromes have been exclusively breastfed, and both conditions may be prevented by administering 1 mg i.m. vitamin K to all neonates. There has been some concern that the administration of intramuscular vitamin K is associated with the development of cancer in childhood, but recent studies provide no evidence for this association.

Liver disease

Liver disease may result in a number of defects in haemostasis:

Vitamin K deficiency
This may occur owing to intrahepatic or extrahepatic cholestasis.

Reduced synthesis
Reduced synthesis of coagulation factors may be the result of severe hepatocellular damage. The use of vitamin K does not improve the results of abnormal coagulation tests, but it is generally given because of the accompanying malabsorption.

Thrombocytopenia
This may result from hypersplenism due to splenomegaly associated with portal hypertension.

Functional abnormalities
Functional abnormalities of platelets and fibrinogen are found in many patients with liver failure.

Disseminated intravascular coagulation
DIC (see below) may occur in acute liver failure.

Disseminated intravascular coagulation (DIC)

There is widespread generation of fibrin within blood vessels, owing to activation of the coagulation cascade by release of coagulant material, and by diffuse endothelial damage or generalized platelet aggregation. Activation of leucocytes, particularly monocytes causing the release of tissue factor and cytokines, may play a role in the development of DIC.

There is consumption of platelets and coagulation factors and secondary activation of fibrinolysis leading to production of fibrin degradation products (FDPs), which may contribute to the coagulation defect by inhibiting fibrin polymerization (Fig 6.32).

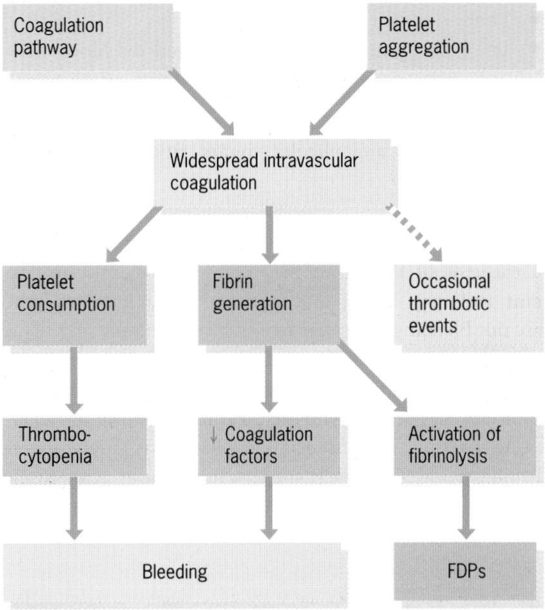

Fig 6.32
Disseminated intravascular coagulation. FDP, fibrin degradation products

CAUSES OF DIC

These include:

- malignant disease
- septicaemia (e.g. Gram-negative and meningococcal)
- haemolytic transfusion reactions
- obstetric causes (e.g. abruptio placentae, amniotic fluid embolism)
- trauma, burns, surgery
- other infections (e.g. falciparum malaria)
- snake bite.

CLINICAL FEATURES

The underlying disorder is usually obvious. The patient is often acutely ill and shocked. The clinical presentation of DIC varies from no bleeding at all to complete haemostatic failure with widespread haemorrhage. Bleeding may occur from the mouth, nose and venepuncture sites and there may be widespread ecchymoses.

Thrombotic events may occur as a result of vessel occlusion by fibrin and platelets. Any organ may be involved, but the skin and kidneys are most often affected.

INVESTIGATIONS

The diagnosis is often suggested by the underlying condition of the patient.

Severe cases with haemorrhage.

- The PT, PTTK and TT are usually very prolonged and the fibrinogen level markedly reduced.
- High levels of FDPs are found owing to the intense fibrinolytic activity stimulated by the presence of fibrin in the circulation.

- There is severe thrombocytopenia.
- The blood film may show fragmented red blood cells.

Mild cases without bleeding. Increased synthesis of coagulation factors and platelets may result in normal PT, PTTK, TT and platelet counts, although the FDPs will be raised.

TREATMENT

Treatment of the underlying condition is most important and may be all that is necessary in patients who are not bleeding. Maintenance of blood volume and tissue perfusion is essential. Transfusions of platelet concentrates, FFP, cryoprecipitate and red cell concentrates may be indicated in patients who are bleeding. The use of heparin to prevent intravascular coagulation is rarely given. Inhibitors of fibrinolysis such as tranexamic acid should not be used in DIC as dangerous fibrin deposition may result.

Excessive fibrinolysis

Activation of fibrinolysis occurs in DIC as a secondary event in response to intravascular deposition of fibrin. It may also occur during surgery involving tumours of the prostate, breast, pancreas and uterus owing to release of tissue plasminogen activators. Such *primary hyperfibrinolysis* is very rare.

The clinical picture is similar to DIC with widespread bleeding. Laboratory investigations are similar with a prolonged PT, PTTK and TT, a low fibrinogen level, and increased FDPs, although fragmented red cells and thrombocytopenia are not seen as disseminated coagulation is not present.

If the diagnosis is certain, fibrinolytic inhibitors such as ε-aminocaproic acid (EACA) or tranexamic acid should be considered. If DIC cannot be excluded, it is safer to treat as for DIC.

Massive transfusion

Stored blood contains few platelets and has reduced levels of factors V and VIII, although there are adequate amounts of the other coagulation factors. During *massive transfusion* (defined as transfusion of a volume of blood equal to the patient's own blood volume within 24 hours, e.g. approximately 10 units in an adult), the platelet count and PT and PTTK should be checked at intervals. Transfusion of platelet concentrates and FFP should be considered if thrombocytopenia or defective coagulation are thought to be contributing to continued blood loss.

Citrate binds ionized calcium and potentially lowers plasma calcium levels. This is rarely a problem as citrate is rapidly metabolized, but neonates and hypothermic patients may have a reduced capacity for removal of citrate. Where there is clinical and ECG evidence of hypocalcaemia, 5 mL of 10% calcium gluconate should be given at 5 minute intervals until the ECG is normal. The plasma potassium content of blood increases during storage but hyperkalaemia is rarely a problem unless very large volumes of blood are transfused rapidly.

Lactic acid is produced by red cell glycolysis in the blood pack and might contribute to the acidosis of hypoxic shocked patients. However, acidosis is usually improved by transfusion because of reversal of hypoxia and improved tissue perfusion.

Hypothermia may result from rapid transfusion of stored blood. Blood warmers should be used if the rate of infusion exceeds 1 unit in 10 minutes in adults and proportionately less in children.

Although it might be expected that massive transfusion of stored blood with high oxygen affinity due to low levels of 2,3-DPG would impair tissue oxygenation, there is little evidence that this occurs. Regeneration of 2,3-DPG is complete within a few hours following transfusion.

The combination of *hyperkalaemia*, *hypocalcaemia*, *hypothermia* and *acidosis* might impair cardiac performance and even cause cardiac arrest. Careful monitoring of the patient's temperature, plasma potassium and ECG for evidence of hypocalcaemia are essential in patients receiving rapid transfusions of large volumes of stored blood.

Inhibitors of coagulation

In addition to the factor VIII:C alloantibodies that are found in up to 10% of severe haemophiliacs, *factor VIII:C autoantibodies* arise occasionally in patients with autoimmune disorders such as SLE, in elderly patients, and sometimes after childbirth. There can be severe bleeding. The antibodies sometimes disappear spontaneously, but treatment with plasma exchange, high-dose intravenous immunoglobulin and immunosuppressive drugs may be required, in addition to any replacement therapy with factor concentrates (see above).

Lupus anticoagulants (p. 490) are autoantibodies directed against phospholipids (anti-phospholipid antibodies). They are found in about 10% of patients with SLE and may also occur in otherwise healthy individuals. They lead to prolongation of phospholipid-dependent coagulation tests, particularly the PTTK, but do not inhibit coagulation factor activity. Bleeding does not occur unless there is coexistent severe immune thrombocytopenia. The main clinical problems are thrombosis and recurrent miscarriages.

Thrombosis

A thrombus is defined as a solid mass formed in the circulation from the constituents of the blood during life. Fragments of thrombi (emboli) may break off and block vessels downstream. Thromboembolic disease is much more common than abnormal bleeding; nearly half of adult deaths in England and Wales are due to coronary artery thrombosis, cerebral artery thrombosis or pulmonary embolism.

A thrombus results from a complex series of events involving coagulation factors, platelets, red blood cells and the vessel wall.

Arterial thrombosis

This usually occurs in association with atheroma, which tends to form at areas of turbulent blood flow such as the bifurcation of arteries. Platelets adhere to the damaged vascular endothelium and aggregate in response to ADP and TXA_2 to form a 'white thrombus'. The growth of the platelet thrombus is limited at its margins by PGI_2. Eventually blood coagulation may be activated at the site of the thrombus, resulting either in complete occlusion of the vessel or embolization that produces distal obstruction. The risk factors for arterial thrombosis are related to the development of atherosclerosis (see p. 686).

Arterial thrombi may form in the heart, as mural thrombi in the left ventricle after myocardial infarction, in the left atrium in mitral valve disease, or on the surfaces of prosthetic valves.

Venous thrombosis

Unlike arterial thrombosis, venous thrombosis often occurs in normal vessels. Important causes are stasis and hypercoagulability. The majority of venous thrombi occur in the deep veins of the leg, originating around the valves as 'red thrombi' consisting mainly of red cells and fibrin. The propagating thrombus is formed of fibrin and platelets and is particularly liable to embolize. Chronic venous obstruction following thrombosis in the deep veins of the leg frequently results in a permanently swollen limb and may lead to ulceration (post-phlebitic syndrome).

Risk factors for venous thrombosis are shown in Table 6.24. Both arterial and venous thrombosis may occur with changes in blood cells such as polycythaemia, thrombocythaemia and sickle cell anaemia, and with coagulation abnormalities (thrombophilia; see below).

The clinical features and diagnosis of venous thrombosis are discussed on p. 742.

Thrombophilia

Thrombophilia is a term describing inherited or acquired defects of haemostasis leading to a predisposition to venous or arterial thrombosis. It should be considered in patients with:

- recurrent venous thrombosis
- venous thrombosis for the first time under age 40 years
- a family history of venous thrombosis
- an unusual venous thrombosis such as mesenteric or cerebral vein thrombosis
- unexplained neonatal thrombosis
- recurrent miscarriages
- arterial thrombosis in the absence of arterial disease.

Table 6.24
Risk factors of venous thromboembolism

Patient factors	Disease or surgical procedure
Age	Trauma or surgery, especially of pelvis, hip or lower limb
Obesity	Malignancy
Varicose veins	Cardiac failure
Immobility (bedrest > 4 days)	Recent myocardial infarction
Pregnancy and puerperium	Infection
High doses of oestrogen	Inflammatory bowel disease
Previous deep vein thrombosis or pulmonary embolism	Nephrotic syndrome
Thrombophilia, e.g. AT-deficiency, factor V Leiden, antiphospholipid antibody	Polycythaemia, thrombocythaemia
	Paroxysmal nocturnal haemoglobinuria
	Sickle cell anaemia
	Homocystinuria

Coagulation abnormalities

Evidence has accumulated on the importantce of a number of factors predisposing to thrombosis:

Factor V Leiden

Before the discovery of factor V Leiden in 1993, the definite diagnosis of thrombophilia was only possible in 5–10% of patients with a tendency to thrombosis. This defect was originally found as an inability of the patient's activated partial thromboplasm time (APTT) to lengthen in the presence of activated protein C (*activated protein C resistance*).

Factor V Leiden is formed by a single nucleotide substitution (arg 506 glu) in the factor V gene and this eliminates the site in the factor V protein which is cleaved by activated protein C. Factor V is a cofactor for thrombin generation (see Fig 6.27) and the failure of activated protein C to inactivate factor V (see Fig 6.28) results in a tendency to thrombosis. Factor V Leiden is found in 3–5% of healthy individuals in the West and in about 20% of patients with venous thrombosis.

The risk of venous thrombosis is increased in women with factor V Leiden who are pregnant or taking oral contraceptives. Consideration has been given to screening for the defect before prescribing oral contraceptives or during pregnancy. However, such a policy would be costly and might deny oral contraception to a substantial number of women who would then be at an increased risk of pregnancy, and therefore thrombosis. In addition, the use of oral anticoagulants in pregnancy carries a risk of fatal maternal bleeding, which may equal the risk of death due to postpartum thrombosis, and the fetus is also at risk of complications from the use of oral anticoagulants (see p. 413).

Antithrombin deficiency
This deficiency can be *inherited* as an autosomal dominant. Many variations have been described that lead to a conformational change in the protein. It can be *acquired* following trauma, with major surgery and with the contraceptive pill. Low levels are also seen in severe proteinuria (e.g. the nephrotic syndrome causing thrombotic episodes). Recurrent thrombotic episodes occur starting at a young age in the inherited variety. Patients are relatively resistant to heparin as AT is required for its action.

Protein C and S deficiency
These autosomal dominant conditions result in venous thrombosis before the age of 40 years.

Antiphospholipid antibody
See pp. 408 and 490.

INVESTIGATIONS

Haemostatic screening tests

- **Full blood count** including platelet count
- **Coagulation screen** including a fibrinogen level.

These tests will detect erythrocytosis, thrombocytosis, and dysfibrinogenaemia and suggest the presence of a lupus anticoagulant.

Testing for specific causes of thrombophilia

- **Assays** for naturally occurring anticoagulants such as AT, protein C and protein S
- **Assay** for activated protein C resistance and molecular testing for factor V Leiden
- **Screen for a coagulation factor inhibitor** including a lupus anticoagulant (see p. 490)
- **Fibrinolytic pathway tests** (see p. 402).

Prevention and treatment of arterial thrombosis

Attempts to prevent or reduce arterial thrombosis are directed mainly at minimizing factors predisposing to atherosclerosis. Treatment of established arterial thrombosis includes the use of antiplatelet drugs and thrombolytic therapy.

Antiplatelet drugs

Platelet activation at the site of vascular damage is crucial to the development of arterial thrombosis, and this can be altered by the following drugs (Table 6.25):

Table 6.25
Drugs used in the treatment of thrombotic disorders

Antiplatelet drugs	Anticoagulant drugs
Aspirin	Heparin
Dipyridamole	unfractionated
	low-molecular-weight, e.g. enoxaparin, tinzaparin, dalteparin
Thrombolytic therapy	Warfarin
Streptokinase	
Anisoylated plasminogen streptokinase activator complex (APSAC or anistreplase)	
Urokinase	
Single-chain urokinase-type plasminogen activator (scu-PA)	
Tissue-type plasminogen activator (rt-PA or alteplase)	
Reteplase	

- *Aspirin* inhibits the enzyme cyclo-oxygenase (see Fig 6.26), resulting in reduced platelet production of TXA_2.
- *Dipyridamole* – which inhibits platelet phosphodiesterase, causing an increase in cyclic AMP with potentiation of the action of PGI_2 – has been used widely as an antithrombotic agent, but there is little evidence that it is effective.
- *Clopidogrel* is a new inhibitor of platelet aggregation induced by ADP. It is similar to ticlopidine, which has not achieved wide use because it causes bone marrow depression, rash and diarrhoea.

A human-murine chimeric monoclonal Fab fragment antibody against the platelet glycoprotein IIb/IIIa receptor (*abciximab*) has been developed as a new strategy for preventing ischaemic complications during and after coronary angioplasty (Fig 6.33). A recent study (EPILOG) of abciximab with low-dose heparin markedly reduced the incidence of acute ischaemic complications in coronary angioplasty patients without increasing the risk of haemorrhage.

The indications for and results of antiplatelet therapy are discussed in the appropriate sections.

Thrombolytic therapy

Streptokinase
Streptokinase is a purified fraction of the filtrate obtained from cultures of haemolytic streptococci. It forms a 1:1 complex with plasminogen, resulting in a conformational change in plasminogen, revealing an active site which activates other plasminogen molecules to form plasmin. Streptokinase is given as an infusion of 1.5 million units over 1 hour in acute myocardial infarction. Laboratory monitoring of such short-term thrombolytic therapy is not necessary.

The main problem with streptokinase is its indiscriminate activation of plasminogen so that both fibrin in clots and free fibrinogen are lysed, leading to low fibrinogen levels and the risk of haemorrhage.

Anisoylated plasminogen streptokinase activator complex (APSAC/anistreplase)

APSAC is a complex of plasminogen and an anisoylated form of streptokinase. The complex binds to any fibrin within intravascular clots where the anisoyl group is hydrolysed and the streptokinase–plasminogen complex produces fibrinolysis. The advantage of APSAC over streptokinase is its more sustained duration of action, and it is given as a single bolus dose.

Urokinase

Urokinase is produced naturally by the kidney. It cleaves plasminogen directly to produce plasmin.

Tissue-type plasminogen activator (t-PA)

Tissue-type plasminogen activator (*alteplase*, *reteplase*) and single-chain urokinase-type plasminogen activator (scu-PA) are produced using recombinant gene technology. They were claimed to be relatively 'clot-specific' (i.e. to have a greater affinity for fibrin-bound plasminogen than circulating plasminogen), and therefore to cause less systemic fibrinolysis and bleeding than streptokinase. However, the use of these newer thrombolytic agents has not yet been shown to produce fewer bleeding episodes than does streptokinase. An accelerated dosage schedule of t-PA seems to produce a more rapid restoration of coronary flow.

INDICATIONS

The use of thrombolytic therapy in myocardial infarction are discussed on p. 695. The combination of aspirin with thrombolytic therapy produces better results than thrombolytic therapy alone. The extent of the benefit depends on how quickly treatment is given.

The main risk of thrombolytic therapy is bleeding. Treatment should not be given to patients who have had recent bleeding, uncontrolled hypertension or a stroke, or surgery or other invasive procedures within the previous 10 days.

Prevention and treatment of venous thromboembolism

Venous thromboembolism is a common problem after surgery, particularly in high-risk patients such as the elderly, those with malignant disease and those with a history of previous thrombosis (Table 6.26). The incidence is also high in patients confined to bed following trauma, myocardial infarction or other illnesses. The prevention and treatment of venous thrombosis includes the use of anticoagulants.

Anticoagulants

Heparin

Heparin is not a single substance but a mixture of polysaccharides. Commercially available unfractionated heparin consists of components with molecular weights varying from 5000 to 35 000 and an average of about 13 000. It was extracted initially from liver – hence its name – but it is now prepared from porcine gastric mucosa.

Heparin has an immediate effect on coagulation by potentiation of the formation of irreversible complexes between antithrombin and activated serine protease coagulation factors (thrombin, XIIa, XIa, Xa, IXa and VIIa).

Low-molecular-weight heparins

These are produced by enzymatic or chemical degradation of standard heparin, producing fractions with molecular weights in the range of 2000–8000. Potentiation of thrombin inhibition (anti-IIa activity) requires a minimum length of the heparin molecule with an approximate molecular weight of 5400, whereas the inhibition of factor Xa requires only a smaller heparin molecule with a molecular weight of about 1700.

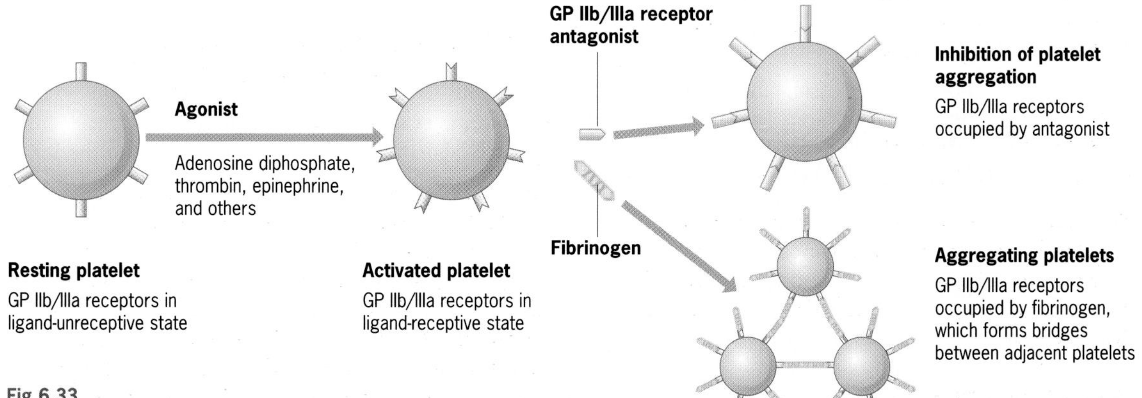

Fig 6.33
The role of glycoprotein IIb/IIIa in platelet aggregation and the inhibition of platelet aggregation by inhibitors of glycoprotein IIb/IIIa receptors. Modified from Lefkovits J, Plow EF, Topol EJ (1995) *New England Journal of Medicine* **332**: 1554, with permission

Table 6.26 Classification of risk of deep vein thrombosis and pulmonary embolism for hospital patients

Low risk (proximal vein thrombosis 0.4%; fatal pulmonary embolism < 0.2%)
Patients <40 years undergoing major surgery (>30 minutes) with no other risk factors
Patients undergoing minor surgery (<30 minutes) with no other risk factors
Patients with minor trauma or illness with no thrombophilia but history of deep vein thrombosis or previous pulmonary embolism
Medium risk (proximal vein thrombosis 2–4%; fatal pulmonary embolism 0.2–0.5%)
Major general, urological, gynaecological, cardiothoracic, vascular, or neurological surgery in patients >40 years or with one or more other risk factor(s)
Major acute medical illness such as myocardial infarction, heart failure, chest infection, cancer, or inflammatory bowel disease
Major trauma
Minor surgery, trauma, or illness in patients with previous deep vein thrombosis, pulmonary embolism, or thrombophilia
Plastercast immobilization of the leg in patients with minor injury
High risk (proximal vein thrombosis 10–20%; fatal pulmonary embolism 1–5%)
Fracture or major orthopaedic surgery of pelvis, hip, or leg
Major pelvic or abdominal surgery for cancer
Major surgery, trauma, or illness in patients with previous deep vein thrombosis, pulmonary embolism, or thrombophilia
Leg paralysis
Critical leg ischaemia or major leg amputation

From Verstraste M *British Medical Journal (*1997) **314**: 124, with permisision

Information

Target INR

2.5	Pulmonary embolism, proximal and calf deep vein thrombosis, recurrence of venous thromboembolism when no longer on warfarin therapy, symptomatic inherited thrombophilia, atrial fibrillation;cardioversion, mural thrombus, cardiomyopathy.
3.5	Recurrence of venous thromboembolism while on warfarin therapy, antiphospholipid syndrome, mechanical prosthetic heart valve, coronary artery graft thrombosis.

Information box 6.1 Indications for oral anticoagulation and target INR (British Society for Haematology 1998)

Low-molecular-weight heparins have the following properties:

- They have greater activity against factor Xa than against factor IIa, suggesting that they may produce an equivalent anticoagulant effect as standard heparin but have a lower risk of bleeding, although this has not generally been confirmed. In addition, low-molecular-weight heparins cause less inhibition of platelet function.
- They have a longer half-life than standard heparin and so can be given as a once-daily subcutaneous injection instead of every 8–12 hours.
- They produce little effect on tests of overall coagulation, such as the PTTK at doses recommended for prophylaxis. They are not fully neutralized by protamine.
- They are widely used for antithrombotic prophylaxis of high-risk surgical patients, and fixed-dose low-molecular-weight heparin regimens are being increasingly used for the treatment of established thrombosis (see p. 742).

The *main complication* of treatment with heparin is bleeding. This is managed by stopping heparin. Very occasionally it is necessary to neutralize unfractionated heparin with protamine. Other complications include osteoporosis with prolonged therapy and thrombocytopenia.

Oral anticoagulants

These act by interfering with vitamin K metabolism. There are two types of oral anticoagulants, the coumarins and indanediones. The coumarin *warfarin* is most commonly used because it has a low incidence of side-effects other than bleeding.

The dosage is controlled by PT tests. Thromboplastin reagents for PT testing are derived from a variety of sources and give different PT results for the same plasma. It is standard practice to compare each thromboplastin with an international reference preparation so that it can be assigned an international sensitivity index (ISI). The international normalized ratio (INR) is the ratio of the patient's PT to a normal control when using the international reference preparation. Therapeutic ranges using the INR for oral anticoagulation in various conditions are shown in Information box 6.1.

Each laboratory can use a chart adapted to the ISI of their thromboplastin to convert the patient's PT to the INR. Suitably selected control plasmas can also be used to achieve the same objective. The use of this system means that PT tests on a given plasma sample using different thromboplastins result in the same INR and that anticoagulant control is comparable in different hospitals across the world.

Contraindications to the use of oral anticoagulants are seldom absolute and include:

- severe hypertension
- non-thromboembolic strokes

- peptic ulceration (unless cured by *Helicobacter pylori* eradication)
- severe liver and renal disease
- pre-existing haemostatic defects.

Oral anticoagulants should be avoided in *pregnancy* because they are teratogenic in the first trimester and may be associated with fetal haemorrhage later in pregnancy. When anticoagulation is considered essential in pregnancy, specialist advice should be sought. Self-administered subcutaneous heparin should be used as an alternative, although this may not be as effective for women with prosthetic cardiac valves.

Many drugs interact with warfarin (see Chapter 14). More frequent PT testing should accompany changes in medication, which should occur with the full knowledge of the anticoagulant clinic.

An increased anticoagulant effect due to warfarin. An increased anticoagulant effect due to warfarin (Emergency box 6.1) is usually produced by one of the following mechanisms.

- drugs causing a reduction in the metabolism of warfarin, including tricyclic antidepressants, cimetidine, sulphonamides, phenothiazines and amiodarone
- drugs such as clofibrate and quinidine which increase the sensitivity of hepatic receptors to warfarin
- drugs interfering with vitamin K absorption (such as broad-spectrum antibiotics and cholestyramine) which also potentiate the action of warfarin
- displacement of warfarin from its binding site on serum albumin by drugs such as sulphonamides (this is not usually responsible for clinically important interactions)
- drugs that inhibit platelet function (such as aspirin) which increase the risk of bleeding
- alcohol excess, cardiac failure, liver or renal disease, thyrotoxicosis and febrile illnesses which result in potentiation of the effect of warfarin.

A decreased anticoagulant effect due to warfarin
This is usually produced by drugs that increase the clearance of warfarin by induction of hepatic enzymes that metabolize warfarin, such as rifampicin and barbiturates.

Prophylaxis to prevent venous thromboembolism

Prophylactic measures to prevent venous thrombosis during surgery are aimed at procedures for preventing stasis, such as early mobilization, elevation of the legs, compression stockings, and possibly calf-muscle stimulation and passive calf-muscle exercises during surgery, and methods for preventing hypercoagulability, usually using heparin.

- *Low-risk patients* (Table 6.26) require no specific measures other than early mobilization.
- *Moderate-risk patients* should receive specific prophylaxis with as low-dose heparin at a dose of 5000 units subcutaneously every 8–12 hours until the patient is ambulatory. No laboratory monitoring is required.
- In *high-risk patients*, such as patients undergoing total hip replacement, low-molecular-weight heparin once daily, such as enoxaparin 40 mg (4000 i.u.), has been shown to be more effective than standard low-dose heparin in preventing thrombosis. There is recent evidence to suggest that it is most effective when administered for a total of a month postoperatively rather than merely during the admission for surgery. However, in general surgical practice there is no clear evidence that low-molecular-weight heparin is superior to standard low-dose heparin and it is more expensive. Before the introduction of low-molecular-weight heparin, other approaches were used in high-risk surgical patients, such as low-dose warfarin and higher doses of subcutaneous heparin to keep the PTTK just prolonged.

Emergency

Life-threatening haemorrhage

Stop warfarin immediately, give vitamin K 5 mg by slow intravenous infusion and either a concentrate of factor II, IX, X with frozen VII concentrate (if these are available) or fresh frozen plasma 15 ml/kg.

Less severe haemorrhage, e.g. haematuria or epistaxis or INR >8 with no bleeding

Withhold warfarin with INR < 5; consider vitamin K 0.5 mg intravenously.

INR of >4.5 without haemorrhage

Withdraw warfarin for 1–2 days and then review.

Unexpected bleeding at therapeutic levels

Investigate possibility of an underlying cause such as unexpected renal or alimentary tract disease.

Emergency box 6.1 Management of over-anticoagulation with warfarin. Modified from the British Society for Haematology (1990).

TREATMENT OF ESTABLISHED VENOUS THROMBOEMBOLISM

The aim of anticoagulant treatment is to prevent further thrombosis and pulmonary embolization while resolution of venous thrombi occurs by natural fibrinolytic activity. Anticoagulation is started with heparin as it produces an immediate anticoagulant effect. There is no evidence that it is necessary to use heparin for any longer than it takes for simultaneously administered warfarin to produce an anticoagulant effect, usually about 3–4 days (see Information box 6.2).

Low-molecular-weight heparin (e.g. tinzaparin 175 units kg^{-1} daily) is equally effective and as safe as unfractionated heparin in the immediate treatment of deep vein thrombosis and pulmonary embolism. This creates the opportunity for treatment of venous thromboembolism without admission to hospital in compliant patients without co-existing risk factors for haemorrhage.

Anticoagulation for six weeks is sufficient for patients after their first thrombosis provided there are no persisting risk factors. Long-term treatment should be given to patients with repeated episodes or continuing risk factors. Outpatient anticoagulation is best supervised in anticoagulant clinics. Patients are issued with national booklets for recording INR results and anticoagulant doses.

The role of *thrombolytic therapy* in the treatment of venous thrombosis is not established. It is sometimes used in patients with massive pulmonary embolism and in patients with extensive deep venous thrombi.

For these conditions it is necessary to give a bolus dose of streptokinase, 250 000 units over 30 minutes, to inactivate antibodies formed by previous streptococcal infection, followed by a continuous infusion, approximately 100 000 units every hour for 24–72 hours. The dose of streptokinase is adjusted to maintain the TT between two and four times the control value.

Thrombolytic therapy should be followed by anticoagulation with heparin for a few days and then by oral anticoagulants for a few months to prevent rethrombosis.

Hirudin is being evaluated as a new antithrombotic agent. It inactivates thrombin bound to fibrin more efficiently than AT-III potentiated by heparin. Clinical studies are required to establish its effectiveness and safety.

i Information

- Obtain objective evidence of thrombosis using e.g. venography, ultrasound imaging or pulmonary ventilation/perfusion scanning as soon as possible (see p. 720).
- Perform a coagulation screen and platelet count before starting treatment to exclude a pre-existing haemostatic effect.
- Give an intravenous loading dose of 5000 units of standard heparin (except in severe pulmonary embolism when 10 000 units should be given.
- Heparinization should be continued with either:
  (a) an intravenous infusion of 1000–2000 units per hour, or
  (b) subcutaneous injections of 15 000 units every 12 hours.
- The dose of intravenous or subcutaneous heparin is adjusted by laboratory monitoring 4–6 hours after the dose of heparin to prolong the PTTK to between 1.5 and 2.5 times the control value. Monitoring should be carried out at least once each day.
- Administer warfarin 5–10 mg (depending on the size and age of the patient) at the time the heparin is started. Give the same dose the next day and check the INR on the third day.
- Heparin is stopped when the INR reaches the therapeutic range (usually 2.0) and the dose of warfarin is adjusted to maintain the INR in the therapeutic range.
- The maintenance dose of warfarin is usually 3–9 mg daily. The INR is measured frequently until stability is achieved. The maximum interval between tests for patients on long-term anticoagulation is 6 weeks.

Information box 6.2 Treatment of established venous thromboembolism

FURTHER READING

British Society for Haematology (1990). Guidelines on oral anticoagulation: second edition. *Journal of Clinical Pathology* **43**: 177–183.

British Society for Haematology (1993). Guidelines on the use and monitoring of heparin: second revision. *Journal of Clinical Pathology* **46**: 97–103.

Diuguid DL (1997) Oral anticoagulant therapy for venous thromboembolism. *New England Journal of Medicine* **336**: 433–434.

Holmes DR (1997) Preventing coronary stenosis and complications. *New England Journal of Medicine* **336**: 1748–1749.

Karpatkin S (1997) Autoimmune (idiopathic) thrombocytopenic purpura. *Lancet* **349**: 1531–1536.

Lip GYH, Lowe GDO (1996) Antithrombotic treatment of atrial fibrillation. *British Medical Journal* **312**: 45–49.

Moake JL (1995) Thrombotic thrombocytopenic purpura. *Thrombosis and Haemostasis* **74**: 240–245.

Schafer AI (1996) Low-molecular-weight heparin: an opportunity for home treatment of venous thrombosis. *New England Journal of Medicine* **334**: 724–725.

CHAPTER BIBLIOGRAPHY

Bain BJ (1995) *Blood Cells: A Practical Guide*. Oxford: Blackwell Science.

Bloom AL, Forbes CD, Thomas DP, Tuddenham EGD (1994) *Haemostasis and Thrombosis*, 2nd edn. Edinburgh: Churchill Livingstone.

Brenner MK, Hoffbrand AV (1996) *Recent Advances in Haematology*, vol 8. London: Churchill Livingstone.

Dacie JV (1992) *The Haemolytic Anaemias*, 3rd edn. Edinburgh: Churchill Livingstone.

Hoffbrand AV, Pettit (1993) *Essential Haematology*, 3rd edn. Oxford: Blackwell Scientific.

Petz LD, Swisher SN, Kleinman S, Spence RK, Strauss RG (1996) *The Clinical Practice of Transfusion Medicine*, 3rd edn. New York: Churchill Livingstone.

Provan D, Henson A (1997) *The ABC of Clinical Haematology*. London: BMJ Publications.

Williams WJ, Beutler E, Erslev AJ, Lichtman MA (1990) *Hematology*, 4th edn. New York: McGraw-Hill.

Medical oncology

7

The term 'malignant disease' encompasses a wide range of illnesses, including common ones such as lung, breast and colon cancer (Table 7.1), as well as rare ones, like the acute leukaemias. Malignant disease is widely prevalent and, in the West, almost a third of the population will develop cancer at some time during their life. It is second only to cardiovascular disease as the cause of death. Although the mortality of cancer is still high, many advances have been made, both in terms of treatment, and in understanding the biology of the disease at the molecular level.

Currently treatment is given with curative or palliative intent, but the situation may change with time. For most people, the word 'cancer' implies certain death, although this is clearly not always the case. Physicians have an obligation to be honest with their patients, combining realism about the prognosis with compassion and understanding.

Table 7.1
Epidemiology of cancer by site of origin in England and Wales

Type	Percentage of all cancers	Percentage of cancer deaths	Sex ratio M:F
Oral cavity/ pharynx	1	1.1	2.1:1
Oesophagus	2.2	3.6	2:1
Stomach	5	5.8	2.4:1
Large bowel	11.6	11.3	1.4:1
Pancreas	2.7	4.2	1.5:1
Lung	16.8	23.7	3.5:1
Melanoma	1.5	0.8	0.6:1
Other skin	12.2	0.3	1.7:1
Breast	11.1	9.6	0.01:1
Cervix	1.8	1.2	
Uterus	1.5	0.7	
Ovary	2.3	2.7	
Prostate	5	6.2	
Bladder	4.6	3.4	3.8:1
Kidney	1.6	1.8	2.2:1
Brain	1.3	1.8	1.5:1
Non-Hodgkin's lymphoma	2.4	2.6	1.5:1
Myeloma	1.1	1.5	1.5:1
Leukaemias	2.1	2.1	1.7:1

Cancers less than 1% have been excluded.

Derived from Doll R, Peto P (1996) In *Oxford Textbook of Medicine*. Oxford: Oxford University Press

Aetiology

In most patients the cause of the illness remains unknown. Several factors have, however, been identified as being associated with the development of malignancy.

Cigarette tobacco

The incidence of lung cancer in both men and women has increased dramatically in the last 25 years. The association of smoking with lung cancer is now indisputable: cigarette tobacco is responsible for one-third of all deaths from cancer in the UK. Smoking not only causes lung cancer, it is also associated with cancer of the mouth, larynx, oesophagus and bladder. As a consequence of public health campaigns, cigarette consumption in the UK is now beginning to decrease.

Alcohol

Alcohol is associated with cancers of the upper respiratory and gastrointestinal tracts (Table 7.2), but it also interacts with tobacco in the aetiology of these tumours. It may be associated with an increased risk of breast cancer.

Diet

Dietary factors have been attributed to account for a third of cancer deaths, although it may be difficult to differentiate these from epidemiological factors. For example, the incidence of stomach cancer is particularly high in the Far East. Although increased dietary fibre may 'protect' against colon cancer, an association between red meat ingestion and carcinomas of the colon has been reported. Food and its role in the causation of gastrointestinal cancer is discussed in Chapter 4.

Table 7.2 Some causative factors associated with the development of cancer at various sites

Smoking	Mouth, pharynx, oesophagus, larynx, lung, bladder, lip
Ultraviolet light	Skin, lip
Alcohol	Mouth, pharynx, larynx, oesophagus, colorectal
Drugs (alkylating agents)	Bladder, bone marrow
Asbestos	Lung, mesothelium
Oestrogens	Endometrium, vagina
Vinyl chloride	Liver (angiosarcoma)
Polycyclic hydrocarbons	Skin, lung
Aromatic amines	Bladder
Aflatoxin	Liver
Biological agents:	
Hepatitis B virus	Liver
Hepatitis C virus	Liver
Schistosoma japonicum	Bladder
Helicobacter pylori	Stomach

Exposure to ultraviolet light

Ultraviolet light is known to increase the risk of skin cancer (basal cell, squamous cell and melanoma). The incidence of melanoma is therefore particularly high in the white population of Australia, New Zealand and South Africa, but exposure to UV light is probably not the only factor.

Occupational factors

In 1775, Percival Pott described the association between carcinogenic hydrocarbons in soot and the development of scrotal epitheliomas in chimney sweeps. Subsequently, other chemicals have been found to be carcinogenic. The principal causes are asbestos (lung and pleural cancer), ionizing radiation (any cancer), and combustion of fossil fuels releasing polycyclic hydrocarbons (skin, lung, bladder cancers).

Infectious agents

Viruses are known to cause cancer in animals. A great deal of time and money has therefore been expended in trying to establish whether they can also cause human cancer. The geographical distribution of a rare malignancy may suggest that it might be caused by, or associated with, an infective agent. For example, a specific type of T-cell leukaemia, seen almost exclusively in the southern island of Japan and in the West Indies, is associated with infection by the retrovirus, HTLV-1 (human T-cell leukaemia virus) which is endemic in these areas. Similarly, hepatocellular cancer is related to hepatitis B and C infection. The Epstein–Barr virus (EBV) has been implicated in Burkitt's lymphoma, and patients with HIV infection have an increased incidence of EBV-related lymphoma and Kaposi's sarcoma. The latter is now known to be associated with herpes virus 8.

The incidence of cervical cancer is increasing, particularly amongst younger women. This suggests an effect of changing social standards with increased sexual freedom and increased use of the oral contraceptive pill. Early sexual activity and multiple sexual partners have both been found to be associated with increased risk. Papilloma virus is thought to be the infectious agent involved in causation.

Helicobacter pylori infection is now recognized as a causative agent in gastric cancer and gastric lymphoma. *Schistosoma japonicum* infection causes bladder cancer.

Drugs

Oestrogens have been implicated in the development of both vaginal and endometrial carcinoma. Alkylating agents and radiotherapy given, for example, for Hodgkin's disease (see later) are themselves associated with an increased incidence of secondary acute myelogenous leukaemia (AML). More recently the epipodophyllotoxin, etoposide, has also been shown to be associated with the development of secondary AML.

Epidemiology

Geographical distribution

The incidence of specific tumours varies with geographical location. England, Scotland and Wales have the highest death rate from malignant disease in the world, mainly because of the very high incidence of lung cancer due to smoking. Breast, colon and prostatic cancer have a relatively low incidence in Asian countries, while liver cancer occurs worldwide but is rare in Europe and North America. Similarly, stomach cancer is particularly prevalent in Japan.

Environmental factors have been clearly implicated. For example, people moving from countries with a low incidence of breast or colon cancer to countries where the incidence is high, eventually acquire the cancer incidence of the country to which they have moved. This suggests that for these specific cancers, environmental factors are more important than genetic ones. For breast cancer, the following have been shown to be associated with a higher incidence: early menarche, late menopause and older age at the time of first pregnancy. Investigation of families with a particularly strong family history has also lead to the identification of two genes, BRCA1 and BRCA2, which confer an increased risk of developing breast cancer at an earlier age.

Age distribution

The majority of common cancers occur in older people. However, in children aged between 3 and 13 years, cancer is the most prevalent cause of death, acute lymphoblastic leukaemia being the cause in most cases (despite high cure rates).

Cancer genetics

The development of cancer is associated with a fundamental genetic change within the cell. There is clear evidence that mutations (see p. 151) can cause cancer. Evidence for the genetic origin of cancer is based on the following:

- Some cancers show a familial predisposition.
- Most known carcinogens induce mutations.
- Susceptibility to some carcinogens depends on the ability of cellular enzymes to convert them to a mutagenic form.
- Genetically determined traits associated with a deficiency in the enzymes required for DNA repair are associated with an increased risk of cancer (see p. 151).
- Some cancers are associated with chromosome 'instability'.
- Malignant tumours represent clonal proliferations of neoplastic cells.
- Some tumours contain mutated oncogenes (p. 152).

Mutations may occur in the germline and can therefore be present in every cell in the body, or they may occur in a single somatic cell and therefore be present only in the tumour following clonal proliferation.

Cytogenetic (chromosome) abnormalities

Genetic changes are often manifest as a chromosome change that can be picked up by examination of dividing cells. Most of these observations have been made in haematological malignancies (leukaemias and lymphomas) because samples of blood can be obtained relatively easily. Chromosome changes are often reciprocal translocations (see below). A non-reciprocal change results in deletion or addition of part of a chromosome; for example, deletion of chromosome 7 is associated with myelodysplasia and the development of acute myeloblastic leukaemia (AML) with a particularly poor prognosis. Examples of specific chromosome changes associated with malignancy are:

- *Chronic myeloid leukaemia*, in which 95% of patients have a reciprocal translocation between part of chromosome 22 and chromosome 9 (see p. 426).
- *Acute promyelocytic leukaemia* (APML), a subtype of acute myelogenous leukaemia. Almost all patients with APML have the t(15;17) reciprocal translocation which occurs at the q25 band on chromosome 15 and the q22 band on chromosome 17. This is of particular interest because the breakpoint on chromosome 17 occurs in the gene encoding the retinoic acid receptor. This is to some extent the explanation for the responsiveness of patients with APML to *all-trans*-retinoic acid (ATRA, see below).
- *Burkitt's lymphoma*, the first tumour in which a cytogenetic change was shown to involve the translocation of a specific gene. The most frequent change is a translocation between chromosomes 8 and 14 in which the *MYC* oncogene moves from chromosome 8 to a position near the constant region of the immunoglobulin heavy chain gene on chromosome 14. It is a reciprocal translocation, so the variable region of the immunoglobulin gene is transferred from chromosome 14 to chromosome 8. Similar rearrangements involving the light chain loci are seen in the alternative Burkitt's lymphoma translocations between chromosome 8 and either chromosome 2 or 22.

DNA repair

Some autosomal recessive diseases associated with abnormalities of DNA repair predispose to the development of cancer:

- xeroderma pigmentosum (XP)
- ataxia telangectasia (AT)

- Bloom's syndrome (BS)
- Fanconi's anaemia (FA).

Patients with XP have a defect in their ability to repair DNA damage caused by ultraviolet light and by some chemicals, leading to a high incidence of skin cancer. The AT mutation results in an increased sensitivity to ionizing radiation and an increased incidence of lymphoid tumours. An increased susceptibility to lymphoid malignancy is also seen in BS and FA. It is not known why these chromosome-break syndromes predispose to tumours of lymphatic tissue.

Inherited cancers

The following are examples of cancer syndromes that exhibit dominant inheritance:

- Retinoblastoma, an eye tumour found in young children. It occurs in both hereditary (40%) and non-hereditary (60%) forms. The 40% of patients with the hereditary form have a germline mutation on the long arm of chromosome 13 that predisposes to retinoblastoma. In addition to the latter, children inheriting this mutation at the so-called *RBL* locus are at risk for developing other tumours, particularly osteosarcoma
- Breast and ovarian cancer. Two genes have been identified – *BRCA1* and *BRCA2*. A strong family history along with germline mutation of these genes accounts for most cases of familial breast cancer and over half of ovarian cancers. Although using these genes to screen family members has been disappointing, *BRCA* genes are crucial to DNA repair. BRCA1 and 2 proteins bind to the DNA repair enzyme Rad51 to make it functional in repairing DNA breaks. Mutations in the *BRCA* genes will lead to accumulation of unrepaired mutations in tumour-suppressor genes and crucial oncogenes.
- Wilm's tumour.
- Familial adenomatous polyposis (p. 273).
- Basal-cell naevus syndrome.
- Neurofibromatosis.
- Multiple-endocrine-adenomatosis syndromes (p. 956).
- Neuroblastoma.
- Family cancer syndrome.

Oncogenes (see also p. 151)

Some malignant T cells have been shown to contain DNA sequences which are complimentary to the sequences of known tumour viruses. This does not in itself imply that the virus has caused the tumour. However, the fact that such sequences can be integrated into the human genome has led to the identification of genes whose function is to regulate (i.e. to 'prevent') the malignant transformation; these are the so-called 'tumour suppressor genes' (e.g. the *p53* molecule). Normal cells also contain genes known as proto-oncogenes, activation of which (for example by a mutation or carcinogen to produce an oncogene) would result in malignant transformation. It has now been demonstrated that specific proto-oncogenes are associated with specific cancers. Some examples are shown in Table 7.3.

Table 7.3
Association of some proto-oncogenes with specific tumours

Proto-oncogene	Tumour
C-Myc	Burkitt's lymphoma Cervical cancer Breast cancer Small-cell lung cancer
L-Myc	Small-cell lung cancer
N-Myc	Small-cell lung cancer
Abl	Chronic myeloid leukaemia
C-Ras	Colon cancer
C-Erb B2	Breast cancer

Molecular genetic techniques are helping to increase understanding of the biology of haematological malignancies, and in some cases they have practical applications. The *bcl*-2 gene encodes a protein that prolongs cell survival by inhibiting apoptosis (programmed cell death). Its expression is altered in 85% of patients with follicular lymphoma who have the translocation t(14;18). The latter leads to an accumulation of clonal cells which are susceptible to additional transforming mutations. Detection of the translocation by PCR amplification provides a marker of minimal residual disease after treatment and a means of identifying occult peripheral blood involvement. It has also been demonstrated that *p53* mutations in follicular lymphoma are associated with transformation to high-grade histology (see p. 435).

FURTHER READING

Healy B (1997) Editorial: *BRCA* genes. *New England Medical Journal* **336**: 1448–1449.

Biology of cancer

Most human neoplasms are monoclonal in origin, i.e. they arise from a single affected cell. Heterogeneity of tumour structure, however, arises during the course of its growth. Normal tissue continues to grow until cell proliferation is balanced by cell loss. In cancer tissue, however, there is a defect in regulatory factors (see p. 151) and the neoplasm increases in size. During growth in normal tissue, the cells become specialized in both structure and function (i.e. differentiation). In cancer cells the tissue is frequently undifferentiated; that is, morphologically the cells have not developed normally, and there is variation in nuclear size and shape. Activity of telomerase (see p. 132), an enzyme that extends telomeric DNA sequences or chromosomal ends, is essential to maintain the neoplastic state in cancer cells.

The *kinetics* of growth appear to be exponential; doubling times of human tumours are enormously variable. For many tumours, there is a progressive slowing of the rate of growth as the tumours become larger. This occurs for many reasons, but outgrowing of the blood supply is paramount. New vessel formation (angiogenesis) is stimulated by a variety of stimulatory peptides produced by both tumour cells and by host inflammatory cells. Angiostatin, a product of plasminogen, is an inhibitor of this process. The infiltration of the tumour mass with new vessels not only provides a stimulus to tumour growth, but also allows access of neoplastic cells to the circulation.

The process of *infiltration* into surrounding tissues occurs with loss of cell–cell cohesion. Cohesion is mediated by active homotypic cell adhesion molecules (CAMs) (see p. 163). The cadherin molecules are transmembrane glycoproteins able to mediate cellular attachment. Epithelial cadherin (E-cadherin) is expressed by many carcinomas and loss of E-cadherin expression is associated with an increase in invasion of the tumour. Invasion is partly determined by the balance of activators to inhibitors of proteolysis. Secretion of proteolytic enzymes, including the matrix metalloproteinases (particularly the collagenases), occurs from adjacent fibroblasts owing to failure of production of tissue inhibitors.

Following invasion, dissemination of tumour cells occurs when they enter the vascular and lymphatic vessels. Here they must survive host–defence mechanisms so as to spread throughout the body (see p. 160). The disseminated cancer cells lodge in distant sites, partly by chance, but also because of specific interactions between receptors/ligands found on endothelial cells and on tumour cells. This accounts for the specific pattern of metastases with certain tumours; for example, breast tumours frequently metastasize to long bones. The attachment of tumour cells to the endothelial cells is partly through adhesion molecules.

Integrins are transmembrane heterodimeric glycoproteins formed by non-covalent association of α and β chains. These cells are normally responsible for cell-substrate adhesive interaction; for example, α_4,β_1 is expressed on normal endothelium and is involved in the binding of lymphocytes to activated endothelium. Patterns of intergrin expression in tumours is complex but, nevertheless, certain tumours demonstrate up-regulation of specific integrins during tumour progression, and this may allow migration of tumour cells through the extracellular matrix substrate and invasion through the basement membrane and formation of a metastatic deposit.

FURTHER READING

Vile RG (ed) (1995) *Cancer Metastasis: From Mechanism to Therapies*. Chichester: John Wiley.

The diagnosis of malignancy

The diagnosis of cancer may be suspected by both patient and doctor but advice about treatment can only be given on the basis of a tissue diagnosis. This may be obtained by surgical biopsy or on the basis of cytology (e.g. lung cancer diagnosed by sputum cytology or cervix cancer diagnosed on the basis of a cervical smear). Malignant lesions can be distinguished from the benign by the pleomorphic nature of the cells, increased numbers of mitoses, nuclear abberation and evidence of invasion into surrounding tissues. The degree of differentiation or conversely of anaplasia of the tumour has prognostic significance: generally speaking, more differentiated tumours have a better prognosis than anaplastic ones. Immunocytochemistry, using monoclonal antibodies against tumour antigens, is very helpful in differentiating between, for example, B- and T-cell lymphomas. It is also useful for diagnosing neuroendocrine tumours and for differentiating between adenocarcinoma, squamous cell cancers and small cell carcinoma of the lung.

Staging

Before a decision about treatment can be made, not only the type of tumour but also its extent and distribution need to be established. Various 'staging investigations' are therefore performed before a treatment decision is made. The staging systems vary according to the type of tumour (see Hodgkin's disease, p. 432). The TNM (Tumour, Node, Metastases) classification shown in Table 7.4 can be applied to most common cancers.

An example of this classification as used for lung cancer is:

- Tx Positive cytology only
- T1 <3 cm
- T2 >3 cm/extends to hilar region/invades visceral pleura/partial atelectasis
- T3 Chest wall, diaphragm, pericardium, mediastinum, pleura, total atelectasis
- T4 heart, great vessels, trachea, oesophagus, malignant effusion
- N1 Peribronchial, ipsilateral hilar
- N2 Ipsilateral mediastinal
- N3 Contralateral mediastinal, scalene or supraclavicular
- M0 No metastases
- M1 Metastases present

Thus a T0/N0/M0 tumour has a much better prognosis than one that is staged as T4/N3/M1.

In addition to anatomical staging, the person's age and general state of health need to be taken into account when planning treatment. The latter has been called 'performance status' and is also of prognostic significance (Table 7.5).

Tumour markers

There are a number of specific tumour markers which are found in serum and are useful in diagnosis:

- α-fetoprotein – hepatocellular carcinoma, and non-seminomatous germ cell testicular tumours
- β human chorionic gonadotrophin (β-HCG) – choriocarcinomas
- prostate-specific antigen (PSA) – carcinoma of prostate.

There are a number of other tumour markers available but these are of little use in diagnosis. Examples include:

- carcinoma embryonic antigen (CEA) – e.g. colonic cancer
- Ca-125 – e.g. ovarian, gut, pancreatic cancer
- Ca-19-9 – e.g. gut, pancreatic cancer.

These markers are nonspecific and should be used only to monitor response to treatment.

Measuring response to treatment

Response to treatment can be subjective or objective. A subjective response is one perceived by the patient in terms of, for example, relief of pain and dyspnoea, or improvement in appetite, weight gain or energy. Quantitative measurements of these subjective symptoms form an increasingly important part of the assessment of response to chemotherapy, especially in those situations where cure is not possible and where the aim of treatment is to provide prolongation of good-quality life. In these circumstances, measures of quality of life enable an estimate of the balance of benefit and side-effects to be made.

Objective response to treatment is measured either as a partial response, which is defined as more than a 50% reduction in the size of the tumour, or complete response, which is a complete disappearance of all detectable disease clinically and radiologically. The terms used to evaluate the responses of tumours are given in Table 7.6. The term remission is often used for haematological malignancies.

Partial response is often associated with a reduction in symptoms and improvement in quality of life. The rate of regrowth of the tumour is dependent on the underlying doubling time of that particular tumour. For more rapidly growing tumours a partial response may not be associated with very much prolongation of life, whereas with more slow-growing tumours responses may continue for a long time. Complete remission is a necessary prerequisite for

Table 7.4
TNM classification

T	Extent of primary tumour
N	Extent of regional lymph node involvement
M	Presence or absence of metastases
Extent of disease	
T0	Excised tumour
T1	Increases in primary tumour size
T2	
T3	
T4	
Increased involvement of nodes	
N0	
N1	Increasing involvement
N2	
N3	
Presence of metastases	
M0	Not present
M1	Present

Table 7.5
Karnowsky performance status

100	Normal; no complaints
90	Able to carry on normal activity Minor symptoms of disease
80	Normal activity with effort Some symptoms of disease
70	Cares for self Unable to carry on normal activity or to work
60	Requires occasional assistance Able to care for most of own needs
50	Requires considerable assistance and frequent medical care
40	Disabled Requires special care and assistance
30	Severely disabled Hospitalization indicated although death not imminent
20	Very sick Hospitalization necessary, active supportive treatment necessary
10	Moribund Fatal processes progressing rapidly

Table 7.6
Definitions of response

Complete response	Complete disappearance of all detectable disease
Partial reponse	More than 50% reduction in the size of the tumour
No response	No change, or less than 50% reduction
Progressive disease	Increase in size of tumour at any site

cure, but unfortunately many patients who achieve complete remission will subsequently relapse because of the presence of residual microscopic disease. Many strategies have been developed to try to increase the proportion of patients with complete remission who go on to long-term remission or cure.

Principles of chemotherapy

The ability to give anticancer treatment via the bloodstream was a major advance as it enabled therapy potentially to reach metastatic disease in any part of the body. However, the toxicity of chemotherapy determined that drugs could be given only intermittently and that time had to be allowed for normal tissues to recover between each administration of new cytotoxic drugs.

Furthermore, it quickly became apparent in the early development of cytotoxic chemotherapy that tumours rapidly developed resistance to single agents given on their own. For this reason the principle of intermittent combination chemotherapy was developed. Several drugs were combined together, chosen on the basis of differing mechanisms of action and non-overlapping toxicities. These drugs were given over a period of a few days followed by a rest of a few weeks, during which time the normal tissues had the opportunity for regrowth. It became apparent that normal tissues repaired more rapidly than cancer cells and it was therefore possible continually to deplete the tumour while allowing the restoration of normal tissues between chemotherapy cycles (Fig 7.1).

In many experimental tumours it has been shown that there is a log–linear relationship between drug dose and number of cancer cells killed. With a chemosensitive tumour a relatively small increase in dose may have a large effect on tumour cell kill. It is therefore apparent that where cure is a realistic option the dose administered may be critical and may need to be maintained despite toxicity. In situations where cure is not a realistic possibility and palliation is the aim, dose is less critical particularly as quality of life becomes paramount.

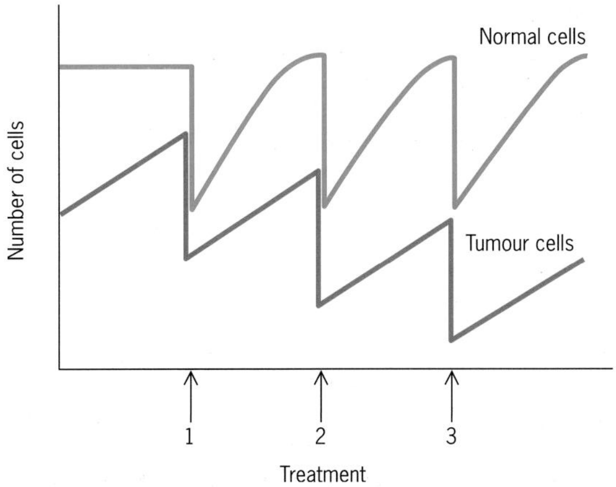

Fig 7.1
Effects of multiple courses of cytotoxic chemotherapy

Classification of cytotoxic drugs (Table 7.7)

Alkylating agents

The alkylating agents act by covalently bonding alkyl groups and their major effect is to cross-link DNA strands, interfering with DNA synthesis. Despite being among the earliest cytotoxic drugs developed they maintain a central position in the treatment of cancer in the 1990s. Common alkylating agents include cyclophosphamide, chlorambucil and busulphan.

Antimetabolites

Antimetabolites are usually structural analogues of naturally occurring metabolites and interfere with normal synthesis of nucleic acids by falsely substituting purines and pyrimidines in metabolic pathways. Antimetabolites can be divided into folic acid antagonists, pyrimidine antagonists and purine antagonists. The classic folic acid antagonist, methotrexate, is structurally very similar to folic acid and binds preferentially to dihydrofolate reductase, the enzyme responsible for the conversion of folic acid to folinic acid. It is used widely in the treatment of solid tumours and haematological malignancies, and also has a role in non-malignant conditions such as rheumatoid arthritis.

The two major pyrimidine antagonists are 5-fluorouracil and cytosine arabinoside (cytarabine). 5-Fluorouracil consists of a uracil molecule with a substituted fluorine atom. It acts by blocking the enzyme thymidylate synthetase which is essential for pyrimidine synthesis. 5-Fluorouracil has a major role in the treatment of solid tumours, particularly gastrointestinal cancers. Cytosine arabinoside is used almost exclusively in the treatment of acute myeloid leukaemia where it remains the backbone of therapy.

6-Mercaptopurine and 6-thioguanine are purine antagonists which are both used almost exclusively in the treatment of acute leukaemia.

Plant alkaloids

Vinca alkaloids

These are isolated from the periwinkle plant and the major drugs in this class are vincristine and vinblastine. They act by binding to tubulin and inhibiting microtubule formation (see p. 127) and have a role in the treatment of haematological and non-haematological cancers. They are perhaps best known for their potential for causing neurotoxicity.

Table 7.7
Antitumour agents

Alkylating agents	
Mustine hydrochloride (HN_2)	
Chlorambucil	
Cyclophosphamide	
Melphalan	
Nitrosoureas (e.g. lomustine)	
Busulphan	
Ifosfamide	
Treosulfan	
Antimetabolites	
Methotrexate	
Mercaptopurine	
Fluorouracil	
Thioguanine	
Cytarabine (cytosine arabinoside)	
Gemcitabine	
Raltitrexed	
Fludarabine	
Antitumour agents derived from plants	
Vinblastine	Vinca alkaloids
Vincristine	Vinca alkaloids
Vindesine	Vinca alkaloids
Etoposide	
Taxanes	
Docetaxel	
Paclitaxel	
Cytotoxic antibiotics	
Dactinomycin	
Daunorubicin	
Doxorubicin	
Idarubicin	
Aclarubicin	
Epirubicin	
Bleomycin	
Mitomycin C	
Mitozantrone	
Miscellaneous drugs of importance	
Cisplatin/carboplatin	
Procarbazine	
Hydroxyurea	
Crisantaspase (L-asparaginase)	
Hormones and antihormones	
Oestrogens	
Progestogens	
Steroids	
Tamoxifen	
Aminoglutethimide	
Buserelin	

Epipodophyllotoxins
These are semi-synthetic derivatives of podophyllotoxin which is an extract from the mandrake plant. Etoposide is a drug used in a wide range of cancers and works by producing DNA strand breaks by acting on the enzyme topoisomerase II. Topoisomerase I inhibitors (e.g. irinotecan) are being tested. Both these enzymes allow unwinding and uncoiling of supercoiled DNA.

Taxanes
Paclitaxel is isolated from the bark of the Western Yew. Docetaxel is a semi-synthetic taxane. They bind to tubulin dimers and prevent their assembly into microtubules and are active drugs against ovarian and breast cancer. Taxanes cause hypersensitivity reactions and patients should be premedicated with steroids, H_1 and H_2 antagonists prior to treatment.

Cytotoxic antibiotics
These drugs act by intercalating adjoining nucleotide pairs on the same strand of DNA. They include doxorubicin and daunorubicin. These drugs have a wide spectrum of activity in haematological and solid tumours. Doxorubicin is one of the most widely used of all cytotoxic drugs.

Platinum analogues
Cisplatin and carboplatin cause interstrand cross-links of DNA and are often regarded as non-classical alkylating agents. They have transformed the treatment of testicular cancer and have a major role against many other tumours, including ovarian cancer and head and neck cancer.

Side-effects of chemotherapeutic drugs

The side-effects of anticancer drugs are legendary and have created fear in both the medical profession and the general public. The situation in the 1990s has improved vastly from the early days of cytotoxic chemotherapy where persistent and prolonged nausea and vomiting were the rule, and life-threatening complications from myelosuppression were not uncommon. Modern cytotoxic chemotherapy has improved out of all recognition from those early days, and newer cytotoxic drugs, often analogues of the original drugs, are frequently associated with significantly fewer side-effects.

Modern antiemetics such as the 5-hydroxytryptamine ($5HT_3$) antagonists can prevent or reduce vomiting to a minimum in a majority of patients. In those intensive chemotherapy regimens where myelosuppression is a major feature, the use of growth factors can now reduce this to a certain extent.

Despite these advances, chemotherapy still carries many potentially serious side-effects and should be used only by practitioners with considerable skill and experience. Listed below are some of the major side-effects.

Nausea and vomiting
This common side-effect can be eliminated or reduced by choice of drugs and by using modern antiemetics. Nausea and vomiting are particular problems with platinum

analogues and with doxorubicin. Antiemetics such as metoclopramide and domperiodone are used initially, but the $5HT_3$ serotonin antagonists (ondansetron and granisetron) have revolutionized the management of vomiting and many patients are now given platinum drugs as an outpatient.

Hair loss

Many but not all cytotoxic drugs are capable of causing hair loss. Scalp cooling can sometimes be used to reduce hair loss with doxorubicin, but in general this side-effect can be prevented only by selection of drugs where this is possible. Hair always regrows on completion of chemotherapy.

Bone marrow suppression

Suppression of the production of haemoglobin, white cell series and platelets may occur with many cytotoxic drugs and is a dose-related phenomenon. Severely myelosuppressive chemotherapy is used only when treatment is given with curative intent. Anaemia and thrombocytopenia are managed by blood or platelet transfusions but white cell transfusions have not been successful. Neutropenic patients are therefore managed by the early introduction of broad-spectrum antibiotics intravenously for the prevention and treatment of infection. Initial 'blind' therapy should be with a third-generation cephalosporin (e.g. ceftazidime), sometimes combined with an aminoglycoside or a broad-spectrum penicillin; therapy should be reviewed following microbiological results. Haemopoietic growth factors can now reduce the duration of neutropenia (see p. 397).

Cardiotoxicity

This is a rare side-effect of chemotherapy, usually associated with doxorubicin. It is dose-related and can largely be prevented by keeping the total dose within the safe range.

Neurotoxicity

This occurs predominantly with the plant alkaloids and platinum analogues. It is dose-related and chemotherapy is usually stopped before the development of a significant polyneuropathy. This is only partially reversible.

Nephrotoxicity

A number of cytotoxic drugs, particularly platinum analogues, can potentially cause renal damage. This can usually be prevented by maintaining an adequate diuresis during treatment.

Sterility

Some anticancer drugs, particularly alkylating agents, may cause sterility, which can be irreversible. In males the storage of sperm is an important consideration when chemotherapy is given with curative intent.

Secondary malignancies

Anticancer drugs have mutagenic potential and the development of secondary malignancies, particularly acute leukaemia, is an uncommon but particularly unwelcome long-term side-effect in patients otherwise cured of their malignancies. The alkylating agents are particularly implicated in this very severe complication.

Drug resistance

Drug resistance is one of the major obstacles to curing cancer with chemotherapy. Some tumours have an inherently low level of resistance to currently available treatment and are often cured. These include testicular teratomas, Hodgkin's disease and childhood acute leukaemia. Solid tumours such as small-cell lung cancer initially appear to be chemosensitive, with the majority of patients responding, but most patients eventually relapse with resistant disease. In other tumours such as melanoma the disease is largely chemoresistant from the start.

It is thought that most resistance occurs as a result of genetic mutation and becomes more likely as the number of tumour cells increases. It has also been shown that anticancer drugs can themselves increase the rate of mutation to resistance. Unfortunately resistance to cytotoxic drugs is often multiple and is then known as multidrug resistance (MDR). An example of this is resistance to anthracyclines (e.g. doxorubicin) which is often associated with resistance to vinca alkaloids and epipodophyllotoxins. This resistance is mediated via increased expression of P-glycoprotein (a 170 kDa membrane phosphoglycoprotein) which mediates an efflux of cytotoxic drugs out of the cells.

A second important mechanism for MDR concerns altered drug binding to topoisomerase II, an enzyme which is important in bringing about DNA strand breaks in association with cytotoxic drugs. Treating patients as early as possible in the disease, using maximal doses of drugs and combination chemotherapy, may help to reduce the likelihood of MDR.

It has become clear that the death of the cancer cell following damage by chemotherapy is not a passive event, but an energy dependent programmed event. This process is called *apoptosis* or programmed cell death (p. 153). The process involves several oncogenes, particularly the tumour suppressor gene *p53*. In tumours that have mutations of *p53* or other oncogenes involved in apoptosis, damage by chemotherapy may not lead to cell death. It is increasingly becoming apparent that failure to undergo apoptosis is a major mechanism of resistance to chemotherapeutic drugs. The search is now on to identify drugs that will induce apoptosis, such as drugs that can mimic the activity of *p53* in tumours where it has mutated. Normal *p53* has also been shown to suppress angiogenesis, which is an important mechanism for tumours to proliferate and metastasize (p. 419).

Adjuvant therapy

When a patient first presents with a tumour, it is possible that small amounts of tumour tissue have already spread to the lungs, liver, bone marrow and other sites. This micrometastatic disease consists of relatively few cells with a good blood supply, and might be particularly amenable to the action of anticancer drugs. Therefore, if the primary tumour is removed and the tumour has a great likelihood of replase, chemotherapy can be given to destroy the residual micrometastatic disease, and the chance of long-term survival and cure might be improved. This was dramatically demonstrated in the childhood renal sarcoma, Wilms' tumour, when the use of actinomycin D given after nephrectomy resulted in a doubling of the number of children who survived. Chemotherapy used in this way is know as 'adjuvant therapy', and has been employed in a number of other childhood tumours. In adults, adjuvant chemotherapy has been shown to be of value in breast and colon cancer.

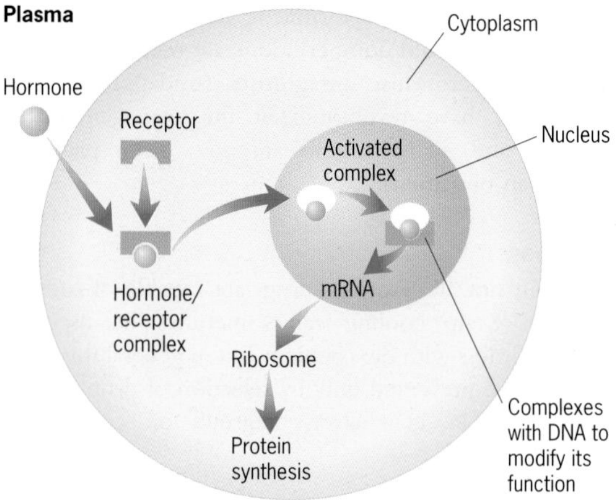

Fig 7.2
Mechanism of the interaction between a steroid hormone and its receptor. This interaction modifies DNA activity and hence cell growth and replication

Treatment of malignancy in sanctuary sites

A 'sanctuary site' is the term used to indicate that metastatic disease has involved a site that is not accessible to conventional drug therapy. An example of this is leukaemic infiltration of the meninges in children with acute lymphoblastic leukaemia. Because of the blood–brain barrier, agents such as vincristine and prednisolone do not enter the subarachnoid space in sufficient quantity to eliminate all the leukaemic cells, and are therefore ineffective in preventing the development of meningeal infiltration. In order to treat these cells, intrathecal chemotherapy and/or cranial irradiation are required.

FURTHER READING

Creaven PJ, Rustum YM, Henderson ES (1996) Chemotherapy: Pharmacologic principles and pharmacology of anti cancer drugs in leukemia. In: Henderson ES, Lister TA, Greaves ME, eds. Leukemia. WB Saunders, Philadelphia, p. 313

Principles of endocrine therapy

It has long been known that oestrogen is capable of stimulating the growth of breast cancer and androgens the growth of prostate cancer. Manipulation of the hormonal environment may result in regression of a number of tumours, particularly breast cancer, endometrial cancer and prostate cancer. Hormonal therapy is in general not curative. It may, however, provide control of a tumour for a period of time often with few side-effects. The presence of cell surface receptors for the hormone in question is a prerequisite for the therapy to be effective. The binding of hormone to receptor and translocation of the hormone–receptor complex into the nucleus, where it reacts with the DNA, is shown diagrammatically in Fig 7.2.

Patients with breast cancer frequently have receptors for oestrogens and progesterones. Hormonal manipulation includes the use of tamoxifen which blocks oestrogen receptors, and the reduction of endogenous oestrogen by oophorectomy or 'medical oophorectomy' via pituitary down-regulation using a luteinizing hormone releasing hormone (LHRH) analogue. Goserelin or buserelin cause tumour regression in 30% of premenopausal women and in more than 50% of patients with oestrogen-receptor-positive tumours.

Progestogens have a direct effect in breast tumour cells as well as effects on the pituitary/ovarian or adrenal axis. In post-menopausal women, androgens are synthesized by the adrenal glands and converted in subcutaneous fat to oestrone by the enzyme aromatase. Aromatase inhibitors, for example formestane, reduce oestrogen levels in tumour cells.

Endometrial tumours also have receptors for both oestrogens and progesterones. These tumours frequently respond to the administration of progesterone and to the anti-oestrogen tamoxifen.

In prostate cancer, orchidectomy is performed which reduces circulating testosterone. LHRH agonists (e.g. buserelin) cause transient stimulation of pituitary LH production followed by down-regulation and a fall in testosterone level. This is often combined with an anti-androgens (e.g. flutamide or bicalutamide) which block the binding of dehydrotestosterone to its receptor, so preventing androgen action.

Principles of biological therapy

This term encompasses a wide range of treatments, most of which are thought to act by an immunologically mediated mechanism rather than by a direct cytotoxic effect. Some examples are discussed below:

Interferons (see also p. 161)

Interferons are naturally occurring cytokines that are normally produced in response to viral infection. The precise mechanism of action in malignant disease remains uncertain; they certainly have antiproliferative activity but can also increase natural killer cell activity and cause other immunological changes that may result in an antitumour effect.

α-Interferon (IFN-α) is commercially available and has been used against several malignancies, such as melanoma, renal cell cancer, myeloma, and chronic myeloid leukaemia. In the latter, it results in a reduction in the number of Philadelphia (Ph) chromosome-positive cells in at least 50% of patients, with total elimination in 10%. Cytogenetic response has been shown to result in prolongation of survival, but interferon is not curative.

Treatment with an IFN has side-effects – 'flu-like symptoms which tend to diminish with time, and fatigue which generally does not. The main disadvantage is that the drug has to be given as a subcutaneous injection.

Colony stimulating factors

Granulocyte (G-CSF) and granulocyte/macrophage colony stimulating factor (GM-CSF) are used:

- to reduce the duration of neutropenia following chemotherapy (particularly in the United States)
- with or without chemotherapy, to stimulate the proliferation of haemopoietic progenitor cells in the marrow so that they enter the circulation and can be collected from the peripheral blood to support high-dose treatment (see p. 437).

Monoclonal antibodies

Monoclonal antibodies directed against tumour cell surface antigens are used as treatment in several experimental settings.

- They are used *in vitro*, in conjunction with complement, to deplete autologous bone marrow of tumour cells in patients with leukaemia and lymphoma receiving high-dose treatment with autologous haemopoietic progenitor cell support.
- They are also used *in vitro* in immunoadsorption columns to select the CD34-positive (stem cell) fraction from peripheral blood progenitor cell or autologous bone marrow collections, to support high-dose treatment in haematological and other malignancies (see below).
- They are used *in vivo*, as treatment for lymphoma (e.g. anti-CD20). This is a chimeric antibody; that is, the molecule comprises a human constant region, with murine heavy and light chain regions. Tumour cell lysis occurs by both complement and antibody-dependent cellular cytotoxicity. The antibody is currently being evaluated as treatment for B-cell non-Hodgkin's lymphomas (NHLs) which express the antigen CD20 on their surface.
- They are also used *in vivo* as a carrier molecule. Anti-CD20 conjugated to radioactive iodine is being used as treatment for NHL. The antibody is here being used to 'carry' radiation to the CD20-bearing tumour cells.

Haematological malignancies (leukaemias)

Leukaemia, lymphoma and myeloma constitute only a small proportion of all malignancies. They are generally responsive to treatment so that many patients with acute leukaemia, Hodgkin's disease, or high-grade non-Hodgkin's lymphoma can be cured. However, most people with haematological malignancy still die as a consequence of the disease, or because of complications of treatment. It is therefore essential to explain the illness, its treatment and the chance of success or failure to the patient and to his or her family.

The leukaemias

These are rare diseases with an annual overall incidence of five per 100 000. Acute lymphoblastic leukaemia (ALL) is predominantly a disease of childhood, whereas acute myelogenous leukaemia (AML) is more frequently seen in older adults, as are the chronic leukaemias.

AETIOLOGY

In the majority of cases the aetiology is unknown. Feline leukaemia virus has been shown to cause leukaemia in cats; there is however no evidence for a viral aetiology in humans, apart from the association of a specific subtype of T-cell leukaemia, found predominantly in the Southern Island of Japan and the Caribbean, with the retrovirus HTLV-1. Although many people in the endemic areas have antibodies to the virus, implying past infection, most of them will never develop leukaemia.

Genetic factors

Leukaemia results from the transformation and clonal expansion of progenitor cells in the bone marrow, but there is much cellular heterogeneity between different types of leukaemia. This heterogeneity may also affect the response to therapy. For example, the response to treatment of acute myelogenous leukaemia is poorer in older than in younger patients. A possible explanation for this is that, in older patients, leukaemia is more likely to have arisen from a pluripotent stem cell than from a lineage-restricted progenitor cell. The former has a high capacity for self-renewal, an active drug-efflux pump mechanism, and a high content of anti-apoptotic proteins, all of which contribute to chemoresistance (see p. 153).

Many patients with leukaemia have a cytogenetic abnormality. When complete remission (CR) is achieved, the chromosomal translocation/deletion usually becomes undetectable, but returns at recurrence. Such a cytogenetic change may imply a worse prognosis but not always: 99% of patients with acute promyelocytic leukaemia (APML) have the t(15;17) translocation; the latter, as well as the t(8;21) translocation in AML, in fact confer a better long-term prognosis once CR has been achieved.

The first non-random chromosomal abnormality to be described was the Philadelphia (Ph) chromosome which is associated with chronic myeloid leukaemia (CML) in 95% of cases. The Ph chromosome is also found in ALL, the incidence in the latter illness increasing with age. The translocation is shown schematically in Fig 7.3. The Ph chromosome is an abnormal chromosome 22, resulting from a reciprocal translocation between part of the long arm of chromosome 22 and chromosome 9. The resulting karyotype is described as t(9;22)(q34;q11). The molecular consequences of the translocation are that the oncogene (*C-ABL*) normally present on chromosome 9 is translocated to chromosome 22, where it comes into juxtaposition with a region of chromosome 22 named the 'breakpoint cluster region' (BCR). The translocation creates a hybrid transcription unit consisting of the 5′ end of the *BCR* gene and the *C-ABL* proto-oncogene. The new gene is capable of being expressed as a chimeric messenger RNA which has been identified in cells from patients with CML. When translated, this produces a fusion protein that has tyrosine kinase activity and enhanced phosphorylating activity compared with the normal protein. The precise contribution of these molecular events to the disease process is at present unclear. The breakpoint differs in CML and Ph-positive ALL, leading to the production of two different tyrosine kinase proteins.

Environmental factors

Environmental factors include *chemicals* (e.g. benzene compounds), *drugs* (e.g. alkylating agents) and *radiation*. The evidence for radiation causing leukaemia comes from three sources:

- The atomic explosions at Hiroshima and Nagasaki resulted in an increased incidence of both AML and, in particular, CML in people living in surrounding areas. There is therefore concern about the population living round Chernobyl.
- In the past, patients with ankylosing spondylitis were treated with radiotherapy, leading to an increased incidence of secondary AML.

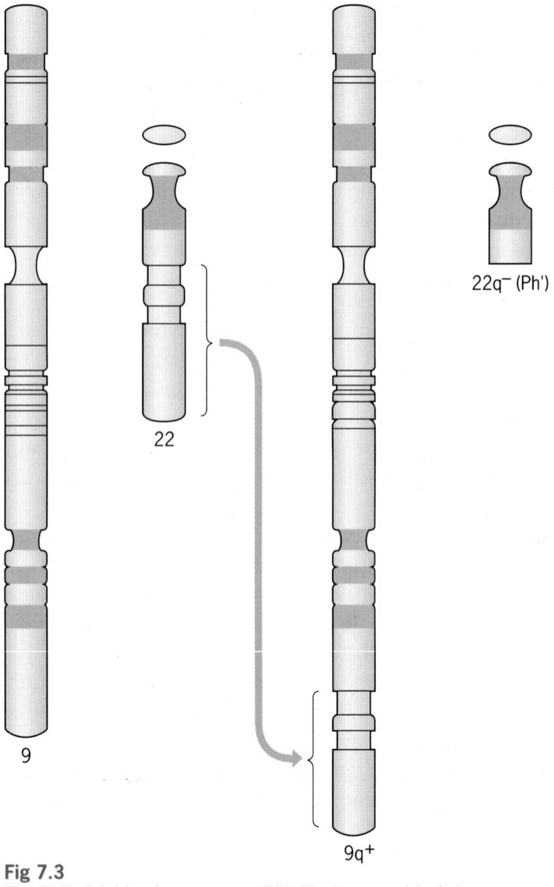

Fig 7.3
The Philadelphia chromosome (Ph). The long arm (q) of chromosome 22 has been shortened by the reciprocal translocation with chromosome 9

- A small proportion of patients with Hodgkin's disease treated with (usually) both chemotherapy and radiotherapy develop secondary AML. Unlike *de novo* AML which is potentially curable, AML developing in relation to previous cytotoxic chemotherapy and/or irradiation is nearly always resistant to treatment.

Classification

Leukaemia can be divided on the basis of the speed of evolution of the disease into *acute* or *chronic*. Each of these is then further subdivided into *myeloid* or *lymphoid*, according to the cell type involved. Hence the terms:

- acute myelogenous leukaemia (AML)
- acute lymphoblastic leukaemia (ALL)
- chronic myeloid leukaemia (CML)
- chronic lymphocytic leukaemia (CLL).

Acute leukaemias

CLINICAL FEATURES

The *symptoms* of acute leukaemia are a consequence of bone marrow failure:

- symptoms of anaemia,such as tiredness, weakness, shortness of breath on exertion

- repeated infections
- bruising and/or bleeding
- occasionally, lymph node enlargement and/or symptoms relating to enlargement of the liver and spleen.

There may be few or no abnormal physical *signs*; but patients often have:

- signs of anaemia
- bruises, petechial haemorrhages, purpura, fundal haemorrhages
- signs of infection
- sometimes, peripheral lymphadenopathy and/or hepatosplenomegaly.

INVESTIGATIONS

The definitive diagnosis is made on the basis of a peripheral blood film and a bone marrow aspirate. Additional investigations such as cytogenetic analysis and immunophenotyping of the leukaemic blast cells are not mandatory but can be helpful. If the patient has a fever, blood cultures and a chest X-ray are essential.

- Blood count typically shows a low haemoglobin (Hb) and a raised white cell count, but this can be decreased or normal. The platelet count is usually low.
- Peripheral blood film shows characteristic leukaemic blast cells (Fig 7.4).
- Bone marrow aspirate shows increased cellularity with abnormal lymphoid or myeloid blast cells (Fig 7.4).

(a)

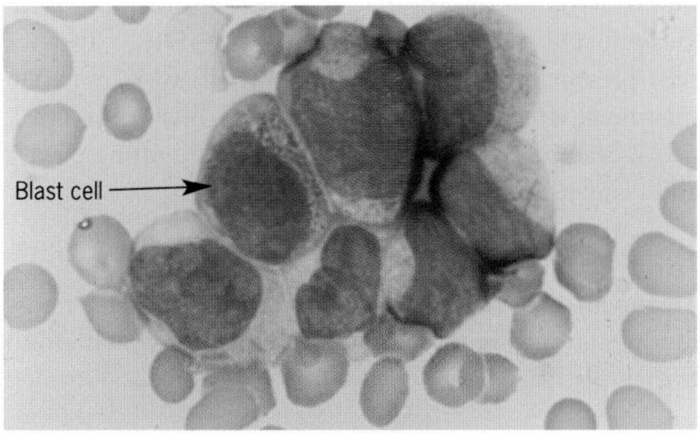

(b)

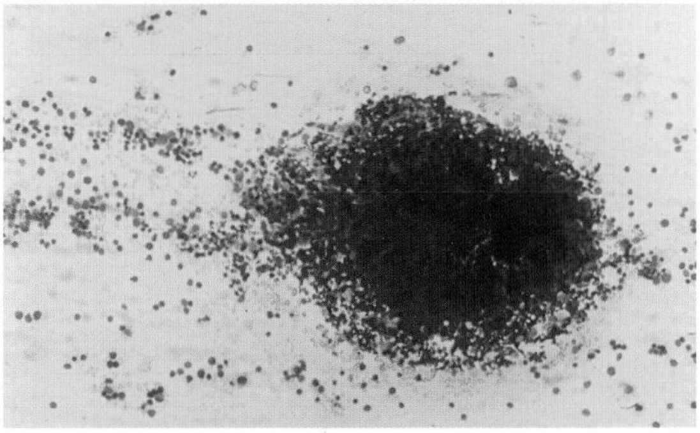

Fig 7.4
(a) Peripheral blood film showing characteristic blast cells. The arrow points to the abnormal blast cell. **(b) Bone marrow aspirate** showing particle with increased cellularity. Courtesy of Dr Manzoor Mangi

GENERAL PRINCIPLES OF MANAGEMENT

The decision to treat a patient with curative intent will depend on the person's age, their general state of health, the time-point in the course of the illness (presentation or recurrence), and the person's wishes. The use of intensive combination chemotherapy may, for example, be inappropriate in an older person. The diagnosis, its implications, treatment options and the likely outcome of such treatment, together with its side-effects, need to be explained to the patient and to the family. People often find it difficult to assimilate all of this information on one occasion; it is therefore essential to give them the opportunity to ask questions, particularly as circumstances change. Before starting treatment, the following points must be considered.

Anaemia and thrombocytopenia need to be corrected by the administration of blood and platelets. Infection should be treated with intravenous antibiotics.

Leukaemic blast cells can infiltrate the brain and lungs, resulting in coma and respiratory failure respectively. If the blast cell count in the peripheral blood is very high ($>100 \times 10^9$/L) the patient may need *leucophoresis*. Blood is collected from a vein and centrifuged so as to remove leukaemic cells, and the red cells and plasma are then returned to the patient via another vein. Leucophoresis can be life-saving.

Hyperuricaemia can be treated or prevented by the administration of allopurinol, a xanthine oxidase inhibitor.

In certain types of leukaemia where the rate of cell division is very fast (e.g. B-cell and T-cell ALL), patients may develop a 'tumour lysis' syndrome when chemotherapy is given. This is characterized by hypercalcaemia and high serum levels of phosphate and potassium, resulting from a high rate of cellular breakdown. This is a potentially life-threatening situation and difficult to treat once it has happened. It can usually be *prevented* by making sure that chemotherapy is not started until the uric acid level is normal. Intravenous fluids need to be given before starting chemotherapy and the relevant biochemical parameters monitored at regular intervals. Patients may require haemodialysis to correct severe metabolic imbalance.

In what follows, specific treatments for the different types of leukaemia will be mentioned only briefly because regimens are evolving continually. Good 'supportive care' (with antibiotics and blood products) is virtually as important as the specific combination of drugs used. Patients with acute leukaemia should therefore be treated in specialist centres where the medical and nursing staff are familiar with the management of neutropenia and thrombocytopenia.

Acute myelogenous leukaemia (AML)

AML is a potentially curable disease. The aim of treatment is to restore the bone marrow to normal and the patient to a normal state of health – complete remission (CR).

AML is classified on the basis of the morphological appearance of the bone marrow into seven subtypes, FAB types M1–M7, which differ by virtue of the predominant cell type involved (Table 7.8).

TREATMENT

Treatment has traditionally been regarded as being in two parts: remission induction and post-remission/consolidation therapy. The rationale for going on with treatment beyond the point of CR is based on data from an experimental mouse model (L1210 leukaemia) and by extrapolation from the situation in children with ALL in whom it has been calculated that, at the time of presentation, the number of leukaemic blast cells is of the order of 10^{12} or 10^{13}. At the point of CR – when there is no morphologically detectable leukaemia – there are still 10^8 or 10^9 leukaemic blast cells present. It is therefore not surprising that if no post-remission therapy is given, the majority of patients develop recurrent leukaemia.

Remission induction therapy usually includes an anthracycline drug such as daunorubicin or doxorubicin (or a newer analogue such as idarubicin), given in conjunction with cytosine arabinoside (cytarabine) with or without another drug such as etoposide. The patient needs to stay in hospital for about four weeks in the first instance owing to the risk of infection and bleeding consequent upon neutropenia and thrombocytopenia. Subsequent cycles of treatment are given on an outpatient basis as much as possible.

There is much debate as to the best *post-remission therapy*. Options include:

- further cycles of chemotherapy, the same as that given to induce remission
- chemotherapy different from that given to induce remission
- myeloablative therapy with allogeneic/autologous bone marrow transplantation (BMT) (see below).

With modern combination chemotherapy, approximately 70% of people aged under 60 years will return to normal health. However, within 1–3 years the disease will recur in at least 60%, the remainder almost certainly having been cured. Treatment has generally become more intensive over the last 25 years with a concomitant improvement in overall survival. Survival curves for patients treated at St Bartholomew's Hospital, London, during three consecutive time periods are shown in Fig 7.5.

Table 7.8
FAB classification of acute myelogenous leukaemia

FAB	Subtype
M1	Myeloblastic (no maturation)
M2	Myeloblastic (with maturation)
M3	Promyelocytic[a]
M4	Myelomonocytic[b]
M5	Monoblastic[c]
M6	Erythroblastic[c]
M7	Megakaryoblastic[c]

[a] Associated with disseminated intravascular coagulation.
[b] Characterized by skin and gum infiltration and a propensity, particularly in children, for CNS involvement with leukaemic blasts in the cerebrospinal fluid.
[c] Very rare.

TREATMENT AT RECURRENCE

Second remissions are more difficult to achieve and are rarely durable. The decision to treat a person at recurrence will therefore again depend on the patient's overall situation and his or her wishes. In younger patients, provided that second remission can be achieved, cure is still a possibility for a proportion, using myeloablative therapy with allogeneic/autologous haemopoietic progenitor cell support.

In older patients the options are further intensive combination chemotherapy or a palliative approach. The aim of palliation is to keep the person as well as possible for as long as possible with supportive measures such as blood transfusions, antibiotics, and the judicious use of orally administered drugs such as hydroxyurea to help lower the number of circulating leukaemic cells.

Acute promyelocytic leukaemia (AML-M3, APML)

Acute promyelocytic leukaemia is associated with the chromosome translocation t(15;17). It warrants separate mention because of its specific association with disseminated intravascular coagulation (DIC). Patients may present with severe bleeding which worsens when treatment is started as the leukaemic blast cells break down, leading to further consumption of clotting factors and platelets.

TREATMENT

Treatment consists of regular, twice-daily platelet transfusions and maintenance of the fibrinogen level with fresh frozen plasma as the chemotherapy is given. Provided

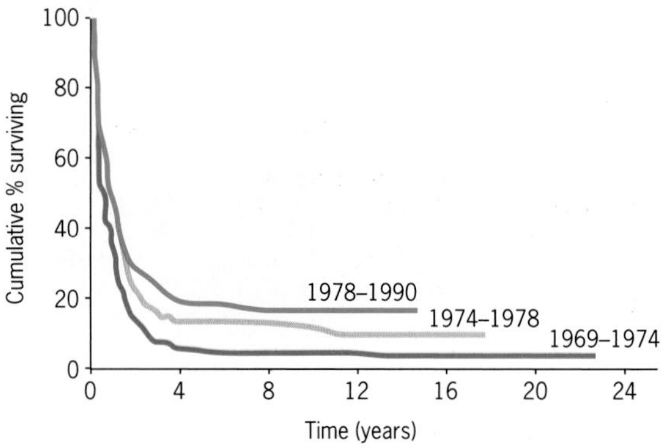

Fig 7.5
Acute myelogenous leukaemia: overall survival over three time periods

remission can be achieved, patients with APML have a somewhat better prognosis overall than patients with other subtypes of AML.

It has been demonstrated that *all-trans*-retinoic acid (ATRA) given orally can lead to achievement of CR in most patients with APML. ATRA has a differentiating effect on leukaemic promyelocytes, both *in vitro* and *in vivo*. It does not appear to be effective in other subtypes of AML. Unfortunately, such remissions are not durable and need to be consolidated with conventional chemotherapy. However, the advantage is that patients receiving ATRA do not usually develop DIC, so there is a concomitant decrease in the risk of fatal haemorrhage. Modern treatment for APML therefore now comprises ATRA with or without chemotherapy, to remission, followed by more chemotherapy.

Acute lymphoblastic leukaemia

Predominantly a disease of children, ALL is potentially curable. Overall, 90% of children respond to treatment and 50–60% are cured. The results in adults are not as good, with only approximately 30% being cured. ALL is classified on the basis of the morphology of the leukaemic blast cells into subtypes L1–L3 (Table 7.9). There is also an immunological classification which is continually evolving as more sophisticated techniques are developed for detecting the B- or T-cell origin of lymphoid cells (Table 7.10).

TREATMENT

The principles of initial treatment are the same as those for AML, the aim being to return the bone marrow to normal and the person to a good state of health. Cyclical combination chemotherapy comprising vincristine, prednisolone, L-asparaginase and an anthracycline such as doxorubicin forms the basis of most treatment regimens. Other drugs such as cyclophosphamide and/or cytosine arabinoside are also being used increasingly in both adults and children considered to be at high risk for recurrence.

The sequence of treatment, however, differs somewhat from that in AML because ALL has a propensity for involvement of the central nervous sytem (CNS). Thus, treatment includes prophylactic intrathecal drugs (a lumbar puncture is performed under local anaesthetic and methotrexate or cystosine arabinoside injected into the cerebrospinal fluid), with or without prophylactic radiotherapy to the cerebral meninges. Most patients also receive oral maintenance therapy for 2–3 years. The sequence of treatment is shown in Fig 7.6.

TREATMENT AT RECURRENCE

A proportion of patients are cured with the initial therapy. In the rest the disease recurs and ultimately proves fatal unless second remission can be achieved, and followed by high dose treatment and some form of transplant procedure. With such treatment, a further 20–30% of patients will survive long-term.

Recurrence occurs most frequently in bone marrow and is associated with a worse prognosis if it occurs while the person is on maintenance therapy. CNS recurrence, detected by the presence of leukaemic blast cells in the cerebrospinal fluid, is now seen less frequently with the regular use of CNS prophylaxis. Treatment for CNS recurrence comprises intrathecal drugs, together with radiotherapy to the meninges surrounding the brain and spinal cord, followed by reinduction chemotherapy if the recurrence is limited to the CNS. Unfortunately, it often occurs in association with bone marrow recurrence, when induction of second CR followed by myeloablative therapy with allogeneic or autologous BMT is the only potentially curative option.

Recurrence may also occur in the testes when it is usually manifest by painless enlargement of one or both testicles. It can occur in isolation, or shortly before or concurrent with

Table 7.9
FAB classification of acute lymphoblastic leukaemia

FAB	Cell type
L1	Homogeneous population of small cells (childhood ALL)
L2	More heterogeneous population of cells (more often seen in adults)
L3	Rare – cells like those in Burkitt's lymphoma

Table 7.10
Immunological categories of acute lymphoblastic leukaemia

	Phenotypic markers				
B lineage	CD10	CD19	TdT	CyIg	SmIg
cALLa positive[a]	+	+	+	–	–
pre-B	+ (usually)	+	+	+	–
B-cell[b]	+	+	–	±	+
T lineage	CD7	CD2	TdT		
pre-T	+	–	+		
T-cell	+	+	+		

[a] Most children and > 50% of adults. [b] Rare.

cALLa, common ALL antigens; CD, cluster designation; CyIg, cytoplasmic immunoglobulin; SmIg, surface membrane immunoglobulin; TdT, terminal deoxynucleotidyl transferase.

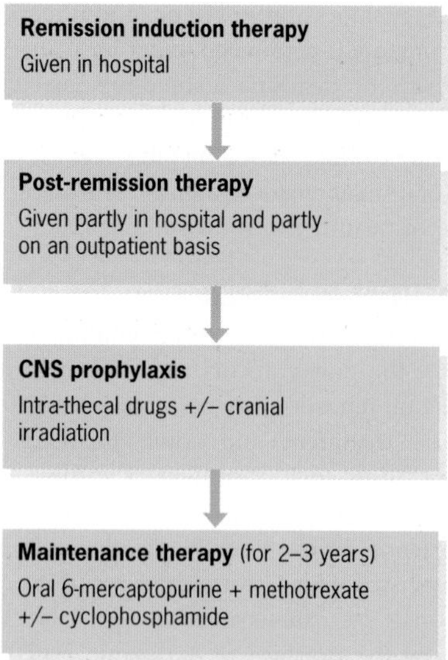

Fig 7.6
Treatment regimen for acute lymphoblastic leukaemia

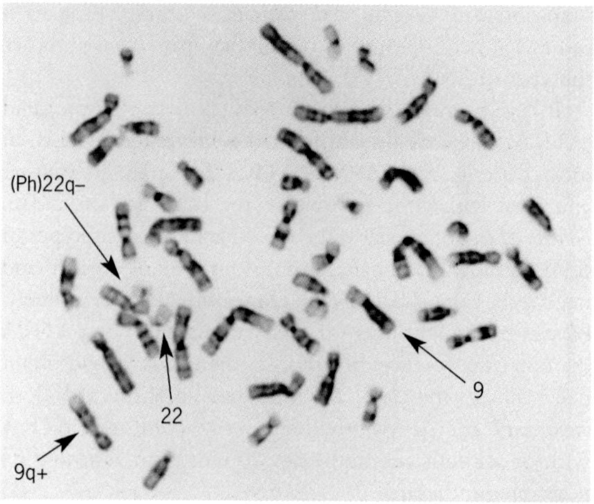

Fig 7.7
Philadelphia chromosome. This is formed by a reciprocal translocation of part of the long arm (q) of chromosome 22 to chromosome 9. It is seen in 90–95% of patients with chronic granulocytic leukaemia. The karyotype is expressed as 46XX, (9;22)(q34;q11)

bone marrow recurrence. Treatment for isolated testicular recurrence involves radiotherapy to the testes, followed by reinduction chemotherapy. If the marrow is also involved, the treatment is reinduction chemotherapy followed by myeloablative therapy with allogeneic or autologous BMT, provided a second remission can be achieved.

Chronic leukaemias

Chronic myeloid leukaemia (CML)

The majority of patients with this disease are older and die within five years of diagnosis. The illness has a progressive clinical course which starts with a chronic phase of 3–4 years' duration. This evolves into an accelerated phase which may be manifest by fever, weight loss, increasing splenomegaly, anaemia, thrombocythaemia and refractory leukocytosis with increasing numbers of blast cells. The duration of the accelerated phase is variable though blastic transformation usually supervenes within a few months.

Unlike *de novo* acute leukaemia, the blastic phase of CML is characterized by the development of acute leukaemia which may be myeloid (60%), lymphoid (30%) or erythroid (10%) in origin. The blastic phase is generally refractory to treatment, the median survival being less than six months. Less frequently, CML transforms into myelofibrosis, death ensuing from bone marrow failure.

CLINICAL FEATURES

The *symptoms* are usually of insidious onset:

- anaemia
- sweating at night, fever, weight loss
- abdominal discomfort owing to splenic enlargement.

The *signs* are those of anaemia, with splenomegaly.

INVESTIGATIONS

- **Blood count**. Hb is low or normal. WCC is raised with, characteristically, the whole spectrum of myeloid precursors, including a few blast cells visible on the blood film.
- **Platelet count**. This may be low, normal or raised.
- **Bone marrow aspirate**. This shows a hypercellular marrow with an increase in myeloid precursors. On cytogenetic analysis, the Ph chromosome t(9;22) is present in most patients (Fig 7.7).

TREATMENT

Until recently, most patients were treated with hydroxyurea. The advent of the interferons (IFNs) has altered this. IFNs have been shown to induce haematological remission in the majority of patients and cytogenetic remission in about 10%. A further proportion of patients will have a reduction in the number of Ph chromosome-containing cells which has been shown to be associated with prolongation of survival. The problems with IFN treatment are (a) that it has to be given by subcutaneous injection and (b) that at the relatively high doses needed to induce a meaningful cytogenetic response, most people experience side-effects (lack of energy and fatigue) which may make it hard to continue with the treatment.

Myeloablative therapy supported by allogeneic BMT can be curative but the approach is limited by donor availability, the age of the patient, and the morbidity and mortality of the transplant procedure (see below). With the development of national and international donor panels, younger patients should now be considered for high-dose treatment with matched unrelated donor marrow. The use of high-dose treatment supported by autologous peripheral blood progenitor cells is also being evaluated.

Chronic lymphocytic leukaemia (CLL)

CLL is an incurable disease of older people, characterized by an uncontrolled proliferation and accumulation of mature B lymphocytes (although T-cell CLL does occur). The symptoms are a consequence of bone marrow failure: anaemia, infection and bleeding. However, a proportion of patients remain asymptomatic and never need any treatment, dying of an unrelated cause. In the remainder, the disease can usually be kept under control for 9–10 years, infection being the predominant cause of death.

Two different staging classifications are in use (Tables 7.11 and 7.12). They are useful because they correlate closely with prognosis. The median survival of patients with stage 0 (or stage A) CLL is eight years, compared with two years for patients presenting with stages III or IV (or stage C) disease.

Table 7.11
RAI staging classification of chronic lymphocytic leukaemia

Stage 0	Lymphocytosis only (in blood and bone marrow)
Stage I	Lymphocytosis with lymphadenopathy
Stage II	Lymphocytosis with hepatic and/or splenic enlargement
Stage III	Lymphocytosis with anaemia (Hb < 11 g dL^{-1})
Stage IV	Lymphocytosis with thrombocytopenia (platelets < 100 × 10^9/L)

Lymphocytosis: white cell count >15 × 10^9/L of which >40% are lymphocytes.

Table 7.12
Binet staging classification of chronic lymphocytic leukaemia

Stage A	< 3 involved lymphoid areas[a]	Hb > 10 g dL^{-1}
Stage B	> 3 involved lymphoid areas	Platelets < 100 × 10^9/L
Stage C	Any number of involved lymphoid areas	Hb < 10 g dL^{-1} Platelets < 100 × 10^9/L

[a] The cervical, axillary and inguinal lymph node groups (whether unilateral or bilateral), the spleen, and the liver each count as one area; therefore, the number of involved areas can be any value between 0 and 5.

CLINICAL FEATURES

In asymptomatic patients, the diagnosis is often a chance finding on the basis of a blood count done for a quite different reason.

The *symptoms* are:

- recurrent infections resulting from neutropenia and reduced immunoglobulin levels
- symptoms of anaemia, which may develop rapidly in the context of haemolysis (usually precipitated by infection)
- painless lymph node enlargement.

The *signs* may be any combination of:

- the signs of anaemia
- lymph node enlargement
- enlarged liver and/or spleen.

INVESTIGATIONS

Blood count:

- **Hb**: low or normal
- **WCC**: >15 × 10^9/L of which at least 40% are lymphocytes
- **Platelets**: low or normal
- **Serum immunoglobulins**: low or normal
- **Coombs' test**: positive if haemolysis is occurring.

TREATMENT

The disease may remain stable for several years. There is no advantage in starting treatment before there is a clinical indication, such as anaemia, recurrent infections, bleeding, 'bulky' lymphadenopathy or in-creasing splenomegaly. Chlorambucil is most often used, with or without prednisolone. Treatment is given intermittently, as and when necessary. Chlorambucil may be effective repeatedly. Haemolysis is a life-threatening situation and is treated in the first instance by high-dose steroids. The purine analogue fludarabine is also useful and much used; it can achieve CR in some patients as opposed to just response. However, such remissions are not durable.

Hairy cell leukaemia (HCL)

HCL is a clonal proliferation of abnormal B (or very rarely T) cells which, as in CLL, accumulate in the bone marrow and spleen. It is a rare disease of late middle age. The bizarre name relates to the appearance of the cells on a blood film – they have an irregular outline owing to the presence of filament-like cytoplasmic projections.

CLINICAL FEATURES

The *symptoms* are:

- those of anaemia
- recurrent infections
- abdominal discomfort owing to splenic enlargement.

The *signs* are:

- those of anaemia
- a palpable spleen.

INVESTIGATIONS

- **Blood count**. Hb is usually low. WCC is usually low, or raised with circulating 'hairy' cells. The platelet count is usually low.
- **Bone marrow**. This shows increased cellularity with characteristic infiltration by 'hairy' cells.

TREATMENT

The drug 2-chloroadenosine acetate (2-CDA) has been shown to have specific activity in this illness, complete remission often being achieved with just one cycle of treatment. The remissions sometimes last for several years and patients can be re-treated.

Prolymphocytic leukaemia

Prolymphocytic leukaemia is another rare B-cell disorder, often mistaken for CLL. It is characterized by bone marrow failure (anaemia, neutropenia and thrombocytopenia) and – as in HCL – splenomegaly. Treatment generally comprises chlorambucil as for CLL, although splenectomy may be indicated and fludarabine can be useful.

FURTHER READING

Goldman JM (1997) Editorial: Optimising treatment for chronic lymphoid leukaemia. *New England Journal of Medicine* **337**: 270–271.

Leukaemia Series. *The Lancet*, starting January 1997.

Kersey JH (1997) Fifty years of the biology and therapy of childhood leukemia. *Blood* **90**: 4243–4251.

Rohatiner A, Lister TA (1996) Acute myelogenous leukemia in adults. In: Henderson ES, Lister TA, Greaves MF, eds. Leukemia. WB Saunders, Philadelphia, p 479

Rozman C, Monserrat E (1995) Chronic lymphocytic leukemia. *New England Journal of Medicine* **333**: 1502–1057

The lymphomas

Lymphomas represent abnormal proliferations of B or T cells and are currently classified on the basis of histological appearance into:

- Hodgkin's disease
- non-Hodgkin's lymphomas.

Hodgkin's disease (HD)

With modern treatment (radiotherapy, chemotherapy or both), HD is now curable in the majority of patients. The choice of treatment is determined largely by the distribution and extent of disease. The staging is shown in Table 7.13.

The Ann Arbor staging classification has been modified to take into account the volume of lymph node masses and the use of modern imaging techniques such as CT scanning.

CLINICAL FEATURES

The *symptoms* are:

- lymph node enlargement, most often of the cervical nodes (other causes are shown in Table 7.14)
- 'B' symptoms: fever, drenching night sweats, weight loss of >10% bodyweight (see Table 7.13).
- other constitutional symptoms, such as pruritus, fatigue, anorexia and, occasionally, alcohol-induced pain at the site of enlarged lymph nodes
- symptoms due to involvement of other organs (e.g. lung, bone, liver).

The signs are:

- peripheral lymph node enlargement
- enlargement of the spleen/liver.

INVESTIGATIONS

- **Blood count** may be normal, or there can be a normochromic, normocytic anaemia.
- **Erythrocyte sedimentation rate** (ESR) is usually raised.
- **Liver biochemistry** is abnormal if the liver is involved.
- **Uric acid** is normal or raised.
- **Chest X-ray** may show mediastinal widening, with or without lung involvement.
- **CT scans** may show involvement of intrathoracic, abdominal or pelvic lymph nodes.
- **Bone marrow aspirate and trephine biopsy** may show involvement in patients with advanced disease.
- **Lymph node biopsy** is required for a definitive diagnosis. Classically, Sternberg–Reed cells are present, together with a characteristic admixture of lymphocytes and histiocytes (Fig 7.8).

A typical chest X-ray and CT scan in one patient are shown in Fig 7.9.

TREATMENT

Initially, treatment is nearly always given with curative intent and consists of radiotherapy, cyclical combination chemotherapy or both. The choice of treatment will depend predominantly on:

- stage
- sites of involvement
- the 'bulk' of lymph node masses
- the presence or absence of 'B' symptoms (Table 7.13).

Table 7.13 Staging classification of Hodgkin's disease (modified Ann Arbor classification)[a, b]

I	Involvement of a single lymph node region (I) or a single extralymphatic organ or site (IE)
II	Involvement of two or more lymph node regions on the same side of the diaphragm (II) or one or more lymph node regions plus an extralymphatic site (IIE)
III	Involvement of lymph node regions on both sides of the diaphragm (III) (the spleen is included in stage III, e.g. splenic involvement plus cervical lymph node enlargement = stage III)
IV	Involvement of one or more extralymphatic organs, e.g. lung, liver, bone, bone marrow, with or without lymph node involvement

[a] All stages are subclassified as A (asymptomatic) or B (fever, night sweats and loss of >10% of bodyweight).

[b] Bulky disease (a lymph node mass >10 cm in diameter, or if involving the mediastinum a mass greater than one-third of the intrathoracic diameter at the level of T10) is denoted by the suffix X.

Stages IA and IIA

The majority of patients are treated with radiotherapy, provided that all the involved sites can be encompassed within a radiation field. Patients with a large mediastinal mass are usually given chemotherapy first, otherwise too much lung tissue would be irradiated with potential long-term damage. Radiotherapy is given subsequently (see below).

Although radiotherapy is highly effective treatment for HD and does not cause some of the side-effects associated with chemotherapy (see below), it is now being recognized that there is an increased risk of breast cancer in patients treated with high doses of radiotherapy for HD many years before. There is also concern about potential impairment of cardiac function.

Stages IIB, IIIA/B and IVA/B

Treatment comprises combination chemotherapy in the first instance, with subsequent radiotherapy to sites of 'bulky' disease to reduce the risk of local recurrence.

The first effective chemotherapy for HD, a regimen comprising mustine, vincristine, procarbazine and prednisolone (MOPP), was used for over 20 years. While this was life-saving, it was also associated with unpleasant immediate side-effects (nausea, vomiting and hair loss) and potential long-term effects, namely infertility and second malignancy. New regimens designed to minimize these long-term effects by reducing the amount of alkylating agent and adding different drugs such as doxorubicin have therefore been developed. The emphasis has been on using alternating, non-cross-resistant drug combinations, given as cycles of treatment (e.g. four-weekly for six months).

Treatment for HD can usually be given on an outpatient basis and most people are able to lead a reasonably normal life while having treatment. The prognosis correlates closely with stage (Fig 7.10). However, survival of patients in whom recurrence occurs is inferior to that of those who remain in continuous remission (Fig 7.11).

Table 7.14
Differential diagnosis of cervical lymph node enlargement

Infections	**Primary lymph node malignancies**
Acute	Hodgkin's disease
Pyogenic infections	Non-Hodgkin's lymphoma
Infective mononucleosis	Chronic lymphocytic leukaemia
Toxoplasmosis	Acute lymphoblastic leukaemia
Cytomegalovirus infection	
Infected eczema	**Secondary malignancies**
Cat scratch fever	Nasopharyngeal
Acute childhood exanthema	Thyroid
Chronic	Laryngeal
Tuberculosis	Lung
Syphilis	Breast
Sarcoidosis	Stomach
HIV infection	
Connective tissue disorders	**Miscellaneous**
Rheumatoid arthritis	Sinus histocytosis
Drug reactions	Kawasaki's syndrome
Phenytoin	

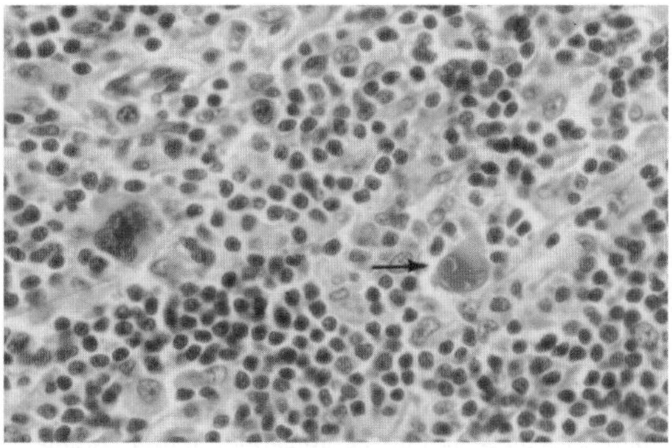

Fig 7.8
Histological appearance of Hodgkin's disease. There is a background rich in small lymphocytes and histocytes together with scattered mononuclear Hodgkin's cells and a classical binucleate Sternberg–Reed cell (arrow) to the right of centre. Courtesy of Dr A J Norton

(a) **(b)**

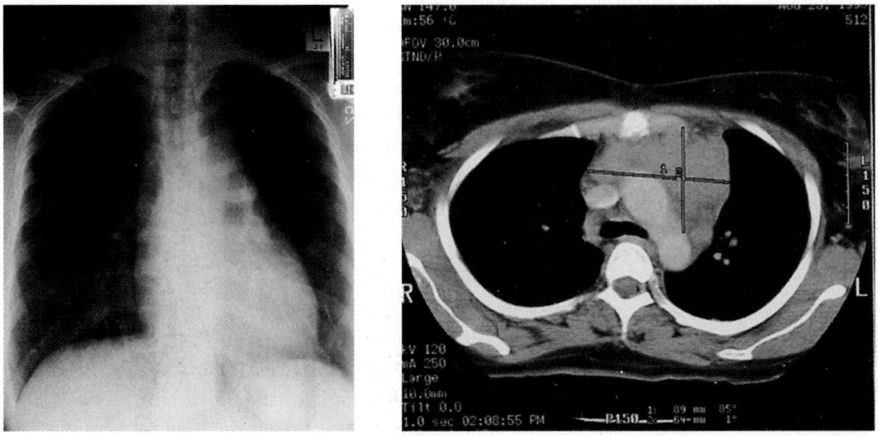

Fig 7.9
(a) Chest X-ray of a large mediastinal mass that is due to Hodgkin's disease. (b) CT scan of the same patient. The mass is indicated here by crossed lines

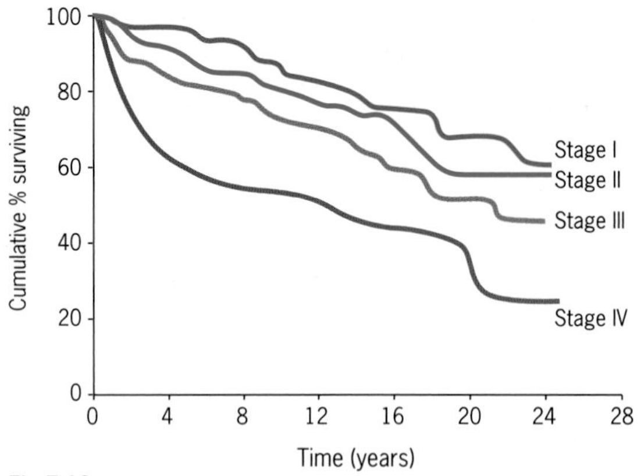

Fig 7.10
Survival in Hodgkin's disease related to stage at presentation

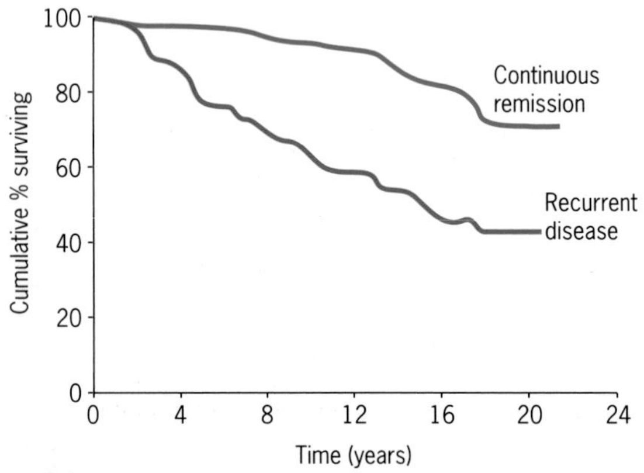

Fig 7.11
Survival of patients with Hodgkin's disease. From Oza AM *et al.* (1993) Patterns of survival in patients with Hodgkin's disease: long follow up in a single centre. *Annals of Oncology* **4**: 385–392

PROGNOSIS AT RECURRENCE

Failure to achieve an initial complete or almost complete response, and recurrence within one year, are both associated with a very poor prognosis. Similarly, patients who develop recurrent HD more than once will almost certainly die of HD eventually. The use of myeloablative therapy with peripheral blood progenitor cell support is now being evaluated in these situations (see p. 436). In contrast, patients who develop recurrent HD (e.g. within the abdomen) a few years after receiving radiotherapy for localized, supradiaphragmatic disease can be given combination chemotherapy and still be cured.

FURTHER READING

Rosenberg SA, Canellos GP (1998) Hodgkins' disease. In: Canellos GP, Lister TA, Sklar JL, eds. The lymphomas. WB Saunders, Philadelphia, p. 305.

Non-Hodgkin's lymphomas (NHLs)

The term 'non-Hodgkin's lymphoma' encompasses many different histological subtypes. Subdivision into *high-grade* and *low-grade* (the Kiel classification) reflects the rate at which the cells are dividing. Ironically, high-grade lymphomas (those in which the cells are dividing quickly) are potentially curable, whereas low-grade lymphomas are generally considered to be incurable with conventional therapy, although patients may live for a number of years and respond to treatment several times. A further subdivision is made on the basis of B- or T-cell origin. Most NHLs are of B-cell phenotype, although T-cell tumours are increasingly being recognized.

Several different histological groupings have been suggested; the two still most widely used at present are the Kiel classification and the 'working formulation'. Both of these were devised prior to observations about cytogenetic abnormalities and immunocytochemistry. A proposal has therefore been made to incorporate the latter into a classification which also recognizes recently described entities, such as lymphomas of mucosa-associated lymphoid tissue (MALT). The proposed REAL (Revised European American Lymphoma Classification) is shown in Table 7.15 with its two counterparts.

CLINICAL FEATURES

Most patients present with peripheral lymph node enlargement, with or without systemic symptoms. NHLs may also involve mediastinal, intra-abdominal and pelvic lymph nodes with resulting symptoms. In contrast, they may involve only an extranodal site, such as part of the gastrointestinal tract.

Low-grade and high-grade lymphomas tend to have a different distribution and behave differently. They are contrasted in Table 7.16.

INVESTIGATIONS

- **Full blood count.** Anaemia, an elevated white cell count or thrombocytopenia are suggestive of bone marrow infiltration.
- **Urea and electrolytes.** Patients may have renal impairment as a consequence of ureteric obstruction secondary to intra-abdominal or pelvic lymph node enlargement.
- **Liver biochemistry.** This may be abnormal if there is hepatic involvement.
- **Chest X-ray.**
- **CT scans** of chest, abdomen and pelvis.
- **Bone marrow aspirate and trephine biopsy.**
- **Lymph node biopsy** (or Trucut needle biopsy in the case of surgically inaccessible nodes).

TREATMENT

As in Hodgkin's disease, treatment will depend on the extent and distribution of disease as well as on the histological subtype. Patients with localized low-grade lymphoma can be cured with radiotherapy alone. Those with more extensive disease require systemic therapy.

Table 7.15
Classifications for non-Hodgkin's lymphoma

Working formulation	Kiel classification	Proposed REAL classification
Small lymphocytic		
(A)	B-cell chronic lymphocytic leukaemia/pro-lymphocytic leukaemia	Small lymphocytic
(A)	Lymphoplasmacytoid	Lymphocytic with plasmacellular differentiation
(A)	Lymphoplasmacytic	Lymphoplasmacytic
Not included	Not included	Marginal zone, low grade
Not included	Not included	Follicle centre, follicular ± diffuse
Follicular small cleaved (B)	Centroblastic/centrocytic, follicular	Follicle centre, follicular, grade I
Follicular mixed (C)	As above	Follicle centre, follicular, grade II
Follicular large cell (D)	Centroblastic, follicular	Follicle centre, follicular, grade III
Diffuse mixed (F)	Centroblastic/centrocytic diffuse	Follicle centre, diffuse, mixed
Diffuse small cleaved (E)	Centrocytic	Mantle cell
Not listed	Monocytoid B-cell	Marginal zone, low grade (low grade B-cell lymphoma of MALT if extranodal)
Diffuse large cell (G)	Centroblastic	Large B-cell
Large cell, immunoblastic (H)	Immunoblastic	Large B-cell
Lymphoblastic (I)	Lymphoblastic B/T	High-grade B-cell lymphoma, Burkitt's-like
Small non-cleaved cell Burkitt's (J)	Burkitt's lymphoma	Burkitt's lymphoma
Not included	Large cell anaplastic (Ki1+)	Anaplastic large cell

Low-grade lymphomas

(Tables 7.15 and 7.16)

Four subtypes will be discussed.

Follicular lymphoma

This is often regarded as the paradigm for low-grade lymphomas. Repeated remissions can usually be achieved with relatively simple treatment, such as with the alkylating agent, chlorambucil. The response rates both at presentation, and at first and second recurrence, are approximately 75%, with a median survival of nine years. Most patients are able to lead a normal life for most of this time. However, the disease remains incurable with conventional therapy. Several new approaches such as fludarabine-containing regimens, myeloablative therapy with peripheral blood progenitor cell (PBPC) support, and immunologically mediated treatments are therefore being investigated.

Lymphoplasmacytoid (LPC) lymphoma

This is generally a disease of older adults. The majority of patients present with advanced disease, the bone marrow frequently being involved. There may be a circulating paraprotein. The prognosis for patients with LPC lymphoma is worse than that for patients with equivalent-stage follicular lymphoma, with a median survival of five years.

Mantle cell lymphoma (centrocytic lymphoma)

Again, this is predominantly a disease of older people. Most present with advanced disease, bone marrow infiltration being almost invariable. Gastrointestinal tract involvement is quite frequently seen. Treatment is unsatisfactory; although patients do respond, the median survival is less than four years.

Low grade T-cell lymphoma (peripheral T-cell lymphoma of low grade)

T-cell lymphomas are less common than their B-cell counterparts. Patients present with lymphadenopathy which, on biopsy and immunophenotyping, shows lymphoma of T-cell origin. Remissions can be achieved (e.g. with chlorambucil) but are usually short; therefore more intensive treatment is generally used. However, with current conventional treatment, recurrence is virtually inevitable.

High-grade lymphomas

High-grade lymphomas may be of B- or T-cell origin. Chemotherapy is given with curative intent. Achievement of remission is a prerequisite for cure. Treatment usually comprises an anthracycline (e.g. doxorubicin hydrochloride) given with cyclophosphamide, vincristine (Oncovin) and prednisolone (CHOP). Variations on the theme of CHOP have since been tried but, thus far, none has been shown to be superior. Between 60% and 70% of patients respond to treatment and about 40% overall are cured. The treatment is myelosuppressive and therefore, particularly in older patients, the main problem is potentially fatal infection.

Table 7.16
Non-Hodgkin's lymphoma: low and high grade

Low grade	High grade
Middle-aged/older people	Any age group
Bone marrow infiltration common	Bone marrow infiltration unusual
Incurable with conventional therapy	Potentially curable

An International Prognostic Index has been derived on the basis of outcome for a large number of patients treated at centres worldwide. When adjusted for age, the index shows three factors to correlate with survival:

- advanced stage (stage III or IV)
- a high serum lactate dehydrogenase (LDH)
- poor performance status (an estimate of the person's general state of health).

Patients who have two or all of these factors at presentation have a worse prognosis. New approaches are therefore being evaluated in this subgroup whose outlook with CHOP is generally poor.

Recurrent high-grade lymphoma has a grave prognosis. However, a proportion of patients who respond to further chemotherapy at recurrence can still be cured with myeloablative therapy with autologous haemopoietic progenitor cell support.

Burkitt's lymphoma

Burkitt's lymphoma was first described in children in West Africa who presented with a jaw tumour (Fig 7.12), extranodal abdominal involvement and ovarian tumours. This type of lymphoma is endemic in West Africa where there is also a high incidence of Epstein–Barr virus (EBV) infection. These are also areas where malaria is common and it has been suggested that the virus is carried from person to person by mosquitoes. Most patients have antibodies to EBV in their serum. The tumour is associated with a chromosome change, most commonly t(18;14) (see p. 417) and can be treated with both radiation and chemotherapy.

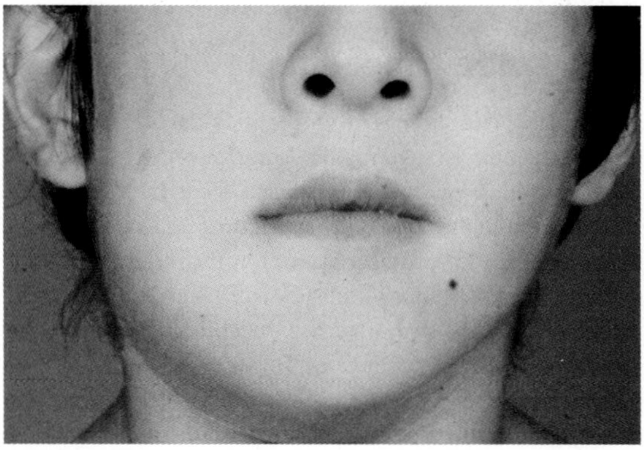

Fig 7.12
A child with Burkitt's lymphoma

A lymphoma pathologically identical to African Burkitt's lymphoma also occurs in the United States and in Europe. However, in these patients it is not usually associated with EBV, but the cytogenetic changes are the same.

With modern intensive chemotherapy regimens, Burkitt's lymphoma can now be cured in most patients, particularly in children.

FURTHER READING

Magrath IT (Ed) (1997) *The Non-Hodgkin Lymphomas*, 2nd edn. Oxford: Oxford University Press.

Myeloablative therapy with haemopoietic progenitor cell support

High doses of chemotherapy and radiotherapy kill dividing cells indiscriminately, so that both normal and malignant cells are killed. Since the bone marrow is a highly dividing tissue, myelosuppression is the main dose-limiting toxicity. Thus, without a 'transplant' as a source of haemopoietic progenitor cells, the person would die of bone marrow failure. The indications for this treatment are shown in Table 7.17.

High-dose treatment may be given using one of the following as a source of haemopoietic progenitor cells:

- allogeneic bone marrow (or allogeneic peripheral blood progenitor cells)
- syngeneic bone marrow
- autologous bone marrow
- autologous peripheral blood progenitor cells.

High-dose treatment with allogeneic BMT (or peripheral blood progenitor cells)

The recipient patient first undergoes a 'conditioning' regimen of myeloablative therapy – drugs, or drug and total body irradiation (TBI) – over a period of several days. The donor, who is usually an HLA-identical brother or sister, then has approximately 1 L of bone marrow aspirated from the posterior iliac crests, and this is given intravenously to the recipient on completion of the myeloablative therapy. Immunosuppressive drugs (usually methotrexate and cyclosporin A) are used to prevent both rejection and graft-versus-host disease (GVHD) (see below). The patient's blood count usually recovers within 3–4 weeks.

Allogeneic BMT can be very effective but has a treatment-related mortality of 20–30%. The main causes of death are infection (bacterial, fungal or viral,

Table 7.17
Possible indications for the use of myeloablative therapy

Allogeneic bone marrow transplantation
Genetic disorders (e.g. thalassaemia)
Aplastic anaemia
AML in first complete remission (patient aged <20 years)
AML and ALL in second complete remission
CML in chronic phase
Myeloablative therapy with autologous BMT/PBPC
This is an experimental treatment in many situations. For example:
AML in first complete remission
Adult ALL in first complete remission
AML and ALL in second complete remission
Low-grade NHL and HD once recurrence has occurred (with regard to HD, either very early recurrence or more than one)
High-grade NHL in first remission in patients at high risk of recurrence
High-grade NHL in second remission

ALL, acute lymphoblastic leukaemia; AML, acute myelogenous leukaemia; BMT, bone marrow transplantation; CML, chronic myeloid leukaemia; HD, Hodgkin's disease; NHL, non-Hodgkin's lymphoma; PBPC, peripheral blood progenitor cells.

cyto-megalo-virus pneumonitis being the greatest problem) and GVHD. The latter is a syndrome in which mature T lymphocytes in the donor marrow infiltrate the skin, gut and liver. Acute GVHD occurs in the first three months but it may also run a chronic course. GVHD can take the form of a mild skin rash and transient impairment of liver function with mild diarrhoea, or the syndrome can be much more severe, patients usually dying of liver failure.

It was noted a number of years ago that patients who develop GVHD have a lower incidence of recurrent leukaemia than those who do not. Thus, not only does the myeloablative chemoradiotherapy have an antileukaemic effect, but T-cells within the donor marrow appear to exert an immunologically mediated 'graft-versus-leukaemia' effect.

The use of allogeneic transplantation is primarily limited by donor availability. The development of donor panels has led to an increased number of transplants being performed using an HLA identical but unrelated donor. Using a 'matched unrelated donor' increases the likelihood of severe GVHD, which, as mentioned above, is the major cause of mortality and long-term morbidity (chronic GVHD). T-cell depletion of the donor marrow has been successful in abrogating the incidence and severity of GVHD but also removes the putative 'graft-versus-leukaemia' effect, resulting in an increased risk of recurrence.

Allogeneic peripheral blood progenitor cells (PBPCs) are currently being evaluated. Granulocyte colony-stimulating factor (G-CSF) is given to the donor; haemopoietic progenitor cells are then collected from a vein. The advantages are that the donor does not have to have a general anaesthetic, and does not have the discomfort associated with collecting marrow from the pelvic bones. Large volumes of blood are phoresed (centrifuged), the PBPCs are separated and collected, and the red cells, granulocytes, platelets and plasma are then returned through another vein. A further advantage is that the incidence and severity of graft-versus-host disease appears to be somewhat lower.

High-dose treatment with autologous BMT

Remission is first induced with chemotherapy. One litre of marrow is then aspirated from the patient's posterior iliac crests under general anaesthetic and cryopreserved in liquid nitrogen. The myeloablative therapy is then given and the thawed marrow reinfused intravenously, as for an allogeneic transplant.

The time to blood count recovery after an autograft is usually longer than after an allograft. Using the patient's own bone marrow also has the potential risk of reinfusing malignant cells; various *in vitro* techniques have therefore been devised to remove them. However, at 5–10% the mortality is considerably lower than with allogeneic BMT. Bacterial, viral and fungal infections are the greatest risk and can continue to be a problem for up to a year later owing to a reversal of the normal T helper:suppressor cell ratio.

High-dose treatment with autologous peripheral blood progenitor cells (PBPC)

Peripheral blood progenitor cells have virtually replaced autologous bone marrow as support for myeloablative therapy. Chemotherapy followed by the growth factor *G-CSF* (see p. 355), or G-CSF alone are administered to stimulate haemopoietic progenitor cells in the marrow to proliferate, so that they can be collected from the peripheral blood as described above. Because the latter are more differentiated cells than those collected directly from the marrow, the time to recovery of the blood count is faster (only 2–3 weeks), with obvious advantages in both human and economic terms. Because the duration of neutropenia is shorter, the treatment is also safer. PBPCs have predominantly been used in patients with Hodgkin's disease, non-Hodgkin's lyphoma, myeloma and breast cancer.

Myeloma

Myeloma is part of a spectrum of diseases characterized by the presence of a paraprotein in the serum that can be demonstrated as a monoclonal band on protein electrophoresis. The paraprotein is produced by abnormal, proliferating plasma cells that produce, most often, IgG or IgA and rarely IgD. The paraproteinaemia may be associated with excretion of light chains in the urine, which are either κ or λ; the excess light chains have for many years been known as Bence–Jones protein.

CLINICAL FEATURES

Myeloma is a disease of the elderly, the median age at presentation being 60 years. It is a complex illness which represents the interrelationship between:

- *bone destruction* causing vertebral collapse (which can cause spinal cord compression) fractures and hypercalcaemia
- *bone marrow infiltration* resulting in anaemia, neutropenia and thrombocytopenia, together with production of the paraprotein which may (rarely) result in symptoms of hyperviscosity
- *renal impairment* owing to a combination of factors – deposition of light chains, hypercalcaemia, hyperuricaemia and (rarely) in patients who have had the disease for some time, deposition of amyloid.

All of this is further complicated by a reduction in the normal immunoglobulin levels, contributing to the tendency for patients with myeloma to have recurrent infections.

PROGNOSIS

Anaemia and renal failure at presentation used to be the two factors associated with a very poor prognosis, 50% of patients dying within nine months. The availability of renal dialysis has reduced the impact of renal failure. In patients without these features at presentation, the median survival with treatment is of the order of two years.

SYMPTOMS

- Bone pain – most commonly backache owing to vertebral involvement.
- Symptoms of anaemia.
- Recurrent infections.
- Symptoms of renal failure.
- Symptoms of hypercalcaemia.
- Rarely, symptoms of hyperviscosity (p. 439) and bleeding resulting from thrombocytopenia.

INVESTIGATIONS

- **Full blood count**. Hb is normal or low. WCC is normal or low. The platelet count is normal or low.
- **ESR**. This is almost always high.
- **Blood film**. There may be rouleaux formation as a consequence of the paraprotein.
- **Urea and electrolytes**. There may be evidence of renal failure (see above).
- **Serum calcium** is normal or raised.
- **Serum alkaline phosphatase** is usually normal.
- **Total protein** is normal or raised.
- **Serum albumin** is normal or low.
- **Protein electrophoresis** characteristically shows a monoclonal band.
- **Uric acid** is normal or raised.
- **Skeletal survey**. This may show characteristic lytic lesions, most easily seen in the skull (Fig 7.13).
- **24 hour urine** – for assessment of light chain excretion.
- **Bone marrow aspirate** shows characteristic infiltration by plasma cells (Fig 7.14).

TREATMENT

General

Anaemia should be corrected and infection treated. Bone pain can be helped most quickly by radiotherapy. Pathological fractures may also be prevented by prompt orthopaedic surgery with pinning of lytic bone lesions seen on the skeletal survey. Renal impairment – often a consequence of hypercalcaemia – requires urgent attention and patients may need to be considered for long-term peritoneal or haemodialysis. The current treatment for hypercalcaemia, in the context of myeloma, is to use biphosphonates such as disodium pamidronate. Biphosphonates may also contribute to the long term control of bone disease. Patients with spinal cord compression due to myeloma are treated with dexamethasone, followed by radiotherapy to the lesion delineated by a magnetic resonance imaging (MRI) scan.

Specific treatment

The use of alkylating agents (melphalan or cyclophosphamide) given in conjunction with prednisolone has improved the median survival of patients with myeloma from seven months to 2.5 years. More intensive doxorubicin-containing regimens have recently been used, and in selected patients, high-dose melphalan supported by autologous BMT or PBPC support. Adjuvant interferon therapy following both standard chemotherapy and high-dose melphalan have been shown to prolong remission.

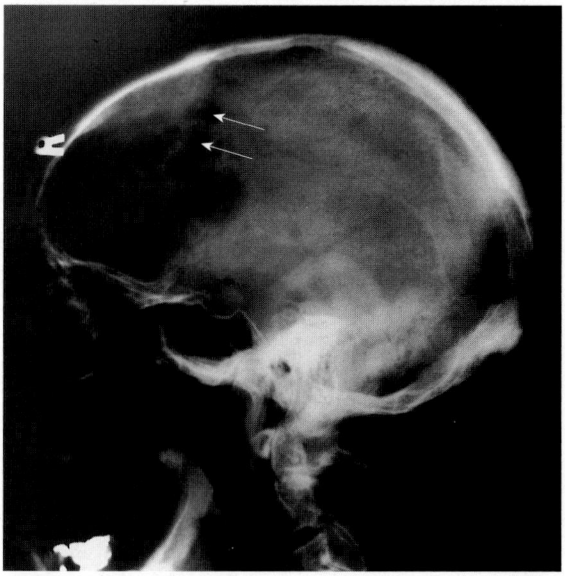

Fig 7.13
Myeloma affecting the skull. Note the rounded lytic translucencies produced by infiltration of the skull with myeloma cells

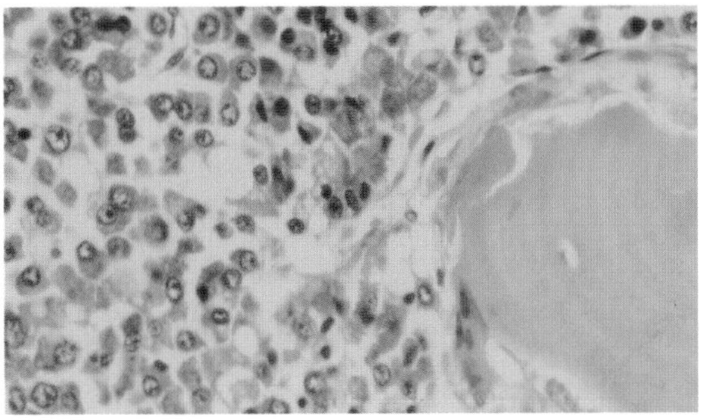

Fig 7.14
Multiple myeloma. Histology shows replacement of the medullary cavity by abnormal plasma cells with some binucleate forms. A residual bony trabeculum is present towards the right. Courtesy of Dr A J Norton

Waldenström's macroglobulinaemia

This is a type of lymphoplasmacytoid lymphoma. Patients tend to be older men and present with peripheral lymph node enlargement and symptoms that are due to bone marrow infiltration. The illness is associated with a paraprotein (IgM) which is responsible for symptoms of hyperviscosity.

CLINICAL FEATURES

- Symptoms of hyperviscosity (headaches, visual disturbance).
- General malaise and weight loss.
- Lymph node enlargement.
- Symptoms of anaemia.
- A tendency to bleed.

INVESTIGATIONS

- **Blood count**. Hb is normal or low. WCC is normal or low. Platelet count is normal or low.
- **ESR**. This is usually raised.
- **Blood film** usually shows rouleaux formation.
- **Bone marrow aspirate** usually shows infiltration with lymphoplasmacytoid cells.
- **Protein electrophoresis** shows an IgM paraprotein ($> 20\ g\ L^{-1}$).

TREATMENT

Alkylating agents and, in younger patients, more intensive doxorubicin-containing regimens produce meaningful responses but recurrence is inevitable. In patients in whom hyperviscosity is the main problem, regular plasmapheresis can be helpful. Death results from progressive bone marrow infiltration and infection.

Monoclonal gammopathy of undetermined significance (MGUS)

This is characteristically seen in older people; a paraprotein is found in the blood but the level is low ($<2\ g\ L^{-1}$). Patients may be quite asymptomatic and the paraprotein detected as a result of investigations for some quite different reason. The blood count is usually normal and there is no renal impairment or bone destruction. In such patients, no specific treatment is required but they should be followed up regularly because they may later develop myeloma or lymphoma.

FURTHER READING

Bataille R, Harousseau J-L (1997). Multiple myeloma. *New England Journal of Medicine* **336**: 1657–1664.

Solid tumours

The treatment of solid tumours involves the combined use of surgery, radiotherapy and chemotherapy. In the earlier stages surgery alone may be curative in many solid tumours, but may fail because of inadequate local excision with residual microscopic disease, or because of disseminated micrometastases present at the time of diagnosis. Radiotherapy, similarly, is a local treatment which can often be used after surgery to reduce the chance of local recurrence. Good examples of this are breast cancer, where the use of surgery plus radiotherapy makes it possible to carry out breast-conserving surgery, and in rectal cancer, where local relapse in the pelvis can be reduced by the addition of radiotherapy. In some solid tumours, such as early laryngeal cancer, radiotherapy can be used on its own with curative intent. It also has an important role in palliative treatment.

Chemotherapy is systemic treatment which can reach any part of the body with an adequate blood supply and is therefore normally used to treat disseminated cancer. Only a minority of metastatic solid cancers can routinely be cured with chemotherapy. These include testicular cancer, choriocarcinoma and childhood solid tumours. In other advanced solid tumours, chemotherapy may cure a small minority but it is usually given with the intention of prolonging life and relieving symptoms. In this situation it may be used to reduce the volume of the tumour without any realistic hope of eradicating disease. When chemotherapy is used without prospect of cure it is essential that care be taken in choosing drugs with the least unpleasant side-effects. The development of new less toxic chemotherapeutic drugs and more effective antiemetics have done much to reduce the side-effects of chemotherapy.

Chemotherapy is increasingly being used in patients who have had surgical clearance of their primary tumour but are at high risk of relapse from metastatic disease at distant sites. When used in this situation as adjuvant chemotherapy, there is a much greater chance of eradicating the tumour than when chemotherapy is given at the time of clinical relapse.

Breast cancer

Breast cancer is the most common cancer in women. Although surgical removal of the primary tumour is usually possible, most women will eventually relapse with metastatic disease.

TREATMENT

Adjuvant therapy

Adjuvant therapy immediately following surgery has reduced the number of women dying from breast cancer by about 25%. A meta-analysis of all randomized trials of adjuvant therapy in breast cancer has shown conclusively that *adjuvant chemotherapy*, most commonly with cyclophosphamide, methotrexate and 5-fluorouracil, for six months reduces the death rate by about 25% in premenopausal node-positive women. *Adjuvant tamoxifen* given for 2–5 years reduces death from breast cancer by a similar amount in postmenopausal patients.

Pilot studies using high-dose chemotherapy and stem cell support (see p. 437) have suggested that this approach may provide a survival advantage in high-risk breast cancer. This is risky and expensive treatment and its value remains unproven. Randomized trials are in progress to answer this important question.

Advanced disease

Patients with established metastatic disease should be treated with hormonal therapy or chemotherapy.

Hormonal therapy

Women who have high levels of oestrogen receptors in their tumour have a greater chance of responding to hormonal treatments. In addition, certain clinical features can predict the likelihood of responding to hormonal manipulations:

- *More likely to respond to hormonal treatment*
  (a) receptor positive
  (b) long interval from initial surgery to time of relapse
  (c) metastatic disease in bone and soft tissue.
- *Less likely to respond to hormonal treatments*
  (a) receptor negative
  (b) short interval from initial surgery to time of relapse
  (c) liver metastases or lymphangitis carcinomatosa.

Endocrine therapy is usually tried first in those patients who have characteristics suggesting they are likely to respond. Useful remissions can be obtained for years, and many elderly patients may live a normal life despite still having residual breast cancer. A range of hormonal manipulations is available:

- *For premenopausal patients*
  (a) cessation of ovarian function by means of oophorectomy, radiation-induced ovarian ablation, or an LHRH analogue with down-regulation of the pituitary
  (b) anti-oestrogen tamoxifen
  (c) progesterone.
- *For postmenopausal patients*
  (a) tamoxifen
  (b) progesterone
  (c) aromatase inhibitors (e.g. formestane, anastrozole).

Chemotherapy

In patients who are unlikely to respond to hormonal treatment or who fail therapy with hormones, chemotherapy is used. If chosen carefully chemotherapy can provide good-quality palliation and prolongation of life. The most common regimens used include:

- CMF (cyclophosphamide, methotrexate, 5-fluorouracil)
- MMM (mitozantrone, methotrexate and mitomycin C)
- doxorubicin and cyclophosphamide
- taxanes used as single agents or in combination with an anthracycline (these may turn out to be the most active drugs available to date for the treatment of breast cancer).

The first two regimens are often very well tolerated and cause little in the way of nausea and vomiting and do not usually cause hair loss. Single-agent mitozantrone is often used in elderly unfit patients and is usually well tolerated.

High-dose chemotherapy with stem cell support is also being explored in advanced disease in a number of randomized trials, after phase-two trials have suggested a possible survival advantage.

Lung cancer (p. 820)

This is the most common cancer in males, and the second most frequent in females (after breast cancer). It is also the most preventable cancer because over 90% is directly related to cigarette smoking.

For practical purposes lung cancer can be divided into small-cell cancer, comprising about 20%, and non-small-cell cancer, comprising the other 80%.

In all cases of *non-small-cell* lung cancer, surgery should be considered, although only a quarter will be operable and only a quarter of those will be cured. Radiotherapy may provide useful palliation in inoperable patients and very good symptom relief in metastatic disease. Chemotherapy is now being used in non-small-cell lung cancer but its role is not yet established (see p. 823).

In *small-cell* lung cancer the disease has almost always disseminated by the time of diagnosis and surgery is thus inappropriate. As opposed to non-small-cell lung cancer, this tumour is very chemosensitive and radiosensitivie and the majority of patients will respond to combination chemotherapy (e.g. etoposide and cisplatin) with good relief of symptoms and modest prolongation of life. A small proportion of limited small-cell lung cancer patients will be cured. In patients with extensive disease, who are incurable, single-agent etoposide orally or intravenously is a possible alternative to combination chemotherapy. As in non-small-cell lung cancer, radiotherapy can provide very useful palliative relief.

Gastrointestinal cancer

Surgery is the primary treatment for gastrointestinal cancer, with radiotherapy sometimes being used after surgery to prevent local relapse. Chemotherapy is also playing an increasing role.

Oesophageal cancer

In early-stage squamous cell carcinoma of the oesophagus, surgery is the treatment of choice. In patients who are inoperable, radiotherapy is given as the primary treatment. More recently it has been shown that chemotherapy, comprising 5-fluorouracil and cisplatin, given concurrently with radiotherapy, improves the cure rate and is now part of standard therapy.

Gastric and colonic cancers

Adjuvant therapy has not yet been shown to be useful in gastric cancer. In contrast, in Dukes' B and C colon cancer, the use of adjuvant chemotherapy following surgery has reduced the number of people relapsing and dying with metastatic disease by about 25%.

For *advanced* metastatic gastric and colonic cancers, relatively mild chemotherapy can provide good-quality palliation and improvement in quality and quantity of life in some patients. Chemotherapy is based on 5-fluorouracil and cisplatin in gastric cancer and 5-fluorouracil and folinic acid in colonic cancer. With the appropriate support these regimens are usually very well tolerated.

New highly active drugs such as irinotecan (a topoisomerase-1 inhibitor) and oxaloplatin have provided the first significant new developments in the treatment of gastrointestinal cancer for many years. The taxanes may also have a role in upper gastrointestinal cancer. The role of these agents in adjuvant therapy and advanced disease will be explored over the next few years.

Ovarian cancer

Surgery has a major role in the treatment of ovarian cancer in all stages. For patients where the disease is confined to the ovary, the surgery can be curative, sometimes without the need for further therapy. For patients with more advanced disease, with spread throughout the pelvis and abdomen, surgery still has a role in improving response and survival from chemotherapy. It has been shown that the response to chemotherapy is much enhanced if the tumour is debulked to leave only small amounts of metastatic disease.

The most important drugs used to treat ovarian cancer are cisplatin and its analogue carboplatin, which is associated with fewer side-effects. Paclitaxel has been shown to have substantial activity in carcinoma of the ovary. Taxanes, alone and in combination with cisplatin, have shown substantial activity and it is hoped that the taxanes may lead to a survival advantage in ovarian cancer.

Testicular cancer

This is the most common cancer in men aged 15–35 years but comprises only 1–2% of all cancers. There are two histological types, seminomas and teratomas.

Seminomas

Seminomas are the least common of these tumours and are very radiosensitive. These can almost always be cured with surgery and radiotherapy to the para-aortic lymph nodes. When there is more widespread disease chemotherapy cures the majority of patients.

Teratomas

This disease often presents with para-aortic and pulmonary metastases. It is very rapidly growing and most patients have a raised α-fetoprotein or human chorionic gonadotrophin (β-HCG) in the peripheral blood which can be used as tumour markers to follow the response of the disease to treatment.

Chemotherapy is the treatment of choice once the disease has spread and radiotherapy has very little role. The great majority of patients can be cured with chemotherapy. The major drugs used include cisplatin, etoposide, bleomycin and ifosfamide.

Management of patients with cancer of an unknown primary site

Approximately 5% of all cancers present with no obvious primary site. The aim of investigation and searching for a primary is to identify tumours that are likely to respond to treatment, and to be able to provide the most appropriate palliative care. It is also important to avoid expensive and unnecessary diagnostic procedures. The most important initial distinction is between *well-differentiated* and *poorly differentiated* carcinomas because a subset of poorly differentiated carcinomas may be extremely responsive to chemotherapy and may occasionally be cured.

Well-differentiated adenocarcinoma

The most important primaries to exclude are those that respond well to the treatment. In females, breast cancer should always be considered, especially if the person has axillary lymphadenopathy. Even in the absence of a clinically palpable mass in the breast, mammography will sometimes detect an unsuspected primary.

Ovarian cancer and thyroid cancer may also respond well to therapy and should be excluded. In men, prostatic carcinoma and thyroid cancer similarly should always be considered.

With improvements in the palliative chemotherapy of advanced gastric and colonic carcinomas, younger fitter patients should also be considered for investigations of the upper and lower gastrointestinal tract to exclude these tumours.

Poorly differentiated carcinomas

In addition to the above investigations, in patients with poorly differentiated carcinomas detailed immunoperoxidase tumour staining is very important as a subgroup of these patients will turn out to have lymphoma, germ cell tumours or neuroendocrine tumours which may all be very reponsive to treatment.

Patients under the age of 50 years, particularly those with peripheral lymphadenopathy or lymph nodes in the mediastinum and retroperitoneum, may have highly responsive tumours that respond well to teratoma-type cisplatin-based chemotherapy. There are a high proportion of complete responders and a minority will achieve long-term remission.

Palliative medicine and symptom control

Palliative care may be defined as the active, total care of patients whose disease is no longer responsive to curative treatment. The goal of this care is to achieve the best possible quality of life for patients and their families by controlling physical symptoms as well as recognizing psychological, social and spiritual problems. Death is accepted as a normal process which should neither be hastened nor postponed, and the need to provide a support system for the family in bereavement is also recognized.

Many symptoms suffered in incurable illness have a complex aetiology in which the physical component may be overlaid by psychosocial issues. For such patients considerable input from a multidisciplinary team of specialist palliative care professionals may be needed to resolve the symptoms. There is now good evidence that integration of palliative care and antitumour management early in the course of disease will reduce long-term distress and difficulty in symptom management. This view moves away from the traditional concentration on the provision of palliative care at the end of life.

The most appropriate first step in providing care in complex situations is often to deal with physical symptoms.

Pain

The symptom most feared by cancer patients is pain, although only two-thirds suffer significant pain throughout the course of their disease. Those patients who suffer pain may present with several pains of differing aetiology, with cancer being directly responsible for about 70%. Pain may be related to associated problems such as rapid weight loss or pressure sores, or may have a separate, non-malignant cause, such as arthritis. The principles of pain relief are careful assessment and diagnosis of the cause of pain, use of analgesics according to the *analgesic ladder*, and regular review of the effectiveness of the prescribed drugs (Fig 7.15).

The analgesic ladder

The cancer pain relief programme of the World Health Organization groups drugs into three main classes:

1. non-opioid drugs, such as paracetamol or aspirin and other non-steroidal anti-inflammatory medications
2. weak opioid drugs, such as codeine, dextropropoxyphene and combinations of codeine with paracetamol
3. strong opiod drugs, such as morphine and diamorphine.

The analgesic ladder states that, if optimal use of a drug from the non-opioid class (e.g. 1000 mg of paracetamol 6-hourly) does not result in satisfactory pain relief, the prescription should be increased up one step to a weak opioid. If the equivalent of codeine 60 mg 4-hourly is not sufficient to control pain, the patient will require a strong opioid. Adjuvant, co-analgesic drugs may be added to each step of the ladder.

Strong opioid drugs

Morphine is the drug of choice and in most circumstances should be given regularly by mouth. The dose can be tailored to the individual patient's needs by the addition of 'as required' doses; morphine has no ceiling analgesic effect. A suitable starting dose of morphine is 10 mg 4-hourly, or 5 mg if the patient is elderly or frail. Patients with renal failure will have impaired excretion of morphine metabolites; they should receive a single dose of

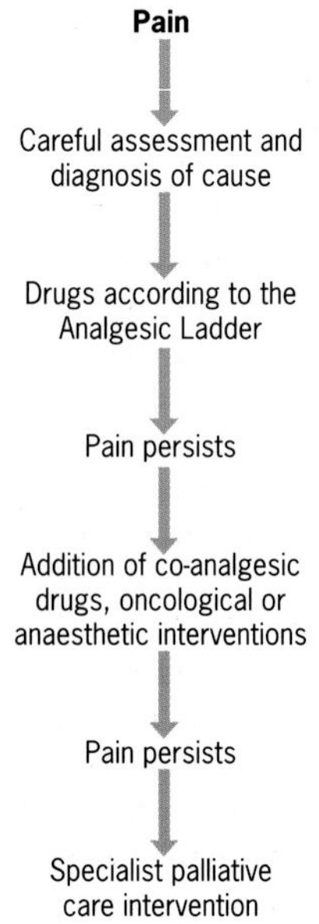

Fig 7.15
Management of cancer pain

morphine and be carefully observed for the return of pain in order to determine the approximate rate of excretion of the metabolites.

If a 10 mg dose of morphine relieves the pain but the relief does not last for four hours, a 50% increase in the dose should be made (i.e. 10, 15, 20, 30, 45, 60, 90, 120, 180 mg) until satisfactory pain control is achieved.

When the patient's 24-hour morphine requirement has been established, the prescription may be converted to a *controlled-release preparation*. There are now both 12-hour and 24-hour release preparations available. The appropriate dose may be calculated by simple addition. For example:

20 mg morphine elixir 4-hourly
= 120 mg morphine per day
= 60 mg twice-daily of a 12-hour preparation
or 120 mg daily of a 24-hour preparation.

If the patient is unable to take oral medication because of nausea or vomiting, gastrointestinal obstruction or altering levels of consciousness, the opioid should be given rectally or parentally. For cancer patients who need long-term analgesia, continuous subcutaneous infusion is the preferred route. Diamorphine is used in this situation because of its greater solubility. By subcutaneous or intramuscular injection, diamorphine is approximately twice as potent as morphine orally. Hence the conversion from oral morphine may be calculated as follows:

30 mg oral morphine 4-hourly
= 180 mg morphine per day
= 90 mg diamorphine subcutaneously over 24 hours.

Side-effects. *Constipation* caused by analgesic drugs is almost universal. The prescription of a stimulant laxative such as co-danthrusate 1–3 capsules at night should be mandatory at the same time as morphine is started. No tolerance develops to this side-effect and laxative medication must be continued as long as analgesics are prescribed.

Nausea or vomiting may occur in 30–60% of patients first started on morphine. However, for those who have worked up the analgesic ladder and who have no other cause for vomiting, the prescription of an 'as required' centrally acting antiemetic (see p. 444) is usually sufficient. Tolerance will develop to this side-effect, usually within 4–5 days.

Confusion, nightmares and *hallucinations* occur in a small percentage of patients. Tolerance to these side-effects does not develop and a change of opiate drug is usually required.

Pain not responsive to opioids

Not all cancer pains are relieved by opioids. In some situations the addition of co-analgesic drugs will result in improved pain control. An increasing number of different classes of drugs have been used in this setting. Some of the most common include the following.

Non-steroidal anti-inflammatory drugs used in addition to a weak or strong opioid for bone pain. Published studies have most frequently used naproxen (500 mg twice-daily) but there is no clear evidence of any one drug being superior in effect. It may be that idiosyncratic side-effects require a trial of a different NSAID.

Pains of nerve destruction called dysaesthetic or deafferentation pain are generally only marginally improved by strong opiates. Several classes of drug, including *steroids*, have been found to be helpful in reducing the symptoms. In cases of constant burning dysaesthesia, the *tricyclic antidepressants* are helpful. Amitriptyline 10 mg at night increasing incrementally to 75–100 mg is usually sufficient (compare with the doses required for mood elevation) and the response, if achieved, can be expected in about a week. *Anticonvulsant drugs* are useful in the management of lancinating, neuropathic pains. Carbamazepine starting at a dose of 100 mg twice-daily is most commonly used, but recent interest has turned to sodium valproate 300 mg twice-daily which may cause fewer adverse side-effects.

In addition to drugs, many *other techniques* such as radiotherapy, anaesthetic and neurosurgical intervention, are employed for the treatment of specific pains.

Regular review of the patient is necessary to achieve optimal pain control. Pain is a complex experience unique to each individual and its perception is modulated by the psychosocial and spiritual situation of the patient. If pain is proving difficult to control, it will be necessary to pay further attention to these other significant factors.

Gastrointestinal symptoms

Anorexia, malaise and weakness are among the most frequently troublesome symptoms in advanced cancer. Current research suggests that endogenously produced cytokines (e.g. tumour necrosis factor and interleukin), are mediators of the anorexia/cachexia syndrome. There is at present no specific therapy, but the approach to treatment depends on adequate management of associated symptoms. Care should be given to addressing the psychological distress caused by a change in body image, with attention to nutrition including dietary advice and the judicious use of steroids.

Nausea and vomiting occur in up to two-thirds of cancer patients in the last six weeks of life. The approach to treatment should be similar to that required for pain, involving careful assessment and diagnosis of the cause. It may, however, be more difficult to reach a diagnosis and a somewhat empirical approach to treatment is often adopted. In order to ensure adequate absorption of the antiemetic, parenteral administration, preferably by the subcutaneous route, may be helpful for the first 24–48 hours.

Antiemetics are classified according to their affinities for neurotransmitter receptor sites. A gastrokinetic dopamine antagonist such as metoclopramide 10 mg 6–8 hourly would be helpful in vomiting related to upper gastrointestinal tract stasis or to liver metastases. Metoclopramide should be avoided in cases of intestinal obstruction as it increases peristalsis in the upper bowel. Centrally acting antiemetics such as the anticholinergic phenothiazine cyclizine 50 mg 8-hourly, or the dopamine antagonist butyrophenone, haloperidol 1.5 mg 8-hourly are the drugs of choice in vomiting caused by drugs or metabolic disturbance. As with the prescription of analgesics, antiemetics will be most effective if prescribed on a regular rather than 'as required' basis.

Bowel obstruction

Bowel obstruction may present acutely or in a more chronic manner and the cause is often multifactorial. A small number of patients may benefit from surgical intervention, so it is important that consideration be given to this modality of treatment in every case. Most patients will not be suitable for surgery and can be managed medically. The active medical management of malignant bowel obstruction includes:

- the relief of intestinal colic using an antispasmodic such as hyoscine butylbromide 60–80 mg daily
- treating continuous pain with adequate analgesia such as diamorphine
- treating vomiting if nausea is a problem with a centrally acting antiemetic such as cyclizine 150 mg daily or haloperidol 5–10 mg daily.

It will be necessary to administer all of these medicines parenterally and the subcutaneous route is most appropriate.

Evidence suggests that the use of corticosteroids or the somatostatin analogue octreotide may shorten the length of episodes of obstruction. Octreotide also reduces the volume of fluids secreted into the bowel, thus reducing the volume of nasogastric aspirate or vomit.

Patients may be allowed to drink and eat low-residue diets which are mostly absorbed in the proximal gastrointestinal tract. It is usually possible, with adequate mouth care, to prevent a sensation of thirst and routine parenteral fluids are not required. A few patients with intractable vomiting due to a high intestinal block may benefit from continuous nasogastric aspiration or gastrostomy drainage.

Respiratory symptoms

Respiratory symptoms, in particular breathlessness, cause great distress to patients and their carers. Management is based on an accurate diagnosis of the cause and active treatment of all potentially reversible situations. Infections should be treated, pleural and pericardial effusions drained and symptomatic anaemic patients transfused. Radiotherapy, cytotoxic agents and local laser therapy or stent insertions may relieve specific areas of bronchial tree obstruction. The place of oxygen in managing breathlessness is not clear, but it may be helpful in patients with correctable hypoxia.

The sensation of breathlessness and a cycle of respiratory panic may be partially relieved by the prescription of regular benzodiazepines. Regular doses of short-acting opioids 5–20 mg 4-hourly are also helpful, as they are postulated to have a local as well as a central effect. Nebulization of a morphine solution may reduce the sensation of breathlessness in a proportion of patients.

Persisitent unproductive cough is a very troublesome symptom. Opiates, codeine, methadone or morphine elixir are helpful as antitussive agents. Antitumour therapy may be required to alleviate pressure on a large airway. Nebulized local anaesthetic may also be helpful in the prevention of cough.

Other physical symptoms

Patients with cancer may develop a large number of physical symptoms. These may be related directly to the presence of the tumour (e.g. vaginal blood loss from a cervix carcinoma), or to the treatment received (e.g. lymphoedema of the arm following breast surgery and radiotherapy). Management of these symptoms will be specific and may require the intervention of other specialists.

Patients may also develop symptoms as a reflection of their debility, such as pressure sores, urinary incontinence, jaundice or recurrent infections. These symptoms may be managed according to the overall expectations and requirements of the patient and their family. These situations of multiple symptomatology in frail patients put considerable demands on the expertise and creativity of clinicians as they present a great challenge for the maintenance of the best possible quality of life.

Psychological symptoms

Effective communication with all patients and their families is a fundamental tenet of clinical practice but is particularly important in the stressful situations which surround fatal disease. Basic communication skills include allowing time for the patient to talk, using language which is appropriate to the circumstances, being prepared to repeat information, and being aware that both the patient and the family may receive bad news by blocking or denying it. It is important to remember that it is not always necessary to have an answer or a solution to every problem that is presented, but that considerable support may be given by sympathetic listening.

Care of cancer patients should be designed to allow them to spend as much time as possible in their own homes. Effective liaison between the cancer centre, the palliative care team and the primary healthcare team is essential to ensure total care. It is especially important to avoid misinterpretation of any information that may be given regarding treatment and prognosis.

Approximately 60% of cancer patients will die in general hospital wards under the care of the physician or surgeon who first diagnosed their tumour, although many are being transferred to hospice care. It is therefore important that every clinician develops some basic skills in symptom control and the ability to recognize those patients who require more specialist intervention. Caring for this group of patients demands detailed attention to alleviating physical symptoms and the establishment of a secure environment for the patient and family to obtain information and support.

The practice of specialist palliative medicine has traditionally been confined to patients with cancer although most services now cover HIV and AIDS and some of the rapidly fatal neurological diseases. These are all conditions in which the clinical situation is changing rapidly and where difficult symptoms exist. There are undoubtedly patients with non-malignant disease such as end-stage renal or cardiac failure who would benefit from a similar multidisciplinary approach to their care. Expansion of specialist palliative medicine into non-malignant situations is currently being actively considered. The patient-orientated principles of palliative medicine can, however, be usefully applied throughout all medical practice.

FURTHER READING

Kaye P Tutorials in palliative medicine. EPL Publications.

Randall F, Downie RS (1996) Palliative care ethics – a good companion. Oxford Medical Publications.

Twycross RG, Lack SA (1990) Therapeutics in terminal cancer, 2nd edn. Churchill Livingstone, Edinburgh.

Rheumatology and bone disease

8

Rheumatological and musculoskeletal disorders

Many of the most common locomotor problems are short-lived and self-limiting or settle with short courses of simple analgesia and/or physiotherapy. They represent 20–30% of the workload of the primary care physician. There is increasing evidence that the early recognition and subsequent treatment of inflammatory arthritis by specialist multidisciplinary teams leads to better symptom control and prevents long-term joint damage and disability. A wide selection of pamphlets offer helpful advice for patients and their use should be encouraged. Most of the musculoskeletal diseases are seen world-wide, although the prevalence of individual conditions varies.

The normal joint

There are two types of joints – synovial and fibrocartilaginous.

Synovial joints (Fig 8.1)

These include the ball-and-socket joints (e.g. shoulder) and the hinge joints (e.g. interphalangeal).

They possess a cavity and permit the opposed cartilaginous articular sufaces to move painlessly over each other. Movement is restricted to a required range,

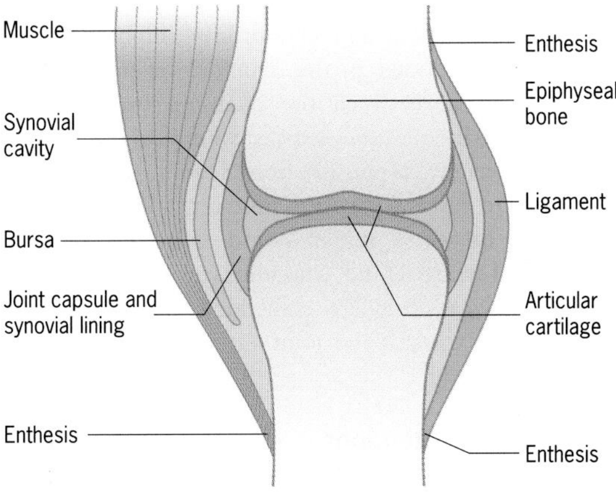

Fig 8.1
The synovial joint

and stability is maintained during use. The load is distributed across the surface, thus preventing damage by overloading or disuse.

Synovium and synovial fluid

Normal synovium is a few cells thick and vascular. Its surface is smooth and non-adherent and is permeable to proteins and crystalloids. As there are no macroscopic gaps, it is able to retain normal joint fluid even under pressure. The surface layer comprises macrophages and fibroblast-like cells. The fibroblasts release hyaluronan into the joint space which helps to retain fluid in the joint. Synovial fluid is a highly viscous fluid secreted by the synovial cells and has a similar constituency to plasma. Glycoproteins ensure a low coefficient of friction between the cartilaginous surfaces. The synovium and synovial fluids also line tendon sheaths and bursae.

Fibrocartilaginous joints

These include the intravertebral discs, the sacro-iliac joints, the pubic symphysis and the costochondral joints.

Bone at joints

The bone which abuts a joint (epiphyseal bone) differs structurally from the shaft (metaphysis). It is highly vascular and comprises a light framework of mineralized collagen enclosed in a thin coating of tougher, cortical bone. The ability of this structure to withstand pressure is low and it collapses and fractures when the normal intra-articular covering of hyaline cartilage is worn away – as, for example, in osteoarthritis (OA). Loss of surface cartilage also leads to the abnormalities of bone growth and remodelling typical of OA (see p. 466).

Hyaline cartilage

This forms the articular surface and is avascular. It relies on diffusion from synovial fluid for its nutrition. It is rich in type II collagen which forms a meshwork enclosing giant macromolecular aggregates of proteoglycan. These heterogeneous macromolecules comprise protein chains (aggrecans) to which are attached side-chains of the carbohydrates keratan and chondroitin sulphate. These molecules retain water in the structure by producing a dynamic tension between the retaining force of the collagen matrix and the expansive effect of osmotic pressure. Intermittent pressure from 'loading' of the joint is essential to normal cartilage function and encourages movement of water, minerals and nutrients between cartilage and synovial fluid. Chondrocytes secrete collagen and proteoglycans and are embedded in the cartilage. They migrate towards the joint surface along with the matrix they produce.

Ligaments and tendons

These structures stabilize joints. Ligaments are variably elastic and this contributes to the degree of stiffness or laxity of joints (see p. 499). Tendons are inelastic and transmit muscle power to bones. The joint capsule is formed by intermeshing tendons and ligaments. The point where a tendon or ligament joins a bone is called an *enthesis* and may be the site of inflammation.

Abnormalities of any of these structures may lead to periarticular or articular symptoms and/or predispose to the development of arthritis.

Joint sensation

The ligaments, periosteum, synovial tissue and capsule of the joint are richly supplied by blood vessels and nerves. Pain usually derives from inflammation of these sites because the synovial membrane is relatively insensitive.

Clinical approach to the patient

Information box 8.1 shows rheumatological terms.

Taking a musculoskeletal history

The following questions are helpful in assessing the problem and making a diagnosis. A history, taken carefully, can often lead to a diagnosis.

Pain

- *Where is it? Is it localized or generalized?* The pattern of joint involvement is an important clue to the diagnosis (e.g. distal interphalangeal joints in osteoarthritis).

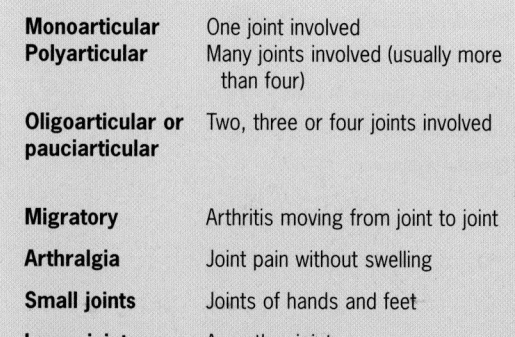

Information

Monoarticular	One joint involved
Polyarticular	Many joints involved (usually more than four)
Oligoarticular or pauciarticular	Two, three or four joints involved
Migratory	Arthritis moving from joint to joint
Arthralgia	Joint pain without swelling
Small joints	Joints of hands and feet
Large joints	Any other joint
Seropositive	Rheumatoid-factor positive
Seronegative	Rheumatoid-factor negative

Information box 8.1 Terms used in rheumatology

- *Is it arising from joints, the spine, muscles or bone?* Soft tissue lesions and inflamed joints are locally tender.
- *Could it be referred from another site?* Joint pain is localized but may radiate distally – shoulder to upper arm; hip to thigh and knee.
- *Is it constant, intermittent or episodic? How severe is it – aching or agonizing?* For example, the pain of gout, or of septic arthritis in a previously fit, non-immunocompromised patient, is agonizing. Alternatively, joint pain lasting a day or so may indicate palindromic rheumatism, whilst longer bouts of a few days are typical of gout. Constant pain, especially pain at night, may be due to an underlying malignancy.
- *Are there aggravating or precipitating factors?* For example:
  Mechanical problems are made worse by activity and eased by rest.
  Inflammatory joint pain and pain from the spine are worse after rest and improve with activity.
  Trauma is a common cause of musculoskeletal pain.
- *Are there any associated neurological features?* Numbness, pins and needles and/or loss of power suggest 'nerve' pain. Consider carpal tunnel syndrome (see p. 456), a spinal problem such as disc prolapse (p. 458) or spondylosis (p. 458), or neurological disease. Nerve root pain, such as that due to a disc prolapse, reflects the anatomical distribution of the affected root.

Stiffness

- *Is it generalized or localized?* Spine or joint stiffness are common after injury.
- *Does it affect the limb girdles or periphery?*
- *Is it worse in the morning and relieved by activity?* Joints which are stiff for more than 15 minutes each morning are usually inflamed – think of rheumatoid arthritis (RA) (see p. 472) or another cause of inflammatory arthritis. Spinal stiffness and pain which is much worse in the morning may indicate ankylosing spondylitis (p. 479), especially in patients in their twenties or thirties. Shoulder and pelvic girdle stiffness and pain which are worse in the morning in a patient over 55 years may be polymyalgia rheumatica (p. 494).

Swelling

- *Is it of one joint, or of several?* Look for symmetry or asymmetry, and/or a peripheral or proximal pattern; these are important clues to the type of arthritis. Rheumatoid arthritis is typically polyarticular. An acute monoarthritis may be due to trauma, gout (in a middle-aged male) or sepsis (fever or immunosuppression).
- *Is it constant or episodic?*
- *Are episodes of swelling short-lived, or longer?*
- *Is there associated inflammation (redness and warmth)?*

Gender

Gout (see p. 482), reactive arthritis (p. 481) and ankylosing spondylitis (p. 479) are more common in men. Rheumatoid arthritis and other autoimmune connective tissue diseases are more common in women.

Age

- *Is the person young, middle-aged or older?* Injury is common in young people but can occur at any age.
- *How old was the patient when the problem first started?* Osteoarthritis (see p. 466) and polymyalgia rheumatica (p. 494) rarely affect the under-fifties. Rheumatoid arthritis is most common in women aged 20–40 years.

General health

- *Is there any associated ill-health or other worrying feature, such as weight loss or fever?* Systemic illness is a common feature of many rheumatic diseases. If there is weight loss and/or fever, think of autoimmune rheumatic disease, sepsis (joint infection may be due to septicaemia and is a medical emergency), or malignancy.
- *Are there other associated medical conditions which may be relevant?* Psoriasis (see p. 1165) or inflammatory bowel disease are associated with asymmetrical arthritis. Charcot's joints (p. 983) are seen in diabetics.

Medication

Could a drug be a cause? Diuretics may precipitate gout in men and older women. Hormone replacement therapy or the oral contraceptive pill may precipitate systemic lupus erythematosus (SLE) (p. 487). Steroids can cause avascular necrosis. Some drugs cause a lupus-like syndrome (p. 489).

Race

Is this relevant? Sickle cell disease causes joint pain in young Africans, but osteoporosis (see p. 506) is uncommon in older Africans.

Past history

Have there been any similar episodes or is this the first? Are there any clues from previous medical conditions? Gout is recurrent; the episodes settle without treatment in about 10 days. Acute episodes of palindromic rheumatism may predate the onset of rheumatoid arthritis (see p. 473).

Family history

Does anyone in the family have a similar problem or another related disorder? Osteoarthritis may be familial. Seronegative spondarthritis (see p. 479) is seen in families with a history of arthritis, psoriasis, ankylosing spondylitis or inflammatory bowel disease. Autoimmunity has a familial tendency.

Occupational history

What job does the patient do? This can be a factor in soft tissue problems and osteoarthritis (e.g. in heavy labourers and dancers). Work-related problems are becoming more common and are complained of more.

Psychosocial history

- *Has there been an injury for which a legal case for compensation is pending?*
- *Has there been any recent major stress in family or working life?* Could these be relevant? Stress rarely causes rheumatic disease but may precipitate a flare-up of inflammatory arthritis. Stress also tends to reduce a person's ability to cope with pain or disability. Remember that the diagnosis of a chronic arthritis has a major influence on the lifestyle of the patient and their family. The extent of disability should be noted.

Examination of the joints

Always observe a patient as he or she walks into the room and sits down, looking for disabilities. General and neurological examinations are often necessary. Guidelines for rapid examinations of the limbs and spine are shown in Practical box 8.1.

Examining an individual joint involves three stages – looking, feeling and moving:

- *Look* at it for swelling, rash or erythema, muscle wasting, deformity such as a distal bone displaced laterally as in knock knees (genu valgus) or bowed legs (genu varus), fixed flexion or hyperextension, loss of range and lack of fluidity of movement, and any pain caused by movement.
- *Feel* it for tenderness, warmth (indicates inflammation) and swelling which may be due to fluid, soft tissue or bone. Common descriptors are 'fluctuant' (fluid), 'firm' or 'boggy' (swelling of the synovium), and 'hard' (bony).
- *Move* it to assess the passive range of movement (e.g. flexion, extension, abduction, adduction and rotation), any instability, or the production of pain and crepitus (grating) seen with cartilage damage.

X-ray of the joint can form an integral part of the examination.

Investigations

Investigations are unnecessary in many of the common regional musculoskeletal problems and osteoarthritis (OA); the diagnosis is clear from the history and examination findings. Tests help to exclude another condition and to reassure the patient or their primary care physician.

Useful blood screening tests

- **Full blood count**
  Haemoglobin: Normochromic, normocytic anaemia occurs in chronic inflammatory and autoimmune diseases. Hypochromic, microcytic anaemia indicates iron deficiency, often due to non-steroidal anti-inflammatory drugs (NSAID) induced gastrointestinal bleeding.

Practical

Rapid examination of the upper limbs

- *Raise arms sideways to the ears (abduction). Reach behind neck and back.* Difficulties with these movements indicates a shoulder or rotator cuff problem.
- *Hold the arms forward, with elbows straight and fingers apart, palm up and palm down.* Fixed flexion at the elbow indicates an elbow problem. Examine the hands for swelling, wasting and deformity.
- *Place the hands in the 'prayer' position with the elbows apart.* Flexion deformities of the fingers may be due to arthritis, flexor tenosynovitis or skin disease. Painful restriction of the wrist limits the person's ability to move the elbows out with the hands held together.
- *Make a tight fist.* Difficulty with this indicates a loss of flexion or grip. Grip strength can be measured.

Rapid examination of the lower limbs

- *Ask the patient to walk* a short distance away from and towards you, and to *stand still.*
- *Move each ankle up and down.* Examine the ankle, the medial arch and toes whilst standing.

Rapid examination of the spine

Stand behind the patient.

- *Ask the patient to (a) bend forwards to touch the toes with straight knees, (b) extend backwards, (c) flex sideways, and (d) look over each shoulder, flexing and extending and side-flexing the neck.* Observe abnormal spinal curves – scoliosis (lateral curve), kyphosis (forward curve) or lordosis (backward curve). A cervical and lumbar lordosis and a thoracic kyphosis are normal. Muscle spasm is worse whilst standing and bending. Leg length inequality leads to a scoliosis which decreases on sitting or lying (the lengths are measured lying).
- *Lie the patient supine.* Examine any restriction of straight-leg raising (see disc prolapse, p. 458).
- *Lie the patient prone.* Examine for anterior thigh pain during a femoral stretch test (flexing knee whilst prone), which indicates a high lumbar disc problem.
- *Palpate* the spine and buttocks for tender areas.

Practical box 8.1 Rapid examinations of the limb and spine

White cell count. Neutrophilia is seen in bacterial infection (e.g. septic arthritis). It also occurs with corticosteroid treatment. Lymphopenia occurs with viral illnesses or active systemic lupus erythematosus (SLE). Neutropenia may reflect drug-induced bone marrow suppression. Eosinophilia is seen in polyarteritis nodosa (p. 495) and Churg–Strauss syndrome (p. 810).
Platelets. Thrombocythaemia occurs with chronic inflammation. Thrombocytopenia is seen in drug-induced bone marrow suppression.

- **Erythrocyte sedimentation rate (ESR) and C-reactive protein (CRP)**. An increase reflects inflammation.
- **Bone and liver biochemistry**. A raised serum alkaline phosphatase may indicate liver or bone disease. A rise in liver enzymes is seen with drug-induced toxicity. For other investigations of bone, see p. 505.

Other blood and urine tests

- *Protein electrophoretic strip and urinary Bence–Jones protein* – to exclude myeloma as a cause of a raised ESR.
- *Serum uric acid* – for gout.
- *Antistreptolysin-O titre* – in rheumatic fever.

Serum autoantibody studies

Rheumatoid factors (RFs)

IgM rheumatoid factors are detected by agglutination tests using IgG-coated latex particles or sheep red cells, the Rose Waaler test or the sheep cell agglutination test (SCAT). They are antibodies (usually IgM, but occasionally IgG or IgA) against the *Fc* portion of immunoglobulin and are detected in 70% of patients with rheumatoid arthritis (RA), but are not diagnostic. A high titre in early RA indicates a poor prognosis. Positive titres occasionally predate the onset of RA (titres may fluctuate). RFs are detected in many autoimmune rheumatic disorders (e.g. SLE), in chronic infections, and in asymptomatic older people (Table 8.1).

Antinuclear antibodies (ANAs)

These are detected by indirect immunofluorescent staining of fresh-frozen sections of rat liver or kidney or Hep-2 cell lines. Different patterns reflect a variety of antigenic specificities which occur with different clinical pictures (e.g. speckled, nucleolar or anticentromere patterns), and are detected in many autoimmune diseases. ANA is used as a screening test for SLE, but low titres occur in RA and chronic infections and in normal individuals, especially the elderly (Table 8.2). The following patterns are seen:

- anti-DNA/histone (homogeneous) antibodies suggest active SLE
- anticentromere antibodies suggest systemic sclerosis.

Table 8.1
Conditions in which rheumatoid factor is found in the serum

Diseases involving joints
Sjögren's syndrome (90%)
Rheumatoid arthritis (70%)
Systemic lupus erythematosus (SLE) (50%)
Systemic sclerosis (30%)
Polymyositis/dermatomyositis (≤50%)
Overlap syndromes
Juvenile chronic arthritis (3%)
Chronic infections (low titres) e.g.
Tuberculosis
Leprosy
Infective endocarditis
Kala-azar
'Normal' population
Elderly
Relatives of patients with rheumatoid arthritis
Miscellaneous
Autoimmune hepatitis
Fibrosing alveolitis
Sarcoidosis
Waldenstrom's macroglobulinaemia

Anti-double-stranded-DNA (dsDNA) antibodies

These are usually detected by a precipitation test (Farr assay), by ELISA, or by an immunofluorescent test using *Crithidia luciliae* (which contains double-stranded DNA). They are diagnostic of active SLE but may be negative in mild or inactive disease. High titres of IgG anti-dsDNA indicate a poor prognosis and are specific to SLE. Anti-single-stranded DNA antibodies are nonspecific.

Anti-extractable nuclear antigen (ENA) antibodies

These produce a speckled ANA fluorescent pattern and can be distinguished by ELISA:

- anti-Ro (SS-A) – SLE + Sjögren's
- anti-La (SS-B) – Sjögren's
- anti-Sm – SLE
- anti-UI-RNP – a range of diseases, including SLE, overlap syndrome.

Table 8.2
Conditions in which antinuclear antibodies are found

Systemic lupus erythematosus (95%)
Systemic sclerosis (80%)
Sjögren's syndrome (60–70%)
Polymyositis and dermatomyositis (30%)
Juvenile chronic arthritis (variable incidence)
Occasionally seen in:
Autoimmune hepatitis
Primary biliary cirrhosis
Infections, e.g. infective endocarditis
Normal elderly people

Anti Jo-1 antibodies

These antibodies to the enzyme histidyl tRNA synthetase block its amino-acylation and are found in polymyositis and dermatomyositis.

Topoisomerase 1 (ScL-70) antibodies

These are seen in systemic sclerosis.

Anti-neutrophil cytoplasmic antibodies (ANCAs)

These are detected on fixed human neutrophils. Two major ANCA patterns are recognized:

- proteinase 3 (PR3-ANCA), formerly called cytoplasmic or cANCA
- myeloperoxidase (MPO-ANCA), formerly called perinuclear or pANCA.

PR3-ANCA is present in up to 90% of serum from patients with Wegener's granulomatosis. MPO-ANCA is found in up to 60% of other vasculitides, such as microscopic polyarthritis (polyangiitis) and Churg–Strauss syndrome. An MPO-ANCA is found in inflammatory bowel disease and rheumatic disease which is not associated with vasculitis.

Antiphospholipid antibodies (aPLs)

These are detected in the antiphospholipid syndrome and SLE.

Joint aspiration (Practical box 8.2)

Examination of joint (or bursa) fluid is used for diagnostic purposes, mainly to diagnose septic or crystal arthritis. The nature of the fluid is also an indicator of the level of inflammation. Clear fluid indicates little inflammation in the joint, whereas translucent or opaque fluid indicates increasing cellularity and underlying inflammation. Purulent fluid is seen in septic arthritis, but crystal arthritis and reactive arthritis may also produce a highly cellular effusion. The procedure is often undertaken in combination with injection of a corticosteroid. Aspiration is therapeutic in crystal arthritis.

Therapeutic injections of soft tissue lesions (e.g. tennis elbow or tenosynovitis) require a similar basic technique.

Practical

This is a sterile procedure which should be carried out in a clean environment

1. Decide on the site to insert the needle and mark it.
2. Clean the skin and your hands scrupulously; remove rings and wristwatch. Gloves are not obligatory, but many prefer to use them.
3. Draw up local anaesthetic (and corticosteroid if being used) and then use a new needle.
4. Warn the patient, insert the needle, injecting local anaesthetic as it advances and, if a joint effusion is suspected, attempt to aspirate as you advance it.
5. If fluid is obtained, change syringes and aspirate fully.
6. Examine the fluid in the syringe and decide whether or not to proceed with a corticosteroid injection.
7. Cover the injection site and advise the patient to rest the affected area for a few days. Warn the patient that the pain may increase initially but to report urgently is this persists beyond a few days, if the swelling worsens, or if they become febrile, since this might indicate an infected joint.

Practical box 8.2 Joint aspiration

Diagnostic imaging and visualization

- **X-rays** can be diagnostic in certain conditions (e.g. rheumatoid arthritis), but remember the following points:
  (a) In acute low back pain, X-rays are indicated only if the pain is persistent, recurrent, associated with neurological symptoms or signs, or worse at night. They should also be performed if the pain is associated with such symptoms as fever or weight loss which might indicate a more sinister underlying pathology.
  (b) Radiological changes are common in older people and may not indicate symptomatic osteoarthritis.
  (c) X-rays are of little diagnostic value in early inflammatory arthritis but are useful as a base line from which to judge later change.
- **Ultrasound** (US) is particularly useful for periarticular structures, soft tissue swellings and tendons. It can be used to guide local injections.
- **Magnetic resonance imaging** (MRI) shows bone changes and intra-articular structures in striking detail. It is more sensitive than X-rays in the early detection of articular disease. It is the investigation of choice for most spinal disorders but is inappropriate in uncomplicated mechanical low back pain.
- **Computerized axial tomography** (CT) is useful for detecting changes in calcified structures.
- **Bone scintigraphy** utilizes radionucleotides, usually ^{99m}Tc, and can detect physiological changes in bone. It detects abnormal bone turnover and blood circulation and, although nonspecific, helps in detecting areas of inflammation, infection or malignancy. It is best used in combination with other anatomical imaging techniques.
- **DEXA scanning** uses very low doses of X-irradiation to measure bone density and is used in the screening and monitoring of osteoporosis.
- **Arthroscopy** is a direct means of visualizing a joint, particularly the knee or shoulder. Biopsies can be taken, surgery performed in certain conditions (e.g. repair of meniscal tears), and loose bodies removed.

Examination of synovial fluid

This is described in Information box 8.2.

Table 8.3
Pain in the neck and shoulder

Trauma (for example, a fall or a whiplash injury)
Mechanical or muscular neck pain
Disc prolapse – nerve root entrapment (p. 1092)
Ankylosing spondylitis
Shoulder lesions
  rotator cuff tendonitis
  calcific tendonitis or bursitis
  impingement syndrome or rotator cuff tear
  adhesive capsulitis (true 'frozen' shoulder)
  inflammatory arthritis or osteoarthritis
Polymyalgia rheumatica
Fibromyalgia
Chronic (work-related) upper limb pain syndrome
Tumour

Information

The fluid can be examined directly in a clear syringe or sterile pot. The characteristics of synovial fluid show a trend from clear to purulent which indicates roughly the type of arthritis.

Colour	Diagnosis	WCC per mm^3
Clear, yellow and viscous	OA	<3000
Translucent and thin	RA	3000–40 000
Very cloudy	Seronegative arthritis	
	Reiter's disease	
	Crystal arthritis	
Purulent	Sepsis	750 000

Polarized light microscopy with a red filter needs to be undertaken by an expert.

- Gout – negatively birefringent, needle-shaped crystals of sodium urate
- Pyrophosphate arthropathy (pseudogout) – rhomboidal, weakly positively birefringent crystals of calcium pyrophosphate

Gram staining is essential if septic arthritis is suspected and may identify the organism immediately. Joint fluid should be cultured and antibiotic sensitivities requested.

RA, rheumatoid arthritis; OA, osteoarthritis

Information box 8.2 Examination of synovial fluid

Common regional musculoskeletal problems

Refer to Fig 8.2 in association with this section. Analgesic and anti-inflammatory drugs used with musculoskeletal problems are discussed in this section on p. 465.

Pain in the neck and shoulder

Table 8.3 shows the many causes of pain. Some of these are discussed below.

Mechanical or muscular neck pain

Unilateral or bilateral muscular-pattern neck pain is common and usually self-limiting. It can follow injury, falling asleep in an awkward position, or prolonged keyboard working.

Worry and stress also cause muscle tension and lead to chronic neck pain which is often burning in quality. Spondylosis (see p. 1097) seen on X-ray increases after the age of 40 years, but it is not always causal as the pain often settles whilst the radiological changes persist. Spondylosis can, however, cause stiffness and increases the risk of mechanical or muscular neck pain. Muscle spasm can be

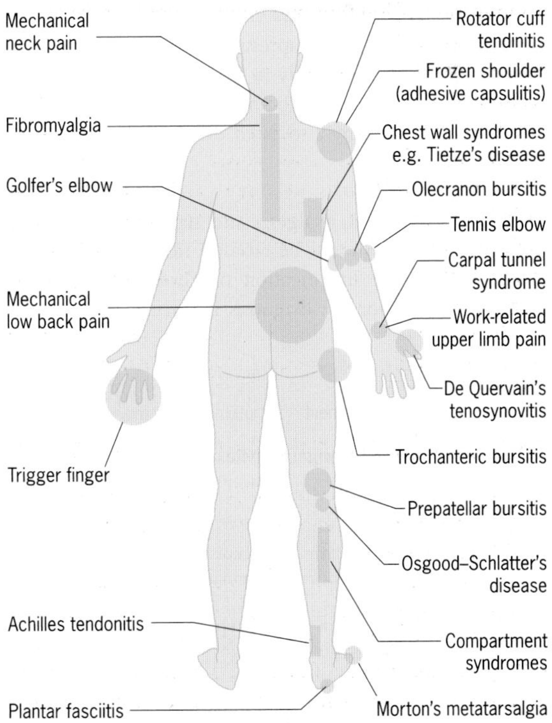

Fig 8.2
Common regional musculoskeletal problems

palpable, is tender and may lead to abnormal neck posture (e.g. acute torticollis). Muscular-pattern neck pain is not localized but affects the trapezius muscle, the C7 spinous process, the paracervical musculature, or all three. Pain often radiates to the occiput but rarely beyond the tip of the shoulder. It is commonly associated with unilateral or bilateral tension headaches; pain over the head to the temple and eye, often described as like a pressure or tight band. These features are also seen in fibromyalgia (see p. 464).

TREATMENT

Patients are given short courses of analgesic therapy along with reassurance and explanation. Physiotherapists can help to relieve spasm and pain, teach exercises and relaxation techniques, and improve posture. An occupational therapist can advise about the ergonomics of the workplace if the problem is work-related (see p. 464).

Nerve root entrapment

This is caused by an acute cervical disc prolapse or pressure on the root from spondylotic osteophytes narrowing the root canal.

Acute cervical disc prolapse presents with pain in the neck, radiating to the interscapular and shoulder regions. This diffuse, aching dural pain is followed by sharp, electric shock-like pain down the arm, in a nerve root distribution, often with pins and needles, numbness, weakness and loss of reflexes (see Table 8.4).

Cervical spondylosis occurs in the older patient with posterior osteophytes compressing the nerve root and causing root pain, commonly in C5/C6, C6/C7; it is seen on oblique radiographs of the neck. An MRI scan shows facet joint OA and any associated disc prolapse clearly.

TREATMENT

A support collar, rest, analgesia and sedation are used as necessary. Patients should be advised not to carry heavy items. MRI is the investigation of choice if surgery is being considered or the diagnosis is uncertain (Fig 8.3).

Table 8.4
Cervical nerve root entrapment – symptoms and signs

Nerve root	Sensory changes	Reflex loss	Weakness
C5	Lateral arm	Biceps	Shoulder abduction Elbow flexion
C6	Lateral forearm Thumb & index finger	Biceps Supinator	Elbow flexion Wrist extension
C7	Middle finger	Triceps	Elbow extension
C8	Medial forearm Little & ring fingers	None	Finger flexion
T1	Medial upper arm	None	Finger AB- & ADduction

Neurosurgical referral is essential if the pain persists or if the neurological signs of weakness or numbness are severe or bilateral. Bilateral root pain is a neurosurgical emergency because a central disc prolapse may compress the cervical spinal cord.

Whiplash injury

This often occurs when a person wearing a seat-belt has their car struck from behind. X-rays are rarely helpful but are essential to exclude a fracture. MRI scans occasionally show severe soft tissue injury. Whiplash injuries commonly lead to litigation.

Treatment is with reassurance (as the patient may be very anxious), analgesia, a short-term collar and physiotherapy.

Pain in the shoulder

The shoulder is a shallow joint with a large range of movement. The humeral head is held in place by the rotator cuff (Fig 8.4), which is part of the joint capsule. It comprises the tendons of infraspinatus posteriorally, supraspinatus superiorally and teres minor and subscapularis anteriorally. The rotator cuff (particularly supraspinatus) prevents the humeral head blocking against the acromion during abduction; the deltoid pulls up and the supraspinatus pulls in to produce a turning moment and permit the greater tuberosity to glide under the acromion without impingement.

Pain in the shoulder can sometimes be due to problems in the neck. The differential diagnosis of this is shown in Information box 8.3. The term 'frozen

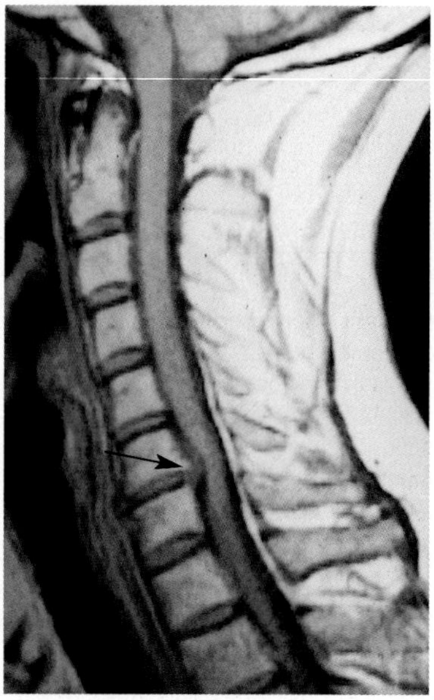

Fig 8.3
MRI of a cervical spine, showing a large central disc prolapse impinging on the spinal cord (arrow) at the C6/C7 level

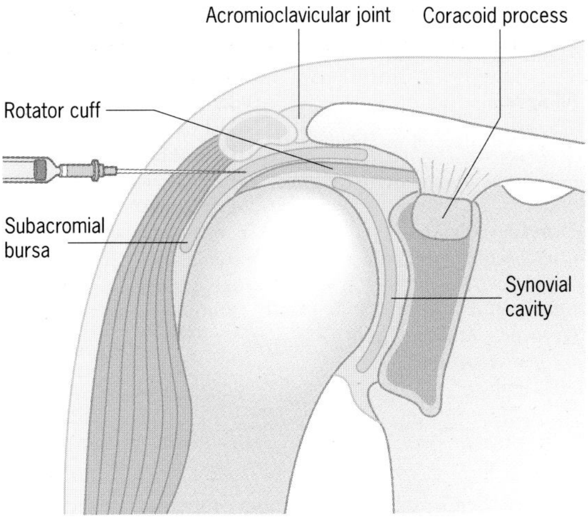

Fig 8.4
The shoulder region, showing site of injection and subacromial space

shoulder' is commonly used for any painful stiff shoulder. True frozen shoulder (adhesive capsulitis) is uncommon – see below. A painful, stiff shoulder can result from rotator cuff lesions and is also seen following hemiplegia, chest or breast surgery or myocardial infarction. Painful shoulders may also be the initial presentation of RA, less commonly a seronegative spondarthritis, and of polymyalgia rheumatica in the elderly.

Rotator cuff (supraspinatus) tendonitis

This is a common cause for the painful restriction of the shoulder at all ages. It follows trauma in 30% of cases and is bilateral in under 5%. The pain radiates to the upper arm and is made worse by arm abduction and elevation, which are often limited. When examined from behind, the scapula rotates earlier during elevation. Passive elevation reduces impingement and is less painful. Severe pain virtually imobilizes the joint, although some rotation is retained (cf. adhesive capsulitis). There is also painful spasm of the trapezius. X-rays are necessary only when rotator cuff tendonitis is persistent or the diagnosis is uncertain.

Information

- Rotator cuff tendonitis pain is worse at night and radiates to the upper arm.
- Painful shoulders produce secondary muscular neck pain.
- Muscular neck pain does not radiate to the upper arm.
- Cervical nerve root pain is usually associated with pins and needles or neurological signs in the arm.

Information box 8.3 Differential diagnosis of 'shoulder' pain

TREATMENT

Analgesics or NSAIDs may suffice, but severe pain responds to an injection of corticosteroid (Fig 8.4). Patients should be warned that 10% will develop worse pain for 24–48 hours after injection. Seventy per cent improve over 5–20 days and mobilize the joint themselves. Physiotherapy helps persistent stiffness but further injections may be needed.

Calcific tendonitis and bursitis

Calcium pyrophosphate deposits in the tendon are visible on X-ray, but they are not always symptomatic. Aspiration of the deposit under X-ray control may be required for persistent pain.

Shedding of crystals into the subacromial bursa causes severe pain and shoulder restriction. The shoulder feels hot and is swollen, and an X-ray will show a diffuse opacity in the bursa. The differential diagnosis of calcific bursitis is gout, pseudogout or septic arthritis.

Aspiration and injection with corticosteroid can help.

Torn rotator cuff

This is caused by trauma in the young but also occurs spontaneously in the elderly and in rheumatoid arthritis (RA). It prevents active abduction of the arm, but patients learn to initiate elevation using the unaffected arm. Once elevated, the arm can be held in place by the deltoid muscle. In younger people, the tear is repaired surgically but this is rarely possible in the elderly or in RA. Repeated trauma of the cuff between humerus and acromion/acromioclavicular joint causes osteophyte and cyst formation.

Shoulder impingement syndrome causes pain and crepitus on abduction and rotation.

Adhesive capsulitis (true 'frozen' shoulder)

This is uncommon. Severe shoulder pain is associated with complete loss of all shoulder movements, including rotation. High doses of NSAIDs and *intra-articular* injections of corticosteroids are helpful. Once the pain settles, a manipulation under anaesthetic is advisable. When untreated, it recovers in 1–2 years.

Pain in the elbow

Pain in the elbow can be due to epicondylitis, inflammatory arthritis or occasionally osteoarthritis.

Epicondylitis

Two common sites where the insertions of tendons into bone become inflamed (*enthesitis*) are the insertions of the wrist extensor tendon into the lateral epicondyle ('tennis elbow') and the wrist flexor tendon into the medial epicondyle ('golfer's elbow'). Both are usually unrelated to either sporting activity.

There is local tenderness. Pain radiates into the forearm on using the affected muscles – typically, holding a heavy bag in tennis elbow or carrying a tray in golfer's elbow. Pain at rest also occurs.

TREATMENT

Advise rest and arrange strapping by a physiotherapist. A local injection of corticosteroid at the point of maximum tenderness is helpful when the pain is severe. Avoid the ulnar nerve when injecting golfer's elbow (Fig 8.5). Both conditions settle spontaneously eventually, but occasionally become disabling.

Pain in the hand and wrist (Table 8.5)

Hand pain is commonly caused by injury or repetitive work-related use. When associated with pins and needles or numbness it suggests a neurological cause arising at the wrist, elbow or neck. Pain and stiffness that are worse in the morning are due to tenosynovitis or inflammatory arthritis. The distribution of hand pain often indicates the diagnosis.

Tenosynovitis

The flexor tendons run through a series of synovial sheaths and under loops which hold them in place. Inflammation occurs with repeated or unaccustomed use, or in inflammatory arthritis when the thickened sheaths are often palpable.

Flexor tenosynovitis causes finger pain when gripping and stiffness in the morning. Occasionally a tendon causes a *trigger finger*, when the finger remains flexed after gripping and has to be pulled straight. A tendon nodule is palpable, usually in the palm.

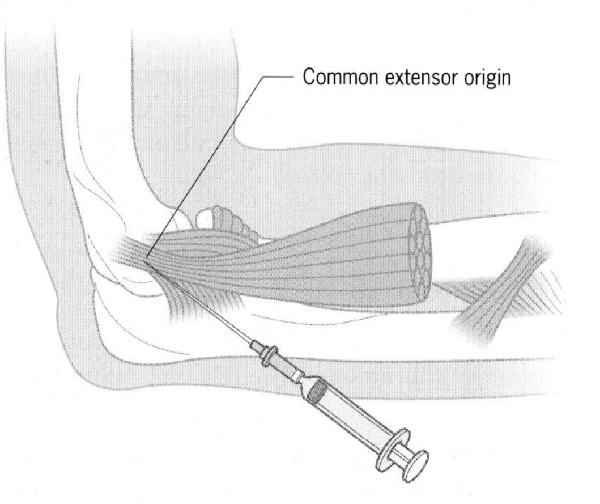

Fig 8.5
Injection for tennis elbow

Table 8.5
Pain in the hand and wrist – causes

All ages	**Older patients**
Trauma/fractures	Nodal OA
Tenosynovitis	DIPs (Heberden's nodes)
flexor with/without triggering	PIPs (Bouchard's nodes)
dorsal	first carpometacarpal
de Quervain's	Trauma – scaphoid fracture
Carpal tunnel syndrome	Pseudogout
Ganglion	Gout
Inflammatory arthritis	acute
Raynaud's syndrome (p. 465)	tophaceous
Reflex sympathetic dystrophy	

DIPs, PIPs = distal and proximal interphalangeal joints.

Dorsal tenosynovitis is less common except in rheumatoid arthritis. The swelling is on the back of the hand and wrist.

De Quervain's tenosynovitis causes pain and swelling around the radial styloid where the abductor policis longus tendon is held in place by a retaining band. There is local tenderness, and the pain at the styloid is worsened by flexing the thumb into the palm.

TREATMENT

Corticosteroids are injected alongside the tendon under low pressure (not into the tendon itself). Occasionally surgery is needed.

Other conditions causing pain

Carpal tunnel syndrome

This is due to thickened tendons or synovitis in the carpal tunnel and is discussed on p. 1092. The history is usually typical and diagnostic with the patient waking with numbness, tingling and pain in a median nerve distribution. The pain radiates to the forearm. The fingers feel swollen but are not.

Treatment is with a splint to hold the wrist in dorsiflexion overnight. This relieves the symptoms and is diagnostic; used nightly for several weeks it may produce full recovery. If it does not, a corticosteroid injection into the carpal tunnel helps in about 70% of cases. Persistent symptoms or nerve damage require nerve conduction studies and surgical release.

Inflammatory arthritis

This may present with pain, swelling and stiffness of the hands. In RA the wrists, proximal interphalangeal (PIP) joints and metacarpophalangeal (MCP) joints are affected symmetrically. In psoriatic arthritis and Reiter's disease a finger may be swollen (*dactylitis*) or the distal interphalangeal (DIP) joints are affected asymmetrically.

Nodal osteoarthritis

This affects the DIP and less commonly PIP joints which are initially swollen and red. The inflammation and pain settle but bony swellings remain. There is often a strong family history and it rarely presents before fifty years of age. Reassurance and local treatment are all that is needed.

First carpometacarpal osteoarthritis

This causes pain at the base of the thumb when gripping, or a painless stiff thumb.

Scaphoid fractures

These cause pain in the anatomical snuff box. They may not be seen immediately on X-ray. Untreated scaphoid fractures eventually cause pain because of failed union.

Ganglion

A ganglion is a jelly-filled, often painless swelling caused by a partial tear of the joint capsule. The wrist is a common site. Treatment is not essential as many resolve or cause little trouble. They rarely respond to injection, and surgical excision is possibly the best option.

Dupuytren's contracture

This is a painless, palpable fibrosis of the palmar aponeurosis. It causes puckering of the skin and gradual flexion of the affected fingers, usually the ring and little fingers. Plastic surgical release is restricted to these with severe deformity.

Pain in the lower back

Low back pain is a common symptom. It is often traumatic and work-related, although lifting apparatus and other mechanical devices are increasingly used to avoid it. Episodes are generally short-lived and self-limiting, and patients attend a physiotherapist or osteopath more often than a doctor. The causes are listed in Table 8.6, and the management of back pain is summarized in Information box 8.4.

INVESTIGATIONS

- **Spinal X-rays** are required only if the pain:
  (a) starts before the age of 20 or after 50 years
  (b) is persistent and a serious cause is suspected
  (c) is worse at night or in the morning, when an inflammatory arthritis (e.g. ankylosing spondylitis) infection or a spinal tumour may be the cause
  (d) is associated with a systemic illness, fever or weight loss
  (e) is associated with neurological symptoms or signs.
- **CT scan** or (better) **MRI** are useful when neurological signs and symptoms are present
- **Bone scans** are useful in infective and malignant lesions but are also positive in degenerative lesions.
- **Full blood count, ESR and biochemical tests** are required only when the pain is likely to be due to malignancy, infection or a metabolic cause.

Table 8.6
Pain in the back (lumbar region) – causes

Trauma
Mechanical
Muscular pain
Postural back pain
Prolapsed disc
Lumbar spondylosis ± spinal stenosis
Disseminated idiopathic skeletal hyperostosis (DISH)
Spondylolisthesis
Fibromyalgia
Inflammatory
Infective lesions of spine
Ankylosing spondylitis/sacroiliitis
Metabolic
Osteoporosis + fracture
Osteomalacia
Paget's disease
Neoplastic
Metastases
Multiple myeloma
Primary bone tumours
Referred pain

Mechanical low back pain

Mechanical low back pain starts suddenly, may be recurrent and is helped by rest. It is often unilateral. Spinal movement occurs at the disc and the posterior facet joints, and stability is normally achieved by a complex mechanism of spinal ligaments and muscles. Any of these structures may be a source of pain. An exact anatomical diagnosis is difficult, but some typical syndromes are recognized. They are often associated with radiological spondylosis (see p. 458).

Postural back pain develops in individuals who sit in poorly designed, unsupportive chairs.

Information

- Most back pain presenting to a primary care physician needs no investigation.
- Pain between ages 20 and 55 years is likely to be mechanical and is managed with analgesia, brief rest and physiotherapy.
- Patients should stay active within the limits of their pain.
- Early treatment of the acute episode, advice and exercise programmes reduce long-term problems and prevent chronic pain syndromes.
- Physical manipulation of uncomplicated back pain produces short term relief and enjoys high patient satisfaction ratings.
- Psychological and social factors may influence the time of presentation.

Information box 8.4 Management of back pain

Fibrositic nodulosis

This causes unilateral or bilateral low back pain, radiating to the buttock and upper posterior thigh. There are tender nodules in the upper buttock and along the iliac crest. Such nodules are relevant only if they are tender and associated with pain. They are probably traumatic. Local, intralesional corticosteroid injections help.

Sway back (back pain of pregnancy)

Low back pain in pregnancy reflects altered spinal posture and increased ligamentous laxity. Weight control and pre- and postnatal exercises are helpful, and the pain usually settles after delivery. Analgesics and NSAIDs are best avoided during pregnancy and breast-feeding. Epidurals during delivery are *not* associated with an increased incidence of subsequent back pain.

Spondylolisthesis

This occurs in adolescents and young adults when bilateral congenital pars interarticularis defects cause instability and permit the vertebra to slip, with or without preceding injury. Rarely a cauda equina syndrome with loss of bladder and anal sphincter control and saddle-distribution anaesthesia develops (p. 1098).

Low back pain in adolescents warrants investigation, and spondylolisthesis requires orthopaedic assessment. A degenerative spondylolisthesis may also develop in older people with lumbar spondylosis.

Lumbar spondylosis

The fundamental lesion in spondylosis is in an intervertebral disc, a fibrous joint whose tough capsule inserts into the rim of the adjacent vertebrae. This capsule encloses a fibrous outer zone and a gel-like inner zone. The disc allows rotation and bending.

Changes in the discs may start in teenage years or early twenties and increase with age. The gel changes chemically, breaks up, shrinks and loses its compliance. The surrounding fibrous zones develop circumferential or radial fissures. In the majority this is initially asymptomatic but visible on MRI as decreased hydration. Later the discs become thinner and less compliant. These changes cause circumferential bulging of disc capsules.

Reactive changes develop in adjacent vertebrae; the bone becomes sclerotic and osteophytes form around the rim of the vertebra (Fig 8.6). The most common sites of spondylosis are L5/S1 and L4/L5. Disc prolapse through an adjacent vertebral endplate to produce a Schmorl's node on X-ray is painless but may accelerate disc degeneration.

Spondylosis may be symptomless, but it can cause:

- episodic mechanical spinal pain
- progressive spinal stiffening
- acute disc prolapse, with or without nerve root irritation
- spinal stenosis
- spondylolisthesis.

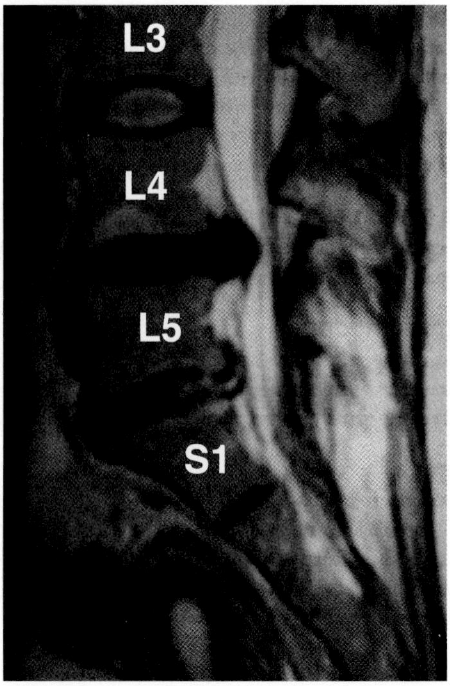

Fig 8.6
MRI of the lumbar spine, showing a central disc prolapse at the L4/L5 level. The signal from the L4/L5 and L5/S1 discs indicates dehydration, while the L3/L4 signal appearance is normal

Facet joint syndrome. Lumbar spondylosis also causes secondary osteoarthritis of the facet joints. Pain is typically worse on bending backwards and when straightening from flexion. It is lumbar in site, unilateral or bilateral and radiates to the buttock. Diagnostic local anaesthetic injections into the joints (under X-ray vision) can be followed by a corticosteroid injection, although the value of this is unclear. Physiotherapy to reduce hyperlordosis and reducing weight are helpful.

Acute lumbar disc prolapse

The central disc gel may extrude into a fissure in the surrounding fibrous zone and cause acute pain and muscle spasm, which in turn leads to a forwards and sideways tilt when standing. These events are often self-limiting. A disc prolapse occurs when the extrusion extends beyond the limits of the fibrous zone (Fig 8.6). The weakest point is posterolateral, where the disc may impinge on emerging spinal nerve roots in the root canal.

The episode starts dramatically during lifting, twisting or bending and produces a typical combination of low back pain and muscle spasm, and severe, lancinating pains, paraesthesia, numbness and neurological signs in one leg (rarely both). The back pain is diffuse, usually unilateral and radiates into the buttock. The muscle spasm leads to a scoliosis which reduces when lying down. The nerve root pain develops with, or soon after, the onset. The site of the pain and other symptoms is determined by the root affected (Table 8.7). A central high lumbar disc prolapse may cause spinal cord compression and long tract signs. Below L2/L3 it produces lower motor neurone lesions.

TREATMENT

Advise bedrest – lying flat for a lower disc but semi-reclining for a high lumbar disc – and prescribe analgesia and muscle relaxants. An X-ray-guided epidural or nerve root injection by a pain specialist reduces pain, although the evidence that it speeds resolution or prevents surgery is unclear. Caudal epidural injections are less effective than lumbar ones but technically easier. Resuscitation equipment must be available for these procedures. Once the pain is tolerable, encourage the patient to mobilize and refer to a physiotherapist for exercises and preventative advice.

Microdiscectomy or hemilaminectomy is necessary if the neurological signs are severe, if the pain persists and is severe for more than 6–10 weeks, or if the disc is central. If bladder or anal sphincter tone is affected it becomes a neurosurgical emergency. Chemical discolysis is still being evaluated.

Spinal and root canal stenosis

Progressive loss of disc height, OA of the facet joints, posterolateral osteophytes and hypertrophy of the ligamentum flavum all contribute to root canal stenosis. This causes nerve root pain or spinal root claudication – pain and paraesthesiae in a root distribution brought on by walking and relieved slowly by rest. The associated sensory symptoms, slow recovery and presence of normal foot pulses distinguishes this from peripheral arterial claudication.

Spinal canal stenosis at more than one level and a congenitally narrow spinal canal cause buttock and bilateral leg pain, paraesthesiae and numbness when walking. Rest helps, as does bending forwards, a manoeuvre which opens the spinal canal. Specialist surgical advice is necessary.

Osteoporotic crush fracture of the spine

Osteoporosis is asymptomatic but leads to an increased risk of fracture of peripheral bones, particularly neck of femur and wrist, and thoracic or lumbar vertebral crush fractures. Such vertebral fractures develop either without trauma, after minimal trauma, or as part of a major accident. They may develop painlessly or cause agonizing localized pain which radiates around the ribs and abdomen. Multiple fractures lead to an increased thoracic kyphosis ('widow's stoop'). The diagnosis is confirmed by X-rays, showing loss of anterior vertebral body height and wedging, with sparing of the vertebral end-plates and pedicles (Fig 8.7).

TREATMENT

Advise bedrest and analgesia until the severe pain subsides over a few weeks, then gradual mobilization. It may warrant hospitalization. There may be some residual pain. Preventative assessment and treatment is helpful (see p. 508).

Table 8.7
Lumbar nerve root entrapment – symptoms and signs

Nerve root	Sensory changes	Reflex loss	Weakness	Usual disc prolapse
L2	Front of thigh	None	Hip flexion/adduction	L2/3
L3	Inner thigh and knee	Knee	Knee extension	L2/3
L4	Inner calf	Knee	Knee extension	L3/4
L5	Outer calf	None	Inversion of foot	L4/5
	Upper, inner foot		Dorsiflexion of toes	
S1	Lateral border and sole of foot	Ankle	Plantar flexion of foot	L5/S1

Diffuse idiopathic skeletal hyperostosis (DISH)

DISH (Forrestier's disease, ankylosing hyperostosis) affects the spine and extraspinal locations. It is an enthesopathy, causing bony overgrowths and ligamentous ossification and is characterized by flowing calcification over the anterolateral aspects of the vertebrae. The spine is usually stiff and but not always painful, despite the dramatic X-ray changes. Ossification at muscle insertions around the pelvis produces radiological 'whiskering'. Similar changes occur at the patella and in the feet.

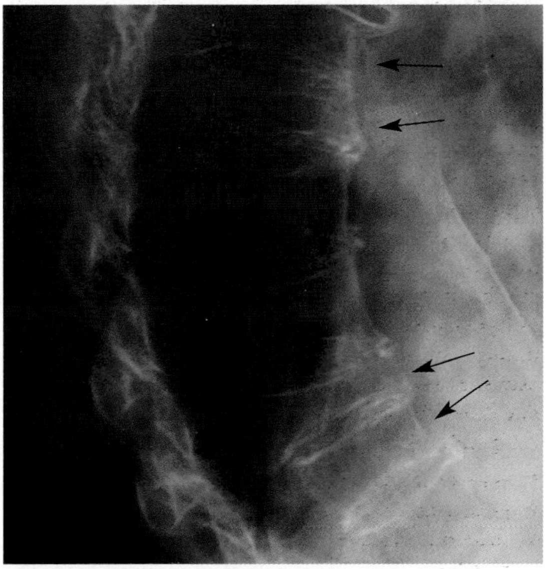

Fig 8.7
X-ray of mid thoracic spine, showing severe osteoporosis with multiple crush fractures (arrows) and biconcave vertebrae

Treatment is with NSAIDs for pain, and exercise to retain movement and muscle strength.

Ankylosing spondylitis (see also p. 479)

Buttock pain and low-back stiffness in a young adult suggests ankylosing spondylitis, especially if it is worse at night and in the morning.

Pain in the hip (Table 8.8)

'Hip' refers to a wide area between the upper buttock, trochanter and groin. It is useful to ask the patient to point to the site of pain and its field of radiation. Pain arising from the hip joint itself is felt in the groin, lower buttock and anterior thigh, and may radiate to the knee. Occasionally and inexplicably, hip arthritis causes pain only in the knee.

Osteoarthritis (OA) (see also p. 466)

OA is the most common cause of hip joint pain in a person over the age of 50 years. It causes pain in the buttock and groin on standing and walking. Stiff hip movements cause difficulty in putting on a sock, or may produce a limp.

Trochanteric bursitis

This may be due to trauma or unaccustomed exercise, but sometimes has an unknown cause. The pain over the trochanter is worse going up stairs and when abducting the hip, and the trochanter is tender to lie on. A local corticosteroid injection on to the surface of the trochanter is helpful.

Meralgia paraesthetica (see also p. 1093)

This causes numbness and burning dysaesthesia (increased sensitivity to light touch) over the anterolateral thigh and may be precipitated by a sudden increase in weight.

Fracture of the femoral neck

This usually occurs after a fall, occasionally spontaneously. There is pain in the groin and thigh, weight-bearing is painful or impossible, and the leg is shortened and externally rotated. Occasionally a fracture is not displaced and remains undetected. X-rays are diagnostic. Anyone with a hip fracture, especially after minimal trauma, should be reviewed for osteoporosis.

Avascular necrosis (osteonecrosis) of the femoral head

This is uncommon but occurs at any age. There is severe hip pain. X-rays are diagnostic after a few weeks, when a well-demarcated area of increased bone density is visible. In the femur this lies at the upper pole of the femoral head. The affected bone may collapse. Early, the X-ray is normal but bone scintigraphy or MRI demonstrate the lesion. Risk factors include treatment with corticosteroids or heparin, exposure to high barometric pressures (divers and tunnellers), excess alcohol consumption, and sickle cell disease.

Table 8.8
Pain in the hip – causes

Hip region	Main site of pain
Osteoarthritis of hip	Groin, buttock, front of thigh to knee
Trochanteric bursitis	Lateral thigh to knee
Meralgia paraesthetica	Anterolateral thigh to knee
Referred from back	Buttock
Fracture of neck of femur	Groin and buttock
Inflammatory arthritis	Groin, buttock, front of thigh to knee
Sacroiliitis (AS)	Buttock(s)
Avascular necrosis	Groin, buttock
Polymyalgia rheumatica	Buttocks, lumbar spine

AS, Ankylosing spondylitis.

Inflammatory arthritis of the hip

This produces pain in the groin and stiffness, which are worse in the morning. *Rheumatoid athritis* (RA) rarely presents with hip pain, although the hip is involved eventually in severe RA. *Ankylosing spondylitis* and other seronegative spondarthritides cause inflammatory hip arthritis in younger people.

Polymyalgia rheumatica (see also p. 494)

Bilateral hip, buttock and thigh pain and stiffness which are worse in the morning in an elderly patient may be attributable to polymyalgia rheumatica.

Pain in the knee (Table 8.9)

The knee depends on ligaments and quadriceps muscle strength for stability. It is frequently injured, particularly during sports. Trauma or overuse of the knee leads to a

Table 8.9
Pain in the knee

- Trauma and overuse
  - Periarticular problems
  - Anterior knee pain or medial knee pain
  - Internal derangements
  - Meniscal tears or cruciate ligament tears
- Popliteal (Baker's) cyst/ruptured cyst
- Osteoarthritis
- Inflammatory arthritis
  - Acute monarthritis
    - Gout, pseudogout Reiter's disease or septic arthritis
  - Pauciarticular (<4 joints)
    - Seronegative spondarthritis or atypical rheumatoid arthritis
  - Polyarticular
  - Rheumatoid arthritis
- Osteochondritis dissecans
- Hypermobility syndrome
- Referred from hip joint

variety of peri- and intra-articular problems. Some are self-limiting, others require physiotherapy, local corticosteroid injections or surgery.

The knee is also a common site of inflammatory arthritis and osteoarthritis. Minor radiographic changes of osteoarthritis (see p. 466) are common in the over-50s and often coincidental, the cause of the pain being peri-articular. Knee pain should not be attributed to osteoarthritis until other causes have been excluded. Symptomatic osteoarthritis of the knee correlates poorly with the severity of the radiological changes.

Common peri-articular knee lesions

Medial knee pain

There may be *medial* (or *lateral*) *ligament strain*, but the medial ligament is more commonly affected. There is pain at the ligament's insertion into the upper medial tibia, which is worsened by standing or stressing the affected ligament.

Anserine bursitis causes pain and localized tenderness 2–3 cm below the posteromedial joint line in the upper part of the tibia at the site of the bursa. It occurs in obese women, often with valgus deformities, and in breast-stroke swimmers.

Treatment is with physiotherapy and a local corticosteroid injection.

Anterior knee pain

Anterior knee pain is common in adolescence. In many cases no specific cause is found despite careful investigation. This is called 'anterior knee pain syndrome' and settles with time. Isometric quadriceps exercises and avoidance of high heels both help the condition. Patient and parents often need firm reassurance.

Pre- and infra-patellar bursitis are caused by unaccustomed kneeling ('housemaid's knee'). There is local pain, tenderness and fluctuant swelling. Avoidance of kneeling and a local corticosteroid injection are helpful. *Septic bursitis* can occur.

Chondromalacia patellae can be diagnosed only arthroscopically. The retropatellar cartilage is fibrillated. In most cases the pain settles eventually. When there is patellar misalignment it may need surgery, as does recurrent patellar dislocation in adolescent girls.

Osgood–Schlatter's disease causes pain and swelling over the tibial tubercle. It is a traction apophysitis of the patellar tendon and occurs in enthusiastic teenage sports players.

Hypermobility of joints causes joint pain (see also p. 499)

Common intra-articular traumatic lesions of the knee

Torn meniscus

The menisci are partially attached fibrocartilages which stabilize the rounded femoral condyles on the flat tibial plateaus. In the young they are resilient but this decreases with age. They can be torn by a twisting injury, commonly in sports which involve twisting and bending or the use of a studded boot. The history is usually diagnostic. There is immediate medial or lateral knee pain and dramatic swelling within a few hours. The affected side is tender. If the tear is large the knee may lock flexed. The immediate treatment is to apply ice to the knee. MRI demonstrates the tear (Fig 8.8). In most circumstances, especially in active sportsmen, early arthroscopic repair or trimming of the torn meniscus is essential. Surgical intervention reduces recurrent pain, swelling and locking but not the risk of secondary osteoarthritis. The long-term benefit of repairing tears is not yet known. Post-surgical quadriceps exercises aid a return to sport.

Torn cruciate ligaments

Torn cruciate ligaments account for around 70% of knee haemarthroses in young people. They often coexist with a meniscal tear. Partial cruciate tears are difficult to diagnose clinically. On flexing the knee to 90 degrees, a torn anterior cruciate allows the tibia to be pulled forwards on the femur. Such injuries need urgent orthopaedic referral. There is a significant incidence of secondary OA.

Osteochonditis dissecans

This occasionally causes knee pain and swelling in adolescents and young adults, more commonly males. It is probably traumatic, possibly with hereditary predisposing factors. A fragment of bone and its attached cartilage detach by shearing, most commonly from the lateral aspect of the medial femoral condyle.

There is aching pain after activity and, if the fragment becomes loose, locking or 'giving way' occurs. The lesion is seen on a tunnel-view X-ray, but MRI is more sensitive, especially if the fragment is undisplaced. Undisplaced lesions are treated with rest, then isometric quadriceps exercises. Loose fragments can be fixed arthroscopically or removed.

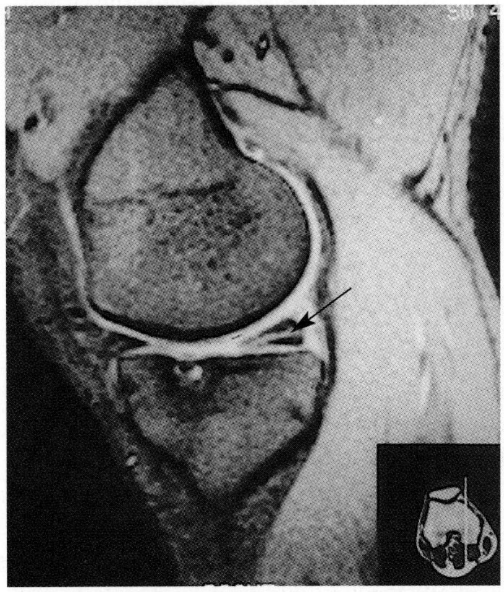

Fig 8.8
MRI of a knee, showing a complete tear of the posterior horn of the medial meniscus, extending to its lower surface (arrow)

Knee joint effusions

An effusion of the knee causes swelling, stiffness and pain. The pain is more severe with an acute onset and with increasing inflammation due to stretching of the capsule which contains the pain receptors. A full clinical history and examination must include a past medical, family and drug history.

Inflammatory arthritis affects the knees by causing warmth and swelling. An acute inflammatory monarthritis of the knee is a common presentation of a seronegative spondarthritis and occasionally is the first sign of RA.

Monarthritis of the knee, associated with severe pain and marked redness, may be due to septic arthritis or gout in the middle-aged male, or to gout or pseudogout in an older male or female. A cool, clear, viscous effusion is frequently seen in elderly patients with moderate or severe OA.

EXAMINATION

A large and tense effusion is easily seen and felt on each side of the patella and in the suprapatellar pouch, and is fluctuant. The effusion delays the patella tapping against the femur when it is pressed firmly (the 'patellar tap' sign). Small effusions also demonstrate the 'bulge' sign when the patient is lying with the quadriceps relaxed. For this, apply a gentle sweeping pressure, first to the medial side of the joint and then, watching the medial dimple, to the lateral side. Slightly delayed bulging of the medial dimple indicates fluid in the joint.

INVESTIGATIONS

These are (a) blood biochemistry, and (b) aspiration and examination of the knee effusion. The basic technique of aspiration is described in Practical box 8.2 on p. 452.

If there is a flexion deformity, externally rotate the leg or support the knee. Approach the joint from the opposite side and insert the needle between the patella, just proximal to its mid point, and the medial femoral condyle. Angle the needle slightly backwards and inject small volumes of local anaesthetic, advancing until aspiration detects fluid. Then change the syringe for a larger one and aspirate as much fluid as possible. Examine the fluid (see Information box 8.2 on p. 453) and decide whether to inject corticosteroid or arrange microbiological tests.

Haemarthrosis of the knee

This is caused by:

- trauma – meniscal, cruciate or synovial lining tear
- clotting or bleeding disorders, such as haemophilia, sickle cell disease or von Willebrand's disease.

Popliteal cyst (Baker's cyst)

In approximately 5% of patients with a knee effusion, a swollen, painful popliteal cyst develops. This is due either to a bursa (usually the semimembranosus bursa), which has a valve-like connection to the knee which allows the effusion to flow into the bursa but not back, or to a synovial herniation through the posterior joint capsule. Some popliteal cysts do not, however, communicate with the knee.

The cyst is best seen and felt in the popliteal fossa with the patient standing.

Ruptured popliteal cyst. A popliteal cyst may rupture if the patient is mobile, particularly on standing up quickly or climbing stairs. Fluid escapes into the soft tissue of the popliteal fossa and upper calf, causing sudden and severe pain, swelling and tenderness of the upper calf. Dependent oedema of ankle develops and the knee effusion reduces dramatically in size and may be undetectable.

A history of previous knee problems, the sudden onset of pain and tenderness high in the calf suggest a ruptured cyst rather than a deep vein thrombosis (DVT). However, the diagnosis is often missed and treated inappropriately with anticoagulants. A diagnostic ultrasound distinguishes a ruptured cyst from a DVT (see p. 742). Analgesics or NSAIDs, rest with the leg elevated, aspiration and injection with corticosteroids into the knee joint are required.

Pain in the foot and heel (Table 8.10)

The feet are subjected to extreme pressures by weight-bearing and inappropriate shoes. They are commonly painful. Broad, deep, thick-soled shoes are essential for sporting activities, prolonged walking or standing, and in people with congenitally flat or arthritic feet.

There are two common types of foot deformity:

- flat feet stress the ankle and throw the hind foot into a valgus (everted) position – a flat foot is rigid and inflexible
- high-arched feet place pressure on the lateral border and ball of the foot.

Table 8.10
Pain in the foot and heel – causes

Structural (flat (pronated) or high arched (supinated))	
Hallux valgus/rigidus (+/– OA)	
Metatarsalgia	
Morton's neuroma	
Stress fracture	
Inflammatory arthritis	
Acute, monarticular – gout	
Chronic, polyarticular – RA	
Chronic, pauciarticular – seronegative spondarthritis	
Tarsal tunnel syndrome	
Heel pain	
Plantar fasciitis	Below heel
Plantar spur	Below heel
Achilles tendonitis/bursitis	Behind heel
Sever's disease	
Arthritis of ankle/subtaloid joints	

The foot is affected by a variety of *inflammatory arthritic conditions*. After the hand, the foot joints are the most commonly affected by rheumatoid arthritis.The diagnosis depends upon careful assessment of the distribution of the joints affected, the pattern of other joint problems, or by finding the associated condition (e.g. psoriasis – see p. 1165).

Hallux valgus

The great toe migrates laterally. In the congenital form the first metatarsal is displaced medially (metatarsus primus varus). Later onset hallux valgus is caused by the shape of modern shoes and is a common complication of RA.

Hallux rigidus

Osteoarthritis of the first MTP joint in a normally aligned or valgus joint causes hallux rigidus – a stiff, dorsiflexed and painful great toe. Careful choice of footwear and the help of a podiatrist suffice for most cases, but some require surgery.

Metatarsalgia

This is common, especially in women who wear high heels, after trauma and in those with hammer toes. The ball of the foot is painful to walk and stand on. Callosities and pressure-induced bursae develop under the metatarsal heads. Rheumatoid arthritis causes misalignment of the metatarsal bones and severe metatarsalgia.

Treatment is with podiatry and the wearing of appropriate shoes. Surgery is occasionally needed, particularly in the rheumatoid forefoot.

Morton's metatarsalgia is due to a neuroma, usually between the third and fourth toes. It causes pain, burning and numbness in the adjacent surfaces of the affected toes when walking. It is helped by wearing wider, cushioned-soled shoes.

Stress (march) fractures

These cause sudden, severe weight-bearing pain in the distal shaft of the fractured metatarsal bone. They occur after unaccustomed walking or with new shoes. There is local tenderness and swelling, but initially X-rays are normal and diagnosis delayed. A radioisotope bone scan reveals the fracture earlier than X-rays. Reduced weight-bearing usually suffices.

Tarsal tunnel syndrome

This is an entrapment neuropathy of the posterior tibial nerve as it rounds the medial maleolus. It produces burning, tingling and numbness of the toes, sole and medial arch. The nerve is tender below the maleolus and, when tapped, produces a shock-like pain (Tinel's sign). A local steroid injection under the retinaculum, between the medial maleolus and calcaneum, is helpful.

Pain under the heel

Plantar fasciitis is an enthesitis at the insertion of the tendon into the calcaneum. It produces localized pain when standing and walking, and tenderness in the midline. It occurs alone or in seronegative spondarthritis.

Plantar spurs are traction lesions at the insertion of the plantar fascia in older people and are usually asymptomatic. They become painful after trauma.

Calcaneal bursitis is a pressure-induced (adventitious) bursa which produces diffuse pain and tenderness under the heel. Compression of the heel pad from the sides is painful, which distinguishes it from plantar fascia pain.

TREATMENT

All of these lesions are treated with heel pads, and reduced walking. A local corticosteroid injection is occasionally helpful. A medial approach is used, rather than through the heel pad, under a posterior tibial nerve block.

Pain behind the heel and leg

Sever's disease is a traction apophysitis of the Achilles tendon in young people (cf. Osgood–Schlatter's disease).

Achilles tendonitis is an enthesitis at the insertion of the tendon into the calcaneum. This is traumatic or it can complicate seronegative spondarthritis. Pain is reduced by raising the shoe heel and a low-pressure corticosteroid injection near the enthesis.

Partial tear of the Achilles tendon causes a painful, tender swelling a few centimetres above its insertion. Advise against walking barefoot and jumping. Therapeutic ultrasound is helpful. (*Caution* – a local injection may cause the tendon to rupture.)

Achilles' bursitis lies clearly anterior to the tendon and can be safely injected with corticosteroid.

Compartment syndromes

The muscles of the lower leg are enclosed in a compartment of fascia, with little room for expansion to occur. Compartment syndromes can be acute and severe, such as following exercise.

In the *anterior tibial syndrome* there is severe pain in the front of the shin, occasionally with foot drop. Immediate surgical decompression to prevent muscle necrosis is sometimes required.

Chronic compartment syndrome produces pain in the lower leg that is aggravated by exercise and may therefore be mistaken for a vascular or neurological disorder.

Pain in the chest

Musculoskeletal conditions are sometimes a cause of chest pain. An example is Tietze's disease. In this condition, pain arises from the costosternal junctions. It is usually unilateral and affects one, two or three joints. There is local tenderness, which helps to make the diagnosis. The condition is benign and self-limiting. It often responds well to anti-inflammatory drugs, or may be treated with local injections of corticosteroid and local anaesthetic.

Chronic pain syndromes

Aches and pains are extremely common with increasing age. Many are minor and self-limiting, but others persist and are often attributed to vague musculoskeletal disorders. These chronic pain syndromes are difficult to manage. It is essential to be objective and non-judgmental when dealing with them, discussing physical, psychological and social factors without assuming which is primary. Chronic pain syndromes are difficult to explain scientifically and it is all too easy for a doctor to 'blame' the patient for this lack of explanation.

Any chronic painful condition can change the way a person copes. Some people with chronic diseases or chronic pain cope well, but others adopt coping strategies and patterns of behaviour which make things worse. They become anxious, depressed or socially isolated, and their quality of life is reduced. In chronic pain syndromes patients need help to lead a more normal life despite their pain, and are best referred to a specialist, multi-disciplinary pain service.

Psychological states such as depression and anxiety produce physical symptoms, of which one is pain, while people with frank physical diseases are often understandably anxious and depressed.

Fibromyalgia (fibrositis syndrome)

'Fibromyalgia' is a controversial diagnosis that is not universally accepted. It is a useful diagnosis of exclusion. Patients value a name to explain symptoms previously dismissed or attributed simply to psychological or social problems. A typical feature of fibromyalgia is tender trigger points. The tenderness is not 'all over', a point which distinguishes it from anxiety states. The patient is usually a middle-aged, middle-class woman who struggles on with her work and/or housework despite the pain. Her complaints are often vocal and her actions reinforced by others: 'She is so brave to carry on despite all her pain!'. Such individuals are difficult to live with and there is often family discord. Many patients have sleep disturbances, so they awake unrefreshed and have poor concentration.

The pain is a widespread, unremitting, aching discomfort. There are often other health problems, such as chronic fatigue syndrome (see below), irritable bowel syndrome, premenstrual syndrome, tension headache, anxiety and depression; doctors sometimes label them 'heart sink' patients. The patient's frustration is compounded by the fact that most tests are normal, and they fear doctors believe it is 'all in their mind'.

TREATMENT

A sympathetic approach is appropriate, with reassurance for the patient that fibromylagia often improves. Encouragement should be given to undertake a graded aerobic exercise regimen. When depression is present, it should be treated, but potentially addictive anxiolytic agents are best avoided. A behavioural psychologist may persuade the person to pace their life more effectively and to cope better, although they often resist referral.

Drugs

- Analgesics or NSAIDs help in some cases but are best used intermittently.
- Low doses of sedative antidepressant drugs, such as amitriptylline or dothiepin, help when taken a few hours before bedtime. It should be explained that these doses are analgesic and not antidepressant, and their side-effects should be outlined.
- Trigger-point injections with local anaesthetic, corticosteroids or acupuncture are sometimes helpful.

Chronic fatigue syndrome

Diffuse muscular pain and stiffness is common in this condition, which is described on p. 66.

Chronic (work-related) upper-limb pain syndrome

This name is preferred to 'repetitive strain injury' (RSI). The predominant symptoms are pain in all or part of one or both arms. A specific lesion, such as tennis elbow or carpal tunnel syndrome, or muscular-pattern neck pain often develops first, and early recognition and treatment may prevent chronicity. After a variable period, the pain becomes more diffuse and no longer simply work-related, and there is often severe distress. It is seen in keyboard workers and others who perform the same task without breaks for prolonged periods, and in musicians. When it arises at work, it is often at a time of changing work practices, shortage of staff or disharmony. Middle managers find it difficult to deal with and this compounds the stress.

It is seen throughout the developed world. It peaked in incidence in Australia in the 1970s and 1980s but has largely disappeared there, apparently because of changes in work practices, improvements in early medical management, changes in workers' compensation legislation, and reduced media discussion of the problem.

TREATMENT

If possible there should be a brief period off work and a gradual return to activity once the pain has settled. Cautious use of analgesia and NSAIDs, with physiotherapy, is helpful during the initial phase to prevent a vicious circle developing.

A review of working practices and the positioning of screen, keyboard and chair are essential, as is the support of the patient by their manager. Musicians are helped by expert advice on playing technique and should reduce playing times temporarily, but not stop completely.

Temporomandibular pain dysfunction syndrome

This is a disorder of the temporomandibular joint associated with abnormalities of bite. It particularly occurs in anxious people who grind their teeth at night. It gives rise to pain and clicking in one or both temporomandibular joints.

Treatment is dental correction of the bite. However, when no dental cause is found, low-dose tricyclic antidepressant therapy may help. Many patients are exposed to much unnecessary dental treatment.

Reflex sympathetic dystrophy (RSD), Sudek's atrophy or chronic regional pain syndrome type I

This is defined as 'a complex disorder or group of disorders that may develop as a consequence of trauma affecting the limbs, with or without obvious nerve lesions'. It may also develop after central nervous system lesions (e.g. strokes), or without cause. Its features are pain and other sensory abnormalities, such as abnormal blood flow and sweating, motor system abnormalities and structural changes of superficial and deep tissues (trophic changes). Not all components need be present. The sensory, motor and sympathetic nerve changes are not restricted to the distribution of a single nerve and may be remote from the site of injury.

- The early phase – with pain, swelling and increased skin temperature – is difficult to diagnose but potentially reversible.
- After a period of weeks or months a second, still painful, dystrophic phase develops, characterized by cold skin and trophic changes, often with localized osteoporosis.
- A late phase involves continued pain, skin and muscle atrophy and muscle contractures and is extremely disabling.

TREATMENT

Management is difficult and the problem often very disabling. Pain relief and general care of the patient are essential. Referral to a pain management clinic is advisable.

Analgesic and anti-inflammatory drugs for musculoskeletal problems

The key to using drugs, particularly in chronic disorders and the elderly, is to balance risk and benefit and constantly to review their appropriateness. Information box 8.5 shows the main drugs available. Adverse drug reactions are discussed in Chapter 14.

Simple and compound analgesic agents

Simple agents such as paracetamol, aspirin, or codeine compounds (or combination preparations), used when necessary or regularly, relieve pain and improve function. Sleep may also be improved. Side-effects are relatively infrequent, although drowsiness and constipation occur with codeine preparations, especially in the elderly.

Stronger analgesics, such as dihydrocodeine or morphine derivatives, should be used only with severe pain.

Non-steroidal anti-inflammatory drugs (NSAIDs)

NSAIDs have anti-inflammatory and centrally acting analgesic properties. They inhibit cyclo-oxygenase (COX), a key enzyme in the formulation of prostaglandins, prostacyclins and thromboxanes. There are two specific cyclo-oxygenase enzymes: COX-1, the constitutive, and COX-2, the inducible form.

- COX-1 is present in many normal tissues, where it stimulates prostaglandin (PGE) production. Inhibition of the enzyme by NSAIDs produces side effects caused, for example, by the loss of gastric mucosal protection and a decrease in renal blood flow.
- COX-2 is induced in response to pro-inflammatory cytokines and is not found in normal tissues. It is associated with oedema and the nociceptive and pyretic effects of inflammation. COX 2-specific NSAIDs may produce fewer side-effects.

Information

Analgesics (in order of potency)

Advise that they be taken *only* if needed. Maximum doses are indicated here.

Paracetamol	500–1000 mg	6-hourly
Paracetamol with codeine	1–2 tablets	6-hourly
Paracetamol with dextropropoxyphene	1–2 tablets	6–8 hourly
Paracetamol with dihydrocodeine	1–2 tablets	6–8 hourly
Dihydrocodeine	30–60 mg	6–8 hourly

Non-steroidal anti-inflammatory drugs (NSAIDs)

Always to be taken with food. Use slow-release preparations in inflammatory conditions or if more regular pain control is needed. Examples:

Ibuprofen	200–400 mg	6–8 hourly
Ibuprofen slow release	600–800 mg	1–3 daily
Diclofenac	25–50 mg	8-hourly
Diclofenac slow release	75–100 mg	1–2 daily
Nabumetone	500–1000 mg	1–2 daily

Information box 8.5 Analgesics and NSAIDs

Uses

- *Short courses* of NSAIDs are used occasionally in *osteoarthritis* and *spondylosis*, even when there is minimal inflammation.
- In *crystal synovitis*, NSAIDs have a true anti-inflammatory effect (see p. 484).
- In *chronic inflammatory synovitis*, NSAIDs do not alter the chronic inflammatory process, nor decrease the risk of joint damage, but they do reduce pain and stiffness.
- Slow-release preparations are useful for *inflammatory arthritis* and when more constant pain control is needed.

Side-effects

The most common side-effects of NSAIDs are indigestion or skin rashes. Gastric erosions and frank peptic ulceration also occur. H_2-blockers, proton-pump inhibitors and prostaglandin-E_2 analogues help as gastroprotective agents for long-term treatment of those at risk of peptic ulceration. In the elderly, NSAIDs may cause peptic ulceration and gastrointestinal bleeding without warning symptoms, thereby causing significant morbidity and mortality. They may also reduce renal function, especially in the elderly.

FURTHER READING

Jayson MIV (ed) (1992) The Lumbar Spine and Back Pain, 4th edn. Churchill Livingstone, London.

Yassi A (1997) Repetitive strain injuries. *Lancet* **349**: 943–947.

Osteoarthritis (OA)

Osteoarthritis is a condition of synovial joints characterized by cartilage loss with an accompanying peri-articular bone response. There is no simple definition of OA as it requires consideration of three overlapping areas – pathological changes, radiological features and clinical consequences. Pathologically, there is an alteration in cartilage structure, radiologically there are osteophytes and joint space narrowing, and clinically patients complain of pain and disability.

EPIDEMIOLOGY

Osteoarthritis is the most common type of arthritis. The prevelance increases with age, and most people over 60 years will have some radiological evidence of it. It occurs world-wide, although OA of the hip is less common in black and Chinese populations than in Caucasians. Most epidemiological studies have been based on radiological evidence, which of course is much more frequent than symptomatic OA. Women over 55 years are affected more commonly than men of a similar age. There is a familial pattern of inheritance in women with distal interphalangeal joint involvement. OA has a variable distribution (Fig 8.9). The resulting disabilities have major socioeconomic resource implications, particularly in the developed world where individuals have ever increasing expectations of health-care.

AETIOLOGY

Osteoarthritis is the result of active, sometimes inflammatory but potentially reparative processes rather than the inevitable result of trauma and ageing. It includes a wide spectrum of idiopathic joint disorders with focal destruction of the articular cartilage as the common pathological feature. The spectrum ranges from *atrophic* disease in which bone destruction occurs without any subchondral bone response, to *hypertrophic* disease in which there is massive new bone formation at the joint margins.

Cartilage is a matrix of collagen fibres (mainly type II – see p. 517), enclosing a mixture of proteoglycans (see below) and water. The properties of this matrix are that it is smooth-surfaced and shock-absorbing. Under normal circumstances there is a dynamic balance between cartilage degradation by wear and its production by chondrocytes. Early in the development of OA the surface of the cartilage becomes fibrillated and fissured as the collagen matrix breaks down. These changes lead to focal erosion of cartilage. Chondrocytes die and, although repair is attempted from adjacent cartilage, the process is

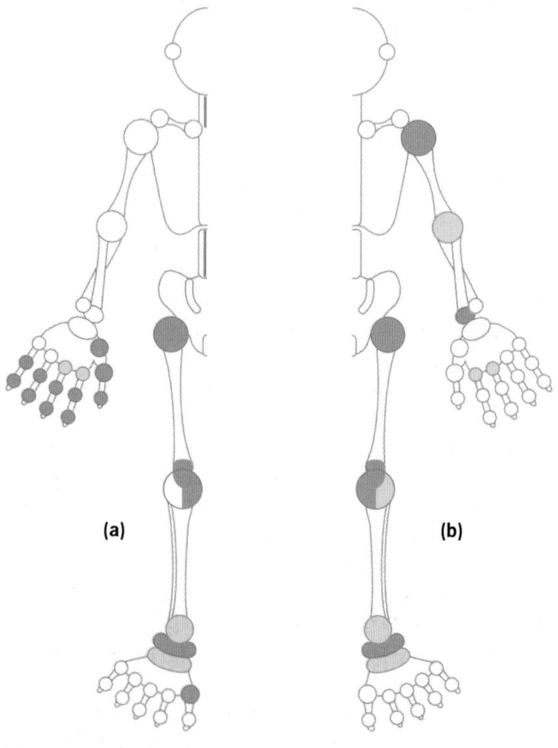

Fig 8.9
Typical distribution of affected joints in (a) generalized nodal OA and (b) pyrophosphate arthropathy (dark circle), more commonly affected; (light circle) less commonly affected

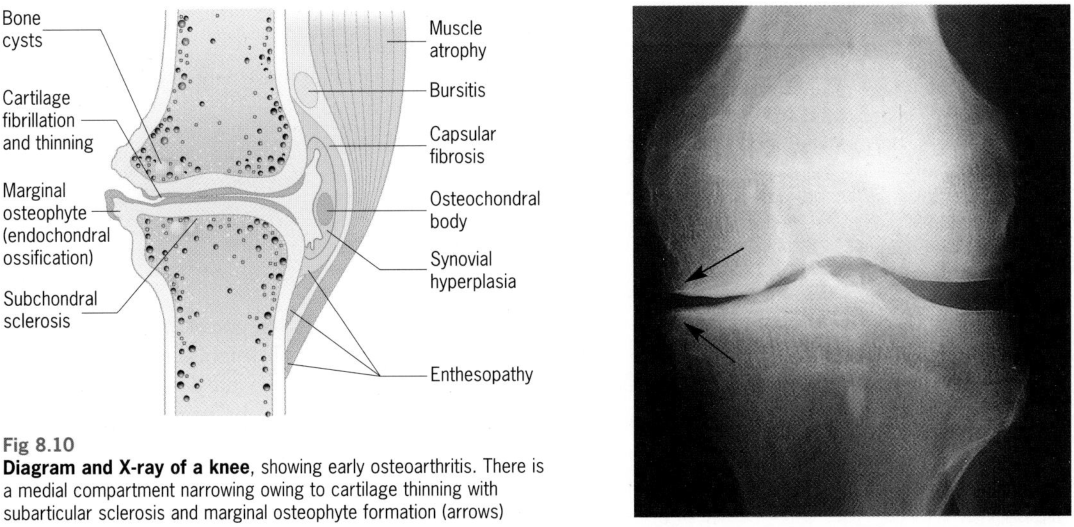

Fig 8.10
Diagram and X-ray of a knee, showing early osteoarthritis. There is a medial compartment narrowing owing to cartilage thinning with subarticular sclerosis and marginal osteophyte formation (arrows)

disordered. Cartilage ulceration exposes underlying bone to increased stress, producing microfractures and cysts. The bone attempts repair but produces abnormal sclerotic subchondral bone and overgrowths at the joint margins, called *osteophytes* (Fig 8.10).

Proteoglycans are present mainly as large molecular aggrecans which consist of a protein core with attached chondroitin and keratan–sulphate chains. The gene for human aggrecan has been cloned and polymorphisms of the gene have been correlated with OA of the hand in older men.

PATHOGENESIS

Several mechanisms have been suggested for the pathogenesis:

- Matrix loss is caused by the action of metalloproteinases such as stromelysin, collagenase and gelatinase which degrade collagen and proteoglycans.
- There is synovial inflammation in OA, producing interleukin-1 (IL-1) and tumour necrosis factor (TNFα). These cytokines stimulate metalloproteinase production and IL-1 inhibits type II collagen production.
- Growth factors, including insulin-like growth factor (IGF-1) and transforming growth factor (TGFβ), are involved in collagen synthesis and may play a role in stimulating collagen repair.
- Mutations in the gene for type II collagen (COL2A1) have been associated with early polyarticular OA.
- Twin studies suggest a strong hereditary element underlying OA, and further studies may reveal genetic markers for the disease.
- In the Caucasian population there is an inverse relationship between the risk of developing OA and osteoporosis.
- A large population study has suggested that a high intake of vitamin C and other antioxidants may reduce the risk of OA. The lack of antioxidants are thought to contribute to many ageing processes.
- In women, weight-bearing sports produce a two- to three-fold increase in risk of OA of the hip and knee.

The term *primary OA* is sometimes used when there is no obvious known predisposing factor.

Information box 8.6 shows some of the predisposing factors for the development of OA, whilst Table 8.11 shows other causes that are sometimes described as secondary arthritis.

CLINICAL FEATURES

Osteoarthritis affects many joints, with diverse clinical patterns. Hip and knee OA is the major cause of disability. However, early OA is rarely symptomatic unless

Table 8.11
Causes of osteoarthritis

Primary OA	No known cause
Secondary OA	Pre-existing joint damage
	rheumatoid arthritis
	gout
	seronegative spondarthritis
	septic arthritis
	Paget's disease
	avascular necrosis, e.g. corticosteroid therapy
	Metabolic disease
	chondrocalcinosis
	hereditary haemochromatosis
	acromegaly
	Systemic diseases
	haemophilia – recurrent haemarthrosis
	haemoglobinopathies, e.g. sickle cell disease
	neuropathies
	Mechanical factors
	trauma and meniscal/cruciate tears
	joint hypermobility
	joint dysplasia

Information

- *Obesity* – Predicts later risk of radiological and symptomatic OA in population studies.
- *Heredity* – Familial tendency to develop nodal and generalized OA.
- *Sex* – Polyarticular OA is more common in women; a higher prevalence after the menopause suggests a role for sex hormones.
- *Hypermobility* (see p. 499) – Increased range of joint motion and reduced stability lead to OA.
- *Osteoporosis* – There is reduced risk of OA.
- Other diseases – See Table 8.11.
- *Trauma* – A fracture through a joint or meniscal and cruciate ligament tears cause OA of the knee.
- *Congenital joint dysplasia* – Alters joint biomechanics and leads to OA. Mild acetabular dysplasia is common and leads to earlier onset of hip OA.
- *Joint congruity* – Congenital dislocation of the hip or a slipped femoral epiphysis or Perthe's disease; osteonecrosis of the femoral head (see p. 460) in children and adolescents cause early-onset OA.
- *Occupation* – Miners develop OA of the hip, knee and shoulder, cotton workers OA of the hand, and farmers OA of the hip.
- *Sport* – Repetitive use and injury in some sports causes a high incidence of lower-limb OA.

Information box 8.6 Factors predisposing to osteoarthritis

accompanied by a joint effusion, whilst advanced radiological and pathological OA is not always symptomatic.

Some flare-ups are due to inflammation but are not associated with an increased ESR or CRP. Focal synovitis is caused by fragments of shed bone or cartilage. Radiological OA is usually, but not inevitably, progressive. This progression may be stepwise or continual. Radiological improvement is uncommon but has been observed, suggesting that repair is possible.

Symptoms

- Joint pain
- Morning stiffness
- Joint gelling
- Joint instability
- Loss of function.

Table 8.12
Features of nodal OA

Familial
Has a higher incidence in women
Typical pattern of polyarticular involvement of the hand joints
Develops in late middle age
Has a generally good long-term functional outcome
Predisposes to OA of the knee, hip and spine

Signs

- Crepitus on movement
- Limitation of range of movement
- Joint instability
- Joint effusion
- Bony swelling
- Wasting of muscles.

CLINICAL SUBSETS

Nodal OA (Table 8.12)

The joints are usually affected one at a time over several years, with the distal interphalangeal joints (DIPs) being more often involved than the proximal interphalangeal joints (PIPs). The onset may be painful and associated with tenderness, swelling and inflammation and impairment of hand function. The inflammation often occurs around the female menopause. PIP-predominant nodal OA has a superficial similarity to early rheumatoid arthritis. A weakly positive rheumatoid factor is occasionally found, but is of no significance. The inflammatory phase settles after some months or years, leaving painless bony swellings posterolaterally with Heberden's nodes (DIPs) and Bouchard's nodes (PIPs), along with stiffness and deformity (Fig 8.11). Functional impairment is slight for most, although PIP osteoarthritis restricts gripping more than DIP involvement. On X-ray, the nodes are marginal osteophytes and there is joint space loss.

Carpometacarpal and metacarpophalangeal OA of the thumb coexist with nodal OA and cause pain which decreases as the joint stiffens. The 'squared' hand in OA is caused by bony swelling of the carpometacarpal joint and fixed adduction of the thumb. Function is rarely severely compromised.

Polyarticular hand OA is associated with a slightly increased frequency of OA at other sites.

Erosive OA

This is rare. The DIPs and PIPs are inflamed and equally affected. In contrast to nodal OA, the functional outcome

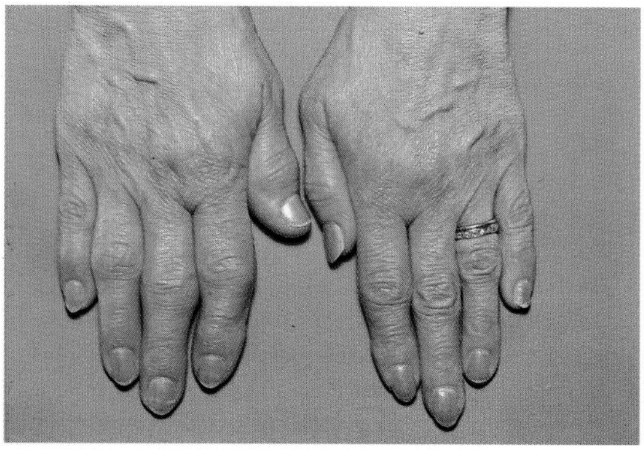

Fig 8.11
Nodal osteoarthritis in the hands showing Heberden's and Bouchard's nodes and squaring of the thumb bases

is poor. Radiologically, there are marked subchondral cysts. Erosive OA may develop into RA and may not be a true subset of OA.

Generalized OA

This is less common than nodal OA of the hands but is usually seen in combination – 'nodal generalized OA' (NGOA). The other joints affected are the knees, first MTP and hip joints. There is a female preponderance and a strong familial tendency. NGOA is associated with immune complex deposition and may have an autoimmune cause.

Large-joint OA

This affects the hips and knees independently as well as in the context of NGOA.

The hips

There are two major subgroups defined by the radiological appearance. The most common is *superior-pole hip OA*, where joint space narrowing and sclerosis predominantly affect the weight-bearing upper surface of the femoral head and adjacent acetabulum. This is most common in men and unilateral at presentation, although both hips may become involved because the disease is progressive. Total hip replacement is a highly successful therapeutic outcome. Less commonly, *medial cartilage loss* occurs. This is most common in women and associated with hand involvement (NSOA), and is usually bilateral and less likely to need surgical replacement.

The knees

The disease is generally bilateral and strongly associated with *polyarticular OA of the hand* in elderly women. The medial compartment is most commonly affected and leads to a varus (bow-legged) deformity. There is often also retropatellar OA. Previous trauma, meniscal and cruciate ligament tears and obesity are risk factors for developing knee OA.

Crystal-associated OA

This is most commonly seen with calcium pyrophosphate deposition in the cartilage (*chondrocalcinosis*). Chondrocalcinosis increases in frequency with age, but is usually asymptomatic. The joints most commonly affected are the knees (hyaline cartilage and fibrocartilage) and wrists (triangular fibrocartilage). There is patchy linear calcification on X-ray (Fig 8.12).

A chronic arthropathy (pseudo-OA) occurs, predominantly in elderly women with severe chondrocalcinosis. There is a florid inflammatory component and marked osteophyte and cyst formation visible on X-rays. The joints affected differ from NGOA – affecting predominantly the knees, then wrists and shoulders, but also elbows, ankles and hips. Chondrocalcinosis is associated with pseudogout, an acute crystal-induced arthritis (see p. 485).

A rare, rapidly destructive arthritis in elderly women, affecting shoulders, hips and knees, is associated with

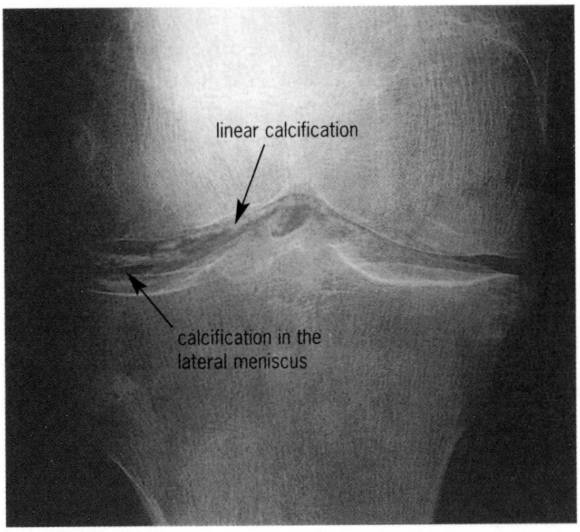

Fig 8.12
Chondrocalcinosis of the knee. Note the linear calcification in the hyaline cartilage and calcification of the lateral meniscus (plus mild secondary OA)

finding crystals of calcium apatite in a bloody joint effusion. The outlook is poor and joints require early surgical replacement.

INVESTIGATIONS IN OA

- **Blood tests**. There is no specific test; the ESR and CRP are normal. Rheumatoid factor and antinuclear antibodies are negative.
- **X-rays** are abnormal only when the damage is advanced.
- **MRI** can demonstrate early cartilage changes.
- **Arthroscopy** can reveal early fissuring and surface erosion of the cartilage.

TREATMENT

The guiding principle is to treat the symptoms and disability, not the radiological appearances. Education of the individual about the disease and its effects reduces pain, distress and disability and increases compliance with treatment. Psychological or social factors alter the impact of the disease.

Physical measures

Weight loss and exercises for strength and stability are useful. Hydrotherapy helps, especially in lower-limb OA. Local heat, ice-packs, massage and rubifacients or local NSAID gels give some relief.

Complementary medicine is commonly used and, despite lack of scientific evidence, little is lost in trying it since a number of patients do seem to be helped.

Medication

Balance the potential benefit against potential side-effects. Patients should be prescribed short courses of simple analgesics before NSAIDs on an intermittent basis (see Information box 8.5). It has been suggested that some NSAIDs may increase the cartilage damage, while others are 'chondroprotective', but these claims remain controversial.

Intra-articular corticosteroid injections produce short-term improvement when there is a painful joint effusion. Frequent injections into the same joint should be avoided.

Surgery

Total replacement arthroplasty has transformed the management of severe OA. The safety of hip and knee replacements is now equal, with a complication rate of about 1%; loosening, and late blood-borne infection are the most serious. These slight but definite risks make it essential that the patient is certain that surgery is wanted, when all else has been tried. For the vast majority, a total hip or knee replacement reduces pain and stiffness and greatly increases function.

Other surgical procedures include realignment osteotomy of the knee or hip, excision arthroplasty of the first MTP and base of the thumb, and fusion of a first MTP joint.

FURTHER READING

Creamer P, Hocberg MC (1997) Osteoarthritis. *Lancet* **350**: 503–508.

Inflammatory arthritis

Inflammatory arthritis includes a large number of arthritic conditions in which the predominant feature is synovial inflammation. This disparate group includes postviral arthritis, rheumatoid arthritis, seronegative spondarthritis, crystal arthritis and Lyme arthritis. The diagnosis of these conditions is helped by the pattern of joint involvement (Table 8.13), along with any nonarticular disease; a past and family history may be helpful. The distribution of the affected joints (symmetrical or asymmetrical; large or small) as well as the periodicity of the arthritis (relapsing, chronic and progressive; single acute) may also help in the diagnosis.

Certain nonarticular disease – for example, psoriasis, iritis, inflammatory bowel disease, nonspecific urethritis or recent dysentery – may suggest a seronegative spondarthritis. There may be evidence of recent viral illness (rubella, hepatitis B or parvovirus), of rheumatic fever, or of a tick bite and skin rash (Lyme disease). In early arthritis it may not be possible to make a specific diagnosis until the disease has evolved.

There is a distinct genetic separation of rheumatoid-pattern synovitis and the seronegative group; RA (p. 471) is associated with a genetic marker in the class II major histocompatibility genes, whilst seronegative spondarthritis shares certain alleles in the B locus of class I MHC genes, usually B27 (see p. 479).

Table 8.13
Pattern of joint involvement in inflammatory arthritis

Diseases presenting as an inflammatory monoarthritis
Crystal arthritis, e.g. gout, pseudogout
Septic arthritis
Palindromic rheumatism
Traumatic ± haemarthrosis
Arthritis due to juxta-articular bone turnover
Occasionally, psoriatic, reactive, rheumatoid may present as monoarthritis
Diseases presenting as an inflammatory polyarthritis
Rheumatoid arthritis
Reactive arthritis
Seronegative arthritis associated with psoriasis or ankylosing spondylitis
Post-viral arthritis
Lyme arthritis
Enteropathic arthritis
Arthritis associated with erythema nodosum

In general the pain and stiffness of inflammatory arthritis are worse in the morning and after rest. This early-morning exacerbation may last several hours, in contrast to the much shorter post-rest gelling of OA. Inflammatory markers (ESR and CRP) are often raised in inflammatory arthritis, and there is often a normochromic normocytic anaemia. Specific types of arthritis are discussed below.

Rheumatoid arthritis (RA)

Rheumatoid arthritis is a chronic symmetrical polyarthritis of unexplained cause. It is a systemic disorder characterized by chronic inflammatory synovitis of mainly peripheral joints. Its course is extremely variable and it is associated with nonarticular features.

AETIOLOGY AND PATHOGENESIS

- *Geographical.* RA has a worldwide distribution and affects 1–3% of the population. It is a significant cause of disability and mortality and carries a high socioeconomic cost.
- *Age.* RA presents from early childhood (when it is rare) to late old age. The most common age of onset is between 30 and 50 years.
- *Sex.* Women before the menopause are affected three times more often than men. After the menopause the frequency of onset is similar between the sexes, suggesting an aetiological role for sex hormones.
- *Familial.* The disease is familial but sporadic. In occasional families it affects several generations. The genetic contribution to its cause is estimated at 15–30%.

(a) (b)

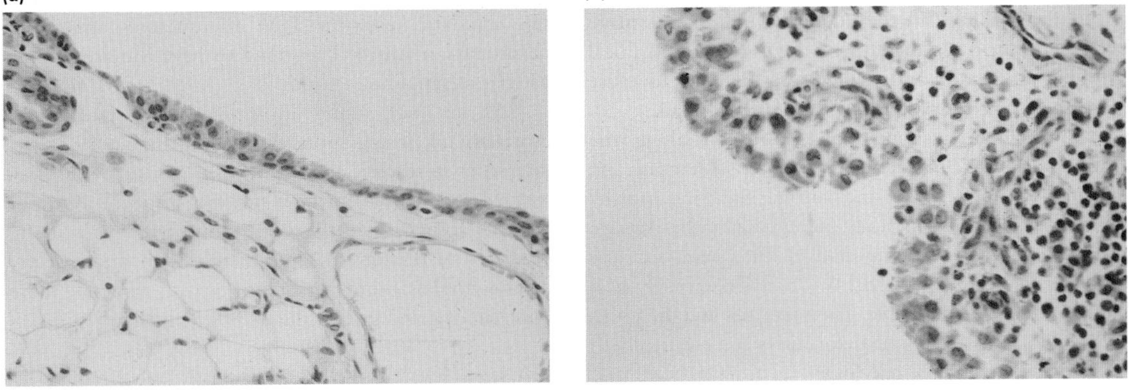

Fig 8.13
Histological appearances of RA synovium.
(a) Normal synovium
(b) Synovial appearances in established RA, showing marked hypertrophy of the tissues with infiltration by lymphocytes and plasma cells (From Shipley M (1993) *Colour Atlas of Rheumatology*, 3rd edn. Wolfe Mosby, with permission

- *HLA types*. There is a strong association between susceptibility to RA and certain HLA haplotypes. HLA-DR4, which occurs in 50–75% of patients, correlates with a poor prognosis and the possession of a specific pentapeptide in the third allelic hypervariable region of HLA-DRβ-1 chain increases susceptibility.

Immunology

The chronic synovial inflammation may be caused by ongoing *T-cell activation* or may be maintained by the local production of rheumatoid factors and continuous *stimulation of macrophages* via IgG *Fc* receptors. Considering the extent of synovial inflammation and lymphocytic infiltration, there are only minimal amounts of the factors produced by T cells (interferon and interleukin-2 and -4). Conversely, the cytokines (IL-1, IL-8, TNFα, granulocyte macrophage colony stimulating factor) and chemoattractive cytokines produced by macrophages (macrophage inflammatory protein, MIP and monocyte chemoattractant protein, MCP) and fibroblasts (IL-6) are abundant. The relevance of these changes is unclear.

CD4-specific antibodies, when used therapeutically, produce a specific helper T-cell lymphopenia but do not significantly alter the disease, raising the possibility that T cells are less important.

Antibodies to *TNFα* or specific blocking agents produce marked short-term improvement in synovitis, indicating the pivotal role of TNFα in the chronic synovitis (see p. 478). They also reduce the malaise felt in active RA.

Synovial fibroblasts have high levels of the *adhesion molecule*, vascular cell adhesion molecule (VCAM-1), a molecule which supports B lymphocyte survival and differentiation, and of delay accelerating factor (DAF), a factor which prevents complement-induced cell lysis. These molecules may facilitate the formation of ectopic lymphoid tissue in synovium.

The *triggering antigen* remains unclear, although it is suggested that the glycosylation pattern of immunglobulins may be abnormal in RA and lead to their becoming potentially antigenic. There is little evidence that collagen type II is the triggering antigen, although it is a cause of arthritis in animal models.

Bacterial or slow virus infections have been implicated but are unproven. It has been suggested that an immune response to any pathogen is to produce autoantibodies by B-cell clonal expansion. In susceptible individuals such clones may persist.

PATHOLOGY

Rheumatoid arthritis is typified by widespread persisting synovitis (inflammation of the synovial lining of joints, tendon sheaths or bursae). The cause of this is unclear, but the production of rheumatoid factors (RFs – see p. 472) by plasma cells in the synovium and the local formation of immune complexes may play a part. In RA, the normal synovium becomes greatly thickened to the extent that it is palpable as a 'boggy' swelling around the joints and tendons. There is proliferation of the synovium into folds and fronds, and it is infiltrated by a variety of inflammatory cells, including polymorphs, which transit through the tissue into the joint fluid, and lymphocytes and plasma cells. The normally sparse surface layer of lining cells becomes hyperplastic and thickened (Fig 8.13). There is marked vascular proliferation. Increased permeability of blood vessels and the synovial lining layer lead to joint effusions which contain lymphocytes and dying polymorphs. Activated lymphocytes and macrophages in the synovium produce a rich mixture of cytokines, including interleukins, prostaglandins and tumour necrosis factor alpha.

The hyperplastic synovium spreads from the joint margins on to the cartilage surface. This 'pannus' of inflamed synovium damages the underlying cartilage by blocking its normal route for nutrition and by the direct effects of cytokines on the chondrocytes. The cartilage becomes thinned and the underlying bone exposed. Local cytokine production and joint disuse combine to cause juxta-articular osteoporosis during active synovitis.

The proliferating synovium also grows along the course of blood vessels between the synovial margins and the epiphyseal bone cavity and damages the bone. Initially this is seen only histologically, but gradually the damage appears on X-rays as diagnostic ill-defined juxta-articular cavities called *erosions* (Fig 8.14). These occasionally heal but are generally irreversible. Their size, site and the joints affected lead to a variety of deformities and eventually to bony collapse or, rarely, ankylosis.

Rheumatoid factors (RFs)

These are circulating autoantibodies which have the *Fc* portion of immunoglobulin as their antigen. The nature of the antigen means that they self-aggregate into immune complexes and thus activate complement and stimulate inflammation, causing chronic synovitis. Transient production of RFs is an essential part of the body's normal mechanism for removing immune complexes, but in RA their production is persistent and occurs into the joints. They may be of any immunoglobulin class (IgM, IgG or IgA), but the most common tests employed clinically detect IgM rheumatoid factor. Around 70% of patients with polyarticular RA have serum IgM rheumatoid factor in the serum.

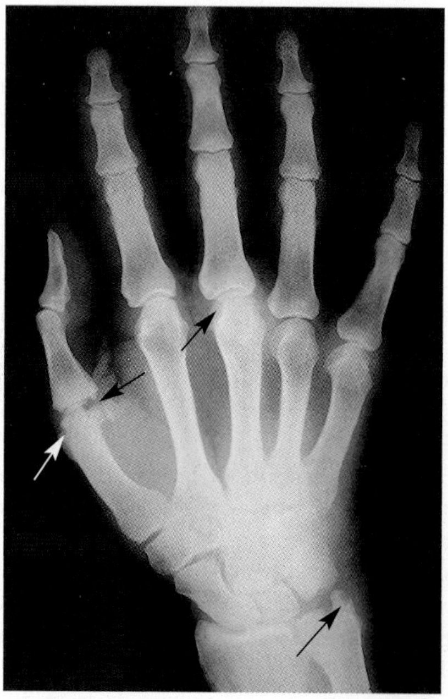

Fig 8.14
X-ray of early RA, showing typical erosions at the thumb and middle MCP joints and at the ulnar styloid

The term *seronegative RA* is used for patients in whom the standard tests for IgM rheumatoid factor are persistently negative. They tend to have a more limited pattern of synovitis.

RFs are not found in synovitis associated with psoriasis, ankylosing spondylitis or inflammatory bowel disease, or in reactive arthritis.

IgM rheumatoid factor is not diagnostic of RA, nor does its absence rule the disease out; but it is a useful predictor of prognosis. A persistently high titre in early disease implies more persistently active synovitis, more joint damage and greater disability eventually.

Clinical features of RA

TYPICAL PRESENTATION

The most typical presentation of rheumatiod arthritis (approximately 70% of cases) begins as a *slowly progressive, symmetrical, peripheral polyarthritis*, evolving over a period of a few weeks or months. Women are affected three times more often than men. The patient is usually in her thirties or forties, but the disease can occur at any age. Less commonly (15%) a *rapid onset* can occur over a few days (or explosively overnight) with a severe symmetrical polyarticular involvement, but surprisingly these patients often have a better prognosis. A worse than average prognosis (with a predictive accuracy of about 80%) is indicated by being female, a gradual onset over a few months, a positive IgM rheumatoid factor, and anaemia within three months of onset.

SYMPTOMS AND SIGNS

The majority of patients complain of pain and stiffness of the small joints of the hands (metacarpophalangeal, MCP), proximal and distal interphalangeal (PIP, DIP) and feet (metatarsophalangeal, MTP). The wrists, elbows, shoulders, knees and ankles are also affected. In most cases many joints are involved, but 10% present with a monoarthritis of the knee or shoulder or with a carpal tunnel syndrome. The hips are rarely affected early in the disease.

The patient feels tired and unwell and the pain and stiffness are significantly worse in the morning and may improve with gentle activity.

The joints are usually warm and tender with some joint swelling. There is limitation of movement and muscle wasting. Deformities develop as the disease progresses. Nonarticular features develop (see below).

OTHER PRESENTATIONS

The presentation and progression of RA can be very variable. Typical presentations are shown in Information box 8.7. There are relapses and remissions, occurring either spontaneously or in response to drug therapy, which slows or halts the progression of the disease. In some patients the disease remains active, producing progressive joint damage, whilst in others the inflammatory process may cease ('burnt-out RA').

A *seronegative, limited synovitis* initially affects the wrists more often than the fingers and has a less symmetrical joint involvement. It has a better long-term prognosis, but some cases progress to severe disability. This form can be confused with psoriatic arthropathy which has a similar distribution. There may be a family history of psoriasis or the patient may develop psoriasis later.

Palindromic rheumatism is unusual (5%) and consists of short-lived (24–48 h) episodes of acute monoarthritis. The joint becomes acutely painful, swollen and red, but resolves completely. Further attacks occur in the same or other joints. About 50% go on to develop typical chronic rheumatoid synovitis after a delay of months or years. The rest remit or continue to have acute episodic arthritis. The detection of IgM rheumatoid factor is a predictor of a change to chronic, destructive synovitis.

COMPLICATIONS (Table 8.14)

Septic arthritis

This is a serious complication with a high mortality. The joint (or joints) may be hot and inflamed with accompanying fever and a neutrophil leucocytosis in the blood. However, these signs are often absent, and any effusion, particularly of sudden onset, should be aspirated. *Staphylococcus aureus* is the most common organism. Treatment is with systemic antibiotics (see p. 485) and drainage.

Amyloidosis

Amyloidosis (see p. 1002) is found in a small number of cases of severe rheumatoid arthritis and this is the most common cause of secondary amyloidosis. Primary amyloidosis causes a polyarthritis that resembles RA in distribution and is also often associated with the carpal tunnel syndrome and subcutaneous nodules.

Information

- **Palindromic** – Monarticular attacks lasting 24–48 hours; 50% progress to other types of RA.
- **Transient** – A self-limiting disease, lasting less than 12 months and leaving no permanent joint damage. Usually seronegative for IgM rheumatoid factor. Some of these may be undetected post viral arthritis.
- **Remitting** – There is a period of several years during which the arthritis is active but then remits, leaving minimal damage.
- **Chronic, persistent** – The most typical form. It may be seropositive or seronegative for IgM rheumatoid factor. The disease follows a relapsing and remitting course over many years. Seropositive patients tend to develop greater joint damage and long-term disability.
- **Rapidly progressive** – The disease progresses remorselessly over a few years and leads rapidly to severe joint damage and disability. It is usually seropositive, has a high incidence of systemic complications and is difficult to treat.

Information box 8.7 Typical presentations of rheumatoid arthritis

Table 8.14
Complications of rheumatoid arthritis

Ruptured tendons
Joint infection
Ruptured joints, e.g. Baker's cysts
Spinal cord compression
Amyloidosis
Side effects of therapy
Anaemia
Marrow hypoplasia
Renal impairment
Gastrointestinal bleeding (dyspepsia)

Joint involvement in RA

Hands and wrists

The impact of RA on the hands is severe. In early disease the fingers are swollen, painful and stiff. Inflamed flexor tendon sheaths increase functional impairment and may cause carpal tunnel syndrome. Joint damage causes a variety of typical deformities. Most typical is a combination of ulnar drift and palmar subluxation of the MCPs (Fig 8.15). This leads to unsightly deformity, but function may be remarkably good once the patient has learned to adapt and pain is controlled. Fixed flexion (buttonhole – Boutonnière's – deformity) or fixed hyperextension (swan-neck deformity) of the PIP joint impair hand function.

Swelling and dorsal subluxation of the ulnar styloid leads to wrist pain and may cause rupture of the finger extensor tendons, leading in turn to a sudden onset of finger drop which needs urgent surgical repair.

Shoulders

The shoulders are commonly affected by RA. Initially the symptoms mimic rotator cuff tendonitis (see p. 455) with a painful arc syndrome and pain in the upper arms at night. As the joints become damaged more global stiffening occurs. Late in the disease rotator cuff tears are common (see p. 455) and interfere with dressing, feeding and personal toilet.

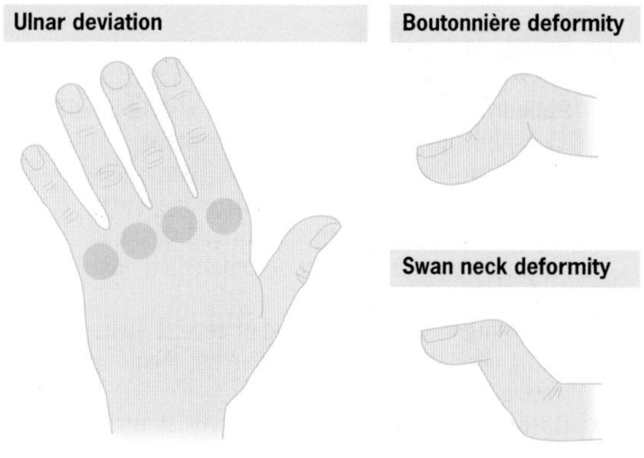

Fig 8.15
Characteristic hand deformities in rheumatoid arthritis

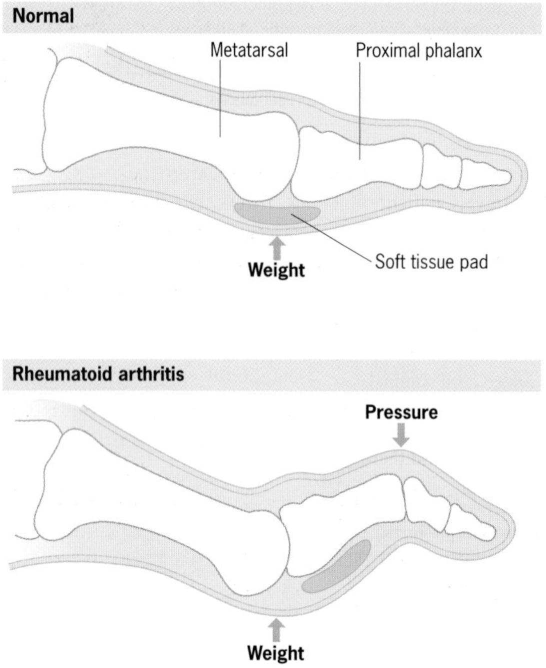

Fig 8.16
The toes in rheumatoid arthritis showing exposure of the metatarsal heads with forward migration of the soft tissue pads

Elbows

Synovitis of the elbows causes swelling and a painful fixed flexion deformity. In late disease flexion may be lost and severe difficulties with feeding result, especially combined with shoulder and hand and wrist deformities.

Feet

One of the earliest manifestations of RA is painful swelling of the MTP joints. The foot becomes broader and a hammer-toe deformity develops. Exposure of the metatarsal heads to pressure by the forwards migration of the protective fibrofatty pad (Fig 8.16) causes pain. Ulcers may develop over the metatarsal heads and the dorsum of the toes. Mid- and hind-foot RA causes a flat medial arch and loss of flexibility of the foot. The ankle often assumes a valgus position. Peripheral oedema is common and compounds the walking difficulties. Appropriate broad, deep shoes are essential but rarely wholly adequate and walking is often painful and limited. Surgery helps sometimes.

Knees

Massive synovitis and knee effusions occur, but respond well to aspiration and injection (see p. 452). A persistent effusion increases the risk of popliteal cyst formation and rupture. In later disease, erosion of cartilage and bone causes loss of joint space on X-ray and damage to the medial and/or lateral and/or retropatellar compartments of the knees. Depending on the pattern of involvement, the knees may develop a varus or valgus deformity. Secondary OA follows. Total knee replacement is often the only way to restore mobility and relieve pain.

Hips

The hips are rarely affected in early RA and are less commonly affected than the knees at all stages of the disease. Pain and stiffness are accompanied by radiological loss of joint space and juxta-articular osteoporosis. Later, secondary OA develops. Hip replacement is usually necessary.

Cervical spine

Painful stiffness of the neck in RA is often muscular, but it may be due to rheumatoid synovitis affecting the synovial joints of the upper cervical spine and the bursae which separate the odontoid peg from the anterior arch of the atlas and from its retaining ligaments. This synovitis leads to bone destruction, damages the ligaments and causes atlantoaxial or upper cervical instability. Subluxation and local synovial swelling may damage the spinal cord, producing pyramidal and sensory signs. MRI is the best way of visualizing this, but plain lateral flexed and extended neck X-rays can demonstrate instability. In late RA, difficulty walking which cannot be explained by articular disease, weakness of the legs or loss of control of bowel or bladder may be due to spinal cord compression and is a neurosurgical emergency.

Other joints

The temporomandibular, acromioclavicular, sternoclavicular, crico-arytenoid and any other synovial joint can be affected.

Nonarticular manifestations (Fig 8.17)

Soft tissue surrounding joints

Subcutaneous nodules are firm, intradermal and generally occur over pressure points, typically the elbows, the finger joints and the Achilles tendon. They occur on the sacrum and occiput in bed-bound patients. They may ulcerate and become infected, but usually resolve when the disease comes under control. The nodules can be removed surgically or injected with corticosteroids if causing a problem. Histologically there is a necrotic centre surrounded by rows of activated macrophages. This resembles synovitis without a synovial space.

The olecranon and other bursae may be swollen (*bursitis*).

Tenosynovitis of affected flexor tendons in the hand can cause a trigger finger. Swelling of the extensor tendon sheath over the dorsum of the wrist is common.

Muscle wasting around joints is common. Muscle enzyme concentrations are normal; myositis is extremely rare. Corticosteroid-induced myopathy is common.

Lungs (see also p. 809)

Peripheral, intrapulmonary nodules are usually asymptomatic but may cavitate. When pneumoconiosis is present (Caplan's syndrome), large cavitating lung nodules develop. Other manifestations are:

- serositis causing pleural effusion
- pleural nodules
- diffuse fibrosing alveolitis
- obstructive bronchiolitis.

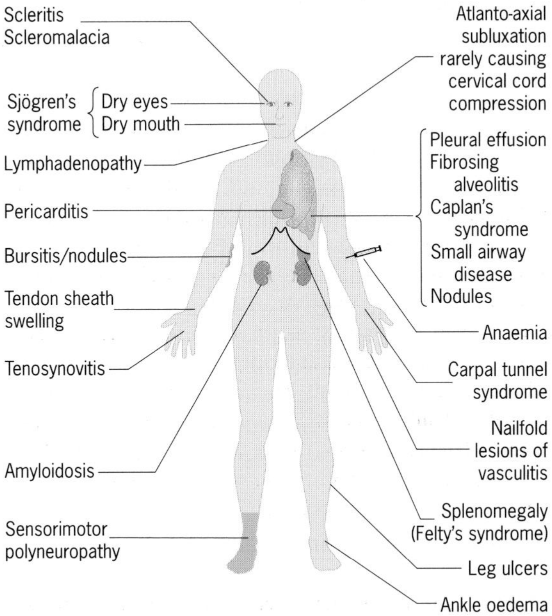

Fig 8.17
Nonarticular manifestations of RA

Vasculitis

Vasculitis (see p. 493) is caused by immune complex deposition in arterial walls. Smoking is a risk factor. Other manifestations are:

- nail-fold infarcts due to cutaneous vasculitis
- widespread cutaneous vasculitis with necrosis of the skin (seen in patients with very active, strongly seropositive disease)
- mononeuritis multiplex (p. 1093)
- bowel infarction due to necrotizing arteritis of the mesenteric vessels (this may be indistinguishable from polyarteritis nodosa).

The heart and peripheral vessels

Clinical pericarditis usually only occurs in strongly seropositive RA (10% of cases). If carefully looked for, for example by echocardiogram or in postmortem studies, 30–40% of patients show pericardial involvement. Constrictive pericarditis is very rare.

Endocarditis and myocardial disease are rarely seen clinically, although found at postmortem in approximately 20% of cases. These are secondary to the vasculitis.

Raynaud's syndrome may occur (see p. 741).

The nervous system

Neuropathies, either mononeuritis multiplex or a sensory loss in a glove and stocking pattern, are due to vasculitis of the vasa nervorum. Compression neuropathies such as carpal or tarsal tunnel syndrome are due to local synovial hypertrophy. Atlanto-axial subluxation can cause serious neurological abnormalities.

The eyes

Scleritis and episcleritis occur in severe, seropositive disease and produce painful red lesions in the eye. Scleritis may lead to perforation of the eye (scleromalacia perforans) and requires active treatment with local and systemic corticosteroids.

Sicca syndrome causes dry mouth and eyes (see Sjögren's syndrome on p. 492).

The kidneys

Amyloidosis causes the nephrotic syndrome and renal failure. Presentation is with proteinuria. It occurs in severe, longstanding rheumatoid disease and is due to the deposition of highly stable serum amyloid A protein (SAP) in the intercellular matrix of a variety of organs. SAP is an acute-phase reactant, produced normally in the liver.

The spleen, lymph nodes and blood

Felty's syndrome is splenomegaly and neutropenia in a patient with RA. Leg ulcers or sepsis are complications. HLA-DRW4 is found in 95% of patients, compared with 70% of patients with RA alone. Skin pigmentation also occurs.

The lymph nodes may be palpable, usually in the distribution of affected joints.

Anaemia is almost universal and is usually the normochromic normocytic of chronic disease. It may be iron-deficient owing to gastrointestinal blood loss from NSAID ingestion, or rarely, haemolytic (Coomb's positive). There may be a pancytopenia due to hypersplenism in Felty's syndrome. A high platelet count occurs with active disease.

Diagnosis and investigations

The diagnosis relies on the clinical features described above. The American College of Rheumatology criteria are shown in Information box 8.8 and are useful for epidemiological and investigative studies.

Initial investigations include:

- **Blood count**. Anaemia may be present. The ESR and/or CRP are raised in proportion to the activity of the inflammatory process
- **Serology**. Rheumatoid factor is present in approximately 70% of cases and ANA at low titre in 30%.
- **X-rays** of the affected joint(s)
- **Aspiration** of the joint if an effusion is present. The aspirate looks cloudy owing to white cells and should be cultured. In a suddenly painful joint septic arthritis should be suspected (see p. 485).

Other investigations will depend on the clinical picture as outlined above. In severe disease extensive imaging of joints may be required (e.g. CT scan and MRI, arthrograms).

Management of RA

The diagnosis of RA inevitably causes concern and fear in the patient and requires a lot of explanation and reassurance. The doctor and therapist should retain a positive approach and remind the patient that most will continue to lead a more or less normal life despite their arthritis, with the help of drugs; 25% will recover completely. The earliest years are often the most difficult. Uncertainty about when the disease will remit and flare, when and if drugs will work, and whether they may produce side-effects, makes planning from day to day difficult. People learn to adjust remarkably but this takes time and support. A rheumatology unit will have a team, including doctors, specialist nurses and physiotherapists, to help the patient learn to cope. Leaflets give helpful advise, as do local patient groups.

Information

- Morning stiffness > 1 hour
- Arthritis of three or more joints
- Arthritis of hand joints and wrists
- Symmetrical arthritis

} For six weeks or more

- Subcutaneous nodules
- A positive serum rheumatoid factor
- Typical radiological changes (erosions and/or periarticular osteopenia)

Four or more criteria are necessary for diagnosis.

Information box 8.8 Criteria for the diagnosis of rheumatoid arthritis (American College of Rheumatology, 1987 revision)

Drug therapy

There is no curative agent available for RA. The approach to treatment has, until recently, been symptom control usually with non-steroidal anti-inflammatory drugs (NSAIDs). The next stage of therapy has involved the use of a disease suppressive or modifying drug (DMARD).

Recent data supports the use of suppressive drugs *early* in the disease to prevent the long-term irreversible damaging effects of inflammation of the joints.

Non-steroidal anti-inflammatory drugs

NSAIDs control the pain and stiffness, but do not reduce the underlying inflammatory relapse or the acute flare reactants in the serum. They all act on the cyclo-oxygenase pathway (see Fig 12.32). The individual response to NSAIDs varies greatly. It is, therefore, desirable to try several different drugs for a particular patient in order to find the best (see Information box 8.5). Each compound should be given for at least a week.

Always start with a familiar drug. It should be cheap, have a low incidence of side-effects, a good safety record and a convenient dosage schedule. Compliance should be encouraged and the effects reviewed in 1–2 weeks. The major side-effects of NSAIDs are gastrointestinal, with haemorrhage being a major problem in the elderly. Patients with previous peptic ulcers should have their *Helicobacter pylori* status checked, followed by eradication therapy if necessary (see p. 237). Gastric cytoprotective treatment (e.g. prostaglandin E analogues, H_2-receptor antagonists or proton-pump inhibitors) can help to reduce the gastrointestinal risks of NSAIDs. Other side-effects include fluid retention, tubulo-intestinal nephritis and problems with drug interactions.

The relief of night pain and morning stiffness is particularly important in rheumatoid arthritis. Slow-release preparations (e.g. slow-release indomethacin or diclofenac, 75 mg, taken after supper) usually work well and can be given in addition to daytime therapy if necessary. For additional relief a simple analgesic can be taken as required (e.g. paracetamol or the combination of dextropropoxyphene and paracetamol). Many patients need night sedation.

Disease-modifying anti-rheumatic drugs

(Table 8.15)

DMARDs, which mainly act through cytokine inhibition, reduce inflammation, as reflected by a reduction of joint swelling, a fall in the acute phase reactants and slowing of

Table 8.15
Disease-modifying anti-rheumatic drugs (DMARDs). Corticosteroids are described on p. 949

Drug	Usual dose	Possible side effects
Sulphasalazine	1–1.5 g twice daily	Rash GI intolerance Marrow suppression Reversible oligospermia
Methotrexate	2.5–15 mg once weekly	Mouth ulcers Hepatotoxicity Bone marrow suppression
Gold oral (auranofin)	3 mg twice daily	Diarrhoea Rash
Intramuscular (sodium aurothiomalate)	50 mg weekly, changing to monthly with disease control	Blood dyscrasias *Severe reaction in up to 5%* Mouth ulcers Skin rash Proteinuria Blood dyscrasia
Penicillamine	250–500 mg daily before food	Loss of taste Thrombocytopenia Proteinuria Rash
Anti-malarials Hydroxychloroquine	400 mg daily	Corneal deposits, rarely retinopathy after 6 years
Less commonly used drugs		
Azathioprine		
Cyclophosphamide		
Cyclosporin		

the development of joint erosions and irreversible damage. Their beneficial effect is not immediate (hence 'slow-acting agents') and may be partial or transient.

Generally DMARDS are used after symptomatic treatment, but in seropositive patients with a poor prognosis they should be used early, before the appearance of erosions on X-rays of hands and feet. DMARDs are usually prescribed by a rheumatologist.

Sulphasalazine

This is a combination of sulphapyridine and 5-aminosalicylic acid. Sulphapyridine is probably the active component. It is well tolerated and for many is the first-choice DMARD. It produces a response in about half the patients in the first 3–6 months. The side-effects are shown in Table 8.15. Serious side-effects are rare, being mainly leukopenia and thrombocytopenia. Blood should be monitored with a full blood count and liver biochemistry regularly.

Methotrexate

This is considered by many to be the drug of choice, given at an initial low weekly dose of 2.5–7.5 mg orally, increased up to 15 mg if necessary. It is well tolerated and it is now suggested that this therapy should be introduced early in the disease. Oral folic acid should be given in addition. Full blood counts and liver biochemistry should be monitored carefully. This regimen usually works within 1–2 months. Side-effects include hepatoxicity (including occasionally cirrhosis), bone marrow suppression, oral ulceration and a potentially life-threatening pneumonitis (in 3%).

There are no firm data that this treatment halts the erosion of cartilage, bone and soft tissue.

Gold

This may be given by intramuscular injection as sodium aurothiomalate or by mouth as auranofin. The oral preparation has fewer side-effects, but its efficacy also seems to be less. Sodium aurothiomalate is given by deep intramuscular injection. A test dose of 10 mg is followed by weekly doses of 50 mg until response occurs, usually in about three months. If there is no remission after a total dose of 1 g, treatment should be stopped. If a response is obtained, the interval between injections is increased to four weeks, continued for up to five years. With relapse the dose frequency is again increased.

Side-effects occur in a third of patients and regular monitoring of white cell count and platelets and urine testing is required. Exfoliative dermatitis and a pruritic skin rash can occur. Other rare side-effects include pulmonary fibrosis, colitis, polyneuropathy and cholestatic jaundice. Gold-induced glomerulonephritis can occur, particularly in patients who are HLA-DR3 positive and routine urinalysis for proteinuria is performed. The diarrhoea produced by the oral preparation can be helped by bran.

Penicillamine

This has to be given for at least three months before improvement occurs. Penicillamine should not be continued if there is no improvement within one year. Patients should be monitored with blood counts and urinalysis for proteinuria and the drug should be stopped, or dosage reduced, if side-effects occur. If proteinuria exceeds 2 g/24 h the drug should be stopped. Loss of taste is reversible. Other rare side-effects include a lupus erythematosus-like syndrome and a myasthenia gravis-like syndrome.

Antimalarials

Hydroxychloroquine has an action similar to penicillamine and gold, but tend to be better tolerated. Retinopathy is the most serious side-effect, but this is rare if the dose given in Table 8.15 is not exceeded. Patients should have six-monthly checks of macular function with an Amsler chart as retinopathy is irreversible. Corneal opacities, headaches, gastrointestinal disturbances and skin rashes occur.

Corticosteroids

The use of oral corticosteroids has a number of problems (Information box 8.9). They are powerful disease-controlling drugs, but must be avoided in the long term because side-effects are inevitable. Early intensive short-term regimens are used in some centres with other DMARDs as maintenance therapy. They are also invaluable in patients with severe disease with extra-articular manifestations such as vasculitis.

Intra-articular injections with semicrystalline preparations have a powerful but sometimes only short-lived effect.

Intramuscular depot injections (40–120 mg depot methylprednisolone) help to control severe flare-up of the disease, or can be used before a holiday or other important life event, but should be used with caution and also infrequently.

Information

- Patients are increasingly anxious about the use of corticosteroids because of adverse publicity about their potential side-effects. This must be discussed frankly and the risks of not treating them be described and balanced against the risks of the drug itself.
- Patients must be warned to avoid sugars and saturated fats and to eat less because of the risk of weight gain.
- The skin becomes thin and easily damaged.
- Monitor for diabetes and hypertension.
- Cataract formation may be accelerated.
- Osteoporosis develops within six months on doses above 7.5 mg daily, and hormone replacement therapy and/or calcium and vitamin D o bisphosphonate is used (see p. 509).

Information box 8.9 Problems associated with the use of corticosteroids

Combinations of DMARDS occasionally with low doses of corticosteroids are being increasingly used and the number of drugs reduced once the synovitis remits. Toxicity, although still a problem, seems to be less with combinations.

Drugs used less commonly

Azathioprine at a dose of 2 mg kg^{-1} and cyclophosphamide 1–2 mg kg^{-1} have been used, usually when other DMARDS have been ineffective. They are often used when extra-articular features are severe, particularly with vasculitis. They are also used in patients who have been treated with corticosteroids and who have developed severe side-effects of those agents.

Cyclosporin 2.5–5 mg kg^{-1} is used for severe active rheumatoid arthritis when conventional therapy has been ineffective.

Newer therapies

Anticytokine therapy is now being used. Blockade of IL-1 and IL-6 with receptor antagonists has been shown to have rapid anti-inflammatory effects.

Therapy against TNFα has been most extensively studied using anti-TNFα monoclonal antibody or soluble *p55* receptor, soluble *p75* receptor and TNF-converting enzyme inhibitors. Early results show a transient reduction in synovitis, but continuous therapy is necessary and further trials are awaited.

Physical measures

Patients with RA need constant advice and support from physiotherapists, especially while they are learning to adjust. A combination of rest for active arthritis and exercises to maintain joint range and muscle power is essential. Exercise in a hydrotherapy pool is popular and effective. Advice about managing activities of daily living despite the arthritis, and about gadgets, seating or structural changes in the home or at work are helpful.

Surgery

This should be considered carefully in the long-term approach to patient management. Its main objectives are prophylactic, to prevent joint destruction and deformity, and reconstructive to restore function.

Single-joint disease can be treated by surgical synovectomy to reduce the bulk of inflamed tissue and prevent damage. Excision arthroplasty of the ulnar styloid reduces pain and the risk of extensor tendon damage. Excision arthroplasties of the metatarsal heads reduce metatarsal pain and relieve pressure points. The major surgical advance has been the development of total replacement arthroplasty of the hip, knee, finger joints, elbows and shoulders. Such procedures need careful planning and preparation, and the expected outcomes and risks should be explined to the patient.

FURTHER READING

Emery P (1997) Rheumatoid arthritis not yet curable with early intensive therapy. *Lancet* **350**: 304–305.

Firestein GS, Zvaifler NJ (1997) Anticytokine therapy in rheumatoid arthritis. *New England Journal of Medicine* **337**: 195–197.

O'Dell JR, Haire CE, Erikson N *et al.* (1996) Treatment of rheumatoid arthritis with methotrexate alone, sulfasalazine and hydroxychloroquine, or a combination of all three medications. *New England Journal of Medicine* **334**: 1287–1291.

Seronegative spondarthritides

This awkward title describes a group of conditions affecting the spine and peripheral joints which cluster in families and are linked to certain type I HLA antigens (Table 8.16). The joint involvement is more limited than that seen in RA and its distribution is different. These diseases occasionally present in childhood.

Histologically the synovitis itself is difficult to distinguish from that of RA, but there is no production of rheumatoid factors – hence 'seronegative'. All are associated with an increased frequency of sacroiliitis and an increased frequency of HLA-B27.

AETIOLOGY

The common aetiological thread of these disorders is their striking association with HLA-B27, particularly ankylosing spondylitis (AS). This was the first demonstrated disease association of any HLA type (B27 is present in >90% of Caucasians with AS but only 8% of controls). Its aetiological relevance remains unclear.

There are clues that infections play a role, possibly by molecular mimicry, with parts of the organism which are structurally similar to the HLA molecule triggering cross-reactive antibody formation. This is unproven.

The types of arthritis that follow a precipitating infection are called *reactive arthritis* (p. 481). *Yersinia enterocolytica* DNA has been found in the synovium in reactive arthritis, as have structures derived from *Chlamydia trachomatis*. These agents are thought to be the trigger for some types of reactive arthritis.

The specialized immune systems of the gut and genitourinary mucous membranes may also play a causal role, perhaps reacting to local infections or to antigens which cross the damaged mucosa.

Table 8.16
Seronegative spondarthritides

Ankylosing spondylitis (AS)
Psoriatic arthritis
Reactive arthritis
Sexually acquired (Reiter's disease)
Post-dysenteric reactive arthritis
Ulcerative colitis/Crohn's (enteropathic) arthritis

Ankylosing spondylitis (AS)

This is an inflammatory disorder of the back affecting mainly young adults. The frequency of AS in different populations is roughly paralleled by the incidence of HLA-B27; Africans and Japanese have a low incidence of both HLA-B27 and ankylosing spondylitis, while the North American Haida Indians have a high incidence of both. The disease is almost as common in women as men, but because the disease is milder in women, men are more likely to present with symptoms of the disease (in a ratio of 4:1).

CLINICAL FEATURES

Episodic inflammation of the sacroiliac joints in the late teenage years or early twenties is the first manifestation of AS. Pain in one or both buttocks and low back pain and stiffness are typically worse in the morning and relieved by exercise. Initially the diagnosis is missed because the patient is asymptomatic between episodes and radiological abnormalities are absent. Non-spinal complications (uveitis or costochondritis) suggest the diagnosis (Information box 8.10). Costochondral junction inflammation causes anterior chest pain.

Peripheral joint involvement is asymmetrical and affects a few, predominantly large joints. Hip involvement leads to fixed flexion deformities of the hips and further deterioration of the posture. Young teenage boys occasionally present with a lower-limb monarthritis (see p. 498).

Acute anterior uveitis is strongly associated with HLA-B27 in AS and related diseases and is occasionally the presenting complaint. Severe eye pain, photophobia and blurred vision is an emergency. Patients with AS should be asked to report eye pain and redness immediately.

INVESTIGATIONS

- **Blood**. The ESR or CRP are usually raised.
- **HLA testing** is rarely of value because of the high frequency of HLA-B27 in the population, but may give supporting evidence in a difficult case.
- **X-rays**. The medial and lateral cortical margins of both sacroiliac joints lose definition owing to erosions and become sclerotic (Fig 8.18). The earliest radiological appearances in the spine are blurring of the upper or lower vertebral rims, owing to an enthesitis at the insertion of the intervertebral ligaments. These changes first appear at the thoracolumbar junction but develop throughout the spine. Persistent inflammatory enthesitis causes bony spurs (syndesmophytes). Syndesmophytes are more vertically oriented than the beak-like osteophytes of spondylosis and the disc is preserved, unlike in spondylosis. Syndesmophytes cause bony ankylosis and permanent stiffening. The sacroiliac joints eventually fuse, as may the costovertebral joints, reducing chest expansion. Calcification of the

Information

- Uveitis, in all types.
- Cutaneous lesions in reactive arthritis (keratoderma blenorrhagica), histologically identical to pustular psoriasis.
- Nail dystrophy, in psoriasis and reactive arthritis.
- Aortitis, occasionally in AS and reactive arthritis.

Information box 8.10 Nonarticular problems in seronegative spondarthritides

intervertebral ligaments and fusion of the spinal facet joints and syndesmophytes leads to what is often called a 'bamboo' spine (Fig 8.19).

TREATMENT

The key to effective management of AS is early diagnosis so that a regimen of preventative exercises is started before syndesmophytes have formed. Morning exercises aim to maintain spinal mobility, posture and chest expansion. Failure to control pain and to encourage regular spinal and chest exercises leads to an irreversible dorsal kyphosis and wasted paraspinal muscles. This, along with stiffening of the cervical spine, makes forward vision difficult.

When the inflammation is active, the morning pain and stiffness are too severe to permit effective exercise. An evening dose of a long-acting or slow-release NSAID or an NSAID suppository improves sleep, pain control and exercise compliance. Peripheral arthritis is managed with NSAIDs or local steroid injections.

Sulphasalazine or methotrexate may help the peripheral arthritis but there is little evidence that they control spinal disease.

PROGNOSIS

With exercise and pain relief, the prognosis is excellent and over 80% of patients are fully employed. The back may be stiff, but disability is minimal unless the hips are involved. HLA-B27 positive offspring have a 30% chance of devloping ankylosing spondylitis.

Psoriatic arthritis

The term 'psoriatic arthritis' describes a variety of different patterns of arthritis and enthesitis seen in people with psoriasis or with a family history of psoriasis. Five to eight per cent of individuals with psoriasis develop one of several different patterns of arthritis for which there is no serological marker.

CLINICAL FEATURES

The arthritis is typically more limited in distribution and less severe than in RA. The skin disease can be mild and may develop after the arthritis. Nail dystrophy is present in 85% of cases (p. 1166).

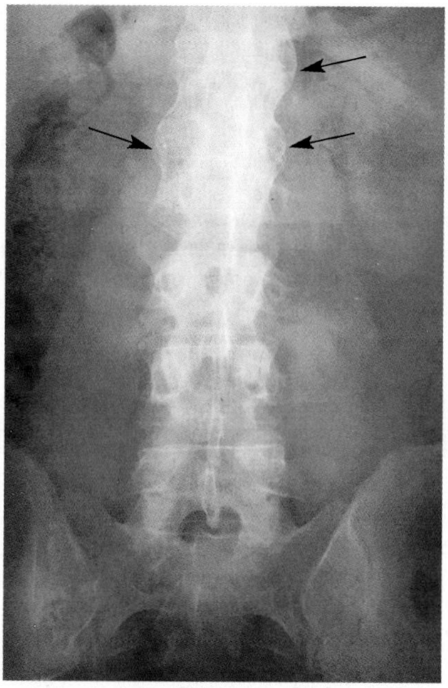

Fig 8.18
X-ray of ankylosing spondylitis. The sacroiliac joints are eroded and show marginal sclerosis. There is bridging syndesmophyte formation at the thoracolumbar junction (arrow)

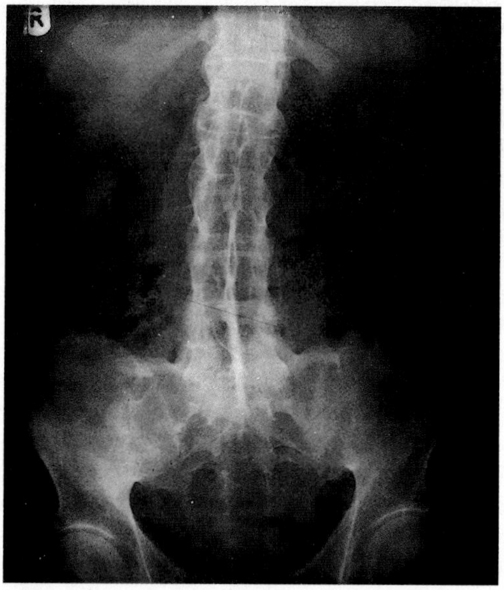

Fig 8.19
X-ray of bamboo spine in ankylosing spondylitis. In advanced disease there is calcification of the interspinous ligaments and fusion of the facet joints as well as syndesmophytes at all levels

The most typical pattern of joint involvement in psoriasis is distal interphalangeal arthritis. It is unsightly, but rarely disabling, and there is often adjacent nail dystrophy. Cutaneous lesions, interphalangeal joint synovitis and tenosynovitis causing a 'sausage' finger or toe (*dactylitis*) is seen in pauci-articular psoriatic arthritis. It is also seen in reactive arthritis.

A seronegative symmetrical polyarthritis similar to rheumatoid arthritis occurs.

Radiologically, psoriatic arthritis is erosive but the erosions are central in the joint, not juxta-articular, and produce a 'pencil in cup' appearance (Fig 8.20).

Arthritis mutilans affects about 5% of patients with psoriatic arthritis and causes marked peri-articular osteolysis and bone shortening ('telescopic' fingers) (Fig 8.21), in which, despite the deformity, pain may be mild and function often surprisingly good.

Individuals with psoriasis may develop unilateral or bilateral *sacroiliitis* and *typical AS*, but with early involvement of the neck; only 50% are HLA-B27 positive.

TREATMENT AND PROGNOSIS

NSAIDs and/or analgesics help the pain, although some NSAIDs may worsen the skin lesions. Local synovitis responds to intra-articular corticosteroid injections.

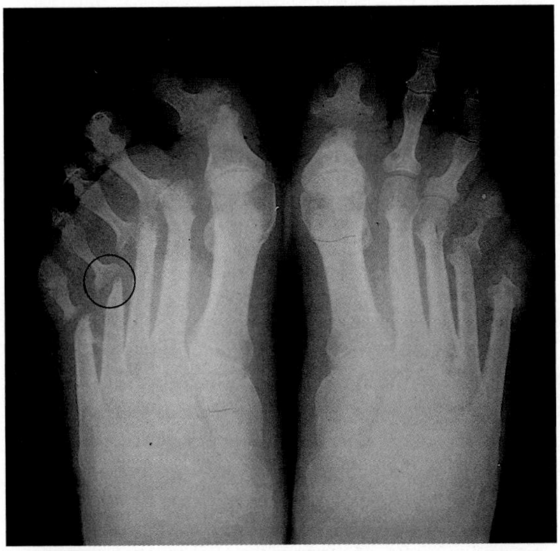

Fig 8.20
X-ray of psoriatic arthritis. There is osteolysis of the metatarsal heads and central erosion of the proximal phalanges to produce the 'pencil cup' appearance (circle). All the lesser toes are subluxed

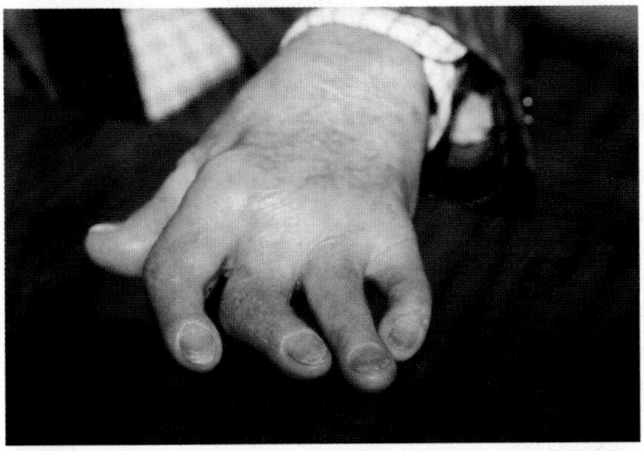

Fig 8.21
Hand showing psoriatic arthritis mutilans. All the fingers are shortened and the joints unstable, owing to underlying osteolysis

In milder, polyarticular cases, sulphasalazine slows the development of joint damage.

When the disease is severe, methotrexate or cyclosporin are given because they control both the skin lesions and the arthritis. Corticosteroids orally may destabilize the skin disease and are best avoided.

The prognosis is good, with only minimal joint impairment in most cases.

Reactive arthritis

Reactive arthritis is a sterile synovitis which occurs following an infection (see also post-streptococcal arthritis on p. 499).

Seronegative spondarthritis, in patients who are B27-positive, follows an acute attack of dysentery, or a sexually acquired infection – nonspecific urethritis (NSU) in the male, nonspecific cervicitis in the female.

AETIOLOGY

A variety of organisms can be the trigger, including some strains of *Salmonella* or *Shigella* spp in bacillary dysentery. *Yersinia entercolitica* causes diarrhoea and a reactive arthritis. In NSU the organisms are *Chlamydia trachomatis* or *Ureasplasma urealyticum*.

Molecules derived from *Chlamydia, Yersinia, Shigella* and *Salmonella* have been found in the inflamed synovium of affected joints, suggesting that this persistent antigenic material is driving the inflammatory process.

There are other organisms which also trigger reactive arthritis, but which have a different genetic basis; see post-streptococcal arthritis (p. 499), gonococcal arthritis (p. 486) and brucellosis (p. 486). In these, the borderline between reactive arthritis and septic arthritis is more indistinct and they can cause both.

CLINICAL FEATURES (Fig 8.22)

The arthritis is typically an acute, asymmetrical, lower-limb arthritis, occurring more commonly in a male, a few days to a couple of weeks after the infection. The arthritis may be the presenting complaint if the infection is mild or asymptomatic. Enthesitis is common, causing plantar fasciitis or Achilles tendinitis (see p. 463).

In susceptible individuals with reactive arthritis, sacroiliitis and spondylitis may also develop. Acute anterior uveitis may complicate more severe or relapsing disease.

The skin lesions resemble psoriasis:

- *Circinate balanitis* in the uncircumcised male causes painless superficial ulceration of the glans penis. In the circumcised male the lesion is raised, red and scaly. Both heal without scarring.
- *Keratoderma blenorrhagica* – the skin of the feet and hands develops painless, red and often confluent raised plaques and pustules histologically similar to pustular psoriasis. This can occur anywhere on the body
- *Nail dystrophy* may occur.

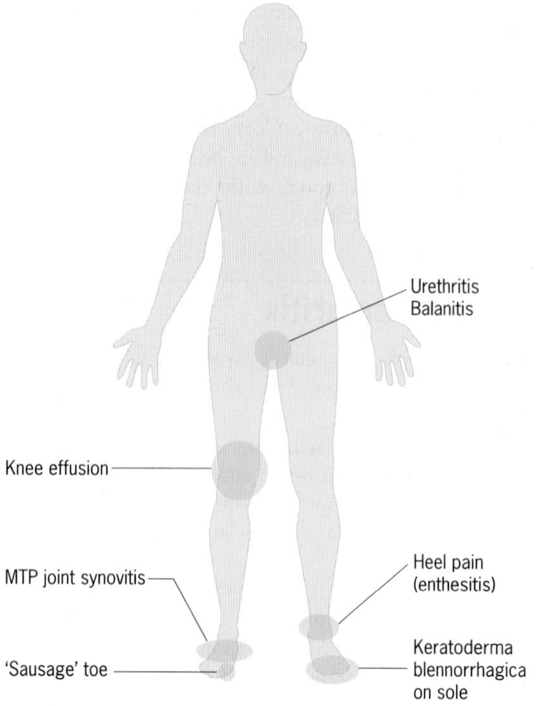

Fig 8.22
Clinical features of reactive arthritis

Other features

These include:

- bilateral conjunctivitis
- the classically described triad of *Reiter's disease* – urethritis, arthritis and conjunctivitis.

TREATMENT

There is little evidence that treating persisting infection with antibiotics will alter the course of the arthritis, once it has developed. Nonetheless, cultures should be taken and any infection treated. Pain responds well to NSAIDs and local corticosteroid injections. The majority of individuals with reactive arthritis have a single attack which settles, but a few develop a disabling relapsing and remitting arthritis. Relapsing cases are sometimes treated with DMARDs (see Table 8.15).

Enteropathic arthritis associated with inflammatory bowel disease

Enteropathic synovitis occurs in approximately 10–15% of patients with ulcerative colitis and Crohn's disease (see p. 264). The link between the bowel disease and the inflammatory arthritis is not clear. Selective mucosal leakiness may expose the individual to antigens which trigger synovitis.

The arthritis is asymmetrical and predominantly affects lower-limb joints. An HLA-B27 associated sacroiliitis or spondylitis is seen in 5% of patients with inflammatory bowel disease and is independent of disease activity. The joint symptoms may predate the development of bowel disease or lead to its diagnosis.

Remission of ulcerative colitis or total colectomy usually lead to remission of the joint disease, but arthritis may persist even in well-controlled Crohn's disease.

TREATMENT

The inflammatory bowel disease is should be treated (see p. 266). In all cases of enteropathic arthritis, the joint disease should be managed symptomatically with NSAIDs, although they may make diarrhoea worse. A monoarthritis is best treated by intra-articular corticosteroids. Sulphasalazine is frequently prescribed as this may help both bowel and joint disease.

FURTHER READING

Nuki G (1998) Ankylosing spondylitis, HLA B27, and beyond. *Lancet* **351**: 767–769.

Crystal arthritis

AETIOLOGY

Two main types of crystal account for the majority of crystal-induced arthritis. They are sodium urate and calcium pyrophosphate and are distinguished by their different shapes and refringence properties under polarized light with a red filter (Fig 8.23). Rarely crystals of calcium apatite (see p. 469) or cholesterol cause acute synovitis.

Neutrophils ingest the crystals and release pro-inflammatory enzymes from their phagosomes into the joint, thus triggering complement activation and attracting more neutrophils. Crystals may be found in asymptomatic joints. Why they initiate an attack is unclear. In pseudogout, crystal shedding from the cartilage causes an attack.

Gout and hyperuricaemia

Gout is an inflammatory arthritis associated with hyperuricaemia.

EPIDEMIOLOGY

The prevelance of gout in Europe and the USA is approximately 0.2%, although hyperuricaemia in this population occurs in about 5%. The prevalence of gout is increasing and it is still mainly seen in developed countries. Gout is seen in men more than women (10:1) and rarely occurs before puberty (when it suggests an enzyme defect), and seldom in premenopausal females.

Uric acid levels start to rise after puberty and are higher in men than women until the female menopause. There is a normal distribution of serum uric acid in the population with a skew distribution at the upper end of the range. Hyperuricaemia is defined as a serum uric acid level greater than two standard deviations from the mean (420 μmol^{-1} in males, 360 μmol^{-1} in females).

Most people with hyperuricaemia are asymptomatic. The range for gouty individuals is higher than for normals, but the distribution curves overlap (Fig 8.24). Serum uric acid levels increase with age, obesity, a high-protein diet, a high alcohol consumption, type IV hyperlipidaemia, diabetes mellitus, ischaemic heart disease and hypertension. There is often a family history of gout.

PATHOGENESIS

Causes of hyperuricaemia are shown in table 8.17. In many patients with gout there is no obvious cause, and in these patients there is often both increased production and decreased excretion of urate.

Uric acid levels in the blood depend on the balance between purine synthesis and the ingestion of dietary purines, and the elimination of urate by the kidney and intestine (Fig 8.25).

Table 8.17
Causes of hyperuricaemia

Impaired excretion of uric acid
Chronic renal disease (clinical gout unusual)
Drug therapy, e.g. thiazide diuretics, low-dose aspirin
Hypertension
Lead toxicity
Primary hyperparathyroidism
Hypothyroidism
Increased lactic acid production from alcohol, exercise, starvation
Glucose-6-phosphatase deficiency (interferes with renal excretion)

Increased production of uric acid
Increased purine synthesis de novo due to:
- Hypoxanthine–guanine–phosoribosyl transferase (HGPRT) reduction (an X-linked inborn error causing the Lesch–Nyhan syndrome)
- Phosphoribosyl–pyrophosphate synthetase overactivity
- Glucose-6-phosphatase deficiency with glycogen storage disease type 1 (patients who survive develop hyperuricaemia due to increased production as well as decreased excretion)

Increased turnover of purines due to:
- Myeloproliferative disorders, e.g. polycythaemia vera
- Lymphoproliferative disorders, e.g. leukaemia
- Others, e.g. carcinoma, severe psoriasis

(a)

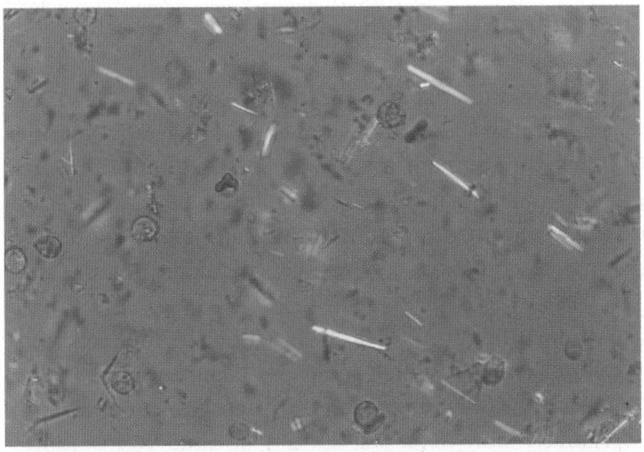

(b)

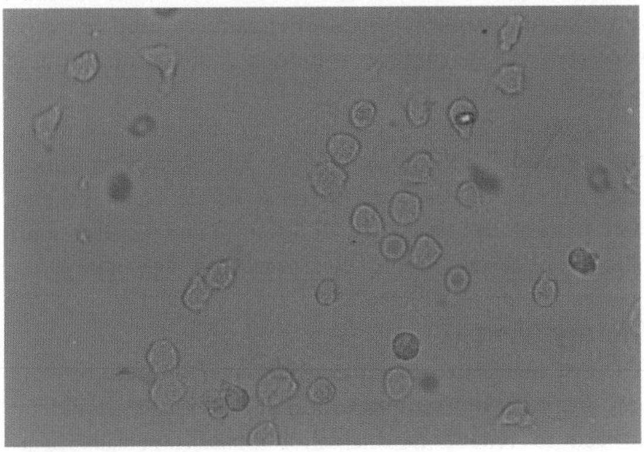

Fig 8.23
(a) Needle-shaped urate crystals, viewed under polarized light with a red filter
(b) A small intracellular pyrophosphate crystal, viewed under polarized light with a red filter

Uric acid synthesis. Uric acid is the last step in the breakdown pathway of purines. The last two steps, the conversion of hypoxanthine to xanthine and of xanthine to uric acid, are catalysed by the enzyme xanthine oxidase.

Uric acid excretion. Uric acid is completely filtered by the glomerulus; 100% is then reabsorbed in the proximal tubule and 75% is secreted by the distal tubule. Some post-secretory reabsorption also takes place. One-third of uric acid is lost in the faeces.

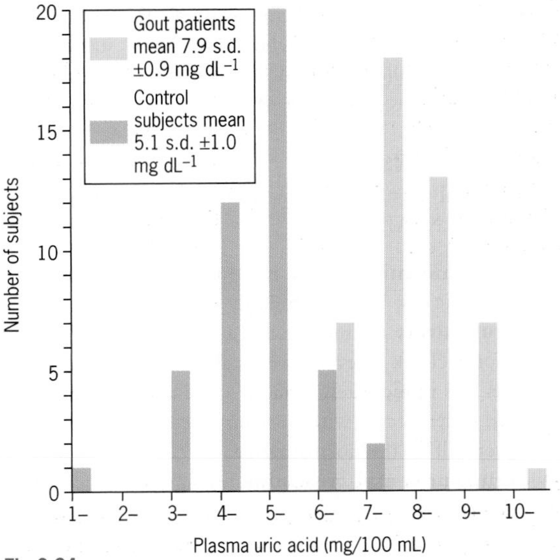

Fig 8.24
Serum uric acid levels in normals and in patients with gout
7.9 mg dL^{-1} is equivalent to 474 μmol L^{-1}, 5.1 mg dL^{-1} is equivalent to 306 μmol L^{-1} (From *Annals of Rheumatic Disease* 1977, with permission)

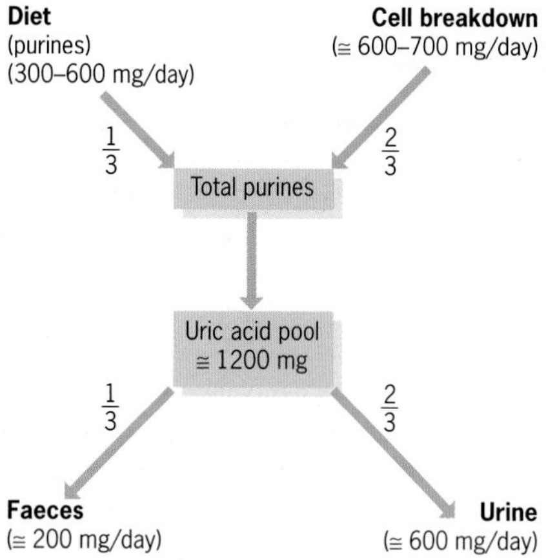

Fig 8.25
Uric acid synthesis (mainly from cell breakdown) and excretion (1 mg ≡ 6 μmol)

CLINICAL FEATURES

Hyperuricaemia causes four clinical syndromes (Information box 8.11).

Acute gout presents typically in a middle-aged male with sudden onset of agonizing pain, swelling and redness of the first MTP joint. The attack occurs at any time, but may be precipitated by too much food or alcohol, by dehydration or by starting a diuretic. Untreated attacks last about seven days. In 25% of attacks, a joint other than the great toe is affected.

In severe attacks, overlying crystal cellulitis makes gout difficult to distinguish clinically from infective cellulitis. A family or personal history of gout and the finding of a raised serum urate suggest the diagnosis but, if in doubt, blood and other cultures should be taken.

Chronic polyarticular gout is unusual, except in elderly people on longstanding diuretic treatment, in renal failure, or occasionally in men who have been started on treatment with allopurinol too soon after an acute attack. *Chronic tophaceous gout* (see p. 485).

INVESTIGATIONS

The clinical picture is often diagnostic, as is the rapid response to NSAIDs.

- **Joint fluid microscopy** is the most specific and diagnostic test but is technically difficult.
- **Serum urate** is usually raised (> 600 μmol L^{-1}). If it is not, recheck it several weeks after the attack as the level falls immediately after an acute attack. Acute gout never occurs with a serum uric acid in the lower half of the normal range.
- **Serum urea and creatinine** for signs of renal impairment.

TREATMENT

The use of NSAIDs in high doses rapidly reduces the pain and swelling. Initial doses, taken with food, are:

Information

- Acute urate synovitis – gout
- Chronic polyarticular gout
- Chronic tophaceous gout
- Urate renal stone formation (p. 556)

Information box 8.11 Hyperuricaemia causes four clinical syndromes

- naproxen: 750 mg immediately, then 500 mg 8–12 hourly
- diclofenac: 75–100 mg immediately, then 50 mg 6–8 hourly
- indomethacin: 75 mg immediately, then 50 mg 6–8 hourly.

After 24–48 hours, reduced doses are given for a further week. In individuals with a history of peptic ulceration, alternative treatments include:

- colchicine: 1 mg immediately, then 0.5 mg every 6–12 hours, but this causes diarrhoea
- corticosteroids: intramuscular or intra-articular depot methylprednisolone.

Treatment with agents which reduce serum urate levels

Only when the attacks are frequent, severe or associated with renal impairment or when the patient finds NSAIDs or colchicine difficult to tolerate should allopurinol or a uricosuric agent be used. They should never be started within a month of an acute attack and always be under cover of a course of NSAID or colchicine for the first 4–6 weeks.

Allopurinol (300–600 mg) blocks the enzyme xanthine oxidase which converts xanthine into urate (see Fig 13.10). It reduces serum urate levels rapidly and is relatively non-toxic but should be used at low doses (50–100 mg) in renal impairment. Skin rashes are the most common side-effect. Bone marrow suppression is very rare. Allopurinol may induce acute gout when it is first introduced.

Uricosuric agents (probenecid) increase urate excretion and are used in individuals who are allergic to allopurinol. They should not be used in renal failure or in patients with urate stones. They may be given in combination with allopurinol in severe tophaceous gout with high urate loads.

Dietary advice

The first attacks may be separated by many months or years and are managed symptomatically. Individuals should be advised to reduce their alcohol intake, especially beer, which is high in purines. A diet which reduces total calorie and cholesterol intake and avoids such foods as offal, some fish and shellfish and spinach, all of which are rich sources of purines, is advised. This can reduce serum urate by 15%.

Chronic tophaceous gout

Individuals with very high levels of urate can present with different clinical pictures. In chronic tophaceous gout sodium urate forms smooth white deposits (tophi) in skin and around joints. They may occur on the ear lobe, the fingers or the Achilles tendon. Large deposits are unsightly and ulcerate. There is chronic joint pain and sometimes superimposed acute gouty attacks.

Peri-articular deposits lead to a halo of radio-opacity and clearly defined ('punched out') bone cysts on X-ray.

Tophaceous gout is often associated with renal impairment and/or the long-term use of diuretics. Whenever possible stop the diuretics or change to less urate-retaining ones, such as bumetamide.

Pseudogout (pyrophosphate arthropathy)

Calcium pyrophosphate deposits in hyaline and fibro-cartilage produce the radiological appearance of chondrocalcinosis (see p. 469). Shedding of crystals into a joint precipitates acute synovitis which resembles gout, except that it is more common in elderly women and usually affects the knee or wrist. The attacks are often very painful.

DIAGNOSIS

The diagnosis is made by detecting rhomboidal, weakly positively birefringent crystals in joint fluid, or deduced from the presence of chondrocalcinosis on X-ray. The joint fluid looks purulent. Septic arthritis must be excluded and joint fluid should be sent for culture.

The attacks may be associated with fever and a raised white blood cell count.

TREATMENT

Aspiration of the joint reduces the pain dramatically but it is usually necessary to use an NSAID or colchicine, as for gout. If infection can be excluded, an intra-articular injection of a corticosteroid helps.

Infective arthritis

Joints may become infected by direct injury or by blood-borne infection from an infected skin lesion or other site.

Chronically inflamed joints (e.g. in rheumatoid arthritis) are more prone to infection than are normal joints. Individuals who are immunosuppressed, by AIDS or by immunosuppressive agents, are particularly at risk, as are the elderly and those who abuse alcohol. Artificial joints are also potential sites for infection.

Septic arthritis

The organism which most commonly causes septic arthritis is *Staphylococcus aureus*. Other organisms include strepto-cocci, other species of *Staphylococcus*, *Neisseria gonorrhoea*, *Haemophilus influenzae* and Gram-negative organisms.

CLINICAL FEATURES

Suspected septic arthritis is a medical emergency. In young and previously fit people, the joint is hot, red, swollen, agonisingly painful and held immobile by muscle spasm. In the elderly and immunosuppressed and in RA the clinical picture is less dramatic, so a high index of suspicion is needed to avoid missing treatable but potentially severely destructive septic arthritis.

INVESTIGATIONS

- **Aspirate** the joint and send the fluid for urgent Gram staining and culture. The fluid is usually frankly purulent. The culture techniques should include those for gonococci and anaerobes.
- **Blood cultures** are often positive.
- **Leucocytosis** is usual, unless the person is severely immunosuppressed.
- **X-rays** are of no value in diagnosis.

TREATMENT

This should be started immediately on diagnosis because joint destruction occurs in days. The joint should be immobilized initially and physiotherapy started early to prevent stiffness and muscle wasting. Intravenous antibiotics should be given for a week. It is usual to give two antibiotics to which the organism is sensitive for six weeks, then one for a further six weeks orally.

Empirical treatment in septic arthritis

This is started *before* the results of culture are obtained. Intravenous flucloxacillin 1–2 g is given six-hourly, plus fusidic acid 500 mg orally eight-hourly. If the patient is allergic to penicillin replace flucloxacillin with erythromycin 1 g i.v. six-hourly or clindamycin 600 mg i.v. eight-hourly. In immunosuppressed patients, flucloxacillin 1–2 g i.v. six-hourly plus gentamycin (to cover anaerobes) should be used. Change the antibiotics if the organism is not sensitive. Drainage of the joint and arthroscopic joint washouts are helpful in relieving pain.

PROGNOSIS

Surgical drainage may be required if there is joint destruction and osteomyelitis. Patients can start weight-bearing as soon as the inflammation subsides. Resolution of the septic arthritis with complete recovery can occur in a few days or weeks.

Specific types of bacterial arthritis

Gonnococcal arthritis

This is the most common cause of a septic arthritis in previously fit young adults, affecting women and homosexual men.

Initially the patient becomes febrile and develops characteristic pustules on the distal limbs. Polyarthralgia and tenosynovitis are common at this stage and about 40% have a gonococcaemia. This phase settles and blood cultures usually become negative. Later, large-joint mono- or pauci-articular arthritis may follow. Culture is usually positive from the genital tract, although the joint fluid may be sterile. It is not clear whether this is simply a septic arthritis – although it responds rapidly to antibiotics – or whether there is also a reactive element to bacterial lipopolysaccharide.

Treatment consists of oral penicillin, ciprofloxacin or doxycycline for two weeks, and joint rest.

Tuberculous arthritis

Around 1% of patients with tuberculosis develop skeletal involvement. It occurs in the primary disease in children. In adults, it is usually due to haematogenous spread from secondary pulmonary or renal lesions.

The organism invades the synovium or intervertebral disc. There are caseating granulomas and rapid destruction of cartilage and adjacent bone.

A hip or knee (30%) is most commonly affected, but around 50% develop spinal disease. The patient is febrile, has night sweats, is anorexic and loses weight. The usual risk factors for tuberculosis apply – debility, alcohol abuse or immunosuppression. HIV-positive/AIDS patients are at particular risk.

Investigations should include culture of fluid, and culture and biopsy of the synovium. *M. tuberculosis* is the usual organism, but atypical mycobacteria are occasionally implicated. A chest X-ray should be performed. Initially joint or spinal X-rays may be normal but joint-space reduction and bone destruction develop rapidly if treatment is delayed.

Treatment is as for tuberculosis (see p. 804). The joint should be rested and the spine immobilized in the acute phase.

Meningococcal arthritis

This may complicate a meningococcal septicaemia and presents as a migratory polyarthritis. Organisms can only rarely be cultured from the joint and most are due to immune complex deposition. *Treatment* is with penicillin.

Infective endocarditis

This may present with arthralgia, polymyalgia rheumatica-like symptoms or an infective arthritis. It is discussed on p. 712.

Lyme arthritis

A person with Lyme disease (see p. 471) develops a fever and headache, and an expanding, erythematous rash called *erythema chronicum migrans*. About 25% of cases develop an acute pauci-articular arthritis. This usually resolves but may relapse.

Diagnosis is by the detection of IgM antibodies against the spirochaete *Borrelia burgdorferi*. *Treatment* is with antibiotics.

Brucellosis

Brucellosis (see p. 28) has a world-wide distribution and the most common cause of chronic brucellosis and of arthritis is *Brucella melitensis*. There is usually a peripheral mono- or oligo-articular arthritis, which may be septic or reactive. Arthritis is more common in chronic infections of more than six months.

Syphilitic arthritis

Congenital syphilis (see p. 102) can cause an acute painful epiphysitis or osteochondritis sometimes associated with para-articular swelling in the first few weeks of life. Later, at age 8–16 years, painless effusion of the knees may occur (Clutton's joints).

In acquired syphilis, arthralgia and arthritis occurs in the secondary stage. Charcot's (neuropathic) joints usually involve the knees in tabes dorsalis (see p. 1074).

Actinomycetes infection

Actinomycetes (see p. 39) can affect the mandible or vertebrae.

Arthritis in viral disease

A transient polyarthritis or arthralgia can occur before, during or after many viral illnesses. These include infectious mononucleosis, chickenpox, mumps, adenovirus, parvovirus and arboviral infections. In most of these it is due to immue complex deposition.

In *rubella* (see p. 59) the virus can occasionally be isolated from the joint. This arthritis occurs most commonly in young adult females a few days after rubella infection. It is a symmetrical polyarthritis involving the MCP or PIP joints most commonly, but many joints can be infected. It closely resembles rheumatoid arthritis, but the ESR is usually normal and rubella antibodies are present. It resolves within a few weeks in most cases; occasionally persistent or recurrent arthralgia occurs. A similar arthritis occurs 2–4 weeks after rubella vaccination in approximately 25% of patients.

In *hepatitis B infection* (see p. 304) a sudden symmetrical polyarticular arthritis of the small joints of the hands occurs in approximately one-third of patients, often in the prodromal phase and mostly resolving before the onset of jaundice.

Arbovirus infections (see p. 59) which are endemic in many parts of the world give rise to an arthralgia and/or arthritis. For example, the Ross River virus has caused an epidemic polyarthritis in Australia and the South Pacific; it involves the small joints of the hands and clears in 2–4 weeks. Other viral infections causing epidemic arthritis include chikungunya (see p. 60) and O'nyong-nyong (p. 59).

Musculoskeletal aspects of infection with human immunodeficiency virus (HIV) and acquired immunodeficiency syndrome (AIDS)

The clinical features seen in these patients are due to a number of causes such as opportunistic infections and drug therapy and are not usually caused by HIV. Infective arthritis seen in these immunosuppressed patients often has minimal symptoms and signs.

Arthralgia is common in AIDS. There is a seronegative, predominantly lower-limb arthritis, similar to psoriasis or Reiter's disease. Spondylitis also occurs. Avascular necrosis, possibly associated with corticosteroids or alcohol, is seen.

Nonarticular diseases such as Sjögren's- and lupus-like syndromes, systemic vasculitis of the necrotizing and hypersensitivity types (see p. 493), and myositis also occur.

Fungal infection

Fungal infections of joints occur rarely. Bone abscesses may be seen. Destructive joint lesions can also occur with blastomycosis. A benign polyarthritis accompanied by erythema nodosum occasionally occurs in coccidioidomycosis and histoplasmosis. Culture of purulent synovial fluid and skin tests for fungi may help the diagnosis.

FURTHER READING

Goldenberg DL (1998) Septic arthritis. *Lancet* **351**: 197–202.

Autoimmune diseases (connective tissue disorders)

Autoimmune diseases are conditions in which the immune system damages specific organs or causes systemic ill-health. Organ-specific autoimmune diseases include Grave's disease, Hashimoto's thyroiditis, pernicious anaemia and insulin-dependent diabetes mellitus. In most of the autoimmune rheumatic diseases it is thought that self-antigens provide the drive, although the trigger may yet prove to be exogenous. They are clinically diverse but are unified by the detection of non organ-specific autoantibodies in the serum and various tissues. Rheumatoid arthritis (RA – see p. 470) is the most common autoimmune rheumatic disease.

This section discusses systemic lupus erythematosus (SLE), polymyositis and dermatomyositis which are also sometimes referred to as *connective tissue disorders* in view of their pathophysiology.

Systemic lupus erythematosus (SLE) and lupus-like diseases

SLE is an inflammatory, multisystem disorder with arthralgia and rashes as the most common clinical features, and cerebral and renal disease as the most serious problems.

EPIDEMIOLOGY

SLE occurs world-wide but the prevalence varies from country to country, with the most common prevalence of 1:250 being in American black women. It is about nine times as common in women than in men, with a peak age of onset between 20 and 40 years.

AETIOLOGY

The cause is unknown but there are several predisposing factors:

- *Heredity*. There is a higher concordance rate in monozygotic twins (up to 85%) compared to dizygotic twins (37%). First-degree relatives have a 3% chance of developing the disease, but approximately 20% have autoantibodies.
- *Genetics*. There is an increased frequency of HLA-B8 and DR3 in caucasians. There is a stronger association with HLA-DR2 in Japanese lupus patients.
- *Complement*. There is an inherited deficiency of C2 and C4 (which are in linkage disequilibrium with HLA-DR3 and DR2).
- *Sex hormone status*. Premenopausal women are affected. In addition, SLE has been seen in males with Klinefelter's syndrome (XXY) (see p. 143). In New Zealand mice, a lupus-like disease is ameliorated by oophorectomy or treatment with male hormones.

Immunological factors

Loss of 'self' tolerance has several consequences:

- *B cell activation* results in increased autoantibody production to a variety of antigens (nuclear, cytoplasmic and plasma membrane) and hypergammaglobulinaemia.
- Development of and failure to remove *immune complexes* from the circulation leads to deposition of complexes in the tissue, causing vasculitis and disease (e.g. glomerulonephritis). Immune complexes also form in situ, e.g. kidney glomerular basement membrane.
- There is *impaired T cell regulation* of the immune response.
- There is *abnormal cytokine production* (IL-1 and IL-2), although its exact role in the pathogenesis is unknown. IL-6 and IL-10 levels are often raised.

Environmental triggers

Drugs such as hydralazine, methyldopa, isoniazid and D-penicillamine can induce lupus not associated with anti-dsDNA. Flare-ups can be induced by the contraceptive pill and hormone replacement therapy (HRT). Ultraviolet light is another well recognized trigger.

A viral agent causing SLE is a possible aetiological factor leading to the production of antibodies to nuclear material.

PATHOGENESIS

Recent evidence suggests that initially there is increased apoptosis of lymphoid cells. Nucleosomes (i.e. the DNA–histone chromatin constituents) are released from these cells and are taken up by antigen-presenting cells via nucleosome receptors. They are presented to T cells that stimulate B cells to produce autoantibodies directed against these nucleosomes and their constituents (e.g. DNA). Different subsets of autoantibodies may be responsible for the various clinical patterns.

PATHOLOGY

SLE is characterized by a widespread vasculitis affecting capillaries, arterioles and venules. Fibrinoid (an eosinophilic amorphous material) is found along blood vessels and tissue fibres. The synovium of joints may be oedematous and also contain fibrinoid deposits which contain immune complexes. Haematoxylin bodies (rounded blue homogeneous haematoxylin-stained deposits) are seen in inflammatory infiltrates and are thought to result from the interaction of antinuclear antibodies and cell nuclei.

Lesions of other organs are described in the appropriate chapters.

CLINICAL FEATURES

SLE is extremely variable in its manifestation and most of the clinical features are due to the consequences of vasculitis. Mild cases may present only with arthralgia, whilst in severe cases there may be multisystem involvement (Fig 8.26).

General features

Fever is common in exacerbations, occurring in up to 50% of cases. Patients complain of marked malaise and tiredness.

The joints

Joint involvement is the most common clinical feature (≥ 90%). Patients often present with symptoms that sound like RA with small joints being involved in a symmetrical fashion. Joints are painful but character-istically appear clinically normal, although sometimes there is slight soft-tissue swelling surrounding the joint. Deformity due to joint capsule and tendon contraction is rare, as are bony erosions. Rarely major joint deformity resembling RA (known as Jaccoud's arthropathy) may be seen. Aseptic necrosis affecting the hip or knee is a rare complication of the disease.

Myalgia is present in up to 50% of patients but a true myositis in < 5%.

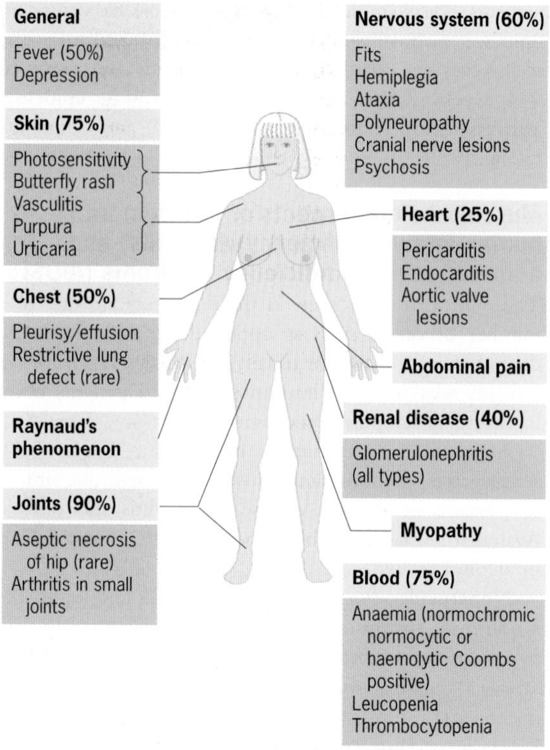

Fig 8.26
Clinical features of systemic lupus erythematosus (SLE)

The skin

This is affected in 75% of cases. Erythema, in a 'butterfly' distribution on the cheeks of the face and across the bridge of the nose, is characteristic. Vasculitic lesions on the fingertips and around the nail-folds, purpura and urticaria occur. In one-third of cases there is photosensitivity and prolonged exposure to sunlight can lead to exacerbations of the disease. Livedo reticularis, palmar and plantar rashes, pigmentation and alopecia may be seen. Raynaud's phenomenon (see p. 741) is common and may precede the development of arthralgia and other clinical problems by years.

Immunofluorescence of 'normal' skin, obtained on biopsy, will show immunoglobulin and complement deposition at the dermo–epidermal junction (known as the positive band test).

Discoid lupus is described on p. 1176.

The lungs

Up to 50% of patients will have lung involvement sometime during the course of the disease. Recurrent pleurisy and pleural effusions (exudates) are the most common manifestations and often are bilateral. Pneumonitis and atelectasis may be seen; eventually a restrictive lung defect develops with loss of lung volumes and raised hemidiaphragms. Rarely, pulmonary fibrosis occurs.

The heart and cardiovascular system

The heart is involved in 25% of cases. Pericarditis, with small pericardial effusions detected by echocardio-graphy, is common. A mild myocarditis also occurs giving rise to arrhythmias. Aortic valve lesions and a cardiomyopathy can rarely be present. A non-infective endocarditis involving the mitral valve (Libman–Sacks syndrome) is very rare. Raynaud's, vasculitis, arterial and venous thromboses can occur.

The kidneys

These invariably show histological changes, but clinical renal involvement occurs in approximately 40% of cases. Most types of glomerulonephritis occur, including mesangial, focal, diffuse and membranous. Proteinuria (> 1 g per 24 h) is common. Hypertension may occur owing to progression to either the nephrotic syndrome or renal failure.

The nervous system

Involvement of the nervous system occurs in up to 60% of cases and symptoms may fluctuate. There may be a mild depression but occasionally more severe psychiatric disturbances occur. Epilepsy, cerebellar ataxia, aseptic meningitis, cranial nerve lesions, cerebrovascular accidents or a polyneuropathy may be seen. These lesions may be due to vasculitis or immune-complex deposition.

The eyes

Retinal vasculitis can cause infarcts (cytoid bodies) which appear as hard exudates, and haemorrhages. There may be episcleritis, conjunctivitis or optic neuritis, but blindness is uncommon. Secondary Sjögren's syndrome may be seen in about 15% of cases.

The gastrointestinal system

SLE causes gastrointestinal symptoms, although these are usually not a major presenting feature. Mesenteric vasculitis can produce inflammatory lesions involving the small bowel (infarction or perforation). Liver involvement is unusual, although lupoid antibodies are described in autoimmune hepatitis. Pancreatitis is uncommon.

Lupus variants

Chronic discoid lupus is a benign variant of the disease in which skin involvement is often the only feature, although systemic abnormalities may occur with time. The rash is characteristic and appears on the face as well-defined erythematous plaques that progress to scarring and pigmentation (see p. 1176). Subacute cutaneous lupus erythematosus, a rare variant, is described on p. 1176.

Drug-induced SLE is usually characterized by arthralgia and mild systemic features, rashes and pericarditis, but seldom renal or cerebral disease. It usually disappears when the drug causing it is stopped. Hydralazine and procainamide are the most likely causes, but other drugs have occasionally been implicated.

Overlap syndrome is discussed on p. 493.

Antiphospholipid syndrome (see below) was originally described in SLE and the presence of antiphospholipid antibodies partially accounts for the increased tendency to thrombosis.

INVESTIGATIONS

- **Blood**:
  (a) *A full blood count* usually shows an anaemia (usually normochromic normocytic), leucopenia and thrombocytopenia. An autoimmune haemolytic anaemia may occur. The ESR is raised in proportion to the disease activity. In contrast, the CRP is normal.
  (b) *Serum antinuclear antibodies* (ANA) are positive in almost all cases. Double-stranded DNA binding is specific for SLE, although it is only present in 50% of cases, particularly those with severe systemic involvement (e.g. renal disease). Antibodies to RNA (ss and ds) anti-Ro and anti-La can also be detected.
  (c) *Rheumatoid factor* is positive in 30–50% of the patients.
  (d) *Serum complement* levels are reduced during active disease.
  (e) *Serological tests* for syphilis – a third of patients have a false-positive test for syphilis.
  (f) *Immunoglobulins* are raised (usually IgG and IgM).
- **Histology**. Characteristic histological and immunofluorescent abnormalities are seen in biopsies from, for example, the kidney and skin.
- **Diagnostic imaging**. CT scans of the brain sometimes show infarcts or haemorrhage with evidence of cerebral atrophy. MRI can detect lesions in white matter which are not seen on CT.

MANAGEMENT

All patients require a caring and sympathetic approach. The disease and its management should be discussed, pointing out that the prognosis is good. Patients with photosensitivity problems should avoid excessive exposure to sunlight.

Drug therapy should be used for active disease. There is no evidence that treatment in remission alters the progression of the disease.

- Arthralgia, arthritis, fever and serositis all respond well to standard doses of NSAIDs.
- Antimalarial drugs (chloroquine or hydroxychloroquine) (see Table 8.15) help mild skin disease, fatigue and arthralgias that cannot be controlled with NSAIDs.
- Corticosteroids orally or as high-dose intravenous boluses and/or immunosuppressive drugs such as azathioprine or cyclophosphamide are essential for more severe disease (glomerulonephritis, vasculitis, cerebral disease or blood dyscrasias) and when the symptoms are poorly controlled.

COURSE AND PROGNOSIS

An episodic course is characteristic, with exacerbations and complete remissions that may last for long periods. These remissions may occur even in patients with renal disease.

A chronic course is occasionally seen. Earlier estimates of the mortality in SLE were exaggerated; 10-year survival rate is about 90%. In most cases the pattern of the disease becomes established in the first ten years; if serious problems have not developed in this time, they are unlikely to do so. The arthritis is usually intermittent. Chronic progressive destruction of joints as seen in RA and OA occurs rarely, but a few patients develop deformities such as ulnar deviation.

Pregnancy and SLE

Fertility is usually normal except in severe disease and there is no major contraindication to pregnancy. Barrier methods of contraception rather than the pill are advisable. Recurrent miscarriages occur and these may be associated with antiphospholipid antibodies. Remission and exacerbations can occur during pregnancy with frequent exacerbations of the disease postpartum. The patient's usual treatment should be continued during pregnancy. Hypertension must be controlled. With severe renal disease and high antiphospholipid antibodies, fetal mortality is high (> 25%).

Antiphospholipid syndrome

This syndrome is due to the presence of antibodies which bind phospholipids. A small proportion of patients have SLE. Recurrent thromboses occur probably due to the inhibition of the phospholipid-dependent coagulation factors. β_2-Glycoprotein (β_2GP1), also known as apolipoprotein H, has been identified as the target for both anticardiolipin antibodies and lupus anticoagulant.

CLINICAL FEATURES

Arterial and venous thromboses

Approximately 20% of strokes occurring under the age of 45 years are thought to be due to the antiphospholipid syndrome. Thromboses of different types occur and cause other features of the disease, including the Budd–Chiari syndrome and Addison's disease

Abortions

Twenty-seven per cent of women who have had more than two abortions have the antiphospholipid syndrome. Antiphospholipid antibodies reduce the levels of annexin V, a protein with potent anticoagulant activity found in the placenta and vascular endothelium

Other features

These include:

- thrombocytopenia
- chorea, migraine and epilepsy
- valvular heart disease
- cutaneous manifestations (e.g. livedo reticularis).

The syndrome may also be important in the development of accelerated atheroma.

INVESTIGATIONS

Anticardiolipin antibodies (detected by ELISA) are diagnostic. Lupus anticoagulant antibodies are found in coagulation assays and these antibodies, directed against β_2GP1, can be detected by ELISA. The ESR is usually normal and antinuclear antibodies are usually negative.

TREATMENT

Anticoagulants are used. Small doses of aspirin are suitable in mild cases, warfarin in severe cases. Heparin and aspirin are given in early pregnancy, however, because warfarin is toxic to the fetus.

Systemic sclerosis (scleroderma)

Systemic sclerosis (SSc) is a multisystem disease of unknown cause. It can be localized to the skin (morphoea – see p. 1175) or more commonly involve the skin and internal organs. Raynaud's phenomenon is seen in 97% of cases.

SSc occurs world-wide with no racial differences. It is more common in women than men (3:1 ratio) with a peak incidence at between 30 and 50 years of age. It is rare in children.

A scleroderma-like disorder has been reported following industrial exposure to the solvent vinyl chloride and after ingestion of cooking oil contaminated with rape seed oil. Drugs such as bleomycin also produce a similar picture. Familial cases have been described, but concordance in twins is rare.

PATHOLOGY AND PATHOGENESIS

Vascular features

An early lesion is widespread vascular damage involving small arteries, arterioles and capillaries. There is initial endothelial cell damage with release of cytokines and endothelin-1, the latter causing vasoconstriction. There is continued intimal damage with increasing vascular permeability, leading to cellular activation, activation of adhesion molecules (E selectin, VCAM, ICAM-1), with migration of cells into the extracellular matrix. Migrating lymphocytes are IL-2 producing cells, expressing surface antigens such as CD3, CD4 and CD5. All these factors cause release of other mediators (e.g. interleukin-1, -4, -6 and -8, TFGβ and PDGF) with activation of fibroblasts.

The damage to small blood vessels also produces widespread obliterative arterial lesions and subsequent chronic ischaemia.

Fibrotic features

Fibroblasts synthesize increased quantities of collagen types I and III, as well as fibrinonectin and glycosaminoglycans, producing fibrosis in the lower dermis of the skin as well as the internal organs.

Humoral immunity

Humoral immunity is also involved because at least 80% of patients have antinuclear antibodies (see below).

CLINICAL FEATURES

Limited cutaneous scleroderma (LcSSc)

This starts initially with Raynaud's phenomenon many years (up to 15) before any skin changes. The skin involvement is usually limited to the hands, face, feet and forearms. The skin is tight, waxy and tethered, often producing flexion deformities of the fingers. Involvement of the skin of the face produces a characteristic 'beak'-like nose and a small mouth (microstomia). Painful digital ulcers and telangectasia with dilated nail-fold capillary loops are seen. Digital ischaemia leads to gangrene. Oesophageal symptoms become more severe, and patients gradually develop pulmonary hypertension and slowly progressive pulmonary interstitial disease.

The CREST syndrome (Calcinosis, Raynaud's phenomenon, Esophageal involvement, Sclerodactyly and skin changes in the fingers, Telangiectasia) was the term previously used to describe this syndrome.

Diffuse cutaneous scleroderma (DcSSc)

The skin is initially oedematous and then becomes tight several months after the patient develops Raynaud's phenomenon. There is telangiectasia and abnormal nail-fold capillaries.

Diffuse swelling and stiffness of the fingers occurs which rapidly becomes more extensive to involve most of the body in the severe cases. Later the skin becomes atrophic.

Early involvement of other organs occurs with general symptoms of lethargy, anorexia and weight loss.

- Heartburn, reflux or difficulty swallowing due to oesophageal involvement are almost invariable. Overflow pneumonia from a dilated oesophageal 'sump' occurs occasionally. Malabsorption from bacterial overgrowth due to dilatation and atony of the small bowel is seen occasionally, and more rarely dilatation and atony of the colon.
- Renal involvement is due to obliterative endarteritis, causing renal failure and malignant hypertension. This used to be the most common cause of death in systemic sclerosis before dialysis and effective anti-hypertensives became available.
- Lower-lobe lung fibrosis causes defects of lung expansion and gas transfer. This is the most common cause of death and produces exertional dyspnoea and cough. Pulmonary hypertension can be primary or secondary to the lung fibrosis.
- Myocardial fibrosis leads to arrythmias and conduction defects. Pericarditis is found occasionally.

Sometimes these systemic features occur without skin involvement (*scleroderma sine scleroderma*). Overlap syndromes with additional features of SLE, RA or inflammatory muscle disorder occur.

INVESTIGATIONS

- **Full blood count**. A normocytic, normochromic anaemia or a microangiopathic haemolytic anaemia can occur.
- **Urea and electrolytes**.
- **Autoantibodies**:
  (a) *In LcSSc*: speckled, nucleolar or anticentromere antibodies (ACAs) occur in 70–80% of cases.
  (b) *In DcSSc*: there are antitopoisomerase-1 antibodies in 30% of cases, and RNA polymerase antibodies I, II and III in 20–25%.
  (c) *Rheumatoid factor* is positive in 30%.
- **Urine**. Microscopy and, if there is proteinuria, a 24-hour urine collection for creatinine clearance.
- **Imaging**:
  (a) CXR – reticular nodular shadowing
  (b) Hands – deposits of calcium around fingers (in severe cases, erosion and absorption of the tufts of the distal phalanges)
  (c) Barium swallow – for impaired oesophageal motility.
  (d) CT – fine cut views to demonstrate lung involvement.
- Other investigations of gastrointestinal tract (e.g. see Fig 4.4), lung, renal and cardiac as appropriate.

MANAGEMENT

These diseases have a variable outlook and rate of progression. There is no cure.

- In severe disease, education, counselling and family support are essential.
- Exercises and lubricants may limit contractures.
- Raynaud's may be improved by hand warmers, oral vasodilators (calcium-channel blockers, ACE inhibitors) and parenteral vasodilators (prostacyclin analogues and calcitonin gene related peptide). Lumbar and digital sympathectomy may help.
- Oesophageal symptoms can be improved by proton-pump inhibitors and prokinetic drugs (cisapride).
- Symptomatic malabsorption requires low-residue diets, nutritional supplements and rotational antibiotics.
- Renal involvement requires intensive hypertensive control (with either ACE inhibitors or calcium antagonists).
- Intravenous prostacyclin may be helpful. High-dose corticosteroids have no place in the management of scleroderma and may precipitate renal crisis.
- Pulmonary vascular disease may initially respond to vasodilators.
- Pulmonary fibrosis does not significantly respond to current therapies.
- Immunosuppressive drugs (e.g. cyclophosphamide) and antifibrotic drugs (e.g D-penicillamine) have been shown to be beneficial only in open studies. Placebo-controlled trials are in progress.

PROGNOSIS

In limited cutaneous scleroderma the disease is often milder, with much less severe internal organ involvement and a 70% ten-year survival. Pulmonary hypertension is a significant but later cause of death. This is in contrast to diffuse disease (55% ten-year survival) where organ involvement is often severe and most patients die of pulmonary, cardiac and/or renal involvement.

Localized forms of scleroderma also occur either in patches (morphea) or linear forms. These are more commonly seen in children and adolescents and do not convert into systemic forms.

Polymyositis and dermatomyositis

Polymyositis is a rare disorder of unknown cause, in which the clinical picture is dominated by non-suppurative inflammation of striated muscle, causing proximal muscle weakness. When the skin is involved it is called 'dermatomyositis'. The aetiology is unknown, although viruses (e.g. Coxsackie, rubella, influenza) have been implicated but not found. An autoimmune mechanism has been suggested owing to the presence of the anti-Jo1 antibody and lymphocyte infiltration in the muscle. Both polymyositis and the anti-Jo1 antibody are HLA-DR3 linked.

CLINICAL FEATURES

The onset can be insiduous over months, but rarely acute. General malaise, weight loss and fever develop during the acute phase.

The major feature of polymyositis is proximal muscle weakness which is progressive. There is wasting of the shoulder and pelvic girdle muscles with pain, weakness and tenderness. Patients have difficulty squatting, going up stairs, rising from a chair and raising their hands above the head.

Respiratory muscles are affected in severe disease (especially those with anti-Jo1 antibodies) and patients may require ventilation. Dysphagia is seen in about 50% owing to oesophageal muscle involvement. Arthralgia is seen in about 25% but is mild.

Cutaneous features include a heliotrope (purple) discolouration of the eyelids and peri-orbital oedema. Scaly, purple-red raised vasculitic patches occur over the extensor surfaces of joints and fingers (*collodion patches*). Ulcerative vasculitis and calcinosis of the subcutaneous tissue are common in the childhood form and occur in 25% of adults. In the long term, muscle fibrosis and contractures of joints occur.

There is an association with other *autoimmune* rheumatic diseases (e.g. SLE, RA and systemic sclerosis) with their associated features (e.g. Raynaud's phenomenon).

There is also an association with malignancy (e.g. lung, ovary, breast, stomach), which can predate the onset of myositis. This occurs particularly in males with dermatomyositis.

INVESTIGATIONS

- **ESR** is raised in about 50%.
- **Muscle enzymes**. Serum creatine phosphokinase (CPK) and aldolase are raised and can be used to follow the progress of the disease during treatment.
- **Anti-Jo1 antibodies** (antibodies to histidyl tRNA synthetase) are positive 30%.
- **Rheumatoid factor** present in up to 50%.
- **Electromyography** (EMG) shows a typical triad of changes: spontaneous fibrillation potentials at rest, polyphasic or short-duration potentials on voluntary contraction, and salvos of repetitive potentials on mechanical stimulation of the nerve.
- **MRI** is used to target abnormal muscle which can then be biopsied.
- **Fine-needle muscle biopsy**. Inflammatory infiltrates with lymphocytes occur around the blood vessels and between the muscle fibres. There is degeneration and abnormal regeneration of fibres and fibre necrosis. The normally peripheral nuclei of skeletal muscle fibres migrate to the centre

TREATMENT

Hospitalization is required during the acute phase for rest, splinting and passive joint movements. Corticosteroids have greatly improved the clinical outlook in children and some adults. Immunosuppressive agents, e.g. azathioprine or methotrexate, are often needed. Muscle disease is monitored by regular formal strength testing and serum CPK measurements. Once the acute phase settles, graded exercises restore strength and avoid contractures.

The disease may persist for years and should be managed with the lowest maintenance doses of corticosteroids possible.

Sjögren's syndrome and keratoconjuctivitis sicca

The syndrome of dry eyes (keratoconjunctivitis sicca) in the absence of rheumatoid arthritis or any of the autoimmune diseases is known as 'primary Sjögren's syndrome'. There is an association with HLA B8 DR3. Dryness of the mouth, skin or vagina may also be a problem. Salivary and parotid gland enlargement is seen.

Associated systemic features include:

- arthralgia and occasional non-progressive polyarthritis, like that seen in SLE (but much less common)
- Raynaud's phenomenon
- dysphagia and abnormal oesophageal motility as seen in systemic sclerosis (but less common)
- other organ-specific autoimmune disease, including thyroid disease, myasthenia gravis, primary biliary cirrhosis and autoimmune hepatitis

- renal tubular defects (uncommon) causing nephrogenic diabetes insipidus and renal tubular acidosis
- pulmonary diffusion defects and fibrosis
- polyneuropathy, fits and depression
- vasculitis
- increased incidence of non-Hodgkins B cell lymphoma.

PATHOLOGY AND INVESTIGATIONS

Biopsies of the salivary gland or of the lip show a focal infiltration of lymphocytes and plasma cells.

- **Schirmer tear test**. This is a standard strip of filter papers placed on the inside of the lower eyelid; wetting of less than < 10 mm in five minutes indicates defective tear production.
- **Rose Bengal staining** of the eyes shows punctate or filamentary keratitis.
- **Laboratory abnormalities**. These included raised immunoglobulin levels, circulating immune complexes and many autoantibodies. Rheumatoid factor is usually positive. Antinuclear antibodies are found in 60–70% of cases and antimitochondrial antibodies in 10%. Anti-Ro (SSA) antibodies are found in 70%, compared with 10% of cases of RA and *secondary* Sjögren's syndrome. This antibody is of particular interest because it can cross the placenta and cause congenital heart block.

Treatment is with artificial tears and saliva replacement solutions.

'Overlap' syndromes

The title 'overlap syndrome' describes patients in whom the clinical features of two or more autoimmune rheumatic diseases occur. They are rare. They are also called '*mixed connective tissue disorders*'. The combinations include:

- RA and SLE
- RA, SLE and Sjögren's syndrome
- polymyositis with scleroderma/systemic sclerosis and/or SLE.

FURTHER READING

Black C (1998) Scleroderma (systemic sclerosis). *Medicine* **26**: 33–40.

Wallace DJ, Hahn BH (eds) (1993) Discoid Lupus Erythematosus, 4th edn. Philadelphia: Lea and Febiger.

Systemic inflammatory vasculitis

Vasculitis is an inflammation of the vessel wall. The classification remains unsatisfactory, but is usually based on the type of artery affected (Fig 8.27 and Table 8.18). There is some overlap and some cases are difficult to classify,

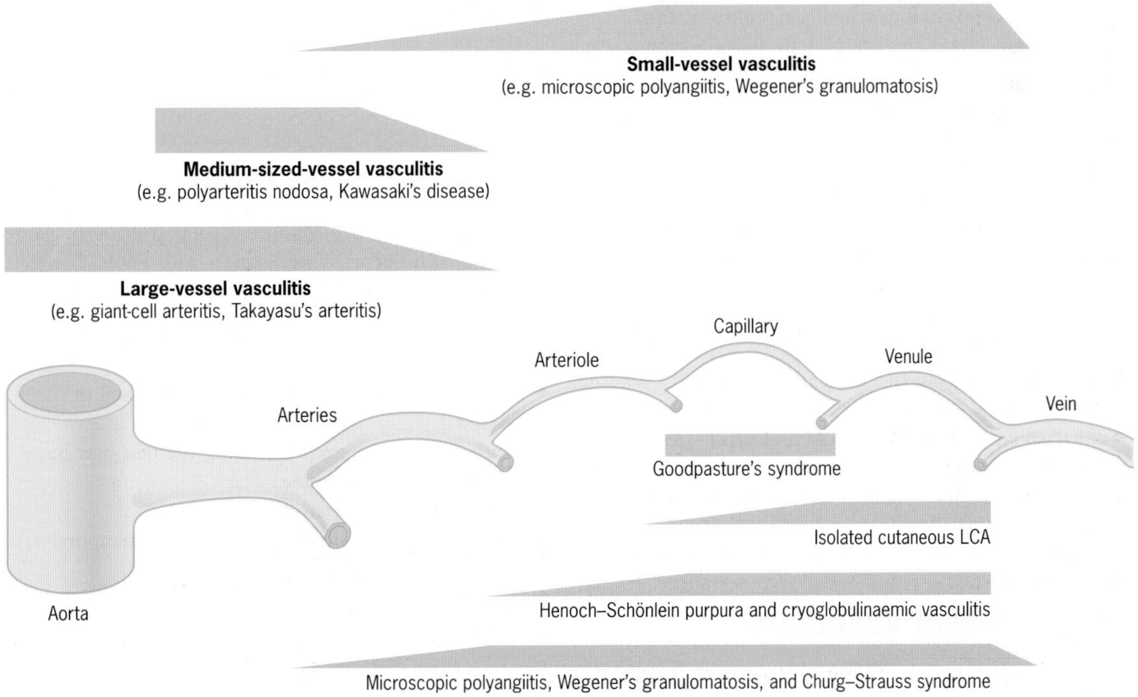

Fig 8.27
Sites of vascular involvement by vasculitides From Jeanette and Falk (1997) *New England Journal of Medicine* **337**: 1512–1523
LCA, leucocyte angiitis

Table 8.18
Types of systemic vasculitis

Non-infective		
Large	Giant cell arteritis Takayasu's arteritis	
Medium	Classical polyarteritis nodosum (PAN) Kawasaki's disease	
Small	Microscopic polyangiitis Wegner's granulomatosis Churg–Strauss syndrome	ANCA associated
	Henoch–Schönlein purpura Cutaneous leucocytoclastic angiitis Essential cryoglobulinaemia	

Table 8.19
Other conditions associated with vasculitis

Infective	e.g. subacute infective endocarditis
Non-infective	Vasculitis with rheumatoid arthritis Systemic lupus erythematosis Scleroderma Polymyositis/dermatomyositis Drug-induced Behçet's disease Goodpasture's syndrome Hypocomplementaemia Serum sickness Paraneoplastic Inflammatory bowel disease

partly because in many conditions there is always some vasculitis histologically. An alternative classification is shown in Table 20.11. Table 8.19 shows other infective and noninfective conditions in which a vasculitis is seen.

The disorders are characterized by inflammation in or through a blood vessel wall, with fibrinoid necrosis or granuloma formation. Histologically there are several different patterns: necrotizing vasculitis, giant cell arteritis and granulomatous angiitis. The clinical manifestations are due to ischaemic necrosis and vary with the size and type of blood vessel affected. Vasculitis is a systemic disease which affects the skin and musculoskeletal, renal and gastrointestinal systems. Skin lesions are palpable and commonly urticarial. Many types of systemic non-autoimmune vasculitis are associated with antineutrophilic cytoplasmic antibody (ANCA – see p. 539).

- *Large vessel* refers to the aorta and its major tributaries.
- *Medium vessel* refers to medium and small-sized arteries and arterioles.
- *Small vessel* refers to small arteries, arterioles, venules and capillaries.

Large vessel vasculitis

Polymyalgia rheumatica (PMR) and giant cell (temporal) arteritis are systemic illnesses of the elderly. Both are associated with the finding of a giant cell arteritis on temporal artery biopsy.

Information

- Polymyositis – proximal pain and weakness
- Polymyalgia rheumatica – proximal morning stiffness and pain
- Myopathy – weakness, but no pain or stiffness

Information box 8.12 Symptom patterns in some muscle disorders

Polymyalgia rheumatica (PMR)

PMR causes a sudden onset of severe pain and stiffness of the shoulders and neck, and of the hips and lumbar spine; a limb girdle pattern. These symptoms are worse in the morning from 30 minutes to several hours. The clinical history is usually diagnostic and the patient is always over 50 years.

Patients develop systemic features of tiredness, fever, weight loss, depression and occasionally nocturnal sweats if it is not diagnosed and treated early. A differential diagnosis is shown in Information box 8.12.

INVESTIGATION OF PMR

- **A raised ESR and/or CRP** is a hallmark of this condition. It is rare to see PMR without an acute-phase response. If it is absent the diagnosis should be questioned and the tests repeated a few weeks later before treatment is started.
- **Serum alkaline phosphatase and γ-glutamyltransferase** may be raised.
- **Anaemia** (mild normochromic, normocytic) is often present.
- **Temporal artery biopsy** shows giant cell arteritis in 10–30% of cases, but is not usually performed.

Giant cell arteritis (GCA)

GCA is inflammatory granulomatous arteritis of large arteries which occurs in association with PMR. It affects only the over-fifties. The patient may have current PMR, a history of recent PMR, or be on treatment for PMR. It may present with the symptoms of GCA which are:

- severe headaches, usually unilateral temporal or occipital
- tenderness of the scalp (combing the hair may be painful) or of the temple
- claudication of the jaw when eating
- tenderness and swelling of one or more temporal or occipital arteries
- systemic manifestations – severe malaise, tiredness and fever.

Involvement of the ophthalmic arteries causes sudden painless temporary or permanent visual loss.

Occasionally GCA presents as a potentially treatable cerebrovascular episode.

If a person with PMR on treatment develops unilateral severe headaches, GCA should be considered. Nevertheless, remember that tension headaches are common.

INVESTIGATION OF GCA

- **ESR** is usually raised (in the region of 50–120 mm h^{-1}) and the **CRP** very high.
- **Liver biochemistry**. Anormalities occur, as in PMR.
- **A temporal artery biopsy** from the affected side is the definitive diagnostic test. This should be taken before, or within 36 hours of starting, high doses of corticosteroids. Start the drug first if the patient is very ill, in severe pain or has experienced visual loss or stroke. The lesions are patchy and the whole length of the biopsy must be examined.

The histological features of CGA are:

- intimal hypertrophy
- inflammation of the intima and sub-intima
- breaking up of the internal elastic lamina
- giant cells in the internal elastic lamina.

TREATMENT OF PMR OR GCA

Corticosteroids produce a dramatic reduction of symptoms within 24–48 hours of starting treatment, provided the dose is adequate. This should reduce the risk of patients with PMR developing GCA. NSAIDs are less effective and should not be used.

In GCA, corticosteroids are obligatory because they significantly reduce the risk of irreversible visual loss and other focal ischaemic lesions, but much higher doses are needed. Both diseases settle after between 12 and 36 months of treatment in about 75% of patients, but the remaining 25% continue to require low doses of corticosteoids for years. Starting doses of prednisolone are:

- PMR: 10–15 mg prednisolone as a single dose in the morning
- GCA: 60–100 mg prednisolone, usually in divided doses.

With GCA it is best to *start* at the higher dose, as the response is more dramatic and diagnostic. The dose should then be reduced gradually in weekly steps. While the dose is above 20 mg the weekly step reductions are 5 mg, reducing the evening doses first. Between 20 mg and 10 mg the reduction can be in 2.5 mg steps, but below 10 mg the rate should be slower and the steps each of 1 mg.

Dose reduction (and increases when necessary) are titrated against the response or recurrence of symptoms and a fall or rise in the ESR or CRP.

Takayasu's arteritis

This is a granulomatous inflammation of the aorta and its major branches and is discussed on p. 741.

Medium-sized vessel vasculitis

Polyarteritis nodosa (PAN)

Classic PAN is a rare condition which, unlike other vasculitic diseases, usually occurs in middle-age men. It is accompanied by severe systemic manifestations, and its occasional association with hepatitis B antigenaemia suggests a vasculitis secondary to the deposition of immune complexes. Pathologically, there is fibrinoid necrosis of vessel walls with microaneurysm formation, thrombosis and infarction.

CLINICAL FEATURES

These include fever, malaise, weight loss and myalgia. These initial symptoms are followed by dramatic acute features that are due to organ infarction.

- *Neurological* – mononeuritis multiplex is due to arteritis of the vaso nervosum.
- *Abdominal* – pain due to arterial involvement of the abdominal viscera, mimicking acute cholecystitis, pancreatitis or appendicitis. Gastrointestinal haemorrhage occurs due to mucosal ulceration.
- *Renal* – presents with haematuria and proteinuria. Hypertension and acute/chronic renal failure occur.
- *Cardiac* – coronary arteritis causes myocardial infarction and heart failure. Pericarditis may occur.
- *Skin* – purpura, subcutaneous haemorrhage and gangrene occur. A persistent livedo reticularis is seen in chronic cases. Chorioretinitis, cutaneous and subcutaneous palpable nodules occur, but are uncommon.
- *Lung* – involvement is rare.

INVESTIGATIONS AND TREATMENT

- **Blood count**. Anaemia, leucocytosis and a raised ESR occur.
- **Biopsy** material from an affected organ.
- **Angiography**. Demonstration of microaneurysms in hepatic, intestinal or renal vessels if necessary.
- Other investigations as appropriate (e.g. ECG and abdominal ultrasound), depending on the clinical problem. ANCA is positive in only 15–20% of cases of classic PAN.

Treatment is with corticosteroids, usually in combination with immunosuppressive drugs such as azathioprine.

Kawasaki's disease

This is an acute systemic vasculitis involving medium-sized vessels, affecting mainly children under five years of age. It is very frequent in Japan, suggesting an infective aetiology, but none has been demonstrated. It occurs world-wide and is also seen in adults.

CLINICAL FEATURES AND TREATMENT

The clinical features are:

- fever lasting five days or more
- bilateral conjunctival congestion 2–4 days after onset
- dryness and redness of the lips and oral cavity three days after onset
- acute cervical lymphadenopathy accompanying the fever
- polymorphic rash involving any part of the body
- redness and an oedema of the palms and soles 2–5 days after onset.

Five of these six features should be present to make the diagnosis, or four of six if coronary aneurysms can be seen on two-dimensional echocardiography or angiography.

Cardiovascular changes in the acute stage include pancarditis and coronary arteritis leading to aneurysms or dilatation. Other features include diarrhoea, albuminuria, aseptic meningitis and arthralgia and, in most, there is a leucocytosis, thrombocytosis and a raised CRP.

Treatment is with high-dose intravenous gamma-globulin which prevents the coronary artery disease, followed after the acute phase by aspirin 200–300 mg daily.

Small vessel vasculitis

This can be separated into those that are positive or negative for antineutrophilic cytoplasmic antibody (ANCA). The role of these antibodies in the pathogenesis is unclear, but there is a correlation between ANCA titres and disease activity. ANCAs are specific for antigens in neutrophil granules and monocyte lysosomes. There are two types (see p. 539):

- antimyeloperoxidase (anti-MPO)
- antiproteinase-3 (anti-PR-3).

Neutrophils activated by ANCA may lead to endothelial injury by interaction between the neutrophils and cytokine activated endothelium which precedes the vasculitic lesions.

The clinical features and diagnosis of small vessel vasculitis are shown in Table 8.20.

ANCA-positive vasculitis

- Wegner's granulomatosis – see p. 810.
- Churg–Strauss granulomatosis – see p. 810.
- Microscopic polyangiitis – see p. 539.

Non-ANCA-positive small-vessel vasculitis

This includes Henoch–Schönlein purpura – see p. 499.

Cutaneous leucocytoclastic angiitis (p. 1186)

This is the characteristic acute purpuric lesion which histologically involves the dermal post-capillary venules. This lesion affects only the skin and should be differentiated from similar lesions produced in systemic vasculitis. The condition can be caused by drugs such as sulphonamides and penicillin.

Cutaneous leucocytoclastic angiitis

This affects mainly patients in their fifties, causing purpura, arthralgia and glomerulonephritis. Hepatitis C infection is common and may be an aetiological agent.

TREATMENT OF SMALL CELL VASCULITIS

Small vessel vasculitis may be self-limiting and requires little treatment. Aggressive therapy with corticosteroids and immunosuppressive agents is required for severe disease.

Table 8.20
Diagnosis and clinical features of small vessel vasculitis

	Wegner's granulomatosis	Churg–Strauss syndrome	Microscopic polyangiitis	Henoch–Schönlein purpura	Cryoglobulinaemic vasculitis
Features					
ANCA (in blood) – PR3	+	+	+	–	–
– MPO	90%	60%	60%		
Necrotizing granulomas	+	+	–	–	–
Cryoglobulins (in blood and vessels	–	–	–	–	–
IgA immune deposits (mainly)	–	–	–	+	–
Asthma and eosinophilia	–	+	–	–	–
Organs involved					
Skin	40	60	40	90	90
Kidneys	80	45	90	50	55
Lungs	90	70	50	<5	<5
ENT	90	50	35	<5	<5
Musculoskeletal	60	50	60	75	70
Neurological	50	70	30	10	40
Gastrointestinal	50	50	50	60	30

Modified from Jeanette JC, Falk RJ (1997) Small vessel vasculitis. *New England Journal of Medicine* **337**: 1512–1523

Behçet's disease

Behçet's disease is a systemic vasculitis of unknown cause. There is a striking geographical distribution, it being most common in Turkey, Iran and Japan. The prevalence per 100 000 is 10–15 in Japan and 80–300 in Turkey. There is a link to HLA-B51, with a relative risk of 5–10; this association is not seen in patients in the USA and Europe.

CLINICAL FEATURES

The cardinal clinical feature is recurrent oral ulceration. The international criteria for diagnosis require any two of the following: genital ulcers, defined eye lesions, defined skin lesions, or a positive skin pathergy test (see below). Oral ulcers can be aphthous or herpetiform. The eye lesions include an anterior or posterior uveitis or retinal vascular lesions. Cutaneous lesions consist of erythema nodosum, pseudofolliculitis and papulopustular lesions.

Other manifestations include a self-limiting peripheral mono- or oligo-arthritis affecting knees, ankles, wrists and elbows; gastrointestinal symptoms of diarrhoea, abdominal pain and anorexia; pulmonary and renal lesions; a brain stem syndrome, organic confusional states and a meningoencephalitis.

The pathergy reaction is highly specific to Behçet's. Skin injury, by a needle prick for example, leads to papule or pustule formation within 24–48 hours.

TREATMENT

Corticosteroids, immunosuppressant agents and cyclosporin-A are used for chronic uveitis and the rare neurological complications. Colchicine helps erythema nodosum and joint pain.

FURTHER READING

Salvarani C et al (1997) Polymyalgia rheumatica. *Lancet* **350**: 43–47.

Savage COS et al (1997) Primary vasculitis. *Lancet* **349**: 553–558.

Jeanette JC, Falk RJ (1997) Small vessel vasculitis. *New England Journal of Medicine* **339**: 1512–1523.

Differential diagnosis of rheumatic complaints in the elderly (Fig 8.28)

Musculoskeletal problems
These are common at all ages. In the elderly, pain arises from a combination of age-related changes and injury.

Back and neck pain
These are commonly associated with spondylosis on X-ray and are more likely to be associated with such complications as spinal stenosis or nerve root claudication.

Osteoporotic fractures
Osteoporotic fractures of the spine cause acute pain or deformity and subsequent postural back pain. *Mechanical back pain* may be worse in the morning, especially when spondylosis is severe or there is marked deformity; there is a normal ESR and CRP, which distinguishes this from polymyalgia rheumatica.

The management of such problems in the elderly is the same as for younger people but a response to treatment is less predictable. Advice about posture, exercise and general fitness is important but must be tempered by the patient's general health and fitness.

Symptomatic osteoarthritis
This increases with increasing age and is uncommon below the age of 50 years. It is necessary to look for possible reversible causes of pain and disability, such as peri-articular lesions or a joint effusion. Caution about drug treatment is necessary because of the increased risk of side-effects in older patients. Joint replacement surgery has transformed the outlook for many older people with OA by offering pain control and increased mobility and independence.

Rheumatoid arthritis
RA may present in the elderly as a dramatic onset of symmetrical polyarthritis. This has a reasonable prognosis and responds well to low doses of prednisolone and other drug therapy. RA may mimic polymyalgia rheumatica; the synovitis becomes apparent as the corticosteroid dose is reduced. Treat with DMARDs as for RA in order to reduce the corticosteroid dose.

Polymyalgia rheumatica and giant cell arteritis
These must be recognized and treated. Failure to respond to adequate doses of prednisolone should trigger a search for an alternative disease, such as RA, vasculitis, infection or malignancy.

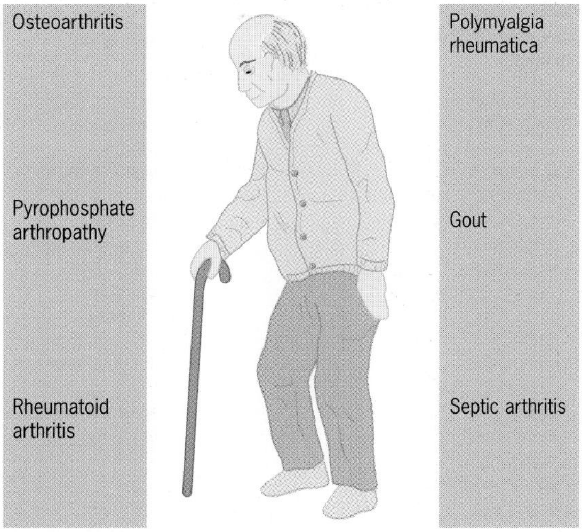

Fig 8.28
The differential diagnosis of arthritis in the elderly

Chondrocalcinosis

This increases with increasing age and is seen on over 40% of knee X-rays in the over-80s. It may produce a variety of arthritic conditions (see p. 469).

Pseudogout

This is an important cause of acute monarthritis of the wrist or knee in older people. It responds well to aspiration and injection and to intra-articular corticosteroids or oral NSAIDs.

Gout

True gout causes acute monarthritis in the elderly but may also present as a polyarticular inflammatory arthritis, especially in elderly women on long-term diuretic treatment, or as tophaceous gout.

Septic arthritis

Septic arthritis in the elderly and frail produces articular symptoms, and signs that may be muted. The patient usually has septicaemia and the best way to ensure its recognition is to retain it in the differential diagnosis of all musculoskeletal presentations in unwell, elderly people.

Arthritis in children

Joint and limb pains are common in children but arthritis is fortunately rare. Babies and young children may present with immobility of a joint or a limp, but the diagnosis can be extremely difficult. Fig 8.29 summarizes the differential diagnosis.

For chronic conditions the child and family often need a great deal of support from physiotherapists, occupational therapists, pyschologists, teachers, social workers and orthopaedic surgeons. These are best obtained in specialist paediatric centres.

Juvenile chronic arthritis

- Systemic arthritis
- Oligoarthritis (persistent)
- Oligoarthritis (extended)
- Polyarticular arthritis (rheumatoid-factor positive)
- Polyarticular arthritis (rheumatoid-factor negative)
- Juvenile spondyloarthropathy
- Psoriatic arthritis
- Unclassified

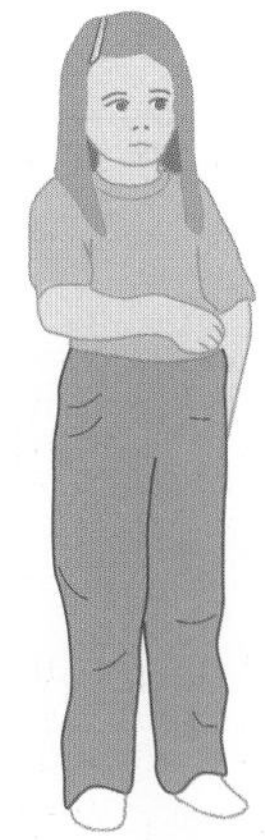

Other types

- Infections, e.g. tuberculosis, rubella
- Rheumatic fever
- Henoch–Schönlein purpura
- Traumatic arthritis
- Hypermobility syndrome
- Leukaemia
- Sickle cell disease
- SLE and connective tissue disorders
- Transient synovitis of the hip

Fig 8.29
The differential diagnosis of arthritis in children

Juvenile chronic (or idiopathic) arthritis (JCA or JIA)

Systemic arthritis

Still's disease (which accounts for 10% of cases of JCA) affects boys and girls equally up to five years of age; then girls are more commonly affected. Adult-onset Still's disease is extremely rare.

Clinical features include a high, swinging, early-evening pyrexia, an evanescent pink maculopapular rash with arthralgia and arthritis, myalgia and generalized lymphadenopathy. Hepatosplenomegaly and pericarditis and pleurisy occur. The differential diagnoses include malignancy, in particular leukaemia and neuroblastoma, and infection. Laboratory tests show a high ESR and CRP, neutrophilia and thrombocytosis. Autoantibodies are negative.

Oligoarthritis (persistent)

This is the most common form of JCA (50–60%) but is still rare. It affects four or fewer joints – especially wrists, knees, ankles – often in an asymmetrical pattern. It affects mainly girls, with a peak age of three years. Uveitis (often with a positive ANA) occurs and requires regular screening by a three-monthly slit-lamp examination; blindness can occur.

Generally the prognosis is good, with remission in 4–5 years.

Oligoarthritis (extended)

This is a chronic arthritis with an oligoarticular onset of the disease, which progresses to involve more than four joints. The joints tend to be stiff rather than hot and swollen.

Polyarticular JCA

This develops with or without a preceding systemic illness at any age after 12 months. It usually occurs in teenagers and produces widespread joint destruction. There is a symmetrical arthritis of hands, wrists, PIPs and occasionally DIPs. Rheumatoid factor is usually negative, but in 3% of cases (often teenage girls) this is strongly positive.

Juvenile spondyloarthropathy

This affects teenage and younger boys, producing an asymmetrical arthritis of lower-limb joints and enthesitis. It is associated with HLA-B27 and acute anterior uveitis and represents the childhood equivalent of adult ankylosing spondylitis. Approximately 60% of these patients will have developed the latter on follow-up.

Psoriatic arthritis

This affects fingers and toes as well as a polyarthritis involving large and small joints. The arthritis can be very erosive. Psoriasis may be present in the child or a first-degree relative.

TREATMENT OF JCA

JCA should always be referred to a specialist paediatric rheumatology unit to avoid long-term disability. These units have facilities for rehabilitation, education and surgical intervention if necessary. Low doses of NSAIDs and paracetamol help the pain and stiffness, but corticosteroids and immunosuppressants (e.g. methotrexate) are often required for systemic disease. Because of the association of Reye's syndrome with aspirin, this drug should not be used under the age of 12 years except for JCA. Growth retardation is a problem with corticosteriod therapy.

PROGNOSIS

This is very variable for JCA, although up to 50% of children will have long-term disability. In severe cases death occurs due to infection, pericarditis or renal amyloidosis.

Other types of arthritis

Henoch–Schönlein purpura (see also p. 535)

This is a common systemic vasculitis seen in children. There is deposition of IgA immune complexes in the arterioles, capillaries and venules. It occurs after an upper respiratory tract infection. Common manifestations include purpura, a transient non-migratory polyarthritis and abdominal pain. Fifty per cent of these patients have haematuria and proteinuria, owing to a glomerulonephritis; *treatment* of this is discussed on p. 535. The prognosis is usually excellent.

Rheumatic fever

Rheumatic fever is still seen in developing countries but is rare in Europe, North America and Australasia where ready access to antibiotics for sore throats prevents it. The incidence was declining before the antibiotic era, possibly due to reduced virulence of the organism and improvements in public health. It predominantly affects children aged 4–15 years, with a peak at 7–8 years. It is triggered by a group-A beta-haemolytic *Streptococcus* infection, usually of the throat, with raised antistreptolysin-O antibody titres. The delayed effects are due to antibodies which cross-react with human sarcolemma, heart or brain tissues and occur 1–5 weeks after the infection, by which time the throat swab may be sterile. Clinical features are described on p. 699.

The fever is persistent but not as high as in Still's disease (see above). The 'flitting' polyarthritis which starts at the same time as the fever is unlike Still's disease, where arthralgia occurs during the febrile period, and joint swelling occurs only later. The arthritis affects larger joints and migrates between joints, each being affected for a few days at a time.

Treatment includes bedrest during the acute phase, paracetamol or NSAIDs for fever and arthritis, and prophylactic penicillin until aged 20 years. Aspirin is now less commonly used because of Reye's syndrome .

Hypermobility syndrome

This occurs in children or young adults with lax joints. Fewer than half of the children with hypermobility will present with recurrent joint pains, mainly affecting the knees, but also other joints. Other problems include joint effusion, dislocation, ligamentous injuries, low back pain and the development of premature osteoarthritis. The condition is benign, but joints become stiffer with age.

Hypermobility is also associated with some rare congenital disorders such as the Ehlers–Danlos syndrome (see pp. 518 and 1187).

Treatment is with exercise directed at improving muscle power.

Miscellaneous conditions

Some children develop *idiopathic musculoskeletal pain* which can become chronic. The management of these children is to exclude the causes shown in Fig 8.29 without doing unnecessary laboratory investigations. *Nocturnal musculoskeletal pains* are episodic, last about thirty minutes and wake the child from sleep. They are often called 'growing pains' – physiotherapy, analgesics and reassurance are given.

Ischaemic bone disease affecting the ossification centre of the ends of bones include *Osgood–Schlatter disease*, which is characterized by localized pain over the tip of the tibial tubercle and is usually seen in athletic teenagers, and *Perthe's disease*. This latter is an idiopathic necrosis of the proximal femoral head epiphysis of unknown aetiology. It presents as a painless limp, usually in boys aged 3–12 years, is occasionally bilateral and, if advanced, may require surgical correction.

A *transient synovitis of the hip* causes painful limitation of the movement of one hip and usually resolves within a few weeks or months. It may cause concern because of the possibility of tuberculosis or other serious conditions.

FURTHER READING

Woo P, Wedderburn LR (1998) Juvenile chronic arthritis. *Lancet* **351**: 969–973.

Arthritis associated with other diseases

Gastrointestinal and liver disease

- *Enteropathic synovitis* – see p. 482.
- *Autoimmune hepatitis* (see p. 213) may be accompanied by an arthralgia similar to that seen in systemic lupus erythematosus. Joint pain occurs in a bilateral, symmetrical distribution, with the small joints of the

hands being prominently affected. Joints usually look normal but sometimes there is a slight soft-tissue swelling. These patients often have positive tests for antinuclear antibodies.

- *Primary biliary cirrhosis* patients occasionally have a symmetrical arthropathy.
- *Hereditary haemochromatosis* is associated with arthritis in 50% of cases; this is often the first sign of the disease and chondrocalcinosis is common.
- *Whipple's disease* (see p. 257) is accompanied by fever and arthralgia.

Malignant disease

It is not uncommon for malignant diseases to present with musculoskeletal symptoms. Bone pain may be due to multiple myeloma, lymphoma, a primary tumour of bone or secondary deposits. The pain is typically unremitting, worse at night and there are other clinical clues such as weight loss or ill-health. Secondary gout occurs in conditions such as chronic myeloid leukaemia.

Hypertrophic pulmonary osteoarthropathy

Hypertrophic osteoarthropathy is most often associated with carcinoma of the bronchus. It is a non-metastatic complication and may be the presenting feature of the disease. It occurs only rarely with other conditions that also cause clubbing. It is seen most often in middle-aged men, who present with pain and swelling of the wrists and ankles. Other joints are involved occasionally.

The diagnosis is made on the presence of clubbing of the fingers, which is usually gross, and periosteal new bone formation along the shafts of the distal ends of the radius, ulna, tibia and fibula seen on X-ray. A chest X-ray usually shows the malignancy.

Treatment should be directed at the underlying carcinoma; if this can be removed, the arthropathy disappears. NSAIDs may help to relieve the symptoms.

Paraneoplastic polyarthritis

This is seen with carcinoma of the breast in women and of the lung in men, and also with renal cell carcinoma. The neoplasm may be occult at onset and the diagnosis is then difficult to make.

Skin disease

Psoriatic arthritis

This is discussed on p. 1166.

Erythema nodosum

This can be due to several conditions (e.g. sarcoidosis) and is accompanied by arthritis in over 50% of cases. The knees and ankles are particularly affected, being swollen, red and tender. The arthritis subsides, along with the skin lesions, within a few months. *Treatment* is with NSAIDs or occasionally steroids.

Neurological disease

Neuropathic joints (Charcot's joints) are joints damaged by trauma as a result of the loss of the protective pain sensation. They were first described by Charcot in relation to tabes dorsalis. They are also seen in syringomyelia, diabetes mellitus and leprosy. The site of the neuropathic joint depends upon the localization of the pain loss:

- in tabes dorsalis, the knees and ankles are most often affected
- in diabetes mellitus, the joints of the tarsus are involved
- in syringomyelia, the shoulder is involved.

Neuropathic joints are not painful, although there may be painful episodes associated with crystal deposition. Presentation is usually with swelling and instability and eventually severe deformities develop.

The characteristic finding is a swollen joint with abnormal but painless movement. This is associated with neurological findings that depend upon the underlying disease (e.g. dissociated sensory loss in syringomyelia or polyneuropathy in diabetes). X-ray changes are characteristic, with gross joint disorganization and bony distortion.

Treatment is symptomatic. Surgery may be required in advanced cases.

Blood disease

Arthritis due to haemarthrosis is a common presenting feature of *haemophilia* (see p. 404).

Attacks begin in early childhood in most cases and are recurrent. The knee is the most common affected joint but the elbows and ankles are sometimes involved. The arthritis can lead to bone destruction and disorganization of joints. Apart from replacement of factor VIII, affected joints require initial immobilization followed by physiotherapy to restore movement and measures to prevent and correct deformities.

Sickle cell crises (p. 378) are often accompanied by joint pain that particularly affects the hands and feet in a bilateral, symmetrical distribution. Affected joints usually look normal but are occasionally swollen. This condition may also be complicated by avascular necrosis (see p. 400) and by *Salmonella osteomyelitis*.

Arthritis can also occur in *acute leukaemia*; it may be the presenting feature in childhood. The knee is particularly affected and is very painful, warm and swollen. Treatment is directed at the underlying leukaemia. Arthritis may also occur in chronic leukaemia, with leukaemic deposits in and around the joints.

Endocrine and metabolic disorders

Hypothyroid patients may complain of pain and stiffness of proximal muscles, resembling polymyalgia rheumatica.

They may also have carpal tunnel syndrome. Less often, there is an arthritis accompanied by joint effusions, particularly in the knees, wrist and small joints of the hands and feet. These problems respond rapidly to thyroxine.

In *acromegaly* an arthritis occurs in about 50% of patients. It resembles osteoarthritis and particularly affects the small joints of the hands and knees. It may be associated with the carpal tunnel syndrome.

In *Cushing's disease*, back pain is common.

Joint disorders related to *diabetes mellitus* are described on p. 985.

Familial hypercholesterolaemia is associated with oligo- or polyarthritis usually with tendon xanthomata. Arthritis also occurs in combined *hyperlipidaemia*.

Miscellaneous arthropathies

Familial Mediterranean fever (FMF)

FMF is inherited as an autosomal recessive condition and occurs in certain ethnic groups, particularly Arabs, Turks, Armenians and Sephardic Jews. The gene, called *MEFV*, has been localized to chromosome 16. It encodes for pyrin or marenostrin which activate the biosynthesis of a chemotatic-factor inactivator. Failure to produce this leads to FMF attacks.

These are characterized by recurrent attacks of fever, arthritis and serositis. Abdominal or chest pain due to peritonitis or pleurisy occur. The arthritis is usually monoarticular and attacks last up to one week. The condition may be mistaken for palindromic rheumatism, but such attacks are not usually accompanied by fever

The diagnosis can be made by PCR, if available, but usually it is based on the clinical picture and exclusion of other conditions.

Treatment regularly with colchicine 1.0–1.5 mg daily can usually prevent the attacks. In general the disorder is benign but in 25% of cases renal amyloidosis develops.

Sarcoidosis (see also p. 806)

The most common type of arthritis is that associated with erythema nodosum, which occurs in 20% of cases of sarcoidosis at or soon after the onset of the disease. The most useful diagnostic test is a chest X-ray, which shows hilar lymphadenopathy in 80% of cases.

Other patterns of arthritis occur later in the disease. These include a transient rheumatoid-like polyarthritis and an acute monarthritis that can be mistaken for gout.

Treatment is with NSAIDs, but if these fail to control the symptoms, corticosteroids are usually very effective.

Osteochondromatosis

In this condition, foci of cartilage form within the synovial membrane. These foci become calcified and then ossified (osteochondromas). They may give rise to loose bodies within the joint. The condition occurs in a single joint of a young adult and X-rays are usually diagnostic. *Treatment* involves removal of loose bodies and synovectomy.

Pigmented villonodular synovitis

This is characterized by exuberant synovial proliferation that occurs either in joints or in tendon sheaths. The main manifestation in joints is recurrent haemarthrosis.

Treatment is synovectomy. In tendons, the condition gives rise to a nodular mass that requires excision.

Relapsing polychondritis

Relapsing polychondritis is a rare inflammatory condition of cartilage. It occurs equally in males and females, usually the elderly. Tenderness, inflammation and eventual destruction of cartilage occurs, mainly in the ear, nose, larynx or trachea. A seronegative polyarthritis occurs, as well as episcleritis and evidence of a vasculitis (e.g. glomerulonephritis). The diagnosis is clinical with laboratory evidence of acute inflammation.

Treatment involves corticosteroids and immunosuppressive agents.

Diseases of bone

Bone is a specialized connective tissue that makes up 25% of the weight of a normal adult. Its major mineral components are calcium, phosphate and some magnesium within a collagen framework. Although major skeletal growth occurs in childhood, adult bone is continuously being remodelled with bone formation and resorption. Bone serves three major functions:

- *mechanical* – for support and attachment of muscles for movement
- *metabolic* – for reserves of calcium and phosphate
- *protective* – for bone marrow and vital organs.

Structure and physiology

There are two major forms of bone – long bones (e.g. femur, tibia, humerus) and flat bones (e.g. skull, scapula, mandible).

Long bones (Fig 8.30) consist of a cylindrical tube of bone with a midshaft (diaphysis), two wider extremities (epiphyses), and a developmental zone (metaphysis) in between. In a growing long bone the epiphyses and metaphysis are separated by a layer of cartilage (epiphyseal cartilage or *growth plate*) where longitudinal growth takes place.

- *Cortical or compact bone* forms the diaphysial shaft and 80–90% of it is calcified. It has a mainly mechanical function and protects the medullary cavity containing haemopoietic bone marrow.

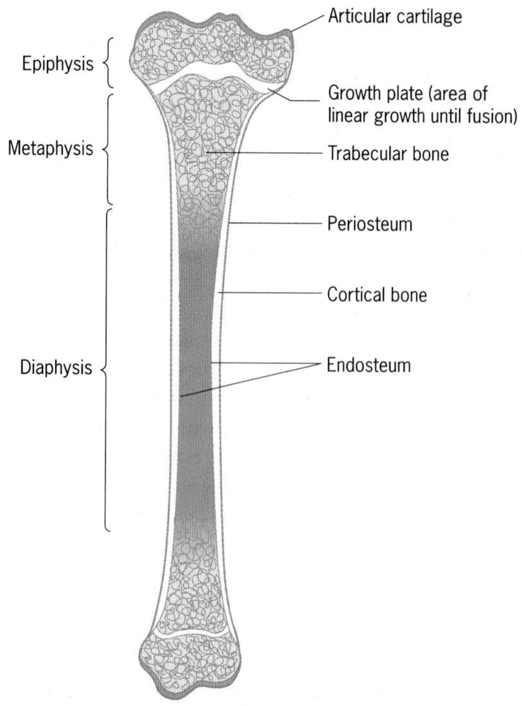

Fig 8.30
Diagram of a longitudinal section of a growing long bone

- *Trabecular or cancellous bone* occurs at the end of long bones towards the metaphysis and inside the cortex of flat bones. It is made up of a network of interconnecting trabecular plates and rods. Only 15–25% is calcified, the remainder consisting of blood vessels, bone marrow and connective tissue. It has a metabolic function and is the major site of bone remodelling.

The *bone matrix* is made up of type I collagen fibres (forming 90% of the total protein) within a ground substance containing primarily glycoproteins and proteoglycans. These substances play an important part in the calcification process where calcium hydroxyapatite crystals are deposited within and on the collagen matrix.

In adult bone, collagen fibres are orientated to give a lamellar structure. The lamellae lie either parallel to each other along trabecular bone and the periosteum, or concentrically around blood vessels to form Haversian canals. The Haversian systems are in communication with each other via transverse canals (Volkmann's canals). When there is increased bone turnover there is no such geometrical arrangement and the bone is then called 'woven bone'.

Numerous *non-collagen proteins* (NCPs) are found in the bone matrix and account for the remaining 10–15% of the total protein content. These consist of vitamin K-dependent gla (glutamyl) proteins consisting of osteocalcin and matrix gla proteins (both made by bone cells) and protein S (primarily made by the liver); osteopontin; osteonectin; fibronectin; bone sialoprotein and thrombospondin.

These NCPs seem to regulate the mineralization process in conjuction with local mediators and systemic hormones (see below).

Bone surfaces and cells

There are two bone surfaces at which remodelling takes place – external periostium and the internal endosteal surface. These surfaces are lined by osteogenic cells organized in layers. Three specialized cells are necessary for bone formation.

Osteoblasts

Osteoblasts are derived from local mesenchymal stem cells. They are found in clusters along the bone surface and are involved in both the synthesis of bone matrix before it is calcified (*osteoid tissue*) and in its mineralization. After performing these functions they line the surfaces or become embedded in calcified bone as *osteocytes*.

Osteoblasts produce type I collagen and the non-collagen protein osteocalcin (bone *gla*-protein). Other factors produced are TGFβ, insulin-like growth factor (IGF), platelet-derived growth factors (PDGFs) and basic fibroblast growth factor which are all part of the family of bone morphogenetic proteins. Osteoblasts are rich in alkaline phosphatase and possess many receptors for compounds such as parathyroid hormone, vitamin D, prostaglandins, interleukins and TGFβ. It now appears that in addition to their primary role in bone synthesis they may also control bone reabsorption, probably through regulation of osteoclast activity. Osteoblasts communicate with each other across gap junctions.

Osteoclasts

Osteoclasts are derived from haemopoetic cells, probably of the macrophage/monocyte lineage. They express colony stimulating factor-1 (CSF-1) receptors similar to mononuclear phagocytes. They also possess receptors for calcitonin, but not for PTH. Lysosomal enzymes are actively synthesized by osteoclasts and secreted into the extracellular bone reabsorbing compartment. The low pH in this compartment dissolves the crystals, exposing the matrix. The enzymes, now at optimal pH, degrade the matrix component. The hydroxyapatite crystals are mobilized by digestion of their link to collagen with any residual fibres being digested by collagenase (see below).

Osteocytes

These are small flattened cells formed from osteoblasts. They have a reduced metabolic activity as, although viable, they are completely encased in bone. Osteocytes possess cytoplasmic processes that ramify throughout the bone matrix and contact other osteocyte processes.

Bone growth and remodelling

In children during growth of the long bone, chondroblasts in the growth plate proliferate and actively synthesize new matrix. This matrix is selectively calcified. This is followed by partial resorption by osteoclasts, and the osteoblasts then form a layer of woven bone on top of the cartilaginous remnants. Growth-plate fusion occurs at puberty leading to a cessation of linear growth.

In adults there is a continuous process of bone remodelling, with bone formation occurring after bone resorption. At the remodelling site, a specific area of the cell membrane of the osteoclasts called the 'ruffled' border attaches to the bone surface via cell-bound proteins (integrins, e.g. vitronectin) sealing off the area undergoing resorption.

In the time between resorption and formation (the *reversal phase*) a cement line is formed marking the limit between the old and the new bone. Osteoblasts now form new bone matrix (osteoid tissue) which calcifies after about ten days.

Regulation of bone remodelling

This is a complex process affecting the osteoblasts and osteoclasts and involves circulating hormones and local factors such as cytokines, growth factors and prostaglandins, synthesized mainly by skeletal cells. These factors affect the replication of undifferentiated cells, the recruitment of cells and the differentiated function of cells.

Bone remodelling takes place in groups of cells called the *basic multicellular units* (BMUs) which turn bone over at multiple bone surfaces; the cycle of activation – resorption/formation – takes about 100 days in the cortical bone and 200 days in the trabecular bone. The resultant effect of remodelling, however, is the maintenance of mineralized bone matrix.

Skeletal mass declines with age after the peak mass is attained after cessation of linear growth (determined by both genetic and environmental factors). This decline is accelerated in postmenopausal women. Nutritional and mechanical factors acting through hormonal and local regulatory factors also affect bone mass.

Hormonal regulation of bone remodelling

- *Parathyroid hormone* (PTH) stimulates bone resorption. This effect is not directly on osteoclasts, and osteoblasts are necessary to mediate the effect.
- *Calcitonin* inhibits bone resorption by direct action on osteoclasts.
- *Insulin* causes a marked stimulation of bone matrix synthesis and cartilage formation. It is also necessary for normal bone mineralization. In part, its action is through increased insulin-like growth factor-1 (IGF-1).
- *Growth hormone* increases IGF-1 in the liver and through this action maintains a normal bone mass. It also increases 1,25-dihydroxy-vitamin-D production which stimulates calcium absorption by the gut.
- *Vitamin D and available calcium* increase bone mineralization. The action on bone is by increasing synthesis of osteocalcin by osteoblasts, by increasing IGF binding proteins, and by other functions that are not yet clearly defined.
- *Glucocorticoids* stimulate bone resorption by decreasing calcium absorption from the gut with a subsequent increase in PTH secretion.
- *Oestrogens* decrease bone resorption indirectly by inhibiting the production of cytokines IL1/IL6. Selective oestrogen receptor modulators have been developed. These agents have been shown to maintain bone mass by regulation of the gene for transforming growth factor-β (TGF-β) acting through the oestrogen receptor. They do not, however, stimulate the oestrogen receptor in the endometrium.
- *Androgens* have an anabolic effect on bone.
- *Thyroid hormones* have a direct effect on osteoclasts via osteoblasts, and stimulate bone resorption and turnover.

Local factors

Bone contains many growth factors synthesized by skeletal and stromal cells. Polypeptide growth factors include PDGF, fibroblast growth factors, the TGFβ family of peptides, as well as interleukins and TNFα, and these all modify the function of osteoblasts and osteoclasts, thereby altering cellular function.

FURTHER READING

Manolagas SC, Jilka BL (1995) Bone marrow, cytokines and bone remodelling. *New England Journal of Medicine* **332**: 305–311.

Calcium homeostasis and its regulation

Calcium homeostasis is regulated mainly by the effects of parathyroid hormone, and 1,25-$(OH)_2$-D_3 on intestinal absorption, renal tubular reabsorption and bone resorption. Calcium-sensing receptors which respond to changes in the extracellular calcium concentrations are present in the parathyroid gland, kidney, brain and other organs.

Calcium absorption and distribution

In a normal Western adult, daily calcium consumption is around 20–25 mmol (800–1000 mg), primarily from dairy foods, though it is much lower in many less affluent countries. Dietary calcium deficiency is, however, rarely a significant cause of bone disease in that absorption of calcium increases in states of calcium deficiency (see vitamin D below). Absorption is sometimes reduced by generalized malabsorption (see p. 254).

Calcium fluxes between gut, plasma, bone and kidney are shown in Fig 8.31.The circulating pool of calcium (about 12 mmol) is tiny compared with the bony 'reservoirs' and small compared with the daily fluxes.

Regulation of calcium homeostasis

Vitamin D metabolism (Fig 8.32)

Vitamin D is produced in the skin as cholecalciferol (vitamin D_3) by sunlight photoactivation of 7-dehydrocholesterol. This, rather than dietary vitamin D, is the *primary* source of vitamin D metabolites in humans, so that sunlight deprivation is normally more important than inadequate nutrition in producing vitamin D deficiency. These metabolites are transported in the circulation, bound to vitamin D-binding protein, to the *liver* where cholecalciferol is converted to 25-hydroxy-cholecalciferol (25-OH-D_3). Measurement of this serum metabolite is a good indicator of vitamin D bioavailability.

25-OH-D_3 is then converted by the *kidney tubule* enzyme, 1α-hydroxylase, to the highly biologically active metabolite 1,25-dihydroxycholecalciferol (1,25-$(OH)_2$-D_3) and a second less active metabolite 24,25-dihydroxy-cholecalciferol (24,25-$(OH)_2$-D_3) if vitamin D supplies are adequate; the regulation of the enzyme is by PTH, phosphate and by feedback inhibition by 1,25-$(OH)_2$-D_3. Extrarenal sources of 1,25-$(OH)_2$-D_3 contribute little under normal cirumstances, but it can be produced by lymphomatous and sarcoid tissue.

Parathyroid hormone (PTH)

PTH, an 84 amino-acid hormone derived from a 115-residue preprohormone, is secreted from the chief cells of the four parathyroid glands. These are normally situated posterior to the thyroid, but occasionally additional glands exist or they may be found elsewhere in the neck or mediastinum. PTH levels rise as serum ionized calcium falls. The latter is detected by specific calcium-sensing receptors on the plasma membrane of the parathyroid cells. PTH has several major actions, all serving to increase plasma calcium by:

- increasing osteoclastic resorption of bone (occurring rapidly)
- increasing intestinal absorption of calcium (a slow response)
- increasing synthesis of 1,25-$(OH)_2$-D_3
- increasing renal tubular reabsorption of calcium
- increasing excretion of phosphate.

PTH effects are mediated at specific membrane receptors on the target cells, resulting in an increase of adenyl cyclase messenger activity (see Chapter 16, p. 896).

Calcitonin

This 32 amino-acid polypeptide is produced by thyroid C-cells. Its physiological relevance to calcium metabolism in man remains unclear, as total thyroidectomy (absent calcitonin) or medullary carcinoma of the thyroid (excess calcitonin, p. 957) have no significant skeletal or other clinical effects. Plasma levels do, however, rise with increasing serum calcium and it is known to inhibit osteoclastic bone resorption and increase the renal excretion of calcium and phosphate. It is used in the treatment of Paget's disease and, rarely, in hypercalcaemia.

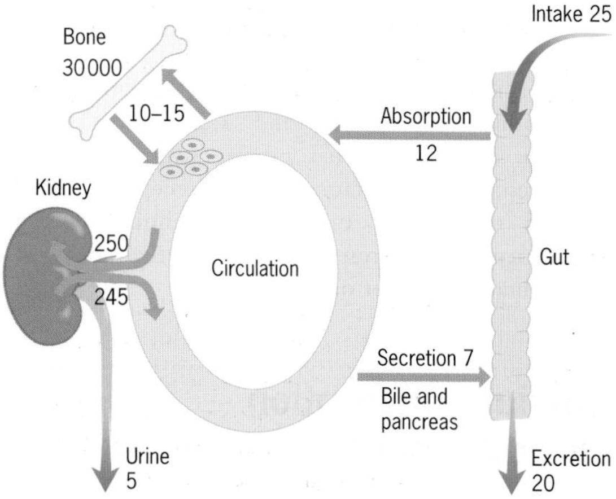

Fig 8.31
Calcium exchange in the normal human. The fluxes are shown in mmol per day

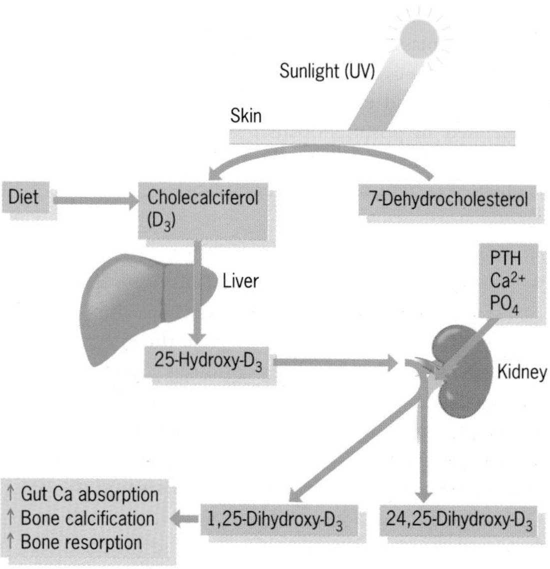

Fig 8.32
The metabolism and actions of vitamin D. PTH, parathyroid hormone

Thyroid hormone

Excess thyroxine (T4) and triiodothyronine (T3) cause increased bone turnover with hypercalcaemia while hypothyroidism leads to growth delay.

Biochemical investigation of bone and calcium disorders (Table 8.21)

Total plasma calcium

The normal range is 2.2–2.6 mmol L^{-1} (8.5–10.5 mg dL^{-1}). Usually only about 40% of this is ionized and physiologically relevant; the remainder is protein-bound, particularly to albumin, or complexed and thus unavailable to the tissues. Ionized calcium is very difficult to measure. Total plasma calcium can, however, be approximately corrected by adding or subtracting 0.02 mmol L^{-1} for every gram per litre of a simultaneous albumin level below and above a standard figure, usually 40 g L^{-1}. Thus a total calcium of 2.22 mmol L^{-1} with an albumin of 35 g L^{-1} becomes a 'corrected' calcium (Ca^{corr}) of 2.32 mmol L^{-1}. For critical measurements samples should be taken in the fasting state and without the use of an occluding cuff on the arm, which may increase local plasma protein concentration.

Plasma phosphate

The normal range is 0. 8–1.4 mmol L^{-1}. Phosphate forms an essential part of most biochemical systems. About 80% of total body phosphate is within bone. Phosphate reabsorption from the kidney is decreased by PTH, so primary hyperparathyroidisim is associated with low levels of plasma phosphate. High levels are found in hypoparathyroidism and when normal excretion does not occur, for example, as in renal failure

25-hydroxy-vitamin D

This is the best indicator of vitamin D status. Levels are higher in summer (owing to increased sunlight) and lower in winter. Measurement is useful in the hypocalcaemic patient (see p. 515) and occasionally in hypercalcaemic patients. Measurements of 1,25-$(OH)_2$-D_3 are seldom helpful clinically.

Urinary calcium

The normal range is 2.5–7.5 mmol/24 h. This is increased with hypercalcaemia and in situations where renal tubular resorption of calcium is decreased. Its main use is in the investigation of renal calculi.

PTH measurements

PTH measurements have been substantially improved by the availability of two-site immunoradiometric assays that measure only the *intact* PTH molecule, and not fragments; interpretation requires a simultaneous calcium measurement and a knowledge of the local assay reference range. Urinary cyclic adenosine monophosphate (cyclic AMP) concentration is an index of the bioactivity of PTH, but is not commonly measured.

Markers of bone formation

- *Serum alkaline phosphatase* is derived from liver, bone, kidney and placenta. Bone-specific alkaline phosphatase is synthesized by osteoblasts, and the excess is spilt over into the serum where it can be measured by monoclonal antibody assays. The levels are raised in the growing child.
- *Serum osteocalcin* is an additional measure of osteoblastic synthetic activity. Osteocalcin levels do not always parallel bone-specific alkaline phosphatase levels, as in some conditions differing amounts are spilt over into the plasma.
- *Type I collagen propeptides* are found in the serum as by-products of collagen synthesis. They are not measured routinely.

Markers of bone resorption

- *Urinary hydroxyproline* is a marker of bone resorption, but as it is affected by diet, lacks specificity to bone collagen and has a tedious assay, it is used infrequently.

Table 8.21
Biochemical changes in the major bone and parathyroid hormone-related diseases

Disorder	Serum Ca^{++}	Serum PO_4^-	Serum alkaline phosphatase	Comments
Osteoporosis	N	N	N	No Ca metabolism abnormality
Osteomalacia	N or ↓	↓	↑	Ca × PO_4 product often more sensitive
Paget's disease	N	N	↑ to ↑↑↑	Ca may be ↑ in immobility
Primary HPT	↑	↓	N or ↑	PTH raised or inappropriately N for ↑ Ca
Secondary HPT	N or ↓	↑ or N	↑ or N	PTH ↑ – compensatory response to ↓ Ca
Tertiary HPT	↑	↑	↑	PTH ↑↑ – autonomous hypertrophy
Hypoparathyroidism	↓	↑	N	PTH ↓ despite hypocalcaemia

HPT, hyperparathyroidism; N, normal

- *Urinary pyridinoline cross-links of collagen* can be measured. They are complex amino acids produced by tissue collagen degradation, and as they are not metabolized they are excreted in the urine. They are not affected by diet and are more sensitive than urinary hydroxyproline.

Diagnostic imaging

- **X-rays**. Plain X-rays are helpful in showing bony lesions such as fracture, tumours and infections. They are also useful in rickets and osteomalacia (see p. 510), severe osteoporosis (p. 508), Paget's disease (p. 511), hyperparathyroidism (p. 514) and inherited disorders of bone (p. 518).
- **Radionucleotide scans**. Technetium-99m-labelled methylene bisphosphonate is given intravenously and gamma camera imaging is performed 2–3 hours later. The uptake of the radionucleotide is predominantly dependent on blood flow. The technique is good at detecting increased bone activity in cases of fracture, infection, metastases or in metabolic bone disease, often when they are not visible on X-ray.

Bone density measurements

A number of techniques can be used to evaluate bone density:

- **Conventional X-rays**. These are of limited value unless there is severe osteopenia. The error rate is 30–50%.
- **Dual energy X-ray absorptiometry** (DEXA). This involves measurements of bone density, usually of the lumbar spine and proximal femur. It is precise, accurate and uses low doses of radiation. It is particularly useful in postmenopausal females and for follow-up of therapy.
- **Quantitative CT scan**. This is less accurate, more expensive and requires higher radiation than other techniques.
- **Quantitative ultrasound measurement**, usually of the calcaneum. This is currently not in routine use.

Bone biopsy

This is performed on the iliac crest under a local anaesthetic. A core of bone is removed (from cortex to cortex) with a trephine, and the non-decalcified specimen is examined for trabecular bone volume, decreased osteoid thickness, mineralization and excessive osteoclastic activity. A fluorochrome, such as tetracycline – which is taken up at the point of mineralization – can be given orally for two days, on two occasions, approximately ten days apart. Its uptake on the mineralization front is demonstrated by fluorescence and is decreased in, for example, osteomalacia.

Osteoporosis

DEFINITION AND INCIDENCE

Osteoporosis is defined as 'a disease characterized by low bone mass and micro-architectural deterioration of bone tissue, leading to enhanced bone fragility and an increase in fracture risk'. Unlike osteomalacia, the defect in osteoporosis is that *the bone that is present is normally mineralized* but is deficient in *quantity, quality and structural integrity* (Fig 8.33).

The World Health Organization (WHO) defines osteoporosis as a bone density more than 2.5 standard deviations (SDs) below the young adult mean value for individuals matched for sex and race. Values between 1 and 2.5 SDs are termed 'osteopenia'.

Osteoporosis and the resultant fractures are a *major* health-care problem, becoming even more so with the rapidly ageing populations in the West. It is estimated that there are over 1.3 million osteoporotic fractures each year in the USA, approximately 50% being vertebral, 25% hip fractures and 25% Colles' fractures. The lifetime risk of hip fracture for a white woman at age 60 is around 15%, compared with 5% for men, with roughly equal risks for Colles' or vertebral fractures. Of the elderly who survive until age 90, approximately 30% of women and 15% of men will have suffered a hip fracture. As can be seen in Fig 8.34(a), the risk of fracture increases exponentially with age.

PATHOGENESIS

The changes in bone mass with age are shown in Fig 8.34(b). Bone mass increases rapidly up to the age of puberty, rises slightly more in the twenties and thirties, and then begins to decline around age 40. In men there is a gradual decline, reaching moderate levels of fracture risk in the seventies and eighties, but a subset of woman show a very accelerated loss in the ten years following the

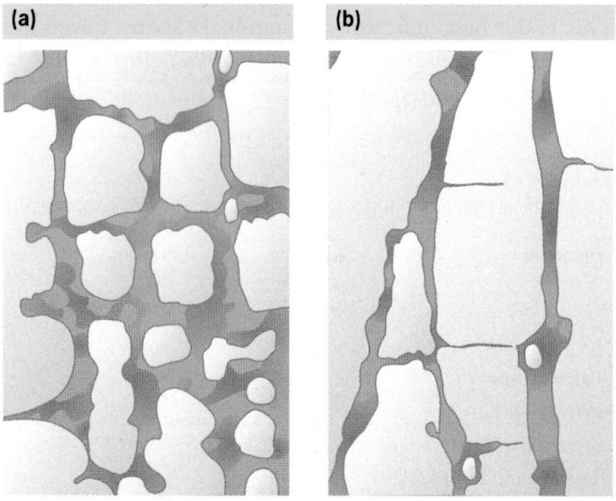

Fig 8.33
The microarchitecture of (a) normal and (b) osteoporotic bone
There is thinning and a loss of trabecular plates

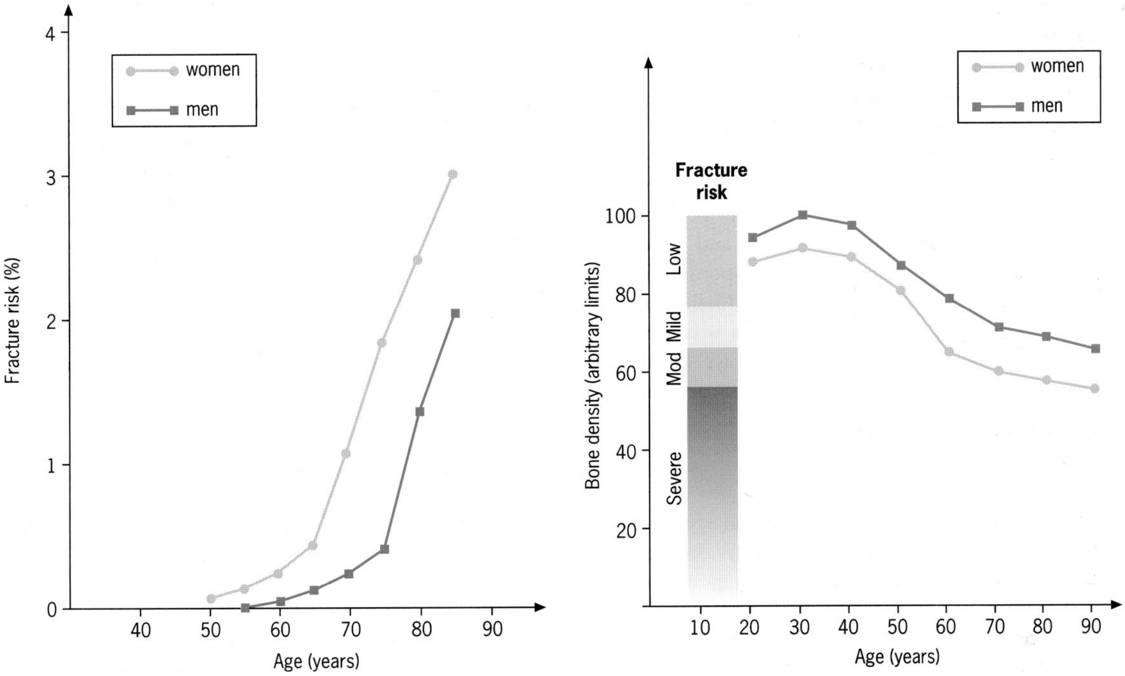

Fig 8.34
Features of osteoporosis according to age and sex
(a) The risk of hip fracture
(b) Schematic diagram showing the decrease in bone density with increasing age, along with an increased fracture risk

menopause and may be at substantial risk of fracture from soon after the menopause. In the event of early (premature) menopause, rapid bone loss begins early.

The female preponderance of fractures has a number of reasons, the most common being the accelerated bone loss in the first ten years after the menopause along with the lower initial bone mass of women. There are, however, several additional factors; non-white ethnic groups have higher peak bone mass and less postmenopausal loss, while other ethnic groups have lower bone density but are still less likely to fracture. Nevertheless, many more women are at risk of fracture than actually have them, so the relationship is not direct.

Osteoporosis arises as the end-result of many years of mismatch between the rates of bone resorption and bone formation during the remodelling process. This can arise either from 'high-turnover' osteoporosis from such conditions as the postmenopausal state, hyperparathyroidism and hyperthyroidism, while others may be due to 'low-turnover' osteoporosis (e.g. as in anorexia nervosa and liver disease).

TYPES

Two major types of osteoporosis are recognized, although such a classification is a gross simplification:

- type I is the typical postmenopausal process
- type II the more gradual senile osteoporosis that occurs in both sexes (Table 8.22).

Osteoporosis does not itself cause symptoms. There are many risk factors for low bone density, listed in Table 8.23, and a number of endocrine and other

Table 8.22
Risk factors and common conditions associated with osteoporosis

	Type I	Type II
Age range for fractures	50–75 Mainly women	Over 70 Both sexes F>M
Major mechanism	Oestrogen deficiency (androgens also)	Age-related changes, possibly decreased calcium absorption
Pathology	Thinning, perforation and disappearance of trabecular bone	Reduction in cortical thickness/trabecular bone
Common fracture types	Vertebral fractures (painful) Distal forearm (Colles)	Hip fractures Vertebral wedge fractures (painless)
Main drug therapy	Oestrogen replacement and bisphosphonates	Calcium and vitamin D Also oestrogens and bisphosphonates

disorders which may induce osteoporosis. Additionally there are other mechanisms which alter fracture risk (e.g. the risk of falling).

The pain of osteoporosis results from fractures. In vertebral crush fractures a typical history would be the onset of severe pain in the dorsal spine which resolves only slowly over a period of around six weeks. Subsequent symptoms include loss of height from collapsed vertebrae, increasing kyphosis and abdominal protuberance. Other typical sites of osteoporotic fracture are the lumbar vertebrae, the distal radius (Colles' fracture) and the neck of the femur. Osteoporosis is common in the elderly and fractures may not always be due to osteoporosis, but can also occur with secondary deposits.

INVESTIGATIONS

Fracture

- **X-rays** may show a fracture and reveal earlier clinically unrecognized fractures. X-rays showing pedicle destruction of vertebrae are suggestive of malignant destruction. Interpretation of these is often difficult because of the poor quality and density of the films which may be due to the osteoporosis itself. *Osteopenia* is often used to describe a nonspecific generalized or regional rarefaction of the skeleton on X-ray.
- **Bone scans** are sometimes useful to demonstrate fractures. An osteoporotic fracture can be distinguished from a metastatic lesion, as the latter is often associated with multiple lesions elsewhere.

X-rays are of limited value in evaluating bone density because up to 30–40% of the bone mineral content has to be lost before any change in radiological bone density is detectable.

Bone density

This is increasingly being measured by bone densitometry (most often by dual-energy X-ray absorption scanning – DEXA) (Fig 8.35). The place of routine scanning of populations remains controversial.

- **CT scanning** can also be used but involves a higher radiation dose.
- **Ultrasound** of the calcaneum is used occasionally.
- **Iliac crest bone biopsy** shows loss of bone trabeculae. This seldom needs to be performed except in treatment trials and when the diagnosis is in doubt.
- **Serum calcium, phosphate and alkaline phosphatase** are normal in osteoporosis alone as no disorder of calcium metabolism is involved.
- **Biochemical markers** of bone resorption (see p. 505) can be used to evaluate treatment.

Appropriate investigations may be needed to exclude other diseases associated with osteoporosis, as shown in Table 8.23.

MANAGEMENT AND PREVENTION

Management of established osteoporosis is unsatisfactory as the bone mass is already substantially reduced. However, trials of therapy have shown substantial improvements in bone density, and accompanying reductions in fracture rate. Optimal therapy in the future will ideally be prophylactic rather than after fractures have occurred.

Fractures should be treated by conventional orthopaedic means. Fresh fractures of the spine often require short-term bedrest with adequate analgesia and, possibly, muscle relaxants. This is followed by rehabilitation and secondary preventative measures, both for the bones and to reduce circumstances favouring falls.

Non-drug therapy

- *Diet.* An adequate intake of calories, calcium and vitamin D is necessary, with at least 1000 mg of calcium daily (ideally 1500 mg postmenopausally) and 400–800 IU of vitamin D. Adequate weight gain in a thin person is necessary as low bodyweight is itself a risk factor for further fractures.
- *Exercise.* A minimum of at least 30 minutes of weight-bearing exercise three times a week has been shown to be beneficial and should be encouraged.
- *Smoking cessation.* Smoking appears to accelerate bone loss and may negate the beneficial effect of oestrogen therapy, possibly by accelerating oestrogen metabolism.
- *Reduction in fall risk.* Physiotherapy and assessment of home safety may be required. Hip protectors may be of value.

These four measures are part of a general health education programme for the over-50s.

Table 8.23
Osteoporosis risk factors, associated diseases and drug therapies

Risk factors	Diseases
Female sex	*Endocrine*
Increasing age	Cushing's syndrome
Early menopause (including ovariectomy)	Hyperparathyroidism
White race	Hypogonadism (including orchidectomy)
Slender habitus	Acromegaly
Lack of exercise/immobility	Type I diabetes mellitus
Smoking	*Joint*
Family history	Rheumatoid arthritis
Excess alcohol	*Other*
Nutrition (very low calcium diet, high protein intake for a long time)	Chronic renal failure
	Chronic liver disease
	Mastocytosis
	Anorexia nervosa
Drug therapy	
Corticosteroids	
Heparin	
Cyclosporin	
Cytotoxic therapy	

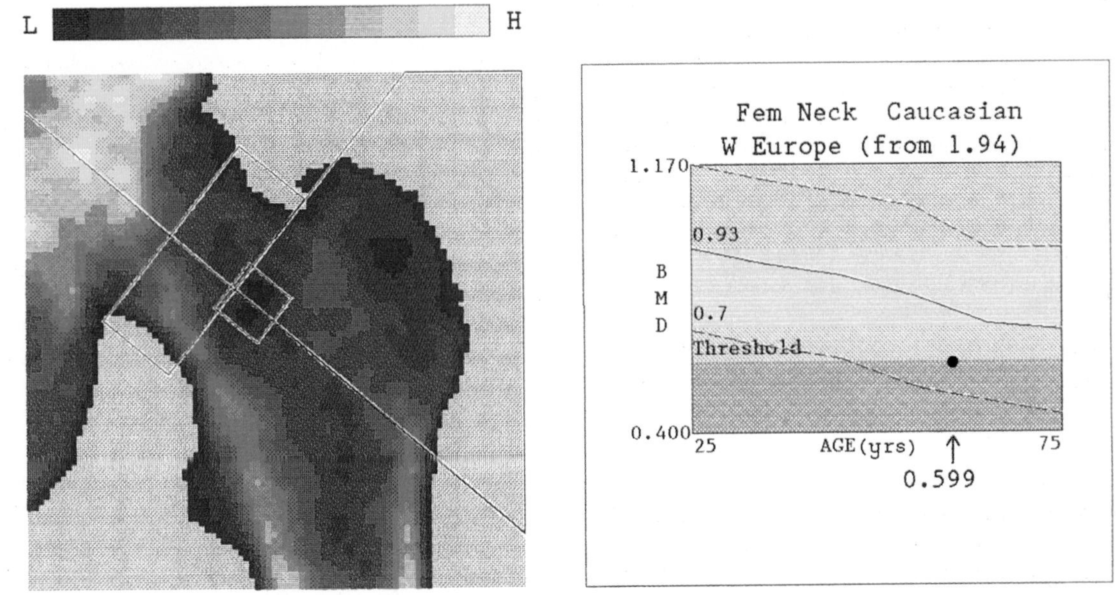

Fig 8.35
DEXA scan of the left femoral neck in a 60-year-old caucasian female (height 153.1 cm, weight 59.8 kg) with osteoporosis.
On the right-hand graph the black dot indicates the patient's BMD (0.599), which is below the threshold level.
BMD, bone mass density
Courtesy of Wellington Regional Bone Density Service

Drug therapy

- *Oestrogen therapy* as hormone replacement therapy (HRT) is of proven value in the prevention of future fractures in postmenopausal women, as discussed in Chapter 16 (p. 913). It is the treatment of choice in this group. The potential side-effects of HRT (breast cancer and thrombosis) remain controversial, but the risk of these is substantially less than those of fractures without HRT. Selective oestrogen-receptor modulators (SERMs) such as raloxifene are under trial; they do not stimulate the endometrium but do stimulate oestrogen receptors in bone (see p. 503), thereby increasing bone mass. They also lower total and LDL cholesterol.
- *Androgens* should be given to hypogonadal men, though prostatic hypertrophy may sometimes be a limiting factor.
- *Bisphosphonates* are increasingly used; they are analogues of normal bone pyrophosphate (Fig 8.36). They adhere to hydroxyapatite and inhibit osteoclastic bone resorption. Alendronate 10 mg daily has been shown to increase bone mass substantially and reduce the incidence of fractures. The only major side-effect of alendronate is oesophageal ulceration which can be minimized if the patient takes the tablets before breakfast with a full glass of water and remains upright for 30 minutes.

Agents used less commonly

- *Combination therapy*, particularly oestrogens and bisphosphonates, are under study and appear promising.
- *Calcitriol.* The active metabolite of vitamin D ($1,25\text{-}(OH)_2\text{-}D_3$) produces some small improvement in bone density, but not as much as HRT or bisphosphonates.
- *Calcitonin.* Nasal calcitonin, or the alternative subcutaneous salmon calcitonin, are recommended by some authorities, especially where vertebral fracture pain is a problem.
- *Fluoride.* Fluoride has been shown to increase bone density, but there is concern about the quality of the bone formed and it is not currently recommended.

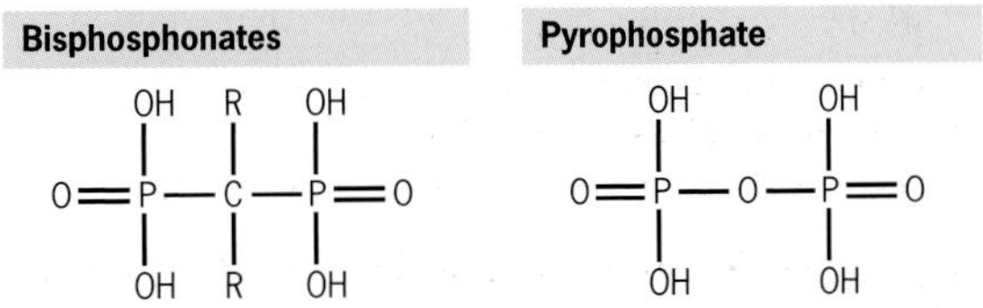

Fig 8.36
Comparative structures of bisphosphonates and pyrophosphate

FURTHER READING

Consensus Development Conference (1993) Diagnosis, prophylaxis and treatment of osteoporosis. *American Journal of Medicine* **94**: 646–648.

Eastell R, Peel N (1998) Osteoporosis. *Journal of the Royal College of Physicians of London* **32**: 14–18.

Hosking D et al (1998) Prevention of bone loss by alendronate in postmenopausal women under 60 years of age. *New England Journal of Medicine* **338**: 485–492.

Smith R (1996) Investigation of osteoporosis. *Clinical Endocrinology* **44**: 371–374.

UK Consensus Group (1998) Management of male osteoporosis: report. *Quarterly Journal of Medicine* **91**: 71–92.

Rickets and osteomalacia

Rickets and osteomalacia result from *inadequate mineralization* of bone matrix (osteoid). Rickets occurs in children and is due to defective mineralization of the epiphyseal growth plate in growing bones. Osteomalacia is the adult counterpart. Both are usually caused by a defect in vitamin D availability or metabolism (see below).

PATHOLOGY

In children the growth plate is elongated with distortion of the arrangement of chondrocytes. Calcification is delayed and vascularization impaired. In adults, osteomalacia is characterized by increased osteoid volume of more than 10% with a widened osteoid seam. Unmineralized osteoid may cover up to 100% of trabecular bone (normal < 27%).

AETIOLOGY (Table 8.24)

Vitamin D deficiency can be *dietary* and/or due to inadequate *sunlight* exposure (see Fig 8.32). This is often seen in Asian immigrant females in Western countries who wear clothing covering virtually all their skin, or seldom go out. This reduces sunlight exposure to a pigmented skin. As many Asians are vegans their diet may contain only small amounts of vitamin D; a high phytate in chapatti flour may also inhibit calcium absorption. The elderly who are immobile and housebound similarly are not exposed to sunlight.

Although malabsorption of vitamin D_3 can be demonstrated in malabsorption syndromes with increased faecal fat excretion, its role in the development of osteomalacia is controversial. Anticonvulsant therapy in epileptics may lead to problems, possibly due to induction of mixed function oxidase systems affecting vitamin D metabolism.

Chronic renal failure results in reduced 1-α hydroxylation of 25-hydroxy vitamin D_3 to its active metabolic 1,25-$(OH)_2$-D_3.

Table 8.24
Causes of rickets and osteomalacia

Vitamin D deficiency
Inadequate synthesis in skin
Low dietary intake
Malabsorption
- Coeliac disease
- Intestinal resection
- Chronic cholestasis, e.g. primary biliary cirrhosis

Renal disease
Chronic renal failure
Renal osteodystrophy
Bone disease due to dialysis
Tubular disorders, e.g. renal tubular acidosis, Fanconi's syndrome

Miscellaneous
Multiple myeloma
Vitamin D-dependent rickets types I and II
X-linked hypophosphataemia (vitamin D-resistant rickets)
Mesenchymal tumours

Vitamin D-dependent rickets type I is a rare condition where there is an abnormality of the renal hydroxylase enzyme. In type II vitamin D-dependent rickets there is a defect in the intracellular 1,25-$(OH)_2$-D_3 receptor.

In the *Fanconi syndrome* and in renal tubular acidosis (p. 999), osteomalacia can develop, mainly owing to the continuous phosphaturia.

X-linked hypophosphataemia (vitamin D-resistant rickets) results in lower-limb deformities and stunted growth rate in the hypophosphataemic affected males.

Rickets/osteomalacia have been associated with many *tumours* – usually those consisting of mesenchymal and giant cells. They release a factor 'phosphatonin' which increases phosphate excretion. Treatment of the tumours results in re-mineralization.

CLINICAL FEATURES

Adult osteomalacia may produce vague symptoms of bone or muscle pain and tenderness, often with subclinical fractures. Occasionally a marked proximal myopathy leads to a characteristic 'waddling' gait. In modern practice many cases are detected biochemically in high-risk patients, especially those with gastrointestinal disease or surgery, before clear symptoms are present. Occasionally, tetany from hypocalcaemia may occur.

Rickets occurs during bone growth in children. At birth, neonatal rickets may present as *craniotabes* (thin deformed skull). In the first few years of life there may be widened epiphyses at the wrists and beading at the costochondrial junctions, producing the 'rickety rosary'. There may be a groove in the rib cage owing to inward pull of the diaphragm (Harrison's sulcus). In older children, bow-leg deformities are seen. A myopathy also occurs.

INVESTIGATIONS

The biochemical and radiological features are often characteristic (see Table 8.21):

- **Serum phosphate** is low, owing to increased PTH-dependent phosphaturia.
- **Plasma calcium** is low or low/normal, leading to secondary hyperparathyroidism and a raised PTH.
- **Serum alkaline phosphatase** is increased (allowing for age), indicating increased osteoblast activity.
- **Serum 25-hydroxy vitamin D_3** is low.
- **X-rays** show defective mineralization, especially in the pelvis, long bones and ribs, often with 'Looser's zones' – linear areas of low density surrounded by sclerotic borders.
- **Iliac crest biopsy** is occasionally necessary if biochemical tests are equivocal. Histological findings reveal increased osteoid seams and reduced mineralization

TREATMENT

Treatment should be directed towards correction of the cause where possible, with increase in dietary vitamin D intake and sunlight exposure.

Multiple formulations of vitamin D and its metabolites are available. When deficiency is nutritional, 'replacement' doses are needed – about 400 IU daily. Much higher pharmacological doses (up to 40 000–100 000) are needed in patients with gastrectomy, malabsorption, liver disease or hypoparathyroidism (see p. 515). Only experts should initiate such treatment and all patients receiving pharmacological doses of vitamin D should have their serum calcium measured regularly; excessive dosage presents with the features of hypercalcemia, often with nausea and vomiting.

PREVENTION

Prevention of both osteomalacia and rickets can follow health education to ensure a balanced diet, adequate exposure to sunlight and, where appropriate in high-risk individuals or communities, dietary vitamin D supplementation.

Paget's disease

Paget's disease (osteitis deformans) is a disorder of bone remodelling. There is excessive resorption with a subsequent compensatory increase in new bone formation. The new bone is structurally abnormal and therefore weak, with secondary phenomena like increased local bone blood flow and fibrous tissue in adjacent bone marrow.

It is a common disorder, most often seen in Europe and particularly northern England, affecting both men and women over age 40 years, with up to 10% of adults radiologically affected by the age of 90. It is relatively rare in North America, Africa and Asia, but epidemiological studies are made more difficult by the asymptomatic nature of most affected patients.

AETIOLOGY AND PATHOGENESIS

There is a significant genetic component with ethnic and geographic clustering of cases. Some evidence suggests a viral aetiology for which canine distemper virus, measles and respiratory syncitial virus have been proposed. The osteoclasts are more numerous than normal and contain an increased number of nuclei. Bone resorption is chaotic and there is a haphazard rather than linear deposition of collagen fibres, leading to 'woven' bone formation. Bone mineralization is normal. The structure of unaffected bone is normal and continues to remain so. Thus, Paget's disease does not spread.

CLINICAL FEATURES

Most patients, possibly 60–80%, with Paget's disease radiologically are entirely asymptomatic. The disease may involve one bone (monostotic) or many (polyostotic). The most common sites of involvement are the femur, pelvis, tibia, skull and lumbosacral spine, and diagnosis often follows the finding of an asymptomatic elevation of serum alkaline phosphatase, or a plain X-ray performed for other indications.

When symptomatic, features can include:

- bone pain, most often in the spine or the pelvis
- apparent joint pain when an involved bone is close to a joint, leading to cartilage damage and osteoarthritis
- deformities, in particular bowed tibia and skull changes (Fig 8.37)
- complications from:
  (a) nerve compression (deafness from VIIIth cranial nerve; also cranial nerves II, V, VII)
  (b) increased bone blood flow (cardiac hypertrophy and high-output cardiac failure)
  (c) weakness of the abnormal bone (pathological fractures)
- rarely osteogenic sarcoma developing in Pagetic bone (fewer than 1% of cases).

INVESTIGATIONS

- **X-rays** show characteristic changes, most often in the pelvis, skull or spine. There is enlargement or expansion of bone, osteolytic lesions, sclerosis and thickening of bone trabeculae in long bones and vertebrae.
- **Bone scans** will show the extent of skeletal involvement, often including largely unsuspected areas; but these and plain X-rays may be difficult to distinguish from metastatic carcinoma, which is sometimes a major clinical differential diagnosis. This is especially the case for the sclerotic secondaries seen with breast and prostate carcinoma.
- **Biochemistry**. The hallmark of Paget's disease is a markedly increased *serum alkaline phosphatase* (the marker of bone formation) with normal *serum calcium and phosphate*, simply reflecting increased bone turnover. Alkaline phosphatase may exceed 1000 U L^{-1}, and levels are normal only when bone involvement is very limited or monostotic – it is a useful marker of progress and treatment. *Mild hypercalcaemia* follows immobilization only when there is very extensive disease.

(a)

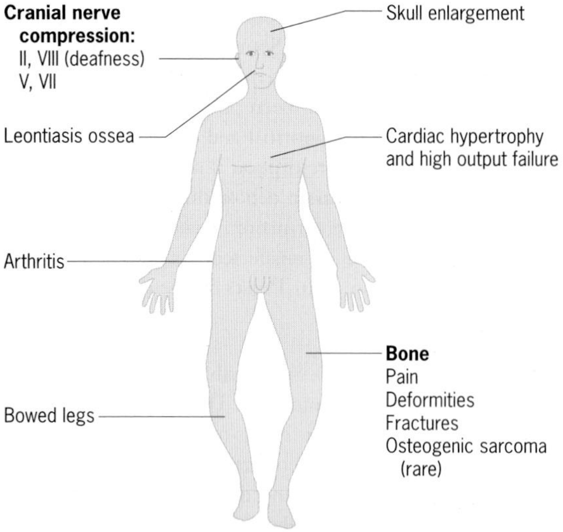

(b)

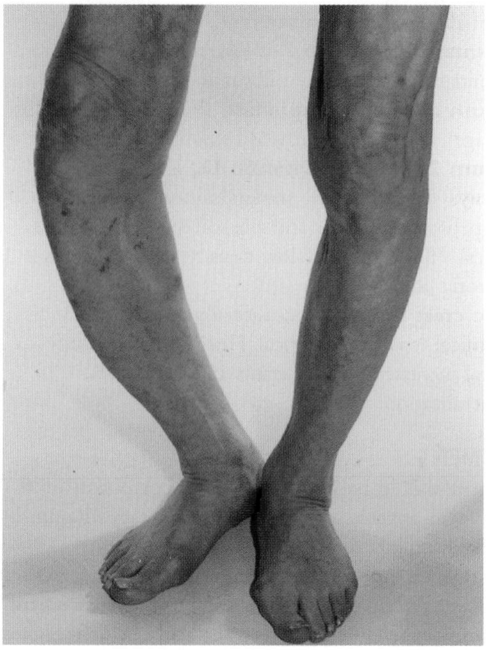

(c)

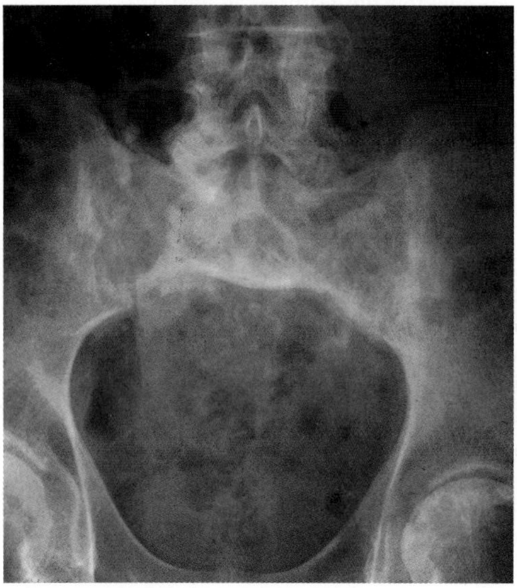

Fig 8.37
Paget's disease
(a) Clinical features
(b) The tibia, showing bowing caused by increased bone growth
(c) X-ray appearance of the pelvis, showing osteolytic and osteosclerotic lesions

- **Measurements of bone resorption** are used in some units, including 24-hour urinary hydroxyproline excretion which is increased, and urinary hydroxyproline/creatinine ratios.

TREATMENT

Treatment depends on the symptomatology, pain being the usual indication. Many patients while asymptomatic require no therapy, and simple analgesics or NSAIDs are sometimes adequate.

Oral bisphosphonates

Oral bisphosphonates, e.g. alendronate 10–40 mg, are given daily for six months. They should be taken with fluid to minimize oesophagitis, on an empty stomach (to increase absorption), and the patient should remain upright for 30 minutes. Alendronate appears to be more effective than cyclical etidronate and does not carry the risk of osteomalacia seen with the latter. Responses to bisphosphonates are long-lasting, with 50–70% reduction in serum alkaline phosphatase activity. The new bone formed is lamellar, not woven.

Other bisphosphonates

Intravenous pamidronate has been used widely as a single or multiple infusion. Other bisphosphonates are available (e.g. clodronate and tiludronate) and new agents are in the development stage.

Calcitonin

Salmon and porcine calcitonin inhibit bone resorption and turnover but are extremely expensive. Moreover, the side-effects of flushing and nausea are frequent problems. Calcitonin nasal spray is available and has a lower incidence of side-effects.

Surgery

Joint replacement or osteotomy are sometimes necessary, or neurosurgery where there is spinal disease. Medical control should be achieved beforehand to prevent excessive bleeding from Pagetic bone.

FURTHER READING

Delmas PD, Meunier PJ (1997) The management of Paget's disease of bone. *New England Journal of Medicine* **336**: 558–566.

Disorders of calcium metabolism

Hypercalcaemia is much more common than hypocalcaemia and is frequently detected incidentally with multichannel biochemical analysers. Mild asymptomatic hypercalcaemia occurs in about 1 in 1000 of the population, with an incidence of 25–30 per 100 000 population. It occurs mainly in elderly females, and is usually due to primary hyperparathyroidism (primary HPT).

Hypercalcaemia

PATHOPHYSIOLOGY AND CAUSES

The major causes of hypercalcemia are listed in Table 8.25; primary hyperparathyrodism and malignancies are by far the most common (>90% of cases). Hyperparathyroidism itself may be primary, secondary or tertiary. Primary hyperparathyroidism is caused by single (>80%) parathyroid adenomas or by diffuse hyperplasia of all the glands (15–20%). Multiple parathyroid adenomas are rare. Some of the latter may be part of a familial syndrome (e.g. multiple endocrine neoplasia (MEN) syndrome type I or II A. Parathyroid carcinoma is rare (less than 1%), though it usually produces severe hypercalcaemia.

The precise cause of *primary hyperparathyroidism* is unclear, though it appears that adenomas at least are monoclonal, as is possibly hyperplasia too. Chromosomal rearrangements in the 5′ regulatory region of the parathyroid hormone gene have been identified as one cause, and there are also suggestions that inactivation of some tumour suppressor genes at a variety of sites may be involved.

Secondary hyperparathyroidism is physiological compensatory hypertrophy of all parathyroids due to hypocalcaemia, such as occurs in renal failure or vitamin D deficiency. PTH levels are raised but calcium levels are low or normal, and PTH falls to normal after correction of the cause of hypocalcaemia where this is possible.

Tertiary hyperparathyroidism is the development of apparently autonomous parathyroid hyperplasia after longstanding secondary hyperparathyroidism, most often in renal failure. Plasma calcium and phosphate are both raised, the latter often grossly so. Parathyroidectomy is necessary at this stage.

Table 8.25
Causes of hypercalcaemia

Excessive parathormone (PTH) secretion Primary hyperparathyroidism (commonest by far), adenoma, hyperplasia or carcinoma Tertiary hyperparathyroidism Ectopic PTH secretion (very rare indeed)	**Other endocrine disease (mild hypercalcaemia only)** Thyrotoxicosis Addison's disease
Excess action of vitamin D Iatrogenic or self-administered excess Granulomatous diseases, e.g. sarcoidosis, TB Lymphoma	**Drugs** Thiazide diuretics Vitamin D analogues Lithium administration (chronic) Vitamin A
Excessive calcium intake 'Milk-alkali' syndrome	**Miscellaneous** Long-term immobility Familial hypocalciuric hypercalcaemia
Malignant disease (second commonest cause) Secondary deposits in bone Production of osteoclastic factors by tumours PTH-related protein secretion Myeloma	

SYMPTOMS AND SIGNS

- *General features.* There is usually tiredness, malaise and depression.
- *Renal features.* There may be renal colic from stones, polyuria or nocturia, haematuria and hypertension. The polyuria results from the effect of hypercalcaemia on renal tubules, reducing their concentrating ability – a form of mild nephrogenic diabetes insipidus. Only 20–40% show any renal involvement. Primary HPT is present in about 5% of stone formers.
- *Bones.* There is bone pain. Hyperparathyrodism mainly affects cortical bone, and bone cysts and locally destructive 'brown tumors' occur but only in advanced disease. Only 5–10% of all cases have definite bony lesions.
- *Abdominal.* There may be abdominal pain, sometimes due to peptic ulceration.
- *Chondrocalcinosis and ectopic calcification.* These are occasional features.
- *Corneal calcification.* This is a marker of longstanding hypercalcemia but causes no symptoms.

There may also be symptoms from the underlying cause. Malignant disease is usually advanced by the time hypercalcaemia occurs, as a result of bony metastases. The common primary tumours are bronchus, breast, myeloma, oesophagus, thyroid, prostate, lymphoma and renal cell carcinoma. True 'ectopic PTH secretion' by the tumour is very rare, and most cases are associated with raised levels of PTH-related protein. This is a 144 amino-acid polypeptide, the initial sequence of which shows an approximate homology with the biologically active part of PTH. Local bone resorbing cytokines and prostaglandins may be involved locally where there are metastatic skeletal lesions, leading to local mobilization of calcium by osteolysis with subsequent hypercalcaemia.

Severe hypercalcaemia (> 3 mmol L^{-1}) is usually associated with malignant disease, hyperparathyroidism, renal dialysis or vitamin D therapy.

INVESTIGATIONS AND DIFFERENTIAL DIAGNOSIS

- **Biochemistry**:
  (a) Several *fasting serum calcium* and *phosphate* samples should be taken. The hallmark of primary hyperparathyroidism is hypercalcaemia and hypophosphataemia with detectable intact PTH levels *during hypercalcaemia*.
  (b) There is often a mild *hyperchloraemic acidosis*.
  (c) *Renal function* is usually normal but should be measured precisely as a baseline.
  (d) The *hydrocortisone suppression test* is much less used with modern PTH assays. Hydrocortisone 40 mg three times daily for 10 days leads to suppression of plasma calcium in sarcoidosis, vitamin D-mediated hypercalcaemia and some malignancies.
  (e) *Protein electrophoresis* is performed to exclude myeloma
  (f) *Serum TSH and T3* are performed to exclude thyrotoxicosis.
- **Imaging**. Abdominal X-rays may show renal calculi or nephrocalcinosis. High-definition hand X-rays may show subperiosteal erosions in the middle or terminal phalanges.

Pre-operative localization investigations are generally indicated only for patients who have undergone previous parathyroid surgery, as they have an overall sensitivity of just 60–70% and a substantial false-positive rate, which is far less accurate than the expert surgical success rate of at least 90%. Methods include:

- ultrasound which, though insensitive for small tumors, is simple and safe
- high-resolution CT scan or MRI (the most sensitive technique)
- radioisotope subtraction scanning – a picture of the parathyroid tissue derived from the difference in uptake between ^{201}Th (taken up by thyroid *and* parathyroid) and ^{99m}Tc (by thyroid only).

TREATMENT OF PRIMARY HYPERPARATHYROIDISM

Details of emergency treatment for severe hypercalcaemia are given in Emergency box 8.1.

Medical management

There are no effective medical therapies at present for primary hyperparathyroidism, but a high fluid intake should be maintained, a high calcium or vitamin D intake avoided, and exercise encouraged. New therapeutic agents that target the calcium-sensing receptors in the kidney may be of value in the future.

Emergency

Acute hypercalcaemia often presents with dehydration, nausea and vomiting, nocturia and polyuria, drowsiness and altered consciousness. The serum Ca^{2+} is over 3 mmol L^{-1} and sometimes as high as 5 mmol L^{-1}. While investigation of the cause is under way, immediate treatment is mandatory if the patient is seriously ill or if the Ca^{+2} is above 3.5 mmol L^{-1}. Specialist help is advised.

- Adequate rehydration is essential – usually at least 4–6 L of saline on day 1, and 3–4 L for several days thereafter. Central venous pressure (CVP) may need to be monitored to control the hydration rate.
- Intravenous bisphosphonates are now the treatment of choice for hypercalcaemia of malignancy. Pamidronate is preferred (15–60 mg as an intravenous infusion in 0.9% saline or dextrose over 2–8 hours or, if less urgent, over 2–4 days).
- Calcitonin (200 units i.v. 6-hourly) has a short-lived action and is now little used.
- Prednisolone (30–60 mg daily) is effective in some instances (e.g. in myeloma, sarcoidosis and vitamin D excess) but in most cases is ineffective.
- Oral phosphate (sodium cellulose phosphate 5 g three times daily) produces diarrhoea. Intravenous phosphate rapidly lowers plasma Ca^{2+} but is dangerous and should not be used.

Emergency box 8.1 Treatment of acute hypercalcaemia

Surgery

Indications for surgery in hyperparathyroidism remain controversial. There is agreement surgery is indicated for:

- patients with renal stones or impaired renal function
- bone involvement or marked reduction in cortical bone density
- unequivocal marked hypercalcaemia (> 2.9–3.0 mmol L^{-1})
- the uncommon younger patient, below age 50 years
- a previous episode of severe acute hypercalcaemia.

The situation where plasma calcium is mildly raised (2.65–3 mmol L^{-1}) is more controversial. Most authorities feel that young patients should be operated on, as should those who have reduced cortical bone density or significant hypercalciuria, as this is associated with stone formation.

In older patients without these problems, or in those unfit for or unwilling to have surgery, conservative management is indicated. Regular measurement of serum and urinary calcium and of renal function is necessary. Bone density of cortical bone should be estimated every 2–3 years.

SURGICAL TECHNIQUE AND COMPLICATIONS

Parathyroid surgery should be performed only by experienced surgeons, as the minute glands may be very difficult to define, and it is difficult to distinguish between an adenoma and normal parathyroid. In expert centres over 90% of operations are successful, involving removal of the adenoma, or removal of all four hyperplastic parathyroids, with implantation of some parathyroid tissue into the forearm to provide residual PTH secretion.

Other than postoperative hypocalcaemia (see below), the other rare complications are those of thyroid surgery – bleeding and recurrent laryngeal nerve palsies (<1%). Vocal cord function should be checked preoperatively.

If initial exploration is unsuccessful, a full work-up including venous catheterization and scanning is essential, remembering that parathyroid tissue can be ectopic.

Postoperative care

The major danger after operation is hypocalcaemia, which is more common in patients with significant bone disease – the 'hungry bone' syndrome. Some authorities pre-treat such patients with alfacalcidol 2 μg daily from two days pre-operatively for 10–14 days. Chvostek's and Trousseau's signs should be checked regularly in all these patients. Plasma calcium measurements are performed daily for at least 2–5 days (more often if low) – a mild transient hypoparathyroidism often continues for 1–2 weeks. Depending on its severity, oral or intravenous calcium (for details see p. 516) should be given temporarily, as only a few patients (<1%) will develop longstanding surgical hypoparathyroidism.

Familial hypocalciuric hypercalcaemia

This uncommon autosomal dominant, and usually asymptomatic, condition demonstrates increased renal reabsorption of calcium despite hypercalcaemia. PTH levels are normal or slightly raised and urinary calcium is low. It is caused by mutations in the calcium-ion-sensing G-protein-coupled receptor gene in the kidney and parathyroid gland. In the past it was frequently detected only after operation when removal of hyperplastic glands was unsuccessful in lowering the hypercalcaemia. Family members are often affected and surgery is not indicated as the course appears benign.

Hypocalcaemia and hypoparathyroidism

PATHOPHYSIOLOGY

Hypocalcaemia may be due to deficiencies of calcium homeostatic mechanisms, secondary to high phosphate levels or other causes of hypocalcaemia (Table 8.26). All forms of hypoparathyroidism, except transient surgical effects, are uncommon.

Table 8.26
Causes of hypocalcaemia

Increased phosphate levels Chronic renal failure (common) Phosphate therapy	**Resistance to PTH** Pseudohypoparathyroidism
Hypoparathyroidism Surgical – after neck exploration (thyroidectomy, parathyroidectomy – common) Congenital deficiency (DiGeorge syndrome) Idiopathic hypoparathyroidism (rare) Severe hypomagnesaemia	**Drugs** Calcitonin Bisphosphonates **Miscellaneous** Acute pancreatitis (quite common) Citrated blood in massive transfusion (not uncommon)
Vitamin D deficiency Osteomalacia Vitamin D resistance	

CAUSES

- Renal failure is the most common cause of hypocalcaemia.
- Hypocalcaemia after thyroid or parathyroid surgery is common but usually transient – fewer than 1% of thyroidectomies leave permanent damage (see above).
- Idiopathic hypoparathyroidism is one of the rarer autoimmune disorders, often accompanied by vitiligo, cutaneous moniliasis and other autoimmune disease.

The *DiGeorge syndrome* is a familial condition where the hypoparathyroidism is associated with intellectual impairment, cataracts and calcified basal ganglia, and occasionally with specific autoimmune disease.

Pseudo-hypoparathyroidism is a syndrome of end-organ resistance to PTH through a defective post-receptor mechanism. It is associated with short stature, short metacarpals and intellectual impairment.

Pseudo-pseudo-hypoparathyroidism describes the phenotypic defects but without any abnormalities of calcium metabolism.

CLINICAL FEATURES

Hypoparathyroidism presents as neuromuscular irritability and neuropsychiatric manifestations. Paraesthesiae, circumoral numbness, cramps, anxiety and tetany (Information box 8.13) are followed by convulsions, laryngeal stridor, dystonia and psychosis. Two signs of hypocalcaemia are Chvostek's sign (gentle tapping over the facial nerve causes twitching of the facial muscles) and Trousseau's sign, where inflation of the sphygmomanometer cuff above systolic pressure for three minutes induces tetanic spasm of the fingers and wrist. Severe hypocalcaemia may cause papilloedema and frequently a prolonged QT interval on the ECG.

Information

In the presence of alkalosis
Hyperventilation
Excess antacid therapy
Persistent vomiting
Hypochloraemic alkalosis, e.g. primary hyperaldosteronism

In the presence of hypocalcaemia
Low plasma albumin, e.g. malnutrition, chronic liver disease
Rickets and osteomalacia
Malabsorption, e.g. coeliac disease
Hypoparathyroidism
Other causes of hypocalcaemia (see Table 8.26)

Information box 8.13 Causes of tetany

INVESTIGATIONS

The *clinical history and picture* is usually diagnostic and is confirmed by a low serum calcium (corrected for any albumin abnormality). Additional tests include:

- **serum and urine creatinine** for renal disease
- **PTH levels** in the serum: absent or inappropriately low
- **parathyroid antibodies** (present in idiopathic hypoparathyroidism)
- **25-hydroxy vitamin D serum level** (low in vitamin D deficiency)
- **X-rays** of metacarpals, showing short fourth metacarpals which occur in pseudohypoparathyroidism.

TREATMENT

Urgency of treatment depends on the severity of the symptoms and the degree of hypocalcaemia. If they are severe with tetany, intravenous calcium is given: 10 mL initially, then 10–40 mL, of 10% calcium gluconate in one litre of 150 mmol L^{-1} saline over 4–8 hours. Oral calcium supplements 2–10 g daily (40–200 mmol calcium) are rarely sufficient alone.

Alpha-hydroxylated derivatives of vitamin D are preferred for their shorter half-life, and especially in renal disease as the others require renal hydroxylation. Usual daily maintenance doses are 0.25–2 μg for alfacalcidol (1α-OH-D_3). During treatment, plasma calcium must be monitored frequently to detect hypercalcaemia.

FURTHER READING

Al Zahrani A, Levine MA (1997) Primary hyperparathyroidism. *Lancet* **349**: 1233–1238.

Pearce SHS (1998) Calcium homeostasis and disorders of the calcium-sensing receptor. *Journal of the Royal College of Physicians of London* **32**: 10–14.

Osteomyelitis

Acute and chronic osteomyelitis

Osteomyelitis can be due either to metastatic haematogenous spread (e.g. from a boil) or to local infection. Malnutrition, debilitating disease and decreased immunity may play a part in the pathogenesis.

Staphylococcus is the organism responsible for 90% of cases of acute osteomyelitis (see p. 20). Other organisms include *Haemophilus influenzae* and *Salmonella*; infection with the latter may occur as a complication of sickle cell anaemia.

Chronic osteomyelitis may follow an acute infection. Another variety of chronic osteomyelitis is due to infection being localized to form a chronic abscess within the bone (Brodie's abscess). Patients may be asymptomatic for months or years or may have intermittent local pain.

Treatment of osteomyelitis is with immobilization and antibiotic therapy with flucloxacillin and fusidic acid.

Tuberculous osteomyelitis

This is usually due to haematogenous spread from a reactivated primary focus in the lungs or gastrointestinal tract. The disease starts in intra-articular bone. The spine is commonly involved (Pott's disease), with damage to the bodies of two neighbouring vertebrae leading to vertebral collapse and later abscess formation ('cold abscess'). Pus can track along tissue planes and discharge at a point far from the affected vertebrae.

Symptoms consist of local pain and later swelling if pus has collected. Systemic symptoms of malaise, fever and night sweats occur.

Treatment is as for pulmonary tuberculosis (see p. 804) together with immobilization.

Neoplastic disease of bone

Malignant tumours of bone are shown in Table 8.27. The most common tumours are *metastases* from the bronchus, breast and prostate. Metastases from kidney and thyroid are less common. Primary bone tumours are rare and usually seen only in children and young adults.

Symptoms are usually related to the anatomical position of the tumour, with local bone pain over the area. Systemic symptoms (e.g. malaise and pyrexia) and aches and pains occur and are sometimes related to hypercalcaemia (see above). The diagnosis of metastases can often be made from the history and examination, particularly if the primary tumour has already been diagnosed. Symptoms from bony metastases may, however, be the first presenting feature.

Table 8.27
Malignant neoplasms of bone

Metastases (osteolytic)
Bronchus
Breast
Prostate (often osteosclerotic as well)
Thyroid
Kidney
Multiple myeloma
Primary bone tumours (rare; seen in the young), e.g.
Osteosarcomas
Fibrosarcomas
Chondromas
Ewing's tumour

INVESTIGATIONS

- **Skeletal isotope scans** can pick up bony metastases as 'hot' areas before radiological changes occur.
- **X-rays** may show metastases as osteolytic areas with bony destruction. Osteosclerotic metastases are characteristic of prostatic carcinoma.
- **Serum alkaline phosphatase** (from bone) is usually raised.
- **Hypercalcaemia** is seen in 10–20% of patients with malignancies. It is associated chiefly with metastases, but can also result from ectopic parathormone or parathyroid hormone-related protein secretion.
- **Serum acid phosphate** is raised in the presence of prostatic metastases.
- **Prostatic specific antigen** (PSA) is raised in presence of prostatic secondaries.

TREATMENT

Treatment is usually with analgesics and anti-inflammatory drugs (e.g. indomethacin). Local radiotherapy over bone metastases may be the best way of relieving pain. Depending on the tumour, cytotoxic chemotherapy is occasionally helpful. Some tumours are hormone-dependent and remission can be obtained by hormonal therapy. Occasionally pathological fractures require internal fixation.

Connective tissue

All connective tissues have a large proportion of extracellular matrix as well as cells. This matrix consists of extracellular macromolecules containing collagens, elastins, non-collagenous glycoproteins and proteoglycans.

COLLAGENS

Collagens consist of three polypeptide chains (α chains) wound around one another in a triple helical confirmation. These α chains contain repeating sequences of *Gly–x–y* triplets, where *x* and *y* are often prolyl and hydroxyprolyl residues. There is much genetic heterogeneity in collagen fibres, and the gene for different chains is located on at least 12 chromosomes.

The majority of collagen in the body is type I; it is the major protein in bones, tendons and ligaments, skin, sclera, cornea, blood vessels and hollow organs. Types III, V and VI are also distributed in most tissues although only a little type III is seen in bone or cartilage. Other collagens are tissue specific, i.e. types II, IX, X and XI are found in hyaline cartilage, type IV in basement membrane and type VII in anchoring fibril structures in the epithelial mesenchymal junctions.

There are several classes of collagen genes, based on their protein structures:

- The fibrillar collagens (e.g. COL1A1–2, COL2A1, COL3, COL5, COL11) which encode collagens types I, II, III, V and XI. Mutations of these produce osteogenesis imperfecta and Ehlers–Danlos syndrome.
- The basement membrane collagen genes, e.g. COL4A1–5 encoding collagen type IV. Mutations lead to Alports' disease.
- Fibril-associated collagens with interrupted triple helices (FACIT), e.g. COL9, COL12 encoding types IX, XII and XIV.
- Filament producing collagen, e.g. COL6A1, 2, 3 encoding type VI.
- Network-forming collagens, e.g. COL8A1, COL10A1 encoding type VIII and X.
- Anchoring fibril collagen, e.g. COL7A1 encoding type VII. Mutations of this gene produce epidermolysis bullosa (p. 1181).

ELASTIN

Elastic fibres in the extracellular matrix consist of elastin and microfibils. Elastin is an insoluble protein polymer and its gene has been characterized. Its precursor, tropoelastin, is synthesized by vascular smooth muscle cells and skin fibroblasts. Elastin fibres are cross-linked with desmosine and isodesmosine which are specific to elastin.

GLYCOPROTEINS

Fibronectin is the major non-collagenous glycoprotein in the extracellular matrix. Its molecule contains a series of functional domains, or cell recognition sites, that bind ligands and are involved in cell adhesion. A synthetic peptide sequence (*Arg–Gly–Asp*), which mimics some of the functions of fibronectin, is also found in other adhesion proteins (e.g. vitronectin, laminin and collagen type VI). Fibronectin plays a major role in tissue remodelling. It is stimulated by interferon-γ and transforming growth factor-β and inhibited by tumour necrosis factor and interleukin-1.

Proteoglycans

These proteins contain glycosaminoglycan side chains. They are of variable forms and sizes. Many have been identified at different sites, e.g. aggrecan, biglycan, fibromodulin, decorin (in extracellular matrix), syndecan,

CD44, fibroglycan (on cell surfaces), cerebroglycan (in brain), serglycan (in intracellular tissues) and perglycan (in basement membranes). In general their function is to bind extracellular matrix together, mediate cell binding and retain soluble molecules in the matrix.

Diseases of collagen

Ehlers–Danlos syndrome

This is a heterogeneous group of disorders of collagen. Ten different types have been recognized with varying degrees of skin fragility, skin hyperextensibility and joint hypermobility. Types I, II and III are inherited in an autosomal dominant fashion; the biochemical basis is unknown. No abnormalities in COL1A1, COL1A2 and COL2A1 genes have been found.

Type IV is also autosomal dominant and involves arteries, the bowel and uterus, as well as the skin. Mutations in COL3A1 gene produce abnormalities in structure, synthesis or secretion of type III collagen.

Type VI is a recessively inherited disorder and results from a mutation in the gene that encodes lysyl hydroxylase.

Type VII is an autosomal dominant disorder where there is a defect in the conversion of procollagen to collagen; COL1A1 and COL1A2 mutations delete the *N*-proteinase cleavage sites.

Other forms of Ehlers–Danlos are very rare and their defects have not been elucidated. The clinical features are described on p. 1187.

Osteogenesis imperfecta (fragilitas ossium brittle bone syndrome)

This is a heterogeneous group of mainly autosomally dominant inherited disorders. In the majority there are mutations in the genes encoding the chains in type I collagen, i.e. COL1A1, COL1A2. There are four types, distinguished by the very variable clinical pictures ranging from death in the perinatal period (type II), severe bone deformity (type III), to a normal lifespan (types I and IV).

The major clinical feature is very fragile and brittle bones but other collagen-containing tissues are also involved, such as tendons, the skin and the eyes. Osteogenesis imperfecta tarda (type I) has mild bony deformities, blue sclerae, defective dentine, early-onset deafness, hypermobility of joints, and heart valve disorders. More severe forms present with multiple fractures and gross deformities. Prognosis is variable, depending on the severity of the disease.

Alport's syndrome (p. 538)

This is inherited in an X-linked fashion. There are mutations in the COL4A5 gene, with the resultant collagen leading to splitting and thinning of the glomerular basement membrane.

Marfan syndrome

This is an autosomal dominant disorder with a frequency of 1:15 000. Mutations on the extracellular matrix glycoprotein, fibrillin, are the cause of the disorder. The fibrillin gene is localized to the long arm of chromosome 15. Clinical features are described on p. 1188.

Skeletal dysplasias

Skeletal dysplasias include a large group of heterogeneous disorders of bone and connective tissue.

Osteopetrosis (marble bone disease)

This condition may be inherited in either an autosomal dominant or an autosomal recessive manner; the recessive type is severe and the dominant type is mild. In addition, another recessive form associated with renal tubular acidosis is due to carbonic anhydrase II deficiency.

In the severe form, bone density is increased throughout the skeleton but bones tend to fracture easily. Involvement of the bone marrow leads to a leucoerythroblastic anaemia. There is mental retardation and early death.

In the mild form there may be only X-ray changes, but fractures and infection can occur. The acid phosphate level is raised.

Hypophosphatasia

This rare autosomal recessive condition is due to a deficiency of alkaline phosphatase and pyrophosphatase. It is not known where the primary defect lies, but it may be in the osteoblasts. It varies in severity from unmineralized bones *in utero* resulting in death, to rickets in infancy or recurrent fractures in adults. Prenatal diagnosis with the measurement of alkaline phosphatase is reliable.

Osteochondrodysplasia

This is a group of heterogeneous disorders that affect the normal development of bone and cartilage. *Achondroplasia* ('dwarfism') is diagnosed in the first years of life. The disease is inherited in an autosomal dominant manner and is caused by a defect in the fibroblast growth factor receptor-3 gene. The trunk is of normal length but the limbs are very short and broad. The vault of the skull is enlarged, the face is small and the nose bridge is flat. Intelligence is normal.

CHAPTER BIBLIOGRAPHY

Dorfman HD, Czerniak B (1998) *Bone Tumors*. St Louis, MO: Mosby.

Favus MJ (ed) (1996) *Primer on the Metabolic Bone Diseases and Disorders of Mineral Metabolism*. Philadelphia: Lippincott–Raven.

Scriver CCR, Beaudet AL, Sly WS, Valle D (eds) (1995) *The Metabolic and Molecular Bases of Inherited Disease*, 7th edn. New York: McGraw–Hill.

Renal disease

9

Renal function

The kidneys' principal role is the elimination of waste material and the regulation of the volume and composition of body fluid (Table 9.1). The kidneys have a unique system involving the free ultrafiltration of water and non-protein-bound low-molecular-weight compounds from the plasma and the selective reabsorption and/or excretion of these as the ultrafiltrate passes along the tubule.

The functioning unit is the *nephron*, of which there are approximately one million in each kidney. A conventional diagrammatic representation is shown in Fig 9.1(a) and a physiological version in Fig. 9.1(b).

An essential feature of renal function is that a large volume of blood – 25% of cardiac output or approximately 1300 mL per minute – passes through the two million glomeruli.

A hydrostatic pressure gradient of approximately 10 mmHg (a capillary pressure of 45 mmHg minus 10 mmHg of pressure within Bowman's space and 25 mmHg of plasma oncotic pressure) provides the driving force for ultrafiltration of virtually protein-free and fat-free fluid across the glomerular capillary wall into Bowman's space and so into the renal tubule (Fig 9.2).

The ultrafiltration rate (glomerular filtration rate; GFR) varies with age and sex but is approximately 120–130 mL min^{-1} per 1.73 m^2 surface area in adults. This means that each day ultrafiltration of 170–180 L of water and unbound small-molecular-weight constituents of blood occurs. The 'need' for this high filtration rate relates to the elimination of compounds present in relatively low concentration in plasma (e.g. urea). If these large volumes of ultrafiltrate were excreted unchanged as urine, it would be necessary to ingest huge amounts of

Table 9.1
Functions of the kidney

Excretory	Excretion of waste products, drugs
Regulatory	Control of body fluid volume and composition
Endocrine	Production of erythropoietin, renin, prostaglandins
Metabolic	Metabolism of vitamin D, small-molecular-weight proteins

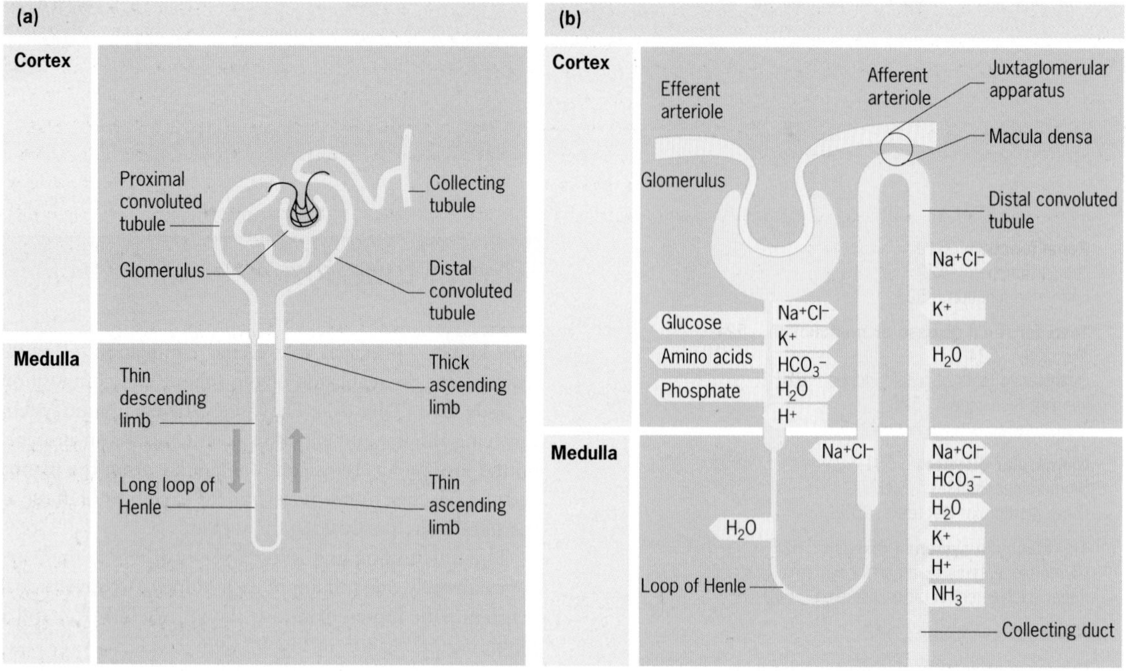

Fig 9.1
(a) Principal parts of the nephron. (b) Sites of removal or addition of electrolytes from or into tubular fluid
Note: The descending limb is permeable to water and impermeable to sodium, whereas in the ascending limb the permeabilities are reversed.

water and electrolytes to stay in balance. This is avoided by the selective reabsorption of water, essential electrolytes and other blood constituents, such as glucose and amino acids, from the filtrate in transit along the nephron. Thus, 60–80% of filtered water and sodium are reabsorbed in the proximal tubule along with virtually all the potassium, bicarbonate, glucose and amino acids (Fig 9.1(b)). Further water and sodium chloride are reabsorbed more distally, and fine tuning of salt and water balance is achieved in the distal and collecting tubules under the influence of aldosterone and antidiuretic hormone (ADH). The final urine volume is thus 1–2 L daily. Calcium, phosphate and magnesium are also selectively reabsorbed in proportion to the need to maintain a normal electrolyte composition of body fluids.

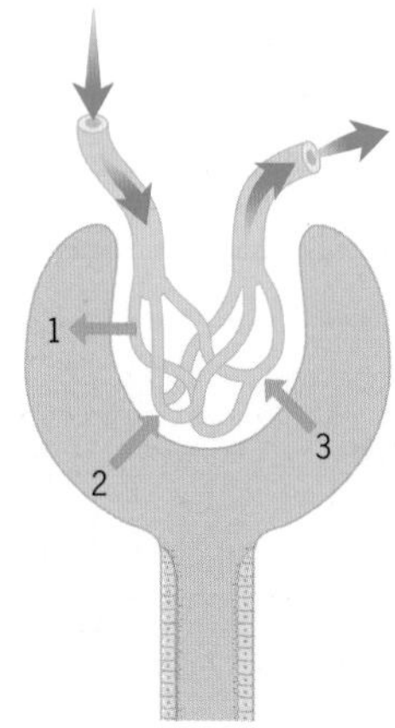

Fig 9.2
Pressures controlling glomerular filtration. 1, capillary hydrostatic pressure (45 mmHg); **2**, hydrostatic pressure in Bowman's space (10 mmHg); **3**, plasma protein oncotic pressure (25 mmHg). Arrows indicate the direction of a pressure gradient

The urinary excretion of some compounds is more complicated. For example, potassium is freely filtered at the glomerulus, almost completely absorbed in the proximal tubule, and excreted in the distal tubule and collecting ducts. An important clinical consequence of this is that the ability to eliminate unwanted potassium is less dependent on GFR than is the elimination of urea or creatinine. Other compounds filtered and reabsorbed or excreted to a variable extent include urate and many organic acids, including many drugs or their metabolic breakdown products. The more tubular secretion of a compound occurs, the less dependent is elimination on the GFR; penicillin and cephradine are examples of compounds secreted by the tubules.

Urine concentration and the countercurrent system

Urine is concentrated by a complex interaction between the loops of Henle, the medullary interstitium, medullary blood vessels (vasa recta) and the collecting tubules. The proposed mechanism of urine concentration is termed 'the countercurrent mechanism'. The countercurrent hypothesis states that a small difference in osmotic concentration at any point between fluid flowing in opposite directions in two parallel tubes connected in a hairpin manner is multiplied many times along the length of the tubes. Tubular fluid moves from the renal cortex towards the papillary tip of the medulla via the proximal straight tubule and the thin descending limb of the loop of Henle which is permeable to water and impermeable to sodium. The tubule then loops back towards the cortex so that the direction of the fluid movement is reversed in the ascending limb, which is impermeable to water but permeable to sodium. This results in a large osmolar concentration difference between the corticomedullary junction and the hairpin loop at the tip of the papilla, and hence countercurrent multiplication. There is an analogy with heat exchangers.

Acid–base balance

Tubular function is also critical to the control of acid–base balance. Thus, filtered bicarbonate is largely reabsorbed and hydrogen ions are excreted mainly buffered by phosphate (see p. 618).

Glomerular filtration rate

In health the GFR remains remarkably constant owing to intrarenal regulatory mechanisms. In disease, with a reduction in intrarenal blood flow, damage to or loss of glomeruli, or obstruction to the free flow of ultrafiltrate along the tubule, the GFR will fall and the ability to eliminate waste material and to regulate the volume and composition of body fluid will decline. This will be manifest as a rise in the blood level of urea or the plasma level of creatinine and in a reduction in *measured* GFR.

Uraemia

The concentration of urea or creatinine in blood or plasma, respectively, represents the dynamic equilibrium between production and elimination. In healthy subjects there is an enormous reserve of renal excretory function, and serum urea and creatinine do not rise above the normal range until there is a reduction of 50–60% in the GFR. Thereafter, the level of urea depends both on the GFR and the production rate (Table 9.2). The latter is heavily influenced by protein intake and tissue catabolism. The level of creatinine is much less dependent on diet but is more related to age, sex and muscle mass. Once it is elevated, serum creatinine is a better guide to GFR than urea and, in general, measurement of serum creatinine is a good way to monitor further deterioration in the GFR.

It must be re-emphasized that a normal serum urea or creatinine is *not* synonymous with a normal GFR.

Table 9.2
Factors influencing serum urea levels

Production	Elimination
Increased by	**Increased by**
High protein diet	Elevated GFR, e.g. pregnancy
Increased catabolism	
Surgery	**Decreased by**
Infection	Glomerular disease
Trauma	Reduced renal blood flow
Corticosteroid therapy	Hypotension
Tetracyclines	Dehydration
Gastrointestinal bleeding	Urinary obstruction
Cancer	Tubulointerstitial nephritis
Decreased by	
Low-protein diet	
Reduced catabolism, e.g. old age	
Liver failure	

GFR, glomerular filtration rate

Measurement of the glomerular filtration rate

Measurement of the GFR is necessary to define the exact level of renal function. It is essential when the serum urea or creatinine are within the normal range.

Inulin clearance – the gold standard of physiologists – is not practical or necessary in clinical practice. The most widely used measurement is the creatinine clearance (Fig 9.3).

The use of creatinine clearance is dependent on the fact that daily production of creatinine (principally from muscle cells) is remarkably constant and little affected by protein intake. Serum creatinine and urinary output thus vary very little throughout the day. This permits the use of 24-hour urine collections, which reduce collection errors, and the measurement of a single serum creatinine value during the 24 hours (Practical box 9.1).

Creatinine excretion is, however, by both glomerular filtration and tubular secretion, although at normal serum

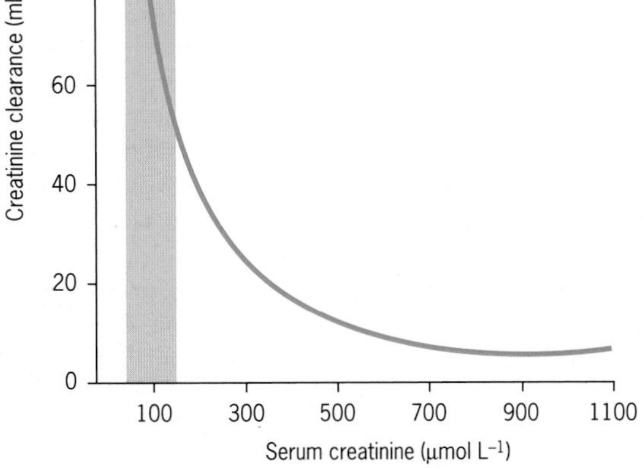

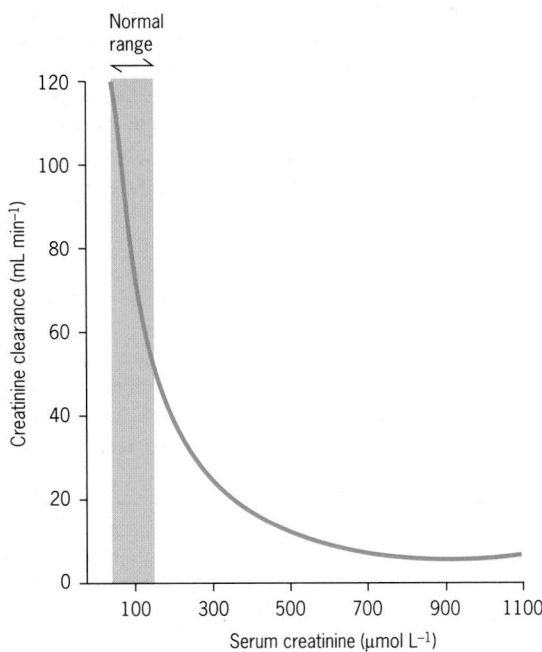

Fig 9.3
Creatinine clearance versus serum creatinine.
Note that the serum creatinine does not rise above the normal range until there is a reduction of 50–60% in the glomerular filtration rate (creatinine clearance)

Practical

1 Empty the bladder at the beginning of the collection period. Discard the urine. Note the time.
2 Collect *all* urine passed (including overnight) during the subsequent 24 hours.
3 Exactly 24 hours after commencement of collection, empty the bladder. Urine thus voided is to be included in collection.

Measurement of creatinine clearance

- Urine is collected over 24 hours for measurement of urinary creatinine; a 24-hour collection diminishes collection errors.
- A plasma level of creatinine is measured sometime during the 24-hour period.
- Given the rate of urine flow (*V*), the urine (*U*) and plasma (*P*) concentrations of creatinine, clearance is obtained from the formula:

$$\frac{U \times V}{P} \times 100$$

where *U* and *P* are measured in mmol L^{-1}, and *V* is measured in mL per minute.
- Normal ranges: men 90–140 mL min^{-1}, women 80–125 mL min^{-1}

Practical box 9.1 To obtain a timed 24-hour urine collection and to measure creatinine clearance

levels the latter is relatively small. As most laboratory methods for measurement of serum creatinine give slight overestimates, the calculation of clearance fortuitously gives a value close to that of inulin.

With progressive renal failure, creatinine clearance may overestimate GFR but, in clinical practice, this is seldom important. Certain drugs – for example cimetidine, trimethoprim, spironolactone and amiloride – reduce tubular secretion of creatinine, leading to a rise in serum creatinine and a fall in measured clearance.

Given these observations, creatinine clearance, nevertheless, is a reasonably accurate measure of GFR in those situations in which it is most required – normal or near normal renal function.

Where urine collections are difficult (e.g. with ileal conduits) or deemed inaccurate, the GFR may be measured by the single injection of compounds such as [^{51}Cr]EDTA (ethylenediaminetetraacetic acid), [^{99m}Tc]DTPA (diethylenetriaminepentaacetic acid) or [^{125}I]iothalamate, their excretion being primarily by glomerular filtration. Following intravenous injection of the compound, three blood samples are obtained at 2, 3 and 4 hours (or rather longer intervals if the patient is oedematous or if renal failure is suspected). The GFR may then be calculated from the slope of the exponential fall in blood level of the compound.

Urea clearance is not an accurate measure of GFR, particularly when urine flow rate is low, and should not be used as a measure of GFR.

Tubular function

The major function of the tubule is the selective reabsorption or excretion of water and various cations and anions to keep the volume and electrolyte composition of body fluid normal (see Chapter 10).

The active reabsorption from the glomerular filtrate of compounds such as glucose and amino acids also takes place. Within the normal range of blood concentrations these substances are completely reabsorbed by the proximal tubule. However, if blood levels are elevated above the normal range, the amount filtered (filtered load = GFR × plasma concentration) may exceed the maximal absorptive capacity of the tubule and the compound 'spills over' into the urine. Examples of this occur with hyperglycaemia in diabetes mellitus or elevated plasma phenylalanine in phenylketonuria.

Conversely, inherited or acquired defects in tubular function may lead to incomplete absorption of a *normal* filtered load, with loss of the compound in the urine (a lowered 'renal threshold'). This is seen in renal glycosuria, in which there is a genetically determined defect in tubular reabsorption of glucose. It is diagnosed by demonstrating glycosuria in the presence of normal blood glucose levels. Inherited or acquired defects in the tubular reabsorption of amino acids, phosphate, sodium, potassium and calcium also occur, either singly or in combination. Examples include cystinuria and the Fanconi syndrome (see p. 999). Tubular defects in the reabsorption of water result in nephrogenic diabetes insipidus. Under normal circumstances, antidiuretic hormone induces an increase in the permeability of water in the collecting tubules by attachment to receptors with subsequent activation of adenyl cyclase. This then activates a protein kinase which induces preformed cytoplasmic vesicles containing water channels (termed 'aquaporins') to move to and insert into the tubular luminal membrane. This allows water entry into tubular cells down a favourable osmotic gradient. Water then crosses the basolateral membrane and enters the bloodstream. When the effect of ADH wears off, water channels return to the cell cytoplasm.

Investigation of tubular function in clinical practice

Proximal tubular function

Five tests of proximal tubular function are employed in clinical practice: measurement of serum potassium and serum phosphorus concentrations and detection of glycosuria, generalized aminoaciduria and 'tubular' proteinuria.

Hypokalaemia in the face of a normal or increased urinary potassium excretion (>40 mmol in 24 hours) is indicative of proximal tubular failure of potassium reabsorption. Unless other explanations exist such as treatment with thiazide diuretics or hyperaldosteronism, the defect can be assumed to lie in the proximal tubule. Similarly, hypophosphataemia may be attributed to a proximal tubular abnormality provided alternative explanations, such as the use of gut phosphorus binders and primary hyperparathyroidism, can be ruled out. Glycosuria in the absence of hyperglycaemia and generalized aminoaciduria are also indicative of failure of proximal tubular reabsorption of glucose and amino acids, respectively. Proteins derived from tubular cells, such as β_2-microglobulin, are reabsorbed in the proximal nephron. If proteinuria is present, and urine electrophoresis shows the characteristic 'tubular' as distinct from 'glomerular' pattern (i.e. albumin), a proximal tubular defect is demonstrated.

Distal tubular function

Two tests of distal tubular function are commonly applied in clinical practice: measurement of urinary concentrating capacity in response to water deprivation, and measurement of urinary acidification. These tests are dealt with on pp. 1208 and 622.

Endocrine function

Renin–angiotensin system (see also p. 953)

The juxtaglomerular apparatus is made up of specialized arteriolar smooth muscle cells that are sited on the afferent glomerular arteriole as it enters the glomerulus (see Fig 9.1(b)). These cells secrete renin, which converts angiotensinogen in blood to angiotensin I. Renin release is controlled by:

- pressure changes in the afferent arteriole
- sympathetic tone
- chloride and osmotic concentration in the distal tubule via the macula densa (Fig 9.1(b))
- local prostaglandin release.

Angiotensin II is generated from angiotensin I by angiotensin-converting enzyme (ACE). Angiotensin II is both a vasoconstrictor and the most important stimulus for the release of aldosterone by the adrenal cortex. It also modifies intrarenal blood flow (see p. 600).

Endothelins

The endothelins ET-1, ET-2 and ET-3 are a family of potent vasoactive peptides that also influence cell proliferation and epithelial solute transport. They do not circulate but act locally. The genes for two of the receptors ET_A and ET_B have been cloned. The vascular actions are mediated by both these receptors whilst the tubular transport and interstitial proliferative actions are mediated by ET_B. Intrarenal levels of ET-1 are raised in acute and chronic renal disease and may play a role in pathogenesis. Antagonists are in the early clinical trial stages.

Erythropoietin (see also p. 356)

Erythropoietin is a glycoprotein produced principally by the kidney and is the major stimulus for erythropoiesis. Loss of renal substance, with decreased erythropoietin production, results in a normochromic, normocytic anaemia. Conversely, erythropoietin secretion may be increased, with resultant polycythaemia, in patients with polycystic renal disease, benign renal cysts or renal cell carcinoma.

Recombinant human erythropoietin has been biosynthesized and is available for clinical use, particularly in patients with renal failure (see p. 579).

Prostaglandins

Prostaglandins are unsaturated fatty acid compounds sythesized from cell membrane phospholipids (see Fig 12.32). They exert their main effects in close proximity to the site of production. The main prostaglandins synthesized in the kidney are PGE_2 (the main renal medullary prostaglandin), PGF_2, PGD_2, prostacyclin (PGI_2, the main renal cortical prostaglandin) and thromboxane A_2.

Prostaglandins are important in the maintenance of renal blood flow and glomerular filtration rate in the face of reductions induced by vasoconstrictor stimuli such as angiotensin II, catecholamines and α-adrenergic stimulation. In the presence of renal underperfusion, inhibition of prostaglandin synthesis by non-steroidal anti-inflammatory drugs results in a further reduction in GFR, sometimes sufficiently severe as to cause acute renal failure. Renal prostaglandins also have a natriuretic renal tubular effect and antagonize the action of antidiuretic hormone. Renal prostaglandins do not regulate salt and water excretion in normal subjects, but in some circumstances, such as chronic renal failure, prostaglandin-induced vasodilatation is important in maintaining renal blood flow. Patients with chronic renal failure are thus vulnerable to further deterioration in renal function on exposure to non-steroidal anti-inflammatory drugs, as are elderly patients in many of whom renal function is compromised by renal vascular disease and/or the effects of ageing upon the kidney.

Kallikrein–kinin system

The role of this system is not fully understood but it too probably plays a part in the control of the distribution of renal blood flow and in salt and water excretion.

The natriuretic-peptide family (see p. 954)

In the early 1980s the discovery of a circulating peptide derived from atrial tissue which had natriuretic, diuretic and vasorelaxant properties confirmed the long-postulated exsitence of a humoral link between heart and kidney. A whole family of such peptides exists. Atrial natriuretic peptide (ANP) mRNA has been found in many tissues, but most abundantly in the cardiac atria. Two other peptides derived from different precursor molecules encoded by different genes have been isolated.

These are brain natriuretic peptide (BNP) and C-natriuretic peptide (CNP). Confusingly, BNP is found in highest concentration in myocardial tissue, whereas CNP is found predominantly in the brain. ANP and BNP have mainly natriuretic and vasorelaxant properties, whereas CNP is not natriuretic. Natriuretic peptide receptors have been cloned for each of the peptides. Natriuretic peptides are cleaved by the enzyme neutral endopeptidase, although this is not the only mechanism of clearance. The affinity of the enzyme for BNP is much less than that for ANP and CNP.

Collectively, natriuretic peptides counterbalance the effects of the renin-angiotensin aldosterone system. In response to volume expansion and pressure overload of the heart, plasma ANP and BNP concentrations increase, and one or both of them antagonize the effects of angiotensin II on the vascular tone, aldosterone secretion, renal tubular sodium reabsorption and vascular cell growth. Intravenous infusion of ANP is followed by a marked natriuresis with a rise in glomerular filtration rate and a fall in blood pressure. Concentrations are elevated in heart failure and renal failure, and a possible therapeutic role for these actions in such conditions has been explored. Currently, interest focuses mainly on the use of neutral endopeptidase inhibitors in the promotion of a salt and water diuresis. Plasma CNP concentrations change little with cardiac overload, and the main role of this peptide appears to be the regulation of vascular tone.

Vitamin D metabolism (see p. 504)

Naturally occurring vitamin D requires hydroxylation in the liver and again by a 1α-hydroxylase enzyme in the kidney to produce the powerfully metabolically active 1,25-dihydroxycholecalciferol (1,25-$(OH)_2D_3$). Reduced 1α-hydroxylase activity in diseased kidneys results in relative deficiency of 1,25-$(OH)_2D_3$. As a result, gastrointestinal calcium absorption is reduced and bone mineralization impaired. Receptors for 1,25-$(OH)_2D_3$ exist in the parathyroid glands and reduced occupancy of the receptors by the vitamin alters the set-point for release of parathyroid hormone (PTH) in response to a given decrement in plasma calcium concentration. Gut calcium malabsorption, which induces a tendency to hypocalcaemia, and relative lack of 1,25-$(OH)_2D_3$, contribute therefore to the hyperparathyroidism seen regularly in patients with renal impairment, even of modest degree.

Protein and polypeptide metabolism

It is clear that the kidney is a major site for the catabolism of many small-molecular-weight proteins and polypeptides, including many hormones such as insulin, PTH and calcitonin. In renal failure the metabolic clearance of these substances is reduced and their half-life is prolonged. This accounts, for example, for the reduced insulin requirements of diabetic patients as their renal function declines.

FURTHER READING

Hendry BM, James AF (1997) Endothelin antagonists in renal disease. *Lancet* **350**: 381–382.

Wilkins MR, Redondo J, Brown LA (1997) The natriuretic-peptide family. *Lancet* **349**: 1307–1311.

Tests for renal disease or malfunction

Renal disease is suspected if there are:

- symptoms referable to the urinary tract
- hypertension
- an elevated serum urea or creatinine concentration
- abnormalities on urinalysis.

The urine

Appearance

This is of little value in the differential diagnosis of renal disease except in the diagnosis of haematuria. Overt 'bloody' urine is usually unmistakable but should be checked using dipsticks (Stix testing). Very concentrated urine may also appear dark or smoky. Other causes of discoloration of urine include cholestatic jaundice, haemoglobinuria, drugs such as rifampicin, use of fluorescein or methylene blue, and ingestion of beetroot. Discoloration of urine after standing for some time occurs in porphyria, alkaptonuria and in patients ingesting the drug L-dopa. In patients with frequency or dysuria the passage of crystal-clear urine usually indicates that significant bacteriuria is absent.

Volume

In health, the volume of urine passed is primarily determined by diet and fluid intake. In temperate climates it lies within the range 800–2500 mL per 24 hours. The minimum amount passed to stay in fluid balance is determined by the amount of solute – mainly urea and electrolytes – being excreted and the maximum concentrating power of the kidneys. On a normal diet, some 800 mOsmol of solute are passed daily. Since the maximum urine concentration is approximately 1200 mOsmol L^{-1}, the minimum volume of urine obligated by excretion of 800 mOsmol of solute would thus be approximately 650 mL (Table 9.3). Fluid intake is generally greater than this, so that larger volumes of more dilute urine are passed. A diet rich in carbohydrate and fat and low in protein and salt results in a lower solute excretion and as little as 300 mL of urine per day may be required. Conversely, a high-salt, high-protein intake obligates a larger urine flow and, via the thirst mechanism, a higher fluid intake. The appropriateness of a given daily urine output must therefore be related to factors such as diet, body size and fluid intake.

In disease, impairment of concentrating ability requires increased volumes of urine to be passed, given the same daily solute output (Table 9.3). An increased solute output, such as in glycosuria or increased protein catabolism following surgery or associated with sepsis, also demands increased urine volumes.

The maximum urine output depends on the ability to produce a dilute urine. Intakes of 10 or even 20 L daily can be tolerated by normal humans but, given a daily solute output of 800 mOsmol, require the ability to dilute to 80 and 40 mOsmol L^{-1}, respectively. Where diluting ability is impaired, the ability to excrete large volumes of ingested water is also impaired.

Oliguria

Oliguria, usually defined as the excretion of less than 300 mL of urine per day, may be 'physiological', as in patients with hypotension and hypovolaemia, where urine is maximally concentrated in an attempt to conserve water. More often, it is due to intrinsic renal disease or obstructive nephropathy (see p. 562).

Anuria (no urine) suggests urinary tract obstruction until proved otherwise; bladder outflow obstruction must always be considered first.

Polyuria

Polyuria is a persistent, large increase in urine output, usually associated with nocturia. It must be distinguished from frequency of micturition with the passage of small volumes of urine. Documentation of fluid intake and output may be necessary. Polyuria is the result of an excessive (hysterical) intake of water, an increased excretion of solute (as in hyperglycaemia and glycosuria), or a defective renal concentrating ability or failure of production of ADH.

Specific gravity and osmolality

Urine specific gravity is a measure of the weight of dissolved particles in urine, whereas urine osmolality reflects the number of such particles. Usually the relationship between the two is close. An exception exists when a relatively small number of relatively large particles are present in urine, such as in multiple myeloma. Measurement of urine specific gravity or osmolality is required only under limited circumstances, such as the differential diagnosis of oliguric renal failure or the investigation of polyuria or inappropriate ADH secretion.

Urinary pH

Measurement of urinary pH is unnecessary except in the investigation and treatment of renal tubular acidosis (see p. 620).

Chemical (Stix) testing

Routine Stix testing of urine for blood, protein and sugar is obligatory in all patients suspected of having renal disease.

Blood

Haematuria may be overt, with bloody urine, or microscopic and found only on chemical testing. Currently used Stix tests for blood are very sensitive, being positive if two or more red cells are visible under the high-power field of a light microscope. Indeed, the test is too sensitive, sometimes giving positive results in normal individuals. A further disadvantage is that Stix testing cannot distinguish between blood and free haemoglobin. A positive Stix test must always be followed by microscopy of fresh urine to confirm the presence of red cells and so exclude the relatively rare conditions of haemoglobinuria or myoglobinuria. In females with a positive Stix test result for blood, it is essential to enquire whether the patient is menstruating.

Bleeding may come from any site within the urinary tract (Fig 9.4):

- *Overt bleeding from the urethra* is suggested when blood is seen at the start of voiding and then the urine becomes clear.
- *Blood diffusely present throughout the urine* comes from the bladder or above.
- *Blood only at the end of micturition* suggests bleeding from the prostate or bladder base.

Table 9.3
Relationship between diet, kidney function and urine volume

Diet	Approximate solute output (mOsmol per 24h)	Minimum urine volume required to excrete solute load (mL per 24h)	
		With normal urine concentration (maximum 1200 mOsmol kg^{-1})	In disease (impaired urine concentration – maximum 300 mOsmol kg^{-1})
Normal	800	667	2667
High-protein/salt	1200	1000	4000
Low-protein/salt	360	300	1200

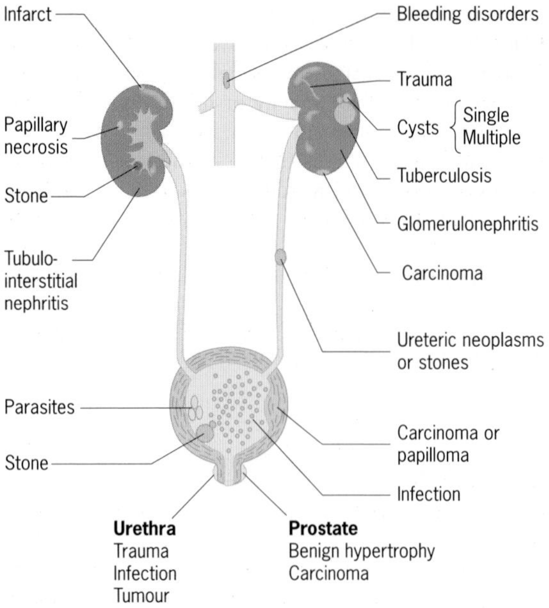

Fig 9.4
Sites and causes of bleeding from the urinary tract

Careful urine microscopy is mandatory as the presence of red-cell casts is diagnostic of bleeding from the kidney itself, most often due to glomerulonephritis. In the absence of red-cell casts, further investigations, such as urine cytology, intravenous urography and cystoscopy, are required to define the site of bleeding. Renal biopsy may be required (see p. 531).

Protein

Proteinuria is one of the most common signs of renal disease. Detection is now primarily by Stix testing. Most reagent strips can detect a concentration of 150 mg L^{-1} or more in urine. They react primarily with albumin and are relatively insensitive to globulin and Bence–Jones proteins.

If proteinuria is confirmed on repeated Stix testing, protein excretion in 24-hour urine collections should be measured. Normal values for urinary protein excretion are dependent on the laboratory methods used and in particular whether or not the method measures Tamm–Horsfall glycoprotein, which is a normal constituent of urine. Results must therefore take account of the laboratory's normal reference range. Given this caveat, healthy adults excrete approximately 60–100 mg of protein daily but up to 150–200 mg daily is within the acceptable range. Slightly higher values – up to 300 mg daily – may be excreted by adolescents. Pyrexia, exercise and adoption of the upright posture all increase urinary protein output. Proteinuria, while occasionally benign, always requires further investigation.

Postural proteinuria. This term is used to refer to proteinuria present on dipstick testing which becomes undetectable after a period of hours lying flat. Typically, a negative dipstick result is obtained on the first urine passed on rising in the morning, whereas subsequent specimens give a positive result. This is regarded by many – including some insurance companies – as a benign condition. Renal biopsy sometimes discloses glomerular abnormalities but progressive renal failure is rare.

Microalbuminuria

The term microalbuminuria is an unfortunate one since the albumin referred to is of normal molecular size and weight. Normal individuals excrete less than 30 μg of albumin per minute (43 mg in 24 hours). Dipsticks, however, detect albumin only in a concentration around 100 mg L^{-1} (150 mg per 24 hours if urine volume is normal). An increase in albumin excretion between these two levels – so-called microalbuminuria – is now known to be an early indicator of diabetic glomerular disease. It is widely used as a predictor of the development of nephropathy in diabetics and may be extended to other conditions.

For example, the majority of patients with systemic lupus erythematosis but without overt renal disease have microalbuminuria and some ultimately develop clinically evident glomerulonephritis. By contrast, patients with minimal-change nephropathy (see p. 535) after remission have normal albumin excretion.

Timed 24-hour urinary excretion rates provide the most precise measure of microalbuminuria. However, in clinical practice it is more convenient to test for microalbuminuria using random urine samples in which albumin concentration is related to urinary creatinine concentration. Kits are now available to test for microalbuminuria.

Glucose

Renal glycosuria is uncommon, so that a positive test for glucose always requires exclusion of diabetes mellitus.

Bacteriuria

Dipsticks are available for testing for bacteriuria based on the detection of nitrite produced from the reduction of urinary nitrate by bacteria and also for the detection of leucocyte esterase, an enzyme specific for neutrophils. Although each test on its own has limitations, a positive reaction with both tests has a high predictive value for urinary tract infection.

Microscopy

An unspun sample of urine may be examined by placing a drop on a slide using a pipettte, covering with a coverslip and examining by low-power and higher power microscopy. Phase-contrast microscopy is a helpful additional tool. Frequently, a spun-urine sample is examined. Urine is centrifuged, the supernatant is discarded and an aliquot of the residuum placed on a glass slide employing a Pasteur pipette. Quantitation of white cells or red cells expressed per high power field by this method is inaccurate.

Urine microscopy should be carried out in all patients suspected of having renal disease. Care must be taken to obtain a 'clean' sample of mid-stream urine (Practical box 9.2).

The presence of numerous skin squames suggests a contaminated, poorly collected sample that cannot be properly interpreted.

If a clean sample of urine cannot be obtained, suprapubic aspiration is required in suspected urinary tract infections.

Most urines are examined by microscopy in hospital practice by microbiology laboratory technicians who must process large numbers of such urines each day. Best results are obtained in nephrological practice if microscopy is carried out by the physician caring for the patient.

White cells

The presence of 10 or more white blood cells (WBCs) per cubic millimetre in fresh unspun mid-stream urine samples is abnormal and indicates an inflammatory reaction within the urinary tract. Most commonly it is due to urinary tract infection (UTI), but it may also be found in sterile urine in patients during antibiotic treatment of urinary infection or within 14 days of treatment. Sterile pyuria also occurs in patients with stones, tubulo-interstitial nephritis, papillary necrosis, tuberculosis, and interstitial cystitis.

Red cells

The presence of one or more red cells per cubic millimetre in unspun urine samples results in a positive Stix test for blood and is abnormal. It is claimed that red cells of glomerular origin can be identified by their dysmorphic appearance, especially on phase-contrast microscopy, but the method is subject to observer error and has not gained wide acceptance.

Practical

Female

1. The patient's bladder should be full ('desperate to go').
2. The patient removes underpants and stands over the toilet pan.
3. The labia are separated using the left hand.
4. The vulva is cleansed front to back with sterile swabs.
5. The patient voids downward into the toilet and continues until 'half-done'.
6. Without stopping the urine flow, the sterile container is plunged into the stream of urine with the right hand. Only a small volume is required.
7. The patient then completes voiding into the toilet.

Male

1. The patient's bladder should be full.
2. The foreskin, if present, is retracted.
3. The glans penis is cleaned with a sterile swab.
4. The patient voids into the toilet until 'half-done'.
5. Without stopping the urine flow, the sterile container is plunged into the stream of urine.
6. The patient then completes voiding into the toilet.

Practical box 9.2 Collection of mid-stream specimens of urine

Casts (see Fig 9.5)

These cylindrical bodies, which are moulded ('cast') in the shape of the distal tubular lumen, may be hyaline, granular or cellular. Hyaline casts and fine granular casts represent precipitated protein and may be seen in normal urine, particularly after exercise. More coarsely granular casts occur with pathological proteinuria in glomerular and tubular disease. Red-cell casts – even one – always indicate renal disease. If red cells degenerate, a rusty coloured 'haemoglobin' granular cast is seen. White cell casts may be seen in acute pyelonephritis. They may be confused with the tubular cell casts that occur in patients with acute tubular necrosis.

Bacteria

The demonstration of bacteria on Gram staining of the centrifuged deposit of a clean-catch mid-stream urine sample is highly suggestive of urinary infection and can be of value in the *immediate* differential diagnosis of UTI. If accompanied by pyuria it may be accepted as evidence of UTI in the ill and febrile patient and treatment should be initiated.

Urine for quantitative culture (see p. 548) must always be obtained prior to starting antibiotic treatment in order to confirm the diagnosis and to allow definition of bacterial antibiotic sensitivities.

Stix testing for blood or protein is of no value in the diagnosis of UTI, as both are absent from the urine of many patients with bacteriuria.

Quantitative tests of renal function

The use of serum urea, creatinine and GFR as measures of renal function is discussed on p. 521. Quantification of proteinuria, including the investigation of selective proteinuria, is discussed on p. 543. Other quantitative tests of disturbed renal function are described under the relevant disorders.

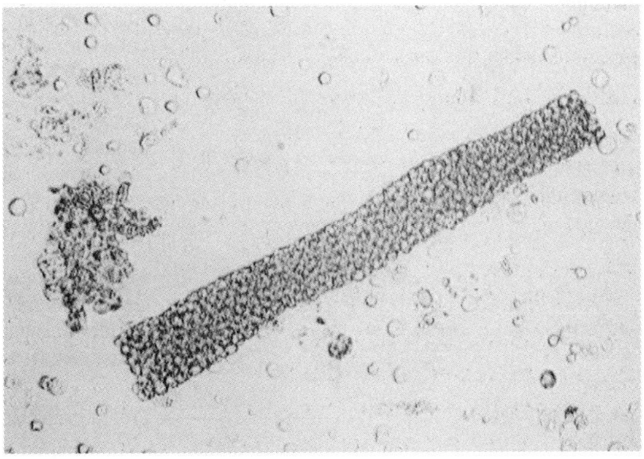

Fig 9.5
Red-cell cast. Note aggregation of red cells as a 'cast' of the tubule

Imaging techniques

Plain X-ray

A plain radiograph of the abdomen is always taken prior to urography. Its main value is to identify renal calcification or radiodense calculi in the kidney pelvis, line of the ureters or bladder (Fig 9.6). Care must be taken in viewing the X-ray in order not to miss calculi obscured by bowel shadows or bone. Renal size and outline are best assessed during excretion urography or by ultrasound.

Excretion urography

This is also known as intravenous urography (IVU) or intravenous pyelography (IVP). If carefully executed and properly interpreted, the urogram is one of the most valuable diagnostic tools for the investigation of renal disease. Carefully timed serial X-rays are taken of the kidneys and the full length of abdomen following a slow intravenous injection of an organic iodine-containing contrast medium. Films taken at the end of the injection show opacification of the parenchyma, allowing definition of size and renal outline. The kidneys are normally smooth in outline. In adults they measure 11–14 cm in length, differing by less than 2 cm. An irregular outline due to cortical scarring is abnormal. Reduction in size indicates chronic disease either primarily of the renal parenchyma or of the renal vasculature.

The application of a compression band to the abdomen, designed partially to obstruct ureteral emptying, helps distension of the upper tracts. Special attention is paid to the size, shape and disposition of the calyces and pelvis for evidence of anatomical abnormality

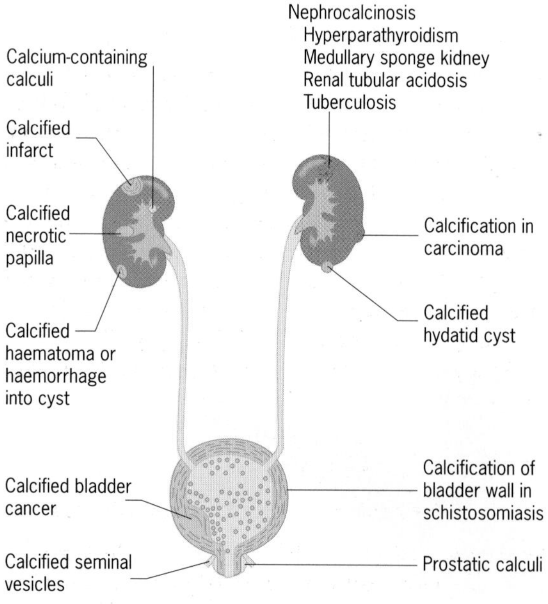

Fig 9.6
Calcification in the renal tract. Calculi can occur at any site

such as calyceal clubbing, abnormal dilatation, cavitation or filling defects. The significance of these are described under the particular diseases.

After 10–20 minutes, the compression bands are removed and full-length films are obtained before and after voiding to study emptying of the upper tract, ureters and bladder.

Reactions to the contrast media include anaphylactic reactions and, rarely, convulsions. Non-ionic contrast media have reduced these complications. Patients with a history of allergy to iodine, those who have had a previous contrast reaction, those with multiple allergies, and asthmatics should receive 60 mg of prednisolone 24 hours before and on the day of the examination. Contrast media may also be nephrotoxic (see p. 541).

Ultrasonography

Ultrasonography of the kidneys, bladder and prostate is extremely useful, but unfortunately it is often used indiscriminately. An ultrasound scan cannot provide the detailed visualization of the calyces and pelvis required to demonstrate pelvicalyceal abnormalities such as reflux nephropathy or papillary necrosis. It does not visualize the greater part of the ureter and gives no functional information on the upper tract. It requires considerable operator skill in performance. In the investigation of haematuria, IVU remains the imaging technique of first choice. If the IVU is normal, ultrasonography should be carried out to exclude the presence of tumours in the renal substance too small to distort the collecting system or be detectable on urography.

The particular value of ultrasound is in defining:

- *renal masses or cystic disease*
- *presence or absence of obstruction* in patients with renal failure when urography is unlikely to provide calyceal detail and the administration of contrast medium may be less safe
- *renal size* in a patient with renal failure
- *bladder emptying* combined with urodynamic studies
- *the prostate* by means of a rectal transducer.

Computed tomography (CT)

CT shows the kidneys, ureters and surrounding tissues in great detail and is useful in the diagnosis of renal tumours. 'Spiral' CT scanning is valuable in producing images in the longitudinal plane, enabling assessment of tumour extension to be made with considerable accuracy. CT is particularly valuable in the diagnosis of retroperitoneal masses and fibrosis and in assessment of renal trauma. It is also valuable in defining the presence and spread of bladder or prostatic tumours and in visualizing uric acid stones which are radiolucent on conventional X-ray. 'Spiral' CT scanning is increasingly being used to image the renal artery (see p. 554).

Magnetic resonance imaging (MRI)

MRI is an imaging system depending upon the manipulation of intrinsic magnetic fields, almost entirely those of protons. A strong uniform magnetic field combined with transient oscillating magnetic fields creates images without the use of ionizing radiation. Its value in nephrology lies in its ability to elucidate the nature of cystic and solid renal masses, and to detect tumour extension into veins. MR angiography of the renal arteries (see p. 554) is increasingly used to screen for renal arterial disease.

Antegrade urography (Fig 9.7)

Antegrade urography involves percutaneous puncture of a renal calyx, with the insertion of a fine catheter and the injection of contrast medium in an antegrade fashion. It is the procedure of choice in patients with upper urinary tract obstruction demonstrated by ultrasound. Not only does it allow definition of the site of obstruction, but also the catheter may be left *in situ* to allow urine drainage in oliguric patients.

Retrograde urography

Following cystoscopy, preferably under screening control, a catheter is either impacted in the ureteral orifice or passed a short distance up the ureter, and contrast medium is injected; this is followed by X-ray filming.

It is mainly used to investigate lesions of the ureter and to define the lower level of ureteral obstruction shown on excretion urography or ultrasound plus antegrade studies. It is invasive, commonly requires a general anaesthetic, and may result in the introduction of infection.

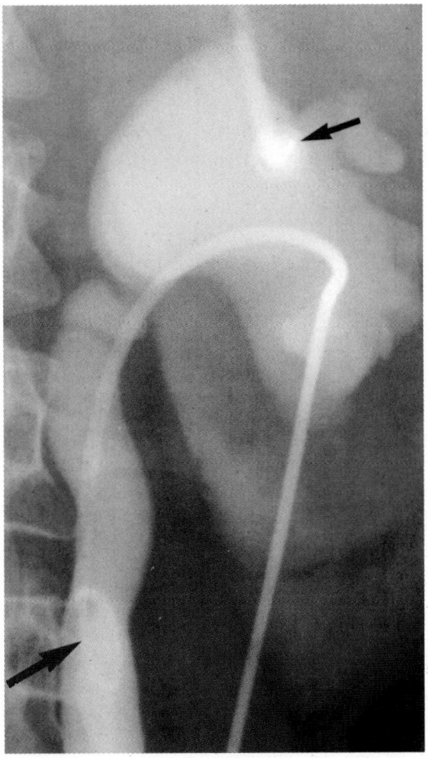

Fig 9.7
Antegrade pyelography via percutaneous catheter (small arrow) **of obstructed system.** Percutaneous drainage catheter (large arrow) has been inserted

Micturating cystourethrography (MCU)

This involves catheterization and the instillation of contrast medium into the bladder. The catheter is then removed and the patient screened and filmed during voiding to demonstrate or exclude vesicoureteric reflux and to study bladder emptying. It is used primarily in children with recurrent infection (see p. 549) and in adults with disturbed bladder function, when it may be combined with urodynamic studies of bladder pressure and urethral flow.

MCU is not an appropriate part of the investigation of the adult female with recurrent bacterial cystitis if the IVU, including an after-micturition bladder film, is normal. This is because vesicoureteric reflux and urinary tract infection cause renal scarring and calyceal distortion in early life, but reflux tends to disappear by the time adulthood is reached. If reflux is detected in an adult with normal renal anatomy, it is thought not to induce kidney damage later. The absence of reflux in an adult does not therefore exclude the diagnosis of chronic atrophic pyelonephritis (reflux nephropathy) and reflux if present in an adult with normal renal anatomy does not require surgical intervention. Therefore whatever the finding on micturating cystourethrography, management is not altered.

The presence or absence of vesicoureteric reflux may also be investigated by scintigraphy (see below).

Arteriography and venography

Conventional or digital subtraction angiography (DSA) are used. The latter allows the use of smaller doses of contrast medium which can be injected via a central venous catheter (venous DSA) or via a fine transfemoral arterial catheter (arterial DSA). Arteriography is used mainly to define extrarenal or intrarenal arterial disease and the presence and extent of renal tumours. Arteriography is still the 'gold standard' method of renal artery imaging but magnetic resonance angiography and spiral CT angiography are being used increasingly (Fig 9.8).

Venography is used occasionally to exclude renal vein thrombosis.

Renal scintigraphy

Renal scintigraphy using a gamma camera is divided into:

- *dynamic studies* in which the function of the kidney is examined serially over a period of time, most often using a radiopharmaceutical excreted by glomerular filtration

- *static studies* involving imaging of tracer that is taken up and *retained* by the renal tubule.

Dynamic scintigraphy

The radiopharmaceutical most often used is technetium-labelled diethylenetriaminepentaacetic acid, [^{99m}Tc]DTPA. It is excreted by glomerular filtration. ^{123}I-labelled *ortho*-iodohippuric acid (Hippuran) is both filtered and secreted by the tubules and is also used but is more expensive and not generally available. Following venous injection of a bolus of tracer, emissions from the kidney can be recorded and stored on computer for analysis of time–activity curves. Analogue images can also be generated at intervals as the study proceeds. This information allows examination of blood perfusion of the kidney, uptake of tracer as a result of glomerular filtration, transit of tracer through the kidney, and the outflow of tracer-containing urine from the collecting system.

Renal blood flow

Dynamic studies can be used to investigate patients in whom renal artery stenosis is suspected as a cause for hypertension and in patients with severe oliguria (post-traumatic, post-aortic surgery, or after a kidney transplant) to establish whether, and to what extent, there is renal perfusion. In patients with unilateral renal artery stenosis there is, typically, a slowed and reduced uptake of tracer with delay in reaching a peak. Studies carried out before and after administration of an ACE inhibitor may demonstrate a fall in uptake that is suggestive of functional arterial stenosis. Both false-positive and false-negative results occur with this test and renal arteriography remains the 'gold standard' in the diagnosis of main renal artery stenosis. In patients with total renal artery occlusion, no kidney uptake of tracers is observed.

Investigation of obstruction

Renography can demonstrate the presence and severity of obstruction. The results obtained from overall uptake and outflow curves must be treated with caution because of the large 'dead space' commonly contributed by dilated calyces and pelves. Dynamic scintigraphy combined with the injection of frusemide can commonly distinguish functional obstruction from a dilated non-obstructed system (Fig 9.9).

Bladder emptying

At the end of dynamic studies, bladder emptying may be investigated and any postmicturition residual measured. Vesicoureteric reflux may be observed, although the sensitivity for detection of this is low. Increased sensitivity can be obtained by direct isotope cystography when a dilute isotope solution is instilled into the bladder by catheter.

Glomerular filtration rate

This is discussed on p. 521.

Static scintigraphy

This is usually performed using [^{99m}Tc]DMSA (dimercaptosuccinic acid), which is taken up by tubular cells. Uptake is proportional to renal function.

Relative renal function

Function is normally evenly divided between the kidneys with a range of 45–55%. Static studies are particularly useful in unilateral renal disease, where the relative uptake of the two kidneys can be calculated.

Kidney visualization

Normal kidneys show a uniform uptake with a smooth renal outline. Scars can be identified as photon-deficient 'bites'. Static scintigraphy is of considerable value in identifying ectopic kidneys or 'pseudotumours' of the kidneys (i.e. normally functioning renal tissue abnormally placed within the kidney).

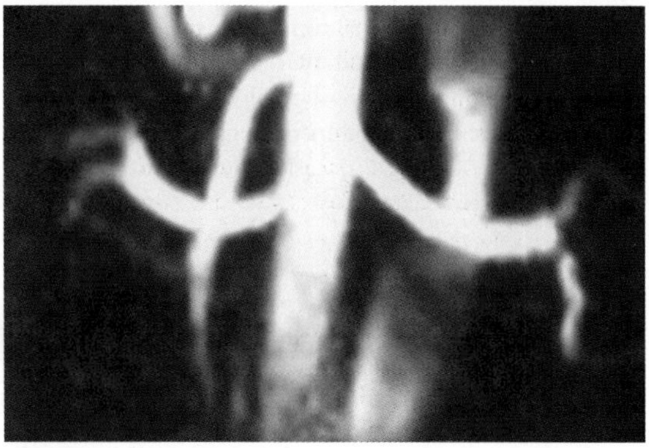

Fig 9.8
Magnetic resonance angiogram of normal renal arteries

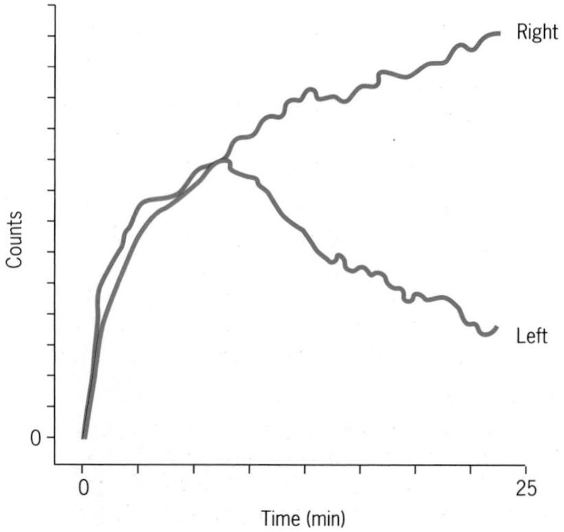

Fig 9.9
Dynamic DTPA scintigram. Note the progressive rise of the right kidney curve to a plateau (in contrast to the normal left kidney curve) owing to urinary tract obstruction on the right side

Localization of infection

The use of citrate labelled with gallium-67 or isotopically labelled leucocytes that are taken up by inflammatory tissue may be of value in defining localized infection, such as renal abscesses or infection within a renal cyst.

Transcutaneous renal biopsy (Practical box 9.3)

Indications for and contraindications to transcutaneous renal biopsy are shown in Table 9.4.

The biopsies are carried out under ultrasound control using a spring-loaded biopsy needle. Native renal biopsy material must be examined by conventional histochemical staining, by electron microscopy, and by immunoperoxidase or immunofluorescence staining. Light microscopy will suffice for some renal transplant biopsies.

The complications of transcutaneous renal biopsy are shown in Table 9.5.

FURTHER READING

Agre P *et al.* (1993) Aquaporin CHIP: the archetypal molecular water channel. *American Journal of Physiology* **265**: F463–476.

Birnbaumer *et al.* (1992) Molecular cloning of the receptor for human antidiuretic hormone. *Nature* **357**: 333–335.

Chantler C, Barrett TM (1972) Estimation of the glomerular filtration rate from the plasma clearance of 51-chromium EDTA. *Archives of Disease in Childhood* **47**: 613–617.

Wrong O, Davies HEF (1959) The excretion of acid in renal disease. *Quarterly Journal of Medicine* **28**: 259–313

Practical

Before biopsy
1. A coagulation screen is performed. It must be normal.
2. The serum is grouped and saved for crossmatching.
3. The patient is given a full explanation of what is involved.

During biopsy
1. The patient lies prone with a hard pillow under the abdomen.
2. The kidney is localized by ultrasound.
3. Local anaesthetic is injected along the biopsy track.
4. The patient holds a breath when the biopsy is performed.

After biopsy
1. A pressure dressing is applied to the biopsy site and the patient rests in bed for 24 hours.
2. The fluid intake is maximized to prevent clot colic.
3. The pulse and blood pressure are checked regularly.
4. The patient is advised to avoid heavy lifting or gardening for two weeks.

Practical box 9.3 Transcutaneous renal biopsy

Table 9.4
Renal biopsy

Indications
Nephrotic syndrome (with some exceptions)
Unexplained renal failure with normal-sized kidneys
Failure to recover from assumed reversible acute renal failure
Diagnosis of systemic disease with renal involvement, such as sarcoidosis, amyloidosis (occasional indication only)
Asymptomatic proteinuria or haematuria (very occasional indication – justified only if knowledge of prognosis is essential)

Contraindications
Uncooperative patient
Single kidney (with the exception of transplant kidney, when biopsy is acceptable)
Small kidneys (technically difficult, histology hard to interpret, prognosis cannot be altered)
Haemorrhagic disorders (unless correctable temporarily or permanently, e.g. by factor VIII administration in haemophilia)
Gross obesity or oedema (technical difficulties)
Uncontrolled hypertension

Table 9.5
Complications of transcutaneous renal biopsy

Macroscopic haematuria – about 20%
Pain in the flank, sometimes referred to shoulder tip
Perirenal haematoma
Arteriovenous aneurysm formation – about 20%, almost always of no clinical significance
Profuse haematuria demanding blood transfusion – 1–3%
Profuse haematuria demanding occlusion of bleeding vessel at angiography or nephrectomy – approximately 1 in 400
Introduction of infection
The mortality rate is about 0.1%

Glomerular diseases

Glomerulonephritides

Glomerulonephritis is a general term for a group of disorders in which:

- there is immunologically mediated injury to glomeruli
- the kidneys are involved symmetrically
- secondary mechanisms of glomerular injury come into play following an initial immune insult (see below)
- the renal lesion may be part of a generalized disease (e.g. systemic lupus erythematosus, SLE).

PATHOGENESIS

Two chief pathogenetic mechanisms are recognized:

- deposition or *in situ* formation of immune complexes (most human glomerulonephritides)

- deposition of antiglomerular basement membrane antibody (fewer than 5% of glomerulonephritides).

Both of these pathogenetic mechanisms activate secondary mechanisms that produce glomerular damage.

Immune complex nephritis

Circulating antigen–antibody complexes (see p. 183) are deposited in the kidney or complexes are formed locally when circulating free antigen has become trapped in the glomerulus. The nature of the antigen involved in the complex formation is important in many instances.
The antigen may be exogenous or endogenous:

- *exogenous* (e.g. bacterial) – for example, a nephritogenic Lancefield group A β-haemolytic *Streptococcus* can cause glomerulonephritis in previously healthy individuals
- *endogenous* – for example, patients with SLE may form antibodies to host DNA, leading to a glomerulonephritis.

Harmful immune complexes can also occur when there is impaired host ability to produce appropriate antibody. Certain strains of black mice regularly develop glomerulonephritis as a result of an impaired ability to produce antibody of appropriate quality or quantity, and it is likely that there are human counterparts of this phenomenon. There is an association between HLA markers and certain nephritides. For example, in Europe there is an increased prevalence of the HLA-A1 B8 DR3 haplotype in patients with membranous glomerulonephritis.

Impaired ability on the part of the host to clear immune complexes from the circulation and deficiencies in the complement system are each associated with an increased incidence of glomerulonephritis.

Antiglomerular basement membrane (anti-GBM) antibody

The major component of the glomerular basement membrane is type 4 collagen (COLIV). This collagen molecule is a heterotrimer containing paired polypeptide α chains.

Anti-GBM antibodies are autoantibodies that bind mainly to the non-collagenous domain of the α-3 chain type IV collagen (COLIVα3). This antigenic target is also present in alveolar basement membrane which accounts for the association of both lung haemorrhage and glomerulonephritis (Goodpasture's syndrome, p. 536). Anti-GBM antibodies are of IgG type.

Secondary mechanisms of glomerular injury

Several events can be triggered by the above immunological insults:

- complement activation
- fibrin deposition
- platelet aggregation
- inflammation with neutrophil-dependent mechanisms
- activation of kinin systems.

Immune complex or anti-GBM antibody deposition trigger these mechanisms to varying degrees, resulting in an increase in capillary permeability and glomerular damage.

In experimentally induced glomerulonephritis in animals, prior anticoagulation, prevention of complement activation, and depletion of polymorphonuclear leucocytes have all been shown to reduce the severity of the induced glomerular injury. However, in humans presenting with most forms of glomerulonephritis these measures do not help.

T-cell dysfunction may play a part in the production of lesions when immune complexes are not seen.

CAUSES

In the majority of patients with immune complex-mediated glomerulonephritis, the cause is unknown; i.e. the nature of the antigen involved is not determined. Antigen derived from viruses, bacteria, parasites, drugs and from the host may be involved (Table 9.6). The reasons for the development of anti-GBM antibody are not known; viral or solvent damage to alveolar capillary basement membrane, rendering it antigenic, has been suggested as a possible cause.

PATHOLOGY

Macroscopic appearances

In acute glomerulonephritis, the kidneys are normal in size or enlarged and oedematous, and the surface of the kidney may show punctate haemorrhages.

In longstanding progressive chronic glomerulonephritis the kidneys may be normal in size or small with finely granular cortical scarring.

Table 9.6
Some causes of immune complex-mediated glomerulonephritis

Viruses	**Parasites**
Mumps	*Plasmodium malariae*
Measles	*Schistosoma*
Hepatitis B and C	Filiariasis
Epstein–Barr	
Coxsackie	**Host antigens**
Varicella	DNA (systemic lupus erythematosus)
HIV	Cryoglobulin
	Malignant tumours
Bacteria	
Lancefield group A β-haemolytic streptococci	**Drugs**
Streptococcus viridans (infective endocarditis)	Penicillamine
Staphylococci	
Treponema pallidum	
Gonococci	
Salmonella	

Microscopic appearances

Different immunological insults may induce similar or identical histological changes. For example, the immune complex-mediated glomerulonephritis in mumps is not distinguishable from that following β-haemolytic streptococcal infection. Conversely, different histological responses may occur in the same disease process in different individuals (e.g. in SLE, see below).

The histological response to immune complex deposition probably depends on the size of the complexes, their rate of deposition, and the efficiency of host clearance mechanisms.

Renal tissue, obtained at transcutaneous renal biopsy, is examined by the following processes:

- *light microscopy* – to assess the extent and histological type of disease
- *electron microscopy* – to define the type of disease and to correlate with immunofluorescence; e.g. to see the exact sites of deposits
- *immunofluorescence* – to assess the type of immunological injury (immunoperoxidase methods may also be applied).

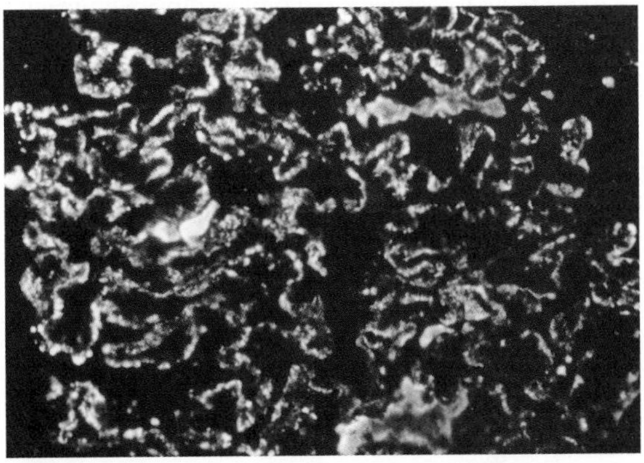

Fig 9.10
Immunofluorescence, showing immune complex deposition in a diffuse granular pattern

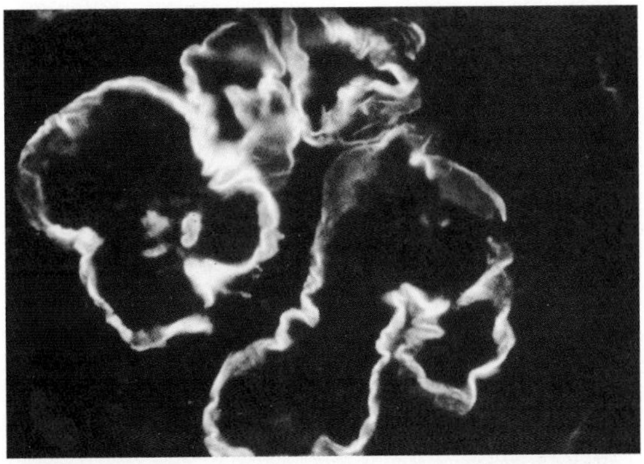

Fig 9.11
Immunofluorescence, showing antiglomerular basement membrane antibody (anti-GBM) deposition in a linear pattern typical of Goodpasture's syndrome

All three methods of examination are necessary for proper histopathological assessment.

Immune complex deposition results in a diffuse granular pattern of staining, with IgG, IgM, IgA, components of the complement system and, in addition, fibrin and fibrinogen all present (Fig 9 10).

The presence of anti-GBM antibody produces a smooth linear pattern of staining for IgG on immunofluorescence (Fig 9.11).

TYPES

There is not a complete correlation between the histopathological types of glomerulonephritides and the clinical features of disease. Table 9.7 shows the most common associations.

Proliferative glomerulonephritis

Proliferative changes occur in many immune complex-mediated nephritides and also in anti-GBM nephritis. It has the following subtypes.

Diffuse proliferative glomerulonephiritis

All the glomeruli are similarly affected. Fig 9.12 shows the typical histological changes, and a normal glomerulus is shown for comparison in Fig 9.13. Immunofluorescence shows granular deposits of immunoglobulin and C3. This type of glomerulonephritis, presenting as an acute nephritis, is commonly seen after a streptococcal infection (see below). Immune complexes are seen as electron-dense deposits on electron microscopy (Fig 9.14).

Focal segmental glomerulonephritis

Only some of the glomeruli here show proliferative changes whilst others are normal; hence the term 'focal'. The affected glomeruli show segmental involvement of the tufts; i.e. changes are present in one or more parts of the glomerulus.

Table 9.7 Correlation between the histological type of glomerulonephritis and the clinical picture

Histological type	Most common clinical presentation
Proliferative glomerulonephritis	
Diffuse	Acute nephritic syndrome
Focal segmental	Haematuria, proteinuria
With crescent formation (rapidly progressive glomerulonephritis)	Progressive renal failure
Mesangiocapillary (membranoproliferative)	Haematuria, proteinuria, acute nephritic or nephrotic syndrome
Membranous glomerulonephritis	Nephrotic syndrome in adults
Minimal-change nephropathy	Nephrotic syndrome, especially in children
IgA nephropathy	Asymptomatic haematuria
Focal glomerulosclerosis	Proteinuria or nephrotic syndrome

This condition may occur as a primary renal disease, but it is also seen in SLE, subacute infective endocarditis, with infected atrioventricular shunts (shunt nephritis), and in disorders with IgA deposits (e.g. Henoch–Schönlein purpura and IgA nephropathy). A severe focal necrotizing form is seen in microscopic polyarteritis and Wegener's granulomatosis. Special subtypes (IgA nephropathy and focal glomerulosclerosis) are discussed below.

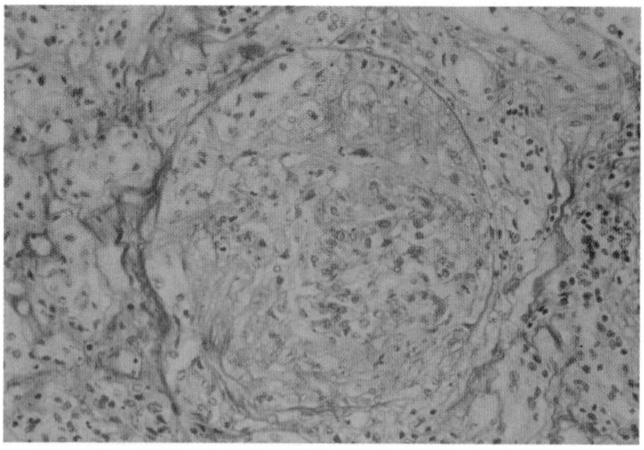

Fig 9.12
A glomerulus showing proliferative glomerulonephritis. The glomerulus is swollen, packed with cells, and bulges into the opening of the proximal tubule. There is proliferation of the endothelial and mesangial cells, and polymorphonuclear leucocytes are present

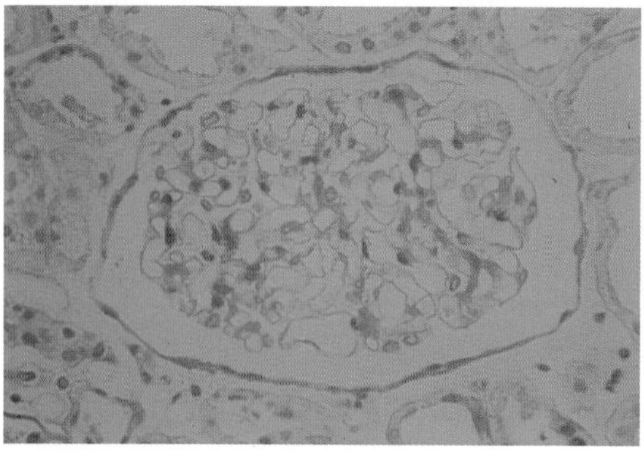

Fig 9.13
A normal glomerulus

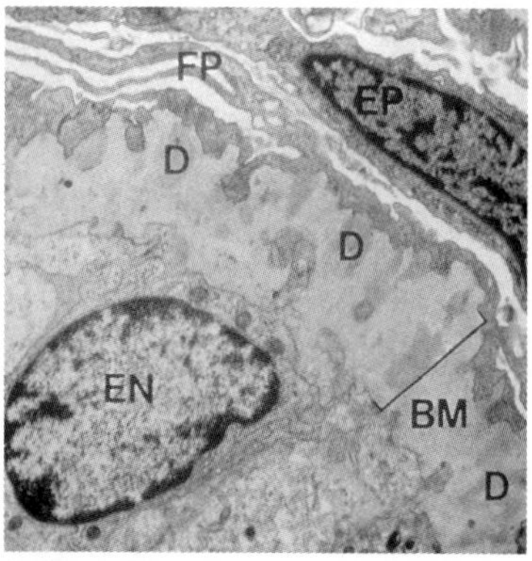

Fig 9.14
Electron micrograph, showing immune complex-mediated glomerulonephritis. BM, basement membrane; D, electron-dense deposits (antigen–antibody complexes); EN, endothelial cell; EP, epithelial podocyte; FP, foot process

Proliferative glomerulonephritis with crescent formation (rapidly progressive glomerulonephritis; RPGN) or crescentic glomerulonephritis

The term 'crescent' is applied to an aggregate of macrophages and epithelial cells in Bowman's space (Fig 9.15). Crescents are associated with severe damage to the glomerular tuft and are seen in occasional glomeruli in several types of glomerulonephritis. However, if most glomeruli show crescents the glomerulonephritis is usually placed in this subtype, as clinical progression to renal failure is rapid.

This condition is seen in both immune complex and anti-GBM antibody-mediated nephritis. It particularly occurs in microscopic polyarteritis, Wegener's granulomatosis and Goodpasture's syndrome.

Mesangiocapillary (membranoproliferative) glomerulonephritis (MCGN)

In *type 1* there is mesangial cell proliferation, with mainly subendothelial immune complex deposition and apparent splitting of the capillary basement membrane, giving a 'tram-line' effect. It may be idiopathic or may occur with shunt nephritis. It can be associated with persistently reduced plasma levels of C3 and normal levels of C4. In some cases hepatitis B and C infection is present and appears to be an aetiological factor.

In *type 2* there is mesangial cell proliferation with electron-dense, linear intramembranous deposits that usually stain for C3 only. This type may be idiopathic or may occur after measles. Partial lipodystrophy (loss of subcutaneous fat in various parts of the body) may be seen. MCGN affects young adults. Patients present with haematuria, proteinuria, the nephrotic syndrome or renal failure. Most patients eventually go on to develop renal failure over several years.

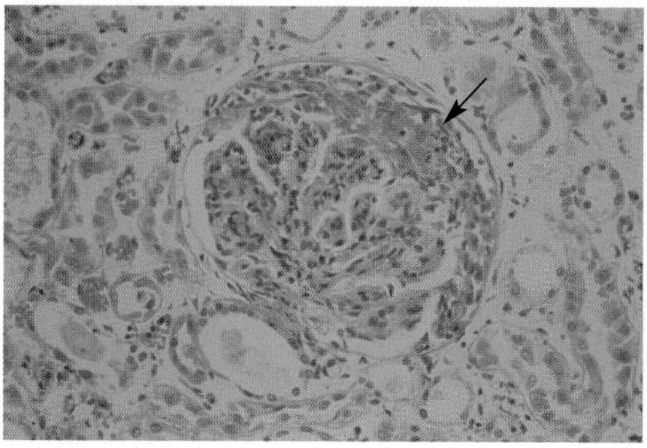

Fig 9.15
Crescentic glomerulonephritis. Note the 'epithelial' crescent at the periphery of the glomerulus (arrow)

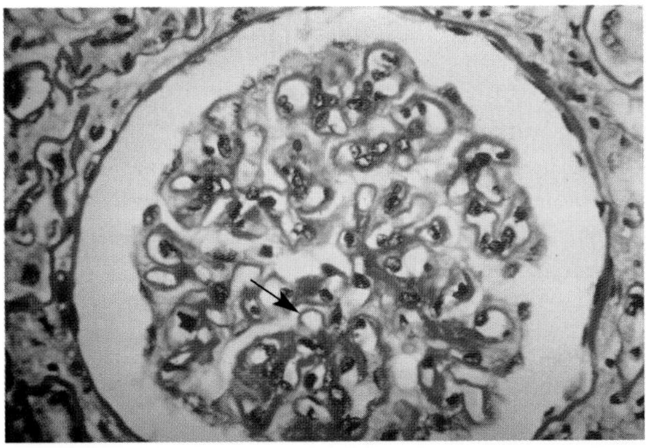

Fig 9.16
Membranous glomerulonephritis showing thickened basement membrane (arrow)

Membranous glomerulonephritis

Thickening of the capillary basement membrane due to immune complex deposition is the main feature of this disease (Fig 9.16). In the majority of patients the antigenic component of the complex is unknown. Associations include SLE (where the antigen is host DNA), malignancy of the bowel and bronchus (tumour-derived antigen), penicillamine therapy, and hepatitis B infection. *Plasmodium malariae* is a common cause in the tropics. A strong association with HLA-DR3 has been found.

This condition occurs mainly in adults, predominantly in males. Patients present with proteinuria or frank nephrotic syndrome. Approximately one-third of patients develop end-stage renal failure within 10–20 years of diagnosis. Younger patients, females and those with asymptomatic proteinuria of modest degree at the time of presentation do best. Spontaneous remission occurs in about one-third of patients, particularly females.

Uncertainty exists as to the place of corticosteroid and immunosuppressive treatment with, for example, chlorambucil, cyclophosphamide or azathioprine in the treatment of membranous glomerulonephritis. Interpretation of controlled trial data in unselected patients with the condition has proved difficult owing to the fact that a significant proportion of patients are destined to do well without specific treatment. There is an increasingly strong consensus (supported by meta-analysis of trial data) that patients with a poor prognosis (those with heavy proteinuria and progressive renal impairment) do benefit from such treatment.

Minimal-change glomerular lesion (minimal-change nephropathy)

This is not a true glomerulonephritis (the suffix 'itis' suggests the presence of inflammation and inflammatory change in glomeruli is not seen in this condition). It is included here for convenience. In this condition the glomeruli appear normal on light microscopy. The only abnormality seen on electron microscopy is fusion of the foot processes of epithelial cells (podocytes). This is a nonspecific finding and is seen in many conditions associated with proteinuria.

Neither immune complexes nor anti-GBM antibody can be demonstrated by immunofluorescence. However, the immunological pathogenesis of this condition is suggested by three factors:

- its response to steroids and immunosuppressive drugs
- its occurrence in Hodgkin's disease, with remission following successful treatment
- patients with the condition and family members having a higher incidence of asthma and eczema; remission following desensitization or antigen avoidance has been described.

A suggested explanation for the proteinuria is the production by T-lymphocytes of a factor that increases glomerular permeability to protein.

Minimal-change nephropathy is most common in children, particularly males, accounting for the large majority of cases of nephrotic syndrome in childhood. The condition accounts for 20–25% of cases of adult nephrotic syndrome. It is often regarded as a condition which does not lead to chronic renal failure (but see focal sclerosis below).

Specific treatment is with corticosteroids, cyclophosphamide and cyclosporin (see p. 586).

IgA nephropathy

This is the most common cause of asymptomatic microscopic haematuria in the developed world. The disease consists of focal proliferative glomerulonephritis and mesangial deposits of IgA. In some cases IgG, IgM or C3 and properdin may also be seen in the glomerular mesangium.

Glomerulonephritis in Henoch–Schönlein purpura has a similar pathological picture and is sometimes regarded as the same condition (see below).

IgA nephropathy tends to occur in children and young males. They present with asymptomatic microscopic haematuria or recurrent macroscopic haematuria, which is sometimes related to upper respiratory infection. Proteinuria occurs and 5% can be nephrotic. The prognosis is usually good especially in those with normal blood pressure, normal renal function and absence of proteinuria at presentation. Surprisingly, recurrent macroscopic haematuria is a good prognostic sign. Meta-analysis has not confirmed the initial evidence suggesting a beneficial effect of fish oil. Up to 20% of patients eventually develop renal failure.

Henoch–Schönlein syndrome

This clinical syndrome comprises a characteristic skin rash, abdominal colic, joint pain and glomerulonephritis. The rash is of purpuric type and the synonym Henoch–Schönlein purpura is often used. It occurs at all ages and in both sexes, but is mainly a disease of early childhood. Males are twice as often affected as females. A recent history of infection, often respiratory, is common. The disease is rare in adults. Serum concentrations of IgA are increased in about half the patients during the first three months of the disease and IgA-containing immune complexes have been detected in serum in a high proportion of cases. The renal lesion is a focal segmental proliferative glomerulonephritis, sometimes with mesangial hypercellularity. Epithelial crescents may be present. Immunoglobulin deposition, mainly of IgA, is seen in the glomerular mesangium and to a lesser extent in the capillary walls on immunofluorescence. IgG, IgM and components of the complement system may also be detectable. Electron-dense deposits, presumably immune complexes, are seen in the mesangium and subendothelial position on electron microscopy. No treatment is of proven benefit.

Goodpasture's syndrome (see also p. 813)

This rare condition is mediated by anti-GBM antibody (p. 532). It presents with recurrent haemoptysis and a severe progressive proliferative, often crescentic, glomerulonephritis. There is a strong association with HLA-DR2. Lung haemorrhage, which occurs more commonly in cigarette smokers, responds to repeated plasma exchange (which removes the anti-GBM antibody) combined with immunosuppressive therapy with cytotoxic drugs and corticosteroids. The effect of this treatment upon the glomerulonephritis is less clear-cut; when oliguria occurs or serum creatinine rises above 0.6–0.7 mmol L^{-1}, renal failure is almost always irreversible.

CLINICAL FEATURES

Glomerulonephritis presents in one of four ways:

- asymptomatic proteinuria and/or microscopic haematuria
- acute nephritic syndrome (see below)
- nephrotic syndrome (p. 542)
- chronic renal failure (p. 573).

Asymptomatic proteinuria and/or microscopic haematuria is discovered incidentally, for example at a routine medical examination. Some causes of haematuria are shown in Fig 9.4. Overt haematuria may occur after exercise.

INVESTIGATIONS

Since false-positives are often obtained using Stix methods, the presence of significant proteinuria must be demonstrated by measuring the 24-hour urinary output of protein on two consecutive occasions (see p. 526).

Urine microscopy is performed to look for haematuria. A positive Stix test for blood may result from haematuria or haemoglobinuria. These can be differentiated on microscopy since red cells are seen only in patients with haematuria. Red cell morphology may provide a guide to diagnosis (see p. 527).

Further investigations will include:

- **urine microscopy** for red-cell casts
- **assessment of renal function** by estimation of serum urea, creatinine and endogenous creatinine clearance
- **renal imaging**, usually by excretion urography.

Acute nephritic syndrome

This comprises:

- haematuria (macroscopic or microscopic) – red cell casts are typically seen on urine microscopy
- proteinuria
- hypertension
- oedema (periorbital, leg or sacral)
- oliguria
- uraemia.

Hypertension and oedema arise from salt and water retention. Causes are shown in Table 9.7.

CLINICAL FEATURES

In classical post-streptococcal glomerulonephritis the patient, usually a child, will have suffered a streptococcal infection 1–3 weeks before the onset of the acute nephritic syndrome. Streptococcal tonsillitis or pharyngitis, otitis media or cellulitis may be responsible.

The infecting organism is a Lancefield group A β-haemolytic *Streptococcus* of a nephritogenic type. The latent interval between the infection and development of symptoms and signs of renal involvement reflects the time taken for immune complex formation and deposition and glomerular injury to occur.

INVESTIGATIONS

A list of investigations is given in Table 9.8.

If the clinical diagnosis of a nephritic illness is clear-cut (e.g. in post-streptococcal glomerulonephritis), renal imaging and renal biopsy are usually unnecessary. A biopsy is required if the diagnosis is uncertain, if the clinical features are unusual, or if renal failure is rapidly progressive, suggesting the presence of crescentic glomerulonephritis (RPGN).

MANAGEMENT

In the majority of patients with glomerulonephritis, neither corticosteroid nor immunosuppressive therapy is of benefit. The same applies to treatment with agents that alter coagulation and platelet function. Important exceptions to this general rule include glomerulonephritis complicating SLE, systemic vasculitides such as microscopic polyarteritis and Wegener's granulomatosis, Goodpasture's syndrome and some forms of rapidly progressive crescentic glomerulonephritis (see later), and probably idiopathic membranous nephropathy with progressive renal impairment.

As spontaneous remissions usually occur in acute glomerulonephritis, the aim of management is to prevent patients dying from pulmonary oedema, uraemia or hypertensive encephalopathy while awaiting improvement in renal function.

Hospital admission is advisable for all children with oliguria and marked hypertension; levels of blood pressure that are of no risk to adults may be associated with hypertensive fits in the young.

Table 9.8
Investigation of acute nephritic syndrome

Investigations	Positive findings
Urine microscopy	Red cells, red-cell casts
Serum urea	May be elevated
Serum creatinine	May be elevated
Culture (throat swab, discharge from ear, swab from inflamed skin)	Nephritogenic organism – not always
Antistreptolysin-O titre	Elevated in poststreptococcal nephritis
C3 and C4 levels	May be reduced
Antinuclear antibody	Present in significant titre in systemic lupus erythematosus
ANCA	Positive in vasculitis
Anti-GBM	Positive in Goodpasture's syndrome
Cryoglobulins	Increased in cryoglobinaemia
Creatinine clearance	Reduced
Urinary protein output	Increased
Chest X-ray	Cardiomegaly, pulmonary oedema (not always)
Renal imaging	Usually normal
Renal biopsy	Glomerulonephritis

Otherwise, hospital admission is not mandatory, provided the general practitioner is able to visit daily to examine the patient and check blood pressure. Blood for measurement of urea or serum creatinine concentrations should be taken every few days.

Management in hospital

Most patients require:

- daily recording of fluid intake and output
- daily weighing (as a check on change in body fluid status)
- regular measurement of blood pressure.

Strict bedrest is unnecessary unless the patient feels ill, is severely hypertensive or has pulmonary oedema.

Dietary protein restriction is required only if severe uraemia occurs, but salt restriction is always necessary. In oliguric patients, fluid restriction is necessary to maintain body weight at a level at which severe hypertension, pulmonary congestion and gross oedema are prevented.

Mild-to-moderate hypertension and oedema may respond to salt restriction and diuretic therapy (e.g. frusemide given orally or parenterally). Other hypotensive agents may be required. β-Adrenergic receptor blocking therapy should be used with caution for hypertension as it may precipitate pulmonary oedema in those on the brink of heart failure.

The prognosis in immune complex-mediated glomerulonephritis is improved if the antigen responsible can be eradicated. In patients with post-streptococcal glomerulonephritis, a course of penicillin should be given.

Management of life-threatening complications

Hypertensive encephalopathy

In this condition the priorities are to maintain the airway and to reduce the blood pressure using a parenteral agent such as hydralazine 5–20 mg by slow intravenous infusion over 20 minutes. Fits should be controlled with parenteral diazepam (10 mg i.v.), but this may induce respiratory depression so that facilities for resuscitation must be available.

Pulmonary oedema

This should be treated in the usual way (see p. 684). Because of the renal failure, high doses of potent diuretics such as frusemide given parenterally may be required. If this fails to produce a diuresis, salt and water may be removed osmotically by peritoneal dialysis, by haemofiltration, by ultrafiltration during haemodialysis (see p. 582).

Severe uraemia

Peritoneal dialysis, haemodialysis or haemofiltration will be required pending recovery of the renal function.

Outbreak of post-streptococcal glomerulonephritis in a closed community

Prophylactic penicillin (phenoxymethylpenicillin 500 mg daily) should be given to all individuals at risk, provided they are not allergic to penicillin. If one member of a family living in overcrowded conditions develops the disorder, other members should be treated prophylactically. Evidence in support of long-term penicillin prophylaxis after the development of glomerulonephritis is lacking.

PROGNOSIS

Post-streptococcal glomerulonephritis. The prognosis in children is excellent. A small number of adults develop hypertension and/or renal impairment later in life. Therefore in older patients, an annual blood pressure check, and less frequently an estimation of serum creatinine, is a reasonable precaution, even after apparent complete recovery.

Acute glomerulonephritis of unknown cause. The prognosis is less good and the need for follow-up is correspondingly greater.

Systemic vasculitides and progressive crescentic glomerulonephritis occurring in isolation. The prognosis is often poor and severe renal failure with oliguria and hypertension often occurs within a few weeks or months of the onset of the illness. This group of conditions constitute a nephrological emergency since specific treatment is beneficial (see p. 538).

Other glomerular disorders

Focal segmental glomerulosclerosis (FSGS)

This is a disease of unknown aetiology. It is particularly prone to recur in kidneys transplanted into affected individuals, sometimes within days of transplantation. A circulating factor may be involved. It presents as proteinuria or nephrotic syndrome and is usually resistant to steroid therapy. All age groups are affected.

On light microscopy, segmental glomerulosclerosis is seen, which later progresses to global sclerosis. The deep glomeruli at the corticomedullary junction are affected first. These may be missed on transcutaneous biopsy, leading to a mistaken diagnosis of a minimal-change glomerular lesion. In addition, some believe that a pathogenetic link exists between minimal-change nephropathy and focal glomerulosclerosis, and that a proportion of cases classified as having the former condition develop progressive renal impairment. Immunofluorescence may show deposits of C3 and IgM in affected portions of the glomerulus, but nonspecific fixation to damaged tissue, rather than immune complex deposition, may well be the explanation for this.

About 50% of patients progress to end-stage renal failure within 10 years of diagnosis.

AIDS-associated nephropathy

A number of renal lesions have been described in association with HIV infection. These include glomerulonephritis of various histological types and haemolytic uraemic syndrome. The most common histological abnormality is a focal glomerulosclerosis. When renal failure supervenes the prognosis is very poor.

Familial glomerular diseases

Alport's syndrome

Alport's syndrome is a rare condition characterized by hereditary nephritis with haematuria, progressive renal failure and high-frequency nerve deafness. It is principally expressed in males and both X-linked (mutation in COLIVα5 gene) and dominant modes of inheritance have been described. Some 15% of cases may have ocular abnormalities such as bilateral anterior lenticonus and macular and perimacular retinal flecks. In families with leiomyomas there is an additional mutation in the COLIVα6 gene. The disease is progressive and accounts for some 5% of cases of end-stage renal failure in childhood or adolescence. Anti-GBM antibody does not adhere normally to the glomerular basement membrane of affected individuals.

Congenital nephrotic syndrome

This syndrome is rare.

Thin glomerular basement membrane disease

The condition is inherited as an autosomal dominant and typically presents with microscopic haematuria. The diagnosis is made by renal biopsy when thinning and splitting of the glomerular capillary basement membrane is seen on electron microscopy. The prognosis for renal function is good. No treatment is of known benefit.

FURTHER READING

Feehally J (1997) IgA nephropathy: a disorder of IgA production? *Quarterly Journal of Medicine* **90**: 387–390.

Gaskin G (1997) Management of rapidly progressive glomerulonephritis. *Journal of the Royal College of Physicians* **31**: 15–18.

Mason PD (1997) The treatment of minimal change nephropathy and focal segmental glomerulosclerosis. *Journal of the Royal College of Physicians* **31**: 137–141.

The kidney in systemic disease

Glomerulonephritis as a part of systemic vasculitis

Systemic lupus erythematosus

(see also p. 487)

The disease is much more common in females than in males and in black rather than white individuals. All varieties of histological abnormality are seen, ranging from a minimal-change lesion to crescentic glomerulonephritis. Serial renal biopsies show that in approximately 25% of patients, histological appearances alter from one histological classification to another during the interbiopsy interval. The prognosis is better in patients with the minimal-change and membranous lesions than in those with proliferative glomerulonephritis.

Pregnancy is associated with significant risk to the lupus patient, not only owing to hypertension and premature delivery, but also to more rapid progression of the glomerular lesion following delivery.

Whilst corticosteroid therapy improves the extrarenal manifestations of SLE, evidence is lacking that this treatment alters the renal prognosis. Both azathioprine and cyclophosphamide improve renal function, but long-term studies suggest that cyclophosphamide is better. There is no consensus as to whether intravenous 'pulse' cyclophosphamide treatment may be safer and more efficacious than continuous oral therapy.

The indications for treatment vary. Those whose urine sediment contains many red cells and red-cell casts and those in whom renal function is impaired or is observed to deteriorate are strong candidates for treatment. A histological diagnosis should be obtained before commencing such potentially hazardous treatment.

Systemic vasculitides (see also p. 493)

In this group of disorders there is considerable overlap between individual varieties. The common feature is an immunologically mediated inflammation of vessels of varying size. Arthralgia or arthritis and a characteristic vasculitic rash (Fig 9.17) may be present.

A major advance in understanding has followed the discovery of autoantibodies directed against constituents of the cytoplasm of normal human granulocytes and monocytes in patients with systemic vasculitis. Antineutrophil cytoplasmic antibodies (ANCA) are now established as a marker for vasculitides involving the kidney with or without signs of systemic disease. Two forms of ANCA can be demonstrated, proteinase-3 PR3-ANCA and myeloperoxidase MPO-ANCA. Binding of PR3-ANCA to neutrophils in indirect immuno-fluorescence assays produces a granular cytoplasmic stain – hence the use of the old term 'cytoplasmic c-ANCA'. MPO-ANCA produces a perinculear stain – hence the old term 'perinuclear p-ANCA'. If ELISA and indirect immuno-fluorescence techniques are combined, diagnostic specificity is 99%.

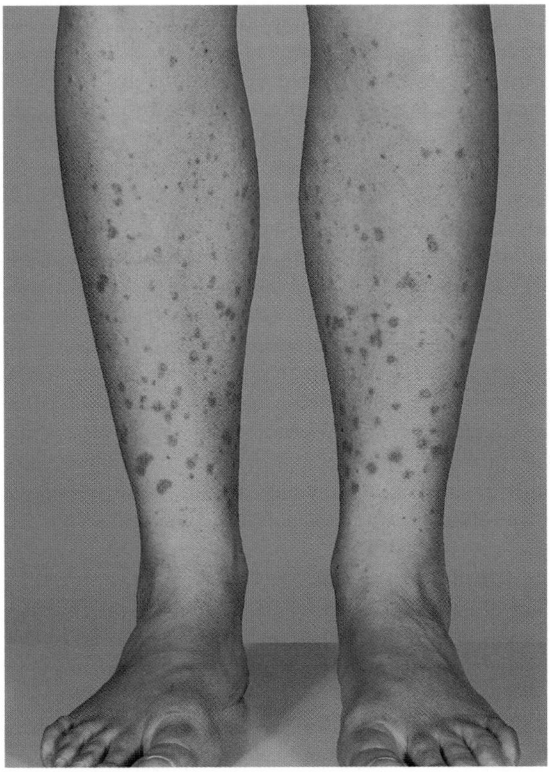

Fig 9.17
Vasculitic rash

PR3-ANCA positivity is found in the large majority of patients with active Wegner's granulomatosis and in up to 50% of patients with microscopic polyarteritis. Anti-MPO positivity is present in the majority of patients with idiopathic crescentic glomerulonephritis and in a variable number of cases of microscopic polyarteritis. Testing for antineutrophil cytoplasmic antibodies should be accompanied by appropriate tests of autoantibodies directed against DNA and the glomerular basement membrane antigen. The simultaneous occurrence of ANCA and anti-GMB antibody is well documented; such patients tend to follow the natural history of Goodpasture's disease. Whether ANCA is only a marker of disease or whether it takes part in the pathogenic process is undetermined. ANCA levels can be measured by enzyme-linked immunosorbent assay (ELISA) and variations in the ANCA titre have been used in the assessment of disease activity.

Polyarteritis nodosa (PAN) (see also p. 495)

Classical PAN is a multisystem disorder. Aneurysmal dilatation of medium-sized arteries may be seen on renal arteriography. The condition is more common in men and in the elderly and, typically, the patient is ANCA-negative. Hypertension and haematuria occur and renal failure is common.

Microscopic polyarteritis

In this condition, crescentic glomerulonephritis without immune complex deposition occurs with both (PR3) and MPO-ANCA positivity. The lungs may be involved but granulomata are not seen.

Hepatitis B infection appears to be an aetiological factor in some cases.

Wegener's granulomatosis (see also p. 810)

In this condition, glomerulonephritis occurs together with necrotizing granulomatous lesions affecting the nasopharynx, lungs and kidneys. The necrotizing glomerular lesions do not appear to be due to immune complex deposition. PR3-ANCA positivity is the rule.

TREATMENT

The sooner treatment is instituted the more chance there is of recovery of renal function. Corticosteroids and cyclophosphamide are of benefit: pulsed high-dose methylprednisolone and plasmapheresis may reverse advanced disease. Once remission has been achieved, azathioprine may be substituted for cyclophosphamide. Relapse after complete cessation of immunosuppressive therapy has been observed relatively frequently, and a consensus appears to be immerging that long-term, albeit relatively low-dose, immunosuppression is appropriate. Long-term follow-up of patients is mandatory. Intravenous immunoglobulin therapy shows promise in the treatment of severe and drug-resistant cases.

Cryoglobulinaemic renal disease

Cryoglobulins are immunoglobulins which precipitate reversibly in the cold. Three types are recognized.

In type 1, the cryoprecipitable immunoglobulin is a single monoclonal type, as is found in multiple myeloma and lymphoproliferative disorders.

Type 2 and 3 cryoglobulinaemias are mixed types. In each, a polyclonal IgG antigen is bound to an antiglobulin. In type 2, the antiglobulin component, which is usually of the IgM class, is monoclonal, while in type 3 it is polyclonal. Glomerular disease is more common in type 2 than type 3 cryoglobulinaemia. In approximately 30% of these 'mixed' cryoglobulinaemias, no underlying or associated disease is found (essential cryoglobulinaemia). Recognized associations include viral infections (hepatitis B and C, cytomegalovirus, Epstein–Barr infection), fungal and spirochaetal infections, malaria, infective endocarditis and autoimmune diseases (SLE, rheumatoid arthritis and Sjögren's syndrome).

Glomerular pathological changes include the following:

- There is endocapillary proliferation caused by leucocyte, mainly monocyte, infiltration.
- There are large, amorphous, PAS-positive, Congo red negative deposits within glomerular capillary lumina and on the inner side of the glomerular capillary membrane. On electron microscopy these have an amorphous or fibrillar appearance and appear to be composed of cryoglobulin.
- There is glomerular basement membrane thickening. There is an interstitial mononuclear leucocyte infiltration without much interstitial fibrosis. Vasculitis of small and medium-sized arteries may be present.

Presentation is usually in the fourth or fifth decades of life and women are more frequently affected than men. The majority of reported cases have been from Mediterranean countries. Systemic features include purpura, arthralgia, leg ulcers, Raynaud's phenomenon, evidence of systemic vasculitis, a polyneuropathy, and hepatic involvement. The glomerular disease presents typically as asymptomatic proteinuria, microscopic haematuria or both, but presentation with an acute nephritic syndrome or features of renal impairment also occurs.

Serological investigation reveals a reduction in concentration of early complement components with an elevation of later components.

Spontaneous remission occurs in about one-third of cases and approximately one-third pursue an indolent course. About 10–20% of patients progress to end-stage renal failure over several years. Corticosteroid and/or immunosuppressive therapy with cyclophosphamide may be of benefit, but evaluation of the efficacy of treatment is difficult owing to the rarity of the disease and the occurrence of spontaneous remissions. Intensive plasma exchange or cryofiltration has been used in selected cases.

Renal involvement in other diseases

Diabetes mellitus

Renal disease is a major complication of diabetes; it is discussed on p. 981.

Systemic sclerosis (see also p. 490)

Interlobular renal arteries are affected with intimal thickening and fibrinoid changes occur in afferent glomerular arterioles. Glomerular changes are non-specific. The pathogenesis is unknown and neither steroid nor immunosuppressive therapy is of value. ANCA are not present. Treatment with ACE inhibitor drugs may be of benefit in reducing proteinuria and in some cases halting or even partially reversing decline in renal function.

Amyloidosis

The kidney is often affected in amyloidosis (see p. 1002). Presentation is with asymptomatic proteinuria, nephrotic syndrome or renal failure.

PATHOLOGY

On light microscopy, eosinophilic deposits are seen in the mesangium, capillary loops and arteriolar walls. Staining with Congo red renders these deposits pink and they show green birefringence under polarized light. Immunofluorescence is unhelpful, but on electron microscopy the characteristic fibrils of amyloid can be seen. Amyloid consisting of immunoglobulin light chains (AL amyloid) can be distinguished by immunological techniques from the protein found in secondary amyloid (amyloid protein A, AA amyloid). AL amyloid is found in disorders associated with lymphoproliferative diseases such as myeloma, Waldenström's macroglobulinaemia or non-Hodgkin's lymphoma. It is also present in cases of so-called primary amyloidosis where an abnormal clone of cells is presumed to be responsible, although at present not identifiable. AA amyloid is found following longstanding inflammatory conditions such as suppurative infections, rheumatoid arthritis and familial Mediterranean fever.

DIAGNOSIS AND TREATMENT

The diagnosis can often be made clinically when features of amyloidosis are present elsewhere. On imaging, the kidneys are often large. Renal biopsy is necessary in doubtful cases.

Treatment of the underlying cause should be undertaken. In primary amyloid, treatment also used in myeloma such as corticosteroids and melphalan and bone marrow transplantation may be of benefit. The success of dialysis and kidney transplantation is dependent upon the extent of amyloid deposition in extrarenal sites, especially the heart.

Haemolytic uraemic syndrome (HUS)

HUS is characterized by intravascular haemolysis with red-cell fragmentation (microangiopathic haemolysis), thrombocytopenia and acute renal failure. The syndrome often follows a febrile illness, particularly gastroenteritis or upper respiratory tract infection. A few particular strains of pathogenic *Escherichia coli*, notably strain O157, have been isolated in many cases and in outbreaks of the disease. It has been suggested that infection triggers endothelial damage and that derangements of the haemostatic coagulation system then occur in susceptible individuals. Recurrent episodes of HUS have been described in the same individual, and familial forms of the disease (with both recessive and dominant inheritance) exist. Fibrin deposition is seen in the vascular endothelium, particularly in the renal arterioles and glomerular capillaries. Most children recover spontaneously, although a proportion never recover normal renal function or, having apparently done so, develop hypertension and renal impairment in later years. Mortality rates are higher in the elderly as was demonstrated during the *E. coli* O157-associated outbreak of haemolytic uraemic syndrome in Scotland in 1996/97.

Treatment with heparin, inhibitors of platelet aggregation, synthetic prostacyclins, infusion of fresh frozen plasma and plasma exchange have been employed, but controlled trials of treatment are lacking.

Thrombotic thrombocytopenic purpura (TTP)

TTP is characterized by the presence of widespread hyaline thrombi in small vessels. Young adults are most commonly affected. Microangiopathic haemolysis, renal failure and evidence of neurological disturbance are characteristically found. The pathogenesis is unknown. Some patients with TTP have underlying SLE or polyarteritis and there is clearly considerable overlap between HUS, TTP and the connective tissue disorders. Corticosteroid therapy and measures employed in HUS may be of benefit.

Multiple myeloma

Acute renal failure is relatively common in myeloma, occurring in 2–8% of affected individuals. Histological appearances may be simply those of acute tubular necrosis; tubular blockage by Tamm–Horsfall glycoprotein, light chains and immunoglobulin may be apparent. Dehydration and the administration of intravenous or intra-arterial contrast medium to the volume-depleted patient with myeloma predispose to the development of acute renal failure.

In myeloma, free κ and λ light chains are excreted. Blockage of tubules by casts composed in part at least of light chains, and their toxic effects upon tubular cells, account for the proteinuria and chronic renal impairment associated with 'myeloma kidney'. Renal amyloid deposition often complicates myeloma, accounting both for proteinuria – sometimes of nephrotic proportions – and chronic renal failure.

Hypercalcaemia, renal sepsis and (rarely) urinary tract obstruction due to bulky myeloma deposits are further causes of renal impairment in myelomatosis.

Contrast nephropathy

Iodinated radiological contrast media are nephrotoxic, possibly by causing renal vasoconstriction. The effect is dose-dependent and therefore more commonly seen in procedures which require large amounts of contrast media such as angiography with or without angioplasty. In many patients the effect is mild, transient, fully reversible and of no clinical significance. The risk and severity of contrast nephropathy is amplified by the presence of coexisting conditions which also cause renal hypoperfusion:

- pre-existing renal impairment
- hypovolaemia
- low cardiac output
- diabetes mellitus
- hyperviscosity (myeloma).

As many as possible of these risk factors should be corrected prior to the use of contrast media. The dose should be minimized. Non-ionic and low osmolality contrast media carry less risk of allergic contrast reactions but *do not* decrease the risk of contrast nephropathy. The most important preventitive measure is prevention of hypovolaemia before administration of contrast. The use of intravenous saline infusion for the 12 hours before and 12 hours after contrast exposure has been suggested, provided volume overload is avoided in susceptible patients.

FURTHER READING

Hawkins PN, Wootton R, Pepys MB (1990) Metabolic studies of radioiodinated serum amyloid P component in normal subjects and patients with systemic amyloidosis. *Journal of Clinical Investigation* **86**: 1862–1869.

Porter G (1983) Gouty nephropathy. Fact or fiction? *American Journal of Kidney Disease* **2**: 553–554.

Savage COS, Harper L, Adu T (1997) Primary systemic vasculitis. *Lancet* **349**: 553–558.

Jennette JC, Falk RJ (1997) Small vessel vasculitis. *New England Journal of Medicine* **337**: 1512–1523.

Nephrotic syndrome

The nephrotic syndrome consists of heavy urinary protein loss, hypoalbuminaemia and oedema. Hypercholesterolaemia is almost always present.

PATHOPHYSIOLOGY

Urinary protein loss of the order 3–5 g daily or more in an adult is required to cause hypoalbuminaemia. In children, proportionately less proteinuria results in hypoalbuminaemia.

The normal dietary protein intake in the UK is of the order 70 g daily and the normal liver can synthesize albumin at a rate of 10–12 g daily. How then does a urinary protein loss of the order of 3–5 g daily result in hypoalbuminaemia? The explanation appears to be that in normal individuals there is some catabolism within the kidney of albumin filtered at the glomeruli. In nephrotic patients with heavy proteinuria, catabolism is substantially increased, limiting the amount of protein appearing in the urine and concealing the extent of protein loss through the glomerulus.

The mechanism of the proteinuria is complex. It occurs partly because structural damage to the glomerular basement membrane leads to an increase in the size and numbers of pores, allowing passage of more and larger molecules. Electrical charge is also involved in glomerular permeability. Fixed negatively charged components are present in the glomerular capillary wall, which repel negatively charged protein molecules. Reduction of this fixed charge occurs in glomerular disease and appears to be an important factor in the genesis of heavy proteinuria.

Pathogenesis of oedema in hypoalbuminaemia

The pathogenesis of the oedema is incompletely understood. A conventional explanation is that a reduction in the concentration of osmotically active albumin molecules in the blood results in a reduction in the oncotic force that retains fluid within blood vessels, and salt and water escapes into the extravascular compartment; i.e. oedema occurs. Such loss of salt and water results in a fall in blood volume and a reduction in pressure within afferent glomerular arterioles. This activates the renin–angiotensin–aldosterone system (see p. 954). The consequent hyperaldosteronism promotes sodium and water reabsorption in the distal nephron, increasing the tendency to oedema.

Unfortunately, this explanation does not fit the facts. Plasma renin activity in nephrotic patients is often normal and measured blood volume may be normal or high in nephrotic patients, even those without renal failure. Moreover, sodium retention by the kidney in minimal-change nephropathy has been shown to occur *before* the development of hypoalbuminaemia. Intrarenal mechanisms of salt retention are presumably involved in this situation.

CAUSES

All types of glomerulonephritis can produce the nephrotic syndrome. Although proliferative glomerulonephritis is more common than membranous disease, the latter is the most common form of glomerulonephritis to cause nephrotic syndrome in adults in the UK (Table 9.9).

Minimal-change glomerular disease accounts for most cases of the nephrotic syndrome in childhood compared with approximately 20% of adult cases. In tropical areas, minimal change is present in fewer than 10% of nephrotic children owing to the high incidence of nephrotic syndrome due to infections such as malaria. Minimal-change disease does not progress to chronic renal failure (see p. 572).

Diabetic glomerular disease (p. 981) can also cause the nephrotic syndrome. The histological lesion seen on light microscopy in diabetes may comprise amorphous nodular deposits (which are not immune complexes) in the glomeruli or a diffuse glomerulosclerosis. There is associated glomerular basement membrane thickening.

Diabetes is also a cause of renal papillary necrosis, but patients with this lesion alone do not have sufficiently heavy proteinuria to become nephrotic.

Drug reactions

Many drugs can cause sufficiently heavy proteinuria to result in the nephrotic syndrome. Penicillamine, which in all probability combines with a plasma protein to form an antigenic hapten, induces an immune complex-mediated membranous glomerulonephritis, as may high-dose captopril. Various metals, whether used therapeutically (e.g. gold) or in industry (e.g. mercury and cadmium), can induce proteinuria severe enough to cause the nephrotic syndrome.

Allergic reactions

Reactions to many allergens such as poison ivy, pollens, bee stings and cows' milk may be associated with the nephrotic syndrome, but evidence of a causal relationship is lacking in most cases.

Most lists of causes of the nephrotic syndrome include renal vein thrombosis, but this is probably a complication rather than a cause of the syndrome. It is particularly likely to complicate membranous glomerulonephritis. In nephrotic patients the blood is more coagulable than normal and the circulation may be sluggish owing to hypovolaemia, both of which are likely to induce

Table 9.9
Causes of the nephrotic syndrome

All glomerulonephritides and minimal-change glomerular lesions
Systemic vasculitides, mainly systemic lupus erythematosus
Diabetic glomerulosclerosis
Amyloidosis
Drugs
Allergies

thrombosis. Estimates of the incidence of this complication range from 5% to approximately 50% in nephrotic syndrome due to membranous glomerulonephritis.

Renal disorders not associated with the nephrotic syndrome

Proteinuria severe enough to cause the nephrotic syndrome is not a feature of reflux nephropathy (chronic atrophic pyelonephritis), chronic tubulo-interstitial nephritis, renal tuberculosis, polycystic disease, or many other renal disorders.

HISTORY

The history may provide clues to the aetiology, such as exposure to a drug or allergen. Patients with a minimal-change lesion may give a history or family history of atopy. There may be a family history of renal disease.

Patients with heavy proteinuria may have noted that their urine has been frothy; the onset of the renal lesion can be timed from this observation.

EXAMINATION

Examination will reveal oedema; ascites may also be present, particularly in children. Genital oedema is sometimes seen. The oedema may involve the face (periorbital oedema) and arms. Neither elevation of the jugular venous pressure nor pulmonary oedema are features of the nephrotic syndrome, though either or both may be present if renal and/or cardiac failure are present in the nephrotic patient.

Features of the underlying disorder may be evident, such as the butterfly facial rash of SLE or the neuropathy and retinopathy associated with diabetes mellitus.

The following must be excluded:

- *primary cardiac failure* – here, the venous pressure is high, oedema is not usually present in the face, and the proteinuria is less severe
- *liver disease*, and other causes of hypoalbuminaemia (Table 9.10), with oedema and ascites.

INVESTIGATIONS

The presence of the nephrotic syndrome is established by measuring:

- **24-hour urinary protein** – usually more than 3–5 g daily in adults
- **serum albumin concentration** – usually less than 30 g L^{-1}.

Increased hepatic albumin synthesis is accompanied by increased cholesterol synthesis and there is an approximate reciprocal relationship between the serum albumin and the serum cholesterol concentration. Low-density lipoprotein (LDL) cholesterol concentrations are elevated, but high-density lipoprotein (HDL) cholesterol is usually normal. Hypertriglyceridaemia is present in about 50% of patients.

Renal function is assessed by measuring:

- **serum urea and creatinine**
- **creatinine clearance**, to determine the GFR.

Further investigations are required to elucidate the cause:

- *Microscopy of the urine* may show red cells and red-cell casts; the latter are virtually diagnostic of glomerulonephritis. Minimal-change lesions do not usually result in red cells or red-cell casts in the urine.
- *Throat swab and serum ASO titre* may show evidence of streptococcal infection.
- *Serum C3 complement concentrations* may be decreased in immune complex-mediated glomerulonephritis.
- *Presence of antinuclear antibody* may suggest SLE. A search for extractable nuclear antigens and/or antibody to double-stranded DNA should be made if antinuclear antibody is detected. A positive test for ANCA (see p. 539) will suggest a systemic vasculitis, and detection of anti-GBM antibody leads to the diagnosis of Goodpasture's syndrome.
- *Screening for hepatitis B surface antigen and hepatitis C antibody.*
- *Cryoglobulinaemia* will be detected if blood is taken and placed immediately in a water bath at 37°C before testing. Cold-precipitable globulins may be found, for example, when nephrotic syndrome is associated with a malignant lymphoproliferative disorder or hepatitis C infection.
- *Serum electrophoresis.* In the nephrotic syndrome there is always a reduced serum albumin, commonly with an increase in the α- and β-globulin fractions (Fig 9.18) on serum electrophoresis. In myeloma, a monoclonal paraprotein band is present and there may be associated immune paresis with reduction in the concentration of one or more of IgG, IgA or IgM proteins. Abnormal protein constituents will be found on electrophoresis of urine. Ten per cent of patients with myeloma have renal amyloid deposition.
- *Raised blood glucose* indicates diabetes mellitus.
- *Selective protein clearance* may be measured. Blood and urine samples are taken at the same time; a timed urine collection is not required. The clearance of large-molecular-weight protein such as IgG is compared with that of a smaller molecule such as albumin or transferrin. A low ratio (selective protein leak) is found in minimal-change glomerulopathy, early diabetes and renal amyloidosis. Severe glomerulonephritides (e.g. diffuse proliferative glomerulonephritis with crescent formation) are more typically associated with an unselective protein leak. Overlap between the

Table 9.10
Causes of hypoalbuminaemia

Inadequate protein intake: protein-energy malnutrition
Failure of protein production: liver disease
Excessive protein loss: nephrotic syndrome, protein-losing enteropathy, extensive burns
Pregnancy

groups exists. Measurement of selective protein clearance is unnecessary if renal biopsy is to be carried out. Its main use is in children in whom a minimal-change lesion is suspected. An unselective protein leak in such a child would bring this diagnosis into question and might prompt renal biopsy (see below).

Renal biopsy (see also p. 531)

Transcutaneous biopsy is performed to make a histological diagnosis when management will be affected, particularly when the major question is whether a steroid-sensitive minimal-change lesion is present or not. It is not indicated in three groups of patients:

- in young children (particularly males) who have a highly selective protein leak, no hypertension and no red cells or red-cell casts in the urine (the diagnosis is almost certain to be a minimal-change lesion, so that a trial of steroids should be instituted first)
- in longstanding, insulin-dependent diabetes with associated retinopathy or neuropathy, since the diagnosis is in little doubt
- in patients on drugs such as penicillamine, which should be stopped first.

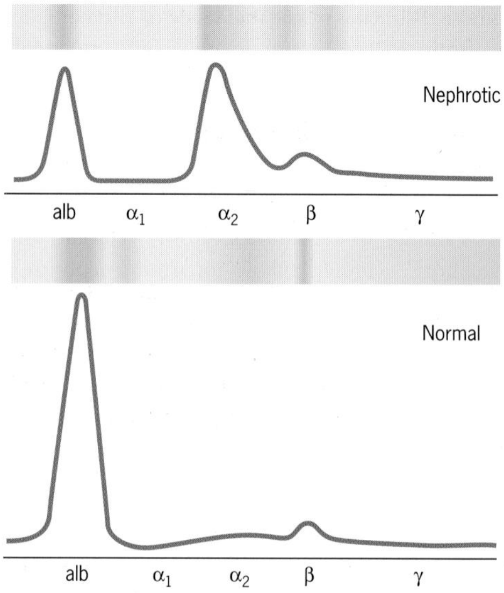

Fig 9.18
Serum electrophoresis in a normal person and in a patient with nephrotic syndrome. Note the reduced albumin and increased α- and β-globulin in the nephrotic patient

MANAGEMENT

General measures

Initial treatment should be with dietary sodium restriction and a thiazide diuretic (e.g. bendrofluazide). Unresponsive patients require frusemide 40–120 mg daily with the addition of amiloride (5 mg daily), but the serum potassium concentration should be monitored carefully. Patients are sometimes hypovolaemic, and moderate oedema may have to be accepted in order to avoid postural hypotension.

A high-protein diet (approximately 80–90 g protein daily) confers no benefit and normal protein intake is advisable.

Infusion of albumin produces only a transient effect and is normally employed only in diuretic-resistant patients and those with oliguria and uraemia in the absence of severe glomerular damage, such as those with minimal-change nephropathy. Such infusion is combined with diuretic therapy. Diuresis, when once initiated in this way, often continues with diuretic treatment alone.

Specific measures

The aim is to reverse the abnormal urinary protein leak.

Minimal-change glomerular lesion

High-dose corticosteroid therapy with prednisolone 60 mg daily (dose corrected to a normal body surface area of 1.73 m^2) for eight weeks corrects the urinary protein leak in more than 95% of children. Response rates in adults are significantly lower and response may occur only after many months of steroid therapy. Spontaneous remission also occurs and steroid therapy should, in general, be withheld if urinary protein loss is insufficient to cause hypoalbuminaemia or oedema.

In both children and adults, if remission lasts for four years after steroid therapy, further relapse is very rare. In children, approximately one-third do not subsequently relapse, but in the remainder further courses of corticosteroids are indicated. One-third of these patients relapse regularly on steroid withdrawal and in these patients remission is induced with steroid therapy once more and a course of cyclophosphamide 3 mg kg^{-1} daily is given for 6–8 weeks. This increases the likelihood of long-term remission. Steroid-unresponsive patients may also respond to cyclophosphamide. No more than two courses of cyclophosphamide should be prescribed in children because of the risk of side-effects, which include azoospermia.

An alternative to cyclophosphamide is cyclosporin, which is effective but must be continued long term to prevent relapse on stopping treatment. Excretory function and cyclosporin blood levels must be monitored carefully as cyclosporin is potentially nephrotoxic.

Membranous glomerulonephritis

This is discussed on p. 535.

Other causes

Remission occurs if the underlying disease can be treated. In patients with SLE, treatment with steroids and cyclophosphamide or azathioprine usually induces long-term remission.

When the glomerular lesion causing the nephrotic syndrome progresses and the GFR declines, the degree of proteinuria often diminishes so that the hypoalbuminaemia and oedema improve.

PREVENTION, AND MANAGEMENT OF COMPLICATIONS

Venous thrombosis

Hypovolaemia and a hypercoagulable state predispose to venous thrombosis. The hypercoaguable state is due to loss of clotting factors (e.g. antithrombin) in the urine and an increased hepatic production of fibrinogen. Prolonged bedrest should therefore be avoided.

Once renal vein thrombosis has occurred, prolonged anticoagulation is required. Thromboembolism is exceptionally common in nephrotic syndrome due to membranous glomerulonephritis, and in the absence of any contraindication, long-term prophylactic anticoagulation is indicated.

Sepsis

Sepsis is an important cause of death in nephrotic patients. The increased susceptibility to infection is partly due to loss of immunoglobulin in the urine. Pneumococcal infections are particularly common and pneumococcal vaccine should be given.

Early detection and aggressive treatment of infections, rather than long-term antibiotic prophylaxis, is the best approach.

Oliguric renal failure

A low blood volume and hypotension may lead to underperfused kidneys. Acute tubular necrosis may therefore readily develop when renal ischaemia occurs from other complications such as blood loss or septicaemia. In some patients, uraemia appears to result from derangements in renal perfusion in the absence of hypotension.

Albumin infusion combined with mannitol or another diuretic may initiate a diuresis in oliguric renal failure.

Lipid abnormalities

It is suggested that these are responsible for an increase in the risk of myocardial infarction or peripheral vascular disease. Treatment of hypercholesterolaemia is best with an HMG-CoA reductase inhibitor (p. 995).

FURTHER READING

Oliveira DBG (1998) Membranous nephropathy: an IgG4-mediated disease. *Lancet* **351**: 617–671.

Ponticelli C *et al.* (1992) Methylprednisolone plus chlorambucil compared with methylprednisolone alone for treatment of idiopathic membranous nephropathy. *New England Journal of Medicine* **327**: 599–603.

Orth SR, Ritz E (1998) The nephrotic syndrome. *New England Journal of Medicine* **338**: 1202–1211.

Urinary tract infection

Urinary tract infection (UTI) is common in women, uncommon in men and of special importance in children. Recurrent infection causes considerable morbidity; if complicated, it can cause severe renal disease including end-stage renal failure. It is also a common source of life-threatening Gram-negative septicaemia.

PATHOGENESIS

Infection is most often due to bacteria from the patient's own bowel flora (Table 9.11). Transfer to the urinary tract may be via the bloodstream, the lymphatics or by direct extension (e.g. from a vesicocolic fistula), but is most often via the ascending transurethral route (Fig 9.19). For the latter route, three important steps are involved.

First, the lower vagina and periurethral area is heavily colonized by uropathogenic bacteria. This is facilitated by the adhesion of bacteria to uroepithelial surfaces by pili or fimbriae present on the bacterial cell surface. Previous UTIs may also predispose to further colonization which may not be eliminated by treatment of the infection, initiating a vicious circle. Important factors contributing to colonization include use of a diaphragm and spermicidal jelly, hormone-deficient vaginal atrophy, and systemic antibiotic treatment for non-urinary tract infections. There is little evidence that personal hygiene affects colonization, but the use of bubblebaths may be a contributory factor.

Second, bacteria are transferred along the urethra to the bladder. This step is facilitated by sexual intercourse or catheterization. Spontaneous transfer along the short female urethra is easy, while the longer male urethra protects against transfer of bacteria to the bladder; in addition, prostatic fluid has defensive bactericidal properties.

The *third* and most important step is the *establishment and multiplication of bacteria within the bladder*. Bladder urine is normally sterile, owing to defence mechanisms within the bladder. These include hydrokinetic and bladder mucosal factors and constituents of urine. A low flow rate and infrequent and poor bladder emptying predispose to infection.

Table 9.11
Organisms causing urinary tract infection in domicilliary practice

Organism	Approximate frequency (%)
Escherichia coli and other 'coliforms'	68+
Proteus mirabilis	12
Klebsiella aerogenes[a]	4
Enterococcus faecalis[a]	6
Staphylococcus saprophyticus or *epidermidis*[b]	10

[a] More common in hospital practice
[b] More common in young women (20–30%)

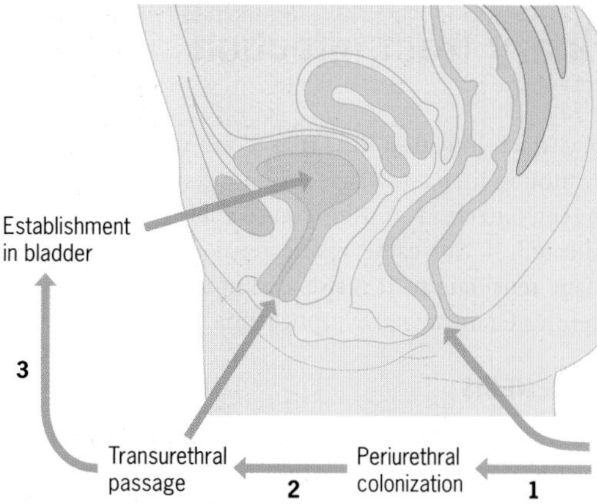

Fig 9.19
Ascending infection of the urinary tract

Mucosal defence mechanisms are poorly understood. The establishment of infection may be facilitated by fimbriated bacteria adhering to the bladder uroepithelium or previous damage to this epithelium. A thin layer of mucopolysaccharide coats the transitional epithelial cells and prevents adhesion of bacteria. Loss or depletion of this layer due to previous infection, bladder trauma from catheterization or vigorous intercourse may predispose to infection. Uromucoid (Tamm–Horsfall protein), present in normal urine, adheres both to bacteria and to uroepithelial cells, and may have a defensive role via uroepithelial cell shedding. The role of urinary immunoglobulins – secretory IgA and IgG – is unclear, but they may have a defensive role.

The first phase in the development of UTI is the entry and establishment of bacteria within the bladder. Extension of infection up the ureters to the kidneys is relatively easy and is facilitated by vesicoureteric reflux and dilated hypotonic ureters. Once infection is established it can pass up or down the system quite readily.

NATURAL HISTORY

UTI is commonly an isolated, never (or rarely) repeated event (Fig 9.20).

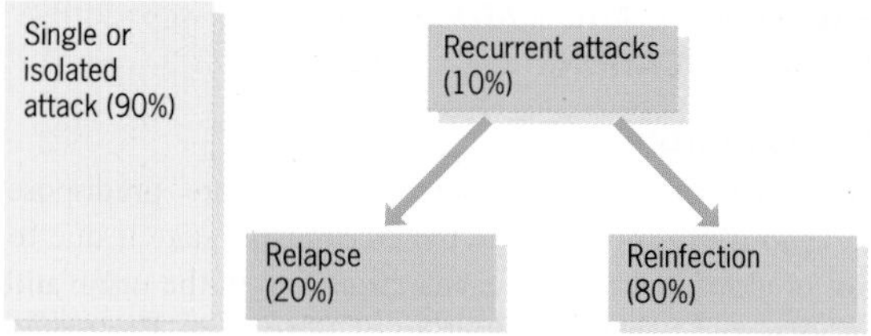

Fig 9.20
The natural history of urinary tract infection

Complicated versus uncomplicated infection

(Fig 9.21)

It is necessary to distinguish between UTI occurring in patients with functionally normal urinary tracts and in those with abnormal tracts.

Functionally normal urinary tracts (with normal excretion urography). Here, persistent or recurrent infection seldom results in serious kidney damage (*uncomplicated* UTI).

Abnormal urinary tracts. Tracts with stones, or associated diseases such as diabetes mellitus which themselves cause kidney damage, may be made worse with infection (*complicated* UTI). UTI, particularly with *Proteus*, may predispose to stone formation. The combination of infection and obstruction results in severe, sometimes rapid, kidney damage (obstructive pyonephrosis) and is an important cause of Gram-negative septicaemia.

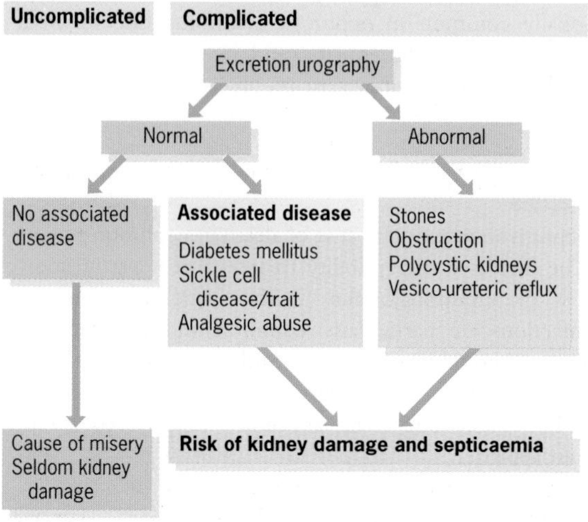

Fig 9.21
Complicated versus uncomplicated urinary tract infection

Acute pyelonephritis

Localization studies have shown that distinguishing between upper and lower urinary tract infection on clinical grounds can be inaccurate. However, the combination of fever, loin pain and tenderness and significant bacteriuria is usually regarded as indicating bacterial infection of the kidney (acute pyelonephritis). Small renal cortical abscesses and streaks of pus in the renal medulla are often present. Histologically there is focal infiltration by polymorphonuclear leucocytes and many polymorphs in tubular lumina.

In the antibiotic era, it appears highly unusual for such infection to cause significant permanent kidney damage in adults with normal urinary tracts. However, the advent of CT scanning has brought to attention the fact that even in such patients wedge-shaped areas of inflammation in the renal cortex may be seen which presumably heal in some instances with fibrosis, and hence some damage to renal function (Fig 9.22). However, it is incorrect to believe that the anatomical appearances referred to as 'chronic pyelonephritis' develop in adults with normal urinary tract anatomy and no complicating conditions (such as diabetes, analgesic abuse or urinary tract obstruction) or as a result of repeated infection of the renal parenchyma. The anatomical abnormalities described in chronic pyelonephritis are acquired as a result of vesicoureteric reflux and infection in infancy and childhood.

Chronic pyelonephritis

Chronic pyelonephritis (also called atrophic pyelonephritis or reflux nephropathy) is now known to result from a combination of:

- vesicoureteric reflux, and
- infection acquired in infancy or early childhood.

Normally the vesicoureteric junction acts as a one-way valve (Fig 9.23), urine entering the bladder from above; the ureter is shut off during bladder contraction, thus preventing reflux of urine. In some infants and children – possibly even *in utero* – this valve mechanism is incompetent, bladder voiding being associated with variable reflux of a jet of urine up the ureter. A secondary consequence is incomplete bladder emptying, as refluxed urine returns to the bladder after voiding. This latter event predisposes to infection, and the reflux of infected urine leads to kidney damage.

Typically there is papillary damage, interstitial nephritis and cortical scarring in areas adjacent to 'clubbed calyces'. Diagnosis is based on excretion urography, which shows irregular renal outlines, clubbed calyces and a variable reduction in renal size. Reflux is confirmed by MCU (see p. 529). The condition may be unilateral or bilateral and affect all or part of the kidney.

Reflux usually ceases around puberty with growth of the bladder base. Damage already done persists and progressive renal fibrosis and further loss of function occurs in severe cases even though there is no further infection. This condition does not develop in the absence of reflux and does not begin in adult life. It is therefore important to reassure adult females with bacteriuria and a normal urogram that kidney damage due to reflux nephropathy will not develop. Chronic pyelonephritis acquired in infancy predisposes to hypertension in later life and, if severe, is a relatively common cause of end-stage renal failure in childhood or adult life. Early detection and treatment of infection, with or without ureteral reimplantation to create a competent valve, can prevent further scarring and allow normal growth of the kidneys.

Reinfection versus relapsing infection

When UTI is recurrent it is important to distinguish between relapse and reinfection.

Relapse is diagnosed by recurrence of bacteriuria with the *same* organism within seven days of completion of antibacterial treatment and implies failure to eradicate infection (Fig 9.24). It usually occurs in conditions in which it is difficult to eradicate the bacteria, such as stones, scarred kidneys, polycystic disease or bacterial prostatitis.

By contrast, in reinfection, bacteriuria is absent after treatment for at least 14 days, usually longer, followed by recurrence of infection with the same or different organisms. This is not due to failure to eradicate infection, but is the result of reinvasion of a susceptible tract with new organisms. Approximately 80% of recurrent infections are due to reinfection.

SYMPTOMS AND SIGNS

The most typical symptoms of UTI are:

- frequency of micturition by day and night
- painful voiding (dysuria)
- suprapubic pain and tenderness
- haematuria
- smelly urine.

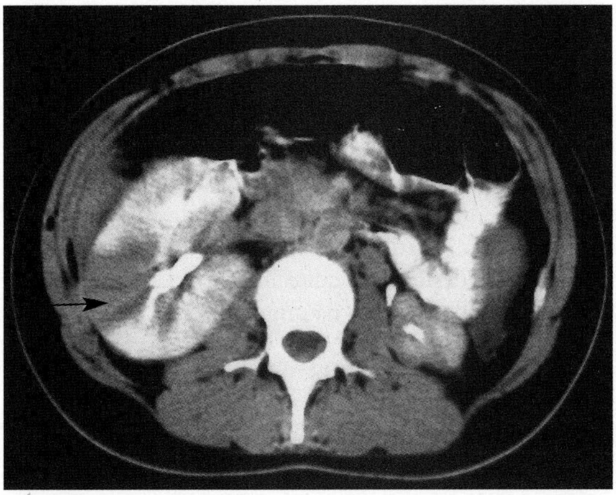

Fig 9.22
CT scan showing a wedge-shaped area of renal cortical loss (arrow) **following acute pyelonephritis**

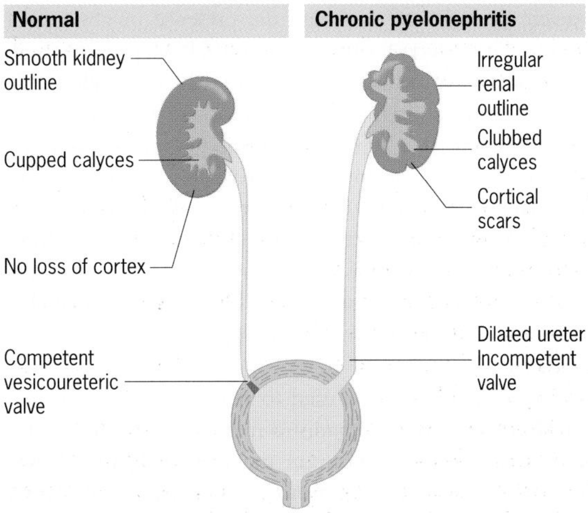

Fig 9.23
Chronic pyelonephritis with vesicoureteric reflux compared with the normal state

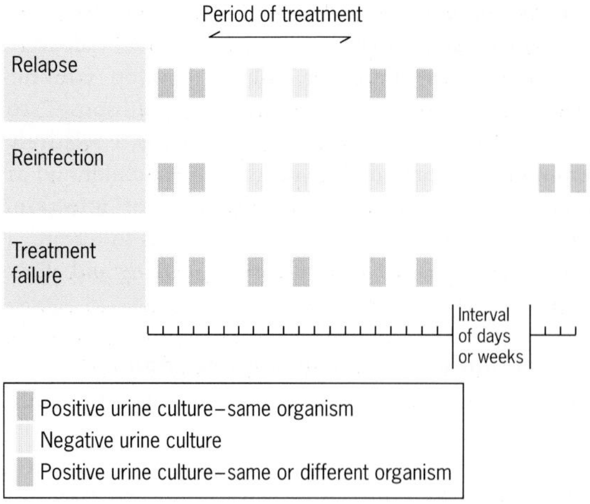

Fig 9.24
A comparison of reinfection, relapse and treatment failure in urinary tract infection

These symptoms relate to bladder and urethral inflammation, commonly called 'cystitis', and suggest lower urinary tract infection. Loin pain and tenderness, with fever and systemic upset, suggest extension of the infection to the pelvis and kidney, known as pyelitis or pyelonephritis. However, localization of the site of infection on the basis of symptoms alone is unreliable.

UTI may also be present with minimal or no symptoms or may be associated with atypical symptoms such as abdominal pain, fever or haematuria in the absence of frequency or dysuria.

In small children, who cannot complain of dysuria, symptoms are often 'atypical'. The possibility of UTI must always be considered in the fretful, febrile sick child who fails to thrive.

DIAGNOSIS

Diagnosis is based on *quantitative* culture of a clean-catch midstream specimen of urine and the presence or absence of pyuria. The criteria for the diagnosis of UTI, particularly in symptomatic women, have changed in the past decade (Table 9.12). Clearly a diagnosis based on rigid adherence to a bacterial count of at least 10^5 organisms per millilitre of urine in these women is incorrect. Diagnosis of 'low count bacteriuria' demands the presence of pyuria. Many laboratories cannot report bacterial counts under 10^4 per mL. In doubtful cases of 'low count bacteriuria', and especially when recurrent, urine should be obtained by suprapubic aspiration when any growth of a uropathogenic organism is evidence of infection.

Dipstick tests can be used to detect nitrates in urine. Most Gram-negative organisms reduce nitrates to nitrites and produce a red colour in the reagent square. False-negative results are common. Dipsticks that detect significant pyuria depend on the release of esterases from leucocytes. Dipstick tests positive for both nitrite and leucocyte esterase are highly predictive of acute infection.

Table 9.12
Criteria for diagnosis of bacteriuria

Symptomatic young women
$\geq 10^2$ coliform organisms/mL urine plus pyuria (> 10 WCC/mm^3)
OR
$\geq 10^5$ any pathogenic organism/mL urine
OR
any growth of pathogenic organisms in urine by suprapubic aspiration
Symptomatic men
$\geq 10^3$ pathogenic organisms/mL urine
Asymptomatic patients
$\geq 10^5$ pathogenic organisms/mL of urine on two occasions

Abacteriuric frequency or dysuria ('urethral syndrome')

Prior to the recognition of 'low count bacteriuria', 50% of symptomatic young women were deemed not to have urinary infection and the term 'urethral syndrome' was coined. With the altered criteria, clearly the majority of these women do indeed have UTI. Alternative causes of truly abacteriuric frequency/dysuria include postcoital bladder trauma, vaginitis, atrophic vaginitis or urethritis in the elderly, and interstitial cystitis (Hunner's ulcer). In symptomatic young women with 'sterile pyuria', *Chlamydia* infection and tuberculosis must be excluded.

Interstitial cystitis is an uncommon but distressing com-plaint, most often affecting women over the age of 40 years. It presents with frequency, dysuria and often severe suprapubic pain. Urine cultures are sterile. Cystoscopy shows typical inflammatory changes with ulceration of the bladder base. The cause is unclear but it is commonly thought to be an autoimmune disorder. Various treatments are advocated with variable success. These include oral prednisolone therapy, bladder instillation of sodium cromoglycate and bladder stretching under anaesthesia.

Careful history-taking will identify a group with predominant frequency and passage of small volumes of urine who have 'irritable bladders', possibly consequent on previous UTI or conditioned by psychosexual factors. Such patients must be distinguished from those with frequency due to polyuria. Repeated courses of antibiotics in patients with genuine abacteriuric frequency or dysuria are quite inappropriate and detract from identifying the true nature of the problem.

SPECIAL INVESTIGATIONS

Excretion urography

Excretion urography is not indicated in women with one or two isolated episodes of UTI if post-treatment urinalysis, including microscopy and urine culture, are normal. If there are further attacks or if post-treatment urinalysis is abnormal, excretion urography should be performed to identify or exclude anatomical or functional abnormalities predisposing to or complicating infection, such as impaired bladder emptying.

Excretion urography should be carried out in all males and children following a first proven episode of bacteriuria to identify complicating factors.

Plain abdominal X-rays and ultrasonography

Plain abdominal X-rays plus renal tomography combined with ultrasonography can identify most renal stones, upper tract obstruction and renal scars, as well as define bladder emptying. This combination of imaging is especially valuable in patients presenting with acute pyelonephritis. Neither it nor DMSA scanning can define calyceal detail or ureteric anatomy, and cannot define conditions such as papillary necrosis or medullary sponge kidney which can affect the course and management of recurrent UTI. Intravenous urography, therefore, remains the investigation of first choice.

Micturating cystourethrography (MCU)

MCU is indicated in children with abnormal excretion urograms and may be required to evaluate abnormal bladder emptying at any age. Otherwise it is of no value in the management of UTI.

Cystoscopy

Cystoscopy in patients with known UTI has a very limited role. It is indicated only to investigate abnormal bladder or ureteral emptying, or haematuria in bacteriuric women over the age of 40 years, since bladder cancer becomes more common with age. It is more appropriately performed in abacteriuric frequency or dysuria to exclude bladder lesions such as carcinoma, tuberculosis or interstitial cystitis (Hunner's ulcer).

TREATMENT

Single isolated attack

Pretreatment urine culture is desirable.

Symptomatic treatment with potassium citrate mixture ('mist pot cit') has largely been abandoned. Treatment is now over 3–5 days with amoxycillin (250 mg thrice daily), nitrofurantoin (50 mg thrice daily), trimethoprim (200 mg twice daily) or an oral cephalosporin. The treatment regimen may be modified in light of the result of urine culture and sensitivity testing, and/or the clinical response. For resistant organisms the alternative drugs are: co-amoxiclav, an oral cephalosporin, or ciprofloxacin.

A high (2 L daily) fluid intake should be encouraged during treatment and for some subsequent weeks. Urinalysis, microscopy and culture should be repeated five days after treatment. 'Single-shot' treatment with 3 g of amoxycillin or 1.92 g of co-trimoxazole can be used for patients with bladder symptoms of less than 36 hours duration who have no previous history of UTI.

If the patient is acutely ill with high fever, loin pain and tenderness (acute pyelonephritis), a broad-spectrum antibiotic is given intravenously, such as aztreonan, cefuroxime, ciprofloxacin or gentamicin (2–5 mg kg^{-1} daily in divided doses) switching to a further seven days' treatment with oral therapy as symptoms improve. Intravenous fluids may be required to achieve a good urine output.

In patients presenting for the first time with high fever, loin pain and tenderness, urgent renal ultrasound examination is required to exclude an obstructed pyonephrosis. If this is present it should be drained by percutaneous nephrostomy.

Recurrent infection

Pretreatment and post-treatment urine cultures are mandatory to confirm the diagnosis and identify whether recurrent infection is due to relapse or reinfection.

In relapse, a search should be made for a cause (e.g. stones or scarred kidneys), and this should be eradicated if possible, for example by the removal of stones. Intense or prolonged treatment – intravenous or intramuscular aminoglycoside for seven days or oral antibiotics for 4–6 weeks – is required. If this fails, long-term antibiotics are required.

Reinfection implies that the patient has a predisposition to periurethral colonization or poor bladder defence mechanisms. Contraceptive practice should be reviewed and the use of a diaphragm and spermicidal jelly discouraged. Atrophic vaginitis should be identified in postmenopausal women who should be treated (see below). All patients must undertake prophylactic measures:

- a 2 L daily fluid intake
- voiding at 2–3 hour intervals with double micturition if reflux is present
- voiding before bedtime and after intercourse
- avoidance of bubblebaths and other chemicals in bathwater
- avoidance of constipation, which may impair bladder emptying.

Evidence of impaired bladder emptying on excretion urography requires urological assessment. If UTI continues to recur, treatment for 6–12 months with low-dose prophylaxis (trimethoprim 100 mg, co-trimoxazole 480 mg, cephalexin 125 mg at night, or microcrystalline nitrofurantoin) is required; it should be taken last thing at night when urine flow is low. An alternative for infrequent attacks is immediate self-treatment with a conventional antibiotic for 3–5 days. When infection is clearly related to coitus, a single dose of microcrystalline nitrofurantoin following intercourse may reduce the total drug usage for prophylaxis. Intravaginal oestrogen therapy has been shown to produce a reduction in the number of episodes of UTI in postmenopausal women.

Urinary infections in the presence of an indwelling catheter

Colonization of the bladder by a urinary pathogen is common after a urinary catheter has been present for more than a few days. So long as the bladder catheter is *in situ*, antibiotic treatment is likely to be ineffective and will encourage the development of resistant organisms. Treatment is indicated only if the patient has symptoms or evidence of infection, and should be accompanied by replacement of the catheter. There may be a place for antibiotic treatment at the time of catheter removal. Bladder stones may form in patients with long-term indwelling catheters, further complicating the situation.

Infection by *Candida* is a frequent complication of prolonged bladder catheterization. Treatment should be reserved for patients with evidence of invasive infection or those who are immunosuppressed, and should consist of removal or replacement of the catheter and possibly intravesical antifungals.

Bacteriuria in pregnancy

The urine of pregnant women must always be cultured as 2–6% have asymptomatic bacteriuria. Whilst asymptomatic bacteriuria in the non-pregnant female seldom leads on to acute pyelonephritis and often does not require treatment, acute pyelonephritis frequently occurs in pregnancy under these circumstances. Failure to treat may thus result in severe symptomatic pyelonephritis later in pregnancy, with the possibility of premature labour. Asymptomatic bacteriuria, in the presence of previous renal disease, may predispose to pre-eclamptic toxaemia, anaemia of pregnancy, and small or premature babies. Therefore bacteriuria must always be treated and be shown to be eradicated. Reinfection may require prophylactic therapy. Tetracycline, trimethoprim, sulphonamides and 4-quinolones must be avoided in pregnancy. Amoxycillin and ampicillin, nitrofurantoin and oral cephalosporins may safely be used in pregnancy.

Bacterial prostatitis

Bacterial prostatitis is a relapsing infection which is difficult to treat. It presents as perineal pain, recurrent epididymo-orchitis and prostatic tenderness, with pus in expressed prostatic secretion. Treatment is for 4–6 weeks with drugs that penetrate the prostate, such as trimethoprim or ciprofloxacin. Long-term low-dose treatment may be required.

Renal carbuncle

Renal carbuncle is an abscess in the renal cortex caused by a blood-borne *Staphylococcus*, usually from a boil or carbuncle of the skin. It presents with a high swinging fever, loin pain and tenderness, and fullness in the loin. The urine shows no abnormality as the abscess does not communicate with the renal pelvis, more often extending into the perirenal tissue. Staphylococcal septicaemia is common. Diagnosis is by ultrasound or CT scanning. Treatment involves antibacterial therapy with flucloxacillin and surgical drainage.

Tuberculosis of the urinary tract

Tuberculous infection is once again on the increase worldwide. Particular dangers are posed by the reservoir of infection in susceptible HIV-infected individuals and by the emergence of drug-resistant strains. Tuberculosis of the urinary tract should be kept in mind in patients presenting with frequency, dysuria or haematuria, particularly in the Asian immigrant population of the UK. Cortical lesions result from haematogenous spread in the primary phase of infection. Most heal, but in some, infection persists and spreads to the papillae, with the formation of cavitating lesions and the discharge of mycobacteria into the urine. Infection of the ureters and bladder commonly follows, with the potential for the development of ureteral stricture and a contracted bladder. Rarely, cold abscessses may form in the loin. In males the disease may present with testicular or epididymal discomfort and thickening.

Diagnosis depends on constant awareness, especially in patients with sterile pyuria. Excretion urography may show cavitating lesions in the renal papillary areas, commonly with calcification. There may also be evidence of ureteral obstruction with hydronephrosis. Diagnosis of active infection depends on culture of mycobacteria from early-morning urine samples. The urogram may be normal in diffuse interstitial renal tuberculosis when diagnosis is made by renal biopsy. Some patients present with small unobstructed kidneys when the diagnosis is easy to miss.

The treatment is as for pulmonary tuberculosis (see p. 804). Renal ultrasonography or excretion urography should be carried out 2–3 months after initiation of treatment as ureteric strictures may first develop in the healing phase.

Xanthogranulomatous pyelonephritis

This is an uncommon chronic interstitial infection of the kidney, most often due to *Proteus*, in which there is fever, weight loss, loin pain and a palpable enlarged kidney. It is usually unilateral and associated with staghorn calculi. CT scanning shows up intrarenal abscesses as lucent areas within the kidney. Nephrectomy is the treatment of choice; antibacterial treatment rarely, if ever, eradicates the infection.

Malakoplakia

This is a rare condition in which plaques of abnormal inflammatory tissue grow within the urinary tract in the presence of urinary infection. The histological appearances are characteristic. It is thought that the condition is caused by an acquired inability of macrophages to kill phagocytosed bacteria. Cholinergic agonists and ascorbic acid may improve macrophage function; ciprofloxacin penetrates the macrophage well and is the antibiotic of choice. Prolonged treatment may be needed.

Viral renal infections

Viruses are present in the urine in a wide range of common viral infections, but very few viruses cause significant renal disease. Secondary immune complex glomerulonephritis may result from chronic viral infections; for instance, membranous nephropathy complicating hepatitis B and cryoglobulinaemic mesangiocapillary glomerulonephritis complicating hepatitis C infection. The role of cytomegalovirus in renal disease is unclear. *Haemorrhagic fever with renal syndrome* is the name given to a spectrum of diseases caused by Hanta viruses (see p. 62); renal failure may be severe, and is caused by an acute haemorrhagic interstitial nephritis. Human immunodeficiency virus infection is associated both with focal glomerulosclerosis and with haemolytic uraemic syndrome, but the pathogenesis of these complications remains uncertain.

FURTHER READING

Cattell WR (ed) (1996) *Infections of the Kidney and Urinary Tract*. Oxford: Oxford University Press.

Tubulointerstitial nephritis

Interstitial inflammation with tubular damage is a regular feature of bacterial pyelonephritis but, contrary to former belief, it rarely, if ever, leads to severe chronic renal damage in the absence of reflux, obstruction or other complicating factors. However, there is growing concern that tubulointerstitial disease due to other causes is more common than was previously diagnosed. The major stimulus for this interest came from recognition that it could be due to analgesic abuse. Subsequently, tubulointerstitial disease due to a variety of drugs has been recognized and this condition should be considered in all patients presenting with otherwise unexplained renal failure. Presentation may be with acute, often oliguric renal failure or more commonly as chronic slowly progressive renal disease.

Table 9.13
Common causes of acute tubulointerstitial nephritis

Penicillins	Cephalosporins
Sulphonamides	Rifampicin
Non-steroidal anti-inflammatory drugs	Diuretics: frusemide, thiazides
Phenindione	Cimetidine
Allopurinol	Phenytoin

Table 9.14
Causes of chronic tubulointerstitial nephritis

Common	Uncommon
Chronic pyelonephritis	Alport's syndrome
Non-steroidal anti-inflammatory drugs	Balkan nephropathy
Diabetes	Irradiation
Sickle cell disease or trait	Sjögren's syndrome
Cadmium or lead intoxication	Hyperuricaemic nephropathy

Acute tubulointerstitial nephritis

Acute tubulointerstitial nephritis is most often due to a hypersensitivity reaction to drugs (Table 9.13), most commonly drugs of the penicillin family and non-steroidal anti-inflammatory drugs (NSAIDs). Patients present with fever, arthralgia, skin rashes and acute oliguric or non-oliguric renal failure. Many have eosinophilia and eosinophiluria. Renal biopsy shows an intense interstitial cellular infiltrate, often including eosinophils, with variable tubular necrosis.

Treatment involves withdrawal of offending drugs. High-dose steroid therapy (prednisolone 60 mg daily) is commonly given but its efficacy has not been proved. Patients may require dialysis for management of the acute renal failure. Most patients have good recovery of kidney function, but some may be left with significant interstitial fibrosis.

Chronic tubulointerstitial nephritis

The major causes of chronic tubulointerstitial nephritis are set out in Table 9.14. In many cases no cause is found.

The patient usually either presents with polyuria and nocturia, or is found to have proteinuria or uraemia. Proteinuria is usually slight (less than 1 g daily). Papillary necrosis with ischaemic damage to the papillae occurs in a number of interstitial nephritides, for example in analgesic abuse, diabetes mellitus, sickle cell disease or trait. The papillae can separate and be passed in the urine. Chronic tubulointerstitial nephritis may be associated with microscopic or overt haematuria or sterile pyuria, and occasionally a sloughed papilla may cause ureteral colic or produce acute ureterial obstruction. The radiological appearances must be distinguished from those of chronic pyelonephritis (Fig 9.25).

Tubular damage to the medullary area of the kidney leads to defects in urine concentration and sodium conservation with polyuria and salt wasting. Fibrosis progressing into the cortex leads to loss of excretory function and uraemia.

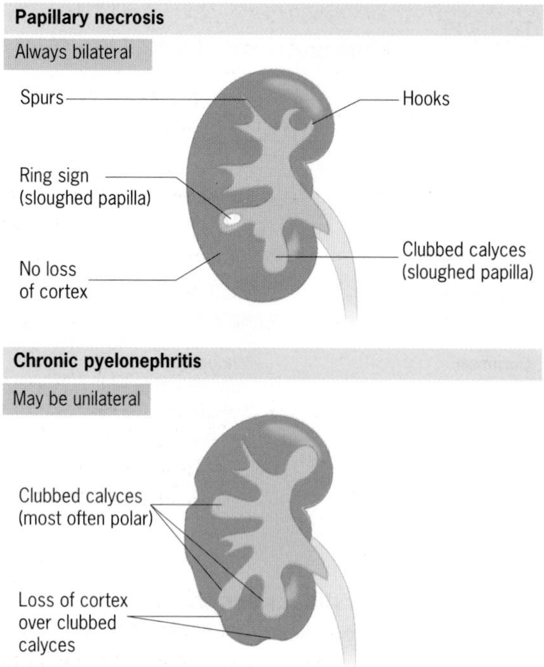

Fig 9.25
A comparison of radiological appearances of papillary necrosis and chronic pyelonephritis

Analgesic nephropathy

The chronic consumption of *large* amounts of analgesics (especially those containing phenacetin) leads to chronic tubulointerstitial nephritis and papillary necrosis. This also seems to be true of NSAIDS. In Australia, the incidence of end-stage renal failure due to analgesic nephropathy has declined as 'over-the-counter' purchase of nephrotoxic analgesics has been reduced by legislation.

CLINICAL FEATURES

Analgesic nephropathy is twice as common in women as in men and presents typically in middle-age. Patients are often depressed or neurotic. Presentation may be with anaemia, chronic renal failure, symptoms of urinary infection (which may be difficult to eradicate), haematuria, or urinary tract obstruction (owing to sloughing of a renal papilla). Salt and water-wasting renal disease may occur.

Chronic analgesic abuse also predisposes to the development of uroepithelial tumours.

MANAGEMENT

The consumption of analgesics should be discouraged. If necessary, dihydrocodeine or paracetamol are reasonable alternative choices. This may result in the arrest of the disease and even in improvement in function.

UTI, hypertension (if present) and saline depletion will require appropriate management.

The development of flank pain or an unexpectedly rapid deterioration in renal function should prompt ultrasonography or urography to screen for urinary tract obstruction due to a sloughed papilla.

Balkan nephropathy

This is a chronic tubulointerstitial nephritis endemic in areas along the tributaries of the River Danube. Inhabitants of the low-lying plains which are subjected to frequent flooding and where the water supply comes from shallow wells are affected, whereas the disease does not occur in hillside villages where surface water provides the water supply.

Its cause is unknown. The disease is insidious in onset, with mild proteinuria progressing to renal failure in three months to 10 years. Patients exhibit a high incidence of uroepithelial tumours. There is no treatment.

Other forms of chronic tubulointerstitial nephritis

These are rare (see Table 9.14). Diagnosis of all forms depends on a careful history being taken, with special attention to drug-taking and industrial exposure to nephrotoxins. In patients with unexplained renal impairment with normal-sized kidneys, renal biopsy must always be undertaken to exclude a treatable interstitial nephritis.

Hyperuricaemic (gouty) nephropathy

Three patterns of renal disease have been described in patients with hyperuricaemia or hyperuricosuria:

- gouty or chronic hyperuricaemic nephropathy
- acute hyperuricaemic nephropathy
- uric acid stone formation (see p. 560).

Chronic hyperuricaemic nephropathy

In severe chronic tophaceous gout, tubulointerstitial nephritis was seen. However there is considerable controversy as to the role of chronic hyperuricaemia causing progressive renal damage. While uric acid 'tophi' may be found in the kidneys of patients with gout, there is no convincing evidence that chronic hyperuricaemia per se causes progressive renal failure, nor that allopurinol treatment improves renal function (see p. 485). There is one important exception: a rare form of familial hyperuricaemia and gout occurring in adolescence is associated with renal impairment and allopurinol therapy both improves and protects kidney function.

Acute hyperuricaemic nephropathy

This is a well-recognized cause of acute renal failure in patients with marked hyperuricaemia that is due to lymphoproliferative or myeloproliferative disorders. It may occur prior to treatment but most often follows on commencement of treatment, when there is rapid lysis of malignant cells, release of large amounts of nucleoprotein and increased uric acid production. Renal failure is due to intrarenal and extrarenal obstruction caused by deposition of uric acid crystals in the collecting ducts, pelvis and ureters. The condition is manifest as oliguria or anuria with increasing uraemia. There may be flank pain or colic. Plasma urate levels are above 0.75 mmol L^{-1} and may be as high as 4.5 mmol L^{-1}. Diagnosis is based on the hyperuricaemia and the clinical setting. Ultrasound may demonstrate extrarenal obstruction due to stones, but a negative scan does not exclude this where there is coexistent intrarenal obstruction.

PREVENTION

Allopurinol 100–200 mg thrice daily for five days is given prior to and continuing throughout treatment with radiotherapy or cytotoxic drugs. A high rate of urine flow must be maintained by oral or parenteral fluid and the urine kept alkaline by the administration of sodium bicarbonate 600 mg four times daily and acetazolamide 250 mg thrice daily, since uric acid is more soluble in an alkaline than an acid medium.

TREATMENT

Allopurinol treatment should be commenced immediately and a forced alkaline diuresis attempted with intravenous 1.26% sodium bicarbonate plus acetazolamide (500 mg orally, then 250 mg thrice daily). In severely oliguric or anuric patients, dialysis is required to lower the plasma urate, which allows urate to diffuse out of the obstructed collecting ducts into the peritubular capillaries. Percutaneous nephrostomy (see p. 529) may be required to relieve extrarenal obstruction caused by stones in the pelvis or ureters. Such stones may subsequently be passed spontaneously or may require surgical removal (p. 559).

FURTHER READING

Nickeleit V, Mihatsch MJ (1997) Uric acid nephropathy and end-stage renal disease: review of a non-disease. *Nephrology Dialysis and Transplantation* **12**: 1832–1838.

Hypertension and the kidney

Hypertension can be the cause or the result of renal disease. It is often difficult to differentiate between the two on clinical grounds. Routine tests as described on p. 732 should be performed on all patients, but IVU is usually unnecessary. A guide to which patients should be fully investigated is given on p. 953.

Essential hypertension

PATHOPHYSIOLOGY

In *benign essential hypertension*, arteriosclerosis of major renal arteries and changes in the intrarenal vasculature (nephrosclerosis) occur as follows:

- *In small vessels and arterioles*, intimal thickening with reduplication of the internal elastic lamina occurs and the vessel wall becomes hyalinized.
- *In large vessels*, concentric reduplication of the internal elastic lamina and endothelial proliferation produce an 'onion skin' appearance.
- *Reduction in size of both kidneys* may occur; this may be asymmetrical if one major renal artery is more affected than the other.
- *The proportion of sclerotic glomeruli is increased* compared with age-matched controls.

Deterioration in excretory function accompanies these changes, but severe renal failure is unusual in Whites. In Afro-Caribbeans, by contrast, such hypertension much more often results in the development of renal failure.

In *accelerated*, or *malignant phase hypertension*:

- *Arteriolar fibrinoid necrosis* occurs, probably as a result of plasma entering the media of the vessel through splits in the intima.
- *Fibrinoid necrosis* in afferent glomerular arterioles is a prominent feature.
- *Fibrin deposition* within small vessels is often associated with thrombocytopenia and red-cell fragmentation seen in the peripheral blood film (microangiopathic haemolytic anaemia).

Microscopic haematuria, proteinuria, usually of modest degree (1–3 g daily), and progressive uraemia occur. If untreated, fewer than 10% of patients survive two years.

MANAGEMENT

The management of benign essential and malignant hypertension is described on p. 733.

If treatment is begun before renal impairment has occurred, the prognosis for renal function is good. Stabilization or improvement in renal function with healing of intrarenal arteriolar lesions and resolution of microangiopathic haemolysis occur with effective treatment of malignant-phase hypertension. Lifelong follow-up of the patient is mandatory.

Renal hypertension

Bilateral renal disease

Hypertension commonly complicates bilateral renal disease such as chronic glomerulonephritis, bilateral reflux nephropathy (chronic atrophic pyelonephritis of childhood), polycystic disease and analgesic nephropathy. Two main mechanisms are responsible:

- activation of the renin–angiotensin–aldosterone system
- retention of salt and water due to impairment in excretory function leading to an increase in blood volume and hence blood pressure.

The second of these assumes greater importance as renal function deteriorates.

Hypertension occurs earlier, is more common and tends to be more severe in patients with renal cortical disorders, such as glomerulonephritis, than in those with disorders affecting primarily the renal interstitium, such as reflux or analgesic nephropathy.

Management is described on p. 733. Meticulous control of the blood pressure is necessary to prevent further deterioration of renal function secondary to vascular changes produced by the hypertension itself. There is good evidence that ACE-inhibitor drug treatment confers an additional reno-protective effect for a given degree of blood pressure control than other hypotensive drugs.

Unilateral renal disease

A small proportion of cases of hypertension are due to unilateral renal disease. The main causes are:

- *unilateral renal artery stenosis* due to fibromuscular hyperplasia (typically in young women) or atheroma in the elderly
- *unilateral reflux nephropathy* (atrophic pyelonephritis).

Mechanism of hypertension

Unilateral renal ischaemia results in a reduction in the pressure in afferent glomerular arterioles. This leads to an increase in the production and release of renin from the juxtaglomerular apparatus (see p. 954) with a consequent increase in angiotensin II.

Physiological changes in renal artery stenosis

In unilateral renal artery stenosis, renal perfusion pressure is reduced and nephron transit time is prolonged on the side of the stenosis; salt and water reabsorption is therefore increased. As a result, urine from the ischaemic kidney is more concentrated but has a lower sodium concentration than urine from the contralateral kidney. Inulin, creatinine and *p*-aminohippuric acid (PAH) clearances are decreased on the ischaemic side.

Screening for unilateral renovascular disease

Intravenous urography. Contrast medium injected intravenously is filtered at the glomerulus more slowly and concentrated within the nephron to a greater extent on the side of the stenosis. Rapid-sequence films taken after injection of contrast may show a small kidney and a delayed and denser pyelogram on the side of the stenosis.

Rapid-sequence intravenous urography, with pictures taken at one-minute intervals for five minutes after contrast injection, has been the traditional screening test for unilateral renovascular disease causing hypertension. The method has a sensitivity of 80% and a specificity of 85% for unilateral renal disease. Increasingly, this method is replaced by radionuclide studies, although the question as to whether these offer superior sensitivity and specificity remains controversial.

Radionuclide studies (see p. 529). Studies using labelled DTPA can demonstrate decreased renal perfusion on the affected side. In unilateral renal artery stenosis, a disproportionate fall in uptake of isotope on the affected side following administration of an ACE inhibitor such as captopril has been claimed to be a useful screening test for significant renal artery stenosis. The value of this investigation has recently been called into question.

Divided renal function studies. These involve ureteric catheterization and are seldom used.

Magnetic resonance imaging. MRI can be used to visualize the renal arteries and a good – though not perfect – correlation between MRI findings and those of renal arteriography has been reported in several studies.

'Spiral' CT scanning. This appears to be a promising alternative to MRI in non-invasive imaging of the renal arteries. It is much less expensive than MRI but does expose the patient to ionizing radiation and to contrast injection.

Renal arteriography (see page 529). This is invasive and requires cannulation of the femoral artery. It involves the injection of contrast medium with the associated risk of contrast-induced kidney damage as well as cholesterol embolization (see p. 555). However, it remains the 'gold standard' investigation.

TREATMENT

Surgical options in renal artery stenosis include transluminal angioplasty to dilate the stenotic region, insertion of stents across the stenosis (sometimes the only endoscopic option when the stenosis occurs close to the origin of the renal artery from the aorta, rendering angioplasty technically difficult or impossible), reconstructive vascular surgery and nephrectomy. With good selection of patients, more than 50% are cured or improved by intervention. In recent years, increasing interest has focused upon the diagnosis and correction of unilateral and bilateral renal arterial disease with a view to improving renal perfusion and excretory function rather than to correcting hypertension alone. Occasional dramatic improvement in renal function ensues but results are generally disappointing. No test can predict the results of vascular surgery and many patients will do well on hypotensive therapy with or without surgery. ACE inhibitors must be avoided as they can lead to acute renal failure in the presence of renal artery stenoses.

Unilateral atrophic pyelonephritis

In this condition, prediction of the outcome after nephrectomy is currently not possible. The case for nephrectomy is strengthened if isotope renography demonstrates the abnormal kidney to be making an insignificant contribution to overall excretory function, particularly if the patient is young and medical treatment has proved unsatisfactory. About one-third of patients with unilateral atrophic pyelonephritis benefit from nephrectomy.

FURTHER READING

Lewis EJ, Hunsicker LG, Bain RP, Rohde RD (1993) The effect of angiotensin-converting enzyme inhibition on diabetic nephropathy. *New England Journal of Medicine* **329**: 1456–1462.

Raine AEG (1996) Hypertension: its effects on the kidney. *Oxford Textbook of Medicine*. Oxford: Oxford University Press, 3247–3250.

Other vascular disorders of the kidney

Renal artery occlusion

This occurs from thrombosis *in situ* usually in a severely damaged atherosclerotic vessel or more commonly from embolization. Both lead to renal infarction, resulting in a wide spectrum of clinical manifestations depending on the size of the artery involved. Occlusion of a small branch artery may produce no effect, but occlusion of larger vessels results in dull flank pain and varying degrees of renal failure.

Embolization may occur from the heart (e.g. in atrial fibrillation).

Cholesterol embolization

Currently this condition is much underdiagnosed. Showers of cholesterol-rich atheromatous material from ulcerated plaques may reach the kidney from the aorta and/or renal arteries, particularly after catheterization of the abdominal aorta or attempts at renal artery angioplasty. Anticoagulants and thrombolytic agents may also precipitate cholesterol embolization. Renal failure from cholesterol emboli may be acute or slowly progressive. Clinical features include fever, eosinophilia, back and abdominal pain, and evidence of embolization elsewhere, for example to the retina or digits. The diagnosis can be confirmed by renal biopsy.

Renal vein thrombosis

This is usually of insidious onset, occurring in the nephrotic syndrome, with a renal cell carcinoma, and in conditions associated with an increased risk of venous thrombosis (e.g. antithrombin deficiency or the presence of anticardiolipin antibodies).

FURTHER READING

Scoble JE (1997) Atherosclerosis and the kidney. *Journal of the Royal College of Physicians* **31**: 19–22.

Calculi and nephrocalcinosis

Renal and vesical calculi

Approximately 2% of the population in the UK have a urinary tract stone at any given time. A much higher prevalence of stone disease has been recorded elsewhere, notably in the Middle East. In the West, most stones occur in the upper urinary tract. The incidence of bladder stones has declined in the UK since the eighteenth and nineteenth centuries, whereas in some developing countries they are still common.

Most stones are composed of calcium oxalate and phosphate; these are more common in men (Table 9.15). Mixed infective stones, which account for about 20% of all calculi, are twice as common in women as in men. The overall male:female ratio of stone disease is 2:1.

Stone disease is frequently a recurrent problem. More than 50% of patients with a calculus will have formed a further stone or stones within 10 years. The risk of recurrence increases if a metabolic or other abnormality predisposing to stone formation is present and is not modified by treatment.

AETIOLOGY

It is in a sense surprising that stones are not universal, since some constituents of urine are at times present in

Table 9.15
Type and frequency of renal stones

Type of renal stone	Approximate frequency (%)
Calcium oxalate	65
Calcium phosphate	15
Magnesium ammonium phosphate	10–15
Uric acid	3–5
Cystine	1–2

Table 9.16
Causes of urinary tract stone formation

Dehydration	Infection
Hypercalcaemia	Cystinuria
Hypercalciuria	Renal tubular acidosis
Hyperoxaluria	Primary renal disease (polycystic kidneys, medullary sponge kidneys)
Hyperuricaemia and hyperuricosuria	

concentrations that exceed their maximum solubility in water. The presence of inhibitors of crystal formation in normal urine appears to be of importance in preventing stones.

Many stone-formers have no detectable metabolic defect, although microscopy of warm, freshly passed urine reveals both more and larger calcium oxalate crystals than are found in normal subjects. Factors predisposing to stone formation in these so-called 'idiopathic stone-formers' are:

- chemical composition of urine that favours stone crystallization
- production of a concentrated urine as a consequence of dehydration associated with life in a hot climate or work in a hot environment
- impairment of (postulated but unidentified) inhibitors that prevent crystallization in normal urine.

Recognized causes of stone formation are listed in Table 9.16.

Hypercalcaemia

If the GFR is normal, hypercalcaemia almost invariably leads to hypercalciuria. The common causes of hypercalcaemia leading to stone formation are:

- primary hyperparathyroidism
- vitamin D ingestion
- sarcoidosis.

Of these, primary hyperparathyroidism (see p. 512) is the most common cause of stones.

Hypercalciuria

This is by far the most common metabolic abnormality detected in calcium stone-formers.

Approximately 8% of men excrete in excess of 7.5 mmol of calcium in 24 hours. Calcium stone formation is more common in this group, but as the majority of even these individuals do not form stones the definition of 'pathological' hypercalciuria is arbitrary. A reasonable definition is 24-hour calcium excretion of more than 7.5 mmol in male stone-formers and more than 6.25 mmol in female stone-formers.

The kidney is the major site for plasma calcium regulation. Approximately 90% of the ionized calcium filtered by the kidney is reabsorbed. Renal tubular reabsorption is a complex process influenced by many hormones, of which parathyroid hormone (PTH) plays the major role.

Approximately 65% of the filtered calcium is absorbed in the proximal convoluted tabule, 20% by the thick ascending limb of the loop of Henle, and 15% by the distal convoluted tubule and collecting ducts. The cells of the thick ascending limb express Ca^{2+} sensing receptors. A high luminal calcium concentration is 'sensed' by these receptors and this triggers a series of events leading to reduced calcium reabsorption; conversely a low luminal concentration leads to avid calcium reabsorption and hypocalciuria.

Causes of hypercalciuria are:

- hypercalcaemia
- an excessive dietary intake of calcium
- excessive resorption of calcium from the skeleton, such as occurs with prolonged immobilization or weightlessness
- idiopathic hypercalciuria.
- There are two main causes of idiopathic hypercalciuria. The majority of patients with idiopathic hypercalciuria can be shown to have increased absorption of calcium from the gut. Dietary calcium restriction in this group markedly reduces urinary calcium excretion. A proportion of patients appear to have a renal tubular calcium leak with secondary compensatory hyperabsorption of calcium from the gut. Calcium restriction has less effect on urinary calcium excretion in this group.

Hyperoxaluria

Two inborn errors of glyoxalate metabolism that cause increased endogenous oxalate biosynthesis are known. Both are inherited in an autosomal recessive manner. In type I (primary hyperoxaluria) there is increased glycolate excretion as well as hyperoxaluria. In type II, L-glycerate excretion is increased. In both types, calcium oxalate stone formation occurs.

The prognosis is poor owing to widespread calcium oxalate crystal deposition in the kidneys. Renal failure typically develops in the late teens or early twenties. Successful liver transplantation has been shown to cure the metabolic defect in type I hyperoxaluria.

Much more common causes of mild hyperoxaluria are:

- excess ingestion of foodstuffs high in oxalate, such as spinach, rhubarb and tea
- dietary calcium restriction, with compensatory increased absorption of oxalate
- gastrointestinal disease (e.g. Crohn's), usually with an intestinal resection, associated with increased absorption of oxalate from the colon.

Dehydration secondary to fluid loss from the gut also plays a part in stone formation.

Hyperuricaemia and hyperuricosuria

Uric acid stones account for 3–5% of all stones in the UK, but in Israel the proportion is as high as 40%.

Uric acid is the end-point of purine metabolism. Hyperuricaemia (see p. 482) can occur as a primary defect in idiopathic gout, and as a secondary consequence of increased cell turnover, for example in myeloproliferative disorders. Increased uric acid excretion occurs in these conditions, and stones will develop in some patients. Some uric acid stone-formers have hyperuricosuria (>4 mmol per 24 hours on a low purine diet) without hyperuricaemia.

Dehydration alone may also cause uric acid stones to form. Patients with ileostomies are at particular risk both from dehydration and from the fact that loss of bicarbonate from gastrointestinal secretions results in the production of an acid urine (uric acid is more soluble in an alkaline than an acid medium).

Some patients with calcium stones also have hyperuricaemia and/or hyperuricosuria; it is believed the calcium salts precipitate upon an initial nidus of uric acid in such patients.

Urinary tract infection

Mixed infective stones are composed of magnesium ammonium phosphate together with variable amounts of calcium. Such stones are often large, forming a cast of the collecting system (staghorn calculus). They are believed to form as a result of infection of the urinary tract with organisms such as *Proteus mirabilis* that hydrolyse urea, with formation of the strong base ammonium hydroxide:

$$\left.\begin{array}{l}NH_2\\NH_2\end{array}\right\rangle C{=}O + HOH \rightleftharpoons 2NH_3 + CO_2$$

$$NH_3 + HOH \rightleftharpoons NH_4OH \rightleftharpoons NH_4^+ + OH^-$$

The availability of ammonium ions and the alkalinity of the urine favour stone formation. An increased amount of mucoprotein resulting from infection also creates an organic matrix on which stone formation can occur.

Cystinuria (see also p. 1000)

Cystinuria results in the formation of cystine stones. About 1–2% of all stones are composed of cystine.

Primary renal diseases

There is a moderate increase in prevalence of stone disease in patients with polycystic renal disease (see p. 588).

Medullary sponge kidney is another primary renal disorder associated with stones. In this congenital (though not inherited) condition there is dilatation of the collecting ducts with associated stasis and calcification (Fig 9.26). Approximately 20% of these patients have hypercalciuria and a similar proportion have a renal tubular acidification defect.

The *renal tubular acidoses*, both inherited and acquired, are associated with nephrocalcinosis and stone formation, owing, in part at least, to the production of a persistently alkaline urine and reduced urinary citrate excretion.

Aetiology of bladder stones

Bladder stones are endemic in some developing countries. The cause of this is unknown but dietary factors are probably important. Stones forming in the bladder do so as a result of:

- bladder outflow obstruction (e.g. urethral stricture, neuropathic bladder, prostatic obstruction)
- the presence of a foreign body (e.g. catheters, nonabsorbable sutures).

Significant bacteriuria is usually found in patients with bladder stones. Some stones found in the bladder have been passed down from the upper urinary tract.

PATHOLOGY

Stones may be single or multiple and vary enormously in size from minute, sand-like particles to staghorn calculi or large stone concretions in the bladder. They may be located within the renal parenchyma or within the collecting system. Pressure necrosis from a large calculus may cause direct damage to the renal parenchyma and stones regularly cause obstruction, leading to hydronephrosis. They may ulcerate through the wall of the collecting system,

Table 9.17
Clinical features of urinary tract stones

Asymptomatic
Pain: renal colic
Haematuria
Urinary tract infection
Urinary tract obstruction

(a) **(b)**

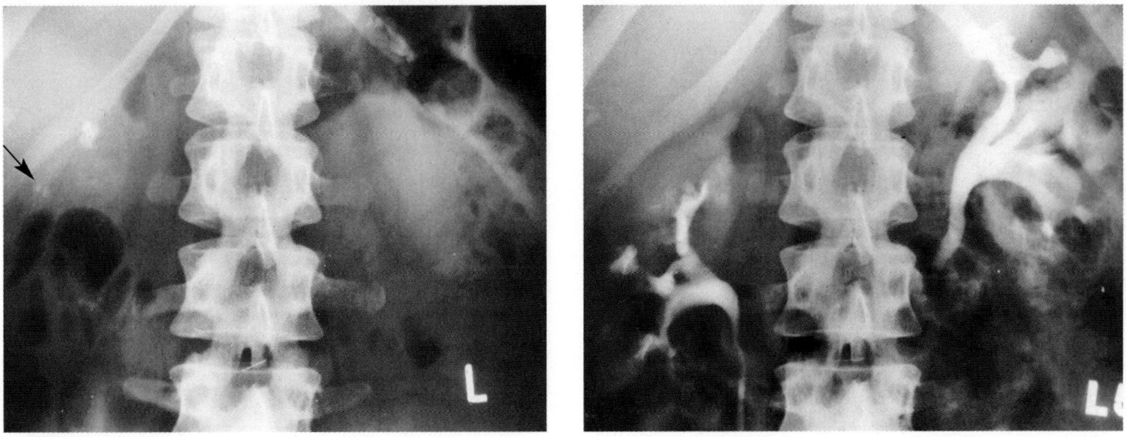

Fig 9.26
Medullary sponge kidney.
(a) Plain film showing 'spotty' calcification in the renal areas (arrow).
(b) After injection of contrast, the calcification is shown to be small calculi in the papillary zones

including the ureter. A combination of obstruction and infection accelerates damage to the kidney.

CLINICAL FEATURES

Most people with urinary tract calculi are asymptomatic. Pain is the most common symptom and may be sharp or dull, constant, intermittent or colicky (Table 9.17).

When urinary tract obstruction is present, measures that increase urine volume, such as copious fluid intake or diuretics, including alcohol, make the pain worse. Physical exertion may cause mobile calculi to move, precipitating pain and, occasionally, haematuria. Calyceal colic – pain resulting from movement of stones within the calyces – is a real entity, but whether small calyceal calculi are the cause of backache or not is often difficult to decide.

Ureteric colic occurs when a stone enters the ureter and either obstructs it or causes spasm during its passage down the ureter. This is one of the most severe pains known. Radiation from the flank to the iliac fossa and testis or labium in the distribution of the first lumbar nerve root is common. Pallor, sweating and vomiting often occur and the patient is restless, tending to assume a variety of positions in an unsuccessful attempt to obtain relief from the pain. Haematuria often occurs. Untreated, the pain of ureteric colic typically subsides after a few hours.

When urinary tract obstruction and infection are present, the features of acute pyelonephritis or of a Gram-negative septicaemia may dominate the clinical picture.

Vesical calculi associated with bladder bacteriuria may present with frequency, dysuria and haematuria; severe introital or perineal pain may occur if trigonitis is present. A calculus at the bladder neck or an obstruction in the urethra may cause bladder outflow obstruction, resulting in anuria and painful bladder distension.

Physical examination should include a search for corneal or conjunctival calcification, gouty tophi and arthritis and features of sarcoidosis.

INVESTIGATIONS AND DIAGNOSIS

A history of possible aetiological factors should be obtained, including:

- occupation and residence in hot countries likely to be associated with dehydration
- a history of vitamin D consumption
- gouty arthritis.

Calcified papillae may mimic ordinary calculi, so that causes of papillary necrosis such as analgesic abuse should be considered.

Investigations should include a mid-stream specimen of urine for culture and measurement of serum urea, electrolyte, creatinine and calcium levels.

Plain abdominal X-ray, and excretion urography are the mainstay of diagnosis. Renal tomography is still sometimes necessary. Ureteric stones can be missed by ultrasound.

Pure uric acid stones are radiolucent. Mixed infective stones in which organic matrix predominates are barely radiopaque. Calcium-containing and cystine stones are radiopaque. Calculi overlying bone are easily missed (Fig 9.27). Staghorn calculi may be missed if the plain abdominal X-ray carried out before contrast injection during urography is not inspected (Fig 9.28). Uric acid

(a) (b)

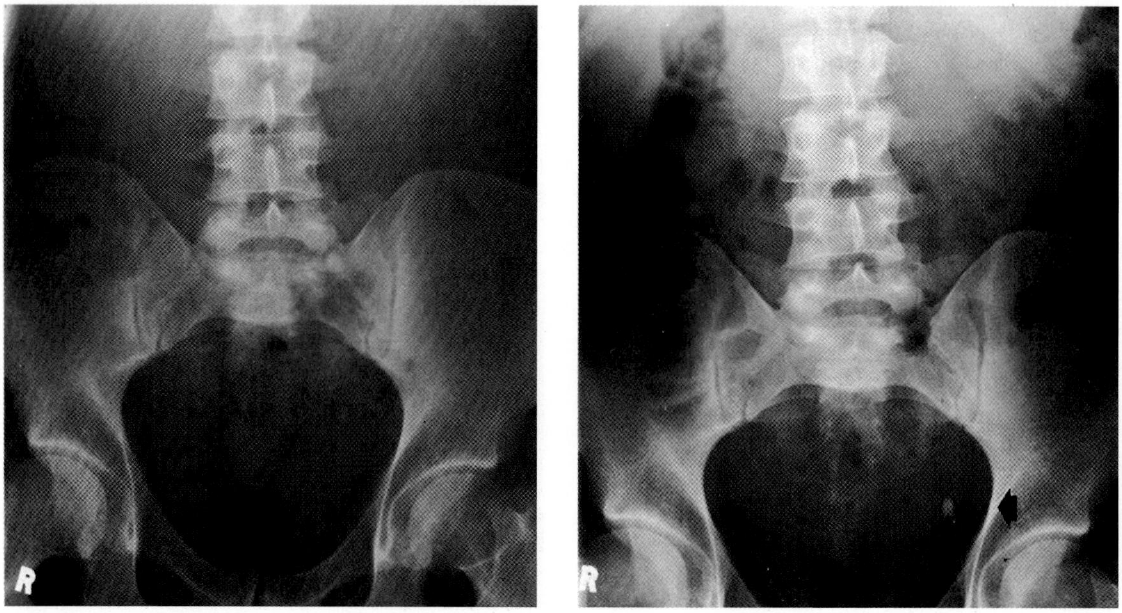

Fig 9.27
X-rays showing calculus.
(a) The calculus is overlying bone on the left (easily missed).
(b) The same patient one week later: the calculus has descended and is easily seen in the pelvis of the left side (arrow)

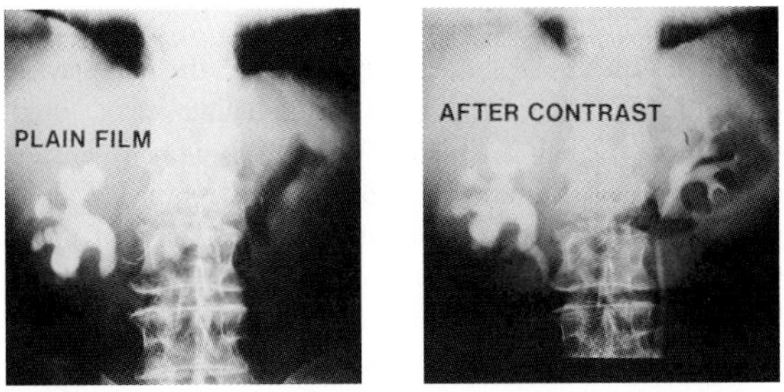

Fig 9.28
Staghorn calculus. X-ray appearances before and after contrast on the right side are identical owing to a staghorn calculus in a non-functioning right kidney. A plain film may be confused with those taken after contrast injection

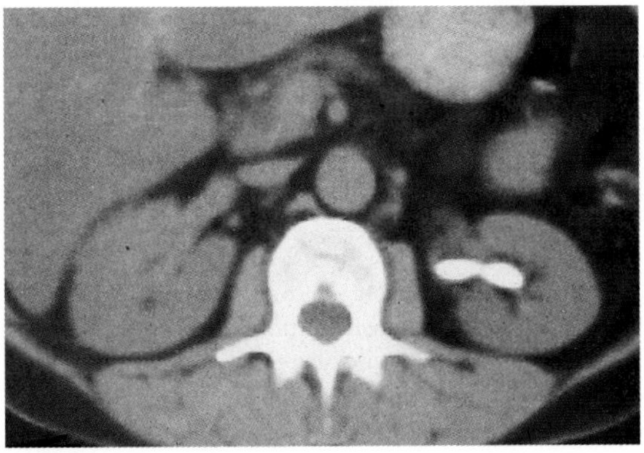

Fig 9.30
CT scan, showing a uric acid stone, which appears as a bright lesion in the left kidney

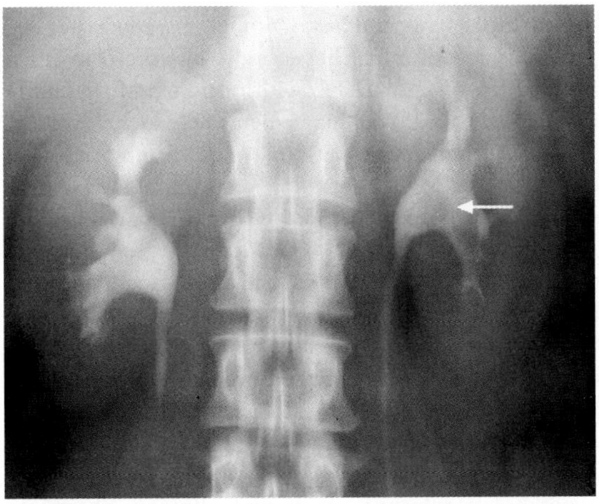

Fig 9.29
Excretion urogram, showing a lucent filling defect (uric acid stone, arrow) in the left renal pelvis. The differential diagnosis includes a sloughed papilla and a transitional cell tumour

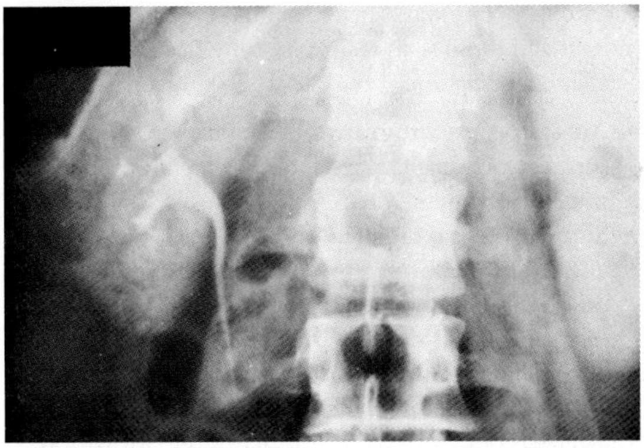

Fig 9.31
X-ray, showing acute left ureteric obstruction. Note the increased density of the nephrogram and the absence of a pyelogram on the left side 15 minutes after contrast injection. From Weatherall DJ, Ledingham JGG, Warrell DA (eds) (1987) *Oxford Textbook of Medicine*, 2nd edn. Oxford: Oxford University Press

stones may present as a filling defect after injection of contrast medium (Fig 9.29). Such stones are readily seen on CT scanning (Fig 9.30).

Excretion urography is carried out during the episode of pain; a normal urogram excludes the diagnosis of pain due to calculous disease. The urographic appearances in a patient with acute left ureteric obstruction are shown in Fig 9.31. The urine of the patient should be passed through a sieve to trap any calculi passed for chemical analysis.

MANAGEMENT

Adequate analgesia should be given, such as intravenous morphine 15–30 mg repeated as necessary. Alternatively an NSAID can be tried. A high fluid intake and, if feasible, increased physical activity are recommended but the efficacy of these measures is doubtful.

Stones less than 0.5 cm diameter usually pass spontaneously and can be left. Stones greater than 1 cm diameter usually require intervention.

Persistent pain, frequent bouts of severe pain, or anuria, are indications for further therapy. Intervention is also required if a stone is not moving though causing only partial obstruction in the absence of infection. With the advent of percutaneous surgery and extracorporeal shock-wave lithotripsy (see below) there has developed a trend towards earlier intervention in such cases. Complete obstruction or the coexistence of UTI with partial obstruction should prompt even earlier intervention owing to the increased risk of permanent kidney damage in these circumstances.

Cutting operations (nephrolithotomy for renal calculi, pyelolithotomy for stones in the renal pelvis, and ureterolithotomy for ureteric stones) can now be avoided by using either percutaneous nephrolithotomy or extra-corporeal shock-wave lithotripsy. In the former, stones in the calyces and renal pelvis are removed by creating a percutaneous track down to the collecting system followed by endoscopic removal along this track. In the latter, shock waves are focused upon the renal calculi, causing them to fragment. Most of the fragments then pass spontaneously via the urethra. Fragments that do not pass can be removed percutaneously.

Ureteric stones may be removed endoscopically or may be pushed up into the upper urinary tract, to allow percutaneous nephrolithotomy or extracorporeal shock-wave lithotripsy.

Large renal stones need to be reduced in bulk by percutaneous means before lithotripsy can be expected to be successful. Some staghorn calculi are best dealt with by open operation.

Bladder stones can be removed endoscopically. They may be dealt with by direct electrohydraulic disintegration at cystoscopy or may be gripped in a lithotrite and crushed, the stone fragments then being washed out. Open cystotomy is required for very large bladder stones.

INVESTIGATING THE CAUSE OF STONE FORMATION

In an elderly patient who has had a single episode with one stone, only limited investigation is required. Younger patients and those with recurrent stone formation require detailed investigation.

- **An excretion urogram** is necessary to define the presence of a primary renal disease predisposing to stone formation.
- **Significant bacteriuria** may indicate mixed infective stone formation, but relapsing bacteriuria may be a consquence of stone formation rather than the original cause.
- **Chemical analysis** of any stone passed may be of great value and may be all that is required to make a diagnosis of cystinuria or uric acid stone formation.
- **Serum calcium concentration** should be estimated and corrected for serum albumin concentration (see p. 505). Hypercalcaemia, if present, should be investigated further (see p. 514).
- **Serum urate concentration** is often, but not invariably, elevated in uric acid stone-formers.
- **A screening test for cystinuria** should be carried out by adding sodium nitroprusside to a random unacidified urine sample; a purple colour indicates that cystinuria may be present. Urine chromatography is required to define the diagnosis precisely.
- **Urinary calcium, oxalate and uric acid output** should be measured in two consecutive carefully collected 24-hour urine samples. After withdrawing aliquots for estimation of uric acid, it is necessary to add acid to the urine in order to prevent crystallization of calcium salts upon the walls of the collection vessel, which would give falsely low results for urinary calcium and oxalate.
- **Plasma bicarbonate** is low in renal tubular acidosis. The finding of a urine pH that does not fall below 5.5 in the face of metabolic acidosis is diagnostic of this condition (see p. 622).

PROPHYLAXIS

The age of the patient and the severity of the problem affect both the need for and the type of prophylaxis.

Idiopathic stone-formers

Where no metabolic abnormality is present, the mainstay of prevention is maintenance of a high intake of fluid throughout the day and night. The aim should be to ensure a daily urine volume of 2-2.5 L, which requires a fluid intake in excess of this, substantially so in the case of those who live in hot countries or work in a hot environment. It is helpful to advise the patient that if his or her urine is deep yellow, fluid intake is inadequate. A large glass of water should be drunk before retiring for the night and on waking during the night if this occurs. Special dietary measures are not warranted, although avoidance of excessive consumption of calcium-rich dairy products seems sensible.

Idiopathic hypercalciuria

Severe dietary calcium restriction is inappropriate (see p. 556). Intake of milk, cheese, and white bread if this is fortified (as it is in the UK) with calcium and vitamin D is reduced. Vitamin D supplements should be avoided. Dietary calcium restriction results in hyperabsorption of oxalate, and so foods containing large amounts of oxalate should also be limited. The advice of a dietitian is helpful. A high fluid intake should be advised as for idiopathic stone-formers. Patients who live in a hard-water area may benefit from drinking softened water.

If hypercalciuria persists and stone formation continues, a thiazide is used (e.g. bendrofluazide 2.5 or 5 mg each morning). Thiazides reduce urinary calcium excretion by a direct effect on the renal tubule. They may precipitate diabetes mellitus or gout and worsen hypercholesterolaemia. Sodium cellulose phosphate reduces calcium absorption from the gut but increases oxalate absorption, causes diarrhoea and has largely been abandoned. Avoidance of excessive sodium intake is also advisable as sodium and calcium excretion are linked.

Mixed infective stones

Recurrent stones should be prevented by maintenance of a high fluid intake and meticulous control of bacteriuria. This will require long-term follow-up and may demand the use of long-term low-dose prophylactic antibacterial agents.

Uric acid stones

Dietary measures are probably of little value and are difficult to implement. Effective prevention can be achieved by the long-term use of the xanthine oxidase inhibitor allopurinol to maintain the serum urate and urinary uric acid excretion in the normal range. A high fluid intake should also be maintained. Uric acid is more soluble at alkaline pH and long-term sodium bicarbonate supplementation to maintain an alkaline urine is an alternative approach in those few patients unable to take allopurinol. However, alkalinization of the urine facilitates precipitation of calcium oxalate and phosphate.

Cystine stones

These can be prevented and indeed will dissolve slowly if there is obsessional attention to maintenance of a high fluid intake – 5 L of water must be drunk each 24 hours, and the patient must wake twice during the night to ingest 500 mL or more of water. Many patients cannot tolerate this regimen. An alternative, though potentially more troublesome, option is the long-term use of the chelating agent penicillamine; this causes cystine to be converted to the more soluble penicillamine–cysteine complex. Side-effects include drug rashes, blood dyscrasias and immune complex-mediated glomerulonephritis and are by no means uncommon. In addition, the drug is expensive. It is, however, especially effective in promoting dissolution of cystine stones already present.

Mild hyperoxaluria with calcium oxalate stones

A high fluid intake and dietary oxalate restriction are required.

Nephrocalcinosis

The term 'nephrocalcinosis' means diffuse renal parenchymal calcification that is detectable radiologically (Fig 9.32). The condition is typically painless. Hypertension and renal impairment commonly occur. The main causes of nephrocalcinosis are listed in Table 9.18.

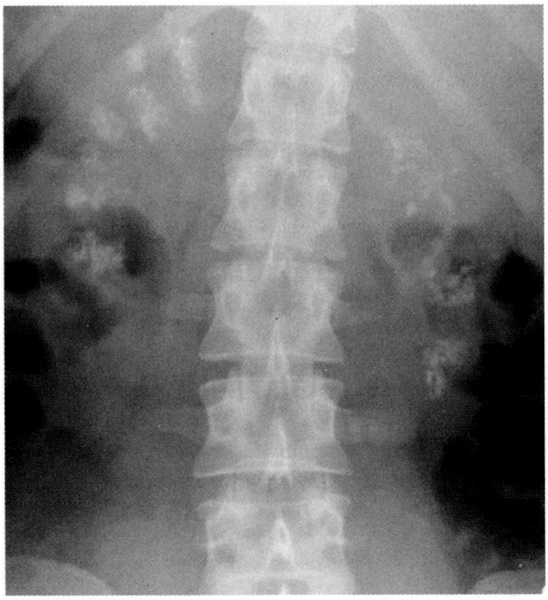

Fig 9.32
X-ray of nephrocalcinosis

Table 9.18
Common causes of nephrocalcinosis

Mainly cortical (rare)
Renal cortical necrosis (tram-line calcification)
Mainly medullary
Hypercalcaemia (primary hyperparathyroidism, hypervitaminosis D, sarcoidosis)
Renal tubular acidosis (inherited and acquired)
Primary hyperoxaluria
Medullary sponge kidney
Tuberculosis

Dystrophic calcification occurs following renal cortical necrosis. In hypercalcaemia and hyperoxaluria, deposition of calcium oxalate results from the high concentration of calcium and oxalate within the kidney.

In renal tubular acidosis (see p. 620) failure of urinary acidification and a reduction in urinary citrate excretion both favour calcium phosphate and oxalate precipitation, since precipitation occurs more readily in an alkaline medium and the calcium-chelating action of urinary citrate is reduced.

Treatment and prevention of nephrocalcinosis consists of treatment of the cause.

FURTHER READING

Coe FL, Parks JH, Asplin JR (1992) Medical progress: the pathogenesis and treatment of kidney stones. *New England Journal of Medicine* **327**: 1141–1152.

Danpure CJ (1994) Molecular and cell biology of primary hyperoxaluria type I. *Clinical Investigation* **72**: 725–727.

Wickhams JEA, Buck AC (1990) Renal tract stone: metabolic basis and clinical practice. Churchill Livingstone, Edinburgh.

Urinary tract obstruction

The urinary tract may be obstructed at any point between the kidney and the urethral meatus. This results in dilatation of the tract above the obstruction. Dilatation of the renal pelvis is known as *hydronephrosis*.

AETIOLOGY

Obstructing lesions may lie within the lumen, or in the wall of the urinary tract, or outside the wall, causing obstruction by external pressure. The major causes of obstruction are shown in Table 9.19. Overall the frequency is the same in men and women. However, in the elderly, urinary tract obstruction is more common in men owing to the frequency of bladder outflow obstruction.

PATHOPHYSIOLOGY

Obstruction with continuing urine formation results in:

- progressive rise in intraluminal pressure
- dilatation proximal to the site of obstruction
- compression and thinning of the renal parenchyma, eventually reducing it to a thin rim and resulting in a decrease in the size of the kidney.

CLINICAL FEATURES

Symptoms of upper tract obstruction

Loin pain occurs which can be dull or sharp, constant or intermittent. It may be provoked by measures that increase

Table 9.19
Causes of urinary tract obstruction

Within the lumen	Pressure from outside
Calculus	Pelviureteric compression (bands; aberrant vessels)
Blood clot	Tumours (e.g. retroperitoneal tumour or glands, carcinoma of colon)
Sloughed papilla (diabetes; analgesia abuse; sickle cell disease or trait)	Diverticulitis
Tumour of renal pelvis or ureter	Aortic aneurysm
Bladder tumour	Retroperitoneal fibrosis
Within the wall	Accidental ligation of ureter
Pelviureteric neuromuscular dysfunction (congenital, 10% bilateral)	Retrocaval ureter (right-sided obstruction)
Ureteric stricture (tuberculosis, especially after treatment; calculus; after surgery)	Prostatic obstruction
Ureterovesical stricture (congenital; ureterocele; calculus; schistosomiasis)	Tumours in pelvis (e.g. carcinoma of cervix)
Congenital megaureter	Phimosis
Congenital bladder neck obstruction	
Neuropathic bladder	
Urethral stricture (calculus; gonococcal; after instrumentation)	
Congenital urethral valve	
Pin-hole meatus	

urine volume and hence distension of the collecting system, such as a high fluid intake or diuretics, including alcohol.

Complete anuria is strongly suggestive of complete bilateral obstruction or complete obstruction of a single kidney.

Conversely, polyuria may occur in partial obstruction owing to impairment of renal tubular concentrating capacity. Intermittent anuria and polyuria indicates intermittent complete obstruction.

Infection complicating the obstruction may give rise to malaise, fever and septicaemia.

Symptoms of bladder outflow obstruction

Symptoms may be minimal. Hesitancy, narrowing and diminished force of the urinary stream, terminal dribbling and a sense of incomplete bladder emptying are typical features. The frequent passage of small volumes of urine occurs if a large volume of residual urine remains in the bladder after urination. Incontinence of such small volumes of urine is known as 'overflow incontinence' or 'retention with overflow'.

Infection commonly occurs, causing increased frequency, urgency, urge incontinence, dysuria and the passage of cloudy smelly urine. It may precipitate acute retention.

Signs

Loin tenderness may be present. An enlarged hydronephrotic kidney may be palpable. In acute or chronic retention the enlarged bladder may be felt or percussed.

Examination of the genitalia, rectum and vagina are essential, since prostatic obstruction and pelvic malignancy are common causes of urinary tract obstruction. However, the apparent size of the prostate on digital examination is a poor guide to the presence of prostatic obstruction.

INVESTIGATIONS

Routine blood and biochemical investigations may be abnormal; for example, there may be a raised serum urea or creatinine, hyperkalaemia, anaemia of chronic disease or blood in the urine. Nevertheless, the diagnosis of obstruction cannot be made on these tests alone and further investigations must be performed.

Ultrasonography (see p. 528)

This is a reliable means of ruling out upper urinary tract dilatation. Ultrasound cannot distinguish a baggy, low-pressure unobstructed system from a tense, high-pressure obstructed one, so that false-positive scans are seen. However, in the hands of an experienced observer, a normal scan does rule out urinary tract obstruction, except in very rare circumstances such as, for example, encasement of the kidney by fibrous or malignant tissue.

Radionuclide studies (see p. 529)

In obstructive nephropathy, the relative uptake may be normal or reduced on the side of obstruction, peak activity may be delayed, and parenchymal (as distinct from pelvic) transit time prolonged. If doubt exists as to whether obstruction at the pelviureteric junction is present, frusemide may be administered; satisfactory 'wash-out' of a radionuclide rules out obstruction, and vice versa. In general, absence of uptake of radiopharmaceuticals indicates renal damage sufficiently severe to render correction of obstruction unprofitable.

Excretion urography

This is the most widely used investigation. Urography can usually exclude obstruction even in the presence of severe renal failure, provided that a high dose of contrast medium, renal tomography and, if necessary, delayed films are employed.

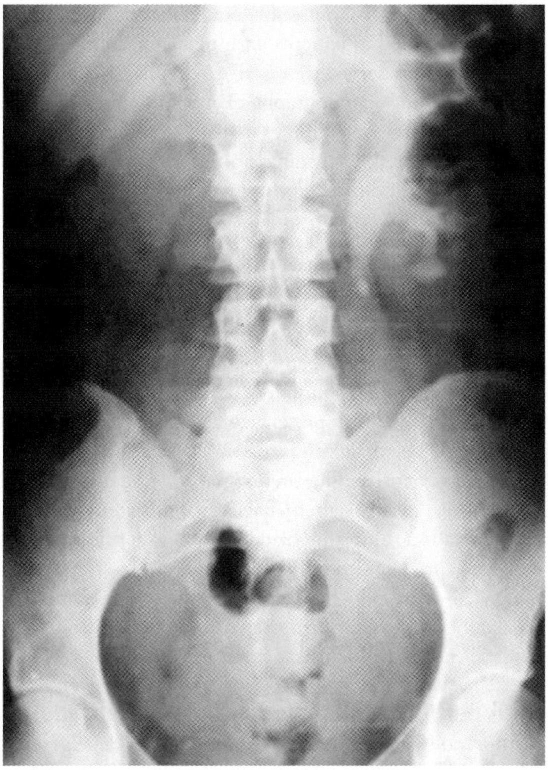

Fig 9.33
X-ray taken 24 hours after injection of contrast, showing a delayed nephrogram and pyelogram on the left side and dilatation of the system to the level of the block. By this time contrast medium has disappeared from the normal right side

A plain film is necessary to detect calcification. However, calculi overlying bone are easily missed.

In recent unilateral obstruction, the affected kidney is enlarged and smooth in outline. The nephrogram is delayed owing to a reduction in the GFR. The calyces and pelvis fill with contrast medium later than on the normal side.

In time the nephrogram on the affected side becomes denser than normal, owing to the prolonged nephron transit time, which allows greater than normal concentration of contrast medium within the tubules. Later, the site of obstruction may be seen, with dilatation of the system proximal to the level of the block (Fig 9.33).

A full-length film should be taken after an attempt at bladder emptying by the patient. Complete emptying indicates either that no obstruction to bladder outflow exists or that intravesical pressure can be raised sufficiently to overcome it. Apparent bladder outflow impairment may be the result of nervousness or embarrassment on the part of the patient, or failure to carry out the X-ray before the bladder has refilled with contrast medium from above, or may be due to an atonic but non-obstructed bladder. Vesicoureteric reflux can result in contrast medium returning to the bladder from above, giving the appearance of a partially full bladder.

Antegrade pyelography and ureterography

(see p. 529)

This defines the site and cause of obstruction. It can be combined with drainage of the collecting system by percutaneous needle nephrostomy.

Retrograde ureterography (see p. 529)

This is indicated if antegrade examination cannot be carried out or if there is the possibility of dealing with ureteric obstruction from below at the time of examination. The technique carries the risk of introducing infection into an obstructed urinary tract.

In obstruction due to neuromuscular dysfunction at the pelviureteric junction or retroperitoneal fibrosis, the collecting system may fill normally from below.

Cystoscopy, urethroscopy and urethrography

Obstructing lesions within the bladder and urethra can be seen directly by endoscopic examination.

Urethrography involves introducing contrast medium into the bladder by catheterization or suprapubic bladder puncture, and taking X-ray films during voiding to show obstructing lesions in the urethra. It is of particular value in the diagnosis of urethral valves and strictures.

Pressure-flow studies

Pressure changes within the bladder during filling and emptying can be recorded. Demonstration that a high voiding pressure is required to maintain urine flow is indicative of bladder outflow obstruction. This may be combined with video cystography and urethrography to define the site of obstruction.

Normally, while the bladder is being filled there is only a small pressure rise before the voluntary initiation of urination. Uninhibited contractions of the detrusor muscle during filling may be seen in upper motor neurone bladder neuropathy, such as occurs in multiple sclerosis. Less commonly, a neuropathic bladder may be 'hypotonic', readily accepting large volumes of fluid before the initiation of weak contractions at a low intravesical pressure. A common cause of such lower motor neurone bladder neuropathy is diabetes mellitus.

Pressure-flow and video studies may enable a logical decision to be taken as to whether surgery to relieve bladder outflow impairment should be carried out.

TREATMENT

Aims

Treatment involves:

- relieving the obstruction
- treating the underlying cause
- preventing and treating infection.

The ultimate aim of treatment is to relieve symptoms and to preserve renal function.

Temporary external drainage of urine by nephrostomy may be valuable, as this allows time for further investigation when the site and nature of the obstructing lesion is uncertain, doubt exists as to the viability of the obstructed kidney, or when immediate definitive surgery would be hazardous.

Recent, complete upper urinary tract obstruction demands urgent relief to preserve kidney function, particularly if infection is present.

In contrast, with partial urinary tract obstruction, particularly if spontaneous relief is expected – such as by passage of a calculus – there is no immediate urgency.

Surgical management

This depends on the cause of the obstruction (see below). Dialysis may be required in the ill patient prior to surgery.

Nephrectomy or nephroureterectomy is justified when obstruction is due to malignant disease or when it is judged that no worthwhile amount of renal excretory function will be conserved by, or will return after, relief of obstruction.

Permanent urinary diversion is required when the obstruction cannot be relieved; in such cases malignant disease is usually present. Ureteric anastomosis to an ileal conduit opening on to the abdominal wall is often a satisfactory method of diversion. In some patients, obstruction is best relieved by the insertion of indwelling catheters or stents into the ureter. An obstruction high in the urinary tract may require a permanent nephrostomy.

In obstruction due to untreatable malignant disease it is wise to consider carefully whether urinary diversion or stent insertion is justified, since this may exchange a pain-free death from renal failure for a painful one with malignant invasion of bones or nerves.

Diuresis usually follows relief of obstruction at any site in the urinary tract. Massive diuresis may occur following relief of bilateral obstruction owing to previous sodium and water overload and the osmotic effect of retained solutes combined with a defective renal tubular reabsorptive capacity (as in the diuretic phase of recovering acute tubular necrosis). This diuresis is associated with increased blood volume and high levels of atrial natriuretic peptide (ANP). Defective renal tubular reabsorptive capacity cannot be the sole mechanism of severe diuresis since this phenomenon is not observed following relief of unilateral obstruction. The diuresis is usually self-limiting, but a minority of patients will develop severe sodium, water and potassium depletion requiring appropriate intravenous replacement. In milder cases oral salt and potassium supplements together with a high water intake are sufficient.

Specific causes of obstruction

Calculi

These are discussed on p. 558.

Pelviureteric junction obstruction (Fig 9.34)

This appears to result from a functional disturbance in peri-stalsis of the collecting system in the absence of mechanical obstruction. Surgical attempts at correction of the obstruction by open or percutaneous pyeloplasty should be limited to patients with recurrent loin pain and those in whom serial excretion urography, background-subtraction isotope renography or measurements of GFR indicate progressive kidney damage. Nephrectomy to remove the risk of developing pyonephrosis and septicaemia is indicated if longstanding obstruction has destroyed kidney function.

Obstructive megaureter

This childhood condition may become evident only in adult life. It results from the presence of a region of defective peristalsis at the lower end of the ureter adjacent to the ureterovesical junction. The condition is more common in males. It presents with UTI, flank pain or haematuria. The diagnosis is made on excretion urography or, if necessary, ascending ureterography.

Excision of the abnormal portion of ureter with reimplantation into the bladder is always indicated in children, and is indicated in adults when the condition is associated with evidence of progressive deterioration in renal function, bacteriuria that cannot be controlled by medical means, or recurrent stone formation.

Retroperitoneal fibrosis (chronic periaortitis)

In this condition the ureters become embedded in dense retroperitoneal fibrous tissue with resultant unilateral or

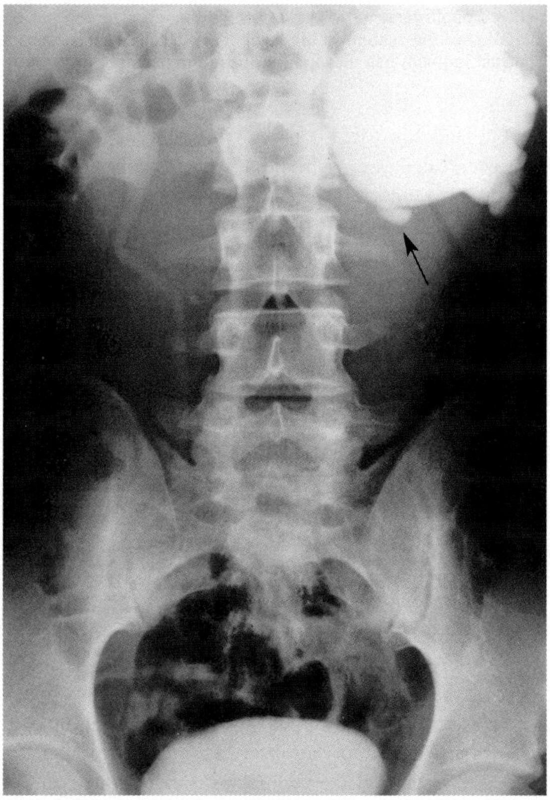

Fig 9.34
X-ray, showing left pelviureteric junction obstruction (arrow)

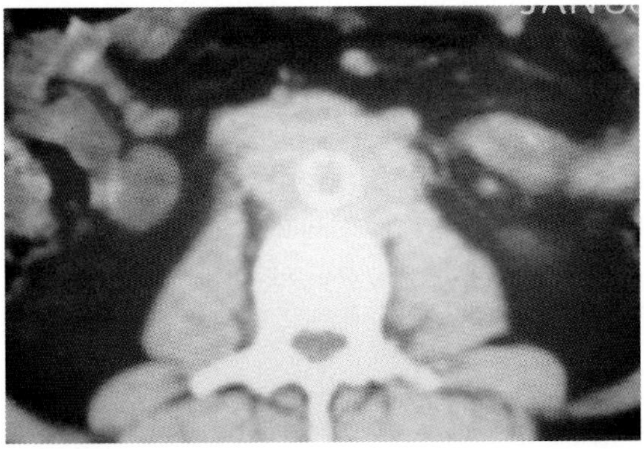

Fig 9.35
Retroperitoneal fibrosis (periaortitis). Note the large mass surrounding the abdominal aorta on this CT scan

bilateral obstruction. The condition may extend from the level of the second lumbar vertebra to the pelvic brim. The incidence of the condition in men is three times that in women. An autoallergic response to leakage of material, probably ceroid, derived from atheromatous plaques is considered to be the underlying cause of the condition. Recognized associations are with abdominal aortic aneurysm and prolonged exposure to the drug methysergide. The differential diagnosis includes retroperitoneal lymphoma or cancer.

Malaise, back pain, normochromic anaemia, uraemia and a raised erythrocyte sedimentation rate (ESR) are typical features. Excretion urography shows bilateral or unilateral ureteric obstruction commencing at the level of the pelvic brim. A periaortic mass may be seen on a CT scan (Fig 9.35).

Obstruction is relieved surgically by ureterolysis. Biopsy should be performed at operation to determine whether there is an underlying lymphoma or carcinoma. Corticosteroids are of benefit, and in bilateral obstruction in frail patients it may be best to free only one ureter and to rely upon steroid therapy to induce regression of fibrous tissue on the contralateral side, since bilateral ureterolysis is a major operation. In some patients, surgery alone or steroid therapy alone may suffice, but in the majority both surgery and subsequent corticosteroid therapy appear to be necessary. An alternative approach is to relieve obstruction by placement of a ureteric stent or stents, and to rely on corticosteroid therapy to induce regression of the periaortic mass, with later stent removal. A disadvantage is that an adequate biopsy of the mass – readily obtainable on open operation – is not easily obtained.

Response to treatment and disease activity are assessed by serial measurements of ESR and GFR supplemented by isotopic and imaging techniques including CT scanning. The latter method enables the size of the retroperitoneal mass to be assessed. Relapse after withdrawal of steroid therapy may occur and treatment may need to be continued for years. Long-term follow-up is mandatory.

Benign prostatic hypertrophy

Benign prostatic hypertrophy is a common cause of urinary tract obstruction. It is described on p. 592.

Prognosis of urinary tract obstruction

The prognosis depends upon the cause and the stage at which obstruction is relieved. In obstruction, four factors influence the rate at which kidney damage occurs, its extent and the degree and rapidity of recovery of renal function after relief of obstruction. These are:

- whether obstruction is partial or complete
- the duration of obstruction
- whether or not infection occurs
- the site of obstruction.

Complete obstruction for several weeks will lead to irreversible or only partially reversible kidney damage. If the duration of complete obstruction is several months, total irreversible destruction of the affected kidney will result. Partial obstruction carries a better prognosis, depending upon its severity.

Bacterial infection coincident with obstruction rapidly increases kidney damage.

Obstruction at or below the bladder neck may induce hypertrophy and trabeculation of the bladder without a rise in pressure within the upper urinary tract, in which case the kidneys are protected from the effects of back-pressure.

FURTHER READING

Baker LRI (1996) Urinary tract obstruction. In: Weatherall DJ, Ledingham JGG, Warrell DA (eds) Oxford Textbook of Medicine, p. 3232–3247.

Ormond JK (1988) Bilateral ureteral obstruction due to envelopment and compression by inflammatory process. *Journal of Urology* **59**: 1072–1079.

Parums DV, Mitchinson MJ (1990) Serum antibodies to oxidised LDL and ceroid in chronic periaortitis. *Archives of Pathology and Laboratory Medicine* **114**: 383–387.

Whitaker RH (1990) The diagnosis of upper urinary tract obstruction. *Postgraduate Medical Journal* **66** (Suppl 1): 25–30.

Drugs and the kidney

Drug-induced impairment of renal function

Prerenal

Impaired perfusion of the kidneys can result from drugs that cause:

- hypovolaemia – for example:

(a) potent loop diuretics such as frusemide, especially in elderly patients
(b) renal salt and water loss, such as from hypercalcaemia induced by vitamin D therapy (since hypercalcaemia adversely affects renal tubular salt and water conservation)

- decrease in cardiac output, which impairs renal perfusion (e.g. β-blockers)
- decreased renal blood flow (e.g. ACE inhibitors).

Renal

Several mechanisms of drug-induced renal damage exist and may coexist.

Acute tubular necrosis produced by direct nephrotoxicity. Examples include prolonged or excessive treatment with aminoglycosides (kanamycin, gentamicin, streptomycin), amphotericin B, cephaloridine, heavy metals or carbon tetrachloride. The combination of aminoglycosides or cephaloridine with frusemide is particularly nephrotoxic.

Acute tubulointerstitial nephritis (see p. 551) **with interstitial oedema and inflammmatory cell infiltration.** This cell-mediated hypersensitivity nephritis occurs with many drugs, including penicillins, particularly methicillin, sulphonamides and some NSAIDS.

Chronic tubulointerstitial nephritis due to drugs. See p. 552.

Immune complex-mediated glomerulonephritis. Examples include penicillamine.

Postrenal

Retroperitoneal fibrosis with urinary tract obstruction may result from the use of methysergide.

Use of drugs in patients with impaired renal function (Information box 9.1)

Many aspects of drug handling are altered in patients with renal impairment.

Absorption

This may be unpredictable in uraemia as nausea and vomiting are frequently present.

Metabolism

Oxidative metabolism of drugs by the liver may be altered in uraemia. This is rarely of clinical significance.

The rate of drug metabolism by the kidney may be reduced as a result of two factors:

- *Reduced drug catabolism.* Insulin, for example, is in part catabolized by the normal kidney. In renal disease, insulin catabolism is reduced. The insulin requirements of diabetics decline as renal function deteriorates for this reason.
- *Reduced conversion of a precursor to a more active metabolite,* such as the conversion of 25-hydroxycholecalciferol to the more active 1,25-$(OH)_2D_3$. The 1α-hydroxylase enzyme responsible for this conversion is located in the kidney. In renal disease, production of the enzyme declines and deficiency of 1,25-$(OH)_2D_3$ results.

Information

Safe prescribing in renal failure demands knowledge of the clinical pharmacology of the drug and its metabolites in normal individuals and in uraemia. The clinician should ask the following questions when prescribing:

1. Is treatment mandatory? Unless it is, it should be withheld.
2. Can the drug reach its site of action? For example, there is little point in prescribing the urinary antiseptic nitrofurantoin in renal failure since bacteriostatic concentrations will not be attained in the urine.
3. Is the drug's metabolism altered in uraemia?
4. Will accumulation of the drug or metabolites occur? Even if accumulation is a potential problem owing to the drug or its metabolites being excreted by the kidneys, it is not necessarily an indication to change the drug given. The size of the loading dose will depend upon the size of the patient and is unrelated to renal function.
   Avoidance of toxic levels of drug in blood and tissues subsequently requires the administration of normal doses of the drug at longer time intervals than usual or smaller doses at the usual time intervals.
5. Is the drug toxic?
6. Are the effective concentrations of the drug in biological tissues similar to the toxic concentrations? Should blood levels of the drug be measured?
8. Will the drug worsen the uraemic state by means other than nephrotoxicity, e.g. steroids, tetracycline?
9. Is the drug a sodium or potassium salt? These are potentially hazardous in uraemia.

Not suprisingly, adverse drug reactions are more than twice as common in renal failure as in normal individuals. Elderly patients, in whom unsuspected renal impairment is common, are particularly at risk. Careful attention to the above and careful titration of the dose of drugs employed should reduce this problem.

The dose may be titrated by:

- observation of its clinical effect, e.g. hypotensive agents
- early detection of toxic effects
- measurement of drug levels in the blood, e.g. gentamicin levels.

Information box 9.1 Safe prescribing in renal disease

Protein binding

Reduced protein binding of a drug potentiates its activity and increases the potential for toxic side-effects. Measurement of the total plasma concentration of such a drug can give misleading results. For example, the serum concentration of phenytoin required to produce an antiepileptic effect is much higher in normal individuals than in those with renal failure, since in the latter proportionately more drug is present in the free form.

Some patients with renal disease are hypoproteinaemic and reduced drug-binding to protein results. This is not the sole mechanism of reduced drug-binding in such patients. For example, hydrogen ions, which are retained in renal failure, bind to receptors for acidic drugs such as sulphonamides, penicillin and salicylates, thus enhancing their potential for causing toxicity.

Volume of distribution

Salt and water overload or depletion may occur in patients with renal disease. This affects the concentration of drug obtained from a given dose.

End-organ sensitivity

The renal response to drug treatment may be reduced in renal disease. For example, mild thiazide diuretics have little diuretic effect in patients with severe renal impairment.

Renal elimination

By far the most important problem in the use of drugs in renal failure concerns the reduced elimination of many drugs normally excreted by the kidneys.

Water-soluble drugs such as gentamicin that are poorly absorbed from the gut, typically given by injection and are not metabolized by the liver, give rise to far more problems than lipid-soluble drugs such as propranolol, which are well absorbed and principally metabolized by the liver. Metabolites of lipid-soluble drugs, however, may themselves be water-soluble and potentially toxic.

Drugs causing uraemia by effects upon protein anabolism and catabolism

Tetracyclines, with the exception of doxycycline, have a catabolic effect and as a result the concentration of nitrogenous waste products is increased. They may also cause impairment of GFR by a direct effect. Corticosteroids have a catabolic effect and so also increase the production of nitrogenous wastes. A patient with moderate impairment of renal function may therefore become severely uraemic if given tetracyclines or corticosteroid therapy.

Drugs and toxic agents causing specific renal tubular syndromes include mercury, lead, cadmium and vitamin D.

Problem patients

Particular problems are presented by patients in whom renal function is altering rapidly, such as those with recovering acute tubular necrosis. In addition, drugs may be removed by dialysis and haemofiltration, which will affect the dosage required.

FURTHER READING

British Medical Association and Royal Pharmaceutical Society of Great Britain (1996) Renal impairment. In: British National Formulary, 35th edn. Bath Press, bath, pp. 592–599.

Golper TA (1991) Drug removal during continuous hemofiltration or hemodialysis. *Contributions to Nephrology* **93**: 110–116.

Acute renal failure

The term 'renal failure' means failure of renal excretory function owing to depression of the glomerular filtration rate. This is accompanied to a variable extent by failure of erythropoietin production (see p. 523), vitamin D hydroxylation (p. 524), regulation of acid–base balance (p. 617), and regulation of salt and water balance and blood pressure (p. 523).

DEFINITION

Acute renal failure means abrupt deterioration in parenchymal renal function which is usually, but not invariably, reversible over a period of days or weeks. In clinical practice, such deterioration in renal function is sufficiently severe to result in uraemia. Oliguria is usually, but not invariably, a feature. Acute renal failure may cause sudden, life-threatening biochemical disturbances and is a medical emergency. The distinction between acute and chronic renal failure may not be readily apparent in a patient presenting with uraemia. Patients with chronic renal impairment are not immune from the development of a superimposed acute-on-chronic renal failure under appropriate circumstances.

Renal failure results in reduced excretion of nitrogenous waste products of which urea is the most commonly measured. A raised serum urea concentration (uraemia) may conveniently be classified as: (i) prerenal, (ii) renal or

Table 9.20 Causes of altered serum urea and creatinine concentration other than altered renal function

	Decreased concentration	Increased concentration
Urea	Low protein intake Liver failure Sodium valproate treatment	Corticosteroid treatment Tetracycline treatment Gastrointestinal bleeding
Creatinine	Low muscle mass	High muscle mass Red meat ingestion Muscle damage (rhabdomyolysis) Decreased tubular secretion (e.g. cimetidine, trimethoprim therapy)

(iii) postrenal. More than one category may be present in an individual patient. Other causes of altered serum urea and creatinine concentration are shown in Table 9.20.

Prerenal uraemia

In prerenal uraemia, there is impaired perfusion of the kidneys with blood. This results either from hypovolaemia, hypotension, impaired cardiac pump efficiency or vascular disease limiting renal blood flow, or combinations of these factors. Usually the kidney is able to maintain glomerular filtration close to normal despite wide variations in renal perfusion pressure and volume status – so-called 'autoregulation'. Further depression of renal perfusion leads to a drop in glomerular filtration and development of prerenal uraemia. Drugs which impair renal autoregulation, such as ACE inhibitors and NSAIDs, increase the tendency to develop prerenal uraemia. All causes of prerenal uraemia may lead to established parenchymal kidney damage and the development of acute renal failure. By definition, excretory function in prerenal uraemia improves once normal renal perfusion has been restored.

A number of criteria have been proposed to differentiate between prerenal and intrinsic renal causes of uraemia (Table 9.21).

- *Urine specific gravity and urine osmolality* are easily obtained measures of concentrating ability but are unreliable in the presence of glycosuria or other osmotically active substances in the urine.
- *Urine sodium* is low if there is avid tubular reabsorption, but may be increased by diuretics or dopamine.
- *Fractional excretion of sodium* (FE_{Na}), the ratio of sodium clearance to creatinine clearance, increases the reliability of this index but may remain low in some 'intrinsic' renal diseases, including contrast nephropathy and myoglobinuria.

Laboratory tests, however, are no substitute for careful clinical assessment. A history of blood or fluid loss, sepsis potentially leading to vasodilatation, or of cardiac disease may be helpful. Hypotension (especially postural), a weak rapid pulse, and low pressure in the great veins of the neck will suggest the possibility that uraemia may be prerenal. In doubtful cases, measurement of central venous pressure is often invaluable.

Table 9.21 Criteria for distinction between prerenal and intrinsic causes of renal dysfunction

	Prerenal	Intrinsic
Urine specific gravity	>1.020	<1.010
Urine osmolality (mOsmol L^{-1})	>500	<350
Urine sodium (mmol L^{-1})	<20	>40
FE_{Na} ($U_{Na} \cdot P_{Cr}/P_{Na} \cdot U_{Cr}$) × 100%	<1%	>1%

FE, fractional excretion; P, plasma; U, urine

MANAGEMENT

If the prerenal uraemia is a result of hypovolaemia and hypotension, prompt replacement with appropriate fluid is essential to correct the problem and prevent development of ischaemic renal injury and acute renal failure. Since prerenal and renal uraemia may coexist, and fluid challenge in the latter situation may lead to volume overload with pulmonary oedema, careful clinical monitoring is vital. Blood pressure should be checked regularly and signs of elevated jugular venous pressure and of pulmonary oedema sought frequently. Central venous pressure monitoring is usually advisable (see p. 839). If the problem relates to cardiac pump insufficiency or occlusion of the renal vasculature, appropriate measures – albeit often unsuccessful – need to be taken.

Postrenal uraemia

Here, uraemia results from obstruction of the urinary tract at any point from the calyces to the external urethral orifice. The causes and presentation of urinary tract obstruction are dealt with on p. 561. Screening for urinary tract obstruction is by renal ultrasonography. Urinary tract obstruction may present in an acute fashion (if obstruction of a single functioning kidney by, for example, a calculus occurs) but typically is of insidious onset.

Acute uraemia due to renal parenchymal disease

CAUSES

Most commonly, patients with acute renal failure are victims of acute renal tubular necrosis (vasomotor nephropathy). Other causes include disease affecting the intrarenal arteries and arterioles as well as glomerular capillaries, such as polyarteritis, Wegener's granulomatosis, accelerated hypertension, cholesterol embolism, haemolytic uraemic syndrome, pre-eclampsia and crescentic glomerulonephritis. Acute tubulointerstitial nephritis, often due to drugs such as non-steroidal anti-inflammatory agents and penicillins, may also cause acute renal failure.

Table 9.22
Some causes of acute tubular necrosis

Haemorrhage	Haemoglobinaemia (due to haemolysis, e.g. in *Falciparum malaria*, 'blackwater fever')
Burns	Hepatorenal syndrome
Diarrhoea and vomiting, fluid loss from fistulae	Radiological contrast agents
Pancreatitis	Drugs, e.g. aminoglycosides, NSAIDS, ACE inhibitors, platinum derivatives
Diuretics	Abruptio placentae
Myocardial infarction	Pre-eclampsia and eclampsia
Congestive cardiac failure	
Endotoxic shock	
Snake-bite	
Myoglobinaemia	

This also occurs when renal tubules are acutely obstructed by crystals, for example following sulphonamide therapy in a dehydrated patient (sulphonamide crystalluria) or after rapid lysis of certain malignant tumours following chemotherapy (acute hyperuricaemic nephropathy). Acute bilateral suppurative pyelonephritis or pyelonephritis of a single kidney can cause acute uraemia.

Acute tubular necrosis

CAUSES

Acute tubular necrosis is common, particularly in hospital practice. It results most often from renal ischaemia but can also be caused by direct renal toxins including drugs such as the aminoglycosides, lithium and platinum derivatives (Table 9.22).

Kidneys appear to be particularly vulnerable to ischaemic injury when cholestatic jaundice is present, and more than one ischaemic factor appears to be present in some situations. For example, disseminated intravascular coagulation complicating Gram-negative septicaemia, snake bite and complications of pregnancy such as placental rupture, pre-eclampsia and eclampsia, may result in occlusion or partial occlusion of intrarenal vessels, exacerbating the ischaemic insult resulting from hypotension associated with the underlying condition.

Myoglobinaemia and haemoglobinaemia consequent upon muscle injury (rhabdomyolysis) complicating trauma, pressure necrosis or heroin use predispose to acute tubular necrosis, perhaps in part owing to occlusion of renal tubules by myoglobin and haemoglobin casts. In liver failure, acute renal failure appears to result from rapidly reversible vasomotor abnormalities within the kidney. A kidney removed from a patient with hepatic cirrhosis and liver failure dying with oliguric renal failure may function normally immediately after transplantation into a normal individual. Efferent glomerular arteriolar dilatation resulting from ACE inhibitor drug therapy, with consequent lowering of glomerular filtration pressure, may cause acute deterioration in excretory function if renal arterial disease is also present. The effect is compounded by concomitant use of non-steroidal anti-inflammatory agents which reduce prostaglandin production, opposing this effect.

The sequence of events involved in the development of acute renal tubular necrosis is complex and incompletely understood. Factors postulated to be involved include: (i) entry of calcium into cells with an increase in cytosolic cell calcium concentration, (ii) induction by hypoxia of nitric oxide synthases with increased production of nitric oxide, (iii) increased production of intracellular proteases such as calpain (fairly strong evidence exists that this mechanism operates in cyclosporin-induced nephrotoxicity), (iv) activation of phospholipase A_2 with increased production of free fatty acids and consequent damage to cell membranes, (v) cell injury resulting from reperfusion with blood after initial ischaemia, (vi) vasoconstriction, (vii) liberation of toxic endothelial factors, (viii) damage from the vasodilator effects of endotoxins, (ix) reduced prostaglandin production, (x) tubular obstruction by desquamated cells and casts.

Whatever the precise mechanisms involved, the decline in the supply of oxygen and essential nutrients to tubular cells and the effect of various toxic factors results in patchy tubular cell necrosis with disruption of the cell membrane, denaturation of intracellular protein, lysosomal disruption and cell necrosis. Tubular cells have the capacity to regenerate rapidly and to reform the disrupted tubular basement membrane, which explains the reversibility of acute tubular necrosis. In established acute tubular necrosis, renal blood flow is much reduced, particularly blood flow to the renal cortex.

Ischaemic tubular damage contributes to a reduction in glomerular filtration by a number of interrelated mechanisms:

- *glomerular contraction* reducing surface area available for filtration
- *reflex afferent arteriolar spasm*
- *'back leak' of filtrate* in the proximal tubule owing to loss of function of the tubular cells
- *obstruction of the tubule* by debris shed from ischaemic tubular cells.

The above notwithstanding, it must be admitted that the exact pathogenesis of acute renal tubular necrosis remains unclear. Reduced glomerular filtration alone appears unlikely to provide a full explanation. In animal experiments of acute tubular necrosis, single-nephron GFR measurements during the acute oliguric phase indicate that GFR is reduced to only 20% of normal or thereabouts. GFR measured by clearance methods in humans with acute oliguric renal failure due to tubular necrosis are of course much lower than this.

COURSE AND PROGNOSIS

The clinical course of acute renal failure associated with acute tubular necrosis is variable depending on the severity and duration of the renal insult. Oliguria is common in the early stages: non-oliguric renal failure is usually a result of a less severe renal insult. Recovery of renal function typically occurs after 7–21 days, although recovery is delayed by continuing sepsis. In the recovery phase, GFR may remain low while urine output increases, sometimes to many litres a day owing to defective tubular reabsorption of filtrate. The clinical course is variable and acute tubular necrosis may last for up to six weeks even after a relatively short-lived initial insult. Eventually renal function usually returns almost to normal or to normal, although exceptions exist (e.g. in renal cortical necrosis – see below). During the recovery phase the kidneys appear relatively insensitive to further insult, such as a recurrence of hypovolaemia.

The overall mortality of acute tubular necrosis is approximately 50% and significantly this has not changed in the last 30 years. This reflects in large measure the effect of the underlying illness on prognosis. An alteration in the case mix of patients with acute renal failure now seen compared with 30 years ago is evident in the United Kingdom. Acute tubular necrosis associated with septic abortion (which carries a good prognosis) is now rare, probably owing to legislative changes, whereas acute renal failure following, for example, major vascular and cardiac surgery in elderly patients is seen more often.

No treatment is, as yet, known which will reduce the duration of acute renal tubular necrosis once it has occurred. Claims that intravenous mannitol, frusemide or 'renal-dose' dopamine may do so are not to-date supported by controlled trial evidence, and none of these treatments is without risk. No overall benefit has been proven from the use of the synthetic analogue of atrial natriuretic factor, anaritide, in reducing the duration of or mortality from acute tubular necrosis. However, oliguric patients did appear to do better whilst non-oliguric ones did worse when treated with this agent in a large clinical trial.

Whether a state of 'incipient' acute tubular necrosis exists in some patients with prerenal uraemia, and whether ATN can be prevented by administration of mannitol, frusemide or dopamine, also remain uncertain. Many nephrologists will administer one or more of these agents if correction of prerenal factors does not initiate a diuresis, but proof of benefit is lacking.

CLINICAL AND BIOCHEMICAL FEATURES

These are the features of the causal condition together with features of rapidly progressive uraemia. The rate at which serum urea and creatinine concentrations increase is dependent upon the rate of tissue breakdown in the individual patient. This is increased in the presence of trauma, sepsis and following surgery. Hyperkalaemia is common, particularly following trauma to muscle and in haemolytic states. Metabolic acidosis is usual unless hydrogen ion loss by vomiting or aspiration of gastric contents is a feature. Hyponatraemia may be present owing to water overload if patients have continued to drink in the face of oliguria, or if overenthusiastic fluid replacement with 5% dextrose has been carried out. Pulmonary oedema owing to salt and water retention is not uncommon, particularly after inappropriate attempts to initiate a diuresis by infusion of normal saline without adequate monitoring of the patient's volume status. Hypocalcaemia due to reduced renal production of 1,25-dihydroxycholecalciferol and hyper-phosphataemia due to phosphate retention are common.

Symptoms of uraemia such as anorexia, nausea, vomiting and pruritis develop, followed by intellectual clouding, drowsiness, fits, coma and haemorrhagic episodes. Epistaxes and gastrointestinal haemorrhage are relatively common. Severe infection may have initiated the acute renal failure or have complicated it owing to the impaired immune defences of the uraemic patient or ill-considered management, such as the insertion and retention of an unnecessary bladder catheter with complicating urinary tract infection and bacteraemia.

INVESTIGATION OF THE URAEMIC EMERGENCY

Investigations are aimed at defining whether the patient has acute or chronic uraemia, whether uraemia results from prerenal, renal or postrenal factors, and establishing the cause.

Acute or chronic uraemia?

The distinction between acute and chronic uraemia depends in part on the history, duration of symptoms and previous urinalysis or measurements of renal function.

A rapid rate of change of serum urea and creatinine with time suggests an acute process. A normochromic, normocytic anaemia suggests chronic disease, but anaemia may complicate many of the diseases which cause acute renal failure owing to a combination of haemolysis, haemorrhage and deficient erythropoietin production.

Ultrasound assessment of renal echogenicity and size is helpful. Small kidneys of increased echogenicity are diagnostic of a chronic process, although the reverse is not true; the kidney may remain normal in size in diabetes and amyloidosis, for instance.

Evidence of renal osteodystrophy (for example, digital subperiosteal erosions due to hyperparathyroid bone disease) is indicative of chronic disease.

Measurement of carbamylated haemoglobin (a product of non-enzymatic reaction between urea and haemoglobin, cf. glycosylated haemoglobin) is not yet widely employed.

Prerenal, renal or postrenal uraemia?

Bladder outflow obstruction is ruled out by insertion of a urethral catheter or flushing of an existing catheter, which should then be removed unless a large volume of urine is obtained. Absence of upper tract dilatation on renal ultrasonography will, with very rare exceptions, rule out urinary tract obstruction.

The distinction between prerenal and renal uraemia may be difficult. Assessment of the patient's volume status is essential and central venous pressure measurement may be extremely helpful. If volume status is low, appropriate corrective measures are indicated. If no diuresis ensues, acute intrinsic renal failure is present. Some believe that an infusion of frusemide or mannitol, or of 'renal-dose' dopamine (1–3 $\mu g\ kg^{-1}$ bodyweight per minute) may induce a diuresis in this situation and prevent progression from prerenal uraemia to established intrinsic renal failure. Proof that this is the case is lacking.

Other investigations

These include urinalysis, urine microscopy, particularly for red cells and red-cell casts (indicative of glomerulonephritis) and urine culture; measurement of serum urea, electrolytes, creatinine, calcium, phosphate, albumin, alkaline phosphatase and urate concentrations; full blood count and examination of the peripheral blood film;

testing, where appropriate, of urine for free haemoglobin and myoglobin; coagulation studies; blood cultures and measurements of nephrotoxic drug blood levels.

MANAGEMENT

The aim of management of acute renal tubular necrosis is to keep the patient alive until spontaneous recovery of renal function occurs. Ideally patients should be managed by a nephrologist or intensivist with access to facilities for blood purification and fluid removal (see p. 572). Early specialist referral is advisable. Poor initial management and late referral results in the arrival in the specialist centre of a patient who is severely uraemic, acidotic and hyperkalaemic, with pulmonary oedema following overenthusiastic intravenous fluid administration and with a Gram-negative septicaemia complicating the presence of an unnecessary indwelling bladder catheter.

General measures

Good nursing and physiotherapy are vital. Regular oral toilet, chest physiotherapy and consistent documentation of fluid intake and output, and where possible measurement of daily body weight to assess fluid balance changes, all have a role. The patient should be confined to bed only if essential.

Emergency measures

Hyperkalaemia

This is a life-threatening complication owing to the risk of cardiac dysrhythmias, particularly ventricular fibrillation. Calcium gluconate (10 mL of 10% solution) should be administered intravenously. This treatment does not alter serum potassium concentration but does reduce cardiac sensitivity to hyperkalaemia, thus reducing the risk of potentially fatal cardiac rhythm disturbance. Reduction in serum potassium is achieved by intravenous administration of 100 mL of 50% dextrose plus 10 units of rapid-acting insulin. A careful watch must be kept for subsequent hypoglycaemia. Correction of acidosis with intravenous sodium bicarbonate will also reduce serum potassium concentration, but administration of sodium may be inappropriate if the patient is salt and water-overloaded. Rapid correction of acidosis in a hypocalcaemic patient may also trigger tetany, since hydrogen ions displace calcium from albumin-binding sites, thus increasing the physiologically active calcium concentration in blood. Ion exchange resins, such as calcium resonium, are given orally (15–30 g two or three times daily), or as a 50 g rectal retention enema. Their action is somewhat delayed and their use is mainly to prevent subsequent hyperkalaemia rather than to deal with the acute emergency. In many patients, hyperkalaemia will be controlled only by dialysis or haemofiltration.

Pulmonary oedema

Unless a diuresis can be induced with intravenous frusemide, dialysis or haemofiltration will be required.

Sepsis

Infections, when detected, should be treated promptly, bearing constantly in mind the need to avoid nephrotoxic drugs and to use drugs excreted by the kidneys with appropriate precautions such as alteration of drug dosage and monitoring of blood levels. Neither the use of prophylactic antibiotics nor barrier-nursing are considered appropriate.

Use of drugs

Great care must be exercised in the use of drugs (see p. 566).

Fluid and electrolyte balance

Twice daily clinical assessment is needed. In general, once the patient is euvolaemic, daily fluid intake should equal urine output plus losses from fistulae and from vomiting, plus an allowance of 500 mL daily for insensible loss. Febrile patients will require an additional allowance. Sodium and potassium intake should be minimized. If abnormal losses of fluid occur, for example in diarrhoea, additional fluid and electrolytes will be required. The development of signs of salt and water overload (peripheral oedema, basal crackles, elevation of jugular venous pressure) or of hypovolaemia should prompt reappraisal of fluid intake. Large changes in daily weight reflecting change in fluid balance status should prompt a reappraisal of the situation.

Diet

With rare exceptions, sodium and potassium restriction are appropriate. The place of dietary protein restriction is controversial. If it is hoped to avoid dialysis or haemofiltration, protein intake is sometimes restricted to approximately 40 g daily. This poses the risk of a negative nitrogen balance despite attempts to reduce endogenous protein catabolism by maintenance of a high energy intake in the form of carbohydrate and fat. Patients treated by blood purification techniques are more appropriately managed by providing 70 g protein daily or more. Hypercatabolic patients will require an even higher nitrogen intake to prevent negative nitrogen balance.

Routes of intake are, in preferred order, enteral by mouth, enteral by nasogastric tube, and parenteral. The last of these is, however, only necessary if vomiting or bowel dysfunction render the enteral route inappropriate.

Vitamin supplements are usually supplied. Vitamin D analogue therapy and pharmacological doses of erythropoetin are not employed routinely.

Dialysis and haemofiltration

The main indications for blood purification and/or excess fluid removal by these techniques are:

- symptoms of uraemia
- complications of uraemia, such as pericarditis
- severe biochemical derangement in the absence of symptoms (especially if a rising trend is observed in an oliguric patient and in hypercatabolic patients)

- hyperkalaemia not controlled by conservative measures
- pulmonary oedema
- severe acidosis
- for removal of drugs causing the acute renal failure, e.g. gentamicin, lithium, aspirin overdose.

The main options are peritoneal dialysis, intermittent haemodialysis combined with ultrafiltration, if necessary, intermittent haemofiltration, continuous arteriovenous or venovenous haemofiltration, and haemodiafiltration. For reasons that are incompletely understood, adverse cardiovascular effects are much less during haemofiltration than during haemodialysis. Continuous treatments are superior to intermittent ones in this respect.

Continuous treatments

Blood flow is achieved either by using the patient's own blood pressure to generate arterial blood flow through a filter or by the use of a blood pump to draw blood from the lumen of a dual-lumen catheter placed in the jugular, subclavian or femoral vein.

Continuous arteriovenous or venovenous haemofiltration. (CAVH, CVVH) refers to the continuous removal of ultrafiltrate from the patient, usually at rates of up to 1000 mL h^{-1}, combined with simultaneous infusion of replacement solution. For instance, in a fluid-overloaded patient one might remove filtrate at 1000 mL h^{-1} and replace at a rate of 900 mL h^{-1}, achieving a net fluid removal of 100 mL h^{-1}.

Continuous haemodiafiltration. (CAVHDF, CVVHDF) is a combination of haemofiltration and haemodialysis, involving both the net removal of ultrafiltrate from the blood and its replacement with a replacement solution, together with the countercurrent passage of dialysate (which may be identical to the replacement solution). Both the ultrafiltrate and the spent dialysate appear as 'waste'.

Acute renal failure in the intensive care unit

In the United Kingdom, increasing numbers of patients with acute renal failure are managed in the setting of an intensive care unit. Many such patients have multiorgan failure, sepsis or both, with associated cardiovascular instability. It is increasingly recognized that continuous methods of blood purification and control of fluid balance, such as venovenous haemofiltration, are preferable to intermittent haemodialysis or peritoneal dialysis in such patients. Advantages include:

- much less disturbance of cardiovascular stability
- the ability to generate as much 'space' for fluid administration as is required, which can be adjusted flexibly to the needs of the patient (many patients require large volumes of fluid to be administered for nutritional and other reasons)
- the removal of potentially harmful substances such as inflammatory cytokines via the more porous membrane employed in haemofiltration.

Acute respiratory distress syndrome (ARDS) is not uncommon in patients with multiorgan failure, including acute renal failure, requiring intensive therapy. In such patients the wish to remove as much fluid from the patient as possible to reduce pulmonary congestion must be balanced against the need of organs, including the kidneys, for an adequate blood flow, if recovery is to occur.

Management of the recovery phase

Usually, after 1–3 weeks, renal function improves as evidenced by an increase in urine volume and improvement in serum biochemistry. Dialysis or haemofiltration, if they have been required, can be discontinued. A careful watch on clinical state, salt and water balance, and serum chemistry is required at this stage, particularly if a major diuretic phase develops owing to recovery of glomerular filtration at a time when renal tubular reabsorptive capacity for sodium, potassium and water remains impaired. Intravenous fluid replacement is sometimes required together with supplements of sodium chloride and potassium. Typically, the diuretic phase lasts for only a few days.

Acute cortical necrosis

Renal hypoperfusion results in diversion of blood flow from the cortex to the medulla, with a drop in GFR. Medullary ischaemic damage is largely reversible owing to the capacity of the tubular cells for regeneration. In contrast, glomerular ischaemic injury heals not with regeneration but with scarring – glomerulosclerosis. Prolonged cortical ischaemia may lead to irreversible loss of renal function termed 'cortical necrosis'. This may be patchy or complete. Any cause of acute tubular necrosis, if sufficiently severe or prolonged, may lead to cortical necrosis. This outcome is particularly common if acute renal failure has been accompanied by derangements of the vascular endothelial system or coagulation system, such as occurs in haemolytic uraemic syndrome and complications of pregnancy.

FURTHER READING

Forni LG, Hilton PJ (1997) Continuous haemofiltration in the treatment of acute renal failure. *New England Journal of Medicine* **336**: 1303–1309.

Hughes HD (1997) Editorial: Acute renal failure: the promise of new therapies. *New England Journal of Medicine* **336**: 870–871.

Klahr S, Muller SB (1998) Acute oliguria. *New England Journal of Medicine* **338**: 671–676

Chronic renal failure

In the UK, the prevalence of chronic renal impairment is approximately 600 individuals per million population per

Table 9.23
Causes of chronic renal failure

Congenital and inherited disease Polycystic kidney disease Alport's syndrome Congenital hypoplasia **Glomerular disease** Primary glomerulonephritides, including focal glomerulosclerosis Secondary glomerular diseases (systemic lupus, vasculitis, diabetic glomerulosclerosis, amyloidosis) **Vascular disease** Arteriosclerosis Main and medium-sized vessel vasculitis Microscopic polyarteritis Systemic lupus Systemic sclerosis with renal involvement	**Tubulointerstitial disease** Tubulointerstitial nephritis (idiopathic, due to drugs, immunologically mediated) Reflux nephropathy Tuberculosis Schistosomiasis Nephrocalcinosis **Urinary tract obstruction** Calculous disease Prostatic disease Pelvic tumours Retroperitoneal fibrosis

year. The incidence of end-stage renal failure is of the order 200 per million population per year.

Chronic renal failure implies longstanding, and usually progressive, impairment in renal function. In many instances, no effective means are currently available to reverse the primary disease process. Exceptions include correction of urinary tract obstruction, immunosuppressive therapy for systemic vasculitis and Goodpasture's syndrome, treatment of accelerated hypertension, and correction of critical narrowing of renal arteries causing renal impairment. A good deal, however, can be done to slow the rate of deterioration in renal function otherwise to be expected (see p. 578). A list of causes of chronic renal failure is given in Table 9.23.

Wide geographical variations in the incidence of disorders causing chronic renal failure exist. For example, the most common cause of glomerulonephritis in sub-Saharan Africa is malaria. Schistosomiasis is a common cause of renal failure due to urinary tract obstruction in parts of the Middle East, including southern Iraq. These disorders are seen in the UK only in those who have resided in endemic areas. The incidence of end-stage renal failure varies between racial groups, as does the relative importance of different causes of chronic renal failure. For example, end-stage renal failure is 3–4 times as common in Afro-Caribbeans in the UK and USA as it is in whites, and hypertensive nephropathy is a much more frequent cause of end-stage renal failure in this group. The prevalence of diabetes mellitus and hence of diabetic nephropathy is higher in some Asian groups than in whites. The age group involved is also of relevance. For example, chronic renal failure due to atherosclerotic renal vascular disease is much more common in the elderly than in the young.

Clinical approach to the patient with chronic renal failure

HISTORY

Particular attention should be paid to:

- *duration of symptoms*
- *drug ingestion*, including non-steroidal anti-inflammatory agents, analgesic and other medications, and unorthodox treatments such as herbal remedies
- *previous medical and surgical history*, e.g. previous chemotherapy, multisystem diseases such as SLE
- *previous occasions* on which urinalysis or measurement of urea and creatinine might have been performed, e.g. pre-employment or insurance medical examinations, new patient checks
- *family history* of renal disease.

SYMPTOMS

The early stages of renal failure are often completely asymptomatic, despite the accumulation of numerous metabolites. Serum urea and creatinine concentrations are measured in renal failure since methods for their determination are available and a rough correlation exists between urea and creatinine concentrations and symptoms. These substances are, however, in themselves not particularly toxic. The nature of the metabolites which are important in the genesis of symptoms is currently unclear. Such metabolites must be products of protein catabolism (since dietary protein restriction may reverse symptoms associated with renal failure) and many of them must be of relatively small molecular size (since haemodialysis employing membranes which allow through only relatively small molecules improves symptoms). Little else is known with certainty.

Symptoms are common when the serum urea concentration exceeds 40 mmol L^{-1}, but many patients develop uraemic symptoms at lower levels of serum urea. Symptoms include:

- malaise, loss of energy
- loss of appetite
- insomnia
- nocturia and polyuria due to impaired concentrating ability (bed-wetting in children may be a result of nocturia rather than emotional disturbance)
- itching
- nausea, vomiting and diarrhoea
- paraesthesiae due to polyneuropathy
- 'restless legs' syndrome (overwhelming need frequently to alter position of lower limbs)
- bone pain due to metabolic bone disease
- paraesthesiae and tetany due to hypocalcaemia
- symptoms due to salt and water retention – peripheral or pulmonary oedema
- symptoms due to anaemia (see p. 358)
- amenorrhoea in women; erectile impotence in men.

In more advanced uraemia (serum urea >50–60 mmol L^{-1}), these symptoms become more severe, and CNS symptoms are common:

- mental slowing, clouding of consciousness, and seizures
- myoclonic twitching.

Severe depression of glomerular filtration can result in oliguria. This can occur with either acute renal failure or in the terminal stages of chronic renal failure.

However, even if the GFR is profoundly depressed, failure of tubular reabsorption may lead to very high urine volumes. For instance, a GFR of 5 mL per minute without any tubular reabsorption would produce a urine output of 300 mL per hour or over 7 L a day! Because tubular dysfunction always accompanies glomerular disease to some extent, the urine output is therefore not a useful guide to renal function.

EXAMINATION

There are few physical signs of uraemia per se. Findings include:

- *short stature* – in patients who have had chronic renal failure in childhood
- *pallor* – due to anaemia
- *increased photosensitive pigmentation* – which may make the patient look misleadingly healthy
- *brown discoloration of the nails*
- *scratch marks* due to uraemic pruritis
- *signs of fluid overload*
- *pericardial friction rub*
- *flow murmurs* – mitral regurgitation due to mitral annular calcification; aortic and pulmonary regurgitant murmurs due to volume overload
- *glove and stocking peripheral sensory loss* (rare).

The kidneys themselves are usually impalpable unless grossly enlarged as a result of polycystic disease, obstruction or tumour. Rectal and vaginal examination may disclose evidence of an underlying cause of renal failure, particularly urinary obstruction, and should always be performed.

In addition to these findings, there may be physical signs of any underlying disease which may have caused the renal failure, for instance:

- cutaneous vasculitic lesions in systemic vasculitides
- retinopathy in diabetes
- evidence of peripheral vascular disease
- evidence of spina bifida or other causes of neurogenic bladder.

An assessment of the central venous pressure, skin turgor, blood pressure both lying and standing and peripheral circulation should also be made. The major symptoms and signs of chronic renal failure are shown in Fig 9.36.

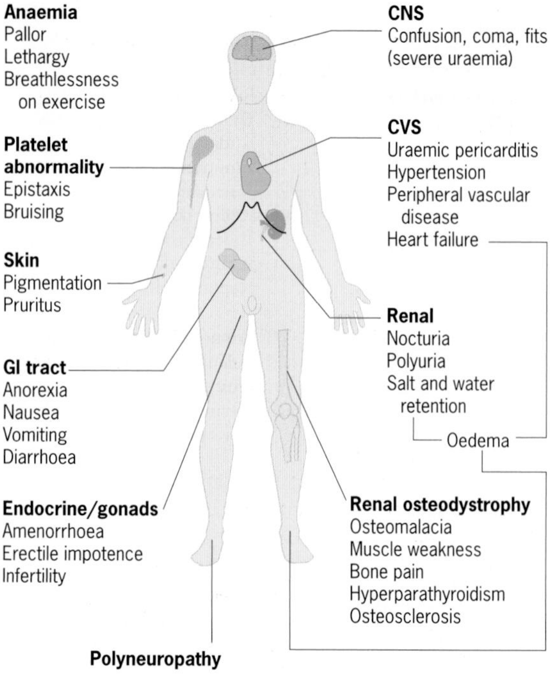

Fig 9.36
Symptoms and signs of chronic renal failure. Oedema may be due to a combination of primary renal salt and water retention and heart failure

INVESTIGATIONS

Urinalysis

- *Haematuria* may indicate glomerulonephritis, but other sources must be considered. Haematuria should not be assumed to be due to the presence of an indwelling catheter.
- *Proteinuria*, if heavy, is strongly suggestive of glomerular disease. Urinary infection may also cause proteinuria.
- *Glycosuria* with normal blood glucose is common in CRF.

Urine microscopy (see p. 526)

- *White cells* in the urine usually indicate active bacterial urinary infection, but this is an uncommon cause of acute renal failure; sterile pyuria suggests papillary necrosis (see p. 551) or renal tuberculosis.
- *Eosinophiluria* is strongly suggestive of allergic tubulointerstitial nephritis or cholesterol embolization.
- *Granular casts* are formed from abnormal cells within the tubular lumen, and indicate active renal disease.
- *Red-cell casts* are highly suggestive of glomerulonephritis.
- *Red cells in the urine* may be from anywhere between the glomerulus and the urethral meatus.

Urine biochemistry

- *24-hour creatinine clearance* is useful in assessing the severity of renal failure.
- *Measurements of urinary electrolytes* are unhelpful in chronic renal failure. The use of urinary sodium concentration in the distinction between prerenal and intrinsic renal disease is discussed on p. 568.
- *Urine osmolality* is a measure of concentrating ability. A low urine osmolality is normal in the presence of a

high fluid intake but indicates renal disease when the kidney should be concentrating urine, such as in hypovolaemia or hypotension.
- *Urine electrophoresis* is necessary for the detection of light chains, which can be present without a detectable serum paraprotein.

Serum biochemistry
- *Urea and creatinine.*
- *Serum electrophoresis* should be performed for myeloma.
- *Extreme elevations of creatine kinase* and a disproportionate elevation in serum creatinine and potassium compared to urea suggest rhabdomyolysis.

Haematology
- *Eosinophilia* suggests vasculitis, allergic tubulointerstitial nephritis, or cholesterol embolism.
- *Markedly raised viscosity or ESR* suggests myeloma or vasculitis.
- *Fragmented red cells and/or thombocytopenia* suggests intravascular haemolysis due to accelerated hypertension or haemolytic uraemic syndrome.
- *Tests for sickle cell* disease should be performed when relevant.

Immunology
- *Complement components* may be low in active renal disease due to SLE, mesangiocapillary glomerulonephritis, poststreptococcal glomerulonephritis, and cryoglobulinaemia.
- *Autoantibody screening* is useful in detection of SLE (p. 487), scleroderma (p. 490), Wegener's granulomatosis and microscopic polyarteritis (p. 539), and Goodpasture's syndrome (p. 536).
- *Cryoglobulins* should be sought in patients with unexplained glomerular disease, particularly mesangiocapillary glomerulonephritis.

Microbiology
- *Urine culture* should always be performed.
- *Early-morning urine samples* should be cultured if tuberculosis is possible.
- *Antibodies to streptococcal antigens* (ASOT, anti-DNAase B) should be sought if poststreptococcal glomerulonephritis is possible.
- *Antibodies to hepatitis B and C* may point to polyarteritis or membranous nephropathy (hepatitis B) or to cryoglobulinaemic renal disease (hepatitis C).
- *Antibodies to HIV* raise the possibility of HIV-associated renal disease.
- *Malaria* is an important cause of glomerular disease in the tropics.

Radiological investigation
- *Ultrasound.* Every patient should undergo ultrasonography (for renal size and to exclude hydronephrosis), and plain abdominal radiography and renal tomography to exclude low-density renal stones or nephrocalcinosis, which may be missed on ultrasound.
- *Intravenous urography* is seldom diagnostic in advanced renal disease.
- *CT* is useful for the diagnosis of retroperitoneal fibrosis and some other causes of urinary obstruction, and may also demonstrate cortical scarring.

Renal biopsy (see p. 531)
This should be considered in every patient with unexplained renal failure and normal-sized kidneys, unless there are strong contraindications. If rapidly progressive glomerulonephritis is possible, this investigation must be performed within 24 hours of presentation if at all possible, to guide immunosuppressive treatment.

Complications of chronic renal failure

Anaemia
Anaemia is present in the great majority of patients with chronic renal failure. Several factors have been implicated:

- *erythropoietin deficiency* (the most important)
- *bone marrow toxins* retained in renal failure
- *bone marrow fibrosis* secondary to hyperparathyroidism
- *haematinic deficiency* – iron, vitamin B_{12}, folate
- *increased red cell destruction*
- *abnormal red cell membranes* causing increased osmotic fragility
- *increased blood loss* – occult gastrointestinal bleeding, blood sampling, blood loss during haemodialysis or due to platelet dysfunction
- *ACE inhibitors* (may cause anaemia in chronic renal failure, probably by interfering with the control of endogenous erythropoietin release).

Red cell survival is reduced in renal failure owing to the hostile biochemical environment in which red cells circulate. Increased red cell destruction may occur during haemodialysis owing to mechanical, oxidant and thermal damage.

Bone disease: renal osteodystrophy
The term 'renal osteodystrophy' embraces the various forms of bone disease which may develop alone or in combination in chronic renal failure – hyperparathyroid bone disease, osteomalacia, osteoporosis and osteosclerosis (Fig 9.37). Covert renal osteodystrophy is present in many patients with moderate renal impairment and in almost all of those with end-stage renal failure.

Pathogenesis of bone disease
Decreased renal production of the 1-hydroxylase enzyme results in reduced conversion of 25-(OH)_2D_3 to the more

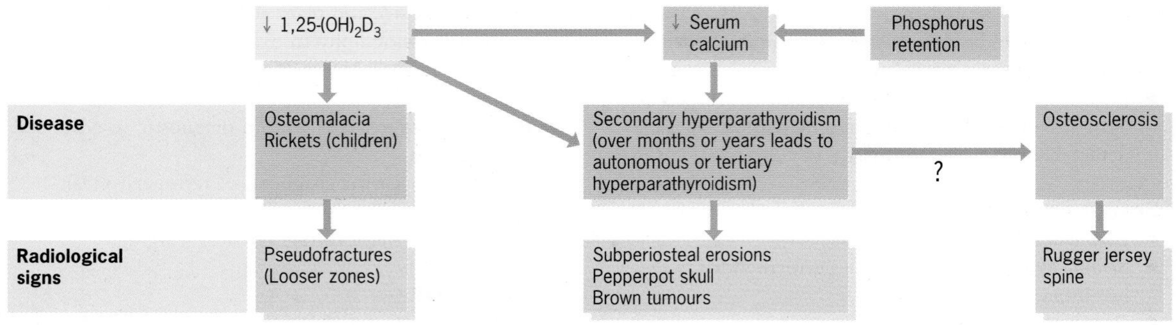

Fig 9.37
Pathogenesis and radiological features of renal osteodystrophy

metabolically active 1,25-$(OH)_2D_3$. Receptors for this exist on the parathyroid glands, failure of occupancy of which leads to increased release of parathyroid hormone. 1,25-dihydroxycholecalciferol deficiency also results in gut calcium malabsorption. Phosphorus retention owing to reduced excretion by the kidneys also indirectly (and probably directly) results in an increase in PTH secretion and release. PTH promotes reabsorption of calcium from bone and increased proximal renal tubular reabsorption of calcium, and this opposes the tendency to develop hypocalcaemia induced by 1,25-$(OH)_2D_3$ deficiency and phosphorus retention. This 'secondary' hyperparathyroidism leads to increased osteoclastic activity, cyst formation and bone marrow fibrosis (osteitis fibrosa cystica). Radiologically, digital subperiosteal erosions and 'pepperpot skull' are seen. Longstanding secondary hyperparathyroidism ultimately leads to hyperplasia of the glands with autonomous or 'tertiary' hyperparathyroidism in which hypercalcaemia is present. Serum alkaline phosphatase concentration is raised in both secondary and tertiary hyperparathyroidism. Longstanding parathyroid hormone excess is also thought to cause increased bone density (osteosclerosis) seen particularly in the spine where alternating bands of sclerotic and porotic bone give rise to a characteristic 'rugger jersey' appearance.

1,25-$(OH)_2D_3$ deficiency and hypocalcaemia result in impaired mineralization of osteoid (osteomalacia). Such impaired mineralization also occurs when osteoblasts are poisoned by, for example, aluminium given as gut phosphorus binders, or accumulated in bone as a result of exposure to aluminium in source water used to make up dialysate for haemodialysis. In this situation, serum alkaline phosphatase concentration tends to be only slightly elevated.

Increasingly, the condition of '*adynamic bone disease*' in which both bone formation and resorption are depressed (in the absence of aluminium bone disease or overtreatment with vitamin D), is recognized in patients with renal failure. The pathogenesis of this condition is unclear and it is not known whether it leads to an increased risk of fractures or other complications. No treatment is of proven benefit.

Many patients with chronic renal failure are found histologically to have mixed bone disease; that is, a combination of hyperparathyroidism and osteomalacia.

Skin disease

Pruritus (itching) is common in severe renal failure and is usually attributed in the main to retention of nitrogenous waste products of protein catabolism. Certainly, marked improvement often follows the institution of dialysis. Other causes of pruritus include:

- hypercalcaemia
- hyperphosphataemia
- elevated calcium × phosphate product
- hyperparathyroidism (even if calcium and phosphate levels are normal)
- iron deficiency.

In dialysis patients, inadequate dialysis is a cause of pruritus. Nevertheless, a significant number of dialysis patients who are well dialysed and in whom other causes of pruritus can be excluded suffer persistent itching. The cause is unknown and no effective treatment exists.

Many patients with renal failure suffer from dry skin for which simple aqueous creams are helpful. Eczematous lesions, particularly in relation to the region of an arteriovenous fistula, are relatively common. Chronic renal failure may also cause pseudoporphyria, a blistering photosensitive skin rash. This results from suppression of hepatic uroporphyrin D-carboxylase combined with a decreased clearance of porphyrins in the urine or by dialysis.

Gastrointestinal complications

These include:

- decreased gastric emptying and increased risk of reflux oesophagitis
- increased risk of peptic ulceration
- increased risk of acute pancreatitis
- constipation – particularly in patients on continuous ambulatory peritoneal dialysis (CAPD).

However, elevations of serum amylase of up to three times normal may be found in chronic renal failure without any evidence of pancreatic disease, owing to retention of high-molecular-weight forms of amylase normally excreted in the urine.

Metabolic abnormalities

Gout. Urate retention is a common feature of chronic renal failure. Treatment of asymptomatic hyperuricaemia does not (as once thought) protect against further deterioration in renal function. Treatment of clinical gout is complicated by the nephrotoxic potential of NSAIDs. Colchicine is useful in treatment of the acute attack, and allopurinol should be introduced later under colchicine cover to prevent further attacks. The dose of allopurinol should be reduced in renal impairment.

Insulin. Insulin is catabolized by and to some extent excreted via the kidneys. For this reason insulin requirements in diabetic patients decrease as renal failure progresses. By contrast, end-organ resistance to insulin is a feature of advanced renal impairment resulting in modestly impaired glucose tolerance when a standard glucose tolerance test is carried out. Insulin resistance may contribute to hypertension and lipid abnormalities.

Lipid metabolism abnormalities. These are common in renal failure, and include:

- impaired clearance of triglyceride-rich particles
- hypercholesterolaemia (particularly in advanced renal failure).

The situation is further complicated in end-stage renal disease, when regular heparinization (in haemodialysis), excessive glucose absorption (in CAPD) and immunosuppressive drugs (in transplantation) may all contribute to lipid abnormalities. Correction of lipid abnormalities by, for example, HMG-CoA reductase inhibitor therapy is increasingly employed in renal failure patients, although without formal proof of benefit derived from prospective controlled trials. Evidence that such treatment is of benefit in lowering the risk of coronary events and death in asymptomatic middle-aged men with normal renal function (see p. 995), and the high incidence of cardiovascular death in renal failure patients, has prompted an active approach to treatment of lipid abnormalities.

Endocrine abnormalities

These include:

- *hyperprolactinaemia*, which may present with galactorrhoea in men as well as women
- *increased luteinizing hormone (LH) levels* in both sexes, and abnormal pulsatility of LH release
- *decreased serum testosterone levels* (only seldom below the normal level); impotence and decreased spermatogenesis are common
- *absence of normal cyclical changes in female sex hormones*, resulting in oligomenorrhoea or amenorrhoea
- *complex abnormalities of growth hormone secretion and action*, resulting in impaired growth in uraemic children (pharmacological treatment with recombinant growth hormone and insulin-like growth factor is being studied)
- *abnormal thyroid hormone levels*, partly due to altered protein binding.

Sensitive assays for thyroid-stimulating hormone are the best way to assess thyroid function. True hypothyroidism occurs with increased frequency in renal failure. Posterior pituitary gland function is normal in renal failure.

Muscle dysfunction

Uraemia appears to interfere with muscle energy metabolism, but the mechanism is uncertain. Decreased physical fitness (cardiovascular deconditioning) also contributes.

Nervous system

Central nervous system

Severe uraemia causes an unusual combination of depressed cerebral function and decreased seizure threshold. However, convulsions in a uraemic patient are much more commonly due to other causes such as accelerated hypertension, thrombotic thrombocytopenic purpura, or drug accumulation. Asterixis, tremor and myoclonus are also features of severe uraemia.

Rapid correction of severe uraemia by haemodialysis leads to 'dialysis disequilibrium' owing to osmotic cerebral swelling. This can be avoided by correcting uraemia gradually by short, repeated haemodialysis treatments or by the use of peritoneal dialysis.

'Dialysis dementia' is a syndrome of progressive intellectual deterioration, speech disturbance, myoclonus and fits which is now known to be due to aluminium intoxication; it may be accompanied by aluminium bone disease and by microcytic anaemia. Low-grade aluminium exposure may also cause more subtle, subclinical deterioration in intellectual function. Prevention involves removal of aluminium from source water used to manufacture dialysis fluid, and restriction or avoidance of aluminium-containing gut-phosphorus binders. Treatment is with the chelating agent desferrioxamine.

Autonomic nervous system

Autonomic dysfunction is common in renal impairment. Findings include:

- increased circulating catecholamine levels associated with down-regulation of α-receptors
- impaired baroreceptor sensitivity
- impaired efferent vagal function.

All of these abnormalities improve to some extent after institution of regular dialysis and resolve after successful renal transplantation.

Peripheral nervous system

Median nerve compression in the carpal tunnel is common, and usually due to β_2-microglobulin-related amyloidosis.

'Restless legs' syndrome is common in uraemia. Patients complain of an irresistible need to move their legs, often interfering with sleep. The syndrome is difficult to treat. Iron deficiency should be treated if present. Attention should be paid to adequacy of dialysis. Symptoms may improve with the correction of anaemia by erythropoietin. Clonazepam and codeine phosphate are sometimes useful. Renal transplantation cures the problem.

A polyneuropathy occurs in patients who are inadequately dialysed.

Cardiovascular disease

Life expectancy remains severely reduced compared with the normal population owing to a greatly increased incidence of cardiovascular disease, particularly myocardial infarction, cardiac failure, sudden cardiac death and stroke.

Hypertension is a frequent complication of renal failure.

Cardiac hypertrophy is common. Risk factors include hypertension, anaemia (causing increased cardiac work), obesity and male sex.

Systolic and diastolic dysfunction are also common. Diastolic dysfunction is largely attributable to left ventricular hypertrophy and contributes to hypotension during fluid removal on haemodialysis. Systolic dysfunction may be due to:

- myocardial fibrosis
- abnormal myocyte function due to uraemia
- calcium overload and hyperparathyroidism
- carnitine and selenium deficiency.

Successful renal transplantation improves some, but not all, of these abnormalities.

Left ventricular hypertrophy is a risk factor for early death in renal failure, as in the general population. Systolic dysfunction is also an important marker for early death in renal failure.

Vascular calcification is frequent in all sizes of vessel in renal failure. In addition to the classical risk factors for atherosclerosis, a raised calcium × phosphate product causes medial calcification. Hyperparathyroidism may also contribute independently to the pathogenesis by increasing intracellular calcium. Diffuse calcification of the myocardium is also common; the causes are similar.

There is no good evidence that dialysis per se results in accelerated atherosclerosis.

Pericarditis is common and occurs in two clinical settings:

- *Uraemic pericarditis* is a feature of severe, preterminal uraemia or of underdialysis. Haemorrhagic pericardial effusion and atrial arrhythmias are often associated. There is a danger of pericardial tamponade and anticoagulants should be used with caution. Pericarditis usually resolves with intensive dialysis.
- *Dialysis pericarditis* occurs as a result of an intercurrent illness or surgery in a patient receiving apparently adequate dialysis.

Progression of chronic renal impairment

Once established, and whatever the initial cause, chronic renal impairment tends to progress inexorably to end-stage renal failure, although the rate of progression may depend upon the underlying nephropathy. Patients with chronic glomerular diseases tend to deteriorate more quickly than those with chronic tubulointerstitial nephropathies. Hypertension and heavy proteinuria are bad prognostic indicators in this context. A nonspecific renal scarring process common to renal disorders of different aetiologies may be responsible for progression. Evidence is accumulating that angiotensin-converting enzyme gene polymorphism may in part account for varying rates of progression between individuals, possession of the DD phenotype carrying a poorer prognosis (see p. 687).

Animal experiments in which one kidney is removed and the other partially removed indicate that progressive loss of renal function follows the initial reduction in nephron mass. A rise in intraglomerular capillary pressure and adaptive glomerular hypertrophy under conditions of reduced nephron mass have been postulated as causes of glomerular scarring in this connection, as has proteinuria per se. Renal interstitial scarring also occurs and is likely to be of major importance. It is not widely appreciated that the prognosis for renal function in chronic glomerular disorders is judged more accurately by interstitial histological appearances than by glomerular morphology. The pathogenesis of progressive interstitial damage is currently uncertain. Slowing of deterioration in renal function in diabetic nephropathy by meticulous control of blood pressure and, in particular, the use of ACE inhibitors, has been proved in a large controlled clinical trial, as has the benefit of tight glycaemic control. In non-diabetics, excellent control of hypertension is of benefit, and ACE inhibitors (which reduce intraglomerular capillary pressure and proteinuria) have been shown to be of particular value. Dietary protein restriction is not of proven benefit in slowing progression. Many other possible approaches to the problem are currently under investigation.

Management of chronic renal failure

The underlying cause of renal disease should be treated aggressively wherever possible.

Blood pressure control

Blood pressure should probably be reduced to around 130/80 mmHg if the patient can tolerate this level of pressure. Adequate control may require a combination of drugs together with large doses of diuretics to correct sodium and water retention. Evidence has accumulated to show that, for a given degree of blood pressure control, ACE inhibitor treatment confers greater protection upon kidney function than does treatment with other hypotensive agents. In the absence of contraindications, initial regimens should consist of or include an ACE inhibitor. Measurement of 24-hour ambulatory blood pressure provides a much more accurate guide to blood pressure control than occasional outpatient clinic recordings. The aim of management is to prevent or reverse left ventricular hypertrophy, which will itself be significantly underdiagnosed if reliance is placed only upon clinical examination and electrocardiography. Echocardiography is essential.

Hyperkalaemia

Hyperkalaemia often responds to dietary restriction of potassium intake. Drugs which cause potassium retention (see p. 613) should be stopped. Occasionally it may be necessary to prescribe ion-exchange resins to remove potassium in the gastrointestinal tract. Emergency treatment of severe hyperkalaemia is described on p. 614.

Acidosis

Correction of acidosis helps to correct hyperkalaemia in chronic renal failure, and may also decrease muscle catabolism. Sodium bicarbonate supplements are often effective, but may cause oedema and hypertension owing to extracellular fluid expansion. Calcium carbonate, also used as a calcium supplement and phosphate binder, has a beneficial effect on acidosis.

Calcium and phosphate

Hypocalcaemia and hyperphosphataemia should be treated aggressively, preferably with regular (e.g. three-monthly) measurements of serum PTH to assess how effectively hyperparathyroidism is being suppressed. Dietary restriction of phosphorus is seldom effective alone, because so many important foods contain it. Oral calcium carbonate acts as a calcium supplement and also reduces bioavailability of dietary phosphorus. Aluminium-containing gut phosphorus binders should be avoided if possible, since absorption of aluminium poses the risk of aluminium bone disease and development of cognitive impairment. Treatment with calcitriol or a vitamin D analogue such as alfacalcidol in early renal impairment has no deleterious effect upon renal function provided hypercalcaemia is avoided. Treatment should probably not be started unless serum PTH level is three times or more the upper limit of normal, in order to prevent the development of adynamic bone disease (see p. 576). Vitamin D therapy has the disadvantage that it increases gut phosphorus absorption and may therefore exacerbate hyperphosphataemia. H2 antagonists decrease the effectiveness of phosphate binders.

Dietary restrictions

In advanced renal disease, reduction of protein intake lessens the amount of nitrogenous waste products generated, and this may delay the onset of symptomatic uraemia. Most patients with renal impairment will require a diet restricted in sodium and potassium. A minority of patients (particularly those with tubulointerstitial disease) manifest impaired capacity to retain salt and water (salt-losing renal disease) and require a high salt intake and/or sodium supplement.

Prolonged dietary protein restriction should be avoided. It is preferable to commence renal replacement therapy a little earlier than to cause malnutrition.

Fluid intake

Fluid depletion and overload should be avoided. Maximum water excretion is approximately 500 mL per 24 hours per mL GFR. It follows that a patient with a GFR of 5 mL per minute cannot usually excrete more than 2.5 L daily. Dilutional hyponatraemia may occur if water intake exceeds the capacity to excrete the water load. Advice to maximize fluid intake in patients with chronic renal failure may thus be misplaced. Conversely, the large majority of patients with moderate chronic renal impairment do not need to restrict fluid intake.

Drug therapy

This should be minimized in patients with chronic renal impairment. Tetracyclines (with the possible exception of doxycycline) should be avoided in view of their antianabolic effect and tendency to worsen uraemia. Drugs excreted by the kidneys, such as gentamicin, should be prescribed with caution and drug levels monitored if feasible. Non-steroidal anti-inflammatory drugs should be avoided. Potassium-sparing agents, such as spironolactone and amiloride, pose particular dangers, as do artificial salt substitutes, all of which contain potassium.

Anaemia

The anaemia of erythropoietin deficiency can be treated with synthetic (recombinant) human erythropoietin, starting at a dose of 25–50 U kg^{-1} three times a week; subcutaneous administration is more effective than intravenous. Blood pressure, haemoglobin concentration and reticulocyte count are measured every two weeks and the dose adjusted to maintain a target haemoglobin of 10–12 g dL^{-1}.

Failure to respond to 300 U kg^{-1} weekly, or a fall in haemoglobin after a satisfactory response, may be due to iron deficiency, bleeding, malignancy or infection. The demand for iron by the bone marrow is enormous when erythropoietin is commenced. Recently available intravenous (rather than oral) iron supplements optimize response to treatment.

Partial correction of anaemia with erythropoietin improves quality of life, exercise tolerance, sexual function and cognitive function in dialysis patients, and leads to regression of left ventricular hypertrophy. Avoidance of blood transfusion also lessens the chance of sensitization to HLA antigens, which may otherwise be a barrier to successful renal transplantation.

The *disadvantages* of erythropoietin therapy are that it is expensive and causes a rise in blood pressure in up to 30% of patients, particularly in the first six months. Peripheral resistance rises in all patients, owing to loss of hypoxic vasodilatation and to increased blood viscosity. A rare complication is encephalopathy with fits, transient cortical blindness and hypertension. Other causes of anaemia should be looked for and treated appropriately (see p. 359).

Male impotence

Testosterone deficiency should be corrected. If vascular or neurological causes exist, intracavernosal injection prostaglandin therapy, the use of a vacuum device or the use of a penile prosthetic implant should be considered. An oral phosphodiesterase inhibitor (sildenafil) is now available in the USA (see p. 984).

Early referral of patients with chronic renal failure

Patients with chronic renal impairment should be referred to a nephrologist with access to facilities for renal replacement therapy at an early stage since late referral has been shown to be associated with increased mortality and morbidity when such patients commence renal replacement therapy. Old age is no bar to referral in the reasonably fit elderly patient.

Referral should be arranged when serum creatinine reaches 350 μmol L^{-1} in non-diabetics and when it reaches 250 μmol L^{-1} in diabetics, who are more prone to require early dialysis owing to impaired cardiac function and consequent pulmonary oedema. Measures aimed at slowing progression of renal failure and limiting its complications can thus be optimized and sufficient time gained to plan replacement therapy if needed.

Patients need time to adjust to the demands of chronic renal failure and its treatment, and to absorb information. Management in the predialysis phase should take account of future needs for vascular access for haemodialysis. Veins required in the future for fashioning of an arteriovenous fistula should not be rendered useless by cannulation (Fig 9.38).

If the patient opts for regular haemodialysis, fashioning of an arteriovenous fistula should be carried out well in advance of the need for dialysis, when serum creatinine is of the order 400–500 μmol L^{-1} in non-diabetics and at an even earlier stage in diabetics with poorer vasculature. Such fistulae require several weeks to mature and become usable for vascular access.

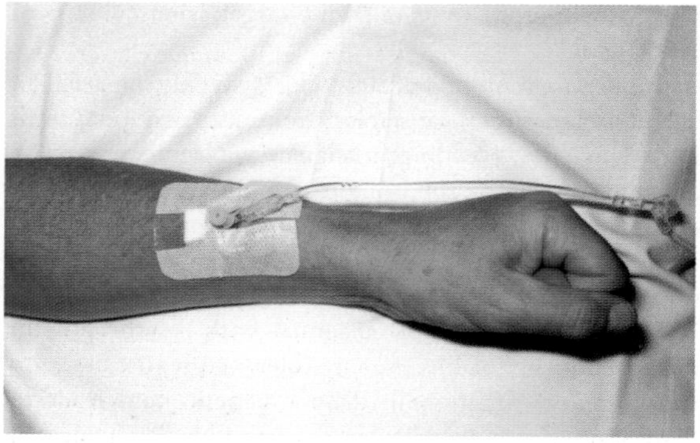

Fig 9.38
Intravenous cannula in exactly the wrong place, in a right-handed patient with chronic renal impairment who will in future need a left (non-dominant arm) radiocephalic fistula.

Renal replacement therapy

Approximately 100 individuals per million population reach end-stage renal failure each year. The aim of all renal replacement techniques is to mimic the excretory functions of the normal kidney, including excretion of nitrogenous wastes, maintenance of normal electrolyte concentrations, and maintenance of a normal extracellular volume.

Haemodialysis

Basic principles

In haemodialysis, blood from the patient is pumped through an array of semipermeable membranes (the dialyser, often called an 'artificial kidney') which bring the blood into close contact with dialysate, flowing countercurrent to the blood. The plasma biochemistry changes towards that of the dialysate owing to diffusion of molecules down their concentration gradients (Fig 9.39).

Table 9.24 Range of concentrations (mmol L^{-1}) in routinely available final dialysates used for haemodialysis

Sodium	130–145
Potassium	0.0–4.0
Calcium	1.0–1.6
Magnesium	0.25–0.85
Chloride	99–108
Bicarbonate	35–40
OR	
Acetate	35–40
Glucose	0–10

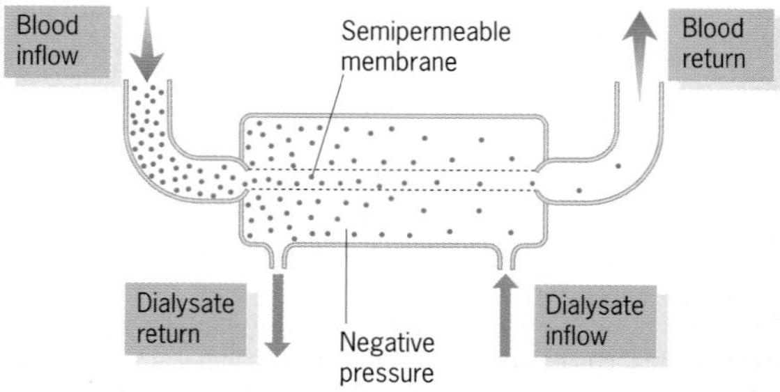

Fig 9.39
Changes across a semipermeable dialysis membrane

The dialysis machine comprises a series of blood pumps, with pressure monitors and bubble detectors and a proportionating unit, also with pressure monitors and blood leak detectors. Blood flow during dialysis is usually 200–300 mL per minute and the dialysate flow usually 500 mL per minute. The efficiency of dialysis in achieving biochemical change depends on blood and dialysate flow and the surface area of the dialysis membrane.

Dialysate is prepared by a proportionating unit which mixes specially purified water with concentrate, resulting in fluid with the composition described in Table 9.24. Newer highly permeable synthetic membranes allow more rapid haemodialysis than with cellulose-based membranes (high-flux haemodialysis).

Access for haemodialysis

Adequate dialysis requires a blood flow of at least 200 mL per minute. The most reliable long-term way of achieving this is surgical construction of an *arteriovenous fistula* (Figs 9.40 and 9.41), using the radial or brachial artery and the cephalic vein. This results in distension of the vein and thickening ('arterialization') of its wall, so that after 6–8 weeks large-bore needles may be inserted to take blood to and from the dialysis machine.

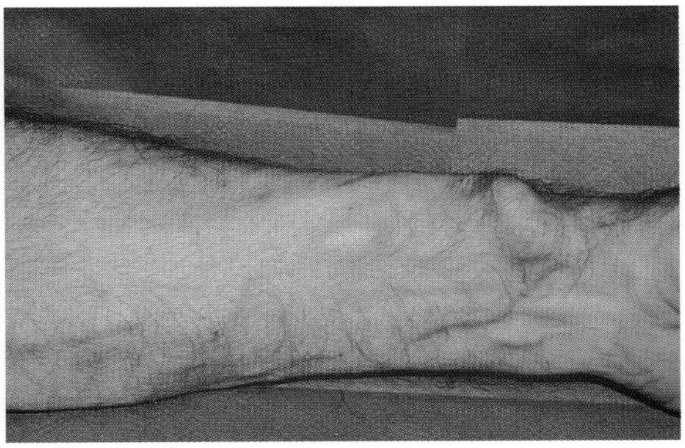

Fig 9.40
Left forearm arteriovenous (radiocephalic) fistula

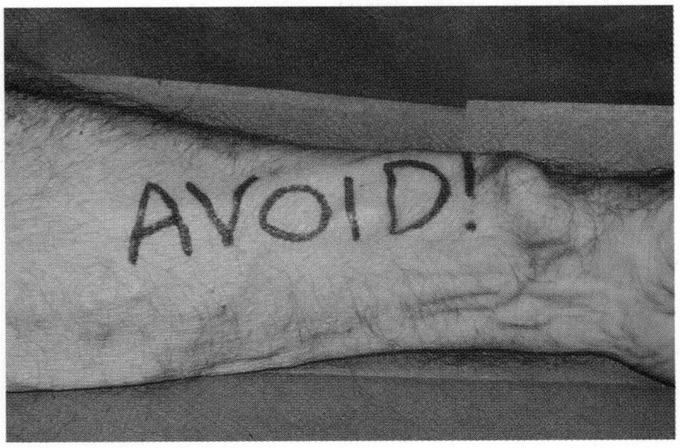

Fig 9.41
One way of reminding the anaesthetic, nursing and surgical team about the presence of an existing arteriovenous fistula in a haemodialysis patient about to undergo surgery. In particular, the fistula should not be compressed during surgery to avoid thrombosis within it

Arteriovenous *shunts* are large-bore plastic cannulae surgically tied into a superficial artery and adjacent vein. These allow direct flow of arterial blood into the dialyser, which is then returned directly into a vein. Between dialysis sessions flow between artery and vein is restored by a plastic connector between the two cannulae, which lie outside the body, usually on the forearm. Disadvantages include a high rate of infection, thrombosis and the potential for disconnection which could result in exsanguination.

If dialysis is needed immediately, a large-bore double-lumen cannula may be inserted into a central vein – usually the subclavian, jugular or femoral. Semipermanent dual-lumen venous catheters may also be inserted with a skin tunnel to lessen the risk of infection. Nevertheless, the risk of local and systemic sepsis with such external devices is substantial and there is much associated morbidity and some increased risk of mortality. Stenosis of the subclavian vein is common when such devices are used and the jugular route is in general to be preferred.

Dialysis prescription

Dialysis must be tailored to an individual patient to obtain optimal results.

Dry weight

This is the weight at which a patient is neither fluid overloaded nor depleted. Patients are weighed at the start of each dialysis session and the transmembrane pressure adjusted to achieve fluid removal equal to the amount by which they exceed their dry weight.

The dialysate buffer

The dialysate buffer is usually acetate or bicarbonate. The sodium and calcium concentrations of the dialysate buffer are carefully monitored. A high dialysate sodium causes thirst and hypertension. A high dialysate calcium causes hypercalcaemia, whilst a low calcium dialysate combined with poor compliance of medication with oral calcium carbonate and vitamin D may result in hyperparathyroidism.

Frequency and duration

Frequency and duration of dialysis is adjusted to achieve adequate removal of uraemic metabolites and to avoid excessive fluid overload between dialysis sessions. An adult of average size usually receives 4–5 hours' treatment three times a week. Twice-weekly dialysis is adequate only if the patient has considerable residual renal function.

Increasingly, short-duration dialysis using very biocompatible high-flux membranes is being employed. Advantages include shorter duration of treatment and hence increased patient convenience. Disadvantages include higher cost of the membranes employed and, in all probability, higher prevalence of hypertension in such patients, requiring hypotensive medication. It should not be forgotten that normal kidneys work for 24 hours a day, seven days a week, and that dialysis is a poor substitute for the natural state.

Underdialysis, which appears to have occurred in the USA in the 1980s, is associated with much increased patient morbidity and mortality. The pendulum appears at present to be swinging back towards longer-duration treatment of patients with end-stage renal failure. All patients are anticoagulated (usually with heparin) during treatment as contact with foreign surfaces activates the clotting cascade. In the UK, a modest minority of patients manage self-supervised home haemodialysis.

COMPLICATIONS

Hypotension during dialysis is the major complication. Contributing factors include: an excessive removal of extracellular fluid, inadequate 'refilling' of the blood compartment from the interstitial compartment during fluid removal, abnormalities of venous tone, autonomic neuropathy, acetate intolerance (acetate acts as a vasodilator), and left ventricular hypertrophy.

Very rarely patients may develop anaphylactic reactions to ethylene oxide, which is used to sterilize most dialysers. Patients receiving ACE inhibitors are at risk of anaphylaxis if polyacrylonitrile dialysers are used.

Other potential, rare, complications include the hard-water syndrome (caused by failure to soften water resulting in a high calcium concentration prior to mixing with dialysate concentrate), haemolytic reactions, and air embolism.

ADEQUACY OF DIALYSIS

Dialysis treatment is empirical since the size, number and nature of 'uraemic toxins' is unclear. The only true measure of adequacy is patient mortality and morbidity. Adequate nutrition of the patient is as important as (perhaps more important than) adequacy of dialysis in reducing morbidity and mortality.

Symptoms of underdialysis are nonspecific and include insomnia, itching, fatigue despite adequate correction of anaemia, restless legs and a peripheral sensory neuropathy.

Adequacy of dialysis may be assessed by computerized calculation of urea kinetics, requiring measurement of the residual renal urea clearance, the rate of rise of urea concentration between dialysis sessions, and the reduction in urea concentration during dialysis.

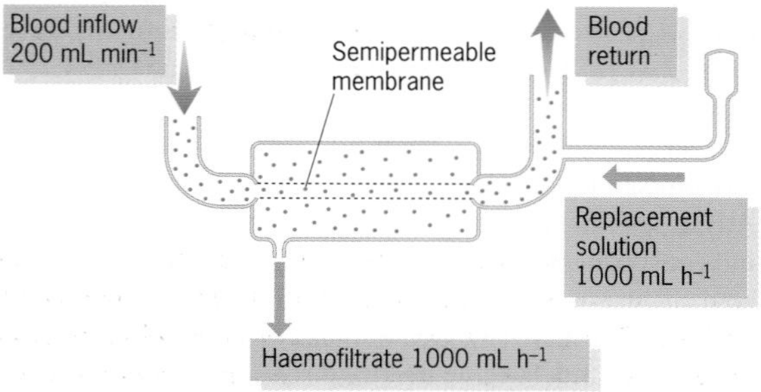

Fig 9.42
Principles of haemofiltration

Machine haemodialysis is the most efficient way of achieving rapid biochemical improvement, for instance in the treatment of acute renal failure or severe hyperkalaemia. This advantage is offset by disadvantages such as haemodynamic instability, especially in acutely ill patients with multiorgan disease, and over-rapid correction of uraemia can lead to 'dialysis disequilibrium'. This is characterized by nausea and vomiting, restlessness, headache, hypertension, myoclonic jerking, and in severe instances seizures and coma owing to rapid changes in plasma osmolality leading to cerebral oedema.

These problems have led to the increasing adoption of gentler continuous methods for the treatment of acute renal failure (see below).

Haemofiltration

This involves removal of plasma water and its dissolved constituents (e.g. K^+, Na^+, urea, phosphate) by convective flow across a high-flux semipermeable membrane, and replacing it with a solution of the desired biochemical composition (Fig 9.42). Lactate is used as buffer in the replacement solution because rapid infusion of acetate causes vasodilatation and bicarbonate may cause precipitation of calcium carbonate.

Haemofiltration can be used for both acute and chronic renal failure. High volumes need to be exchanged in order to achieve adequate small molecule removal; typically a 22 L exchange three times a week for maintenance treatment and 1 L per hour in acute renal failure. Financial costs of disposable items (such as filters and replacement fluid) are high and only a tiny minority of patients with end-stage renal failure are managed in this way. However, nursing costs are reduced when acute renal failure is managed in an intensive care unit setting since haemofiltration can be managed by ITU nursing staff rather than renal unit nurses.

Peritoneal dialysis

Peritoneal dialysis utilizes the peritoneal membrane as a semipermeable membrane, avoiding the need for extracorporeal circulation of blood. This is a very simple,

Table 9.25 Range of concentrations (mmol L^{-1}) in routinely available CAPD dialysate[a]

Sodium	130–134
Potassium	0
Calcium	1.0–1.75
Magnesium	0.25–0.75
Chloride	95–104
Lactate	35–40
Glucose	77–236
Total osmolality	356–511

[a]Glucose content is often expressed as g dL^{-1} of anhydrous glucose (e.g. 1.36% = 77 mmol L^{-1}. An even more hypertonic dialysate (6.36%) is available for acute (intermittent) peritoneal dialysis

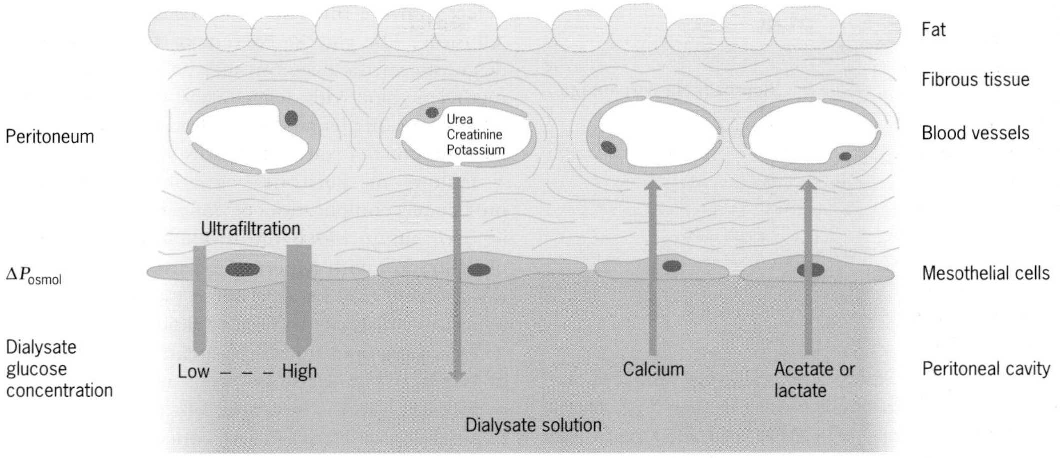

Fig 9.43
Principles of peritoneal dialysis

low-technology treatment compared to haemodialysis. The principles are simple (Fig 9.43).

1. A tube is placed into the peritoneal cavity through the anterior abdominal wall.
2. Dialysate is run into the peritoneal cavity, usually under gravity.
3. Urea, creatinine, phosphate, and other uraemic toxins pass into the dialysate down their concentration gradients.
4. Water (with solutes) is attracted into the peritoneal cavity by osmosis, depending on the osmolarity of the dialysate. This is determined by the dextrose content of the dialysate (Table 9.25).
5. The fluid is changed regularly to repeat the process.

Chronic peritoneal dialysis requires insertion of a soft catheter, with its tip in the pelvis, exiting the peritoneal cavity in the midline and lying in a skin tunnel with an exit site in the lateral abdominal wall (Fig 9.44).

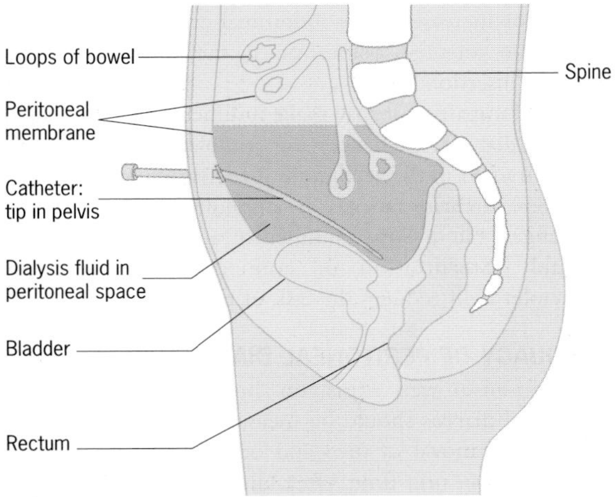

Fig 9.44
The siting of a Tenckhoff peritoneal dialysis catheter

This form of dialysis can be adapted in several ways.

- **Continuous ambulatory peritoneal dialysis** (CAPD). Dialysate is present within the peritoneal cavity continuously, except when dialysate is being exchanged. Dialysate exchanges are performed 3–5 times a day, using a sterile no-touch technique to connect 1.5–3 L bags of dialysate to the peritoneal catheter; each exchange takes 20–40 minutes. This is the technique most often used for maintenance peritoneal dialysis in patients with end-stage renal failure.
- **Nightly intermittent peritoneal dialysis** (NIPD) An automated device is used to perform exchanges each night while the patient is asleep. Sometimes dialysate is left in the peritoneal cavity during the day in addition, to increase the time for which biochemical exchange is occurring.
- **Tidal dialysis**. A residual volume is left within the peritoneal cavity with continuous cycling of smaller volumes in and out.

Osmotic removal of excess plasma water and solutes is achieved using hypertonic dialysate, which exerts an osmotic 'drag'. Depending on the patient's fluid intake and residual urine output, it may be necessary to use one or more hypertonic dialysate bags daily to achieve fluid balance in CAPD. Fluid overload is a relatively common problem in CAPD, and is due to failure of transport across the peritoneal membrane.

COMPLICATIONS

Peritonitis

Bacterial peritonitis is the most common serious complication of CAPD and other forms of peritoneal dialysis. Clinical presentations include abdominal pain of varying severity (guarding and rebound tenderness are unusual), and a cloudy peritoneal effluent – without which the diagnosis cannot be made. Microscopy reveals a

Table 9.26
Some causes of CAPD peritonitis[a]

	Approximate percentage of cases
Staphylococcus epidermidis	40–50
Esherichia coli, Pseudomonas and other Gram-negative organisms	25
Staphylococcus aureus	15
Mycobacterium tuberculosis	2
Candida and other fungal species	2

[a]In approximately 20%, no bacteria are found

neutrophil count of above 100 cells per mL. Nausea, vomiting, fever and paralytic ileus may be seen if peritonitis is severe. The incidence of CAPD-associated peritonitis has been much reduced (to about one episode every three patient years) by use of a Y-disconnect system in preference to previous methods.

CAPD peritonitis must be investigated with culture of peritoneal effluent. Empirical antibiotic treatment is started thereafter, with a spectrum which covers both Gram-negative and Gram-positive organisms. Antibiotics may be given by the oral, intravenous or intraperitoneal route; most centres rely on intraperitoneal antibiotics. Common causative organisms are listed in Table 9.26.

Staph. aureus peritonitis should lead to a search for nasal carriage of this organism and *Staph. epidermidis* peritonitis may indicate contamination from the patient's (or helper's) skin. Relapsing *Staph. epidermidis* peritonitis with an organism with the same antibiotic sensitivity pattern on each occasion may indicate that the Tenckhoff catheter has become colonized: often this is difficult to eradicate without replacement of the catheter under antibiotic cover.

Gram-negative peritonitis may complicate septicaemia from urinary or bowel infection. A mixed growth of Gram-negative and anaerobic organisms strongly suggests bowel perforation, and is an indication for laparotomy.

Fungal peritonitis often follows antibacterial treatment but may occur de novo. Clinical presentation is very variable. It is rare to be able to cure fungal peritonitis without catheter removal as well as antifungal treatment. Intraperitoneal amphotericin has been associated with the formation of peritoneal adhesions.

Infection around the catheter site

Infection where the catheter exits through the skin is relatively common. It should be treated aggressively (with systemic and/or local antibiotics) to prevent spread of the infection into the subcutaneous tunnel and the peritoneum. The most common causative organisms are staphylococci.

Other complications

CAPD is often associated with constipation, which in turn may impair flow of dialysate in and out of the pelvis. Occasionally dialysate may leak through a diaphragmatic defect into the thoracic cavity, causing a massive pleural 'effusion'. The glucose content of the effusion is usually diagnostic, or the diagnosis may be made by instillation of methylene blue with dialysate and the demonstration of a blue colour on pleural tap. Dialysate may also leak into the scrotum down a patent processus vaginalis.

Failure of peritoneal membrane function is a predictable complication of long-term CAPD, resulting in worsening biochemical exchange and decreased ultrafiltration with hypertonic dialysate. It is thought that this problem may be accelerated by excessive reliance on hypertonic dialysate to remove fluid.

Sclerosing peritonitis is a potentially fatal complication of CAPD. The cause is often unclear, but recurrent peritonitis, and exposure of the peritoneum to unphysiological high glucose concentrations, is probably responsible in most cases. Progressive thickening of the peritoneal membrane occurs in association with adhesions and strictures, turning the small bowel into a mass of matted loops and causing repeated episodes of small bowel obstruction. CAPD should be abandoned. Improvement may follow renal transplantation or treatment with prednisolone or azathioprine.

CONTRAINDICATIONS

There are few absolute contraindications apart from unwillingness or inability on the patient's part to learn the technique.

Previous peritonitis causing peritoneal adhesions may make peritoneal dialysis impossible: but the extent of adhesions is difficult to predict, and it may be worth an attempted surgical placement of a dialysis catheter.

The presence of a stoma (colostomy, ileostomy, ileal urinary conduit) makes successful placement of a dialysis catheter extremely unlikely.

Active intra-abdominal sepsis, for instance due to diverticular abscesses, is an absolute contraindication to peritoneal dialysis although diverticular disease per se is not.

Abdominal hernias may often expand during CAPD as a result of increased intra-abdominal pressure, and should ideally be repaired before or at the time of CAPD catheter insertion.

Visual impairment may make it difficult for a patient to perform dialysate exchanges, but completely blind patients can be trained in the technique if adequately motivated.

Severe arthritis makes it difficult to perform the exchanges, but a large number of mechanical aids are available. Sterilization of connections by heat or ultraviolet light reduces the risk of peritonitis.

ADEQUACY OF PERITONEAL DIALYSIS

No consensus yet exists on how the adequacy of peritoneal dialysis should be measured and the optimum degree of removal of urea and other waste products to be obtained in unit time. Urea kinetic modelling may be employed, as with haemodialysis. However, it is increasingly appreciated that patient prognosis improves with greater degrees of waste product removal than were hitherto considered acceptable, and that peritoneal dialysis inadequacy is common when residual renal function declines to zero. With increasing time on treatment, adequacy may become impaired owing to alterations in the efficiency of the peritoneal membrane in transporting waste products, fluid and electrolytes. Under these circumstances conversion to haemodialysis is necessary.

COMPLICATIONS OF LONG-TERM DIALYSIS

Cardiovascular disease (see p. 578) and sepsis are the leading causes of death in long-term dialysis patients.

Causes of fatal sepsis include peritonitis complicating peritoneal dialysis and *Staph. aureus* infection (including endocarditis) complicating the use of indwelling access devices for haemodialysis.

Dialysis amyloidosis

This is the accumulation of amyloid protein (p. 1002) as a result of failure of clearance of β_2-microglobulin, a molecule of 11.8 kDa. This protein is the light chain of the class I HLA antigens and is normally freely filtered at the glomerulus but is not removed by cellulose-based haemodialysis membranes. Complement activation resulting from the use of cellulose-based membranes may increase the generation rate of the protein. The protein polymerizes to form amyloid deposits, which may cause median nerve compression in the carpal tunnel or a dialysis arthropathy – a clinical syndrome of pain and disabling stiffness in the shoulders, hips, hands, wrists and knees. β_2-Microglobulin-related amyloid may be demonstrated in the synovium. There is little inflammation and the pathogenesis is not well understood. Rapid improvement after renal transplantation is probably due to steroid therapy. Low-dose prednisolone alone can also cause an improvement. A change to a biocompatible synthetic membrane has also been reported to be of benefit: again, the mechanism for this improvement is not clear. Amyloid deposits can also cause pathological bone cysts and fractures, pseudotumours and gastrointestinal bleeding caused by amyloid deposition around submucosal blood vessels.

The extent of amyloid deposition is best assessed by nuclear imaging, either using [^{99m}Tc]DMSA, or, more specifically, by the use of radiolabelled serum amyloid P component.

Surgery in patients with chronic renal failure

To reduce the risk of worsening renal failure and the risk of morbidity and mortality, the following measures are important:

- Ensure that blood volume is normal, employing measurement of central venous pressure if necessary.
- Ensure an adequate diuresis in the perioperative period, using intravenous fluid infusion as necessary.
- Avoid hypotension using inotropes if necessary.
- Delay surgery if hyperkalaemia (serum potassium >5.5 mmol L^{-1}) or fluid overload is present preoperatively until these have been corrected.
- Monitor urea, electrolyte and creatinine concentrations carefully. Serum potassium should be checked immediately postoperatively (or intraoperatively if surgery is prolonged) and 4–6 hours later, and urea, electrolyte and creatinine concentrations should be checked daily thereafter. If possible weigh the patient daily to monitor fluid balance.
- Prior mannitol infusion may reduce the risk of acute renal tubular necrosis in patients with extrahepatic cholestatic jaundice.
- The action of some anaesthetic agents such as muscle relaxants and opiates are prolonged in renal impairment. Appropriate precautions should be taken. Anaesthetic agents that are safe in renal failure and can be used without alteration in dosage include fentanyl, atropine, diazepam, halothane and nitrous oxide.

Patients near to end-stage renal failure who may be precipitated into the need for dialysis by surgery should be operated on only if essential. For example, coronary bypass surgery in a patient with a serum creatinine of 600 μmol L^{-1} should, if possible, be deferred until the patient is safely established on regular dialysis and is stable. All possible attempts should be made to avoid breaching the peritoneum in patients on CAPD or damaging an arteriovenous fistula in haemodialysis patients (see Fig 9.41).

Transplantation

Successful renal transplantation offers the potential for almost complete rehabilitation in end-stage renal failure. It allows freedom from dietary and fluid restriction, anaemia and infertility are corrected, and the need for parathyroidectomy is reduced.

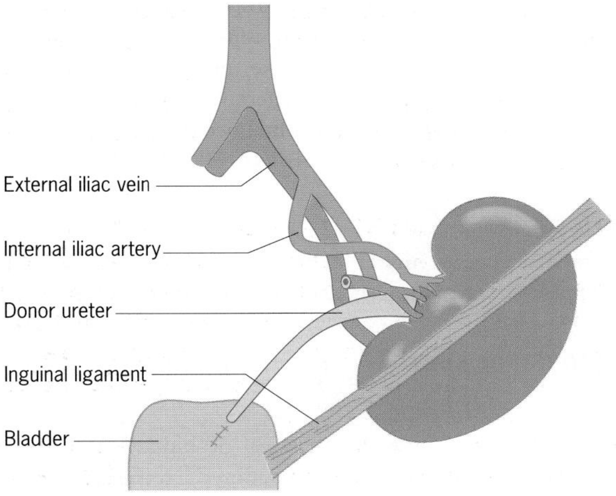

Fig 9.45
Anatomy of a renal transplant operation

The technique involves the anastomosis of an explanted human kidney, either from a cadaveric donor or, less frequently, from a living close relative, on to the iliac vessels of the recipient (Fig 9.45). The donor ureter is placed into the recipient's bladder. Unless the donor is genetically identical (i.e. an identical twin), immunosuppressive treatment is needed, for as long as the transplant remains in place, to prevent rejection. Eighty per cent of grafts now survive for 5–10 years in the best centres, and 60% for 10–30 years.

In the future, attention may turn increasingly to the induction of immunological tolerance to grafted organs and perhaps to the use of organs from genetically modified animals (xenotransplantation). In respect of the latter, formidable problems in overcoming rejection remain and there is considerable disquiet about the potential for transmission from animal to human species of viral infections which may be highly pathogenic to man.

Factors affecting success

Success of transplantation is affected by numerous factors, apart from ABO (blood group) compatibility.

Matching donor and recipient for HLA type

Matching for HLA-DR antigens appears to have the most impact on survival, followed by the B and, least importantly, the A locus antigens. Complete compatibility at A, B and DR offers the best chance of success, followed by a single HLA mismatch (i.e. antigen possessed by the donor and not possessed by the recipient). The effect of further degrees of mismatching upon graft survival in first transplants is of modest degree. Nationwide matching schemes for kidneys retrieved from cadaver donors are in existence.

Adequate immunosuppressive treatment

See below.

Preoperative blood transfusion

Before the introduction of cyclosporin as an immunosuppressive agent, preoperative transfusion appeared to exert a nonspecific immunosuppressive effect, decreasing the incidence of rejection. The effect is no longer clearly evident. Blood transfusion, less often necessary in the current erythropoietin era, carries the risk of HLA sensitization.

The 'centre effect'

Graft survival is higher in those centres with extensive experience of management of transplant recipients.

The donor kidney

Cadaveric donation

Most countries allow the removal of kidneys and other organs from patients who have suffered irretrievable brain damage ('brainstem death') while their hearts are still beating (see p. 858).

Living related donation

A close relative may volunteer as a potential donor. A sibling donor may be HLA identical or share one or no haplotypes with the potential recipient. Most transplant centres accept one-haplotype matches as well as HLA-identical donors. Some avoid using child-to-parent donation unless the circumstances are exceptional.

Potential living related donors are subjected to an intensive preoperative evaluation, including clinical examination and measurement of renal function, tests for carriage of hepatitis B, C, HIV and cytomegalovirus, and detailed imaging of renal anatomy with IVU and then arteriography, to be sure that transplantation will be technically feasible.

Unrelated living donors may be accepted provided no inducement (financial or otherwise) is involved. Paid live non-related donor transplantation is illegal in the UK.

Immunosuppression for transplantation

Long-term drug treatment for the prevention of rejection is employed in all cases apart from living related donation from an identical twin. Some degree of immunological tolerance does develop, and the risk of rejection is highest in the first three months after transplantation. In the early months rejection episodes occur in 30–50% of cadaver kidney recipients. Most are reversible. A combination of immunosuppressive drugs is usually used.

Corticosteroids. Corticosteroids have a nonspecific immunosuppressive action. High-dose methylprednisolone is used as the primary treatment for acute rejection.

Azathioprine. Azathioprine prevents cell-mediated rejection by interfering with nucleic acid synthesis and preventing replication of lymphocytes. Adverse effects include suppression of red cell and platelet production, an increased incidence of infections (particularly viral), and hepatotoxicity.

Cyclosporin, tacrolimus and mycophenolate mofetil. Cyclosporin, a fungal metabolite, prevents the activation of T lymphocytes in response to new antigens and is highly effective in preventing rejection, while leaving the functioning of the rest of the immune system largely intact. Its introduction has revolutionized organ transplantation. Disadvantages include variable bioavailability, high cost and nephrotoxicity. Even with careful adjustment of the dose in response to trough blood levels, renal function may be adversely affected. A new microemulsion preparation is more consistently absorbed.

Tacrolimus, a macrolide, blocks T-cell activation by a mechanism very similar to that of cyclosporin but with fewer rejection episodes.

Mycophenolate mofetil is metabolized to mycophenolic acid and may supplant azathioprine as an immunosuppressant, as trials have shown a reduction in rejection episodes.

Antilymphocyte and antithymocyte globulin. These are potent immunosuppressive agents. Antibodies may be polyclonal or monoclonal, derived from mouse, rabbit, horse, or 'humanized', and directed against any of a number of lymphocycte surface marker proteins, enabling neutralization or killing of lymphocytes with certain functions (e.g. T cells, activated T cells, cells expressing adhesion molecules, cells expressing the interleukin-2 receptor). Basiliximab is a chimeric (human and mouse) CD25 monoclonal antibody, which binds to IL-2 receptors inhibiting IL-2-driven proliferative responses. Recent trials have shown its safety, and when given prophylactically it reduces first-time rejection by 40%. The risk of long-term infections and virus-associated malignancy (e.g. lymphoma) remain to be evaluated.

COMPLICATIONS

Technical failures

There may be occlusion or stenosis of the aterial anastomosis, occlusion of the venous anatomosis, and urinary leaks owing to damage to the lower ureter, or defects in the anastomosis between ureter and recipient bladder.

Immunosuppression

- Corticosteroid therapy (see p. 831) can lead to weight gain, 'mooning' of the face, skin striae, increased skin fragility with ecchymoses, diabetes, osteoporosis and fractures, particularly of the femoral neck owing to avascular necrosis of bone.
- Cyclosporin therapy can produce nephrotoxicity, rash, tremor, increased hairiness and diabetes.
- Tacrolimus therapy can lead to neurotoxicity and nephrotoxicity that appear to be greater than with cyclosporin. Abnormalities of glucose metabolism and also cardiomyopathy occur.
- Azathioprine therapy can lead to bone marrow depression.

Both corticosteroid and cyclosporin treatment contribute to post-transplant hypertension. Cyclosporin and azathioprine may cause liver damage. Treatment with corticosteroids, cyclosporin and azathioprine alone or in combination increase the risk of skin tumours, including basal and squamous cell carcinomata, and the risk appears to have increased markedly since the introduction of cyclosporin. In white recipients, exposure to ultraviolet light should be minimized and sun-block creams employed. All immunosuppressive agents used, including antilymphocyte and antithymo-cyte globulin, increase the risk of infections, particularly opportunistic infections such as *Pneumocystis carinii* and cytomegalovirus infection. Malignancy, particularly lymphomas and skin cancers, may often be attributable to viral induction of malignancy.

Other complications

Recurrence of the disease which caused renal failure, although uncommon, may occur in specific diseases. Examples are primary oxalosis, mesangiocapillary glomerulonephritis, focal segmental glomerulosclerosis, and Goodpasture's syndrome.

Other possibilities are that there may be de novo glomerulonephritis in the grafted kidney, or lipid abnormalities and a high risk of cardiovascular events.

Choice of renal replacement therapy

For many patients with end-stage renal failure a renal transplant is the treatment of choice, but because of the limited availability of donor organs many patients remain on dialysis for years whilst waiting for a transplant. Sensitization to HLA antigens, for instance by pregnancy, blood transfusion or a previous failed transplant, makes finding a compatible organ more difficult. In addition, there are a number of factors rendering patients less suitable for transplantation, such as:

- previous malignancy
- severe non-renal disease likely to limit survival and the degree of rehabilitation after transplantation
- vascular disease (especially in diabetes) rendering vascular anastomoses difficult and compromising blood flow to the lower limb.

Age in itself is no bar to transplantation, so policies which limit transplantation to, for example, the under-70 age group may be criticized. Conversely, if the choice is between allocating a precious donor kidney to a fit 25-year-old or a fit 75-year-old recipient, it is difficult to criticize a decision to transplant the former. The problem can be resolved only by a better match between demand and supply of donor organs.

Combined renal and pancreatic transplantation is appropriate in carefully selected patients with diabetes mellitus.

The choice between CAPD and haemodialysis is influenced by medical, social, psychological and other factors. Unless specific indications or contraindications exist, patients should be offered a free choice of modality of treatment.

FURTHER READING

El Nahas AE, Coles EA (1997) Progressive renal failure. *Journal of the Royal College of Physicians* **31**: 27–31.

Lewis H *et al.* (1993) The effect of angiotensin converting enzyme inhibitor on diabetic nephropathy. *New England Journal of Medicine* **329**: 1456–1462.

Lightstone L *et al.* (1995) High incidence of end-stage renal disease in Indo-Asians in the UK. Quarterly Journal of Medicine 88: 191–195.

GISEN trial (1997) Randomized placebo-controlled trial of effect of ramipril on decline in glomerular filtration rate and risk of terminal renal failure in proteinuric, non-diabetic nephropathy. *Lancet* **349**: 1857–1863. Also, editorial: 1852–1853.

Klahr S (1991) Chronic renal failure: management. *Lancet* **338**: 423–427.

Cystic, congenital and familial disease

Cystic renal disease

Solitary or multiple renal cysts are common, especially with advancing age: 50% of those aged 50 years or more have one or more such cysts. They have no special significance except in the differential diagnosis of renal tumours (see p. 591). Such cysts are often asymptomatic and are found on excretion urography or ultrasound examination performed for some other reason. Occasionally they may cause pain and/or haematuria owing to their large size, or bleeding may occur into the cyst. Cystic degeneration (the formation of multiple cysts which enlarge with time) occurs regularly in the kidneys of patients with end-stage renal failure treated by dialysis and/or transplantation. Malignant tumour formation seems to be more common in such kidneys than in the general population.

Autosomal-dominant polycystic kidney disease

Autosomal-dominant polycystic kidney disease (ADPKD) is an inherited disorder usually presenting in adult life. It is characterized by the development of multiple renal cysts, variably associated with extrarenal (mainly hepatic and cardiovascular) abnormalities. ADPKD is by far the most common inherited nephropathy, with a prevalence rate ranging from 1:400 to 1:1000 in white populations. It accounts for 3–10% of all patients commencing regular dialysis in the West.

In about 85% of cases, the gene responsible (PKD1) has been located on chromosome 16. A second gene, PKD2, which has been mapped on chromosome 4, accounts for the vast majority of other cases. A third polycystic gene may exist. These genetic abnormalities are distinct from the autosomal recessive form of polycystic disease which is often lethal in early life. The protein corresponding to PKD1 gene, polycystin I, appears to be an integral membrane glycoprotein involved in cell-to-cell and/or cell-to-matrix interaction. The protein corresponding to the PKD2 gene appears to function as an ion channel or pore. Polycystin could act as the regulator of the PKD2 channel activity. How mutations in PKD1 and PKD2 lead to cyst development and other abnormalities is unclear. It is hoped that elucidation of the mechanism involved may pave the way to intervention which prevents or, at any rate, arrests or slows the manifestations of the disease.

CLINICAL FEATURES

Clinical presentation may be at any age from the second decade. Presenting symptoms include:

- acute loin pain and/or haematuria owing to haemorrhage into a cyst, cyst infection or urinary tract stone formation
- loin or abdominal discomfort owing to the increasing size of the kidneys
- subarachnoid haemorrhage associated with berry aneurysm rupture
- complications of hypertension
- complications of associated liver cysts
- symptoms of uraemia and/or anaemia associated with chronic renal failure.

Erythraemia is a rare complication and presentation of ADPKD.

The natural history of the disease is one of progressive renal impairment, sometimes punctuated by acute episodes of loin pain and haematuria, and commonly associated with the development of hypertension. The rate of progression to renal failure is variable. The determinants of progression are both genetic and non-genetic. In the PKD2 form, renal cysts develop more slowly and end-stage renal failure (ESRF) occurs 10–15 years later than in the PKD1 form. Gender affects renal prognosis, males with ADPKD reaching end-stage renal failure 5–6 years earlier than females. There is a large variability in the age at ESRF within families, even between affected monozygotic twins.

COMPLICATIONS AND ASSOCIATIONS

Pain

A minority of patients suffer chronic renal pain resistant to common analgesics, presumably owing to the pressure effect of large cysts. Surgical decompression of such cysts appears to be of benefit in about two-thirds of patients. Laparoscopic cyst decortication is a promising minimally-invasive alternative technique.

Cyst infection

The response to standard antibacterial therapy is often poor owing to poor penetration of conventional antibiotics across the cyst wall. Lipophilic antibiotics active against Gram-negative bacteria, such as cotrimoxazole and fluoroquinolones, penetrate into the cysts better and their use has greatly improved the treatment of this complication.

Renal calculi

These are diagnosed in about 10–20% of patients with ADPKD. Frequently they are composed of uric acid and hence radiolucent. Obstructing or painful stones are treated no differently than are stones in patients with normal urinary tracts. Percutaneous stone removal and extracorporeal lithotripsy may safely be employed.

Hypertension

Hypertension is an early and very common feature of ADPKD. Elevation of blood pressure, still within the normal range, is detectable in young affected individuals and is associated with an increase in left ventricular mass. It appears that left ventricular hypertrophy occurs to a greater degree for a given rise in blood pressure in ADPKD compared with other renal disorders and with essential hypertension. Intrarenal activation of the renin angiotensin system is, in all probability, of central importance in pathogenesis and ACE inhibitors are logical first-line agents in treatment. Early control of blood pressure is essential as cardiovascular complications are a major cause of death in ADPKD.

Progressive renal failure

This is the most serious complication of ADPKD. At glomerular filtration rates below 50 mL per minute, the rate of decline in GFR averages 5 mL per minute each year, which is more rapid than in other primary renal disorders. The probability of being alive without requiring dialysis or transplantation by the age of 70 years is of the order 30%. Survival rates on regular haemodialysis and after renal transplantation in ADPKD are similar to those of patients with other primary renal diseases.

Hepatic cysts

Approximately 30% of patients have hepatic cysts and in a minority of patients massive enlargement of the polycystic liver is seen. Pain, infection of cysts and, more rarely, compression of the bile duct, portal vein or hepatic venous outflow may occur. Rarely, percutaneous drainage of painful cysts, laparoscopic fenestration or even partial hepatectomy may be necessary. Infected cysts may require drainage.

Intracranial aneurysm formation

About 8% of ADPKD patients have an asymptomatic intracranial aneurysm and the prevalence is twice as high in the subgroup of patients with a family history of such aneurysms or of subarachonoid haemorrhage. Such haemorrhage is preceded in from 20–40% of cases by premonitory headaches from a few hours up to two weeks before the onset of subarachnoid bleeding. Headache of sudden onset or unusual character or severity in a patient with ADPKD should prompt investigation. Contrast-enhanced spiral CT is the best investigation. Screening for intracranial aneurysm in ADPKD is currently recommended for patients aged 18–40 years who have a positive family history. Screening is performed either by magnetic resonance angiography or spiral CT.

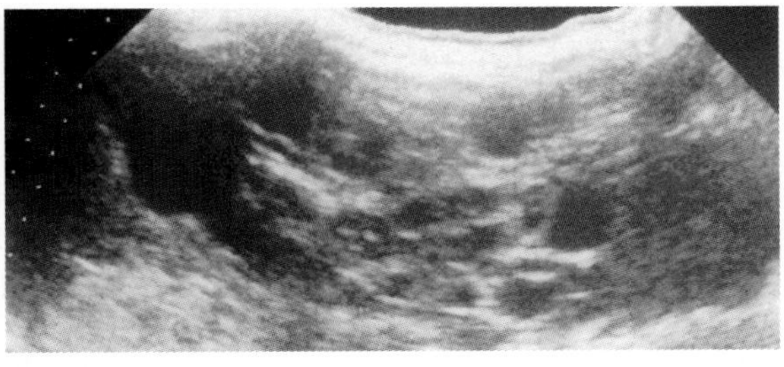

Fig 9.46
Ultrasound scan of a polycystic kidney, showing an enlarged kidney with many cysts of varying size

Mitral valve prolapse

This is found in 20% of individuals with ADPKD, whereas it is present in only 2–3% of the general population.

DIAGNOSIS

Physical examination commonly reveals large, irregular kidneys and possibly hepatomegaly. Definitive diagnosis is established by ultrasound examination (Fig 9.46). However, such renal imaging techniques may be equivocal, especially in subjects under the age of 20 years.

SCREENING

The children and siblings of patients with established ADPKD should, in general, be offered screening. Affected individuals should have regular blood pressure checks and should be offered genetic counselling. Screening by ultrasonography should not be carried out before the age of 20 years, as excluding the condition may be difficult and hypertension is unusual before this age. Even at age 20, renal ultrasonography may give a false-negative result. Gene linkage analysis can be utilized in many families.

Medullary cystic disease ('juvenile nephronophthisis')

Developing early in childhood, juvenile nephronophthisis is commonly inherited in an autosomal recessive manner. A similar condition developing later in childhood (medullary cystic disease) is inherited as an autosomal dominant trait, but sporadic cases occur in both conditions. Despite its name, the dominant histological finding is interstitial inflammation and tubular atrophy, with later development of medullary cysts. Progressive glomerular failure is a secondary consequence.

The dominant features are polyuria, polydipsia and growth retardation. Diagnosis is based on the family history and renal biopsy, the cysts rarely being visualized by imaging techniques.

Medullary sponge kidney

Medullary sponge kidney is an uncommon but not rare condition that usually presents with renal colic or haematuria. Although it is most often sporadic, a few affected families have been reported. The condition is characterized by dilatation of the collecting ducts in the papillae, sometimes with cystic change. In severe cases the medullary area has a sponge-like appearance. The condition may affect one or both kidneys or only part of one kidney. Cyst formation is commonly associated with the development of small calculi within the cyst. In about 20% of patients there is associated hypercalciuria or renal tubular acidosis (see p. 620). Hemihypertrophy of the skeleton has been described in this condition.

The diagnosis is made by excretion urography, which shows small calculi in the papillary zones with an increase in radiodensity around these following injection of contrast medium as the dilated or cystic collecting ducts are filled with contrast (see Fig 9.26).

The natural history is one of intermittent colic with passage of small stones or haematuria. Renal function is usually well maintained and renal failure is unusual, except where obstructive nephropathy develops owing to the presence of stones in the pelvis or ureters.

Congenital abnormalities

Agenesis

Agenesis may be bilateral or unilateral. Unilateral agenesis ('solitary kidney') occurs in 1 in 1000 of the population. It is usually associated with compensatory hypertrophy of the single kidney and normal renal function. Save for the potential hazard of trauma to this solitary kidney, it has no clinical significance.

Hypoplasia

Renal hypoplasia (failed development) of one kidney is uncommon, and hypoplasia of both kidneys is rare. It may be difficult to distinguish unilateral renal hypoplasia from a small kidney due to renal artery stenosis, obstruction or reflux nephropathy in early life. Clinical interest in the condition most often arises in patients with hypertension, where the small kidney may be considered the cause. If the small kidney is shown by radioisotope studies to contribute no useful renal function, and if the hypertension has developed in a young subject or is difficult to control by medical treatment, nephrectomy should be undertaken.

Ectopic kidneys

Defects in embryological renal development may lead to ectopic or maldeveloped renal systems. At the risk of oversimplification, the kidneys may be thought of as developing in the embryo as one structure in the 'pelvic' area, migrating upwards and separating with growth. Failure in normal development may result in failure of the kidneys to migrate normally and indeed they may fail to separate. This results in a 'pelvic kidney' when one or both remain in the pelvis, a 'crossed ectopic kidney' when both have moved to the same side of the spine, a horseshoe or discoid kidney when there is partial (usually fusion of the lower poles) or total failure of separation.

In clinical practice the main problem associated with ectopic kidneys usually relates to impaired urinary drainage with secondary obstruction or stone formation. This may be compounded if infection supervenes, the poor drainage making eradication of infection difficult and predisposing to stone formation. Pelvic kidneys may interfere with parturition.

Renal tubular transport defects

Renal tubular transport defects include cystinuria, Hartnup disease, adult Fanconi syndrome, galactosaemia and fructosaemia. They are discussed in more detail on p. 999.

Animal experiments now suggest that X-linked hypophosphataemia ('vitamin D-resistant rickets'), formerly regarded as an intrinsic proximal renal tubular transport defect, results from the effect of a distant mediator upon renal tubular phosphate handling. A mouse model of X-linked hypophosphataemia exists and transplantation of a kidney from an affected animal into a normal bi-nephrectomized mouse does not confer a renal tubular phosphate leak on the recipient. Conversely, transplantation of a normal mouse kidney into a bi-nephrectomized mouse with X-linked hypophosphataemia does not correct the renal tubular phosphate leak.

Renal glycosuria

Renal glycosuria, in which there is glucose in the urine in subjects demonstrated to have normal blood glucose levels, who are not starved and who have no other urinary abnormality, is uncommon. Such patients have either a defect in the tubular threshold for reabsorption of glucose in the proximal tubule (a 'splayed' reabsorption curve) or a defect in the maximal tubular reabsorption of glucose. Both autosomal dominant and recessive inheritance have been postulated. It has no clinical significance except in the differential diagnosis of patients with diabetes mellitus or other tubular disorders such as the Fanconi syndrome.

FURTHER READING

Pirson Y (1996) Recent advances in the clinical management of autosomal-dominant polycystic kidney disease. *Quarterly Journal of Medicine* **89**: 803–806.

Tumours of the kidney and genitourinary tract

Malignant renal tumours

These comprise 1–2% of all malignant tumours, and the male/female ratio is 2:1.

Renal cell carcinoma

Renal cell carcinomas (previously called hypernephromas or Grawitz tumours) arise from proximal tubular epithelium. They are the most common renal tumour in adults. They rarely present before the age of 40 years, the average age of presentation being 55 years.

The pathogenesis of some malignant tumours, including renal cell carcinoma, is currently in the process of being clarified by the techniques of modern cytogenetics. In von Hippel–Lindau disease, an autosomal dominant disorder, bilateral renal cell carcinomas are common and haemangioblastomas, phaeochromocytomas and renal cysts are also found. Polymorphic probes from chromosome 3p, the region implicated in renal cell carcinoma, have demonstrated genetic linkage between them and von Hippel–Lindau disease. It seems likely, therefore, that mutation of the same tumour suppressor gene may be responsible for both renal cell carcinoma and von Hippel–Lindau disease.

PATHOLOGY

The tumours may be solitary, multiple or occasionally bilateral. The tumour lies within the kidney but it may eventually penetrate the capsule. Macroscopically, its cut surface appears as a yellow mass, sometimes containing areas of haemorrhage and cystic degeneration. Local invasion of renal veins and spread to the opposite kidney may occur, as may metastasis to lymph nodes, liver, bone and lung (often as an apparently solitary metastasis). Renal cell carcinomas are highly vascular tumours. Microscopically the tumour is composed of large cells containing clear cytoplasm.

CLINICAL FEATURES

Patients present with haematuria, loin pain and a mass in the flank. Malaise, anorexia and weight loss may occur, and occasionally patients present with polycythaemia (see p. 389). Pyrexia is present in about one-fifth of patients and approximately one-quarter present with metastases. Rarely, a left-sided varicocele may be associated with left-sided tumours that have invaded the renal vein and caused obstruction to drainage of the left testicular vein.

DIAGNOSIS

Excretion urography will reveal a space-occupying lesion in the kidney; 10% of these show calcification.

Ultrasonography is used to demonstrate the solid lesion and to examine the patency of the renal vein and inferior vena cava. CT scanning can also be used to identify the renal lesion and involvement of the renal vein or inferior vena cava. MRI is better than CT for tumour staging. Renal arteriography will reveal the tumour's circulation (Fig 9.47) but is now seldom employed. Urine cytology for malignant cells is of no value. The ESR is usually raised.

TREATMENT

Treatment is by nephrectomy unless bilateral tumours are present or the contralateral kidney functions poorly, in which case conservative surgery such as partial nephrec-tomy may be indicated. If metastases are present, nephrectomy may still be warranted since regression of metastases has been reported after removal of the main tumour mass. Severe flank pain may also demand nephrectomy despite the presence of metastases. Radiotherapy has no proven value.

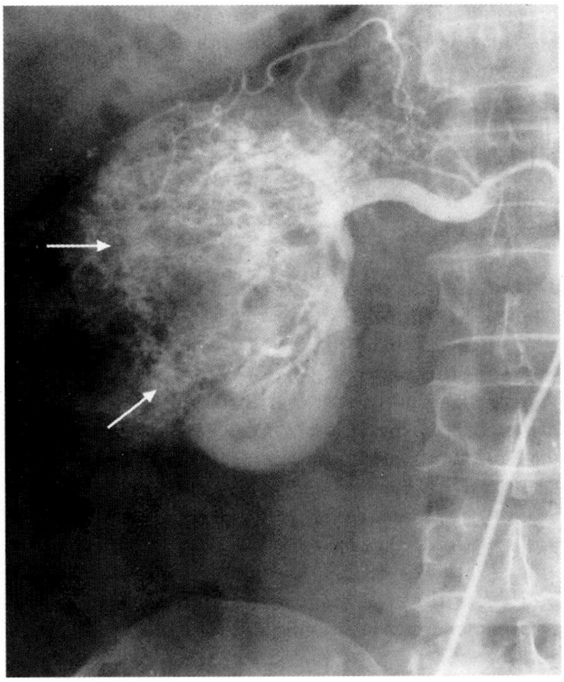

Fig 9.47
Renal arteriogram in a patient with renal carcinoma. Note the abnormal tumour circulation

Medroxyprogesterone acetate is of some value in controlling metastatic disease. Treatment with α-interferon produces up to a 20% response rate in the short term.

PROGNOSIS

The prognosis depends upon the degree of differentiation of the tumour and whether or not metastases are present. The five-year survival rate is 60–70% with tumours confined to the renal parenchyma, 15–35%, with lymph node involvement, and only approximately 5% in those who have distant metastases.

Nephroblastoma (Wilms' tumour)

This tumour is seen mainly within the first three years of life and may be bilateral. It presents as an abdominal mass, rarely with haematuria. Diagnosis is established by excretion urography followed by arteriography. A combination of nephrectomy, radiotherapy and chemotherapy has much improved survival rates, and the majority of children, even those with metastatic disease, are cured.

Benign renal tumours

Renal adenoma

Benign adenomas are usually an incidental finding, presenting as a space-occupying lesion on excretion urography. They seldom cause symptoms. On urography they may be difficult to distinguish from a renal cell carcinoma.

Simple cysts

Simple cysts are common. They are discussed in more detail on p. 588.

Differentiation of benign renal cyst from malignant tumour

If a space-occupying lesion is a chance finding on excretion urography in a patient with no relevant symptoms and no haematuria, ultrasonography should be carried out. If the lesion is transonic with no features suggesting a tumour, no further investigation is required. If haematuria has been present, a needle should be inserted into the transonic lesion and cyst fluid aspirated and examined for malignant cells. Contrast medium may be injected to delineate the walls of the cyst. Lesions shown to be solid or non-homogeneous on ultrasonography require further investigation by CT or MRI.

Urothelial tumours

The calyces, renal pelvis, ureter, bladder and urethra are lined by transitional cell epithelium. Transitional cell tumours account for about 3% of deaths from all forms of malignancy. Such tumours are uncommon below the age of 40 years, and the male/female ratio is 4:1. Bladder tumours are about 50 times as common as those of the ureter or renal pelvis.

Predisposing factors include:

- cigarette smoking
- exposure to industrial carcinogens such as β-naphthylamine and benzidene (workers in the chemical, cable and rubber industries are at particular risk)
- exposure to drugs (e.g. phenacetin, cyclophosphamide)
- chronic inflammation (e.g. schistosomiasis, usually associated with squamous carcinoma).

PRESENTATION

Painless haematuria is the most common presenting symptom of bladder malignancy, although pain may occur owing to clot retention. Symptoms suggestive of UTI may develop in the absence of significant bacteriuria. In patients with bladder cancer, pain may also result from local nerve involvement.

Presenting symptoms may result from local metastases.

Transitional cell carcinomas in the kidney and ureter may present with haematuria. They may also give rise to flank pain, particularly if urinary tract obstruction is present.

INVESTIGATIONS

- **Cytological examination** of urine for malignant cells.
- **Excretion urography**.
- **Cystoscopy** if no evidence of upper urinary tract pathology has been found.

Cystoscopy may be omitted in men under 20 and women under 30 years if significant bacteriuria accompanies the haematuria and ceases following control of the infection, provided urine cytology and excretion urography are normal. With these exceptions, haematuria should always be investigated.

In cases where the tumour is not clearly outlined on excretion urography, abdominal CT scanning and/or retrograde ureterography may be helpful.

TREATMENT

Pelvic and ureteric tumours

These are treated by nephroureterectomy. Radiotherapy and chemotherapy appear to be of little or no value. Subsequently cystoscopy should be regularly carried out, since about half the patients will develop bladder tumours.

Bladder tumours

Treatment depends upon the stage of the tumour (in particular whether it has penetrated the bladder muscle) and its degree of differentiation. Treatment options include local cystodiathermy and/or resection with follow-up check cystoscopies, cytological examination of urine/cystoscopy, cystectomy, radiotherapy, or local and systemic chemotherapy.

PROGNOSIS

The prognosis ranges from a five-year survival rate of 80% for lesions not involving bladder muscle to 5% for those presenting with metastases.

Diseases of the prostate gland

Benign enlargement of the prostate gland

Benign prostatic enlargement occurs most often in men over the age of 60 years. Such enlargement is much less common in African and Asian individuals. It is unknown in eunuchs. The aetiology of the condition is unknown.

Microscopically, hyperplasia affects the glandular and connective tissue elements of the prostate. Enlargement of the gland stretches and distorts the urethra, obstructing bladder outflow. The bladder musculature hypertrophies so that a higher than usual pressure is generated within the bladder in order to overcome the obstruction and allow voiding of urine. Bands of muscle fibre are seen at cystoscopy (trabeculation). Eventually the bladder becomes dilated and the muscle hypotonic. The sphincter mechanism at the vesicoureteric junction may be impaired and reflux of urine from the bladder into the ureters and upper urinary tract may occur.

CLINICAL FEATURES

Frequency of urination, usually first noted as nocturia, is a common early symptom. Difficulty or delay in initiating urination, with variability and reduced forcefulness of the urinary stream and post-void dribbling, are often present. Suprapubic pain occurs if bladder bacteriuria is present, if a bladder calculus has formed as a result of stagnation of urine within the bladder, or in acute retention of urine. Flank pain may accompany dilatation of the upper tracts. Acute retention of urine (see below) or retention with overflow incontinence may occur. Occasionally, severe haematuria results from rupture of prostatic veins or as a consequence of bacteriuria or stone disease. Some patients present with severe renal failure.

Abdominal examination for bladder enlargement together with examination of the rectum are essential. A benign prostate feels smooth. An accurate impression of prostatic size cannot be obtained on rectal examination.

INVESTIGATIONS

These should include urine culture, assessment of renal function by measuring serum urea and creatinine concentrations, measurement of prostate-specific antigen (markedly raised in prostatic cancer), a plain abdominal X-ray, and renal ultrasonography to define whether upper tract dilatation is present. Excretion urography is not usually necessary. The completeness of bladder emptying after an act of voiding can be assessed by ultrasonography or by inspection of the after-voiding radiograph carried out during excretion urography if this is performed. Cystourethroscopy is essential.

MANAGEMENT AND PROGNOSIS

Patients with mild-to-moderate symptoms should be managed by 'watchful waiting', because symptoms following therapy are sometimes greater than those with no therapy at all.

Patients with moderate prostatic symptoms can be treated medically. A number of drugs have been employed, including α-blockers such as doxazosin. Finasteride is a competitive inhibitor of 5α-reductase, which is the enzyme involved in the conversion of testosterone to dihydrotestosterone. This is the androgen primarily responsible for prostatic growth and enlargement. Finasteride decreases prostatic volume with an increase in urine flow.

Deterioration in renal function or the development of upper tract dilatation requires surgery. Transurethral resection is usually successful unless the gland is very large. It carries a lower morbidity and mortality with a shorter stay in hospital than open prostatectomy. Microwave hyperthermia, balloon dilatation and prostatic stents are all being tried, but evidence from long-term randomized prospective controlled trials is not yet available. Very large glands require open transvesical prostatectomy.

In acute retention or retention with overflow, the first priorities are to relieve pain and to establish urethral catheter drainage. If urethral catheterization is impossible, suprapubic catheter drainage should be carried out. The choice of further management is then between immediate prostatectomy, a period of catheter drainage followed by prostatectomy, or the acceptance of a permanent indwelling suprapubic or urethral catheter.

Prostatic carcinoma

Prostatic carcinoma accounts for 7% of all cancers in men and is the fourth most common cause of death from malignant disease in men in England and Wales. Malignant change within the prostate becomes increasingly common with advancing age. By the age of 80 years, 80% of men have malignant foci within the gland, but most of these appear to lie dormant. Histologically, the tumour is an adenocarcinoma. Hormonal factors are thought to play a role in the aetiology.

CLINICAL FEATURES

Presentation is usually with symptoms of lower urinary tract obstruction or of metastatic spread, particularly to bone. The diagnosis may be made by the incidental finding of a hard irregular gland on rectal examination, or as an unexpected histological result after prostatectomy for what was believed to be benign prostatic hypertrophy.

INVESTIGATIONS

Investigations are as for benign enlargement of the prostate gland, with, in addition, measurement of prostate-specific antigen level, supplemented by transrectal ultrasound of the prostate and prostatic biopsy. Prostate-specific antigen levels are unaffected by the presence of renal failure.

A histological diagnosis is essential before treatment is considered. This may be obtained by:

- cytological staining of biopsy material from the prostate
- histological examination of biopsy material or material obtained at transurethral or open prostatectomy.

If metastases are present, serum prostate-specific antigen levels are usually markedly elevated; it is a myth that elevated levels occur as a result of rectal examination.

Ultrasonography and transrectal ultrasonography are of value in defining the size of the gland and staging any tumour present. The upper renal tracts can be examined by ultrasonography for evidence of dilatation. Bone metastases may appear as osteosclerotic lesions on X-ray or may be detected by isotopic bone scans.

TREATMENT
Microscopic, not clinically palpable, tumour can be managed expectantly. Treatment for disease confined to the gland is radical prostatectomy (provided the patient is fit for the procedure) or radiotherapy. Evidence is accumulating that radical prostatectomy is the treatment of choice in younger patients with poorly differentiated tumours. There have, however, been no controlled trials of this therapy and survival may be good without therapy. Locally extensive disease is managed with radiotherapy. Metastatic disease can be treated with orchidectomy, but many men refuse. Luteinizing hormone-releasing hormone (LHRH) analogues such as buserelin or goserelin are equally effective and preferred by many. Non-hormonal chemotherapy is unhelpful.

PROGNOSIS
The duration of survival depends on the age of the patient and the degree of differentiation and extent of the tumour.

SCREENING
The value or otherwise of screening for prostate cancer is debated and the place, if any, of screening is unclear. Undoubtedly an annual measurement of prostate-specific antigen in asymptomatic men results in earlier diagnosis. It is not clear, however, that any benefit ensues in terms of increased survival; and the financial cost of screening, emotional impact upon the patient of a positive result, and complications of treatment of any abnormality found have to be set against any possible benefit. Large-scale trials are in progress.

Testicular tumours

Testicular tumours, though uncommon, are the most common malignant disease in men between the ages of 29 and 34 years. All such tumours should nowadays be regarded as curable. Patient survival depends upon early diagnosis, accurate staging of the tumour and appropriate treatment and follow-up. The expertise of a specialist centre is invaluable.

More than 96% of testicular tumours arise from germ cells. Two main types of tumour exist:

- seminomas (about one-third)
- teratomas (about two-thirds).

AETIOLOGY
The aetiology is unknown. The risk of malignant change is much greater in undescended testes and there is a history of orchidopexy in about 10% of patients. Previous testicular biopsy appears to be associated with an increased risk of malignant change.

CLINICAL FEATURES
Common presenting symptoms are:

- testicular swelling, which may be painless or painful
- symptoms from metastases.

DIFFERENTIAL DIAGNOSIS
The differential diagnosis includes:

- epididymo-orchitis
- torsion
- chronic infection (e.g. tuberculosis, syphilitic gumma).

INVESTIGATIONS
Diagnosis may only be possible after surgical exploration of the testis through the groin. Scrotal exploration and scrotal testicular biopsy should be avoided owing to the high incidence of tumour implantation.

Staging of the tumour will require:

- chest X-ray to look for metastases
- estimation of α-fetoprotein and β-human chorionic gonadotrophin concentrations (tumour markers)
- abdominal CT scanning.

TREATMENT
Seminomas are radiosensitive, so tumours confined to the testis or with metastases below the diaphragm only are treated by radiotherapy. More widespread tumours require chemotherapy.

Teratomas are treated by orchidectomy if the growth is confined to the testis. Chemotherapy is required for more widespread disease (see p. 441).

FURTHER READING

Diasko JC, Lange PH (1997) Prostate cancer. *New England Journal of Medicine* **337**: 340–341.

Frydenberg M, Stricker PD, Kaye KW (1997) Prostate cancer diagnosis and management. *Lancet* **349**: 1681–1685.

Motzer RJ, Bander NH, Nanus DM (1996) Medical progress: renal cell carcinoma. *New England Journal of Medicine* **335**: 865–875.

Renal disease in the elderly

Renal disease and renal failure are common in the elderly. Acceptance of patients aged 65 years and over for renal replacement therapy approximately doubles the number of such patients in whom renal replacement is initiated.

Renal failure in the elderly more often results from renal vascular disease or urinary tract obstruction than in younger age groups. In males, obstruction is most often due to benign or malignant prostatic enlargement, while in females it results from pelvic cancer.

Progressive sclerosis of glomeruli occurs with ageing and this, together with the development of atheromatous renal vascular disease, accounts for the progressive reduction in GFR seen with advancing years. A GFR of 50–60 mL per minute (about half the normal value for a young adult) may be regarded as 'normal' in patients in their eighties. The reduction in muscle mass often seen with ageing may mask this deterioration in renal function in that the serum creatinine concentration may be less than 0.12 mmol L^{-1} in an elderly patient whose GFR is 50 mL per minute or lower. The use of serum creatinine as a measure of renal function in the elderly must take this into account. This is especially important in the elderly when prescribing drugs whose excretion is in whole or in part by the kidney.

Urinary tract infections

UTIs are more common in the elderly, in whom impaired bladder emptying due to prostatic disease in males and neuropathic bladder – especially common in females – is frequently found. Symptoms may be atypical, the major complaints being incontinence, nocturia, smelly urine or vague change in well-being with little in the way of dysuria. Demonstration of significant bacteriuria in the presence of such symptoms requires treatment.

Urinary incontinence

This is one of the major disabilities of the elderly. Correctable factors, such as chronic constipation, diuretic therapy, infections and treatable bladder outflow impairment need to be excluded. Often there is a combination of factors including, for example, difficulty in getting to the toilet, and dementia. An expert and committed incontinence advisory and treatment service combining nursing and medical skills is invaluable for elderly patients with this distressing problem. Home visits to ensure the availability of commodes and toilets is essential. For established incontinence, catheterization may be necessary.

Incontinence and its treatment is a matter of major importance and by no means solely in the elderly.

FURTHER READING

Fliser D, Franek E, Ritz E (1997) Renal function in the elderly: is the dogma of an inexorable decline of renal function correct? *Nephrology, Dialysis, Transplantation* **12**: 1553–1555.

Tropical nephrology

This chapter approaches nephrology from the perspective of a nephrologist practising in a developed Western country, the climate of which is temperate. Inevitably, an unbalanced view is therefore provided of nephrological problems worldwide. Wide geographical variations exist in the incidence and prevalence of diseases affecting the kidneys in developing and tropical countries.

For example, in some parts of southern Iraq the onset of macroscopic haematuria in pubescent males is regarded as almost a normal development – akin to the onset of menstruation in females – owing to the wide prevalence of infection with *Schistosoma haematobium*. In Nigeria, the most common causes of acute renal failure are typhoid and snake-bite, usually envenomation from a puff adder bite. In sub-Saharan Africa, malarial infection remains an extremely common cause of glomerulonephritis. In black Africans living in urban (as distinct from rural) areas, hypertension is exceptionally common, being characterized by relatively low levels of renin and normal levels of aldosterone in blood. Such hypertension has a particular predeliction for inducing kidney damage and it is likely – although data are scant – that end-stage renal failure due to hypertensive nephropathy in urban blacks is extremely common. Certainly in the United Kingdom and USA, end-stage renal failure is reached at about four times the rate in blacks compared with whites and hypertension is a major cause of this. It appears that less efficient renal excretion of sodium in blacks versus whites explains some of these observations. In rural sub-Saharan Africa, dietary salt intake is in general very low and in a hot country where sodium intake is low, reduced renal capacity to excrete sodium might well have been an evolutionary advantage. Exposure to the higher dietary salt intake in cities may well account, in part at least, for the high prevalence of hypertension in urban blacks.

The vast majority of black individuals reaching end-stage renal failure in sub-Saharan Africa die untreated since facilities for dialysis and transplantation are, by comparison with developed countries, minimal.

CHAPTER BIBLIOGRAPHY

Cameron JS, Davison AM, Grunfeld JP, Kerr DNS, Ritz E (eds) (1997) *Oxford Textbook of Clinical Nephrology.* Oxford: Oxford University Press.

Schrier RW (ed) (1997) *Renal Electrolyte Disorders,* 5th edn. Philadelphia, Lippincott Raven.

Weatherall DJ, Ledingham JGG, Warrell JDA (eds) (1996) *Oxford Textbook of Medicine*, 3rd edn. Oxford: Oxford University Press.

Current Opinions in Nephrology and Hypertension is a monthly journal with review articles: each issue devoted to one or two topics.

Journal of Royal College of Physicians has a series on renal disease, starting Jan/Feb 1997.

Nephrology, Dialysis, Transplantation is the major European journal devoted to the subject, with review articles, editorial comments and original papers.

Water, electrolytes and acid–base homeostasis

10

In health, the volume and biochemical composition of both extracellular and intracellular fluid compartments in the body remains remarkably constant. Many different disease states result in changes of control either of extracellular fluid *volume*, or of the *electrolyte composition* of extracellular fluid. An understanding of these abnormalities is therefore essential for the management of a wide range of clinical disorders.

Distribution and composition of body water

In normal persons, the total body water constitutes 50–60% of lean bodyweight in men and 45–50% in women. In a healthy 70 kg male, total body water is approximately 42 L. This is contained in three major compartments:

- the intracellular fluid (28 L, about 35% of lean bodyweight)
- the interstitial fluid that bathes the cells (9.4 L, about 12%)
- plasma (4.6 L, about 4–5%).

In addition, small amounts of water are contained in bone, dense connective tissue, and epithelial secretions, such as the digestive secretions and cerebrospinal fluid.

The intracellular and interstitial fluids are separated by the cell membrane; the interstitial fluid and plasma are separated by the capillary wall (Fig 10.1). In the absence of solute, water molecules move randomly and in equal numbers in either direction across a permeable membrane. However, if solutes are added to one side of the membrane, the intermolecular cohesive forces reduce the activity of the water molecules. As a result, water tends to stay in the solute-containing compartment because there is less free diffusion across the membrane. This ability to hold water in the compartment can be measured as the osmotic pressure.

Osmotic pressure

Osmotic pressure is the primary determinant of the distribution of water between the three major compartments. The concentrations of the major solutes in these fluids differ, and each compartment has one solute that is primarily limited to that compartment and therefore determines its osmotic pressure: K^+ salts in the intracellular

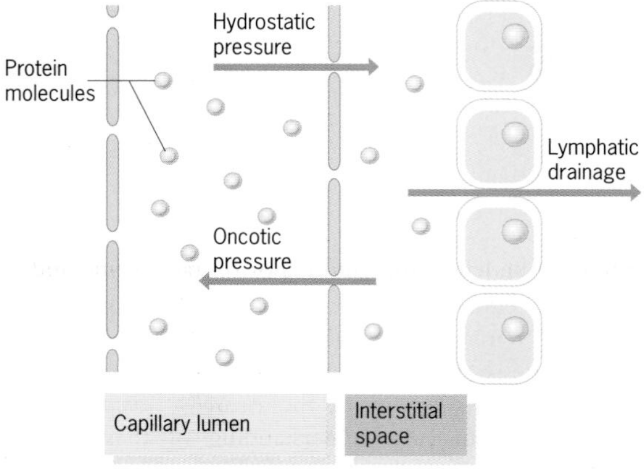

Fig 10.1
Distribution of water between the vascular and extravascular (interstitial) spaces. This is determined by the equilibrium between hydrostatic pressure, which tends to force fluid out of the capillaries, and oncotic pressure, which acts to retain fluid within the vessel. The net flow of fluid outwards is balanced by 'suction' of fluid into the lymphatics, which returns it to the bloodstream. Similar principles govern the volume of the peritoneal and pleural spaces

fluid (most of the cell Mg^{2+} is bound and osmotically inactive), Na^+ salts in the interstitial fluid, and proteins in the plasma. Regulation of the plasma volume is somewhat more complicated because of the tendency of the plasma proteins to hold water in the vascular space by an osmotic effect which is in part counterbalanced by the hydrostatic pressure in the capillary that is generated by cardiac contraction (Fig 10.1). The composition of intracellular and extracellular fluids is shown in Table 10.1.

A characteristic of an osmotically active solute is that it cannot freely leave its compartment. The capillary wall, for example, is relatively impermeable to plasma proteins, and the cell membrane is 'impermeable' to Na^+ and K^+ because the Na^+–K^+-ATPase pump largely restricts Na^+ to the extracellular fluid and K^+ to the intracellular fluid. By contrast, Na^+ freely crosses the capillary wall and achieves similar concentrations in the interstitium and plasma; as a result, it does not contribute to fluid distribution between these compartments. Similarly, urea crosses both the capillary wall and the cell membrane and is osmotically inactive. Thus, the retention of urea in renal failure does not alter the distribution of the total body water.

A conclusion from these observations is that body Na^+ stores are the primary determinant of the extracellular fluid volume. Thus the extracellular volume – and therefore tissue perfusion – are maintained by appropriate alterations in Na^+ excretion. For example, if Na^+ intake is increased, the extra Na^+ will initially be added to the extracellular fluid. The associated increase in extracellular osmolality will cause water to move out of the cells, leading to extracellular volume expansion. Balance is restored by excretion of the excess Na^+ in the urine.

Table 10.1
Electrolyte composition of intracellular and extracellular fluids

	Plasma (mmol L^{-1})	Interstitial fluid (mmol L^{-1})	Intracellular fluid (mmol L^{-1})
Na^+	142	144	10
K^+	4	4	160
Ca^{2+}	2.5	2.5	1.5
Mg^{2+}	1.0	0.5	13
Cl^-	102	114	2
HCO_3^-	26	30	8
PO_4^{2-}	1.0	1.0	57
SO_4^{2-}	0.5	0.5	10
Organic acid	3	4	3
Protein	16	0	55

Distribution of different types of replacement fluids

Figure 10.2 shows the relative effects of the addition of identical volumes of water, saline and colloid solutions on the compartments. Thus, 1 L of water given intravenously as 5% dextrose is distributed equally into all compartments, whereas the same amount of 0.9% saline remains in the extracellular compartment. The latter is thus the correct treatment for extracellular water depletion – sodium keeping the water in this compartment. The addition of 1 L of colloid with its high oncotic pressure stays in the vascular compartment and is the treatment for hypovolaemia.

Regulation of extracellular volume (Fig 10.3)

The extracellular volume is determined by the sodium concentration. The regulation of extracellular volume is dependent upon a tight control of sodium balance which is exerted by normal kidneys. Renal Na^+ excretion varies directly with the effective circulating volume. In a 70 kg man, plasma fluid constitutes one-third of extracellular volume (4.6 L), of which 85% (3.9 L) lies in the venous side and only 15% (0.7 L) resides in the arterial circulation. The unifying hypothesis of extracellular volume regulation in health and disease proposed by Schrier states that the fullness of the arterial vascular compartment – or the so-called effective arterial blood volume (EABV) – is the primary determinant of renal sodium and water excretion. Thus effective arterial blood volume constitutes effective circulatory volume for the purposes of body fluid homeostasis. The fullness of the arterial compartment depends upon a normal ratio between cardiac output and peripheral arterial resistance. Thus diminished EABV is initiated by a fall in cardiac output or a fall in peripheral arterial resistance (an increase in the holding capacity of the arterial vascular tree). When the effective arterial volume is expanded, the urinary Na^+ excretion is increased and can exceed 100 mmol L^{-1}. In contrast, the urine can be rendered virtually free of Na^+ in the presence of volume depletion and normal renal function.

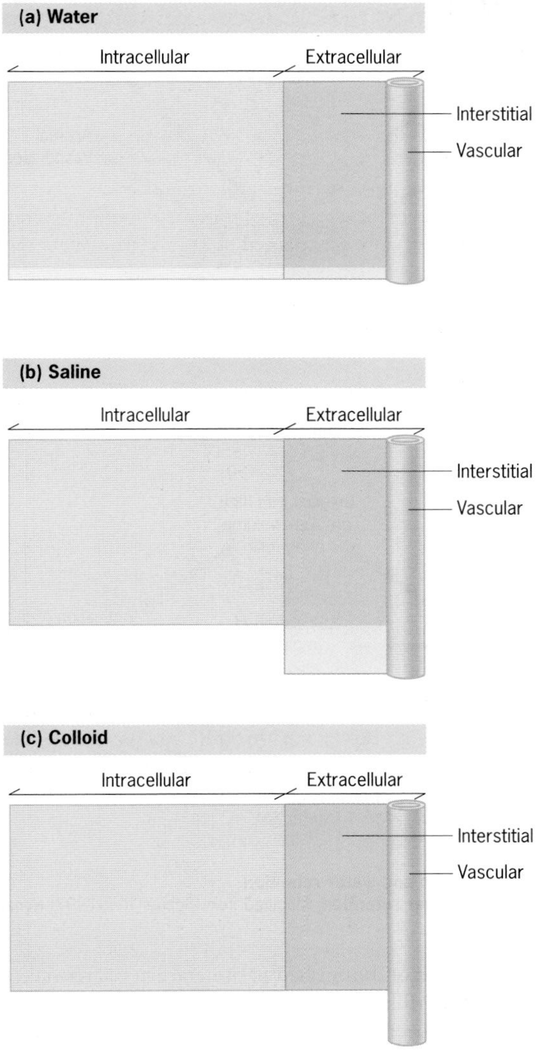

Fig 10.2
Relative effects of the addition of (a) 1 L of water, (b) saline 0.9%, and (c) a colloid solution

These changes in Na^+ excretion can result from alterations both in the filtered load, determined primarily by the glomerular filtration rate (GFR), and in tubular reabsorption, which is affected by multiple factors. In general, it is changes in tubular reabsorption that constitute the main adaptive response to fluctuations in the effective circulating volume. How this occurs can be appreciated from Table 10.2, which depicts the sites and determinants of segmental Na^+ reabsorption. Although the loop of Henle and distal tubule make an important overall contribution to net Na^+ handling, transport in these segments primarily varies with the amount of Na^+ delivered; that is, reabsorption is flow-dependent. In comparison, the neurohumoral regulation of Na^+ reabsorption according to body needs occurs primarily in the proximal and collecting tubules.

Neurohumoral regulation of extracellular volume

This is mediated by volume receptors which sense changes in the effective circulatory volume rather than alterations in the sodium concentration. These receptors are distributed in both the cardiovascular and renal tissues.

- *Extrarenal receptors.* These are located in the vascular tree in the left atrium and major thoracic veins, and in the carotid sinus body and aortic arch. These volume receptors respond to a slight reduction in effective circulating volume and result in increased sympathetic nerve activity and a rise in catecholamines. In addition, volume receptors in the cardiac atria control the release of a powerful natriuretic hormone – atrial natriuretic peptide (ANP) – from granules located in the atrial walls.
- *Intrarenal receptors.* Receptors in the walls of the afferent glomerular arterioles respond, via the juxtaglomerular apparatus, to changes in renal perfusion, and control the activity of the renin–angiotensin–aldosterone system (p. 953). In addition, sodium concentration in the distal tubule and sympathetic nerve activity alter renin release from the juxtaglomerular cells. Prostaglandins I_2 and E_2 are also generated within the kidney in response to angiotensin II, acting to maintain glomerular filtration rate and sodium and water excretion, modulating the sodium-retaining effect of this hormone.

The receptors distributed in the thoracic tissues (cardiac atria, right ventricle, thoracic veins, pulmonary vessels) are low-pressure volume receptors and must be of some importance in the volume regulatory system. However, there is now considerable evidence that high-pressure arterial receptors (carotid, aortic arch, juxtaglomerular apparatus) predominate over low-pressure volume receptors in volume control in mammals.

It seems likely that aldosterone and possibly atrial natriuretic peptide (or related peptides such as urodilatin) are responsible for day-to-day variations in Na^+ excretion, by their respective ability to augment and diminish Na^+ reabsorption in the collecting tubules. A salt load, for example, leads to an increase in the effective circulatory and extracellular volume, raising both renal perfusion pressure, atrial and arterial filling pressure. The increase in the renal perfusion pressure reduces the secretion of renin, and subsequently that of angiotensin II and aldosterone, whereas the rise in atrial and arterial filling pressure increases the release of ANP. These factors combine to reduce Na^+ reabsorption in the collecting duct, thereby promoting excretion of excess Na^+. In contrast, in patients on low Na^+ intake or in those who become volume-depleted as a result of vomiting and diarrhoea, the ensuing decrease in effective volume enhances the activity of the renin–angiotensin–aldosterone system and reduces the secretion of ANP. The net effect is enhanced Na^+

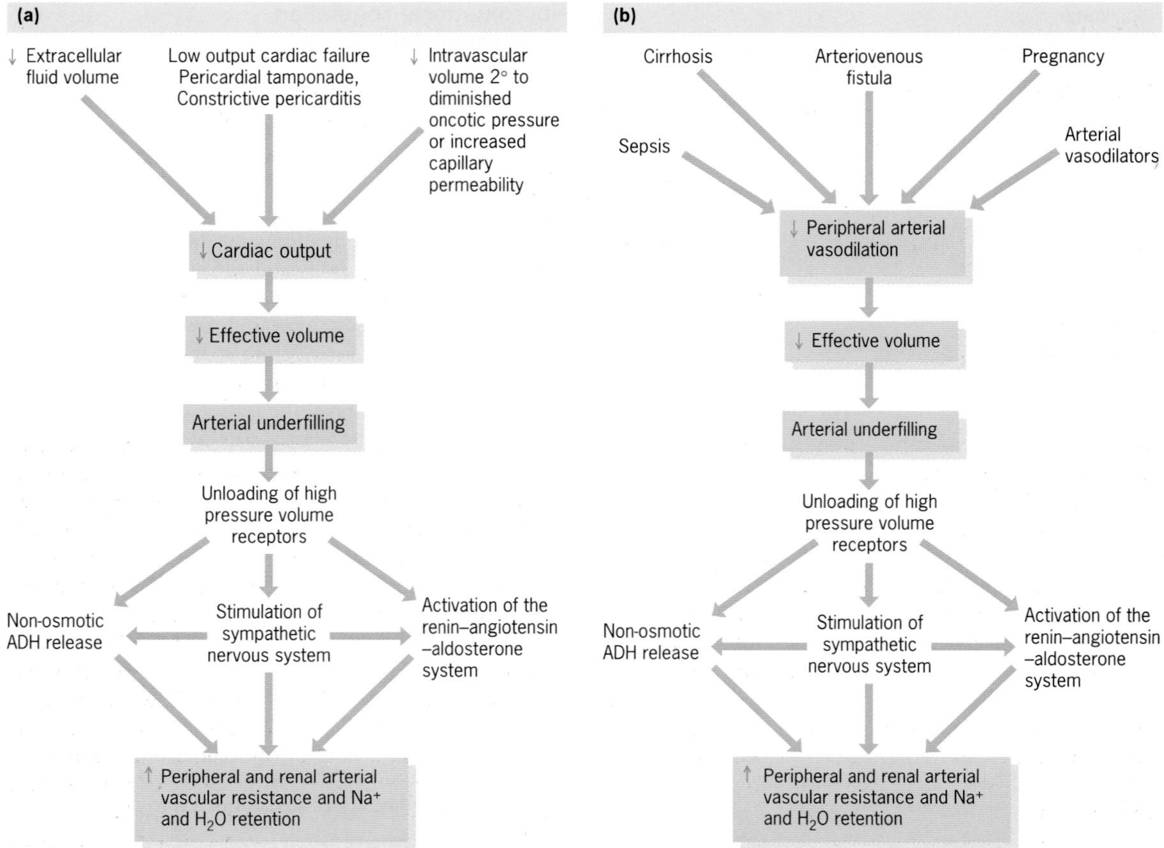

Fig 10.3
(a) Sequence of events in which a decrease in cardiac output initiates renal sodium and water retention.
(b) Sequence of events in which arterial vasodilation initiates renal sodium and water retention. Modified from Schrier RW (1997) *Renal and Electrolyte Disorders*, 5th edn

reabsorption in the collecting tubules, which seems to account for the appropriate fall in Na^+ excretion in this setting, which tends to increase the extracellular volume towards normal.

With more marked hypovolaemia, a decrease in GFR and increase in proximal and thin ascending limb Na^+ reabsorption also contribute to Na^+ retention. This is brought about by enhanced sympathetic activity acting directly on kidneys and indirectly by stimulating the secretion of renin/angiotensin II and nonosmotic release of antidiuretic hormone. The pressure natriuresis phenomenon may be the final defence against changes in the effective circulating volume. Marked persistent hypovolaemia leads to systemic hypotension and increased salt and water absorption in the proximal tubules and ascending limb of Henle. This process may be mediated by changes in renal interstitial hydrostatic pressure and local prostaglandin and nitric oxide production.

Sodium and water are retained despite increased extracellular volume in oedematous conditions such as cardiac failure, hepatic cirrhosis and hypoalbuminaemia. Here the principal mediator of salt and water retention is the concept of arterial underfilling due to either reduced cardiac output or diminished peripheral arterial resistance. Arterial underfilling in these settings leads to reduction of pressure or stretch (i.e. 'unloading' of arterial volume receptors) which results in the activation of the sympathetic nervous system, activation of the renin–angiotensin–aldosterone system and nonosmotic release of antidiuretic hormone (ADH). These neurohumoral mediators promote salt and water retention in the face of increased extracellular volume. The common nature of the degree of arterial fullness and neurohumoral pathway in the regulation of extracellular volume in health and disease states forms the basis of Schrier's unifying hypothesis of volume homeostasis (Fig 10.3).

Regulation of water excretion

Body water homeostasis is effected by thirst and the urine concentrating and diluting functions of the kidney. These in turn are controlled by intracellular osmoreceptors, principally in the hypothalamus, to some extent by volume receptors in capacitance vessels close to the heart, and via the renin–angiotensin system. Of these, the major and best-understood control is via *osmoreceptors*. Changes in the plasma Na^+ concentration and osmolality are

Table 10.2
Mechanisms of sodium transport in the various nephron segments

Tubule segment	Filtered Na^+ reabsorbed (%)	Major mechanism of luminal Na^+ entry	Major factors regulating transport
Proximal tubule	60–70	Na^+–H^+ exchange and cotransport of Na^+ with glucose, phosphate and other organic solutes	Angiotensin II Noradrenaline
Loop of Henle	20–25	Na^+–K^+–$2Cl^-$ cotransport	Flow dependent Pressure natriuresis mediated by nitric oxide
Distal tubule	5	Na^+–Cl^- cotransport	Flow dependent
Collecting tubules	4	Na^+ channels	Aldosterone Atrial natriuretic peptide

sensed by osmoreceptors that influence both thirst and the release of ADH (also called vasopressin) from the supraoptic and paraventricular nuclei.

ADH plays a central role in urinary concentration by increasing the water permeability of the normally impermeable cortical and medullary collecting tubules. The ability of ADH to increase the urine osmolality is related indirectly to transport in the ascending limb of the loop of Henle, which reabsorbs NaCl without water. This process, which is the primary step in the countercurrent mechanism, has two effects: it makes the tubular fluid dilute and the medullary interstitium concentrated. In the absence of ADH, little water is reabsorbed in the collecting tubules, and a dilute urine is excreted. In contrast, the presence of ADH promotes water reabsorption in the collecting tubules down the favourable osmotic gradient between the tubular fluid and the more concentrated interstitium. As a result, there is an increase in urine osmolality and a decrease in urine volume.

The cortical collecting tubule has two cell types with very different functions:

- *Principal cells* (about 65%) have sodium and potassium channels in the apical membrane and, as in all sodium reabsorbing cells, Na^+–K^+-ATPase pumps in the basolateral membrane.
- *Intercalated cells*, in comparison, do not transport NaCl, since they have a lower level of Na^+–K^+-ATPase activity. They appear to play an important role in hydrogen and bicarbonate handling and in potassium reabsorption in states of potassium depletion.

The ADH-induced increase in collecting tubule water permeability occurs primarily in the principal cells. ADH acts on V2 (vasopressin) receptors located on the basolateral surface of principal cells resulting in the activation of adenyl cyclase. This initiates a sequence of events in which a protein kinase is activated, leading to preformed cytoplasmic vesicles that contain unique water channels (called aquaporins) moving to and then being inserted into the luminal membrane. The water channels span the luminal membrane and permit water movement into the cells down a favourable osmotic gradient (Fig 10.4). This water is then rapidly returned to the systemic circulation across the basolateral membrane. When the ADH effect has worn off, the water channels aggregate within clathrin-coated pits, from which they are removed from the luminal membrane by endocytosis and returned to the cytoplasm. A defect in any step in this pathway, such as attachment of ADH to its receptor or the function of the water channel, can cause resistance to the action of ADH and an increase in urine output. This disorder is called *nephrogenic diabetes insipidus*.

In addition to influencing the rate of water excretion, ADH plays a central role in osmoregulation because its release is directly affected by the plasma osmolality. At a plasma osmolality of less than 275 mOsm kg^{-1}, which usually represents a plasma Na^+ concentration of less than 135–137 mmol L^{-1}, there is essentially no circulating ADH. As the plasma osmolality rises above this threshold, however, the secretion of ADH increases progressively.

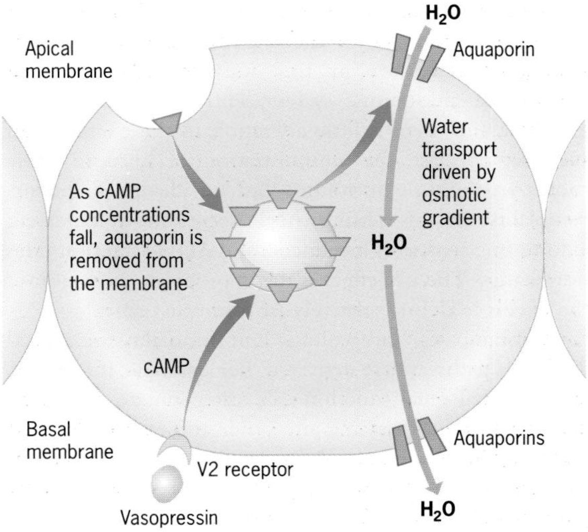

Fig 10.4
Aquaporin-mediated water transport in the renal collecting duct. Stimulation of the vasopressin 2 receptor causes cAMP-mediated insertion of the aquaporin into the apical membrane, allowing water transport down the osmotic gradient. Adapted from Connolly DL, Shanahan CM, Weissberg PL (1996) *Lancet* **347**: 211.

Two simple examples will illustrate the basic mechanisms of osmoregulation, which is so efficient that the plasma Na^+ concentration is normally maintained within 1–2% of its baseline value. Ingestion of a water load leads to an initial reduction in the plasma osmolality, thereby diminishing the release of ADH. The ensuing reduction in water reabsorption in the collection tubules allows the excess water to be excreted in a dilute urine. By contrast, water loss resulting from sweating is followed by, in sequence, a rise on both plasma osmolality and ADH secretion, enhanced water reabsorption, and the appropriate excretion of a small volume of concentrated urine. This renal effect of ADH minimizes further water loss but does not replace the existing water deficit. Thus, optimal osmoregulation requires an increase in water intake, which is mediated by a concurrent stimulation of thirst. The importance of thirst can also be illustrated by studies in patients with central diabetes insipidus, who are deficient in ADH. These patients often complain of marked polyuria, which is caused by the decline in water reabsorption in the collecting tubules. However, they do not typically become hypernatraemic, because urinary water loss is offset by the thirst mechanism.

Osmoregulation versus volume regulation

A common misconception is that regulation of the plasma Na^+ concentration is closely correlated with the regulation of Na^+ excretion. However, it is related to volume regulation, which has different sensors and effectors (volume receptors) from those involved in water balance and osmoregulation (osmoreceptors).

The roles of these two pathways should be considered separately when evaluating patients. A water load, for example, is rapidly excreted (in 4–6 hours) by inhibition of ADH release. This process is normally so efficient that volume regulation is not affected and there is no change in ANP release or in the activity of the renin–angiotensin–aldosterone system. Thus, a dilute urine is excreted, and there is little alteration in the excretion of Na^+. In contrast, the administration of isotonic saline causes an increase in volume but no change in plasma osmolality. In this setting, ANP secretion is increased, aldosterone secretion is reduced, and ADH secretion does not change. The net effect is the appropriate excretion of the excess Na^+ in a relatively iso-osmotic urine.

In some cases, both volume and osmolality are altered and both pathways are activated. For example, if a person with normal renal function eats salted potato chips and peanuts without drinking any water, the excess Na^+ will increase the plasma osmolality, leading to osmotic water movement out of the cells and increased extracellular volume. The rise in osmolality will stimulate both ADH release and thirst (the main reason why many restaurants and bars supply free salted foods), whereas the hypervolaemia will enhance the secretion of ANP and suppress that of aldosterone. The net effect is increased excretion of Na^+ without water.

This principle of separate volume and osmoregulatory pathways is also evident in the syndrome of inappropriate ADH secretion (SIADH). Patients with SIADH have impaired water excretion and hypo-natraemia caused by the persistent presence of ADH; but the release of ANP and aldosterone is not impaired; thus, Na^+ handling remains intact. These findings have important implications for the correction of the hyponatraemia in this setting and require restriction of water intake.

However, there is convincing evidence that ADH is also secreted by non-osmotic stimuli such as stress (e.g. surgery, trauma), markedly reduced effective circulatory volume (cardiac failure, hepatic cirrhosis), psychiatric disturbance, and nausea, irrespective of plasma osmolality. This is mediated by the effects of sympathetic overactivity on supraoptic and paraventricular nuclei. In addition to water retention, ADH release in these conditions promotes vasoconstriction owing to the activation of V1 (vasopressin) receptors distributed in the vascular tissue.

Regulation of cell volume

Maintenance of a constant volume in the face of extracellular and intracellular osmotic alterations is a critical problem faced by all cells. Most cells respond to swelling or shrinkage by activating specific metabolic or membrane-transport processes that return cell volume to its normal resting state. Within minutes after exposure to hypotonic solutions and resulting cell swelling, a common feature of many cells is the increase in plasma membrane potassium and chloride conductance. Although extrusion of intracellular potassium certainly contributes to a regulatory volume decrease, the role of chloride efflux itself is modest, given the relatively low intracellular chloride concentration. Indeed other intracellular osmolytes, such as taurine and other amino acids, are transported out of the cell to achieve a regulatory volume decrease. In contrast, these regulatory mechanisms are operative in reverse to protect cell volume under hypertonic conditions, as is the case in the renal medulla. The tubular cells at the tip of renal papillae which are constantly exposed to hypertonic extracellular milieu maintain their cell volume on a long-term basis by actively taking up smaller molecules, such as betaine, taurine and myoinositol, and by synthesizing more sorbitol and glycerophosphocholine. These changes are mediated by the transcription of a specific enzyme or transporter gene. The limitations or alterations of these adaptive responses in various disease states will be the focus of future research.

Increased extracellular volume

Increased extracellular volume occurs in numerous disease states. The physical signs depend on the distribution of excess volume and on whether the increase is local or systemic. According to Starling principles, distribution depends on:

- venous tone, which determines the capacitance of the blood compartment and thus hydrostatic pressure
- capillary permeability
- oncotic pressure – mainly dependent on serum albumin
- lymphatic drainage.

Depending on these factors, fluid accumulation may result in expansion of interstitial volume, blood volume, or both.

CLINICAL FEATURES

Peripheral oedema is caused by expansion of the extracellular volume by at least 2 L (15%). The ankles are normally the first part of the body to be affected, although the ankles may be spared in patients with lipodermatosclerosis (where the skin is tethered and cannot expand to accommodate the oedema). Oedema may be noted in the face, particularly in the morning. In a patient in bed, oedema may accumulate in the sacral area. Expansion of the interstitial volume also causes pulmonary oedema, pleural effusion, pericardial effusion and ascites. Expansion of the blood volume causes a raised jugular venous pressure, cardiomegaly, added heart sounds, and a raised arterial blood pressure in certain circumstances.

CAUSES

Extracellular volume expansion is due to *sodium chloride retention*. Increased salt intake does not normally cause volume expansion because of rapid homeostatic mechanisms which increase salt excretion. However, a rapid intravenous solution of a large volume of saline will cause volume expansion. Thus most causes of extracellular volume expansion are associated with renal sodium chloride retention.

Heart failure

Reduction in cardiac output and the consequent fall in effective circulatory volume and arterial filling leads to activation of the renin–angiotensin–aldosterone system, non-osmotic release of ADH, and increased activity of the renal sympathetic nerves via volume receptors and barorecetors (Fig 10.3). Sympathetic overdrive also indirectly augments ADH and renin–angiotensin–aldosterone response in these conditions. The cumulative effect of these mediators results in increased peripheral and renal resistance and water and sodium retention. These factors result in extracellular volume expansion and increased venous pressure, causing oedema formation.

Hypoalbuminaemia

The major mechanism is loss of plasma oncotic pressure leading to loss of water from the vascular space to the interstitial space. Reduction in effective circulatory volume and the consequent fall in cardiac output and arterial filling leads to a chain of events as in cardiac failure (see above). These factors result in extracellular volume expansion and increased venous pressure, causing oedema formation. However, other factors may be involved. There is some evidence that the nephrotic syndrome itself alters renal sodium handling.

Hepatic cirrhosis

The mechanism is again complex, but involves peripheral vasodilatation, possibly owing to increased nitric oxide generation resulting in reduced effective volume and arterial filling. This leads to an activation of a chain of events common to cardiac failure, hypoalbuminaemia and other conditions with marked peripheral vasodilatation (Fig 10.3). The cumulative effect of these mediators results in increased peripheral and renal resistance and water, sodium retention, and oedema formation.

Sodium retention

A decreased GFR decreases the renal capacity to excrete sodium. This may be acute, as in the acute nephritic syndrome (p. 536), or may occur as part of the presentation of chronic renal failure. In end-stage renal failure, extracellular volume is controlled by the balance between salt intake and its removal by dialysis.

Mild sodium retention can also be caused by oestrogens which have a weak aldosterone-like effect. This produces weight gain in the premenstrual phase.

Numerous other drugs may cause renal sodium retention, particularly in patients whose renal function is already impaired:

- *mineralocorticoids and liquorice* (the latter potentiates the sodium-retaining action of cortisol), which have aldosterone-like actions
- *NSAIDs* cause sodium retention in the presence of activation of the renin–angiotensin–aldosterone system by heart failure, cirrhosis and in renal artery stenosis.

Substantial amounts of sodium and water may accumulate in the body without clinically obvious oedema or evidence of raised venous pressure. In particular, several litres may accumulate in the pleural space or as ascites; these spaces are then referred to as 'third spaces'. Bone may also act as a 'sink' for sodium and water.

Other causes of oedema

- Initiation of insulin treatment for type 1 diabetes and refeeding after malnutrition are both associated with the development of transient oedema. The mechanism is complex.
- Oedema may result from increased capillary pressure owing to relaxation of precapillary arterioles. The best example is the peripheral oedema caused by dihydropyridine calcium-channel blockers such as nifedipine.
- Oedema may be caused by increased interstitial oncotic pressure as a result of increased capillary permeability to proteins. This can occur as part of a rare

complement-deficiency syndrome; with therapeutic use of interleukin-2 in cancer chemotherapy; or in ovarian hyperstimulation syndrome.

Idiopathic oedema of women

This, by definition, occurs in women without heart failure, hypoalbuminaemia, renal or endocrine disease. Oedema is intermittent and often worse in the premenstrual phase. The condition remits after the menopause. Patients complain of swelling of the face, hands, breasts and thighs, and a feeling of being bloated. Sodium retention during the day and increased sodium excretion during recumbency are characteristic; an abnormal fall in plasma volume on standing caused by increased capillary permeability to proteins may be the cause of this. The oedema may respond to diuretics, but returns when they are stopped. A similar syndrome of diuretic-dependent sodium retention can be caused by abuse of diuretics, for instance as part of an attempt to lose weight; but not all women with idiopathic oedema admit to having taken diuretics, and the syndrome was described before diuretics were introduced for clinical use.

Local increase in oedema

This does not reflect disturbances of extracellular volume control *per se*, but can cause clinical confusion. Examples are ankle oedema due to venous damage following thrombosis or surgery, ankle or leg oedema due to immobility, oedema of the arm due to subclavian thrombosis, and facial oedema due to superior vena caval obstruction. Local loss of oncotic pressure may result from increased capillary permeability to proteins, caused by inflammatory mediators such as histamine and interleukins (e.g. a bee sting). Lastly, local loss of lymphatic drainage causes lymphoedema (see p. 1187).

TREATMENT

The underlying cause should be treated where possible. Heart failure, for example, should be treated, and offending drugs such as NSAIDs withdrawn.

Sodium restriction has only a limited role, but is useful in patients who are resistant to diuretics. Sodium intake can easily be reduced to approximately 100 mmol daily; reductions below this are often difficult to achieve without affecting the palatability of food.

Manoeuvres which increase venous return stimulate salt and water excretion by effects on cardiac output and ANP release. This is the rationale for strict bedrest in congestive cardiac failure. Water immersion also causes redistribution of blood towards the central veins, but is seldom of practical use. Venous compression stockings or bandages may help to mobilize oedema in heart failure.

The mainstay of treatment is the use of diuretic agents, which increase sodium, chloride and water excretion in the kidney (Table 10.3). These agents act by interfering with membrane ion pumps which are present on numerous cell types; but most achieve specificity for the kidney by being secreted into the proximal tubule, resulting in much higher concentrations in the tubular fluid than in other parts of the body.

Clinical use of diuretics

Loop diuretics

These potent diuretics, which are used widely, are useful in the treatment of any cause of systemic extracellular volume overload. They stimulate excretion of both sodium chloride and water, and are useful in stimulating water excretion in states of relative water overload. They also act by causing increased venous capacitance, resulting in rapid clinical improvement in patients with left ventricular failure, preceding the diuresis. Unwanted effects include:

- urate retention causing gout
- hypokalaemia
- hypomagnesaemia
- decreased glucose tolerance
- allergic tubulo-interstitial nephritis and other allergic reactions
- myalgia – especially with bumetanide
- ototoxicity (due to an action on sodium pump activity in the inner ear) – particularly with frusemide
- interference with excretion of lithium, resulting in toxicity.

In most situations there is little to choose between the drugs in this class. Ethacrynic acid is now very seldom used because of ototoxicity. Bumetanide has a better oral bioavailability, particularly in patients with severe peripheral oedema, and may have more beneficial effects than frusemide on venous capacitance in left ventricular failure. It may cause severe muscle cramps when used in high doses.

Thiazide diuretics

These are weaker than loop diuretics. They cause relatively more urate retention, glucose intolerance and hypokalaemia. They interfere with water excretion and may cause hyponatraemia, particularly if combined with amiloride or triamterene. This effect is clinically useful in diabetes insipidus. Thiazides reduce peripheral vascular resistance by mechanisms which are not completely understood but which do not appear to depend on their diuretic action, and are widely used in the treatment of essential hypertension. They are also used extensively in mild to moderate cardiac failure. Thiazides reduce calcium excretion. This effect is useful in patients with idiopathic hypercalciuria, but may cause hypercalcaemia. Numerous agents are available, with varying half-lives but little else to choose between them. Metolazone is not dependent for its action on glomerular filtration, and therefore retains its potency in renal impairment.

Table 10.3
Types and clinical uses of diurectics

Class	Major action	Examples	Clinical uses	Potency
Carbonic anhydrase inhibitors	↓ Na^+ HCO_3^- reabsorption in proximal tubule ↓ Aqueous humour formation	Acetazolamide	Metabolic alkalosis Glaucoma	+
Loop diuretics	↓ Na^+ Cl^- K^+ cotransport in thick ascending limb	Frusemide Bumetanide Torasemide	Volume overload (CCF, nephrotic syndrome, CRF) Sodium-dependent hypertension Hypercalcaemia ?Acute renal failure SIADH	+++
Thiazide and related diuretics	↓ Na^+ Cl^- cotransport in early distal tubule	Bendrofluazide Hydrochloro-thiazide Metolazone Indapamide	Hypertension Volume overload (CCF) Hypercalciuria	++
Potassium sparing	↓ Na^+ reabsorption (in exchange for K^+) in collecting duct	Aldosterone antagonist e.g. oral spironolactone or i.v. potassium canrenoate Others: Amiloride Triamterene	Hyperaldosteronism (primary and secondary) Bartter's syndrome Prevention of K^+ deficiency in combination with loop or thiazide Cirrhosis with fluid overload	+

CCF, congestive cardiac failure; CRF, chronic renal failure; SIADH, syndrome of inappropriate antidiuretic hormone secretion

Potassium-sparing diuretics

These are relatively weak and are most often used in combination with thiazides or loop diuretics to prevent potassium depletion.They are of two types. Spironolactone, an aldosterone antagonist, competes with aldosterone in the collecting ducts, so reducing sodium absorption. Amiloride and triamterene inhibit sodium uptake in collecting duct epithelial cells and reduce renal potassium excretion.

Carbonic anhydrase inhibitors

These are relatively weak diuretics and are seldom used except in the treatment of glaucoma. They may cause metabolic acidosis and hypokalaemia.

Resistance to diuretics

Resistance may occur as a result of:

- poor bioavailability
- reduced GFR, which may be due to decreased circulating volume despite oedema (e.g. nephrotic syndrome, local causes of oedema) or intrinsic renal disease
- activation of sodium-retaining mechanisms, particularly aldosterone.

Intravenous administration may establish a diuresis. High doses of loop diuretics may be required to achieve adequate concentrations in the tubule if GFR is depressed. However, the daily dose of frusemide must be limited to a maximum of 2 g for an adult, because of ototoxicity. Intravenous albumin solutions restore plasma oncotic pressure temporarily in the nephrotic syndrome and may allow mobilization of oedema.

Combinations of various classes of diuretics are extremely helpful in patients with resistant oedema. A loop diuretic plus a thiazide inhibits two major sites of sodium reabsorption; this effect may be further potentiated by addition of a potassium-sparing agent. Metolazone in combination with a loop diuretic is particularly useful in refractory congestive cardiac failure, because its action is less dependent on glomerular filtration. However, this potent combination can cause severe electrolyte imbalance.

Both aminophylline and dopamine increase renal blood flow and may be useful in refractory cardiogenic sodium retention.

Effects on renal function

All diuretics may increase plasma urea concentrations by increasing urea reabsorption in the medulla. Thiazides may also promote protein breakdown. In certain situations diuretics may also decrease GFR:

- Excessive diuresis may cause volume depletion and prerenal failure.
- Diuretics may cause allergic tubulo-interstitial nephritis.

- Thiazides may directly cause a drop in GFR; the mechanism is complex.

Decreased extracellular volume

Deficiency of sodium and water causes shrinkage both of the interstitial space and of the blood volume and may have profound effects on organ function.

CLINICAL FEATURES

Symptoms are variable. Thirst, muscle cramps, nausea and vomiting, and postural dizziness may occur. Severe depletion of circulating volume causes hypotension and impairs cerebral perfusion, causing confusion and eventual coma.

Signs can be divided into those due to loss of interstitial fluid and those due to loss of circulating volume.

- Loss of interstitial fluid leads to loss of skin elasticity ('turgor') – the rapidity with which the skin recoils to normal after being pinched. Skin turgor decreases with age, particularly at the peripheries. The turgor over the anterior triangle of the neck or on the forehead is a very useful sign in all ages.
- Loss of circulating volume leads to decreased pressure in the venous and (if severe) arterial compartments. Loss of up to 1 L of extracellular fluid in an adult may be compensated for by venoconstriction and may cause no physical signs. Loss of more than this causes the following.

Postural hypotension

Normally the blood pressure rises if a subject stands up, as a result of increased venous return due to venoconstriction (this maintains cerebral perfusion). Loss of extracellular fluid prevents this and causes a fall in blood pressure. This is one of the earliest and most reliable signs of volume depletion, as long as the other causes of postural hypotension are excluded (Table 10.4).

Low jugular venous pressure

In hypovolaemic patients, the jugular venous pulsation can be seen only with the patient lying completely flat, or even head down, because the left atrial pressure is lower than 5 cmH_2O.

Peripheral venoconstriction

This causes cold skin with empty peripheral veins, which are difficult to cannulate just when the patient needs intravenous therapy the most! This sign is often absent in sepsis, where peripheral vasodilatation contributes to effective hypovolaemia.

Tachycardia

This is not always a reliable sign. Beta-blockers and other antiarrhythmics may prevent tachycardia, and hypovolaemia may activate vagal mechanisms and actually cause bradycardia.

CAUSES

Salt and water may be lost from the kidneys, from the gastrointestinal tract, or from the skin. Examples are given in Table 10.5.

In addition, there are a number of situations where signs of volume depletion occur despite a normal or increased body content of sodium and water.

- Septicaemia causes vasodilatation of both arterioles and veins, resulting in greatly increased capacitance of the vascular space. In addition, increased capillary permeability to plasma proteins leads to loss of fluid from the vascular space to the interstitium.
- Diuretic treatment of heart failure or nephrotic syndrome may lead to rapid reduction in plasma volume. Mobilization of oedema may take much longer.
- There may be inappropriate diuretic treatment of oedema (e.g. when the cause is local rather than systemic).

Table 10.4 Postural hypotension: some causes of a fall in blood pressure from lying to standing

Decreased circulating volume (hypovolaemia)	**Interference with peripheral vasoconstriction by drugs** Nitrates Calcium-channel blockers Alpha-adrenergic receptor antagonists
Autonomic failure Diabetes Systemic amyloidosis Shy–Drager syndrome	**Prolonged bedrest (cardiovascular deconditioning)**
Interference with autonomic function by drugs Ganglion blockers Tricyclic antidepressants	

Table 10.5
Causes of extracellular volume depletion

Haemorrhage External Concealed, e.g. leaking aortic aneurysm	**Renal losses** Diuretic use Impaired tubular sodium conservation Reflux nephropathy Papillary necrosis Analgesic nephropathy Diabetes Sickle cell disease
Burns	
Gastrointestinal losses Vomiting Diarrhoea Ileostomy losses Ileus	

INVESTIGATIONS

Blood tests are in general not helpful in the assessment of extracellular volume. Plasma urea may be raised owing to increased urea reabsorption and, later, to prerenal failure (when the creatinine rises as well), but this is very nonspecific. Urinary sodium is low if the kidneys are functioning normally, but is misleading if the cause of the volume depletion involves the kidneys (e.g. diuretics, intrinsic renal disease). Urine osmolality is high in volume depletion (owing to increased water reabsorption), but may also often mislead.

TREATMENT

The overriding principle is to aim to replace what is missing.

Haemorrhage

This involves the loss of whole blood. The rational treatment of acute haemorrhage is therefore the infusion of whole blood, or a combination of red cells and a plasma substitute. (Chronic anaemia causes salt and water retention rather than volume depletion by a mechanism common to conditions with peripheral vasodilatation.)

Loss of plasma

Loss of plasma, as occurs in burns or severe peritonitis, should be treated with human plasma or a plasma substitute (see p. 844).

Loss of water and electrolytes

Loss of water and electrolytes, as occurs with vomiting, diarrhoea, or excessive renal losses, should be treated by replacement of the loss. If possible, this should be done with oral water and sodium salts. These are available as slow sodium (600 mg, approximately 10 mmol NaCl per tablet), the usual dose of which is 6–12 tablets per day with 2–3 L of water. It is used in mild or chronic salt and water depletion, such as that associated with renal salt wasting.

Sodium bicarbonate (500 mg, 6 mmol $NaHCO_3$ per tablet) is used in doses of 6–12 tablets per day with 2–3 L of water. This is used in milder chronic sodium depletion with acidosis (e.g. chronic renal failure, postobstructive renal failure, renal tubular acidosis). Sodium bicarbonate is less effective than sodium chloride in causing positive sodium balance.

Oral rehydration solutions are described in Table 1.19 (see p. 32). Intravenous fluids may sometimes be required (Table 10.6). Rapid infusion (e.g. 1000 mL per hour or even faster) is necessary if there is hypotension and evidence of impaired organ perfusion (e.g. oliguria, confusion); in these situations, plasma expanders (colloids) are often used in the first instance to restore an adequate circulating volume (see p. 843). Repeated clinical assessments are vital in this situation, usually complemented by frequent measurements of central venous pressure (see p. 839 in Chapter 13 for the management of shock). Severe hypovolaemia induces venoconstriction, which maintains venous return; over-rapid correction does not give time for this to reverse, resulting in signs of circulatory overload (e.g. pulmonary oedema) even if a total body ECF deficit remains. In less severe ECF depletion (such as in a patient with postural hypotension complicating acute tubular necrosis), the fluid should be replaced at a rate of 1000 mL every 4–6 hours, again with repeated clinical assessment. If all that is required is avoidance of fluid depletion during surgery, 1–2 L may be given over 24 hours, remembering that surgery is a stimulus to sodium and water retention and that over-replacement may be as dangerous as under-replacement. Regular monitoring by fluid balance charts, bodyweight and plasma biochemistry is mandatory.

Loss of water alone

This causes extracellular volume depletion only in severe cases, because the loss is spread evenly between all the compartments of body water. In the rare situations where there is a true deficiency of water alone, as in diabetes insipidus in a patient who is unable to drink (after surgery, for instance), the correct treatment is to give water. If intravenous treatment is required, water is given as 5% dextrose, because pure water would lead to osmotic lysis of blood cells.

FURTHER READING

Connolly DL, Shanahan CM, Weissberg PL (1996) Water channels in health and disease. *Lancet* **347**: 210–212.

Editorial (1988) What causes oedema? *Lancet* **i**: 1028–1030.

McManus LM, Churchwell KB, Strange K (1995) Regulation of cell volume in health and disease. *New England Journal of Medicine* **333**: 1260–1266.

Schrier RW (1992) A unifying hypothesis of body fluid regulation. *Journal of the Royal College of Physicians, London* **26**: 295–299.

Disorders of sodium concentration

These are best thought of as disorders of body water content. As discussed above, sodium content is regulated by volume receptors; water content is adjusted to maintain, in health, a normal osmolality and (in the absence of abnormal osmotically active solutes) a normal sodium concentration. Disturbances of sodium concentration are caused by disturbances of water balance.

Table 10.6
Intravenous fluids in general use for fluid and electrolyte disturbances

	Na^+ (mmol L^{-1})	K^+ (mmol L^{-1})	HCO_3^- or equivalent (mmol L^{-1})	Ca^{2+} (mmol L^{-1})	Ca_2^+ (mmol L^{-1})	Indication (see footnote)
Normal plasma values	142	4.5	26	103	2.5	
Sodium chloride 0.9%	150	–	–	150	–	1
Sodium chloride 0.18% + glucose 4%	30	–	–	30	–	2
Glucose 5% + potassium chloride 0.3%	–	40	–	40	–	3
Sodium bicarbonate 1.26%	150	–	150	–	–	4
Compound sodium lactate (Hartmann's)	131	5	29	111	2	5

1. Volume expansion in hypovolaemic patients. Rarely to maintain fluid balance when there are large doses of sodium. The sodium (150 mmol L^{-1}) is greater than plasma and hypernatraemia can result. It is often necessary to add KCl 20–40 mmol L^{-1}.
2. Maintenance of fluid balance in normovolaemic, normonatraemic patients.
3. To replace *water*. Can be given with or without potassium chloride. May be alternated with normal saline as an alternative to (2).
4. For volume expansion in hypovolaemic, acidotic patients alternating with (1). Occasionally for maintenance of fluid balance combined with (2) in salt-wasting, acidotic patients. To induce forced alkaline diuresis, e.g. in severe salicylate poisoning.
5. Used for maintenance of fluid balance after surgery. The potassium content may be dangerous in renal failure but occasionally useful in the diuretic phase of acute tubular necrosis where hypokalaemia occurs.

Hyponatraemia

Hyponatraemia is one of the most common abnormalities detected in biochemistry laboratories. It may be associated with normal extracellular volume (Table 10.7) and total body sodium content. The differential diagnosis of hyponatraemia depends on an assessment of extracellular volume (see also Tables 10.8 and 10.10).

Rarely, hyponatraemia may be pseudo-hyponatraemia, where in hyperlipidaemia or hyperproteinaemia there is a spuriously low measured sodium concentration, the sodium being confined to the aqueous phase but having its concentration expressed in terms of the total volume of plasma. In this situation, plasma osmolality is normal and therefore treatment of 'hyponatraemia' is unnecessary. It is also important to exclude artefactual 'hyponatraemia' caused by taking blood from the limb into which fluid of low sodium concentration is being infused.

Table 10.7
Causes of hyponatraemia with normal extracellular volume

Abnormal ADH release
Vagal neuropathy (failure of inhibition of ADH release)
Deficiency of adrenocorticotrophic hormone (ACTH) or glucocorticoids (Addison's disease)
Hypothyroidism
Severe potassium depletion

Syndrome of inappropriate antidiuretic hormone

Stress
Surgery
Nausea

Major psychiatric illness
'Psychogenic polydipsia'
Nonosmotic ADH release?
Antidepressant therapy

Increased sensitivity to ADH
Chlorpropamide
Tolbutamide

ADH-like substances
Oxytocin
1-Deamino-D-arginine vasopressin (DDAVP)

Unmeasured osmotically active substances stimulating osmotic ADH release
Glucose
Alcohol
Mannitol
Sick-cell syndrome (leakage of intracellular ions)

Salt-deficient hyponatraemia

This is due to salt loss in excess of water; the causes are listed in Table 10.8. In this situation, ADH secretion is initially suppressed (via the hypothalamic osmoreceptors); but as fluid volume is lost, volume receptors override the osmoreceptors and stimulate both thirst and the release of ADH. This is an attempt by the body to defend circulating volume at the expense of osmolality.

Table 10.8
Causes of hyponatraemia with decreased extracellular volume

Gut
Vomiting
Diarrhoea
Haemorrhage

Kidney
Osmotic diuresis (e.g. hyperglycaemia, severe uraemia)
Excessive use of diuretics
Adrenocortical insufficiency
Tubulo-interstitial renal disease
Unilateral renal artery stenosis
Recovery phase of acute tubular necrosis

Table 10.9
Average concentrations and potential daily losses of water and electrolytes from the gut

	Na^+ (mmol L^{-1})	K^+ (mmol L^{-1})	Cl^- (mmol L^{-1})	Volume (mL in 24 hours)
Stomach	50	10	110	2500
Small intestine				
Recent ileostomy	120	5	110	1500
Adapted ileostomy	50	4	25	500
Bile	140	5	105	500
Pancreatic juice	140	5	60	2000
Diarrhoea	130	10-15	95	1000–2000+

With extrarenal losses and normal kidneys, the urinary excretion of sodium falls in response to the volume depletion, as does water excretion, leading to concentrated urine containing less than 10 mmol L^{-1} of sodium. However, in salt-wasting kidney disease, renal compensation cannot occur and the only physiological protection is increased water intake in response to thirst.

CLINICAL FEATURES

With sodium depletion the clinical picture is usually dominated by features of volume depletion (see p. 606). The diagnosis is usually obvious where there is a history of gut losses, diabetes mellitus or diuretic abuse.

Table 10.9 shows the potential daily losses of water and electrolytes from the gut. Losses due to renal or adrenocortical disease may be less easily identified and are suggested by a urinary sodium concentration of more than 20 mmol L^{-1} in the presence of clinically evident volume depletion.

TREATMENT

This is directed at the primary cause whenever possible. Increased salt intake as slow sodium 60–80 mmol daily is all that is required in the relatively healthy patient who can take this by mouth. In the face of vomiting or severe volume depletion, intravenous infusion of normal saline is given. Potassium supplements and correction of acid–base abnormalities may also be required.

Hyponatraemia due to water excess

This results from an intake of water in excess of the kidney's ability to excrete it. It is uncommon with normal kidney function, requiring an intake of approximately 1 L per hour. Overgenerous infusion of 5% glucose into postoperative patients is one of the most common causes, and in this situation it is exacerbated by an increased ADH secretion in response to stress. Some degree of hyponatraemia is usual in acute oliguric renal failure, while in chronic renal failure it is most often due to ill-given advice to 'push' fluids.

The most common presentation of hyponatraemia due to water excess is in patients with severe cardiac failure, hepatic cirrhosis or the nephrotic syndrome in which there is evidence of volume overload (Table 10.10). In all these conditions there is usually an element of reduced glomerular filtration rate with avid reabsorption of sodium and chloride in the proximal tubule. This leads to reduced delivery of chloride to the 'diluting' ascending limb of Henle's loop and a reduced ability to generate 'free water', with a consequent inability to excrete dilute urine. This is commonly compounded by the administration of diuretics that block chloride reabsorption and interfere with the dilution of filtrate either in Henle's loop (loop diuretics) or distally (thiazides).

CLINICAL FEATURES

Symptoms are common with dilutional hyponatraemia when this develops acutely. They are principally neurological and are due to the movement of water into brain cells in response to the fall in extracellular osmolality. Symptoms rarely occur until the serum sodium is less than 120 mmol L^{-1} and are more usually associated with values around 110 mmol L^{-1} or lower. Symptoms and signs of hyponatraemia are nonspecific and include headache, confusion, and restlessness leading to drowsiness, myoclonic jerks, generalized convulsions, and eventually coma. Other features depend on the cause, such as signs of congestive cardiac failure or liver disease.

INVESTIGATIONS

No further investigation of hyponatraemia is usually necessary if it is associated with clinically detectable

Table 10.10
Causes of hyponatraemia with increased extracellular volume

Heart failure
Liver failure
Oliguric renal failure
Hypoalbuminaemia

extracellular volume excess. The cause of hyponatraemia with apparently normal extracellular volume is usually less obvious, and this category requires careful investigations to:

- exclude Addison's disease
- exclude hypothyroidism
- consider 'syndrome of inappropriate ADH secretion' (SIADH) and drug-induced water retention

It should be remembered that potassium and magnesium depletion potentiate ADH release and are causes of diuretic-associated hyponatraemia.

The syndrome of inappropriate ADH secretion is often over-diagnosed. Some causes are associated with a lower set point for ADH release, rather than completely autonomous ADH release; an example is chronic alcohol abuse.

TREATMENT

The underlying cause should be corrected where possible. Most cases are simply managed by restriction of water intake (to 1000 or even 500 mL per day) with review of diuretic therapy. Magnesium and potassium deficiency must be corrected. The use of hypertonic saline is restricted to patients with acute water retention in whom there are severe neurological signs, such as fits or coma. It must be given slowly (not more than 70 mmol per hour), the aim being to increase the serum sodium to more than 125 mmol L^{-1}. If hyponatraemia has developed slowly, as it does in the majority of patients, the brain will have adapted by decreasing intracellular osmolality. A rapid rise in extracellular osmolality, particularly if there is an 'overshoot' to high serum sodium and osmolality, will result in severe shrinking of brain cells, and in the syndrome of 'central pontine myelinolysis', which may be fatal. Hypertonic saline must not be given to patients who are already fluid overloaded because of the risk of acute heart failure; in this situation, 100 mL of 20% mannitol may be infused in an attempt to increase renal water excretion.

Syndrome of inappropriate ADH secretion

This is described in Chapter 16.

Hypernatraemia

This is much rarer than hyponatraemia and nearly always indicates a water deficit. This may be due to (Table 10.11):

- pituitary diabetes insipidus (see p. 951) (failure of ADH secretion)
- nephrogenic diabetes insipidus (failure of response to ADH)
- osmotic diuresis
- excessive loss of water through the skin or lungs.

Excessive administration of hypertonic sodium may also contribute; for example:

- excessive reliance on 0.9% (150 mmol L^{-1}) saline for volume replacement
- administration of drugs with a high sodium content (e.g. piperacillin)
- use of 8.4% sodium bicarbonate after cardiac arrest.

Hypernatraemia is always associated with increased plasma osmolality, which is a potent stimulus to thirst. None of the above causes hypernatraemia unless thirst sensation is abnormal or access to water limited. For instance, a patient with diabetes insipidus will maintain a normal serum sodium concentration by maintaining a high water intake until an intercurrent illness prevents this. Thirst is frequently deficient in elderly people, making them more prone to water depletion. Hypernatraemia may occur in the presence of normal, reduced or expanded extracellular volume, and does not necessarily imply that total body sodium is increased.

CLINICAL FEATURES

Symptoms of hypernatraemia are nonspecific. Nausea, vomiting, fever and confusion may occur. A history of longstanding polyuria, polydipsia and thirst suggests diabetes insipidus. There may be clues to a pituitary cause. A drug history may reveal ingestion of nephrotoxic drugs. Assessment of extracellular volume status is important in guiding resuscitation. Mental state should be assessed. Convulsions occur in severe hypernatraemia.

INVESTIGATIONS

Simultaneous urine and plasma osmolality and sodium should be measured. Serum osmolality is high in hypernatraemia. Passage of urine with an osmolality lower than that of plasma in this situation is clearly abnormal and indicates diabetes insipidus. In pituitary diabetes insipidus, urine osmolality will increase after administration of desmopressin; the drug (a vasopressin analogue) has no

Table 10.11
Causes of hypernatraemia

ADH deficiency Diabetes insipidus	**Osmotic diuresis** Total parental nutrition Hyperosmolar diabetic coma
Iatrogenic Administration of hypertonic sodium solutions	**PLUS** Deficient water intake
Insensitivity to ADH (nephrogenic diabetes insipidus) Lithium Tetracyclines Amphotericin B Acute tubular necrosis	

effect in nephrogenic diabetes insipidus. If urine osmolality is high this suggests either an osmotic diuresis due to an unmeasured solute (e.g. in parenteral feeding) or excessive extrarenal loss of water (e.g. heat stroke).

TREATMENT

Treatment is that of the underlying cause: in ADH deficiency, replacement of ADH in the form of desmopressin, a stable nonpressor analogue of ADH; withdrawal of nephrogenic drugs where possible; and replacement of water either orally, if possible, or intravenously. In *severe* (>170 mmol L^{-1}) hypernatraemia, 0.9% saline (150 mmol L^{-1}) should be used initially, to avoid too rapid a drop in serum sodium concentration; the aim is correction over 48 hours, as over-rapid correction may lead to cerebral oedema. In *less severe* (e.g. >150 mmol L^{-1}) hypernatraemia the treatment is 5% dextrose or 0.45% saline; the latter is obviously preferable in hyperosmolar diabetic coma. Very large volumes – 5 L a day or more – may need to be given in diabetes insipidus.

If there is clinical evidence of volume depletion (see p. 606), this implies that there is a sodium deficit as well as a water deficit. Treatment of this is discussed on p. 607.

FURTHER READING

Arieff AI (1993) Management of hyponatraemia. *British Medical Journal* **307**: 305–308.

Disorders of potassium content and concentration

Regulation of serum potassium concentration

The usual dietary intake varies between 80 and 150 mmol daily, depending upon fruit and vegetable intake. Most of the body's potassium (3500 mmol in an adult man) is intracellular. Serum potassium levels are controlled by:

- uptake of K^+ into cells
- renal excretion
- extrarenal losses (e.g. gastrointestinal).

Uptake of potassium into cells is governed by the activity of the Na^+–K^+-ATPase in the cell membrane and by H^+ concentration. Uptake is *stimulated* by:

- insulin
- β-adrenergic stimulation
- theophyllines

and is *decreased* by:

- α-adrenergic stimulation
- acidosis – K^+ exchanged for H^+ across cell membrane
- cell damage or cell death – resulting in massive K^+ release.

Excretion of potassium is increased by aldosterone, which stimulates K^+ and H^+ secretion in exchange for Na^+ in the collecting duct. Because H^+ and K^+ are interchangeable in the exchange mechanism, acidosis decreases and alkalosis increases the secretion of K^+. Aldosterone secretion is stimulated by hyperkalaemia and increased angiotensin II levels, as well as by some drugs, and this acts to protect the body against hyperkalaemia and against extracellular volume depletion. The body adapts to dietary deficiency of potassium by reducing aldosterone secretion. However, because aldosterone is also influenced by volume status, conservation of potassium is relatively inefficient, and significant potassium depletion may therefore result from prolonged dietary deficiency.

A number of drugs affect K^+ homeostasis by affecting aldosterone release (e.g. heparin, NSAIDs) or by directly affecting renal potassium handling.

Normally only about 10% of daily potassium intake is excreted in the gastrointestinal tract. Vomit contains around 5–10 mmol L^{-1} of K^+, but prolonged vomiting may cause hypokalaemia by inducing sodium depletion, stimulating aldosterone, which increases renal potassium excretion. Potassium may be secreted by the colon, and diarrhoea contains 10–50 mmol L^{-1} of K^+; profuse diarrhoea can therefore induce marked hypokalaemia. Villous adenomas may rarely produce profuse diarrhoea and K^+ loss.

Hypokalaemia

CAUSES

The most common causes of chronic hypokalaemia are diuretic treatment (particularly thiazides) and hyperaldosteronism. Acute hypokalaemia is more often caused by intravenous fluids without potassium and redistribution into cells. The common causes are shown in Table 10.12.

Rare causes

Bartter's syndrome

This consists of hypokalaemia, alkalosis, hypercalciuria, normal blood pressure, and elevated plasma renin and aldosterone. The primary defect in this disorder appears to be an impairment in sodium and chloride reabsorption in the thick ascending limb. Mutation in the genes encoding either the sodium–potassium–chloride cotransporter (NKCC2) or the ATP-regulated potassium channel cause loss of function of these channels, with consequent impairment of sodium and chloride reabsorption. There is also an increased intra-renal production of prostaglandin E_2.

This tubular defect in sodium chloride transport is thought to initiate the following sequence, which is almost identical to those seen with chronic ingestion of a loop diuretic. The initial salt loss leads to mild volume depletion, resulting in activation of the

Table 10.12
Causes of hypokalaemia

Increased renal excretion	**Severe dietary deficiency**
Diuretics	
Thiazides	**Redistribution into cells**
Loop diuretics	β-Adrenergic stimulation
Increased aldosterone secretion	Acute myocardial infarction
Liver failure	Beta-agonists: fenoterol, salbutamol
Heart failure	Insulin treatment, e.g. treatment of diabetic ketoacidosis
Nephrotic syndrome	Correction of megaloblastic anaemia, e.g. B_{12} deficiency
Cushing's syndrome	Alkalosis
Conn's syndrome	Hypokalaemic periodic paralysis
ACTH-producing tumours	
Exogenous mineralocorticoid	**Gastrointestinal losses**
Corticosteroids	Vomiting
Carbenoxolone	Severe diarrhoea
Liquorice (potentiates renal actions of cortisol)	Purgative abuse
Renal disease	Villous adenoma
Renal tubular acidosis types 1 and 2	Ileostomy or uterosigmoidostomy
Renal tubular damage (diuretic phase)	Fistulae
Acute leukaemia	Ileus/Intestinal obstruction
Cytotoxic treatment	
Nephrotoxicity	
Amphotericin	
Aminoglycosides	
Release of urinary tract obstruction	
Bartter's syndrome	
Liddle's syndrome	

renin–angiotensin–aldosterone system. The combination of hyperaldosteronism and increased distal flow (owing to the reabsorptive defect) enhances potassium and hydrogen secretion at the secretory sites in the collecting tubules, leading to hypokalaemia and metabolic alkalosis.

Diagnostic pointers include high urinary potassium and chloride despite low serum values, increased plasma renin (differential diagnosis; primary aldosteronism renin levels are low), hyperplasia of the juxtaglomerular apparatus on renal biopsy, and careful exclusion of diuretic abuse. Magnesium wasting may also occur. Treatment is with combinations of potassium supplements, amiloride and indomethacin.

Liddle's syndrome

This is characterized by potassium wasting, hypokalaemia, and alkalosis, but is associated with low renin and aldosterone production, and high blood pressure. There is a mutation in the gene encoding for the amiloride-sensitive epithelial sodium channel in the distal tubule/collecting duct. This leads to excessive sodium reabsorption with coupled potassium and hydrogen secretion.

Therapy in Liddle's syndrome consists of sodium restriction along with amiloride or triamterene administration, both potassium-sparing diuretics which directly close the sodium channels. The mineralocorticoid antagonist spironolactone is ineffective, since the increase in sodium-channel activity is not mediated by aldosterone in this disorder.

Hypokalaemic periodic paralysis

This condition may be precipitated by carbohydrate intake, suggesting that insulin-mediated potassium influx into cells may be responsible. This syndrome also occurs in association with hyperthyroidism in Chinese patients.

CLINICAL FEATURES

Hypokalaemia is usually asymptomatic, but severe hypokalaemia may cause muscle weakness. Potassium depletion may also cause symptomatic hyponatraemia (see p. 609).

Hypokalaemia is associated with an increased frequency of atrial and ventricular ectopic beats. This association may not always be causal, because adrenergic activation (for instance after myocardial infarction) causes both hypokalaemia and increased cardiac irritability. Hypokalaemia in patients without cardiac disease is unlikely to lead to serious arrhythmias.

Hypokalaemia seriously increases the risk of digoxin toxicity by increasing binding of digoxin to cardiac cells, potentiating its action, and decreasing its clearance.

Chronic hypokalaemia is associated with interstitial renal disease, but the pathogenesis is not completely understood.

TREATMENT

The underlying cause should be identified and treated where possible. Table 10.13 shows some examples.

Acute hypokalaemia may correct spontaneously. In most cases, withdrawal of oral diuretics or purgation, accompanied by the oral administration of potassium supplements in the form of slow-releasing potassium or effervescent potassium, is all that is required. Intravenous potassium replacement is

Table 10.13
Treatment of hypokalaemia

Cause	Treatment
Dietary deficiency	Increase intake of fresh fruit/vegetables or oral potassium supplements (20–40 mmol daily) (Potassium supplements can cause gastrointestinal irritation)
Hyperaldosteronism	Spironolactone or, in heart failure, ACE inhibitors
Thiazides	Co-prescription of a potassium-sparing diuretic with a similar onset and duration of action
Bartter's syndrome	Amiloride with or without indomethacin

required only in conditions such as cardiac arrhythmias, muscle weakness or severe diabetic ketoacidosis when the potassium is <2.5 mmol L^{-1}. When using intravenous therapy in the presence of poor renal function, replacement rates >20 mmol per hour should be used only with hourly monitoring of serum potassium and ECG changes.

The treatment of adrenal disorders is described on p. 955.

Failure to correct hypokalaemia may be due to concurrent hypomagnesaemia. Serum magnesium should be measured and any deficiency corrected.

Hyperkalaemia

CAUSES

Acute self-limiting hyperkalaemia occurs normally after vigorous exercise and is of no pathological significance. Hyperkalaemia in all other situations is due either to increased release from cells or to failure of excretion (Table 10.14). The most common causes are renal impairment and drug interference with potassium excretion. The combination of ACE inhibitors with potassium-sparing diuretics or NSAIDs is particularly dangerous.

Rare causes

Hyporeninaemic hypoaldosteronism

This is also known as type 4 renal tubular acidosis (see p. 620).

Pseudo-hypoaldosteronism

This is a disease of infancy apparently due to resistance to the action of aldosterone. It is characterized by hyperkalaemia and evidence of sodium wasting (hyponatraemia, extracellular volume depletion).

Hyperkalaemic periodic paralysis

This is precipitated by exercise, and is caused by an autosomal dominant mutation of the skeletal muscle sodium channel gene.

Gordon's syndrome

This appears to be a mirror-image of Bartter's syndrome (see above), in which primary renal retention of sodium causes hypertension, volume expansion, low renin/aldosterone, hyperkalaemia and acidosis.

Suxamethonium and other depolarizing muscle relaxants

These cause release of potassium from cells. Induction of muscle paralysis during general anaesthesia may result in a rise of plasma potassium of up to 1 mmol L^{-1}. This is not usually a problem unless there is pre-existing hyperkalaemia.

CLINICAL FEATURES

Serum potassium of greater than 7.0 mmol L^{-1} is a medical emergency and is associated with ECG changes (Fig. 10.5). Severe hyperkalaemia may be asymptomatic and may predispose to sudden death from asystolic cardiac arrest. Muscle weakness is often the only symptom, unless (as is commonly the case) the hyperkalaemia is associated with metabolic acidosis, causing Kussmaul respiration. Hyperkalaemia causes hyperpolarization of cell membranes, leading to decreased cardiac excitability, hypotension, bradycardia, and eventual asystole.

TREATMENT

Treatments for hyperkalaemia are summarized in Practical box 10.1 and should also include treatment of the cause.

Calcium ions protect the cell membranes from the effects of hyperkalaemia but do not alter the potassium concentration. Insulin drives potassium into the cell, but *must* be accompanied by glucose to avoid hypoglycaemia. Regular measurements of blood glucose must be used for at least 6 hours after use of insulin in this situation, and extra glucose must be available for immediate use. Alternatively, glucose can be given (without insulin) as this stimulates endogenous insulin and avoids problems with hypoglycaemia.

Table 10.14
Causes of hyperkalaemia

Decreased excretion	**Increased extraneous load**
Renal failure	Potassium chloride
Drug: direct effect on potassium handling	Iatrogenic
Amiloride	Salt substitutes
Triamterene	Potassium citrate
Spironolactone	Transfusion of stored blood
Aldosterone deficiency	
Hyporeninaemic hypoaldosteronism (RTA type 4)	**Spurious**
Addison's disease	Increased *in vitro* release from abnormal cells
ACE inhibitors	Leukaemia
NSAIDs	Infectious mononucleosis
Cyclosporin treatment	Thrombocytosis
Heparin treatment	Familial pseudohyperkalaemia
Acidosis	Increased release from muscles
Gordon's syndrome	Vigorous fist clenching during phlebotomy
Increased release from cells (decreased Na^+–K^+-ATPase activity)	
Acidosis	
Diabetic ketoacidosis	
Rhabdomyolysis/tissue damage	
Tumour lysis	
Succinylcholine (amplified by muscle denervation)	
Digoxin poisoning	
Vigorous exercise (α-adrenergic; transient)	

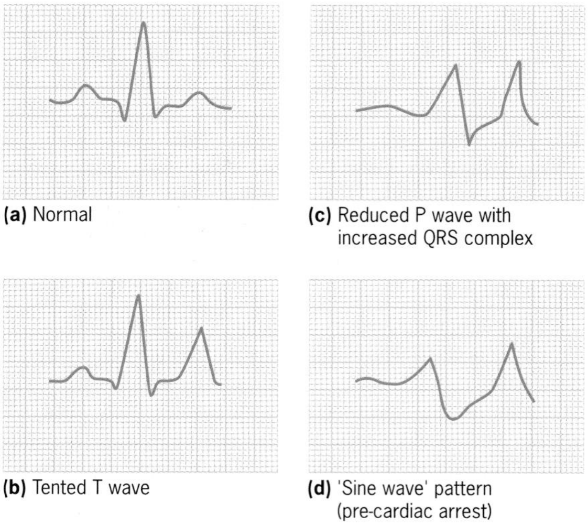

Fig 10.5
Progressive ECG changes with increasing hyperkalaemia

Intravenous salbutamol has not yet found widespread acceptance and may cause disturbing muscle tremor at the doses required. Correction of acidosis with hypertonic (8.4%) sodium bicarbonate causes volume expansion and should not be used, particularly in renal failure. Gastric aspiration will remove potassium and leads to alkalosis.

Cation exchange resins (sodium and calcium resonium) make use of the ion fluxes which occur in the gut to remove potassium from the body, and are the only way short of dialysis of removing potassium from the body. They may cause sodium (extracellular fluid) overload and hypercalcaemia respectively.

In general, all of these measures are simply ways of buying time either to correct the underlying disorder or to arrange removal of potassium by dialysis, which is the definitive treatment for hyperkalaemia.

All of these measures may cause digoxin toxicity in patients receiving digoxin, in whom cardiac monitoring is essential.

+ Practical

Protect myocardium

10 mL of 10% calcium gluconate given in the presence of ECG change

Effect is temporary but dose can be repeated

Drive K^+ into cells

Insulin 10 units + 50 mL of 50% glucose followed by regular checks of blood glucose and plasma K^+

Repeat as necessary

and/or correction of severe acidosis – $NaHCO_3$ (1.26%)

and/or salbutamol 0.5 mg in 100 mL of 5% glucose over 15 min (rarely used)

Deplete body K^+

Calcium or sodium resonium:

- 15 g orally up to three times daily with laxatives
- 30 g rectally followed 3–6 hours later by an enema

Haemodialysis or peritoneal dialysis

Practical box 10.1 Correction of hyperkalaemia

FURTHER READING

Ackerman MJ, Clapham DE (1997) Ion channels – basic science and clinical disease. *New England Journal of Medicine* **336**: 1575–1586.

Disorders of magnesium concentration

Plasma magnesium levels are normally maintained within the range 0.7–1.1 mmol L^{-1}. Magnesium balance is a function of intake and excretion. The average daily magnesium intake is 15 mmol. One-third of this magnesium is absorbed, principally in the small bowel. In the healthy adult, there is no net gain or loss of magnesium from bone, so that balance is achieved by the urinary excretion of the net magnesium absorbed.

Primary disturbance of magnesium balance is uncommon, hypo- or hypermagnesaemia usually developing on a background of more obvious fluid and electrolyte disturbances. Disturbance in magnesium balance should always be suspected in association with other fluid and electrolyte disturbances when the patient develops unexpected neurological signs or symptoms.

Renal handling of magnesium

Magnesium transport differs from that of most other ions in that the proximal tubule is not the major site of reabsorption. Only 15–25% of the filtered magnesium is reabsorbed passively in the proximal tubule and 5–10% in the distal tubule. The major site of magnesium transport is the thick ascending limb of the loop of Henle, where 60–70% of the filtered load is reabsorbed. Loop magnesium reabsorption varies with changes in the plasma magnesium concentration, which is the main physiological regulator of urinary magnesium excretion. Hypermagnesaemia inhibits loop transport, while hypomagnaesemia stimulates magnesium transport. Hypercalcaemia inhibits magnesium loop transport by an unknown mechanism.

Another factor that can influence loop magnesium transport is the rate of sodium chloride reabsorption. This effect is relatively unimportant in normal subjects, but decreased reabsorption and magnesium wasting can be induced by the administration of a loop diuretic.

Hypomagnesaemia

This most often develops as a result of deficient intake, defective gut absorption, or excessive gut or urinary loss (see Table 10.15). It can also occur with acute pancreatitis, possibly due to the formation of magnesium soaps in the areas of fat necrosis. Calcium deficiency usually develops with hypomagnesaemia.

CLINICAL FEATURES

Symptoms and signs include irritability, tremor, ataxia, carpopedal spasm, hyperreflexia, confusional and hallucinatory states, and epileptiform convulsions. The serum magnesium is usually <0.7 mmol L^{-1}. An ECG may show a prolonged QT interval, broad flattened T waves, and occasional shortening of the ST segment.

TREATMENT

This involves the withdrawal of precipitating agents such as diuretics or purgatives and the parenteral infusion of 50 mmol of magnesium chloride in 1 L of 5% dextrose or other isotonic fluid over 12–24 hours. This should be repeated daily until the plasma magnesium level is normal.

Table 10.15
Causes of hypomagnesaemia

Decreased magnesium absorption	**Gut losses**
Malabsorption (severe)	Prolonged nasogastric suction
Malnutrition	Excessive purgation
Alcohol excess	Gastrointestinal/biliary fistulae
	Severe diarrhoea
Increased renal excretion	
Drugs	**Miscellaneous**
Loop diuretics	Acute pancreatitis
Thiazide diuretics	
Digoxin	
Diabetic ketoacidosis	
Bartter's syndrome	
Hyperaldosteronism	
SIADH	
Alcohol excess	
Hypercalciuria	
1,25-(OH)-vitamin D deficiency	
Drug toxicity	
Amphotericin	
Aminoglycosides	
Cisplatinum	
Cyclosporin	

Hypermagnesaemia

This primarily occurs in patients with acute or chronic renal failure given magnesium-containing laxatives or antacids. It can also be induced by magnesium-containing enemas. Mild hypermagnesaemia may occur in patients with adrenal insufficiency. Causes are given in Table 10.16.

CLINICAL FEATURES

Symptoms and signs relate to neurological and cardiovascular depression, and include weakness with hyporeflexia proceeding to narcosis, respiratory paralysis and cardiac conduction defects. Symptoms usually develop when the plasma magnesium level exceeds 2 mmol L^{-1}.

TREATMENT

Treatment requires withdrawal of any magnesium therapy. An intravenous injection of 10 mL of calcium gluconate 10% (2.25 mmol calcium) is given to antagonize the effects of hypermagnesaemia, along with dextrose and insulin (as for hyperkalaemia) to lower the plasma magnesium level. Dialysis may be required in patients with severe renal failure. Respiratory failure requires artificial ventilation until the plasma magnesium level returns to normal level.

Table 10.16
Causes of hypermagnesaemia

Impaired renal excretion
Chronic renal failure
Acute renal failure
Increased magnesium intake
Purgatives, e.g. magnesium sulphate
Antacids, e.g. magnesium trisilicate
Haemodialysis with high [Mg^+] dialysate

Disorders of phosphate concentration

Phosphate forms an essential part of most biochemical systems, from nucleic acids downwards. About 80% of all body phosphorus is within bone, plasma phosphate normally ranging from 0.80 to 1.40 mmol L^{-1}. Phosphate reabsorption from the kidney is decreased by PTH, thus hyperparathyroidism is associated with low plasma levels of phosphate.

The regulation of plasma phosphate level is closely linked to calcium.

Table 10.17
Causes of hypophosphataemia

Redistribution	**Decreased intake/absorption**
Respiratory alkalosis	Dietary
Treatment of diabetic ketoacidosis	Malabsorption
Carbohydrate administration after fasting	Vomiting
Cellular uptake syndrome	Gut phosphate binders, e.g. aluminium hydroxide
After parathyroidectomy	Vitamin D deficiency or resistance
Renal losses	Alcohol withdrawal
Hyperparathyroidism	
Renal tubular defects	
Diuretics	

Hypophosphataemia

Significant hypophosphataemia may occur in a number of clinical situations, due to redistribution into cells, to renal losses, or to decreased intake (Table 10.17). It may cause:

- muscle weakness – diaphragmatic weakness, decreased cardiac contractility, skeletal muscle rhabdomyolysis
- a left-shift in the oxyhaemoglobin dissociation curve (reduced 2,3-diphosphoglycerate (2,3-DPG))
- confusion, hallucinations and convulsions.

Mild hypophosphataemia often resolves without specific treatment. However, diaphragmatic weakness may be severe in acute hypophosphataemia, and may impede weaning a patient from a ventilator. Interestingly, chronic hypophosphataemia (in X-linked hypophosphataemia) is associated with normal muscle power.

Treatment of acute hypophosphataemia, if warranted, is with intravenous phosphate at a maximum rate of 9 mmol every 12 hours, with repeated measurements of calcium and phosphate, as over-rapid administration of phosphate may lead to severe hypocalcaemia, particularly in the presence of alkalosis. Chronic hypophosphataemia can be corrected, if warranted, with oral effervescent sodium phosphate.

Hyperphosphataemia

Hyperphosphataemia is common in patients with chronic renal failure (see p. 579) (Table 10.18). Hyperphosphataemia is usually asymptomatic but may result in precipitation of calcium phosphate, particularly in the presence of a normal or raised calcium or of alkalosis. Uraemic itching may be caused by a raised calcium × phosphate product. Prolonged hyperphosphataemia causes hyperparathyroidism, and periarticular and vascular calcification.

Usually no treatment is required for acute hyperphosphataemia, as the causes are self-limiting. Treatment of chronic hyperphosphataemia is with gut phosphate binders and dialysis (see p. 579).

Table 10.18
Causes of hyperphosphataemia

Chronic renal failure
Phosphate-containing enemas
Tumour lysis
Myeloma-abnormal phosphate-binding protein
Rhabdomyolysis

Acid–base disorders

The concentration of hydrogen ions in both extracellular and intracellular compartments is extremely tightly controlled, and very small changes may lead to major cell dysfunction. The blood pH is tightly regulated and is normally maintained at between 7.38 and 7.42. Any deviation from this range indicates a change in the hydrogen ion concentration $[H^+]$ because blood pH is the negative logarithm of $[H^+]$ (Table 10.19). The $[H^+]$ at a physiological blood pH of 7.40 is 40 nmol L^{-1}. An increase in the $[H^+]$ – a fall in pH – is termed acidaemia. A decrease in $[H^+]$ – a rise in the blood pH – is termed alkalaemia. The disorders that cause these changes in the blood pH are acidosis and alkalosis, respectively.

Normal acid–base physiology

The normal adult diet contains an excess of 70–100 mmol of acid. Throughout the body, there are buffers that minimize any changes in blood pH that these ingested hydrogen ions might cause. Such buffers include intracellular proteins (e.g. haemoglobin) and tissue components (e.g. the calcium carbonate and calcium phosphate in bone) as well as the bicarbonate–carbonic acid buffer pair generated by the hydration of carbon dioxide. This buffer pair is clinically most important, in part because its contribution can be measured and because alterations in this buffer pair reveal changes in all other

Table 10.19
Relationship between $[H^+]$ and pH

pH	$[H^+]$ (nmol L^{-1})
6.9	126
7.0	100
7.1	79
7.2	63
7.3	50
7.4	40
7.5	32
7.6	25

buffer systems. Bicarbonate ions (HCO_3^-) and carbonic acid (H_2CO_3) exist in equilibrium; and in the presence of carbonic anhydrase, carbonic acid dissociates to carbon dioxide and water, as expressed in the following equation:

$$H^+ + HCO_3^- \rightleftharpoons H_2CO_3 \xrightleftharpoons{\text{carbonic anhydrase}} CO_2 + H_2O$$

The addition of hydrogen ions drives the reaction to the right, decreasing the plasma bicarbonate concentration [HCO_3^-] and increasing the arterial carbon dioxide pressure (P_aCO_2). As shown in the following Henderson–Hasselbach equation, a fall in the plasma [HCO_3^-] increases [H^+] and thus lowers blood pH:

$$[H^+] = 181 \times P_aCO_2/[HCO_3^-]$$

where [H^+] is expressed in nmol per litre, P_aCO_2 in kilopascals, [HCO_3^-] in mmol per litre, and 181 is the dissociation coefficient of carbonic acid. Alternatively the equation can be expressed as:

$$pH = pK + \log [HCO_3^-] / [H_2CO_3]$$

where pK = 6.1. Thus, the bicarbonate used in the buffering process must be regenerated to maintain normal acid–base balance.

Although the acidaemia stimulates an increase in ventilation, which blunts this change in pH, increased ventilation does not regenerate the bicarbonate used in the buffering process. Consequently, the kidney must excrete hydrogen ions to return the plasma [HCO_3^-] to normal. Maintenance of a normal plasma [HCO_3^-] under physiological conditions depends not only on daily regeneration of bicarbonate but also on reabsorption of all bicarbonate filtered across the glomerular capillaries.

Renal reabsorption of bicarbonate

The plasma [HCO_3^-] is normally maintained at approximately 25 mmol L^{-1}. In individuals with a normal glomerular filtration rate (120 mL min^{-1}), about 4500 mmol of bicarbonate is filtered each day. If this filtered bicarbonate were not reabsorbed, the plasma [HCO_3^-] would fall, along with blood pH. Thus, maintenance of a normal plasma [HCO_3^-] requires that essentially all of the bicarbonate in the glomerular filtrate be reabsorbed.

The proximal convoluted tubule reclaims 85–90% of filtered bicarbonate; in contrast, the distal nephron reclaims very little. This difference is caused by the greater quantity of luminal carbonic anhydrase in the proximal tubule than in the distal nephron. As a result of these quantitative differences, bicarbonate that escapes reabsorption in the proximal tubule is excreted in the urine.

Proximal tubular bicarbonate reabsorption is catalysed by the Na^+–K^+-ATPase pump located in the peritubular cell membrane. By exchanging peritubular potassium ions for intracellular sodium ions, the pump keeps the intracellular sodium concentration low, allowing sodium ions to enter the cell by moving down the sodium concentration gradient from the tubule lumen to the cell interior. Hydrogen ions are transported in the opposite direction (at the Na^+–H^+ antiporter), thereby maintaining electroneutrality. Before bicarbonate enters the proximal tubule, it combines with secreted hydrogen ions, forming carbonic acid. In the presence of luminal carbonic anhydrase, carbonic acid rapidly dissociates into carbon dioxide and water, which can then rapidly enter the proximal tubular cell. In the cell, carbon dioxide is hydrated, ultimately forming bicarbonate, which is then transported down an electrical gradient from the cell interior, across the membrane into the peritubular fluid, and into the blood. In this process, each hydrogen ion secreted into the proximal tubule lumen is reabsorbed and can be resecreted; there is no net loss of hydrogen ions or net gain of bicarbonate ions (Fig. 10.6).

Renal excretion of [H^+] (Fig 10.7)

More acid is secreted into the proximal tubule (up to 4500 nmol of hydrogen ions each day) than into any other nephron segment. However, the hydrogen ions secreted into the proximal tubule are almost completely reabsorbed with bicarbonate; consequently, proximal tubular hydrogen ion secretion does not contribute significantly to hydrogen ion elimination from the body. The excretion of the daily acid load requires hydrogen ion secretion in more distal nephron segments.

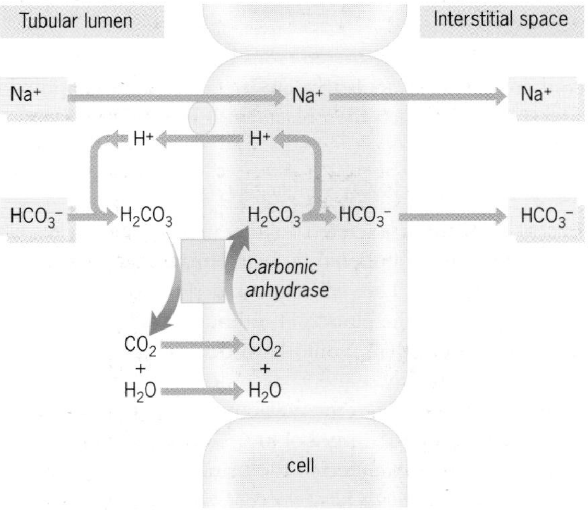

Fig 10.6
Resorption of sodium bicarbonate in the renal (mainly proximal) tubule.
Bicarbonate is reclaimed by the secretion of H^+ into the tubule in exchange for Na^+. This results in the formation of H_2CO_3 which is then broken down to CO_2. This is reabsorbed and converted back to H_2CO_3, which now dissociates into H^+ and HCO_3^-. The net result is reabsorption of Na^+ and HCO_3^-. This process is dependent on carbonic anhydrase within the cells and on the luminal surface of the tubular cell

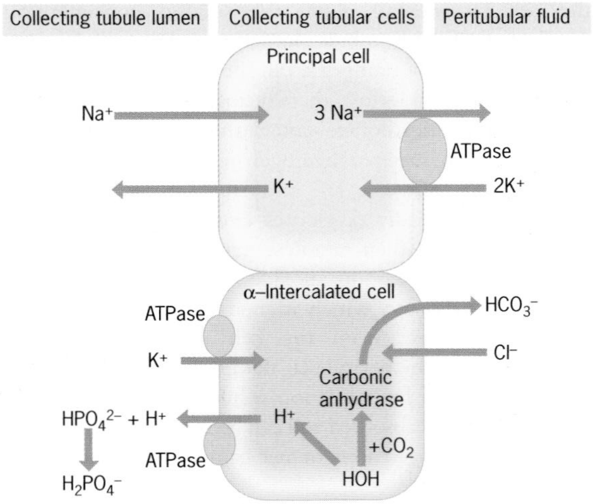

Fig 10.7
Renal excretion of H^+.
Secretion of H^+ from the cortical collecting tubule is indirectly linked to Na^+ reabsorption. Intracellular potassium is exchanged for sodium in the principal cell. Aldosterone stimulates H^+ secretion by entering the principal cell, where it opens Na^+ channels in the luminal membrane and increases Na^+–K^+-ATPase activity. The movement of cationic Na^+ into the principal cells then creates a negative charge within the tubule lumen. K^+ moves from the electrochemical gradient and into the lumen. Aldosterone apparently also stimulates the H^+-ATPase directly in the intercalated cell, further enhancing H^+ secretion. When the urinary pH falls to 4.0–4.5, further H^+ secretion by the alpha-intercalated cells ceases. The filtration of titratable acids (e.g. phosphoric acid) raises the intraluminal pH and permits this process to continue. Secreted H^+ binds to the conjugate anion of a titratable acid (HPO_4^{2-}, in this case) and is excreted in the urine. The H^+ to be secreted arises from the reassociation of H_2O and CO_2 in the presence of carbonic anhydrase; thus, a bicarbonate molecule is regenerated each time an H^+ is eliminated in the urine

Most dietary hydrogen ions come from sulphur-containing amino acids that are metabolized to sulphuric acid (H_2SO_4), which then reacts with sodium bicarbonate as follows:

$$H_2SO_4 + 2NaHCO_3 \rightarrow Na_2SO_4 + 2CO_2 + 2H_2O.$$

Excess sulphate is excreted in the urine, whereas excess hydrogen ions are buffered by bicarbonate and depress the plasma [HCO_3^-]. This fall in plasma [HCO_3^-] leads to a slight decrease in the blood pH, although a smaller decrease in the blood pH than would have occurred if buffer were unavailable. The subsequent excretion of hydrogen ions takes place primarily in the collecting tubule and results in the regeneration of 1 mmol of bicarbonate for every mmol of hydrogen ions excreted in the urine.

The *collecting tubule* has two types of cells:

- the principal cell with an aldosterone-sensitive Na absorption site
- the α-intercalated cell which possesses the proton pump for the active secretion of hydrogen ions.

Secretion of hydrogen ions from the cortical collecting tubule is indirectly linked to sodium reabsorption. Aldosterone has several facilitating effects on hydrogen ion secretion. Aldosterone opens sodium channels in the luminal membrane of the principal cell and increases Na^+–K^+-ATPase activity. The subsequent movement of cationic sodium into the principal cell creates a negative charge within the tubule lumen. Potassium ions from the principal cells and hydrogen ions from the intercalated cells move out from the cells down the electrochemical gradient and into the lumen. Aldosterone also stimulates directly the H^+-ATPase in the intercalated cell, further enhancing hydrogen ion secretion.

When hydrogen ions are secreted into the lumen of the collecting tubule, a tiny, but physiologically critical, fraction of these excess hydrogen ions remains in solution. Here, they increase the urinary [H^+] and lower urinary pH below 4.0. Nevertheless, below this urine pH, inhibition of proton-secreting pumps such as H^+-ATPase severely restrict kidney secretion of more hydrogen ions. Consequently, secretion of hydrogen ions depends on the presence of buffers in the urine that maintain the urine pH at a level higher than 4.0.

Two *buffer systems* are important in acid excretion: the titratable acids such as phosphate and the ammonia system. Each system is responsible for excreting about half of the daily acid load of 50–100 mmol under physiological conditions (Fig 10.7).

Titratable acid

A titratable acid is a filtered buffer substance having a conjugate anion that can be titrated within the pH range occurring physiologically in the urine. Phosphoric acid (pK_a 6.8) is the usual titratable urinary buffer. Hydrogen ions bind to the conjugate anions of the titratable acids and are excreted in the urine. For each hydrogen ion excreted in this form, a bicarbonate ion is regenerated within the cell and returned to the blood (Fig 10.7).

Ammonium (NH_4^+)

Although half of dietary hydrogen ions are excreted as titratable acid and the other half as ammonium, in pathophysiological conditions the ammonia (NH_3) buffer system is far more important than titratable acids. In the setting of metabolic acidosis, titratable acids cannot increase significantly because availablity of the titratable acid is fixed by the plasma concentration of the buffer and by the GFR. The ammonia buffer system, in contrast, can increase several hundred-fold when necessary. Consequently, impaired renal excretion of hydrogen ions is always associated with a defect in ammonium excretion (Fig 10.8).

All ammonia used to buffer urinary hydrogen ions in the collecting tubule is synthesized in the proximal convoluted tubule. Glutamine is the primary source of ammonia. It undergoes deamination catalyzed by glutaminase, resulting in α-ketoglutaric acid (see Fig 10.8) and ammonia. Once formed, ammonia can diffuse into the proximal tubule lumen and become acidified, forming ammonium. Once in

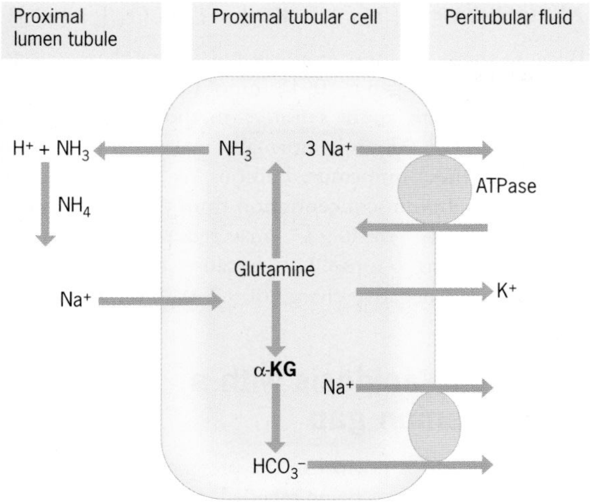

Fig 10.8
The ammonia buffering system in the kidney.
All ammonia used to buffer H^+ in the collecting tubule is synthesized in the proximal convoluted tubule, and glutamine is the main source of this ammonia. As glutamine is metabolized, α-ketoglutarate (α-KG) is formed, which ultimately breaks down to bicarbonate that is then secreted into the peritubular fluid at an Na^+–HCO_3^- cotransporter

the proximal tubule lumen, ammonium flows along the tubule to the thick ascending limb of Henle's loop. Here, it is transported out of the tubule into the medullary interstitium. Ammonium then dissociates to ammonia, leading to a high interstitial ammonia concentration. Ammonia diffuses down its concentration gradient into the lumen of the collecting tubule. Here, it reacts with the hydrogen ions secreted by the collecting tubular cell to form ammonium. Because ammonium is not lipid-soluble, it is trapped in the lumen and excreted in the urine as ammonium chloride. Controversy still exists about whether glutamine metabolism in the liver plays a role in acid–base homeostasis.

Two conditions are more important than others in promoting ammonia synthesis by the proximal tubular cell: systemic acidosis and hypokalaemia.

CAUSES OF ACID–BASE DISTURBANCE

Acid–base disturbance may be caused by:

- abnormal CO_2 removal in the lungs ('respiratory' acidosis and alkalosis)
- abnormalities in the regulation of bicarbonate and other buffers in the blood ('metabolic' acidosis and alkalosis).

Both may, and usually do, coexist. For instance, metabolic acidosis causes hyperventilation (via medullary chemoreceptors, see p. 750), leading to increased removal of CO_2 in the lungs and partial compensation for the acidosis. Conversely, respiratory acidosis is accompanied by renal bicarbonate retention, which could be mistaken for primary metabolic alkalosis. The situation is even more complex if a patient has both respiratory disease and a metabolic disturbance.

Table 10.20
Changes in arterial blood gases

	pH	P_aCO_2	HCO_3^-
Respiratory acidosis	N or ↓	↑↑	↑
Respiratory alkalosis	N or ↑	↓↓	↓ (slight)
Metabolic acidosis	N or ↓	↓	↓↓
Metabolic alkalosis	N or ↑	↑ (slight)	↑↑

DIAGNOSIS

Clinical history and examination usually point to the correct diagnosis. Table 10.20 shows the typical changes, but in complicated patients the acid–base nomogram (Fig 10.9) is invaluable. The H^+ and P_aCO_2 are measured in arterial blood (for precautions see p. 850) as well as the bicarbonate. If the values from a patient lie in one of the bands in the diagram, it is likely that only one abnormality is present. If the $[H^+]$ is high (pH low) but the P_aCO_2 is normal, the intercept lies between two bands: the patient has respiratory dysfunction, leading to failure of CO_2 elimination, but this is partly compensated for by metabolic acidosis, stimulating respiration and CO_2 removal (this is the most common 'combined' abnormality in practice).

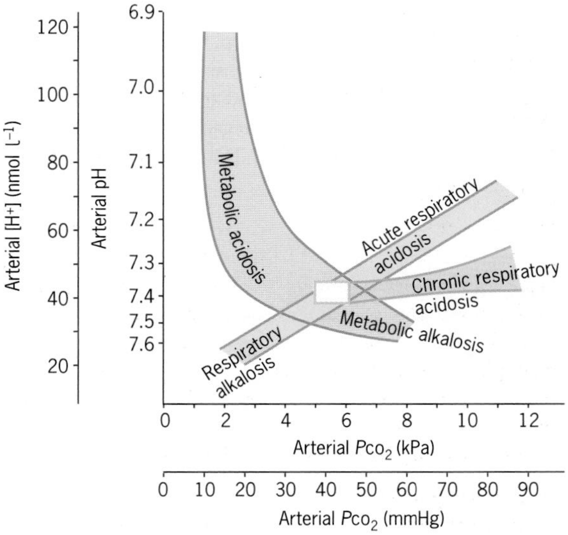

Fig 10.9
The Flenley acid–base nomogram.
This was derived from a large number of observations in patients with 'pure' respiratory or metabolic disturbances. The bands show the 95% confidence limits representing the individual varieties of acid–base disturbance. The central white box shows the approximate limits of arterial pH and Pco_2 in normal individuals

Respiratory acidosis and alkalosis

Respiratory acidosis

This is caused by retention of CO_2. The P_aCO_2 and $[H^+]$ rise. Renal retention of bicarbonate may partly compensate, returning the $[H^+]$ towards normal (see p. 850).

Respiratory alkalosis

Increased removal of CO_2 is caused by hyperventilation, so there is a fall in P_aCO_2 and $[H^+]$ (see p. 850).

Metabolic acidosis

This is due to the accumulation of any acid other than carbonic acid and there is a primary decrease in the plasma $[HCO_3^-]$. Several disorders can lead to metabolic acidosis: acid administration, acid generation (e.g. lactic acidosis during shock or cardiac arrest), impaired acid excretion by the kidneys, or bicarbonate losses from the gastrointestinal tract or kidneys. From a diagnostic viewpoint, calculation of the plasma anion gap is extremely useful in narrowing this differential diagnosis.

The anion gap

The first step is to identify whether the acidosis is due to retention of H^+Cl^- or to another acid. This is achieved by calculation of the anion gap. The principles underlying this calculation are straightforward:

- The normal cations present in plasma are Na^+, K^+, Ca^{2+}, Mg^{2+}.
- The normal anions present in plasma are Cl^-, HCO_3^-, negative charges present on albumin, phosphate, sulphate, lactate, and other organic acids.
- The sum of the positive and negative charges are equal.
- Measurement of $[Na^+]$, $[K^+]$, $[Cl^-]$ and $[HCO_3^-]$ are usually easily available.

$$\text{ANION GAP} = \{[Na^+] + [K^+]\} - \{[HCO_3^-] + [Cl^-]\}.$$

Because there are more unmeasured anions than cations, the normal anion gap is 10–18 mmol L^{-1}, although recent calculations with more sensitive methods place this at 6–12 mmol L^{-1}. Albumin normally makes up the largest portion of these unmeasured anions. As a result, a fall in the plasma albumin concentration from the normal value of about 40 g L^{-1} to 20 g L^{-1} may reduce the anion gap by as much as 6 mmol L^{-1}, because each 1 g L^{-1} of albumin has a negative charge of 0.2–0.28 mmol L^{-1}.

Metabolic acidosis with a normal anion gap

If the anion gap is normal in the presence of acidosis, this suggests that H^+Cl^- is being retained or that $Na^+HCO_3^-$ is being lost. Causes of a normal anion gap acidosis are given in Table 10.21. In these conditions, plasma bicarbonate decreases and is replaced by chloride to maintain electroneutrality. Consequently, these disorders are sometimes referred to collectively as hyperchloraemic acidoses.

Renal tubular acidosis

This term refers to systemic acidosis caused by impairment of the ability of the renal tubules to maintain acid–base balance. This group of disorders is uncommon and only rarely a cause of significant clinical disease. Renal tubular acidosis may be secondary to immunological, drug-induced or structural damage to the tubular cells, an inherited abnormality, or an isolated ('primary') abnormality. As with most disorders which are not well understood, the nomenclature is confusing.

Type 4 renal tubular acidosis

Also called 'hyporeninaemic hypoaldosteronism', this is probably the most common of these disorders. The cardinal features are hyperkalaemia and acidosis occurring in a

Table 10.21
Causes of metabolic acidosis with a normal anion gap

Increased gastrointestinal bicarbonate loss	**Decreased renal hydrogen ion excretion**
Diarrhoea	Distal (type 1) renal tubular acidosis
Ileostomy	Type 4 renal tubular acidosis (aldosterone deficiency)
Ureterosigmoidostomy	
Increased renal bicarbonate loss	**Increased HCl production**
Acetazolamide	Ammonium chloride ingestion
Proximal (type 2) renal tubular acidosis	Increased catabolism of lysine, arginine
Hyperparathyroidism	
Tubular damage, e.g. drugs, heavy metals, paraproteins	

Table 10.22 Diagnosis of hyporeninaemic hypoaldosteronism (type 4 renal tubular acidosis)

Hyperkalaemia
(In the absence of drugs known to cause hyperkalaemia)
low plasma bicarbonate and hyperchloraemia

Normal ACTH stimulation test

Low basal 24 hour urinary aldosterone

Subnormal response of plasma renin and plasma aldosterone to stimulation
Samples taken over 2 hours supine and again after 40 mg frusemide (80 mg if creatinine > 120 μmol L^{-1}) and 4 hours upright posture

Correction of hyperkalaemia by fludrocortisone 0.1 mg daily

patient with mild chronic renal insufficiency, usually caused by tubulo-interstitial disease (e.g. reflux nephropathy) or diabetes. Plasma renin and aldosterone are found to be low even after measures which would normally stimulate their secretion (Table 10.22). An identical syndrome may be caused by chronic ingestion of NSAIDs, which impair renin and aldosterone secretion. In the presence of acidosis, urine pH may be low. Treatment is with fludrocortisone, sodium bicarbonate, diuretics, or ion exchange resins to remove potassium, or some combination of these. Dietary potassium restriction alone is ineffective.

Type 3 renal tubular acidosis

This condition is vanishingly rare, and represents a combination of type 1 and type 2.

Type 2 ('proximal') renal tubular acidosis

This is very rare in adult practice (Table 10.23). It is caused by failure of sodium bicarbonate reabsorption in the proximal tubule. The cardinal features are acidosis, hypokalaemia, an inability to lower the urine pH below 5.5 despite systemic acidosis, and the appearance of bicarbonate in the urine despite a subnormal plasma bicarbonate. This disorder normally occurs as part of a generalized tubular defect, together with other features such as glycosuria and amino-aciduria. Treatment is with sodium bicarbonate: massive doses may be required to overcome the renal 'leak'.

Type 1 ('distal') renal tubular acidosis

This is due to a failure of H^+ excretion in the distal tubule (Table 10.24). It consists of:

- acidosis
- hypokalaemia (few exceptions – see Table 10.24)
- inability to lower the urine pH below 5.5 despite systemic acidosis
- low urinary ammonium production.

These features may be present only in the face of increased acid production; hence the need for an acid load test in diagnosis (Practical box 10.2). Other features include:

- low urinary citrate
- hypercalciuria.

These abnormalities result in osteomalacia, renal stone formation and recurrent urinary infections. Osteomalacia is caused by buffering of H^+ by Ca^{2+} in bone, resulting in depletion of calcium from bone. Renal stone formation is caused by hypercalciuria, hypocitraturia (citrate inhibits calcium phosphate precipitation), and alkaline urine (which favours precipitation of calcium phosphate).

Recurrent urinary infections are caused by renal stones. Treatment is with sodium bicarbonate, potassium supplements and citrate. Thiazide diuretics are useful by causing volume contraction and increased proximal sodium bicarbonate reabsorption. Diagnosis of renal tubular acidosis requires logical steps as summarized in Practical box 10.2.

Table 10.23
Causes of proximal renal tubular acidosis

Cystinosis **Tyrosinaemia** **Wilson's disease** **Glycogen storage disease, type I** **Pyruvate carboxylase deficiency** **Multiple myeloma**	**Vitamin D deficiency/ hyperparathyroidism** **Toxins and drugs** Carbonic anhydrase inhibitors Lead Cadmium Mercury Uranium Copper Outdated tetracycline Streptozocin

Urinary anion gap

Another useful tool in the evaluation of metabolic acidosis with a normal anion gap is the urinary anion gap:

$$\text{URINARY ANION GAP} = \{\text{urinary } [Na^+] + \text{urinary } [K^+]\} - \text{urinary } [Cl^-].$$

This calculation can be used to distinguish the normal anion gap acidosis caused by diarrhoea (or other gastrointestinal alkali loss) from that caused by distal renal tubular acidosis. In both disorders, the plasma $[K^+]$ is characteristically low. In patients with renal tubular acidosis, urinary pH is always greater than 5.3. Although excretion of urinary hydrogen ions in the patient with diarrhoea should acidify the urine, hypokalaemia leads to enhanced ammonia synthesis by

Table 10.24
Causes of distal renal tubular acidosis

Primary Idiopathic **Genetic** Familial Marfan syndrome Ehlers–Danlos syndrome **Nephrocalcinosis** Chronic hypercalcaemia Medullary sponge kidney **Hypergammaglobulinaemic states** Amyloidosis* Cryoglobulinaemia Cirrhosis **Drugs and toxins** Amphotericin B Lithium carbonate	**Autoimmune diseases** Sjögren's syndrome* Thyroiditis Autoimmune hepatitis Primary biliary cirrhosis **Urinary tract obstruction** **Sickle cell anaemia** **Systemic lupus erythematosus** **Renal transplant rejection***

*May also cause proximal renal tubular acidosis

Practical

Plasma HCO_3^- < 21 mmol L^{-1}, urine pH > 5.3: renal tubular acidosis

To differentiate between proximal (very rare) and distal (rare) requires bicarbonate infusion test

Plasma HCO_3^- > 21 mmol L^{-1} but suspicion of partial renal tubular acidosis (e.g. nephrocalcinosis associated diseases): **acid load test** required as follows

- Give 100 mg kg^{-1} ammonium chloride by mouth
- Check urine pH hourly and plasma HCO_3^- at 3 hours
- Plasma HCO_3^- should drop below 21 mmol L^{-1} unless the patient vomits
  - (in which case the test should be repeated with an antiemetic)
- If urine pH remains > 5.3 despite a plasma HCO_3^- of 21 mmol L^{-1}, the diagnosis is confirmed

Practical box 10.2 Diagnosis of renal tubular acidosis

Table 10.25
Causes of metabolic acidosis with an increased anion gap

Renal failure (sulphate, phosphate)

Accumulation of organic acids

Lactic acidosis
L-lactic
- Type A – anaerobic metabolism in tissues
  - Hypotension/cardiac arrest
  - Sepsis
  - Poisoning – ethylene glycol, methanol, others
- Type B – decreased hepatic lactate metabolism
  - Insulin deficiency (decreased pyruvate dehydrogenase activity)
  - Metformin accumulation (chronic renal failure)
  - Haematological malignancies
  - Other drugs
  - Rare inherited enzyme defects

D-lactic (fermentation of glucose in bowel by abnormal bowel flora, complicating abnormal small bowel anatomy, e.g. blind loops)

Ketoacidosis
Insulin deficiency
Alcohol excess
Starvation

Exogenous acids
Salicylate

the proximal tubular cells. Despite acidaemia, the excess urinary buffer increases the urine pH to a value above 5.3 in some patients with diarrhoea.

Whenever urinary acid is excreted as ammonium chloride, the increase in urinary chloride excretion decreases the urinary anion gap. Thus, the urinary anion gap should be negative in the patient with diarrhoea regardless of the urine pH. On the other hand, although hypokalaemia may result in enhanced proximal tubular ammonia synthesis in distal renal tubular acidosis, the inability to secrete hydrogen ions into the collecting tubule in this condition limits ammonium chloride formation and excretion; thus, the urinary anion gap is positive in distal renal tubular acidosis.

Metabolic acidosis with a high anion gap

If the anion gap is increased, one may conclude that an unmeasured anion is present in increased quantities. This may be either one of the acids normally present in small, but unmeasured quantities, such as lactate, or an exogenous acid. Causes of a high anion gap acidosis are given in Table 10.25.

Lactic acidosis

Increased lactic acid production occurs when cellular respiration is abnormal, due either to lack of oxygen in the tissues ('type A') or to a metabolic abnormality, such as drug-induced ('type B') (Table 10.25). The most common cause in clinical practice is type A lactic acidosis, occurring in septic or cardiogenic shock. Significant acidosis can occur despite a normal blood pressure and P_aO_2, owing to splanchnic and peripheral vasoconstric-tion. Acidosis worsens cardiac function and vasocon-striction further, contributing to a downward spiral and fulminant production of lactic acid.

Diabetic ketoacidosis (see p. 974)

This is a high-anion-gap acidosis resulting from the accumulation of organic acids, acetoacetic acid and hydroxybutyric acid, owing to increased production and some reduced peripheral utilization.

Uraemic acidosis

Kidney disease may cause acidosis in several ways. Reduction in the number of functioning nephrons decreases the capacity to excrete ammonia and H^+ in the urine. In addition, tubular disease may cause bicarbonate wasting. Acidosis is a particular feature of those types of chronic renal failure in which the tubules are particularly affected, such as reflux nephropathy and chronic obstructive uropathy.

Chronic acidosis is most often caused by chronic renal failure, where there is a failure to excrete fixed acid. Up to 40 mmol of hydrogen ions may accumulate daily. These are buffered by *bone*, in exchange for calcium. Chronic acidosis is therefore a major risk factor for renal osteodystrophy and hypercalciuria.

Chronic acidosis has also been shown to be a risk factor for muscle wasting in renal failure, and may also contribute to the inexorable progression of some types of renal disease.

Uraemic acidosis should be corrected because of the effects of chronic acidosis on growth, muscle turnover and bones. Oral sodium bicarbonate 2–3 mmol kg^{-1} daily is usually enough to maintain serum bicarbonate above 20 mmol L^{-1}, but may contribute to sodium overload. Calcium carbonate improves acidosis and also acts as a phosphate binder and calcium supplement, and is increasingly used. Acidosis in end-stage renal failure is usually fully corrected by adequate dialysis.

Mixed metabolic acidosis

Both types of acidosis may coexist. For instance, cholera would be expected to cause a normal-anion-gap acidosis owing to massive gastrointestinal losses of bicarbonate, but the anion gap is often increased owing to renal failure and lactic acidosis as a result of hypovolaemia.

CLINICAL FEATURES

Clinically the most obvious effect is stimulation of respiration, leading to the clinical sign of 'air hunger', or Kussmaul's sign. Interestingly, patients with profound hyperventilation may not complain of breathlessness, although in others it may be a presenting complaint.

Acidosis increases delivery of oxygen to the tissues by shifting the oxyhaemoglobin dissociation curve to the right, but it also leads to inhibition of 2,3-DPG production, which returns the curve towards normal (see Chapter 13). Cardiovascular dysfunction is common in acidotic patients, although it is often difficult to dissociate the numerous possible causes of this. There is no doubt that acidosis is negatively inotropic. Severe acidosis causes venoconstriction, resulting in redistribution of blood from the peripheries to the central circulation, and increased systemic venous pressure, which may worsen pulmonary oedema caused by myocardial depression. Arteriolar vasodilatation also occurs, further contributing to hypotension.

Cerebral dysfunction is variable. Severe acidosis is often associated with confusion and fits, but numerous other possible causes are usually present.

As mentioned earlier, acidosis stimulates potassium loss from cells, which may lead to potassium deficiency if renal function is normal, or to hyperkalaemia if renal potassium excretion is impaired.

TREATMENT

In lactic acidosis caused by poor tissue perfusion ('type A'), treatment should be aimed at maximizing oxygen delivery to the tissues; this usually requires inotropic agents, mechanical ventilation and invasive monitoring. In 'type B' lactic acidosis, treatment is that of the underlying disorder; e.g.

- insulin in diabetic ketoacidosis
- treatment of methanol and ethylene glycol poisoning with ethanol
- removal of salicylate by dialysis.

The question of whether severe acidosis should be treated with bicarbonate is extremely controversial. Severe acidosis ($[H^+]$ > 100 nmol L^{-1}, pH < 7.0) is associated with a very high mortality, which makes many doctors keen to correct it. Since acidosis is known to impair cardiac contractility, it would seem sensible to correct acidosis with bicarbonate in a sick patient. However:

- Rapid correction of acidosis may result in tetany and fits owing to a rapid decrease in ionized calcium.
- Administration of sodium bicarbonate may lead to extracellular volume expansion, exacerbating pulmonary oedema.
- Bicarbonate therapy increases CO_2 production and will therefore correct acidosis only if ventilation can be increased to remove the added CO_2 load.
- The increased amounts of CO_2 generated may diffuse more readily into cells than bicarbonate, worsening intracellular acidosis.

Administration of sodium bicarbonate (50 mmol, as 50 mL of 8.4% sodium bicarbonate intravenously) is still occasionally given during cardiac arrest and is often necessary before arrhythmias can be corrected. Correction of hyperkalaemia associated with acidosis is also of undoubted benefit. In other situations there is no clinical evidence to show that correction of acidosis improves outcome, but it is standard practice to administer sodium bicarbonate when $[H^+]$ is above 126 nmol L^{-1} (pH < 6.9), using intravenous 1.26% (150 mmol L^{-1}) bicarbonate.

Metabolic alkalosis

Renal excretion of excess bicarbonate is normally very efficient, and for this reason metabolic alkalosis is much rarer than acidosis. A number of factors stimulate bicarbonate reabsorption and hydrogen ion excretion despite the presence of alkalosis:

- extracellular volume depletion
- potassium deficiency
- excess mineralocorticoids
- thiazide and loop diuretics.

All of these may be thought of as increasing secretion of H^+ in exchange for Na^+ in the distal tubule.

Vomiting causes alkalosis both by causing volume depletion and by causing loss of gastric acid.

Exogenous alkalis, such as those found in effervescent preparations of analgesics or in proprietary antacids, may also contribute to metabolic alkalosis, particularly if combined with another contributory factor.

CLINICAL FEATURES

These include tetany (see p. 516), apathy, confusion and drowsiness. The oxyhaemoglobin dissociation curve is shifted to the left. Respiration may be depressed.

TREATMENT

Replacement of sodium, potassium and chloride allows renal excretion of bicarbonate. Clearly sodium chloride administration should be avoided in patients on diuretics as appropriate treatment for heart failure. Acetazolamide may be useful in patients without sodium depletion.

FURTHER READING

Atkinson DE, Bourke E (1987) Metabolic aspects of the regulation of systemic pH. *American Journal of Physiology* **252**: F947–F956.

Cameron et al (eds) (1993) Water, electrolyte or acid–base disorders. In *Oxford Textbook of Clinical Nephrology.* Oxford: Oxford University Press, 867–917.

Field MJ, Giebisch GJ (1985) Hormonal control of renal potassium excretion. *Kidney International* **27**: 379–387.

Schrier RW (eds) (1997) In *Renal and Electrolyte Disorders.* New York: Lippincott–Raven, 1–240.

Adrogue HJ, Madias NE (1998) Management of life-threatening acid–base disorders *New England Journal of Medicine* **338**:26–34 and 107–111.

Cardiovascular disease

11

The age-adjusted incidence of heart disease has started to decline in Western Europe and North America, but poses an increasing threat in Eastern Europe and in developing countries. Worldwide, ischaemic heart disease is believed to cause around 6.3 million deaths annually, more than any other single cause. Cerebrovascular disease accounts for a further 4.4 million deaths annually. Many of these deaths might be prevented by reducing tobacco consumption, by altering diets and by treating hypercholesterolaemia and hypertension. Rheumatic fever is now rare in industrialized countries, but remains common worldwide. Infective causes of heart failure, such as Chagas' disease, typhoid fever and diphtheria, are also important in developing countries.

Congenital heart disease is important in the young and is responsible for approximately 1% of deaths in patients below 15 years of age.

Lastly, pulmonary heart disease is common in countries with a high incidence of smoking.

Essential anatomy, physiology and embryology of the heart

The cellular basis of myocardial contraction

Myocardial cells (myocytes) contain bundles of parallel myofibrils. Each myofibril is made up of a series of sarcomeres (Fig 11.1). A sarcomere is bound by two transverse Z lines, to each of which is attached a perpendicular filament of the protein actin. The actin filaments from each of the two Z bands overlap with thicker parallel protein filaments known as myosin. Actin and myosin filaments are attached to each other by cross-bridges that contain ATPase.

During cardiac contraction the length of the actin and myosin monofilaments does not change. Rather, the actin filaments slide between the myosin filaments when a high-energy bond of ATP is split by ATPase. To supply the ATP, the myocyte (which cannot stop for a rest) has an extraordinarily high mitochondrial density (35% of the cell volume). Calcium ions initiate contraction by inactivating another protein called troponin C, which ordinarily inhibits the actin–myosin interaction. Calcium is made available during the plateau phase (phase 2) of the

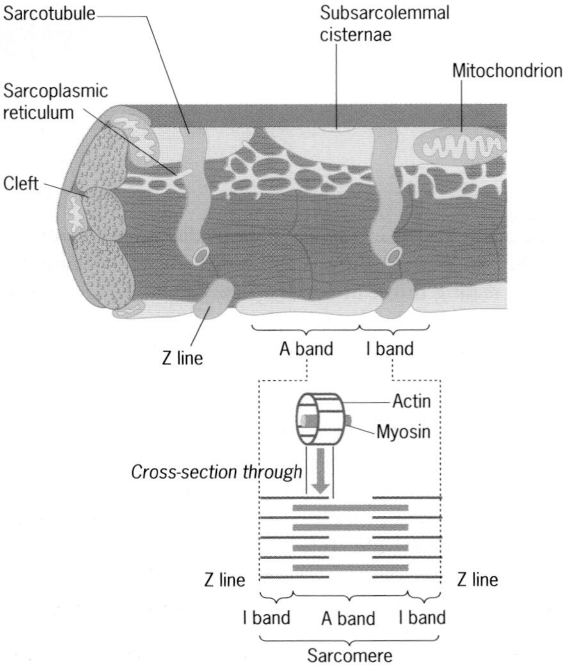

Fig 11.1
Schematic showing the structure of a myofibril within a myocyte. The myofibrils are made up of a series of sarcomeres joined at the Z line

action potential (see Fig 11.32 on p. 658) by calcium ions entering the cell and by being mobilized in mass from the sarcoplasmic reticulum. The force of cardiac muscle contraction ('inotropic state') is thus regulated by the influx of calcium ions into the cell through calcium channels (Fig 11.2). T (transient) calcium channels open when the muscle is more depolarized, whereas L (long-lasting) calcium channels require less depolarization.

Starling's law of the heart

The contractile function of an isolated strip of cardiac tissue can be described by the relationship between the velocity of muscle contraction, the load that may be moved by the contracting muscle, and the extent to which the muscle is stretched before contracting. As with all other types of muscle, the velocity of contraction of myocardial tissue is reduced by increasing the load against which the tissue must contract. However, in the non-failing heart, prestretching of cardiac muscle improves the relationship between the force and velocity of contraction (Fig 11.3).

This phenomenon was described in the intact heart as an increase of stroke volume (ventricular performance) with an enlargement of the diastolic volume (preload), and is known as 'Starling's law of the heart' or the 'Frank–Starling relationship'. It has been transcribed into more clinically relevant indices. Thus, stroke work (aortic pressure × stroke volume) is increased as ventricular end-diastolic volume is raised. Alternatively, within certain limits, cardiac output rises as pulmonary capillary wedge pressure increases. This clinical relationship is described by the ventricular function curve (Fig 11.3, which also shows the effect of sympathetic stimulation).

The law of Laplace

This is also relevant to the contractile function of the heart. Laplace stated that the pressure within a sphere is proportional to wall stress (in the heart this is equivalent to afterload) and inversely proportional to its radius. Thus, as the heart enlarges beyond the point at which Starling's law confers an advantage, the wall stress increases and cardiac output falls.

The conduction system of the heart

Each natural heart beat begins in the heart's pacemaker – the sinoatrial (SA) node. This is a crescent-shaped structure that is located around the medial and anterior aspect of the junction between the superior vena cava and the right atrium (Fig 11.4). Progressive loss of the diastolic resting membrane potential is followed, when the threshold potential has been reached, by a more rapid depolarization of the sinus node tissue. This depolarization triggers depolarization of the atrial myocardium. The atrial tissue is activated like a 'forest fire', but the activation peters out when the insulating layer between the atrium and the ventricle – the annulus fibrosus – is reached.

The depolarization continues to conduct slowly through the atrioventricular (AV) node. This is a small, bean-shaped structure that lies beneath the right atrial endocardium within the lower interatrial septum. The AV node continues as the His bundle, which penetrates the annulus fibrosus and conducts the cardiac impulse rapidly towards the ventricle. The His bundle reaches the crest of the interventricular septum and divides into the right bundle branch and the main left bundle branch.

The right bundle branch continues down the right side of the interventricular septum to the apex, from where it radiates and divides to form the Purkinje network, which spreads throughout the subendocardial surface of the right ventricle.

The main left bundle branch is a short structure which fans out into many strands on the left side of the interventricular septum. These strands can be grouped into an anterior superior division (the anterior hemibundle) and a posterior inferior division (the posterior hemibundle). The anterior hemibundle supplies the subendocardial Purkinje network of the anterior and superior surfaces of the left ventricle, and the inferior hemibundle supplies the inferior and posterior surfaces. Impulse conduction through the AV node is slow and depends on action potentials largely produced by slow transmembrane calcium flux. In the

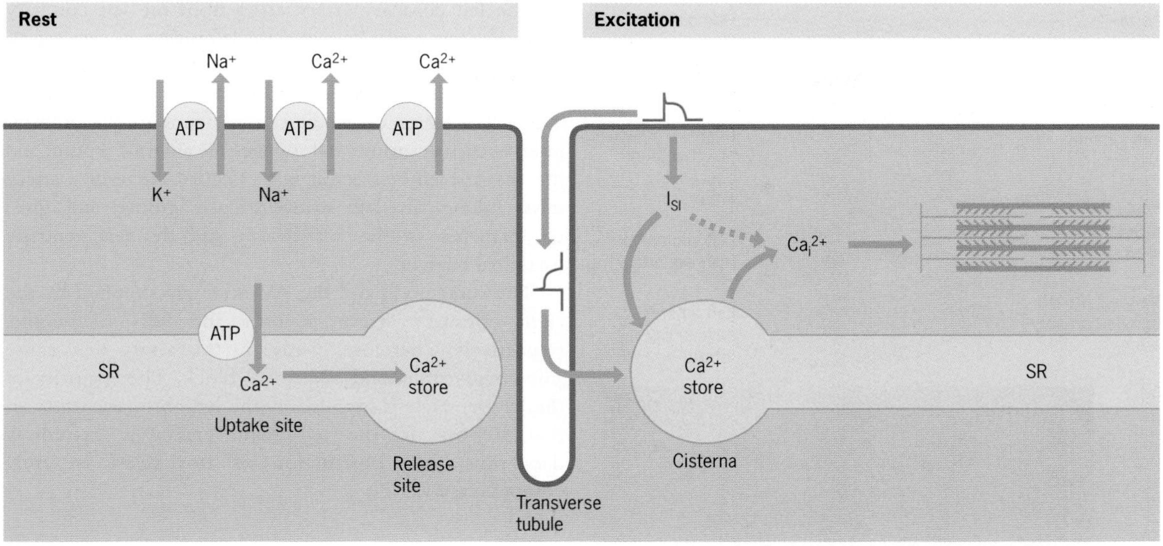

Fig 11.2
The calcium cycle
Right: Ca^{2+} ions stored in the cisternae of the sarcoplasmic reticulum (SR) are released when the depolarization spike travels into the cell along the transverse tubule. A second inward current (I_{SI}) causes release of extra calcium
Left: Calcium levels are restored by sarcolemmal Na^+–Ca^{2+} pump and SR pump. From Levick et al (1995) *Introduction to Cardiovascular Physiology*

atria, ventricles and His–Purkinje system conduction is rapid and is due to action potentials generated by rapid transmembrane sodium diffusion.

Nerve supply of the cardiovascular system

Adrenergic nerves supply atrial and ventricular muscle fibres as well as the conduction system. β_1-Receptors predominate in the heart with both adrenaline and noradrenaline having positive inotropic and chronotropic effects. β_2-Receptors predominate in the vascular smooth muscle.

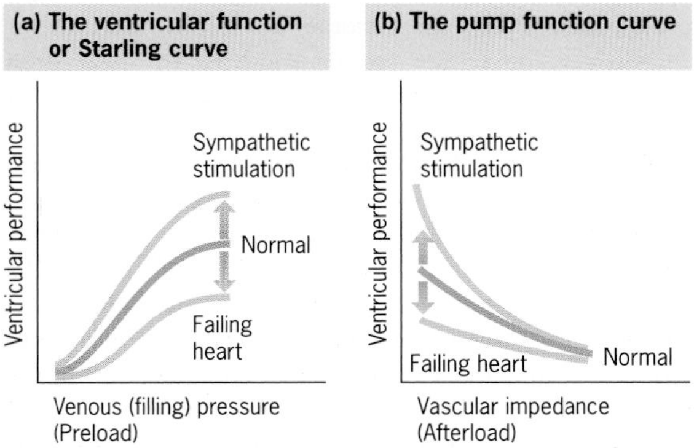

Fig 11.3
The Frank–Starling mechanism, showing the effect on ventricular contraction of alteration in filling pressures and outflow impedance in the normal, failing and sympathetically stimulated ventricle

Cholinergic nerves from the vagus supply mainly the SA and AV nodes via M2 muscarinic receptors. The ventricular myocardium is sparsely innervated by the vagus.

Under basal conditions, vagal inhibitory effects predominate over the sympathetic excitatory effects, resulting in a slow heart rate.

The coronary circulation

The coronary arterial system (Fig 11.5) consists of the right and left coronary arteries. The right coronary artery arises from the right coronary sinus and courses through the right side of the atrioventricular groove, giving off vessels that supply the right atrium and the right ventricle. The vessel usually continues as the posterior descending coronary

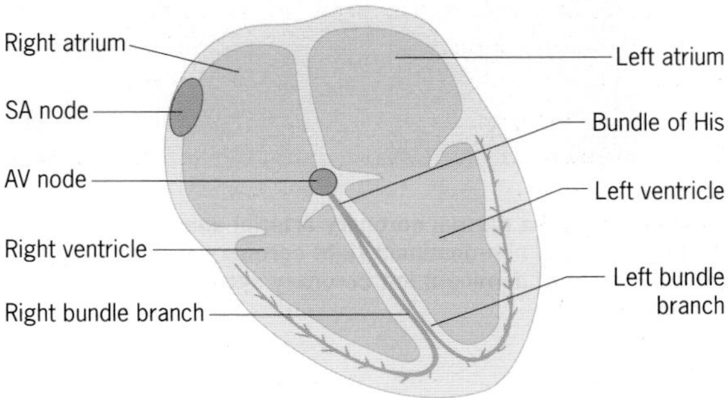

Fig 11.4
The normal cardiac conduction system
AV, atrioventricular; SA, sinoatrial

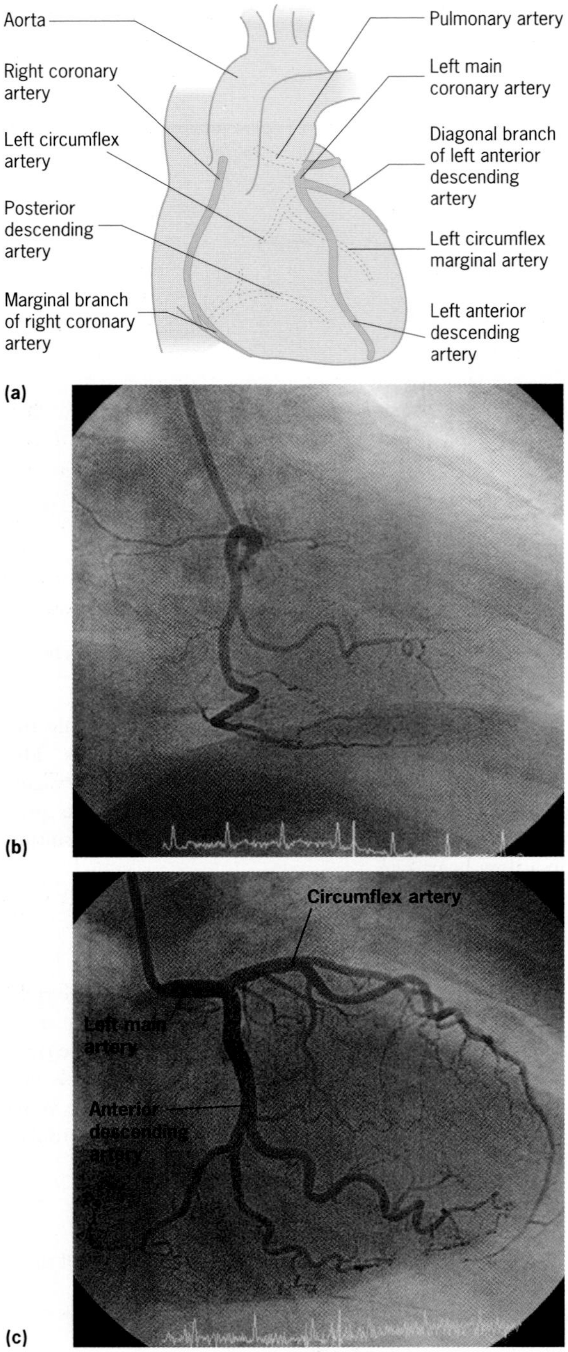

Fig 11.5
(a) Diagram of the normal coronary arterial anatomy
(b) Angiogram of non-dominant right coronary system
(c) Angiogram of dominant left coronary system from the same patient

artery, which runs in the posterior interventricular groove and supplies the posterior part of the interventricular septum and the posterior left ventricular wall.

The left coronary artery arises from the left coronary sinus. The first part is known as the left main coronary artery, and is usually not more than 2.5 cm long. It then divides into the left anterior descending and the left circumflex arteries. The left anterior descending artery runs in the anterior interventricular groove and supplies the anterior septum and the anterior left ventricular wall. The left circumflex artery travels along the left atrioventricular groove and gives off branches to the left atrium and the left ventricle (marginal branches).

The sinus node and the AV node are supplied by the right coronary artery in 60% and 90% of people, respectively. Therefore, disease in this artery may cause sinus bradycardia and AV nodal block. The majority of the left ventricle is supplied by the left coronary artery, so that stenosis in the left main artery is extremely dangerous; total obstruction of this vessel is rarely compatible with life.

Functions of the vascular endothelium

The vascular endothelium is a cardiovascular endocrine organ which occupies a strategic interface between blood and other tissues, and has many regulatory roles:

- modulation of immunoresponses
- regulation of vascular cell growth
- vasomotor control
- pro- and antithrombotic mechanisms.

Enzymes located on the endothelial surface control the level of circulating compounds, such as bradykinin, serotonin, angiotensin and adenine nucleotides. In addition, the endothelium releases substances which affect vascular tone and platelet function. Many endothelium-derived substances have been characterized and play an important role in the physiological control of the coronary circulation through the production of endothelium-derived relaxing and contracting factors. The most potent of these factors are nitric oxide (NO), prostacyclin (PGI_2) and endothelin.

Nitric oxide release can be triggered by sheer stress (flow) and by a number of transmitters, including bradykinin, histamine, noradrenaline, substance P (neurokinin), platelet-derived products, serotonin and thrombin. NO evokes relaxation of vascular smooth muscle and inhibits platelet function through activation of soluble guanylate cyclase, which leads to an increase in the intracellular levels of cyclic 3,5-guanosine monophosphate. The potent vasomotor and antiplatelet properties of NO indicate a functional role of the endothelium in the maintenance of an adequate organ blood flow.

The normal endothelium is a non-thrombogenic surface, which under physiological circumstances does not react with platelets or blood constituents. NO inhibits platelet aggregation, adhesion and secretion.

Several other factors contribute to the anti-aggregatory activity of the endothelium. Endothelial cells offer a negatively charged surface which repels the negatively charged platelets. Prostacyclin (PGI_2) is formed by the endothelial lining of blood vessels. It inhibits platelet aggregation and formation of platelet-derived growth factors.

In addition to their inhibitory effects on platelet function, prostacyclin and NO act together to antagonize procoagulant factors such as thrombin and thromboxane A2.

Endothelin is a 21-amino-acid peptide, the secretion of which is inhibited by increased shear stress. Endothelin promotes vasconstriction and hypertrophy of vascular smooth muscle, counteracting the effects of NO and PGI_2. An imbalance between these opposing forces is an early feature of hypertension and atheroma, where increased production of endothelin and reduced secretion of NO may contribute to the increased vascular tone.

Other endothelium-derived compounds are also specific antagonists of the procoagulant activity of thrombin. Endothelial cells generate specific thrombin inhibitors that remove thrombin from the circulation. Examples of these are thrombomodulin, a surface receptor, and heparin sulphate, a glycosaminoglycan, which activates antithrombin. The endothelium also modulates fibrinolysis by generation of fibrinolytic components.

The fetal circulation

In utero, the pulmonary circulation is largely unnecessary because fetal blood is oxygenated by placental blood flow, a parallel and integral element in the systemic circulation. In the fetus, systemic venous blood returning to the right atrium is partly deflected through the foramen ovale to the left atrium. Blood that passes through the right ventricle is diverted from the pulmonary artery to the aorta through the ductus arteriosus. Thus, the systemic venous return, which is a mixture of oxygenated and deoxygenated blood, is mostly returned to the systemic arterial system.

At birth, inspiration dilates the pulmonary arterioles, resulting in a dramatic reduction of pulmonary vascular resistance. Blood therefore flows through the pulmonary circulation. The increased oxygen tension and reduced levels of prostaglandins trigger closure of the ductus arteriosus, and the reduced right atrial pressure and increasing left atrial pressure tend to close the foramen ovale. Thus, the circulation is divided into two separate circuits connected in series.

In the fetus the left and right heart both propel blood from the systemic veins to the systemic arteries; thus, severe abnormalities of the heart may not compromise fetal blood flow.

The cardiac cycle (Fig 11.6)

The first event in the cardiac cycle is atrial depolarization (a P wave on the surface ECG) followed by right atrial and then left atrial contraction. Ventricular activation (the QRS complex on the ECG) follows after a short interval (the PR interval). Left ventricular contraction starts and shortly thereafter right ventricular contraction begins. The increased ventricular pressures exceed the atrial pressures, and close first the mitral and then the tricuspid valves. Until the aortic and pulmonary valves open, the ventricles contract with no change of volume (isovolumetric contraction). When ventricular pressures rise above the aortic and pulmonary artery pressures, the pulmonary valve and then the aortic valve open and ventricular ejection occurs. As the ventricles begin to relax, their pressures fall below the aortic and pulmonary arterial pressures, and aortic valve closure is followed by pulmonary valve closure. Isovolumetric relaxation then occurs. After the ventricular pressures have fallen below the right atrial and left atrial pressures, the tricuspid and mitral valves open.

The cardiac cycle can be graphically depicted as the relationship between the pressure and volume of the ventricle. This is shown in Fig 11.7, which illustrates the changing pressure–volume relationships in response to increased contractility and to exercise.

FURTHER READING

Levick JRS (1995) An Introduction to Cardiovascular Physiology, 2nd edn. London: Butterworth-Heinemann

Symptoms of heart disease

Patients even with severe heart disease may be asymptomatic. However, symptoms include the following.

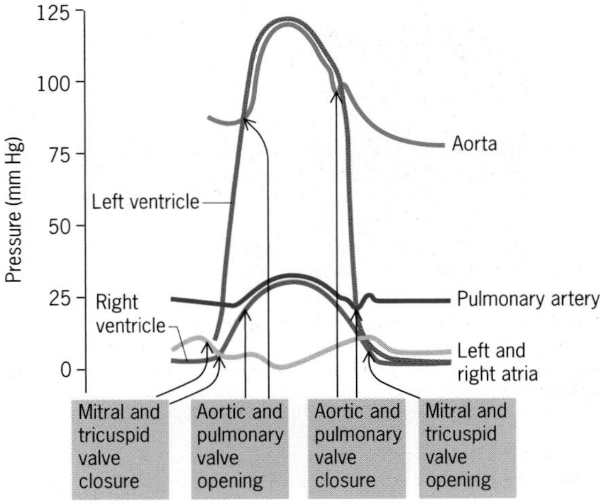

Fig 11.6
The cardiac cycle

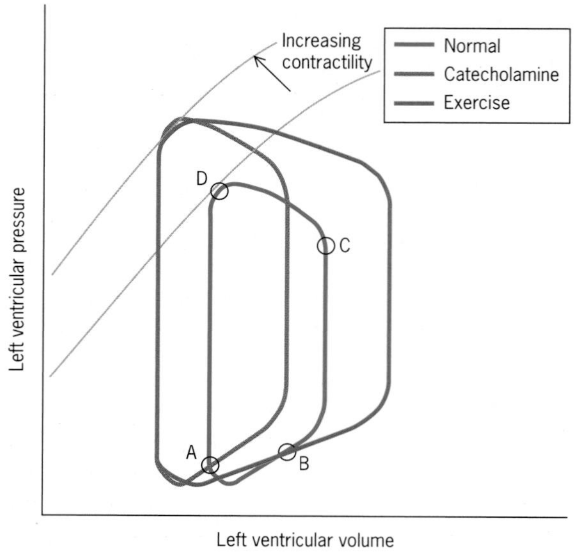

Fig 11.7
Pressure–volume loop
AB, diastole-ventricular filling;
BC, systole-isovolumetric ventricular contraction;
CD, systole-ventricular emptying;
DA, diastole-isovolumetric ventricular relaxation

Dyspnoea

Dyspnoea is an awareness of breathlessness. It can be due to cardiac or respiratory causes. It is also a symptom during exercise in healthy people.

Breathlessness may occur only on exercise or may be present at rest. The New York Heart Association has graded this symptom (Table 11.1), but this classification, although often used, has now been officially discontinued and is replaced by a very similar grading known as 'cardiac status' (Table 11.2).

It is also clinically valuable to grade dyspnoea by the amount of physical exertion possible before breathlessness occurs – for example, climbing 14 stairs or walking 200 yards on the flat.

Table 11.1 The New York Heart Association functional and therapeutic classification applied to dyspnoea

Grade 1	No breathlessness
Grade 2	Breathlessness on severe exertion
Grade 3	Breathlessness on mild exertion
Grade 4	Breathlessness at rest

Table 11.2
The New York Heart Association grading of 'cardiac status'

Grade 1	Uncompromised
Grade 2	Slightly compromised
Grade 3	Moderately compromised
Grade 4	Severely compromised

Left ventricular failure causes dyspnoea because of a rise in left atrial pressure and pulmonary capillary pressure leading to interstitial and alveolar oedema. This makes the lung stiff (less compliant), which increases the amount of respiratory effort necessary to breathe. Usually a fast breathing rate (tachypnoea) is also present due to stimulation of the pulmonary stretch receptors.

Orthopnoea

This is a form of breathlessness that occurs when the patient lies flat. Orthopnoea occurs because lying flat results in the redistribution of blood, leading to an increased central and pulmonary blood volume. Recumbency also causes the abdominal contents to press up against the diaphragm. Both factors increase the difficulty of breathing. Patients usually cope with orthopnoea by propping themselves up with pillows.

Paroxysmal nocturnal dyspnoea (PND)

This occurs when there is an accumulation of fluid in the lungs (pulmonary oedema) at night. The mechanism is similar to orthopnoea, but because sensory awareness is depressed during sleep, severe interstitial and alveolar oedema can accumulate (see p. 684). The patient is woken from sleep fighting for breath, a dramatic and frightening experience. The breathlessness may be relieved by sitting on the side of the bed or getting up. Sometimes the patient will get up and open a window to gasp for fresh air. Wheezing, due to bronchial endothelial oedema, is common (cardiac asthma), and a cough, often productive of frothy or blood-tinged sputum, usually occurs. Initially these episodes terminate spontaneously. Episodes of 'PND', often with coughing, can occur in asthma, but conventionally the term is reserved for cardiac problems.

Cheyne–Stokes respiration (see also p. 1045)

In very severe heart failure, alternate hyperventilation and apnoea known as Cheyne–Stokes respiration may occur. This may also develop in the elderly without obvious heart failure. It is related to depression of the respiratory centre, which is partly due to prolonged circulation time and cerebrovascular disease. This type of respiration is also seen after morphine administration.

Chest pain

Pain in the chest is the most common symptom associated with ischaemic heart disease.

Angina pectoris

Angina pectoris literally means a strangling sensation (angina) in the chest (pectoris). It is a gripping or crushing central chest pain (or discomfort) that may be felt around the whole chest or deep within the chest. The pain may radiate into the neck or jaw and, rarely, into the teeth, back or abdomen. It is associated with heaviness, paraesthesia or pain in one (usually the left) or both arms. It is typically provoked by exercise and is promptly relieved by rest. A pain of similar distribution and type also occurs at rest in myocardial infarction (see p. 693). The mechanism of the pain is myocardial hypoxia secondary to inadequate coronary blood flow. Sharp pains over the heart are not usually angina. Angina should be classified according to the Canadian Cardiovascular Society grading of angina of effort (Table 11.3), although most physicians find that a verbal description is adequate.

Table 11.3
The Canadian Cardiovascular Society grading of angina of effort

Grade 1	Ordinary physical activity does not cause angina (strenuous physical activity provokes angina)
Grade II	Slight limitations of ordinary physical activity (climbing more than one flight of stairs or walking uphill provokes angina)
Grade III	Marked limitation of ordinary physical activity (walking on the level or climbing one flight of stairs provokes angina)
Grade IV	inability to carry on any physical activity (angina may be present at rest)

Other causes of chest pain

The pain of pericarditis is felt in the centre of the chest and, like that of pleurisy, is aggravated by movement, posture, respiration and coughing. It is sharp and severe.

Central chest pain that radiates to the back is characteristic of a dissecting or enlarging aortic aneurysm (see p. 740) and can mimic the pain of myocardial infarction. It is important to consider and exclude a dissection since the administration of a thrombolytic agent in this circumstance would be catastrophic.

Left, submammary stabbing pain – known as 'precordial catch' – is usually associated with anxiety and is sometimes known as effort (Da Costa's) syndrome. Occasionally, cardiac conditions such as mitral valve prolapse cause similar pain. Central chest pain similar to angina can occur with oesophageal disease and can be difficult to differentiate (see p. 228).

Other causes of chest pain are pulmonary embolism, pulmonary hypertension, costochondritis, pleurisy, pneumothorax and mediastinitis.

Palpitations

A palpitation is an increased awareness of the normal heart beat or the sensation of slow or rapid heart rate or an irregular heart rhythm. The normal heart beat is sensed when the patient is anxious, excited, exercising, or lying on the left side. The most common arrhythmias to be felt as palpitations are premature ectopic beats and paroxysmal tachycardias.

Premature beats

These are usually felt as 'missed beats' because the premature beat is followed by a pause before the next normal beat, which is rather forceful because of the longer diastolic filling period. Premature beats often occur in clusters and may cause the patient much anxiety.

Paroxysmal tachycardias

These start abruptly and may terminate equally suddenly. Often, however, the tachycardia slows before terminating and therefore seems to fade away. Paroxysmal atrial fibrillation is noticeably irregular, whereas other forms of paroxysmal supraventricular or ventricular tachycardia are regular. Paroxysms of rapid tachycardia, especially when prolonged, may be associated with syncope, presyncope, dyspnoea or chest pain. Palpitations can be graded in a similar way to the grading of dyspnoea or angina. Supraventricular tachycardias, such as atrial fibrillation or junctional tachycardias, may produce polyuria.

Bradycardias

An unduly slow heart rate may be appreciated as slow, regular, 'heavy' or forceful beats. Most often bradycardias are not felt as palpitations.

Syncope

Syncope can be due to many causes (see p. 1060), the most common of which is situational or vasovagal syncope. These attacks may be provoked by fright, anxiety, phobias or other situations such as micturition or coughing. The basic mechanism is vasodilatation leading to venous pooling followed by emptying of the heart. Vigorous contraction of the near-empty heart stimulates mechanoreceptors in the inferoposterior wall of the left ventricle. Consequent reflexes via the central nervous system leads to further vasodilatation and sometimes profound bradycardia. This is known as 'neurocardiogenic' syncope. The episodes are usually associated with a prodome that consists of dizziness, nausea, sweating, ringing in the ears, a sinking feeling and yawning. Recovery occurs within a few seconds.

Cardiovascular syncope is usually sudden and brief. The classical variety is known as a Stokes–Adams attack and is due to a disturbance of cardiac rhythm (e.g. a profound bradycardia related to complete heart block). Without warning the patient falls to the ground, pale and deeply unconscious. The pulse is usually very slow or absent. After a few seconds the patient flushes brightly and recovers consciousness as the pulse quickens. If the period of unconsciousness is prolonged the patient may suffer a generalized convulsion but this is not usual. Often there are no sequelae, but patients may injure themselves during falls.

Other causes of syncope due to heart disease can be grouped as cardiac arrhythmias or valvular or vascular obstruction (Table 11.4).

Table 11.4
Cardiac causes of syncope

Arrhythmias	
Ventricular tachycardia	
Rapid supraventricular tachycardia	
Sinus arrest	
Atrioventricular block	
Artificial pacemaker failure	
Obstruction	
Aortic/pulmonary stenosis	
Hypertrophic obstructive cardiomyopathy	
Fallot's tetralogy	
Pulmonary hypertension/embolism	
Atrial myxoma	
Atrial thrombus	
Defective prosthetic valve	
Situational	
Neurocardiogenic (vasovagal)	

Fatigue

This symptom, which consists of tiredness and lethargy, is associated with heart failure, persistent cardiac arrhythmias and cyanotic heart disease. It is due to poor cerebral and peripheral perfusion and poor oxygenation. When severe cardiac disorders are not present, an active infection such as infective endocarditis may be responsible. However, disorders of most systems may produce this nonspecific symptom. Drugs prescribed for angina or hypertension, particularly β-blockers, may cause fatigue.

Oedema

Heart failure results in salt and water retention. Retained fluid accumulates in the feet and ankles of ambulant patients and over the sacrum of bed-bound patients. The oedema associated with heart failure becomes progressively worse during the day and is often absent on initial rising as the fluid is reabsorbed on lying down. When severe, the calf and thigh may become oedematous and ascites or a pleural effusion may develop.

Examination of the cardiovascular system

General examination

General features of the patient's well-being should be noted as well as the presence of anaemia, obesity, jaundice and cachexia.

Clubbing (see also p. 757)

The most common cardiac causes of severe clubbing are subacute infective endocarditis and congenital cyanotic heart disease, particularly Fallot's tetralogy. Clubbing takes many months to develop and is therefore not seen in acute endocarditis or in neonates or infants with cyanotic heart disease. Clubbing seen in cor pulmonale is due to the underlying pulmonary disease (e.g. bronchiectasis or fibrosing alveolitis).

Splinter haemorrhages

These small, subungual linear haemorrhages are most frequently due to trauma, but are also seen in infective endocarditis – when they may be florid.

Cyanosis

This is a dusky blue discoloration of the skin (particularly at the extremities) or of the mucous membranes. It is due to the presence of unoxygenated haemoglobin (traditionally at least 5 g dL^{-1} of blood) and occasionally of other reduction products of haemoglobin such as sulphaemoglobin or methaemoglobin. Cyanosis is more readily provoked in the presence of polycythaemia and is uncommon when anaemia is present.

Central cyanosis

This is present when the tongue is cyanosed. It is caused by cardiac failure or respiratory disorders. The central cyanosis of pulmonary or cardiac failure is improved by breathing oxygen if the degree of shunting is small.

Peripheral cyanosis

This is due to vasoconstriction and stasis of blood in the extremities, and increased oxygen extraction by peripheral tissues. Peripheral cyanosis occurs in congestive heart failure, shock, exposure to cold temperatures and with abnormalities of the peripheral circulation.

The arterial pulse

A pulse is felt by compressing an artery against a bone. The first pulse to be examined is the right radial pulse. The timings of the left radial and femoral pulses are then compared with that of the right radial pulse. Delayed femoral pulsation occurs because of a proximal stenosis, particularly of the aorta (coarctation).

Pulse rate

The pulse rate should be between 60 and 80 beats per minute (b.p.m.) when an adult patient is lying quietly in bed. Young children may have higher pulse rates and athletes and elderly adults may have slower rates. The exact rate is unimportant but changes (seen on a pulse chart) are helpful. When the pulse is irregular, not all beats may be transmitted to the wrist and it is therefore best to count the pulse whilst at the same time listening to the heart beat with a stethoscope. An apex-radial (pulse) deficit is common in atrial fibrillation.

Rhythm

In normal subjects the pulse is regular except for a slight quickening in early inspiration and a slowing in expiration (sinus arrhythmia). Irregularities of the pulse rhythm are usually due to premature beats, intermittent heart block or atrial fibrillation.

Premature beats occur as occasional or repeated irregularities superimposed on a regular pulse rhythm. Similarly, intermittent heart block is revealed by occasional beats dropped from an otherwise regular rhythm. A more irregular pattern (irregularly irregular) of heart beats occurs in atrial fibrillation. This irregular pattern persists when the pulse quickens in response to exercise, in contrast to pulse irregularity due to ectopic beats, which usually disappears on exercise. However, this is not a reliable way to distinguish ectopic beats from other causes of pulse irregularity.

Carotid pulse

The amplitude and shape of the carotid pulse is examined. Usually carotid pulsation is not visible, but a very large-volume pulse may be apparent as pulsation of the neck (Corrigan's sign). A large-volume pulse occurs in high output states and in aortic regurgitation. The carotid pulse is also visible when the carotid artery is aneurysmal or kinked. The right carotid is palpated lightly in order to detect a thrill.

A large-volume pulse with a brisk rise and fall is known as a 'collapsing' or 'waterhammer' pulse (Fig 11.8). It is found in the elderly when the aorta is rigid, or when the cardiac output is high, such as in thyrotoxicosis, anaemia or fever. Aortic valvular regurgitation or a persistent ductus arteriosus also cause a collapsing pulse. A large-volume pulse that is not collapsing in nature is associated with the large stroke volume that is necessary if bradycardia is present.

A small-volume pulse is seen in cardiac failure, shock and obstructive vascular or valvular disease. It is also present when tachycardia occurs. The pulse of aortic stenosis is not only small in volume but is slow in rising to a peak (plateau pulse) and is often associated with a notch on the upstroke (anacrotic pulse) or a systolic shudder or thrill (Fig 11.8).

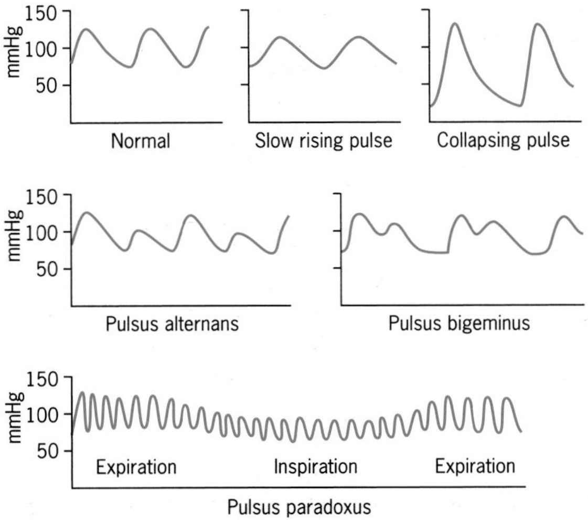

Fig 11.8
Various arterial waveforms

Other changes in arterial pulse

Paradoxical pulse (pulsus paradoxus)

Paradoxical pulse is a misnomer as it is actually an exaggeration of the normal pattern (Fig 11.8). In normal subjects, the systolic pressure and the pulse pressure (the difference between the systolic and diastolic blood pressures) fall during inspiration. The normal fall of systolic pressure is less than 10 mmHg and this can be measured using a sphygmomanometer. The reason for this fall in pressure is that the right heart responds directly to changes in intrathoracic pressure while the filling of the left depends on the pulmonary intravascular volume. Thus as the return of blood to the left ventricle falls there is a drop in systolic pressure. At high respiratory rates this is exaggerated with the volumes of the right and left ventricles being unequal. In severe airflow limitation (especially severe asthma) there is an increased and sudden negative intrathoracic pressure on inspiration and this will enhance the normal fall in blood pressure. In patients with cardiac tamponade the fluid in the pericardium increases the intrapericardial pressure, thereby reducing the heart's filling capacity. The inspiratory increase in the right ventricle occurs very much at the expense of the left ventricle as both ventricles are confined within a relatively 'fixed' pericardium. Through a similar mechanism, paradox can occur in constrictive pericarditis but is less common.

Alternating pulse (pulsus alternans)

This is characterized by alternate beats that are weak and strong but with a regular rhythm. It is a feature of severe myocardial failure and is due to the prolonged recovery time of damaged myocardium; it indicates a very poor prognosis. It is easily noticed when taking the blood pressure because the systolic blood pressure may vary from beat to beat by as much as 50 mmHg. Pulsus alternans may also occur when there is rapid, abnormal tachycardia. In this case it acts as a compensatory mechanism and does not indicate a poor prognosis. Pulsus alternans should be distinguished from a bigeminal pulse (see below).

Bigeminal pulse (pulsus bigeminus)

This is due to premature ectopic beats following every sinus beat. The rhythm is not regular (Fig 11.8) because every weak pulse is premature.

Pulsus bisferiens

This is a pulse that is found in hypertrophic obstructive cardiomyopathy and in aortic regurgitation combined with aortic stenosis. The first systolic wave is the 'percussion' wave produced by the transmission of the left ventricular pressure in early systole. The second peak is the 'tidal' wave caused by recoil of the vascular bed. This normally happens in diastole (the dicrotic wave), but when the left ventricle empties slowly or is obstructed from emptying completely, the tidal wave occurs in late systole. The result is a palpable double pulse.

Blood pressure (Practical box 11.1)

The peak systemic arterial blood pressure is produced by transmission of left ventricular systolic pressure. The diastolic blood pressure is maintained by vascular tone and an intact aortic valve.

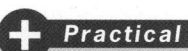

Practical

1 The blood pressure is taken in the (right) arm with the patient relaxed and comfortable.
2 The sphygmomanometer cuff is wrapped around the upper arm with the inflation bag placed over the brachial artery.
3 The cuff is inflated until the pressure exceeds the arterial pressure – when the radial pulse is no longer palpable.
4 The diaphragm of the stethoscope is positioned over the brachial artery just below the cuff.
5 The cuff pressure is slowly reduced until sounds (Korotkoff sounds) can be heard (phase 1). This is the **systolic pressure**.
6 The pressure is allowed to fall further until the Karotkoff sounds become suddenly muffled (phase 4).
7 The pressure is allowed to fall still further until they disappear (phase 5).

The **diastolic pressure** is usually taken as phase 5 because this phase is more reproducible and nearer to the intravascular diastolic pressure. The Korotkoff sounds may disappear (phase 2) and reappear (phase 3) between the systolic and diastolic pressures. It is important not to mistake phase 2 for the diastolic pressure or phase 3 for the systolic pressure.

Practical box 11.1 Taking the blood pressure

The normal blood pressure

There is no single blood pressure or limited range of blood pressures that is normal in all subjects and circumstances. However:

- *In a resting adult* the systolic blood pressure does not usually exceed 150 mmHg and the diastolic pressure does not exceed 90 mmHg.
- *In children or young adults* the pressures are correspondingly less.
- *In the elderly* the rigidity of the arterial vessels produces an increase, predominantly in the systolic blood pressure.

There is a *diurnal variation* of blood pressure, the pressure during the day being greater than at night. *Anxiety* (for example when consulting a physician – 'white coat' hypertension, see p. 732) and exertion increase the blood pressure.

Note that a cuff that is too small leads to overestimation of the pressure. For example, if a standard arm cuff size (12 cm) is used in an obese patient, the pressure measured will be too high. Similarly, if an arm cuff is used on the thigh (with the diaphragm of the stethoscope applied over the popliteal artery), the femoral pressure will be overestimated. The usual thigh cuff is 15 cm wide. Smaller cuff sizes are available for children and thin adults.

Variations in blood pressure

The systolic blood pressure varies by up to 10 mmHg between the right and left brachial arteries. Standing usually causes a slight reduction of the systolic pressure (<20 mmHg) and an increase in the diastolic blood pressure (<10 mmHg). In postural (orthostatic) hypotension, a large postural fall of both the systolic and diastolic pressures is associated with dizziness. When an irregular heart rhythm such as atrial fibrillation is present, the blood pressure is variable. Because the blood pressure is normally liable to variation, it must be estimated on several occasions before it can be declared elevated.

Jugular venous pulse (JVP)

(Practical box 11.2)

There are no valves between the internal jugular vein and the right atrium and observation of the column of blood in the internal jugular system is therefore a good measure of right atrial pressure. The external jugular cannot be relied upon because of its valves and because it may be obstructed by the fascial and muscular layers through which it passes; it can only be used if typical venous pulsation is seen, indicating no obstruction to flow.

An abnormally low jugular venous pressure cannot be measured clinically. Causes include haemorrhage and other forms of hypovolaemia.

Elevation of the jugular venous pressure occurs in heart failure. It is also produced by:

- constrictive pericarditis
- cardiac tamponade
- renal disease with salt and water retention
- overtransfusion or excessive infusion of fluids
- superior vena caval obstruction (but in this case pulsation is absent).

In constrictive pericarditis or cardiac tamponade, ventricular filling is reduced during inspiration because the ventricles are squeezed by the pericardial fluid or non-compliant pericardium, which tightens as the diaphragm descends. Thus, the level of venous pressure increases during inspiration (Kussmaul's sign). Other causes of an increased jugular pressure also distort the shape of the pressure wave and are considered below.

The jugular venous pressure wave

This consists of three peaks and two troughs (Fig 11.9). The peaks are described as *a*, *c* and *v* waves and the troughs are known as *x* and *y* descents:

- The ***a* wave** is produced by atrial systole.
- The ***x* descent** occurs when the atrial contraction finishes.
- As the pressure falls there is a small transient increase that produces a positive deflection called the ***c* wave**. This is caused by transmission of the rapidly increasing right ventricular pressure before the tricuspid valve closes.
- The ***v* wave** develops as the venous return fills the right atrium during continued ventricular systole.
- The ***y* descent** follows the *v* wave when the tricuspid valve opens.

The *a* wave can be distinguished from the *v* wave by observing the venous pulse while palpating the carotid artery. The *a* wave occurs immediately before carotid pulsation and the *v* wave occurs simultaneously with carotid pulsation.

The main abnormalities of the shape of the jugular venous pressure wave are elevations of the *a* and *v* waves and steepness of the *y* descent (Fig 11.9).

Large *a* waves

These are caused by increased resistance to ventricular filling, as seen with right ventricular hypertrophy due to pulmonary hypertension or pulmonary stenosis. They may also be caused by tricuspid stenosis, but this is unusual because patients with tricuspid stenosis are usually in atrial fibrillation and therefore do not have *a* waves.

A very large *a* wave occurs when the atrium contracts against a closed tricuspid valve. This is known as a 'cannon wave'. Cannon waves occur irregularly in complete heart block and in ventricular tachycardia. In both these situations there is atrioventricular dissociation, and by random chance there is occasional simultaneous atrial and

Practical

1. The patient is positioned at about 45° to the horizontal (between 30° and 60°, wherever the top of the venous pulsation can be seen in a good light).
2. The head is supported by a pillow and the neck is slightly flexed to allow the skin and muscle overlying the vein to relax.
3. The jugular venous pressure is measured as the vertical distance between the manubriosternal angle and the top of the venous column.
4. The normal jugular venous pressure is usually less than 3 cmH_2O, which is equivalent to a right atrial pressure of 8 cmH_2O when measured with reference to a point midway between the anterior and posterior surfaces of the chest. The venous pulsations are not usually palpable (except for the forceful venous distension associated with tricuspid regurgitation).

Notes

- Pulsations should be looked for before touching the neck.
- Gentle pressure at the root of the neck may abolish visible venous pulsation and may make a vein visible by causing distension above the occlusion.
- *Hepatojugular reflex*. Abdominal compression causes a temporary increase in central and hence jugular venous pressure. It is a simple way of confirming the venous nature of a pulsation in the neck.

Practical box 11.2 Measurement of the jugular pressure

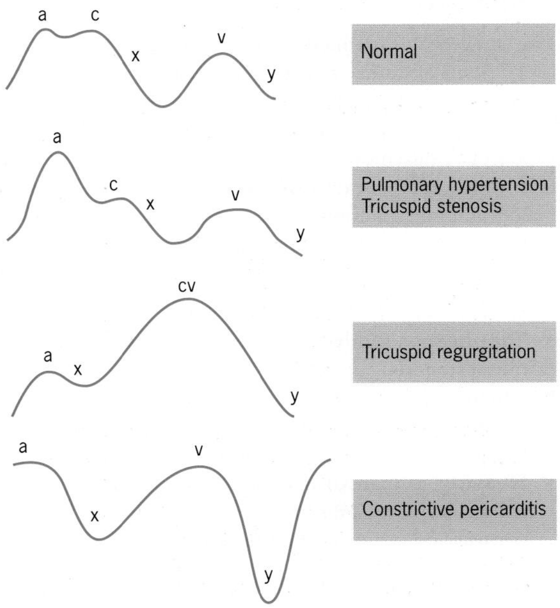

Fig 11.9
Various jugular venous waveforms

ventricular contraction. In junctional rhythms the atria and ventricles usually contract simultaneously and rapid, regular cannon waves are produced.

Large *v* waves

Tricuspid regurgitation results in giant *v* waves (systolic waves) because the right ventricular pressure is transmitted directly to the right atrium and the great veins.

Steep *y* descent

Diastolic collapse of elevated venous pressure can occur in right ventricular failure but is more dramatic in constrictive pericarditis and tricuspid regurgitation. At the end of ventricular systole the elevated atrial pressure suddenly falls when the tricuspid valve opens. However, the ventricles are stiff and cannot be distended. The venous pressure therefore rapidly rises again. This rapid fall and rise of the jugular venous pulse is known as Friedreich's sign.

Examination of the precordium

Inspection

Deformities should be looked for as they can mimic cardiac abnormalities. For example, pectus excavatum (funnel chest) or kyphoscoliosis may cause an ejection systolic murmur. The position of the apex beat and other cardiac pulsations should be noted; a left ventricular aneurysm may produce an eccentric and abnormal pulsation.

Palpation

The apex beat is defined as the most inferior and most lateral point of cardiac pulsation. It is usually felt just inside the mid-clavicular line at the level of the fourth or fifth left intercostal space. Cardiac enlargement, particularly left ventricular dilatation, displaces the apex beat to the left. The apex beat may also be displaced by a pneumothorax, pulmonary collapse or skeletal abnormalities such as scoliosis. The apex beat is normally just palpable and confined to a point that can be covered by one finger. There are several abnormal forms:

- **Tapping** is a sudden but brief cardiac impulse felt in mitral stenosis.
- **Thrusting** (hyperdynamic) is vigorous but non-sustained pulsation typical of 'volume overload' due to mitral or aortic regurgitation.
- **Heaving** (sustained) is a vigorous and sustained pulsation due to 'pressure overload' as in aortic stenosis and systemic hypertension.

There is often confusion about the terms *thrusting* and *heaving*.

- **Impalpable** This occurs in emphysema, pleural effusion, obesity and pericardial effusion.
- **Double** pulsation – two apical pulsations with each heart beat – may be felt in hypertrophic cardiomyopathy. This may be due to a palpable atrial impulse. A double apex can also be due to accentuated outward movement in late systole in a ventricular aneurysm.

A *parasternal sustained impulse* (heave) is elicited by pressing the outstretched hand flat against the sternum or against the costal cartilages just to the left of the sternum. It occurs because of right ventricular hypertrophy. An enlarged left atrium may also cause a parasternal heave. Left atrial pulsation can be distinguished from pulsation due to right ventricular hypertrophy because it occurs before the apex beat or carotid pulsation. Vigorous pulmonary artery pulsation may be appreciated by palpation in the second left interspace. This is usually due to pulmonary hypertension.

Thrills are palpable murmurs that are most easily appreciated with the flat or ulnar border of the hand rather than with the fingers. A thrill implies a definite abnormality. Systolic thrills in the aortic area are usually due to aortic stenosis, whereas at the apex a systolic thrill is due to mitral regurgitation. A diastolic thrill is usually caused by mitral stenosis; a diastolic thrill due to aortic regurgitation is uncommon.

Heart sounds that are very loud may also be palpated. In systemic hypertension the aortic second sound may be felt, and in pulmonary hypertension the pulmonary component of the second sound may be felt. Occasionally a third or fourth heart sound may be palpated.

Percussion

Percussion is not usually undertaken, but it may allow the approximate position and size of the heart to be determined.

Auscultation

The sounds best heard with the bell or the diaphragm of the stethoscope are shown in Table 11.5.

There are four traditional areas where the heart sounds and valvular murmurs are best heard:

- The **mitral area or apex** is the point at which the apex beat is felt. The first heart sound and mitral murmurs are loudest here, and aortic regurgitation and third and fourth left ventricular sounds are often heard best at this point.
- The **tricuspid area** is in the fourth interspace to the left of the sternum (left sternal edge). Not only is this close to the tricuspid valve but is also over the ventricles. Therefore, as well as the murmurs and sounds from the tricuspid valve, the murmurs of pulmonary and aortic regurgitation and third and fourth right ventricular sounds are also heard well here.

Table 11.5
Use of the stethoscope

Bell (for low-frequency sounds)	Diaphragm (for high-frequency sounds)
Mid-diastolic rumbles of mitral stenosis and tricuspid stenosis	Early diastolic murmurs of aortic and pulmonary regurgitation
Third and fourth heart sounds	Second heart sound Systolic clicks and opening snaps

- The **pulmonary area** is in the second interspace just to the left of the sternum. This is the closest point to the pulmonary valve, where the murmur of pulmonary stenosis and the pulmonary component of the second heart sound are loudest.
- The **aortic area** is in the second intercostal space immediately to the right of the sternum. The aorta arches upwards and forwards from the aortic valve and the murmur of aortic stenosis is transmitted best to this area.

The sequence of cardiac auscultation is summarized in Table 11.6.

Table 11.6
Summary of the auscultation procedure

The mitral, tricuspid, pulmonary and aortic areas should be auscultated in turn	**Sitting forward** Aortic diastolic murmur – tricuspid and mitral areas
Supine First heart sound – mitral area Second heart sound – pulmonary and aortic areas, during inspiration and expiration Third and fourth heart sounds – mitral and tricuspid areas Clicks, snaps – mitral and tricuspid areas Systolic murmurs – all four auscultation areas, also the neck, axilla and back	**Lying on the left side** Mitral diastolic murmur – mitral area (exactly over the apex beat) **During inspiration and expiration** – see Table 11.8 **Exercise, Valsalva manoeuvres** Can be used to accentuate murmurs

Heart sounds

The first heart sound

This is caused by the closure of the mitral and tricuspid valves and is best heard at the cardiac apex. The sound is usually single but may be slightly split. If split, this 'double' sound at the beginning of systole must be distinguished from the combination of the first heart sound with a fourth heart sound or with an ejection click.

The first heart sound is loud when the patient is thin and when the circulation is hyperdynamic (e.g. due to anaemia or thyrotoxicosis). The sound is also loud if the valve is still open when ventricular systole begins (e.g. in mitral stenosis).

A soft first heart sound occurs in patients with obesity, emphysema or pericardial effusion. It is also present when the valve leaflets are immobile (e.g. in severe calcific mitral stenosis), or when the leaflets are partly closed when systole begins, which occurs when the PR interval is long. A soft first heart sound also occurs when the valve does not close properly, as in mitral regurgitation. Heart failure and cardiogenic shock are also associated with a soft first heart sound.

The intensity of the first heart sound is variable when the relationship between atrial and ventricular systole is not constant (e.g. during ventricular tachycardia or complete heart block). When the PR interval is short the sound is loud, and when the PR interval is long the sound is soft.

The second heart sound

This is caused by the closure of the aortic and pulmonary valves. Unless excessively loud, the pulmonary component of the second sound is heard only in the pulmonary area. Left heart emptying is usually finished just before right heart emptying; therefore the pulmonary component of the second sound closely follows the aortic component. Inspiration results in increased venous return to the right heart, which further delays right heart emptying. The pulmonary sound is therefore delayed further on inspiration and the second heart sound becomes audibly split (Fig 11.10). Splitting of the second heart sound on inspiration is known as *normal* or *physiological* splitting and is most commonly heard in children or young adults.

Reversed splitting of the second heart sound (when the aortic component follows the pulmonary component) occurs on expiration. It is due to a fixed delay in left heart emptying caused by aortic stenosis, left bundle branch block or left ventricular failure. Thus, when right heart emptying is delayed during inspiration, the two sounds move together, and when the right heart empties more quickly during expiration, the sounds move apart.

The fixed delay in the emptying of the right ventricle – produced, for example, by right bundle branch block or pulmonary stenosis – will result in wide splitting of the second heart sound. With an atrial septal defect there is usually some degree of right bundle branch block, and because of shunting of blood from the left to the right atrium the right-sided cardiac output is high and ventricular emptying is further delayed. The second heart sound is therefore widely split. Because communication at atrial level prevents differential changes of the venous return during inspiration and expiration, the wide splitting of the second heart sound is not varied by respiration. This is called *fixed splitting*.

The aortic second sound is louder in systemic hypertension and when a hyperdynamic circulation is present. It is soft in aortic stenosis because the valve is relatively immobile, and it is soft in cardiac failure because of low

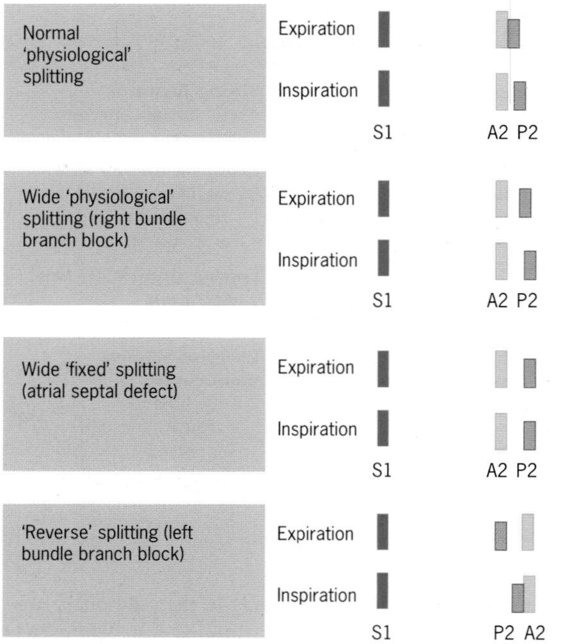

Fig 11.10
Variations of the second heart sound.
A2, aortic component; P2, pulmonary component

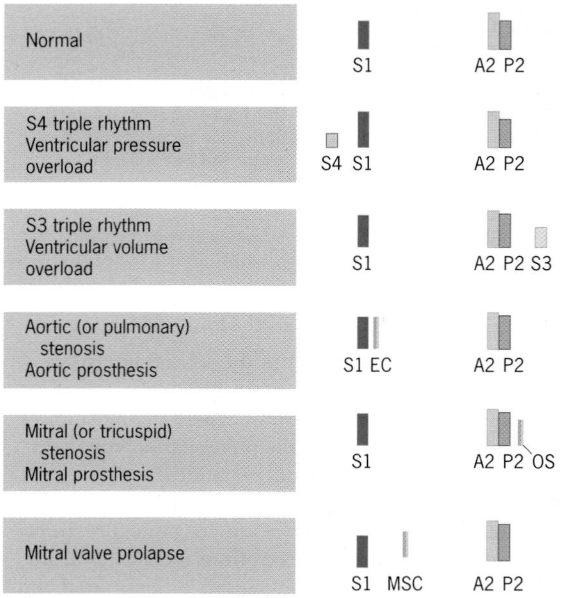

Fig 11.11
Normal and additional heart sounds and the conditions in which they are found
A2, aortic component of the second sound;
EC, ejection click;
MSC, mid-systolic click;
OS, opening snap;
P2, pulmonary component of the second sound;
S1, first heart sound; S3, third heart sound; S4, fourth heart sound

blood flow. Similarly, the pulmonary component of the second heart sound is loud in pulmonary hypertension and soft in pulmonary stenosis.

Additional heart sounds (Fig 11.11)

Third and fourth heart sounds are diastolic in timing, representing ventricular filling, and are heard as soft 'thudding' noises immediately before the first sound (fourth sound) or after the second sound (third sound). The presence of a third or fourth sound produces a triple rhythm that, when associated with sinus tachycardia, sounds like a galloping horse – a *gallop rhythm*. The cadence of a gallop rhythm due to a third heart sound has been likened to 'Kentucky', whilst that due to a fourth heart sound resembles 'Tennessee'. When both third and fourth heart sounds occur there is usually a marked sinus tachycardia, which results in a short diastolic period so that third and fourth sounds occur simultaneously. This is known as a *summation gallop*.

The third sound

This is due to rapid ventricular filling as soon as the mitral and tricuspid valves open. It is a normal finding in children and young adults when it is heard at the apex, especially in the left lateral position. In those over 40 years it represents heart failure or volume overload, for example due to mitral regurgitation. It is therefore sometimes referred to as a sound of 'distress'. A right ventricular third sound is heard best at the left sternal edge, and a left ventricular third sound is heard at the apex.

The fourth sound

This is caused by the surge of ventricular filling that accompanies atrial systole. It therefore occurs in late diastole. It may be a normal finding in an elderly subject, but in younger patients it usually indicates increased ventricular stiffness associated with hypertension, aortic stenosis or acute myocardial infarction. It is called the sound of cardiac 'stress', and can sometimes be felt.

Abnormal heart valves

These may cause an audible signal when opening. An *ejection click* sound occurs immediately following the first heart sound. It is produced by the sudden opening of a deformed but mobile aortic or pulmonary valve. It is most commonly heard in association with a bicuspid aortic valve when it is easily heard throughout the respiratory cycle. A stenotic pulmonary valve also produces an ejection click, but this is best heard on expiration. A dilated aorta or pulmonary artery may also give rise to an ejection click.

A stenotic mitral or tricuspid valve

This may produce a high-frequency opening *snap* that occurs just after the second heart sound. It can be distinguished from a split second sound or a third sound by the site at which it is best heard, its higher frequency and its lack of respiratory variation.

A mid-systolic click (or clicks)
This is due to sudden prolapse of the mitral valve into the left atrium during ventricular systole. It occurs when the mitral valve is congenitally deformed or has undergone myxomatous degeneration, as in the mitral valve prolapse syndrome. These auscultatory features are inconsistent and wax and wane with time.

Prosthetic sounds

Mechanical replacement heart valves produce loud clicks owing to the opening and closing of the valve. These prosthetic sounds may be muffled or absent if valve movement is impeded by thrombus or vegetations.

Heart murmurs

Turbulent blood flow causes heart murmurs. Turbulence may be produced when there is high blood flow through a normal valve, or when there is normal blood flow through an abnormal valve or into a dilated chamber. Turbulence is also caused by the regurgitation of blood through a leaking valve. Murmurs produced by high-velocity blood flow (e.g. the systolic murmur of mitral regurgitation) are high frequency and are often described as 'blowing' in quality. The intensity of murmurs is determined not only by the blood velocity but also by the volume of blood producing the murmur and the distance of the source of the murmur from the stethoscope. Right-sided murmurs tend to become louder on inspiration because inspiration increases the venous return to the right heart.

Heart murmurs may occur with a normal or near-normal heart (innocent murmurs). They are usually soft and short, and occur early in systole. Murmurs also occur in the following situations:

- *Anaemia, thyrotoxicosis, pregnancy and other causes of a high cardiac output* produce flow murmurs, which are usually brief systolic ejection murmurs heard best at the left sternal edge or in the pulmonary area. These murmurs are believed to emanate from the pulmonary or aortic valve. Similar murmurs are heard in association with skeletal abnormalities such as kyphoscoliosis or funnel chest.
- *A very small ventricular septal defect* may produce a short early systolic murmur, heard well at the left sternal edge. The murmur is short because contraction of the ventricle closes the small defect early in systole.

Murmurs are classified as *systolic, diastolic* or *continuous* (another functional classification divides systolic murmurs into *ejection* or *regurgitant*). Murmurs should be assessed carefully; a summary of the auscultation procedure is shown in Table 11.6. The intensity of cardiac murmurs can be graded as indicated in Table 11.7, and Table 11.8 lists some common structural causes.

Table 11.7
The grading of murmur intensity

Grade	Systolic murmurs	Diastolic murmurs
1	Very soft (heard only in good circumstances)	Very soft (heard only in good circumstances)
2	Soft	Soft
3	Moderate	Moderate
4	Loud	Loud or associated with palpable thrill
5	Very loud	–
6	Very loud (no stethoscope needed) or associated with palpable thrill	–

Table 11.8
Some common structural causes of murmurs

Murmur	Position where murmur is best heard
Systolic	
Ejection (mid-)systolic	
Aortic stenosis	Aortic area, clavicles and carotids
Pulmonary stenosis / Atrial septal defect	Left sternal edge on inspiration
Left (e.g. hypertrophic cardiomyopathy, HOCM) and right (e.g. Fallot's tetralogy) outflow tract obstruction may also cause mid-systolic murmurs	
Pansystolic	
Mitral regurgitation (blowing)	Apex to axilla
Tricuspid regurgitation (low-pitched)	Left sternal edge
Ventricular septal defect (loud and rough)	Left sternal edge
Late systolic	
Dynamic outflow tract obstruction (HOCM)	Accentuated on standing
Mitral valve prolapse	Apex
Coarctation of the aorta	Left sternal edge
Diastolic	
Mid-diastolic	
Mitral stenosis (low-frequency rumbling)	Apex, patient on left side, accentuated on exertion
Tricuspid stenosis	Left sternal edge, accentuated on inspiration
Austin Flint murmur	Apex
Early diastolic	
Aortic regurgitation (blowing, high-pitched)	Left sternal edge and apex, patient sitting forward and in expiration
Pulmonary regurgitation (blowing, variable pitch)	Right of sternum, louder on inspiration
Graham–Steell in pulmonary hypertension (due to mitral stenosis)	Left sternal edge
Combined systolic and diastolic	
Patent ductus arteriosus	Left sternal edge
Aortic stenosis and regurgitation	

Systolic murmurs

Systolic murmurs occur synchronously with carotid pulsation. There are three main varieties of pathological systolic murmur:

- *Ejection mid-systolic murmurs* are heard separately from the first and second heart sounds. Their intensity rises then falls, being greatest in mid-systole.
- *Pansystolic murmurs* extend from the first to the second heart sound and tend to be of constant intensity throughout the whole of systole.
- *Late systolic murmurs* are separated from the first sound but extend up to the second sound.

Diastolic murmurs

Diastolic murmurs are always associated with cardiac disease. They are of two types:

- *Mid-diastolic murmurs* usually arise from the mitral and tricuspid valves. In aortic regurgitation the flow of blood back into the left ventricle may partially close and obstruct the mitral valve, producing a mitral mid-diastolic murmur (Austin Flint murmur).
- *Early diastolic murmurs* usually result from aortic regurgitation and rarely from pulmonary regurgitation. These murmurs begin with the second heart sound and are blowing (high-pitched) in quality. Pulmonary hypertension secondary to mitral stenosis may lead to pulmonary valve regurgitation (Graham–Steell murmur).

Continuous murmurs

A continuous murmur may occur because of a combination of systolic and diastolic murmurs, owing to connections between the aorta and pulmonary artery (e.g. in patent ductus arteriosus) or owing to arteriovenous anastomoses and collateral circulations (such as those associated with coarctation of the aorta). High venous flow, especially in young children, can produce a continuous venous hum in the neck. This is reduced by occluding the vein or by lying the child flat. Similarly, high mammary blood flow in pregnant or lactating women can produce a continuous murmur known as a 'mammary souffle'.

Extra cardiac sounds

Bruits, usually due to arterial stenoses, are murmurs arising from a peripheral artery, including the distal aorta.

A *pericardial friction rub* is a scratching or crunching noise produced by the movement of inflamed pericardium. Since it is relatively high frequency, it is best heard with the diaphragm. It is most obvious in systole but may also be heard in early diastole or synchronously with atrial contraction. It should be listened for during both held inspiration and expiration.

FURTHER READING

Perloff JK (1990) Physical Examination of the Heart and Circulation, 2nd edn. Philadelphia, WB Saunders.

Cardiac investigations

Chest X-ray

This is taken in the postero-anterior (PA) direction at maximum inspiration with the heart close to the X-ray film to minimize magnification with respect to the thorax. A lateral may give additional information if the PA is abnormal. The cardiac structures and great vessels that can be seen on these X-rays are indicated in Fig 11.12.

Heart size

Heart size can be reliably assessed only from the PA chest film; the maximum transverse diameter of the heart is compared with the maximum transverse diameter of the chest measured from the inside of the ribs.

The cardiothoracic ratio (CTR) is usually less than 50%, except in neonates, infants, athletes and patients with skeletal abnormalities such as scoliosis and funnel chest. A transverse cardiac diameter of more than 15.5 cm is abnormal. Pericardial effusion or cardiac dilatation causes an increase in the ratio.

A pericardial effusion produces a globular, sharp-edged shadow. This enlargement may occur quite suddenly and, unlike heart failure, there is no associated change in the pulmonary vasculature. The echocardiogram is more specific than the chest X-ray for the diagnosis of pericardial effusion, particularly because at least 250 mL of fluid must accumulate before X-ray changes are apparent.

Certain patterns of specific chamber enlargement may be seen on the chest X-ray:

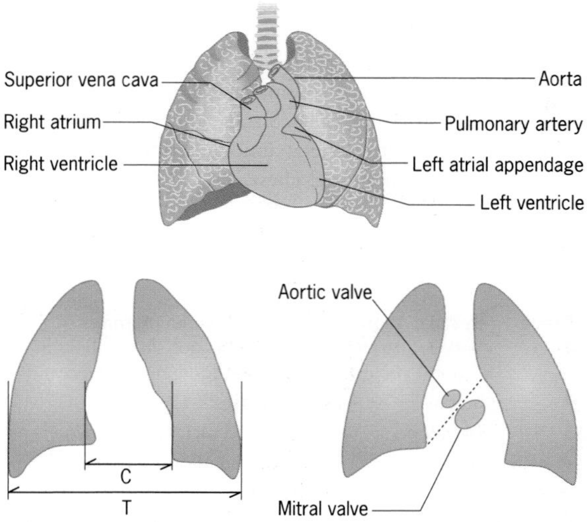

Fig 11.12
Diagrams to show the heart silhouette on the chest X-ray, measurements of the cardiothoracic ratio (CTR) and the location of the cardiac valves
CTR = (C/T) 100%; normal CTR <50%

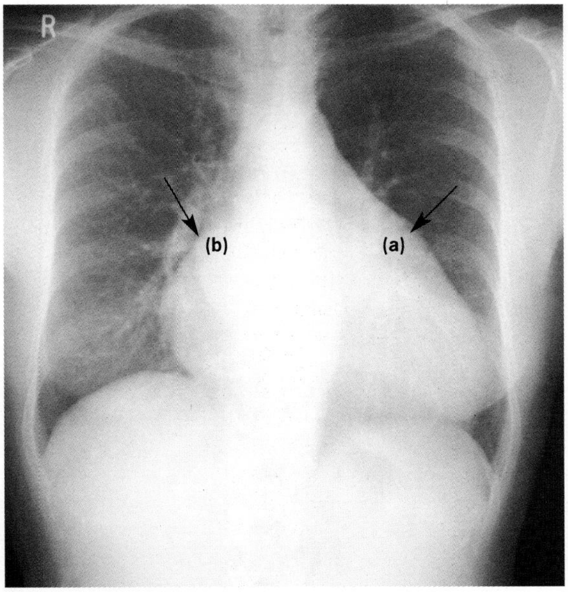

Fig 11.13
Plain PA chest X-ray taken from a patient with mixed mitral valve disease. The left atrium is markedly enlarged **(a)**. Note the large bulge on the left heart border (left atrium) and the 'double shadow' (border of the right and left atria) **(b)** on the right side of the heart. There is cardiac (left ventricular) enlargement due to mitral regurgitation

Left atrial dilatation. This results in prominence of the left atrial appendage on the left heart border, a double atrial shadow to the right of the sternum, and splaying of the carina because a large left atrium elevates the left main bronchus (Fig 11.13). On a lateral chest X-ray an enlarged left atrium bulges backwards, impinging on the oesophagus.

Left ventricular enlargement. This results in an increase in the CTR and a smooth elongation and increased convexity of the left heart border. A left ventricular aneurysm may produce a distinct bulge or distortion of the left heart border.

Right atrial enlargement. This results in the right border of the heart projecting into the right lower lung field.

Right ventricular enlargement. This is due to congenital heart disease. It results in an increase of the CTR and an upward displacement of the apex of the heart because the enlarging right ventricle pushes the left ventricle leftwards, upwards and eventually backwards. Differentiation of left from right ventricular enlargement may be difficult from the shape of the left heart border alone, but the lateral view shows enlargement anteriorly for the right ventricle and posteriorly for the left ventricle.

Ascending aortic dilatation or enlargement. This is seen as a prominence of the aortic shadow to the right of the mediastinum between the right atrium and superior vena cava.

Dissection of the ascending aorta. This is seen as a widening of the mediastinum, although it is often difficult to assess on an AP chest X-ray. A left-sided pleural effusion may be evident if the aneurysm is leaking or there may be blood around the apex of the lung ('capping').

Enlargement of the pulmonary artery. Enlargement of the pulmonary artery in pulmonary hypertension, pulmonary artery stenosis and left-to-right shunts produces a prominent bulge on the left-hand border of the mediastinum below the aortic knuckle.

Calcification

Calcification in the cardiovascular system occurs because of tissue degeneration. Calcification is visible on a lateral or a penetrated PA film, but is best studied by fluoroscopy or CT scanning. Various types of calcification can occur.

Pericardial calcification. This may be seen as plaque-like opacities over the surface of the heart, but particularly concentrated in the atrioventricular groove. Such calcification often results from tuberculous pericarditis and may be associated with pericardial constriction.

Valvular calcification. This may result from longstanding rheumatic or bicuspid aortic valve disease. The aortic and mitral valves are most commonly affected. On the lateral film, a calcified aortic valve is seen on or above a line joining the carina to the sternophrenic angle. Mitral valvular calcification is seen below and behind this line (see Fig 11.12).

Myocardial calcification. This may occur after myocardial infarction, especially in association with a left ventricular aneurysm (Fig 11.14).

Calcification of the aorta. Calcification of the aorta is a common, normal finding in patients over the age of 40 years and appears as a curvilinear opacity around the circumference of the aortic knuckle. Calcification in the

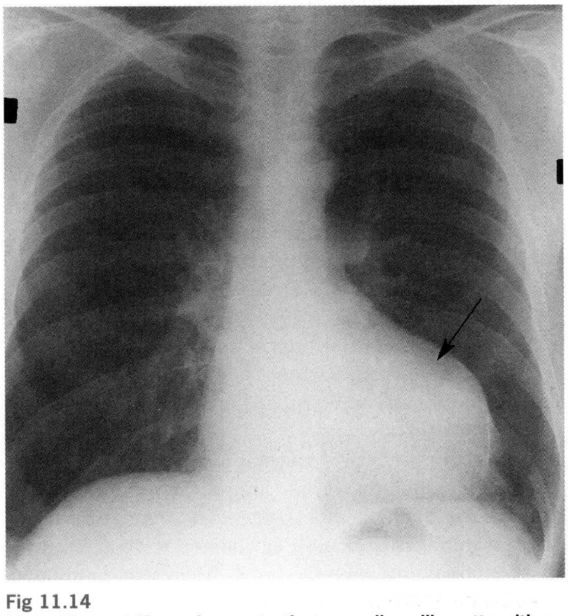

Fig 11.14
Plain PA chest X-ray demonstrating a cardiac silhouette with a 'bulge' on the left lateral border. This bulge is due to aneurysm formation of many years following a myocardial infarction. A thin line of calcification can be seen along the edge of this bulge

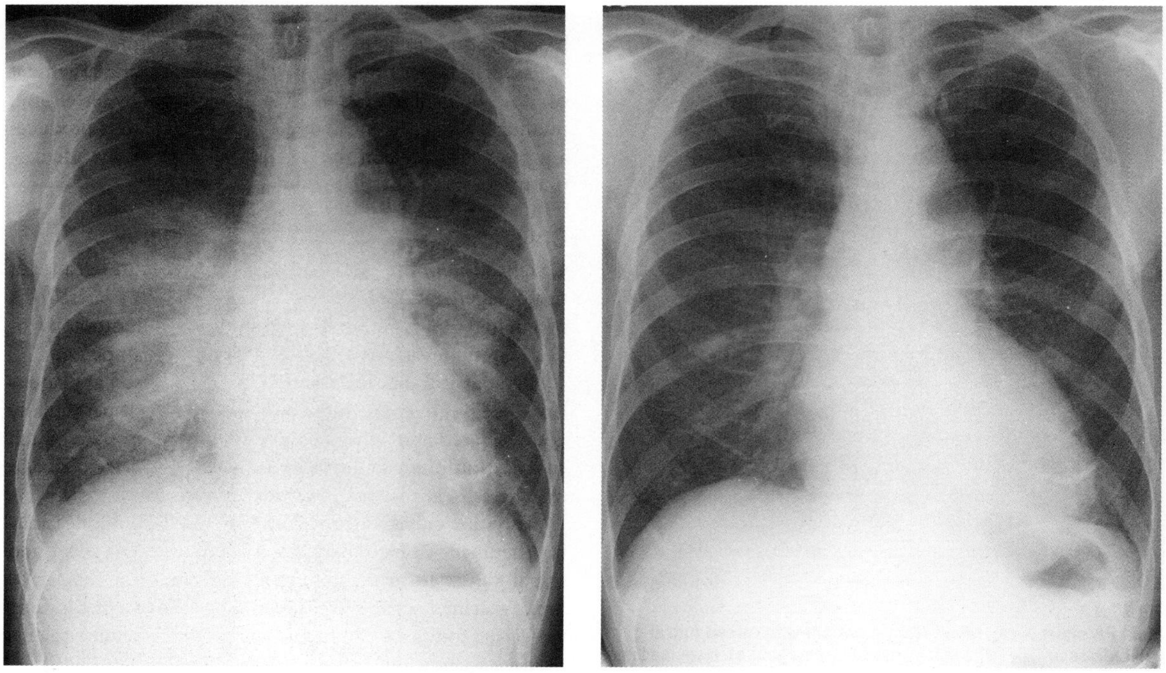

Fig 11.15
This pair of chest X-rays were taken from a patient before (left) and after (right) treatment of acute pulmonary oedema. The chest X-ray taken when the oedema was present demonstrates hilar haziness, Kerley B lines, upper lobe venous engorgement and fluid in the right horizontal interlobar fissure. These abnormalities are resolved on the film taken after successful treatment

ascending aorta usually denotes syphilitic aortitis, whereas in the descending aorta it is due to atheroma or, in the younger patient, to nonspecific aortitis.

Coronary arterial calcification. Coronary arterial calcification, especially of the proximal left coronary artery, is associated with coronary atheroma but does not necessarily correspond to the site of maximal stenosis.

Lung fields

Pulmonary plethora results from left-to-right shunts (e.g. atrial or ventricular septal defects). It is seen as a general increase in the vascularity of the lung fields and as an increase in the size of hilar vessels (e.g. in the right lower lobe artery), which normally should not exceed 16 mm diameter.

Pulmonary oligaemia is a paucity of vascular markings and a reduction in the width of the arteries. It occurs in situations where there is reduced pulmonary blood flow, such as pulmonary embolism, severe pulmonary stenosis and Fallot's tetralogy.

Pulmonary arterial hypertension may result from pulmonary embolism, chronic lung disease or chronic left heart disease, such as shunts due to a ventricular septal defect or mitral valve stenosis. In addition to X-ray features of these conditions, the pulmonary arteries are prominent close to the hili but are very reduced in size (pruned) in the peripheral lung fields. This pattern is usually symmetrical.

Pulmonary venous hypertension occurs in left ventricular failure or mitral valve disease. Normal pulmonary venous pressure is 5–14 mmHg at rest. Mild pulmonary venous hypertension (15–20 mmHg) produces isolated dilatation of the upper zone vessels. Interstitial oedema occurs when the pressure is between 21 and 30 mmHg. This manifests as fluid collections in the interlobar fissures, interlobular septa (Kerley B lines) and pleural spaces. This gives rise to indistinctness of the hilar regions and haziness of the lung fields. Alveolar oedema occurs when the pressure exceeds 30 mmHg, appearing as areas of consolidation and mottling of the lung fields (Fig 11.15) and pleural effusions. Patients with longstanding elevation of the pulmonary venous pressure have reactive thickening of the pulmonary arteriolar intima, which protects the alveoli from pulmonary oedema. Thus, in these patients the pulmonary venous pressure may increase to well above 30 mmHg before frank pulmonary oedema develops.

Fluoroscopy

Fluoroscopy has been largely superseded by echocardiography. However, it is still essential for the insertion of cardiac catheters and pacemaker electrodes.

Electrocardiography

The electrocardiogram (ECG) is a recording of the electrical activity of the heart. It is the vector sum of the depolarization and repolarization potentials of all myocardial cells (see Fig 11.32). At the body surface these generate potential differences of about 1 mV and the fluctuations of these potentials create the familiar P-QRS-T pattern. At rest the intracellular voltage of the myocardium is polarized at −90 mV compared with that of the extracellular space. This diastolic voltage difference occurs because of the high intracellular potassium concentration, which is maintained by the sodium–potassium pump despite the free membrane permeability to potassium. Depolarization of cardiac cells occurs when there is a sudden increase in the permeability of the membrane to sodium. Sodium rushes into the cell and the negative resting voltage is lost (stage 0 in Fig 11.32). The depolarization of a myocardial cell causes the depolarization of adjacent cells and, in the healthy heart, the entire myocardium is depolarized in a coordinated fashion. During repolarization, cellular electrolyte balance is slowly restored (stages 1, 2 and 3). Slow diastolic depolarization (stage 4) follows until the threshold potential is reached. Another action potential then follows.

The ECG is recorded from two or more simultaneous points of skin contact (electrodes). When cardiac activation proceeds towards the positive contact, an upward deflection is produced on the ECG. Correct representation of a three-dimensional spatial vector requires recordings from three mutually perpendicular (orthogonal) axes. The shape of the human torso does not make this easy, so the practical ECG records 12 projections of the vector, called 'leads' (Fig 11.16 and Practical box 11.3).

Six of the leads are obtained by recording voltages from the limbs (I, II, III, AVR, AVL and AVF). The other six leads record potentials between points on the chest surface and an average of the three limbs: RA, LA and LL. These are designated V_1–V_6 and aim to select activity from the right ventricle (V_1–V_2), interventricular septum (V_3–V_4) and left ventricle (V_5–V_6). Note that leads AVR and V_1 are oriented towards the cavity of the heart, leads II, III and AVF face the inferior surface, and leads I, AVL

Practical

Standard leads (bipolar) are derived:

Lead I	Right arm (–ve) to left arm (+ve)
Lead II	Right arm (–ve) to left leg (+ve)
Lead III	Left arm (–ve) to left leg (+ve)

Augmented leads (augmented bipolar) are derived:

AVR	Right arm (+ve) to left arm and left leg (–ve)
AVL	Left arm (+ve) to left leg and right arm (–ve)
AVF	Left leg (+ve) to left arm and right arm (–ve)

Chest leads (unipolar) are derived by connecting the V lead against the three extremity leads – the exploring electrodes are placed as follows:

V_1	4th intercostal space just to the right of the sternum
V_2	4th intercostal space just to the left of the sternum
V_3	Halfway between V_2 and V_4
V_4	5th intercostal space in the left mid-clavicular line
V_5	On same horizontal as V_4 in anterior axillary line
V_6	On same horizontal as V_4 in mid-axillary line

Practical box 11.3 ECG leads

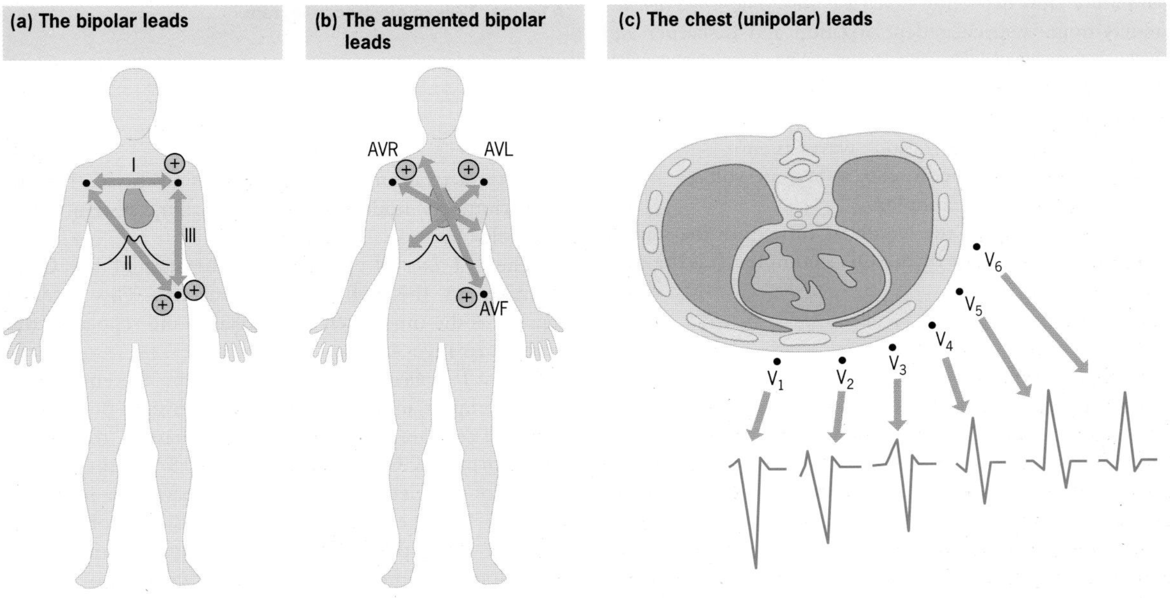

Fig 11.16
The connections or directions that comprise the 12-lead electrocardiogram

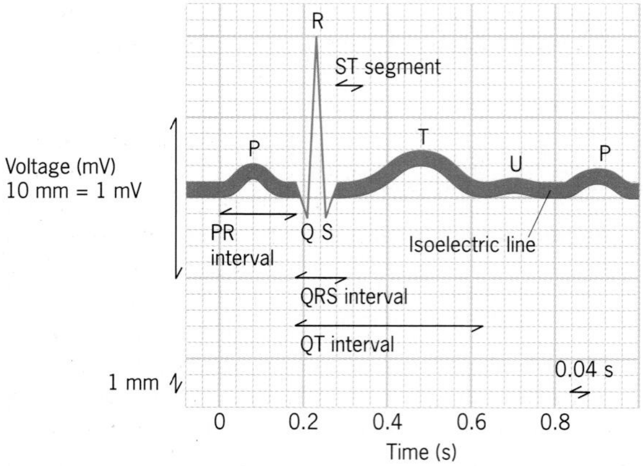

Fig 11.17
The waves and elaboration of the normal electrocardiogram.
From Goldman MJ (1976) Principles of Clinical Electrocardiography, 9th edn. Los Altos: Lange

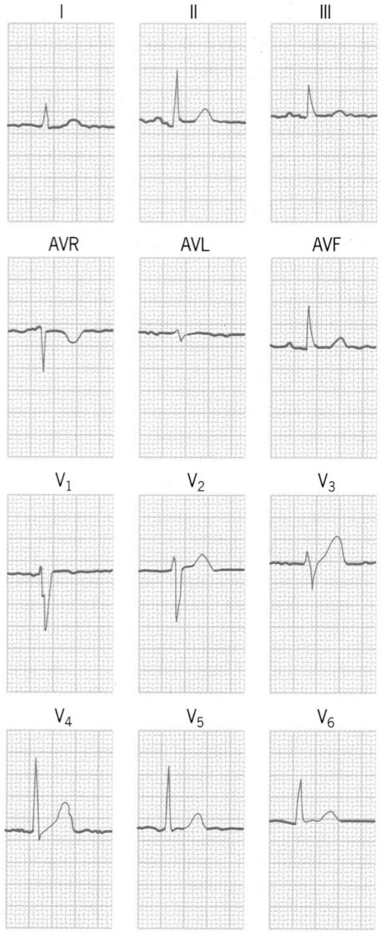

Fig 11.18
A normal 12-lead electrocardiogram

and V_6 face the lateral wall of the left ventricle. A V_4 on the right side of the chest (V_4R) is occasionally useful.

Most ECG machines are simultaneous three-channel recorders with output either as a continuous strip or with automatic channel switching. Many ECG machines also analyse the recordings and print the analysis on the record. Usually the machine interpretation is correct, but many arrhythmias still defy automatic analysis.

The ECG waveform

The shape of the normal ECG waveform (Fig 11.17) has important similarities, whatever the orientation. The first deflection is caused by atrial depolarization, and it is a low-amplitude slow deflection called a *P wave*. The *QRS complex* results from ventricular depolarization and is sharper and larger in amplitude than the P wave. The *T wave* is another slow and low-amplitude deflection that results from ventricular repolarization.

The atrial repolarization wave is not seen in a conventional ECG because it is low in voltage and is hidden by the QRS complex.

The *PR interval* is the length of time from the start of the P wave to the start of the QRS complex. It is the time taken for activation to pass from the sinus node, through the atrium, AV node and the His–Purkinje system to the ventricle.

The *QT interval* extends from the start of the QRS complex to the end of the T wave. This interval represents the time taken to depolarize and repolarize the ventricular myocardium.

The *ST segment* is the period between the end of the QRS complex and the start of the T wave. In the normal heart, all cells are depolarized by this phase of the ECG.

A normal ECG is shown in Fig 11.18, and the normal values for the electrocardiographic intervals are indicated in Table 11.9. Leads that face the lateral wall of the left ventricle have predominantly positive deflections, and leads looking into the ventricular cavity are usually negative. Detailed patterns depend on the size, shape and rhythm of the heart and the characteristics of the torso.

Table 11.9
Normal ECG intervals

P wave duration	≤ 0.12 s
PR interval	0.12–0.22 s
QRS Complex duration	≤ 0.10 s
Corrected QT (QT_c)	≤ 0.44 s (male) ≤ 0.46 s (female)
$QT_c = \frac{QT}{\sqrt{RR\ interval}}$	(Bajett's correction)

Cardiac vectors

At any point in time during depolarization and repolarization, electrical potentials are being propagated in different directions. Most of these cancel each other out and only the net force is recorded. This net force in the frontal plane is known as the *cardiac vector*.

The mean QRS vector can be calculated from the six standard leads (Fig 11.19); it normally lies between –30° and +90°. Left axis deviation lies between –30° and –90° and right axis deviation between +90° and +150°. Calculation of this vector is useful in the diagnosis of some cardiac disorders.

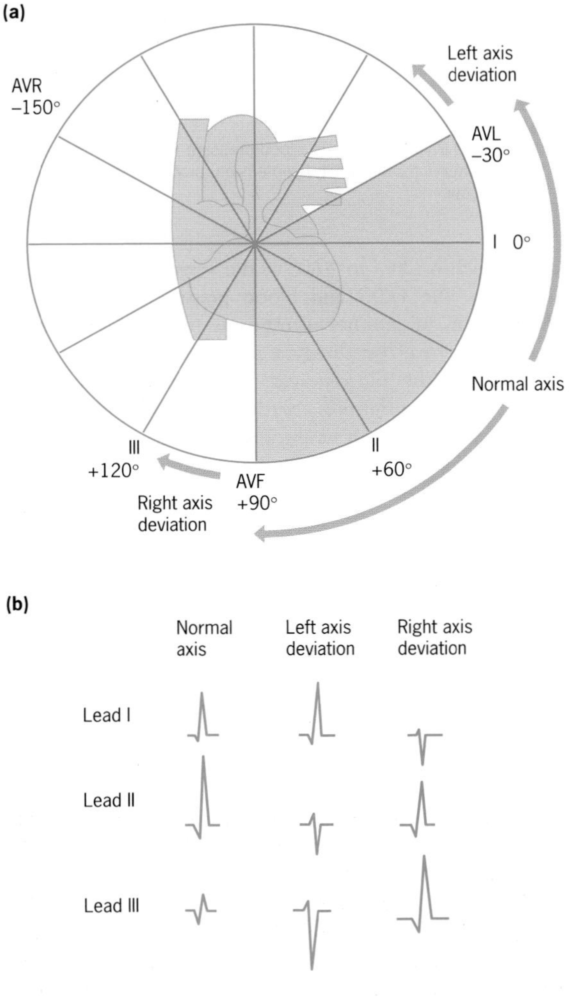

Fig 11.19
(a) The hexaxial reference system, illustrating the six leads in the frontal plane, e.g. lead I is 0°, lead II is +60°, lead III is +120°
(b) Calculating the direction of the cardiac vector. In the first column the QRS complex with zero net amplitude (i.e. when the positive and negative deflections are equal) is seen in lead III. The mean QRS vector is therefore perpendicular to lead III and is either –150° or +30°. Lead I is positive, so the axis must be +30°, which is normal. In left axis deviation (second column) the main deflection is positive (R wave) in lead I and negative (S wave) in lead III. In right axis deviation (third column) the main deflection is negative (S wave) in lead I and positive (R wave) in lead III. The frontal plane QRS axis is normal only if the QRS complexes in leads I and II are predominantly positive

Exercise electrocardiography

This is a technique used to assess the cardiac response to exercise. The ECG is recorded whilst the patient walks or runs on a motorized treadmill or cycles on a stationary cycle ergometer. Recording the ECG after the exercise is not an adequate form of stress test. Normally there is little change in the T wave or ST segment.

Myocardial ischaemia provoked by exertion results in ST segment depression (>1 mm) in leads facing the affected area. Although most abnormalities are detected in leads V_5 (anterior and lateral ischaemia) or AVF (inferior ischaemia), it is best to record a full 12-lead ECG. The form of ST segment depression provoked by ischaemia is characteristic: it is either planar or shows down-sloping depression (Fig 11.20). Up-sloping depression is a nonspecific finding. During an exercise test the exercise tolerance, blood pressure and rhythm responses to exercise are also assessed. Exercise causes an increase in heart rate and blood pressure. A sustained fall in blood pressure indicates severe coronary artery disease.

The usual indications and contraindications for the test are shown in Table 11.10. Its use in angina is described on p. 688.

24-hour ambulatory taped electrocardiography

This is a technique for recording transient changes such as a brief paroxysm of tachycardia, an occasional pause in the rhythm, or intermittent ST segment shifts. A conventional 12-lead ECG is recorded in less than a minute and usually samples less than 20 complexes. In a 24-hour period over 100 000 complexes are recorded. Such a large amount of data must be analysed by automatic or semi-automatic methods. This technique is called 'Holter' electrocardiography after its inventor.

Table 11.10
Indications and contraindications for exercise electrocardiography

Indications
Investigation of chest pain
Evaluation of treatment of ischaemia
Provocation of arrhythmia
Assessment of exercise tolerance
Risk assessment after myocardial infarction

Contraindications
Recent myocardial infarction (within 1 week)
Unstable angina
Hypertrophic cardiomyopathy
Severe aortic stenosis
Malignant hypertension

Provided that adequate precautions are observed (doctor and resuscitation facilities available, continuous ECG and blood pressure monitoring), the mortality from exercise testing is less than 0.01%. Myocardial infarction occurs in less than 0.05%.

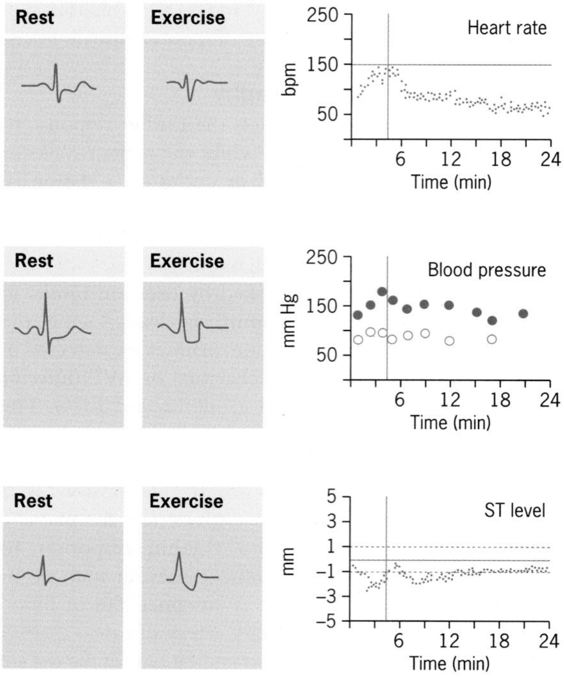

Fig 11.20
Electrocardiographic, heart rate and blood pressure changes on exercise. The middle (planar) and lower (downsloping) depression are characteristic in response to 4 minutes of exercise in a patient with myocardial ischaemia. The top exercise ECG shows upsloping depression which is nonspecific. The end of the exercise period is indicated by the vertical line in the graphs

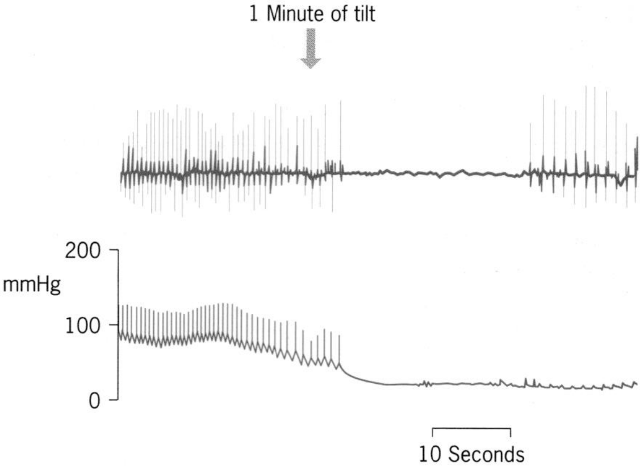

Fig 11.21
Tilt test
The ECG (top trace) and arterial blood pressure recorded during a tilt test. After 1 minute of tilt, hypotension, bradycardia and syncope occur

Event recording is another technique that may be used to record rare arrhythmias. The patient is provided with a pocket-sized device that can record and store a short segment of the ECG. The device may be kept for several days or weeks until the arrhythmia is recorded. Most units of this kind will also allow transtelephonic ECG transmission so that the physician can determine the need for treatment or the continued need for monitoring.

A very small event recorder can also be implanted subcutaneously, triggered by events or a magnet and interrogated by the physician.

Heart rate variability (HRV) can be assessed from a 24-hour ECG. HRV is decreased in some patients following myocardial infarction and represents an abnormality of autonomic tone or cardiac responsiveness. Low HRV is a major risk factor for sudden death and ventricular arrhythmias in patients discharged following myocardial infarction.

Ambulatory ECG recordings may also be used to monitor the level of the ST segment and to record transient ST segment depression.

Tilt testing

Patients with suspected neurocardiogenic syncope should be investigated by upright tilt. The patient is secured to a table which is tilted to +60° to the vertical for 45 minutes or more. The ECG and blood pressure are monitored throughout. If neither symptoms nor signs develop, isoprenaline may be slowly infused or glyceryl trinitrate inhaled and the tilt repeated. A positive test results in hypotension, sometimes bradycardia (Fig 11.21) and presyncope/syncope. If symptoms and signs appear, they can be quickly reversed by placing the patient flat. The effect of treatment can be evaluated by repeating the tilt test.

Carotid sinus massage

Carotid sinus massage (see p. 666) may lead to asystole (≥ 3 s) and/or fall of blood pressure (> 50 mmHg). This hypersensitive response occurs in many of the normal (especially elderly) population, but may also be responsible for loss of consciousness in some patients with carotid sinus syndrome (see p. 663). In one-third of cases carotid sinus massage is only positive when the patient is standing.

Phonocardiography

The application of a sensitive microphone to the chest wall allows heart sounds and murmurs to be recorded. Usually cardiac, carotid or jugular pulsations are recorded at the same time. The technique is difficult and, except for research purposes, has been largely superseded by echocardiography and other noninvasive techniques.

Echocardiography

Echocardiography uses echoes of ultrasound waves to map the heart and study its function. To provide detailed images, ultrasound wavelengths of 1 mm or less are used, which correspond to frequencies of 2 MHz (2 million cycles per second) or more. At such high frequencies, the ultrasound waves behave more like light and can be focused into a 'beam' and aimed at a particular region of the heart. The waves are generated in very short bursts or pulses a few microseconds long by a crystal transducer, which also detects returning echoes and converts them into electrical signals.

When the crystal transducer is placed on the body surface, the emitted ultrasound pulses encounter interfaces between various body tissues as they pass through the body. In crossing each interface, some of the wave energy is reflected, and if the beam path is approximately at right angles to the plane of the interface, the reflected waves return to the transducer as an echo. Since the velocity of sound in body tissues is almost constant (1550 m s^{-1}), the time delay for the echo to return measures the distance of the reflecting interface. Thus, if a single ultrasound pulse is transmitted, a series of echoes return, the first from the closest interface, and so on, until the distance becomes too great for further echoes to be detected.

To document in detail the motion patterns of individual structures, a technique called M-mode is used. The echo signals from a particular beam direction are recorded as a column of dots on a roll of photosensitive paper which is pulled past the cathode-ray tube display at constant speed. Stationary structures thus generate straight lines, the distances of which from the top of the paper indicate their depths, and movements, such as those of heart valves, are indicated by zig-zag lines (Fig 11.22(c)).

Calibration markers indicate depth at 1 cm intervals and lines along the edges of the paper show time intervals of 0.04 s. It is customary to add an ECG trace as an aid to identifying the phases of the heart cycle.

Alternatively a series of views from different positions can be obtained in the form of a two-dimensional image (cross-sectional 2-D echocardiography) (Figs 11.22(a), (b) and (d)). This method is useful for delineating anatomical structures.

Transoesophageal echocardiography (TOE)

In this technique a transducer, mounted on a flexible tube, is placed in the oesophagus. This avoids the problem of small windows (see below) in the transthoracic echo technique. High-quality images can be obtained in both longitudinal (vertical) and horizontal planes because of the close proximity to the heart. It is particularly useful for studying the atria, the interatrial septum, the right ventricular outflow tract, prosthetic valves and the aorta. This technique is obviously more invasive than the transthoracic approach.

Intracardiac and intravascular (coronary) ultrasound probes are now used to image intracardiac structures and coronary abnormalities.

Doppler echocardiography

Echocardiography imaging utilizes echoes from tissue interfaces. Using high amplification, it is also possible to detect weak echoes scattered by small targets, including those from red blood cells. If the blood is moving relative to the direction of the ultrasound beam, the frequency of the returning echoes will be changed according to the Doppler phenomenon. The Doppler shift frequency is directly proportional to the blood velocity.

Blood velocity data can be acquired and displayed in several ways. Continuous-wave (CW) Doppler collects all the velocity data from the path of the beam and analyses it to generate a spectral display. The outline of the envelope of the spectral display shows the value of peak velocity throughout the cardiac cycle. Normal velocities are of the order of 1 m s^{-1}, but if there is an obstructive lesion, such as a stenotic valve, velocities of 5 m s^{-1} or more can occur. These velocities are generated by the pressure gradient that exists across the lesion. According to the Bernoulli equation:

$$\text{Pressure gradient} = 4 \times (\text{velocity})^2$$

This equation has been validated in a wide variety of clinical situations, including valve stenoses, and ventricular septal defects, and makes it unnecessary to resort to invasive methods to measure intracardiac pressure gradients in many cases.

CW Doppler does not provide any depth information. Pulsed-wave (PW) Doppler extracts velocity data from the pulse echoes used to form a two-dimensional image and gives useful qualitative information. It can be thought of as a small intracardiac 'stethoscope' the location of which can be determined precisely. Doppler colour flow imaging uses one colour for blood flowing towards the transducer and another colour for blood flowing away. This technique allows the direction, velocity and timing of the flow to be measured with a simultaneous view of cardiac structure and function.

The echocardiographic examination

Echocardiography is a 'noninvasive' procedure that causes the patient no discomfort and is harmless. Studies are performed by a physician or technician and a comprehensive examination takes 15–30 minutes.

The major problem of echocardiography is that access to the heart is restricted by the lungs and rib cage, both of which form impenetrable barriers to ultrasound in the adult subject. Small 'windows' can usually be found in the third and fourth left intercostal spaces (termed left parasternal); just below the xiphoid process of the sternum (subcostal); and, with the subject turned to the left and exhaling, from the point where the apical beat is palpated (apical). By positioning the transducer successively over these sites and angling and rotating it to align the scan plane, a series of standard sectional views is obtained. In children, and some adults, the aortic arch can be visualized from a suprasternal position.

The standard nomenclature for two-dimensional echocardiographic images is shown in Fig 11.22(a). The left parasternal position gives access to the long-axis and short-axis planes. The apical approach gives a second view of the long-axis plane, but with the apex in the

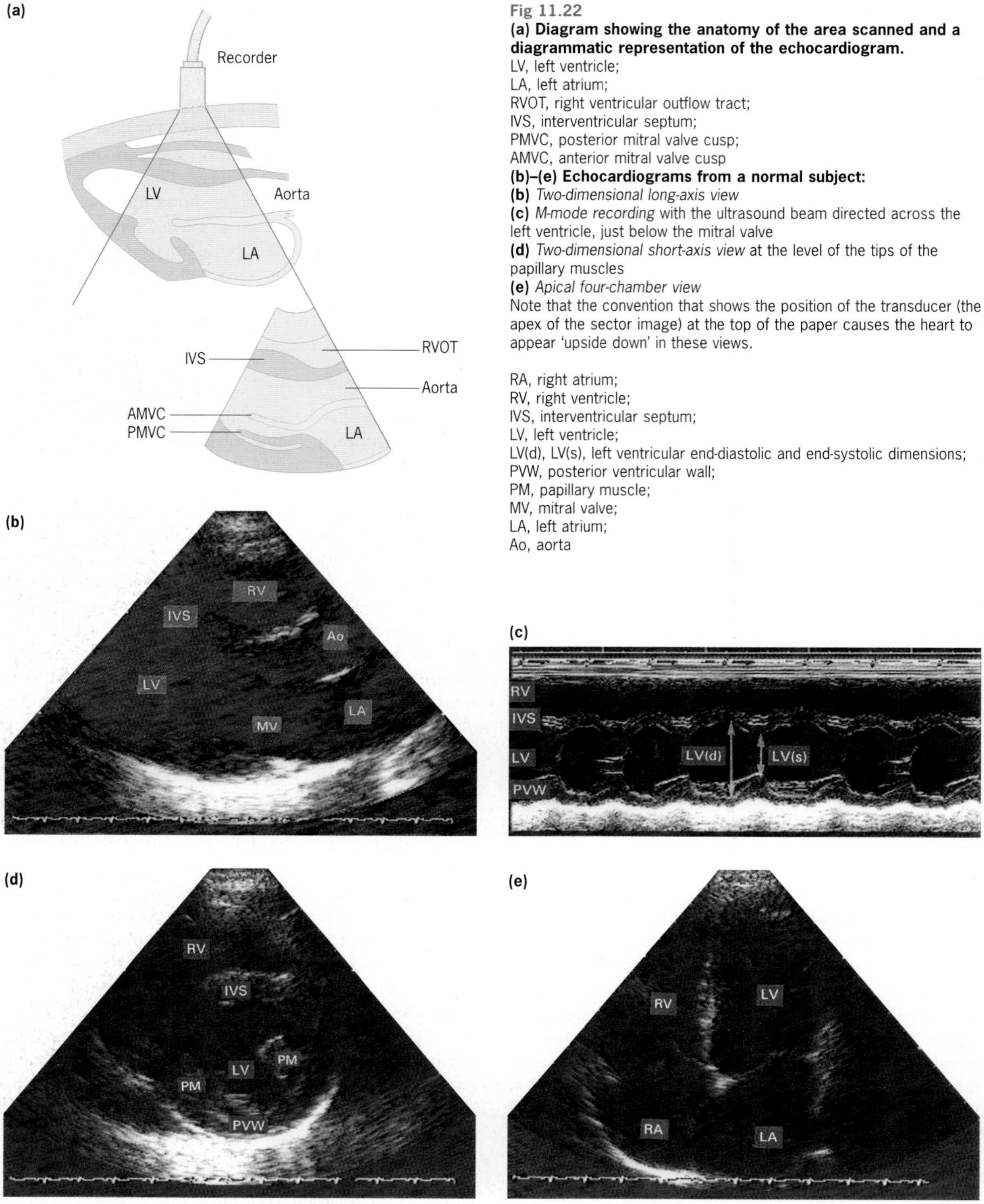

Fig 11.22
(a) Diagram showing the anatomy of the area scanned and a diagrammatic representation of the echocardiogram.
LV, left ventricle;
LA, left atrium;
RVOT, right ventricular outflow tract;
IVS, interventricular septum;
PMVC, posterior mitral valve cusp;
AMVC, anterior mitral valve cusp
(b)–(e) Echocardiograms from a normal subject:
(b) *Two-dimensional long-axis view*
(c) *M-mode recording* with the ultrasound beam directed across the left ventricle, just below the mitral valve
(d) *Two-dimensional short-axis view* at the level of the tips of the papillary muscles
(e) *Apical four-chamber view*
Note that the convention that shows the position of the transducer (the apex of the sector image) at the top of the paper causes the heart to appear 'upside down' in these views.

RA, right atrium;
RV, right ventricle;
IVS, interventricular septum;
LV, left ventricle;
LV(d), LV(s), left ventricular end-diastolic and end-systolic dimensions;
PVW, posterior ventricular wall;
PM, papillary muscle;
MV, mitral valve;
LA, left atrium;
Ao, aorta

foreground, and also shows the four-chamber plane (Fig 11.22(e)). Note that the convention of showing the transducer position at the top of the image results in these views being 'upside-down'.

M-mode recordings are obtained from the parasternal position to document motion patterns of the aorta, aortic valve and left atrium, the mitral valve, and the left and right ventricles (Fig 11.22(c)).

The 1 cm calibration markers on M-mode recordings permit measurement of cardiac dimensions at any point in the cardiac cycle with an accuracy typically of ±2–3 mm.

Comparison of end-diastolic and end-systolic values allows some parameters of cardiac function to be derived. For example, the percentage reduction in the left ventricular cavity size ('shortening fraction' – SF) is given by:

$$SF = \frac{LVDD - LVSD}{LVDD} \times 100\%$$

where LVDD is left ventricular diastolic diameter and LVSD is left ventricular systolic diameter. The normal range is 30–45%.

The echocardiographic findings in particular conditions are discussed in relevant sections, but a brief overview is given below.

Valve stenosis. Congenitally abnormal aortic or pulmonary valves show a characteristic 'dome' shape in systole because the cusps cannot separate fully and a bicuspid configuration may be demonstrated. The presence of calcium in a valve gives rise to intense echoes that generate multiple, parallel lines on M-mode recordings. CW Doppler directed from the apex measures velocity of the jet crossing the diseased valve, from which the pressure gradient can be calculated (Fig 11.23).

In mitral stenosis, the M-mode shows restriction and reversal of direction of the posterior leaflet motion (Fig 11.24). A short-axis view shows the shape of the mitral orifice in diastole and its area can be measured directly from the image. Peak, mean and end-diastolic pressure gradients can be obtained from CW Doppler. Additional imaging views indicate the size of the left atrium, and may show the presence of left atrial thrombus.

Valve regurgitation. Doppler is extremely sensitive for detecting valve regurgitation and, indeed, demonstrates mild physiological regurgitation through the tricuspid and pulmonary valves in the majority of normal subjects. It is hard to quantify the amount of regurgitation with echo Doppler techniques, but echocardiography is an excellent way to determine the underlying cause of valve regurgitation, such as rheumatic disease or mitral valve prolapse.

Aortic aneurysms and dissections. Dilatation of the aortic root can be measured accurately and the presence of a reflecting structure within the lumen of the aorta is strongly suggestive of an intimal flap associated with dissection. Transoesophageal views are particularly suitable for detecting pathology in the ascending and descending aorta. In many hospitals this is the investigation of first choice when aortic dissection is suspected.

Prosthetic heart valves. Each type of heart valve prosthesis has characteristic echocardiographic features. Irregularity or restriction of movement can be shown on M-mode recordings. The presence of stenosis or regurgitation may be documented by Doppler. Prosthetic valves cast acoustic shadows which obscure the area behind the valve. A transoesophageal approach is often used to inspect a prosthetic mitral valve for evidence of endocarditis or thrombosis.

(a)

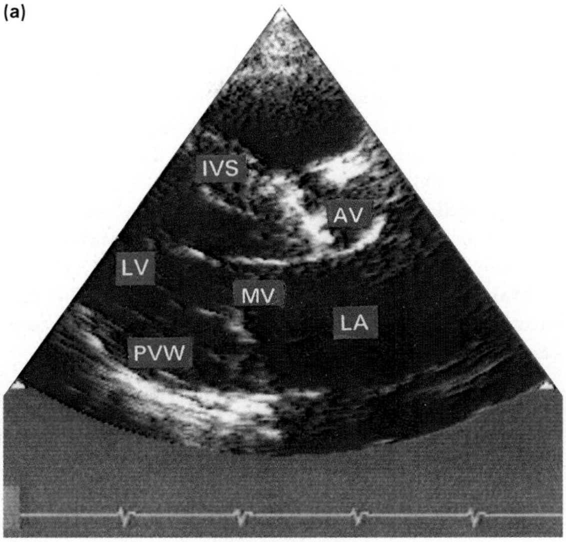

(b)

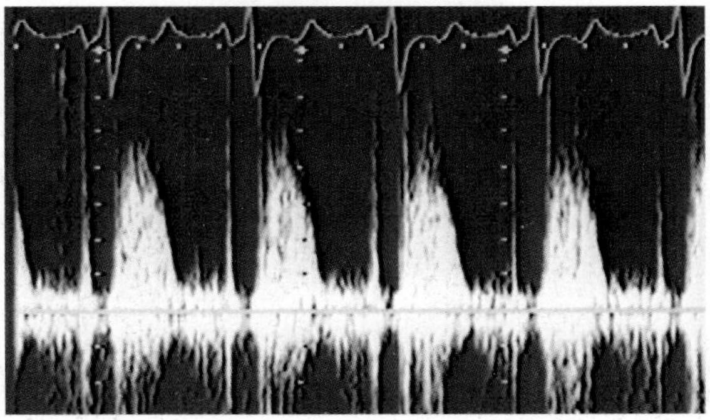

Fig 11.23
(a) Two-dimensional echocardiogram (long-axis view) in a patient with calcific aortic stenosis. The calcium in the valve generates abnormally intense echoes. There is some evidence of the associated left ventricular hypertrophy
(b) Continuous-wave (CW) Doppler signals obtained from the right upper parasternal edge, where the high velocity jet from the stenotic valve is coming towards the transducer. The peak jet velocity is 5 m s^{-1}, corresponding to a pressure gradient of 100 mmHg
AV, aortic valve;
LA, left atrium;
MV, mitral valve;
LV, left ventricle;
IVS, interventricular septum;
PVW, posterior ventricular wall

Infective endocarditis. Vegetations >2 mm can be detected (see Fig 11.77 on p. 713).

Cardiac failure. Left ventricular function and response to treatment is readily assessed and should be performed in all patients with heart failure.

Cardiomyopathies. Dilated cardiomyopathy is characterized by an enlarged, globular-shaped, thin-walled left ventricle with poor function and low stroke output shown by reduced movements of the valves (see Fig 11.90 on p. 725).

In hypertrophic cardiomyopathy (see Fig 11.92 on p. 726), the left ventricle is small, with a grossly thickened, immobile interventricular septum (asymmetric septal hypertrophy – ASH). There is a characteristic, though poorly understood, displacement of the mitral valve apparatus towards the septum in systole (systolic anterior motion – SAM).

Pericardial effusion. Fluid in the pericardial cavity shows as an echo-free region between the myocardium and the intense echo of the parietal pericardium (Fig 11.25).

Masses within the heart. Echocardiography is a sensitive method for detecting masses within the heart (see Fig 11.88 on p. 723).

Ischaemic disease. Coronary arteries cannot be imaged adequately using echo techniques, but images may be useful for the diagnosis of complications related to myocardial infarction, such as mitral papillary muscle rupture, tamponade or ventricular septal rupture.

In the postinfarction period, echocardiography and Doppler are used to diagnose left ventricular aneurysm, left ventricular thrombus, mitral regurgitation and pericardial effusion as well as to assess left ventricular function (ejection fraction).

Congenital heart disease. Echocardiography has largely replaced cardiac catheterization and angiography.

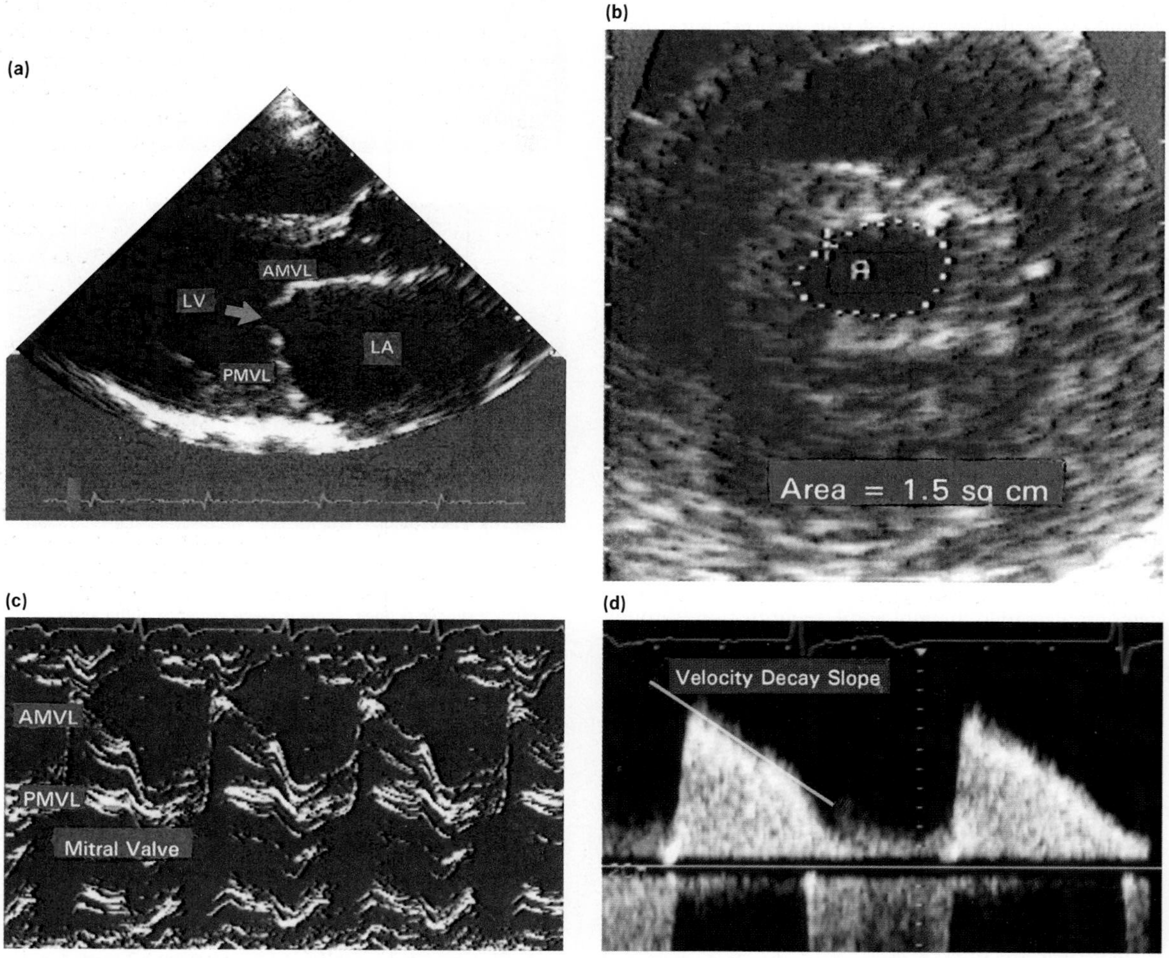

Fig 11.24
Echocardiograms in rheumatic mitral valve disease
(a) *Two-dimensional long-axis view* showing enlarged left atrium and 'hooked' appearance of the mitral valve leaflets resulting from commisural fusion
(b) *Magnified short axis view* showing the mitral valve orifice as seen from the direction of the arrow in (a). The orifice area can be planimetered to assess the severity; in this case it is 1.5 cm^2, indicating moderately severe disease
(c) *M-mode recording* of the mitral valve showing restricted motion of the thickened leaflets
(d) *Continuous-wave (CW) Doppler recording* showing slow rate of decay of flow velocity from the left atrium to the left ventricle during diastole. It is also possible to derive the valve orifice area from the velocity decay rate
LA, left atrium;
LV, left ventricle,
AMVL, PMVL, anterior and posterior mitral valve leaflets;

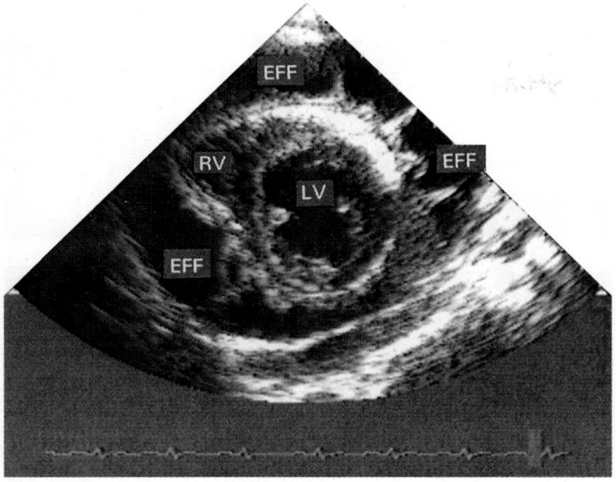

Fig 11.25
Two-dimensional echocardiogram (short-axis view) from a patient with a large pericardial effusion associated with pulmonary tuberculosis. The exudate is seen between the visceral and parietal layers of the pericardium and would give a false impression of cardiomegaly on a chest X-ray. Note the multiple fibrous strands within the effusion, showing that it is consolidating and will probably lead to constriction of cardiac function
LV, left ventricle;
RV, right ventricle;
EFF, effusion

The aim of the examination is first to establish the sequence of blood flow through the heart, and to define anatomical abnormalities.

Nuclear imaging

Nuclear imaging may be used to detect myocardial infarction or to measure myocardial function, perfusion or viability, depending on the radiopharmaceutical used and the technique of imaging. These data are particularly valuable when used in combination.

Image type

Gamma cameras produce a planar image in which structures are superimposed as in a standard radiograph. Single-photon-emission computed tomography (SPECT) imaging uses similar raw data to construct tomographic images, just as a CT image is reconstructed from X-rays. This gives finer anatomical resolution, but is technically demanding. These methods may be used with any of the radiopharmaceuticals.

Myocardial perfusion and viability

Thallium-201 is rapidly taken up by the myocardium, so an image taken immediately after injection reflects the distribution of blood flow to the myocardium. Areas of ischaemia or infarction receive less ^{201}Tl and appear dark. Between 2 and 24 hours after injection, ^{201}Tl is redistributed so that all cardiac myocytes contain a comparable concentration. Images at this time show dark areas where the myocardium has infarcted, but normal density in ischaemic areas. Comparison of the early and late images is one method of predicting whether an ischaemic area of myocardium contains enough viable tissue to justify coronary bypass or angioplasty.

Technetium-99 labelled sestamibi (Fig 11.26) is also taken up rapidly by cardiac myocytes, but does not undergo redistribution. When this substance is injected during exercise, its distribution in the myocardium reflects the distribution of blood at the time of the exercise, even if the image is taken several hours later. This is a sensitive method of detecting myocardial viability. Images produced following injection of ^{99m}Tc-sestamibi during exercise can be compared to images produced following injection at rest to decide which areas of ischaemia are reversible (p. 688).

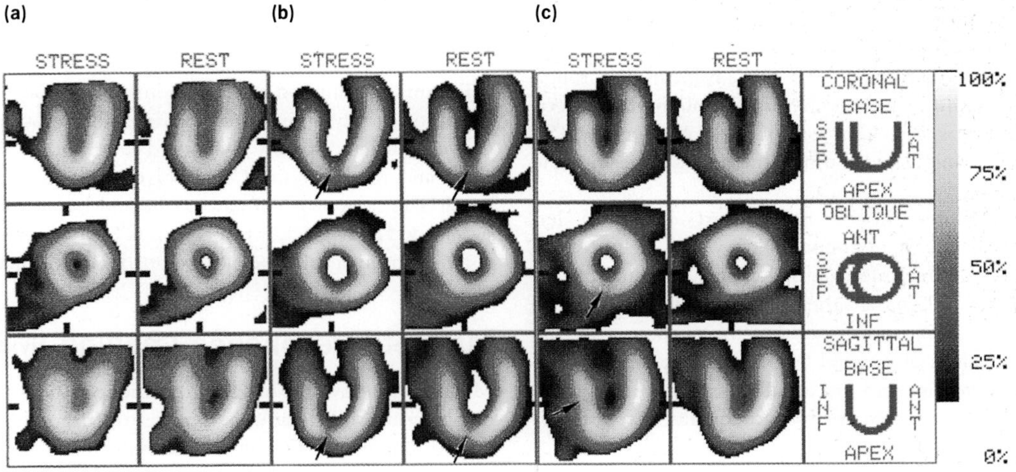

Fig 11.26
Thallium or sestamibi myocardial scintigram during stress and afterwards at rest in three patients
(a) *Normal perfusion* at rest and during stress
(b) *Similar (fixed) defect at rest and during stress.* This is due to a previous myocardial infarction
(c) *Poor reperfusion* in the inferior wall during stress which is largely resolved at rest due to 'reversible ischaemia'

Infarct imaging

Perfusion images produced using compounds labelled with ^{201}Tl or ^{99m}Tc-sestamibi show a myocardial infarction as a perfusion defect or 'cold spot'. These methods are sensitive for detecting and localizing the infarct, but give no information about its chronicity. ^{99m}Tc pyrophosphate is preferentially taken up by myocardium which has undergone infarction within the previous few days. Images are difficult to interpret because the isotope is also concentrated by bone and cartilage.

Radionuclide ventriculography

Two methods are used to obtain blood pool images:

- A *MUGA* (multigated acquisition) or equilibrium image is obtained by intravenous injection of ^{99m}Tc which attaches to the patient's own red cells *in vivo* and which is therefore retained in the vascular space. Over 200 heart beats are imaged. Comparison of the study with the ECG allows systolic and diastolic points of the cycle to be identified.
- A *first-pass study* images the heart as a bolus of isotope makes a single pass through the circulation.

These techniques are complementary, but both outline the cardiac chambers, particularly the left ventricle, by imaging the isotope within the central circulation during systole and diastole. The percentage of the left ventricular volume ejected with each systole (the ejection fraction) can be measured accurately, and any section of the left ventricular wall that contracts abnormally (a wall motion defect) can be visualized (Fig 11.27).

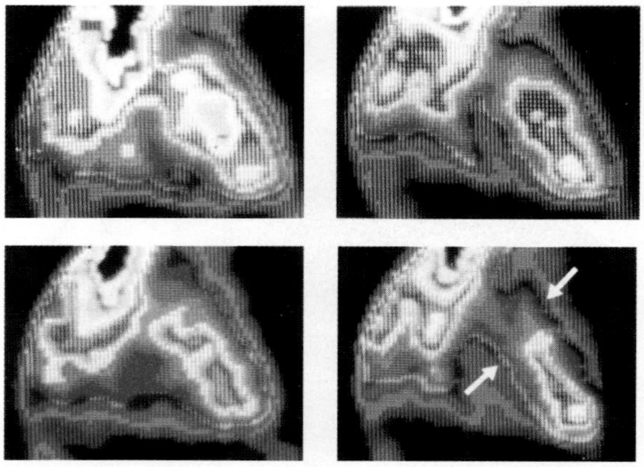

Fig 11.27
MUGA scan of patient with left ventricular aneurysm. End-diastolic (ed) and end-systolic (es) images were recorded before administration of sublingual nitrate (above) and again after administration (below). The apical aneurysm is not altered by administration of nitrate, although the remainder of the left ventricle shows a reduced end-systolic size (arrows)

Cardiac catheterization

Cardiac catheterization is the introduction of a thin radiopaque tube (catheter) into the circulation.

The right heart is catheterized by introducing the catheter into a peripheral vein and advancing it through the right atrium and ventricle into the pulmonary artery. The left heart is reached by way of a peripheral artery. The catheter is manipulated through the aortic valve into the left ventricle.

The pressures in the right heart chambers, left ventricle, aorta and pulmonary artery can be measured directly. An indirect measure of left atrial pressure can be obtained by 'wedging' a catheter into the distal pulmonary artery (see p. 842). In this position the pressure from the right ventricle is obstructed by the catheter and only the pulmonary venous and left atrial pressures are recorded. Pressure measurements are used to quantify stenoses or measure contractile function.

During cardiac catheterization, blood samples may be withdrawn to measure the concentration of ischaemic metabolites (e.g. lactate) and the oxygen content. These estimations are used to gauge ischaemia, quantify intracardiac shunts, and measure cardiac output.

Contrast cine-angiograms are also taken during catheterization. Radiopaque contrast material is injected into the cardiac chambers. Fig 11.28 presents a normal angiogram showing normal left ventricular function. Coronary angiography is described on p. 688.

Digital subtraction angiography

This technique permits the injection of small volumes of radiocontrast agents during cardiac catheterization with the production of computer-analysed high-quality angiograms.

Unfortunately, peripheral injection of contrast does not give adequate visualization of the coronary arteries, but aortic lesions can be visualized.

CT scanning

CT scanning is limited because an image must be obtained in approximately 50 ms to eliminate cardiac motion. Both conventional and spiral CT are used to image the thoracic aorta and mediastinum. CT involves ionizing radiation, requires intravascular contrast media and has been largely superseded by MRI. Electron-beam CT, which produces a faster beam image, has been developed, but is expensive.

Magnetic resonance imaging (MRI)

MRI is a noninvasive imaging technique which does not involve harmful radiation. A powerful magnetic field is used to line up the protons in the hydrogen atoms of the body, each of which can be thought of as a tiny magnet. A radiofrequency emission distorts this line-up, but when the radio waves are turned off, the atoms return to their previous position and give off energy. This energy can be reconstituted as an image.

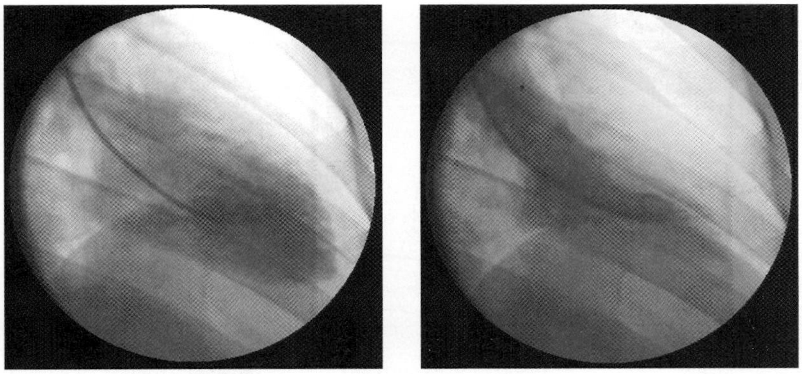

Fig 11.28
Diastolic (left) and systolic (right) frames recorded after X-ray contrast was injected into the left ventricle (contrast left ventriculogram). Normal left ventricular function is demonstrated

Synchronization with the ECG allows cardiac images in systole and diastole to be obtained (Fig 11.29). MRI is occasionally useful in congenital heart disease, intracardiac masses and pericardial disease. Its main use is in imaging thoracic aneurysms either for surveillance or in the diagnosis of acute dissection. Apart from structure, images can also be obtained for flow velocity.

FURTHER READING

Uretsky BF (1997) Diagnostic Cardiac Catheterization. Oxford: Blackwell.

Peterson KL, Nicol P (1996) Cardiac Catheterization. Methods, Diagnosis and Therapy. Philadelphia: WB Saunders.

Therapeutic procedures

Cardiac resuscitation

No matter where cardiac arrest occurs it is essential that someone close to the victim institutes basic life support. The longer the period of respiratory and circulatory arrest, the less the possibility of restoring healthy life. After three minutes there will be permanent cerebral dysfunction. Because sudden unexpected cardiac arrest is relatively common in the hospital, medical students and all doctors must know what to do. A cardiac arrest usually causes a great deal of excitement and some panic. Therefore, it is very important that the basic procedure is well known. A standard procedure must be used in order that a variety of personnel may work easily together.

Basic life support (BLS)

The first step is to establish whether the victim is unconscious (shake and shout at the patient) and whether there is a pulse. It is best to feel the carotid pulse by pressing backwards just to the side of the thyroid cartilage. If there is no pulse, immediately call for help. Quickly place the victim in an accessible position with firm underlying support (e.g. on his/her back on the floor), and begin basic life support. This can be remembered as A (airway) and B (breathing) and C (circulation) (see Emergency box 11.1).

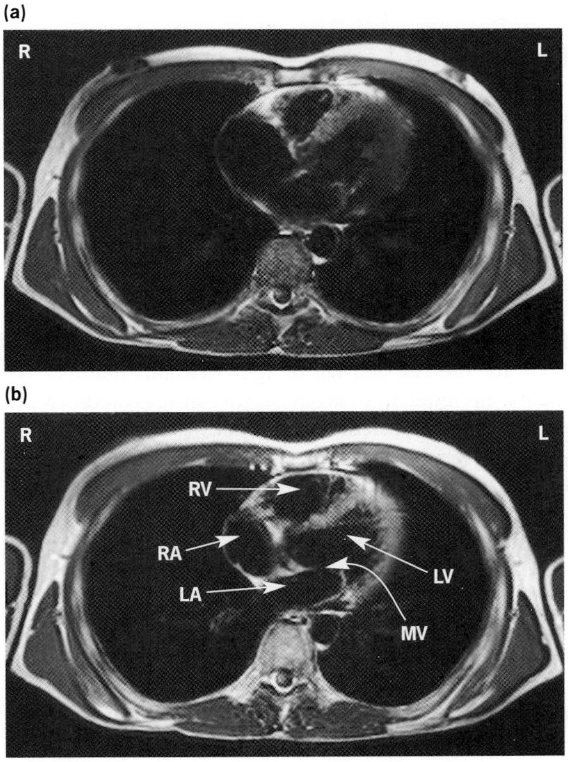

Fig 11.29
Magnetic resonance image (MRI), showing a pair of axial images taken through the mid-thorax at the level of the mitral valve
(a) A view of end-systole
(b) Taken at end-diastole. Note the clear differentiation between the atria and ventricles. This is a normal study
LA, left atrium;
LV, left ventricle;
MV, mitral valve;
RA, right atrium;
RV, right ventricle

Emergency

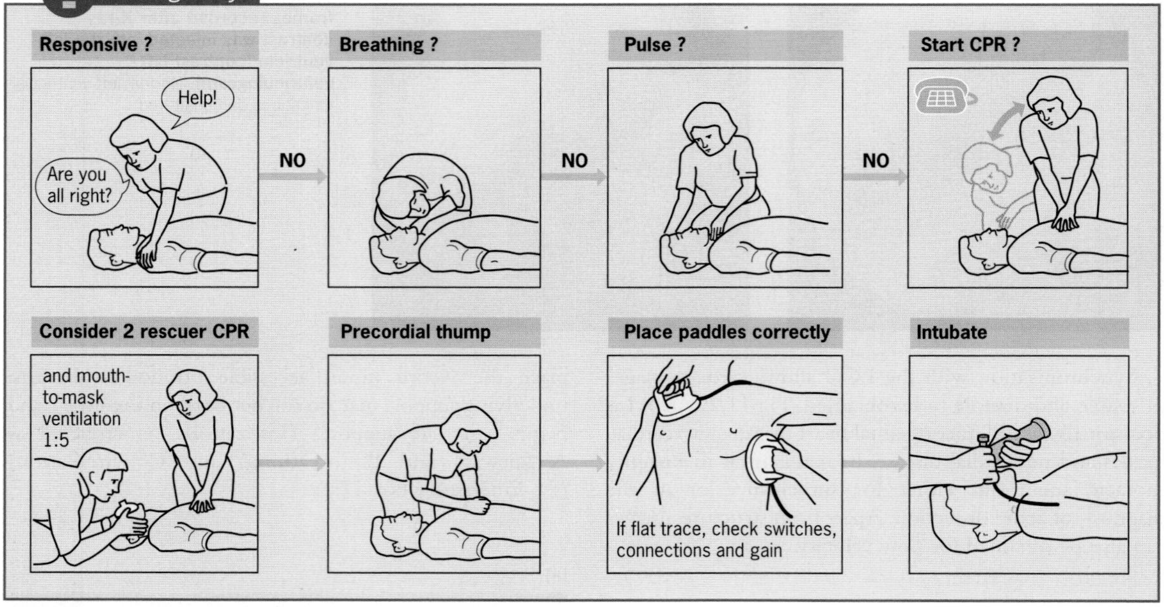

Emergency box 11.1 Basic life support

Airway

Any loose obstruction (e.g. blood and mucus) in the mouth and pharynx should be quickly removed. Unless already detached, leave false teeth in place because they give form and support to the oral cavity. Open the airway by flexing the neck and extending the head ('sniffing the morning air' position).

Breathing

Look for the rise and fall of the chest and abdomen. If there is no respiration, begin expired air respiration. With the head of the victim tilted backwards and the chin pulled forward, the rescuer takes a deep breath and seals his/her lips around the mouth or nose of the victim. Four quick puffs are given. Expired air respiration is the only method of artificial respiration that successfully ventilates the patient. The mechanical methods of Holger and Neilson, Shaeffer and Sylvester are completely useless because they result in the movement of less air than is required to fill the dead space.

If the airway is obstructed, the head, neck and jaw are readjusted and another check is made for debris in the mouth. If obstruction persists, any foreign body stuck in the larynx or upper airway should be removed by a firm thrust to the epigastrium (the Heimlich manoeuvre, see p. 774).

Circulation

Circulation is achieved by external chest compression. The heel of one hand is placed over the lower half of the victim's sternum and the heel of the second hand is placed over the first with the fingers interlocked. The arms are kept straight and the sternum is rhythmically depressed by 2–5 cm. Chest compression does not massage the heart. The thorax acts as a pump and the heart provides a system of one-way valves to ensure forward circulation.

Respiration and compression is now continued as follows:

- *single rescuer* – compression at a rate of 80 b.p.m. with two respirations after 15 compressions.
- *two rescuers* – continuous compressions at a rate of 60 b.p.m. and one respiration given after every five compressions.

If possible, it is better to give compressions without interruption. This maintains adequate cerebral and coronary perfusion pressures. Ventilation can easily be achieved despite continued chest compression.

Advanced cardiac life support

By the time effective life support has been established, more help should have arrived and advanced cardiac life support can begin. This consists of ECG monitoring, endotracheal intubation and setting up an intravenous infusion in a large peripheral vein or a central vein. Immediate therapy includes defibrillation, oxygen and cardioactive drugs. It is not possible to recommend an exact sequence of management because it will depend on the arrival of skilled personnel and equipment and the nature of the cardiac arrest. However, as soon as possible the ECG should be connected. At first this is easily achieved by monitoring the ECG through the paddles of a defibrillator. Later, electrodes, leads and specific ECG scopes can be set up. If the ECG shows ventricular fibrillation, no time should be lost before defibrillating the patient. If initial defibrillation attempts are unsuc-cessful, time can then be spent intubating the patient and setting up an intravenous infusion whilst the circulation is supported by external chest compression. If there is any difficulty in intubating the patient, ventilation should be continued by means of an airway, a ventilating bag and oxygen.

There are two main mechanisms of sudden unexpected cardiac arrest (Information box 11.1):

- ventricular fibrillation/ventricular tachycardia (VF/VT)
- non-VF/VT (asystole or electromechanical dissociation).

Three-quarters of arrests are due to ventricular fibrillation or rapid ventricular tachycardia. Only a very small proportion are due to electromechanical dissociation, and the remainder are due to asystole. In patients dying of other causes, such as terminal pneumonia, the heart rhythm is described as being *agonal*. This is characterized by an inexorable slowing and widening of the QRS complexes associated with falling blood pressure and cardiac output. This type of arrhythmia is very difficult to reverse and usually no attempt should be made because it is the result rather than the cause of death.

Arrests are treated in the following ways:

- *Ventricular fibrillation* is readily treated with defibrillation, antiarrhythmic drugs and cardiac stimulants.
- *Asystole* is more difficult to treat but the heart may respond to atropine or adrenaline (epinephrine). If there is any sign of electrocardiographic activity, emergency pacing should be used.
- *Electromechanical dissociation* is often due to a severe mechanical problem such as pericardial tamponade or massive pulmonary embolism. These conditions should be treated urgently. Toxic levels of cardiodepressant drugs, such as β-blockers, may also cause electromechanical dissociation. If there is an antidote, such as adrenaline, it should be administered.

Information

Each year in the UK there are approximately 100 000 unexpected deaths occurring within 24 hours of the development of cardiac symptoms. About half of these deaths are almost instantaneous. There are several causes:

- cardiac arrhythmias (e.g. ventricular fibrillation)
- sudden pump failure (e.g. acute myocardial infarction)
- acute circulatory obstruction (e.g. pulmonary embolism)
- cardiovascular rupture (e.g. aortic dissection, myocardial rupture)
- vasomotor collapse (e.g. in pulmonary hypertension)

Most deaths are due to ventricular fibrillation or rapid ventricular tachycardia, and a small proportion are due to severe bradyarrhythmias. Although coronary disease is frequent in these victims, acute coronary occlusion and myocardial infarction is relatively uncommon (about 40%).

Information box 11.1 Causes of unexpected cardiac arrest

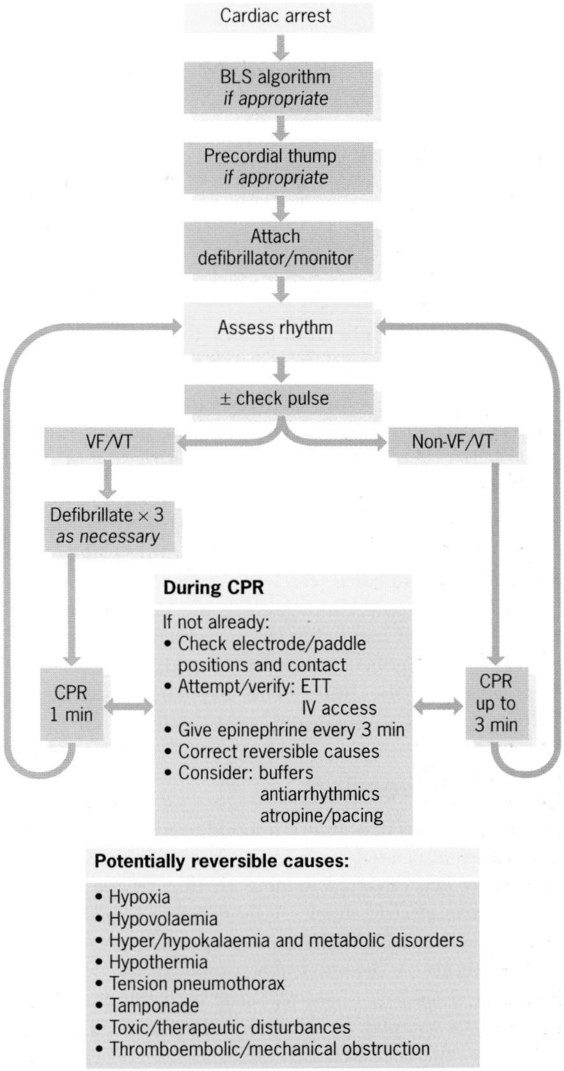

Fig 11.30
Universal advanced life-support algorithm
BLS, basic life support (see Emergency box 11.1);
CPR, cardiopulmonary resuscitation;
ETT, endotracheal tube
Epinephrine = adrenaline

Figure 11.30 shows the treatments recommended by the European Resuscitation Council and the Resuscitation Council UK.

Defibrillation

This technique is used for the conversion of ventricular fibrillation into sinus rhythm. Electrical energy is discharged through two paddles placed on the chest wall. Initially 200 J is used for defibrillation.

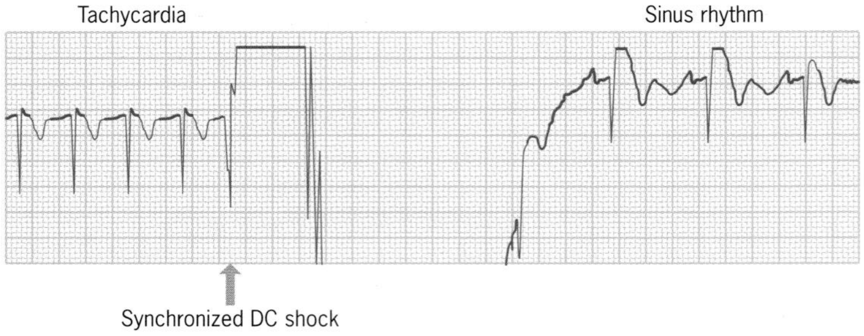

Fig 11.31
DC-cardioversion of a supraventricular tachycardia to sinus rhythm. The direct current shock is delivered synchronously with the QRS complex

The paddles are placed in one of two positions:

1. One paddle is placed to the right of the upper sternum and the other over the cardiac apex.
2. One paddle is placed under the tip of the left scapula and the other is placed over the anterior wall of the left chest.

Electrode jelly or electrolyte gel pads should be used to ensure good contact between the electrode paddles and the skin. Jelly smeared carelessly across the chest may cause short-circuits and arcing of the charge. All personnel should stand clear of the patient.

When the defibrillator is discharged, a high-voltage field envelopes the heart. This depolarizes the whole heart and allows an organized heart rhythm to emerge.

DC-cardioversion

Tachyarrhythmias that do not respond to medical treatment or that are associated with severe haemodynamic disturbance may be converted to sinus rhythm by the use of a transthoracic electric shock. A short-acting general anaesthetic is used. Muscle relaxants are not usually given. When the arrhythmia has definite QRS complexes, the delivery of the shock should be timed to occur with the downstroke of the QRS complex (synchronization) (Fig 11.31). This is the major difference between defibrillation and cardioversion, since a non-synchronized shock is used to defibrillate.

Indications for cardioversion are atrial fibrillation and atrial flutter, and ventricular tachycardia. Occasionally, sustained junctional tachycardias may have to be DC-cardioverted to sinus rhythm.

If the arrhythmia, especially atrial fibrillation, has been present for more than a few days, it is necessary to anticoagulate the patient for three weeks before and four weeks after elective cardioversion to reduce the risk of embolization.

Digoxin toxicity may lead to ventricular arrhythmias or asystole following cardioversion. Therapeutic digitalization does not increase the risks of cardioversion, but it is conventional to omit digoxin several days prior to elective cardioversion in order to be sure that toxicity is not present.

Repeated cardioversion leads to an enzyme rise because of damage to the muscles of the chest wall. Specific cardiac enzymes increase very slightly because of myocardial damage produced by the shock.

Temporary pacing

Symptomatic bradycardias unresponsive to atropine are treated with a cardiac pacemaker. A temporary pacemaker (external unit) may be connected to the myocardium by a thin (French gauge 5 or 6), bipolar pacing electrode wire inserted via a subclavian or internal jugular vein and manipulated into the right ventricular apex using cardiac fluoroscopy. The energy needed for successful pacing (the pacing threshold) is assessed by reducing the energy until the pacemaker fails to stimulate the tissue (loss of capture). The output energy is then set at three times the threshold value to prevent inadvertent loss of capture. If the threshold increases above 5 V, the pacemaker wire should be re-sited. A temporary pacemaker unit is almost always set to work 'on demand' – to fire only when a spontaneous beat has not occurred. The rate of temporary pacing is usually 60–80 b.p.m.

Permanent pacing

Permanent pacemakers are fully implanted in the body and connected to the heart by one or two electrode leads. The pacemaker is powered by solid-state lithium batteries, which usually last 5–10 years. Modern pacemakers are 'programmable'. This means that their operating characteristics (e.g. the pacing rate) can be changed by a programmer that transmits specific electromagnetic signals through the skin. The pacemaker leads are passed transvenously to the right heart chambers.

Most pacemakers are designed to pace and sense the ventricles. Such pacemakers are described as 'VVI' units because they pace the ventricle (V), sense the ventricle (V) and are inhibited (I) by a spontaneous ventricular signal. Occasionally (e.g. in symptomatic sinus bradycardia), an atrial pacemaker (AAI) may be implanted. Pacemakers that are connected to both the right atrium and ventricle ('dual chamber' pacemakers) are used to simulate the natural pacemaker and activation sequence of the heart. This form of pacemaker is called DDD because it paces the two (Dual) chambers, senses both (D) and reacts in two (D) ways – pacing in the same chamber is inhibited by spontaneous atrial and ventricular signals, and ventricular pacing is triggered by spontaneous atrial events. Another form of 'physiological' pacemaker is the 'rate-responsive' system, which, by measuring activity, respiration, biochemical or electrical indicators with one or more biosensors, changes its rate of pacing so that it is appropriate to the level of exertion.

The choice of pacemaker mostly depends on the underlying condition (e.g. sick sinus syndrome must be treated with a dual-chamber device) and the general condition of the patient (inactive or infirm patients do not usually benefit from the most sophisticated units).

Permanent pacemakers are inserted under local anaesthetic using fluoroscopy to guide the insertion of the electrode leads. The pacemaker is usually positioned subcutaneously in front of the pectoral muscle. Following surgery, which usually takes 30–60 minutes, the patient rests in bed for 6–24 hours before being discharged. Patients may not drive until the pacemaker has been shown to be working correctly for at least one month after implantation, and must inform the licensing authorities and their motor insurers. Antibiotics may be prescribed prophylactically.

Complications are few but include the following:

- *Infection*. When a pacemaker system is infected, antibiotic treatment is not sufficient and the pacemaker must usually be removed before antibiotics will subdue the infection. Another pacemaker is fitted later.
- *Erosion*. The pacemaker may erode through the skin. This is usually due to a low-grade infection. Mechanical factors may also be responsible.
- *Lead displacement*. In most cases the pacing lead is securely wedged into the trabeculae of the right ventricle. It rarely displaces but when it does it may lead to sudden loss of pacing and a recurrence of prepacing symptoms.
- *Pacemaker malfunction*. This is now a very uncommon complication but requires replacement of the pacemaker.
- *Electromagnetic interference*. This is not common with modern pacemakers. High-tension cables, high-energy radars, arc-welding equipment and some medical equipment, such as MRI machines and lithotripters, may transiently inhibit the output of a pacemaker or convert it to interference mode (continuous pacing despite an adequate underlying rhythm). Digital cellular telephones may cause similar problems, but only when the telephone is held within 30 cm of the pacemaker.

Pericardiocentesis

A pericardial effusion is an accumulation of fluid between the parietal and visceral layers of pericardium. Fluid is removed to relieve symptoms that are due to haemodynamic embarrassment or for diagnostic purposes.

Pericardial aspiration or pericardiocentesis is performed by inserting a needle into the pericardial space, usually via a subxiphisternal route under ultrasound guidance. If a large volume of fluid is to be removed, a wide-bore needle and cannula are inserted. The needle may be removed and the cannula left *in situ* to drain the fluid. Fluid that is removed is sent for chemical analysis, microscopy, including cytology, and culture. If a reaccumulation of pericardial fluid is anticipated, the cannula may be left in place for several days or an operation can be performed to cut a window in the parietal pericardium (fenestration) or to remove a large section of the pericardium.

Right-heart bedside catheterization

Bedside catheterization of the pulmonary artery with a Swan–Ganz catheter may be performed in patients with:

- cardiac failure
- cardiogenic shock
- doubtful fluid status.

The catheter is used to measure cardiac output, pulmonary artery pressure, right atrial pressure and the pulmonary artery wedge pressure (an indirect measurement of left atrial pressure). The measurement of these pressures and the cardiac output allows appropriate therapy to be prescribed and the effects of that therapy to be monitored. The catheter also provides a route for the delivery of drugs to the central circulation (see Fig 13.16).

Intra-aortic balloon pumping

This is a technique used to assist temporarily the failing left ventricle. A catheter with a long sausage-shaped balloon at its tip is introduced percutaneously into the femoral artery and manipulated under X-ray control so that the balloon lies in the descending aorta just below the aortic arch. The balloon is rhythmically deflated and inflated with carbon dioxide gas. Using the ECG or intra-aortic pressure changes, the inflation is timed to occur during ventricular diastole to increase diastolic aortic pressure and consequently to improve coronary and cerebral blood flow. During systole the balloon is deflated, resulting in a reduction in the resistance to left ventricular emptying.

Improving cardiac output. Balloon pumping is used when there is a transient or reversible depression of left ventricular function, such as in a patient with severe mitral valve regurgitation who is awaiting surgical replacement of the mitral valve, or in a patient with a ventricular septal defect that is due to septal infarction.

Treating unstable angina pectoris. Balloon pumping is used to treat unstable angina pectoris by improving coronary flow and decreasing myocardial oxygen consumption by reducing the 'afterload'. This technique may be successful, even when medical therapy has failed. It is followed by early arteriography and appropriate definitive therapy such as surgery or coronary angioplasty.

Contraindications and complications

Balloon pumping should not be used when there is no remediable cause of cardiac dysfunction. It is also unsuitable in patients with aortic valve regurgitation or dissection of the aorta.

Complications of balloon pumping occur in about 20% of patients and include aortic dissection, leg ischaemia, emboli from the balloon, and balloon rupture. Embolic complications are reduced by anticoagulation with heparin.

FURTHER READING

Morley-Davis A, Cobbes M (1997) Cardiac pacing. *Lancet* **349**: 41–46

Skinner DV (1996) Cardiopulmonary Resuscitation, 2nd edn. Oxford: OUP.

Cardiac arrhythmias

An abnormality of the cardiac rhythm is called a *cardiac arrhythmia*. Such a disturbance of rhythm may cause sudden death, syncope, heart failure, dizziness, palpitations or no symptoms at all. There are two main types of arrhythmia:

- *bradycardia*, where the heart rate is slow (<60 b.p.m.) – the slower the heart rate the more likely the arrhythmia will be symptomatic
- *tachycardia*, where the heart rate is fast (>100 b.p.m.).

Tachycardias are more symptomatic when the arrhythmia is fast and sustained. Tachycardias are subdivided into supraventricular tachycardias, which arise from the atrium or the atrioventricular junction, and ventricular tachycardias, which arise from the ventricles.

Ventricular tachyarrhythmias tend to be more symptomatic than supraventricular tachycardias. Some arrhythmias occur in patients with apparently normal hearts, and in others arrhythmias reflect underlying cardiac abnormalities. When myocardial function is poor, ventricular arrhythmias tend to be more symptomatic and are potentially life-threatening.

Mechanisms of arrhythmia production

Abnormalities of automaticity, which could arise from a single cell, and abnormalities of conduction, which requires abnormal interaction between cells, account for both bradycardia and tachycardia. Sinus bradycardia is a result of abnormally slow automaticity while bradycardia due to AV block is caused by abnormal conduction within the AV node or the distal AV conduction system. The mechanisms of tachycardia production are shown in Fig 11.32.

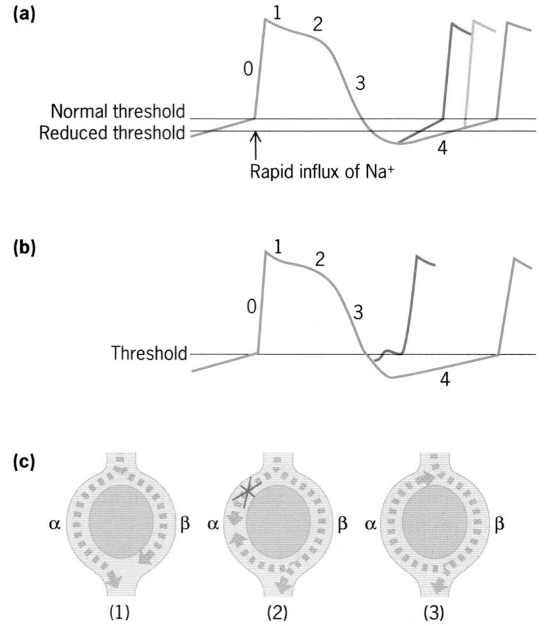

Fig 11.32
Mechanisms of arrhythmogenesis
(a) and (b) Action potentials (i.e. the potential difference between intracellular and extracellular fluid) of ventricular myocardium after stimulation
(a) Increased automaticity due to a reduced threshold potential or an increased slope of phase 4 depolarization (see p. 643)
(b) Triggered activity due to 'after' depolarizations reaching threshold potential
(c) Mechanism of circus movement or re-entry. In panel (1) the impulse passes down both limbs of the potential tachycardia circuit. In panel (2) the impulse is blocked in the pathway but proceeds slowly down the pathway and returns along the pathway. In panel (3) the impulse travels so slowly along the pathway that when it returns along the pathway to its starting point it is able to travel again down the pathway, producing a circus movement tachycardia

Accelerated automaticity (Fig 11.32a)

The normal mechanism of cardiac rhythmicity is slow depolarization of the transmembrane voltage during diastole until the threshold potential is reached and the action potential of the pacemaker cells takes off. This mechanism may be accelerated by increasing the rate of diastolic depolarization or changing the threshold potential. Such changes are thought to produce sinus tachycardia, escape rhythms and accelerated AV nodal rhythms.

Triggered activity (Fig 11.32b)

Myocardial damage can result in oscillations of the transmembrane potential at the end of the action potential. These oscillations may reach threshold potential and produce an arrhythmia. The abnormal oscillations can be exaggerated by pacing and by catecholamines and these stimuli can be used to trigger this abnormal form of automaticity. The atrial tachycardias produced by digoxin toxicity are due to triggered activity. The initiation of ventricular arrhythmia in the long QT syndrome may

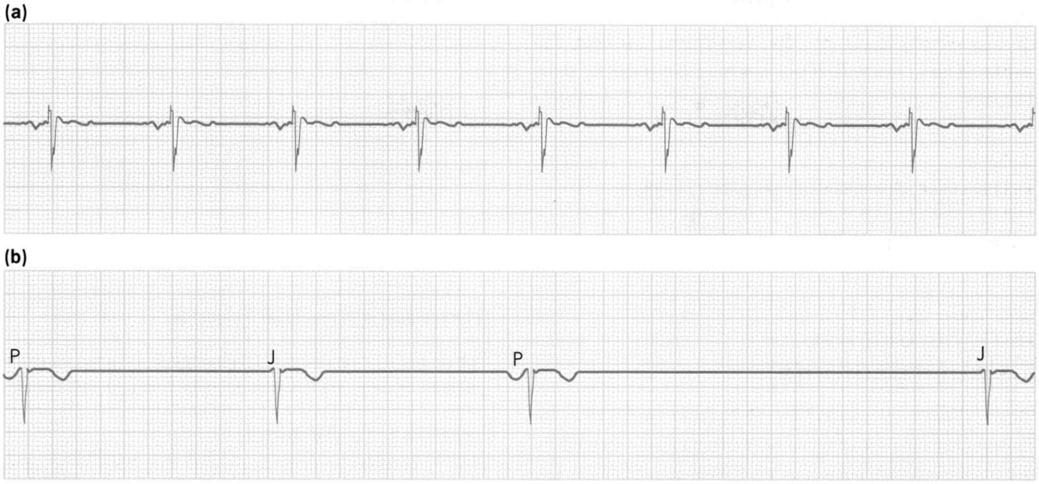

Fig 11.33
(a) An ECG showing normal sinus rhythm (PR interval <0.2 s). P wave preceding each QRS complex
(b) A patient with sick sinus syndrome. This shows sinus arrest (only occasional sinus P waves) and junctional escape beats (J). P waves are inverted in the cavity leads that are shown here

be caused by this mechanism, but re-entry may also be involved in the perpetuation of the arrhythmia.

Re-entry (or circus movement) (Fig 11.32c)

A wave of depolarization may be forced to travel in one direction around a ring of cardiac tissue. If the time to conduct around the ring is longer than the recovery of any tissue within the ring, circus movement will result, producing a tachycardia. The majority of regular paroxysmal tachycardias are thought to be produced by this mechanism.

Sinus rhythms

The normal cardiac pacemaker is the sinus node and, like most cardiac tissue, it depolarizes spontaneously. Its rate of discharge is controlled by the autonomic nervous system. Normally the parasympa-thetic system predomi-nates, resulting in slowing of the spontaneous discharge rate from approximately 100 to 70 b.p.m. A reduction of parasympathetic tone or an increase in sympathetic stimulation leads to tachycardia; con-versely, increased parasympathetic tone and decreased sympathetic stimulation produces bradycardia. The sinus rate in women is slightly faster than in men. Normal sinus rhythm is characterized by P waves that are upright in leads I and II of the ECG (see Fig 11.18 on p. 644), but are inverted in the cavity leads AVR and V_1 (Fig 11.33).

Sinus arrhythmia

Fluctuations of autonomic tone result in phasic changes of the sinus discharge rate. Thus, during inspiration, parasympathetic tone falls and the heart rate quickens, and on expiration the heart rate falls. This variation is normal, particularly in children and young adults.

Sinus bradycardia

A sinus rate of less than 60 b.p.m. during the day or less than 50 b.p.m. at night is known as *sinus bradycardia*. It is usually asymptomatic unless the rate is very slow. It is normal in athletes and in elderly patients. Causes include:

- hypothermia, hypothyroidism, cholestatic jaundice and raised intracranial pressure
- drug therapy with β-blockers, digitalis and other antiarrhythmic drugs
- acute ischaemia and infarction of the sinus node
- chronic degenerative changes such as fibrosis of the atrium and sinus node.

TREATMENT

Treatment of acute symptomatic sinus bradycardia is with intravenous atropine 600 μg. If the symptomatic arrhythmia persists and there is no reversible cause, a permanent cardiac pacemaker is required.

Sinus tachycardia

Sinus rate acceleration to more than 100 b.p.m. is known as *sinus tachycardia*. Causes include:

- fever
- exercise
- emotion
- pregnancy
- anaemia
- cardiac failure with compensatory sinus tachycardia
- thyrotoxicosis
- catecholamine excess
- primary sinus tachycardia (rare).

TREATMENT

This involves correction of the condition causing the tachycardia. If necessary, β-blockers may be used to slow the sinus rate.

Pathological bradycardias

There are two main forms of severe bradycardia: sinus node disease and atrioventricular block.

Sinus node disease (sick sinus syndrome)

Sinus node disease is caused by ischaemia, infarction or degenerative disease of the sinus node. It is characterized by long intervals between consecutive P waves (>2 s) on the ECG (Fig 11.33). These sinus pauses may be an exact multiple of the basic sinus interval (sinoatrial exit block) or not (sinus arrest). Both conditions have a similar prognosis.

Sinus pauses and sinus bradycardia may allow cardiac tachyarrhythmias to emerge. A combination of fast and slow supraventricular rhythms is known as the tachycardia-bradycardia ('tachy-brady') syndrome.

TREATMENT

Treatment of chronic symptomatic sick sinus syndrome requires permanent pacing, with additional antiarrhythmic drugs to manage any tachycardia element. Thromboembolism is common in tachy-brady syndrome and patients should be anticoagulated unless there is a contraindication.

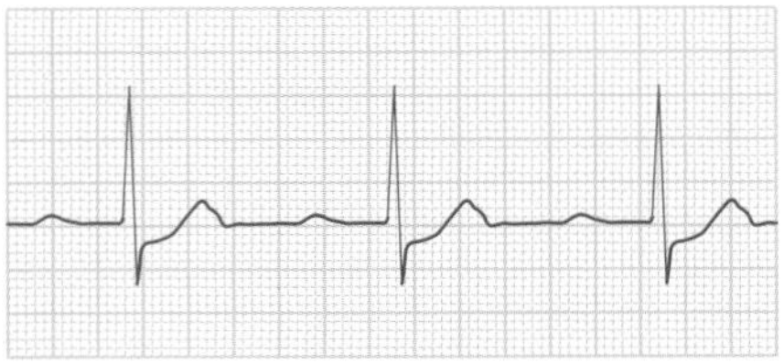

Fig 11.34
An ECG showing first-degree atrioventricular block with a prolonged PR interval. In this trace coincidental ST depression is also present

Atrioventricular block

There are three forms: first-degree block, second-degree (partial) block, and third-degree (complete) block.

First-degree AV block

This is simple prolongation of the PR interval to more than 0.22 s. Every atrial depolarization is followed by conduction to the ventricles but with delay (Fig 11.34).

Second-degree (partial) AV block

This occurs when some P waves conduct and others do not. There are several forms of second-degree AV block (Fig 11.35).

- *Mobitz I block* (Wenckebach block phenomenon) is progressive PR interval prolongation until a P wave fails to conduct. The PR interval before the blocked P wave is much longer than the PR interval after the blocked P wave.
- *Mobitz II block* occurs when a dropped QRS complex is not preceded by progressive PR interval prolongation.

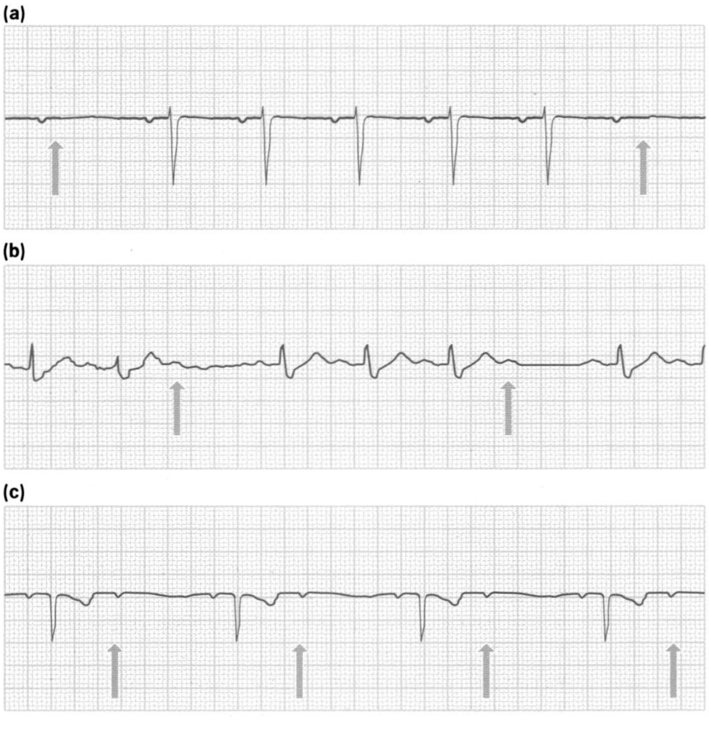

Fig 11.35
Three varieties of second-degree atrioventricular (AV) block
(a) *Wenckebach (Mobitz type I) AV block.* The PR interval gradually prolongs until the P wave does not conduct to the ventricles (arrows)
(b) *Mobitz type II AV block.* The P waves that do not conduct to the ventricles (arrows) are not preceded by gradual PR interval prolongation
(c) *Two P waves to each QRS complex.* The PR interval prior to the dropped P wave is always the same. It is not possible to define this type of AV block as type I or type II Mobitz block and it is, therefore, a third variety of second-degree AV block (arrows show P waves)

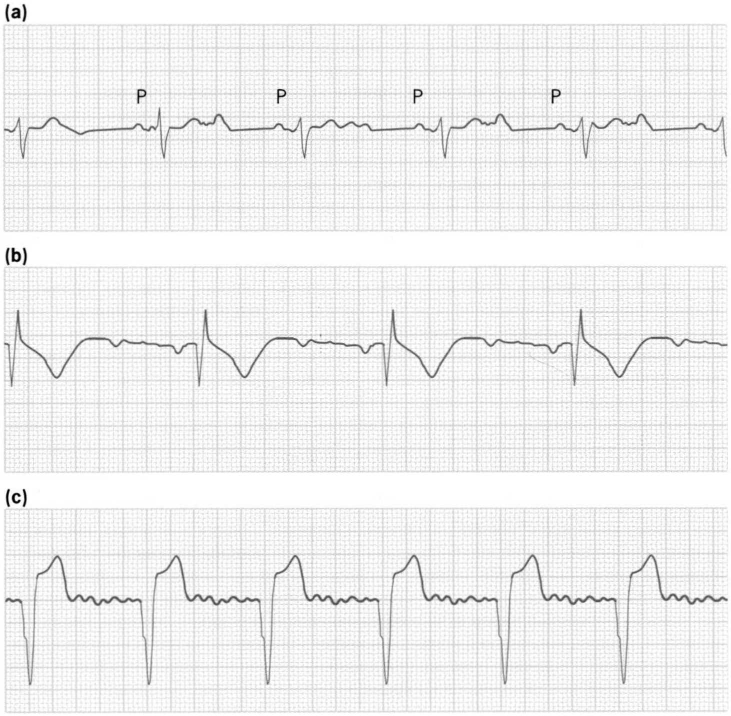

Fig 11.36
Three examples of complete heart block
(a) Congenital complete heart block. The QRS complex is narrow (0.08 s) and the QRS rate is relatively rapid (52 b.p.m.)
(b) Acquired complete heart block. The QRS complex is broad (0.13 s) and the QRS rate is relatively slow (38 b.p.m.)
(c) Drug-induced complete heart block in a patient with atrial fibrillation rather than sinus rhythm (note the undulating baseline but the regular and slow ventricular rate)

- *2:1 or 3:1 (advanced) block* occurs when every second or third P wave conducts to the ventricles. This form of second-degree block is neither Mobitz I nor II. A 4:1 block or 5:1 block can also occur.

Wenckebach block is more benign than other forms of second-degree block. Patients with 2° block are usually asymptomatic. A close watch should be kept on them, although no treatment may be necessary unless more serious or symptomatic heart block develops. Patients with Mobitz II or advanced AV block may need pacing.

Third-degree (complete) AV block

This occurs when no P waves conduct to the ventricles (Fig 11.36). In this situation life is maintained by a spontaneous escape rhythm that has either broad (≥0.12 s) or narrow (<0.12 s) QRS complexes.

Narrow complex escape rhythm

This is due to disease in the AV node or the proximal His bundle. The escape rhythm occurs with an adequate rate (50–60 b.p.m.) and is relatively reliable. It occurs in association with:

- congenital heart disease (such as transposition of the great arteries)
- an isolated congenital problem (congenital heart block)
- myocardial infarction
- diphtheria
- rheumatic fever
- toxic concentrations of drugs such as digitalis, verapamil or β-blockers
- aortic calcification
- endocarditis.

Treatment is often unnecessary except for the eradication of toxic causes. Recent-onset narrow-complex AV block due to acute myocardial infarction may respond to intravenous atropine, but a temporary pacemaker may be necessary. Chronic narrow-complex AV block requires permanent pacing if it is symptomatic or associated with heart disease.

Increasingly, permanent pacing is advocated for asymptomatic, isolated, congenital AV block.

Broad complex escape rhythm

This occurs because of disease in the Purkinje system. The escape pacemaker arises from the distal Purkinje network or the ventricular myocardium. The resulting rhythm is slow (15–40 b.p.m.) and relatively unreliable. Dizziness and blackouts (Stokes–Adams attacks) often occur. In the elderly, it is usually caused by degenerative fibrosis and calcification of the distal conduction system (Lenegre's disease) or the more proximal conduction system (Lev's disease). In younger patients, broad-complex AV block may be caused by ischaemic heart disease.

A permanent pacemaker should always be inserted, as the mortality from the condition, even when asymptomatic, is considerably reduced by pacing.

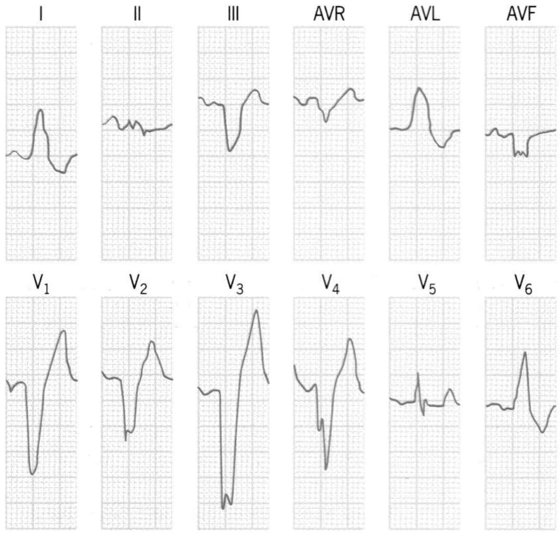

Fig 11.37
A 12-lead ECG showing left bundle branch block. The QRS duration is greater than 0.12 s. Note the broad notched R waves with ST depression in leads I, AVL, and V_6, and the broad QS waves in V_1–V_3

Intraventricular conduction disturbances

The intraventricular conduction system consists of the His bundle, the right and left bundle branches and the antero-superior and postero-inferior divisions of the left bundle branch. Various conduction disturbances can occur:

His bundle delay. This may produce a long PR interval but it is often too small a delay to be noticed on the surface ECG.

Blocked His bundle conduction. This produces AV block.

Bundle branch conduction delay. This produces trivial widening of the QRS complex (up to 0.11 s). It is known as incomplete bundle branch block.

Complete block of a bundle branch. This is associated with a wider QRS complex (0.12 s or more). The shape of the QRS depends on whether the right or the left bundle is blocked. Right bundle branch block (an example is shown in Fig 11.66 on p. 697) produces late activation of the right ventricle. This is seen as deep S waves in leads I and V_6 and as a tall late R wave in lead V_1 (see Fig 11.87 on p. 721) (late activation moving towards right and away from left-sided leads). Left bundle branch block (Fig 11.37) produces the opposite – a deep S wave in lead V_1 and a tall late R wave in leads I and V_6. Because left bundle branch conduction is normally responsible for the initial ventricular activation, left bundle branch block also produces abnormal Q waves.

Delay or block in the divisions of the left bundle branch produces a swing in the direction of depolarization (electrical axis) of the heart. When the anterosuperior division is blocked, the left ventricle is activated from inferior to superior. This produces a superior (leftwards) movement of the axis. Delay or block in the posteroinferior division swings the QRS axis inferiorly.

Bisfascicular block (see Fig 11.66). This is a combination of a block of any two of the following: the right bundle branch, the left anterosuperior division and the left posteroinferior division. Block of the remaining fascicle will result in complete AV block.

Table 11.11 Causes of right bundle branch block. It is also a normal finding in 1% of young adults and 5% of elderly adults

Congenital heart disease Atrial septal defect Fallot's tetralogy Pulmonary stenosis Ventricular septal defect	**Myocardial disease** Acute myocardial infarction Cardiomyopathy Conduction system fibrosis
Pulmonary disease Cor pulmonale Recurrent pulmonary embolism Acute pulmonary embolism (transient)	**Drugs and electrolytes** Hyperkalaemia Class 1a drugs **Right ventriculotomy**

Table 11.12
Causes of left bundle branch block

Left ventricular outflow obstruction Aortic stenosis Hypertension	**Cardiomyopathy** **Conduction system fibrosis**
Coronary artery disease Acute myocardial infarction Severe coronary disease (two- to three-vessel disease)	

CLINICAL FEATURES

Intraventricular conduction disturbances other than complete block of the His bundle are usually asymptomatic. Sometimes the onset of left bundle branch block actually seems to provoke chest pain.

Right bundle branch block causes wide but physiological splitting of the second heart sound. Left bundle branch block may cause reverse splitting of the second sound. Patients with intraventricular conduction disturbances may complain of syncope. This is due to intermittent complete heart block or to ventricular tachyarrhythmias. ECG monitoring and electro-physiological studies are needed to determine the cause of syncope in these patients.

CAUSES

Right bundle branch block (Table 11.11) occurs as an isolated congenital anomaly or is associated with right ventricular overload. Left bundle branch block (Table 11.12) is almost always caused by disease of the left ventricle. All forms of intraventricular conduction disturbance may be caused by ischaemic heart disease and cardiomyopathy.

Table 11.13
Causes of atrial arrhythmias

Hypertension
Ischaemic heart disease
Rheumatic heart disease
Thyrotoxicosis
Cardiomyopathy
Lone atrial fibrillation (i.e. no cause discovered)
Junctional tachycardia (e.g. Wolff–Parkinson-White syndrome)
Pneumonia
Atrial septal defect
Carcinoma of the bronchus
Pericarditis
Pulmonary embolus
Acute and chronic alcohol abuse
Cardiac surgery

Conduction system fibrosis and calcification (Lenegre's disease and Lev's disease, see above) are progressive conditions that may present with bundle branch block or bifascicular block and eventually lead to complete heart block, when a pacemaker will be required.

Bradycardic syndromes

Carotid sinus syndrome (which occurs predominantly in the old) and neurocardiogenic syndrome (which often occurs in the young) both present with recurrent syncope and presyncope. These two autonomic syndromes are characterized by bradycardia (AV block and/or sinus arrest) and hypotension. Carotid sinus syndrome is usually bradycardic and the neurocardiogenic syndrome is usually hypotensive. Fainting in the carotid sinus syndrome is due to stimulation of the carotid sinus by turning the neck, wearing stiff collars or coughing. In neurocardiogenic syndrome, syncope results from a variety of situations that affect the autonomic nervous system.

Carotid sinus syndrome often requires treatment with a dual-chamber pacemaker. Neurocardiogenic syncope may be ameliorated by pacemaker treatment. Compression of the lower legs with hose and drugs such as β-blockers, α-agonists or myocardial negative inotropes (such as disopyramide) may be helpful. Symptomatic bradycardia (sinus bradycardia) or AV nodal block generally requires implantation of a permanent pacemaker unless a reversible cause is found.

Pathological tachycardias

Atrial tachyarrhythmias

Ectopic beats, tachycardia, flutter and fibrillation may all arise from the atrial myocardium. They share common aetiologies, which are listed in Table 11.13.

Atrial ectopic beats

These often cause no symptoms although they may be sensed as an irregularity or heaviness of the heart beat.

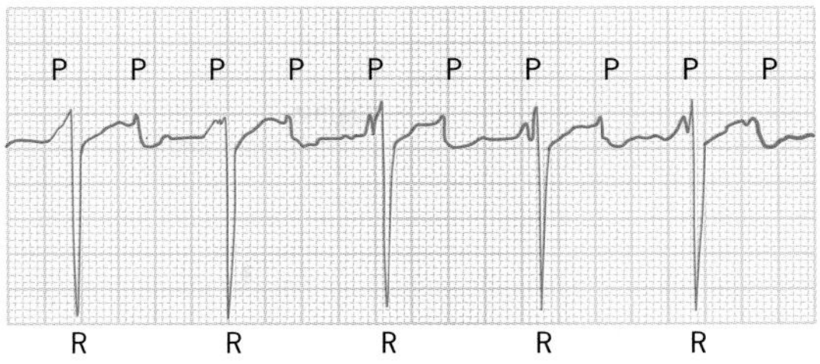

Fig 11.38
Atrial tachycardia with second-degree atrioventricular block. Note the fast atrial (P wave) rate of 150 per minute and the slower ventricular (R wave) rate of 75 per minute. This arrhythmia is most commonly due to digoxin toxicity

On the ECG they appear as early and abnormal P waves, and are usually, but not always, followed by normal QRS complexes (see Fig 11.39(a)).

Treatment is not normally required unless the ectopic beats provoke more significant arrhythmias, when β-blockade may be effective.

Atrial tachycardia

This is an uncommon arrhythmia. (Previously, arrhythmias arising from the AV junction were wrongly called 'atrial tachycardias'). There are three varieties of true atrial tachycardia:

- paroxysmal tachycardia
- incessant tachycardia
- atrial tachycardia with AV block.

Most are associated with heart disease, but incessant atrial tachycardia may occur in young children with no obvious heart disease. Atrial tachycardia with block is often a result of digitalis poisoning.

Figure 11.38 demonstrates an atrial tachycardia at an atrial rate of 150 per minute. The P waves are abnormally shaped and occur in front of the QRS complexes. Carotid sinus massage may increase AV block during tachycardia but does not usually terminate the arrhythmia. Treatment with class Ia, Ic or III drugs (see p. 670) is usually successful (e.g. disopyramide 2 mg kg^{-1} over 10 minutes).

Atrial flutter

This is a rhythm disturbance that is usually associated with organic heart disease. The atrial rate varies between 280 and 350 per minute but is usually around 300 per minute.

Symptoms are largely related to the degree of AV block. Most often, every second flutter beat conducts, giving a ventricular rate of 150 per minute. Occasionally, every beat conducts, producing a heart rate of 300 b.p.m. More often, especially when patients are receiving treatment, AV conduction block reduces the heart rate to approximately 75 b.p.m.

The ECG shows regular sawtooth-like atrial flutter waves (F waves) between QRST complexes (Figs 11.39(b) and (c)). If they are not clearly visible, AV conduction may be transiently impaired by carotid sinus

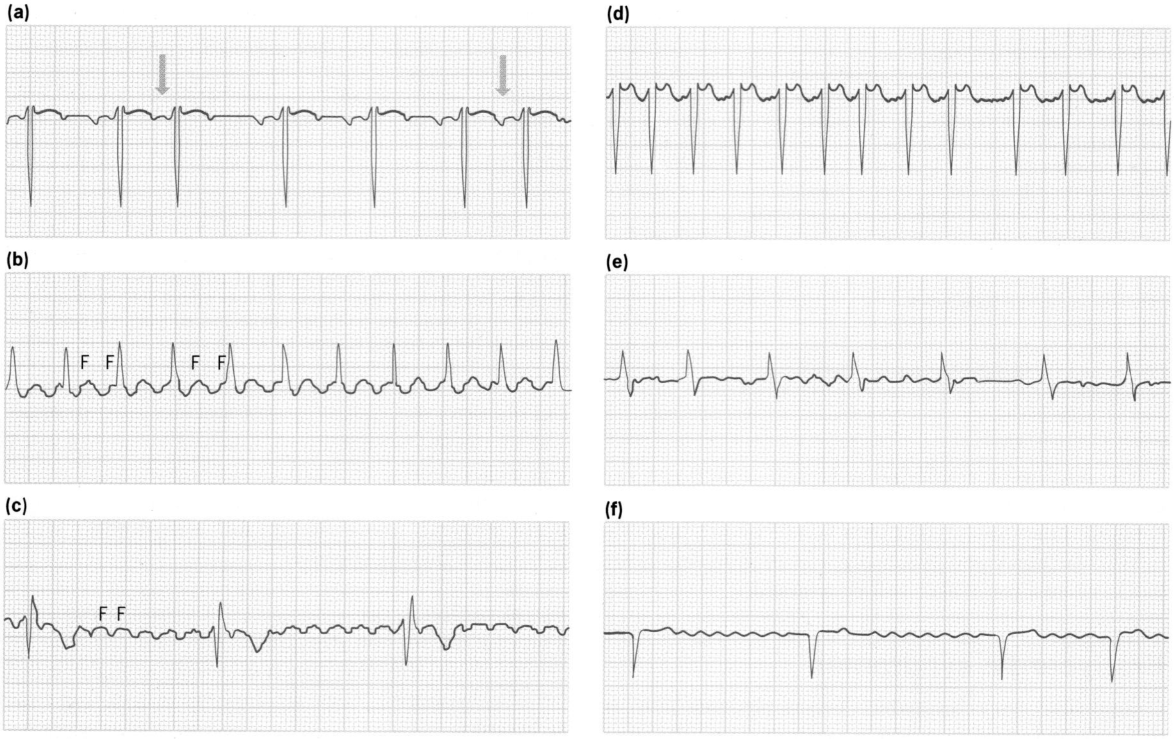

Fig 11.39
ECGs of a variety of atrial arrhythmias
(a) Atrial premature beats (arrows). The premature P wave is different to the sinus P wave and conducts to the ventricle with a slightly prolonged PR interval
(b) Atrial flutter. Some flutter waves are marked with an F. In this case the flutter frequency is 270 per minute. Every second flutter wave is transmitted to the ventricles, and the ventricular rate is therefore 135 per minute
(c) Atrial flutter at a frequency of 305 per minute. The ventricular rate is approximately 38 per minute. Therefore, only one in eight flutter waves is transmitted to the ventricles
(d) Irregular ventricular response. This is typical of rapidly conducted atrial fibrillation
(e) Moderate conduction of atrial fibrillation. The underlying baseline undulations can now be appreciated
(f) So-called 'slow' atrial fibrillation. The ventricular response rate is slow and the underlying atrial fibrillation is seen as minor fluctuations of the baseline

massage or by the administration of AV nodal blocking drugs such as verapamil.

Treatment of a symptomatic acute paroxysm is electrical cardioversion (50 J, 100 J, then 360 J) and Class III drugs are also often effective. Prophylaxis is achieved with class Ia, Ic or III drugs (see p. 670). AV nodal blocking drugs (classes II or IV or digitalis) may be used to control the ventricular rate if the arrythmia persists. However, the treatment of choice for patients with frequent episodes of, or with, persistent typical atrial flutter is now radiofrequency catheter ablation (see p. 673). This technique offers patients whose only arrhythmia is typical atrial flutter an almost certain chance of a cure.

Atrial fibrillation

This is a common arrhythmia, occurring in 5–10% of patients over 65 years of age. It also occurs, particularly in a paroxysmal form, in younger patients. It is caused by a raised atrial pressure, increased atrial muscle mass, atrial fibrosis, or inflammation and infiltration of the atrium.

Atrial fibrillation is continuous, rapid (400 per minute) activation of the atria by multiple meandering wavelets. The atria respond electrically at this rate but there is no coordinated mechanical action and only a proportion of the impulses are conducted.

AETIOLOGY

This includes most cardiac disorders, but in some patients no cause can be found – 'lone atrial fibrillation'. Thyrotoxicosis may provoke atrial fibrillation, sometimes as virtually the only feature of the disease. Thyroid function tests are mandatory in any patient with unaccounted atrial fibrillation.

SYMPTOMS AND SIGNS

Symptoms attributable to atrial fibrillation are highly variable. In some patients it is an incidental finding whilst others attend hospital as an emergency following the onset of atrial fibrillation. Most patients experience some deterioration on exercise capacity or well-being, but this may only be appreciated once sinus rhythm is restored. When caused by rheumatic mitral stenosis, the onset of atrial fibrillation results in considerable worsening of cardiac failure.

The patient has a very irregular pulse, as opposed to a basically regular pulse with an occasional irregularity (e.g. extrasystoles) or recurring irregular patterns (e.g. Wenckebach block). The irregular nature of the pulse in atrial fibrillation is maintained during exercise.

The ECG shows fine oscillations of the baseline (so-called fibrillation or F waves) and no clear P waves. The QRS rhythm is rapid and irregular. Untreated, the ventricular rate is usually 120–180 per minute, but it slows with treatment (Figs 11.39(d), (e) and (f)).

MANAGEMENT

When atrial fibrillation is due to an acute precipitating event such as alcohol toxicity, chest infection or thyrotoxicosis, the provoking cause should be treated. Strategies for the acute management of AF are ventricular rate control or cardioversion (± anticoagulation). Ventricular rate control is achieved by drugs which block the AV node (see below) while the cardioversion is achieved electrically by DC shock (see p. 656) or medically by intravenous infusion of an anti-arrhythmic drug of class Ia, Ic or amiodarone. The choice depends upon:

- how well the arrhythmia is tolerated (is cardioversion urgent?)
- whether anticoagulation is required before considering elective cardioversion (to minimize the excess risk of thromboembolism associated with cardioversion of AF which is more than 1–2 days' duration)
- whether spontaneous cardioversion is likely (previous history? reversible cause?).

Conversion to sinus rhythm can then be achieved by electrical DC cardioversion 200 J, then 2 × 360 J (see p. 656) in about 80% of patients. Recurrent paroxysms may be prevented by oral medication with class Ia, Ic or III drugs.

If the arrhythmia is chronic and cannot be converted to sinus rhythm, AV nodal blocking drugs should be used to control the ventricular response rate. This should generally be below 90 b.p.m. at rest. The most usual drug used for this purpose is digoxin. However, β-blockers and verapamil are commonly required to control the ventricular response rate during activity. Catheter ablation (see p. 673) of the AV node in conjunction with implantation of a permanent pacemaker may also be used to control the ventricular rate during atrial fibrillation. This technique may be particularly useful where there is impairment of ventricular function which limits the use of drugs other than digitalis. Modification of AV nodal function (partial ablation) may allow control of the ventricular rate without the need for a pacemaker.

Anticoagulation (INR 2.5) is essential when atrial fibrillation is associated with valvular heart disease, left ventricular dysfunction, old age (>75 years) or hypertension. Anticoagulation is also advised if there has been a previous thromboembolus, if the left atrium is enlarged or if the left ventricle does not function well. In most other patients aspirin is prescribed. Young patients (< 60 years) with no heart disease (lone AF) may not require any treatment unless the cause is alcoholic heart disease, thyrotoxicosis or sick sinus syndrome.

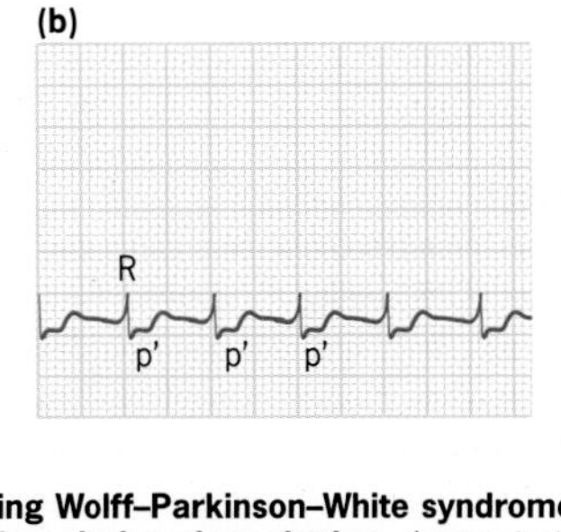

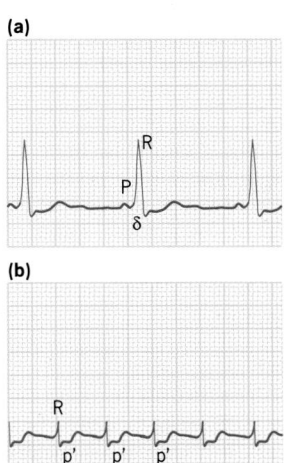

Fig 11.40
An ECG showing Wolff–Parkinson–White syndrome
(a) A trace taken during sinus rhythm, demonstrating a short PR interval (0.09 s) and broad QRS complex (0.12 s)
(b) Paroxysmal junctional tachycardia associated with this syndrome. Note the tachycardia p' waves, which closely follow each QRS complex δ wave (a slurred upstroke)

Junctional re-entrant tachycardia

Almost all junctional tachycardia is paroxysmal in nature. There is usually no associated structural heart disease but there may be demonstrable electrophysiological or electrocardiographic abnormalities such as the Wolff–Parkinson–White syndrome (Fig 11.40) (see p. 665) or the Lown–Ganong–Levine syndrome (in which there is an anomalous connection between the atrium and the bundle of His).

There are two main varieties of junctional tachycardia:

- intra-AV nodal re-entry tachycardia (AVNRT)
- atrioventricular re-entry tachycardia (AVRT).

In the intra-AV nodal re-entry tachycardia the entire tachycardia circuit is confined to the AV node and its surrounding myocardium. In atrioventricular re-entry tachycardia there is a large circuit comprising the AV node, the His bundle, the ventricle, an abnormal connection and the atrium. The abnormal connection linking the ventricle to the atrium completes the circuit necessary to sustain the tachycardia.

Clinically, the tachycardia often strikes suddenly without obvious provocation, but exertion, coffee, tea and alcohol

Practical

Carotid sinus massage is performed for three reasons:

- to break junctional tachycardia by blocking AV nodal conduction
- to reveal on the ECG the P wave pattern of an atrial arrhythmia by reducing the frequency of AV nodal conduction during the tachycardia so that the QRS complexes do not mask the artrial activity
- to test for carotid sinus hypersensitivity, which is a severe fall in blood pressure or heart rate in response to carotid sinus stimulation

The carotid sinus is stimulated by firm rotary pressure of the carotid sinus against the transverse processes of the third cervical vertebrum. Provided that there is no carotid bruit, each carotid should be tried in turn. In general, right carotid pressure tends to slow the sinus rate and left carotid pressure tends to impair AV nodal conduction.

Practical Box 11.4 Carotid sinus massage

may aggravate or induce the arrhythmia. The rhythm is rapid (140–280 per minute) and regular. An attack may stop spontaneously or may continue indefinitely until medical intervention. The predominant symptom is palpitations, but chest pain, dyspnoea, pure syncope and polyuria may develop. The polyuria occurs because tachycardia leads to an elevated atrial pressure and the release of atrial natriuretic peptide and other hormones.

The rhythm is recognized by normal QRS complexes at a rate of 140–280 per minute. Sometimes the QRS complexes will show typical bundle branch block (aberration). In the Wolff–Parkinson–White syndrome, the tachycardia is occasionally pre-excited whereby conduction from the atria to the ventricles proceeds via the accessory pathway. The P waves are often obscured, but generally occur simultaneously with the QRS complex (AV nodal tachycardia) or just after the QRS in the ST segment or the T wave (atrioventricular tachycardia).

Treatment of acute supraventricular tachycardia

An acute paroxysm of tachycardia is easy to treat.

Vagotonic manoeuvres

Most supraventricular arrhythmias require conduction through the AV node for their continuation or their expression at ventricular level. An intense efferent vagal discharge increases AV nodal conduction time and the AV nodal recovery time. Thus, atrial arrhythmias may be revealed on the ECG by vagotonic stimulation, which blocks the transmission of these arrhythmias to the ventricles, and junctional tachycardias that involve the AV node may be terminated by these manoeuvres.

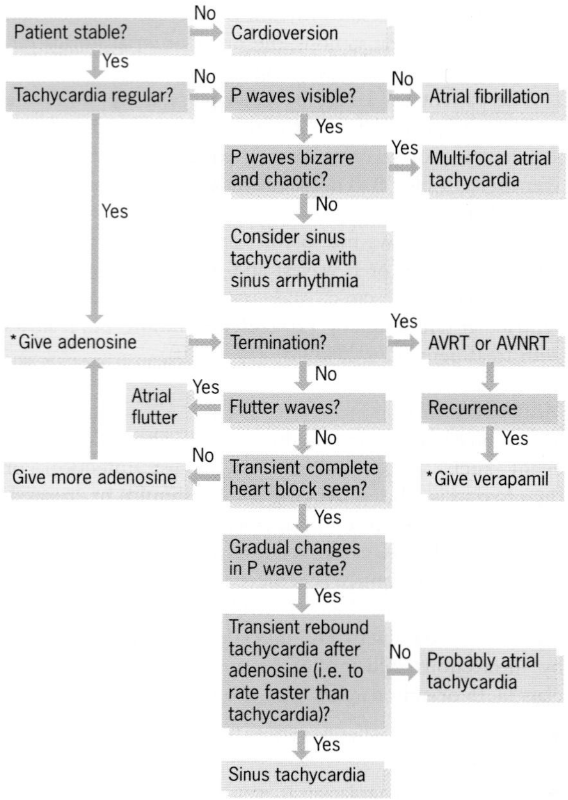

Fig 11.41
Management of tachycardia. Narrow complex
AVRT, atrioventicular re-entry tachycardia
AVNRT, intra-AV nodal re-entry tachycardia
*if haemodynamic instability develops proceed to immediate cardioversion

Carotid sinus massage (Practical box 11.4), ocular pressure, immersion of the face in water (diving reflex) and the Valsalva manoeuvre may be used to stimulate the vagal efferent discharge. Of these techniques the Valsalva manoeuvre is the best and often easier for the patient to perform successfully. It should be undertaken when the patient is resting in the supine position (thus avoiding elevated background sympathetic tone). Several seconds after the release of strain, the resulting intense vagal effect may terminate a junctional re-entry tachycardia or may produce sufficient AV block to reveal an underlying atrial tachyarrhythmia.

Drug treatment (Fig 11.41)

If physical manoeuvres have not been successful, intravenous adenosine (up to 0.25 $mg\,kg^{-1}$) should be tried. This is a very short-acting (half-life <10 s) naturally occurring purine nucleoside that causes complete heart block for a fraction of a second following i.v. administration. It is highly effective at terminating junctional tachycardias or revealing atrial tachycardias. It rarely affects ventricular tachycardia. The side-effects of adenosine are very brief but include bronchospasm, chest pain and heaviness of the limbs. It is contraindicated in patients with a history of asthma.

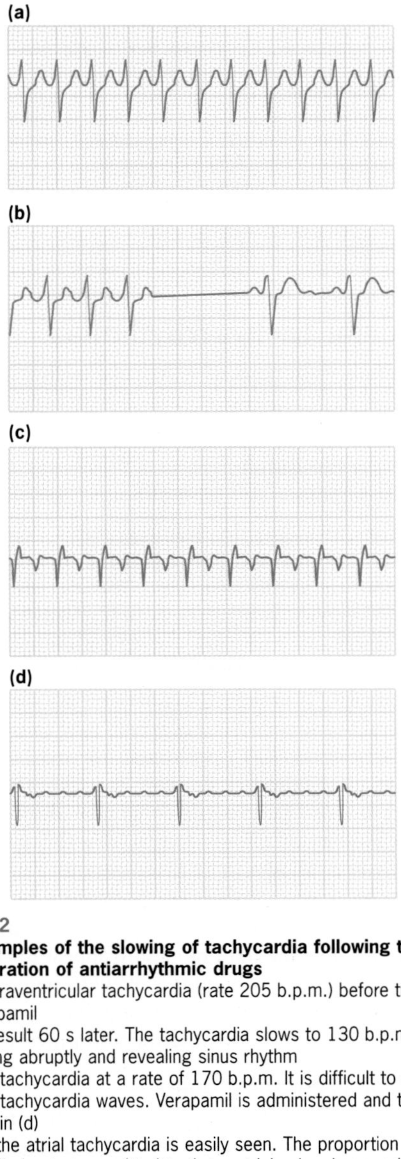

Fig 11.42
Two examples of the slowing of tachycardia following the administration of antiarrhythmic drugs
(a) A supraventricular tachycardia (rate 205 b.p.m.) before treatment with verapamil
(b) The result 60 s later. The tachycardia slows to 130 b.p.m. before terminating abruptly and revealing sinus rhythm
(c) Atrial tachycardia at a rate of 170 b.p.m. It is difficult to discern the atrial tachycardia waves. Verapamil is administered and the result is shown in (d)
(d) Now the atrial tachycardia is easily seen. The proportion of atrial tachycardia beats transmitted to the ventricles has been reduced following the administration of verapamil

An alternative treatment is verapamil 10 mg i.v. over 5–10 minutess (Fig 11.42). It is important not to give verapamil if β-blockers have been previously administered or if the tachycardia presents with broad (>0.14 s) QRS complexes.

Other treatments

Rarely, medical therapy fails to terminate a tachycardia and rapid atrial pacing (directly or via the oesophagus) or DC cardioversion may be considered.

Prophylaxis

To prevent recurrences, drugs may be used to impair AV nodal conduction (classes II and IV and digoxin), impair abnormal connection conduction (classes Ia and III), or suppress the ectopic beats that initiate the arrhythmia (classes I, II and III) (see p. 670). In most cases, however, AV nodal modification, by a radiofrequency ablation technique, is used to destroy the tachycardia circuit and prevent recurrences. This technique involves introducing catheters from a large vein or artery into the heart and identifying the atrial or ventricular insertion site of the accessory pathway by recording the electrograms at the tip of the catheter. Once the ablation catheter is in position, radiofrequency energy is delivered to its tip to achieve a local tissue temperature of around 60°C.

Table 11.14 Causes of prolonged repolarization syndrome (long QT interval and torsades de pointes tachycardia)

Congenital syndromes
Jervell–Lange–Nelson (autosomal recessive)
Romano–Ward (autosomal dominant)
Electrolyte abnormalities
Hypokalaemia
Hypomagnesaemia
Hypocalcaemia
Drugs
Quinidine (and other class Ia antiarrhythmic drugs)
Sotalol (and other class III antiarrhythmic drugs)
Amitriptyline (and other tricyclic antidepressants)
Chlorpromazine (and other phenothiazine drugs)
Terfenadine and astemizole
Terodiline
Erythromycin and the macrolides
Cisapride
Poisons
Organophosphate insecticides
Miscellaneous
Bradycardia
Mitral valve prolapse
Acute myocardial infarction
Prolonged fasting and liquid protein diets (long term)
Central nervous system diseases

Wolff–Parkinson–White (WPW) syndrome

This is a congenital condition caused by an abnormal myocardial connection between atrium and ventricle (bundle of Kent). During sinus rhythm the electrical impulse can conduct quickly over this abnormal connection to depolarize part of the ventricles abnormally. This results in the typical ECG pattern of WPW syndrome – a short PR interval and a wide QRS complex that begins as a slurred part known as the δ wave (see Fig 11.40). About half of those with WPW pattern on the ECG have tachycardias (Fig 11.40(b)). The tachycardias are of two sorts.

Atrioventricular re-entry. This is a circus movement tachycardia in which a depolarization wave travels from the atrium to the ventricle, usually through the AV node, and from the ventricle to the atrium through the abnormal pathway. Intravenous adenosine will terminate most of these tachycardias.

(a)

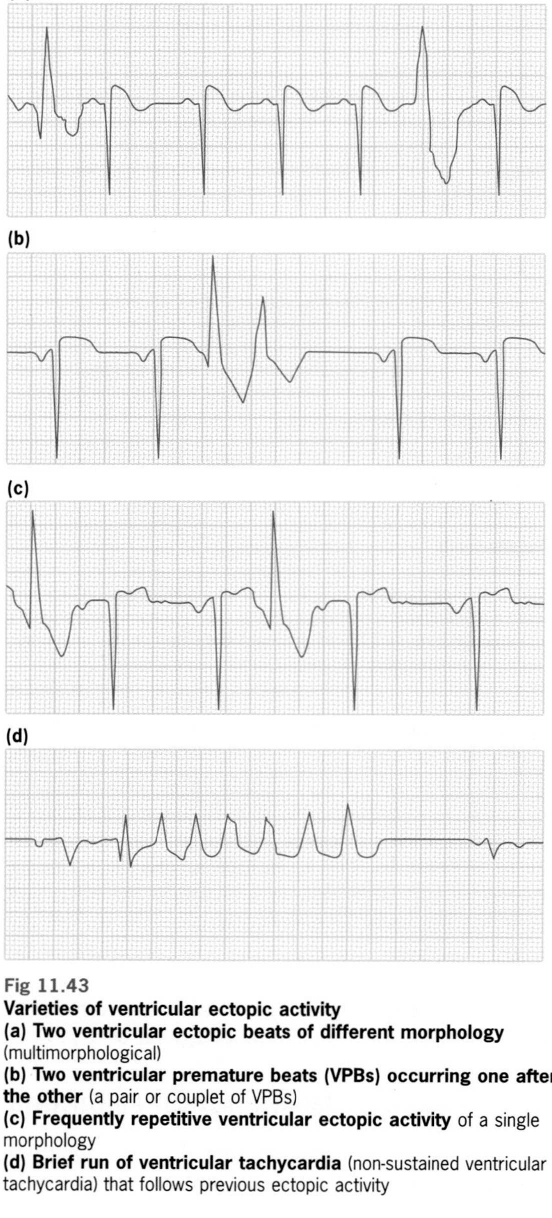

Fig 11.43
Varieties of ventricular ectopic activity
(a) Two ventricular ectopic beats of different morphology (multimorphological)
(b) Two ventricular premature beats (VPBs) occurring one after the other (a pair or couplet of VPBs)
(c) Frequently repetitive ventricular ectopic activity of a single morphology
(d) Brief run of ventricular tachycardia (non-sustained ventricular tachycardia) that follows previous ectopic activity

Atrial fibrillation. During atrial fibrillation the ventricles may be depolarized by impulses travelling over both the abnormal and the normal pathways. The conduction ability of the abnormal pathway is depressed by drugs that affect the atrium (e.g. classes I and III) but not by verapamil and digoxin, which may allow a higher rate of conduction over the abnormal pathway. Therefore, neither verapamil nor digoxin should be used to treat atrial fibrillation associated with the WPW syndrome.

Symptomatic patients should be treated by radiofrequency ablation of the abnormal pathway. Drugs, such as classes Ia, Ic and III, may be used if ablation is (rarely) unsuccessful or not wanted.

Table 11.15 Grading system for ventricular premature beats (VPBs) following acute myocardial infarction, as proposed by Lown

Grade	Description
0	No VPBs
1	Occasional VPBs (< 30 hour^{-1}, not > 1 min^{-1})
2	Frequent VPBs (≥ 30 hour^{-1})
3	Multiform VPBs
4A	Couplets (two consecutive VPBs)
4B	Repetitive VPBs (3 or more)
5	Early VPBs (R-on-T)

Ventricular tachyarrhythmias

There are four main types of ventricular tachyarrhythmia:

- ventricular premature beats
- ventricular tachycardia
- ventricular fibrillation
- torsades de pointes (twisting of points).

Except for torsades de pointes, most ventricular arrhythmias are caused by coronary heart disease, hypertension or cardiomyopathy. Torsades de pointes arises when ventricular repolarization is greatly prolonged (long QT interval). The causes of QT prolongation and torsades de pointes are listed in Table 11.14.

Congenital QT prolongation may be associated with syncope, and torsades de pointes which may cause sudden death. Congenital QT prolongation may (Jervell–Lange–Nielsen syndrome) or may not (Romano–Ward syndrome) be associated with congenital deafness. The molecular biology of the congenital long QT syndromes has recently been shown to be heterogenous; a number of mutations in genes coding for potassium or sodium channels have been identified and linked to several chromosomes. The different mutations appear to correlate with different phenotypes and it is likely to be possible to improve therapy for the congenital long QT syndrome on the basis of identification of the mutation involved.

Ventricular premature beats

These may be uncomfortable, especially when frequent. The patient may complain of extra beats, missed beats or heavy beats because it may be the premature beat, the post-ectopic pause or the next sinus beat that is noticed by the patient. The pulse is irregular owing to the premature beats. Some early beats may not be felt at the wrist. When a premature beat occurs regularly after every normal beat, 'pulsus bigeminus' may occur.

On the ECG (Fig 11.43) the premature beat has a broad (>0.12 s) and bizarre QRS complex because it arises from an abnormal (ectopic) site in the ventricular myocardium. Following the premature beat there is usually a complete compensatory pause because the AV node or ventricle is refractory to the next sinus impulse. Early 'R-on-T' ventricular premature beats (occurring simultaneously with the upstroke or peak of the T wave of the previous beat) may induce ventricular fibrillation, particularly in patients following myocardial infarction.

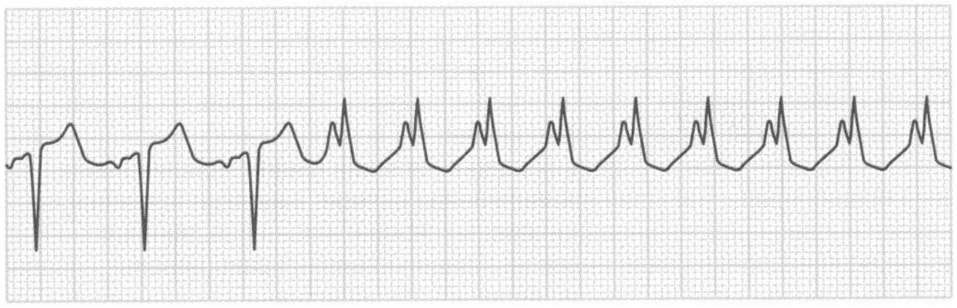

Fig 11.44
Ventricular tachycardia at a rate of 140 b.p.m. following three sinus beats at a rate of 92 b.p.m.

Ventricular premature beats have been graded in order of severity. The 'Lown Classification' (Table 11.15) is designed for premature beats occurring in the setting of acute myocardial infarction, but has been wrongly applied to other situations. This is particularly true of R-on-T ventricular premature beats (occurring simultaneously with the upstroke or peak of the T wave of the previous beat). Following myocardial infarction, such premature beats may induce ventricular fibrillation. This is extremely uncommon in other circumstances.

Treatment of ventricular ectopics may be advised because of symptoms or because they may provoke or threaten to provoke more serious arrhythmias. If structural heart disease is present and premature beats are frequent or run together (three or more beats at a time), treatment is offered. Drugs from classes I, II or III (see p. 670) are used. In the absence of heart disease, ventricular premature beats may safely be ignored.

Ventricular tachycardia

This is defined as three or more ventricular beats occurring at a rate of 120 b.p.m. or more. Often the patient will be hypotensive and ill but some ventricular tachycardias are well tolerated.

Examination reveals a pulse rate of 120–220 b.p.m. Usually there are clinical signs of atrioventricular dissociation (i.e. intermittent cannon *a* waves and variable intensity of the first heart sound).

The ECG shows a rapid ventricular rhythm with broad (often 0.14 s or more), abnormal QRS complexes. Dissociated P wave activity may be seen (Fig 11.44). Supraventricular tachycardia with bundle branch block (aberration) may resemble ventricular tachycardia on the ECG; the diagnostic features are indicated in Table 11.16. In all cases of doubt, a ventricular tachycardia should be diagnosed.

Table 11.16 ECG distinction between supraventricular tachycardia (SVT) with bundle branch block and ventricular tachycardia (VT)

VT is more likely than SVT with bundle branch block when there is:

- a very broad QRS (> 0.14 s)
- atrioventricular dissociation
- a bifid, upright QRS with a taller first peak in V_1
- a deep S wave in V_6
- a concordant (same polarity) QRS direction in all chest leads (V_1–V_6)

Treatment may be urgent depending on the haemodynamic situation (Fig 11.45). If the cardiac output and the blood pressure are very depressed, emergency DC cardioversion must be considered. On the other hand, if the blood pressure and cardiac output are well maintained, intravenous therapy with class I drugs is usually advised.

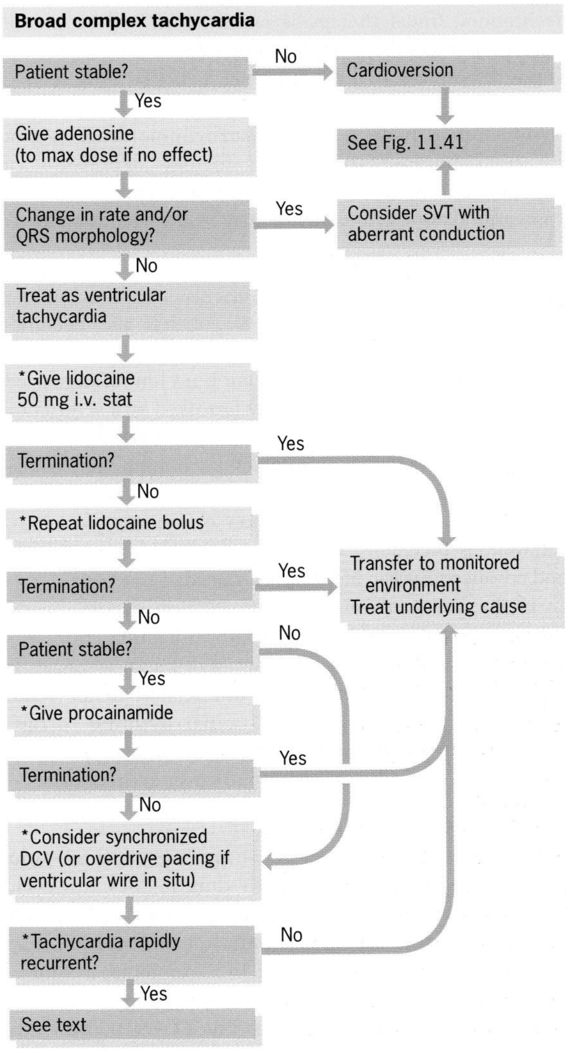

*If haemodynamic instability develops, proceed to immediate cardioversion.

Fig 11.45
Management of tachycardia. Broad complex DCV, DC cardioversion

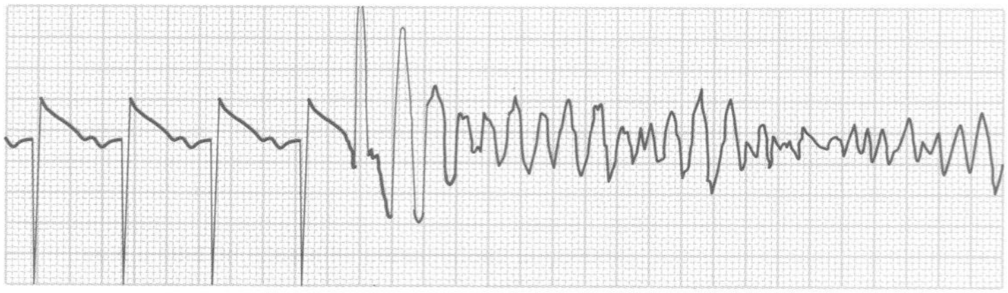

Fig 11.46
Four beats of sinus rhythm followed by a ventricular ectopic beat that initiates ventricular fibrillation. The ST segment during sinus rhythm is elevated owing to acute myocardial infarction

First-line drug treatment consists of lidocaine (50–100 mg i.v. over 5 minutes) followed by a lidocaine infusion (2–4 mg i.v. per minute). DC cardioversion may be necessary if medical therapy is unsuccessful. The administration of multiple antiar-rhythmic drugs should be avoided.

Prophylaxis against relapse is extremely important. If possible, the likely success of therapy should be judged by Holter monitoring, exercise testing or other provocative techniques. Initial therapy is usually with a β-blocker if exercise induces the arrhythmia, or a class I drug if exercise is not responsible. If these drugs fail, a class III drug such as amiodarone or sotalol is tried. When severe left ventricular dysfunction is present, most antiarrhythmic drugs cannot be used because they cause further depression of myocardial function (negative inotropic effect). In such cases amiodarone or mexiletine may be the agent of choice.

Ventricular fibrillation

This is very rapid and irregular ventricular activation with no mechanical effect. The patient is pulseless and becomes rapidly unconscious, and respiration ceases. The ECG shows shapeless, rapid oscillations and there is no hint of organized complexes (Fig 11.46). It is usually provoked by a ventricular ectopic beat (especially in acute myocardial infarction), ventricular tachycardia or torsades de pointes. Ventricular fibrillation rarely reverses spontaneously. The only effective treatment is electrical defibrillation or, on rare occasions, intravenous bretylium 5–10 mg kg^{-1} over 5 minutes. Basic and advanced cardiac life support is needed (see p. 654).

If the attack of ventricular fibrillation occurs during the first day or two of an acute myocardial infarction, it is probable that prophylactic therapy will be unnecessary. If the ventricular fibrillation was not related to an acute infarction, prophylaxis with antiarrhythmic drugs, especially amiodarone or β-blockers, and possibly an implantable defibrillator (see p. 673) may be necessary.

Torsades de pointes (see Table 11.14)

This arrhythmia is usually short in duration and spontaneously reverts to sinus rhythm. It does, however, give rise to presyncope or syncope and occasionally converts to ventricular fibrillation, and sudden death may occur. It is characterized on the ECG by rapid, irregular, sharp complexes that continuously change from an upright to an inverted position (Fig 11.47(a)). Between spells of tachycardia the ECG shows a prolonged QT interval; the corrected QT (see Table 11.9) is equal to or greater than 0.44 s. Fig 11.47(b) shows a further example of a prolonged QT interval.

The arrhythmia is treated as follows:

1 Any electrolyte disturbance is corrected.
2 Causative drugs are stopped.
3 The heart rate is maintained with atrial or ventricular pacing.
4 Intravenous isoprenaline may be effective when QT prolongation is acquired.
5 β-Blockade or left stellectomy is advised if the QT prolongation is congenital. (Isoprenaline is contraindicated for congenital long-QT syndrome.)

Managements available for arrhythmias

Many cardiac arrhythmias are symptomatic, and some are life-threatening. Usually arrhythmias can only be suppressed, but occasionally – for example with surgical treatment – a complete cure can be effected.

Arrhythmias such as ventricular tachycardia must be terminated, but others, such as atrial fibrillation, may not easily convert to sinus rhythm. In this case, control of the ventricular rate response is the best treatment available.

Arrhythmias can be managed by a wide variety of means (Table 11.17), ranging from simple techniques that increase

Table 11.17
Management of arrhythmias

Aims	Techniques available
Cure	Vagotonic methods
Prevention (suppression)	DC cardioversion
Termination	Antiarrhythmic drugs
Reduction of ventricular rate	Pacemakers and other electronic devices
	Catheter ablation
	Surgery

Table 11.18
Vaughan Williams' classification of antiarrhythmic drugs

Class Ia	Quinidine, procainamide, disopyramide
Class Ib	Lidocaine, mexiletine, tocainide
Class Ic	Flecainide, propafenone
Class II	β-Adrenergic blocking drugs
Class III	Amiodarone, sotalol, bretylium, ibutilide, dofetilide
Class IV	Verapamil, diltiazem
(Other	Adenosine, digoxin)

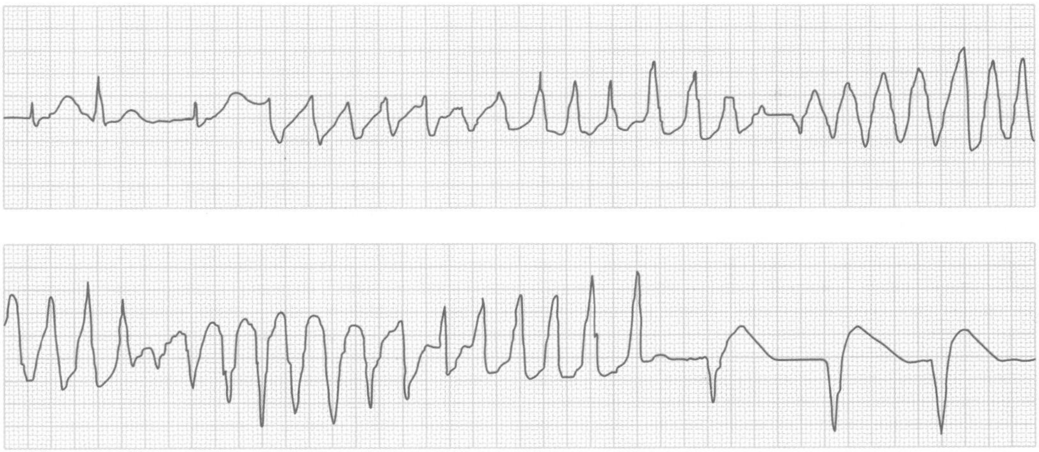

Fig 11.47
(a) An ECG demonstrating a supraventricular rhythm with a long QT interval giving way to atypical ventricular tachycardia (torsades de pointes). The tachycardia is short-lived and is followed by a brief period of idioventricular rhythm

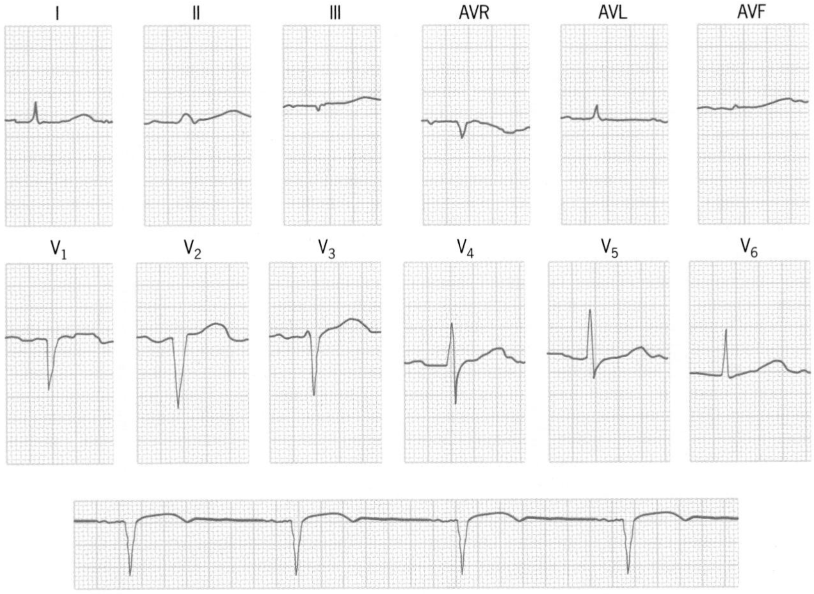

Fig 11.47
(b) A 12-lead ECG from an 11-year-old child with a history of syncope, demonstrating sinus bradycardia with a long QT interval (560 ms). The ECG is typical of a form of hereditary long-QT syndrome

vagal tone to expensive and sophisticated treatments such as surgery or implantable electronic devices. Antiarrhythmic drugs remain the most important form of treatment.

Antiarrhythmic drugs

Drugs that modify the rhythm and conduction of the heart are used to prevent cardiac arrhythmias. All such drugs may aggravate or produce arrhythmias and they may also depress ventricular contractility and must therefore be used with caution. There are more than 30 antiarrhythmic drugs. They are classified according to their effect on the action potential (Vaughan Williams' classification; Fig 11.48 and Table 11.18).

The features of the major antiarrhythmic drugs are given in Table 11.19.

Class I drugs

These are membrane-depressant drugs that reduce the rate of entry of sodium into the cell. They may slow conduction, delay recovery or reduce the spontaneous discharge rate of myocardial cells. Class Ia drugs (e.g. disopyramide) lengthen the action potential, Class Ib drugs (e.g. lidocaine) shorten the action potential, and Class Ic (flecainide, propafenone) do not affect the duration of the action potential.

In one post-infarction study in the USA (cardiac arrhythmia suppression trial – CAST), mortality in the patient group receiving flecainide was twice that of the control group. In view of this, flecainide and other class I drugs should be reserved for intractable life-threatening ventricular arrhythmias or supraventricular arrhythmias

Table 11.19
Details of antiarrhythmic drugs. For class II drugs (β-blockers) see Table 11.43. Adenosine 0.05–0.25 mg kg^{-1} (see p. 666) is given only intravenously

	Quinidine	Disopyramide	Lidocaine	Mexiletine	Flecainide	Propafenone	Amiodarone	Sotalol	Verapamil	Diltiazem	Digoxin
Class	Ia	Ia	Ib	Ib	Ic	Ic	III	II/III	IV	IV	N/A
Daily dose	250–500 mg orally	100–250 mg × 3 orally	1–4 mg min^{-1} (50–150 mg i.v. loading dose)	400–800 mg orally loading, 150–300 mg maintenance	100 mg × 2 orally	150 mg × 3 300 mg × 2 or 300 mg × 3	200 mg × 1–2 orally	80–160 mg × 2–3 orally	0.1 mg kg^{-1} i.v. 40–160 mg × 3–4 orally	60–120 mg × 3–4 orally	0.25 mg × 1 orally
Protein binding	75%	40–90%	50–80%	70%	50%	85%	98%	<10%	90%	80%	25%
Half-life	6 hours	5 hours	1.5–2 hours	15 hours	18 hours	6 hours	50 days +	24 hours	6 hours	2–8 hours	36 hours
Plasma therapeutic range	2–5 μg mL^{-1}	3–6 μg mL^{-1}	2–6 μg mL^{-1}	0.5–2.0 μg mL^{-1}	0.2–0.8 μg mL^{-1}	0.2–1.5 μg mL^{-1}	0.2–5.0 μg mL^{-1}	0.3–1.5 μg mL^{-1}	0.1–0.3 μg mL^{-1}	0.02–0.16 μg mL^{-1}	1.3–2.6 nmol L^{-1}
Indication	AF PSVT VT VPBs WPW	AF PSVT VT VPBs WPW	VT/VF associated with myocardial infarction VPBs	VT, especially after myocardial infarction	VT PSVT WPW	VT/VF PSVT WPW	VT/VF WPW PSVT AF	VT WPW PSVT	PSVT	PSVT	AF/AFL PSVT
Side-effects	Nausea Diarrhoea Rash Fever Cinchonism Syncope Blood dyscrasia	Hypotension Anticholinergic effects Dry mouth Urinary hesitancy Blurred vision Heart failure	Confusion Convulsions	Confusion Tremor Bradycardia Hypotension	Dizziness Visual disturbance Arrhythmo-genesis	Light-headedness Unusual taste Headache Constipation Arrhythmo-genesis	Corneal deposits Photosensitivity Skin pigmentation Thyroid disturbance Pulmonary alveolitis Nightmares Liver disease Neurological	Ventricular arrhythmias Bradycardia Heart failure Bronchospasm Hypotension	Nausea Vomiting Constipation Flushing Headache Bradycardia Fluid retention Hypotension	Nausea Vomiting Constipation Flushing Headache Bradycardia Fluid retention Hypotension	Nausea Anorexia Vomiting Visual disturbance Bradycardia Gynaecomastia

AF, atrial fibrillation; AFL, atrial flutter; N/A, not applicable; PSVT, paroxysmal supraventricular tachycardia; VF, ventricular fibrillation; VPBs, ventricular premature beats; VT, ventricular tachycardia; WPW, Wolff–Parkinson–White syndrome.

causing disabling symptoms in patients who do not have significant left ventricular dysfunction or a previous myocardial infarction or acute coronary ischaemia.

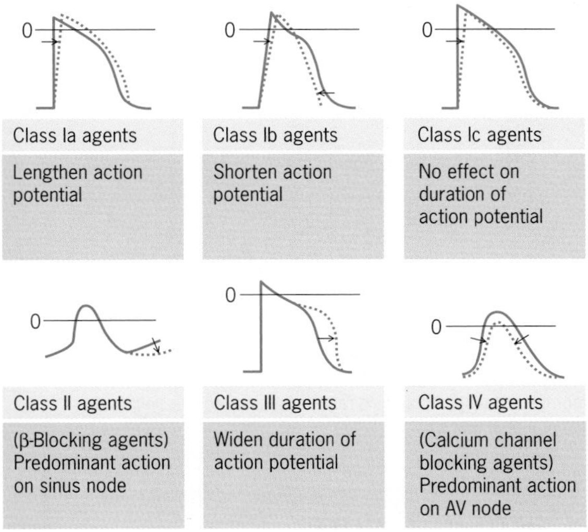

Fig 11.48
Vaughan Williams' classification of antiarrhythmic drugs based on their effect on cardiac action potentials. 0, 0 mV. The dotted curves indicate the effects of the drugs

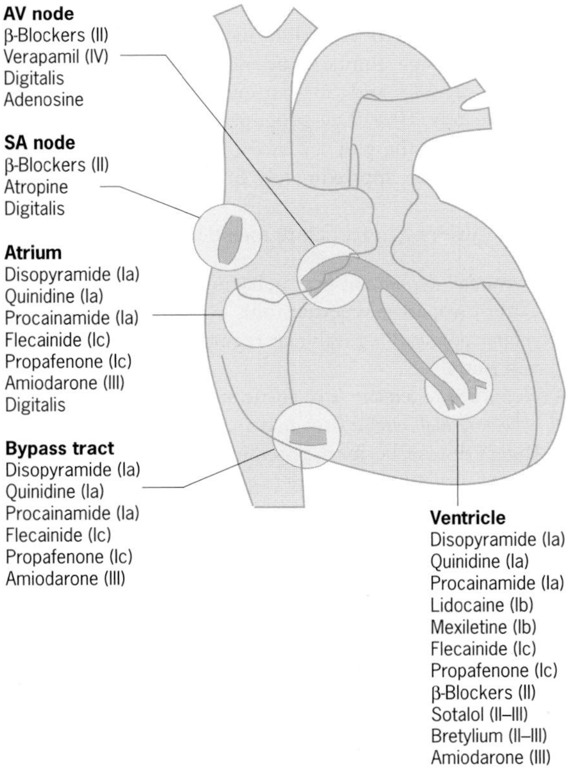

Fig 11.49
Drugs that affect various parts of the heart. The Vaughan Williams' class is given in parentheses

Class II drugs

These antisympathetic drugs prevent the effects of catecholamines on the action potential. Most are β-adrenergic antagonists. Cardioselective β-blockers (β_1) include metoprolol, atenolol and acebutalol.

Class III drugs

These prolong the action potential and do not affect sodium transport through the membrane. There are two major drugs in this class: amiodarone and sotalol. Sotalol is also a β-blocker.

Several new drugs, such as ibutilide and dofetilide, will be available soon. Recent trials with amiodarone for prophylaxis against sudden death (EMIAT, CAMIAT, CHESTAT, GESICA) have shown discordant results (no effect or benefit) but overall a meta-analysis has shown a 12% reduction in morbidity and a 29% reduction in sudden mortality associated with amiodarone treatment.

Class IV drugs (see also Table 11.27)

The non-dihydropyridine calcium antagonists that reduce the plateau phase of the action potential are particularly effective at slowing conduction in nodal tissue. Verapamil and diltiazem are the most important drugs in this group.

Another clinical classification is based on the part of the heart that is affected by the antiarrhythmic drug (Fig 11.49).

Other management techniques

Steerable electrode catheters can be used to deliver radiofrequency energy to any part of the heart responsible for the generation or continuation of tachycardias. Atrial tachycardia, AV nodal tachycardia and the abnormal pathways responsible for WPW syndrome can be successfully treated. The catheter ablation technique is very successful and safe.

The AV node or His bundle may also be destroyed by radiofrequency energy delivered through a catheter electrode placed close to the AV conduction system. This procedure effectively prevents the AV conduction of atrial arrhythmias, such as atrial fibrillation. A ventricular pacemaker is then needed to prevent ventricular bradycardia.

Ventricular tachycardia can be stopped by surgical removal of the focus of the arrhythmia and atrial fibrillation may be eradicated by multiple incisions in the atria. However, such operations carry considerable risk and are reserved for very serious problems.

Implantable automatic cardioverter–defibrillator

Serious ventricular arrhythmias (ventricular fibrillation or rapid ventricular tachycardia with hypotension) carry a mortality within one year of up to 40%. Antiarrhythmic drug therapy, particularly with amiodarone, may reduce the mortality. Another important therapy is the implantable cardioverter–defibrillator (ICD), which can

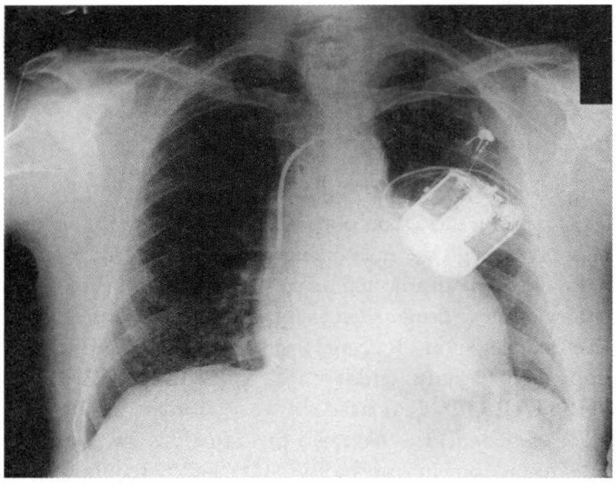

Fig 11.50
PA X-ray of an 'ICD' in a left pectoral position with a single lead on which are mounted defibrillation electrodes in the superior vena cava and in the right ventricle

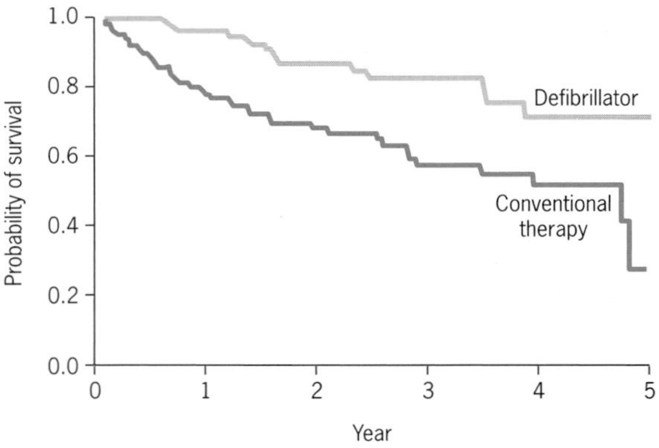

Fig 11.51
Survival curves of the Multicentre Automatic Defibrillator Implantation Trial (MADIT) following myocardial infarction. Patients with left ventricular ejection fractions of ≤0.35 and documented asymptomatic non-sustained ventricular tachycardia and inducible ventricular tachycardia were randomized to receive an ICD or conventional therapy

recognize ventricular tachycardia or fibrillation and automatically deliver pacing or a shock to the heart to cause cardioversion to sinus rhythm.

Modern ICDs are only a little larger than a pacemaker and may be implanted in a pectoral position (Fig 11.50). The device may have leads to sense and pace both the right atrium and ventricle, and the lithium batteries employed are able to provide energy for over 100 shocks each of around 30 J. When an arrythmia develops that requires treatment by a shock, the device takes up to 15 s to recognize the arrythmia and charge its capacitors. It then delivers the defibrillating discharge which may be painful if the patient is conscious. However, ventricular tachycardia may often be cardioverted by pacing of the heart, which is painless.

The use of this device has cut the sudden death rate in patients with a history of serious ventricular arrhythmias to 1–2% in the first year, but because of its expense it is not widely available. It is being applied successfully to patients with risk factors for arrhythmic death such as those with a cardiomyopathy or those with significant impairment of left ventricular function and non-sustained ventricular tachycardia on ambulatory monitoring following myocardial infarction (Fig 11.51).

Several new trials (AVID, CIDS and CASH) have also shown that ICD treatment reduces mortality in patients with resuscitated or spontaneously recovered VT/VF.

FURTHER READING

Ackerman MS, Clapham DE (1997) Ion channels: basic science and chemical disease. *New England Journal of Medicine* **336**: 1575–1580.

Narayan SM, Cain ME, Smith JM (1997) Atrial fibrillation. *Lancet* **350**: 943–950.

Zimetbaum P, Josephson ME (1998) Evaluation of patients with palpitations. *New England Journal of Medicine* **338**: 1369–1373.

Cardiac failure

Cardiac failure occurs when, despite normal venous pressures, the heart is unable to maintain sufficient cardiac output to meet the demands of the body. The incidence of heart failure increases with advancing age. The average annual incidence between 35 and 64 years is 2–4%, and in patients over 65 years is approximately 10%. The prognosis of heart failure has improved over the past ten years, but the mortality rate is still high with approximately 50% of patients dead at five years.

The causes of heart failure include:

- *myocardial dysfunction* (e.g. ischaemic heart disease, cardiomyopathy, hypertension)
- *volume overload* (e.g. valvular regurgitation – aortic and mitral)
- *obstruction to outflow* (e.g. aortic stenosis)
- *obligatory high output* (e.g. anaemia, thyrotoxicosis, Paget's disease, beriberi, systemic-to-pulmonary shunts)
- *compromised ventricular filling* (e.g. constrictive pericarditis, pericardial tamponade, restrictive cardiomyopathy)
- *altered rhythm* (e.g. atrial fibrillation).

Factors aggravating or precipitating heart failure

Any factor that increases myocardial work may aggravate existing heart failure or initiate failure. These factors must be carefully considered in patients who present with heart failure. The most common are arrhythmias, anaemia, thyrotoxicosis, pregnancy, infective endocarditis, pulmonary infection or adjustment of heart failure therapy.

Table 11.20
Pathophysiological changes in heart failure

Ventricular dilatation
Myocyte hypertrophy
Increased collagen synthesis
Altered myosin gene expression
Altered sarcoplasmic Ca^{2+}–ATPase density
Increased ANP secretion
Salt and water retention
Sympathetic stimulation
Peripheral vasoconstriction

Pathophysiology

When the heart fails, considerable changes occur to the heart and peripheral vascular system in response to the haemodynamic changes associated with heart failure (Table 11.20). These physiological changes are compensatory and maintain cardiac output and peripheral perfusion. However, as heart failure progresses, these mechanisms are overwhelmed and become pathophysiological. The development of pathophysiological peripheral vasoconstriction and sodium retention in heart failure reflects loss of beneficial compensatory mechanisms and represents cardiac decompensation manifested by the onset of clinical heart failure. Factors involved are the venous return, the outflow resistance, the contractility of the myocardium, and salt and water retention.

Myocardial remodelling in heart failure

Myocardial hypertrophy is one of the major adaptations to haemodynamic overload of the left ventricle. As cardiac myocytes are terminally differentiated, this occurs by an increase in myocyte size and the growth of non-myocyte components such as vascular smooth muscle cells and fibroblasts. Collagen synthesis may also be increased. These structural changes result in an increase in myocardial volume and mass, impaired systolic and diastolic function, and impaired coronary blood flow.

Changes in myocardial gene expression. Haemodynamic overload of the ventricle stimulates changes in cardiac contractile protein gene expression. The overall effect is to increase protein synthesis, but many proteins also switch to fetal and neonatal isoforms. Human myosin is composed of a pair of heavy chains (MHC) and two pairs of light chains. Myosin heavy chains (MHC) exist in two isoforms, α and β, that have different contractile properties and ATPase activity. $\alpha\alpha$-MHC predominates in the atria and $\beta\beta$-MHC in the ventricles. In animal models, pressure overload results in a shift from $\alpha\alpha$- to $\beta\beta$-MHC in the atria, in parallel with atrial size. This results in reduction in atrial contractility but reduced energy demands. This shift is less important in the human ventricle as the $\beta\beta$-MHC isoform already predominates. Other genes affected in heart failure include those encoding Na^+–K^+-ATPase, Ca^{2+}-ATPase and β_1-adrenoceptors.

Abnormal calcium homeostasis. Calcium ion flux within myocytes plays a pivotal role in the regulation of contractile function. Excitation of the myocyte cell membrane causes the rapid entry of calcium into myocytes from the extracellular space via calcium channels. This triggers the release of *intracellular* calcium from the sarcoplasmic reticulum and initiates contraction (see Fig 11.2). Relaxation results from the uptake and storage of calcium by the sarcoplasmic reticulum. In heart failure, there is a prolongation of the calcium current in association with prolongation of contraction and relaxation. One mechanism may be a decrease in sarcolemmal Ca^{2+}-ATPase density.

Apoptosis (see also p. 153). Apoptosis (or 'programmed cell death') is the process by which cells self-destruct following the induction of endonucleases that degrade DNA. It is a normal feature in the developing fetus and in some adult tissues (e.g. thymus). Apoptosis has been demonstrated in animal models of ischaemic reperfusion, rapid ventricular pacing, mechanical stretch, and pressure overload. Preliminary work in humans suggests that apoptosis occurs in patients with idiopathic dilated cardiomyopathy, and it is proposed that the spiral of ventricular dysfunction characteristic of heart failure may result from the initiation of apoptosis by cytokines, free radicals and other triggers.

Cardiac hormones

Atrial natriuretic peptide (ANP) is released from atrial myocytes in response to stretch. ANP induces diuresis, natriuresis, vasodilation and suppression of the renin-angiotensin system. Levels of circulating ANP are increased in congestive cardiac failure and correlate with functional class, prognosis and haemodynamic state. The renal response to ANP is attenuated in heart failure, probably secondary to reduced renal perfusion, receptor down-regulation, increased peptide breakdown, renal sympathetic activation, and excessive renin–angiotensin activity. The potential therapeutic benefits of the natriuretic peptides have been investigated by the administration of i.v. ANP and the inhibition of the enzyme responsible for breakdown of the peptic (neutral endopeptidase – NEP). Initial results suggest that these drugs might have a therapeutic role in the future.

Endothelial function in heart failure

The endothelium has a central role in the regulation of vasomotor tone. In patients with heart failure, endothelium-dependent vasodilation in peripheral blood vessels is impaired and may be one mechanism of exercise limitation. The cause of abnormal endothelial responsiveness is complex but relates to abnormal release of both nitric oxide and vasconstrictor substances, such as endothelin (ET). Endothelin secretion from a variety of tissues is stimulated by many factors, including hypoxia, catecholamines, angiotensin II and sheer stress. Although most of the endothelin produced by the vascular endothelium in response to these stimuli is secreted abluminally, endothelin is also found circulating in plasma. Plasma ET concentration is elevated in patients with heart failure, and levels correlate with the severity of haemodynamic disturbance. Preliminary data indicate that the major source of circulating ET in heart failure is the pulmonary vascular bed.

Endothelin has many actions that potentially contribute to the pathophysiology of heart failure: vasoconstriction, sympathetic stimulation, renin–angiotensin system activation and left ventricular hypertrophy. Experimental data suggest that the acute intravenous administration of endothelin antagonists improves haemodynamic abnormalities in patients with congestive cardiac failure, and oral endothelin antagonists are now being developed.

Venous return (preload)

In the intact heart, myocardial failure leads to a reduction of the volume of blood ejected with each heart beat and an increase in the volume of blood remaining after systole. This increased diastolic volume stretches the myocardial fibres and, as Starling's law of the heart would suggest, myocardial contraction is restored. However, the failing myocardium results in depression of the ventricular function curve (cardiac output plotted against the ventricular diastolic volume) (see Fig 11.3 on p. 627).

Slight myocardial depression is not associated with a reduction in cardiac output because it is maintained by an increase in venous pressure (and hence diastolic volume). However, the proportion of blood ejected with each heart beat (ejection fraction) is reduced early in heart failure. Sinus tachycardia also ensures that any reduction of stroke volume is compensated for by the increase in heart rate; cardiac output (stroke volume × heart rate) is therefore maintained.

When there is more severe myocardial dysfunction, cardiac output can be maintained only by a large increase in venous pressure and/or marked sinus tachycardia. This eventually results in further depression of the ventricular function curve and reduced contractility; the resultant increased venous pressure contributes to the development of dyspnoea, owing to the accumulation of interstitial and alveolar fluid, and to the occurrence of hepatic enlargement, ascites and dependent oedema, owing to increased systemic venous pressure. Despite symptoms due to increased venous pressure, the cardiac output at rest may not be much depressed, but myocardial and haemodynamic reserve is so compromised that a normal increase in cardiac output cannot be produced by exercise.

In very severe heart failure the cardiac output at rest is depressed, despite high venous pressures. The inadequate cardiac output is redistributed to maintain perfusion of vital organs, such as the heart, brain and kidneys, at the expense of the skin and muscle.

Outflow resistance (afterload) (see Figs 13.2 and 13.4)

This is the load or resistance against which the ventricle contracts. It is formed by:

- pulmonary and systemic resistance
- physical characteristics of the vessel walls
- the volume of blood that is ejected.

An increase in afterload decreases the cardiac output. This decrease in function with further increase of end-diastolic volume and dilatation of the ventricle itself further exacerbates the problem of afterload. This is expressed by Laplace's law: the tension of the myocardium (*T*) is proportional to the intraventricular pressure (*P*) multiplied by the radius of the ventricular chamber (*R*): i.e. $T \propto PR$ (see p. 626).

Myocardial contractility (inotropic state)

The state of the myocardium also influences performance. Increased contractility (positive inotropism) can result from increased sympathetic drive, and this is a normal part of the Frank–Starling relationship (see Fig 11.3 on p. 627). Conversely, myocardial depressants (e.g. hypoxia) decrease myocardial contractility (negative inotropism).

Salt and water retention

The increase in venous pressure that occurs when the ventricles fail leads to retention of salt and water and their

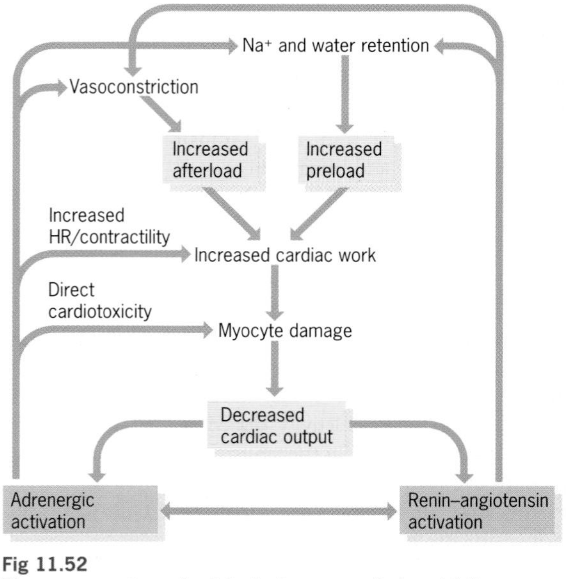

Fig 11.52
The compensatory physiological response to heart failure. Chronic activation of the renin–angiotensin and adrenergic systems results in a 'vicious cycle' of cardiac deterioration that further exacerbates the physiological response

accumulation in the interstitium, producing many of the physical signs of heart failure. Reduced cardiac output also leads to diminished renal perfusion, activating the renin–angiotensin system and enhancing fluid retention (see p. 600). This increased salt and water retention further increases venous pressure (Fig 11.52) which, in the early stages of heart failure, improves cardiac output by the Starling mechanism. In severe heart failure the ventricular function curve plateaus such that further increases in venous pressure do not provoke an increase in cardiac output. This retention of sodium is in part compensated by the action of circulating atrial natriuretic peptides. These are short-chain peptides secreted by the atria in response to distension. These atrial peptides are potent vasodilators with natriuretic properties and levels rise considerably in heart failure. The effect of their action may represent a beneficial, albeit inadequate, compensatory response tending to reduce cardiac load (preload and afterload) by vasodilatation and by enhancing sodium and water excretion.

The precise way in which haemodynamic and neurohumoral factors interact and contribute to the progression of heart failure remains unclear. Both increase ventricular wall stress which promote ventricular dilatation and further worsen contractile efficiency. In addition, prolonged activation of the sympathetic nervous and renin–angiotensin–aldosterone systems exert direct toxic effects on myocardial cells. The realization over recent years that heart failure was not just a mechanical disorder but involved considerable pathophysiological changes has improved our understanding of many clinical aspects of the heart failure syndrome and also has provided a more rational basis for treatment.

Clinical syndromes of heart failure

It is clinically useful to divide heart failure into the syndromes of right, left and biventricular (congestive) cardiac failure, but it is rare for any part of the heart to fail in isolation.

Right heart failure

This syndrome occurs in association with:

- chronic lung disease (cor pulmonale)
- pulmonary embolism or pulmonary hypertension
- tricuspid valve disease
- pulmonary valve disease
- left-to-right shunts (e.g. atrial or ventricular septal defects)
- isolated right ventricular cardiomyopathy
- mitral valve disease with pulmonary hypertension.

The most frequent cause of right heart failure is secondary to left heart failure.

SYMPTOMS AND SIGNS

Symptoms include fatigue, breathlessness, anorexia and nausea. They relate to distension and fluid accumulation in areas drained by the systemic veins.

Physical signs are usually more prominent than the symptoms, with:

- jugular venous distension (± *v* waves of tricuspid regurgitation)
- tender smooth hepatic enlargement
- dependent pitting oedema
- development of free abdominal fluid (ascites)
- pleural transudates (commonly right-sided).

Dilatation of the right ventricle produces cardiomegaly and may give rise to functional tricuspid regurgitation. Tachycardia and a right ventricular third heart sound are usual.

Left heart failure

Causes include:

- ischaemic heart disease (the most common cause)
- systemic hypertension (chronic or 'malignant')
- mitral and aortic valve disease
- cardiomyopathies.

Mitral stenosis causes left atrial hypertension and signs of left heart failure but does not itself cause failure of the left ventricle.

SYMPTOMS AND SIGNS

Symptoms are predominantly fatigue, exertional dyspnoea, orthopnoea and paroxysmal nocturnal dyspnoea.

Physical signs are few and not prominent until a late stage or if the ventricular failure is acute. Cardiomegaly is demonstrable with a displaced and often sustained apical impulse. Auscultation reveals a left ventricular third or fourth heart sound that, with tachycardia, is described as a gallop rhythm. Dilatation of the mitral annulus results in functional mitral regurgitation. Crackles are heard at the lung bases. In severe left heart failure the patient has pulmonary oedema. In this circumstance a chest X-ray is the most useful investigation. Rarely the cause of left ventricular failure is apparent, such as a ventricular aneurysm at the site of previous infarction.

Systolic versus diastolic heart failure

The most common cause of systolic ventricular dysfunction is coronary artery disease, usually following myocardial infarction. The left ventricle is usually dilated and fails to contract normally. Diastolic ventricular dysfunction is usually due to hypertension. There is left ventricular hypertrophy with failure of ventricular relaxation. Diastolic dysfunction appears to carry a better prognosis. Systolic and diastolic dysfunction often coexist.

Cardiac cachexia

The term *cardiac cachexia* describes the loss of lean (non-oedematous) body mass that occurs in some patients with moderate to severe heart failure. Most patients with cachexia are over 40 years of age, have had heart failure for at least five years and are in NYHA (p. 630) functional class II/IV. Its presence is associated with increased morbidity and mortality.

Several mechanisms are thought to contribute to wasting in heart failure, including malabsorption, anorexia caused by intestinal oedema and drugs, and loss of nutrients through the gastrointestinal and renal tracts. Patients with heart failure also have an increased metabolic rate secondary to increased sympathetic activity in association with reduced anabolic metabolism. The cytokine tumour necrosis factor α (TNFα) is increased in patients with cardiac cachexia and may also contribute to the phenomenon. Possible stimuli to TNFα release include reduced peripheral blood flow, failing myocardium and prostaglandin release.

Biventricular failure (congestive)

This term is used variously but is best restricted to cases where right heart failure is a result of pre-existing left heart failure. The physical signs are thus a combination of the above syndromes.

Acute heart failure

Acute failure of the heart most commonly occurs in the setting of acute myocardial infarction when there is extensive loss of ventricular muscle. The condition may also occur with rupture of the interventricular septum producing a ventricular septal defect, or be due to acute valvular regurgitation. Common examples of valvular regurgitation are papillary or chordal rupture producing mitral regurgitation, or sudden aortic valve regurgitation in infective endocarditis. Other causes of acute heart failure include obstruction of the circulation by acute pulmonary embolus and cardiac tamponade. In each case severe cardiac failure can occur with a relatively normal heart size.

High-output heart failure

The heart may not be able to meet the demands placed on it in conditions such as anaemia, thyrotoxicosis, beriberi and Gram-negative septicaemia. This form of heart failure presents in much the same manner as low-output states but is associated with tachycardia and a gallop rhythm. Patients are often warm with distended superficial veins. Unlike low-output failure, the oxygen content of systemic venous blood is high owing to the delivery of large amounts of arterial blood to non-metabolizing tissues.

Investigations

A clinical diagnosis of heart failure should always be confirmed using objective measures of left ventricular structure and function (usually echocardiography). Similarly, the underlying cause of heart failure should be established in all patients.

General/diagnostic investigations

- **Chest X-ray/ECG** for cardiac size and evidence of ischaemia or hypertension.
- **Echocardiography**. Two-dimensional and Doppler echocardiography establishes the presence of systolic and/or diastolic impairment of the left or right ventricle, may reveal the aetiology (valve disease, regional wall motion abnormalities in ischaemic heart disease, cardiomyopathy, amyloid), and may detect intracardiac thrombus. An ejection fraction of <0.45 is generally accepted as evidence for systolic dysfunction.
- **Blood tests**:
  (a) Full blood count, liver biochemistry, urea and electrolytes
  (b) Cardiac enzymes in acute heart failure to diagnose myocardial infarction
  (c) Thyroid function
- **Cardiac catheterization** – see p. 652.

Functional/prognostic investigations

- **Cardiopulmonary exercise testing** and a 6-minute exercise walk.
- **Resting and stress radionuclide angiography** (MUGA) – ejection fraction, regional wall motion abnormality.
- **Ambulatory ECG monitoring** for 24–48 hours – if arrhythmia is suspected.
- **Serum ANP levels** are over 70% sensitive and specific for detecting left ventricular systolic dysfunction.

Treatment of heart failure

Treatment of chronic heart failure is aimed at relieving symptoms, retarding disease progression and improving survival. The management of heart failure requires that any factor aggravating the failure should be identified and treated. Similarly the cause of heart failure must be elucidated and where possible corrected. Nursing care of the mouth and pressure areas is necessary and patients should be nursed in a comfortable upright position.

The prevention of heart failure is also of great importance. Specific measures include cessation of smoking, effective treatment of hypertension and hypercholesterolaemia, and pharmacological therapy following myocardial infarction.

Table 11.21
Treatment of heart failure: drugs and non-pharmacological options

Drugs	
Diuretics	
Angiotensin-converting enzyme (ACE) inhibitors	
Digitalis glycosides	
Vasodilator combinations (hydralazine and nitrate)	
β-Adrenoceptor blockers	
Antiarrhythmics	
Anticoagulants	
Positive inotropes	
Devices and surgery	
Coronary artery bypass grafting	
Pacemaker/implantable cardioverter–defibrillator	
Heart transplantation	
Cardiomyoplasty	

Table 11.22
Effects of vasodilator drugs used in heart failure

	Reduction in:	
	Preload	**Afterload**
Nitroprusside	+	+++
Glyceryl trinitrate	+++	+
Isosorbide di/mono nitrate	+++	+
Prazosin	+	++
ACE inhibitors/antagonists	++	++
Hydralazine	0	+++
Calcium antagonists	+	++

ACE, angiotensin-converting enzyme

General treatment

Physical activity

For patients with exacerbations of congestive cardiac failure, bedrest reduces the demands of the heart and is useful for a few days. Migration of fluid from the interstitium promotes a diuresis, reducing heart failure. Prolonged bedrest may, however, lead to development of deep vein thrombosis; this can be avoided by daily leg exercises, low-dose subcutaneous heparin and elastic support stockings. Low-level endurance exercise (e.g. 20–30 minute walking three or five times per week, or 20 minutes cycling at 70–80% of peak heart rate five times per week) is actively encouraged in patients with compensated heart failure in order to reverse 'deconditioning' of peripheral muscle metabolism. Strenuous isometric activity should be avoided.

Dietary modifications

Large meals should be avoided and if necessary weight reduction instituted. Salt restriction is important and foods rich in salt or added salt in cooking and at the table should be avoided. A low-sodium diet is unpalatable and of questionable value. Alcohol has a negatively inotropic effect and patients should abstain.

Vaccination

While prospective clinical trials are lacking, it is recommended that patients with heart failure be vaccinated against pneumococcal disease and influenza.

Drug management

The pharmacological management of heart failure relies on the following categories of drugs: diuretics, vasodilators, positive inotropic agents including digitalis glycosides, and antiarrhythmic agents (Table 11.21).

Diuretics (see Table 10.2)

These act by promoting the renal excretion of salt and water by blocking tubular reabsorption of sodium and chloride. The resulting loss of fluid reduces ventricular filling pressures (preload) and produce consistent haemodynamic and symptomatic benefits in patients with heart failure and rapidly relieve dyspnoea and peripheral oedema. The intravenous administration of loop diuretics such as frusemide relieves pulmonary oedema rapidly by means of arteriolar vasodilatation reducing afterload, an action that is independent of its diuretic effect.

Diuretics act in various ways.

Loop diuretics

Loop diuretics such as frusemide and bumetanide act by reducing sodium and chloride reabsorption in the ascending limb of the loop of Henle. They cause a brisk and generally short-lived diuresis as the concentrating power of the kidney is reduced. These agents also produce marked potassium loss and promote hyperuricaemia.

Thiazide diuretics

Thiazide diuretics such as bendrofluazide have a mild diuretic effect and act on the distal convoluted tubule, reducing sodium reabsorption. Potassium excretion is enhanced. Thiazides are less effective in patients with reduced glomerular filtration rates. Metolazone is a

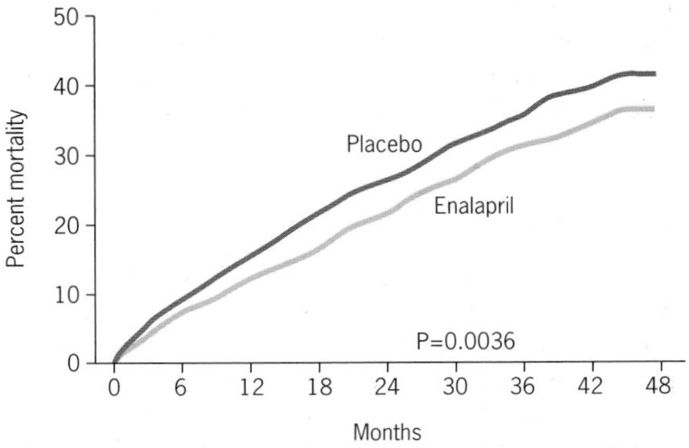

Fig 11.53
Survival in patients with symptomatic heart failure taking placebo and enalapril (the SOLVD treatment trial). Modified from *New England Journal of Medicine* (1991) **325**: 293–302

powerful thiazide producing profound diuresis acting synergistically with loop diuretics. This combination is useful in treating severe and resistant heart failure.

Potassium-sparing diuretics

Spironolactone is a specific competitive antagonist to aldosterone, producing a weak diuresis but with a potassium-sparing action. Amiloride and triamterene act at the distal tubule preventing potassium secretion in exchange for sodium. These drugs are weak diuretics but are useful in combination with more powerful loop diuretics. They should be avoided in the presence of renal failure and in patients taking ACE inhibitors unless there is persistent hypokalaemia.

Summary. Although heart failure symptoms are improved by diuretic treatment alone, they do not provide any survival benefit. In addition, their use may be complicated by over-diuresis and electrolyte depletion (potassium and magnesium), which may predispose to the development of lethal ventricular arrhythmias, hyper-kalaemia (potassium-sparing diuretics) and other metabolic disturbances (hyperuricaemia and dyslipidaemia) and gynaecomastia.

Vasodilator therapy (see Table 11.22)

Diuretics and sodium restriction serve to activate the renin–angiotensin system, promoting formation of angiotensin (a potent vasoconstrictor) and an increase in afterload. A variety of other neural and hormonal reactions also serve to increase preload and afterload. These compensatory mechanisms are initially beneficial in maintaining blood pressure and redistributing blood flow, but in the later stages of heart failure they are deleterious and reduce cardiac output. The high venous pressures found in heart failure are also related to the activation of the sympathetic nervous system and the presence of circulating vasoconstrictors, thus shifting the Starling curve to the right.

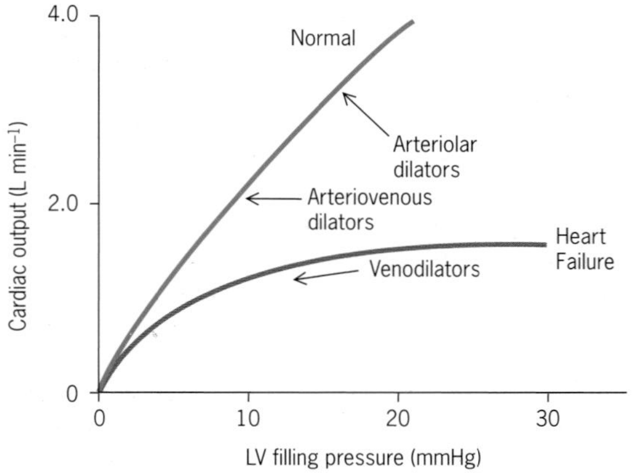

Fig 11.54
Effect of vasodilators on cardiac output and left ventricular filling pressure. Agents with arteriolar and arteriovenous dilating properties reduce the afterload and increase cardiac output. Venodilators reduce the left ventricular filling pressure (and pulmonary oedema) but do not increase cardiac output

Several large controlled trials (e.g. CONSENSUS and SOLVD), have established the benefit of vasodilator therapy in heart failure (Fig 11.53). The trials have shown that in addition to producing considerable symptomatic improvement in patients with symptomatic heart failure, vasodilators markedly improve prognosis and limit the development of progressive heart failure. The SAVE study has confirmed the benefit of ACE inhibitor therapy in patients with asymptomatic heart failure following myocardial infarction in whom the development of overt heart failure was reduced by this treatment.

Arteriolar vasolidators (Fig 11.54)

Drugs such as α-adrenergic blockers (e.g. prazosin) and direct smooth-muscle relaxants (e.g. hydralazine) are potent arteriolar vasodilators. Calcium-channel blockers also reduce afterload, but first generation calcium antagonists (diltiazem, nifedipine) may have a detrimental effect on left ventricular function in patients with heart failure. The PRAISE trial suggests that the second-generation calcium antagonist amlodipine is safe in heart failure and of possible prognostic benefit in patients with non-ischaemic aetiology. The reduction in afterload causes an increase in cardiac output. Any tendency to hypotension is usually offset by the increased output.

Venodilators (Fig 11.54)

Short- and long-acting nitrates (e.g. glyceryl trinitrate and isosorbide mononitrate) act by reducing preload and lowering venous pressure with resulting reduction in pulmonary and dependent oedema. Reduction of filling pressure does not significantly enhance cardiac output because the heart is operating on the flat portion of the ventricular filling curve. With chronic use, tolerance develops with loss of efficacy and consequent worsening of heart failure. Combined therapy with hydralazine and oral nitrates has been shown to improve mortality and exercise performance, and may be useful when ACE inhibitors are contraindicated.

Angiotensin-converting enzyme inhibitors (Fig 16.28)

ACE inhibitors lower systemic vascular resistance and venous pressure and reduce levels of circulating catecholamines, thus improving myocardial performance. The beneficial haemodynamic effect of these drugs appears to be independent of their inhibition of ACE as they are equally effective when plasma renin activity is normal.

These drugs should be carefully introduced to patients with heart failure because of the risk of first-dose hypotension. This is a particular risk in patients who are receiving large doses of diuretics and in the presence of hyponatraemia (<130 mmol L^{-1}). In such cases a test dose of ACE inhibitor should be commenced and the preceding diuretic doses omitted. Some of these agents are prodrugs (e.g. enalapril) and require conversion to the active metabolite (enalaprilat) by liver enzymes; these drugs have a delayed onset of action and first-dose hypotension may not occur for several hours. Prodrugs are best avoided if heart failure results in significantly altered hepatic function. Serious hypotension may result in acute renal failure. Concomitant potassium-sparing diuretics should be discontinued, as ACE inhibitors tend to promote potassium retention. Creatinine levels rise by approximately 10–15% during ACE therapy. ACE inhibitors are contraindicated in patients with bilateral renal artery stenosis. Between 10 and 15% of patients develop a cough, owing to the inhibition of bradykinin metabolism.

Angiotensin II receptor antagonist

Angiotensin II receptor antagonists (e.g. Losartan) have similar haemodynamic effects to ACE inhibitors, but do not affect bradykinin metabolism or produce a cough. A recent trial in elderly patients with heart failure (ELITE) has shown that Losartan has a beneficial effect on functional class and the combined end-point of death and/or progressive heart failure.

β-Adrenoceptor blocking agents

Studies using a variety of drugs (metoprolol, bisoprolol) have shown that β-blockers improve symptomatic class, exercise tolerance and left ventricular function in patients with heart failure of any cause. A recent study (US Carvedilol Studies) using carvedilol, a non-selective vasodilator β-blocker with additional vasodilator and antioxidant properties, has demonstrated a significant improvement in mortality. Following the administration of β-blockers, ejection fraction may decline, but it usually returns to baseline within a month and then increases after three months. Thus, initial doses should be low, and should be titrated slowly over a period of months rather than days. As yet, there is no general agreement on the timing of β-blocker therapy. Until ongoing randomized trials confirm the mortality benefit, they should at present be used only in patients who remain symptomatic despite treatment with diuretics, vasodilators and digoxin.

Inotropic agents

Intravenous inotropes are frequently used to support myocardial function in patients with acute left ventricular failure and following cardiac surgery. Several orally active agents have been tested in patients with chronic congestive cardiac failure, but most have been associated with increased mortality and so are not widely used.

Digitalis glycosides

Digitalis glycosides have been used for many years in patients with heart failure and atrial fibrillation, but their use in patients in sinus rhythm is controversial. While several small placebo-controlled trials have shown that digoxin improves exercise tolerance, increases left ventricular ejection fraction and alleviates the symptoms and signs of congestive cardiac failure, other studies have indicated that digoxin may increase mortality in patients with myocardial infarction. However, this effect is not significant when other factors such as the severity of heart failure are taken into account. A recent large prospective trial (Digoxin Investigation Group (DIG) trial) has shown that when combined with ACE inhibitors and diuretics, digoxin reduces death and hospitalization resulting from progressive heart failure. A small increase in deaths presumed to be secondary to myocardial infarction and/or arrhythmia meant that the effect on overall mortality was neutral. The half-life of digoxin is approximately 36 hours. It is partly protein bound, making it liable to drug interaction. As 90% is excreted unchanged in urine, accumulation can occur in renal failure. Digoxin acts as a positive inotrope by competitive inhibition of Na^+–K^+-ATPase, producing high levels of intracellular sodium. This is then exchanged for extracellular calcium. High levels of intracellular calcium result in enhanced actin–myosin interaction and increased contractility (see Fig 11.2). Digoxin also improves baroreceptor responsiveness, and reduces sympathetic activity and circulating renin.

Digoxin is administered orally (1 mg loading and 0.125–0.25 mg daily according to body mass and renal function). Trough serum levels should be monitored (1.3–2.6 nmol L^{-1}) and hypokalaemia should be avoided. The elderly and patients with hyperthyroidism are more prone to digoxin toxicity. In patients with fluctuating renal function, digoxin, which is metabolized by the liver, may be preferable.

With improvement in formulation, *digoxin toxicity* has become less problematic but is prone to occur in the elderly and in patients with renal impairment. The most common features of digoxin toxicity are:

- anorexia, nausea, altered vision
- arrhythmia (e.g. ventricular premature beats especially bigeminy, ventricular tachycardia and AV block)
- digoxin levels >2.5 nmol L^{-1}.

Digoxin toxicity is treated by discontinuing the drug, restoration of serum potassium levels and management of arrhythmias. Digoxin antibodies (Fab fragments) are a specific antidote that are useful for life-threatening toxicity.

β-Adrenergic agonists

Based on the demonstration that inotropic state of the failing myocardium is impaired and that the myocardial response to adrenergic stimulation is reduced, several adrenergic agonists have been tested in heart failure.

Xamoterol, the only oral β-adrenoreceptor agonist to be extensively tested, improves exercise intolerance and symptoms in patients with mild heart failure, but has not gained widespread use as it increases mortality in patients with moderate to severe heart failure.

Dobutamine, dopexamine and dopamine are intravenous adrenergic agonists. Dobutamine is a selective agonist of the β_1-adrenoreceptor increasing intracellular cyclic AMP which, in turn, increases calcium availability for myocardial contraction. Dobutamine also causes peripheral vasodilatation by an α-adrenergic effect. Dopexamine is a selective β_2 agonist with an additional action on peripheral dopamine receptors that theoretically results in improved renal perfusion. Dopamine is a less selective inotrope that is often used in a low dose to improve renal perfusion (via dopaminergic receptors).

β-Adrenergic agents are used in patients with acute left ventricular failure and in patients with end-stage heart failure as a bridge to transplantation. Intermittent dobutamine therapy may produce long-lasting improvements in symptoms and exercise performance at the cost of increased mortality.

Phosphodiesterase inhibitors

Amrinone, milrinone and enoximone are in a class of so-called 'inodilator' drugs that act by inhibiting phosphodiesterase, thus preventing breakdown of cyclic AMP. Accumulation of cAMP produces an increase in contractility and also peripheral vasodilatation. The Starling curve is shifted upwards. Although these agents are effective in improving myocardial performance acutely, there is evidence that they have a deleterious effect on myocardial cells when administered in the long term with an increased mortality. They are not often used.

Ibopamine

Ibopamine is an orally active dopamine agonist, its active metabolite *N*-methyldopamine acting on both DA-1 and DA-2 receptors to produce renal and peripheral vasodilatation without a major inotropic effect. Preliminary data demonstrated that ibopamine improved symptoms and exercise tolerance in patients with mild-to-moderate heart failure, but the recent PRIME-II study revealed increased mortality in patients taking concomitant antiarrhythmics.

Vesarinone/Pimobendan

These drugs have several mechanisms of action including increased sensitivity of troponin C for calcium and weak phophodiesterase inhibition. Both have been shown to increase mortality (Vesarinone Evaluation of Survival Trial (VEST) and Pimobendan in Congestive Cardiac Failure trial (PICO)) and are unlikely to have a major role in the treatment of heart failure.

Anticoagulants

Heart failure is associated with a fourfold increase in the risk of a stroke. Oral anticoagulants are recommended in patients with atrial fibrillation, a previous history of thromboembolism or endocardial thrombus, but their role in patients in sinus rhythm is less certain.

Antiarrhythmic agents

Arrhythmias are frequent in heart failure and are implicated in sudden death. Although treatment of complex ventricular arrhythmias might be expected to improve survival, there is conflicting evidence that this is so. This may be related to the diverse mechanisms of death in patients with heart failure, death commonly being associated with bradyarrhythmias, particularly in patients with non-ischaemic heart failure. Patients with sustained episodes of ventricular tachycardia should undergo electrophysiological study and serial drug testing or receive empirical treatment, usually with amiodarone or sotalol.

The use of class I agents may result in deterioration of heart failure owing to their negative inotropic effect. In patients with a history of myocardial infarction, they may increase mortality (Cardiac Arrhythmia Suppression Trial (CAST)).

Two trials (Grupo de Estudio de la Sobrevida en la Insurficiencia Cardiaca en Argentina (GESICA) and Survival Trial of Antiarrhythmic Therapy in Congestive Heart Failure (CHF-STAT)) have evaluated the class III drug, amiodarone, in heart failure. GESICA, but not CHF-STAT, demonstrated improved survival. The discrepancy may relate to the differing aetiology of heart failure in the two studies, analysis suggesting that patients with dilated cardiomyopathy benefited most.

It should be noted that ACE inhibitors probably exert an indirect antiarrhythmic effect by reducing high circulating levels of noradrenaline and improving cardiac function. In the future the use of the ICD is likely to improve the survival prospects of patients with serious ventricular arrhythmias.

Summary. It is now recommended that all patients with clinical heart failure should receive treatment with diuretics and an ACE inhibitor. Patients in atrial fibrillation should be digitalized but patients in sinus rhythm may also be improved by the addition of digoxin or a β-blocker. Patients with asymptomatic left ventricular dysfunction are at risk of progressive deterioration and should be treated with prophylactic ACE inhibitor therapy. Patients with ischaemic heart failure and ongoing ischaemia, and patients intolerant of ACE inhibitors or in whom they are contraindicated (hypotension, renal insufficiency or hyperkalaemia), may benefit from nitrate/hydralazine therapy.

Non-pharmacological treatment of heart failure

Revascularization

While coronary artery disease is the most common cause of heart failure, the role of revascularization in patients with heart failure is unclear. Patients with angina and left ventricular dysfunction have a higher mortality from surgery (10–20%), but probably have the most to gain in terms of improved symptoms and prognosis. Factors that must be considered before recommending surgery include age, symptoms and evidence for reversible myocardial ischaemia (and/or the presence of viable heart muscle that may recover after revascularization, i.e. 'hibernating' myocardium). Myocardial hibernation is persistent ventricular dysfunction due to reduced myocardial perfusion, which is just sufficient to maintain viability of the heart muscle, i.e. blood flow matches function. Recent studies suggest that myocardial hibernation may result from repetitive episodes of cardiac stunning that occur, for example, with repeated exercise in a patient with coronary artery disease. Myocardial stunning is reversible ventricular dysfunction that persists following an episode of ischaemia when the blood flow has returned to normal, i.e. there is a mismatch between flow and function.

The clinical relevance of the hibernating and stunned myocardium is that in the past these were wrongly ascribed to myocardial necrosis and scarring. Myocardial viability can be assessed using echocardiography and nuclear techniques, as well as positron emission tomography (PET). Cardiac function can be restored by coronary revascularization.

Pacemaker or implantable cardioverter–defibrillator (p. 656)

Pacemakers are indicated in patients with sino-atrial disease and atrioventricular conduction block. The use of pacemakers in patients without AV block is more controversial, but they may have a role in a minority of patients with prolonged PR intervals, left bundle branch block and severe mitral regurgitation.

In patients with a history of sustained ventricular tachycardia or ventricular fibrillation, implantable cardioverter–defibrillators (ICDs) (p. 673) are effective in terminating further episodes of ventricular arrhythmia. Their effect on survival in relation to established drug therapies requires further study.

Cardiac transplantation

Since the advent of cyclosporin in the late 1970s and improved immunosuppression regimens, cardiac transplantation has become the treatment of choice for younger patients with severe intractable heart failure, whose life expectancy is less than six months. With careful recipient selection, the expected one-year survival for patients following transplantation is over 80%, and is 70% at five years. Irrespective of survival, quality of life is dramatically improved for the majority of patients.

Heart allografts do not function normally. Cardiac denervation results in a high resting heart rate, loss of diurnal blood pressure variation and impaired renin–angiotensin–aldosterone regulation. Some patients develop 'stiff heart' syndrome, thought to be caused by rejection, denervation and ischaemic injury during organ harvest and implantation. Transplantation of an inappropriately small donor heart can also result in elevated right and left heart pressure.

The complications of heart transplantation are summarized in Table 11.23. Many (infection, malignancy, hypertension and hyperlipidaemia) are related to immunosuppression. Allograft coronary atherosclerosis is the major cause of long-term graft failure and is present in 30–50% of patients at five years. It is thought to be caused by a 'vascular' rejection process in conjunction with hypertension and hyperlipidaemia.

While there are specific contraindications to cardiac transplantation (Table 11.24), the principal limitation to its use is the shortage of donor hearts. Several alternatives to transplantation are being investigated: cardiomyoplasty (augmentation of left ventricular contraction by wrapping a latissimus dorsi muscle flap around the ventricle), artificial hearts and left ventricular assist devices. In the future, xenografts may supplant human hearts as donor organs. A new operation, the Babista procedure, that surgically reduces the size of the left ventricular activity is currently undergoing evaluation.

Table 11.23
Complications of cardiac transplantation

Allograft rejection 'Humoral' 'Vascular' 'Cell-mediated'	**Allograft vascular disease**
	Malignancy
	Hypertension
Infections Early: nosocomial organisms, staphylococci, Gram-negatives Late (2–6 months): opportunistic (toxoplasmosis, cytomegalovirus, fungi, *Pneumocystis*)	**Hypercholesterolaemia**

Pulmonary oedema

This is a very frightening, life-threatening emergency characterized by extreme breathlessness. The dyspnoea may first occur at night in the form of paroxysmal dyspnoea due to pulmonary congestion. This occurs because of reabsorption of dependent oedema when lying flat, and the relative insensitivity of the respiratory centre at night allows pulmonary congestion to develop. In more severe cases the patient is severely breathless at all times of the day.

Table 11.24
Contraindications for cardiac transplantation

Age > 60 years (some variations between centres)
Alcohol/drug abuse
Uncontrolled psychiatric illness
Uncontrolled infection
Severe renal/liver failure
High pulmonary vascular resistance
Systemic disease with multiorgan involvement
Treated cancer in remission but with <5 years' follow-up
Recent thromboembolism
Other disease with a poor prognosis

PATHOPHYSIOLOGY

Left ventricular failure and mitral valve disease cause pulmonary oedema because of increased pulmonary capillary pressure. A pressure above 20 mmHg causes increased filtration of fluid out of the capillaries into the interstitial space (interstitial oedema). Further accumulation of fluid disrupts intercellular membranes, leading to the collection of fluid in the alveolar spaces (alveolar oedema). Alveolar oedema occurs when the capillary pressure exceeds the total oncotic pressures (approximately 30 mmHg).

CLINICAL FEATURES

Patients with alveolar oedema are acutely breathless, wheezing, anxious and perspiring profusely. In addition, they usually have a cough productive of frothy, blood-tinged (pink) sputum, which can be copious. The patient is tachypnoeic with peripheral circulatory shutdown. There is a tachycardia, a raised venous pressure and a gallop rhythm. Crackles and wheeze are heard throughout the chest. The arterial PO_2 falls and initially the P_aCO_2 also falls owing to overbreathing. Later, however, the P_aCO_2 increases because of impaired gas exchange. The chest X-ray shows diffuse haziness owing to alveolar fluid and the Kerley B lines of interstitial oedema (see Fig 11.15). The abnormality can be unilateral, giving the appearance of a tumour that disappears on treatment (a pseudotumour).

TREATMENT

The patient should be placed in a sitting position. High-concentration oxygen (60% via a variable performance mask) is given unless it is suspected that there is a coexisting chronic hypercapnia due to longstanding respiratory failure. In severe cases it may be necessary to ventilate the patient (see p. 651).

Intravenous diuretic treatment with frusemide or bumetanide is given. These diuretics produce immediate vasodilatation in addition to the more delayed diuretic response.

Morphine (10–20 mg i.v. depending on the size of the patient) together with an antiemetic such as metoclopramide (10 mg i.v.) or cyclizine (50 mg i.v.) is given. Morphine sedates the patient and causes systemic vasodilatation; it must be *avoided* if the systemic arterial pressure is less than 90 mmHg. Respiratory depression occurs with large doses of morphine.

Venous vasodilators, such as glyceryl trinitrate, may produce prompt relief by reducing the preload. Cardiac output may be increased by using arterial vasodilatation, such as occurs with hydralazine (see Table 11.22 and Fig 11.54).

Aminophylline (250–500 mg or 5 mg kg^{-1} i.v.) is infused over 10 minutes. Aminophylline is a phosphodiesterase inhibitor that causes bronchodilatation, vasodilatation and increased cardiac contractility. It must be given slowly because of the risk of precipitating ventricular arrhythmias. It is now only used when bronchospasm is present.

Venesection and mechanical methods of reducing venous return (e.g. sphygmomanometer cuffs inflated to 10 mmHg below diastolic blood pressure and placed around the thighs) are inefficient and rarely used.

In a severe case, after the acute emergency is controlled, a pulmonary artery balloon catheter may be inserted to monitor progress and treatment. Any factor that precipitated the heart failure, such as cardiac arrhythmias or chest infection, should be corrected. The underlying cardiac problem should be diagnosed and treated.

Cardiogenic shock

Shock is a severe failure of tissue perfusion, usually characterized by hypotension, a low cardiac output and signs of poor tissue perfusion such as oliguria, cold extremities and poor cerebral function. *Cardiogenic shock* (pump failure) is an extreme type of cardiac failure with a high mortality of approximately 90%. Its most common cause is myocardial infarction.

Cardiogenic shock must be differentiated from other forms of shock. Cardiogenic shock is diagnosed when the shock syndrome occurs despite an adequate or elevated pulmonary capillary wedge pressure and in the absence of mechanical circulatory obstruction. An essential element in this diagnosis is the measurement of the pulmonary capillary wedge pressure (see p. 841). In situations where the vascular capacity has expanded or the circulatory fluid volume has decreased, the wedge pressure will be low. In cardiogenic shock the wedge pressure is normal or elevated.

The mortality rate in cardiogenic shock is so high because of the vicious downward spiral that occurs: hypotension due to pump failure results in a reduction of coronary flow, which results in further impairment of pump function, and so on.

TREATMENT (see also p. 842)

Patients require intensive care, as described in Chapter 13. General measures such as complete rest, continuous 60% oxygen administration and pain relief are essential.

The infusion of fluid is necessary if the pulmonary capillary wedge pressure is below 18 mmHg, which is probably the optimal 'filling pressure' with which to prime a failing heart.

Short-acting venous dilators such as glyceryl trinitrate or sodium nitroprusside should be administered intravenously if the wedge pressure is 25 mmHg or more.

Cardiac inotropes such as dobutamine and dopamine may be used to increase aortic diastolic pressure (coronary perfusion pressure). Dopamine also selectively increases renal perfusion.

Mechanical assist devices such as an intra-aortic balloon pump may be used (see p. 657). Although leading to a temporary improvement, long-term prognosis is not improved unless there is a surgically correctable cause, such as a ruptured interventricular septum or acute mitral regurgitation.

FURTHER READING

Cohn JN (1996) The management of chronic heart failure. *New England Journal of Medicine* **335**: 490–498.

Marwick TH (1998) The viable myocardium. *Lancet* **341**: 815–816.

Task Force of the Working Group on Heart Failure of the European Society of Cardiology (1997) Treatment of heart failure. *European Heart Journal* **18**: 736–753.

Ischaemic heart disease

Myocardial ischaemia occurs when there is an imbalance between the supply of oxygen (and other essential myocardial nutrients) and the myocardial demand for these substances. The causes are as follows:

- The coronary blood flow to a region of the myocardium may be reduced by a mechanical obstruction that is due to:
  atheroma
  thrombosis
  spasm
  embolus
  coronary ostial stenosis
  coronary arteritis (e.g. in SLE).
- There can be a decrease in the flow of oxygenated blood to the myocardium that is due to:
  anaemia
  carboxyhaemoglobulinaemia
  hypotension causing decreased coronary perfusion pressure.
- An increased demand for oxygen may occur owing to an increase in cardiac output (e.g. thyrotoxicosis) or myocardial hypertrophy (e.g. from aortic stenosis or hypertension).

In the United Kingdom, myocardial ischaemia most commonly occurs as a result of obstructive coronary disease in the form of coronary atherosclerosis. In addition to this fixed obstruction, variations in the tone of smooth muscle in the wall of a coronary artery may add an important element of dynamic or variable obstruction.

Coronary artery disease is the largest single cause of death in the UK. There are approximately 60 deaths per 100 000 (giving a standardized mortality rate of about 200 per 100 000).

Coronary atherosclerosis

Coronary atherosclerosis is a complex process characterized by the accumulation of lipid, macrophages and smooth muscle cells in intimal plaques in the large and medium-sized epicardial coronary arteries. The vascular endothelium plays a critical role in maintaining vascular in-tegrity and homeostasis. Mechanical shear stresses, biochemical abnormalities and immunological factors may contribute to the initial endothelial 'injury' which is believed to trigger atherogenesis. The resultant endothelial dysfunction allows accumulation of oxidized lipoproteins which are taken up by macrophages to produce lipid-laden foam cells. Release of a host of cytokines such as platelet-derived growth factor and transforming growth factor-β promote further accumulation of macrophages as well as smooth muscle cell migration and proliferation.

A 50% reduction in luminal diameter (producing a reduction in luminal cross-sectional area of approximately 70%) causes a haemodynamically significant stenosis. At this point the smaller distal intramyocardial arteries and arterioles are maximally dilated (coronary flow reserve is near zero), and any increase in myocardial oxygen demand provokes ischaemia.

(a)

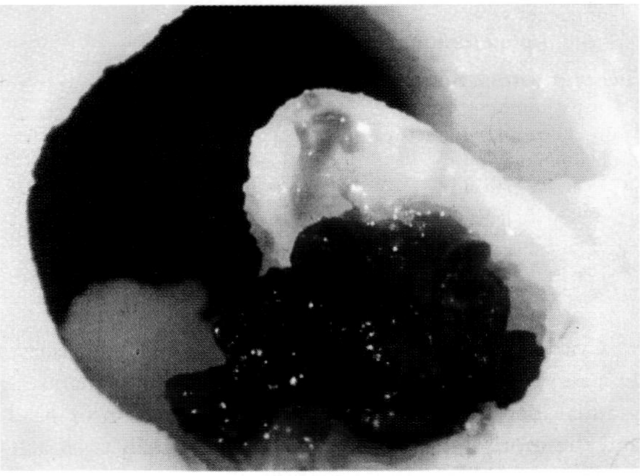

(b)

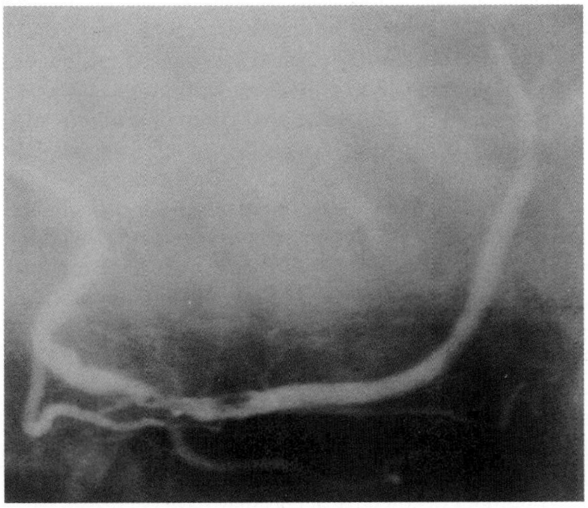

Fig 11.55
Acute coronary thrombi
(a) Cross-section (× 30) of the epicardial coronary artery, demonstrating a rupture of the shoulder region of the plaque with a luminal thrombus
(b) Angiogram demonstrating a severe proximal right coronary artery stenosis and a fresh semi-occlusive thrombus extending about 2 cm distal to the stenosis

Table 11.25
Risk factors for coronary disease

Fixed	
Age	
Male sex	
Positive family history	
Deletion polymorphism in the ACE gene (DD)	
Potentially changeable with treatment	
Strong association	
Hyperlipidaemia	
Cigarette smoking	
Hypertension	
Diabetes mellitus	
Weak association	
Personality	
Obesity	
Gout	
Soft water	
Lack of exercise	
Contraceptive pill	
Heavy alcohol consumption	
Recent associations	
Plasma homocysteine	
Blood coagulation factors	
Fibrinogen	
C-reactive protein	
Chlamydia pneumoniae	

ACE, angiotensin-converting enzyme

Coronary atherosclerosis is a progressive disease. Disease progression occurs by two basic mechanisms: gradual increase in plaque size by incorporation of lipid, and the more unpredictable changes in lumen encroachment as a result of plaque rupture.

Plaque rupture results from fissuring of the fibrous cap leading to exposure of the extracellular matrix (in particular, tissue factor) which triggers platelet adhesion, aggregation and activation. Plaques that are vulnerable to rupture are those with large lipid cores, thin fibrous caps (with high densities of activated macrophages and low density of smooth muscle cells). The resultant platelet activation leads to the release of active mediators (including thromboxane A2, 5-hydroxytryptamine and adenosine diphosphate) which trigger further platelet activation and activation of the coagulation cascade. As a result thrombus forms, reducing the lumen further (Fig 11.55). In addition, vasoactive substances, such as 5-hydroxytryptamine and thromboxane A2, released from aggregating platelets, cause transient local vasoconstriction, and dysfunctional endothelium produces less vasodilatory substances such as nitric oxide and prostacyclin.

A number of infective agents may have been associated with coronary atherosclerosis, including *Helicobacter pylori* and *Chlamydia pneumoniae*. Further studies are required in order to establish if they contribute directly to the pathogenesis of this chronic inflammatory disease.

Coronary artery disease gives rise to a wide variety of clinical presentations. These range from relatively stable angina through to the acute coronary syndromes of unstable angina and myocardial infarction. These will be discussed in detail below.

Risk factors for coronary artery disease

The aetiology of coronary artery disease is multifactorial, and a number of 'risk' factors are known to predispose to the condition (Table 11.25). Some of these – such as age, gender, race and family history – cannot be changed, whereas other major risk factors, such as serum cholesterol, smoking habits, diabetes and hypertension, can be modified.

Age

Coronary artery disease rates increase with age. Atherosclerosis is rare in childhood, except in familial hyperlipidaemia, but is often detectable in young men between 20 and 30 years of age. It is almost universal in the elderly in the West.

Gender

Men have a higher incidence of coronary artery disease than premenopausal women. However, after the menopause, the incidence of atheroma in women approaches that in men. The reasons for this gender difference is not clearly understood, but probably relates to the loss of the protective effect of oestrogen.

Family history

Coronary artery disease is often found in several members of the same family. Because the disease is so prevalent and because other risk factors are familial, it is uncertain whether family history, *per se*, is an independent risk factor. A positive family history is generally accepted to refer to those in whom a first-degree relative has developed ischaemic heart disease before the age of 50 years.

Hyperlipidaemia (see p. 991)

A high serum cholesterol, especially when associated with low values of high-density lipoproteins (HDLs), is strongly associated with coronary atheroma. There is increasing evidence that high triglycerides are also independently linked with coronary atheroma.

Familial hypercholesterolaemia, familial combined with hyperlipidaemia and remnant hyperlipidaemia are also associated with increased risk of coronary atherosclerosis.

Measurement of the fasting lipid profile (total cholesterol, low- and high-density lipoproteins and triglycerides) should be performed on all patients. Angiographic studies have shown that lowering the serum cholesterol can not only slow the progression of coronary atherosclerosis, but can cause regression of disease. Large clinical trials have shown that lipid-lowering can decrease total mortality and new coronary events, and reduce the need for revascularization. Management is described on p. 995.

Smoking

In men, the risk of developing coronary artery disease is directly related to the number of cigarettes smoked. This relationship is less certain (but still important) in women and cigar and pipe smokers. The risk from smoking declines to almost normal after ten years of abstention.

Hypertension

Both systolic and diastolic hypertension are associated with an increased risk of coronary artery disease. The risk is the same for men and women. Whilst reduction of blood pressure reduces the risk of a cerebrovascular event, it does not appear to affect the risk of cardiac events such as myocardial infarction.

Diet

Diets high in fats are associated with ischaemic heart disease, as are those with low intakes of anti-oxidants. Supplementation may be helpful (see p. 201).

Other factors

Diabetes mellitus, or even just an abnormal glucose tolerance test, is strongly associated with vascular disease. Obesity, particularly central obesity, is associated with coronary artery disease, but it is not certain whether obesity itself is independently linked to the condition.

Coronary artery disease rates also vary among different ethnic groups, by socioeconomic status and geographical region.

Lack of exercise is thought to increase the risk of coronary artery disease, and regular exercise probably protects against its development.

A number of genetic factors have been linked with coronary artery disease. The angiotensin-converting enzyme (ACE) gene contains an insertion/deletion (I/D) polymorphism, the DD genotype of which has been associated with a predisposition to coronary artery disease and myocardial infarction.

High levels of coagulation factor VII and fibrinogen are associated risk factors. Polymorphisms of the factor VII gene may increase the risk of myocardial infarction.

Elevated plasma homocysteine levels are a risk factor for coronary heart disease and a strong predictor of mortality in this group. Its effects are thought to be due to an interference with coagulation and the vasodilator and antithrombotic effects of nitric oxide. A raised C-reactive protein is also a risk factor.

It is clear that many factors influence the development of coronary atheroma. Modification of some of these can help reduce both the development of the coronary artery disease (primary prevention) and slow the progression of established disease (secondary prevention). In addition, for primary prevention for men with high risk factors, aspirin 75 mg per day should be given.

Angina (see also p. 630)

The diagnosis of angina is largely based on the clinical history. The chest pain is generally described as 'heavy', 'tight' or 'gripping'. Typically, the pain is central/retrosternal and may radiate to the jaw and/or arms. Angina can range from a mild ache to a most severe pain that provokes sweating and fear. There may be associated breathlessness. Angina is common with a prevalence of approximately 2%. The incidence of new cases each year is approximately 1 per 1000.

Classical or exertional angina pectoris is provoked by physical exertion, especially after meals and in cold, windy weather, and is commonly aggravated by anger or excitement. The pain fades quickly (usually within minutes) with rest. Occasionally it disappears with continued exertion ('walking through the pain'). Whilst in some patients the pain occurs predictably at a certain level of exertion, in most patients the threshold for developing pain is variable. The severity of pain can be graded according to the Canadian Cardiovascular Society as in Table 11.3.

Decubitus angina is that occurring on lying down. It usually occurs in association with impaired left ventricular function, as a result of severe coronary artery disease. Nocturnal angina is that occurring at night and may wake the patient from sleep. It may be provoked by vivid dreams. It tends to occur in patients with critical coronary artery disease and may be the result of vasospasm.

Variant (Prinzmetal's) angina refers to an angina that occurs without provocation, usually at rest, as a result of coronary artery spasm. It occurs more frequently in women. Characteristically, there is ST segment elevation during the pain. Specialist investigation using provocation tests (e.g. hyperventilation, cold-pressor testing or ergometrine challenge) may be required to establish the diagnosis. Arrhythmias, both ventricular tachyarrhythmias and heart block, can occur during the ischaemic episode.

Cardiac syndrome X refers to those patients with a good history of angina, a positive exercise test and angiographically normal coronary arteries. This forms a heterogeneous group in whom there may be functional abnormalities of the coronary microcirculation. It is much more common in women than in men. Whilst they have a good prognosis, they are often highly symptomatic and can be difficult to treat.

Unstable angina refers to angina of recent onset (less than one month), worsening angina or angina at rest, and will be described in more detail below.

EXAMINATION AND DIAGNOSIS

There are usually no abnormal findings in angina, although occasionally a fourth heart sound may be heard. Signs to suggest anaemia, thyrotoxicosis or hyperlipidaemia (e.g. lipid arcus, xanthelasma, tendon xanthoma) should be sought. It is essential to exclude aortic stenosis (i.e. slow-rising carotid impulse and

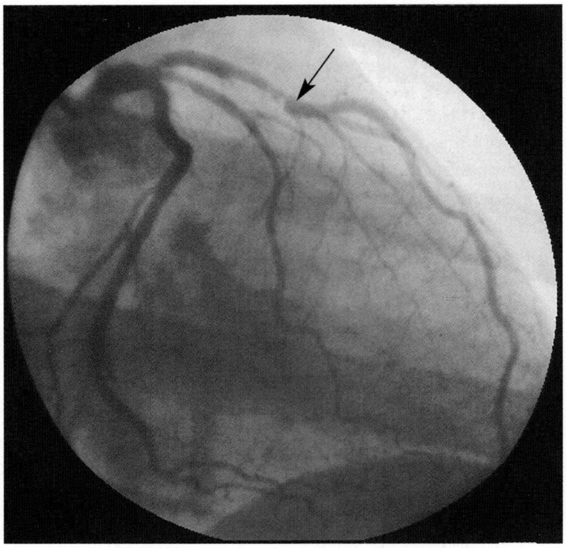

Fig 11.56
Left coronary angiogram. X-ray contrast material is injected into the ostium of the left main coronary artery. In this example, the left main artery divides into three vessels: left anterior descending (top) diagonal and circumflex (bottom) vessels. In the proximal part of the left anterior descending artery is a severe narrowing due to an atherosclerotic plaque (arrow)

ejection systolic murmur radiating to the neck) as a possible cause for the angina. The blood pressure should be taken to identify coexistent hypertension.

INVESTIGATIONS FOR ANGINA

Resting ECG

This is usually normal between attacks. Evidence of old myocardial infarction (e.g. pathological Q waves), left ventricular hypertrophy or left bundle branch block may be present. During an attack, transient ST depression, T-wave inversion or upright T waves may appear.

Exercise ECG

Exercise testing can be very useful both in confirming the diagnosis of angina and in giving some indication as to the severity of the coronary artery disease. ST segment depression of greater than or equal to 1 mm suggests myocardial ischaemia, particularly if typical chest pain occurs at the same time (Fig 11.20).

Approximately 75% of patients with significant coronary artery disease will give a positive test. A strongly positive test (within six minutes of starting the Bruce protocol) suggests 'prognostic' disease (see surgical management below) and helps to identify patients who should be considered for coronary angiography. Exercise testing, however, can be misleading:

- A normal test does not exclude coronary artery disease (so-called false-negative test) although these patients, as a group, have a good prognosis
- Up to 20% of patients with positive exercise tests are subsequently found to have no evidence of coronary artery disease (so-called false-positive test).

Table 11.26
Indications for coronary angiography

Angina refractory to medical therapy
Strongly positive exercise test
Unstable angina
Angina occurring after myocardial infarction
Patients under 50 years with angina or myocardial infarction
Where the diagnosis of angina is uncertain

Cardiac scintigraphy

Myocardial perfusion scans (see p. 651) both at rest and after stress, can be obtained using various contrast agents (e.g. thallium-201 or technetium-99 MIBI – methoxyisobutylisonitrile). When a patient is unable to exercise, the heart can be 'stressed' with drugs such as dipyridamole or dobutamine. Redistribution of the contrast agent is a sensitive indicator of ischaemia and can be particularly useful in deciding if a stenosis seen at angiography is giving rise to ischaemia. Again a normal perfusion scan makes significant coronary artery disease unlikely.

Echocardiography

This can be used to assess ventricular wall involvement and ventricular function. Regional wall motion abnormalities at rest reflect previous ventricular damage. Stress echocardiography, although technically difficult, is useful especially in women with coronary artery disease.

Coronary angiography

This is occasionally useful in patients with chest pain where the diagnosis is unclear. More often, the test is performed to delineate the exact coronary anatomy (Fig 11.56) in patients being considered for revascularization (i.e. coronary artery bypass grafting or coronary angioplasty). Coronary angiography should be performed only when the benefit in terms of diagnosis and potential treatment outweighs the small risk of the procedure (a mortality rate of less than one in 1000 cases). The indications for coronary angiography are outlined in Table 11.26.

Lesions with complex morphology (irregular borders, overhanging edges, thrombus or ulceration) appear to identify a subgroup of stenoses associated with disease progression and adverse clinical outcomes.

TREATMENT OF ANGINA

General management

Patients should be informed as to the nature of their condition and reassured that, in general, the prognosis is good (annual mortality less than 2%). Underlying problems, such as anaemia or hyperthyroidism, should be treated. Managment of coexistent conditions, such as diabetes and hypertension, should be optimized. Risk

Table 11.27
Calcium-channel blockers

	Class 1 (non-dihydropyridine) (e.g. verapamil, diltiazem	Class 2 (dihydropyridine) (e.g. nifedipine, nicardipine, amlodipine)
Effects		
Sinus node suppression	+++	+
AV node suppression	+++	+
Myocardial depression	++	++
Arteriolar vasodilation	+	+++
Side-effects		
Flushing, ankle oedema, palpitations	+	++
Bradycardia, impaired AV conduction	++	+
Aggravation of heart failure	++	+
Combination with β-blockers	No	Yes

AV, atrioventricular

factors should be evaluated and steps made to correct them where possible; for example, smoking must be stopped, hypercholesterolaemia should be identified and treated (see below), weight loss where appropriate and regular exercise should be encouraged.

Choosing between medical therapy and revascularization (coronary artery bypass grafting and angioplasty) can be difficult and will depend on a number of factors including symptoms, angiographic anatomy and patient/physician preference. The various treatment options are not mutually exclusive and should be considered as complementary.

Medical treatment

In recent years there has been a change in emphasis to encompass the concept of medication that alters prognosis and medication used to control symptoms.

Prognostic therapies

There is good evidence that aspirin reduces the risk of coronary events in patients with coronary artery disease. All patients with angina, therefore, should take aspirin (75 mg daily is probably adequate) unless contraindicated.

Lipid-lowering therapy should be considered in patients with total cholesterol above 4.8 mmol L^{-1} (particularly if the LDL is >3.3 mmol L^{-1} and the HDL is <1.0 mmol L^{-1}), despite a low fate diet. If the triglycerides (TGs) are under 3.5 mmol L^{-1} then one of the statins (HMG CoA reductase inhibitors) should be used. If the TGs are above 3.5 mmol L^{-1} a fibrate should be considered. If simple therapy fails to reduce the LDL adequately, then the patient should be referred to a lipidologist. Lipid-lowering therapy can be expected to prevent 20–30 deaths or myocardial infarcts per 1000 patient-years.

Symptomatic treatment

Glyceryl trinitrate (GTN) used sublingually, either as a tablet or as a spray, gives prompt relief (in a few minutes) and can also be used prior to performing activities that the patient knows will provoke angina.

All but the most mildly affected patients will probably require regular prophylactic therapy. The choice of drugs is between β-blockers, nitrates and calcium-channel blockers. There is no commonly accepted algorithm and treatment needs to be tailored to the individual patient. Some patients will require combination therapy, but there

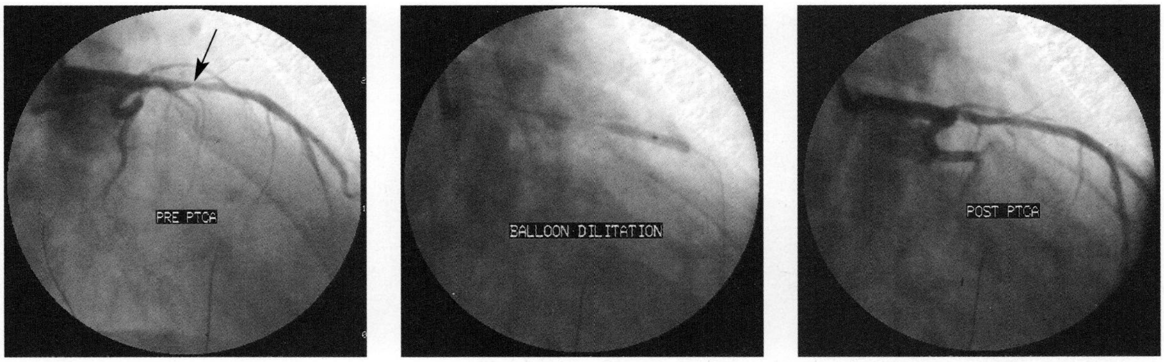

Fig 11.57
Percutaneous transluminal coronary angioplasty (PTCA) demonstrated in a sequence of three films in a patient with a 90% stenosis in the proximal left anterior descending coronary artery (left film taken during coronary angiogram). The middle X-ray shows the inflated angioplasty balloon across the arterial lesion. The right film is taken from the post-PTCA coronary angiogram. It shows virtually complete alleviation of the stenosis

is little evidence that adding a third drug is of benefit. Patients not controlled adequately on medical therapy should be considered for revascularization (see below).

β-Blockers reduce the heart rate (negative chronotropic effect) and the force of ventricular contraction (negative inotropic effect), both of which reduce the myocardial oxygen demand, especially on exertion. They are the drug of choice in patients with previous myocardial infarction because of their proven benefit in secondary prevention. Atenolol, 50–100 mg daily, is the most commonly prescribed. Metoprolol, 25–50 mg twice daily, is often used if renal function is impaired. β-Blockers may aggravate coronary artery spasm.

Long-acting nitrates (e.g. isosorbide mononitrate) are particularly useful in patients who gain relief from sublingual GTN. They reduce venous return and hence intracardiac diastolic pressures, reduce the impedence to the emptying of the left ventricule and relax the tone of the coronary arteries. Once-daily preparations are available which have a smooth pharmacokinetic profile and avoid the problem of tolerance. Nitrates should be given with care to patients on other hypotensive agents. Sildenafil should not be given to patients taking nitrates.

Calcium-channel blockers block calcium flux into the cell and the utilization of calcium within the cell (Table 11.27). They relax coronary arteries, cause peripheral vasodilation and reduce the force of left ventricular contraction, thereby reducing the oxygen demand of the myocardium. The non-dihydropyridine calcium antagonists (e.g. diltiazem and verpamail) also reduce the heart rate and are particularly useful anti-anginal agents, but should be used with caution in combination with β-blockers. Short-acting dihydropyridines (e.g. nifedipine) can cause reflex tachycardia when used alone. Case-control studies have suggested that high-dose nifedipine is associated with adverse outcome. Slow-release formulations and the third-generation agents (e.g. amlodipine) can be used once daily and have a smooth profile of action with no significant effect on the heart rate and no significant negative inotropic effect.

Specific T (transient) channel blockers are being developed. Mibefradil was introduced in 1997 but has been withdrawn because of drug interactions.

Nicorandil is a relatively new drug that combines nitrate-like activity with potassium-channel blockade. Whilst not used as a first-line drug, it may be useful when there are contraindications to the above agents.

Observational studies suggest that *hormone replacement therapy* (HRT) is cardioprotective. Exogenous oestrogen increases HDL, decreases oxidation of LDL and has beneficial effects on vasomotion. However, side-effects such as vaginal bleeding, and adverse effects such as the possible increase in risk of breast cancer, have limited its use. HRT is likely to be of benefit in women with a high risk of developing ischaemic heart disease and should be considered for all women with established coronary artery disease who are not at high risk of breast carcinoma. Data from long-term randomized trials regarding the risks and benefits of HRT are awaited.

Coronary angioplasty

Percutaneous transluminal coronary angioplasty (PTCA) refers to the technique of dilating coronary atheromatous obstructions by inflating a balloon within the obstruction (Fig 11.57). The balloon, which is mounted on the tip of a very thin catheter, is inserted through the obstruction using X-ray fluoroscopy and is then inflated with dilute contrast material. Multiple inflations of the balloon using a pressure of several atmospheres usually relieves the obstruction.

A number of different mechanisms have been postulated, including fracturing and compression of the plaque, and stretching of the artery. Endothelial denudation, local dissection and distal embolization also occur and may account for some of the complications of the procedure. Whilst PTCA is ideally suited to single, discrete stenoses, multiple lesions may be treated and repeat procedures can be undertaken.

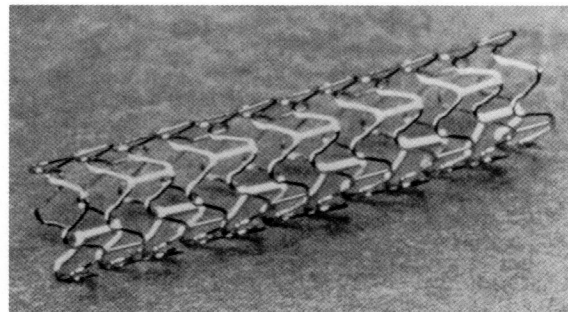

Fig 11.58
Intra-coronary stents

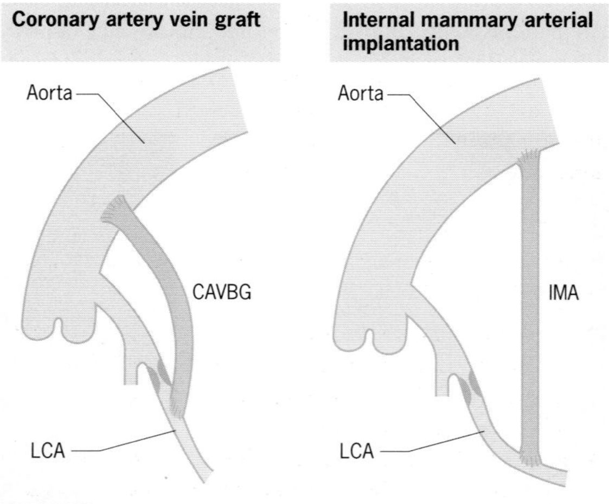

Fig 11.59
Relief of coronary obstruction by surgical techniques: coronary artery vein bypass grafting (CAVBG) or internal mammary arterial implantation (IMA). In both of these examples, the graft bypasses a coronary obstruction in the left coronary artery (LCA)

Table 11.28
Risk stratification in patients with unstable angina

High risk	Intermediate risk	Low risk
Prolonged, ongoing (> 20 min) rest pain	Rest angina (< 20 min or relieved with GTN)	Increased angina severity frequency or duration
Pulmonary oedema or angina with hypotension	New-onset angina (<4 weeks) Nocturnal angina	Angina provoked at a lower threshold, but no rest pain
Rest angina with dynamic ST changes >1 mm	Angina with dynamic T wave changes	Normal/unchanged ECG
Raised troponin (I/T)	Age >65 years	Normal troponin I/T

Acute coronary occlusion occurs in a small proportion of cases (2–4%), and local dissection of the coronary artery is frequently observed. PTCAs improve symptoms of angina, but confer no signficant prognostic benefit. The risks associated with PTCA are often understated and comprise: mortality (1%), acute myocardial infarction (2%), and the need for urgent coronary artery bypass grafting (CABG) (2%).

A number of trials have compared PTCA with medical therapy for stable angina. PTCA may provide more complete relief from angina, but is associated with higher rates of myocardial infarction or bypass surgery (as a result of this procedure).

An increasing number of intracoronary stents (Fig 11.58) are being used both to 'bale out' in cases of dissection and for the primary treatment of stenoses in: large vessels (>3 mm; for example, proximal lesions in big left anterior descending arteries and dominant right coronary arteries), in coronary vein grafts, and in restenotic lesions following PTCA. Stents have a lower incidence of restenosis which still complicates up to 30% of PTCAs (usually within the first six months post-procedure), but are more expensive. Aspirin plus other antiplatelet agents (e.g. ticlopidine) are routinely prescribed following stent insertion. The use of monoclonal antibodies to the glycoprotein IIb/IIIa platelet receptor (the final common pathway of aggregation) in selected high-risk cases may reduce periprocedural complications. Ongoing studies of new stents and optimal antithrombotic therapies may improve both the short-term success of the procedure and longer-term outcome (incidence of restenosis).

Surgical management (Fig 11.59)

There are two principal indications for coronary artery bypass grafting (CABG):

- *Symptom control* in patients who remain symptomatic despite optimal medical therapy and whose disease is not suitable for PTCA. Surgery provides dramatic relief from angina in about 90% of cases.
- *Prognostic disease* in patients with severe three-vessel coronary artery disease (significant proximal stenoses in all three main coronary vessels), particularly those with impaired left ventricular function, and those with left main stem artery disease. These patients obtain prognostic benefit from CABG, irrespective of symptoms.

Where possible, the left internal mammary artery (LIMA) is used to bypass proximal stenoses in the left anterior descending artery. Similarly, the right internal mammary artery is increasingly being used to bypass stenoses in the right coronary artery. Reverse saphenous vein grafts are still commonly used in addition to arterial grafts, although the long-term patency is less good with atheromatous occlusion occurring in up to 10% of cases per year. Operative mortality is well below 1% in patients with normal left ventricular function. Perioperative strokes occur in up to 2% of cases, and more subtle neurological deficits are common.

Minimally invasive operative procedures for bypass grafting ('MIDCAB') are being developed which do not require the use of extracorporeal circulatory support. These include laparoscopic approaches and may be of use in certain subgroups of patients (e.g. previous CABG and those with coexistent medical conditions which would increase the operative risks of 'full' CABG).

Aggressive lowering of LDL (to less than 2.5 mmol L^{-1}) has been shown to be of benefit in patients who have had coronary artery bypass surgery.

PTCA versus bypass surgery

Several studies have compared PTCA with bypass surgery. Both provide excellent symptomatic relief with a similar incidence of major ischaemic complications. The major short-term advantage of PTCA is the avoidance of major open heart surgery (and a shorter hospital stay). However, up to 50% of patients will require a repeat revascularization procedure within the next two years. There is some evidence that diabetic patients have a better five-year survival after treatment with bypass surgery than with PTCA.

Patients with intractable angina

Some patients remain symptomatic despite medication and are not suitable for (further) revascularization. Transmyocardial laser revascularization (TMR), whereby a laser is used to form channels in the myocardium to allow direct perfusion of the myocardium from blood within the ventricular cavity, is being developed in some centres.

Spinal cord stimulation (SCS) is accomplished using a flexible electrode in the epidural space at the mid-thoracic level. Stimulation via a pacemaker-like generator reduces angina and has been shown to reduce indices of ischaemia. Similarly, transcutaneous electrical nerve stimulation has been shown to reduce angina and increase exercise capacity in selected patients.

Unstable angina

Unstable angina is a medical emergency which, untreated, will progress to myocardial infarction in over 10% of cases. Standard therapy (see below) reduces this rate to less than 5%. However, death within one year still occurs in 5–15%.

Patients require admission for bedrest, aspirin and heparin as well as standard medical anti-anginal therapy (see above). Aspirin decreases the incidence of both death and myocardial infarction. Heparin, traditionally given intravenously, should be given for at least three days and probably confers additional benefit to that given by aspirin alone. There is increasing evidence that low-molecular-weight heparin (LMWH) is at least as effective as standard unfractionated heparin and has the advantage of being able to be given subcutaneously and of not requiring monitoring. Recent trials have shown that infusion of glycoprotein IIb/IIIa receptor inhibitors (e.g. abciximab) may have an additional advantage over heparin plus aspirin. These receptors are activated in the final common pathway of platelet aggregation.

In terms of the short-term risk of death or myocardial infarction, it is possible to risk-stratify patients with unstable angina into high risk, intermediate risk and low risk (Table 11.28).

Those at high risk should proceed promptly to angiography, with a view to proceeding to revascularization, where appropriate, during that admission. Those at low risk can be discharged and then assessed electively as outpatients. In between, there is much controversy regarding the optimal management of patients at intermediate risk, and in particular those who settle on initial medical therapy. Early intervention does not convincingly appear to influence the medium- and long-term outcomes. Attention is increasingly being directed at therapies which can favourably influence the proco-agulant/thrombogenic state that seems to persist for several months following presentation. In particular, the prolonged use (weeks to months) of subcutaneous low-molecular-weight heparin and oral glycoprotein IIb/IIIa antagonists are under investigation.

Irrespective of the immediate success of treatment, early coronary angiography and, depending on the results, referral for revascularization are usually advised.

Thrombolytic therapy has not been shown to be of benefit in patients with unstable angina. Occasionally, intra-aortic balloon pumping (see p. 657) can be helpful in stabilizing the patient, and to enable angiography (± PTCA) to be undertaken.

Myocardial infarction

Myocardial infarction is the most common cause of death in the UK. There are approximately 300 000 new myocardial infarctions per year and only half of these survive the acute event. A further 10% die in hospital and up to 20% more die in the first two years. Fifty per cent of initial survivors are alive at ten years.

Myocardial infarctions almost always occur in patients with coronary atheroma as a result of plaque rupture with superadded thrombus. This occlusive thrombus consists of a platelet-rich core ('white clot') and a bulkier surrounding fibrin-rich ('red') clot. About six hours after the onset of infarction, the myocardium is swollen and pale, and at 24 hours the necrotic tissue appears deep red owing to haemorrhage. In the next few weeks, an inflammatory reaction develops and the infarcted tissue turns grey and gradually forms a thin, fibrous scar.

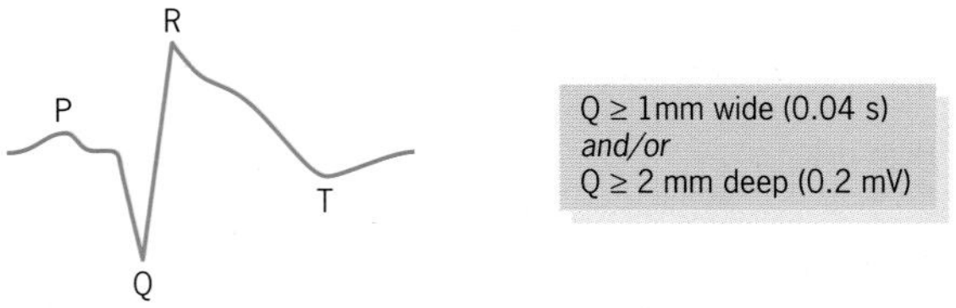

Fig 11.60
Electrocardiographic features of myocardial infarction, showing a Q wave, ST elevation and T wave inversion

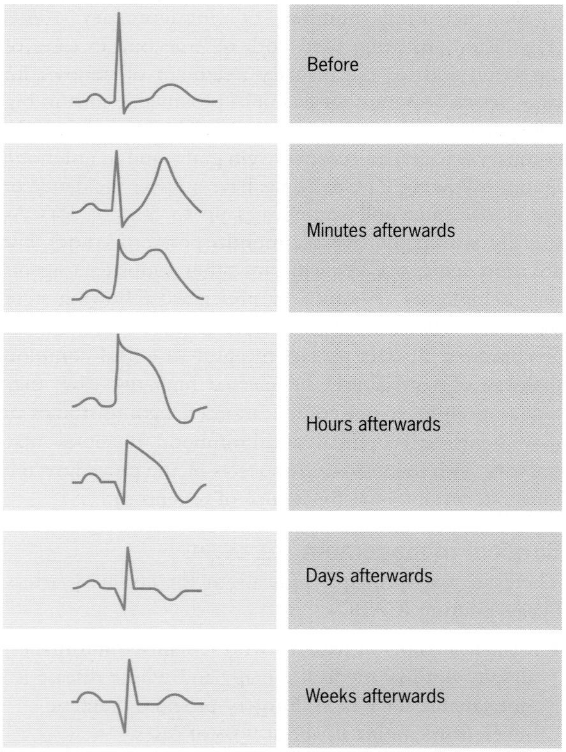

Fig 11.61
Electrocardiographic evolution of myocardial infarction. After the first few minutes the T waves become tall, pointed and upright and there is ST segment elevation. After the first few hours the T waves invert, the R wave voltage is decreased and Q waves develop. After a few days the ST segment returns to normal. After weeks or months the T wave may return to upright but the Q wave remains

Remodelling refers to the alteration in size, shape and thickness of both the infarcted myocardium (which thins and expands) and the compensatory hypertrophy that occurs in other areas of the myocardium. The resultant global ventricular dilatation may help maintain the stroke volume of the heart.

The use of thrombolysis (see below) has transformed the acute management of patients with myocardial infarction. Thrombolysis recanalizes the thrombotic occlusion by lysing the fibrin-rich elements, resulting in restoration of coronary blood flow. Many large trials have established benefits in reducing infarct size, improving myocardial function and improving survival. Paramedic and hospital services should be organized to ensure its prompt administration. GPIIb/IIIa antagonists which disaggregate the white clot are currently being investigated.

CLINICAL FEATURES

Myocardial infarction typically presents with severe chest pain, similar in character to exertional angina. The onset is usually sudden, often occurring at rest, and persists fairly constantly for some hours (often it continues until diamorphine is given). Whilst the pain may be so severe that the patient fears imminent death, it can be less severe, and as many as 20% of patients with myocardial infarction have no pain. So-called 'silent' myocardial infarctions are more common in diabetics and the elderly. Myocardial infarction is often accompanied by sweating, breathlessness, nausea, vomiting and restlessness.

Patients with acute myocardial infarction appear pale, sweaty and grey. There may be no specific physical sign unless complications develop (see below). A sinus tachycardia, fourth heart sound and a raised JVP are common. A modest fever (up to 38°C) due to myocardial necrosis often occurs over the course of the first five days.

Diagnosis requires *at least two* of the following:

Table 11.29
Typical ECG changes in myocardial infarction

Infarct site	Leads showing main changes
Anterior	
Small	V_3–V_4
Extensive	V_2–V_5
Anteroseptal	V_1–V_3
Anterolateral	V_4–V_6, I, AVL
Lateral	I, II, AVL
Inferior	II, III, AVF
Posterior	V_1, V_2 (reciprocal)
Subendocardial	Any lead

- a history of ischaemic-type chest pain
- evolving ECG changes
- a rise and fall in cardiac enzymes.

These will be discussed in detail below.

INVESTIGATIONS

ECG

A Q wave is a broad (>1 mm) and deep (>2 mm or more than 25% of the amplitude of the following R wave) negative deflection that starts the QRS complex (Fig 11.60). It may occur normally in leads AVR and V_1 (and sometimes in lead III) but, in other leads, it is abnormal. Abnormal Q waves are produced by several abnormalities such as left bundle branch block, ventricular tachycardia and the WPW syndrome. The gradual development of Q waves over minutes or hours suggests the occurrence of a full-thickness (as opposed to a subendocardial) myocardial infarction. They develop because the electrical silence of infarcted cardiac tissue results in a so-called 'window' through which the

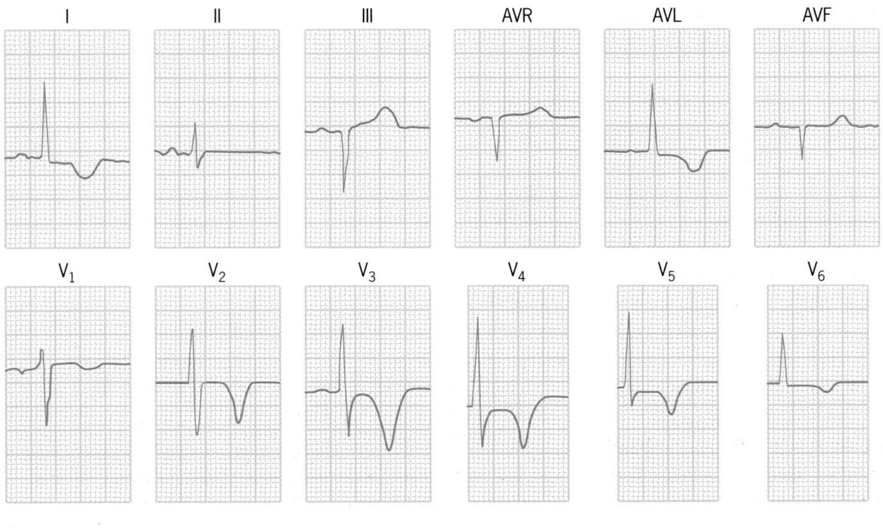

Fig 11.62
A widespread (anterolateral) subendocardial myocardial infarction shown by a 12-lead ECG. Note the deeply inverted, symmetrical T waves in addition to ST depression

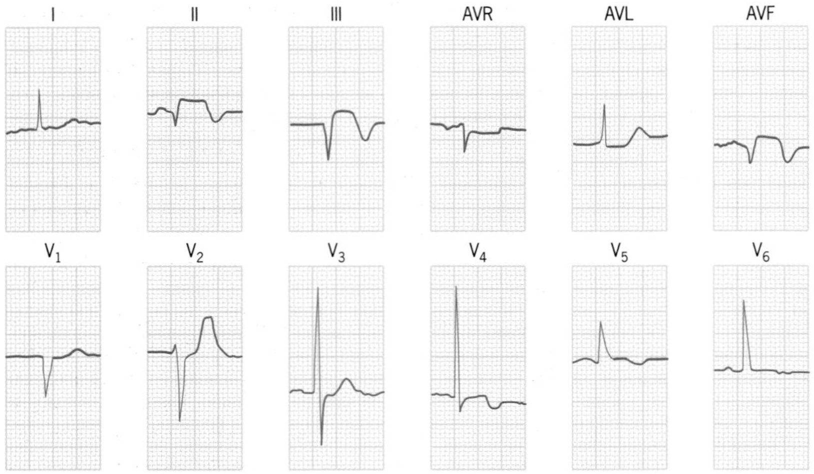

Fig 11.63
An acute inferior wall myocardial infarction shown by a 12-lead ECG. Note the raised ST segment and Q waves in the inferior leads (II, III and AVF). The additional T wave inversion in V_4 and V_5 probably represents anterior wall ischaemia

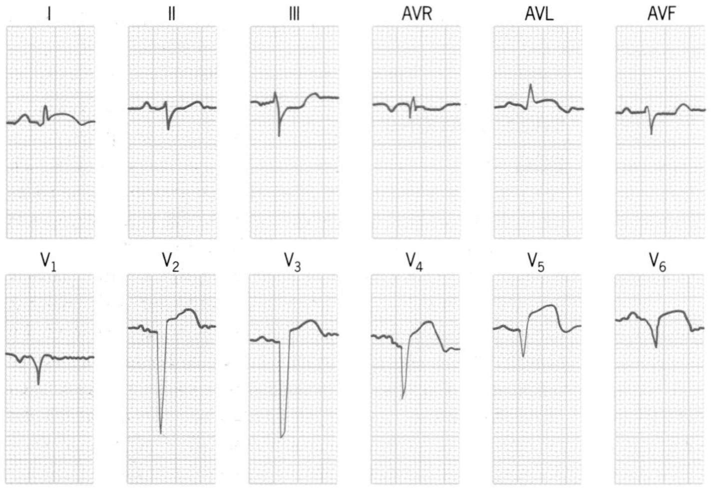

Fig 11.64
An acute anterolateral myocardial infarction shown by a 12-lead ECG. Note the ST segment elevation in leads I, AVL, and V_2–V_6. The T wave is inverted in leads I, AVL and V_3–V_6. Pathological Q waves are seen in leads V_2–V_6

normal endocardial-to-epicardial activation of the opposite non-infarcted ventricular wall is 'seen', resulting in an unopposed depolarization front moving away from an electrode situated over the epicardial surface of the infarct. Q waves are usually permanent echocardiographic features following full-thickness myocardial infarction.

T wave and ST segment changes result from ischaemia and injury. They are therefore often transient, occurring only during the acute attack. The progressive changes or evolution of the ECG during the course of a full-thickness myocardial infarction are illustrated in Fig 11.61.

With subendocardial infarction (Fig 11.62) only the endocardial surface is infarcted and Q waves do not develop (so-called 'non-Q-wave MI'). ST segment and T wave changes are therefore the only ECG features of a subendocardial infarction. Because the injury is endocardial rather than predominantly epicardial, ST segment depression rather than elevation is usual.

Typically, ECG changes (Table 11.29) are usually confined to the ECG leads that 'face' the infarction. Therefore, an inferior wall myocardial infarction is diagnosed when the ECG findings are seen in leads II, III and AVF (Fig 11.63). Lateral infarction produces changes in leads I, AVL and $V_{5/6}$. In anterior infarction, leads V_2–V_5 may be affected. Changes seen in an anterolateral infarction are demonstrated in Fig 11.64. Because there are no posterior leads, a true posterior wall infarct is usually diagnosed by the appearance of a mirror image or reciprocal changes in leads V_1 and V_2 (i.e. the development of a tall initial R wave, ST segment depression and tall, upright T waves). These reciprocal changes can also be seen in association with other infarctions. For example, in an inferior wall myocardial infarction, anterior ST segment depression may be seen.

Cardiac enzymes (Fig 11.65)

Necrotic cardiac tissue releases several enzymes as follows:

- *Creatinine kinase* (CK). This peaks within 24 hours and is usually back to normal by 48 hours. It is also produced by damaged skeletal muscle and brain. Cardiac-specific isoforms can be measured (CK-MB) allowing greater diagnostic accuracy. The size of the enzyme rise is broadly proportional to the infarct size.

Table 11.30
Criteria for thrombolysis in acute myocardial infarction

Indications	Chest pain consistent with myocardial infarction, within 12 hours AND ST segement elevation (>1 mm in two or more contiguous leads) or new left bundle branch block
Contraindications	Stroke or active bleeding in last two months Systolic blood pressure > 200 mmHg Proliferative diabetic retinopathy Pregnancy
Relative contraindications	Prolonged or traumatic resuscitation Recent (>2 weeks) surgery or trauma Known bleeding diathesis or current use of anticoagulants

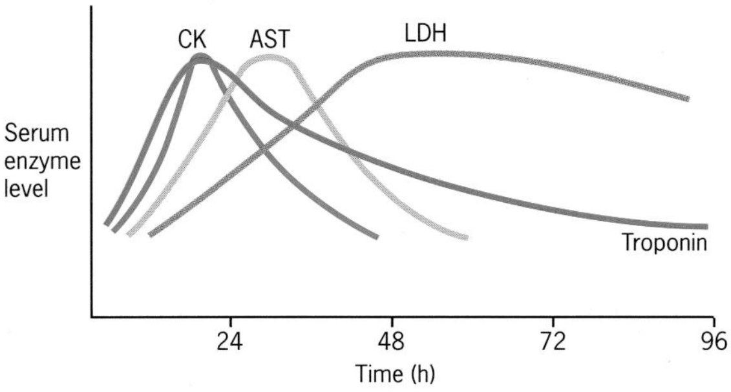

Fig 11.65
The enzyme profile in acute myocardial infarction
CK, Creatinine kinase; AST, Aspartate aminotransferase; LDH, Lactic dehydrogenase

- *Cardiac-specific troponins.* Troponin T and troponin I are regulatory proteins with a very high specificity for cardiac injury. They are released early (2–4 hours) and can persist for up to seven days. Measurement of these enzymes is becoming more widely available.
- *Aspartate aminotransferase* (AST) and *lactate dehydrogenase* (LDH). These nonspecific enzymes are rarely used now for the diagnosis of myocardial infarction. LDH peaks at 3–4 days and remains elevated for up to 10 days and can be useful in confirming myocardial infarction in patients presenting several days after an episode of chest pain.
- *Serial cardiac enzymes.* These should be measured in all patients presenting with suspected myocardial infarction. Levels greater than twice the upper limit of normal are confirmatory in patients with a good history and/or ECG changes. With successful reperfusion, the enzyme rise should be curtailed.

MANAGEMENT OF MYOCARDIAL INFARCTION

Acute management

If the diagnosis of myocardial infarction is suspected, an ECG should be obtained immediately. If diagnostic ST elevation is present (see below), thrombolysis should be commenced without delay (unless contraindicated) and aspirin given (150 mg, chewed). The beneficial effects of aspirin and thrombolysis are synergistic. Adequate analgesia (diamorphine 5–10 mg i.v. combined with antiemetics such as cyclizine 50 mg i.v. or metoclopramide 10 mg i.v.) should be given if required.

Thrombolytic treatment can achieve reperfusion in 50–70% of patients (compared with a spontaneous rate of 20–30%). Many large trials have shown that thrombolysis within 12 hours reduces the extent of ventricular damage and mortality rate. The criteria for thrombolysis are outlined in Table 11.30.

Streptokinase (1.5 million units over one hour) is the agent used most commonly. Front-loaded tissue-type plasminogen activator (t-PA) achieves higher reperfusion rates but is more expensive than streptokinase and is associated with a higher risk of stroke. t-PA tends to be given in preference to streptokinase in patients under 50 years of age with anterior MIs, where the blood pressure is low (systolic below 100 mmHg), and in those patients who have previously received streptokinase. t-PA must be followed by intravenous heparin. t-PA is considerably more effective than streptokinase if it can be given within four hours of the onset of chest pain.

There is an approximate 1% risk of stroke and a 0.7% risk of major haemorrhage associated with the use of thrombolysis. Allergic reactions occur in under 2% of patients receiving streptokinase, and hypotension in 10%.

Following initiation of thrombolysis, the patient should be transferred to the coronary care unit. An i.v. β-antagonist such as metoprolol 5–10 mg should be given, particularly if the heart rate is above 100 b.p.m. with persistent pain. Intravenous nitrates are also given for persistent pain or pulmonary oedema (only if the systolic blood pressure is above 100 mmHg). Oxygen 60% is given routinely, by face mask or nasal cannula.

If the ECG is normal or shows only minor or nonspecific changes, then take a careful history, examine the patient, and repeat the ECG after one hour. Alternative diagnoses should be considered during this period (e.g. aortic dissection, see p. 740).

Whilst thrombolytic therapy is effective in restoring antegrade flow, improving left ventricular function and reducing mortality, reperfusion is unsuccessful in approximately 25% of patients, and early re-occlusion occurs in a further 10%. An increasing number of interventional centres are performing 'primary PTCA' – immediate cardiac catheterization and PTCA – in patients with evolving myocardial infarction. Primary PTCA can be attempted when thrombolysis is contraindicated (see below), when initial ECG changes are equivocal, and when thrombolysis has failed. However, it requires experienced operators and, ideally, cardiothoracic surgical backup, a scenario that is not widely available in the UK.

Subsequent management in hospital

The patient should be monitored in the coronary care unit for 48 hours (this is the at-risk time for cardiac arrests secondary to ventricular arrhythmias) to enable prompt resuscitation by specially trained staff as necessary.

Aspirin 150 mg daily is given unless contraindicated. β-Blockers have been shown to reduce the incidence of sudden death following MI by 20–25% (about 10 lives saved per 1000 patients yearly). All patients – except those with very poor ejection fraction – should be treated with β-blockers unless contraindicated (e.g. COPD).

Patients with clinical evidence of pulmonary oedema or reduced ejection fraction on the echocardiogram (which all patients should have, ideally) should be commenced on an angiotensin-converting enzyme inhibitor (ACE). There is good evidence from several large trials that ACEs have prognostic benefit in these patients. Patients with large anterior Q-wave infarcts should also be anticoagulated with warfarin, usually for three months.

Gradual mobilization is commenced on the second day and the patient should be pain-free and fully ambulant before discharge – six days in uncomplicated cases. Prior to discharge patients should undergo submaximal exercise testing. Risk stratification can be aided by 24-hour Holter monitoring (for arrhythmia profile, ST depression and heart rate variability) together with signal-averaged ECG. All high-risk patients should have coronary angiography. Patients with non-Q-wave myocardial infarcts should also be evaluated.

All patients should be seen by a rehabilitation nurse and dietitian. Risk factors should be modified (see above). Patients should be advised that they cannot drive for one month, and heavy goods and public service driving licences are withdrawn prior to special assessment.

Follow-up

Structured psychological and physical rehabilitation should be available to all patients after myocardial infarction. Most will be fully recovered at two months and able to return to work.

Most patients should be reviewed as outpatients at 6–8 weeks. All should be considered for lipid-lowering therapy if the fasting lipid profile is unfavourable, despite a low-fat diet. Aspirin should be continued indefinitely. Consideration can be given to withdrawing β-blockers after three years in low-risk, normotensive patients. ACE inhibitors should be continued indefinitely in patients with persistent impairment of left ventricular function (i.e. an ejection fraction <40%).

COMPLICATIONS

In the acute phase – the first two or three days following myocardial infarction – cardiac arrhythmias, cardiac failure and pericarditis are the most common complications. Later, recurrent infarction, angina, thromboembolism, mitral valve regurgitation and ventricular septal or free wall rupture may occur. Late complications include the post-myocardial infarction syndrome (Dressler's syndrome), ventricular aneurysm, and recurrent cardiac arrhythmias. Cardiac arrhythmias are described in detail on p. 658.

Ventricular extrasystoles. These commonly occur after myocardial infarction. Their occurrence may precede the development of ventricular fibrillation, particularly if they are frequent (more than five per minute), multiform (different shapes) or R-on-T (falling on the upstroke or peak of the preceding T wave). Treatment has not been shown to reduce the likelihood of subsequent ventricular tachycardia or fibrillation.

Ventricular tachycardia. This may degenerate into ventricular fibrillation or may itself produce serious haemodynamic consequences. It can be treated with intravenous lignocaine or, if haemodynamic deterioration occurs, synchronized cardioversion (initially 200 J).

Ventricular fibrillation. This may occur in the first few hours or days following a myocardial infarction in the absence of severe cardiac failure or cardiogenic shock. It is treated with prompt defibrillation (200–360 J). Recurrences of ventricular fibrillation can be treated with lignocaine infusion or, in cases of poor left ventricular function, amiodarone. When ventricular fibrillation occurs in the setting of heart failure, shock or aneurysm (so-called 'secondary ventricular fibrillation'), the prognosis is very poor unless the underlying haemodynamic or mechanical cause can be corrected. It is prudent to ensure the serum potassium is above 4.5 mmol L^{-1}.

Atrial fibrillation. This occurs in about 10% of patients with myocardial infarction. It is due to atrial irritation caused by heart failure, pericarditis and atrial ischaemia or infarction. It may be managed with intravenous digoxin or intravenous amiodarone and by treatment of the underlying pathology. It is not usually a longstanding problem.

Table 11.31 Progression from different types of fascicular block to complete heart block in patients with acute myocardial infarction

Type of fascicular block	Percentage progressing to complete heart block
LAH	4
LPH	8
Long PR interval	10
LBBB	10
RBBB	20
RBBB + LAH	30
RBBB + LPH	40
RBBB + (LPH or LAH) + Long PR interval	40

LAH, left anterior hemiblock; LPH, left posterior hemiblock; RBBB, right bundle branch block; LBBB, left bundle branch block

Table 11.32 Killip (clinical) classification of heart failure in patients with acute myocardial infarction

Class	Description	Incidence (%)	Mortality (%)
I	No heart failure	40	5
II	Mild left ventricular failure	40	20
III	Pulmonary oedema	10	40
IV	Cardiogenic shock	10	90

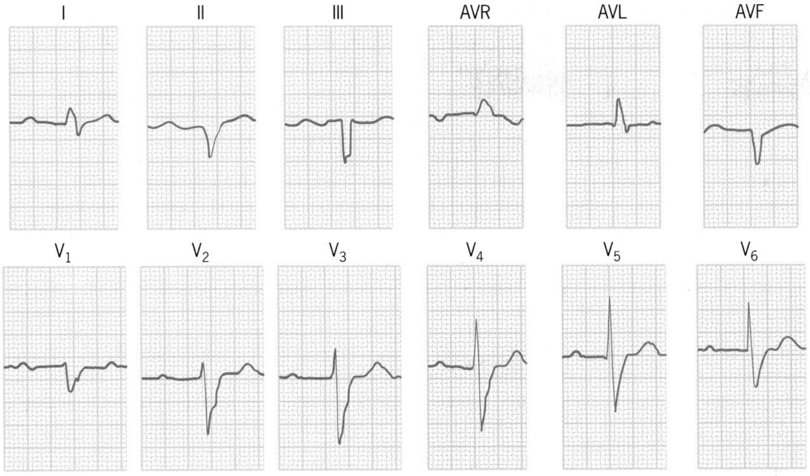

Fig 11.66
Electrocardiographic picture consistent with bifascicular block with delay in the AV node on the third fascicle. There is a prolonged PR interval (0.32 s), a broad QRS complex with a deep S wave in leads I and V_6 (right bundle branch block) and left axis deviation (–75°)

Sinus bradycardia. This is especially associated with acute inferior wall myocardial infarction. Symptoms emerge only when the bradycardia is severe. When symptomatic, the treatment consists of elevating the foot of the bed and giving intravenous atropine, 600 μg if necessary. When sinus bradycardia occurs, an escape rhythm such as idioventricular rhythm (wide QRS complexes with a regular rhythm at 50–100 b.p.m.) of idiojunctional rhythm (narrow QRS complexes) may occur. Usually no specific treatment is required. It has been suggested that sinus bradycardia following myocardial infarction may predispose to the emergence of ventricular fibrillation. Severe sinus bradycardia associated with symptoms or the emergence of unstable rhythms may need treatment with temporary pacing.

Sinus tachycardia. This is produced by heart failure, fever and anxiety. Usually, no specific treatment is required.

Conduction disturbances. These are common following myocardial infarction. AV nodal delay (first-degree AV block) or higher degrees of block may occur during acute myocardial infarction, especially of the inferior wall (the right coronary artery usually supplies the SA and AV nodes). Complete block, when associated with haemodynamic compromise, may need treatment with atropine or a temporary pacemaker. Such blocks may last for only a few minutes, but frequently continue for several days. Permanent pacing may need to be considered if complete heart block persists for over two weeks.

Acute anterior wall myocardial infarction may produce damage to the distal conduction system (the His bundle or bundle branches). The development of complete heart block usually implies a large myocardial infarction and a poor prognosis. The ventricular escape rhythm is slow and unreliable, and a temporary pacemaker is necessary. This form of block is often permanent.

The development of complete AV block (Table 11.31) can be expected in 20–30% of cases where progressive bundle branch block (right bundle branch block and then right bundle branch block with a QRS axis shift) has already occurred (Fig 11.66).

Cardiac failure and cardiogenic shock

Heart failure after acute myocardial infarction is graded according to a clinical classification (Table 11.32).

Mild left heart failure (a few basal crackles that persist after coughing, an extra heart sound and upper lobe blood diversion on chest X-ray) occur in about 40% of patients with acute myocardial infarction. Treatment for a few days with low-dose diuretics is usually all that is needed for symptomatic relief, but an ACE inhibitor should be given for prognostic benefit (see p. 680).

A large myocardial infarction may lead to severe heart failure and pulmonary oedema. In such cases more prolonged and powerful diuretics and vasodilator treatment is necessary. In very severe cases a pulmonary artery balloon catheter is used to measure the pulmonary artery and indirectly the left atrial pressures and the cardiac output. Treatment is with loop diuretics, vasodilators (see p. 680) and, occasionally, digoxin.

The Amiodarone Trials Meta-Analysis has shown that amiodarone therapy reduces both arrhythmic deaths and all-cause mortality in high-risk patients (i.e. after myocardial infarction and left ventricular dysfunction) (see also p. 673).

Hypotension and raised right-heart filling pressures are characteristically seen in right ventricular infarction which may accompany inferior infarcts. ST segment elevation is seen in V4R. Echocardiography should be performed to exclude pericardial effusion. Initial treatment is with volume expansion (p. 843).

Severe heart failure may also follow ventricular septal rupture or mitral valve papillary muscle rupture. Both of these conditions present with worsening heart failure, a systolic thrill and a loud pansystolic murmur, widely heard over the precordium. Often, echocardiography and right heart catherization with a balloon catheter is needed to differentiate between these two conditions. Both are associated with a poor prognosis, but vigorous treatment, including early surgical correction, can be successful in selected cases.

Cardiogenic shock is an extreme form of cardiac failure or circulatory collapse. Its features and management are described on p. 684. The mortality from this condition is about 90%. The majority of those rescued (usually with the help of intra-aortic balloon counterpulsation) have a complication that can be treated surgically, such as left ventricular aneurysm, torrential mitral regurgitation or ventricular septal perforation.

Cardiac rupture results in almost immediate cardiac tamponade and is usually fatal within a few minutes. Electromechanical dissociation – no pulse or cardiac output, but a persistently normal rhythm on ECG – is the classical presentation. Treatment is rarely successful.

Ventricular asynergy and papillary muscle dysfunction (not rupture) may produce mild mitral regurgitation in association with heart failure. This causes a transient, soft, pansystolic murmur in up to half of those with acute myocardial infarction. In these cases, no specific treatment is necessary for the mitral regurgitation.

Thromboembolism

Bedrest and cardiac failure contribute to the common occurrence of thrombosis and embolism associated with myocardial infarction. Only 10% of patients have clinical features of thromboembolism, but in almost 50% of patients who die, there is evidence of emboli. Deep venous thrombosis (p. 742) is the most common manifestation and pulmonary embolism may result from this.

Left ventricular mural thrombus may form on the endocardial surface of the infarcted region. Systemic embolization may occur in over 10% of patients. A review of over 2000 patients with left ventricular dysfunction following myocardial infarction found a five-year stroke rate of 8.1%. A decreased ejection systolic fraction and older age were both independent predictors of an increased risk of stroke. Anticoagulant therapy appears to protect against stroke and should be considered in a patient with documented mural thrombus and in those patients with significant left ventricular dysfunction.

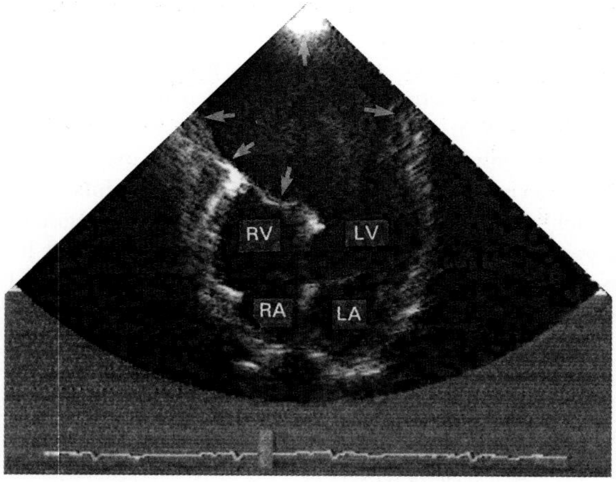

Fig 11.67
Two-dimensional echocardiogram (apical four-chamber view) showing a very large apical left ventricular aneurysm (arrowed). The relatively static blood in the aneurysm produces a swirling 'smoke' effect. This aneurysm was successfully resected surgically
LV, left ventricle; LA, left atrium; RV, right ventricle; RA, right atrium

Other complications

Pericarditis. This is characterized by sharp chest pain, aggravated by movement and respiration. It is characteristically worse on lying down. There may be a pericardial rub. It is common in the first few days, particularly in anterior wall infarction. ECG shows generalized ST segment elevation (concave upward) with upright, peaked T waves. Anti-inflammatory drugs are usually effective. Anticoagulation should be avoided.

Post-myocardial infarction syndrome (Dressler's syndrome). This occurs weeks or months after an acute myocardial infarction and consists of pericarditis, fever and a pericardial effusion. It is caused by an autoimmune response to damaged cardiac tissue. Anti-inflammatory medication, including systemic corticosteroids, may be necessary.

Left ventricular aneurysm. This is a late complication. Patients may present with heart failure, arrhythmias or systemic emboli. It is characterized by ventricular asynergy (often palpable as a double impulse) and ECG shows persistent ST segment elevation. Diagnosis is confirmed by echocardiography (Fig 11.67). Treatment comprises anticoagulation, ACE inhibitors and antiarrhythmic drugs as necessary. Surgical removal (aneurysectomy) may be helpful in selected cases.

PROGNOSIS

Prognosis following myocardial infarction is variable. The main prognostic indicators are advanced age and large infarcts (e.g. reduced left ventricular function, large heart on chest X-ray, heart failure). Left ventricular dysfunction, residual myocardial ischaemia and a susceptibility to ventricular arrhythmias are the three main determinants of survival. Patency of the infarct-related artery is associated with a significantly lower long-term mortality.

Overall, approximately 25% of patients surviving the initial heart attack die in the first two years, with the five-year mortality approaching 30%. In young patients (<50 years) the absolute risk of death is below 3% per year, compared with over 15% in those over 70 years old.

Sudden cardiac death

(see also Information box 11.1 on p. 654)

Sudden cardiac death is generally defined as death due to cardiac causes which occurs within six hours of the onset of symptoms. Post-mortem studies have revealed that coronary atheroma is present in 80–90% of cases. Forty per cent of all deaths due to coronary atherosclerosis occur suddenly in this way, although up to 50% of patients dying suddenly due to coronary atheroma have no preceding history of coronary disease. The majority of cases of sudden death due to atheroma appear to be due to fatal ventricular arrhythmia, sometimes triggered by acute myocardial ischaemia.

FURTHER READING

Alexander JH, Harrington RA (1997) Antiplatelet and antithrombin therapies in the acute coronary syndromes. *Current Opinion in Cardiology* **12**: 427–437.

Anderson WD, King SB (1996) A review of randomized trials comparing coronary angioplasty and bypass grafting. *Current Opinion in Cardiology* **11**: 583–590.

Bittl JA (1996) Advances in coronary angioplasty. *New England Journal of Medicine* **335**: 1290–1311.

Braunwald E et al (1994) Diagnosing and managing unstable angina. *Circulation* **90**: 613–622.

Collins R, Peto R, Baigent C, Sleight P (1997) Aspirin, heparin and fibrinolytic therapy in suspected myocardial infarction. *New England Journal of Medicine* **336**: 847–866.

Coronary Heart Disease (1996) Supplement to *Lancet* **348**: 1–31.

Davies MJ (1996) Stability and instability: two faces of coronary atherosclerosis. *Circulation* **94**: 2013–2020.

Davies MJ (1997) The composition of coronary artery plaques. *New England Journal of Medicine* **336**: 1312–1314.

Falk E, Shah PK, Fuster V (1995) Coronary plaque disruption. *Circulation* **92**: 657–671.

Greenbaum AB, Ohman EM (1997) An update on acute myocardial infarction from recent clinical trials. *Current Opinion in Cardiology* **12**: 418–426.

Kanagasaby RR, Parker DJ (1996) Long term results of coronary bypass grafting. *Current Opinion in Cardiology* **11**: 568–573.

McGorisk GM, Treasure CB (1996) Endothelial dysfunction in coronary artery disease. *Current Opinion in Cardiology* **11**: 341–350.

Narins CR, Topol EJ (1997) Attention shifts to the white clot. *Lancet* **350** (Suppl 3): 2.

Rheumatic fever

Rheumatic fever is an inflammatory disease that occurs in children and young adults (the first attack usually occurs at between 5 and 15 years of age) as a result of infection with group A streptococci. It affects the heart, skin, joints and central nervous system. It is common in the Middle and Far East, eastern Europe and South America. It is rare in the UK, western Europe and North America, but there is a suggestion of a recent resurgence of the disease. This decline in the incidence of rheumatic fever (from 10% of children in the 1920s to 0.01% today) parallels the reduction in all streptococcal infections and is largely due to improved sanitation and the use of antibiotics.

Pharyngeal infection with group A *Streptococcus* may be followed by the clinical syndrome of rheumatic fever. This is thought to develop because of an autoimmune reaction triggered by the infecting *Streptococcus*. The condition is not due to direct infection of the heart or to the production of a toxin.

PATHOLOGY

All three layers of the heart may be affected. The characteristic lesion of rheumatic carditis is the Aschoff nodule, which is a granulomatous lesion with a central necrotic area occurring in the myocardium, particularly in the subendocardium of the left ventricle. Small, warty vegetations may develop on the endocardium, particularly on the heart valves. This leads to some degree of valvular regurgitation. A serofibrinous effusion characterizes the acute pericarditis that occurs.

The synovial membranes are acutely inflamed during rheumatic fever, and subcutaneous nodules (which are also granulomatous lesions) are seen in the acute stage of the disease.

CLINICAL FEATURES

The disease presents suddenly, with fever, joint pains, malaise and loss of appetite. The clinical features depend on the organs that are involved. Diagnosis relies on the presence of two or more major clinical manifestations or one major manifestation plus two or more minor features. These are known as the Duckett Jones criteria (Table 11.33).

Carditis manifests as:

- new or changed heart murmurs
- development of cardiac enlargement or cardiac failure
- appearance of a pericardial effusion and ECG changes of pericarditis (raised ST segments) or myocarditis (inverted or flattened T waves), first-degree or greater AV block or other cardiac arrhythmias
- transient diastolic mitral (Carey–Coombs) murmur due to mitral valvulitis.

Non-cardiac features include the following:

- There is usually a fever with an apparently excessive tachycardia.
- The arthritis associated with rheumatic fever is classically a fleeting polyarthritis affecting large joints such as the knees, elbows, ankles and wrists. The joints are swollen, red and tender. As the inflammation in one joint recedes, another becomes affected. Once the acute inflammation disappears, the rheumatic process leaves the joints normal.
- Sydenham's chorea (or St Vitus' dance, see p. 1066) is involvement of the central nervous system that develops late after a streptococcal infection. Sufferers are noticeably 'fidgety' and display spasmodic, unintentional movements. Speech is often affected.
- Skin manifestations include erythema marginatum, a transient pink rash with slightly raised edges, which occurs in 20% of cases. The erythematous areas found

Table 11.33 Revised Duckett Jones criteria for the diagnosis of rheumatic fever. The diagnosis is made on the basis of two or more major criteria or one major plus two or more minor criteria

Major criteria
Carditis
Polyarthritis
Chorea
Erythema marginatum
Subcutaneous nodules

Minor criteria
Fever
Arthralgia
Previous rheumatic fever
Raised ESR/C-reactive protein
Leucocytosis
Prolonged PR interval on ECG

Plus evidence of antecedent streptococcal infection, e.g. positive throat cultures for group A streptococci, elevated antistreptolysin O titre (> 250 U) or other streptococcal antibodies, or a history of recent scarlet fever

ESR, erythrocyte sedimentation rate.

Table 11.34
Rheumatic valvular lesions

Valves involved	Percentage of cases
Mitral valve alone	50
Mitral and aortic valves	40
Mitral, aortic and tricuspid	5
Aortic valve alone	2
All other combinations	3

mostly on the trunk and limbs coalesce into crescent- or ring-shaped patches. Subcutaneous nodules, which are painless, pea-sized, hard nodules beneath the skin, may also occur, particularly over tendons, joints and bony prominences.

INVESTIGATIONS

- **Throat swabs** are cultured for the group A Streptococcus.
- **Serological changes** may indicate a recent streptococcal infection. The antistreptolysin O titre, and sometimes others such as the antistreptokinase titre, are performed.
- **Nonspecific indicators of inflammation** such as the ESR and the C-reactive protein levels are usually elevated.

TREATMENT

Patients with fever, active arthritis or active carditis should be completely rested in bed. When the clinical syndrome has subsided (e.g. no pyrexia, normal pulse rate, normal ESR, normal white count) the patient may be mobilized.

Residual streptococcal infections should be eradicated with a single intramuscular injection of 916 mg of benzathine penicillin or oral phenoxymethylpenicillin 500 mg four times daily for one week. This therapy should be administered even if nasal or pharyngeal swabs do not culture the streptococci.

High-dose salicylate (preferably acetylsalicylate, i.e. aspirin) therapy is given to the limit of tolerance determined by the development of tinnitus. If carditis is present, systemic corticosteroids may be given. Prednisolone 60–120 mg in four divided doses each day is administered until the clinical syndrome is improved and the ESR has fallen to normal. Steroids are then tapered off over 2–4 weeks. However, the efficacy of steroids is in doubt.

Recurrences are most common when persistent cardiac damage is present, and are prevented by the continued administration of oral phenoxymethylpenicillin 250 mg daily or by monthly injections of 916 mg of benzathine penicillin until the age of 20 years or for five years after the latest attack (see p. 10). A sulphonamide (e.g. sulfadiazine) may be used if the patient is allergic to penicillin. Any streptococcal infection that does develop should be treated very promptly.

Chronic rheumatic heart disease

More than 50% of those who suffer acute rheumatic fever with carditis will later (after 10–20 years) develop chronic rheumatic valvular disease, predominantly affecting the mitral and aortic valves (Table 11.34).

FURTHER READING

Stollerman GH (1997) Rheumatic fever. *Lancet* **349**: 935–942.

Valvular heart disease

Mitral stenosis

Almost all mitral stenosis is due to rheumatic heart disease:

- At least 50% of sufferers have a history of rheumatic fever or chorea.
- The single most common valve lesion due to rheumatic fever is pure mitral stenosis (50%).
- The mitral valve is affected in over 90% of those with rheumatic valvular heart disease.
- Rheumatic mitral stenosis is much more common in women.
- The pathological process results after some years in valve thickening, cusp fusion, calcium deposition, a narrowed (stenotic) valve orifice and progressive immobility of the valve cusps.

Other causes

- Lutembacher's syndrome is the combination of acquired mitral stenosis and an atrial septal defect.

Table 11.35
Complications of mitral stenosis

Atrial fibrillation
Systemic embolization
Pulmonary hypertension
Pulmonary infarction
Chest infections
Infective endocarditis (rare)
Tricuspid regurgitation
Right ventricular failure

- A rare form of congenital mitral stenosis can occur.
- In the elderly, a syndrome similar to mitral stenosis can develop because of calcification and fibrosis of the valve, valve ring and subvalvular apparatus (chordae tendineae).

PATHOPHYSIOLOGY

When the normal valve orifice area of 5 cm^2 is reduced to approximately 1 cm^2, severe mitral stenosis is present. In order that sufficient cardiac output will be maintained, the left atrial pressure increases and left atrial hypertrophy and dilatation occurs. Consequently, pulmonary venous, pulmonary arterial and right heart pressures also increase. The increase in pulmonary capillary pressure is followed by the development of pulmonary oedema. This is partially prevented by alveolar and capillary thickening and pulmonary arterial vasoconstriction (reactive pulmonary hypertension). Pulmonary hypertension leads to right ventricular hypertrophy, dilatation and failure. Right ventricular dilatation results in tricuspid regurgitation. Mitral stenosis is frequently associated with complications (Table 11.35).

SYMPTOMS

Usually there are no symptoms until the valve orifice is moderately stenosed (i.e. has an area of 2 cm^2). In Europe this does not usually occur until several decades after the first attack of rheumatic fever, but in the Middle or Far East children of 10–20 years of age may have severe calcific mitral stenosis.

Because of pulmonary venous hypertension and recurrent bronchitis, progressively severe dyspnoea develops. A cough productive of blood-tinged, frothy sputum is quite common, and occasionally frank haemoptysis may occur. The development of pulmonary hypertension eventually leads to right heart failure and its symptoms of weakness, fatigue and abdominal or lower limb swelling.

The large left atrium favours atrial fibrillation, giving rise to symptoms such as palpitations. Atrial fibrillation may result in systemic emboli, most commonly to the cerebral vessels resulting in neurological sequelae, but mesenteric, renal and peripheral emboli are also seen. Clinical pulmonary embolism as a result of mitral stenosis associated with atrial fibrillation is less commonly seen, but it is likely that subclinical pulmonary emboli occur.

SIGNS (see Clinical memo in Fig 11.68)

Face

Severe mitral stenosis with pulmonary hypertension is associated with the so-called mitral facies or malar flush. This is a bilateral, cyanotic or dusky pink discoloration over the upper cheeks that is due to arteriovenous anastomoses and vascular stasis.

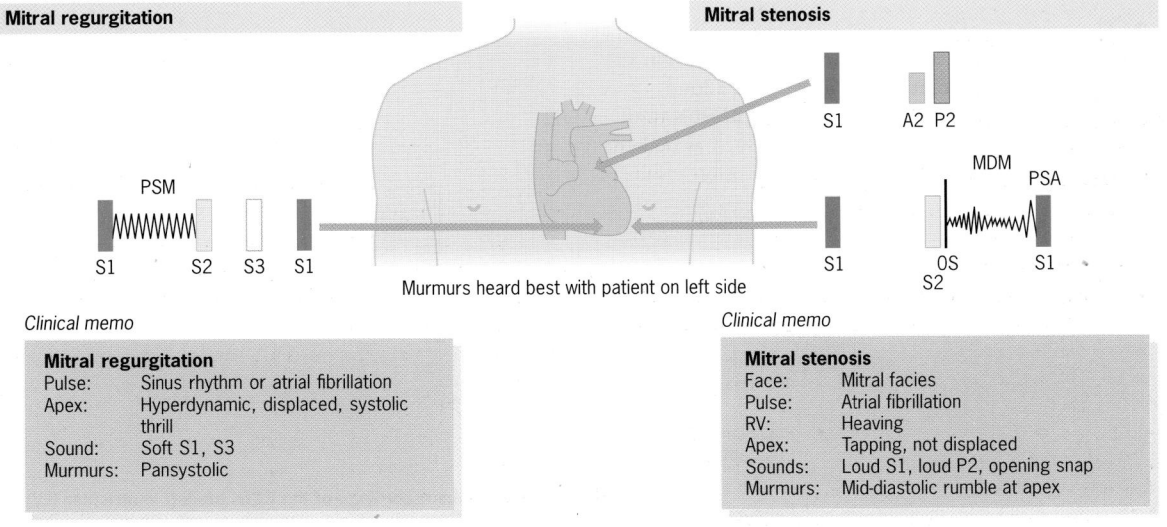

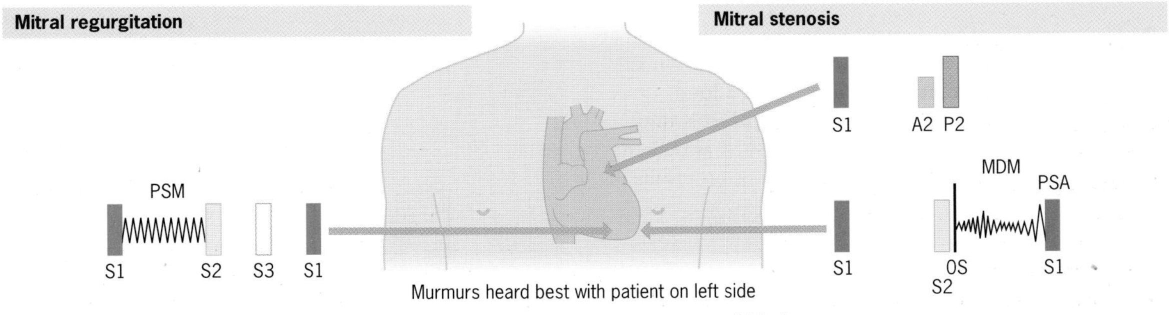

Clinical memo

Mitral regurgitation

Pulse:	Sinus rhythm or atrial fibrillation
Apex:	Hyperdynamic, displaced, systolic thrill
Sound:	Soft S1, S3
Murmurs:	Pansystolic

Clinical memo

Mitral stenosis

Face:	Mitral facies
Pulse:	Atrial fibrillation
RV:	Heaving
Apex:	Tapping, not displaced
Sounds:	Loud S1, loud P2, opening snap
Murmurs:	Mid-diastolic rumble at apex

Fig 11.68
Auscultatory features associated with mitral regurgitation and mitral stenosis. A2, aortic component of the second heart sound; MDM, mid-diastolic murmur; OS, opening snap; P2, pulmonary component of the second heart sound; PSA, presystolic accentuation; PSM, pansystolic murmur; S1, first heart sound; S2, second heart sound; S3, third heart sound

Pulse

Mitral stenosis may be associated with a small volume pulse which is usually regular early on in the disease process when most patients are in sinus rhythm. However, as the severity of the disease progresses, many patients develop atrial fibrillation resulting in an irregularly irregular pulse. The development of atrial fibrillation in patients with mitral stenosis often causes a dramatic clinical deterioration.

Jugular veins

If right heart failure develops there is obvious distension of the jugular veins. If pulmonary hypertension or tricuspid stenosis is present, the *a* wave will be prominent provided that atrial fibrillation has not supervened.

Apex beat

The apex beat is 'tapping' in quality. This is the result of a palpable first heart sound combined with left ventricular backward displacement produced by an enlarging right ventricle. A parasternal sustained impulse due to right ventricular hypertrophy may also be felt.

Auscultation

Auscultation (Fig 11.68) reveals a loud first heart sound if the mitral valve is pliable, but will not occur in calcific mitral stenosis. As the valve suddenly opens with the force of the increased left atrial pressure, an 'opening snap' will be heard. This is followed by a low-pitched 'rumbling' mid-diastolic murmur best heard with the bell of the stethoscope held lightly at the apex with the patient lying on the left side. If the patient is in sinus rhythm, the murmur becomes louder at the end of diastole as a result of atrial contraction (pre-systolic accentuation).

The severity of mitral stenosis is judged clinically on the basis of several criteria:

- The presence of pulmonary hypertension implies that mitral stenosis is severe. Pulmonary hypertension is recognized by a right ventricular heave, a loud pulmonary component of the second heart sound, and signs of right-sided heart failure, such as oedema and hepatomegaly. Pulmonary hypertension results in pulmonary valvular regurgitation which causes an early diastolic murmur in the pulmonary area known as a Graham–Steell murmur.
- The closeness of the opening snap to the second heart sound is proportional to the severity of mitral stenosis.
- The length of the mid-diastolic murmur is proportional to the severity.

As the valve cusps become immobile, the loud first heart sound softens and the opening snap disappears. When

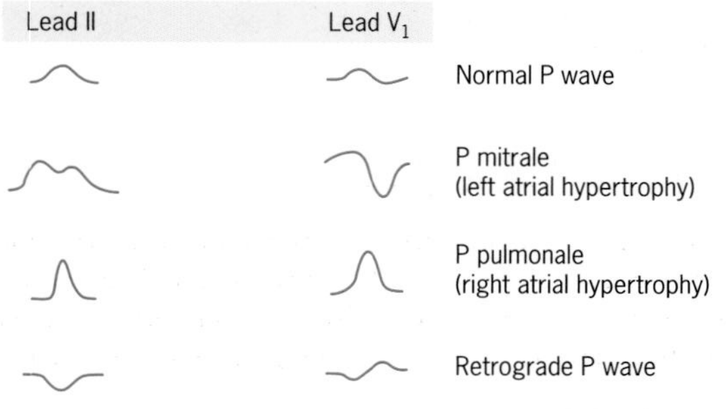

Fig 11.69
A bifid P wave as seen on the ECG in mitral stenosis (P mitrale). Also shown for comparison are other P wave abnormalities

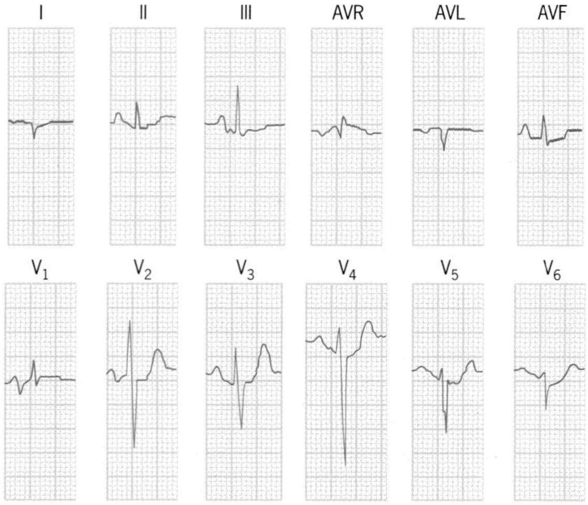

Fig 11.70
Severe mitral stenosis shown by a 12-lead ECG. Note the right axis deviation (frontal plane axis = +120°), the left atrial conduction abnormality (large terminal negative component of the P wave in V_1) and the right ventricular hypertrophy (R wave in V_1 and right axis deviation)

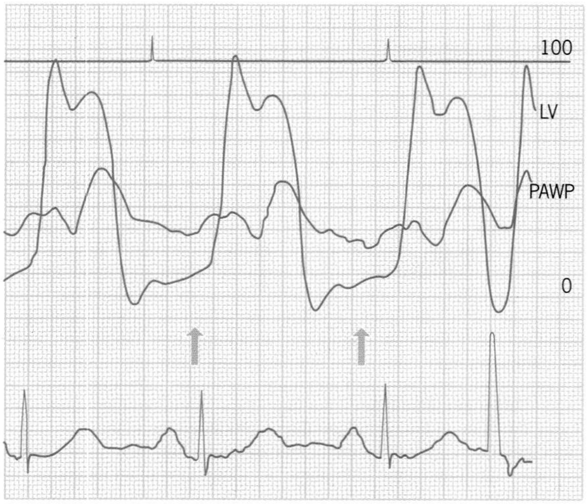

Fig 11.71
Simultaneous recordings of the ECG, the left ventricular (LV) and the pulmonary arterial wedge pressure (PAWP). The PAWP is almost equivalent to the left atrial pressure. Thus at end-diastole (the onset of the QRS complex) the PAWP is significantly higher than the LV pressure (arrows). The pressure gradient is due to mitral valve stenosis. PAWP is also known as PAOP (occlusion pressure)

pulmonary hypertension occurs, the pulmonary component of the second sound is increased in intensity and the mitral diastolic murmur may become quieter because of the reduction of cardiac output.

INVESTIGATIONS

Chest X-ray

The chest X-ray usually shows a generally small heart with an enlarged left atrium (see Fig 11.13 on p. 641). Pulmonary venous hypertension is usually also present. Late in the course of the disease a calcified mitral valve may be seen on a penetrated or lateral view. The signs of pulmonary oedema or pulmonary hypertension may also be apparent when the disease is severe.

ECG

In sinus rhythm the ECG shows a bifid P wave due to delayed left atrial activation (Fig 11.69). However, atrial fibrillation is frequently present. As the disease progresses, the ECG features of right ventricular hypertrophy (right axis deviation and perhaps tall R waves in lead V_1) may develop (Fig 11.70).

Echocardiogram (Fig 11.24)

On M-mode echocardiography, instead of the anterior and posterior valve leaflets separating normally during diastole, they move forward together as a result of fusion of the commissures. Continous wave (CW) is used to estimate valve area which can also be measured by direct visualization of the valve on 2-D echocardiography. Pulmonary artery pressure can be estimated by measuring the degree of tricuspid regurgitation. In many cases, echocardiography is sufficient to judge the severity of mitral stenosis such that decisions regarding surgery can be made.

Cardiac catheterization

This is required only if an adequate echocardiogram (transthoracic or transoesophageal) is impossible to obtain or if coexisting cardiac problems (e.g. mitral regurgitation or coronary artery disease) are suspected. The typical findings in mitral stenosis are a diastolic pressure that is higher in the left atrium than in the left ventricle (Fig 11.71). This gradient of pressure is usually proportional to the degree of the stenosis.

TREATMENT

Mild mitral stenosis may need no treatment other than prompt therapy of attacks of bronchitis. Although infective endocarditis in pure mitral stenosis is uncommon, antibiotic prophylaxis is advised (see p. 10). Early symptoms of mitral stenosis such as mild dyspnoea can usually be treated with low doses of diuretics. The onset of atrial fibrillation requires treatment with digoxin and anticoagulation to prevent atrial thrombus and systemic embolization. If pulmonary hypertension develops or the symptoms of pulmonary congestion persist despite therapy, surgical relief of the mitral stenosis is advised. There are four operative measures.

Trans-septal balloon valvotomy

A catheter is introduced into the right atrium via the femoral vein. The interatrial septum is then punctured and the catheter advanced into the left atrium and across the mitral valve. A balloon is passed over the catheter to lie across the valve, and then inflated briefly to split the valve commisures. The procedure is performed under local anaesthesia in the cardiac catheter laboratory. As with other valvotomy techniques, significant regurgitation may result, necessitating valve replacement (see below). This procedure is ideal for patients with pliable valves in whom there is little involvement of the subvalvular apparatus and in whom there is minimal mitral regurgitation. The procedure cannot be performed when there is heavy calcification or more than mild mitral regurgitation. Transoesophageal echocardiography must be performed prior to this technique in order that left atrial thrombus can be excluded.

Closed valvotomy

This operation is advised for patients with mobile, non-calcified and non-regurgitant mitral valves. The fused cusps are forced apart by a dilator introduced through the apex of the left ventricle and guided into position by the surgeon's finger inserted via the left atrial appendage. Cardiopulmonary bypass is not needed for this operation. Closed valvotomy may produce a good result for 10 years or more. The valve cusps often re-fuse and eventually another operation may be necessary.

Open valvotomy

This operation is often preferred to closed valvotomy. The cusps are carefully dissected apart under direct vision. Cardiopulmonary bypass is required. Open dissection reduces the likelihood of causing traumatic mitral regurgitation.

Mitral valve replacement

Replacement of the mitral valve is necessary if:

- mitral regurgitation is also present
- there is a badly diseased or badly calcified stenotic valve that cannot be reopened without producing significant regurgitation.

Artificial valves (see p. 710) may work successfully for more than 20 years. Anticoagulants are generally necessary to prevent the formation of thrombus, which might obstruct the valve or embolize.

Mitral regurgitation

Of the many causes of mitral valve regurgitation, rheumatic heart disease (50%) and the prolapsing mitral valve are the most common. Any disease that causes dilatation of the left ventricle may cause mild mitral regurgitation; for example:

- aortic valve disease
- acute rheumatic fever
- myocarditis

- dilated cardiomyopathy
- hypertensive heart disease
- ischaemic heart disease.

Other causes

- *Infective endocarditis* – mitral regurgitation may result from destruction of the mitral valve leaflets.
- *Hypertrophic cardiomyopathy* – left ventricular contraction is disorganized and mitral regurgitation often results.
- *Connective tissue disorders* – systemic lupus erythematosus (SLE) may cause mitral regurgitation.
- *Collagen abnormalities* – Marfan's syndrome and Ehlers–Danlos syndrome may cause mitral regurgitation.
- *Degeneration of the valve cusps or mitral annular calcification* – this may result in mitral regurgitation
- *Rupture of the chordae tendineae* (due to myocardial infarction, infective endocarditis or trauma) – this may result in acute and very severe mitral regurgitation.

PATHOPHYSIOLOGY

Regurgitation into the left atrium produces left atrial dilatation but little increase in left atrial pressure if the regurgitation is longstanding, as the regurgitant flow is accommodated by the large left atrium. With acute mitral regurgitation the normal compliance of the left atrium does not allow much dilatation and the left atrial pressure rises. Thus, in acute mitral regurgitation the left atrial *v* wave is greatly increased and pulmonary venous pressure rises to produce pulmonary oedema.

Since a proportion of the stroke volume is regurgitated, the stroke volume increases to maintain the forward cardiac output and the left ventricle therefore enlarges.

SYMPTOMS

Mitral regurgitation can be present for many years and the cardiac dimensions may be greatly increased before any symptoms occur. The increased stroke volume may be sensed as a 'palpitation'. Dyspnoea and orthopnoea may develop owing to pulmonary venous hypertension occurring as a direct result of the mitral regurgitation and secondarily to left ventricular failure. Fatigue and lethargy develop because of the reduced cardiac output. In the late stages of the disease the symptoms of right heart failure also occur and eventually lead to congestive cardiac failure. Cardiac cachexia may develop. Thromboembolism is less common than in mitral stenosis, but subacute infective endocarditis is much more common.

SIGNS (see Clinical memo in Fig 11.68)

The physical signs of uncomplicated mitral regurgitation are:

- a laterally displaced, thrusting (hyperdynamic), diffuse apex beat and a systolic thrill
- a soft first heart sound, owing to the incomplete apposition of the valve cusps and their partial closure by the time ventricular systole begins
- a pansystolic murmur, owing to the occurrence of regurgitation throughout the whole of systole, being loudest at the apex but radiating widely over the precordium and into the axilla
- a prominent third heart sound, owing to the sudden rush of blood back into the dilated left ventricle in early diastole (sometimes a short mid-diastolic flow murmur may follow the third heart sound).

The signs related to atrial fibrillation, pulmonary hypertension, and left and right heart failure may develop later in the disease. The onset of atrial fibrillation has a much less dramatic effect on symptoms than in mitral stenosis.

INVESTIGATIONS

Chest X-ray

The chest X-ray may show left atrial and left ventricular enlargement. There is an increase in the CTR, and valve calcification may be seen.

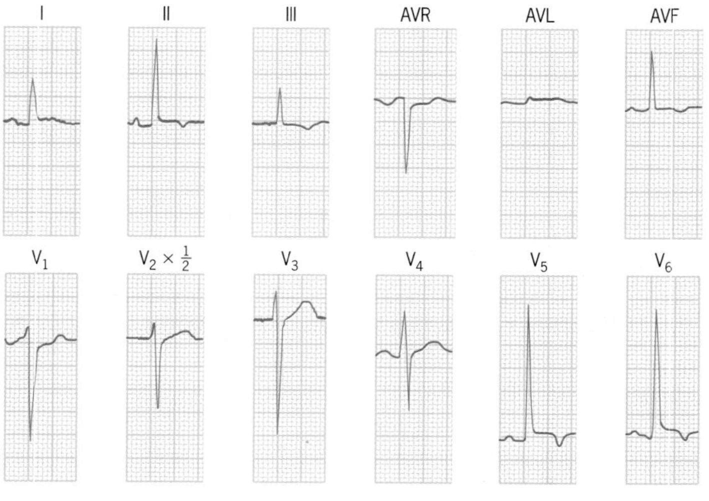

Fig 11.72
Left ventricular hypertrophy shown in a 12-lead ECG. Note the size of the S wave seen in V_1 (21 mm); S in V_1 + R in V_6 = >35 mm

ECG

The ECG shows the features of left atrial delay (bifid P waves) and left ventricular hypertrophy (Fig 11.72) as manifested by tall R waves in the left lateral leads (e.g. leads I and V_6) and deep S waves in the right-sided precordial leads, (e.g. leads V_1 and V_2). (Note that SV_1 plus RV_5 or RV_6 >35 mm indicates left ventricular hypertrophy.) Left ventricular hypertrophy occurs in about 50% of patients with mitral regurgitation. Atrial fibrillation may be present.

Echocardiogram

The echocardiogram shows a dilated left atrium and left ventricle. There may be specific features of chordal or papillary muscle rupture. CW Doppler can determine the velocity of the regurgitant jet.

The echocardiogram is not as definitive in mitral regurgitation as in mitral stenosis. However, useful information regarding the severity of the condition can be obtained indirectly by observing the dynamics of ventricular function in the condition.

Cardiac catheterization

This demonstrates a prominent left atrial systolic pressure wave, and when contrast is injected into the left ventricle it may be seen regurgitating into an enlarged left atrium during systole.

TREATMENT

Mild mitral regurgitation in the absence of symptoms can be managed conservatively by following the patient with serial echocardiograms. Prophylaxis against endocarditis is required (see p. 10). Any evidence of progressive cardiac enlargement generally warrants early surgical intervention by either mitral valve repair or replacement. The advantages of surgical intervention are diminished in more advanced disease. In patients who are not considered appropriate for surgical intervention, or in whom surgery will be considered at a later date, management usually involves treatment with ACE inhibitors, diuretics and possibly anticoagulants. Sudden torrential mitral regurgitation, as seen with chordal or papillary muscle rupture or infective endocarditis, may necessitate emergency mitral valve replacement.

Prolapsing (billowing) mitral valve

This is also known as Barlow's syndrome or floppy mitral valve. It is due to excessively large mitral valve leaflets, an enlarged mitral annulus, abnormally long chordae or disordered papillary muscle contraction. Histology may demonstrate myxomatous degeneration of the mitral valve leaflets. It is more commonly seen in young women than in men or older women and it has a familial incidence. Its cause is unknown but it may be associated with Marfan's syndrome, thyrotoxicosis, rheumatic or ischaemic heart disease. It also occurs in association with atrial septal defect and as part of hypertrophic cardiomyopathy. Mild mitral valve prolapse is so common that it should be regarded as a normal variant.

PATHOPHYSIOLOGY

During ventricular systole, a mitral valve leaflet (most commonly the posterior leaflet) prolapses into the left atrium. This may result in abnormal ventricular contraction, papillary muscle strain and some mitral regurgitation. Usually the syndrome is not haemodynamically serious. Thromboembolism may occur.

SYMPTOMS

Atypical chest pain is the most common symptom. Usually the pain is left submammary and stabbing in quality. Sometimes it is substernal, aching and severe. Rarely it is similar to typical angina pectoris. Palpitations may be experienced because of the abnormal ventricular contraction or because of the atrial and ventricular arrhythmias that are commonly associated with mitral valve prolapse.

SIGNS

The most common sign is a mid-systolic click, which is produced by the sudden prolapse of the valve and the tensing of the chordae tendineae that occurs during systole. This may be followed by a late systolic murmur owing to some regurgitation. Sometimes, pansystolic mitral regurgitation occurs. The signs typically fade quickly but return later.

INVESTIGATIONS

Chest X-ray

The chest X-ray is usually normal unless significant mitral regurgitation is present.

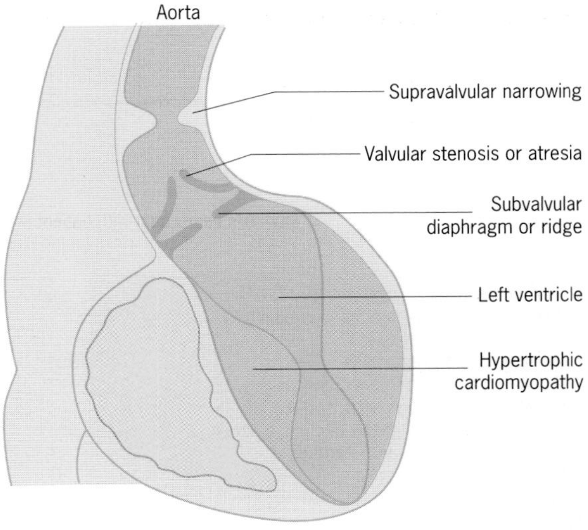

Fig 11.73
Several forms of left ventricular outflow tract obstruction

ECG

Nonspecific ST/T wave changes have been described in 15–30% of cases, but there is no evidence that this is more than in the general population.

Echocardiogram

The diagnosis is confirmed on M-mode echocardiography, which typically shows posterior movement of one or both mitral valve cusps into the left atrium during systole.

Cardiac catheterization

Contrast angiograms performed during cardiac catheterization reveal the systolic prolapse of the mitral valve into the left atrium, and mitral regurgitation, if present, is seen. This investigation is not normally required.

TREATMENT

Usually, β-blockade is effective for the treatment of the atypical chest pain and palpitations. Sometimes more specific antiarrhythmic drug treatment is necessary. When a prolapsing mitral valve is associated with significant mitral regurgitation and atrial fibrillation, anticoagulation is advised to prevent thromboembolism. Very occasionally, mitral valve replacement may be necessary for severe regurgitation, although many surgeons prefer to repair rather than replace such valves. Prophylaxis against endocarditis (see p. 10) is advised if there is significant mitral valve regurgitation.

Aortic stenosis

There are three causes of aortic valve stenosis:

- Congenital aortic valve stenosis develops progressively because of turbulent blood flow through a congenitally abnormal (usually bicuspid) aortic valve. Most congenitally abnormal aortic valves occur in men.
- Rheumatic fever results in progressive fusion, thickening and calcification of a previously normal three-cusped aortic valve. In rheumatic heart disease the aortic valve is affected in about 40% of cases and there is usually associated mitral valve disease.
- The wear and tear of age may lead to arteriosclerotic degeneration and calcification of the aortic valve.

Valvular aortic stenosis should be distinguished from other causes of obstruction to left ventricular emptying (Fig 11.73), which include:

- *supravalvular obstruction* – a congenital fibrous diaphragm above the aortic valve often associated with mental retardation and hypercalcaemia (William's syndrome)
- *hypertrophic cardiomyopathy* – septal muscle hypertrophy obstructing left ventricular outflow
- *subvalvular aortic stenosis* – a congenital condition in which a fibrous ridge or diaphragm is situated immediately below the aortic valve

PATHOPHYSIOLOGY

Obstructed left ventricular emptying leads to increased left ventricular pressure and compensatory left ventricular hypertrophy. In turn, this results in relative ischaemia of the left ventricular myocardium, and consequent angina, arrhythmias and left ventricular failure. The obstruction to left ventricular emptying is relatively more severe on exercise. Normally, exercise causes a many-fold increase in cardiac output, but when there is severe narrowing of the aortic valve orifice the cardiac output can hardly increase.

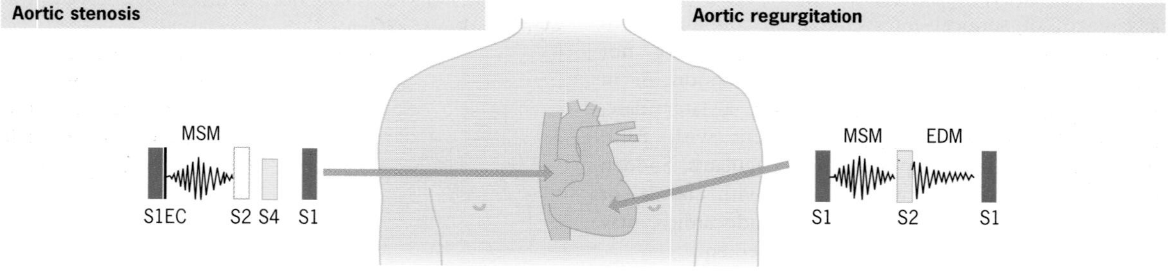

Murmurs heard best with patient leaning forwards and breath held in expiration

Clinical memo

Aortic stenosis	
Pulse:	Sinus rhythm, low volume, slow rising
Aortic area:	Systolic thrill
Apex:	Not displaced, sustained
Sounds:	Ejection click, soft A2, S4
Murmurs:	Systolic, low pitched, ejection, radiating to carotids

Clinical memo

Aortic regurgitation	
Pulse:	Sinus rhythm, large volume, collapsing
Blood pressure:	Wide pulse pressure
Apex:	Displaced, diffuse, hyperdynamic
Murmurs:	(1) High pitched, early diastolic at LSE (2) Ejection systolic at base and into neck (3) Mid-diastolic rumble at apex (Austin-Flint)

Fig 11.74
Auscultatory features of aortic stenosis and aortic regurgitation
EC, ejection click; EDM, early diastolic murmur; MSM, mid-systolic murmur; S1, first heart sound

Thus, the blood pressure falls, coronary ischaemia worsens, the myocardium fails and cardiac arrhythmias develop.

SYMPTOMS

There are usually no symptoms until aortic stenosis is moderately severe (when the aortic orifice is reduced to one-third of its normal size). At this stage, exercise-induced syncope, angina and dyspnoea may develop. When symptoms occur, the prognosis is poor – on average, death occurs within 2–3 years if there has been no surgical intervention.

SIGNS (see Clinical memo in Fig 11.74)

Aortic stenosis is characterized by abnormalities of the pulse, precordial pulsation and auscultation.

Pulse

The carotid pulse is of small volume and is slow-rising or plateau in nature (see p. 633).

Precordial palpation

The apex beat is not usually displaced because hypertrophy (as opposed to dilatation) does not produce noticeable cardiomegaly. However, the pulsation is sustained and obvious. A double impulse is sometimes felt because the fourth heart sound or atrial contraction ('kick') may be palpable. A systolic thrill may be felt in the aortic area.

Auscultation

The most obvious auscultatory finding in aortic stenosis is an ejection systolic murmur that is usually 'diamond-shaped' (crescendo–decrescendo). The murmur is usually longer when the disease is more severe as a longer ejection time is needed. The murmur is usually rough in quality and best heard in the aortic area. It radiates into the carotid arteries and also the precordium. The intensity of the murmur is usually not a good guide to the severity of the condition because it is lessened by a reduced cardiac output. In severe cases, the murmur may be inaudible.

Other findings

- There is a *systolic ejection* click (see p. 639), unless the valve has become immobile and calcified.
- There is a *soft or inaudible aortic second heart sound* when the aortic valve becomes immobile.
- There is *reversed splitting of the second heart sound* (splitting on expiration) (see p. 637).
- There is a *prominent fourth heart sound* (see p. 638), unless coexisting mitral stenosis prevents this.

Degenerative disease of the aortic valve (*aortic sclerosis*) results in a loud mid-systolic murmur but, because there is little stenosis, there are no signs of left ventricular hypertrophy or of a slow-rising pulse. This murmur can be ignored.

INVESTIGATIONS

Chest X-ray

The chest X-ray usually reveals a relatively small heart with a prominent, dilated, ascending aorta. This occurs because turbulent blood flow above the stenosed aortic valve produces so-called 'post-stenotic dilatation'. The aortic valve may be calcified. When heart failure occurs, the CTR increases.

ECG

The ECG shows left ventricular hypertrophy and left atrial delay. A left ventricular 'strain' pattern due to 'pressure overload' (depressed ST segments and T wave inversion in leads orientated towards the left ventricle, i.e. leads I, AVL, V_5 and V_6) is common when the disease is severe. Usually, sinus rhythm is present, but ventricular arrhythmias may be recorded.

Echocardiogram

The echocardiogram readily demonstrates the thickened, calcified and immobile aortic valve cusps. Left ventricular hypertrophy may also be seen. The gradient across the valve can be estimated by CW Doppler, provided the left ventricular function is reasonable (see Fig 11.23 on p. 649).

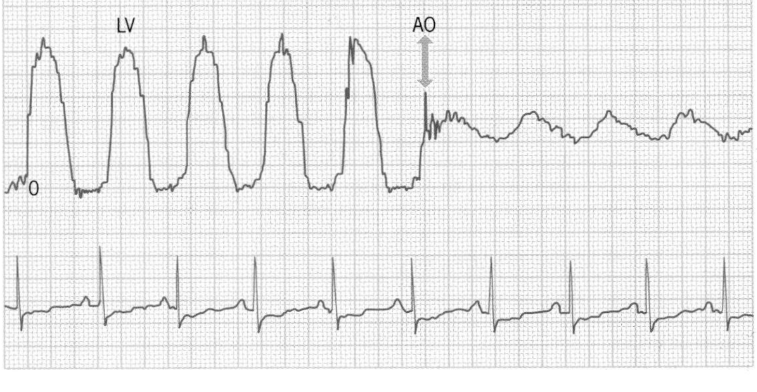

Fig 11.75
ECG and pressure trace as a cardiac catheter is withdrawn from the left ventricle (LV) to the aorta (AO). Note that the peak systolic pressure changes from 250 to 130 mmHg (arrow). The 120 mmHg peak-to-peak systolic gradient indicates severe aortic valvular stenosis

Table 11.36
Causes and associations of aortic regurgitation

Acute aortic regurgitation	Chronic aortic regurgitation
Acute rheumatic fever	Rheumatic heart disease
Infective endocarditis	Syphilis
Dissection of the aorta	Arthritides
Ruptured sinus of Valsalva aneurysm	Reiter's syndrome
Failure of prosthetic heart value	Ankylosing spondylitis
	Rheumatoid arthritis
	Hypertension (severe)
	Bicuspid aortic valve
	Aortic endocarditis
	Marfan's syndrome
	Osteogenesis imperfecta

Cardiac catheterization

Cardiac catheterization is used to document the systolic pressure difference (gradient) between the aorta and the left ventricle (Fig 11.75). A gradient of 50 mmHg or more is usually sufficient to advise surgery. A trivial degree of aortic regurgitation that is undetectable clinically is often demonstrated by contrast aortography. Coronary angiography is important before recommending surgery.

TREATMENT

Patients with aortic stenosis should not overly exert them-selves, and in particular they should not compete in stren-uous physical games. Angina is best treated with β-blockade because vasodilators such as glyceryl trinitrate or isosorbide dinitrate may aggravate exertional syncope. ACE inhibitors are relatively contraindicated and should be prescribed only by experienced physicians. Antibiotic prophylaxis against infective endocarditis is essential (see p. 10).

Irrespective of symptoms, aortic valve replacement with a prosthetic or tissue valve is recommended when aortic stenosis is severe. Cardiopulmonary bypass is necessary to achieve this. Provided that the valve is not severely deformed or heavily calcified, critical aortic stenosis in childhood or adolescence can be treated by valvotomy (performed under direct vision by the surgeon or by balloon dilatation using X-ray visualization). This produces temporary relief from the obstruction. Aortic valve replacement will usually be needed a few years later. Balloon dilatation (valvuloplasty) has been tried in adults, especially in the elderly, as an alternative to surgery. Generally results are poor and such treatment is reserved for patients unfit for surgery or as a 'bridge' to surgery (i.e. to improve them for surgery).

Aortic regurgitation

The most common causes of aortic regurgitation are rheumatic fever and infective endocarditis complicating a previously damaged valve. This can be a congenitally abnormal valve (e.g. a bicuspid valve) or one damaged by rheumatic fever. There are numerous other causes and associations (Table 11.36). The majority of patients with aortic regurgitation are men (75%), but rheumatic aortic regurgitation occurs more commonly in women.

PATHOPHYSIOLOGY

Aortic regurgitation is reflux of blood from the aorta through the aortic valve into the left ventricle during diastole. If net cardiac output is to be maintained, the total volume of blood pumped into the aorta must increase, and consequently the left ventricular size must enlarge. Because of the aortic run-off during diastole, diastolic blood pressure falls and coronary perfusion is decreased. In addition, the larger left ventricular size is mechanically less efficient so that the demand for oxygen is greater and cardiac ischaemia develops.

SYMPTOMS

In aortic regurgitation, significant symptoms occur late and do not develop until left ventricular failure occurs. As with mitral regurgitation, a common symptom is 'pounding of the heart' because of the increased left ventricular size and its vigorous pulsation. Angina pectoris is a frequent complaint. Varying grades of dyspnoea occur depending on the extent of left ventricular dilatation and dysfunction. Arrhythmias are relatively uncommon.

SIGNS (see Clinical memo in Fig 11.74)

The signs of aortic regurgitation are many and are due to the hyperdynamic circulation, reflux of blood into the left ventricle and the increased left ventricular size.

The pulse is bounding or collapsing (see p. 633). The following signs, which are rare, also indicate a hyper-dynamic circulation:

- *Quincke's sign* – capillary pulsation in the nail beds
- *De Musset's sign* – head nodding with each heart beat
- *Duroziez's sign* – a to-and-fro murmur heard when the femoral artery is auscultated with pressure applied dis-tally (if found, it is a sign of severe aortic regurgitation)
- *pistol shot femorals* – a sharp bang heard on auscultation over the femoral arteries in time with each heart beat.

The apex beat is displaced laterally and downwards and is thrusting (hyperdynamic) in quality. On auscultation, there is a high-pitched early diastolic murmur best heard at the left sternal edge in the fourth intercostal space with the patient leaning forward and the breath held in expiration.

Because of the volume overload there is commonly an ejection systolic flow murmur. The regurgitant jet can impinge on the anterior mitral valve cusp, causing a mid-diastolic murmur (Austin Flint).

INVESTIGATIONS

Chest X-ray

The chest X-ray features are those of left ventricular enlargement and possibly of dilatation of the ascending aorta. The ascending aortic wall may be calcified in syphilis and the aortic valve may be calcified if valvular disease is responsible for the regurgitation.

ECG

The ECG appearances are those of left ventricular hypertrophy due to 'volume overload' – tall R waves and deeply inverted T waves in the left-sided chest leads, and deep S waves in the right-sided leads. Normally, sinus rhythm is present.

Echocardiogram

The echocardiogram demonstrates vigorous cardiac contraction and a dilated left ventricle. The aortic root may also be enlarged. Diastolic fluttering of the mitral leaflets or septum occurs in severe aortic regurgitation (producing the Austin Flint murmur, see p. 640). The regurgitant jet can be detected by CW Doppler.

Cardiac catheterization

During cardiac catheterization, injection of contrast medium into the aorta (aortography) will outline aortic valvular abnormalities and allow assessment of the degree of regurgitation.

TREATMENT

The underlying cause of aortic regurgitation (e.g. syphilitic aortitis or infective endocarditis) may require specific treatment. The treatment of aortic regurgitation usually requires aortic valve replacement but the timing of surgery is important.

Because symptoms do not develop until the myocardium fails and because the myocardium does not recover fully after surgery, it is important to operate before significant symptoms occur. The timing of the operation is best determined according to haemodynamic, echocardiographic or nuclear angiographic criteria.

Both mechanical prostheses and tissue valves are used. Tissue valves are preferred in the elderly and when anticoagulants must be avoided, but are contraindicated in children and young adults because of the rapid calcification and degeneration of the valves.

Antibiotic prophylaxis against infective endocarditis (see p. 10) is necessary even if a prosthetic valve replacement has been performed.

Tricuspid stenosis

This uncommon valve lesion, which is seen much more often in women than in men, is usually due to rheumatic heart disease and is frequently associated with mitral and/or aortic valve disease. Tricuspid stenosis is also seen in the carcinoid syndrome.

PATHOPHYSIOLOGY

Tricuspid valve stenosis results in a reduced cardiac output, which is restored towards normal when the right atrial pressure increases. The resulting systemic venous congestion produces hepatomegaly, ascites and dependent oedema.

SYMPTOMS

Usually, patients with tricuspid stenosis complain of symptoms due to the associated left-sided rheumatic valve lesions. The abdominal pain (due to hepatomegaly) and swelling (due to ascites) and peripheral oedema that occur are relatively severe when compared with the degree of dyspnoea.

SIGNS

If the patient remains in sinus rhythm, which is unusual, there is a prominent jugular venous *a* wave. This presystolic pulsation may also be felt over the liver. There is usually a rumbling mid-diastolic murmur, which is heard best at the lower left sternal edge and is louder on inspiration. It may be missed because of the murmur of coexisting mitral stenosis. A tricuspid opening snap may occasionally be heard.

Hepatomegaly, abdominal ascites and dependent oedema may be present.

INVESTIGATIONS

Chest X-ray

On the chest X-ray there may be a prominent right atrial bulge.

ECG

The enlarged right atrium may be manifested on the ECG by peaked, tall P waves (≥3 mm) in lead II.

Echocardiogram

The echocardiogram may show a thickened and immobile tricuspid valve, but this is not so clearly seen as an abnormal mitral valve.

Cardiac catheterization

This demonstrates a diastolic pressure gradient between the right atrium and the right ventricle. Contrast injection will demonstrate a large right atrium.

TREATMENT

Medical management consists of diuretic therapy and salt restriction. Tricuspid valvotomy is occasionally possible, but tricuspid valve replacement is often necessary. Other valves usually also need replacement because tricuspid valve stenosis is rarely an isolated lesion.

Tricuspid regurgitation

Functional tricuspid regurgitation may occur whenever the right ventricle dilates, e.g. in cor pulmonale, myocardial infarction or pulmonary hypertension.

Organic tricuspid regurgitation may occur with rheumatic heart disease, infective endocarditis, carcinoid syndrome, Ebstein's anomaly (a congenitally malpositioned tricuspid valve) and other congenital abnormalities of the atrioventricular valves.

SYMPTOMS AND SIGNS

The valvular regurgitation gives rise to high right atrial and systemic venous pressure. Patients may complain of the symptoms of right heart failure (see p. 677).

Physical signs include a large jugular venous *cv* wave and a palpable liver that pulsates in systole. Usually a right ventri-cular impulse may be felt at the left sternal edge, and there is a blowing pansystolic murmur, best heard on inspiration at the lower left sternal edge. Atrial fibrillation is common.

TREATMENT

Functional tricuspid regurgitation usually disappears with medical management. Severe organic tricuspid regurgitation may require operative repair of the tricuspid valve (annuloplasty or plication). Very occasionally, tricuspid valve replacement may be necessary. In drug addicts with infective endocarditis of the tricuspid valve, surgical removal of the valve is recommended to eradicate the infection. This is usually well tolerated in the short term. The insertion of a prosthetic valve for this condition is considered on p. 710.

Pulmonary stenosis

This is usually a congenital lesion, but it may rarely result from rheumatic fever or from the carcinoid syndrome. Congenital pulmonary stenosis may be associated with an intact ventricular septum or with a ventricular septal defect (Fallot's tetralogy).

Pulmonary stenosis may be valvular, subvalvular or supra-valvular. Multiple congenital pulmonary arterial stenoses are usually due to infection with rubella during pregnancy.

SYMPTOMS AND SIGNS

The obstruction to right ventricular emptying results in right ventricular hypertrophy which in turn leads to right atrial hypertrophy. Severe pulmonary obstruction may be incompatible with life, but lesser degrees of obstruction give rise to fatigue, syncope and the symptoms of right heart failure. Mild pulmonary stenosis may be asymptomatic.

The physical signs are characterized by a harsh mid-systolic ejection murmur, best heard on inspiration, to the left of the sternum in the second intercostal space. This murmur is often associated with a thrill. The pulmonary closure sound is usually delayed and soft. There may be a pulmonary ejection sound if the obstruction is valvular. A right ventricular fourth sound and a prominent jugular venous *a* wave are present when the stenosis is moderately severe. A right ventricular heave (sustained impulse) may be felt.

INVESTIGATIONS

Chest X-ray

The chest X-ray usually shows a prominent pulmonary artery due to poststenotic dilatation.

ECG

The ECG demonstrates both right atrial and right ventricular hypertrophy, although it may sometimes be normal even in severe pulmonary stenosis.

Cardiac catheterization

The passage of a catheter through the right heart allows the level and degree of the stenosis to be established by measuring the systolic pressure gradient.

TREATMENT

Treatment of severe pulmonary stenosis requires pulmonary valvotomy (balloon valvotomy or direct surgery).

Pulmonary regurgitation

This is the most common acquired lesion of the pulmonary valve. It results from dilatation of the pulmonary valve ring, which occurs with pulmonary hypertension. It is characterized by a decrescendo diastolic murmur beginning with the pulmonary component of the second sound that is difficult to distinguish from the murmur of aortic regurgitation. Pulmonary regurgitation usually causes no symptoms and treatment is rarely necessary.

Prosthetic heart valves

There are two types of prosthetic heart valve: tissue and mechanical. *Tissue valves* are usually fashioned from a pig aortic valve (xenograft); occasionally a human aortic valve is used (homograft). *Mechanical valves* are of various types, the most common being a ball-and-cage design (Starr–Edwards valve), a tilting disc (Björk–Shiley valve), or a double tilting disc (St Jude valve).

The disadvantage of the mechanical valve over the tissue valve is that formal anticoagulation is required. However, mechanical valves are much harder wearing; a tissue valve tends to degenerate after about 10 years. Unlike a tilting disc valve, the ball of a ball-and-cage valve presents some obstruction to flow through the valve. Although ball-and-cage valves have always been mechanically satisfactory, some tilting disc valves have been mechanically insecure.

Prosthetic valves may become detached from the valve ring, thrombose, stick, degenerate or become infected. Echocardiography is often helpful, but echoes are scattered from the mechanical valve making assessment of the structure of the valve rather difficult. This is particularly troublesome with the mitral valve, but the advent of transoesophageal echocardiography has largely overcome this problem. Transoesophageal echocardiography is the investigation of choice when prosthetic valve endocarditis is suspected.

FURTHER READING

Carabello BA, Crawford FA (1997) Medical progress: valvular heart disease. *New England Journal of Medicine* **337**: 32–41.

Infective endocarditis

Infective endocarditis is an infection of the endocardium or vascular endothelium. The disease may occasionally occur as a fulminating or acute infection, but more commonly runs an insidious course and is known as subacute (bacterial) endocarditis (SBE). The annual incidence in the UK is 6–7 per 100 000, but it is much more common in developing countries.

Endocarditis occurs most commonly on rheumatic or congenitally abnormal valves as well as in mitral valve prolapse and calcified aortic valve disease. It also occurs in association with congenital lesions such as ventricular septal defect or persistent ductus arteriosus. A very similar disease may occur from infection of arteriovenous fistulae. Prosthetic valves or prosthetic vascular material may be similarly infected and this is one of the reasons for the increasing incidence of endocarditis in developed countries. The organisms are often non-virulent.

Virulent organisms may infect normal valves, especially when the victim is generally debilitated or immunologically incompetent.

The term 'infective endocarditis' is preferred because not all the infecting organisms are bacteria.

AETIOLOGY

Many organisms cause infective endocarditis. Currently the three most common organisms are *Streptococcus viridans*, *Enterococcus faecalis*, and *Staphylococcus aureus*. It can also be caused by *Staph. epidermidis*, *Histoplasma*, *Brucella*, *Candida* and *Aspergillus*, or by *Coxiella burnetii*. However, although Gram-negative bacteraemia/septicaemia frequently occur with these latter organisms, endocarditis is unusual.

- *Str. viridans* (e.g. *Str. viridans mitis* and *Str. viridans sanguis*) (50% of cases). These organisms are part of the bacterial flora of the pharynx and upper respiratory tract, and the infection may follow dental extraction or cleaning, tonsillectomy or bronchoscopy.
- *Enterococcus faecalis* (found in perineal and faecal bacterial flora). Infections with this organism are more usual in older men with prostatic disease, in women with genitourinary infections, or following pelvic surgery.

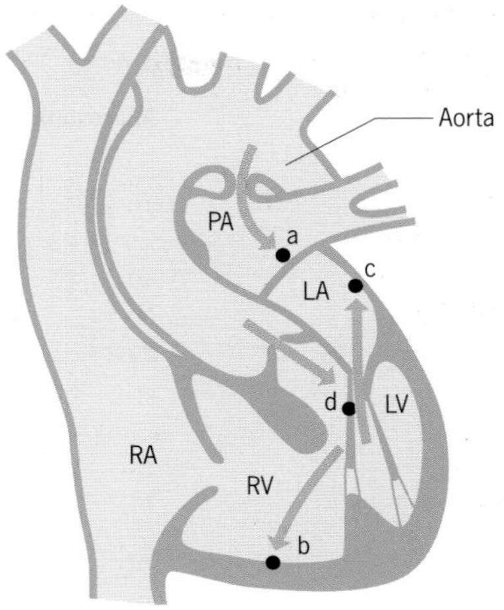

Fig 11.76
Jet lesions produced in infective endocarditis
a: Lesion in the pulmonary artery (PA) because of a ductus arteriosus
b: Lesion in the right ventricle (RV) due to a ventricular septal defect
c: Lesion in the left atrium (LA) due to mitral regurgitation
d: Lesion in the left ventricle (LV) and on the mitral valve chordae tendineae due to aortic regurgitation
RA, right atrium

- *Staph. aureus.* This organism may cause subacute endocarditis and is responsible for 50% of the acute forms. Patients with central venous catheters used for parenteral feeding, temporary pacemaker electrode catheters or pulmonary artery (Swan–Ganz) catheters are prone to this infection. Cellulitis or skin abscesses are often the origin of the infection, particularly in drug addicts who 'mainline'.
- *Staph. epidermidis, Histoplasma, Brucella, Candida* and *Aspergillus.* Infections with these organisms are particularly common in intravenous drug addicts, alcoholics and patients with prosthetic heart valves.
- *C. burnetii* (the causative organism of Q fever, see p. 49). This may cause a subacute infection.

PATHOLOGY

Infection occurs along the edges of the heart valves. It is more common on the left side, with mitral and aortic regurgitation being the most common valve lesions complicated by endocarditis. In i.v. drug addicts the valves in the right heart are usually affected.

The endocardium on the low-pressure side of a shunt such as ventricular septal defect is infected and it is the pulmonary artery that is infected when a persistent ductus arteriosus is present; in both instances the lesions are 'jet lesions' produced on the wall opposite the shunt (Fig 11.76).

Hypertrophic cardiomyopathy, syphilitic aortic regurgitation, prolapsing mitral valve and arteriosclerotic valve lesions may also rarely be complicated by endocarditis.

The lesion of infective endocarditis is a mass of fibrin, platelets and infecting organisms known as a *vegetation*. The chance of an organism sticking to a vegetation is increased

Table 11.37
Clinical features of infective endocarditis

	Approximate %
General systems	
Malaise	95
Clubbing	10
Cardiac	
Murmurs	90
Cardiac failure	50
Arthralgia	25
Pyrexia	90
Skin lesions	
Osler's nodes	15
Splinter haemorrhages	10
Janeway lesions	5
Petechiae	50
Eyes	
Roth spots	5
Conjunctival splinter haemorrhages	Rare
Splenomegaly	40
Neurological	
Cerebral emboli	20
Mycotic aneurysm	10
Renal	
Haematuria	70

because of the clumping together of bacteria caused by agglutinating antibodies. These can develop because of repeated infection with the bacterium over a period of years. In acute endocarditis, vegetations may be very large and may embolize. Virulent micro-organisms may rapidly destroy the valve cusp, producing ulceration and regurgitation.

The extracardiac manifestations result either from embolization or from the deposition of immune complexes. The latter is thought to be responsible for arthralgia, Roth spots and Janeway lesions, focal glomerulonephritis and acute vasculitis (see below).

Splenic and renal infarcts are produced by emboli. Myocardial infarction can result from coronary emboli, and pulmonary infarction may occur if right-sided lesions embolize.

PRESENTATIONS

Subacute endocarditis

The patient presents with fever, night sweats, weight loss, weakness and symptoms due to cardiac failure or embolism. Another important presentation is the combination of renal failure and a heart murmur. It is not usually possible to date the onset of the illness.

Acute endocarditis

In intravenous drug abusers or following an acute suppurative illness such as pneumonia or meningitis, the development of acute endocarditis is suggested by the persistence of fever and the development of heart murmurs, vasculitis (with petechial haemorrhage) and emboli, including metastatic abscesses. The onset of severe heart failure may indicate chordal rupture or acute valvular destruction.

Prosthetic endocarditis

There are two varieties: the first develops soon after surgery and is due to infection of the prosthesis at surgery, and the second occurs late and follows a bacteraemia. In both cases it is the valve ring that is infected. This produces myocardial abscesses and damage, for example to the conduction system. Vegetations in the valve may prevent it from opening and closing properly. Emboli are common.

CLINICAL FEATURES

Table 11.37 lists the clinical features of infective endocarditis. The patients are often elderly. They appear pale (often anaemic) and ill. They are intermittently pyrexial and may complain of myalgia and arthralgia. Some of the following signs and symptoms may be present, but endocarditis must always be suspected in a patient with a heart murmur and a fever.

Cardiac findings

The signs of any underlying heart disease should be obvious, but occasionally only trivial lesions such as mild aortic regurgitation or a bicuspid aortic valve are present. The development of a new murmur or a change in the character of an existing murmur may warn of the presence of endocarditis.

Vascular lesions

Small petechial or mucosal haemorrhages occur because of vasculitis. They are usually small and red, with a pale centre. They frequently appear on the mucosa of the pharynx and conjunctivae. Sometimes they are seen on the retinae (Roth spots). Small, flat, erythematous, non-tender macules are seen mainly on the thenar and hypothenar eminences (Janeway lesions); these blanch with pressure. Subungual splinter haemorrhages may develop.

Embolic lesions such as hard, painful, tender, subcutaneous swellings occur in the fingers, toes, palms and soles (Osler's nodes).

Clubbing of the fingers

Mild clubbing of the fingers and toes appears late in the disease, and thus it occurs only in subacute endocarditis. It is rare nowadays because of relatively rapid diagnosis and treatment of the endocarditis.

Splenomegaly

Slight splenomegaly is common. If a splenic infarct has occurred, the spleen may be painful and tender and a friction rub may be heard over it.

Renal lesions

Haematuria is common, usually owing to infarction as a result of emboli. Renal abscesses and acute glomerulonephritis also occur.

(a)

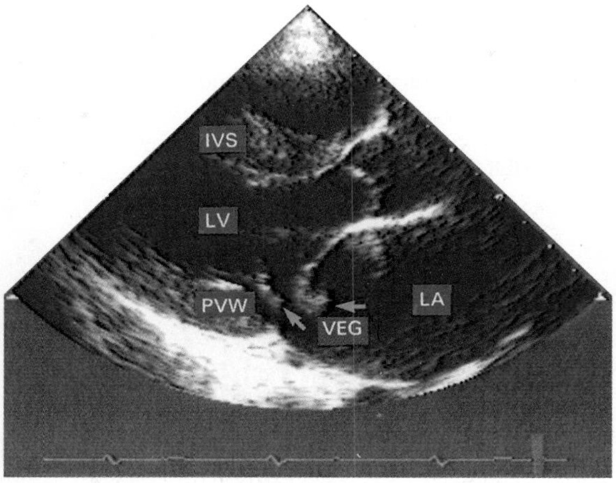

(b)

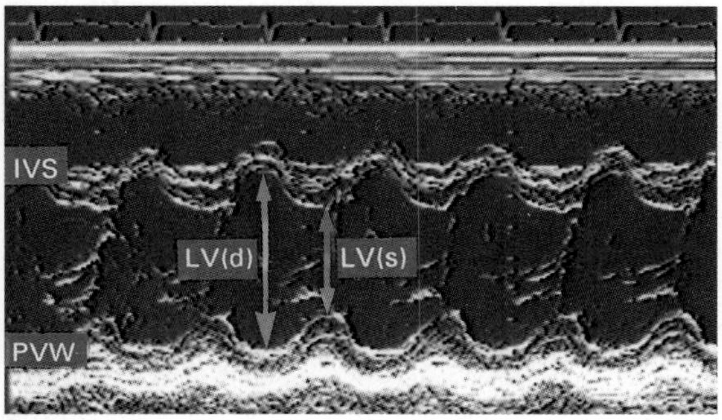

Fig 11.77
Upper: Two-dimensional echocardiogram (long-axis view) showing vegetations (arrowed) attached to both the anterior and posterior leaflets of the mitral valve in a patient with infective endocarditis
Lower: M-mode echocardiogram of the left ventricle in the same patient, showing hyperdynamic contraction associated with volume overloading from the associated severe mitral regurgitation. Compare with Fig 11.22(c)
IVS, interventricular septum; LV, left ventricle;
LV(d) and LV(s), diastolic and systolic left ventricular dimensions;
PVW, posterior ventricular wall; LA, left atrium; VEG, vegetation

Arthritis

Arthritis of the major joints is frequently seen.

Other embolic phenomena

Cerebral emboli can occur, usually to the middle cerebral artery or its branches. Mycotic infected aneurysms are seen and may present after the endocarditis has healed. Peripheral arterial, pulmonary and coronary infarcts may also occur.

INVESTIGATIONS

Laboratory tests

- **Blood**. A normochromic normocytic anaemia is usual and C-reactive protein and the ESR are increased. A polymorphonuclear leucocytosis is common and thrombocytopenia can occasionally occur.
- **Liver biochemistry** is often mildly disturbed with, in particular, an increased serum alkaline phosphatase.
- **Immunoglobulins and complement**. Serum immunoglobulins are increased, but total complement and C3 complement are decreased owing to immune complex formation. Circulating immune complexes are present in more than 70% of cases but are not routinely measured.
- **Urine**. Proteinuria may occur and microscopic haematuria is nearly always present.
- **Blood cultures** are positive in about three-quarters of cases. At least six sets of samples are usually taken and cultured in aerobic and anaerobic conditions. Special culture techniques may be necessary for unusual micro-organisms such as *Brucella* and *Histoplasma*. Serological tests are needed to incriminate *Coxiella* and *Chlamydia*, and may be helpful for *Candida* and *Brucella*.

Echocardiography

Echocardiography (particularly using the transoesophageal approach) is used to visualize vegetations (Fig 11.77), but small vegetations typical of the subacute disease can be missed. Echocardiography is useful to document valvular dysfunction and to identify patients in need of urgent surgery.

Transthoracic echocardiography cannot exclude the diagnosis of infective endocarditis, and in 20% of cases vegetations will be missed. Transoesophageal echocardiography (TOE) is a more accurate method of investigating infective endocarditis and is being used increasingly for this purpose, particularly in cases of suspected prosthetic valve endocarditis when it is the investigation of choice. Aortic root abscess, a dangerous complication of infective endocarditis, can be accurately excluded only with TOE.

Despite the greater accuracy of transoesophageal compared to transthoracic echocardiography in the investigation of infective endocarditis, the technique is by no means 100% sensitive and the diagnosis remains a clinical one.

Chest X-ray

This may show evidence of heart failure or emboli in right-sided endocarditis.

ECGs

These may show evidence of myocardial infarction (emboli) or conduction defects.

TREATMENT

Drug therapy

Any underlying infection should be treated (e.g. a dental abscess should be drained). The endocarditis is treated with bactericidal antibiotics chosen on the basis of the results of the blood culture and antibiotic sensitivity assessment. The treatment should continue for 4–6 weeks.

Serum levels are measured and 'back titration' is performed to ensure that sufficient bactericidal antibiotic activity is present to inhibit growth of the organism.

Str. viridans is usually treated with benzylpenicillin 2.4 g i.v. 6-hourly and low-dose gentamicin 1 mg kg^{-1} 8-hourly for the first two weeks because of the additive effects of gentamicin and penicillin against *Str. viridans*. Oral amoxycillin 6 g daily can replace intravenous therapy after two weeks.

Str. faecalis (enterococcus) is managed with penicillin and gentamicin (3 mg kg^{-1} in divided 8-hourly doses). The dosage of penicillin should be higher (up to 24 g daily) than for *Str. viridans* because *Str. faecalis* is relatively insensitive to penicillin and ampicillin 8 g daily is often substituted. The exact dose of gentamicin depends on renal function and efficacy, and blood levels should be measured at least twice each week.

It is more difficult to choose antibiotics when the infecting organism has not been isolated. However, in the acute form of the disease this is likely to be *Staphylococcus*, and treatment should include flucloxacillin and fusidic acid. In the subacute form, unless it is highly likely that the infecting organism is *Str. viridans*, it is usual to begin treatment with a broad-spectrum combination of antibiotics such as gentamicin and ampicillin. The treatment is adjusted if it is not successful.

The recurrence of fever may suggest that the antibiotic therapy is inadequate, but may also signal a drug reaction. The antibiotics may be omitted for 24–72 hours to test this.

Surgery

There are several situations in which surgery is necessary:

- extensive damage to a valve
- early infection of prosthetic material
- worsening renal failure
- persistent infection but failure to culture an organism
- embolization
- large vegetations
- progressive cardiac failure.

The timing of surgery is important. On the one hand the infection should, if possible, be eradicated before surgery is undertaken, but on the other hand the heart should not be left in a badly compromised haemodynamic state. In general, early surgery is preferable.

PROGNOSIS

The prognosis is worse when the organism cannot be isolated, when cardiac failure is present, when infection occurs on a prosthetic valve, and when the micro-organisms found are resistant to therapy. In general, 70% of those affected are treated effectively, but greater awareness of the subacute form of the disease will improve the success rate.

PROPHYLAXIS (see also p. 10)

Those at risk of developing endocarditis should receive antibiotic therapy before undergoing a procedure likely to result in a bacteraemia. The form of the prophylaxis depends on the procedure and on the likelihood of endocarditis. High-risk patients are those with a prosthetic heart valve or a previous history of endocarditis.

FURTHER READING

Weinstein L, Brusch JL (1996) Infective endocarditis. Oxford: OUP.

Congenital heart disease

A congenital cardiac malformation occurs in about 1% of live births. There is an overall male predominance, although some individual lesions (e.g. atrial septal defect and persistent ductus arteriosus) occur more commonly in females. The aetiology of congenital cardiac disease is often unknown, but recognized associations include:

- *maternal rubella infection* (persistent ductus arteriosus, and pulmonary valvular and arterial stenosis)
- *maternal alcohol abuse* (septal defects)
- *maternal drug treatment and radiation*
- *genetic abnormalities* (e.g. the familial form of atrial septal defect and congenital heart block)
- *chromosomal abnormalities* (e.g. septal defects and mitral and tricuspid valve defects are associated with Down's syndrome (trisomy 21) or coarctation of the aorta in Turner's syndrome (45, XO)).

Some symptoms and signs are common in congenital heart disease:

- *Central cyanosis* occurs because of right-to-left shunting of blood or because of complete mixing of systemic and pulmonary blood flow.
- *Pulmonary hypertension* results from large left-to-right shunts. The persistently raised pulmonary flow leads to the development of increased pulmonary artery vascular resistance and consequent pulmonary hypertension. This is known as the Eisenmenger

Table 11.38
Common congenital lesions

	Percentage of congenital lesions	Occurrence in first-degree relatives (%)
Ventricular septal defect	39	4
Atrial septal defect	10	2
Persistent ductus arteriosus	10	4
Pulmonary stenosis	7	
Coarctation of the aorta	7	2
Aortic stenosis	6	4
Fallot's tetralogy	6	4
Others	15	

reaction (or the Eisenmenger syndrome when due specifically to a ventricular septal defect). The development of pulmonary hypertension significantly worsens the prognosis.

- *Clubbing of the fingers* may occur in congenital cardiac conditions associated with prolonged cyanosis.
- *Paradoxical embolism* of thrombus from the systemic veins to the systemic arterial system may occur when a communication exists between the right and left heart.
- *Growth retardation* is common in children with cyanotic heart disease.
- *Syncope* is common when severe right or left ventricular outflow tract obstruction is present. Exertional syncope, associated with deepening central cyanosis, may occur in Fallot's tetralogy. Exercise increases resistance to pulmonary blood flow but reduced systemic vascular resistance. Thus, the right-to-left shunt increases and cerebral oxygenation falls.
- *Squatting* is the posture adopted by children with Fallot's tetralogy. It results in obstruction of venous return of desaturated blood and an increase in the peripheral systemic vascular resistance. This leads to a reduced right-to-left shunt and improved cerebral oxygenation.

Table 11.38 lists the most common congenital lesions and their occurrence in first-degree relatives.

Genetic factors should be considered in all patients presenting with congenital heart disease. For example, parents with a child suffering from Fallot's tetralogy stand a 4% chance of conceiving another child with the disease, and so fetal ultrasound screening of the mother during pregnancy is essential.

Ventricular septal defect (VSD)

VSD is the most common congenital cardiac malfor-mation (1 in 500 live births). It may occur as an isolated abnormality or in association with other anomalies. Left ventricular pressure is higher than right ventricular pressure; blood therefore moves from left to right and pulmonary blood flow increases. When pulmonary blood flow is very large, progressive obliteration of the pulmonary vas-culature changes eventually causes the pulmonary arterial pressure to equal the systemic pressure (Eisenmenger's syndrome). Consequently, the shunt is reduced or reversed (becoming right-to-left) and central cyanosis may develop.

CLINICAL FEATURES

A small VSD ('maladie de Roger') presents with a loud and sometimes long systolic murmur in an asymptomatic patient. Such VSDs usually close spontaneously. Moderate VSDs produce some fatigue and dyspnoea. Physical signs include cardiac enlargement and a prominent apex beat. There is often a palpable systolic thrill at the lower left sternal edge. A loud 'tearing' pansystolic murmur is heard at the same position.

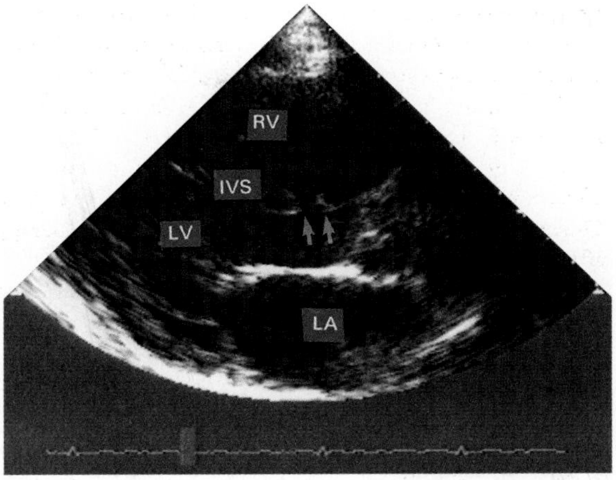

Fig 11.78
Two-dimensional echocardiogram (long-axis view) showing a ventricular septal defect (arrowed). Colour Doppler would provide graphic demonstration of the left to right shunt
RV, right ventricle; IVS, interventricular septum; LV, left ventricle; LA, left atrium

Large VSDs eventually cause pulmonary hypertension (right ventricular parasternal heave and a loud, pulmonary component of the second heart sound). The murmur may be soft. It is important to note that the increased right ventricular pressure may be nearly equal to the left ventricular pressure, so that flow across the VSD is small.

INVESTIGATIONS

A small VSD produces no abnormal X-ray or ECG findings. On the chest X-ray, larger defects show a prominent pulmonary artery owing to increased pulmonary blood flow. In Eisenmenger's syndrome the radiological signs of pulmonary hypertension (i.e. 'pruned' pulmonary arteries) can be seen. Cardiomegaly occurs when a moderate or a large VSD is present. The ECG shows features of both left and right ventricular hypertrophy. The size and location of the VSD, and its haemodynamic consequences, can be assessed by 2-D echocardiography and CW Doppler (Fig 11.78).

TREATMENT

Moderate and large VSDs should be surgically repaired before the development of severe pulmonary hyper-tension. Infective endocarditis prophylaxis should be advised.

Information

Sternal impulse:	Right ventricular heave
Sounds:	Loud P2 Fixed split S2(A2–P2)
Murmurs:	Mid-systolic ejection in pulmonary area

Information box 11.2 Atrial septal defect

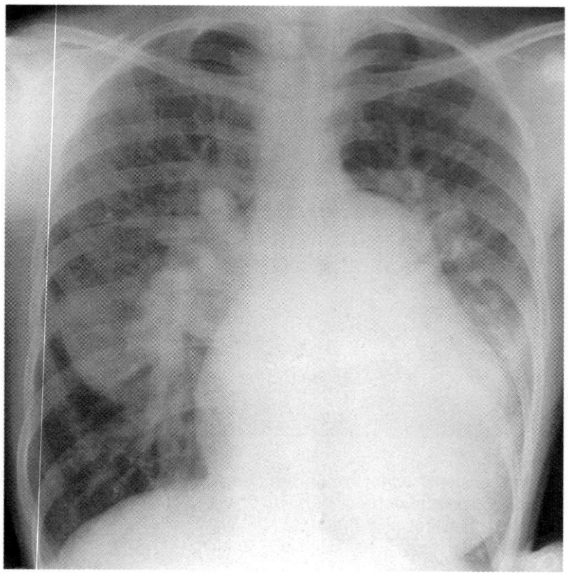

Fig 11.79
Atrial septal defect shown by a PA chest X-ray from a young woman. The film shows a prominent main pulmonary artery and pulmonary arterial plethora. The heart is increased in size

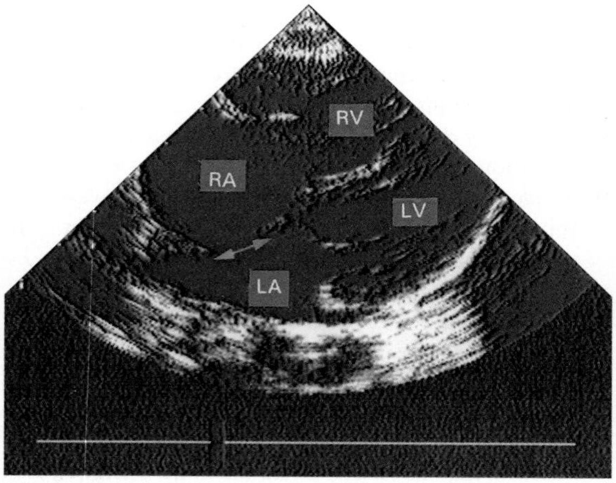

Fig 11.80
Ostium secundum atrial septal defect (arrowed) in a young girl, shown by a two-dimensional echocardiogram subcostal four-chamber view (similar to Fig 11.78, but rotated clockwise). Colour Doppler can demonstrate the left-to-right shunt
LA, left atrium; RA, right atrium; LV, left ventricle; RV, right ventricle

Atrial septal defect (ASD)

This congenital condition is often first diagnosed in adults. It is more common in women than in men. There are two types of ASD, ostium secundum and ostium primum. The common form is ostium secundum. Communication at the level of the atria allows left-to-right shunting of blood. Because the pulmonary vascular resistance is low and the right ventricle is easily distended (i.e. it is compliant), there is a considerable increase in right heart output. Above the age of 30 years there may be an increase in pulmonary vascular resistance, which gives rise to pulmonary hypertension. Atrial arrhythmias, particularly atrial fibrillation, are common at this stage.

CLINICAL FEATURES (Information box 11.2)

Most children with ASDs are asymptomatic, although they are prone to pulmonary infection. Some complain of dyspnoea and weakness. Palpitations due to atrial arrhythmias are not uncommon. Right heart failure may develop in later life.

The physical signs of ASD reflect the volume overloading of the right ventricle. Therefore, the splitting of the second sound is wide and fixed (see p. 637). The increased flow through the right heart produces a loud ejection systolic pulmonary flow murmur, and sometimes a diastolic tricuspid flow murmur may be heard. A right ventricular heave can usually be felt.

INVESTIGATIONS

Chest X-ray

This reveals a prominent pulmonary artery and pulmonary plethora. Fig 11.79 shows a more severe case with pulmonary hypertension. There may be noticeable right ventricular enlargement.

ECG

This usually shows some degree of right bundle branch block (because of dilatation of the right ventricle) and right axis deviation.

Echocardiogram

This is usually abnormal if a significant defect is present. Indirect evidence includes right ventricular hypertrophy and pulmonary arterial dilatation, and abnormal motion of the interventricular septum. Sometimes the ASD is part of a major developmental abnormality and may also involve the ventricular septum and the mitral and tricuspid valves. In this case there is left axis deviation on the ECG. Subcostal views may demonstrate the ASD (Fig 11.80), and transoesophageal echocardiography may sometimes be necessary.

Doppler

Flow disturbance can be assessed by colour Doppler.

TREATMENT

A significant ASD (i.e. a pulmonary flow that is more than 50% increased when compared with systemic flow) should be repaired before the age of 10 years or as soon as possible if first diagnosed in adulthood. There is a good result from surgery unless pulmonary hypertension has developed. Angiographic closure is now becoming possible.

Persistent ductus arteriosus (PDA)

The ductus arteriosus connects the pulmonary artery at its bifurcation to the descending aorta immediately distal to the subclavian artery. In fetal life the ductus diverts blood away from the unexpanded, and hence high-resistance, pulmonary circulation into the systemic circulation, where the blood is reoxygenated as it passes through the placenta. At birth, the high oxygen in the lungs and the reduced pulmonary vascular resistance triggers closure of the duct. If the duct is malformed (i.e. it does not contain sufficient elastic tissue) it will not close. This is more common in females and is sometimes associated with maternal rubella. Premature babies are often born with persistent ducts that are anatomically normal but are immature in that they lack the mechanism to close.

Because aortic pressure exceeds pulmonary artery pressure throughout the cardiac cycle, a persistent duct produces continuous aorta-to-pulmonary artery shunting. This leads to an increased pulmonary venous return to the left heart and an increased left ventricular volume load.

CLINICAL FEATURES

If the shunt is large, the left heart volume overload results in severe left heart failure. However, there are often no symptoms until later in life when heart failure or infective endocarditis develop.

The characteristic physical sign is a continuous 'machinery' murmur (due to turbulent aortic-to-pulmonary artery shunting in both systole and diastole), best heard below the left clavicle in the first interspace or over the first rib. A thrill may often be felt. The peripheral pulse is large in volume ('bounding') because of the increased left heart blood flow and the decompression of the aorta into the pulmonary artery.

INVESTIGATIONS

The aorta and pulmonary arterial system are prominent radiologically. There is both a left atrial abnormality and left ventricular hypertrophy on the ECG. The echocardiogram shows a dilated left atrium and left ventricle.

TREATMENT

Premature infants with a persistent duct may be treated medically with indomethacin, which inhibits prostaglandin production and stimulates duct closure. In other cases the duct can be ligated surgically or angiographically with very little risk. Surgery should be performed as soon as possible and not later than the age of five years.

Coarctation of the aorta

Coarctation of the aorta occurs twice as commonly in men as in women. It is also associated with Turner's syndrome. The coarctation is a narrowing of the aorta at, or just distal to, the insertion of the ductus arteriosus (Fig 11.81). In 80% of cases coarctation of the aorta is associated with a bicuspid (and potentially stenotic) aortic valve.

Severe narrowing of the aorta encourages the formation of a collateral arterial circulation involving the

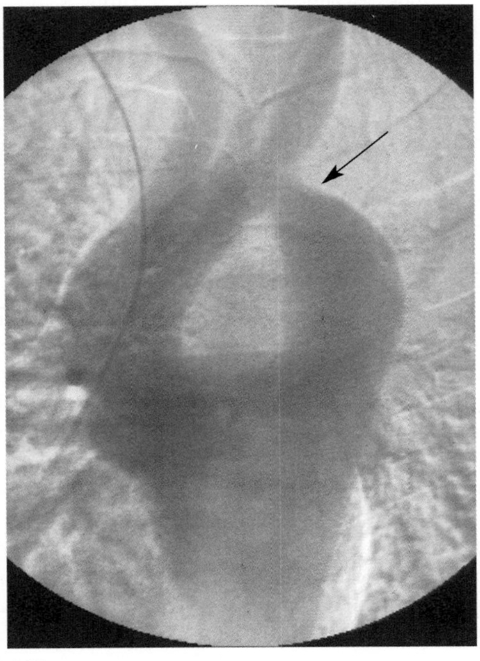

Fig 11.81
This aortogram demonstrates a coarctation of the aorta. Contrast outlines the left ventricle, aorta (ascending, arch and descending) and three major arteries arising from the aorta (right subclavian, right carotid and innominate). Immediately after the innominate artery the aorta is very markedly narrowed owing to a coarctation of the aorta

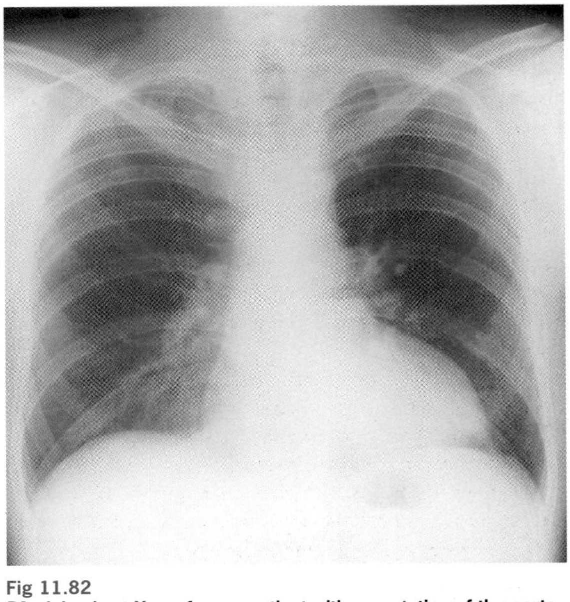

Fig 11.82
PA plain chest X-ray from a patient with coarctation of the aorta. The prominent abnormality on this film is the 'erosion' ('scalloping') of the lower margins of the 5th, 6th and 7th ribs owing to collateral flow in the intercostal arteries. On the upper mediastinal border is a small calcified bulge due to calcification of post-stenotic dilatation

periscapular and intercostal arteries. Decreased renal perfusion can lead to the development of systemic hypertension that persists even after surgical correction.

CLINICAL FEATURES

Coarctation of the aorta is often asymptomatic for many years. Headaches and nose bleeds (due to hypertension) and claudication and cold legs (due to poor blood flow in the lower limbs) may be present.

Physical examination reveals hypertension in the upper limbs, and weak, delayed (radiofemoral delay) pulses in the legs.

A mid-to-late systolic murmur due to turbulent flow through the coarctation may be heard over the upper precordium or the back. Vascular bruits from the collateral circulation may also be heard.

INVESTIGATIONS

The chest X-ray may reveal a dilated aorta indented at the site of the coarctation. This is manifested by an aorta (seen in the upper right mediastinum) shaped like a figure '3'. In adults, tortuous and dilated collateral intercostal arteries may erode the undersurfaces of the ribs ('rib notching') (Fig 11.82).

The ECG demonstrates left ventricular hypertrophy. Echocardiography sometimes shows the coarctation and other associated anomalies. Aortography will show the defect, and digital vascular imaging allows the coarctation to be visualized after the intravenous injection of contrast. MRI can accurately demonstrate the coarctation and quantify flow.

TREATMENT

The treatment is surgical excision of the coarctation and end-to-end anastomosis of the aorta. If the coarctation is extensive, prosthetic vascular grafts may be needed. When surgery is performed in childhood, hypertension usually resolves completely. However, when the operation is performed on adults the hypertension persists in 70% because of previous renal damage. Balloon dilatation is used in some centres.

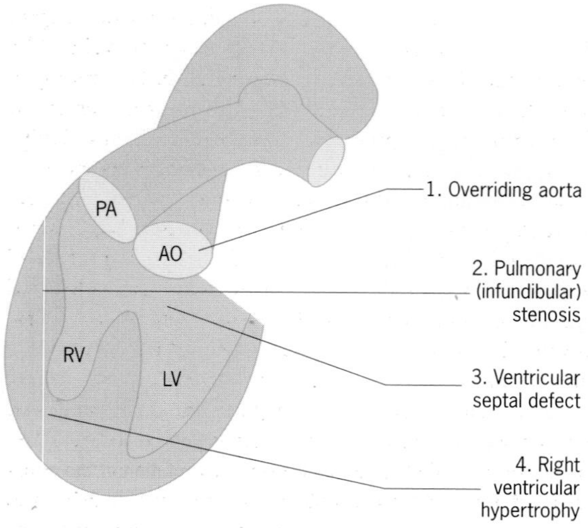

Fig 11.83
The four features of Fallot's tetralogy

Fallot's tetralogy

This is the most common cyanotic congenital heart abnormality in children who survive beyond the neonatal period. It consists of the following four features (Fig 11.83):

- a ventricular septal defect (VSD)
- positioning of the aorta above the VSD ('overriding aorta')
- a right ventricular outflow obstruction
- right ventricular hypertrophy.

The level of the right ventricular outflow obstruction may be subvalvular, valvular or supravalvular. The most common obstruction is subvalvular, either alone (50%) or in combination with valvular stenosis (25%).

This combination of lesions leads to a high right ventricular pressure and right-to-left shunting of blood through the VSD. Thus the patient is centrally cyanosed.

CLINICAL FEATURES

Children with this condition may present with dyspnoea or fatigue, or with hypoxic episodes on exertion (Fallot's spells) – deep cyanosis and possible syncope. Squatting is common.

Physical signs include a parasternal sustained heave and a systolic ejection murmur, often associated with a thrill in the second left interspace close to the sternum. The second heart sound is usually single because the pulmonary component is too soft to be heard. Central cyanosis is commonly present from birth, and finger clubbing and polycythaemia are obvious after about 12 months. Growth may be retarded.

INVESTIGATIONS

The chest X-ray shows a large right ventricle and a small pulmonary artery. The ECG reveals right ventricular hypertrophy, and the echocardiogram demonstrates discontinuity between the aorta and the anterior wall of the ventricular septum. Cardiac catheterization is performed to evaluate the size and degree of the right ventricular outflow obstruction.

TREATMENT

Complete surgical correction of this combination of lesions is possible even in infancy. Occasionally a palliative procedure – an anastomosis between a subclavian artery and a pulmonary artery (Blalock shunt) – is performed on very young infants.

This operation results in an increased blood supply to the lungs. Fallot's spells may need treatment with β-blockade or, when severe, with diamorphine to relax the right ventricular outflow obstruction.

Adolescent congenital heart disease

As more children with structural heart disease survive into adulthood there is a need for an increased awareness amongst general physicians and cardiologists of the problems posed by these young adults. Both atrial and ventricular arrhythmias are common sequels of longstanding structural heart disease and are often quite resistant to treatment. Sudden cardiac death is not uncommon. End-stage heart failure secondary to congenital heart disease can now be managed by heart or heart-lung transplantation.

FURTHER READING

Perloff JK (1994) Congenital Heart Disease, 4th edn. Philadelphia: WB Saunders.

Pulmonary heart disease (cor pulmonale)

The term 'cor pulmonale' means right heart disease arising secondary to pulmonary hypertension. In some ways it is an unsatisfactory term, in that the causes of cor pulmonale are very diverse and mostly represent very different disease processes. The approach to treatment varies according to the aetiology, as well as specific therapy often being required for the causative disease. The reason for continued use of the term is that most clinically relevant right heart diseases arise secondary to a problem downstream in the circulation from it, and the term 'right heart failure' is therefore also unsatisfactory in this context. Equally, the diseases in question do not inevitably lead to cor pulmonale.

As long as it is remembered that cor pulmonale is not a disease but a final common pathway, then it is still a useful term. Where possible, the two diagnoses should be given together; for example, cystic fibrosis complicated by cor pulmonale, cor pulmonale secondary to multiple pulmonary emboli, etc.

Pure right heart failure does occur, but is rare. Examples include right ventricular myocardial infarction and isolated right-sided heart valve disease.

The causes of acute and chronic cor pulmonale are numerous but, in clinical practice, one disorder of each type predominates. These are *pulmonary embolism* in the case of acute cor pulmonale and *chronic obstructive pulmonary disease* (COPD) in the latter. The causes of cor pulmonale are shown in Table 11.39.

Table 11.39
The causes of cor pulmonale

Pulmonary vascular disorders
Acute pulmonary thromboembolism (rarely tumour emboli)
Primary pulmonary hypertension
Multiple pulmonary artery stenoses
Pulmonary veno-occlusive disease
Recurrent pulmonary emboli

Disease of the lung and parenchyma
COPD
All other chronic lung disorders (Chapter 12)

Musculoskeletal disorders (causing chronic underventilation)
Kyphoscoliosis
Poliomyelitis
Myasthenia gravis

Disturbance of respiratory control
Morbid obesity (Pickwickian syndrome)
Obstructive sleep apnoea
Cerebrovascular disease

Left heart disorders
Mitral stenosis
Left artrial myxoma
Left ventricular failure

Miscellaneous
Appetite suppressant drugs (e.g. dexfenfluramine)

Acute cor pulmonale (pulmonary embolism)

Thrombus, usually formed in the systemic veins or rarely in the right heart (less than 10% of cases) may dislodge and embolize into the pulmonary arterial system. Postmortem studies indicate that this is a very common condition (microemboli are found in up to 60% of autopsies) but it is not usually diagnosed this frequently in life. Ten per cent of clinical pulmonary emboli are fatal.

Most clots which cause clinically relevant pulmonary emboli actually come from the pelvic and abdominal veins, but femoral deep venous thrombosis, and even occasionally axillary thrombosis, can be the origin of the clot. Clot forms as a result of a combination of sluggish blood flow, local injury or compression of the vein and a hypercoagulable state. Risk factors include prolonged bedrest, pelvic and lower limb fractures, pelvic or abdominal surgery, pregnancy and childbirth, any debilitating systemic disease (cardiac failure, malignancy, etc.) advanced age, smoking, excess oestrogen (e.g. oral contraception) and inherited hypercoagulable states). Factor V Leiden and deficiency of protein S, protein C and of antithrombin are examples of inherited hypercoagulable states (p. 409), and testing for these should be considered where no other cause for pulmonary emoblism is found in a young patient.

After pulmonary embolism, lung tissue is ventilated but not perfused, resulting in impaired gas exchange. After some hours surfactant is no longer produced by the non-perfused lung. Alveolar collapse occurs and exacerbates hypoxaemia. The haemodynamic consequence of pulmonary embolism is an elevation of pulmonary arterial pressure and a reduction in cardiac output. The zone of lung that is no longer perfused by the pulmonary artery may infarct, but often does not do so because oxygen continues to be supplied by the bronchial circulation and the airways.

CLINICAL FEATURES

Many pulmonary emboli occur silently, but there are three typical clinical presentations. A clinical deep venous thrombosis is not commonly observed, although detailed investigation of the lower limb and pelvic veins will reveal thrombosis in more than half of the cases.

Small/medium pulmonary embolism

In this situation an embolus has impacted in a terminal pulmonary vessel. Symptoms are pleuritic chest pain and breathlessness. Haemoptysis occurs in 30%, often three or more days after the initial event. On examination, the patient may be tachypnoeic with a localized pleural rub and often coarse crackles over the area involved. A pleural effusion (occasionally blood-stained) can develop. The patient may have a fever and cardiovascular examination is normal.

Massive pulmonary embolism

This is a much rarer condition where sudden collapse occurs due to an acute obstruction of the right ventricular outflow tract. The patient has severe central chest pain (cardiac ischaemia due to lack of coronary blood flow) and becomes shocked, pale and sweaty. Syncope may result if the cardiac output is transiently but dramatically reduced, and death may occur. On examination, the patient is tachypnoeic, has a tachycardia with hypotension and peripheral shutdown. The jugular venous pressure (JVP) is raised with a prominent 'a' wave. There is a right ventricular heave, a gallop rhythm and a widely split second heart sound. There are usually no abnormal chest signs.

Multiple recurrent pulmonary emboli

This leads to increased breathlessness, often over weeks or months. It is accompanied by weakness, syncope on exertion and occasionally angina. The physical signs are due to the pulmonary hypertension that has developed from multiple occlusions of the pulmonary vasculature. On examination, there are signs of right ventricular overload with a right ventricular heave and loud pulmonary second sound.

DIAGNOSIS

The symptoms and signs of small and medium-sized pulmonary emboli are often subtle and nonspecific, so the diagnosis is often delayed or even completely missed. Pulmonary embolism should be considered if patients present with symptoms of new-onset atrial fibrillation (or other tachycardia), unexplained breathlessness or cough, if no other obvious cause is present.

INVESTIGATIONS

Small/medium pulmonary emboli

- **Chest X-ray** is often normal, but linear atelectasis or blunting of a costophrenic angle (due to a small effusion) is not uncommon. Sometimes these features develop only after some time and a raised hemidiaphragm is present in some patients. More rarely, a wedge-shaped pulmonary infarct, the abrupt cut-off of a pulmonary artery or a transluncency of an underperfused distal zone is seen. Previous infarcts may be seen as opaque linear scars.
- **ECG** is usually normal, except for sinus tachycardia, but sometimes atrial fibrillation or another tachycardia occur. There may be evidence of right ventricular strain.
- **Blood tests**. If pulmonary infarction has occurred, there will be a polymorphonuclear leucocytosis, an elevated ESR and increased lactate dehydrogenase levels in the serum.
- **Plasma D-dimer** (see p. 400). If this is undetectable, it excludes a diagnosis of pulmonary embolism.
- **Radionucleotide ventilation perfusion scan** (V/Q scan) is a good and widely available diagnostic investigation. The pulmonary ^{99m}Tc scintigram demonstrates underperfused areas (Fig 11.84) which, if not accompanied by a ventilation defect on a ventilation scintigram performed after inhalation of radioactive xenon gas (see p. 761), is highly suggestive of a pulmonary embolus. There are limitations to the test, however. For example, a matched defect may arise with a pulmonary embolus which causes an infarct or from emphysematous bullae. This test is therefore conventionally reported as a probability of pulmonary embolus and should be interpreted in the context of the history, examination and other investigations.

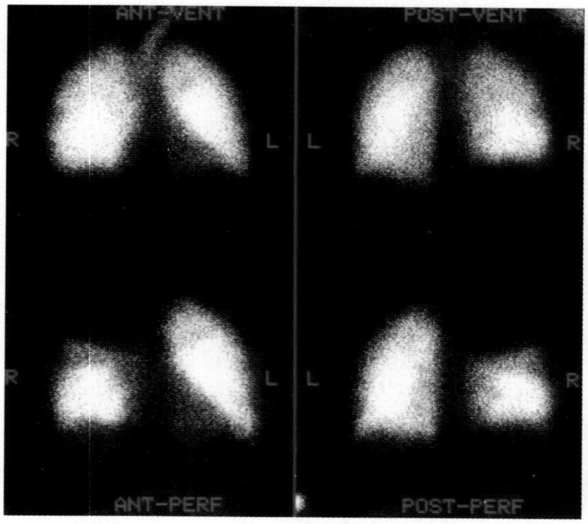

Fig 11.84
Ventilation (top) **and perfusion** (bottom) **lung scans** which demonstrate absence of perfusion but normal ventilation in the right upper lobe

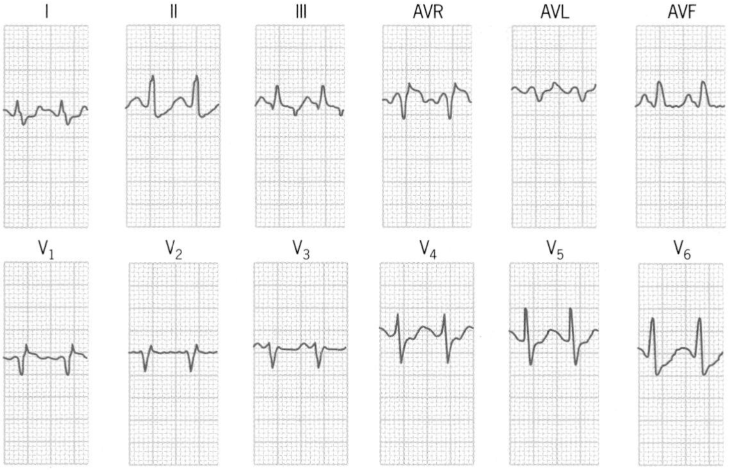

Fig 11.85
Acute pulmonary embolism shown by a 12-lead ECG. There is an S wave in lead I, a Q wave in lead III and an inverted T wave in lead III (the S1, Q3, T3 pattern). There is sinus tachycardia (160 b.p.m.) and an incomplete right bundle branch block pattern (an R wave in AVR and V_1 and an S wave in V_6)

- **Ultrasound** can be performed for the detection of clots in pelvis or ileofemoral veins (see p. 742).
- **Spiral CT scans** with intravenous contrast show good sensitivity and specificity for medium-sized pulmonary emboli. They do not exclude pulmonary emboli in small arteries.
- **MR imaging** gives similar results and is used if CT angiography is contraindicated.

Massive pulmonary emboli

- **Chest X-ray** may show pulmonary oligaemia, sometimes with dilatation of the pulmonary artery in the hila. Often there are no changes.
- **ECG** shows right atrial dilatation with tall peaked T waves in lead II. Right ventricular strain and dilatation give rise to right axis deviation, some degree of right bundle branch block, and T wave inversion in the right precordial leads (Fig 11.85). The 'classic' ECG pattern with an S wave in lead I, and a Q wave and inverted T waves in lead III (S1, Q3, T3), is rare.
- **Blood gases** show hypoxia and hypocapnia.
- **Echocardiogram** shows a vigorously contracting left ventricule and occasionally a clot in the right ventricular outflow tract.
- **Pulmonary angiography** is sometimes undertaken if surgery is considered in acute massive embolism. The test is performed by injecting contrast material through a catheter inserted into the main pulmonary artery. Filling defects or obstructed vessels can be

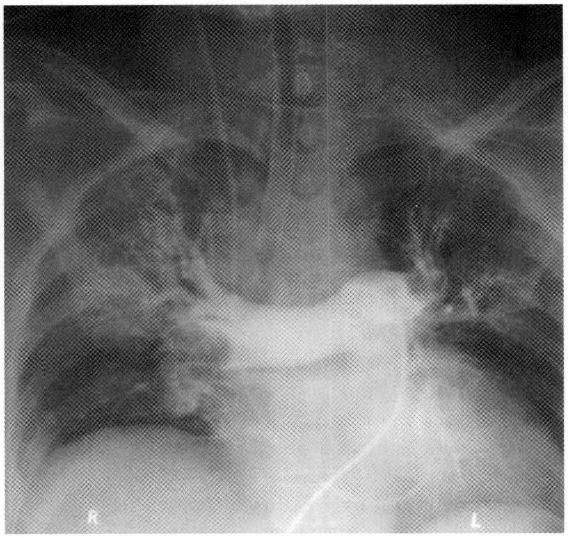

Fig 11.86
Contrast injected directly into the main pulmonary artery (pulmonary angiogram) demonstrates a large filling defect in the interlobar segment of the right pulmonary artery and extensive occlusion in the proximal left pulmonary artery

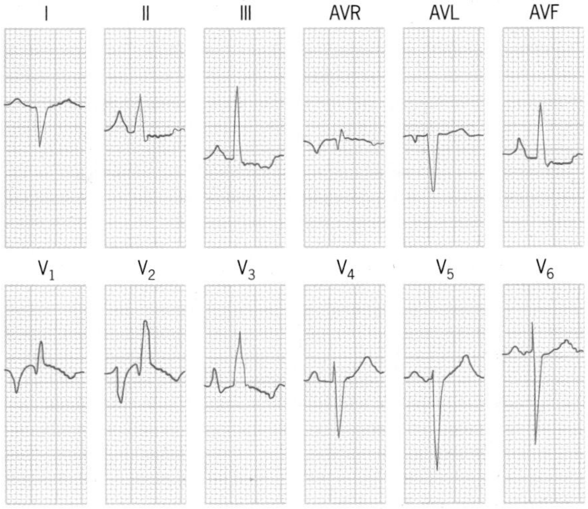

Fig 11.87
Pulmonary hypertension shown by a 12-lead ECG. There is right axis deviation (+120°), right ventricular hypertrophy (dominant secondary R wave [R′] in V_1) and a combination of left and right atrial conduction abnormalities

delineated (Fig 11.86). Angiography is hazardous but the risk may be reduced if contrast is injected into each pulmonary artery separately. If the patient is in extremis and the diagnosis is obvious, surgery should proceed without prior angiography.

Multiple recurrent pulmonary emboli

- **Chest X-ray** may be normal. Enlarged pulmonary arterioles with oligaemic lung fields indicate advanced disease.
- **ECG** can be normal or show signs of pulmonary hypertension (Fig 11.87).
- **Leg imaging** with ultrasound and venography may show thrombi.
- **V/Q scan** may show evidence of pulmonary infarcts.
- **Further tests** looking for exercise-induced hypoxaemia and catheter studies to estimate pulmonary artery pressures may be required.

TREATMENT

Acute management

All patient should receive high-flow oxygen (60–100%) unless they have significant chronic lung disease. Patients with pulmonary infarcts require bedrest and analgesia. In severe cases, intravenous fluids and even inotropic agents to improve the pumping of the right heart are sometimes required, but very ill patients will require care on the intensive therapy unit (p. 833).

Prevention of further emboli

The basis of therapy is intravenous heparin. This can be with a bolus of 10 000 units of unfractionated heparin followed by the continuous infusion of 1000–2000 units per hour. A comparison of low molecular weight heparin (LMWH) with unfractionated heparin has shown no difference. As LMWHs simplify treatment (p. 412) they are being increasingly used, although they are more expensive. Oral anticoagulants are usually begun after 48 hours and the heparin is tapered off as the oral anticoagulant becomes effective. Oral anticoagulants are continued for six weeks to six months, depending on the likelihood of recurrence of venous thrombosis or embolism. In some situations, such as after recurrent embolism, lifelong treatment is indicated.

Occasionally, physical methods are required to prevent further emboli. This is usually because recurrent emboli occur despite adequate anticoagulation, but is also indicated in high-risk patients in whom anticoagulation is absolutely contraindicated. The most common method by which pulmonary embolism is treated in this situation is by insertion of a filter in the inferior vena cava above the level of the renal veins.

Dissolution of the thrombus

Fibrinolytic therapy such as streptokinase (250 000 units by i.v. infusion over 30 minutes, followed by streptokinase 100 000 i.v. hourly) is often used following a major embolism.

Surgery

Surgical embolectomy is rarely necessary, but there may be no alternative when the haemodynamic circumstances are very severe.

Chronic cor pulmonale

PATHOPHYSIOLOGY

The precise mechanism varies according to the cause of cor pulmonale, but chronic obstructive pulmonary disease (COPD), which is discussed here, is illustrative. Pulmonary vascular resistance is increased because loss of pulmonary vascular tissue and because of pulmonary vasoconstriction caused by hypoxia and acidosis. The increased pulmonary vascular resistance leads to pulmonary hypertension, which initially occurs only during an acute respiratory infection. Eventually, the pulmonary hypertension becomes persistent and progressively more severe. The pulmonary vascular bed is gradually obliterated by muscular hypertrophy of the arterioles and thrombus formation. Right ventricular function is progressively compromised because of the increased pressure load. Hypoxia further impairs right ventricular function and, as it develops, left ventricular function is also depressed.

CLINICAL FEATURES

Chest pain, exertional dyspnoea, syncope and fatigue are common symptoms, and sudden death may occur. Other symptoms are due to the cause of the pulmonary hypertension.

On physical examination, there is a prominent a wave in the jugular venous pulse, a right ventricular (parasternal) heave, and a loud pulmonary component to the second heart sound. Other findings include a right ventricular fourth heart sound, a systolic pulmonary ejection click, a mid-systolic ejection murmur, and an early diastolic murmur due to pulmonary regurgitation (Graham–Steell murmur). If tricuspid regurgitation develops, there is a pansystolic murmur and a large jugular venous wave.

INVESTIGATIONS

- **Chest X-ray** may show right ventricular enlargement and right atrial dilatation. The pulmonary artery is usually prominent and the enlarged proximal pulmonary arteries taper rapidly. Peripheral lung fields are oligaemic.
- **ECG** demonstrates right ventricular hypertrophy (right axis deviation, possibly a dominant R wave in lead V_1, and inverted T waves in right precordial leads) and a right atrial abnormality (tall peaked P waves in lead II) (Fig 11.87).
- **Echocardiography** will usually demonstrate right ventricular dilatation and/or hypertrophy. It is often possible to measure the peak pulmonary artery pressure indirectly with Doppler echocardiography. The echocardiogram may also reveal the cause of pulmonary hypertension, such as an intracardiac shunt.

Other investigations may also be required to evaluate the cause of pulmonary hypertension. It is particularly important to look for treatable conditions, such as left-to-right shunts, mitral stenosis or left atrial tumours. Direct measurement of pulmonary artery pressure and pulmonary wedge pressure by cardiac catheterization may be warranted in some patients with severe pulmonary hypertension of unknown cause. Pulmonary angiography may be indicated if multiple pulmonary emboli are suspected, but is dangerous.

If no other cause is found, then a diagnosis of *primary pulmonary hypertension* is made. This disease typically affects young females (20–35 years).

TREATMENT

Treatment is determined by the condition underlying pulmonary hypertension. Diuretic treatment may be used for right ventricular failure, but care should be taken to avoid excessive fluid depletion as this will result in reduced output from the impaired right ventricle. Hypoxia is avoided by the use of oxygen therapy when safe and necessary. In those with COPD and some others, long-term oxygen therapy (LTOT) improves symptoms and prognosis. In contrast to their enormous value in those with left ventricular impairment, angiotensin-converting enzyme inhibitors are seldom useful and may make matters worse.

Primary pulmonary hypertension is treated with anticoagulation (because the possibility of recurrent thromboembolism can seldom be fully excluded). Vasodilators, such as the calcium antagonist, verapamil, are sometimes of symptomatic benefit, and continuous prostacyclin infusions delay deterioration for some patients. Usually there is a progressive downhill course, however. Heart and lung transplantation is recommended for young patients.

FURTHER READING

British Thoracic Society (1997). Suspected acute pulmonary embolism: a practical approach. *Thorax* **52** (Suppl): 1–24.

Atrial myxoma

This is the most common primary cardiac tumour. A myxoma usually develops in the left atrium and is a polypoid, gelatinous structure attached by a pedicle to the atrial septum. The tumour may obstruct the mitral valve or may be a site of thrombi that then embolize. It is also associated with constitutional symptoms: the patient may present with dyspnoea, syncope or a mild fever. The most important physical signs are a loud first heart sound, a tumour 'plop' (a loud third heart sound produced as the pedunculated tumour comes to an abrupt halt), a mid-diastolic murmur, and signs due to embolization. A raised ESR is usually present.

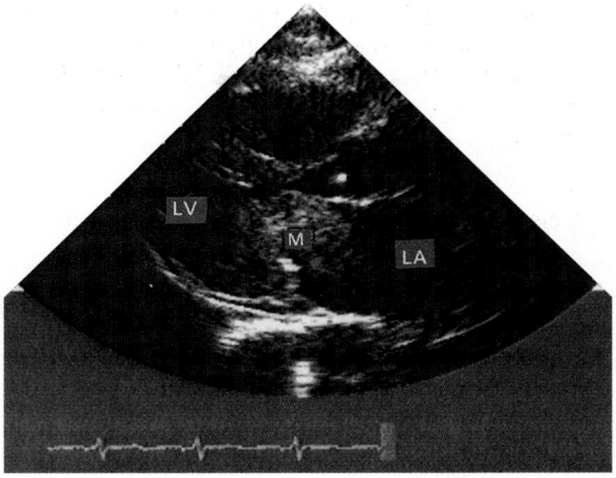

Fig 11.88
Atrial myxoma shown by a two-dimensional echocardiogram (long-axis view). The myxoma is an echo-dense mass obstructing the mitral valve orifice. It was removed surgically
LV, left ventricle; LA, left atrium; M, mass

The diagnosis is easily made by echocardiography because the tumour is demonstrated as a dense space-occupying lesion (Fig 11.88). Surgical removal usually results in a complete cure.

Myxomas may also occur in the right atrium or in the ventricles. Other primary cardiac tumours include rhabdomyomas and sarcomas.

Myocardial disease

Myocardial disease that is not due to a specific heart muscle disorder or a known infiltrative, metabolic/toxic or neuromuscular disorder may be caused by:

- an acute or chronic inflammatory pathology (myocarditis)
- idiopathic myocardial disease (cardiomyopathy).

Myocarditis

Myocarditis, whether idiopathic or infective, is the most common form of inflammatory endomyocardial disease. A definitive aetiology with isolation of viruses or bacteria is uncommon. Causative factors include:

- *viruses*, particularly Coxsackie, influenza, rubella, polio, adenovirus, echovirus and rarely HIV
- *protozoa*, e.g. *Trypanosoma cruzi*, cause of Chagas' disease endemic in central and South America, and *Toxoplasma gondii*, a common cause of myocarditis in the newborn or in immunologically compromised adults
- *radiation*, *chemicals* and *drugs*, e.g. lead poisoning, emetine and chloroquine

- *bacterial infection*, e.g. diphtheria, which is due to an exotoxin produced by *Corynebacterium*, *Rickettsia*, *Chlamydia*, *Coxiella* – the causative agent of Q fever
- *autoimmunity*, occasionally myocarditis may be a continuing autoimmune disease, and many patients have circulating cardiac antibodies.

CLINICAL FEATURES

Patients present with an acute illness, often characterized by fever and cardiac failure. There may be a history of previous respiratory or febrile illness. Physical examination reveals soft heart sounds, a prominent third sound and tachycardia (gallop rhythm). Often a pericardial friction rub may be heard.

INVESTIGATIONS

- **Chest X-ray** may show some cardiac enlargement, depending on the stage and virulence of the disease.
- **ECG** demonstrates ST and T wave abnormalities and arrhythmias. Heart blocks may be seen with diphtheritic myocarditis, while Chagas' disease produces both heart block and ventricular tachyarrhythmias.
- **Cardiac enzymes** are elevated.
- **Endomyocardial biopsy** shows acute inflammation.
- **Viral antibody titres** may be increased.

TREATMENT

General management includes bedrest and the eradication of any acute infection. Therapy is aimed towards the management of cardiac failure and the treatment of cardiac arrhythmias. The prognosis depends on aetiology and is usually good, although a chronic cardiomyopathy may ensue.

Cardiomyopathy

Cardiomyopathy is a general term indicating disease of the cardiac muscle. Diseases are classified on predominant clinical presentations:

- dilated cardiomyopathy – ventricular dilatation

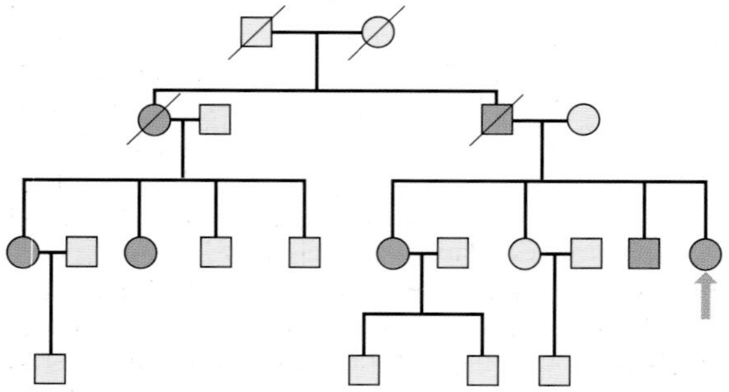

Fig 11.89
Pedigree of a family with dilated cardiomyopathy. Blue symbols are affected family members. The arrow indicates the index case

- hypertrophic cardiomyopathy – myocardial hypertrophy
- restrictive cardiomyopathy – impaired ventricular filling.

Dilated cardiomyopathy (DCM)

DCM is characterized by dilatation and impaired systolic function of the left ventricle and/or right ventricle. The aetiology of idiopathic DCM is unknown.

DCM is familial (autosomal dominant) in at least 20% of the families and a role for autoimmunity has been proposed in the pathogenesis of this disease. Pedigree analysis reveals a significant number of affected relatives either with full-blown disease or asymptomatic ventricular enlargement (25–30%) (Fig 11.89). Many such relatives have cardiac antibodies. About 30–40% of patients with DCM have organ-specific antibodies and these may become negative with disease progression. The disease may be associated with HLA DR-4.There is an association with viral (Coxsackie or HIV) infection and this may be immune-mediated.

Many cases of systemic heart muscle disease present with clinical features of DCM, and they include:

- cardiovascular disease (ischaemic, rheumatic, congenital, systemic hypertension)
- generalized disease, e.g. haemochromatosis, sarcoidosis
- connective tissue disorders, e.g. systemic lupus erythematosus, systemic sclerosis
- neuromuscular disease, e.g. muscular dystrophy, Friedreich's ataxia, mitochondrial myopathies
- glycogen storage disease, e.g. Pompe's disease
- primary heart muscle disease, e.g. amyloidosis
- alcohol excess
- cytotoxic drug therapy, e.g. doxorubicin, cyclophosphamide.

CLINICAL FEATURES

Symptoms depend on the relative degree of right and left heart failure and the incidence of cardiac arrhythmias and emboli.

Physical signs reflect heart failure – cardiomegaly, tachycardia, jugular venous pressure elevation, third or fourth heart sounds and basal crackles. Ventricular dilatation leads to functional mitral or tricuspid valvular regurgitation.

INVESTIGATIONS

- **Chest X-ray** demonstrates generalized cardiac enlargement
- **ECG** shows diffuse nonspecific ST segment and T wave changes. Sinus tachycardia, conduction abnormalities and arrhythmias (i.e. atrial fibrillation, ventricular premature contractions or ventricular tachycardia) may also be seen.
- **Echocardiogram** reveals dilatation of the left ventricle and/or right ventricle with poor global contraction function (Fig 11.90).

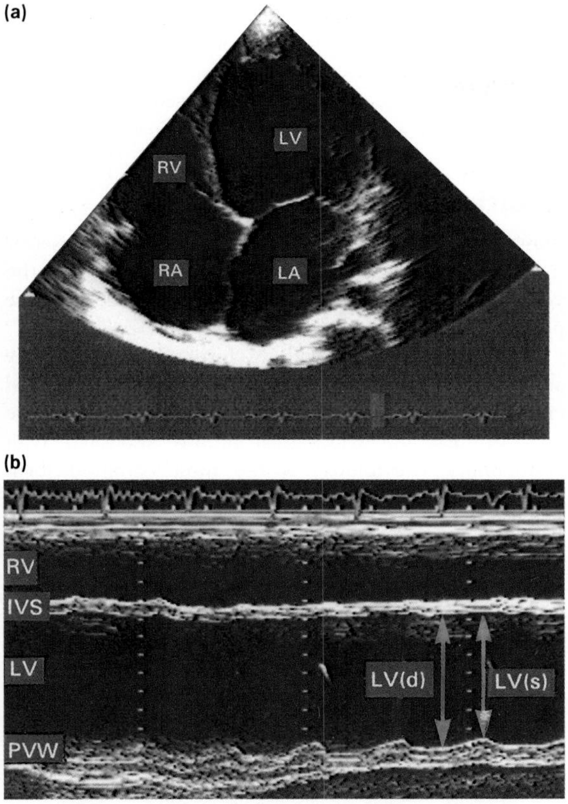

Fig 11.90
Dilated cardiomyopathy shown in two-dimensional (apical four-chamber view) and M-mode echocardiograms. The heart has a 'globular' appearance with all four chambers dilated. The extremely impaired left ventricular function can be appreciated from the M-mode recording. Compare the systolic shortening fraction with that of Figs 11.22 and 11.74
LA, left atrium; RA, right atrium; LV, left ventricle;
LV(d) and LV(s), diastolic and systolic left ventricular dimensions;
IVS, interventricular septum; PVW, posterior ventricular wall

Table 11.40
Various mutations causing HCM

CMH1	Chromosome 14 (β-myosin)
CMH2	Chromosome 1 (troponin-T)
CMH3	Chromosome 15 (α-tropomyosin)
CMH4	Chromosome 11 (myosin binding protein-C)

CMH, cardiac myosin heavy chain

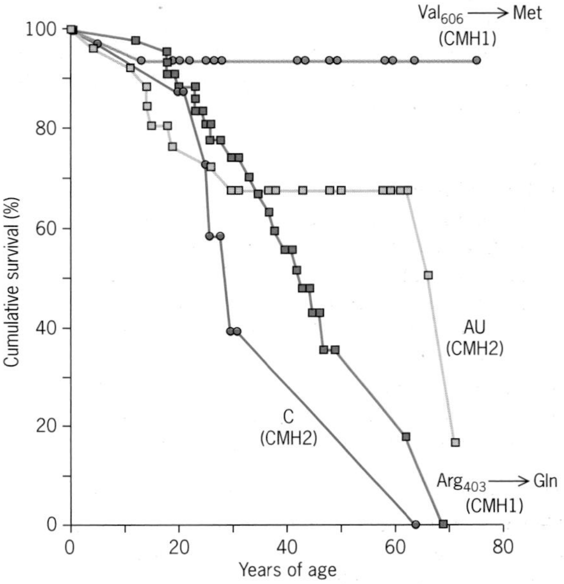

Fig 11.91
Hypertrophic cardiomyopathy: Kaplan–Meir cumulative survival curves in families with various mutations, some of which are associated with poor survival (Arg–Gln), whereas others are not (Val→Met). AU and C indicate families with troponin-T mutations (CMH2), who have a poor prognosis

TREATMENT

Management involves the conventional treatment of heart failure and arrhythmias. Documented atrial fibrillation or a history of embolization is an indication for anticoagulant treatment. Prolonged bedrest, avoidance of alcohol, and nutritional supplements may be indicated in special cases. Metoprolol has been shown to improve haemodynamic and clinical function in some patients. Growth hormone therapy may be useful in some cases of severe heart failure. Severe cardiomyopathy is treated with cardiac transplantation.

Hypertrophic cardiomyopathy (HCM)

An inherited disorder of heart muscle, this condition is characterized by variable hypertrophy of the left and/or right ventricle, without a cardiac or systemic cause. Massively thickened (hypertrophied) interventricular septum is characteristic but not invariably present, and results in distorted ventricular contraction with abnormal mitral valve movement during systole. A degree of mitral regurgitation may develop. Apposition of the anterior mitral leaflet to the thickened septum causes obstruction to left ventricular emptying. Histology shows the characteristic myocyte disarray.

The majority of cases are familial, autosomal dominant, and due to mutations in the genes coding for sarcomeric proteins. Several mutations of β-myosin (chromosome 14) have been identified. Mutations in genes of other sarcomeric proteins are also responsible (Table 11.40).

Families with certain of these mutations have a high incidence of sudden death (Fig 11.91). Increased frequency of D allele (DD genotype of ACE gene polymorphism) occurs in families with a high incidence of sudden death. It has been suggested that one of the D alleles (with increased ACE plasma levels) interacts with growth regulators (e.g. C-*myc*); this, along with the different mutations, may account for the variable presentation of HCM. The hypertrophy may not manifest before completion of the adolescent growth spurt, making the diagnosis in children difficult. Sporadic cases of HCM occur, but the aetiology is unknown. HCM may also be associated with Noonan's syndrome, Friedrich's ataxia, glycogen storage disease, and mitochondrial myopathies.

CLINICAL FEATURES

Patients with HCM present with chest pain, dyspnoea, syncope or pre-syncope (typically with exertion), cardiac arryhythmias and sudden death. Sudden death typically occurs in asymptomatic young adults or adolescents. Family history of suddent death, recurrent syncope, non-sustained ventricular tachycardia and blood pressure response during exercise are recognized clinical risk factors. Dyspnoea is common and is due to the inability of the heart muscle to relax. Left ventricular filling – and therefore left ventricular emptying – are impaired, compounded by outflow obstruction in about one-third of cases. Systolic ventricular function remains good until the very late stages of disease.

The classical physical findings are:

- *double apical pulsation* (forceful atrial contraction producing a fourth heart sound)
- *jerky carotid pulse* because of rapid ejection and sudden obstruction to left ventricular outflow during asystole
- *ejection systolic murmur* due to left ventricular outflow obstruction late in systole. It can be increased by manoeuvres that decrease the afterload, e.g. standing or Valsalva, and decreased by manoeuvres that increase afterload and venous return, e.g. squatting.
- *pansystolic murmur* due to mitral regurgitation
- *fourth heart sound.*

INVESTIGATIONS

- **Chest X-ray** is usually unremarkable.
- **ECG** demonstrates left ventricular hypertrophy (see Fig 11.72) and ST and T wave changes.
- **Echocardiogram** is diagnostic as it shows left ventricular hypertrophy (especially septal hypertrophy greater than that of the posterior wall), systolic anterior motion of the mitral valve, and a very vigorously contracting ventricle (Fig 11.92).
- **Pedigree analysis** provides important clues.
- **Genetic analysis** provides confirmation of the diagnosis.
- **Exercise test and ECG ambulatory recording** provide prognostic information.

TREATMENT

Firstly, sudden death must be avoided by antiarrhythmic therapy or devices (implantable defibrillators). Long-term amiodarone treatment is effective. Chest pain and dyspnoea may be treated with β-blockers and verapamil, either singly or in combination. In selected cases with significant left outflow obstruction and recalcitrant symptoms, dual-chamber pacing may be of use. Alcohol (non-surgical) ablation of the septum may also be useful and its long-term effect is under investigation. Occasionally, resection of septal myocardium may be indicated. Vasodilators should be avoided because they may aggravate left ventricular outflow obstruction and also cause refractory hypotension.

Restrictive cardiomyopathy

Some cardiomyopathies do not present with muscular hypertrophy or ventricular dilatation. Instead, the ventricular filling is restricted (as with constrictive pericarditis), resulting in features of heart failure.

Conditions associated with this form of cardiomyopathy are amyloidosis, sarcoidosis, Loeffler's endocarditis and endomyocardial fibrosis; in the latter two conditions there is myocardial and endocardial fibrosis associated with eosinophilia. Amyloidosis is the most common form

(a)

(b)

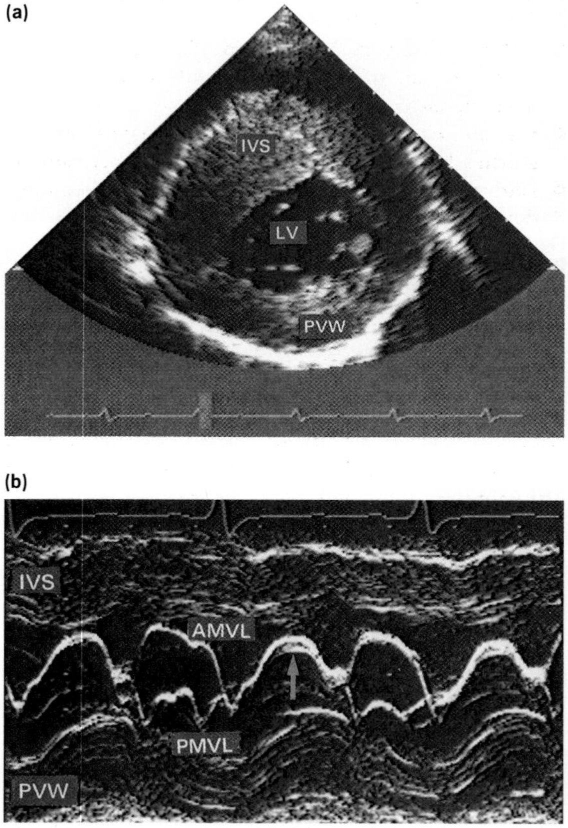

Fig 11.92
Hypertrophic cardiomyopathy of the mitral valve shown by a two-dimensional echocardiogram (short-axis view) and M-mode recording. The grossly thickened interventricular septum is shown, resulting in a small left ventricular cavity. This condition is associated with an abnormal anterior motion of the mitral valve during systole (arrowed) IVS, interventricular septum; LV, left ventricle; PVW, posterior ventricular wall; AMVL, PMVL, anterior and posterior mitral valve leaflets

of restrictive cardiomyopathy. The idiopathic form of restrictive cardiomyopathy may be familial. Dilatation of the atria and thrombus formation are common in restrictive cardiomyopathy.

CLINICAL FEATURES

Dyspnoea, fatigue and embolic symptoms may be the presenting features. Restriction to ventricular filling (espcially right) results in persistently elevated venous pressures, consequent hepatic enlargement, ascites, and dependent oedema.

Physical signs are similar to those of constrictive pericarditis – a high jugular venous pressure with diastolic collapse (Friedreich's sign) and elevation of venous pressure with inspiration (Kussmaul's sign). Cardiac enlargement with a third or fourth heart sound is common. In idiopathic restrictive cardiomyopathy, however, cardiac size may be normal.

INVESTIGATIONS

- **Chest X-ray** confirms the cardiac enlargement.
- **ECG** usually has low-voltage and ST segment and T wave abnormalities.
- **Echocardiogram** shows symmetrical myocardial thickening and often a normal systolic ejection fraction, but impaired ventricular filling.
- **Cardiac catheterization and haemodynamic studies** help distinction from constrictive pericarditis.
- **Endomyocardial biopsy** may be useful for a more detailed diagnosis.

TREATMENT

There is no specific treatment. Cardiac failure and embolic manifestations should be treated. Cardiac transplantation should be considered in some severe cases, especially the idiopathic variety. In primary amyloidosis, combination therapy with melphalan plus prednisolone with or without colchicine may improve survival. However, patients with cardiac amyloidosis have a worse prognoses than those with other forms of the disease, and the disease may recur after transplantation.

FURTHER READING

Maron BJ (1997) Hypertrophic cardiomyopathy. *Lancet* **350**: 127–133.

Pericardial disease

The normal pericardium lubricates the surface of the heart, prevents sudden deformation or dislocation of the heart, and acts as a barrier to the spread of infection. There are three common presentations of pericardial disease:

- acute pericarditis
- pericardial effusion
- constrictive pericarditis

Acute pericarditis

Acute pericarditis has numerous aetiologies, but Coxsackie viral infections and myocardial infarction are the most common causes in the UK.

Viral pericarditis

This is often sudden in onset and tends to affect young adults. Usually, the illness lasts only a few weeks and the prognosis is good. However, recurrences as well as sudden death do occur.

Pericarditis following myocardial infarction

This occurs in about 20% of patients, especially with anterior myocardial infarction. A pericardial friction rub, recurrence of chest pain and fever are typical.

Dressler's syndrome. This form occurs one month to one year after an acute myocardial infarction (see p. 698).

Uraemic pericarditis

This is seen usually in the terminal stages of uraemia and is often asymptomatic.

Bacterial pericarditis

Purulent pericarditis may rarely occur with septicaemia or pneumonia. *Staphylococcus* and *Haemophilus influenzae* account for two-thirds of such cases. Antibiotics are the mainstay of treatment and surgical drainage may be indicated. This form of pericarditis, especially staphylococcal, is usually fatal.

Tuberculous pericarditis

Typical presentation is with chronic low-grade fever, particularly in the evening, associated with features of acute pericarditis, malaise and weight loss. Pericardial aspiration is often required to make the diagnosis. The effusion may be bloodstained, but is usually serous. Antituberculous chemotherapy is needed.

Malignant pericarditis

Carcinoma of the bronchus, carcinoma of the breast and Hodgkin's disease are the most common causes. Leukaemia and malignant melanoma are also associated with pericarditis. Pericardiocentesis may be useful in establishing the diagnosis.

CLINICAL FEATURES

Pericardial inflammation gives rise to chest pain that is substernal and sharp. It is relieved by sitting forward and made worse by lying down and, like pleurisy, is aggravated by movement and respiration. It may be referred to the neck or shoulders.

The cardinal clinical sign is a pericardial friction rub. It is characteristically a leathery triphasic sound heard best with the patient leaning forward. There is usually a fever when pericarditis is due to viral or bacterial infection, rheumatic fever or myocardial infarction.

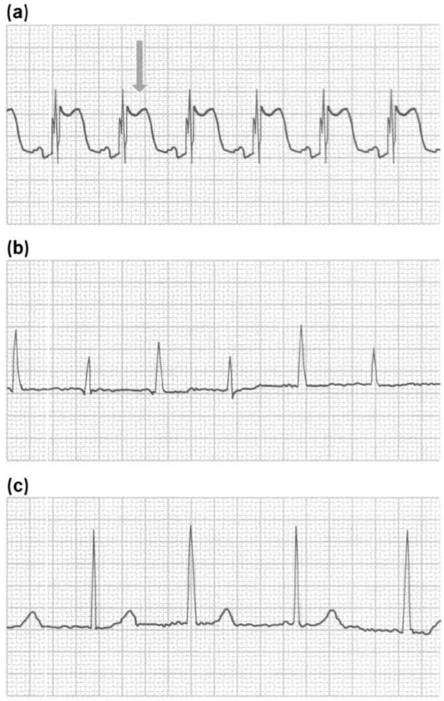

Fig 11.93
ECGs associated with pericarditis
(a) Acute pericarditis. Note the raised ST segment, concave upwards (arrow)
(b) Chronic phase of pericarditis associated with a pericardial effusion. Note the T wave flattening and inversion and the alternation of the QRS amplitude (QRS alternans)
(c) The same patient after evacuation of the pericardial fluid. Note that the QRS voltage has increased and the T waves have returned to normal

INVESTIGATIONS

The ECG is diagnostic. During the first week there is ST segment elevation, concave upwards, in all leads facing the epicardial surface – i.e. the anterior, lateral and inferior leads (Fig 11.93). Only cavity leads AVR, V_1 and rarely V_2 show ST depression. Later ST segment normalizes and T wave inversion may be seen. As the illness improves the T waves become normal.

Cardiac enzymes may be elevated if there is associated myocarditis.

TREATMENT

Treatment consists of anti-inflammatory drugs such as aspirin, naproxen or indomethacin and rest. Occasionally, if pericarditis is severe or recurrent, systemic corticosteroids may be needed.

Pericardial effusion

Acute pericarditis is initially dry and fibrinous. However, almost all aetiologies of this condition also induce the formation of a pericardial effusion. The effusion collects in the closed pericardium, and when the pericardium can distend no further this produces mechanical embarrassment to the circulation by preventing ventricular filling. This is called cardiac tamponade.

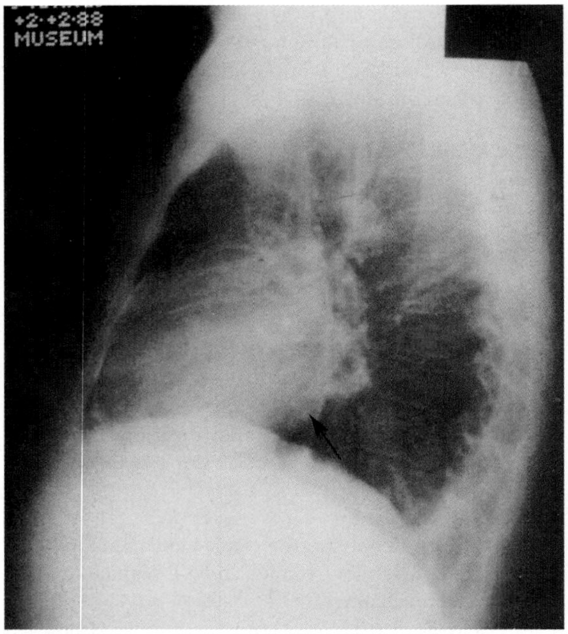

Fig 11.94
Chest X-ray showing pericardial calcification (arrow)

CLINICAL FEATURES

The effusion obscures the apex beat and the heart sounds are soft and distant. Although a friction rub may be heard in the early stages, it may be quieter once the fluid accumulates as this separates the visceral and parietal pericardium. Features of cardiac tamponade include a raised jugular venous pressure with sharp diastolic collapse, y descent (Friedreich's sign), a paradoxical pulse (systolic blood pressure falls during inspiration), increased neck vein distension during inspiration (Kussmaul's sign), and reduced cardiac output.

INVESTIGATIONS

ECG shows low voltages and the chest X-ray may demonstrate a large globular heart with sharp outlines. Typically, the pulmonary veins are not distended. Echocardiography is the most useful technique for demonstrating the effusion (see Fig 11.25 on p. 651).

TREATMENT

Cardiac tamponade is a medical emergency and the effusion must be tapped. Pericardiocentesis is also indicated when a malignant, tuberculous or a purulent pericarditis is suspected. In the UK, malignancy is the most common cause of re-accumulation of pericardial effusion. Re-accumulation may require pericardial fenestration (i.e. the creation of a pericardial window), either transcutaneously via a balloon pericardiotomy under local anaesthesia, or by using a conventional surgical approach.

Constrictive pericarditis

Following certain forms of pericarditis (tuberculous effusion, haemopericardium or bacterial infection or rheumatic heart disease), the pericardium may become thick, fibrous and calcified (Fig 11.94). The heart is then encased in a solid shell and cannot fill properly.

CLINICAL FEATURES

Typical signs are of systemic venous congestion – ascites, dependent oedema, hepatomegaly and jugular venous distension, without much breathlessness or pulmonary venous distension. There are signs of impaired ventricular filling (Kussmaul's sign), Friedreich's sign and pulse paradoxus. Fatigue and exercise intolerance are common symptoms.

Atrial fibrillation is common (30%), and a loud third heart sound (a *pericardial knock*) due to rapid ventricular filling may be heard. This is an early third heart sound.

Other causes of ascites must be excluded. Restrictive cardiomyopathy is a close mimic.

INVESTIGATIONS

The chest X-ray shows a relatively small heart with obvious calcification seen on a lateral film or by using fluoroscopy (see Fig 11.94 on p. 728). The ECG may show low QRS voltages and T wave inversion.

The echocardiogram may demonstrate the thickened pericardium with relative immobility of the heart. Typically, the ventricular cavities are small with normal wall thickness and dilated atria. CT is also good for detecting the thickness and the calcification of the pericardium.

Cardiac catheterization and MRI scan may be useful in difficult cases. Typically, the diastolic pressures are equal in all four chambers; the left and right ventricular end-diastolic pressures, the left and right atrial pressures are all equal or differ by less than 5 mmHg.

TREATMENT

Surgical removal of a substantial portion of the thickened pericardium provides a cure in about half the cases. In others, persistent constriction, atrial fibrillation and myocardial fibrosis prevent full recovery.

FURTHER READING

Zales VR, Wright KL (1997) Endocarditis, pericarditis and myocarditis. *Paediatric Annals* **26**: 116–121.

The cardiovascular system in systemic disease

The heart can be involved in many diseases (Table 11.41)

Table 11.41
Cardiac involvement in some systemic disorders

Disease	Cardiac involvement
Endocrine disorders	
Diabetes mellitus	Coronary artery disease
Thyrotoxicosis	Atrial fibrillation Cardiomyopathy
Hypothyroidism	Bradycardia Heart failure Coronary disease Pericardial effusion
Acromegaly	Cardiomegaly Hypertension Cardiac arrhythmias
Cushing's syndrome	Hypertension
Conn's syndrome	Hypertension
Phaeochromocytoma	Hypertension
Connective-tissue disorders	
Systemic lupus erythematosus	Non-infective endocarditis (Libman–Sachs) Myocarditis Pericarditis
Systemic sclerosis	Myocarditis Pericarditis Arrhythmias
Polyarteritis nodosa	Hypertension Pericarditis Arrhythmias
Rheumatoid disease and ankylosing spondylitis	Aortic and mitral regurgitation Pericarditis
Miscellaneous	
Renal failure	Hypertension Heart failure Pericarditis Infective endocarditis
Morbid obesity	Hypertension Cardiomegaly Associated with atherosclerotic coronary artery disease
Gout	Hypertension
Carcinoid syndrome	Pulmonary stenosis Tricuspid stenosis
Alcohol	Cardiomyopathy Atrial arrhythmias
Syphilis	Aortic regurgitation Coronary arterial stenosis (ostial) Ascending aortic aneurysm

Systemic hypertension

DEFINITIONS OF NORMOTENSION AND HYPERTENSION

Blood pressure is a characteristic of each individual, like height and weight, with marked interindividual variation.

The blood pressure within a population is therefore distributed around a mean level with an asymmetrical curve as more individuals have high blood pressure than low. The levels of blood pressure observed will depend on the characteristics of the population studied – in particular, the age and ethnic background. Blood pressure rises with age, certainly up to the seventh decade. This rise is more marked for systolic pressure and is more pronounced in men. Diastolic pressure may start to decline in the seventies. There is some evidence that the black population in the USA has higher blood pressure levels than the Caucasian population; it remains unclear whether this ethnic difference is seen in the UK.

The definition of an abnormal blood pressure remains a controversial issue. The risk of mortality or morbidity rises progressively with increasing systolic and diastolic pressures, with each measure having independent prognostic value; for example, isolated systolic hypertension is associated with a two- to threefold increase in cardiac mortality. The level at which blood pressure becomes associated with a significant increase in risk will also depend on the age, sex, race and other environmental factors of the population being studied. It is also clear that a single reading of elevated blood pressure may be misleading; in most patients, blood pressure will fall with repeated measurements as the patient becomes more comfortable with the technique.

The World Health Organization's criterion for the definition of hypertension is 160/95 mmHg. In contrast, the Framingham Study (a long-term study being carried out on a population in the USA, and which has been the basis for much of our knowledge about the natural history of hypertension) a blood pressure of 160/95 mmHg is deemed to be definitely hypertensive, and between 140/90 mmHg and 160/95 mmHg as borderline. Recent guidelines from the USA recommend a definition of hypertension as 140/90 mmHg, based on at least two readings on separate occasions. Lower criteria will clearly lead to a higher apparent prevalence of hypertension in the population; and using the latter criteria, 36% of US males in the age range 18–74 years are defined as having hypertension. Of more clinical relevance are the criteria used for initiation of drug treatment, and these will be discussed later.

CAUSES

Hypertension can be either primary ('essential') or secondary. Over 90% of cases are primary.

Essential hypertension

Essential hypertension has a multifactorial aetiology. The recognized factors are discussed here.

Genetic factors

Blood pressure levels tend to correlate within a family and adoption studies have confirmed that this must be partly due to genetic factors. The genes that contribute to essential hypertension have not yet been identified.

Fetal factors

Studies have consistently shown a relationship between lower birthweight and subsequent higher blood pressure. This relationship may be due to fetal adaptation to intrauterine undernutrition with long-term changes in blood vessel structure or in the function of crucial hormonal systems. These observations have been the basis for a large body of ongoing research.

Environmental factors

Amongst the several environmental factors that have been proposed, the following seem to be the most significant:

- *Obesity.* Blood pressure is associated with overall body mass and more closely with 'central obesity' (as measured by an increased waist-to-hip ratio). This is independent of the error in measurement of blood pressure that arises in obesity (cuff artefact).
- *Alcohol intake.* Heavy alcohol intake (greater than six units per day) is associated with an increase in blood pressure, and reduction in intake can reduce blood pressure.
- *Sodium intake.* The role of salt in hypertension remains controversial. Some smaller studies suggested a positive association between salt intake and blood pressure levels, although a larger study found the relationship to be weak. Studies of the restriction of salt intake have shown a mild beneficial effect in hypertensives. There is some evidence that a high potassium diet can protect against the effects of a high sodium intake.
- *Stress.* Whilst acute pain or stress can raise blood pressure, it has been difficult to study the relationship between chronic stress and blood pressure and, therefore, it remains uncertain whether chronic 'job strain' can be implicated in hypertension.

Humoral mechanisms

The autonomic nervous system, as well as the renin–angiotensin, natriuretic peptide and kallikrein–kinin system, plays a role in the physiological regulation of blood pressure and has been implicated in the pathogenesis of essential hypertension. However, there is no convincing evidence that any of these systems is directly involved.

Insulin resistance

An association between diabetes and hypertension has long been recognized, but more recently a syndrome has been described of hyperinsulinaemia, glucose intolerance, reduced levels of HDL cholesterol, hypertriglyceridaemia and central obesity (all of which are related to insulin resistance) in association with hypertension. This association (also called the 'metabolic syndrome' or 'syndrome X') is a major risk factor for cardiovascular disease. However, it has been difficult to define the mechanism linking the insulin resistance with hypertension.

Secondary hypertension

It is important to consider secondary forms of hypertension since these cases may be amenable to curative treatment. In addition, in some cases drug treatment may be dangerous (e.g. an ACE inhibitor in renovascular disease). In particular, one should be vigilant in those who present at a young age (<35 years). The causes can be broadly considered in the following categories.

Renal causes

Renal diseases account for over 80% of the cases of secondary hypertension. The common causes are diabetic nephropathy, chronic glomerulonephritis, adult polycystic disease, chronic tubulointerstitial nephritis, and renovascular disease. Hypertension can itself cause renal disease. The mechanism of this blood pressure elevation is primarily due to sodium and water retention, although there is also an inappropriate elevation of plasma renin levels.

Endocrine causes

These include:

- Conn's syndrome
- adrenal hyperplasia
- phaeochromocytoma
- Cushing's syndrome
- acromegaly.

Cardiovascular causes

The most important cardiovascular cause of hypertension is coarctation of the aorta.

Drugs

The oral contraceptive pill, other steroids, carbenoxolone and vasopressin may all cause hypertension. Patients taking monoamine oxidase inhibitors, who consume tyramine-containing foods, may develop paroxysms of severe hypertension.

Hypertension in pregnancy

Cardiac output rises in pregnancy but, owing to a relatively greater fall in peripheral resistance, blood pressure in pregnant women is usually lower than in those not pregnant.

Hypertension detected in the first half of pregnancy is usually due to pre-existing essential hypertension. Hypertension presenting in the second half of pregnancy – or 'pregnancy-induced hypertension' – usually resolves after delivery. Pre-eclampsia is a syndrome consisting of pregnancy-induced hypertension with proteinuria. The primary pathology is unknown, but involves a disturbance of the uteroplacental circulation. The syndrome may advance to the critical condition of eclampsia with severe hypertension, convulsions, cerebral and pulmonary oedema, jaundice, clotting abnormalities and fetal death. Eclampsia requires immediate treatment

PATHOPHYSIOLOGY

The pathogenesis of essential hypertension remains unclear. In some young hypertensive patients, there is an early increase in cardiac output, in association with increased pulse rate and an increase in circulating catecholamines. This could result in changes in baroreceptor sensitivity, which would then operate at a higher blood pressure level. However, this mechanism has not been confirmed.

In chronic hypertension, the cardiac output is normal and it is an increased peripheral resistance that maintains the elevated blood pressure. The resistance vessels (the small arteries and arterioles) show structural changes in hypertension. These are an increase in wall thickness with a reduction in the vessel lumen diameter. There is also some evidence for rarefaction (decreased density) of these vessels. These mechanisms would result in an increased overall peripheral vascular resistance.

Hypertension also causes changes in the large arteries. There is thickening of the media, an increase in collagen and the secondary deposition of calcium. These changes result in a loss of arterial compliance, which in turn leads to a more pronounced arterial pressure wave. Atheroma develops in the large arteries owing to the interaction of these mechanical stresses and low growth factors (see p. 686).

Left ventricular hypertrophy develops as a result of the increased peripheral vascular resistance, and the increased left ventricular load.

Changes in the renal vasculature eventually lead to a reduced renal perfusion, reduced glomerular filtration rate and, finally, a reduction in sodium and water excretion. The decreased renal perfusion may lead to activation of the renin–angiotensin system (renin converts angiotensinogen to angiotensin I, which is in turn converted to angiotensin II by the angiotensin-converting enzyme) with increased secretion of aldosterone and further sodium and water retention.

COMPLICATIONS

Cerebrovascular disease and coronary artery disease are the most common causes of death in hypertension, although these patients are also prone to renal failure and peripheral vascular disease.

In the Framingham study, hypertensives had a six-fold increase in stroke compared with normotensives. This was due to both cerebral haemorrhage (pressure-related) and infarction (atheroma-related). In the same study, there was a three-fold increase in cardiac death (due either to coronary events or to cardiac failure). Peripheral artery disease is twice as common in hypertensives.

Malignant hypertension

Malignant hypertension is said to occur when blood pressure rises rapidly and is considered with severe hypertension (diastolic blood pressure >140 mmHg). The characteristic histological change is fibrinoid necrosis of the vessel wall. These changes in the renal circulation result in rapidly progressive renal failure, proteinuria and haematuria. There is also a high risk of cerebral oedema and haemorrhage. There are marked changes in the retinal vessels and these are diagnostic of malignant hypertension. Without effective treatment there is a one-year survival of less than 20%. Hypertensive encephalopathy is the clinical condition of fluctuating neurological signs in association with very high blood pressure and, usually, advanced retinal changes.

ASSESSMENT OF PATIENTS

The management of patients should be considered in three stages: assessment, non-pharmacological treatment, and drug treatment. During the assessment period, secondary causes of hypertension should be excluded, the target-organ effect of the blood pressure should be evaluated, and any concomitant conditions (e.g. dyslipidaemia or diabetes) identified.

History

The patient with mild hypertension is usually asymptomatic. Features in the history such as attacks of sweating and palpitations in phaeochromocytoma might suggest secondary hypertension. Higher levels of blood pressure may be associated with headaches, epistaxis or nocturia. Breathlessness may be present owing to left ventricular hypertrophy or cardiac failure, whilst angina or peripheral claudication may represent atheromatous disease. Maligant hypertension may present with severe headaches, visual disturbances, fits, transient loss of consciousness or symptoms of heart failure.

Examination

The elevated blood pressure is usually the only abnormal sign. Signs of an underlying cause should be sought, such as renal artery bruit in renovascular hypertension, or radio-femoral delay in coarctation of the aorta. The cardiac examination may also reveal features of left ventricular hypertrophy and a loud aortic second sound. If cardiac failure develops, there may be a sinus tachycardia and a third heart sound.

Fundoscopy is an essential part of the examination of any hypertensive patient (Fig 11.95). The abnormalities are graded according to the Keith–Wagener classification:

- Grade 1 – tortuosity of the retinal arteries with increased reflectiveness (silver wiring)
- Grade 2 – grade 1 plus the appearance of arterovenous nipping produced when thickened retinal arteries pass over the retinal veins
- Grade 3 – grade 2 plus flame-shaped haemorrhages and soft ('cotton wool') exudates actually due to small infarcts
- Grade 4 – grade 3 plus papilloedema (blurring of the margins of the optic disc).

Grades 3 and 4 are diagnostic of malignant hypertension.

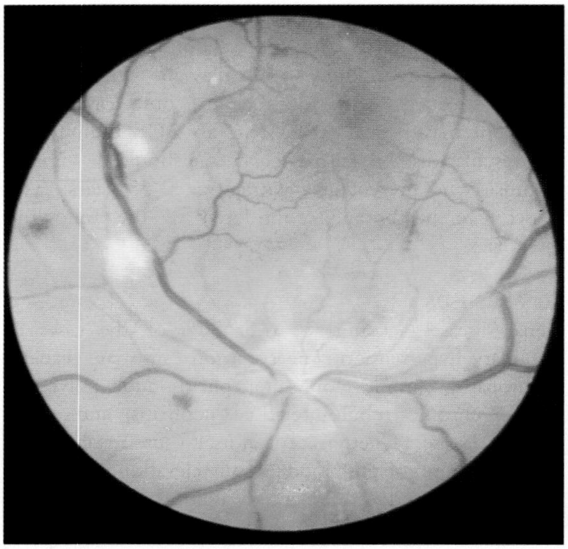

Fig 11.95
Fundus showing hypertensive changes: Grade 4 retinopathy

Ambulatory blood pressure monitoring

Indirect automatic blood pressure measurements can be made usually over a 24-hour period using a measuring device worn by the patient. The clinical role of such devices remains uncertain, although they are used to confirm the diagnosis in those patients with 'white-coat' hypertension – those who have a blood pressure increase that is due solely to the presence of a doctor or nurse (Fig 11.96a). These patients do not have any evidence of target-organ damage and unnecessary treatment can be avoided. These devices may also be used to monitor the response of patients to drug treatment and, in particular, can be used to determine the adequacy of 24-hour control with once-daily medication (Fig 11.96, band C).

Ambulatory blood pressure recordings seem to be better predictors of cardiovascular risk than measurements in a clinic. It is possible to analyse the diurnal variation in blood pressure, and some evidence suggests that those hypertensives with a loss of the usual nocturnal fall in blood pressure ('non-dippers') have a worse prognosis than those who retain this pattern.

INVESTIGATIONS

Routine investigation of the hypertensive patient should include:

- chest X-ray
- ECG
- echocardiogram
- urinalysis
- fasting blood for lipids and glucose
- serum urea, creatinine and electrolytes.

If the urea or creatinine are elevated, more specific renal investigations are indicated – creatinine clearance, renal ultrasound and renal isotope scans. A low serum

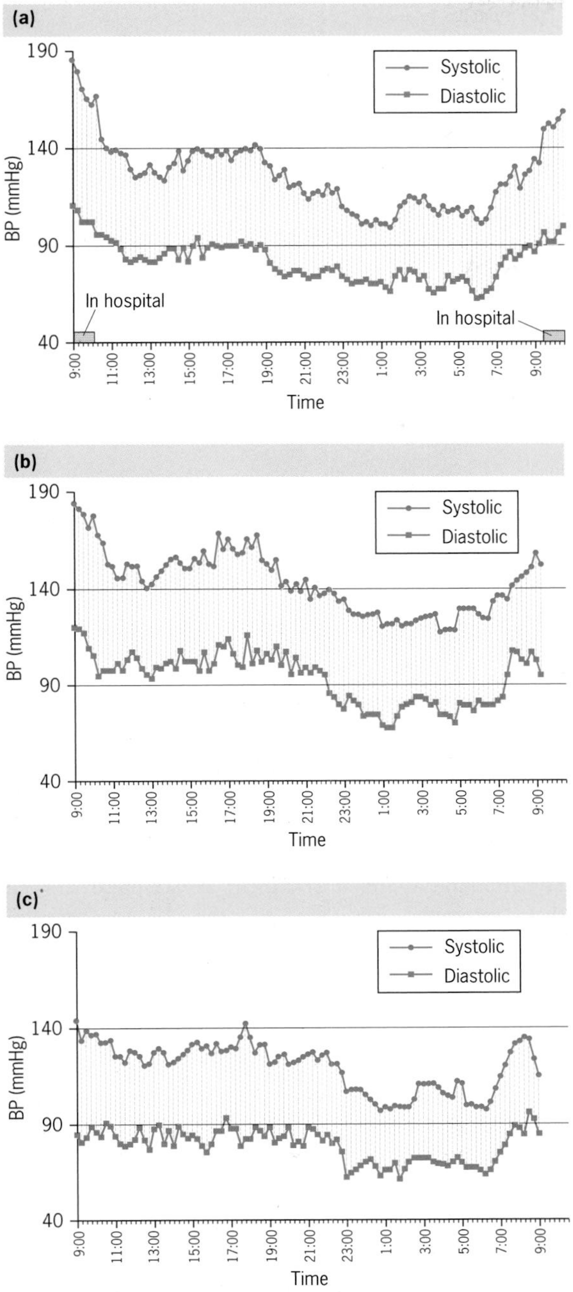

Fig 11.96
24-hour ambulatory blood pressure monitoring, showing:
(a) white-coat hypertension;
(b) pre-treatment;
(c) after three months' treatment

potassium may indicate an endocrine disorder, and aldosterone, cortisol and renin measurements must then be made. Clinical suspicion of phaeochromocytoma should be investigated further with measurement of urinary metanephrines and plasma catecholamines.

The ECG may show evidence of coronary artery disease or left ventricular hypertrophy, although echocardiography is a far more sensitive method for detection of left ventricular hypertrophy. The chest X-ray may show cardiomegaly or pulmonary congestion if heart failure is developing. Rib notching on the X-ray may be a sign of coarctation of the aorta and should be investigated further with an MRI scan.

TREATMENT

Unless the patient has severe or malignant hypertension, there should be a period of assessment with repeated blood pressure measurements, combined with advice and non-pharmacological measures prior to the initiation of drug therapy. The guidelines of the British Hypertension Society are illustrated in Fig 11.97.

General measures

All patients should be given advice on non-pharmacological measures that may lead to some reduction in blood pressure levels.

- *Weight reduction.* A number of trials have confirmed that weight reduction in overweight patients leads to a true fall in blood pressure
- *Reduction of heavy alcohol intake.* This can lead to a fall in blood pressure of 5–10 mmHg.
- *Salt restriction.* Moderate salt restriction has been shown to be of benefit in some patients and seems to enhance the blood-pressure lowering effects of some medication, particularly the ACE inhibitors, β-blockers and diuretics. The patient should be advised not to add salt to their food at the table or eat high salt-containing foods.
- *Regular exercise.* Moderate exercise in the form of jogging or brisk walking produces a beneficial effect on blood pressure that is independent of any reduction in weight.
- *Biofeedback and behavioural therapy.* There is some evidence for a positive short-term effect of these techniques in hypertensive patients, although long-term results are disappointing.

The individual's overall cardiovascular risk should be addressed. Patients should be advised to avoid smoking, and hyperlipidaemia treated appropriately.

Drug treatment (Table 11.42)

The decision to commence specific drug therapy should usually be made only after a careful period of assessment, of up to six months, with repeated measurements of blood pressure. The aim of drug treatment to reduce the risk of complications of hypertension should be carefully explained to the patient. All of the drugs used to treat hypertension can be associated with side-effects and, since the benefits of drug treatment are not immediately apparent to the patient, compliance is a major problem.

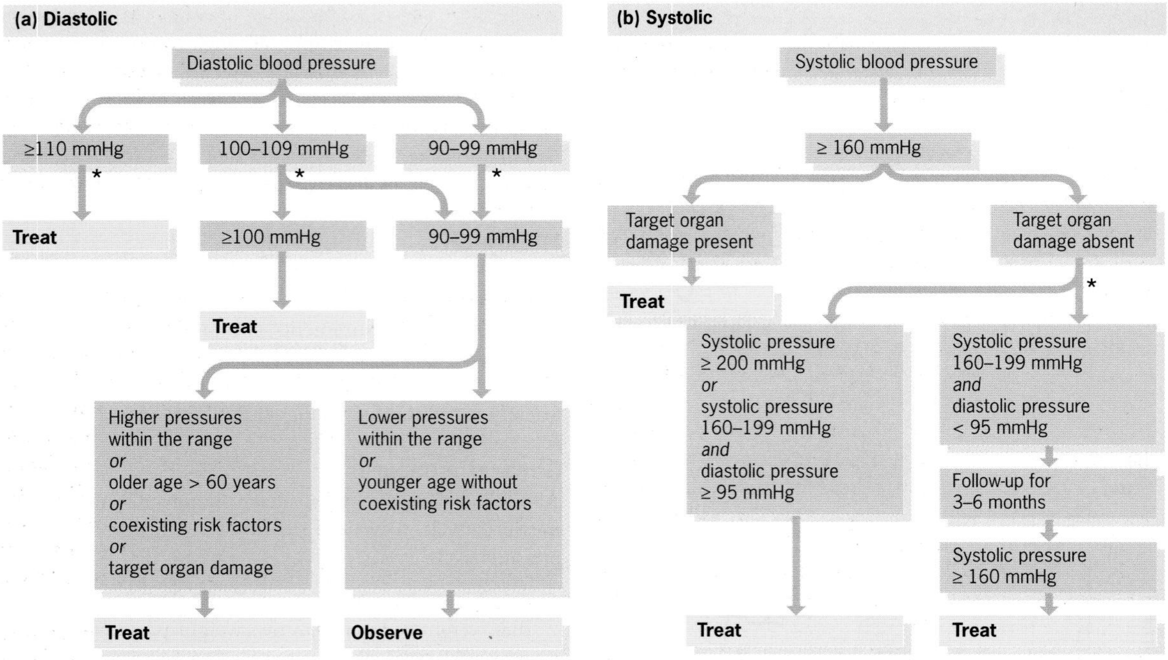

Fig 11.97
Thresholds for treatment of (a) diastolic and (b) systolic hypertension as recommended by the British Hypertension Society. Asterisks indicate repeated measurements. From Sever P et al (1993) *British Medical Journal* **306**: 983–987

The British Hypertension Society recommends the initiation of drug therapy if the diastolic blood pressure exceeds 100 mmHg during the assessment period. If the diastolic pressure is in the range 90–100 mmHg during the assessment period, treatment should be initiated if there is evidence of target organ damage, if there are other risk factors (e.g. diabetes), or if the patient is above 60 years of age.

Patients with isolated systolic hypertension (systolic blood pressure >160 mmHg and diastolic of <90 mmHg) are at increased cardiovascular risk; indeed, in the elderly, systolic blood pressure is a better predictor of cardiovascular risk than the diastolic blood pressure. It is therefore recommended that all patients with a persistent systolic blood pressure above 160 mmHg should commence drug treatment. The recent Hypertension Optimal Treatment (HOT) trial showed that intensive lowering of the blood pressure (82.6 mmHg) with aspirin was associated with a low rate of cardiovascular events.

Treatment of hypertension in the very elderly (>80 years) remains controversial, but it is probably inappropriate to apply a strict age limit in deciding on treatment.

Table 11.42
Advantages and disadvantages of drugs used in hypertension with respect to associated conditions

	Diuretic	β-Blocker	ACE inhibitor/Angiotensin II receptor antagonist	Calcium channel blockers	α-Blocker
Diabetes	Care[a]	Care[a]	Yes	Yes	Yes
Gout	No	Yes	Yes	Yes	Yes
Dyslipidaemia	Care[b]	Care[b]	Yes	Yes	Yes
Ischaemic heart disease	Yes	Yes	Yes	Yes	Yes
Heart failure	Yes	Care[c]	Yes	Care[d]	Yes
Asthma	Yes	No	Yes	Yes	Yes
Peripheral vascular disease	Yes	Care	Care[e]	Yes	Yes
Renal artery stenosis	Yes	Care	No	Yes	Yes
Pregnancy	Caution	Not in late pregnancy	No	No	Caution

[a] Diuretics may aggravate diabetes: β-blockers worsen glucose intolerance and mask symptoms of hypoglycaemia.
[b] Both diuretics and β-blockers disturb the lipid profile.
[c] There is some evidence for beneficial effects of some β-blockers when used cautiously in heart failure.
[d] Verapamil and diltiazem may exacerbate heart failure, although amlodipine appears to be safe.
[e] Patients with peripheral vascular disease may also have renal artery stenosis; therefore ACE inhibitors should be used cautiously.

Available drugs

Several classes of drugs are available to treat hypertension. The most appropriate 'first-line' treatment depends on the individual patient characteristics.

Diuretics

Thiazide diuretics such as bendrofluazide (2.5–5 mg daily) and cyclopenthiazide (0.25–0.5 mg daily) are well-established agents which have been shown to reduce the risk of stroke in hypertension. The lower doses seem to be as effective as higher doses in the reduction of blood pressure and most have a duration of 12–24 hours. The major concern with these agents is their adverse metabolic effects, and in particular an increased serum cholesterol, impaired glucose intolerance, hyperuricaemia (which may precipitate gout) and hypokalaemia. The latter may require the concomitant use of oral potassium or a potassium-sparing diuretic. However, combination diuretics should be used with caution as they may cause profound biochemical disturbances, particularly in the elderly.

Loop diuretics such as frusemide (40 mg daily) do have a hypotensive effect, but are not routinely used in the treatment of essential hypertension. Potassium-sparing diuretics such as amiloride (5–10 mg daily) or spironolactone (50–200 mg daily) are not effective agents when used alone, with the exception of spironolactone in hyperaldosteronism.

β-Blockers

The β-blockers have been shown to improve the prognosis of hypertensives, although their mechanism of action remains unclear. They reduce the force of cardiac contraction, some reduce renin secretion and some reduce anxiety. There are major differences between the agents (Table 11.43):

- *Cardioselectivity*. Some have less effect on the β_2 (non-cardiac) receptors and are therefore said to be relatively cardioselective. These include atenolol and bisoprolol.
- *Intrinsic sympathomimetic activity*. Some agents have partial agonist activity and cause less bradycardia. These include oxprenolol and pindolol.
- *Lipid solubility*. The agents that are less lipid-soluble are less likely to cause central nervous system side-effects. These include atenolol.

The major side effects of this class of agents are bradycardia, bronchospasm, cold extremities, fatigue, bad dreams and hallucinations. They initially aggravate cardiac failure but this is usually short-term. They also have adverse metabolic effects, and in particular an increase in triglycerides and a reduction in HDL cholesterol. These agents are especially useful in patients with both hypertension and angina.

Angiotensin-converting enzyme (ACE) inhibitors

These drugs block the conversion of angiotensin I to angiotensin II which is a potent vasoconstrictor. They also block the degradation of bradykinin, a potent vasodilator. They are generally safe and effective drugs for reduction of blood pressure, although there are no long-term trials to demonstrate a reduction in complications. There is also some evidence that the African population do not respond as well to ACE inhibitors. They are particularly useful in diabetics with nephropathy where they have been shown to slow disease progression and in diabetics with depressed left ventricular function, where they improve survival.

The major potential side-effects are profound hypotension following the first dose and deterioration of renal function in those with critical renovascular disease (in whom the production of angiotensin II is critical for maintaining renal perfusion). A common mild side-effect is a chronic dry cough, owing to the accumulation of bradykinin.

These are now several ACE inhibitors available and there are no significant differences between them in terms of blood pressure effect. However, those with the longest duration of action may be taken once-daily, which is clearly a benefit in terms of compliance. The agents include captopril (50–150 mg daily in divided doses), enalapril (10–20 mg daily), and trandolapril (1–4 mg daily).

Angiotensin II receptor antagonists

This is a new group of agents that selectively block the receptors for angiotensin II. They share many of the actions of ACE inhibitors but, since they do not have any effect on bradykinin, do not cause a cough. They are currently used for patients who cannot tolerate ACE inhibitors because of persistent cough. The agents

Table 11.43
Main properties of the β-blockers commonly used for hypertension

	Cardiac selectivity	Intrinsic sympathomimetic activity	Lipid solubility	Plasma half-life (hours)	Usual dosage
Acebutalol	+	+	0	5	400 mg once or twice daily
Atenolol	+	0	0	6	50 mg once daily
Bisoprolol	++	0	0	10–12	10–20 mg once daily
Oxprenolol	0	++	+	1.5	20–80 mg thrice daily
Propranolol	0	0	+++	5	80–160 mg twice daily
Timolol	0	0	+	5	5–20 mg twice daily

include losartan (50–100 mg daily) and valsartan (80–160 mg daily).

Calcium channel blockers

These agents effectively reduce blood pressure by casuing arteriolar dilatation, and some also reduce the force of cardiac contraction. Like the β-blockers, they are especially useful in patients with concomitant ischaemic heart disease. The major side-effects are seen in the short-acting agents and include headache, sweating, palpitations and flushing. Many of these side-effects can be lessened by the co-administration of a β-blocker. The short-acting agents, such as nifedipine (10–20 mg thrice daily) are being replaced by once-daily agents which are very well tolerated and include amlodipine (5–10 mg daily).

α-Blockers

These agents cause postsynaptic α_1-receptor blockade with resulting vasodilatation and blood pressure reduction. Earlier short-acting agents caused serious first-dose hypotension, but the newer longer-acting agents are far better tolerated. These include doxazosin (1–4 mg daily). Labetalol is an agent that has combined α- and β-blocking properties, but is not commonly used, except in pregnancy-induced hypertension.

Other vasodilators

These include hydralazine (up to 100 mg daily) and minoxidil (up to 50 mg daily). Both are extremely potent vasodilators that are reserved for patients resistant to other forms of treatment. Hydralazine can be associated with tachycardia, fluid retention and a systemic lupus erythematosus-like syndrome. Minoxidil can cause severe oedema and excessive hair growth. If these agents are used, it is usually in combination with a β-blocker.

Indapamide (2.5 mg daily) is a thiazide-related agent that causes vasodilatation. It produces fluid retention and can aggravate glucose intolerance and is therefore used rarely.

Sodium nitroprusside is a potent arterial and venous dilator. It is now only used intravenously, in hypertensive crises when blood pressure has to be reduced immediately (e.g. dissecting aortic aneurysm).

Centrally acting drugs

Moxonidine, a selective imidazoline-I_1-receptor agonist, acts in the medulla by reducing central sympathetic drive and attenuating peripheral vascular resistance. It results in lower plasma concentrations of catecholamines and renin. Its selectivity reduces the adverse side-effects seen with the first-generation drugs, α-methyldopa and clonidine. It is useful when ACE inhibitors have failed and, because it has little effect on glucose metabolism, is being used in the metabolic syndrome (syndrome X; see p. 978).

Other agents

Adrenergic neurone blocking drugs, such as guanethidine, are used extremely rarely.

Drug selection

Treatment is normally commenced with a single agent (monotherapy). The target of therapy should be to maintain diastolic blood pressure in the range of 80–90 mmHg with systolic blood pressure below 160 mmHg. Some experts have suggested that in diabetics the diastolic blood pressure should be reduced even further.

The most appropriate first-line agent will depend on the patient's age, ethnic background, sex and any concomitant illnesses. Conventionally, thiazide diuretics and β-blockers have been used as first-line agents with the other agents reserved for those in whom these prove ineffective. However, as our understanding of the adverse metabolic actions of these traditional agents increases, more patients are being prescribed calcium antagonists and ACE inhibitors as first-line treatment. There is some evidence that the drugs differ in their ability to reverse left ventricular hypertrophy (with the ACE inhibitors, β-blockers and diuretics being the most effective) although larger long-term studies are required to confirm these findings.

If monotherapy is unsuccessful, it is appropriate to move to combination therapy and certain combinations have been found to be particularly effective. These include the combination of an ACE inhibitor or β-blocker with a diuretic, and the combination of a calcium antagonist with a β-blocker.

Resistant hypertension is most commonly due to non-compliance with medication, although it may reflect an unrecognized underlying cause (e.g. coarctation of the aorta), or may genuinely be due to refractory hypertension requiring more potent agents.

Management of severe or malignant hypertension

Patients with severe hypertension (diastolic pressure >140 mmHg), malignant hypertension (grades 3 or 4 retinopathy), hypertensive encephalopathy or with severe hypertensive complications, such as cardiac failure, should be admitted to hospital for immediate initiation of treatment. However, it is unwise to reduce the blood pressure too rapidly since this may lead to cerebral, renal, retinal or myocardial infarction, and the blood pressure response to therapy must be carefully monitored. In most cases, the aim is to reduce the diastolic blood pressure to 100–110 mmHg over 24–48 hours. This can often be achieved with oral medication. The blood pressure can then be normalized over the next two to three days.

When rapid control of blood pressure is required (e.g. in an aortic dissection), the agent of choice is intravenous sodium nitroprusside. Alternatively, an infusion of labetalol can be used. The infusion dosage must be titrated against the blood pressure response.

Management of hypertension in pregnancy

Many antihypertensive agents are contraindicated in pregnancy. Mild hypertension can be treated with methyldopa, which has been established as being safe in pregnancy, or labetalol. Pre-eclamptic hypertension can be treated with the same agents, or nifedipine, although the only method for reversal of overt pre-eclampsia is delivery. More severe hypertension or eclampsia requires treatment with intravenous hydralazine and may require termination of the pregnancy.

PROGNOSIS

The prognosis from hypertension depends on a number of features:

- the level of blood pressure
- the presence of target-organ changes (retinal, renal, cardiac or vascular)
- coexisting risk factors for cardiovascular disease, such as hyperlipidaemia, diabetes, smoking, obesity, male sex
- age at presentation.

Several studies have confirmed that the treatment of hypertension, even mild hypertension, will reduce the risk of stroke dramatically and of coronary artery disease to a lesser extent.

FURTHER READING

British Hypertension Society Working Party (1993) Management guidelines in essential hypertension: report of the second working party. *British Medical Journal* **306**: 983–987.

Hansson L *et al.* (1998) Hypertension Optimal Treatment (HOT) randomised trial. *Lancet* **351**: 1755–1762.

Medical Research Council Working Party (1985) MRC trial of treatment of mild hypertension: principal results. *British Medical Journal* **291**: 97–104.

Swales JD (1994) *Textbook of Hypertension*. Oxford: Blackwell Scientific.

Heart disease in the elderly

As the average age of the population increases, cardiac disease predominates. The elderly population are vulnerable to most forms of heart disease, especially coronary artery disease, hypertension, arrhythmias and degenerative pathologies.

NORMAL FINDINGS

Diagnosis of mild forms of heart disease may be difficult in the elderly. The wear and tear of age results in some features that would be regarded as abnormal in the young. For example, a fourth heart sound and a systolic aortic ejection murmur are common findings on examining normal elderly adults. The ECG often shows slight PR interval prolongation (to 0.22 s), left axis deviation and T wave flattening. On the chest X-ray there may be some aortic, valvular or coronary arterial calcification, but the cardiac silhouette is usually normal. The echocardiogram may show mild myocardial hypertrophy and buckling of the ventricular septum.

It is particularly difficult to diagnose and define hypertension in the elderly. Cuff blood pressure usually overestimates intravascular pressure if the old arterial wall is stiff (pseudohypertension). Normally, blood pressure steadily increases with age, at least up to the age of 70 years, and blood pressure is particularly labile in the elderly. In the very old (>80 years) there is only a weak association between 'hypertension' and diseases such as stroke, myocardial infarction and heart failure.

DISEASE PRESENTATION

Cardiac disease may present in unexpected ways in an old person. It is not unusual for significant bradycardia to present as a fractured hip because the fall that caused the fracture resulted from transient asystole. Left heart failure may present as an acute confusional state due to poor cerebral perfusion, rather than with the classical symptom of breathlessness. Myocardial infarction may not cause any chest pain ('silent' myocardial infarction) but may present as weakness or abdominal pain.

TREATMENT

The principles of treatment of heart disease in old people are usually no different from those governing treatment in the young. However, it is important to remember that drug pharmacokinetics are changed in the elderly: absorption is reduced, renal and hepatic clearance are delayed, body fat increases and lean body mass decreases. Old people may forget to take their medications or be confused about the correct dose.

Some therapies seem inappropriate or futile in the elderly. For example, it is probably unnecessary to inflict a spartan lifestyle or rigorous uncomfortable drug therapy on an old person in an attempt to modify the risk of developing coronary disease. However, there are treatments that have emerged in recent years that are extremely useful for old people; for example, hypertension should be treated. Coronary angioplasty, and perhaps mitral/aortic valvuloplasty, can be undertaken in patients too frail to consider for surgery. Cardiac surgery does carry a much greater (approximately two to five times) risk in the elderly but, as with younger patients, the absolute risk is dependent upon the state of the myocardium, the extent of cardiac disease and the condition of other organ systems. Age is no bar to effective treatment of heart disease.

SPECIFIC HEART PROBLEMS IN THE ELDERLY

There are a few cardiac conditions that are largely confined to the elderly.

Aortic sclerosis

Aortic sclerosis results from fibrosis and calcification on the aortic side of an otherwise normal tricuspid aortic valve. This may result in an obstruction to left ventricular outflow but it is often trivial. Aortic valve replacement may be necessary if the obstruction is severe.

Mitral annulus calcification

Mitral annulus calcification occurs predominantly in old women. It is diagnosed from the chest X-ray and it is not usually responsible for any symptoms.

Endocarditis

A non-infective form of endocarditis may occur in the elderly. It is a hypercoagulable state that presents with cachexia, thrombosis and embolization. Anticoagulation may be needed.

Lev's disease

Disruption of His–Purkinje conduction by fibrosis and calcification is most common in the old when it is known as Lev's disease. It presents with Stokes–Adams attacks and must be treated by pacemaker insertion.

Atrial fibrillation

Atrial fibrillation is much more common in the old but it is often well tolerated and may not need any active treatment for control of heart rate. Anticoagulation is usually advised (see p. 665), except in the very elderly.

FURTHER READING

Martin A, Camm AJ (1994) Heart Disease in the Elderly. Chichester: John Wiley.

The heart in pregnancy

In pregnancy the cardiac output and blood volume increase from the second month up to the thirtieth week to 30–50% above the normal levels. This, along with the increased metabolic work, produces the physical signs of warm extremities, a tachycardia with a large-volume pulse and a slight rise in venous pressure. The apex beat is displaced, owing partly to cardiomegaly and partly to a raised diaphragm. The increased blood flow produces a pulmonary systolic murmur and a third heart sound. The diastolic blood pressure is lower owing to vasodilatation.

The added burden of pregnancy on the cardiovascular system can make underlying, otherwise latent, disease clinically apparent. Ten per cent of maternal deaths in England and Wales are due to heart disease. This is usually rheumatic or congenital in origin, but any heart disease can be seen in pregnancy. Moderate-to-severe mitral stenosis can cause breathlessness early in pregnancy and may lead to pulmonary oedema later in pregnancy. Pregnancy should be avoided in severe mitral stenosis or delayed until after valvotomy. Termination may be necessary in a severe case occurring before the sixteenth week. Most cases of congenital heart disease have been corrected by the time women reach the reproductive age. However, patients with small and uncomplicated septal defects usually tolerate pregnancy well. Patients with prosthetic valves are usually on anticoagulant therapy. This may require a change to heparin because warfarin can cause fetal abnormalities. Patients with pulmonary hypertension of any aetiology have an extremely high mortality (up to 50%) either during or immediately after delivery, and termination should be considered.

In Marfan's syndrome, with aortic disease, there is a high rate of aortic dissection.

Postpartum, or late in pregnancy, a cardiomyopathy of uncertain aetiology is sometimes seen. There is also a rise in thromboembolic complications of cardiac disease owing to the hypercoagulability that exists postpartum. Sepsis is a risk during delivery, and patients with heart disease may be at risk of developing infective endocarditis.

FURTHER READING

Oakley C (ed) (1997) Heart Disease in Pregnancy. London: BMJ.

Peripheral vascular disease

Arterial disease

Arterial disease can be due to a number of pathological processes.

Arteriosclerosis

This is the term applied to generalized, age-related arterial changes, which are exaggerated in hypertension. In arteries down to 1 mm diameter these changes initially take the form of compensatory muscular hypertrophy of the media, which is followed by fibrosis and dilatation of the lumen. In hypertensive vessels of this size, atheroma is often superadded.

Smaller arteries show different changes that are usually most marked in the viscera, especially in the kidneys. Here, although there is medial hypertrophy, the predominant change is intimal thickening by concentric layers of connective tissue, with luminal narrowing.

Arterioles undergo hyaline thickening of their walls and luminal narrowing. The narrowing of small vessels in the kidney due to hypertension causes renal ischaemia, which further promotes hypertension.

In malignant hypertension, arterioles also show fibrinoid necrosis of their walls.

Möncкeberg's sclerosis

This is a degenerative disease of unknown cause, characterized by dystrophic calcification of the media. It is especially common in the major lower limb arteries of the elderly, and there is an increased incidence of this degeneration in diabetics.

Cystic medial necrosis or degeneration

This describes mucoid degeneration of the collagen and elastic tissue of the media, often with cystic changes. It occurs mainly in elderly hypertensives. Dissecting aneurysms of the thoracic aorta are often due to this process. Cystic medial degeneration also occurs in inherited defects of collagen tissue formation (e.g. Marfan's syndrome, Ehlers–Danlos syndrome), again resulting in dissecting aneurysms.

Atherosclerosis

The pathogenesis of this condition is described on p. 685. The various vessels that may be involved are shown in Table 11.44. Atheroma seldom involves arteries of less than 2 mm diameter. Most arterial disease is due to atherosclerosis.

Table 11.44 Common sites of clinically significant atherosclerosis, in order of frequency

Abdominal aorta and iliac arteries
Proximal coronary arteries
Femoral and popliteal arteries, and thoracic aorta
Internal carotid arteries
Vertebrobasilar system

Chronic ischaemia of the legs

This is due to atherosclerosis involving the aorta, iliac and/or any other peripheral vessels. It consequently occurs over the age of 50 years, chiefly in men who are smokers. The incidence of intermittent claudication is approximately 0.2% per year for men, 35–45 years of age, rising to 1% per year for men over 65 years of age.

SYMPTOMS

Often both limbs are affected, but usually one is more severely affected than the other. There is cramp-like pain, usually in the calves during exercise and relieved by rest (intermittent claudication). The thighs and buttocks are sometimes involved. The *Leriche syndrome* is due to severe atheromatous disease of the distal aorta leading to thigh claudication and male impotence.

Rest pain, which is often worse at night, is sometimes relieved by dangling the legs over the edge of the bed. The feet are cold, sometimes with discoloration due to peripheral cyanosis.

Non-healing leg ulcers or gangrene occur which may be painful (but, in diabetes, are usually not).

SIGNS

- A cold limb with dry skin and lack of hair.
- Diminished or absent pulses to diseased areas.
- Ulceration.
- Gangrene; dark discoloration, usually starting at the toes.

INVESTIGATIONS

Doppler ultrasound

Measurement of the cuff pressure at which blood flow is detectable by Doppler in the peripheral arteries is a good guide to the severity of arterial disease. It is expressed as a ratio of ankle/brachial pressure. With intermittent claudication, the ratio is about 0.5. After exercise there is a further fall in the pressure ratio in patients with arterial disease and this is a highly sensitive test.

B-mode ultrasonography and Doppler combined (duplex imaging) gives a detailed image of the lower limb arteries from the aorta to the pedal vessels with detection of any stenotic areas and also the direction of blood flow.

MRI and spiral CT angiography

These are used in some centres. MRI avoids exposure to X-rays and is accurate in detecting arterial stenosis.

Intravascular ultrasonography and angioscopy are invasive techniques that are being used for intraluminal visualization, particularly after angioplasty and stenting.

Angiography

This is performed via a percutaneous catheter inserted into the brachial or other artery. With digital subtraction imaging, an intravenous injection has been used with good definition using only small doses of contrast. These investigations are now less often required because of good Doppler images.

MANAGEMENT

General

Risk factors should be reduced. In particular, smoking should be stopped, diabetes and hypertension treated, and a weight-reduction programme introduced. Hypercholesterolaemia should be treated (see p. 995).

The limbs should be kept warm but local heat should not be applied. Foot care should be introduced to avoid infection and trauma of the feet. Elderly patients often need regular visits to a chiropodist. Supervised exercise programmes significantly increase walking distances and quality of life.

Low-dose aspirin should be given to reduce the risk of myocardial infarction and stroke, with a possible reduction in the rate of re-occlusion following angioplasty. Vasodilators should not be used. Anticoagulants are of no benefit.

Surgery

Surgery should not be considered for three months after intermittent claudication has developed, to allow time for collaterals to develop. In 75% of patients the disease remains static.

Aorto-iliac bypass grafts give good results, but reconstructive surgery for blockages below the inguinal ligament is less successful. In the short term, percutaneous transluminal angioplasty via a catheter inserted into the artery is useful for local iliac or femoral stenoses; over 2–5 years, the results are similar to those of medical therapy.

Amputation is necessary for severely ischaemic limbs, usually those with gangrene. Rehabilitation may take months in the elderly and is often unsuccessful.

Many of the patients have generalized atheromatous conditions, with 50% having symptomatic ischaemic heart disease. Thus, the overall prognosis often dictates the outcome of localized disease; many die from a myocardial infarction or stroke.

Acute ischaemia of the legs

Like chronic ischaemia of the legs, this is mainly due to atherosclerosis with an acute thrombosis. It can also occur from an embolism from the heart (e.g. in atrial fibrillation) or from an atheromatous central vessel.

The clinical picture is of an acutely painful, pale, paralysed, pulseless limb.

Treatment is surgical, with removal of the clot. Anticoagulants with heparin can help some patients. Intra-arterial thrombolysis, usually with streptokinase, provides successful recannulization in about 50% of patients. Further revascularization surgery is usually required later. If gangrene develops, amputation is necessary.

Aortic aneurysm

An aortic aneurysm refers to a permanent localized dilatation of the aorta with a diameter of at least 1.5 times that of the expected diameter.

Abdominal aneurysms

The most common aortic aneurysms are abdominal between the renal and iliac arteries. They are usually due to atherosclerosis. The incidence increases with age, with men being affected four to five times more frequently.

Asymptomatic aneurysms may be found as a pulsatile mass on examination or as calcification on an X-ray. A CT scan or ultrasound of the abdomen will demonstrate the size of the aneurysm, the thickness of the aortic wall and whether any leak has occurred. An expanding aneurysm may cause epigastric or back pain. Rupture presents with epigastric pain radiating through to the back. A pulsatile mass is felt and the patient is shocked. Treatment of symptomatic aneurysms is surgical. A ruptured aneurysm requires emergency surgery, but even then the mortality is high.

Large, asymptomatic aneurysms should also be treated surgically (except in the very old) because those larger than 5 cm diameter have a high risk of rupture. Follow-up with ultrasound is required with small aneurysms and surgery offered when the aneurysm reaches 5 cm.

Thoracic aneurysms

These can be divided into ascending, arch or descending aortic aneurysms (the most common).

Ascending thoracic aortic aneurysms most often result from cystic medial degeneration necrosis (see p. 739). Descending thoracic aortic and arch aneurysms are usually due to atherosclerosis. Syphilis as a cause of aneurysms is now rare.

Forty per cent are asymptomatic at diagnosis, but when large they can give rise to chest pain or to evidence of pressure on other organs, such as the superior vena cava or the oesophagus. They can rupture. Transoesophageal echocardiography is accurate in diagnosis. Asymptomatic aneurysms should probably be resected when they reach 6–7 cm, possibly smaller if the patient has Marfan's syndrome. Arch aneurysms are technically the most difficult to deal with and carry a higher mortality.

Dissecting aortic aneurysms

Aortic dissection usually begins with a tear in the intima. Blood penetrates the diseased medial layer and then cleaves the lamina plain of the intima in two, leading to a dissection of variable length. In a small number of cases no tear is found and it is proprosed that a haemorrhage within the media is the first step.

Aortic dissections are three types:

- DeBakey I – originates in the ascending aorta, propagates at least to the aortic arch and often beyond
- DeBakey II – originates in, and is confined to, the ascending aorta
- DeBakey III – originates in the distal aorta and extends distally down the aorta.

The major symptom is severe and central chest pain, often radiating to the back. The pain radiates down the arms and into the neck and can be difficult to distinguish from myocardial infarction.

On examination, the patient is usually shocked and there may be neurological signs owing to the involvement of the spinal vessels. The peripheral pulses may be absent, but this is not invariable. Half of the patients are hypertensive and this should be controlled immediately.

The diagnosis is suggested by the presence of back pain in addition to chest pain and no ECG or enzyme changes of myocardial infarction. The chest X-ray may show a wide mediastinum, and CT scanning and ultrasonography with transoesophageal echocardiography (if available) are diagnostic (Fig 11.98). MRI is highly accurate and is the gold standard. Aortography is now rarely necessary to confirm the diagnosis.

Emergency surgery is necessary for acute proximal dissections. Acute distal aortic dissections are best treated medically to control pain and hypertension. Five-year survival in both groups is in the region of 70–80%.

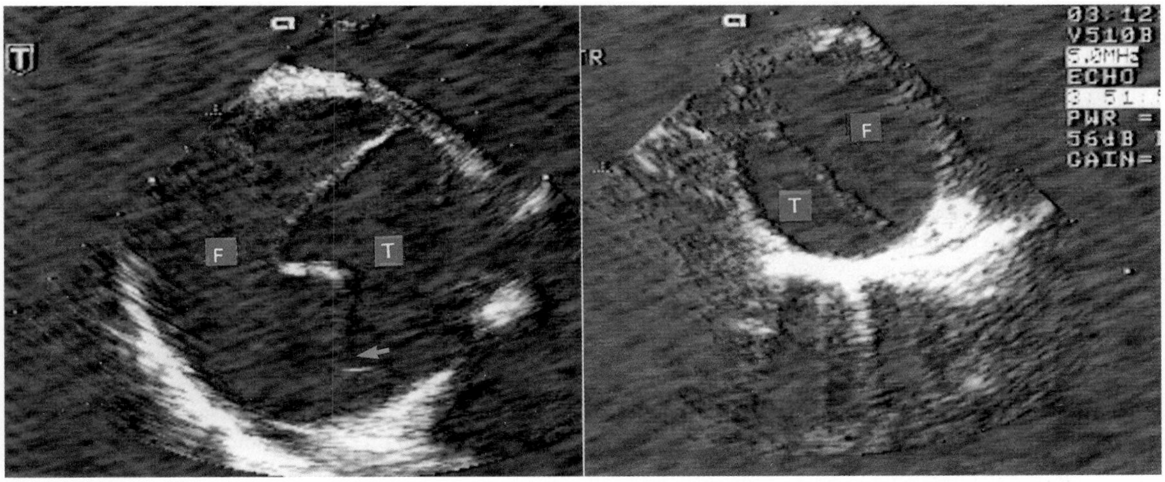

Fig 11.98
Two-dimensional transoesophageal echocardiograms from a patient with Marfan's syndrome resulting in dissection of the aorta. From its position in the oesophagus, the transducer can be aimed forward to visualize the greatly enlarged ascending aorta (left), or backwards to show the descending thoracic aorta (right). In both views the dissected intima is seen within the aortic lumen. The main entry point to the false lumen is seen in the ascending aorta (arrowed), just above the aortic valve
T, true lumen; F, false lumen

Thromboangiitis obliterans (Buerger's disease)

This disease, involving the small vessels of the lower limbs, occurs in young men who smoke. It is thought by some workers to be indistinguishable from atheromatous disease. However, pathologically there is inflammation of the arteries and sometimes veins that may indicate a separate disease entity. Clinically it presents with severe claudication and rest pain leading to gangrene. A thrombophlebitis is sometimes present. Treatment is as for all peripheral vascular disease, but patients must stop smoking.

Takayasu's syndrome

This is rare, except in Japan. It is known as 'pulseless disease' or the aortic arch syndrome. It is of unknown aetiology and occurs in young females. There is a vasculitis involving the aortic arch as well as other major arteries. There is also a systemic illness, with pain and tenderness over the affected arteries. Absent peripheral pulses and hypertension are usually found. Corticosteroids help the constitutional symptoms. Heart failure and cerebrovascular accidents eventually occur, but most patients survive for at least five years.

Kawasaki disease (mucocutaneous lymph node syndrome) (p. 495)

This is an uncommon acute febrile illness of early childhood. There is a generalized vasculitis with involvement of the coronary arteries and lymphadenopathy.

Cardiovascular syphilis

This gives rise to:

- uncomplicated aortitis
- aortic aneurysms, usually in the ascending part
- aortic valvulitis with regurgitation
- stenosis of the coronary ostia.

The diagnosis is confirmed by serology. Treatment is with penicillin. Aneurysms and valvular disease are treated as necessary by the usual methods.

Connective tissue disorders

These cause vasculitis and can give rise to peripheral vascular disease. They are discussed on p. 487.

Raynaud's disease and phenomenon

Raynaud's phenomenon consists of spasm of the arteries supplying the fingers or toes and is usually precipitated by cold and relieved by heat. When Raynaud's phenomenon occurs without any underlying disorder, it is then known as Raynaud's disease. This is a common disease affecting 5% of the population and occurring predominantly in young women.

The disorder is usually bilateral and fingers are affected more commonly than toes. There is an initial pallor of the skin resulting from vasoconstriction and this is followed by cyanosis due to sluggish blood flow. Redness finally occurs owing to hyperaemia. The duration of the attacks can be variable and can sometimes last for hours. Numbness and burning of the fingers usually occurs and pain can be severe, particularly in the rewarming phase.

Between the attacks the pulses and the digits appear normal, but trophic changes with small areas of gangrene can occur in severe and persistent cases.

DIAGNOSIS

Primary Raynaud's disease must be differentiated from secondary causes of Raynaud's phenomenon, which are chiefly disorders of connective tissue, particularly systemic sclerosis. It can also occur in cryoglobulinaemia and as a side-effect of drug treatment, especially with β-blocking agents.

TREATMENT (see also p. 491)

No treatment is usually required for the attacks but any underlying disease must be looked for. The hands and feet should be kept warm, and smoking should be avoided. β-Blockers should be stopped. Nifedipine 10 mg three times daily may be helpful.

Venous disease

Varicose veins

Varicose veins are a common problem, sometimes giving rise to pain. They are treated by injection or surgery.

Venous thrombosis

Thrombosis can occur in any vein, but the veins of the leg and the pelvis are the most common sites.

Superficial thrombophlebitis

This commonly involves the saphenous veins and is often associated with varicosities. Occasionally the axillary vein is involved, usually as a result of trauma. There is local superficial inflammation of the vein wall, with secondary thrombosis.

The clinical picture is of a painful, tender, cord-like structure with associated redness and swelling.

The condition usually responds to symptomatic treatment with rest, elevation of the limb and analgesics (e.g. non-steroidal anti-inflammatory drugs). Anticoagulants are not necessary, as embolism does not occur from superficial thrombophlebitis.

Deep-vein thrombosis

A thrombus forms in the vein, and any inflammation of the vein wall is secondary to this.

Thrombosis commonly occurs after periods of immobilization, but it can occur in normal individuals for no obvious reasons. The precipitating factors are discussed on p. 409.

A deep-vein thrombosis in the legs occurs in 50% of patients after prostatectomy or following a cerebral vascular accident. In addition, one-third of patients with a myocardial infarct have a deep-vein thrombosis.

Thrombosis can occur in any vein of the leg, but is particularly found in veins of the calf. It is often undetected; autopsy figures give an incidence of over 60% in hospitalized patients.

Axillary vein thrombosis occasionally occurs, sometimes related to trauma, but usually for no obvious reason. Anticoagulation is not required.

CLINICAL FEATURES

The individual may be asymptomatic, presenting with clinical features of pulmonary embolism (see p. 720).

A major presenting feature is pain in the calf, often with swelling, redness and engorged superficial veins. The affected calf is often warmer and there may be ankle oedema. Homan's sign (pain in the calf on dorsiflexion of the foot) is often present, but is not diagnostic and occurs with all lesions of the calf.

Thrombosis in the iliofemoral region can present with severe pain, but there are often few physical signs apart from occasional swelling of the thigh and/or ankle oedema.

Complete occlusion, particularly of a large vein, can lead to a cyanotic discoloration of the limb and severe oedema, which can very rarely lead to venous gangrene.

Pulmonary embolism can occur with any deep-vein thrombosis but is more frequent from an iliofemoral thrombosis and is rare with thrombosis confined to veins below the knee. In 20–30% of patients, spread of thrombosis can occur proximally without clinical evidence, so careful monitoring of the leg, usually by ultrasound, is required.

INVESTIGATIONS

Clinical diagnosis is unreliable and confirmation of an iliofemoral thrombosis can usually be made with ultrasound or Doppler ultrasound. Below-knee thromboses can be detected reliably only by venography. A venogram is performed by injecting a vein in the foot with contrast which will detect virtually all thrombi that are present.

TREATMENT

The main aim of therapy is to prevent pulmonary embolism, and all patients with thrombi above the knee must be anticoagulated. Anticoagulation of below-knee thrombi is controversial, but as it reduces proximal extension it is usually recommended for six weeks. Bedrest is advised until the patient is fully anticoagulated. The patient should then be mobilized, with an elastic stocking giving graduated pressure over the leg.

Heparin is given normally for at least 2–3 days, whilst warfarin, which is started immediately, becomes effective. Low-molecular-weight heparins (see p. 412) are replacing unfractionated heparin as they are more effective, they do not require monitoring and there is less risk of bleeding. DVTs are now being treated at home with low-molecular-weight heparin. The duration of warfarin treatment is debatable – three months is the period usually recommended, but four weeks is long enough if a definite risk factor (e.g. bedrest) has been present. The target INR should be at 2.5. Anticoagulants do not lyse the thrombus that is already present.

Thrombolytic therapy (see p. 410) is occasionally used for patients with a large iliofemoral thrombosis.

PROGNOSIS

Destruction of the deep-vein valves produces a clinically painful, swollen limb that is made worse by standing and is accompanied by oedema and sometimes venous eczema. It occurs in approximately half of the patients with a clinically symptomatic deep-vein thrombosis, and it means that elastic support stockings are then required for life.

PREVENTION

Subcutaneous low-dose heparin (see p. 412) should be given to patients with cardiac failure, a myocardial infarct or surgery to the leg or pelvis.

Early ambulation is indicated as most thromboses occur within the first 72 hours following surgery. Leg exercises should be encouraged and patients should *not* sit in a chair with their legs immobilized on a stool. An elastic support stocking should be given to patients at high risk (e.g. those with a history of thrombosis or with obesity).

FURTHER READING

Rosendaal FR (1997) Risk factors for venous thrombosis. *Seminars in Haematology* **34**: 171–187.

Low molecular weight heparins for venous thromboembolism. *Drugs and Therapeutics Bulletin* **36**: no 4, April 1998.

Adam J, van der Vliet, Boll APM (1997) Abdominal aortic aneurysm. *Lancet* **349**: 863–866.

Kouchoukos NT, Dougenis D (1997) Surgery of the thoractic aorta. *New England Journal of Medicine* **336**: 1876–1888.

Golledge J (1997) Lower limb arterial disease. *Lancet* **350**: 1459–1465.

Ginsberg JS (1996) Management of venous thromboembolism. *New England Journal of Medicine* **335**: 1816–1828.

GENERAL READING

Bennet DH (1997) Cardiac Arrhythmias, 5th edn. Oxford: Butterworth-Heinemann.

Braunwald E (1997) Heart Disease. Philadelphia: WB Saunders.

Coronary Heart Disease (1996) Supplement to *Lancet* **348**: 1–31.

Respiratory disease

12

Structure of the respiratory system

The nose

The anterior one-third of the nasal cavity is divided into right and left halves by the nasal septum (Fig 12.1). The nasal vestibule leads to the internal ostium (a) which is the narrowest part of the nasal cavity. This causes a 50% increased resistance to airflow when breathing through the nose rather than through the mouth. The respiratory region (b) is divided by three folds arising from the lateral wall, termed the superior, middle and inferior turbinates. Behind these turbinates are situated the openings of the nasolacrimal duct and the frontal, ethmoidal and maxillary sinuses. The olfactory region for smell is found above the superior turbinate. The nasal cavities communicate with the nasopharynx via the posterior nasal apertures (the choanae (c)), and the eustachian tube opens into this area just above the soft palate.

The pharynx and larynx

The pharynx is divided by the soft palate into an upper nasopharyngeal and lower oropharyngeal region. There are numerous collections of lymphoid tissue arranged in a

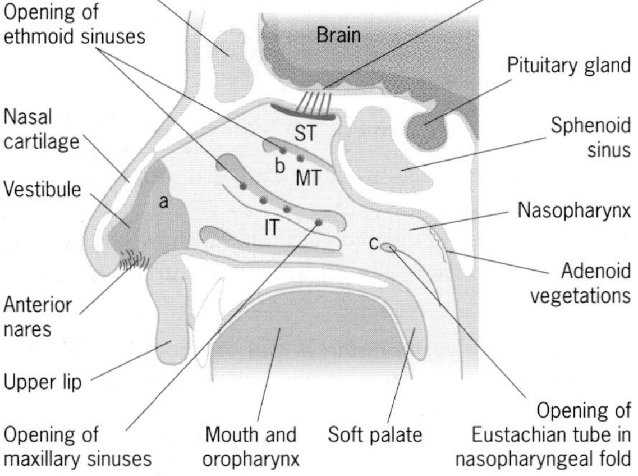

Fig 12.1
The anatomy of the nose in longitudinal section. IT, inferior turbinate; MT, middle turbinate; ST, superior turbinate; a, internal ostium; b, respiratory region; c, choanae

circular fashion around the nasopharynx; these include the adenoids. The tonsils lie between the anterior and posterior fauces, separating the mouth from the oropharynx.

The larynx consists of a number of articulated cartilages, vocal cords, muscles and ligaments, all of which serve to keep the airway open during breathing and occlude it during swallowing.

The main motor nerve to the larynx is the recurrent laryngeal nerve. The left recurrent laryngeal nerve leaves the vagus at the level of the aortic arch, hooking round it to run upwards through the mediastinum between the trachea and the oesophagus; it can be affected by disease in these areas. The principal tensor of the vocal cords is the external branch of the superior laryngeal nerve, which can be injured during thyroidectomy.

The trachea, bronchi and bronchioles

The trachea is 10–12 cm in length. It lies slightly to the right of the midline and divides at the carina into right and left main bronchi. The carina lies under the junction of the manubrium sternum and the second right costal cartilage. The right main bronchus is more vertical than the left and, hence, inhaled material is more likely to pass into it.

The right main bronchus divides into the upper lobe bronchus and the intermediate bronchus, which further subdivides into the middle and lower lobe bronchi. On the left the main bronchus divides into upper and lower lobe bronchi only. Each lobar bronchus further divides into segmental and subsegmental bronchi. There are about 25 divisions in all between the trachea and the alveoli. Of the first seven divisions the bronchi have:

- walls consisting of cartilage and smooth muscle
- epithelial lining with cilia and goblet cells
- submucosal mucus-secreting glands
- endocrine cells – Kulchitsky or APUD (amine precursor and uptake decarboxylation) containing 5-hydroxytryptamine.

In the next 16–18 divisions the bronchioles have:

- no cartilage and a muscular layer that progressively becomes thinner
- a single layer of ciliated cells but very few goblet cells
- granulated Clara cells that produce a surfactant-like substance.

The ciliated epithelium is an important defence mechanism. Each cell contains approximately 200 cilia beating at 1000 beats per minute in organized waves of contraction. Each cilium consists of nine peripheral parts and two inner longitudinal fibrils in a cytoplasmic matrix (Fig 12.2). Nexin links join the peripheral pairs. Dynein arms consisting of ATPase protein project towards the adjacent pairs. Bending of the cilia results from a sliding movement between adjacent fibrils powered by an ATP-dependent shearing force developed by the dynein arms. Absence of dynein arms leads to immotile cilia. Mucus, which contains macrophages, cell debris, inhaled particles and bacteria, is moved by the cilia towards the larynx at about 1.5 cm min^{-1} (the 'mucociliary escalator', see below).

The bronchioles finally divide within the acinus into smaller respiratory bronchioles that have alveoli arising from the surface (Fig 12.3). Each respiratory bronchiole supplies approximately 200 alveoli via alveolar ducts. The term 'small airways' refers to bronchioles of less than 2 mm; there are 30 000 of these in the average lung.

The alveoli

There are approximately 300 million alveoli in each lung. Their total surface area is 40–80 m^2. The epithelial lining consists largely of *type I pneumocytes* (Fig 12.4). These cells

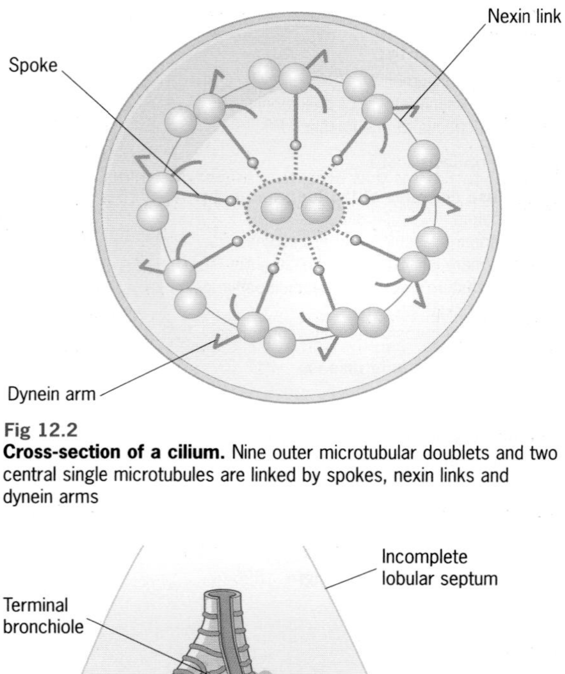

Fig 12.2
Cross-section of a cilium. Nine outer microtubular doublets and two central single microtubules are linked by spokes, nexin links and dynein arms

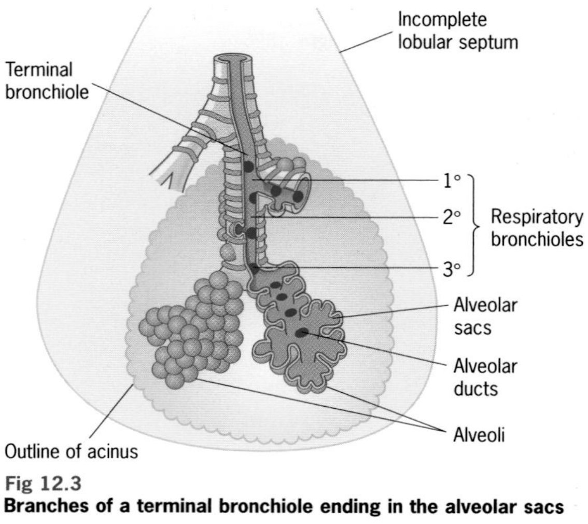

Fig 12.3
Branches of a terminal bronchiole ending in the alveolar sacs

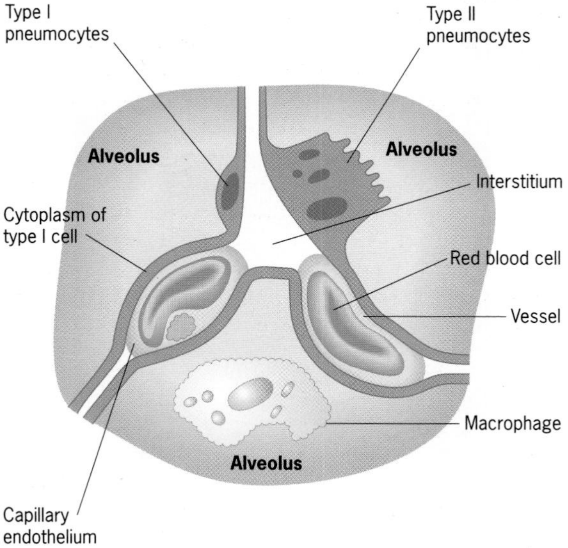

Fig 12.4
The structure of alveoli, showing the pneumocytes and capillaries

have an extremely attenuated cytoplasm, and thus provide only a thin barrier to gas exchange. They are derived from type II pneumocytes. *Type I cells* are connected to each other by tight junctions that limit the fluid movements in and out of the alveoli. *Type II pneumocytes* are slightly more numerous than type I cells but cover less of the epithelial lining. They are found generally in the borders of the alveolus and contain distinctive lamellar vacuoles, which are the source of surfactant. Macrophages are also present in the alveoli and are involved in the defence mechanisms of the lung.

The pores of Kohn are holes in the alveolar wall allowing communication between alveoli of adjoining lobules.

The lungs

The lungs are separated into lobes by invaginations of the pleura, which are often incomplete. The right lung has three lobes, whereas the left lung has two. The position of the oblique fissures and the right horizontal fissure are shown in Fig 12.5. The upper lobe lies mainly in front of the lower lobe and therefore signs on the right side in the front of the chest found on physical examination are due to lesions mainly of the upper lobe or part of the middle lobe.

Each lobe is further subdivided into bronchopulmonary segments by fibrous septa that extend inwards from the pleural surface. Each segment receives its own segmental bronchus.

The bronchopulmonary segment is further divided into individual lobules approximately 1 cm in diameter and generally pyramidal in shape, the apex lying towards the bronchioles supplying them. Within each lobule a terminal bronchus supplies an acinus and within this structure further divisions of the bronchioles eventually give rise to the alveoli.

A chest X-ray (Fig 12.6) illustrates the above features.

The pleura

The pleura is a layer of connective tissue covered by a simple squamous epithelium. The visceral pleura covers the surface of the lung, lines the interlobar fissures, and is continuous at the hilum with the parietal pleura, which

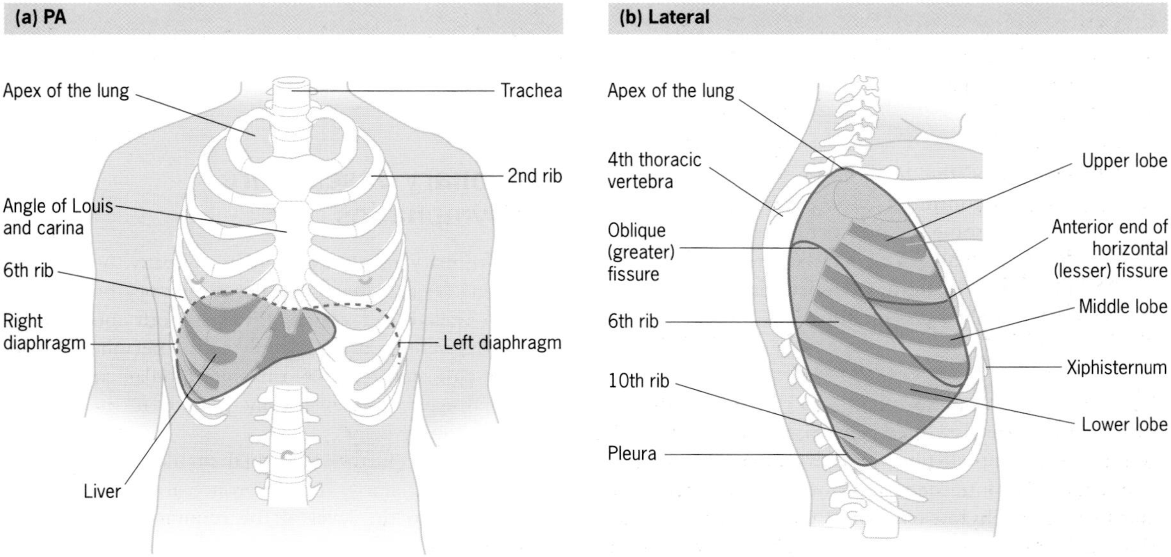

Fig 12.5
Surface anatomy of the chest. (a) PA; **(b)** lateral

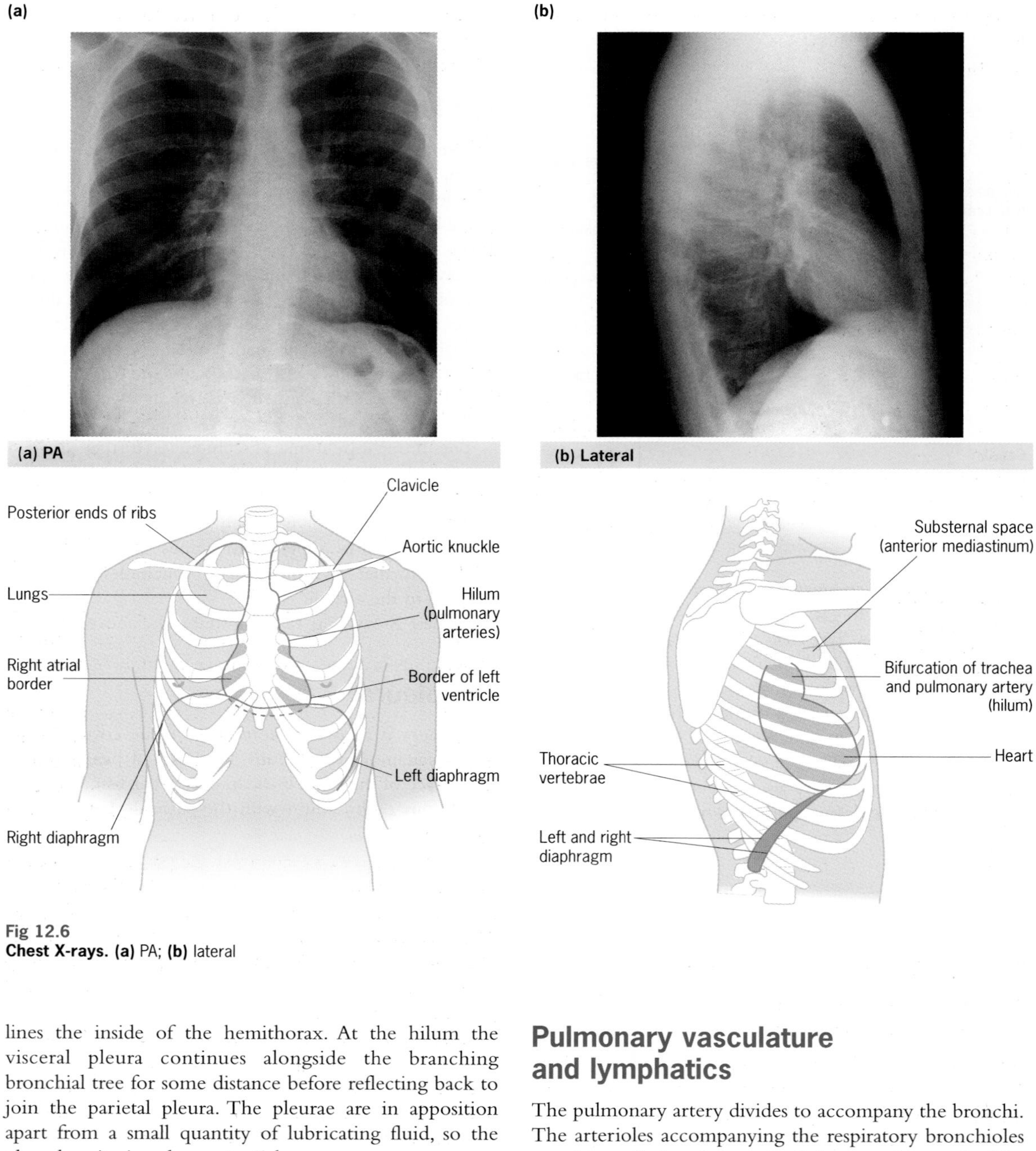

Fig 12.6
Chest X-rays. (a) PA; **(b)** lateral

lines the inside of the hemithorax. At the hilum the visceral pleura continues alongside the branching bronchial tree for some distance before reflecting back to join the parietal pleura. The pleurae are in apposition apart from a small quantity of lubricating fluid, so the pleural cavity is only a potential space.

The diaphragm

The diaphragm is lined by parietal pleura and peritoneum. Its muscle fibres arise from the lower ribs and insert into the central tendon. Motor and sensory nerve fibres go separately to each half of the diaphragm via the phrenic nerves. Fifty per cent of the muscle fibres are of the slow-twitch type with a low glycolytic capacity; they are relatively resistant to fatigue.

Pulmonary vasculature and lymphatics

The pulmonary artery divides to accompany the bronchi. The arterioles accompanying the respiratory bronchioles are thin-walled and contain little smooth muscle. The pulmonary venules drain laterally to the periphery of the lobules, pass centrally in the interlobular and inter-segmental septa, and eventually join to form the four main pulmonary veins.

In addition, a further bronchial circulation arises from the descending aorta. These bronchial arteries supply tissues down to the level of the respiratory bronchiole. The bronchial veins drain into the pulmonary vein, forming part of the physiological shunt observed in normal individuals.

Lymphatic channels lie in the potential interstitial space between the alveolar cells and the capillary endothelium of the pulmonary arterioles.

Nerve supply to the lung

The innervation of the lung remains incompletely understood. Parasympathetic (from the vagus) and sympathetic (from the adjacent sympathetic chain) nerve supplies entwine in a plexus at the nerve root and branches accompany the pulmonary arteries and the airways. Airway smooth muscle is innervated by vagal afferents, postganglionic cholinergic vagal efferents and vagally derived non-adrenergic non-cholinergic (NANC) fibres. Neurotransmitters (peptides and purines) may be involved. Three muscarinic receptor subtypes have been identified: M_1 receptors on parasympathetic ganglia, a smaller number of M_2 receptors on cholinergic nerve terminals, and M_3 receptors on airway smooth muscle. The parietal pleura is innervated from intercostal and phrenic nerves but the visceral pleura has no innervation.

FURTHER READING

Brewis RAL, Corrin B, Gibson GJ, Geddes DM (1995) Respiratory medicine, 2nd edn, vols 1 and 2. WB Saunders, London.

Physiology of the respiratory system

The nose

The major functions of nasal breathing are:

- to heat and moisten the air
- to remove particulate matter.

About 10 000 L of particle-laden air are inhaled daily. Deposited particles are removed from the nasal mucosa within 15 minutes, compared with 60–120 days from the alveolus. The relatively low flow rates and turbulence of inspired air are ideal for particle deposition, and few particles greater than 10 μm pass through the nose. For this reason nasal secretion contains many protective proteins in the form of antibodies, lysozymes and interferon. In addition, the cilia of the nasal epithelium move the mucous gel layer rapidly back to the oropharynx where it is swallowed. Bacteria have little chance of settling in the nose.

Mucociliary protection against viral infections is more difficult because viruses bind to receptors on epithelial cells. The majority of rhinoviruses bind to an adhesion molecule, intercellular adhesion molecule 1 (ICAM-1), shared by neutrophils and eosinophils. Many noxious gases, such as SO_2, are almost completely removed by nasal breathing.

Breathing

Lung ventilation can be considered in two parts:

- the mechanical process of inspiration and expiration
- the control of respiration to a level appropriate for the metabolic needs.

Mechanical process

Inspiration is an active process and results from the descent of the diaphragm and movement of the ribs upwards and outwards under the influence of the intercostal muscles. In resting healthy individuals, contraction of the diaphragm is responsible for most inspiration. Respiratory muscles are similar to other skeletal muscles but are less prone to fatigue. However, weakness may play a part in respiratory failure resulting from neurological and muscle disorders and possibly with severe chronic airflow limitation.

Expiration follows passively as a result of gradual lessening of contraction of the intercostal muscles, allowing the lungs to collapse under the influence of their own elastic forces.

Inspiration against increased resistance may require the use of the accessory muscles of ventilation, such as the sternomastoid and scalene muscles. Forced expiration is also accomplished with the aid of accessory muscles, chiefly those of the abdominal wall, which help to push up the diaphragm.

The lungs have an inherent elastic property that causes them to tend to collapse away from the thoracic wall, generating a negative pressure within the pleural space. The strength of this retractive force relates to the volume of the lung; for example, at higher lung volumes the lung is stretched more, and a greater negative intrapleural pressure is generated.

Lung compliance is a measure of the relationship between this retractive force and lung volume. It is defined as the change in lung volume brought about by unit change in transpulmonary (intrapleural) pressure and is measured in litres per kilopascal (L kPa^{-1}). At the end of a quiet expiration, the retractive force exerted by the lungs is balanced by the tendency of the thoracic wall to spring outwards. At this point respiratory muscles are resting and the volume of the lung is known as the *functional residual capacity* (FRC).

Diseases that can affect the movement of the thoracic cage and diaphragm can have a profound effect on ventilation. These include diseases of the thoracic spine such as ankylosing spondylitis and kyphoscoliosis, neuropathies (e.g. the Guillain–Barré syndrome), injury to the phrenic nerves, and myasthenia gravis.

The control of respiration

Coordinated respiratory movements result from rhythmical discharges arising in an anatomically ill-defined group of interconnected neurones in the reticular substance of the brain stem known as the *respiratory centre*. Motor discharges from the respiratory centre travel via the phrenic and intercostal nerves to the respiratory musculature.

The pressures of oxygen and carbon dioxide in arterial blood are closely controlled. In a typical normal adult at rest:

- The pulmonary blood flow of 5 L min^{-1} carries 11 mmol min^{-1} (250 mL min^{-1}) of oxygen from the lungs to the tissues.
- Ventilation at about 6 L min^{-1} carries 9 mmol min^{-1} (200 mL min^{-1}) of carbon dioxide out of the body.
- The normal pressure of oxygen in arterial blood (P_aO_2) is between 11 and 13 kPa (83 and 98 mmHg).
- The normal pressure of carbon dioxide in arterial blood (P_aCO_2) is 4.8–6.0 kPa (36–45 mmHg).

Neurogenic and chemical factors are involved in the control of ventilation (Fig 12.7).

Breathlessness on physical exertion is normal and not considered a symptom unless the level of exertion is very light, such as when walking slowly. Although breathlessness is a very common symptom, the sensory and neural mechanisms underlying it remain obscure. The sensation of breathlessness is derived from at least three sources:

- *Changes in lung volume*. These are sensed by receptors in thoracic wall muscles signalling changes in their length.
- *The tension developed by contracting muscles*. This can be sensed by Golgi tendon organs. The tension developed in normal muscle can be differentiated from that developed in muscles weakened by fatigue or disease.
- *Central perception of the sense of effort*.

The airways of the lungs

From the trachea to the periphery, the airways become smaller in size (although greater in number). The cross-sectional area available for airflow increases as the total number of airways increases. The flow of air is maximum in the trachea and slows progressively towards the periphery (as the velocity of airflow depends on the ratio of flow to cross-sectional area). In the terminal airways, gas flow occurs solely by diffusion. The resistance to airflow is very low (0.1–0.2 kPa L^{-1} in a

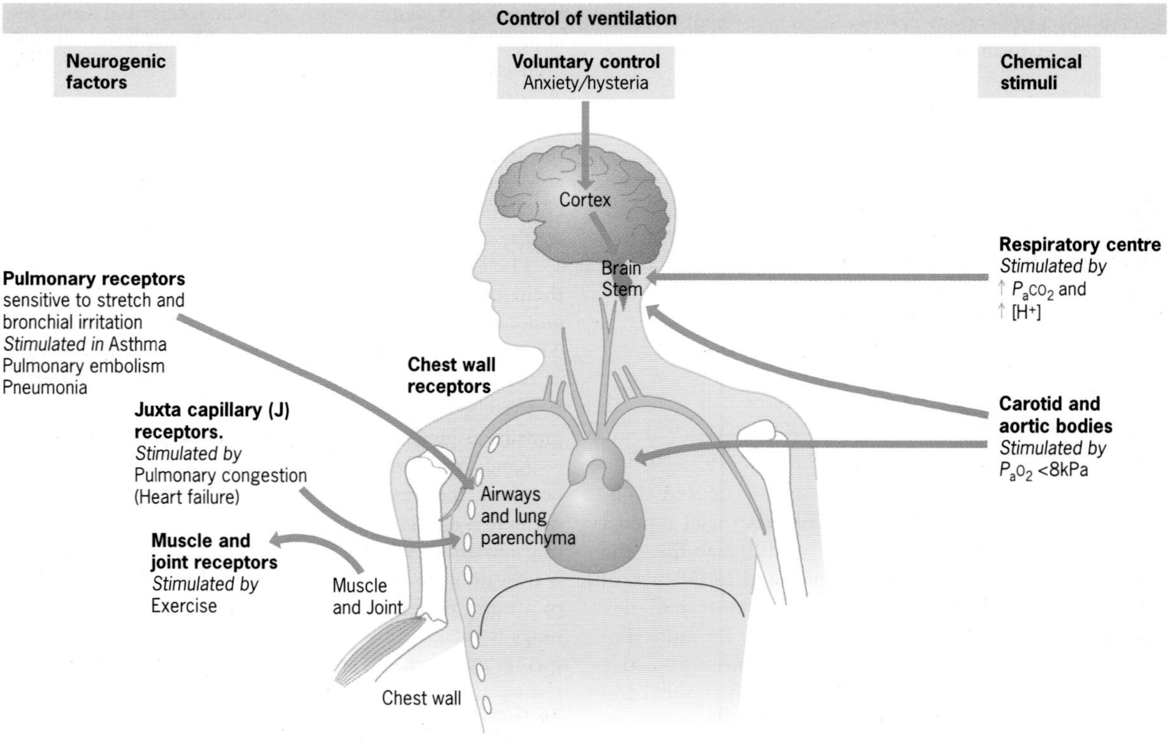

Fig 12.7
Chemical and neurogenic factors in the control of ventilation. The strongest stimulant to ventilation is a rise in P_aCO_2 which increases [H+] in CSF. Sensitivity to this may be lost in COPD. In these patients hypoxaemia is the chief stimulus to respiratory drive; oxygen treatment may therefore reduce respiratory drive and lead to a further rise in P_aCO_2. An increase in [H+] due to metabolic acidosis as in diabetic ketoacidosis will increase ventilation with a fall in P_aCO_2 causing deep sighing (Kussmaul) respiration. The respiratory centre is depressed by severe hypoxaemia and sedatives (e.g. opiates) and stimulated by doxapram, large doses of aspirin and pyrexia. COPD = Chronic obstructive pulmonary disease. (From Manning HL, Schwartzstein RM (1995) *New England Journal of Medicine* **333**: 1547–1553, with permission.)

normal tracheobronchial tree), steadily increasing from the small to the large airways.

Airways expand as lung volume is increased, and at full inspiration (total lung capacity, TLC) they are 30–40% larger in calibre than at full expiration (residual volume, RV). In chronic bronchitis and emphysema, which principally affect the smaller airways, the airway narrowing is partially overcome by breathing at a larger lung volume.

Control of airway tone

This is under the autonomic nervous system. Bronchomotor tone is maintained by vagal efferent nerves and, even in a normal subject, is reduced by atropine or β-adrenoreceptor agonists. The many adrenoreceptors on the surface of bronchial muscles respond to circulating catecholamines; sympathetic nerves do not directly innervate them. Airway tone shows a *circadian rhythm*, which is greatest at 04.00 and lowest in the mid-afternoon. Tone can be increased briefly by inhaled stimuli acting on epithelial nerve endings, which trigger reflex bronchoconstriction via the vagus.

These stimuli include cigarette smoke, inert dust, and cold air; airway responsiveness to these increases following respiratory tract infections even in healthy subjects. In asthma, the characteristic increased airway responsiveness is an exaggeration of this normal response and, as the circadian rhythm remains the same, asthmatic symptoms are worst in the early morning.

Air flow

Movement of air through the airways results from a difference between the pressure in the alveoli and the atmospheric pressure; a positive alveolar pressure occurs in expiration and a negative pressure occurs in inspiration. During quiet breathing the subatmospheric pleural pressure throughout the breathing cycle slightly distends the airways. With vigorous expiratory efforts (e.g. cough), although the central airways are compressed by positive pleural pressures exceeding 10 kPa, the airways do not close completely because the driving pressure for expiratory flow (alveolar pressure) is also increased. *Alveolar pressure* P_{ALV} *is equal to the elastic recoil pressure* (P_{EL}) *of the lung plus the pleural pressure* (P_{PL}). When there is no airflow (i.e. during a pause in breathing) the tendency of the lungs to collapse (the positive recoil pressure) is exactly balanced by an equivalent negative pleural pressure.

As air flows from the alveoli towards the mouth there is a gradual loss of pressure owing to flow resistance. In forced expiration, as mentioned above, the driving pressure raises both the alveolar pressure and the intrapleural pressure. Between the alveolus and the mouth, a point will occur (C in Fig 12.8) where the airway pressure will equal the intrapleural pressure, and airway compression will occur. However, this compression of the airway is temporary, as the transient occlusion of the airway results in an increase in pressure behind it (i.e. upstream) and this raises the intra-airway pressure so that the airways open and flow is restored. The airways thus tend to vibrate at this point of 'dynamic compression'.

The elastic recoil pressure of the lungs decreases with decreasing lung volume and the 'collapse point' moves upstream (i.e. towards the smaller airways – see Fig 12.8(c)). Where there is pathological loss of recoil pressure (as in chronic obstructive pulmonary disease, COPD), the 'collapse point' starts even further upstream and these patients are often seen to 'purse their lips' in order to increase airway pressure so that their peripheral airways do not collapse. The expiratory airflow limitation is the disordered physiology that underlies chronic airflow limitation. The measurement of the forced expiratory volume in one second (FEV_1) is a useful clinical index of this phenomenon.

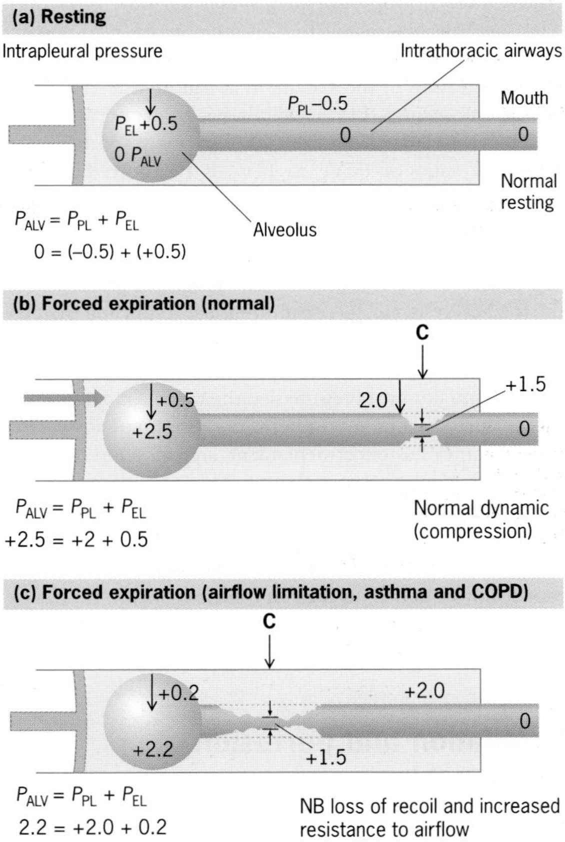

Fig 12.8
Diagrams showing ventilatory forces.
(a) During resting at functional residual capacity.
(b) During forced expiration in normal subjects.
(c) During forced expiration in a patient with COPD.
The respiratory system is represented as a piston with a single alveolus and the collapsible part of the airways within the piston (see text). C, compression point; P_{ALV}, alveolar pressure; P_{EL}, elastic recoil pressure; P_{PL}, pleural pressure

On inspiration the intrapleural pressure is always less than the intraluminal pressure within the intrathoracic airways, so there is no limitation to airflow with increasing effort. Inspiratory flow is limited only by the power of the inspiratory muscles.

Flow–volume loops

The relationship between maximal flow rates on expiration and inspiration is demonstrated by the maximal flow–volume (MFV) loops. Figure 12.9(a) shows this in a normal subject.

In subjects with healthy lungs the clinical importance of flow limitation will not be apparent, since maximal flow rates are rarely achieved even during vigorous exercise. However, in patients with severe COPD, limitation of expiratory flow occurs even during tidal breathing at rest (see Fig 12.9(b)). To increase ventilation these patients have to breathe at higher lung volumes and also allow more time for expiration by increasing flow rates during inspiration, where there is proportionately much less flow limitation. This explains the clinical phenomenon of a prolonged expiratory time in patients with severe airflow limitation.

The measure of the volume that can be forced in from RV in one second (FIV_1) will always be greater than that which can be forced out from TLC in one second (FEV_1). Thus, the ratio of FEV_1 to FIV_1 is below 1. The only exception to this occurs when there is significant obstruction to the airways outside the thorax, such as with a tumour mass in the upper part of the trachea. Under these circumstances expiratory airway narrowing is prevented by the tracheal resistance (a situation similar to pursing the lips) and expiratory airflow becomes more effort-dependent. During forced inspiration this same resistance causes such negative intraluminal pressure that the trachea is compressed by the surrounding atmospheric pressure. Inspiratory flow thus becomes less effort-dependent, and the ratio of FEV_1 to FIV_1 becomes greater than 1. This phenomenon, and the characteristic flow–volume loop, is used to diagnose extrathoracic airways obstruction (Fig 12.9(c)).

When obstruction occurs in large airways within the thorax (lower end of trachea and main bronchi), expiratory flow is impaired more than inspiratory flow but a characteristic plateau to expiratory flow is seen (Fig 12.9(d)).

Ventilation and perfusion relationships

For efficient gas exchange it is important that there is a match between ventilation of the alveoli ($\dot{V}_A$) and their perfusion ($\dot{Q}$). There is a wide variation in the $\dot{V}_A/\dot{Q}$ ratio throughout both normal and diseased lung. In the normal lung the extreme relationships between alveolar ventilation and perfusion are:

- ventilation but no perfusion (physiological deadspace)
- perfusion but no ventilation (physiological shunting).

These and the 'ideal' match are illustrated in Fig 12.10. In normal lungs there is a tendency for ventilation not to be matched by perfusion towards the apices, with the reverse occurring at the bases.

An increased physiological shunt results in arterial hypoxaemia. The effects of an increased physiological deadspace can usually be overcome by a compensatory increase in the ventilation of normally perfused alveoli. In advanced disease this compensation cannot occur, leading to increased alveolar and arterial $P\text{CO}_2$, together with hypoxaemia.

Hypoxaemia occurs more readily than hypercapnia because of the different ways in which oxygen and carbon dioxide are carried in the blood. Carbon dioxide can be considered to be in simple solution in the plasma, the

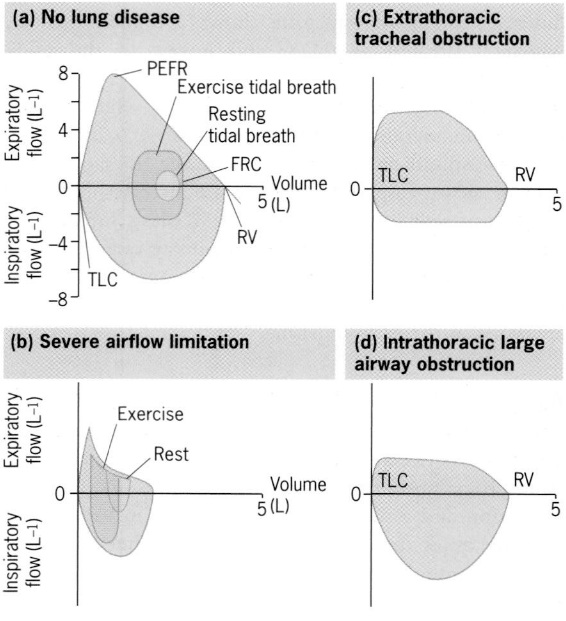

Fig 12.9
(a and b) Maximal flow-volume loops, showing the relationship between maximal flow rates on expiration and inspiration.
(a) In a normal subject.
(b) In a patient with severe airflow limitation.
Flow–volume loops during tidal breathing at rest (starting from the functional residual capacity (FRC)) and during exercise are also shown. The highest flow rates are achieved when forced expiration begins at total lung capacity (TLC) and represent the peak expiratory flow rate (PEFR). As air is blown out of the lung, so the flow rate decreases until no more air can be forced out, a point known as the residual volume (RV). Because inspiratory airflow is only dependent on effort, the shape of the maximal inspiratory flow–volume loop is quite different, and inspiratory flow remains at a high rate throughout the manoeuvre.
(c and d) Flow–volume loops of patients with large airway (tracheal) obstruction, showing plateauing of maximal expiratory flow high in the lung volume.
(c) Extrathoracic tracheal obstruction with a proportionally greater reduction of maximal inspiratory (as opposed to expiratory) flow rate.
(d) Intrathoracic large airway obstruction; the expiratory plateau is more pronounced and inspiratory flow rate is less reduced than in (c). In severe airflow limitation the ventilatory demands of exercise cannot be met (cf. a and b), greatly reducing effort tolerance

volume carried being proportional to the partial pressure. Oxygen is carried in chemical combination with haemoglobin in the red blood cells, and the relationship between the volume carried and the partial pressure is not linear (see Fig 13.5). Alveolar hyperventilation resulting in a low alveolar $P\text{CO}_2$ and a high alveolar $P\text{O}_2$ will therefore lead to a marked reduction in the carbon dioxide content of the resulting blood but no increase in the oxygen content. The hypoxaemia of even a small amount of physiological shunting cannot therefore be compensated for by hyperventilation.

The $P_a\text{O}_2$ and $P_a\text{CO}_2$ of some individuals who have mild disease of the lung causing slight $\dot{V}_A/\dot{Q}$ mismatch may still be normal. Increasing the requirements for gas exchange by exercise will widen the $\dot{V}_A/\dot{Q}$ mismatch and the $P_a\text{O}_2$ will fall. $\dot{V}_A/\dot{Q}$ mismatch is by far the most common cause of arterial hypoxaemia.

Alveolar stability

The alveoli of the lung are essentially hollow spheres. Surface tension acting at the curved internal surface tends to cause the sphere to decrease in size. The surface tension within the alveoli would make the lungs extremely difficult to distend were it not for the presence of surfactant. The type II cells within the alveolus secrete an insoluble lipoprotein largely consisting of dipalmitoyl lecithin, which forms a thin monomolecular layer at the air–fluid interface. Surfactant reduces surface tension so that alveoli remain stable.

Fluid surfaces covered with surfactant exhibit a phenomenon known as hysteresis; that is, the surface-tension-lowering effect of the surfactant can be improved by a transient increase in the size of the surface area of the alveoli. During quiet breathing, small areas of the lung undergo collapse, but it is possible to re-expand these rapidly by a deep breath; hence the importance of sighs or deep breaths as a feature of normal breathing. Failure of such a mechanism – which can occur, for example, in patients with fractured ribs – gives rise to patchy basal lung collapse. Surfactant levels may be reduced in a number of diseases that cause damage to the lung (e.g. pneumonia). Lack of surfactant plays a central role in the respiratory distress syndrome of the newborn. Severe reduction in perfusion of the lung causes impairment of surfactant activity and may well account for the characteristic areas of collapse associated with pulmonary embolism.

FURTHER READING

Manning HL, Schwartzstein RM (1995) Pathology of dyspnea. *New England Journal of Medicine* **333**: 1547–1553.

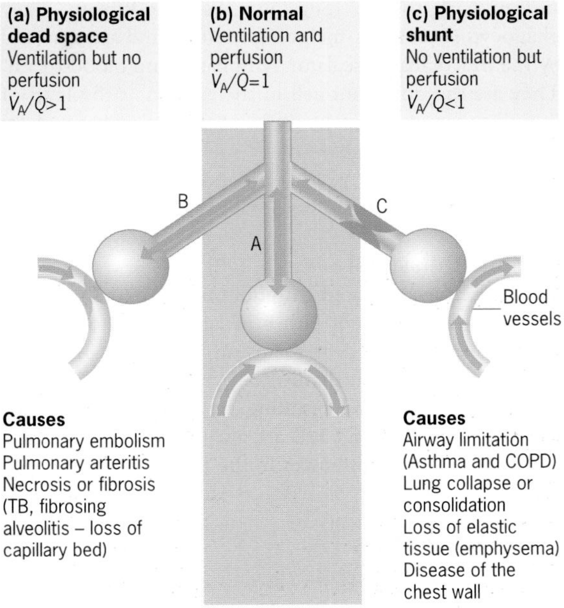

Fig 12.10
Relationships between ventilation and perfusion: a schematic diagram showing the alveolar–capillary interface. The centre shows normal ventilation and perfusion. On the left there is a block in perfusion (physiological deadspace), while on the right there is reduced ventilation (physiological shunting)

Defence mechanisms of the respiratory tract

Pulmonary disease often results from a failure of the many defence mechanisms that usually protect the lung in a healthy individual (Fig 12.11). These can be divided into physical and physiological mechanisms and humoral and cellular mechanisms.

Physical and physiological mechanisms

HUMIDIFICATION

This prevents dehydration of the epithelium.

PARTICLE REMOVAL

Over 90% of particles greater than 10 μm diameter are removed in the nostril or nasopharynx. Of the remainder, 5–10 μm particles become impacted in the carina and 1–2 μm particles are deposited in the distal lungs. Most pollen grain (>20 μm) particles are deposited in the nose and conjunctiva.

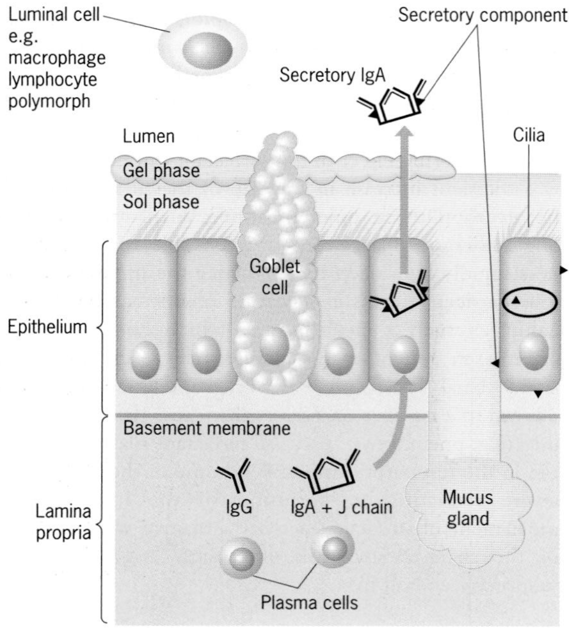

Fig 12.11
Defence mechanisms present at the epithelial surface

PARTICLE EXPULSION

This is effected by coughing, sneezing or gagging.

RESPIRATORY TRACT SECRETIONS

The mucus of the respiratory tract is a gelatinous substance consisting chiefly of acid and neutral polysaccharides. The mucus consists of a 5 μm thick gel that is relatively impermeable to water. This floats on a liquid or sol layer that is present around the cilia of the epithelial cells. The gel layer is secreted from goblet cells and mucous glands as distinct globules that coalesce increasingly in the central airways to form a more or less continuous mucus blanket. Under normal conditions the tips of the cilia are in contact with the undersurface of the gel phase and coordinate their movement to push the mucus blanket upwards. Whilst it may only take 30–60 minutes for mucus to be cleared from the large bronchi, there may be a delay of several days before clearance is achieved from respiratory bronchioles. One of the major long-term effects of cigarette smoking is a reduction in mucociliary transport. This contributes to recurrent infection and in the larger airways it prolongs contact with carcinogens. Air pollutants, local and general anaesthetics and bacterial and viral infections also reduce mucociliary clearance.

Congenital defects in mucociliary transport occur. In the 'immotile cilia' syndrome there is an absence of the dynein arms in the cilia themselves, and in cystic fibrosis an abnormal mucus is associated with ciliary dyskinesia. Both diseases are characterized by recurrent infections and eventually with the development of bronchiectasis.

Humoral and cellular mechanisms

Nonspecific soluble factors

- *α_1-Antitrypsin* (α_1-antiprotease, see p. 327) is present in lung secretions derived from plasma. It inhibits chymotrypsin and trypsin and neutralizes proteases and elastase.
- *Lysozyme* is an enzyme found in granulocytes that has bacteriocidal properties.
- *Lactoferrin* is synthesized from epithelial cells and neutrophil granulocytes and has bacteriocidal properties.
- *Interferon* (see p. 166) is produced by most cells in response to viral infection. It is a potent modulator of lymphocyte function. It renders other cells resistant to infection by any other virus.
- *Complement* is present in secretions and is derived by diffusion from plasma. In association with antibodies, it plays an important cytotoxic role.
- *Surfactant protein A* (SP_A) is one of four species of surfactant proteins which opsonizes bacteria/particles, enhancing phagocytosis by macrophages.
- *Defensins* are bactericidal peptides present in the azurophil granules of neutrophils.

Pulmonary alveolar macrophages

These are derived from precursors in the bone marrow and migrate to the lungs via the bloodstream. They phagocytose particles, including bacteria, and are removed by the mucociliary escalator, lymphatics and bloodstream. They are the dominant cell in the airways at the level of the alveoli and comprise 90% of all cells obtained by bronchoalveolar lavage.

Macrophages (see p. 174) process antigens and play a part in both cellular and humoral immunity.

Lymphoid tissue (see also p. 172)

The bronchus-associated lymphoid tissue (BALT) consists of lymphocytes present either in aggregates (tonsils and adenoids) or scattered. It forms an important immunological defence mechanism. Lymphocytes become sensitized to antigens, resulting in local production of secretory IgA. IgG and IgE are also present in secretions derived from B lymphocytes in the lamina propria.

FURTHER READING

Stockley RA (1998) Role of bacteria in the pathogenesis and progression of acute and chronic lung infection. *Thorax* **53**: 58–62.

Wanner A, Salathé M, O'Riordan TG (1996) Mucociliary clearance in the airways. *American Journal of Respiratory and Critical Care Medicine* **154**: 1868–1882.

Symptoms

Runny, blocked nose and sneezing

Nasal symptoms are extremely common. The differentiation between the common cold or allergic rhinitis as a cause of 'runny nose' (rhinorrhoea), nasal blockage and attacks of sneezing is difficult. In allergic rhinitis, symptoms may be seasonal, following contact with grass pollen, or perennial, when the house-dust mite is the important allergen. Colds are frequent during the winter but, if more than three occur, the patient is probably suffering from perennial rhinitis rather than from infection due to a virus. Patients may be able to identify the cause of their symptoms if, for example, they sneeze whilst walking in the park in summer or after making beds.

Nasal secretions are usually thin and runny in rhinitis but thicker and yellowish green in the common cold. Nose bleeds and blood-stained nasal discharge are common occurrences and are not as serious as haemoptysis. Nevertheless, a blood-stained nasal discharge associated with nasal obstruction and pain may be the presenting feature of a nasal tumour. Total nasal blockage with loss of smell is often a feature of nasal polyps.

Cough

Cough is the most common manifestation of lower respiratory tract disease. Smokers often have a morning cough with little sputum. Cough is the cardinal feature of chronic bronchitis, while sputum production and coughing, particularly at night, can be symptoms of asthma. Cough also occurs in asthmatics after mild exertion or following a forced expiration. A cough can also occur for psychological reasons.

A worsening cough is the most common presenting symptom of a bronchial carcinoma. The explosive character of a normal cough is lost when laryngeal paralysis is present – a bovine cough – usually resulting from carcinoma of the bronchus infiltrating the left recurrent laryngeal nerve. Cough may be accompanied by stridor in whooping cough and in the presence of laryngeal or tracheal obstruction.

Despite the popularity of cough mixtures, the correct treatment of this symptom is to identify and treat the underlying cause. Cough may persist in some individuals for many weeks following a respiratory tract infection, perhaps as the result of persisting bronchial inflammation and increased airway responsiveness, a process that may settle with inhaled corticosteroid treatment.

Sputum

Approximately 100 mL of mucus is produced daily in a healthy, non-smoking individual. This flows at a regular pace up the airways, through the larynx, and is swallowed. Excess mucus is expectorated as sputum. The most common cause of excess mucus production is cigarette smoking.

Mucoid sputum is clear and white but can contain black specks resulting from the inhalation of carbon. Yellow or green sputum is due to the presence of cellular material, including bronchial epithelial cells, or neutrophil or eosinophil granulocytes. Yellow sputum is not necessarily due to infection, as eosinophils in the sputum, as seen in asthma, can give the same appearance. The production of large quantities of yellow or green sputum is characteristic of bronchiectasis.

Haemoptysis (blood-stained sputum) varies from small streaks of blood to massive bleeding. The following should be borne in mind.

- The most common cause of haemoptysis is acute infection, particularly in exacerbations of chronic obstructive pulmonary disease (COPD) but it should not be attributed to this without investigation.
- Other common causes are pulmonary infarction, bronchial carcinoma and tuberculosis.
- In lobar pneumonia, the sputum is rusty in appearance when blood is present.
- Pink, frothy sputum is seen in pulmonary oedema.
- In bronchiectasis, the blood is often mixed with purulent sputum.
- Massive haemoptyses (>200 mL of blood in 24 hours) are usually due to bronchiectasis or tuberculosis.
- Uncommon causes of haemoptyses are idiopathic pulmonary haemosiderosis, Goodpasture's syndrome, microscopic polyarteritis, trauma, blood disorders and benign tumours.

Haemoptysis should always be investigated. Often, the diagnosis can be made from a chest X-ray.

Firm plugs of sputum may be coughed up by patients suffering from an exacerbation of allergic bronchopulmonary aspergillosis. Sometimes such sputum may appear as firm threads representing casts from inflamed bronchi.

Breathlessness (Table 12.1)

Breathlessness should be assessed in relation to the patient's lifestyle. For example, a moderate degree of breathlessness may be totally disabling if the patient has to climb many flights of stairs to reach home. A grading for breathlessness is given on p. 630.

Dyspnoea should be used to describe a sense of awareness of increased respiratory effort that is unpleasant and that is recognized by the patient as being inappropriate. It is highly unlikely that this term will be used by the patient. Patients may complain of tightness in the chest; this must be differentiated from angina. Respiratory sensations described by patients with different chest diseases are shown in Table 12.1.

Table 12.1
Respiratory sensations described by patients with different chest diseases

Sensation	Asthma	Chronic obstructive pulmonary disease (COPD)	Pulmonary fibrosis	Chest wall disease	Congestive heart failure	Pulmonary vascular visease
Rapid breathing					✓	✓
Shallow breathing	✓					
Incomplete exhalation	✓					
Increased effort	✓	✓	✓	✓		
Feeling of suffocation (heavy breathing)	✓	✓				
Chest tightness	✓					

Orthopnoea (see p. 630) is breathlessness on lying down and is partly due to the weight of the abdominal contents pushing the diaphragm further into the thorax. Such patients are also made uncomfortable by bending over.

Tachypnoea and *hyperpnoea* refer, respectively, to an increased rate of breathing and an increased level of ventilation, which may be appropriate to the situation (e.g. during exercise).

Hyperventilation is overbreathing and results in a lowering of the alveolar and arterial $P\text{CO}_2$ (see p. 1129).

Paroxysmal nocturnal dyspnoea is described on p. 630.

Respiratory diseases can cause breathlessness over differing time periods:

- Sudden
  - (a) Inhaled foreign body
  - (b) Pneumothorax
  - (c) Pulmonary embolism
- Over a few hours
  - (a) Asthma
  - (b) Pneumonia
  - (c) Pulmonary oedema
  - (d) Extrinsic allergic alveolitis
- Intermittent
  - (a) Asthma
  - (b) Pulmonary oedema
- Over days
  - (a) Pleural effusions
  - (b) Carcinoma of the bronchus/trachea
- Over months or years
  - (a) Chronic obstructive pulmonary disease (COPD)
  - (b) Cryptogenic fibrosing alveolitis
  - (c) Occupational fibrotic lung disease
  - (d) Non-respiratory causes – anaemia, hyperthyroidism.

Wheezing

Wheezing is a common complaint and is the result of airflow limitation due to any cause. The symptom of wheezing is *not* diagnostic of asthma; it may be absent in the early stages of this disease, and may also occur in patients with chronic obstructive pulmonary disease.

Chest pain

The most common type of chest pain encountered in respiratory disease is a localized sharp pain, often referred to as pleuritic. It is made worse by deep breathing or coughing and can be precisely localized by the patient. Localized anterior chest pain may be accompanied by tenderness of a costochondral junction as a symptom of costochondritis. Pain in the shoulder tips suggests irritation of the diaphragmatic pleura, whereas central chest pain radiating to the neck and arms is typically of cardiac origin. Retrosternal soreness may occur in patients with tracheitis, and a constant, severe, dull pain may be the result of invasion of the thoracic wall by carcinoma.

FURTHER READING

Pasterkamp H, Kraman SS, Wodicka GR (1997) Respiratory sounds. Advances beyond the stethoscope. *American Journal of Respiratory and Critical Care Medicine* **156**: 974–987.

Examination of the respiratory system

The nose

The anterior part of the nose can be examined using a nasal speculum and light source. In allergic rhinitis the mucosa lining the nasal septum and inferior turbinate appears swollen and a dark red or plum colour. Nasal polyps can also be identified, as can a frequent site of nasal haemorrhage (Little's area).

The chest (Table 12.2)

Radiology is an essential part of examination of the chest. Diseases such as tuberculosis or lung cancer may not be detectable on clinical examination but are obvious on the chest X-ray. Conversely, the abnormal physical signs in asthma or chronic bronchitis may be associated with a normal chest X-ray.

EXAMINATION OF THE CHEST

Inspection

The patient should be observed carefully, paying particular attention to mental alertness, cyanosis, breathlessness at rest, use of accessory muscles and any deformity or scars on the chest. A coarse tremor or flap of the outstretched hands indicates CO_2 intoxication. Prominent veins on the chest may imply obstruction of the superior vena cava. The jugular venous pressure should be assessed.

Central cyanosis (see p. 632) is assessed on the colour of the tongue and lips, and indicates a P_aO_2 below 6 kPa. *Peripheral cyanosis* is noted on the fingernails and skin of the extremities and in the absence of central cyanosis is due to a reduced peripheral circulation.

Finger clubbing is present when the normal angle between the base of the nail and the nail fold is lost. The base of the nail is fluctuant owing to increased vascularity, and there is an increased curvature of the nail in all directions, with expansion of the end of the digit. Some causes of clubbing are given in Table 12.3. Clubbing is not seen in chronic bronchitis.

Table 12.2
Physical signs of respiratory disease

Pathological process	Chest wall movement	Mediastinal displacement	Percussion note	Breath sounds	Vocal resonance	Added sounds
Consolidation (i.e. lobar pneumonia)	Reduced on affected side	None	Dull	Bronchial	Increased	Fine crackles
Collapse						
Major bronchus	Reduced on affected side	Towards lesion	Dull	Diminished or absent	Reduced or absent	None
Peripheral bronchus	Reduced on affected side	Towards lesion	Dull	Bronchial	Increased	Fine crackles
Fibrosis						
Localized	Reduced on affected side	Towards lesion	Dull	Bronchial	Increased	Coarse crackles
Generalized (e.g. cryptogenic fibrosing alveolitis)	Reduced on both sides	None	Normal	Vesicular	Increased	Fine crackles
Pleural effusion (>500 mL)	Reduced on affected side	Away from lesion (in massive effusion)	Stony dull	Vesicular reduced or absent	Reduced or absent	None
Large pneumothorax	Reduced on affected side	Away from lesion	Normal or hyperresonant	Reduced or absent	Reduced or absent	None
Asthma	Reduced on both sides	None	Normal	Vesicular Prolonged expiration	Normal	Expiratory polyphonic wheeze
Chronic obstructive pulmonary disease	Reduced on both sides	None	Normal	Vesicular Prolonged expiration	Normal	Expiratory polyphonic wheeze and coarse crackles

Table 12.3
Some causes of finger clubbing

Respiratory	Cardiovascular
Bronchial carcinoma, especially epidermoid (squamous cell) type (major cause)	Cyanotic heart disease
Chronic suppurative lung disease	Subacute infective endocarditis
Bronchiectasis	
Lung abscess	**Miscellaneous**
Empyema	Congenital - no disease
Pulmonary fibrosis (e.g. cryptogenic fibrosing alveolitis)	Cirrhosis
Pleural and mediastinal tumours (e.g. mesothelioma)	Inflammatory bowel disease
Cryptogenic organizing pneumonia	

Palpation

The position of the mediastinum should be ascertained by checking whether the trachea is central and whether the cardiac apex is in the fifth intercostal space. The supraclavicular fossa is examined for enlarged lymph nodes. The distance between the sternal notch and the cricoid cartilage (three to four finger breadths in full expiration) is reduced in patients with severe airflow limitation. Movement of the upper and lower parts of the chest should be assessed. Compression of the chest laterally and anteroposteriorly may produce a localized pain suggestive of a rib fracture.

Percussion

This should be performed symmetrically on both sides for comparison. Liver dullness is usually detected anteriorly at the level of the sixth rib. Liver and cardiac dullness are lost with over-inflated lungs. The percussion note is dull over consolidation and stony dull over a pleural effusion.

Auscultation

The diaphragm of the stethoscope should be used. The patient is asked to take deep breaths through the mouth. Inspiration sounds more prolonged than expiration. Healthy lungs filter off most of the high-frequency component, mainly due to turbulent flow in the larynx. Normal breath sounds are harsher anteriorly over the upper lobes (particularly on the right) and described as vesicular. Vesicular sounds may be loud in a thin healthy subject or soft in patients with emphysema. Breath sounds are reduced or absent in a pneumothorax, over a pleural effusion, or when the bronchus to a lobe is obstructed by a carcinoma.

Bronchial breathing

These abnormal breath sounds are heard best over consolidated or collapsed lung and sometimes over areas of localized fibrosis or bronchiectasis. Such areas conduct the high-frequency hissing component of breath sounds well. Characteristically, the noise heard during inspiration and expiration is equally long but separated by a short silent phase. Bronchial breathing can be imitated by listening over the larynx, particularly if the subject breathes with the vocal cords in a position to sound a whispered 'eee'. Whispering pectoriloquy (whispered, and therefore higher-pitched, sounds heard distinctly) invariably accompanies bronchial breathing.

Added sounds

The terms 'rhonchi', 'rales' and 'crepitations' are best discarded and replaced with the simple terms *wheezes* and *crackles*.

Wheeze. Wheeze is usually heard during expiration and results from vibrations in the collapsible part of the airways when apposition occurs as a result of the flow-limiting mechanisms. Wheezes are heard in asthma and in chronic obstructive pulmonary disease, but are not invariably present. In the most severe cases of asthma a wheeze may not be heard, as the airflow may be insufficient to generate the sound. Wheezes may be monophonic (single large airway obstruction) or polyphonic (narrowing of many small airways).

Crackles. These brief crackling sounds are probably produced by opening of previously closed bronchioles, and their timing during breathing is of significance – early inspiratory crackles are associated with diffuse airflow limitation, whereas late inspiratory crackles are characteristically heard in pulmonary oedema, fibrosis of the lung and bronchiectasis. They may be described as fine or coarse but this is of no significance.

Pleural rub. This is a creaking or groaning sound that is usually well localized. It is indicative of inflammation and roughening of the pleural surfaces, which normally glide silently over one another.

Vocal resonance and fremitus. Healthy lung attenuates high-frequency notes, leaving the booming low-pitched components of speech. Consolidated lung has the reverse effect, transmitting the high frequencies; the spoken word then takes on a bleating quality. Whispered (and therefore high-pitched) speech can barely be heard over healthy lung, whereas consolidation allows its clear transmission. Sonorous sounds such as 'ninety-nine' are well transmitted across healthy lung to produce vibration that can be felt over the chest wall. Consolidated lung transmits these low-frequency noises less well, and pleural fluid severely dampens or obliterates the vibrations altogether.

Additional bedside tests

Since so many patients with respiratory disease have airflow limitation, airflow should be routinely measured at the bedside using a peak flow meter. This will provide a much more accurate assessment of airflow limitation than any physical sign.

Investigation of respiratory disease

Routine haematological and biochemical tests

These should include tests for:

- haemoglobin, to detect the presence of anaemia
- packed cell volume (PCV) (secondary polycythaemia occurs with COPD)
- routine biochemistry.

Other blood investigations sometimes required include (α_1-antitrypsin levels, autoantibodies, and, in asthma, IgE to specific allergens (RAST; radioallergosorbent test) and *Aspergillus* antibodies.

Sputum

Sputum should be inspected for colour:

- yellowish green indicates inflammation (infection or allergy)
- the presence of blood suggests neoplasm or pulmonary infarct.

Microbiological studies (Gram stain and culture) are not helpful in upper respiratory tract infections or in acute or chronic bronchitis. They *are* of value in:

- pneumonia
- the diagnosis of tuberculosis (Ziehl–Nielsen stain)
- unusual clinical problems
- *Aspergillus* lung disease.

Cytology

This is extremely useful in the diagnosis of bronchial carcinoma. Advantages are:

- a quick result
- cheapness
- it is non-invasive.

However, its value depends on the production of sputum and the presence of a reliable cytologist. Sputum can be induced following the inhalation of nebulized hypertonic saline (5%). This is unpleasant and for important samples it is better to proceed to transtracheal aspiration or more usually bronchoscopy and bronchial washings (see p. 766).

Transtracheal aspiration

This technique involves pushing a needle through the cricothyroid membrane, through which a catheter is threaded to a position just above the carina. This procedure induces coughing, and specimens are collected by aspiration or by the introduction and subsequent aspiration of sterile saline. It is an excellent technique (although not often required) for assessing infection in the lower respiratory tract because it obviates any possibility of contamination of the specimen with bacteria from the pharynx and mouth.

Imaging

CHEST X-RAY

The following must be taken into account when viewing films:

- *Centring of the film.* The distance between each clavicular head and the spinal processes must be equal.
- *Penetration.*
- *The view.* Postero-anterior (PA) is the routine film. Antero-posterior (AP) films are taken only in very ill patients who are unable to stand up or be taken to the radiology department; the cardiac outline appears bigger and the scapulae cannot be moved out of the way.

The following should be noted:

- the shape and bony structure of the chest wall
- whether the trachea is central
- whether the diaphragm is elevated or flat
- the shape, size and position of the heart
- the shape and size of the hilar shadows
- the vascular shadowing and the size and shape of any abnormalities of the lungs.

X-ray abnormalities

Collapse and consolidation

A diagram showing the X-ray changes in collapse of a whole lung is given in Fig 12.12 and causes are shown in Table 12.4.

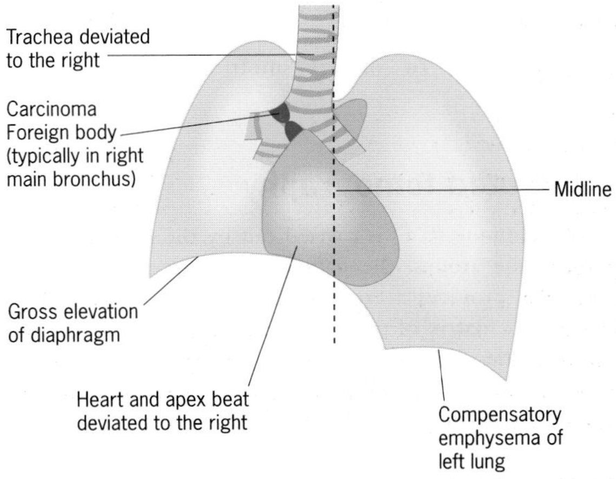

Fig 12.12
Collapse of the right lung. Diagram showing a raised right diaphragm and compensatory emphysema of the left lung

Table 12.4
Causes of collapse of the lung

Tumours Enlarged tracheobronchial lymph nodes due to: Malignant disease Tuberculosis Inhaled foreign bodies (e.g. peanuts) in children, usually in the right main bronchus	Bronchial casts or plugs (e.g. allergic bronchopulmonary aspergillosis) Retained secretions - postoperatively and in debilitated patients

Pleural effusion

Pleural effusions need to be more than 500 mL to cause much more than blunting of the costophrenic angle. On an erect film they produce a characteristic shadow with a curved upper edge rising into the axilla. If very large, the whole of one side of the thorax may be opaque, with shift of the mediastinum to the opposite side.

Fibrosis

Localized fibrosis causes streaky shadowing and the accompanying loss of lung volume causes mediastinal structures to move to the same side. More generalized fibrosis in the lung can lead to a honeycomb appearance (see p. 813), seen as diffuse shadows containing multiple circular translucences a few millimetres in diameter.

Round shadows

The causes of round shadows (> 3 cm) are shown in Table 12.5.

Miliary mottling

This term describes numerous minute opacities, 1–3 mm in size, which are caused by many pathological processes. The most common causes are miliary tuberculosis, pneumoconiosis, sarcoidosis, fibrosing alveolitis and pulmonary oedema, though the latter is usually perihilar and accompanied by larger, fluffy shadows. A rare but striking cause of miliary mottling is pulmonary microlithiasis.

Table 12.5
Causes of round shadows (>3 cm) in the lung

Carcinoma Metastatic tumours (usually multiple shadows) Tuberculoma (may be calcification within the lesion) Lung abscess (usually with fluid level) Encysted interlobar effusion (usually in horizontal fissure) Hydatid cysts (rare and often with a fluid level) Arteriovenous malformations (usually adjacent to a vascular shadow)	Aspergilloma Rheumatoid nodules Rare causes: Bronchial carcinoid Cylindroma Chondroma Lipoma Other shadows related to mediastinum: Pericardium, Oesophagus, Spinal cord } Seen on lateral chest X-ray

Computed tomography

This technique (CT) is carried out by the rotation of an X-ray tube around the patient in a series of complete circles. It provides a cross-sectional image consisting of 512 × 512 matrix of picture elements (pixels). Each pixel records the X-ray absorption of the corresponding volume element (voxel) in the patient. CT differentiates tissues by their relative densities, with air and fat being of low density and bone of high density.

The computerized image is manipulated such that scans can be viewed at different settings to show lung parenchymal tissue (90% air, 10% soft tissue) with the trachea and main bronchi, or centred at soft tissue density to show mediastinal structures (Fig 12.13). Demonstration of mediastinal structures is facilitated by injection of intravenous contrast to enhance the vascular structures. Vessels and nodes can be distinguished and the enhancement characteristics of a mass aids diagnosis.

The advent of rapid volumetric or 'spiral' scanning means that scans can be obtained rapidly (within seconds) during contrast injection. This is a useful technique for directly demonstrating pulmonary emboli within pulmonary vessels.

CT is valuable in bronchial carcinoma staging to demonstrate mediastinal, pleural or chest wall invasion and to determine operability. Enlarged mediastinal nodes (>1 cm) may be either malignant or reactive and may require biopsy. Scanning should include assessment of liver, adrenals and brain, which are likely sites for metastatic disease.

High-resolution CT scanning involves sampling the lung parenchyma with thin 1–2 mm thickness scans at 10–20 mm intervals throughout the lungs. This technique allows assessment of diffuse lung parenchymal processes, particularly interstitial disease. It is valuable in the following situations:

- Detection of diffuse interstitial pulmonary involvement in any type of interstitial lung disease, including sarcoidosis, cryptogenic and extrinsic allergic alveolitis, occupational lung disease, and any other form of interstitial pulmonary fibrosis.
- Bronchiectasis. High-resolution CT has a sensitivity and specificity of greater than 90%. Inspiratory and expiratory scans may allow demonstration of air trapping in small airway disease. This technique has replaced bronchography.
- Distinguishing emphysema from interstitial lung disease or pulmonary vascular disease as a cause of a low gas transfer factor with otherwise normal lung function
- Diagnosis of lymphangitis carcinomatosa.

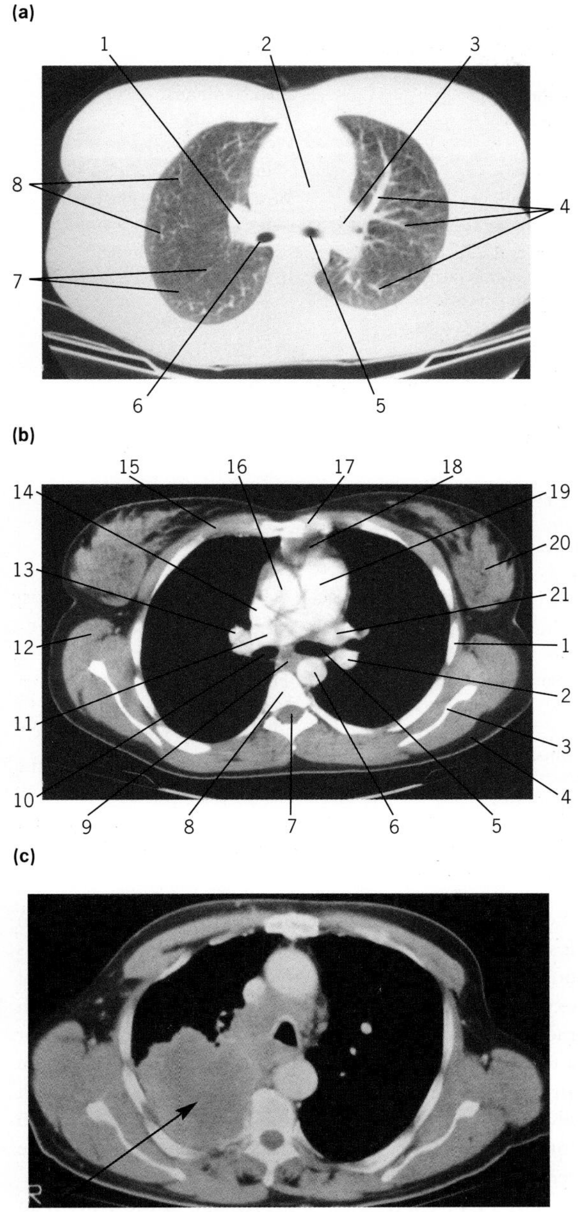

Fig 12.13
CT scan of the lung.
(a) Lung setting – showing normal lung markings. 1, right hilum; 2, mediastinum; 3, left hilum; 4, lung vessels; 5, L. main bronchus; 6, R. main bronchus; 7, position of oblique fissure; 8, peripheral lung vessels
(b) Mediastinal (soft tissue) setting – showing normal mediastinal structures following intravenous contrast enhancement. 1, rib; 2, descending L. pulmonary artery; 3, scapula; 4, subcutaneous fat; 5, L. main bronchus; 6, descending aorta; 7, spinal canal; 8, vertebral body; 9, oesophagus; 10, R. main bronchus; 11, R. pulmonary artery; 12, muscle; 13, R. superior pulmonary vein; 14, superior vena cava; 15, costal cartilage; 16, ascending aorta; 17, sternum; 18, thymic remnant; 19, pulmonary trunk; 20, breast tissue; 21, L. superior pulmonary vein
(c) Post contrast scan showing large right upper zone carcinoma with enlarged lymph nodes in the mediastinum surrounding the trachea

Magnetic resonance imaging

Problems with motion artefact, both respiratory and cardiac, make MRI less valable than CT in assessment of lung parenchyma. These problems are partially overcome in the mediastinum by appropriate gating and the advent of fast acquisition scanning. The main strength of MRI in staging lung cancer is in the assessment of mediastinal, chest wall and particularly apical invasion of tumour, by virtue of its ability to produce images easily in the sagittal and coronal planes. Vascular structures are clearly differentiated as flowing blood produces a signal void on MRI.

Scintigraphic imaging

This technique is used widely for the detection of pulmonary emboli.

Perfusion scan

Macro-aggregated human albumin labelled with technetium-99m is injected intravenously. The particles are of such a size that they impact in pulmonary capillaries, where they remain for a few hours. A gamma camera is then used to detect the position of the macro-aggregated human albumin. The resultant pattern indicates the distribution of pulmonary blood flow; cold areas occur where there is defective blood flow (e.g. in pulmonary emboli).

Ventilation–perfusion scan

Xenon-133 gas is inhaled into the lung and its distribution is detected at the same time. On using the two scans, a pulmonary embolus can be seen to cause a striking diminution of perfusion relative to ventilation. Other lung diseases (e.g. asthma or pneumonia) impair both ventilation and perfusion. Unfortunately, however, a pulmonary embolus often produces substantial changes in the lung substance (e.g. atelectasis) so that such a clear distinction is not always obvious. Nevertheless, this is a better technique than perfusion scan alone.

Respiratory function tests (Table 12.6)

In practice, airflow limitation can be assessed by use of relatively simple tests that have good intrasubject repeatability. Normal values are required for their interpretation since these tests vary considerably, not only with sex, age and height, but also within individuals of the same age, sex and height. The standard deviation about the mean for a group of individuals is therefore very high; for example, the standard deviation for the peak expiratory flow rate is approximately 50 L min^{-1}, and for the FEV_1 it is approximately 0.4 L. Repeated measurements of lung function are required for assessing the progression of disease in an individual patient.

Table 12.6
Respiratory function tests and exercise tests

Test	Use	Advantages	Disadvantages
PEFR	Monitoring changes in airflow limitation in asthma	Portable Can be used at the bedside	Effort-dependent Poor measure of airflow limitation
FEV, FVC, FEV_1/FVC	Assessment of airflow limitation The best single test	Reproducible Relatively effort-independent	Bulky equipment but smaller portable machines available
Flow–volume curves	Assessment of flow at lower lung volumes Detection of large airway obstruction both intra- and extra-thoracic (e.g tracheal stenosis, tumour)	Recognition of patterns of flow–volume curves for different diseases	Sophisticated equipment needed
Airways resistance	Assessment of airflow limitation	Sensitive	Technique difficult to perform
Lung volumes	Differentiation between restrictive and obstructive lung disease	Essential adjunct to FEV_1	Sophisticated equipment needed
Gas transfer	Assessment and monitoring of extent of interstitial lung disease and emphysema	Non-invasive (compared with lung biopsy or radiation from repeated chest X-rays and CT)	Sophisticated equipment needed
Blood gases	Assessment of respiratory failure	Can detect early lung disease when measured during exercise	Invasive
Pulse oximetry	Postoperative, sleep studies and respiratory failure	Continuous monitoring Non-invasive	Measures saturation only
Exercise tests (6 min walk)	Practical assessment for disability and effects of therapy	No equipment required	Time consuming Learning effect At least two walks required
Cardiorespiratory assessment	Early detection of lung/heart disease Fitness assessment	Essential in differentiating breathlessness due to lung or heart disease	Expensive and complicated equipment required

Tests of ventilatory function

These tests are used mainly to assess the degree of airflow limitation present during expiration.

Peak expiratory flow rate (PEFR)

This is an extremely simple and cheap test. Subjects are asked to take a full inspiration to total lung capacity and then blow out forcefully into the peak flow meter (Fig 12.14), which is held horizontally. The lips must be placed tightly around the mouthpiece. The best of three tests is recorded.

Although reproducible, PEFR is not a good measure of airflow limitation since it measures the expiratory flow rate only in the first 2 ms of expiration and overestimates lung function in patients with moderate airflow limitation. PEFR is best used to monitor progression of disease and its treatment. Regular measurements of peak flow rates on waking, during the afternoon, and before bed demonstrate the wide diurnal variations in airflow limitation that characterize asthma and allow an objective assessment of treatment to be made (Fig 12.15).

Spirometry

The Vitalograph spirometer measures the FEV_1 and the forced vital capacity (FVC). Both the FEV_1 and FVC are related to height, age and sex. The instrument used is shown in Fig 12.16. The technique involves a maximum inspiration followed by a forced expiration (for as long as possible) into the dry bellows spirometer. The act of expiration triggers the moving record chart, which measures volume against time. The record chart moves for a total of 5 s, but expiration should continue until all the air has been expelled from the lungs, as patients with severe airflow limitation may have a very prolonged forced expiratory time. This is demonstrated on the record chart in Fig 12.16.

The FEV_1 expressed as a percentage of the FVC is an excellent measure of airflow limitation. In normal subjects it is around 75%. With *increasing airflow limitation* the FEV_1 falls proportionately more than the FVC, so that the FEV_1/FVC ratio is reduced. With *restrictive lung disease* the FEV_1 and the FVC are reduced in the same proportion and the FEV_1/FVC ratio remains normal or may even increase because of the enhanced elastic recoil.

In chronic airflow limitation (particularly in emphysema and asthma) the total lung capacity (TLC) is usually increased, yet there is nearly always some reduction in the FVC. This is the result of disease in the small airways causing obstruction to airflow before the normal RV is reached. This trapping of air within the lung (giving an increased RV) is a characteristic feature of these diseases.

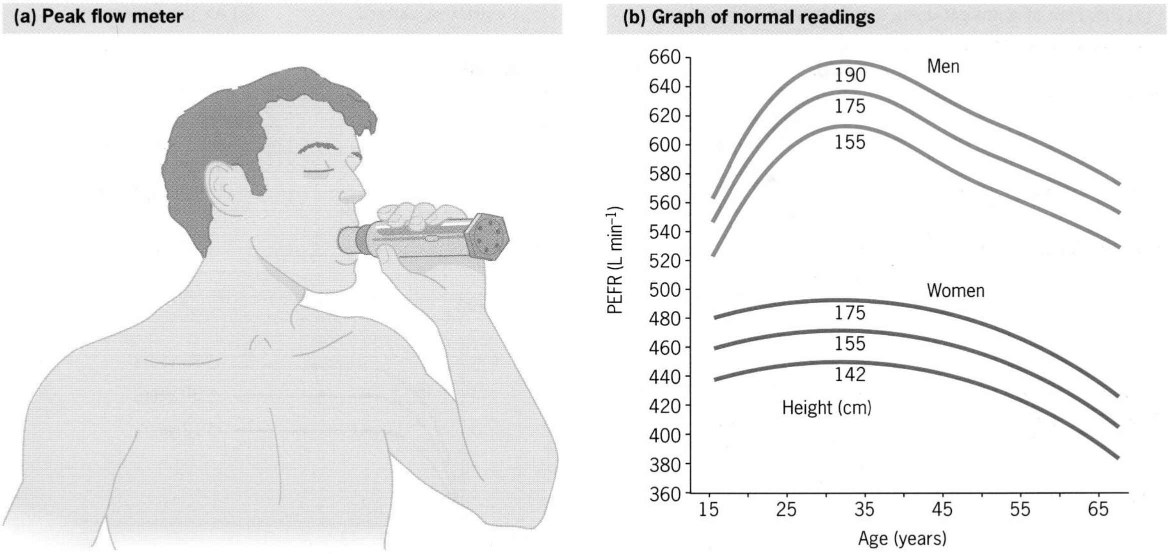

Fig 12.14
Peak flow measurements.
(a) Peak flow meter: the lips should be tight around the mouthpiece
(b) Graph of normal readings for men and women

Other tests

Tests such as the measurement of airways resistance in a body plethysmograph are more sensitive but the equipment is expensive and the necessary manoeuvres are too exhausting for many patients with chronic airflow limitation.

Flow–volume loops

The ability to measure flow rates against volume (flow–volume loops; see Fig 12.9) enables a more sophisticated analysis to be made of the site of airflow limitation within the lung. At the start of expiration from TLC, the site of maximum resistance is the large airways, and this accounts for the flow reduction in the first 25% of the curve. As the lung volume reduces further, so the elastic pressures within the lung holding open the smaller airways reduce, and disease either of the lung parenchyma or the small airways themselves becomes readily apparent. For example, in diseases such as chronic obstructive pulmonary disease (COPD), where the brunt of the disease falls upon the smaller airways, expiratory flow rates at 50% or 25% of the vital capacity may be disproportionately reduced when compared with flow rates at larger lung volumes.

Lung volume

The subdivisions of the lung volume are shown in Fig 12.17. Tidal volume and vital capacity can be measured using a simple spirometer, but the TLC and RV need to be measured by an alternative technique. TLC is measured by connecting the lungs to a reservoir containing a known amount of non-absorbable gas (helium) that can readily be measured. If the concentration of the gas in the reservoir is known at the start of the test and is measured after equilibration of the gas has occurred (when the patient has breathed in and out of the reservoir), the dilution of the gas will reflect the TLC. This technique is known as *helium dilution*. RV can be calculated by subtracting the vital capacity from the TLC.

The TLC measured using this technique is inaccurate if large cystic spaces are present in the lung, because the helium cannot diffuse into them. Under these circumstances the thoracic gas volume can be measured more accurately using a body plethysmograph. The difference between the two measurements can be used to define the extent of non-communicating air space within the lungs.

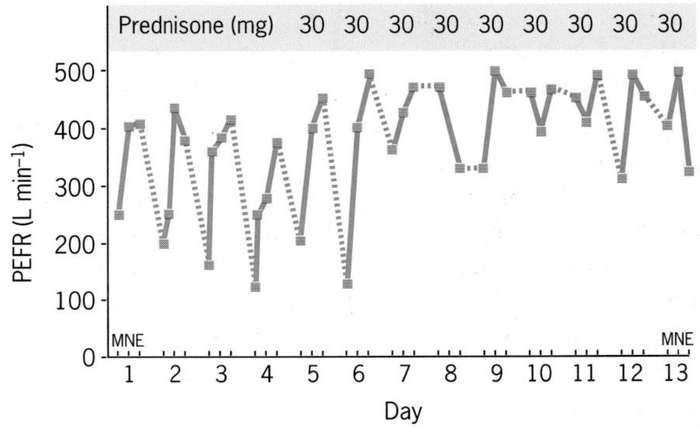

Fig 12.15
Diurnal variability in airflow limitation, showing the effect of steroids. M, morning; N, noon; E, evening

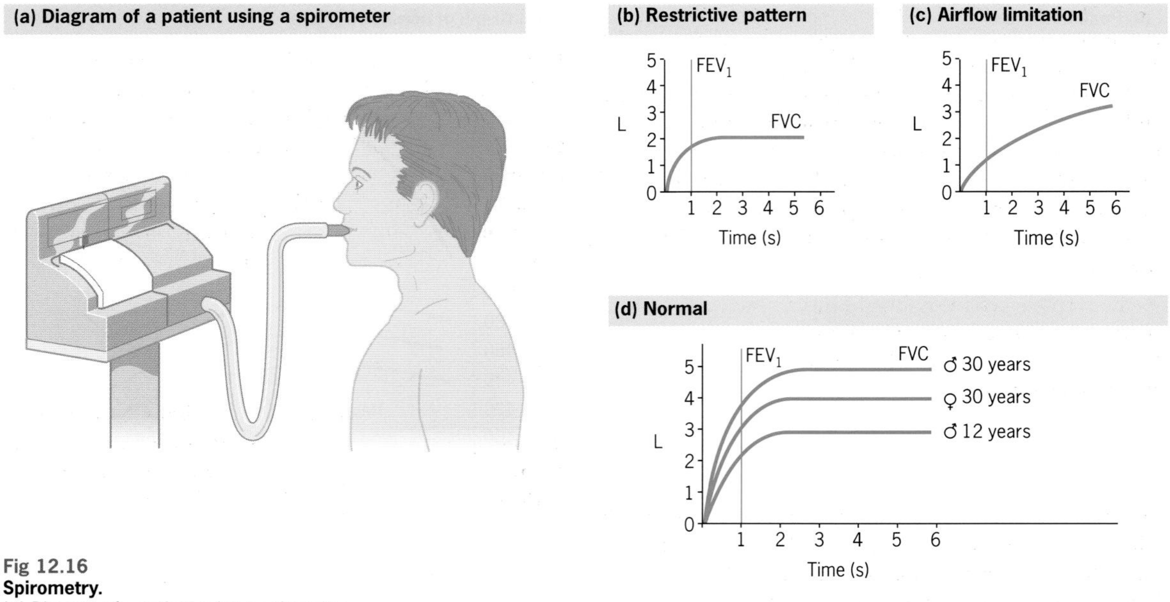

Fig 12.16
Spirometry.
(a) Diagram of a patient using a spirometer
(b)-(d) Graphs showing **(b) restrictive pattern** (FEV_1 and FVC reduced), **(c) airflow limitation** (FEV_1 only reduced), and **(d) normal patterns** for age and sex

Transfer factor

This measures the transfer of gas across the alveolar–capillary membrane and reflects the uptake of oxygen from the alveoli into the red cells. A low concentration of carbon monoxide is inhaled and is avidly taken up in a linear fashion by circulating haemoglobin, the amount of which must be known when the test is performed. In normal lungs the transfer factor is a true measure of the diffusing capacity of the lungs for oxygen and depends on the thickness of the alveolar–capillary membrane. In lung disease the diffusing capacity (D_{CO}) also depends on the $\dot{V}_A/\dot{Q}$ relationship as well as on the area and thickness of the alveolar membrane. To control for differences in lung volume, the uptake of carbon monoxide is related to the lung volume; this is known as the transfer coefficient (K_{CO}).

Gas transfer is usually reduced in patients with severe degrees of emphysema and fibrosis. Overall gas transfer can be thought of as a relatively nonspecific test of lung function but one that can be particularly used in the early detection and assessment of progress of diseases affecting the lung parenchyma (e.g. cryptogenic pulmonary fibrosis, sarcoidosis, asbestosis).

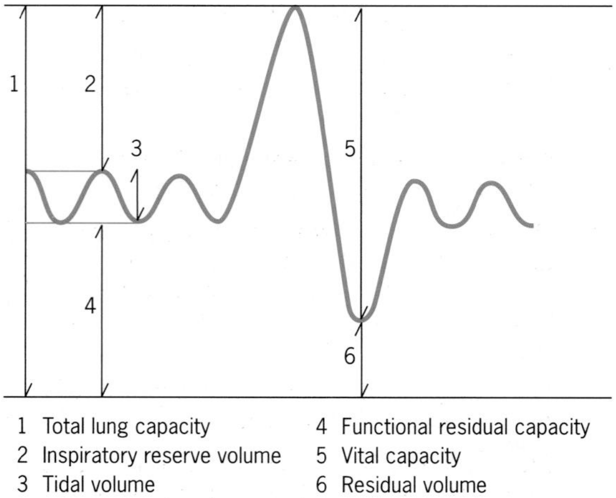

Fig 12.17
The subdivisions of the lung volume. 1, total lung capacity; 2, inspiratory reserve volume; 3, tidal volume; 4, functional residual capacity; 5, vital capacity; 6, residual volume.

Measurement of blood gases

This technique is described on p. 849.

Measurement of the partial pressures of both oxygen and carbon dioxide within arterial blood is an extremely useful test in diseases of the respiratory and circulatory systems. It is essential in the management of cases of respiratory failure and severe asthma, when repeated measurements are often the best guide to therapy.

Arterial oxygen saturation (S_aO_2) can be continuously measured using an oximeter with either ear or finger probes. The oximeter measures the differential absorption of light by oxy- and deoxyhaemoglobin and measures saturation to within 5% of that obtained by blood gas analysis.

Exercise tests

The predominant symptom in respiratory medicine is that of breathlessness. The degree of disability produced by breathlessness can be assessed before and after treatment by asking the patient to walk for six minutes along a measured track. This has been shown to be a reproducible and useful test once the patient has undergone an initial training walk to overcome the learning effect.

Exercise tests incorporating assessment of both lung and heart function are of particular value in the investigation of breathlessness. Such tests involve the use of sophisticated equipment enabling measurement of uptake of oxygen ($\dot{V}O_2$), work performed, heart rate and blood pressure together with serial ECGs. Correlation of these variables allows:

- the early detection of lung disease
- the detection of myocardial ischaemia
- the distinction between lung and heart disease
- assessment of fitness.

Pleural aspiration

Diagnostic aspiration is necessary for all but very small effusions. A needle attached to a 20 mL syringe is inserted through an intercostal space over an area of dullness. Fluid is withdrawn and the presence of any blood is noted. Samples are sent for protein estimation, cytology and bacteriological examination, including culture and Ziehl–Nielsen stain for tuberculosis. Large amounts of fluid can be aspirated through a large needle to help relieve extreme breathlessness. Because of the risk of introducing infection into the pleural space, with the subsequent development of an empyema, this technique must be performed using full aseptic precautions (see Practical box 12.2).

Pleural aspiration, drainage and biopsy are often performed under ultrasound or X-ray localization of the fluid.

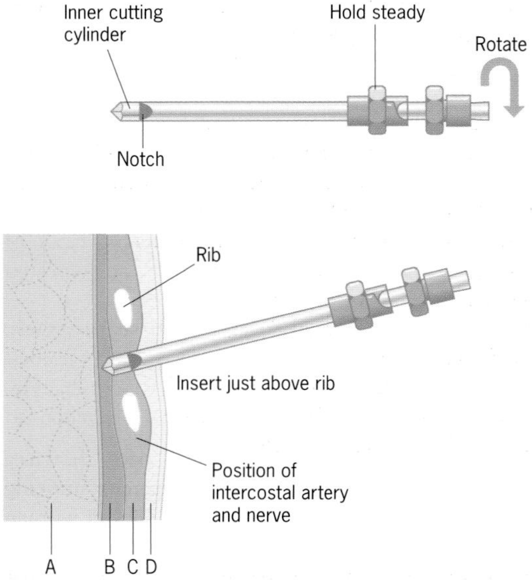

Fig 12.18
Technique of pleural biopsy. The biopsy needle is shown penetrating the chest wall. A, lung parenchyma; B, pleural space; C, muscle; D, skin and subcutaneous tissue

Pleural biopsy

Experienced operators obtain tissue in nearly all patients and, provided multiple specimens are taken, positive results may be expected in up to 80% of cases of tuberculosis and in 60% of cases of malignancy. The technique is illustrated in Fig 12.18. If tissue is not obtained by blind pleural biopsy, the pleura can be examined by fibreoptic thoracoscopy and any lesions biopsied, yielding results in a further 80% (see Practical box 12.1).

Pleural drainage

This is carried out when large effusions are present producing severe breathlessness or for drainage of an empyema (see Practical box 12.2). Pleurodesis is performed for recurrent/malignant effusion.

Mediastinoscopy and scalene node biopsy

This technique can be used in the management of carcinoma of the bronchus. It involves inspection of the mediastinal structures using a mediastinoscope inserted by blunt dissection downwards from behind the proximal end of the clavicle. Subsequent biopsy of tissue will reveal the presence or absence of malignant cells in enlarged lymph nodes previously detected by CT, allowing accurate staging of the disease.

Practical

1. Pleural biopsy is usually performed at the end of the aspiration of fluid.
2. A small skin incision is made, as the end of the Abrams' pleural biopsy needle is fairly blunt.
3. Once in place through the pleura, the back part of the needle is rotated to open the notch; this is kept pointing forward.
4. With lateral pressure the needle is withdrawn so that the notch will snag against the pleura.
5. The needle is held firmly and the hexagonal grip is twisted clockwise to cut the biopsy. To avoid damage to the intercostal vessel or nerve, the notch should never be directed upwards when the biopsy is taken.
6. Several biopsies should be taken at different angles by repeated insertion of the needle.
7. Specimens should be put in sterile saline for culture for tuberculosis and into 10% formol saline for histological examination.

Practical box 12.1 Pleural biopsy

Practical

1. Carefully sterilize the skin over the aspiration site. Sterile gloves, cap, gown and mask must be worn.
2. Anaesthetize the skin, muscle and pleura with 2% lignocaine.
3. Make a small incision, then push a 28 French gauge Argyle catheter into the pleural space.
4. Attach to three-way tap and 50 mL syringe.
5. Aspirate up to 1000 mL. Stop aspiration if patient becomes uncomfortable – shock may ensue if too much fluid is withdrawn too quickly.
6. A silastic pigtail catheter can be inserted under X-ray/ultrasound control and attached to tubing and bag for slower aspiration. For drainage and effusions, an 8–12 French gauge pigtail is inserted using the Seldinger technique in which the needle used to enter the pleural space is withdrawn over a control wire along which the catheter is then passed. A 14–16 French gauge pigtail catheter is used for drainage of empyema.

For pleurodesis

Tetracycline 500 mg or bleomycin 15 units in 30–50 mL sodium chloride 0.9% solution is instilled into the pleural cavity to achieve pleurodesis in recurrent/malignant effusion.

Practical box 12.2 Pleural drainage

Fibreoptic bronchoscopy (Practical box 12.3)

Central bronchial lesions can be biopsied readily. Washings can be taken from lobes containing more peripheral lesions for cytological examination for malignant cells, and appropriate staining and culture for bacteria including *Mycobacterium* and *Pneumocystis carinii*.

Diffuse parenchymal lung disease can be investigated using transbronchial biopsy. The biopsy forceps are pushed as far as possible to the periphery of the lung, the patient is asked to breathe in, and the jaws of the forceps are closed, removing a small piece of peripheral airway and surrounding lung parenchyma. Biplanar screening allows isolated peripheral lesions to be biopsied in the same way. A histological diagnosis can be made in 95% of central lung cancers but in only 50–75% of peripheral lesions biopsied during fibreoptic bronchoscopy.

Peripheral lesions are best biopsied percutaneously using a fine needle under X-ray or CT control.

Bronchoalveolar lavage

This technique can be used both in patients who have disease confined to one lobe and in those with more diffuse lung disease. The tip of the fibreoptic bronchoscope is lodged in the segmental orifice and 20 mL of 0.9% sterile saline is squirted down the suction port of the bronchoscope and immediately aspirated. This is repeated five times; about 40–60% of the total volume is recovered. Fluid is strained through two layers of surgical gauze and the volume is noted. The cells are then spun down and resuspended at a concentration of 1×10^7 cells/mL for differential counting. Since there is a considerable overlap in the distribution of cells seen in bronchoalveolar wash specimens in different diseases, this technique has no value in diagnosis. However, it can be used to monitor progression of disease, since improvement is characterized by a reduction in the number of cells and a return towards the normal proportions of different cell types.

Skin-prick tests

The tip of a fine needle is placed through a drop of allergen solution on the volar surface of the forearm into the epidermis, which is gently pricked with an upward lifting motion. A separate needle should be used for each allergen. If the patient is sensitive to the allergen, a weal develops and the diameter of the induration (not the erythema) should be measured after 15 minutes. A weal of at least 2 mm diameter and greater than the reaction to the control solution is a positive test. The results should be interpreted in the light of the history (see p. 771).

Skin tests can be inhibited by concurrent administration of antihistamines, so these should be stopped 48 hours before testing. They are not inhibited by bronchodilators or corticosteroids.

FURTHER READING

Armstrong P, Wilson AG, Dee P, Hansell DM (1994) Imaging of diseases of the chest, 2nd edn. Chicago, Mosby Year Book.

Smoking and air pollution

Smoking

Prevalence

General household surveys in the UK have shown a continuing decline in the prevalence of cigarette smoking in men but not women: 44% of men and 34% of women aged 16 years and over have smoked tobacco in some form. Manufactured cigarettes were smoked by an equal proportion of both sexes (34%). Cigarette smoking is now most common between the ages of 16 and 24 years (42% in both sexes). At the age of 15 more girls (27%) than boys

Practical

This enables the direct visualization of the bronchial tree as far as the subsegmental bronchi under a local anaesthetic.

Indications

- Lesions requiring biopsy seen on chest X-ray
- Haemoptysis
- Stridor
- Positive sputum cytology for malignant cells with no chest X-ray abnormality
- Collection of bronchial secretions for bacteriology, especially tuberculosis
- Recurrent laryngeal nerve paralysis of unknown aetiology
- Infiltrative lung disease (to obtain a transbronchial biopsy)
- Investigation of collapsed lobes or segments and aspiration of mucus plugs

Procedure

1. The patient is starved overnight.
2. Atropine 0.6 mg i.m. is given 30 min before the procedure.
3. Topical anaesthesia (lignocaine 2% gel) is applied to the nose, nasopharynx and pharynx.
4. Intravenous sedation (e.g. diazepam 10 mg or midazolam 2.5–10 mg) may be needed.
5. The bronchoscope is passed through the nose, nasopharynx and pharynx under direct vision to minimize trauma.
6. Lignocaine (2 mL of 4%) is dropped through the instrument on to the vocal cords.
7. The bronchoscope is passed through the cords into the trachea.
8. All segmental and subsegmental orifices should be identified.
9. Biopsies and brushings should be taken of macroscopic abnormalities or occasionally from peripheral lesions under radiographic control.

Disadvantages

- All patients require sedation to tolerate the procedure.
- Minor and transient cardiac dysrhythmias occur in up to 40% of patients on passage of the bronchoscope through the larynx.
- Oxygen supplementation is required in patients with P_aO_2 below 8 kPa.
- Fibreoptic bronchoscopy should be performed with care in the very sick and transbronchial biopsies avoided in ventilated patients owing to the increased risk of pneumothorax.
- Massive bleeding may occur on accidental biopsy of vascular lesions or carcinoid tumours. Rigid bronchoscopy may be required to allow adequate access to the bleeding point and haemostasis.

Practical box 12.3 Fibreoptic bronchoscopy

(18%) smoke cigarettes. A greater proportion of professional workers than manual workers have given up smoking. In the USA the proportion of adult males and females who smoke is less than 30%. However, cigarette consumption is rising in Central and Eastern Europe and China.

Toxic effects

Cigarette smoke contains polycyclic aromatic hydrocarbons and nitrosamines, which are potent carcinogens and mutagens in animals. It causes release of enzymes from neutrophil granulocytes and macrophages that are capable of destroying elastin and leading to lung damage. Pulmonary epithelial permeability increases even in symptomless cigarette smokers, and correlates with the concentration of carboxyhaemoglobin in blood. This altered permeability possibly allows easier access to carcinogens.

The dangers

Cigarette smoking is addictive. Smoking nearly always begins in adolescence for psychosocial reasons and, once it is a regular habit, the pharmacological properties of nicotine play an important part in persistence, conferring some advantage to the smoker's mood. Very few cigarette smokers (less than 2%) can limit themselves to occasional or intermittent smoking. The dangers are listed in Table 12.7.

There is a significant dose–response relationship between the smoking of 0–40 cigarettes daily and lung cancer mortality (Table 12.8). Sputum production and airflow limitation increase with daily cigarette consumption, and effort tolerance decreases, partly owing to high levels of carboxyhaemoglobin in bronchitis patients. Smoking and asbestos exposure are synergistic in producing bronchial carcinoma, increasing the risk in asbestos workers by up to five to eight times that of non-smokers exposed to asbestos.

Cigarette smokers who change to other forms of tobacco can reduce the risk, even if they continue to inhale, and are better off changing to cigars or pipes. All pipe and cigar smokers have a greater risk of lung cancer than lifelong non-smokers or former smokers.

Environmental tobacco smoke ('passive smoking') has been shown to cause more frequent and more severe attacks of asthma in children and possibly increases the number of cases of asthma. It is also associated with a small but definite increase in lung cancer.

Table 12.7
The dangers of cigarette smoking

General	Passive smoking
Lung cancer COPD Carcinoma of the oesophagus Ischaemic heart disease Peripheral vascular disease Bladder cancer An increase in abnormal spermatozoa Memory problems	Risk of asthma, pneumonia and bronchitis in infants of smoking parents An increase in cough and breathlessness in smokers and non-smokers with COPD and asthma Increased cancer risk
Maternal smoking	
A decrease in birthweight of the infant An increase in fetal and neonatal mortality An increase in asthma	

Table 12.8
Effects of smoking on the lung

Large airways	Small airways
Increase in submucosal gland volume Increase in number of goblet cells Chronic inflammation Metaplasia and dysplasia of the surface epithelium	Increase in number and distribution of goblet cells Airway inflammation and fibrosis Epithelial metaplasia/dysplasia Carcinoma
	Parenchyma
	Proximal acinar scarring Increase in alveolar macrophage numbers Emphysema (centri-acinar, pan-acinar)

Stopping smoking

If the entire population could be persuaded to stop smoking, the effect on healthcare provision would be enormous. National campaigns, bans on advertising and a substantial increase in the cost of cigarettes are the most certain ways of achieving this. Only one in five general practitioners actively encourage their patients to give up smoking, yet simple advice and follow-up can motivate some 50% of their patients to stop. In smoking withdrawal clinics, success rates of 80% can be achieved in the first month, though only 15–20% of patients remain abstinent in the long term. Nicotine chewing gum has been advocated but is probably no better than verbal advice. Nicotine patches are available over the counter and are better than placebo in helping smokers to stop, though they must not be used by those suffering from heart disease. Chest symptoms usually have to be severe to stop patients from smoking.

Air pollution

Atmospheric air pollution, an unwanted product of the industrial revolution caused by the burning of coal for energy and heat, has been a characteristic of urban living in developed countries for two centuries. It consists of black smoke and sulphur dioxide (SO_2). Air pollution of this type (I) peaked in the 1950s in the UK, until legislation led to restrictions on coal burning. Such pollution continues to increase in newly industrialized countries (India, China) and continues in Eastern Europe and Russia. The combustion of petroleum and diesel oil in motor vehicles has led to new air pollution (type II), consisting of primary pollutants such as the oxides of nitrogen (NO and NO_2), diesel particulates, polyaromatic hydrocarbons and the secondary pollutant ozone (O_3) generated by incompletely understood photochemical reactions in the atmosphere. Levels of NO_2 can be higher in poorly ventilated kitchens and living rooms where gas is used for cooking and in fires. Seventy per cent of the particulates present in urban air results from the combustion of diesel fuel. Very small particles (<2.5 μm, $PM_{2.5}$) remain airborne for long periods and are carried into rural areas. In the UK, ozone concentrations are highest in sunny rural areas.

Epidemiology

Classical studies in the 1950s showed that winter-time episodes of severe air pollution (smog – type I pollution) were associated with up to 4000 excess deaths in one week, particularly from respiratory disease when temperature inversion trapped black smoke and SO_2 over urban areas. Air pollution of this type continues to cause excess deaths from respiratory and cardiovascular disease in older populations, and symptoms of bronchitis in children. Pollution resulting primarily from motor vehicles has been shown to cause:

- increased deaths from respiratory and cardiovascular causes in the elderly – diesel particulates less than 10 μm in diameter (PM_{10})
- increased respiratory symptoms, hospital admissions and reduced lung function in children and younger adults – SO_2, NO_2, O_3, PM_{10}
- increase in lung cancer – polyaromatic hydrocarbons.

Frequently there is a lag of 1–2 days between peaks in air pollution and disease effects.

The evidence that air pollutants are one of the causes of the dramatic increase in asthma and other allergic diseases (Table 12.9) remains controversial. However, both NO_2 and ozone have been shown to enhance the airway response (both nose and lung) to inhaled allergen.

Table 12.9
Air pollutants and their health effects

	Average concentration	Poor air quality	Susceptible individuals	Mechanism of health effects
Sulphur dioxide (SO_2)	5–15 ppb	> 125 ppb	Asthmatics	Bronchoconstriction through neurogenic mechanism
Ozone (O_3)	10–30 ppb	> 90 ppb	All affected, particularly during exercise	Restrictive lung defect Airway inflammation Enhanced response to allergen
Nitrogen dioxide (NO_2)	25–40 ppb	> 100 ppb	Allergic individuals	Airway inflammation Enhanced response to allergen
Diesel particulates (PM_{10})	25-30 $\mu g\ m^{-3}$	> 70 $\mu g\ m^{-3}$	Elderly Allergic individuals	Airway and alveolar inflammation Enhanced production selectively of the allergy antibody (IgE)

Management

Asthmatics are advised not to exercise outdoors during periods of poor air quality and to increase their anti-inflammatory medication (i.e. inhaled sodium cromoglycate/nedocromil or inhaled corticosteroids).

Short- and long-term measures are required to reduce air pollution, particularly diesel particulates (which are predicted to increase as more diesel engines are used). Such measures include increased motor engine efficiency, catalytic converters, diesel particulate traps and decreased reliance on cars and trucks.

FURTHER READING

Davies RJ, Magnussen W (1997) Is pollution a cause or trigger for the increase in allergic disease? *Allergy* **38** (Suppl): 5–66.

Diseases of the upper respiratory tract

The common cold (acute coryza)

This highly infectious illness comprises a mild systemic upset and prominent nasal symptoms. It is due to infection by rhinoviruses, the majority of which belong to the picornavirus group and exist in at least 100 different antigenic strains. Infectivity from close personal contact (nasal mucus on hands) or droplets is high in the early stages of the infection, and spread is facilitated by overcrowding and poor ventilation. On average, individuals suffer two to three colds per year; but the incidence lessens with age, presumably as a result of accumulating immunity to the causative virus strains. The incubation is from 12 hours to an upper limit of 5 days.

The clinical features are tiredness, slight pyrexia, malaise and a sore nose and pharynx. Profuse, watery nasal discharge, eventually becoming thick and mucopurulent, persists for up to a week. Sneezing is present in the early stage. Secondary bacterial infection occurs only in a minority.

Sinusitis

Sinusitis is an infection of the paranasal sinuses that often complicates upper respiratory tract infections (e.g. coryza and allergic rhinitis). Acute infections are usually caused by *Streptococcus pneumoniae* and *Haemophilus influenzae*. Symptoms include frontal headache and facial pain and tenderness, usually with nasal discharge, but are often difficult to differentiate from symptoms of the common cold.

Treatment is with antibiotics. Many strains of *H. influenzae* are resistant to amoxycillin so co-amoxiclav or cefaclor are preferred. In addition, nasal treatment with decongestants such as xylometazoline or anti-inflammatory therapy with topical corticosteroids such as fluticasone propionate nasal spray should be given to reduce swelling of the mucosa and unblock the sinus openings. Rare complications include local and cerebral abscesses. Chronic sinusitis can be a cause of headaches, but often these headaches are due to tension.

Rhinitis

Rhinitis is present if sneezing attacks, nasal discharge or blockage occur for more than an hour on most days for:

- a limited period of the year (seasonal rhinitis)
- throughout the whole year (perennial rhinitis).

Seasonal rhinitis

This is often called 'hay fever' and is the most common of all allergic diseases. It is better described as seasonal allergic rhinitis. Worldwide prevalence rates vary from 2% to 20%. Prevalence is maximum in the second decade, when up to 30% of young people suffer symptoms in June and July.

Nasal irritation, sneezing and watery rhinorrhoea are the most troublesome symptoms, but many also suffer from itching of the eyes and soft palate and occasionally even itching of the ears due to the common innervation of the pharyngeal mucosa and the ear. In addition, approximately 20% suffer from attacks of asthma. The common seasonal allergens are shown in Fig 12.19.

Perennial rhinitis

Patients with perennial rhinitis rarely have symptoms that affect the eyes or throat. Half have symptoms predominantly of sneezing and watery rhinorrhoea, whilst the other half complain mostly of nasal blockage. The patient may lose the sense of smell and taste. A swollen mucosa can obstruct drainage from the sinuses, causing sinusitis in half of the patients. Perennial rhinitis is most frequent in the second and third decades, decreasing with age, and can be divided into four main types.

Perennial allergic rhinitis

The major cause of this is an allergen called Der p1 contained in the faecal particles of the house-dust mite *Dermatophagoides pteronyssinus*; these particles are approximately 20 µm in diameter (Fig 12.20), not dissimilar in size to pollen grains. The house-dust mite itself is under 0.5 mm in size, invisible to the naked eye (Fig 12.20), and is found in dust throughout the house, particularly in older, damp dwellings. It depends for nourishment on desquamated human skin scales and is found in abundance (4000 mites per gram of surface dust) in human bedding.

The next most common allergens come from domestic pets and are proteins derived from urine or saliva spread over the surface of the animal as well as skin protein. Allergy to urinary protein from small mammals is a major cause of morbidity amongst laboratory workers.

Industrial dust, vapours and fumes are more likely to cause occupationally related perennial rhinitis than asthma.

The presence of perennial rhinitis makes the nose more reactive to nonspecific stimuli such as cigarette smoke, washing powders, household detergents, strong perfumes and traffic fumes; these are *not* acting as allergens.

Perennial non-allergic rhinitis with eosinophilia

No extrinsic allergic cause can be identified in these patients, either from the history or on skin testing; but, as in patients with perennial allergic rhinitis, eosinophilic granulocytes are present in nasal secretions.

Vasomotor rhinitis

These patients with perennial rhinitis have no demonstrable allergy or eosinophilia in nasal secretions. They may be suffering from nonspecific nasal hyperreactivity that is due to an imbalance of the autonomic nervous system innervating the erectile tissue (sinusoids) in the nasal mucosa.

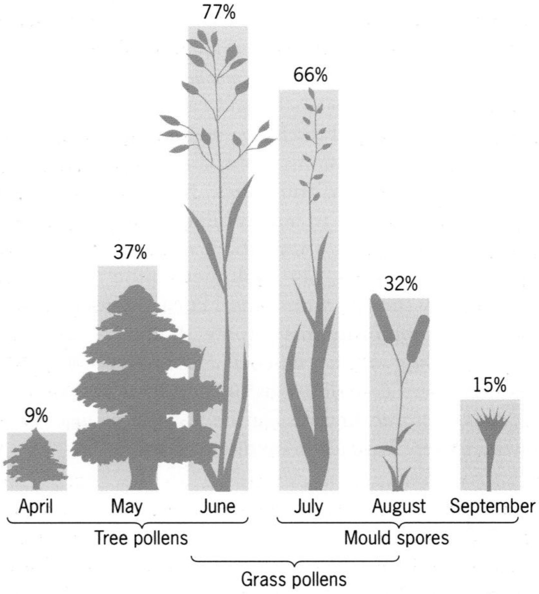

Fig 12.19
Seasonal allergic rhinitis. Bar graph showing the proportion of patients whose symptoms are worst in the month or months indicated. The causative agents are also shown

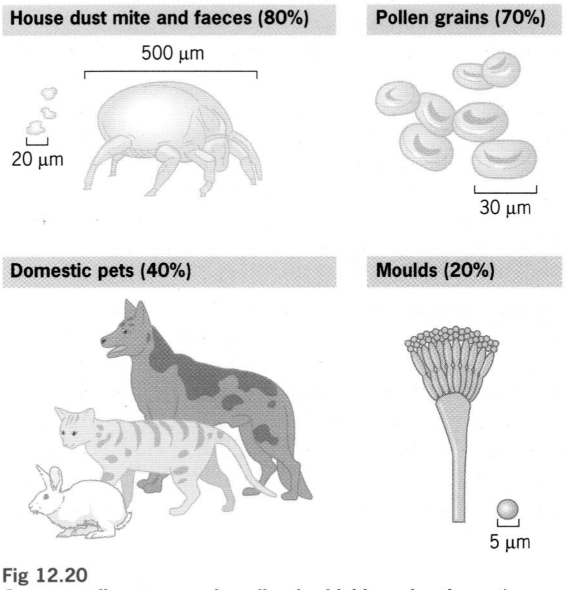

Fig 12.20
Common allergens causing allergic rhinitis and asthma: the house-dust mite, faeces of house-dust mites, pollen grains, domestic pets and moulds. Percentages are those of positive skin-prick tests to these allergens in patients with allergic rhinitis

Nasal polyps
These are round, smooth, soft, semi-translucent, pale or yellow, glistening structures attached to the sinus mucosa by a relatively narrow stalk or pedicle, occuring in patients with both allergic and vasomotor rhinitis. They cause nasal obstruction, loss of smell and taste, and mouth breathing, but rarely sneezing, since the mucosa of the polyp is largely denervated.

PATHOGENESIS

Sneezing, increased secretion and changes in mucosal blood flow are mediated both by efferent nerve fibres and by released mediators (see p. 789). Mucus production results largely from parasympathetic stimulation, whilst blood vessels are under both sympathetic and parasympathetic control. Sympathetic fibres maintain tonic contraction of blood vessels, keeping the sinusoids of the nose partially constricted with good nasal patency. Stimulation of the parasympathetic system dilates these blood vessels. This stimulation varies spontaneously in a cyclical fashion so that air intake alternates slowly over several hours from one nostril to the other. The erectile cavernous nasal sinusoids can be influenced by emotion, which, in turn, can affect nasal patency.

Allergic rhinitis develops as a result of interaction between the inhaled allergen and adjacent molecules of IgE antibody present on the surface of mast cells found in nasal secretions and within the nasal epithelium. Release of preformed mediators, in particular histamine, causes an increase in permeability of the epithelium, allowing allergen to reach IgE-primed mast cells in the lamina propria. Sneezing results from stimulation of afferent nerve endings and begins within minutes of the allergen entering the nose. This is followed by nasal secretion and eventually nasal blockage at a maximum of 15–20 minutes after contact with the allergen.

Although the mast cell contains or can generate many other potent vasomotor and chemotactic factors (see Fig 12.34), the exact role for each of these has still to be evaluated. It is likely that histamine plays a more important role in the development of allergic rhinitis than of asthma, since antihistamines are a useful and effective treatment for allergic rhinitis but are of little value in the everyday management of asthma. More mast cells are present in the nasal mucosa of individuals with rhinitis compared with those without rhinitis, and increase as allergen stimulation continues, accounting for the increasing responsiveness of the nose to lower amounts of grass pollen as the season progresses. The mechanisms for recruitment of mast cells under these circumstances probably involves the release of interleukin-3 from T lymphocytes.

INVESTIGATIONS AND DIAGNOSIS

A detailed history is mandatory for the diagnosis of allergic factors in rhinitis.

Skin-prick testing indicates that the mechanisms leading to allergic rhinitis (or asthma) are present in human skin. It does not necessarily mean that the particular allergen producing the weal causes the respiratory disease. However, if there is a positive clinical history for that allergen, a causative role is likely.

Specific serum IgE antibody against the particular allergen provides the same information as the skin-prick test.

TREATMENT

Allergen avoidance

Removal of a household pet or total enclosure of industrial processes releasing sensitizing agents can lead to cure of rhinitis and, indeed, asthma.

Pollen avoidance is impossible. Contact may be diminished by wearing sunglasses, driving with the car windows shut, avoiding walks in the countryside (particularly in the late afternoon when the number of pollen grains is highest at ground level), and keeping the bedroom window shut at night. These measures are rarely sufficient in themselves to control symptoms. Exposure to pollen is generally lower at the seaside, where sea breezes keep pollen grains inland.

The house-dust mite infests most areas of the house, but particularly the bedroom. Mite counts are extremely low in hospitals where carpets are absent, floors are cleaned frequently and mattresses and pillows are covered in plastic sheeting that can be wiped down. Such conditions need to be reproduced in the home if mite counts are to be reduced to levels that can diminish symptoms. Avoidance is best achieved by enclosing bedding in fabric specifically designed to prevent the passage of mite allergen, though allowing water vapour through. This is both comfortable and reduces symptoms. Acaricides are less effective.

Antihistamines

Antihistamines remain the most common therapy for rhinitis, and many can be purchased directly over the counter in the UK. They are particularly effective against sneezing, but are less effective against rhinorrhoea and have little influence on nasal blockage. The first-generation antihistamines cause sedation. Second-generation drugs such as astemizole (10 mg daily), cetirizine (10 mg once daily), loratidine (10 mg once daily) and terfenadine (60 mg twice daily) are highly specific for H_1 receptors; they do not cross the blood–brain barrier and are therefore not associated with sedation. Fatal cardiac arrhythmias (torsade de points) have been described, particularly with terfenadine and astemizole, so the recommended dose must not be exceeded nor must they be prescribed with erythromycin or ketoconazole (which reduce their hepatic metabolism). The active metabolite of terfenadine, fexofenadine, is being used instead, with careful monitoring. Although rarely sufficient for the treatment of rhinitis, antihistamines will control itching in the eyes and palate.

Decongestants

Drugs with sympathomimetic activity (α-adrenergic agents) are widely used for the treatment of nasal obstruction. They may be taken orally or more commonly as nasal drops or sprays (e.g. ephedrine nasal drops). Xylometazoline and oxymetazoline are widely used because they have a prolonged action and tachyphylaxis does not develop. Secondary nasal hyperaemia can occur some hours later as a rebound effect and rhinitis medicamentosa can develop if patients subsequently take increasing quantities of the local decongestant to overcome this phenomenon. Local decongestants may be the only effective treatment for vasomotor rhinitis, but patients must be warned about rebound nasal obstruction and must use the drug carefully. Usually, such preparations should be prescribed for only a limited period to open the nasal airways for administration of other therapy, particularly topical corticosteroids.

Anti-inflammatory drugs

These drugs, sodium cromoglycate and nedocromil sodium, previously considered to act primarily by preventing release of mediators from mast cells and called therefore anti-allergic compounds, are known to influence a number of aspects of inflammation, including mast cell and eosinophil activation and nerve function, and are best labelled 'anti-inflammatory drugs'. They act by blocking an intracellular chloride channel and preventing cell activation. Sodium cromoglycate applied topically in spray or powder form is of limited value in the treatment of allergic rhinitis, though is very effective in the management of allergic conjunctivitis.

Corticosteroids

The most effective treatment for rhinitis is the use of small doses of topically administered corticosteroid preparations (e.g. beclomethasone spray twice daily or fluticasone propionate spray once daily). The amount used is insufficient to cause systemic effects and the effect is primarily anti-inflammatory. Preparations should be started prior to the beginning of seasonal symptoms. The combination of a topical corticosteroid with a non-sedative antihistamine taken regularly is particularly effective.

Seasonal and perennial rhinitis respond readily to a short course (two weeks) of treatment with oral prednisolone 5–10 mg daily if other therapy has failed. Nasal polyps respond well to such oral doses of corticosteroids and their recurrence may be prevented by continuous application of topical corticosteroids.

Pharyngitis

The most common viruses causing pharyngitis are those of the adenovirus group, which consists of about 32 serotypes. Endemic adenovirus infection causes the common sore throat, in which the oropharynx and soft palate are reddened and the tonsils are inflamed and swollen. Within 1–2 days the tonsillar lymph nodes enlarge. Occasionally, localized epidemics occur, particularly in schools in the summer-time, with episodes of fever, conjunctivitis, pharyngitis and lymphadenitis of the neck glands; these are due to adenovirus serotype 8. These diseases are self-limiting, and symptomatic treatment is all that is required.

Only about one-third of sore throats are due to bacterial infections, e.g. haemolytic streptococcus, but this proportion appears to be falling. Persistent and severe tonsillitis requires antibiotic therapy. Phenoxymethyl penicillin (500 mg four times a day) or cefaclor (250 mg three times daily) can be used. Avoid amoxycillin if there is a possibility of infectious mononucleosis.

Acute laryngotracheobronchitis

Acute laryngitis is an occasional but striking complication of upper respiratory tract infections, particularly those caused by viruses of the parainfluenza group and the measles virus. Inflammatory oedema extends to the vocal cords and the epiglottis, causing considerable narrowing of the airway; in addition, there may be associated tracheitis or tracheobronchitis. Children under the age of three years are most severely affected. The voice becomes hoarse, the cough assumes a barking quality (croup) and there is audible laryngeal stridor. Progressive airways obstruction may occur, with recession of the soft tissue of the neck and abdomen during inspiration, and in severe cases central cyanosis may occur. Inhalation of steam may be helpful; in severe cases endotracheal intubation may be necessary. Oxygen and adequate fluids should be given. Rarely, a tracheostomy may be required.

Acute epiglottitis

This is caused by *H. influenzae* type B. Since the advent of the Hib immunization there has been an 88% reduction in notification in England and Wales (Fig 12.21). However, where the vaccine is not available, *H. influenzae* type B can cause life-threatening infection of the epiglottis, a condition that is rare over the age of 5 years. The young child becomes extremely ill with a high fever, and severe airflow obstruction may rapidly occur. This is a life-threatening emergency and requires urgent endotracheal intubation and intravenous ceftazidime (25–150 mg kg^{-1} in children). Chloramphenicol (50–100 mg kg^{-1} in children) can also be used. The epiglottis, which is red and swollen, should not be inspected until facilities to maintain the airways are available.

Other manifestations of *H. influenzae* type b (Hib) are meningitis, septic arthritis and osteomyelitis. Immunization is achieved with a purified polyribosylribitol phosphate from the capsule of Hib linked to a non-toxic diphtheria toxin PRP-T to increase immunogenicity. It is highly

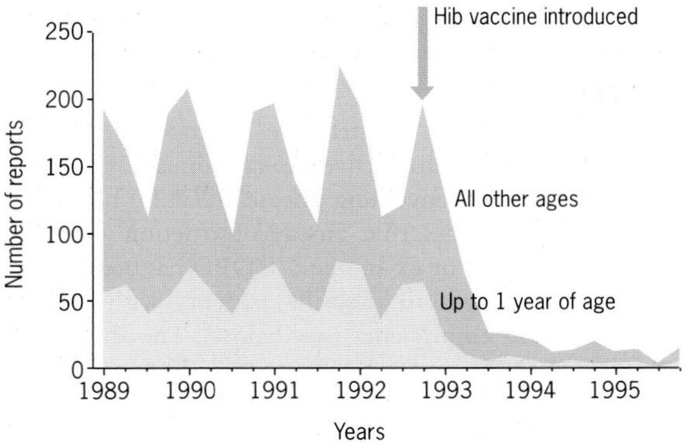

Fig 12.21
Laboratory reports of *Haemophilus influenzae* type b by age, England and Wales 1989-95. From Salisbury DM, Begg NT (1996), with permission.

effective when given to infants at two, three and four months with primary immunization against diphtheria, tetanus and pertussis (DTP), reducing death rates from Hib infections virtually to zero.

Influenza (see also p. 62)

The influenza virus belongs to the orthomyxovirus group and exists in two main forms, A and B. Influenza B is associated with localized outbreaks of milder nature, whereas influenza A is the cause of worldwide pandemics. Influenza A has a capacity to develop new antigenic variants at irregular intervals. Human immunity develops against the haemagglutinin (H) antigen and the neuraminidase (N) antigen on the viral surface. Major shifts in the antigenic make-up of influenza A viruses provide the necessary conditions for major pandemics, whereas minor antigenic drifts give rise to less severe epidemics because immunity in the population is less blunted.

The most serious pandemic of influenza occurred in 1918, and was associated with more than 20 million deaths worldwide. In 1957, a major shift in the antigenic make-up of the virus led to the appearance of influenza A2 type H2-N2, which caused a worldwide pandemic. A further pandemic occurred in 1968 owing to the emergence of Hong Kong influenza type H3-N2, and minor antigenic drifts have caused outbreaks around the world ever since. In 1997, avian H5N1 strain of influenza A was found in humans and represented a major change in viral surface antigens. Its worldwide impact is being monitored.

CLINICAL FEATURES

The incubation period of influenza is usually 1–3 days. The illness starts abruptly with a fever, shivering and generalized aching in the limbs. This is associated with severe headache, soreness of the throat and a persistent dry cough that can last for several weeks. Influenza viruses can cause a prolonged period of debility and depression that may take weeks or months to clear; this is known as the postviral syndrome.

COMPLICATIONS

Secondary bacterial infection, particularly with *Strep. pneumoniae* and *H. influenzae*, is common following influenza virus infection. Rarer, but more serious, is the development of pneumonia caused by *Staph. aureus*, which has a mortality of up to 20%. Postinfectious encephalomyelitis rarely occurs after infection with influenza virus.

DIAGNOSIS AND TREATMENT

Laboratory diagnosis of all cases is not necessary. Definitive diagnosis can be established by demonstrating a fourfold increase in the complement-fixing antibody or the haemagglutinin antibody when measured before and after an interval of 1–2 weeks. Viral cultures are still a research procedure.

Treatment is bedrest and paracetamol, together with antibiotics for individuals with chronic bronchitis, or heart or renal disease.

PROPHYLAXIS

Protection by influenza vaccines is only effective in up to 70% of people and is of short duration, usually lasting for only a year. Influenza vaccine should not be given to individuals who are allergic to egg protein as some are manufactured in chick embryos. New vaccines have to be prepared to cover each change in viral antigenicity and are therefore in limited supply at the start of an epidemic. Routine vaccination is reserved for susceptible people with chronic heart disease, chronic lung disease (including asthma), chronic renal failure, diabetes mellitus and those who are immunosuppressed. In pandemics key hospital and health service personnel are also vaccinated.

Amantadine hydrochloride 100–200 mg daily may attenuate influenza A infection and should be reserved for individuals with chronic respiratory or cardiovascular disease who have not previously been immunized.

Inhalation of foreign bodies

Children inhale foreign bodies, frequently peanuts, more commonly than adults. In the adult, inhalation often occurs after an excess of alcohol or under general anaesthesia (loose teeth or dentures).

When the foreign body is large it may impact in the trachea. The person chokes and then becomes silent; death occurs unless the material is quickly removed (see Emergency box 12.1).

Impaction usually occurs in the right main bronchus and produces:

- choking
- persistent monophonic wheeze
- later, persistent suppurative pneumonia
- lung abscess (common).

Emergency

Emergency

The Heimlich manoeuvre is used to expel the obstructing object:

1. Stand behind the patient.
2. Encircle your arms around the upper part of the abdomen just below the patient's rib cage.
3. Give a sharp, forceful squeeze, forcing the diaphragm sharply into the thorax. This should expel sufficient air from the lungs to force the foreign body out of the trachea.

Non-emergency

Fibreoptic bronchoscopy should be performed.

Emergency box 12.1
Treatment of inhaled foreign bodies (Heimlich manoeuvre)

FURTHER READING

Rusznak C, Davies RJ (1998) ABC of allergies. Diagnosing allergy. *British Medical Journal* **316**: 686–689.

Salisbury DM, Begg NT (1996) *Immunisation Against Infectious Disease:* Haemophilus influenzae *type B.* London: HMSO, 77–83.

Diseases of the lower respiratory tract

Acute bronchitis

Acute bronchitis in previously healthy subjects is often viral. Bacterial infection with organisms such as *Strep. pneumoniae* and *H. influenzae* is a common sequel to viral infections, and is more likely to occur in individuals who are cigarette smokers and in those with chronic obstructive pulmonary disease (COPD).

The illness begins with an irritating, unproductive cough, together with discomfort behind the sternum. This may be associated with tightness in the chest, wheezing and shortness of breath. The cough becomes productive, the sputum being yellow or green. There is a mild fever and a neutrophil leucocytosis; wheeze with occasional crackles can be heard on auscultation. In otherwise healthy adults the disease improves spontaneously in 4–8 days without the patient becoming seriously ill. Treatment with antibiotics may be given (e.g. amoxycillin 250 mg thrice daily), though it is not known whether this hastens recovery in otherwise healthy individuals.

Chronic obstructive pulmonary disease (COPD)

The terms 'chronic obstructive pulmonary disease' (COPD), 'chronic obstructive airways disease' (COAD), and 'chronic obstructive lung disease' (COLD) have been variously used to describe 'airway obstruction' occuring mainly in smokers or ex-smokers. COPD has become the most popular term to describe patients with chronic bronchitis and emphysema (see below). The distinction between COPD and asthma (see p. 790) is blurred because most patients with COPD have some reversible airflow obstruction.

As the common tests for 'airway obstruction', the FEV_1 and PEFR, actually measure airflow limitation (caused by both loss of elastic recoil and/or narrowing of airways), the term 'airflow limitation' is the preferred terminology to describe the functional and physiological abnormality in these diseases (Table 12.10).

Definitions in COPD

Chronic bronchitis is defined on the basis of the *history* as:

- Cough productive of sputum on most days for at least three months of the year for more than one year.

Emphysema, on the other hand, is defined *pathologically* as:

- Dilatation and destruction of the lung tissue distal to the terminal bronchioles.

Clinical observations led to the suggestion that there were two distinct types of patient, types A and B:

- The type A fighter is *pink and puffing*. Although the person is very breathless, arterial tensions of oxygen and carbon dioxide are relatively normal and there is no cor pulmonale. These individuals were thought to be suffering predominantly from emphysema with little bronchitis.
- The type B non-fighter, on the other hand, is *blue and bloated*. The person does not appear to be breathless, but has marked arterial hypoxaemia, carbon dioxide retention, secondary polycythaemia and cor pulmonale. These patients were thought to be suffering predominantly from chronic bronchitis.

Although this was an attractive concept with some clinical usefulness, it is not supported by CT or post-mortem studies that have shown no difference in the degree of mucous gland hyperplasia (i.e. bronchitis) or in the amount of emphysema in patients with type A compared with type B disease. On this basis the two are considered together as COPD since both conditions may coexist to a greater or lesser degree in each patient.

Autopsy studies have shown that substantial numbers of centri-acinar emphysematous spaces are found in the lungs of 50% of British smokers over the age of 60 years

Table 12.10
Causes of airflow limitation

Reversible	
• Asthma	
• Acute bronchitis and bronchiolitis.	
Partially reversible	
• COPD (chronic bronchitis and emphysema)	
Irreversible	
• Bronchiolitis obliterans	
	Connective tissue disease
	Exposure to toxic fumes
	Post lung transplantation
• Long-standing left heart failure.	

(From Lamb D, Wallace WAH (1995) *Medicine* 302–304, with permission)

and are unrelated to the diagnosis of significant respiratory disease before death.

EPIDEMIOLOGY AND AETIOLOGY

COPD, diagnosed on the basis of a reduction in FEV_1 of two standard deviations below predicted, occurs in 18% of male and 14% of female smokers and in 7% and 6% of never smokers. In the USA similar prevalence figures have been obtained and many developing countries are showing an increased prevalence.

There is no doubt that cigarette smoking is a major factor in the development of COPD. Not only is this disease virtually confined to cigarette smokers, it is also related to the number of cigarettes smoked per day. The risk of death from COPD in patients smoking 30 cigarettes daily is 20 times that of a non-smoker. The bronchitis mortality amongst male doctors in relation to the number of cigarettes smoked is shown in Fig 12.22.

Climate and air pollution are of less importance; nevertheless, there is a great increase in mortality from COPD during periods of heavy atmospheric pollution (p. 768). The effect of urbanization, social class and occupation may also play a part in aetiology, but these effects are difficult to separate from that of smoking.

Diet appears to be a risk factor for COPD; fresh fruit and vegetables may be preventative as studies in rats show that retinoic acid can prevent lung damage.

The socio-economic burden of COPD is considerable. In the UK, COPD causes approximately 18 million lost working days for men and 2.1 million lost working days for women per year, accounting for some 7% of all days of sickness absence from work. Nevertheless, the number of patients discharged from hospitals in the UK with this disease has been steadily falling; the death rate has also fallen in the last 20 years from 200 to 70 per 100 000.

PATHOPHYSIOLOGY

In COPD there are mixed pathological changes of bronchitis and emphysema. In this section we have separated them for clarity.

Chronic bronchitis

The most consistent pathological finding in chronic bronchitis is hypertrophy of the mucus-secreting glands of the bronchial tree. The hypertrophy of these mucous glands is evenly distributed throughout the lung, and is mainly seen in the larger bronchi. In addition, the number of the mucus-secreting goblet cells increases. This leads to increased mucus production and the regular expectoration of sputum.

In more advanced cases, the bronchi themselves are obviously inflamed and pus is seen in the lumen. Microscopically there is infiltration of the walls of the bronchi and bronchioles with acute and chronic inflammatory cells. The epithelial layer may become ulcerated and, when the ulcers heal, squamous epithelium may replace the columnar cells. The inflammation leads to widespread narrowing in the small airways.

The small airways are particularly affected early in the disease, initially without the development of any significant breathlessness. This initial inflammation of the small airways is reversible and accounts for the improvement in airway function if smoking is stopped early.

Further progression of the disease leads to progressive squamous cell metaplasia, and fibrosis of the bronchial walls. The physiological consequences of these changes is the development of airflow limitation. If the airway narrowing is combined with emphysema (causing loss of the elastic recoil of the lung) the resulting airflow limitation is even more severe.

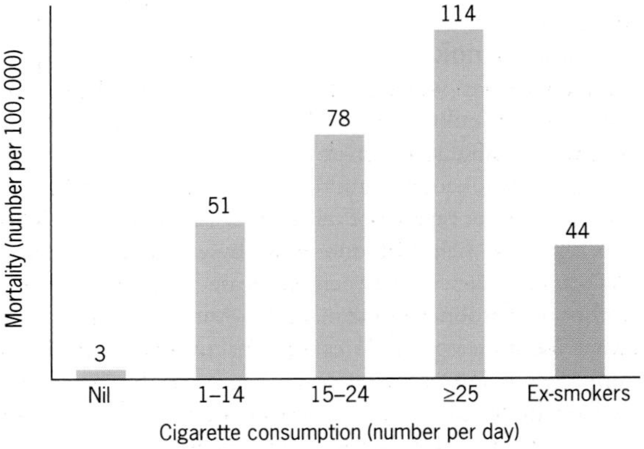

Fig 12.22
Bronchitis death rates per 100 000 British male doctors according to their smoking habits. From Doll R, Peto R (1976) *British Medical Journal* **2**: 1525

Emphysema (Fig 12.23)

Emphysema can be classified according to the site of damage:

- *Centri-acinar emphysema.* Distension and damage of lung tissue is concentrated around the respiratory bronchioles, whilst the more distal alveolar ducts and alveoli tend to be well preserved. This form of emphysema is extremely common; when of modest extent, it is not necessarily associated with disability. Severe centri-acinar emphysema is associated with substantial airflow limitation.
- *Pan-acinar emphysema.* This is less common. Here, distension and destruction appear to involve the whole of the acinus, and in the extreme form the lung becomes a mass of bullae. Severe airflow limitation and $\dot{V}_A/\dot{Q}$ mismatch occur. This type of emphysema occurs in α_1-antitrypsin deficiency (see p. 327).
- *Irregular emphysema.* There is scarring and damage affecting the lung parenchyma patchily without particular regard for acinar structure.

Emphysema leads to expiratory airflow limitation and air trapping. The loss of lung elastic recoil results in an increase in TLC while the loss of alveoli with emphysema results in decreased gas transfer.

$\dot{V}_A/\dot{Q}$ mismatch occurs partly because of damage and mucus plugging of smaller airways from chronic bronchitis, and partly because of the rapid expiratory closure of the smaller airways owing to loss of elastic recoil from emphysema. This leads to a fall in P_aO_2 and a subsequent rise in P_aCO_2.

Carbon dioxide is normally the major stimulant of the respiratory centre. In the face of a prolonged high P_aCO_2 this sensitivity is diminished and hypoxaemia becomes the chief drive to respiration. In this situation an attempt to abolish hypoxaemia by administration of oxygen can result in an increase in P_aCO_2 by decreasing the respiratory drive, worsening respiratory failure.

PATHOGENESIS

Cigarette smoking

Bronchoalveolar washes have shown that smokers have neutrophil granulocytes present within the lumen of the lung that are absent in non-smokers. Additionally, the small airways of smokers are infiltrated by granulocytes. These granulocytes are capable of releasing elastases and proteases, which possibly help to produce emphysema. It is suggested that an imbalance between protease and antiprotease activity may produce the damage. α_1-Antitrypsin is a major serum antiprotease which can be inactivated by cigarette smoke (see below).

The hypertrophy of mucous glands in the larger airways is thought to be a direct response to persistent irritation resulting from the inhalation of cigarette smoke. The smoke has an adverse effect on surfactant, favouring overdistension of the lungs.

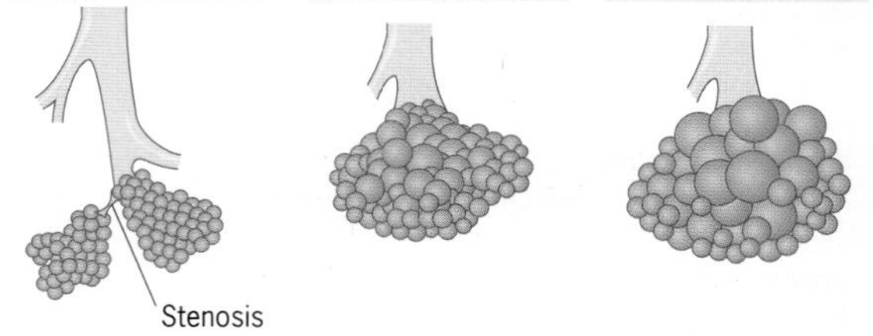

Fig 12.23
Pathological features of chronic bronchitis and emphysema

Infections

Infections are frequent and are often the precipitating cause of acute exacerbations of the disease. However, the role of infection in the development of the progressive airflow limitation that characterizes disabling COPD is far less clear. Nevertheless, release of enzymes from the excess neutrophil granulocytes found in infections probably adds to the lung damage.

α_1-Antitrypsin deficiency (see also p. 327)

α_1-Antitrypsin inhibitor is an antiproteinase inhibitor produced in the liver, secreted into the blood and which diffuses into the lung. Here it functions as an antiprotease that inhibits neutrophil elastase, a proteolytic enzyme capable of destroying alveolar wall connective tissue.

More than 75 alleles of the α_1-antitrypsin inhibitor gene have been described. The three main phenotypes are MM (normal), MZ (heterozygous deficiency) and ZZ (homozygous deficiency); these groups are defined by the serum level of α_1-antitrypsin inhibitor. About one child in 5000 in Britain is born with the homozygous deficiency, but not all develop chest disease. Those who do develop breathlessness under the age of 40 years have radiographic evidence of basal emphysema and are usually, but not always, cigarette smokers. Hereditary deficiency of α_1-antitrypsin inhibitor accounts for about 2% of emphysema cases and a few develop liver disease (see p. 327).

CLINICAL FEATURES

SYMPTOMS

The characteristic symptoms of COPD are cough with the production of sputum, wheeze and breathlessness following many years of a smoker's cough. Colds seem to 'go down to the chest' and frequent infective exacerbations occur, giving purulent sputum. Symptoms can be worsened by factors such as cold, foggy weather and atmospheric pollution. With advanced disease, breathlessness becomes severe even after mild exercise such as dressing.

SIGNS

In mild disease there are no signs apart from 'wheeze' throughout the chest. In severe disease, the patient is tachypnoeic, with prolonged expiration. The accessory muscles of respiration are used and there may be intercostal indrawing on inspiration and pursing of the lips on expiration (see p. 751). Chest expansion is poor, the lungs are hyperinflated, and there is loss of the normal cardiac and liver dullness.

The 'pink puffer' is always breathless and is not usually cyanosed. Rarely oedema or heart failure may be seen.

The 'blue bloater' is oedematous, deeply cyanosed, with hypoventilation and often little respiratory effort. These patients are likely to have hypercapnia, which gives the following physical findings:

- peripheral vasodilatation
- a bounding pulse
- later, a coarse flapping tremor of the outstretched hands.

More severe hypercapnia leads to:

- confusion
- progressive drowsiness and coma with papilloedema.

There is often considerable overlap between these two clinical patterns.

COMPLICATIONS

Respiratory failure

The later stages of COPD are characterized by the development of respiratory failure. For practical purposes this is said to occur when there is either a P_aO_2 of less than 8 kPa (60 mmHg) or a P_aCO_2 of more than 7 kPa (55 mmHg) (see Chapter 13).

The persistence of chronic alveolar hypoxia and hypercapnia leads to constriction of the pulmonary arterioles and subsequent pulmonary arterial hypertension.

Cor pulmonale

Patients may develop cor pulmonale (see p. 722), which is defined as heart disease secondary to disease of the lung. It is characterized by pulmonary hypertension, right ventricular hypertrophy, and eventually right heart failure. On examination, the patient is centrally cyanosed (owing to the lung disease) and, when heart failure develops, the patient becomes more breathless and ankle oedema occurs. Initially a prominent parasternal heave may be felt that is due to right ventricular hypertrophy and a loud pulmonary second sound may be heard. In very severe pulmonary hypertension there is incompetence of the pulmonary valve. With right heart failure, tricuspid incompetence may develop with a greatly elevated jugular venous pressure (JVP), ascites and upper abdominal discomfort owing to swelling of the liver.

DIAGNOSIS

This is usually clinical. There is a history of breathlessness and sputum production in a lifetime smoker. It is unwise to make a diagnosis of COPD in the absence of a history of cigarette smoking unless there is a family history of lung disease suggestive of a deficiency of α_1-antitrypsin inhibitor.

In clinical practice, emphysema is often incorrectly diagnosed on signs of overinflation of the lungs (e.g. loss of liver dullness on percussion), since this may occur with other diseases such as asthma. Furthermore, centri-acinar emphysema may be present without signs of overinflation. Some elderly men develop a barrel-shaped chest as a result of osteoporosis of the spine, and a consequent decrease in height. This should not be attributed to emphysema.

In many patients the airflow limitation is reversible to some extent (usually a change in FEV_1 of <15%), and the distinction between asthma and COPD can be difficult.

INVESTIGATIONS

- **Lung function tests** show evidence of airflow limitation (see Figs 12.9 and 12.16). The ratio of the FEV_1 to the FVC is reduced and the PEFR is low. Lung volumes may be normal or increased, and the gas transfer coefficient of carbon monoxide is low when significant emphysema is present.
- **Chest X-ray** is often normal, even when the disease is advanced. The classic features are the presence of bullae, severe overinflation of the lungs with low, flattened diaphragms, and a large retrosternal air space on the lateral film. There may also be a deficiency of blood vessels in the peripheral half of the lung fields compared with relatively easily visible proximal vessels.
- **Haemoglobin level and PCV** can be elevated as a result of persistent hypoxaemia (secondary polycythaemia, see p. 389).
- **Blood gases** are often normal. In the advanced case there is evidence of hypoxaemia and hypercapnia.
- **Sputum** examination is unnecessary in the ordinary case as *Strep. pneumoniae* or *H. influenzae* are the only common organisms to produce acute exacerbations. Occasionally *Moraxella catarrhalis* may be the causative bacterium for the infection.
- **Electrocardiogram**. In cor pulmonale the P wave is taller (P pulmonale) and there may be right bundle branch block (RSR complex) and the changes of right ventricular hypertrophy (see p. 721).
- **Echocardiogram** is performed to assess cardiac function.
- **α_1-Antitrypsin**. The normal range is 2–4 g L^{-1}.

TREATMENT

The single most important aspect in the management of COPD is to persuade the patient to stop smoking. Even at a late stage of the disease this may slow down the rate of deterioration and prolong the time before disability and death occur (Fig 12.24). Accompanying heart failure should be treated (see p. 679).

Drug therapy

This is used both for the short-term management of exacerbations and for the long-term relief of symptoms. In some cases the therapy is similar to that used in asthma (see p. 791).

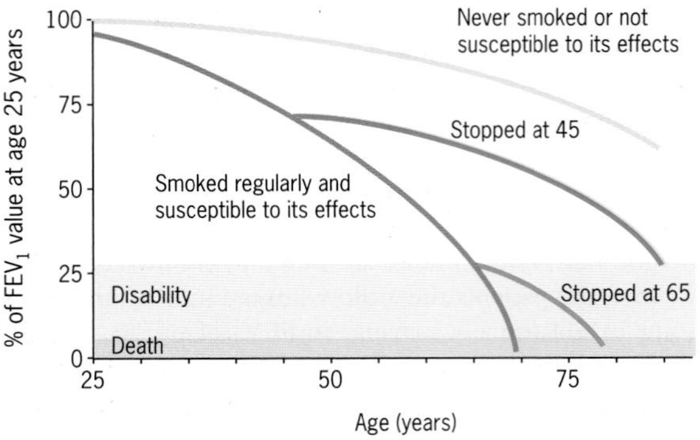

Fig 12.24
Influence of smoking on airflow limitation. From Fletcher CM, Peto R (1977) *British Medical Journal* **1**: 1645

Bronchodilators

Many patients feel less breathless following the inhalation of a β-adrenoceptor agonist such as salbutamol (200 μg every 4–6 hours). More prolonged and greater bronchodilatation results from the use of antimuscarinic agents: ipratropium bromide 40 μg four times daily or oxitropium bromide 200 μg twice daily. Objective evidence of improvement in the peak flow or FEV_1 may be small, but with severe disability it may be of considerable help. Long-acting preparations of theophylline are of little benefit.

Corticosteroids

In symptomatic patients with COPD, a trial of corticosteroids is always indicated, since a proportion of patients have a large, unsuspected, reversible element to their disease and airway function may improve considerably. Prednisolone 30 mg daily should be given for two weeks, with measurements of lung function before and after the treatment period. If there is objective evidence of a substantial degree of improvement in airflow limitation (>15%), prednisolone should be gradually reduced and replaced by inhaled corticosteroids (beclomethasone 100–500 μg thrice daily). The long-term value of regular inhaled corticosteroids in all patients with COPD awaits evaluation.

Antibiotics

Prompt antibiotic treatment shortens exacerbations and should always be given in acute episodes as it may prevent subsequent further lung damage. Patients can be given a supply of antibiotics to keep at home to start as soon as their sputum turns yellow or green. Amoxycillin-resistant *H. influenzae* is an increasing problem, occurring in 10–20% of isolates from sputum. Resistance to cefaclor 500 mg 8-hourly or cefixime 400 mg once daily is significantly less frequent and they are the antibiotics of choice.

Long-term treatment with antibiotics remains controversial. They were once thought to be of no value, but eradication of infection and keeping the lower respiratory tract free of bacteria may help to prevent deterioration in lung function.

Diuretic therapy (see p. 605)

This is necessary for all oedematous patients.

α_1-Antitrypsin replacement

Weekly or monthly infusions of α_1-antitrypsin have been recommended for patients with serum levels of this compound below 310 mg L^{-1} and abnormal lung function. Whether this modifies the long-term progression of the disease has still to be determined.

Mucolytics and vaccines

There is little evidence that mucolytics are of any benefit, though it is vital that patients be encouraged to cough up sputum, initially with the help of a physiotherapist. Symptomatic treatment with steam inhalations may help to liquefy the sputum so that it can be more easily coughed up. Influenza vaccines should be given yearly to patients with disabling COPD. These patients should also receive one dose of the polyvalent pneumococcal polysaccharide vaccine.

Treatment of respiratory failure

There are many causes of respiratory failure (Fig 12.25) but by far the most common is COPD. In this type II respiratory failure the P_aCO_2 is elevated and the P_aO_2 is reduced. Hypercapnia is intoxicating, but hypoxaemia is potentially lethal. The primary aim of the management of respiratory failure is to improve the P_aO_2 by continuous oxygen therapy. This nearly always leads to a rise in the P_aCO_2 (see p. 851). Small increases in P_aCO_2 can be tolerated but not if the pH falls dramatically. The pH should not be allowed to fall below 7.25; under such circumstances, increased ventilation must be achieved either by the use of a respiratory stimulant or by artificial ventilation.

Fig 12.26 shows a fixed-performance mask (Venturi mask) for the administration of oxygen. This style of mask is used when only low concentrations of oxygen can be given. It should be compared with the variable-performance face mask (see Fig 13.18).

Initially, 24% oxygen is given, which is only slightly greater than the concentration of oxygen in air. However, because of the shape of the oxygen–haemoglobin dissociation curve, this small increase in oxygen is valuable. Gradually, the concentration of inspired oxygen can be increased if there is no dramatic rise in the P_aCO_2.

Additional measures

- *Removal of retained secretions.* The patient should be encouraged to cough to remove secretions. Physiotherapy is helpful. If this fails, bronchoscopy and/or aspiration via an endotracheal tube may be necessary. A tracheostomy is only rarely required.

- *Secondary polycythaemia.* Venesection is recommended if the packed cell volume is greater than 55%.
- *Respiratory stimulants.* Doxapram, 1.5–4.0 mg min^{-1} by slow i.v. infusion, may help in the short term to arouse the patient and to stimulate coughing, with clearance of some secretions.
- *Respiratory support* (see p. 851). Non-invasive techniques using tight-fitting facial masks, e.g. bilevel positive airway pressure ventilatory support, are now being used prior to considering endotracheal intubation (p. 852). Assisted ventilation is occasionally used for patients with COPD with severe respiratory failure when there is a definite precipitating factor and the overall prognosis is reasonable. This can be a difficult ethical problem.
- *Corticosteroids, antibiotics and bronchodilators* should also be administered (see above).

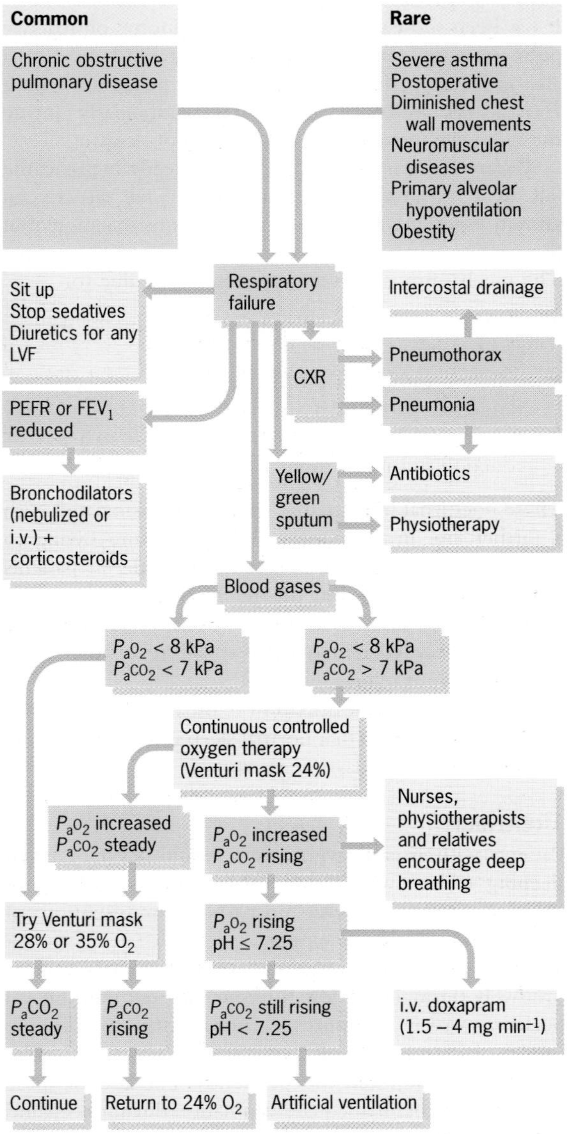

Fig 12.25
Algorithm for the treatment of respiratory failure. LVF, left ventricular failure

Further management at home

Oxygen

Two controlled trials (chiefly in men) have indicated that the continuous administration of oxygen at 2 L min^{-1} via nasal prongs to achieve an oxygen saturation of greater than 90% for large proportions of the day and night can prolong life. Survival curves from these two studies are shown in Fig 12.27.

Only 30% of those not receiving long-term oxygen therapy survived for more than five years. A fall in pulmonary artery pressure was achieved if oxygen was given for 15 hours daily, but substantial improvement in mortality was only achieved by the administration of oxygen for 19 hours daily. These results suggest that

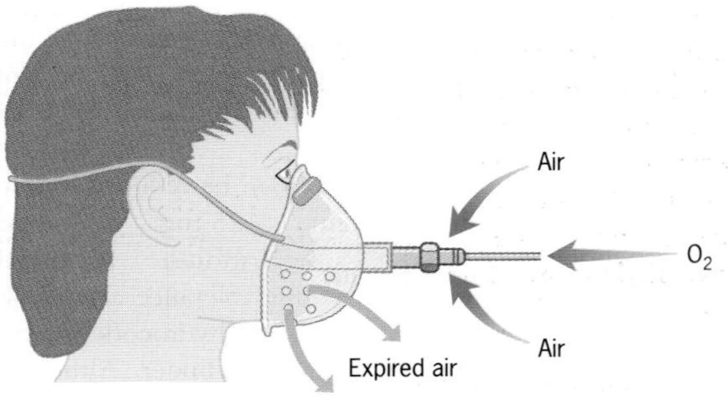

Fig 12.26
'Fixed-performance' device for administration of oxygen to spontaneously breathing patients (Venturi mask). Oxygen is delivered through the injector of the Venturi mask at a given flow rate. A fixed amount of air is entrapped and the inspired oxygen can be predicted accurately. Masks are available to deliver 24%, 28% and 35% oxygen

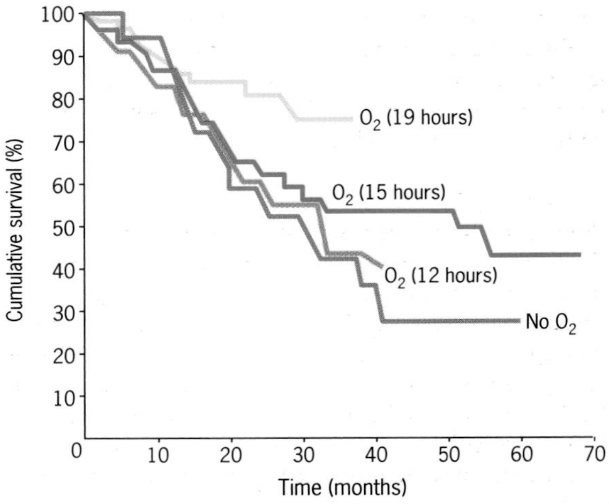

Fig 12.27
Cumulative survival curves for patients receiving oxygen. Oxygen doses are in hours per day

long-term continuous domiciliary oxygen therapy will benefit patients who have:

- COPD with an FEV_1 of less than 1.5 L
- a P_aO_2 on air on two occasions three weeks apart of less than 7.3 kPa (55 mmHg) with or without hypercapnoea
- carboxyhaemoglobin of less than 3% (i.e. patients who have stopped smoking).

Measurements should be taken on two occasions at least three weeks apart after appropriate bronchodilator therapy. The provision of 19 hours of oxygen daily at a flow rate of 1–3 L min^{-1}, using a 28% oxygen mask to increase the arterial oxygen saturation to over 90%, needs 20 oxygen cylinders per week. This is extremely expensive. Oxygen concentrators are cheaper and are available through the health service in the UK for patients who fulfil the above criteria.

Drugs

Pulmonary hypertension can be partially relieved by the use of oral β-adrenoceptor stimulants such as salbutamol (4 mg thrice daily), but whether this is useful in the long term is unknown.

The sensation of breathlessness can be reduced by the use of either promethazine 125 mg daily or dihydrocodeine 1 mg kg^{-1} by mouth. Reduced breathlessness and increased exercise tolerance also result from the combined administration of dihydrocodeine and oxygen delivered from a portable cylinder. Although opiates are the most effective treatment for intractable breathlessness they depress ventilation and carry risk of increasing respiratory failure.

Surgery

Some patients with large emphysematous bullae (which reduce lung capacity) can benefit from bullectomy, enabling adjacent areas of pulmonary collapse to re-expand and function again. In addition, carefully selected patients with severe COPD (FEV_1 <1 L), often awaiting lung transplantation, can benefit from *lung volume reduction surgery*. This increases elastic recoil, reducing the expiratory collapse of the airway and also reducing expiratory airflow limitation. It also enables the diaphragm to work at a better advantage. Overall, ventilation is improved and patients are less breathless.

Single lung transplantation (see p. 785) is used for end-stage emphysema, with 3-year survivals of 75%. This, however, does not statistically improve survival but may improve quality of life.

Exercise training

A modest increase in exercise capacity with diminution in the sense of breathlessness and improved general well-being can result from exercise training. Regular training periods can be instituted at home; climbing stairs or walking fixed distances combined with regular clinic visits for encouragement. Breathing exercises are probably of less value. Quality of life though not life expectancy or decline in lung function can be improved by a multidisciplinary approach emphasizing physiotherapy, exercise, education and smoking cessation.

PROGNOSIS

In general, 50% of patients with severe breathlessness die within five years (Fig 12.27), but even in the severe group stopping smoking helps the prognosis.

Nocturnal hypoxia

It has been shown that patients with chronic obstructive pulmonary disease who show severe arterial hypoxaemia also suffer from profound nocturnal hypoxaemia with a P_aO_2 as low as 2.5 kPa (19 mmHg), particularly during the rapid eye movement (REM) phase of sleep.

Because patients with COPD are already hypoxic, the fall in P_aO_2 produces a much larger fall in oxygen saturation (owing to the steepness of the oxyhaemoglobin dissociation curve) and desaturation of up to 50% occurs. The mechanism is alveolar hypoventilation due to:

- inhibition of intercostal and accessory muscles in REM sleep
- shallow breathing in REM sleep, which reduces ventilation, particularly in severe COPD
- an increase in upper airway resistance due to a reduction in muscle tone.

These nocturnal hypoxaemic episodes are associated with a further rise in pulmonary arterial pressure owing to vasoconstriction, and the majority of deaths in patients with COPD occur during the night, possibly from cardiac arrhythmias. These patients additionally show severe secondary polycythaemia, partly as a result of the severe nocturnal hypoxaemia.

Each episode of desaturation is usually terminated by arousal from sleep, so that normal sleep is reduced and the patient suffers from daytime sleepiness.

TREATMENT

Patients with arterial hypoxaemia should never be given sleeping tablets, which will further depress respiratory drive. Treatment is with nocturnal administration of oxygen and ventilatory support.

Positive pressure ventilation can be administered non-invasively through a tightly fitting nasal mask with bilevel positive airway pressure – inspiratory to provide inspiratory assistance and expiratory to prevent alveolar closure, each adjusted independently. The use of these devices to maintain adequate ventilation during sleep and to allow respiratory muscles to rest at night are effective in chronic chest wall disease (e.g. kyphoscoliosis) or neuromuscular disease (e.g. previous poliomyelitis). These devices, however, have not led to improvement in respiratory function, respiratory muscle strength, exercise tolerance or breathlessness in patients with COPD.

Obstructive sleep apnoea

This condition occurs most often in overweight middle-aged men and affects 1–2% of the population. It can occur in children, particularly those with with enlarged tonsils. The major symptoms and their frequency are listed in Table 12.11.

Apnoeas occur when the airway at the back of the throat is sucked closed when breathing in during sleep. When awake this tendency is overcome by the action of opening muscles of the upper airway – the genioglossus and palatal muscles, which become hypotonic during sleep (Fig 12.28). Partial narrowing results in snoring, occlusion in apnoea and critical narrowing in hypopnoeas. Patients are woken by the struggle to breathe against the blocked throat. The awakenings are so brief that the patient remains unaware of them but is woken thousands of times per night leading to daytime sleepiness and impaired performance. Important contributory factors are obesity, a small pharyngeal opening and COPD.

Correctable factors occur in about one-third of cases and include:

- encroachment on pharynx – obesity, acromegaly, enlarged tonsils
- nasal obstruction – nasal deformities, rhinitis, polyps, adenoids
- respiratory depressant drugs – alcohol, sedatives, strong analgesics.

DIAGNOSIS

The diagnosis can usually be made by non-invasive ear or finger oximetry, best performed at home, accompanied by observation of the pattern of the snore-silence-snore cycle by the patient's family. Arterial oxygen saturation falls significantly in a cyclical manner. However, false-negative or equivocal results may occur in 50%, necessitating full polysomnographic studies. These involve:

- electroencephalography to record patterns of sleep and arousal
- recording of thoracoabdominal movements to assess breathing

Table 12.11
Signs of obstructive sleep apnoea

Loud snoring (95%)	Nocturnal choking (30%)
Daytime sleepiness (90%)	Reduced libido (20%)
Unrefreshed sleep (40%)	Morning drunkenness (5%)
Restless sleep (40%)	Ankle swelling (5%)
Morning headache (30%)	

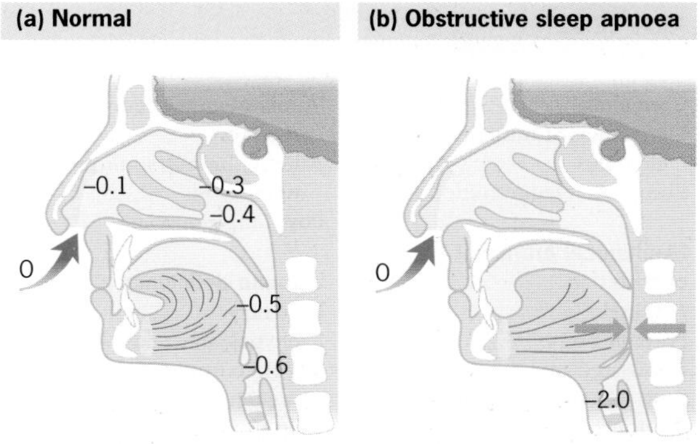

Fig 12.28
Section through head, showing pressure changes (in kPa) in (a) the normal situation and (b) obstructive sleep apnoea. There is a pressure drop during inspiration as air is sucked through the turbinates. In patients with obstructive sleep apnoea this is sufficient to collapse the pharynx, obstructing inspiration

- oronasal flow
- oximetry.

The diagnosis of sleep apnoea/hypopnoea is made if there are more than 15 apnoeas or hypopnoeas in any 1 hour of sleep.

MANAGEMENT

Management consists of correction of treatable factors (see above) with, if necessary, nasal continuous positive airway pressure (CPAP) delivered by a nasal mask during sleep. Such systems raise the pressure in the pharynx by about 1 kPa, keeping the walls apart.

Bronchiectasis

The term 'bronchiectasis' is used to describe abnormal and permanently dilated airways. Bronchial walls become inflamed, thickened and irreversibly damaged. The mucociliary transport mechanism is impaired and frequent bacterial infections ensue. Clinically, the disease is characterized by cough production of large amounts of sputum and dilated and thickened bronchi, detected on CT scanning of the thorax.

AETIOLOGY

The causes are shown in Table 12.12. Cystic fibrosis is now the most common cause in developed countries.

CLINICAL FEATURES

Patients with mild bronchiectasis only produce yellow or green sputum after an infection. Localized areas of the lung may be particularly affected, when sputum production will depend on position. As the condition worsens, the patient suffers from persistent halitosis, recurrent febrile episodes with malaise, and episodes of pneumonia. Clubbing occurs, and coarse crackles can be heard over the infected areas, usually the bases of the

Table 12.12
Causes of bronchiectasis

Congenital Deficiency of bronchial wall elements Pulmonary sequestration	**Immunological over-response** Allergic bronchopulmonary aspergillosis Post-lung transplant
Mechanical bronchial obstruction **Intrinsic** Foreign body Inspissated mucus Post-tuberculous stenosis Tumour **Extrinsic** Lymph node Tumour	**Immune deficiency** **Primary** Panhypogammaglobulinaemia Selective immunoglobulin deficiencies (IgA and IgG_2) **Secondary** HIV and malignancy
Postinfective bronchial damage Bacterial and viral pneumonia, including pertussis, measles and aspiration pneumonia	**Mucociliary clearance defects** **Genetic** Primary ciliary dyskinesia (Kartagener's syndrome with dextrocardia and situs inversus) Cystic fibrosis
Granuloma and fibrosis Tuberculosis, sarcoidosis and fibrosing alveolitis	**Acquired** Young's syndrome – azoospermia sinusitis

lungs. When the condition is severe there is continuous production of foul-smelling, thick, khaki-coloured sputum. Haemoptysis, either as blood-stained sputum or as a massive haemorrhage, can occur. Breathlessness may result from airflow limitation.

INVESTIGATIONS

- **Chest X-ray** may be normal or may show dilated bronchi with thickened bronchial walls and sometimes multiple cysts containing fluid.
- **High-resolution CT scanning** (see p. 760) shows bronchial dilatation and wall thickening and is the investigation of choice (Fig 12.29).
- **Bronchography** is rarely required except if the diagnosis is in doubt or where there is reason to believe that the disease may be localized and therefore amenable to surgical treatment. The left lower lobe and lingula are the most common sites for localized disease. The investigation is uncomfortable and can be performed during fibreoptic bronchoscopy.
- **Sputum** examination with culture and sensitivity of the organisms is essential for adequate treatment. The major pathogens are *Staph. aureus*, *Pseudomonas aeruginosa*, *H. influenzae* and anaerobes. Other pathogens include *Strep. pneumoniae* and *Klebsiella pneumoniae*. *Aspergillus fumigatus* can be isolated from 10% of sputum specimens in cystic fibrosis, but the role of this organism is uncertain.
- **Sinus X-rays**. Thirty per cent have concomitant purulent rhinosinusitis.
- **Serum immunoglobulins**. Ten per cent of adults have immune deficiency.
- **Sweat electrolytes** – if appropriate (see p. 784).
- **Mucociliary clearance** (nasal clearance of saccharin). A 1 mm cube of saccharin is placed on the inferior turbinate and the time to taste measured (normally less than 30 minutes).

TREATMENT

Postural drainage

Postural drainage is of vital importance and patients must be trained by physiotherapists to tip themselves into a position in which the lobe to be drained is uppermost at least three times daily for 10–20 minutes. Most patients find that lying over the side of the bed with head and thorax down is the most effective position.

Antibiotics

Experience from the treatment of cystic fibrosis suggests that bronchopulmonary infections should be eradicated if progression of the disease is to be halted. In mild cases, intermittent chemotherapy with cefaclor 500 mg thrice daily or ciprofloxacin 500 mg twice daily may be the only therapy needed. Flucloxacillin 500 mg 6-hourly is the best treatment if *Staph. aureus* is isolated.

If the sputum remains yellow or green despite regular physiotherapy and intermittent chemotherapy, or if lung function deteriorates despite treatment with bronchodilators, it is likely that there is infection with *Ps. aeruginosa*. Treatment requires parenteral or aerosol chemotherapy at regular three-month intervals. Ceftazidime 2 g intravenously 8-hourly or by inhalation (1 g twice daily) has been shown to be effective. Ciprofloxacin 750 mg twice daily orally may be equally effective but rapid development of resistance is a problem. High sputum levels of some antibiotics can be achieved by inhalation. A treatment regimen of ticarcillin 1 g and gentamicin

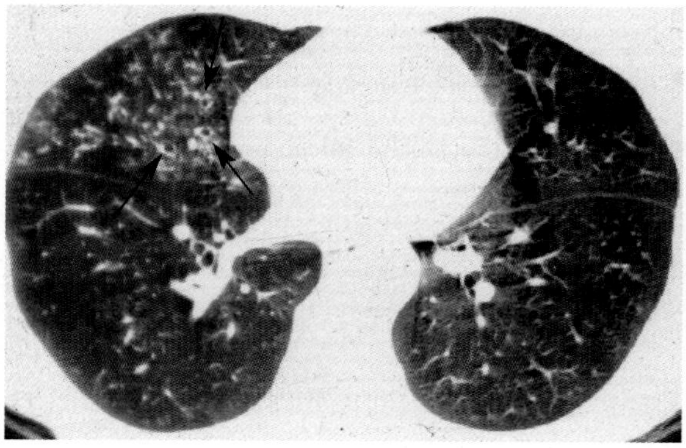

Fig 12.29
CT scan showing bronchiectasis in the right middle lobe. Note dilated bronchi with thickened wall and adjacent artery giving a signet ring appearance

80 mg given by a compressor-driven nebulizer twice daily is useful in young adult patients with chronic *Pseudomonas* infection, but many physicians prefer intravenous therapy with ceftazidime.

Bronchodilators

Bronchodilators are useful in patients with demonstrable airflow limitation.

Anti-inflammatory agents

Inhaled or oral steroids can decrease the rate of progression.

Surgery

Unfortunately, bronchiectasis is rarely sufficiently localized for surgery to be of any value. Lung–heart lung transplantation is sometimes required.

COMPLICATIONS

The incidence of complications has fallen with antibiotic therapy. Pneumonia, pneumothorax, empyema and metastatic cerebral abscess can occur. Severe, life-threatening haemoptysis can also occur, particularly in patients with cystic fibrosis.

PROGNOSIS

The advent of effective antibiotic therapy has greatly improved the prognosis, improving life expectancy from less than 40 years to approximately 55 years.

Massive haemoptysis originates from the high-pressure systemic bronchial arteries and has a mortality of 25%. Other causes, apart from bronchiectasis, include pulmonary tuberculosis (most common), aspergilloma, lung abscess and infection, and primary and secondary malignant tumours.

Treatment of the haemoptysis consists of bedrest and antibiotics when most stop bleeding. Blood transfusion is given if required. Urgent fibreoptic bronchoscopy is occasionally necessary to detect the source of bleeding. If the haemoptysis does not settle rapidly the affected area must be surgically resected. Bronchial artery embolization is the treatment of choice in those not fit for surgery.

Cystic fibrosis

In cystic fibrosis (CF) there is an alteration in the viscosity and tenacity of mucus production at epithelial surfaces. The classical form of the syndrome includes bronchopulmonary infection and pancreatic insufficiency, with a high sweat sodium and chloride concentration. It is an autosomal recessive inherited disorder with a carrier frequency in Caucasians of 1 in 22 (see p. 154). There is a gene mutation on the long arm of chromosome 7 (7q 21.3 → 7q 22.1). A specific deletion in the coding region – the codon for phenylalanine at position 508 in the amino acid sequence [ΔF_{508}] – results in a defect in a transmembrane regulator protein (see p. 157). This is the cystic fibrosis transmembrane conductance regulator (CFTR) which represents a critical chloride channel (Fig 12.30). The mutation alters the secondary and tertiary structure of the protein, leading to a failure of opening of the chloride channel in response to elevated cyclic AMP in epithelial cells. This results in a decreased excretion of chloride into the airway lumen and a threefold increase in the reabsorption of sodium into the epithelial cells. With less excretion of salt there is less excretion of water and increased viscosity and tenacity of airway secretions. A possible reason for the high salt content of sweat is that there is a CFTR-independent mechanism of chloride secretion in the sweat gland with an impaired reabsorption of sodium chloride in the distal end of the duct.

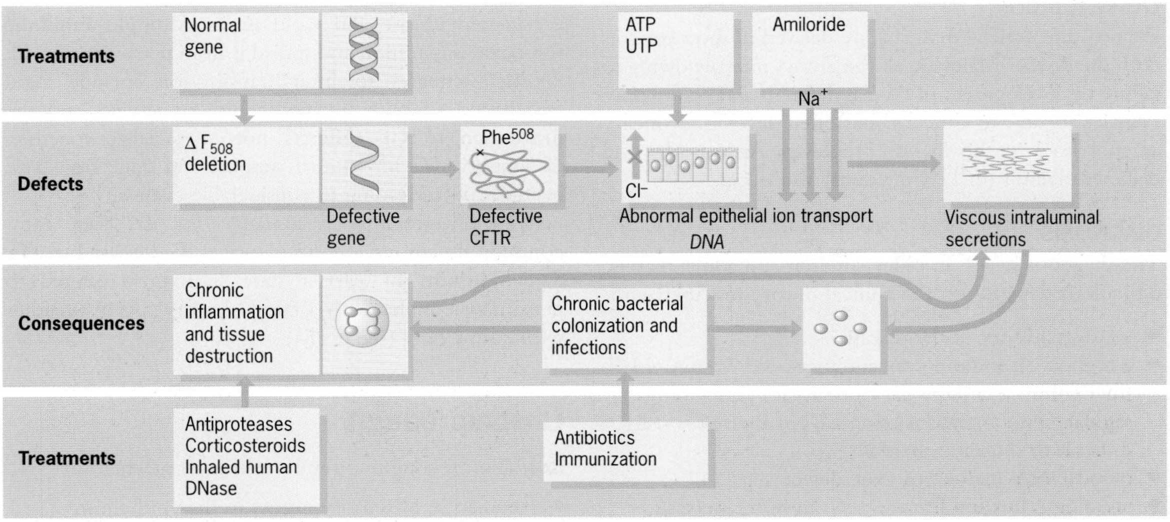

Fig 12.30
Cystic fibrosis: abnormalities and recent therapeutic advances (see text)

The frequency of ΔF_{508} mutation in CF is 70% in the USA and UK, under 50% in southern Europe and 30% in Ashkenazi families.

CLINICAL FEATURES

Respiratory effects

Although the lungs of babies born with CF are structurally normal at birth, respiratory symptoms are usually the presenting feature. CF is now the most common cause of recurrent bronchopulmonary infection in childhood, and is an important cause in early adult life.

Sinusitis is almost inevitable and finger clubbing universal. Haemoptysis is frequent and breathlessness occurs in the later stages as airflow limitation develops. Older children may also develop nasal polyps. Spontaneous pneumothorax may occur. Respiratory failure and cor pulmonale eventually develop.

Gastrointestinal effects

About 85% of patients have symptomatic steatorrhoea owing to pancreatic dysfunction (see p. 350). Children may be born with meconium ileus owing to the viscoid consistency of meconium in CF, and later in life develop the meconium ileus equivalent (MIE) syndrome, an important cause of small intestinal obstruction unique to CF. Cholesterol gallstones appear to occur with increased frequency. Cirrhosis develops in about 5% of older patients. Other associations include an increased incidence of peptic ulceration and gastrointestinal malignancy.

Nutritional effects

Many patients suffer from malnutrition resulting mainly from anorexia associated with pulmonary sepsis. Reduced absorption due to pancreatic insufficiency is another contributory factor.

Other features

Puberty and skeletal maturity are delayed in most patients with the disease. Males are almost always infertile owing to failure of development of the vas deferens and epididymis. Females are able to conceive, but often develop secondary amenorrhoea as the disease progresses. Arthropathy and diabetes mellitus (in 11% of adults) also occur.

DIAGNOSIS

The diagnosis of CF in older children and adults may be difficult. It depends on the clinical history together with:

- a family history of the disease
- a high sweat sodium concentration over 60 mmol L^{-1} (meticulous technique by laboratories performing regular sweat analysis is essential, but the test is still difficult to interpret in adults)
- blood DNA analyses of gene defect
- radiology showing features seen in bronchiectasis (see p. 782).
- absent vas deferens and epididymis
- blood immunoreactive trypsin levels are not useful diagnostically but may be useful in screening.

TREATMENT

Antibiotic treatment for the respiratory disease is described under bronchiectasis on p. 782 and treatment of pancreatic insufficiency and malnutrition is described on p. 370.

Better understanding of the basic abnormality in CF has led to dramatic changes in treatment. Potential treatments to improve hydration of secretions include blocking of Na^+ reabsorption with amiloride or stimulating Cl^- secretion with a triphosphate nucleotide (adenosine or uridine triphosphates, ATP and UTP) which stimulate nucleotide receptors by a pathway independent of cAMP. Viscosity of secretions is contributed to by macromolecules such as DNA from dead inflammatory cells. Human DNase capable of degrading DNA has been cloned, sequenced and expressed by recombinant techniques. Inhalation of this material has been shown to improve FEV_1 by 20%. Similarly, inhaled or oral corticosteroids and antiproteases such as inhaled α_1-antitrypsin inhibitor help to reduce inflammation and improve lung function.

Human experimental studies have been conducted on the delivery to the epithelium of the normal CFTR gene using, as a vector, a replication-deficient adenovirus containing normal human CFTR complementary DNA which is trophic for epithelial cells.

Lung transplantation should be considered (p. 785).

PROGNOSIS AND COUNSELLING

The prognosis has consistently improved; 90% of children survive into their teens and the median survival for those born after 1990 is 40 years. Progressive respiratory failure almost inevitably occurs. Of particular concern is the finding in sputum of *Burkholderia* (previously *Pseudomonas*) *cepacia*, a plant pathogen previously considered a harmless commensal. Its acquisition can be associated with accelerated disease and rapid death. Multiple antibiotic resistance is common and spread is from person to person. Drastic strategies to limit transmission include rigid segregation of both inpatients and outpatients and the instruction to CF sufferers not to socialize together. Groups formed for mutual support and education have been disrupted leading to considerable distress.

Genetic screening is available for the four most common mutations and this identifies 85–95% of carriers. Screening for the carrier state should be offered to persons or couples with a family history of CF, together with counselling (see p. 154).

Chronic cough

Pathological coughing results from two mechanisms:

- stimulation of sensory nerves in the epithelium by secretions, foreign bodies, cigarette smoke and tumours

- sensitization of the cough reflex in which there is an abnormal increase in the sensitivity of the cough receptors demonstrable by inhalation of the tussive agents capsaicin or low chloride solutions

Sensitization of the cough reflex presents clinically as a persistent tickling sensation in the throat with paroxysms of coughing induced by changes in air temperature, aerosol sprays, perfumes and cigarette smoke. It is found in association with viral infections, oesophageal reflux, postnasal drip, cough variant asthma, idiopathic cough, and in 15% of patients taking angiotensin converting enzyme (ACE) inhibitors. The association with the latter implicates neuroactive peptides – prostaglandins E_2 and $F_{2\alpha}$ and bradykinin as a cause of the cough. In the absence of chest X-ray abnormalities, investigations should include:

- ENT examination and sinus CT for postnasal drip
- lung function tests and histamine bronchial provocation testing for cough variant asthma
- ambulatory oesophageal pH monitoring for oesophageal reflux
- CT scan of thorax for interstitial lung disease
- $\dot{V}_A/\dot{Q}$ scans for recurrent pulmonary embolism
- fibreoptic bronchoscopy for inhaled foreign body or tumour
- ECG, echocardiography and exercise testing for cardiac causes
- hyperventilation testing and psychiatric appraisal

Treatment in the absence of any pathology makes the management of cough difficult. Morphine will depress the sensitized cough reflex but its unwanted effects limit its use in the long term. Dihydrocodeine linctus may be of value in some patients. Demulcent preparations and cough sweets provide temporary relief only. Patients on ACE inhibitors should be changed to an angiotensin-II receptor antagonist, e.g. losartan (see p. 680).

Lung and heart–lung transplantation

INDICATIONS AND DONOR SELECTION

Indications for this treatment are patients under 60 years with a life expectancy of less than 18 months, no underlying cancer and no serious systemic disease. The main diseases treated by transplantation are:

- pulmonary fibrosis
- primary pulmonary hypertension
- cystic fibrosis
- bronchiectasis
- emphysema – particularly α_1-antitrypsin inhibitor deficiency
- Eisenmenger's syndrome.

Donor selection includes age under 40 years, good cardiac and lung function, and chest measurements slightly smaller than the recipient's. Matching for ABO blood group compatibility but not rhesus blood group is essential. Since donor material is limited, single lung transplantation is preferred to double lung or heart–lung transplantation and can be successfully undertaken in pulmonary fibrosis, pulmonary hypertension and emphysema. Bilateral lung transplantation is required in infective conditions to prevent spillover of bacteria from the diseased lung to a single lung transplant. Eisenmenger's syndrome requires heart–lung transplant.

COMPLICATIONS AND THEIR TREATMENT

- *Early* – post-transplant pulmonary oedema requires diuretics and respiratory support by ventilation.
- *Infections*, particularly within first three months:
  Bacterial pneumonia – antibiotics
  Cytomegalovirus – ganciclovir
  Herpes simplex – acyclovir
  P. carinii – prophylactic co-trimoxazole.
- *Immunosuppression* is with cyclosporin, azathioprine and prednisolone.
- *Rejection:*
  Early (first few weeks) – high-dose i.v. corticosteroids
  Late (after three months) – in obliterative bronchiolitis, high-dose i.v. corticosteroids are sometimes effective.

Prognosis. There is a two-year survival of 75% and five-year survival of almost 50%.

FURTHER READING

Lamb D, Wallace WAH (1995) Pathology of chronic obstructive pulmonary disease. *Medicine* **23**: 303–305.

Wood AJJ (1996) Management of pulmonary disease in cystic fibrosis *New England Journal of Medicine* **335**:179–188.

Wright J, Johns R, Watts I, Melville A, Sheldon T (1997). Health effects of obstructive sleep apnoea and the effectiveness of continuous positive airways pressure: a systemic review of the research evidence. *British Medical Journal* **314**: 851–860.

Asthma

Asthma is a common chronic inflammatory condition of the lung airways whose cause is incompletely understood. Symptoms are cough, wheeze, chest tightness and shortness of breath, often worse at night. It has three characteristics:

- *airflow limitation* which is usually reversible spontaneously or with treatment
- *airway hyperresponsiveness* to a wide range of stimuli (see below)
- *inflammation of the bronchi* with eosinophils, T lymphocytes and mast cells with associated plasma exudation, oedema, smooth muscle hypertrophy, mucus plugging and epithelial damage.

In chronic asthma, inflammation may lead to irreversible airflow limitation.

The underlying pathology in preschool children may be different, in that they may not exhibit appreciable bronchial hyperreactivity. There is no evidence that chronic inflammation is the basis for the episodic asthma associated with viral infections.

PREVALENCE

In many countries the prevalence of asthma is increasing, particularly in the second decade of life where this disease affects 10–15% of the population. There is also a geographical variation, with asthma being common in, for example, New Zealand, but being much rarer in Far Eastern countries such as China and Malaysia. Long-term follow-up in developing countries suggests that the disease may become more frequent as individuals become more 'Westernized'. Studies of occupational asthma suggest that a high percentage of the workforce, perhaps up to 20%, may become asthmatic if exposed to potent sensitizers.

CLASSIFICATION

Asthma can be divided into:

- *extrinsic* – implying a definite external cause
- *intrinsic or cryptogenic* – when no causative agent can be identified.

Extrinsic asthma occurs most frequently in atopic individuals who show positive skin-prick reactions to common inhaled allergens. Positive skin tests to inhalant allergens are shown in 90% of children with asthma, whereas only 50% of adults show this phenomenon. Eczema is often seen in childhood (see p. 1160).

Intrinsic asthma often starts in middle age. Nevertheless, many show positive skin tests and on close questioning give a history of respiratory symptoms compatible with childhood asthma.

However, this classification is of little value in clinical practice. Non-atopic individuals may develop asthma in middle age from extrinsic causes such as sensitization to occupational agents or aspirin intolerance, or because they were given β-adrenoreceptor-blocking agents for concurrent hypertension or angina. Extrinsic causes must be considered in all cases of asthma and, where possible, avoided.

AETIOLOGY AND PATHOGENESIS

There are two major factors involved in the development of asthma and many other stimuli that can precipitate attacks (Fig 12.31).

Atopy and allergy

The term 'atopy' was used by clinicians at the beginning of the century to describe a group of disorders, including asthma and hay fever, that appeared:

- to run in families
- to have characteristic wealing skin reactions to common allergens in the environment
- to have circulating antibody in their serum that could be transferred to the skin of non-sensitized individuals.

The term is now best used to describe those individuals who readily develop antibodies of IgE class against common materials present in the environment. Such antibodies are present in 30–40% of the population, and there is a link between serum IgE levels and both the prevalence of asthma and airway responsiveness to histamine or methacholine. Genetic and environmental factors affect serum IgE levels. The use of candidate groups for linkage and DNA microsatellite markers to scan the entire genome has uncovered 14–15 separate linkages so far. Some of these, in combination with environmental factors, may turn out to play a key role in the development of asthma. The genes controlling the production of the cytokines IL-3, IL-4, IL-5, and GM-CSF – which in turn affect mast and eosinophil cell development and longevity as well as IgE production – are present on chromosome 5.1q. Early childhood exposure to allergens and maternal smoking have an important influence on IgE production.

The allergens involved are similar to those in rhinitis, though the particle size of pollens (>20 μm) means that they are much more likely to cause conjunctivitis, rhinitis and pharyngitis than asthma. Allergens from the faecal particles of the house-dust mite are the most important extrinsic cause of asthma worldwide. Recently cockroach allergy has been implicated in asthma in inner-city

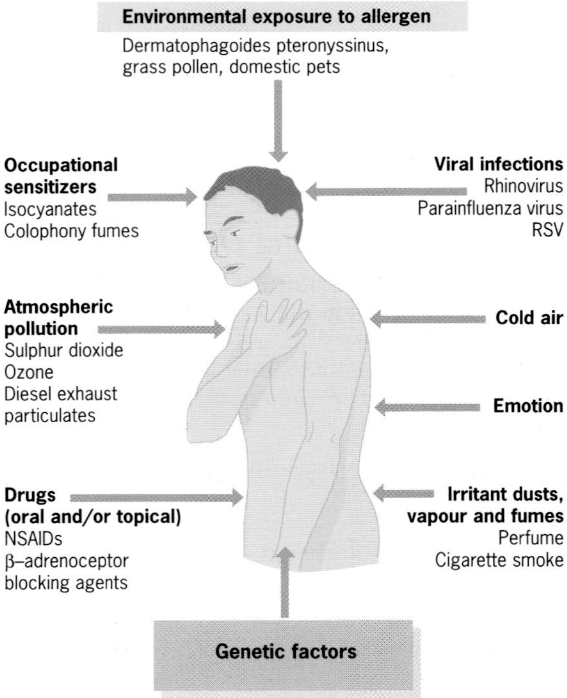

Fig 12.31
Causes and triggers of asthma. RSV, respiratory syncytial virus; NSAIDs, non-steroidal anti-inflammatory drugs

children. The fungal spores from *A. fumigatus* give rise to a complex series of lung disease, including asthma (see p. 811).

Increased responsiveness of the airways of the lung (airway hyperreactivity)

Bronchial reactivity can be demonstrated by asking the patient to inhale gradually increasing concentrations either of histamine or methacholine (*bronchial provocation tests*). This induces a transient episode of airflow limitation in susceptible individuals (approximately 20% of the population); the dose of the agonist (provocation dose) necessary to produce a 20% fall in FEV_1 is known as the $PD_{20}FEV_1$. Patients with clinical symptoms of asthma respond to very low doses of methacholine; i.e. they have a low $PD_{20}FEV_1$ (<11 μmol). In general, the greater the degree of hyperreactivity, the more persistent the symptoms and the greater the need for treatment.

Some patients also react to methacholine but at *higher doses* and include those with:

- attacks of asthma only on extreme exertion
- wheezing or prolonged periods of coughing following a viral infection
- cough variant asthma
- problems with asthma only during the pollen season
- allergic rhinitis, but not complaining of any lower respiratory symptoms until specifically questioned
- some subjects with no respiratory symptoms.

Although the degree of hyperreactivity can itself be influenced by allergic mechanisms (see p. 788 and Fig 12.34), its pathogenesis and mode of inheritance remain to be elucidated.

PRECIPITATING FACTORS

Occupational sensitizers

Over 200 materials encountered at the workplace are known to give rise to occupational asthma. The important causes are recognized occupational diseases in the UK, and patients in insurable employment are therefore eligible for statutory compensation provided they apply within 10 years of leaving the occupation in which the asthma developed (Table 12.13). The development of asthma following exposure to some of these materials is linked to the development of specific IgE antibody in serum in some cases, whilst in others the cause has yet to be determined.

The proportion of employees developing occupational asthma depends primarily upon the level of exposure. Proper enclosure of industrial processes or appropriate ventilation can greatly reduce the risk. Atopic individuals develop occupational asthma more rapidly when exposed to agents causing the development of specific IgE antibody. Non-atopic individuals can also develop asthma when exposed to such agents, but usually after a longer period.

Nonspecific factors

The characteristic feature of bronchial hyperreactivity in asthmatics means that as well as reacting to specific antigens their airways will also respond to a wide variety of nonspecific stimuli.

Cold air and exercise

Most asthmatics experience an attack of wheezing after prolonged and continuous exercise. Typically, the attack does not occur during the exercise period but at its conclusion. The inhalation of cold, dry air will also precipitate an attack. In both cases the wheezing is thought to be precipitated by the cooling and drying of the epithelial lining of the bronchi. Exercise and cold air provocation tests can be performed.

Atmospheric pollution and irritant dusts, vapours and fumes

Many patients with asthma experience worsening of symptoms on contact with cigarette smoke, car exhaust fumes, strong perfumes or high concentrations of dust in the atmosphere. Further minor epidemics of the disease have occurred during periods of heavy atmospheric pollution in industrial areas, caused by the presence of high concentrations of sulphur dioxide, ozone and nitrogen dioxide in the air.

Diet

Increased intakes of fresh fruit and vegetables may be preventative.

Emotion

It is well known that emotional factors may influence asthma, but there is no evidence that patients with the disease are any more psychologically disturbed than their non-asthmatic peers.

Table 12.13
Occupational asthma in the UK

Cause	Source
Non-IgE related	
Isocyanates	Polyurethane varnishes Industrial coatings Spray painting
Colophony fumes	Soldering/welders Electronics industry
IgE related	
Allergens from animals and insects	Laboratories
Allergens from flour and grain	Farmers Millers/bakers Grain handlers
Proteolytic enzymes	Manufacture (but not use) of 'biological' washing powders
Complex salts of platinum	Metal refining
Acid anhydrides and polyamine hardening agents	Industrial coatings

Drugs

Non-steroidal anti-inflammatory drugs (NSAIDs), particularly aspirin, have a major role in the development and precipitation of attacks in approximately 5% of patients with asthma. This effect is almost universal in those individuals who have both nasal polyps and asthma. The precise mechanism involved is unknown, but it is thought that treatment with these drugs leads to an imbalance in the metabolism of arachidonic acid. NSAIDs inhibit arachidonic acid metabolism via the cyclooxygenase (COX) pathway, preventing the synthesis of prostaglandins. It is suggested that under these circumstances arachidonic acid is preferentially metabolized via the lipoxygenase pathway, resulting in the production of leukotrienes, previously known as the slow-reacting substances for anaphylaxis (Fig 12.32).

The airways of the lung have a direct parasympathetic innervation that tends to produce bronchoconstriction. There is no direct sympathetic innervation of the smooth muscle of the bronchi, and antagonism of parasympathetically induced bronchoconstriction is critically dependent upon circulating adrenaline acting through β_2-receptors on the surface of smooth muscle cells. Inhibition of this effect by β-adrenoreceptor-blocking drugs such as propranolol leads to bronchoconstriction and airflow limitation, but only in asthmatic subjects. The so-called selective β_1-adrenoceptor-blocking drugs such as atenolol may still induce attacks of asthma; their use in asthmatic patients for hypertension or angina should be questioned.

Allergen-induced asthma

The experimental inhalation of allergen by atopic asthmatic individuals leads to the development of four types of reaction, as illustrated in Fig 12.33.

Immediate asthma

This is the most common reaction, in which airflow limitation begins within minutes of contact with the allergen, reaches its maximum in 15–20 minutes and subsides by 1 hour.

Dual asthmatic resonse

This is a combination of an immediate reaction followed by a late reaction.

Late-phase reactions

Following an immediate reaction many asthmatics subsequently develop a more prolonged and sustained attack of airflow limitation that responds poorly to inhalation of bronchodilator drugs such as salbutamol. Alternatively, the inhalation of some materials, particularly occupational sensitizers such as the isocyanates, usually causes the development of an *isolated late reaction* with no preceding immediate response.

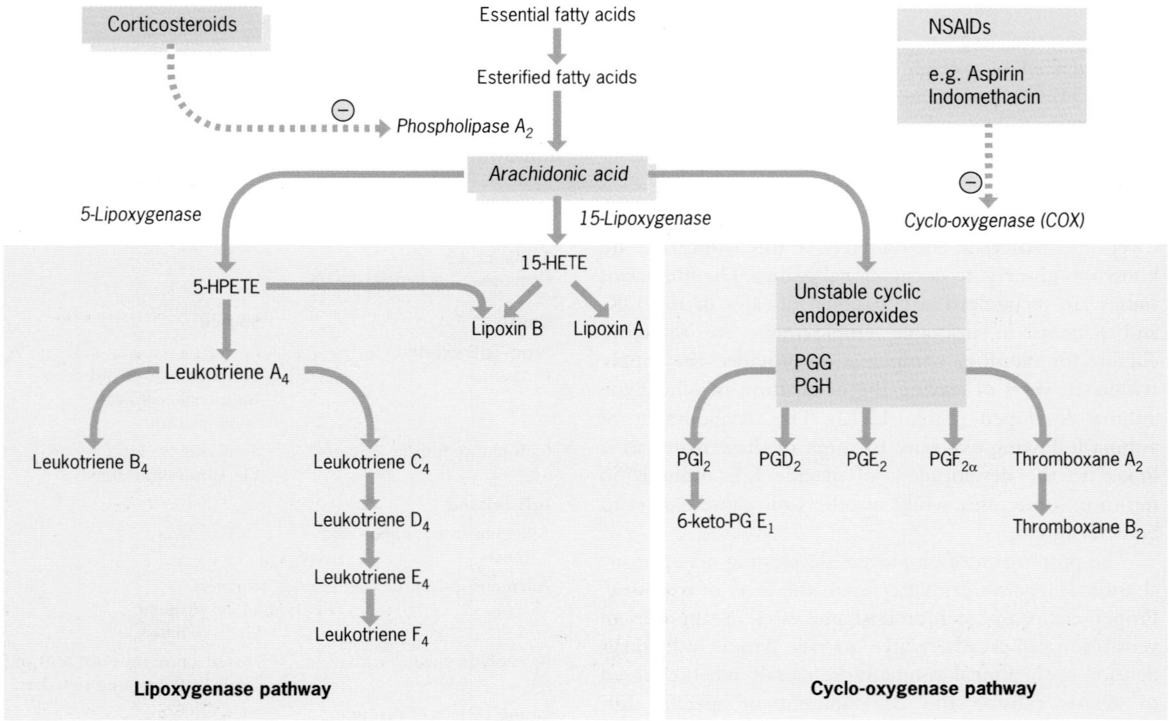

Fig 12.32
Arachidonic acid metabolism and the effect of drugs
The enzyme cyclo-oxygenase occurs in two isoforms, COX-1 (constitutive) and COX-2 (inducible)

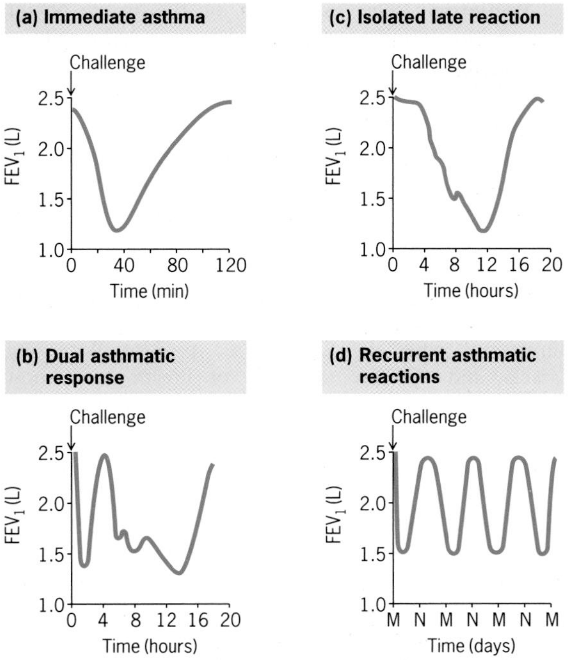

Fig 12.33
Different types of asthmatic reactions following challenge with allergen. (a) Immediate asthma. **(b)** Dual asthmatic response. **(c)** Isolated late reaction. **(d)** Recurrent asthmatic reactions. M, midnight; N, noon

Recurrent asthmatic reactions

The development of the late-phase reaction is associated with an increase in the underlying level of airway hyperreactivity such that individuals may show continuing episodes of asthma on subsequent days.

PATHOGENESIS

The pathogenesis of asthma is complex and not fully understood. It involves a number of cells, mediators, nerves and vascular leakage that can be activated by several different mechanisms, of which exposure to allergens is the most important (Fig 12.34). It is now appreciated that there are differences in the underlying pathogenesis of *intermittent and mild asthma*, which is mast cell driven, and *severe asthma* in which the lymphocyte is the prime driving cell.

Mast cells (see also p. 164). These are increased in both the epithelium and surface secretions of asthmatics and can generate and release powerful smooth muscle and vasoactive mediators, such as histamine, prostaglandin D_2 (PGD_2) and leukotriene C_4 (LTC_4), which cause the immediate asthmatic reaction. Since potent β_2-adrenoceptor agonists such as salbutamol have little effect on airway inflammation or hyperreactivity but inhibit mast cell mediator release, many other factors are involved in the pathogenesis of late and recurrent asthmatic reactions leading to more severe asthma.

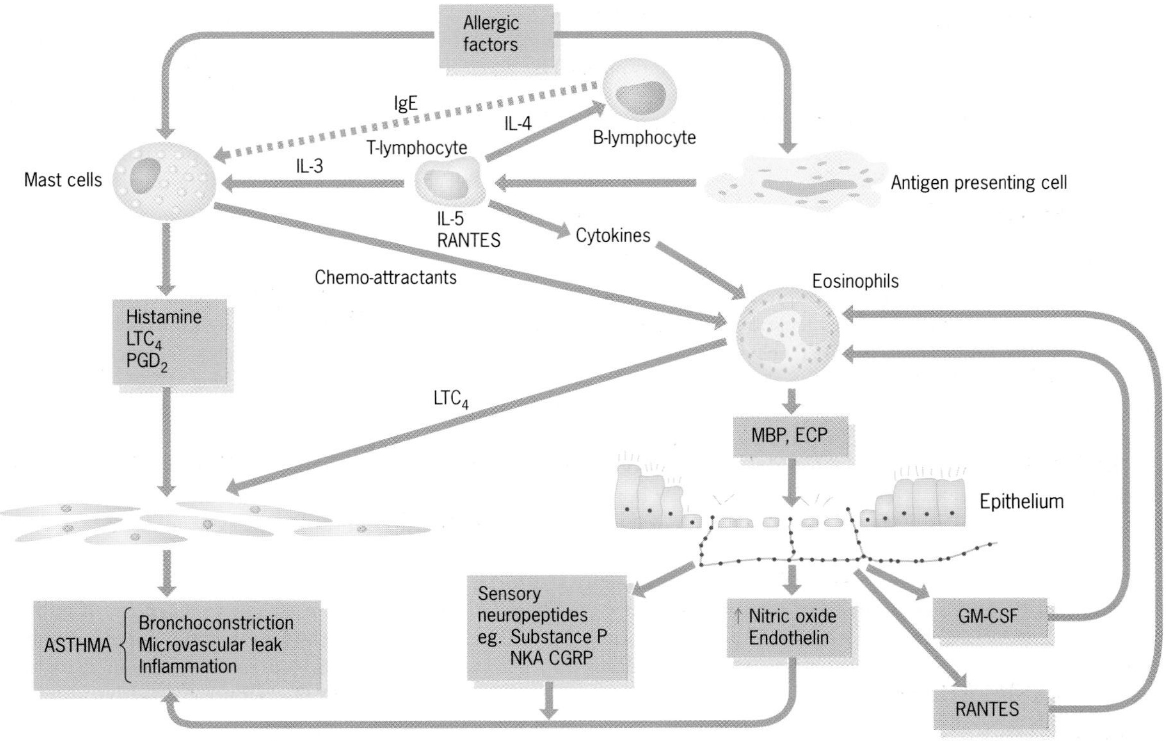

Fig 12.34
Pathogenesis of asthma. ECP, eosinophil cationic protein; MBP, major basic protein; CGRP, calcitonin gene-related peptide; NKA, neurokinin A

Epithelium. Epithelial cells are shed during exacerbations of asthma (they can readily be identified in sputum), causing increased permeability of airways to inhaled allergens, exposure of afferent nerve endings, and release of neutral endopeptidases capable of breaking down sensory neuropeptides. There is also generation of eosinophil chemoattractant factors such as the chemokine RANTES (Regulated upon activation of normal T cell expressed and secreted). Epithelial cells also produce cytokines, particularly granulocyte macrophage colony stimulating factor (GM-CSF) which prolongs the life of tissue eosinophils, tumour necrosis factor-α (TNF-α) and interleukin-1β, both of which up-regulate expression of intercellular adhesion molecule-1 (ICAM-1) which plays a crucial role in capturing inflammatory cells within the epithelium, and interleukin 8 (IL-8) which is a chemoattractant for neutrophils.

Basement membrane. Biopsy studies have shown that the subbasement membrane region, the lamina reticularis, is widened even in the mildest asthmatics owing to increased deposition of collagen types III and V and fibronectin, indicating that inflammation occurs at the earliest stages of the disease.

Nerves. There is a complex interaction between the neural control of airways and inflammation. Damage or loss of epithelial cells exposes C-fibre afferent nerve endings that can release the sensory neuropeptides substance P, neurokinin (NK) A and calcitonin gene-related peptide (CGRP). Substance P and neurokinin A, members of the tachykinin family, act through the transmembrane receptor NK-1R to increase the inflammatory process. This contributes towards bronchoconstriction, microvascular leakage and mucus secretion. Vasoactive intestinal peptide (VIP) and nitric oxide, both potent neurotransmitters, are rapidly degraded in inflammation, leading to bronchoconstriction.

Macrophages and lymphocytes. These cells are abundant in the mucous membranes of the airways and the alveoli. Macrophages may have a role in the initial uptake and presentation of allergens to lymphocytes. They can release prostaglandins, thromboxanes, leukotriene B_4 (LTB_4) and platelet activating factor (PAF). T-helper lymphocytes (CD4) show evidence of activation and the release of their cytokines may play a part in the migration and activation of mast cells (IL-3) and eosinophils (IL-5). In addition production of IL-4 leads to the switching of antibody production by B lymphocytes to IgE. The activity of both macrophages and lymphocytes is influenced by corticosteroids but not β_2-adrenoceptor agonists.

Eosinophils. These cells are found in large numbers in the bronchial secretions of asthmatics. When activated, they release LTC_4, PAF and basic proteins such as major basic protein (MBP) and eosinophil cationic protein (ECP) that are toxic to epithelial cells. Both the number and activation of eosinophils is rapidly decreased by corticosteroids.

Mediators. The exact role of the many potent smooth muscle and vasoactive mediators, including LTC_4, LTD_4, thromboxanes and the sensory neuropeptides, as well as the chemoattractants LTB_4 and PAF, awaits the introduction of effective and specific antagonists. Studies with potent selective H_1 antagonists have shown that histamine plays only a small role in the pathogenesis of the persisting airflow limitation of asthma.

CLINICAL FEATURES

Patients suffering from asthma exhibit symptoms that are virtually identical to those suffering from airflow limitation caused by COPD (see p. 776). Wheezing attacks and episodic shortness of breath are almost universal. Symptoms are usually worst during the night. Cough is a frequent symptom that sometimes predominates and is often misdiagnosed as being due to bronchitis. Nocturnal cough can be a presenting feature.

There is a tremendous variation in the frequency and duration of the attacks. Some patients have only one or two attacks a year that last for a few hours, whilst others have attacks lasting for weeks. Some patients can have chronic symptoms. Attacks may be precipitated by all the factors illustrated in Fig 12.31. The signs of asthma are listed in Table 12.2 on p. 756.

INVESTIGATIONS

There is no single satisfactory diagnostic test for all asthmatic patients.

Lung function tests

The diagnosis of asthma is based on the demonstration of a greater than 15% improvement in FEV_1 or PEFR following the inhalation of a bronchodilator. However, this is often not present if the asthma is in remission or in very severe chronic disease, when little reversibility can be demonstrated.

Peak flow charts

Measurements of PEFR on waking, in the middle of the day, and before bed are particularly useful in demonstrating the variable airflow limitation that characterizes the disease. An example is shown in Fig 12.15 on p. 763. This technique is also of help in the longer-term assessment of the patient's disease and its response to treatment. Peak flows need to be measured over several days and preferably over a weekend or short holiday if the effect of work exposure is also being studied.

Exercise tests

These have been widely used in the diagnosis of asthma in children. Ideally, the child should run for six minutes on a treadmill at a workload sufficient to increase the heart rate above 160 beats per minute. A negative test does not rule out asthma.

Histamine or methacholine bronchial provocations test (see p. 787)

This test indicates the presence of airway hyperreactivity, a feature found in all asthmatics, and can be particularly useful in investigating those patients whose main symptom is cough. The test should *not* be performed on individuals who have poor lung function (FEV_1 < 1.5 L).

Trial of corticosteroids

Prednisolone 30 mg orally should be given daily for two weeks to all patients who present with severe airflow limitation. A substantial improvement (>15%) confirms the presence of an asthmatic element and that the administration of steroids will prove beneficial to the patient. The dose is slowly reduced over several weeks and is replaced by inhaled corticosteroids in those who will benefit.

Blood and sputum tests

Patients with asthma may have an increase in the number of eosinophils in peripheral blood ($>0.4 \times 10^9$/L). This is rarely helpful in the diagnosis. The presence of large numbers of eosinophils, particularly when present in clumps in sputum, is helpful in the differential diagnosis of asthma from COPD.

Chest X-ray

There are no diagnostic features of asthma on the chest X-ray. A chest X-ray may be helpful in excluding a pneumothorax, which can occur as a complication, or in detecting the pulmonary shadows associated with allergic bronchopulmonary aspergillosis.

Skin tests

Skin-prick tests should be performed in all cases of asthma to help identify extrinsic causes. Experimentally, the inhalation of an allergen that gives rise to a large weal on skin testing will almost always produce an attack of asthma in patients with the disease, but whether this occurs in everyday life depends on the concentrations encountered in the atmosphere.

Allergen provocation tests

These are seldom, if ever, required in the clinical investigation of patients. An exception is the investigation of food allergy causing asthma. This diagnosis is difficult; blind oral challenges with the food disguised in opaque gelatine capsules are necessary to confirm or refute a causative link (see p. 213).

MANAGEMENT

Asthma is an extremely common disease producing considerable morbidity. The aim of treatment must be:

- to abolish symptoms
- to restore normal or best possible long-term airway function
- to reduce the risk of severe attacks
- to enable normal growth to occur in children
- to minimize absence from school or employment.

This involves:

- patient and family participation
- avoidance of identified causes where possible
- use of the lowest effective doses of convenient medications to minimize short-term and long-term side-effects.

Many asthmatics belong to self-help groups whose aim is to further their understanding of the disease and to foster self-confidence and fitness.

Control of extrinsic factors

Measures must be taken to avoid causative allergens such as the house-dust mite, pets, moulds and certain foodstuffs (see allergic rhinitis), particularly in childhood.

Avoidance of the house-dust mite is now possible with effective and comfortable covers for bedding and changes to living accommodation. Active and passive smoking should be avoided, as should β-blockers in either tablet or eyedrop form.

Individuals intolerant to aspirin may benefit, though are rarely cured, by avoiding salicylates. Other agents (e.g. preservatives and colouring materials such as tartrazine) should be avoided if shown to be a causative factor. Fifty per cent of individuals sensitized to occupational agents may be cured if they are kept permanently away from exposure. The remaining 50% continue to have symptoms as severe as when exposed to materials at work. This is particularly so if they had been symptomatic for a long time before the diagnosis was made.

All the foregoing underline two points:

- the importance of the rapid identification of extrinsic causes of asthma and their removal wherever possible (e.g. the family pet)
- once extrinsic asthma is initiated, it may become self-perpetuating.

Drug treatment

The mainstay of asthma therapy is the use of therapeutic agents delivered as aerosols or powders directly into the lungs (Practical box 12.4). The advantages of this method of administration are obvious. Drugs are delivered direct to the lung and the first-pass metabolism in the liver is avoided; both these factors mean that much lower doses are necessary and unwanted effects are slight.

Both national and international guidelines have been published on the stepwise treatment of asthma (Information box 12.1) based on three important factors:

- asthma self-management with regular asthma monitoring using peak flow meters and individual treatment plans discussed with each patient

Practical

Use of an inhaler

1. The canister is shaken.
2. The patient exhales to functional residual capacity (not residual volume), i.e. normal expiration.
3. The aerosol nozzle is placed to the open mouth.
4. The patient simultaneously inhales rapidly and activates the aerosol.
5. Inhalation is completed.
6. The breath is held for 10 seconds if possible.

Even with good technique only 15% of the contents is inhaled and 85% is deposited on the wall of the pharynx and ultimately swallowed.

Spacers

These are plastic conical spheres inserted between the patient's mouth and the inhaler. They are designed to reduce particle velocity so that less drug is deposited in the mouth. Spacers also diminish the need for coordination between aerosol activation and inhalation. They are useful in children and in the elderly.

Practical box 12.4 Inhaled therapy

- the appreciation that asthma is an inflammatory disease and that anti-inflammatory therapy should be started even in mild cases
- a diminution in the role of bronchodilators (e.g. salbutamol) since they are not anti-inflammatory and regular treatment with these drugs on their own may be associated with worsening of asthma and even asthma deaths.

β_2-Adrenoceptor agonists

The bronchodilator preparations contain selective β_2-adrenoceptor agonists for the respiratory tract and do not stimulate the β_1-adrenoceptors of the myocardium. These drugs are potent bronchodilators in that they cause relaxation of bronchial smooth muscle. Such treatment is very effective in relieving symptoms but does little for the underlying inflammatory nature of the disease. Inhalants such as salbutamol (100 μg) or terbutaline (250 μg) should be prescribed as two puffs as required.

Salmeterol (50–100 μg), a highly selective and potent β_2-adrenoceptor agonist, is effective by inhalation for up to 12 hours, reducing the need for administration to twice daily. Only the mildest asthmatics with intermittent attacks should rely on bronchodilator treatment alone. Some patients use nebulizers at home for self-administration of salbutamol or terbutaline. Such treatment is very effective owing to the high dose delivered, but patients must not rely on repeated home administration of nebulized β_2-adrenoceptor agonists for worsening asthma, and must be encouraged to seek medical advice urgently if their condition does not improve. Tablets of β_2-adrenoceptor agonists are less effective than when the drug is inhaled. To help those who cannot coordinate activation of the aerosol and inhalation, devices that are breath-activated have been developed.

Anticholinergic bronchodilators

Muscarinic receptors are found in the respiratory tract; large airways contain mainly M3 receptors whereas the peripheral lung tissue contains M3 and M1 receptors (see p. 749). Non-selective muscarinic antagonists – ipratropium bromide (20–40 mg three or four times daily) or oxitropium bromide (200 mg twice daily) – by aerosol inhalation are useful bronchodilators, particularly in COPD, and may be additive to β_2-adrenoceptor stimulants.

Information

Step	PEFR	Treatment
1 Occasional symptoms, less frequent than daily	100% predicted	As-required bronchodilators If used more than once daily, move to step 2
2 Daily symptoms	≤ 80% predicted	Anti-inflammatory drugs Sodium cromoglycate or low-dose inhaled corticosteroids up to 800 μg If not controlled move to step 3
3 Severe symptoms	50–80% predicted	High-dose inhaled corticosteroids up to 2000 μg daily
4 Severe symptoms uncontrolled with high-dose inhaled corticosteroids	50–80% predicted	Add regular long-acting β_2-agonists (e.g. salmeterol)
5 Severe symptoms deteriorating	≤ 50% predicted	Add prednisolone 40 mg daily
6 Severe symptoms deteriorating in spite of prednisolone	≤ 30% predicted	Hospital admission

Short-acting bronchodilator treatment taken at any step on as-required basis

Information box 12.1 The stepwise management of asthma

Anti-inflammatory drugs

Sodium cromoglycate and nedocromil sodium prevent activation of many inflammatory cells, particularly mast cells, eosinophils and epithelial cells, but not lymphocytes, by blocking a specific chloride channel which in turn prevents calcium influx. These drugs are particularly effective in patients with milder asthma. Sodium cromoglycate is taken regularly either in the form of a Spincap containing 20 mg or in aerosol form from a metered-dose inhaler delivering 5 mg per puff. The dose should be two puffs four times daily from an inhaler, or one Spincap three or four times daily. Nedocromil sodium is taken as an aerosol at a dose of 4 mg (two puffs) two to four times daily.

Inhaled corticosteroids

All patients who have regular persisting symptoms in spite of treatment with as-required β_2-adrenoceptor agonists, sodium cromoglycate or nedocromil need regular treatment with inhaled corticosteroids. Beclomethasone dipropionate is available in doses of 50, 100 and 250 μg per puff, budesonide is available in doses of 200 μg per metered inhalation and fluticasone propionate 50, 100 and 250 μg per inhalation. Fluticasone propionate is twice as potent as beclomethasone dipropionate with considerably less systemic bioavailability. High-dose beclomethasone, budesonide and fluticasone should be reserved for patients who have not responded to lower dose inhaled corticosteroids. The unwanted effects of inhaled corticosteroids are oral candidiasis, which may develop in 5% of patients, and hoarseness due to the effect of corticosteroids on the laryngeal muscles. Subcapsular cataract formation can occur. Abnormalities of bone metabolism can be detected when inhaled steroids are needed at high dose (> 800 μg daily). In children, inhaled steroids at doses greater than 400 μg daily have been shown to retard growth at least in the short term. Asthma itself retards growth. Catch-up growth may occur when asthma improves and doses of inhaled steroids can be reduced.

Oral corticosteroids

Use of oral corticosteroids is necessary for those individuals not controlled on inhaled corticosteroids. The dose should be kept as low as possible to avoid side-effects. The effect of short-term treatment with prednisolone 30 mg daily is shown in Fig 12.15 on p. 763. Some patients require continuing treatment with oral corticosteroids.

Studies suggest that treatment with low doses of methotrexate (15 mg weekly) can significantly reduce the dose of prednisolone needed to control the disease in some patients, and cyclosporin also improves lung function in some steroid-dependent asthmatics.

Antibiotics

There is no evidence that antibiotics are helpful in the management of patients who suffer from properly diagnosed asthma. However, wheezing frequently occurs in exacerbations of COPD associated with infected sputum.

Yellow or green sputum containing eosinophils and bronchial epithelial cells may be coughed up in acute exacerbations of asthma. This is not due to bacterial infection and antibiotics are not required.

Leukotriene receptor antagonists

Montelukast is now available. It is given as a single tablet daily. It improves control when used with an inhaled steroid in mild to moderate asthma. It may also be useful as a steroid-sparing drug.

MANAGEMENT OF SEVERE ASTHMA

Refer to Emergency box 12.2.

Although this condition is often called 'status asthmaticus', it is better considered as severe asthma that has not been controlled by the patient's use of medication. Patients with severe asthma have:

- inability to complete a sentence in one breath
- respiratory rate ≥ 25 breaths per minute
- tachycardia ≥ 110 beats min^{-1} (pulsus paradoxus – p. 633 – is not useful as it is only present in 45% of cases)
- PEFR <50% of predicted normal or best.

Life threatening features are:

- a silent chest, cyanosis or feeble respiratory effort
- exhaustion, confusion or coma
- bradycardia or hypotension
- PEFR <30% of predicted normal or best (approximately 150 L min^{-1} in adults).

Arterial blood gases should always be measured in patients requiring admission to hospital. Pulse oximetry is useful in further monitoring oxygen saturation and reduces the need for repeat arterial puncture. Patients with very severe life-threatening attacks have:

- a high P_aCO_2 > 6 kPa
- severe hypoxaemia P_aO_2 < 8 kPa irrespective of treatment with oxygen
- a low and falling arterial pH.

Treatment is commenced with 5 mg of nebulized salbutamol or 10 mg terbutaline with oxygen as the driving gas. A chest X-ray is taken to exclude a pneumothorax. If no improvement occurs with nebulized therapy, 250 μg of salbutamol or terbutaline should be administered by intravenous infusion over 10 minutes. Intravenous aminophylline is sometimes used for severe asthma but has a narrow therapeutic index. Hydrocortisone 200 mg i.v. should be administered four-hourly for 24 hours, and 60 mg of prednisolone should be given orally daily. Patients who do not respond to this regimen may require ventilation.

Patients should be kept in hospital for at least five days, since the majority of sudden deaths occur 2–5 days after admission. During this time oxygen saturation should be monitored by oximetry. Oral corticosteroids can be reduced from 60 mg to 30 mg once improvement occurs. Further reduction should be gradual on an

Emergency

At home

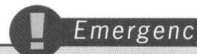

1. The patient is assessed. Tachycardia, a high respiratory rate and inability to speak in sentences indicate a severe attack.
2. If the PEFR is less than 150 L min^{-1} (in adults), an ambulance should be called. (All doctors should carry peak flow meters.)
3. Nebulized salbutamol 5 mg or terbutaline 10 mg is administered.
4. Hydrocortisone sodium succinate 200 mg i.v. is given.
5. Oxygen 40–60% is given if available.
6. Prednisolone 60 mg is given orally.

At hospital

1. The patient is reassessed.
2. Oxygen 40–60% is given.
3. The PEFR is measured using a low-reading peak flow meter, as an ordinary meter measures only from 60 L min^{-1} upwards. Measure O_2 saturation with pulse oximeter.
4. Nebulized salbutamol 5 mg or terbutaline 10 mg is repeated and administered 4-hourly.
5. Add nebulized ipratropium bromide 0.5 mg to nebulized salbutamol/terbutaline.
6. Hydrocortisone 200 mg i.v. is given 4-hourly for 24 hours.
7. Prednisolone is continued at 60 mg orally daily for 2 weeks.
8. Arterial blood gases are measured; if the P_aCO_2 is greater than 7 kPa, ventilation should be considered.
9. A chest X-ray is performed to exclude pneumothorax.
10. One of the following intravenous infusions is given if no improvement is seen:
salbutamol 3–20 μg min^{-1}, or
terbutaline 1.5–5.0 μg min^{-1}.

Emergency box 12.2 Treatment of severe asthma

outpatient basis until an appropriate maintenance dose or substitution by inhaled corticosteroid aerosols can be achieved.

If the PEFR is greater than 150 L min^{-1}, patients may improve dramatically on nebulized therapy and may not require hospital admission. Their regular treatment should be increased, probably to include treatment for two weeks with 30 mg of prednisolone followed by a gradual reduction in the oral dose and substitution by an inhaled corticosteroid preparation.

MANAGEMENT OF CATASTROPHIC SUDDEN SEVERE (BRITTLE) ASTHMA

This is an unusual variant of asthma in which patients are at risk from sudden death in spite of the fact that their asthma may have been well controlled. Severe life-threatening attacks occur within hours or even minutes. Such patients require a carefully worked out management plan agreed by respiratory physician, primary care physician and patient, and require:

- Medic Alert bracelet
- emergency supplies of medications at home, in the car and at work
- oxygen and resuscitation equipment at home and at work
- nebulized β_2-agonists at home and at work
- autoinjectors of adrenalin: two Epi-pens of 0.3 mg adrenalin at home, at work and to be carried by patient at all times
- prednisolone 60 mg.

Attend the nearest hospital immediately. Admission to intensive care may be required.

PROGNOSIS OF ASTHMA

Although asthma often improves in children as they reach their teens, it is now realized that the disease frequently returns in the second, third and fourth decades. Overall, in adults, there is a tendency for asthma to improve with age.

FURTHER READING

Barnes PJ, Karim M (1997) Mechanisms of disease: nuclear factor kB – a pivotal transcription factor in chronic inflammatory diseases. *New England Journal of Medicine* **336**: 1066–1071.

British Thoracic Society (1997) The British guidelines on asthma management. *Thorax* **52** (Suppl 1): S1–S21.

Holgate ST (1998) Asthma and allergy. *Quarterly Journal of Medicine* **91**: 171–184.

Inhaled beta-agonists. *New England Journal of Medicine* (1996) **335**: 886–888.

Lancet (1997) Asthma. *Lancet* **350**: (Suppl 11) 1–27

Venables KM, Chan-Yeung M (1997) Occupational asthma. *Lancet* **349**: 1465–1469.

Pneumonia

Pneumonia may be defined as an inflammation of the substance of the lungs. It is usually caused by bacteria. Clinically it presents as an acute illness characterized in the majority of cases by the presence of cough, purulent sputum and fever together with physical signs or radiological changes compatible with consolidation of the lung.

The advent of antibiotics might have been expected to decrease dramatically the mortality from pneumonia.

However, mortality statistics obtained from death certificates show the reverse. This is because the dramatic decrease in deaths from pneumonia in children under 10 years has been counterbalanced by an increase in deaths from pneumonia in individuals over the age of 70 years. Bacterial pneumonia is more frequent in HIV-infected individuals than in the general population, particularly in HIV infected intravenous drug users. The causative agents are the same as found in non-HIV community-acquired pneumonia.

Classification

Pneumonia can be classified both anatomically and on the basis of the aetiology.

Classification by site

Pneumonias are either localized, such as when the whole of one lobe is affected, or diffuse, when they primarily affect the lobules of the lung, often in association with the bronchi and bronchioles – a condition referred to as 'bronchopneumonia'.

Classification by aetiology

An aetiological factor can be discovered in approximately 75% of patients. The term 'atypical pneumonia' was used to describe pneumonia caused by agents such as *Mycoplasma*, influenza A virus, *Chlamydia* and *Coxiella burnetii*. These types of pneumonia alone account for almost one-fifth of the cases of pneumonia (Table 12.14), and the term 'atypical' has been dropped. Pneumonias may also result from:

- chemical causes, such as in the aspiration of vomit (see p. 799)
- radiotherapy (see p. 816)
- allergic mechanisms (see p. 811).

Mycobacterium tuberculosis is an important cause of pneumonia; it is considered separately, since both its mode of presentation and its treatment are very different from the other infective agents.

PRECIPITATING FACTORS

- *Strep. pneumoniae* – often follows influenza or parainfluenza viral infection.
- Hospitalized 'ill' patients – often infected with Gram-negative organisms.
- Cigarette smoking.
- Alcohol excess.
- Bronchiectasis (e.g. in cystic fibrosis).
- Bronchial obstruction (e.g. carcinoma) – occasionally associated with infection with 'non-pathogenic' organisms.
- Immunosuppression (e.g. AIDS or treatment with cytotoxic agents) – organisms include *P. carinii*, *Mycobacterium avium intracellulare*, cytomegalovirus.
- Intravenous drug abuse – frequently associated with *Staph. aureus* infection.
- Inhalation from oesophageal obstruction – often associated with infection with anaerobes.

CLINICAL FEATURES

The clinical presentation varies according to the immune state of the patient and the infecting agent. In the most common type of pneumonia – caused by *Strep. pneumoniae* – there is often a preceding history of a viral infection. The patient rapidly becomes more ill with a high temperature (up to 39.5°C), pleuritic pain and a dry cough. A day or two later, rusty-coloured sputum is produced and at about the same time the patient may develop labial herpes simplex. The patient breathes rapidly and shallowly, the affected side of the chest moves less, and signs of consolidation may be present together with a pleural rub.

INVESTIGATIONS

Chest X-ray confirms the area of consolidation (Fig 12.35), but radiological changes lag behind the clinical course so that X-ray changes may be minimal at the start of the illness. Conversely, consolidation may remain on the chest X-ray for several weeks after the patient is clinically cured. The chest X-ray should always return to normal by six weeks, except in patients with severe airflow limitation. Persistent changes on the chest X-ray after this time suggest a bronchial abnormality, usually a carcinoma, with persisting secondary pneumonia. Chest X-rays should rarely be repeated more frequently than at weekly intervals during the acute illness and then at six weeks after discharge from hospital.

In *Strep. pneumoniae* pneumonia, there is often a white blood cell count that is greater than 15×10^9/L (90% polymorphonuclear leucocytosis) and an erythrocyte sedimentation rate (ESR) greater than 100 mm h^{-1}.

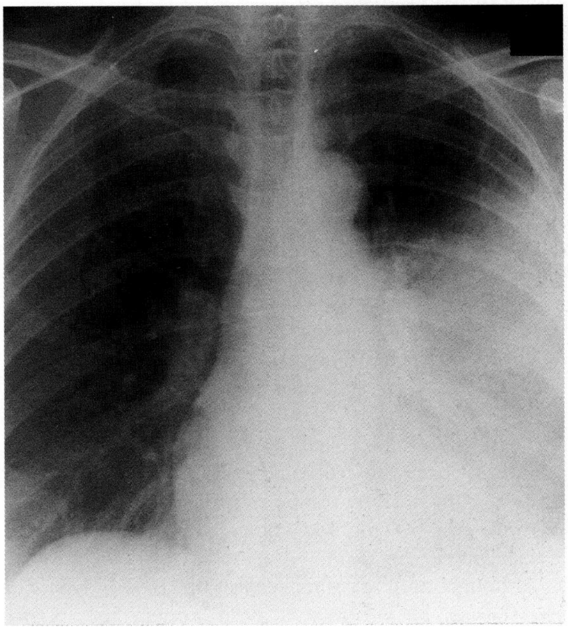

Fig 12.35
Chest X-ray to show lobar pneumonia

Table 12.14
The aetiology of pneumonia in the UK

Infecting agent	Frequency as a cause of pneumonia (%)	Clinical circumstances
Streptococcus pneumoniae	50	Community pneumonia patients usually previously fit
Mycoplasma pneumoniae	6	As above
Influenza A virus (usually with a bacterial component)	5	As above
Haemophilus influenzae	5	Pre-existing lung disease: COPD
Chlamydia pneumoniae	5	Community-acquired pneumonia
Chlamydia psittaci	3	Contact with birds (though not inevitable)
Staphylococcus aureus	2	Children, intravenous drug abusers, associated with influenza virus infections
Legionella pneumophilia	2	Institutional outbreaks (hospitals and hotels), sporadic, endemic
Coxiella burnetti	1	Abattoir and animal-hide workers
Pseudomonas aeruginosa	<1	Cystic fibrosis
Pneumocytis carinii *Actinomyces israelli* *Nocardia asteroides* Cytomegalovirus *Aspergillus fumigatus*	<1	AIDS, lymphomas, leukaemias, use of cytotoxic drugs and corticosteroids
Anaerobic organisms	<1	Inhalation pneumonia, alcohol abuse, postoperative
None isolated	20	–

Types of pneumonia

The individual features of various pneumonias are given below. The overall investigation and management is shown in Fig 12.36 and discussed on p. 800.

Mycoplasma pneumonia

This is a common cause of pneumonia. It often occurs in patients in their teens and twenties, frequently amongst those living in boarding institutions. Generalized features such as headaches and malaise often precede the chest symptoms by 1–5 days. Cough may not be obvious initially and physical signs in the chest may be scanty.

On chest X-ray, usually only one of the lower lobes is involved but sometimes there may be dramatic shadowing in both lower lobes. There is frequently no correlation between the X-ray appearances and the clinical state of the patient.

The white blood cell count is not raised. Cold agglutinins occur in half of the cases. The diagnosis is confirmed by a rising antibody titre. Treatment is with erythromycin 500 mg four times daily for 7–10 days. Tetracycline is effective.

Although most patients recover in 10–14 days, the disease can be protracted, with cough and X-ray appearance lasting for weeks and relapses occurring. Lung abscesses and pleural effusions are rare.

Extrapulmonary complications can occur at any time during the illness and occasionally dominate the clinical picture. Most are rare but they include:

- myocarditis and pericarditis
- rashes and erythema multiforme
- haemolytic anaemia and thrombocytopenia
- myalgia and arthralgia
- meningoencephalitis and other neurological abnormalities
- gastrointestinal symptoms (e.g. vomiting, diarrhoea).

Viral pneumonia

Viral pneumonia is uncommon in adults, bacteria being the usual cause of the pneumonia *per se*. Influenza A virus or adenovirus infection can occasionally produce pneumonia.

Other pneumonias

Haemophilus influenzae

H. influenzae is frequently identified in the yellow-green sputum produced during exacerbation of chronic bronchitis. It is therefore not surprising that this organism may be the cause of pneumonia in people suffering from COPD. The pneumonia can be diffuse or confined to one lobe. There are no special features to separate it from other bacterial causes of pneumonia. It responds well to treatment with oral cefaclor 500 mg 8-hourly.

Chlamydia psittaci (see also p. 50)

Typically the individual has been working with infected birds, especially parrots, but a history of contact is not always elicited. The incubation period is 1–2 weeks and the disease may pursue a very low-grade course over several months. Symptoms include malaise, high fever, cough and muscular pains. The liver and spleen are occasionally enlarged and scanty 'rose spots' may be seen on the abdomen. The chest X-ray shows segmental or a diffuse pneumonia. Occasionally the illness presents with a high, swinging fever and dramatic prostration with photophobia and neck stiffness that can be confused with meningitis. The diagnosis is confirmed by the demonstration of a rising titre of complement-fixing antibody. Erythromycin or tetracycline are the antibiotics of choice.

Chlamydia pneumoniae

Outbreaks of *Chlamydia pneumoniae* have been reported in institutions and within families, suggesting person-to-person spread without any avian or animal reservoir. Serological tests on patients admitted to hospital with community-acquired pneumonia suggest that 5–10% may be the result of *C. pneumoniae* infection. In general, disease is mild with 50% of *C. pneumoniae* infections presenting as pneumonia, 28% as acute bronchitis, 10% with a 'flu-like illness and 12% with upper respiratory illnesses. Type-specific microimmunofluorescence tests are required to distinguish *C. pneumoniae* from *C. psittaci* and *C. trachomatis*. Treatment is with erythromycin or tetracycline.

Staphylococcus aureus

Staph. aureus normally causes a pneumonia only after a preceding influenzal viral illness. The infection starts in the bronchi, leading to patchy areas of consolidation in one or more lobes, which break down to form abscesses. These may appear as cysts on the chest X-ray.

Pneumothorax, effusion and empyemas are frequent. Septicaemia develops with metastatic abscesses in other organs.

Fulminating staphylococcal pneumonia occurring in influenza epidemics can lead to death in hours. All patients with this type of pneumonia are very ill; intravenous antibiotics must be administered promptly, but are not always effective.

Areas of pneumonia (septic infarcts) are also seen in staphylococcal septicaemia. This is frequently seen in intravenous drug abusers, and in patients with central catheters being used for parenteral nutrition. The infected puncture site is the source of the *Staphylococcus*. Pulmonary symptoms are often few but breathlessness and cough occur and the chest X-ray reveals areas of consolidation. Abscess formation is frequent.

Diagnosis and treatment are shown in Fig 12.36.

Coxiella burnetii (Q-fever) (see also p. 49)

The patient develops systemic symptoms of fever, malaise and headache, often associated with multiple lesions on the chest X-ray. The illness may run a chronic course and is occasionally associated with endocarditis. Diagnosis is made by an increase in the titre of complement-fixing antibody. Treatment is usually with erythromycin or tetracycline. Severe cases can be treated with rifampicin.

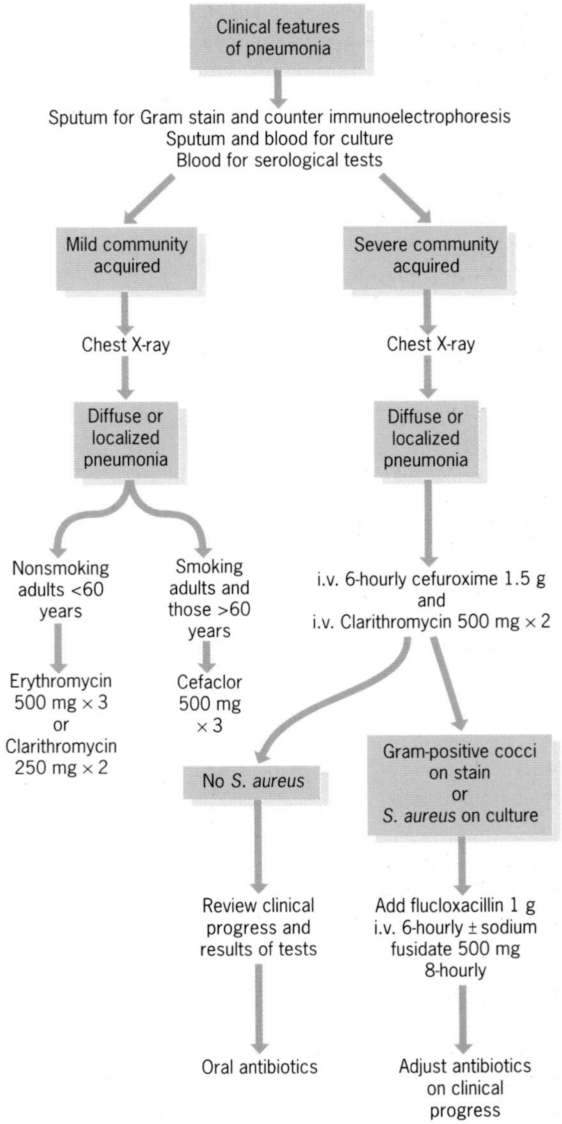

Fig 12.36
Algorithm for the management of pneumonia (see also p. 800)

Legionella pneumophila (see also p. 38)

Three epidemiological patterns of this disease are recognized:

- outbreaks among previously fit individuals staying in hotels, institutions or hospitals where the shower facilities or cooling systems have been contaminated with the organism
- sporadic cases occurring in many parts of the world where the source of the infection is unknown; most

cases involve middle-aged and elderly men who are smokers, but it is now being seen in children.
- outbreaks occur in immunocompromised patients, e.g. on corticosteroid therapy.

Legionella grows well in water up to 40°C in temperature, and the infection is almost certainly spread by the aerosol route. Adequate chlorination and temperature control of the water supply are important factors in the prevention of the disease.

The incubation period is 2–10 days. Males are affected twice as commonly as females. The infection may be mild, but the characteristic picture is of malaise, myalgia, headache and a fever with rigors and a pyrexia of up to 40°C. Half of the patients have gastrointestinal symptoms, with nausea, vomiting, diarrhoea and abdominal pain. Patients may be acutely ill, with mental confusion and other neurological signs. Haematuria occurs and occasionally renal failure.

The patient is tachypnoeic with initially a dry cough that later may become productive and purulent. The chest X-ray usually shows lobar and then multilobar shadowing, sometimes with a small pleural effusion. Cavitation is rare.

A strong presumptive diagnosis of *L. pneumophila* infection is possible in the majority of patients if they have three of the four following features:

- a prodromal virus-like illness
- a dry cough, confusion or diarrhoea
- lymphopenia without marked leucocytosis
- hyponatraemia.

Hypoalbuminaemia and high serum levels of liver aminotransferases are also common in this disease.

Diagnosis is confirmed by a fourfold increase in antibody titre in the blood, but the quickest way is by the direct immunofluorescent staining of the organism in the pleural fluid, sputum or bronchial washings. A Gram stain does not detect the organism. Culture on special media is possible but takes up to three weeks. A urinary antigen test is commercially available and is highly specific.

Treatment is with an antibiotic. The organism is sensitive to the macrolides, clarithromycin now being the drug of choice. Ciprafloxacin is also effective and rifampicin can be used in addition in ill patients. Mortality can be up to 30% in elderly patients but most patients recover spontaneously.

Prevention is important, with chlorination and sealing of water supplies.

Gram-negative bacteria

These are the cause of many hospital-acquired pneumonias but they are occasionally responsible for cases in the community.

Klebsiella pneumoniae

Pneumonia that is due to *Klebsiella* usually occurs in the elderly with a history of heart or lung disease, diabetes, alcohol excess or malignancy. The onset is often sudden, with severe systemic upset. The sputum is purulent, gelatinous or blood-stained. The upper lobes are more commonly affected and the consolidation is often extensive. There is often swelling of the infected lobe so that on the lateral chest X-ray there is bulging of the fissures. The organism can be found in the sputum or in the blood.

Treatment is dependent on the sensitivity of the organism, but a cephalosporin is usually required. The mortality is high, partly owing to the presence of an underlying condition.

Pseudomonas aeruginosa

Pneumonia due to this organism is of considerable significance in patients with cystic fibrosis, since it correlates with a worsening clinical condition and mortality. It is also seen in patients with neutropenia following cytotoxic chemotherapy. The isolation of *P. aeruginosa* must be interpreted with care because the organism grows well on bacterial culture medium and may simply represent contamination from the upper airways.

Pseudomonal and other Gram-negative infections respond well to treatment with the 4-quinolone antibiotic ciprofloxacin (200–400 mg i.v. over 30–60 minutes twice daily) or ceftazidime (2 g bolus i.v. 8-hourly). Azlocillin (2 g i.v. 8-hourly), ticarcillin (15–20 g daily i.v. infusion) and piperacillin are active against these bacilli. Tobramycin 3–5 mg kg^{-1} i.v. or i.m. daily in 8-hourly doses together with one of the above penicillins are synergistic. Tobramycin and ticarcillin can be inhaled direct into the lung via nebulizers in patients with CF (see p. 782).

Modifications may have to be made in the light of sensitivity testing. Tobramycin is nephrotoxic and also produces vestibular damage, so that blood levels should be monitored.

Moraxella catarrhalis

This organism has been found to be associated with exacerbations of COPD and occasionally with fatal pneumonia. Some strains produce a β-lactamase capable of destroying amoxycillin. The exact role of this organism in bronchopulmonary infection remains to be determined.

Anaerobic bacteria

Infections with these organisms usually occur in patients with an underlying condition, such as diabetes, and are often associated with aspiration. *Bacteroides* is the most common organism and is sensitive to metronidazole. The prognosis depends largely on the precipitating cause.

Pneumonias due to opportunistic infections

These are commonly recognized in the immunocompromised patient.

Pneumocystis carinii

This is by far the most common opportunistic infection, accounting for 50% of the cases of pneumonia in patients with acquired immunodeficiency syndrome (AIDS) (see p. 115) particularly when the CD4 lymphocyte count is ≤200/mm^3. It is also seen in patients receiving immunosuppressive therapy. In the developing world, however, *Pneumocystis carinii* pneumonia (PCP) is not infrequently found in malnourished children.

P. carinii is a fungus found in the air and pneumonia arises from reinfection rather than reactivation of persisting organisms acquired in childhood. Clinically the pneumonia is associated with a high fever, breathlessness and dry cough. In patients with AIDS, the clinical features are described on p. 115.

The typical radiographic appearance of PCP is of a diffuse bilateral alveolar and interstitial shadowing beginning in the perihilar regions and spreading out in a butterfly pattern. Other chest X-ray appearances include a localized infiltrate, nodule, cavity or a pneumothorax. In patients receiving aerosolized pentamidine for prophylaxis, infiltrates may be localized to the upper zones. For CT appearances see p. 115. Investigation includes induction of sputum with hypertonic saline or fibreoptic bronchoscopy with bronchoalveolar lavage; the diagnosis can be made in 90% of cases by staining sputum using indirect immunofluorescence with monoclonal antibodies.

Shadowing on the chest X-ray in AIDS patients, though most commonly due to *P. carinii*, can result from:

- cytomegalovirus
- *M. avium intracellulare*
- *M. tuberculosis*
- *L. pneumophila*
- *Cryptococcus*
- pyogenic bacteria
- Kaposi's sarcoma
- lymphoid interstitial pneumonia
- nonspecific interstitial pneumonitis.

Treatment of PCP is with high-dose co-trimoxazole. It is discussed along with prophylaxis on p. 115.

Actinomyces israeli (see also p. 39)

The clinical picture is that of severe pneumonia, lung abscess or empyema. Treatment is surgical drainage when appropriate, with high-dose intravenous penicillin for 4–6 weeks.

Nocardia asteroides

This produces a similar picture to *Actinomyces*, though of greater severity. The chest X-ray often shows irregular opacities in one or both lungs, particularly in the mid-zones. Treatment is with sulphadiazine in doses up to 9 g daily.

Cytomegalovirus (see also p. 53)

Bronchitis and pneumonia may occur but these are usually a more minor part of the generalized systemic illness.

Aspergillus fumigatus (see also p. 811)

This fungus gives rise to a widespread invasion of lung tissue in patients who are immunocompromised. It is a serious pneumonia that is usually rapidly fatal. Treatment is with amphotericin and flucytosine.

Mycobacterium avium intracellulare (MAI)

This bacterium causes lung disease in patients with AIDS primarily as part of disseminated disease when CD4 lymphocyte counts are ≤100/mm^3 with the pulmonary complications being of less significance than the extra-pulmonary involvement. Therapeutic regimens include combinations of rifabutin or rifampicin, ethambutol and clofazimine. Clarithromycin and azithromycin may prove to be particularly efficacious.

Cryptococcus

Infection with this fungus is usually disseminated but pulmonary involvement includes intrathoracic lymph node enlargement and effusions.

Kaposi's sarcoma (see also p. 118 and p. 1185)

This is the most common malignancy affecting one-third of HIV-infected homosexual men. Intrathoracic involvement usually follows cutaneous manifestations and includes nodules or infiltrates in the lungs with lymph node enlargement and endobronchial lesions. Symptoms are those of progressive dyspnoea and cough. Chest X-ray appearances are nonspecific. Bronchoscopy reveals multiple red or purple flat lesions which are not biopsied because of difficulty with histological diagnosis in crushed fragments and risk of haemorrhage. Treatment is with chemotherapy, vincristine 2 mg and bleomycin 10 mg m^{-2} every three weeks.

Lymphoid interstitial pneumonia

Infiltration with lymphocytes, plasma cells and immunoblasts characterizes this disease which is more common in children than in adults. It is thought to be a viral pneumonia and causes diffuse reticulonodular infiltrates on the chest X-ray. Corticosteroid therapy appears to be of benefit, as is zidovudine.

Rare causes of pneumonia

Pneumonia may be seen in the course of infection by *Bordetella pertussis*, typhoid and paratyphoid bacillus, brucellosis, leptospirosis and a number of viral infections including measles, chickenpox and glandular fever. It is not usually a major feature. Details of these infections are described in Chapter 1.

Aspiration pneumonia

The acute aspiration of gastric contents into the lungs can produce an extremely severe and sometimes fatal illness owing to the intense destructiveness of gastric acid – the Mendelson syndrome. It can complicate anaesthesia, particularly during pregnancy.

In the absence of a tracheo-oesophageal fistula, aspiration occurs only during periods of impaired consciousness (e.g. during sleep), in reflux oesophagitis or oesophageal stricture, or in bulbar palsy. Because of the bronchial anatomy, the most usual site for spillage is the posterior segment of the right lower lobe. The persistent pneumonia is often due to anaerobes and it may progress to lung abscess or even bronchiectasis. It is vital to identify any underlying problem, since appropriate corrective measures can lead to resolution of the pulmonary problems.

Cryptogenic organizing pneumonia (COP)

This condition is an organizing pneumonia of unknown aetiology although probably not infective. In the USA this is called bronchiolitis obliterans organising pneumonia (BOOP). Clinical features are a short history of feeling unwell with cough, breathlessness, fever and sometimes pleuritic chest pain. Finger clubbing is rare. There is a raised ESR, a normal white blood count and patchy or confluent shadows are seen bilaterally on the chest X-ray. Lung function tests show a restrictive defect. Pathologically there are characteristic buds of connective tissue in alveolar ducts and respiratory bronchioles which are diagnostic, and there is an absence of any detectable microorganism. The diagnosis is usually clinical and the disease responds rapidly to corticosteroid treatment.

Diffuse pneumonia (bronchopneumonia)

Diffuse pneumonia is very common. It is differentiated from severe bronchitis by signs of bronchial breathing or patchy shadows on the chest X-ray.

Widespread diffuse pneumonia is a common terminal event, largely resulting from an inability of patients dying from other conditions (e.g. cancer) to cough up retained secretions, allowing infection to develop throughout the lungs. Treatment in this situation is rarely appropriate.

General management of pneumonia

Refer to the algorithm given in Fig 12.36.

Sputum should always be sent for culture. In *mild* cases, treatment should be started immediately with oral erythromycin or, preferably, clarithromycin in patients under 60 who do not smoke. Smokers and patients over 60 should be given cefaclor, usually with erythromycin.

More severe cases need to be admitted to hospital and a chest X-ray performed. Other investigations required are:

- **sputum** – Gram stain and culture
- **white blood-cell count** is raised above 15×10^9/L (with a high neutrophil count) in more than 50% of patients with pneumococcal pneumonia but only in 10% of cases of *Legionella* or *Mycoplasma* pneumonia
- **arterial blood gases**
- **blood culture.**

Further investigations may be necessary for the diagnosis of certain types of pneumonia:

- ***Mycoplasma* antibodies** (IgM and IgG) – in acute and convalescent samples. Cold agglutinins present in 50%
- ***Legionella* and *Chlamydia* antibodies** – immunofluorescent tests
- **Pneumococcal antigen** – counterimmunoelectrophoresis (CIE) of sputum, urine and serum (three to four times more sensitive than sputum or blood cultures)
- *urine antigen* – for legionella.

A high percentage of organisms causing pneumonia (e.g. *Mycoplasma pneumoniae*, *H. influenzae* and *L. pneumophila*) will not respond to penicillin or ampicillin/amoxycillin. These drugs should no longer be prescribed and should be replaced by bactericidal antibiotics that cover the most common organisms. In severe cases treatment is commenced with cefuroxime 750 mg to 1.5 g i.v. 6-hourly together with a macrolide, e.g. clarithromycin 500 mg i.v. 12-hourly. The purpose of this programme is to treat pneumonia with sufficient doses of appropriate antibiotics at the earliest stage. The treatment can later be reviewed in the light of clinical progress and subsequent bacteriological and serological findings. The chances of identifying a causative organism are greatly decreased in individuals who have received antibiotics in the week prior to their admission to hospital.

The overall mortality for pneumonia is currently 5% but for pneumonia due to *Staph. aureus* it is in excess of 25%. Patients who die from pneumonia usually have not received the appropriate antibiotics in sufficient doses before or during the early stages of hospital admission. Severe community-acquired pneumonia has a high mortality particularly in those over 65 years. The presence of a respiratory rate ≥ 30 min^{-1}, a diastolic blood pressure ≤ 60 mmHg and a serum urea >7 mmol L^{-1} indicates a poorer prognosis and the need for intensive care. In spite of treatment in the intensive care unit approximately 50% of such patients will die.

General measures

These include care of the mouth and skin. Fluids should be encouraged, to avoid dehydration. The patient is normally nursed sitting up or in the most comfortable position. Cough should normally be encouraged, but if it is unproductive and distressing, suppressants such as codeine linctus can be given. Physiotherapy is needed to help and encourage the patient to cough.

Pleuritic pain may require analgesia, but powerful analgesia (e.g. opiates) should be used with care because they cause respiratory depression.

In severe hypoxia, oxygen therapy should be given. However, since the hypoxia is often due to a physiological shunt, it may make little difference to the hypoxaemia.

Severe hospital-acquired pneumonias

These should be treated in the same way as severe community-acquired pneumonias once appropriate samples for culture and sensitivities have been taken. Gram-negative bacteria are common and treatment should include i.v. ciprofloxacin or ceftazidime. Immunosuppressed patients may require very high-dose broad-spectrum antibiotics as well as antifungal and antiviral agents.

Complications of pneumonia

Lung abscess

This term is used to describe severe localized suppuration in the lung associated with cavity formation on the chest X-ray, often with the presence of a fluid level, and not due to tuberculosis.

Causes of lung abscesses are many, but the most common is aspiration, particularly amongst alcohol abusers following aspiration pneumonia. Lung abscesses also frequently follow the inhalation of a foreign body into a bronchus and occasionally occur when the bronchus is obstructed by a bronchial carcinoma.

Abscesses may develop during the course of specific pneumonias, particularly when the infecting agent is *Staph. pyogenes* or *Klebsiella pneumoniae*. Septic emboli, usually staphylococci, result in multiple lung abscesses. Infarcted areas of lung may occasionally cavitate and rarely become infected. Amoebic abscesses may occasionally develop in the right lower lobe following transdiaphragmatic spread from an amoebic liver abscess.

The clinical features are those of persisting and worsening pneumonia associated with the production of large quantities of sputum, which is often foul-smelling owing to the growth of anaerobic organisms. There is usually a swinging fever. Chronic or subacute lung abscesses follow an inadequately treated pneumonia. Fever, malaise and weight loss occur. The chest signs may be few but clubbing often develops. The patient is often anaemic with a high ESR.

Empyema

Empyema means the presence of pus within the pleural cavity. This usually arises after the rupture of a lung abscess into the pleural space or from bacterial spread from a severe pneumonia. Typically an empyema cavity becomes infected with anaerobic organisms and the patient is severely ill with a high fever and a neutrophil granulocytosis.

INVESTIGATIONS

Bacteriological investigation of lung abscess and empyema is best conducted on specimens obtained by transtracheal aspiration, bronchoscopy or percutaneous transthoracic aspiration with ultrasound or CT guidance.

TREATMENT

Although anaerobic organisms are found in up to 70% of lung abscesses and empyemas, there is usually a mixed flora, often with aerobes, particularly *Strep. milleri*. Anaerobic cocci, black-pigmented bacteroids and fusobacteria are the anaerobes found most commonly.

Antibiotics should be given to cover both aerobic and anaerobic organisms; prolonged courses are often necessary. Treatment should be cefuroxime 1 g i.v. 6-hourly and metronidazole 500 mg i.v. 8-hourly for five days, followed by oral cefaclor and metronidazole for a prolonged period depending on bacterial sensitivities. Abscesses occasionally require surgery.

Empyemas should in addition be treated by prompt tube drainage or by rib resection and drainage of the empyema cavity under ultrasound control. Appropriate antibiotic treatment is given for up to six weeks.

FURTHER READING

Bartlett JG, Mundy LM (1995) Community-acquired pneumonia. *New England Journal of Medicine* **333**: 1618–1624.

Miller R (1996) HIV-associated respiratory disease. *Lancet* **348**: 307–312.

Stout JE, Yu VL (1997) Legionellosis. *New England Journal of Medicine* **337**: 682–687.

Tuberculosis (see also p. 40)

Tuberculosis is on the increase in developed countries, particularly where immunosuppressive drugs have altered the host defence mechanisms, or in AIDS. In developing countries it is 20–50 times more common and remains a problem partly because of inadequately supervised treatment and cost.

EPIDEMIOLOGY

Tuberculosis is the world's leading cause of death from a single infectious disease, with two million deaths (without HIV infection) in 1990. This is the result of:

- inadequate programmes for disease control
- multiple drug resistance
- co-infection with HIV
- a rapid rise in the world's population of young adults – the age group with the highest mortality from tuberculosis.

In the UK there has been no decline in the number of cases, with 7000 new cases per year. In the UK the incidences of tuberculosis in immigrants from the Asian subcontinent and from the West Indies are respectively forty and four times as common as in the native white population. This has led to great variation in the frequency of the disease in different areas of the UK. Tuberculosis is a notifiable disease.

PATHOLOGY

The first infection with *M. tuberculosis* is known as primary tuberculosis. It is usually subpleural, often in the mid to upper zones. Within an hour of reaching the lung, tubercle bacilli reach the draining lymph nodes at the hilum of the lung and a few escape into the bloodstream.

The initial reaction comprises exudation and infiltration with neutrophil granulocytes. These are rapidly replaced by macrophages that ingest the bacilli. These interact with T lymphocytes, with the development of cellular immunity that can be demonstrated 3–8 weeks after the initial infection by a positive reaction in the skin to an intradermal injection of protein from tubercle bacilli (tuberculin).

At this stage the classical pathology of tuberculosis can be seen. Granulomatous lesions consist of a central area of necrotic material of a cheesy nature, called caseation, surrounded by epithelioid cells and Langhans' giant cells with multiple nuclei, both cells being derived from the macrophage. Lymphocytes are present and there is a varying degree of fibrosis. Subsequently the caseated areas heal completely and many become calcified. It is known that at least 20% of these calcified primary lesions contain tubercle bacilli, initially lying dormant but capable of being activated by depression of the host defence system. Reactivation leads to typical post-primary pulmonary tuberculosis with cavitation, usually in the apex or upper zone of the lung. 'Post-primary tuberculosis' refers to all forms of tuberculosis that occur after the first few weeks of the primary infection when immunity to the mycobacterium has developed.

CLINICAL FEATURES AND INVESTIGATIONS

Primary tuberculosis is symptomless in the great majority of individuals. Occasionally there may be a vague illness, sometimes associated with cough and wheeze. A small transient pleural effusion or erythema nodosum may occur occasionally, both representing allergic manifestations of the infective process.

Enlargement of lymph nodes compressing the bronchi can give rise to collapse of segments or lobes of the lung. Apart from cough and a monophonic wheeze, the individual remains remarkably well and the collapse disappears as the primary complex heals. Occasionally, persistent collapse can give rise to subsequent bronchiectasis, often in the middle lobe (Brock's syndrome).

The manifestations of primary and post-primary tuberculosis are shown in Fig 12.37, together with the times when they usually occur. Extrapulmonary manifestations are summarized on p. 40. Miliary tuberculosis can occur within a year of the primary infection, or can occasionally occur much later as a manifestation of reactivation or, rarely, reinfection with tubercle bacillus.

Reactivation in the lung, or indeed in any extrapulmonary location, can occur as immunity wanes, usually with age and chronic ill-health. All manifestations are shown in Fig 12.37.

Miliary tuberculosis

This disease is the result of acute diffuse dissemination of tubercle bacilli via the bloodstream. It can be a difficult diagnosis to make, especially in older people, where it is particularly covert. This form of disseminated tuberculosis is universally fatal without treatment.

It may present in an entirely nonspecific manner with the gradual onset of vague ill-health, loss of weight and then fever. Occasionally the disease presents as tuberculosis meningitis. Usually there are no abnormal physical signs in the early stages, although eventually the spleen and liver become enlarged. Choroidal tubercles are seen in the eyes. These lesions are about one-quarter of the diameter of the optic disc and are yellowish and slightly shiny and raised in nature, later becoming white in the centre. There may be one or many in each eye.

The chest X-ray may be entirely normal in miliary tuberculosis as the tubercles are not visible until uniform miliary shadows 1–2 mm in diameter are seen throughout the lung; they have a hard outline. The lesions can increase in size up to 5–10 mm. Sarcoidosis and staphylococcal or *Mycoplasma* pneumonia can mimic the chest X-ray appearance of miliary tuberculosis. CT scanning may reveal lung parenchymal abnormalities at an earlier stage.

The Mantoux test is positive but is occasionally negative in people with very severe disease. Transbronchial biopsies are frequently positive before any abnormality is visible on the chest X-ray.

Biopsy and culture of liver and bone marrow may be necessary in patients presenting with a pyrexia of unknown origin (PUO). A trial of antituberculous therapy can be used in individuals with a PUO. The fever should settle within two weeks of starting chemotherapy if it is due to tuberculosis. This approach is used in susceptible individuals when a diagnosis cannot be confirmed.

Adult post-primary pulmonary tuberculosis

Typically there is gradual onset of symptoms over weeks or months. Tiredness, malaise, anorexia and loss of weight together with a fever and cough remain the outstanding features of pulmonary tuberculosis. Drenching night sweats are now rather uncommon and are more usually due to anxiety. Sputum in tuberculosis may be mucoid, purulent or blood-stained. Many patients suffer a dull

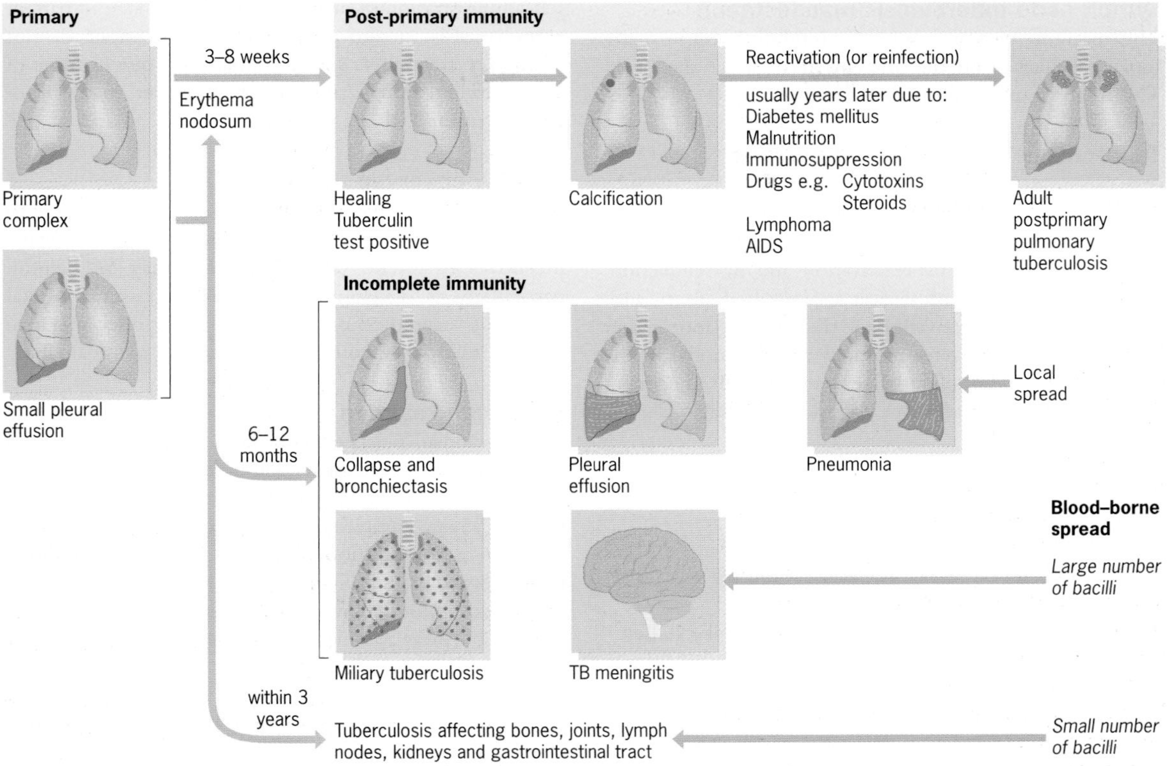

Fig 12.37
Manifestations of primary and post-primary tuberculosis

ache in the chest and it is not uncommon for patients to complain of recurrent colds. A pleural effusion or pneumonia can be the presenting feature of tuberculosis.

Physical examination reveals little. Finger clubbing is only present if the disease is advanced and associated with considerable production of purulent sputum. There are often no physical signs in the chest even in the presence of extensive radiological changes, though occasionally persistent crackles may be heard. Physical signs of an associated effusion, pneumonia or fibrosis may be present.

Chest X-ray

An abnormal chest X-ray is often found with no symptoms, but the reverse is extremely rare – pulmonary tuberculosis is unlikely in the absence of any radiographic abnormality. The chest X-ray (Fig 12.38) typically shows patchy or nodular shadows in the upper zones, loss of volume, and fibrosis with or without cavitation. Calcification may be present. The X-ray appearances alone may strongly suggest tuberculosis, but every effort must be made to obtain microbiological evidence. A single X-ray does not give an indication of the activity of the disease. Very similar chest X-ray appearances occur in histoplasmosis and other fungal infections of the lung, including cryptococcosis, coccidioidomycosis and aspergillosis.

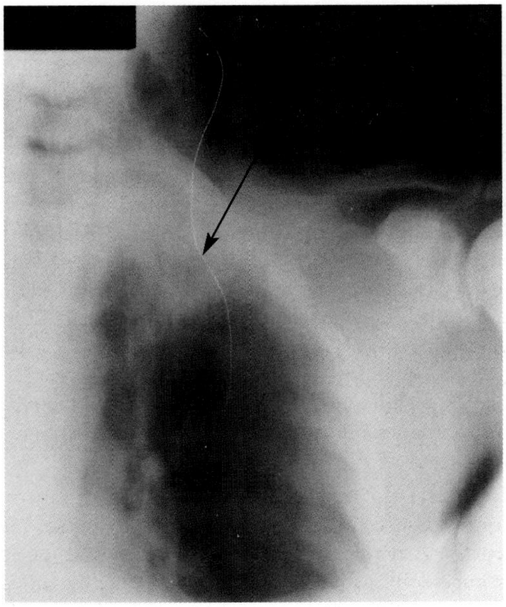

Fig 12.38
Chest X-ray showing tuberculosis of left upper lobe with cavitation

Lymph node tuberculosis manifestation

The patient presents with a tender lump, usually supraclavicular or in the anterior triangle of the neck. This form of tuberculosis is discussed on p. 40.

Tuberculosis in HIV-infected persons

(see also p. 117)

Tuberculosis in an HIV-infected person is an AIDS-defining illness and disease may arise from rapid progression of primary infection, by reactivation and by reinfection. The clinical pattern of disease is described on p. 117. Treatment is with conventional therapy but four rather than three drugs. Adverse reactions are common and the prognosis poor. Multiple drug resistance (MDR) occurs in 3% of cases of tuberculosis in HIV-positive individuals.

DIAGNOSIS

The diagnosis is made on the basis of the following investigations:

- **Imaging**. Chest X-ray (see above), and CT scan if necessary.
- **Staining**. The sputum is stained with Ziehl–Nielsen (ZN) stain for acid and alcohol-fast bacilli (AAFB).
- **Culture**. The sputum is cultured on Dover's or Lowenstein–Jensen medium for 4–8 weeks. Cultures to determine the sensitivity of the bacillus to antibiotics take a further 3–4 weeks.
- **Fibreoptic bronchoscopy** with washings from the affected lobes is useful if no sputum is available. This has replaced techniques such as gastric washings. Transbronchial biopsies can be obtained.
- **Biopsies** of the pleura, lymph nodes and solid lesions within the lung (tuberculomas) may be required to confirm the diagnosis.

The slow growth of *M. tuberculosis* in culture has hindered the ability to make a rapid definitive diagnosis. Radio-labelled DNA probes specific for various mycobacterial species can identify organisms in culture. The sensitivity of these methods has been enhanced by amplifying target DNA using the polymerase chain reaction. This allows direct testing of sputum and other fluids to provide a laboratory diagnosis within 48 hours. This is still not entirely reliable and should not be accepted as a final diagnosis, particularly in the difficult case when it is most likely to be used.

ELISA techniques have been developed which have high specificities, but unfortunately low sensitivity.

TREATMENT

Bedrest does not affect the outcome of the disease. Some patients will require hospitalization for a brief period; these include ill patients, those in whom the diagnosis is uncertain and those individuals from whom it is essential to gain cooperation. The most important factor in the successful treatment of tuberculosis lies in the continual self-administration of drugs for six months; lack of patient compliance is a major reason why 5% of patients do not respond to treatment. *In vitro* resistance to one or more of the antituberculous drugs occurs in fewer than 1% of patients in the UK.

Directly observed therapy (DOT)

In order to improve compliance, special clinics are used to supervise treatment regimens directly. In this group, incentives to attend (e.g. free meals) may be helpful, particularly in developing countries. Long-stay hospital treatment is required only for persistently uncooperative patients, many of whom are homeless and abuse alcohol.

Six-month regimen

This is standard practice for patients with pulmonary and lymph node disease: daily administration of rifampicin 600 mg and isoniazid 300 mg. (For those whose bodyweight is below 55 kg, rifampicin is reduced to 450 mg daily.) These are given as combination tablets and are taken 30 minutes before breakfast, since the absorption of rifampicin is influenced by food. This is supplemented for the first two months by pyrazinamide at a dose of 1.5 g (bodyweight <55 kg) or 2.0 g daily. Studies have indicated that pyrazinamide is of particular value in treating mycobacteria present within macrophages, and for this reason it may have a very valuable effect on preventing subsequent relapse.

Longer regimens

Treatment of bone tuberculosis should be continued for a total of nine months and of tuberculous meningitis for one year. The drugs used are the same as for pulmonary tuberculosis, with pyrazinamide prescribed for the first two months only.

Drug-resistant organisms

The development of resistance after initial drug sensitivity (secondary drug resistance) occurs in patients who do not comply with the treatment regimens. Primary drug resistance is seen in immigrants to the UK and those exposed to others infected with resistant organisms. Multidrug resistance occurring particularly in patients with HIV infection is a major therapeutic problem with a high mortality. Nosocomial transmission of multidrug-resistant tuberculosis to healthcare workers and to other patients is recognized and poses a major public health problem. The drug treatment of suspected drug resistance in HIV-positive and HIV-negative patients is as follows:

- with multiple drug resistance use at least three drugs to which the organism is sensitive
- with resistance to one of the four main drugs, use the other three.

Therapy should be continued for up to two years and in HIV-positive patients for at least 12 months after negative cultures. Second-line drugs available for treatment of resistant *M. tuberculosis* are capreomycin, cycloserine, clarithromycin, azithromycin, ciprofloxacin and ofloxacin.

Unwanted effects of drug treatment

Rifampicin. This drug induces liver enzymes, which may be transiently elevated in the serum of many patients. The drug should be stopped only if the serum bilirubin becomes elevated, which is extremely rare. Thrombocytopenia has been reported. Rifampicin stains body secretions pink and the patients should be warned of the change in colour of their urine, tears and sweat. Induction of liver enzymes means that concomitant drug treatment may be made less effective (see Chapter 14). Oral contraception will not be effective, so alternative birth control methods should be used.

Isoniazid. This gives rise to very few unwanted effects. At high doses it may produce a polyneuropathy but this is extremely rare when the normal dose of 200–300 mg is given daily. Nevertheless, it is customary to prescribe pyridoxine 10 mg daily to prevent this effect (see Fig 3.6). Occasionally, isoniazid gives rise to allergic reactions in the form of a skin rash and fever, with hepatitis occurring in fewer than 1% of cases. The latter, however, may be fatal if the drug is continued.

Pyrazinamide. The main unwanted effect of this drug is severe hepatic toxicity, though recent experience suggests that this is much rarer than initially thought using present dosage schedules. Gout may occur owing to hyperuricaemia.

Ethambutol. This drug can cause a dose-related retrobulbar neuritis that presents with colour blindness for green, reduction in visual acuity and a central scotoma. It usually reverses provided the drug is stopped when symptoms develop; patients should therefore be warned of its effects. Because of this problem ethambutol is rarely used unless resistance of *M. tuberculosis* is present to one or more of the other drugs. All patients prescribed the drug should be seen by an ophthalmologist prior to treatment.

Streptomycin. The main unwanted effect of streptomycin is irreversible damage to the vestibular nerve. It is more likely to occur in the elderly and in those with renal impairment. Allergic reactions to streptomycin are more common than to rifampicin, isoniazid and pyrazinamide. This drug is used only if patients are very ill and not responding adequately to therapy.

Follow-up

Patients should be seen regularly for the duration of chemotherapy and once more after three months, since relapse, though very unlikely, usually occurs within this period of time.

Chemoprophylaxis

Patients who have any chest X-ray changes compatible with previous tuberculosis and who are about to undergo long-term treatment that has an immunosuppressive effect, such as renal dialysis or treatment with corticosteroids, should receive chemoprophylaxis with isoniazid 200–300 mg daily.

PREVENTION

BCG vaccination

Vaccination with BCG (Bacille Calmette–Guérin) has been given to schoolchildren in the UK since 1954. BCG is a bovine strain of *M. tuberculosis* that lost its virulence after growth in the laboratory for many years. Early trials showed that it decreases the risk of developing tuberculosis by about 70%. With the continuing decrease in the incidence of tuberculosis it is becoming less cost-effective to administer this vaccine, and the procedure is being stopped in certain areas of the UK. However, in other areas of the UK with a high immigrant population, the vaccine is being administered six weeks after birth rather than at the traditional age of 13 years. This is to prevent the disease from developing in young children, where it can progress extremely rapidly and in whom any delay in diagnosis can be fatal. BCG has been shown to be particularly effective in preventing miliary tuberculosis and tuberculous meningitis.

The efficacy of BCG vaccination throughout the world varies from zero to 94% protection and appears to depend on latitude, being most beneficial in Norway, Sweden and Denmark (80–94%) and least so in the southern states of the USA and in India (0–20%). The lack of efficacy is thought to be related to the frequency of infection with environmental mycobacteria (e.g. *M. fortuitum*, *M. kansasii*), which may induce a degree of protection similar to but not enhanced by BCG. The high frequency of *M. tuberculosis* in India and Africa is the result of the overwhelming effect of poor nutrition, overcrowding and lack of control measures.

BCG is given only to individuals who are tuberculin-negative; those with positive tests are further screened by a chest X-ray. BCG should be given at a dose of 0.1 mL intradermally to children and adults, but at a dose of 0.05 mL to infants. The practice of BCG vaccination in the UK, thereby producing cellular immunity and a positive tuberculin test, is an important reason why the Mantoux test is of little value in clinical practice for subsequent diagnosis of active disease.

Contact tracing

Tuberculosis is spread from person to person and effective tracing of close contacts has helped to limit spread of the disease as well as to identify diseased individuals at an early stage. Screening procedures involve screening all close family members or other individuals who share the same kitchen and bathroom facilities. Occasionally, close contacts at work or school may also be screened. Contacts who are ill should be thoroughly investigated for tuberculosis. If they are well, a chest X-ray is taken and a tuberculin test is performed (Practical box 12.5).

In adults, even if the tuberculin test is positive, provided the chest X-ray is negative nothing more need be done. In patients with HIV infection, who have not had BCG, chemoprophylaxis with isoniazid is given. In children, a positive tuberculin test is usually taken as evidence of infection, and treatment is instituted. If the tuberculin test is negative in children and young adults (<35 years) it is repeated at six weeks, and if it remains negative then BCG is administered. If it has become positive (without BCG), this is again taken as an indication of active disease and the individual is treated.

Children under the age of 1 year who have a family member with tuberculosis are given chemoprophylaxis with a daily dose of isoniazid 5–10 mg kg^{-1} for six months together with immunization with a strain of BCG that is resistant to isoniazid.

Practical

Mainly used for:

- Contact tracing
- BCG vaccination programmes.

It is rarely of any value in the diagnosis of tuberculosis.

Patients are tested with:

- Purified protein derivative (PPD) of *Myobacterium tuberculosis*.

The test is based on cell-mediated immunity with the development of induration and inflammation at the site of infection due to infiltration with mainly T lymphocytes. In patients with AIDS the test may be falsely negative owing to impairment of delayed hypersensitivity.

The Mantoux test

This is used for individual patients.

1. 0.1 mL of a 1:1000 strength PPD (equivalent to 10 tuberculin units) is injected intradermally.
2. The induration is measured (not the erythema) after 72 hours. The test is positive if the induration is 10 mm or more in diameter.

The Heaf test

This is a simple test used for large-scale screening.

1. A small amount of PPD (100 000 IU mL^{-1}) is placed on the flexor surface of the left forearm.
2. The 6-point disposable apparatus is actuated through the solution.
3. The Heaf reaction is graded 0–4 depending on the degree of induration: 0 and 1 (where there is only discrete induration at the puncture site) is a negative result after 3–10 days.

Practical box 12.5 Tuberculin testing

In general, in the UK much greater emphasis is placed on contact tracing and investigation of those under the age of 35 years and in some immigrant groups (Irish and Asian) in whom the disease is more virulent and prevalent.

Other mycobacteria

M. kansasii occurs in water and milk, though not in soil. Disease caused by this mycobacterium has mainly been described in Europe and the USA. It rarely causes a relatively benign type of human pulmonary disease, usually in middle-aged males. Men working in dusty jobs (e.g. miners) appear to be especially at risk, as are those who have underlying COPD. *M. avium intracellulare* is an important cause of pulmonary infection in AIDS patients (see p. 117).

FURTHER READING

Fine PEM (1995) Variation in protection by BCG: implications of and for heterologous immunity. *Lancet* **346**: 1339–1345.

Enarson DA, Grosser J, Mwinga A *et al.* (1995) The challenge of tuberculosis: Statements on global control and prevention. *Lancet* **346**: 809–819.

Diffuse diseases of the lung parenchyma

Granulomatous lung disease

A granuloma is a mass or nodule composed of chronically inflamed tissue formed by the response of the mononuclear phagocyte system (macrophage/histiocyte) to a slowly soluble antigen or irritant. If the foreign substance is inert (e.g. an inhaled dust), the phagocytes turn over slowly; if the substance is toxic or reproducing, the cells turn over faster, producing a granuloma.

A granuloma is characterized by epithelioid multinucleate giant cells, as seen in tuberculosis. Granulomas are also seen in other infections, including fungal and helminthic, in sarcoidosis, and in extrinsic allergic alveolitis, and can also be due to foreign bodies (e.g. talc). Granulomatosis with pulmonary vasculitis is discussed on p. 809.

Sarcoidosis

Sarcoidosis is a multisystem granulomatous disorder, commonly affecting young adults and usually presenting with bilateral hilar lymphadenopathy, pulmonary infiltration and skin or eye lesions. The diagnosis is confirmed on the histological evidence of widespread, non-caseating, epithelioid granulomas in more than one organ. Poisoning with beryllium can rarely produce a clinical and histological picture identical to sarcoidosis, though contact with this element is now strictly controlled.

EPIDEMIOLOGY AND AETIOLOGY

Sarcoidosis is a common disease that is often detected by mass X-ray studies. The aetiology remains unknown. There is great geographical variation. The prevalence in the UK is approximately 19 in 100 000 of the population. It is common in the USA but is uncommon in Japan. The course of the disease is much more severe in American Blacks than in Whites. There is no relation with any histocompatibility antigen, but cases of sarcoidosis are seen within families, possibly suggesting an environmental factor. Other aetiological factors suggested are an atypical mycobacterium or fungus, the Epstein–Barr virus, and occupational, genetic, social or other environmental factors (a higher incidence occurs in rural than in urban populations). None of these has been substantiated.

IMMUNOPATHOLOGY

- Typical sarcoid granulomas consist of focal accumulations of epithelioid cells, macrophages and lymphocytes, mainly T cells.
- There is depressed cell-mediated reactivity to tuberculin and other antigens such as *Candida albicans*.
- There is overall lymphopenia: circulating T lymphocytes are low but B cells are slightly increased.
- Bronchoalveolar lavage shows a great increase in the number of cells; lymphocytes (particularly CD4 helper cells) are greatly increased.
- The number of alveolar macrophages is increased but they represent a reduced percentage of the total number of cells.
- Transbronchial biopsies show infiltration of the alveolar walls and interstitial spaces with leucocytes, mainly T cells, prior to granuloma formation.

It seems likely that the decrease in circulating T lymphocytes and changes in delayed hypersensitivity responses are the result of sequestration of lymphocytes within the lung. There is no evidence to suggest that patients with sarcoidosis suffer from an overall defect in cellular immunity, since the frequency of fungal, viral and bacterial infections is not increased and there is no substantiated evidence of a greater risk of developing malignant neoplasms.

CLINICAL FEATURES

The peak incidence is in the third and fourth decades, with a female preponderance. Sarcoidosis can affect many different organs of the body. The most common presentation is with respiratory symptoms or abnormalities found on chest X-ray (50%). Fatigue or weight loss occurs in 5%, peripheral lymphadenopathy in 5% and a fever in 4%. A chest X-ray may be negative in up to 20% of non-respiratory cases, though lesions may be detected later.

Bilateral hilar lymphadenopathy

This is a characteristic feature of sarcoidosis. It is often symptomless and simply detected on a routine chest X-ray. Occasionally, the bilateral hilar lymphadenopathy is associated with a dull ache in the chest, malaise and a mild fever.

Although the chest X-ray may not show any evidence of infiltration in the lung fields, evidence from CT scanning (Fig 12.39), transbronchial biopsies and bronchoalveolar lavage indicate that the lung parenchyma is nearly always involved.

The differential diagnosis of the bilateral hilar lymphadenopathy includes:

- lymphoma – though it is rare for this to affect only the hilar lymph nodes
- pulmonary tuberculosis – though it is rare for the hilar lymph nodes to be symmetrically enlarged
- carcinoma of the bronchus with malignant spread to the contralateral hilar lymph nodes – again it is rare for this to give rise to a typical symmetrical picture.

In the early stages it may be difficult to distinguish enlarged lymph nodes on the chest X-ray from the pulmonary arteries, and lymph node enlargement is not always symmetrical. It is for these reasons that, in the absence of additional erythema nodosum (see below), histological confirmation of the disease process is advisable.

Pulmonary infiltration

This type of sarcoidosis may be progressive and may lead to increasing effort dyspnoea and eventually cor pulmonale and death. The chest X-ray shows a mottling in the mid-zones proceeding to generalized fine nodular shadows. Eventually, widespread pulmonary line shadows develop, reflecting the underlying fibrosis. A honeycomb appearance can occasionally occur. Pulmonary function tests show a typical restrictive lung defect (see below).

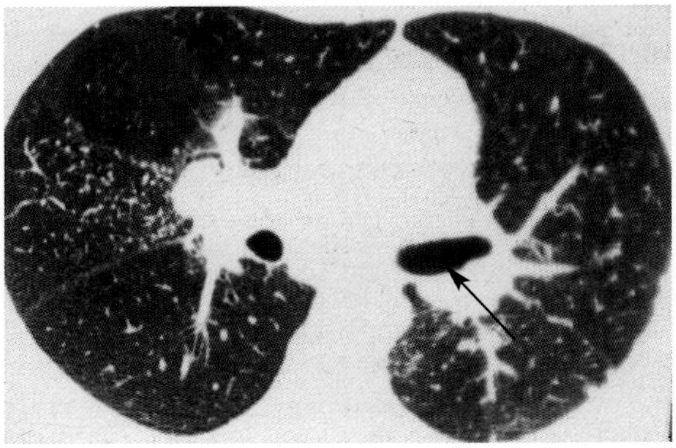

Fig 12.39
CT scan in sarcoidosis. Note enlarged glands at the hilum (arrow) and nodular shadowing, particularly in right middle lobe

It is possible to have a normal chest X-ray with abnormal lung function tests. Conversely, lung infiltration may be present on the X-ray with lung function tests in the normal range.

Extrapulmonary manifestations

Skin and ocular sarcoidosis are the most common extrapulmonary presentations.

Skin lesions. In 10% of cases; apart from erythema nodosum, a chilblain-like lesion known as lupus pernio is seen, as are nodules (see p. 1177). Sarcoidosis is the most common cause of erythema nodosum (see p. 1174). The association of bilateral symmetrical hilar lymphadenopathy with erythema nodosum occurs only in sarcoidosis.

Ocular and associated effects. Anterior uveitis is common and may present with misting of vision, pain and a red eye, but posterior uveitis may present simply as progressive loss of vision. Although ocular sarcoidosis accounts for about 5% of uveitis presenting to ophthalmologists, evidence of asymptomatic uveitis may be found in up to 25% of patients with sarcoidosis. Conjunctivitis may occur and retinal lesions have been recognized recently.

Keratoconjunctivitis sicca and lacrimal gland enlargement may also occur. *Uveoparotid fever* is a syndrome of bilateral uveitis and parotid gland enlargement together with occasional development of facial nerve palsy and is sometimes seen with sarcoidosis.

Metabolic manifestations. It is rare for sarcoidosis to present with problems of calcium metabolism, though hypercalcaemia is found in 10% of established cases. Hypercalcaemia and hypercalciuria can lead to the development of renal calculi and nephrocalcinosis. The cause of the hypercalcaemia is due to the high circulating 1,25-dihydroxy vitamin D_3, with the 1α-hydroxylation occurring in sarcoid macrophages in the lung in addition to that taking place in the kidney.

The central nervous system. Involvement of the central nervous system (CNS) is rare (2%) but can lead to severe neurological disease (see p. 1077).

Bone and joint involvement. Arthralgia without erythema nodosum is seen in 5% of cases. Bone cysts are found, particularly in the digits, with associated swelling. In the absence of swelling, routine X-rays of the hands are unnecessary.

Hepatosplenomegaly. Sarcoidosis is a cause of hepatosplenomegaly, though it is rarely of any clinical consequence.

Cardiac involvement. Cardiac involvement is rare (3%). Ventricular dysrhythmias, conduction defects and cardiomyopathy with congestive cardiac failure may be seen.

INVESTIGATIONS

- **Imaging.** Chest X-ray (see above). CT is useful for assessment of diffuse lung involvement.
- **Full blood count.** There is mild normochromic, normocytic anaemia with raised ESR.
- **Serum biochemistry.** There is raised serum calcium and hypergammaglobulinaemia.
- **Transbronchial biopsy** is the most useful investigation. Positive results are seen in 90% of cases of pulmonary sarcoidosis with or without X-ray evidence of lung involvement. The test provides positive histological evidence of a granuloma in approximately one-half of patients with clinically extrapulmonary sarcoidosis in whom the chest X-ray is normal.
- **Serum level of angiotensin converting enzyme** (ACE) is two standard deviations above the normal mean value in over 75% of patients with untreated sarcoidosis. Raised (but lower) levels are also seen in patients with lymphoma, pulmonary tuberculosis, asbestosis and silicosis, rendering the test of no diagnostic value. However, it is a simple test and is of use in assessing the activity of the disease and therefore as a guide to treatment with corticosteroids. Reduction of serum ACE during treatment with corticosteroids has not, however, been proved to reflect resolution of the disease.
- **Lung function tests** show a restrictive lung defect with pulmonary infiltration. There is a decrease in TLC, a decrease in both FEV_1 and FVC, and a decrease in gas transfer.
- **The Kveim test**, which involved an intradermal injection of sarcoid tissue, was regularly used for confirmation of the diagnosis. It should not be used because of the risk of transmission of infection. It is less sensitive and less specific than transbronchial biopsy which has superseded it.
- **Tuberculin test** is negative in 80% of patients with sarcoidosis; it is of no diagnostic value.

TREATMENT

Both the need to treat and the value of corticosteroid therapy are contested in many aspects of this disease.

Hilar lymphadenopathy on its own with no evidence of chest X-ray involvement of the lungs or decrease in lung function tests does not require treatment. Persisting infiltration on the chest X-ray or abnormal lung function tests are unlikely to improve without corticosteroid treatment. If the disease is not improving spontaneously six months after diagnosis, treatment should be started with prednisolone 30 mg for six weeks, reducing to alternate-day treatment with prednisolone 15 mg for 6–12 months. Although there have been no controlled trials that have proved the efficacy of such treatment, it is difficult to withhold corticosteroids when there is continuing deterioration of the disease.

Topical or systemic prednisolone should be given for patients suffering from involvement of the eyes or the presence of persistent hypercalcaemia. If the erythema nodosum of sarcoidosis is severe or persistent it will respond rapidly to a two-week course of prednisolone 5–15 mg daily.

Myocardial sarcoidosis and neurological manifestations are also treated with prednisolone, and uveoparotid fever responds rapidly to steroids.

PROGNOSIS

Sarcoidosis is a much more severe disease in certain racial groups, particularly American Blacks, where death rates of up to 10% have been recorded. It is probable that the disease is fatal in fewer than 1 in 20 individuals in the UK, most often as a result of respiratory failure and cor pulmonale but, rarely, from myocardial sarcoidosis and renal damage.

The chest X-ray provides a guide to prognosis. The disease remits by two years in over two-thirds of patients with hilar lymphadenopathy alone, in approximately one-half with hilar lymphadenopathy plus chest X-ray evidence of pulmonary infiltration, but in only one-third of patients with X-ray evidence of infiltration without any demonstrable lymphadenopathy.

Langerhans' cell histiocytosis (LCH)

This rare disease (a prevalence of 1 per 50 000) was previously known as histiocytosis X. It is characterized histologically by proliferation of LCH cells identified by the presence of Birbeck granules on electron-microscopy or the CD_{1a} antigen on the surface of the cells. There is a wide variation in clinical presentation, from uni-focal bone lesions in older children (which may regress spontaneously), to more disseminated disease in younger children (with a high mortality). Chest X-rays show multiple small cysts (honeycomb lung), fibrosis or widespread nodular shadows. Etoposide treatment is justified for advanced progressive disease.

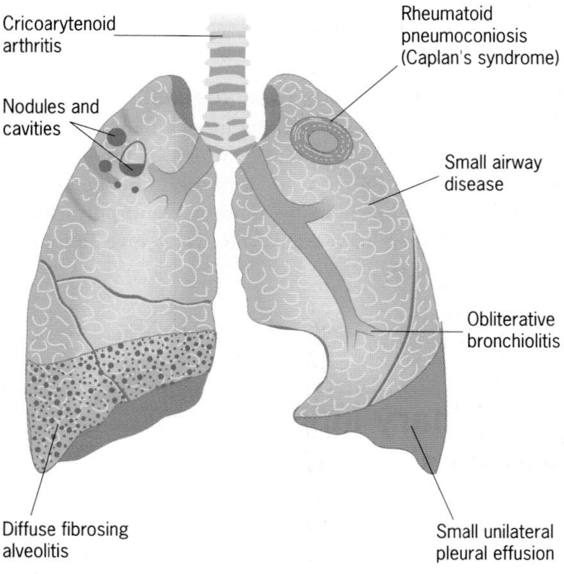

Fig 12.40
Respiratory manifestations of rheumatoid disease

Pulmonary vasculitis and granulomatosis

In this section diseases associated with both granulomas and vasculitis are described. The classification is unsatisfactory. Here the first main subsection contains the respiratory manifestations of systemic connective tissue diseases, whilst the second subsection contains disorders associated with the presence of anti-neutrophil cytoplasmic antibodies (ANCAs)

Pulmonary vasculitis with connective tissue disease

Rheumatoid disease (see also p. 475)

The features of respiratory involvement in rheumatoid disease are illustrated in Fig 12.40.

Pleural adhesions, thickening and effusion are the most common lesions. The effusion is often unilateral and tends to be chronic. It has a low glucose content but this can occur in any chronic pleural effusion.

Rheumatoid diffuse fibrosing alveolitis can be considered as a variant of the cryptogenic form of the disease (see p. 475). The clinical features and gross appearance are the same but the disease is often more chronic.

Rheumatoid nodules appear on the chest X-ray as single or multiple nodules ranging in size from a few millimetres to a few centimetres. The nodules frequently cavitate. They usually produce no symptoms but can give rise to a pneumothorax or pleural effusion.

Obliterative disease of the small bronchioles is rare. It is characterized by progressive breathlessness and irreversible airflow limitation. Corticosteroids may prevent progression.

Involvement of the cricoarytenoid joints gives rise to dyspnoea, stridor, hoarseness and occasionally severe obstruction necessitating tracheostomy. Caplan's syndrome is due to a combination of dust inhalation and the disturbed immunity of rheumatoid arthritis. It occurs particularly in coal-worker's pneumoconiosis but it can occur in individuals exposed to other dusts, such as silica and asbestos. Typically the lesions appear as rounded nodules 0.5–5.0 cm in diameter, though sometimes they become incorporated into large areas of fibrosis that are indistinguishable radiologically from progressive massive fibrosis. There may be little evidence of simple pneumoconiosis prior to the development of the nodule.

These lesions may precede the development of the arthritis. Rheumatoid factor is always present in the serum.

Systemic lupus erythematosus (see also p. 487)

The most common respiratory manifestation of this disease, occurring in up to two-thirds of cases, is the development of pleurisy, with or without an effusion. Effusions are usually small and bilateral. Basal pneumonitis is often present, perhaps as a result of poor movement of the diaphragm, or restriction of chest movements because of pleural pain. Pneumonia also occurs, due either to infection or to the disease process itself. Unlike rheumatoid arthritis, diffuse pulmonary fibrosis is rare.

Systemic sclerosis

Autopsy studies have indicated that there is almost always some evidence of diffuse fibrosis of alveolar walls and obliteration of capillaries and the alveolar space. Severe changes result in nodular then streaky shadowing on the chest X-ray, followed by cystic changes, ending up with a honeycomb lung. Lung function tests indicate a restrictive lesion and poor gas transfer.

Pneumonia may occur owing to inhalation from the dilated oesophagus (see p. 230). Breathlessness may be worsened by restriction of chest wall movement owing to thickening and contraction of the skin and trunk.

Granulomatous vasculitides

Anti-neutrophil cytoplasmic antibodies

(see also p. 452 and p. 539)

Anti-neutrophil cytoplasmic antibodies (ANCAs) are found in the acute phase of vasculitides, particularly Wegener's granulomatosis, Churg–Strauss syndrome and microscopic polyangiitis (polyarteritis) associated with neutrophil infiltration of the vessel wall.

Two major ANCA reactivities are recognized:

- proteinase-3 (PR3) ANCA which in neutrophil indirect immunofluorescence assays produces a typical granular cytoplasmic stain
- myeloperoxidase (MPO) ANCA which produces a perinuclear stain.

About 10% of all vasculitis patients are ANCA-negative: this is more common in Wegener's granulomatosis limited to the upper respiratory tract. 10–15% of cases of progressive glomerulonephritis with anti-glomerular basement membrane (GBM) antibodies are MPO ANCA-positive and these are the most likely to suffer pulmonary haemorrhage.

Wegener's granulomatosis

This granulomatous disease of unknown aetiology is one of the primary systemic vasculitides (the other is the Churg–Strauss syndrome, see below) in which the small arteries are predominantly affected. It is characterized by lesions involving the upper respiratory tract, the lungs and the kidneys. Often the disease starts with severe rhinorrhoea with subsequent nasal mucosal ulceration followed by cough, haemoptysis and pleuritic pain. Occasionally there may be involvement of the skin and nervous system. A chest X-ray usually shows single or multiple nodular masses or pneumonic infiltrates with cavitation. The most remarkable radiographic feature is the migratory pattern, with large lesions clearing in one area and new lesions appearing in another.

The typical histological changes are usually best seen in the kidneys, where there is a necrotizing microvascular glomerulonephritis.

This disease responds well to treatment with cyclophosphamide 150–200 mg daily. A variant of Wegener's granulomatosis called 'mid-line granuloma' particularly affects the nose and paranasal sinuses and is particularly mutilating; it has a poor prognosis

The Churg–Strauss syndrome

This condition occurs in patients, usually male, in their fourth decade who have a triad of rhinitis and asthma, eosinophilia and systemic vasculitis. It probably represents an unusual progression of allergic disease in a subset of predisposed individuals.

The pathology of this condition is dominated by an eosinophilic infiltration with a characteristic high blood eosinophil count, vasculitis of small arteries and veins, and extravascular granulomas. The lungs, peripheral nerves and skin are most often affected and kidney involvement is uncommon. Transient patchy pneumonia-like shadows may occur, but sometimes these can be massive and bilateral. Skin lesions include tender subcutaneous nodules as well as petechial or purpuric lesions. ANCA is usually positive. The disease responds well to corticosteroids.

Microscopic vasculitis (polyangiitis)

This involves the kidneys and the lungs where it results in recurrent haemoptysis. ANCA is usually positive. In the early literature there was confusion between this condition, the Churg–Strauss syndrome and polyarteritis nodosa. The latter, however, is ANCA-negative and rarely involves the lungs.

Pulmonary infiltration with eosinophilia

The common types and characteristics of these diseases are shown in Table 12.15. They range from very mild, simple, pulmonary eosinophilias to the often fatal polyarteritis nodosa.

Simple and prolonged pulmonary eosinophilia

Simple pulmonary eosinophilia is a relatively mild illness with a slight fever and cough and usually lasting for less than two weeks. It is probably due to a transient allergic reaction in the alveolus. Many allergens have been implicated, including *Ascaris lumbricoides*, *Ankylostoma*, *Trichuris*, *Trichinella*, *Taenia* and *Strongyloides*. Drugs such as *p*-aminosalicylic acid, aspirin, penicillin, nitrofurantoin and sulphonamides have been implicated. Often, no allergen is identified. No treatment is required and the disease is self-limiting.

Occasionally, the disease becomes more prolonged, with a high fever lasting for over a month. There is usually an eosinophilia in the blood and this condition is then called *prolonged pulmonary eosinophilia*. In both conditions the chest X-ray shows either localized or diffuse opacities. Where appropriate, worms are treated and possible drugs stopped. Corticosteroid therapy is indicated, with resolution of the disease over the ensuing weeks.

Asthmatic bronchopulmonary eosinophilia

This is characterized by the presence of asthma, transient fleeting shadows on the chest X-ray, and blood or sputum eosinophilia. By far the most common cause worldwide is allergy to *A. fumigatus* (see below), although *Candida albicans* and other mycoses may be the allergen in a small number of patients. In many, the appropriate allergen has still to be identified.

Diseases caused by *Aspergillus fumigatus*

The various types of lung disease caused by *A. fumigatus* are illustrated in Fig 12.41.

The spores of *A. fumigatus* (diameter 5 μm) are readily inhaled and are present in the atmosphere throughout the year, though they are at their highest concentration in the late autumn. They can be grown from the sputum in up to 15% of patients with chronic lung disease in whom they do not produce disease. They are an important cause of extrinsic asthma in atopic individuals.

Allergic bronchopulmonary aspergillosis

In this rare disease, *Aspergillus* actually grows in the walls of the bronchi and eventually produces proximal bronchiectasis. There are episodes of eosinophilic pneumonia throughout the year, particularly in late autumn and winter. The episodes present with a wheeze, cough, fever and malaise. They are associated with expectoration of firm sputum plugs containing the fungal mycelium, which results in the clearing of the pulmonary infiltrates on the chest X-ray. Occasionally the large mucus plugs obliterate the bronchial lumen, causing collapse of the lung.

Repeated episodes of eosinophilic pneumonia left untreated can result in progressive pulmonary fibrosis that is often seen in the upper zones and can give rise to a similar chest X-ray appearance to that produced by tuberculosis.

The peripheral blood eosinophil count is usually raised, and total levels of IgE are extremely high (both that specific to *Aspergillus* and nonspecific). Skin-prick testing

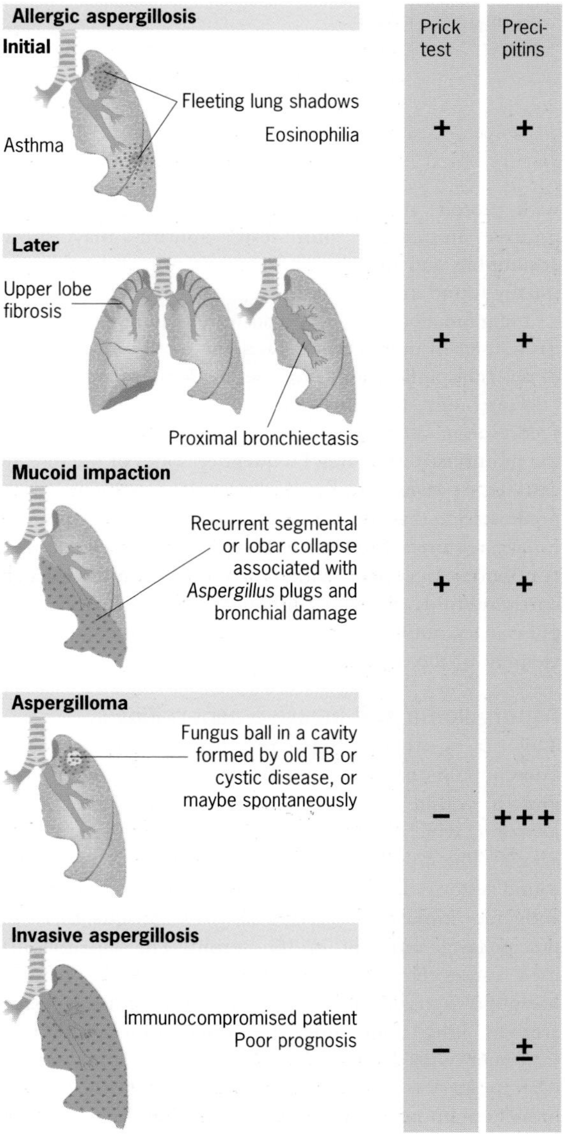

Fig 12.41
Diseases caused by *Aspergillus fumigatus*

Table 12.15
Common types and characteristics of pulmonary infiltration with eosinophilia

Disease	Symptoms	Blood eosinophils (%)	Multisystem involvement	Duration	Outcome
Simple pulmonary eosinophilia	Mild	10	None	<1 month	Good
Prolonged pulmonary eosinophilia	Mild/ moderate	>20	None	>1 month	Good
Asthmatic bronchopulmonary eosinophilia	Moderate/ severe	5–20	None	Years	Fair
Tropical pulmonary eosinophilia	Moderate/ severe	>20	None	Years	Fair
Hypereosinophilic syndrome	Severe	>20	Always	Months/ years	Poor

with protein allergens from *A. fumigatus* gives rise to positive immediate skin tests. Sputum may show eosinophils and mycelia, and precipitating antibodies are usually found in the serum.

Lung function tests show a decrease in lung volumes and gas transfer in more chronic cases, but in all cases evidence of reversible airflow limitation can be demonstrated.

Treatment for this allergic pneumonia is with prednisolone 30 mg daily, which readily causes clearing of the pulmonary infiltrates. Frequent episodes of the disease can be prevented by long-term treatment with prednisolone, but doses as high as 10–15 mg daily are usually required. Moderately severe asthma itself requires continuous treatment with oral corticosteroids. Inhaled corticosteroids do not influence the occurrence of pulmonary infiltrates but are useful for the asthmatic element of the disease.

Aspergilloma and invasive aspergillosis

This is a totally separate disease from allergic bronchopulmonary aspergillosis. It simply represents the growth within previously damaged lung tissue of *A. fumigatus*, which forms a ball of mycelium within lung cavities. The typical appearance on the chest X-ray is of a round lesion with an air 'halo' above it. The continuing antigenic stimulation gives rise to large quantities of precipitating antibody in the serum. The aspergilloma itself causes little trouble, though occasionally massive haemoptysis may occur, requiring resection of the damaged area of lung containing the aspergilloma. Although treatment with antifungal agents, such as amphotericin (250 $\mu g\ kg^{-1}$ i.v.), has been tested in both allergic bronchopulmonary aspergillosis and aspergilloma, this has had little success. However, it remains the only treatment for invasive aspergillosis, when it is often combined with flucytosine (200 mg kg^{-1} i.v. daily in four doses).

Tropical pulmonary eosinophilia

This term is reserved for an allergic reaction to microfilaria from *Wuchereria bancrofti*. The condition is seen in the Asian subcontinent and presents with cough and wheeze together with fever, lassitude and weight loss. The typical appearance of the chest X-ray is of bilateral hazy mottling that is frequently uniformly distributed in both lung fields. The individual shadows may be as large as 5 mm or may become more confluent, giving the appearance of pneumonia.

The disease is characterized by a very high eosinophil count in peripheral blood. The filarial complement fixation test is positive in almost every case, although the microfilaria are seldom found. The treatment of choice is diethylcarbamazine at a dose of 5 mg kg^{-1} bodyweight for 10–14 days; this usually produces a good response.

The hypereosinophilic syndrome

This disease is characterized by eosinophilic infiltration in various organs, sometimes associated with an eosinophilic arteritis. The heart muscle is particularly involved, but pulmonary involvement in the form of a pleural effusion or interstitial lung disease occurs in about 40% of cases. Typical features are fever, weight loss, recurrent abdominal pain, persistent non-productive cough and congestive cardiac failure. Corticosteroid treatment may be of value in some cases.

Goodpasture's syndrome and idiopathic pulmonary haemosiderosis

Goodpasture's syndrome (see also p. 536)

The disease often starts with an upper respiratory tract infection followed by cough and intermittent haemoptysis, tiredness and eventually anaemia, though massive bleeding may occur. The chest X-ray shows transient blotchy shadows that are due to intrapulmonary haemorrhage. These features usually precede the development of an acute glomerulonephritis by several weeks or months. The course of the disease is variable; some spontaneously improve while others proceed to renal failure.

The disease usually occurs in individuals over 16 years of age. It is thought to be due to a type II cytotoxic hypersensitivity reaction, the hypothesis being that there may be a shared antigen between a virus and the basement membrane of both kidney and lung. Anti-GBM antibodies are found in the serum and ANCA may be positive. An association with influenza A2 virus has been reported.

Treatment is with corticosteroids, but plasmapheresis to remove the antibodies has led to dramatic improvement in some cases.

Idiopathic pulmonary haemosiderosis

This is a disease similar to Goodpasture's syndrome, but the kidneys are less frequently involved. Most cases occur in children under seven years of age. Characteristically, haemosiderin-containing macrophages are found in the sputum. The child develops a chronic cough and anaemia and the chest X-ray shows diffuse shadows that are due to intrapulmonary bleeding, and eventually miliary nodulation. There is an association with a sensitivity to cows' milk, and an appropriate diet is usually tried.

The prognosis in general is poor and treatment with corticosteroids or azathioprine is usually given.

Pulmonary fibrosis and honeycomb lung

Pulmonary fibrosis is the end result of many diseases of the respiratory tract. It may be:

- localized (e.g. following unresolved pneumonia)
- bilateral (e.g. in tuberculosis)
- widespread (e.g. in cryptogenic fibrosing alveolitis, in industrial lung disease, or due to drugs such as busulphan, bleomycin and cyclophosphamide).

Sometimes with widespread fibrosis a typical radiological appearance is seen that is known as 'honeycomb lung'. This refers to the presence, often diffusely in both lungs, of cysts 0.5–2.0 cm diameter that are thick-walled and do not fill with opaque material on bronchography. The cystic air spaces probably represent dilated and thickened terminal and respiratory bronchioles. The main causes are shown in Table 12.16.

Cryptogenic fibrosing alveolitis (CFA)

This relatively rare disorder causes diffuse fibrosis throughout the lung fields, usually in late middle age. It is thought that the disease, at least in some, is the result of occupational exposure to metal or wood dust and that the term 'cryptogenic' should be dropped in these cases.

PATHOGENESIS

The pathogenesis of damage and fibrosis is complex and several factors are involved (Fig 12.42).

Macrophages activated by several factors (see p. 161) produce growth factors. These include fibronectin, platelet-derived growth factor, transforming growth factor β, and insulin-like growth factor 1. This leads to the deposition of collagens type I and III. Histologically there are two main features:

- cellular infiltration with lymphocytes and plasma cells and thickening and fibrosis of the alveolar walls
- alveolitis – increased cells within the alveolar space (mainly shed type II pneumocytes and macrophages).

CLINICAL FEATURES

The cardinal features are progressive breathlessness and cyanosis, which eventually lead to respiratory failure, pulmonary hypertension and cor pulmonale. Gross clubbing occurs in two-thirds of cases and bilateral fine end-inspiratory crackles are heard on auscultation. An acute form known as the Hamman–Rich syndrome occurs in about 20%. The chest X-ray appearance initially is of ground-glass appearance, progressing to obvious small nodular shadows with streaky fibrosis and finally a honeycomb lung.

Table 12.16
The main causes of honeycomb lung

Localized	Diffuse
Systemic sclerosis	Crytogenic fibrosing alveolitis
Sarcoidosis	Rheumatoid lung
Tuberculosis	Langerhans' cell histiocytosis
Asbestosis	Tuberous sclerosis
Berylliosis	Neurofibromatosis

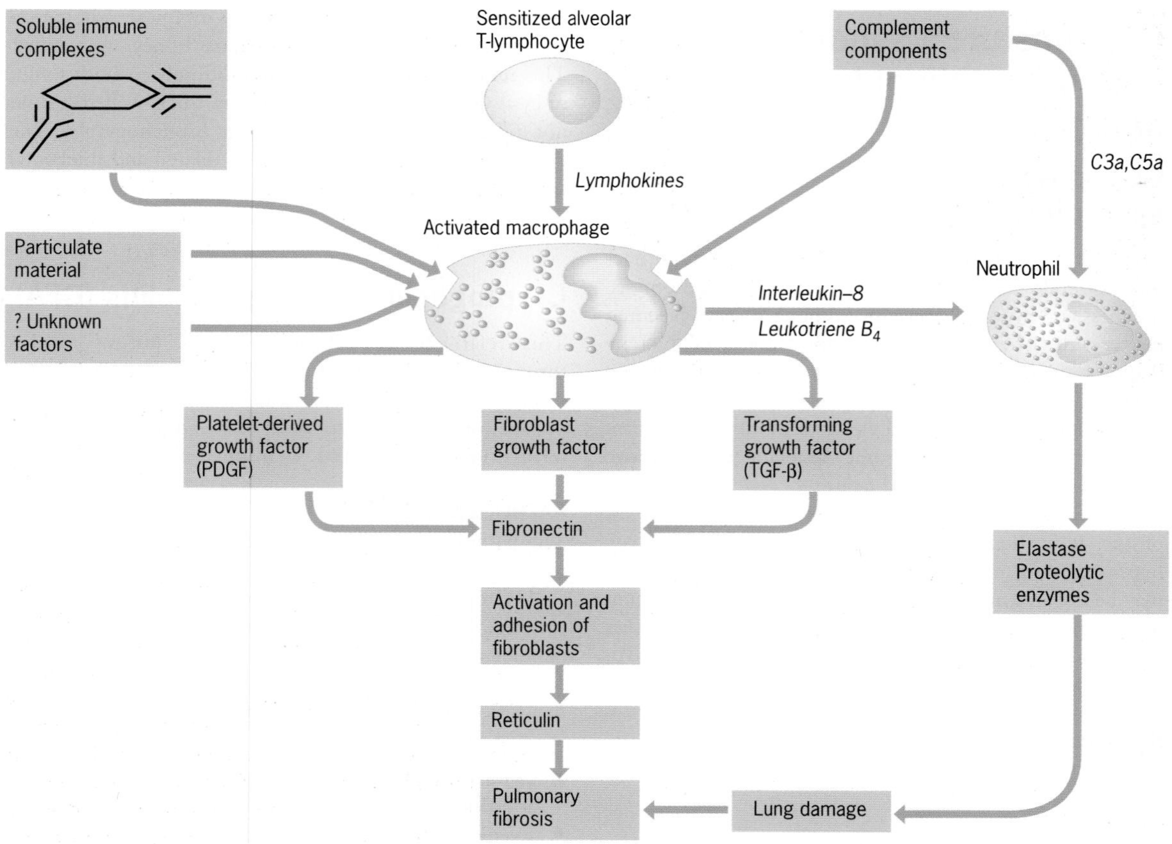

Fig 12.42
Pathogenesis of pulmonary fibrosis. Macrophages can be activated by several factors, such as soluble immune complexes and sensitized T-lymphocytes, resulting in the release of various cytokines leading to fibrosis

A number of autoimmune diseases are seen in association with this condition. For example, autoimmune hepatitis occurs in 5–10% of cases.

Similar lung changes are also seen in rheumatoid arthritis, systemic sclerosis and Sjögren's syndrome, often associated with Raynaud's phenomenon.

CFA has also been reported in association with coeliac disease, ulcerative colitis and renal tubular acidosis.

INVESTIGATIONS

- **Chest X-ray** shows irregular reticulonodular shadowing, maximal in the lower zones.
- **High-resolution CT scan** shows characteristic changes of peripheral reticular and ground-glass opacification, seen best in the basal regions but extending all over the lungs (Fig 12.43).
- **Respiratory function tests** show a restrictive ventilatory defect – the lung volumes are reduced, the FEV_1 and FVC ratio is normal to high (with both values being reduced), and gas transfer is reduced. Peak flow rates may be normal.
- **Blood gases** show an arterial hypoxaemia with normal P_aCO_2.
- **Blood tests** The antinuclear factor and rheumatoid factor are positive in one-third of patients. The ESR is mildly elevated.
- **Bronchoalveolar lavage** shows increased numbers of cells (particularly neutrophils).
- **Histological confirmation** is necessary in some patients, requiring a transbronchial lung biopsy or even an open lung biopsy to obtain a larger specimen.

DIFFERENTIAL DIAGNOSIS

The diagnosis of CFA is usually made in a patient presenting with the above signs and characteristic CT changes. The differential diagnosis of chest X-ray appearance includes extrinsic allergic alveolitis, bronchiectasis, chronic left heart failure, sarcoidosis, industrial lung disease, and lymphangitis carcinomatosa.

PROGNOSIS AND TREATMENT

The median survival time for patients with CFA is approximately five years, although mortality is very high with the acute form. Treatment with prednisolone (30 mg

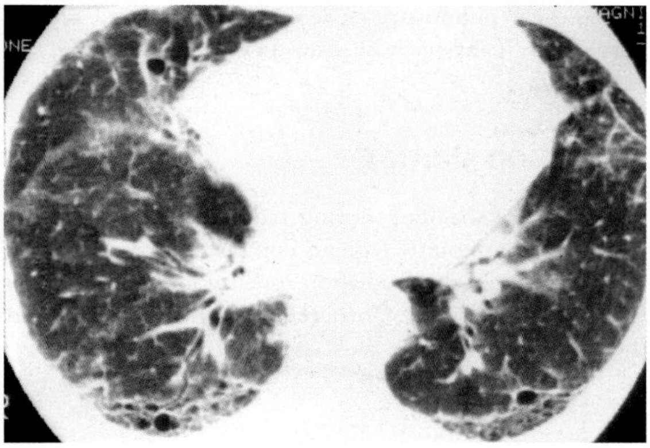

Fig 12.43
CT scan showing cryptogenic fibrosing alveolitis

daily) is usually prescribed for disabling disease, though its benefit has still to be proved by appropriate controlled trials. Azathioprine or cyclophosphamide may be added if there is no response. Supportive treatment includes domiciliary oxygen therapy. In severe disease, single lung transplantation can be offered.

Extrinsic allergic alveolitis

In this disease there is a widespread diffuse inflammatory reaction in both the small airways of the lung and alveoli. It is due to the inhalation of a number of different antigens, the most common being microbial spores contaminating vegetable matter (e.g. straw, hay, mushroom compost). Some examples are illustrated in Table 12.17. By far the most common of these diseases worldwide is farmer's lung, which affects up to 1 in 10 of the farming community in poor, wet areas around the world. In the West the incidence is almost certainly declining as more mechanized farming procedures are introduced.

Table 12.17
Extrinsic allergic (bronchiolar) alveolitis – some causes

Disease	Situation	Antigens
Farmer's lung	Forking mouldy hay or any other mouldy vegetable material	Thermophilic actinomycetes and *Micropolyspora faeni*
Bird fancier's lung	Handling pigeons, cleaning lofts or budgerigar cages	Proteins present in the 'bloom' on the feathers and in excreta
Maltworker's lung	Turning germinating barley	*Asperigillus clavatus*
Humidifier fever	Contaminated humidifying systems in air conditioners or humidifiers in factories (especially in printing works)	Possibly a variety of bacteria or amoeba (e.g. *Naegleria gruberi*)
Mushroom workers	Turning mushroom compost	Thermophilic actinomycetes

PATHOGENESIS

Histologically there is an initial infiltration of the small airways and alveolar walls with neutrophils followed by lymphocytes and macrophages, leading to the development of non-caseating granulomas. These comprise multinucleated giant cells, occasionally containing the inhaled antigenic material. The major allergic response to the inhaled antigens is through cellular immunity, though there is evidence in some cases of an additional immediate hypersensitivity reaction involving specific IgE antibody and the deposition of immune complexes. All these mechanisms can attract and activate alveolar macrophages, so that continued antigenic exposure results in the development of pulmonary fibrosis.

CLINICAL FEATURES

The typical history is that of the onset of fever, malaise, cough and shortness of breath several hours after exposure to the causative antigen. For example, a farmer forking hay in the morning may notice symptoms only during the late afternoon and evening that resolve by the following morning. On examination the patient may have a fever, tachypnoea and coarse end-inspiratory crackles and wheezes throughout the chest. Cyanosis may be severe even at rest. Continuing exposure leads to a chronic illness characterized by severe weight loss, effort dyspnoea and cough, and the features of fibrosing alveolitis (see p. 813).

INVESTIGATIONS

- **Chest X-ray** shows fluffy nodular shadowing with the subsequent development of streaky shadows, particularly in the upper zones. In very advanced cases, honeycomb lung is seen.
- **Polymorphonuclear leucocyte count** is raised in acute cases.
- **Precipitating antibodies** are present in the serum. One-quarter of pigeon fanciers have precipitating antibody against pigeon protein and droppings in their serum, but only a small proportion have lung disease. Precipitating antibodies are evidence of *exposure*, not disease.
- **Lung function tests** show a restrictive ventilatory defect with a decrease in gas transfer.
- **Bronchoalveolar lavage** shows increased cells (lymphocytes and granulocytes).

DIFFERENTIAL DIAGNOSIS

Although an extrinsic allergic bronchiolar alveolitis due to inhalation of the spores of *Micropolyspora faeni* is common among farmers, it is probably more common for these individuals to suffer from asthma related to inhalation of antigens from a variety of mites that infest stored grain and other vegetable material. The common ones are *Lepidoglyphus domesticus*, *L. destructor* and *Acarus siro*. Symptoms of asthma resulting from inhalation of these allergens are often mistaken for farmer's lung.

Pigeon fancier's lung is quite common, but alveolitis from budgerigars is very rare.

MANAGEMENT

Prevention is the aim. This can be achieved by changes in work practice, with the use of silage for animal fodder and the drier storage of hay and grain. It is difficult to control pigeon fancier's lung, since individuals remain addicted to their hobby.

Prednisolone, initially in large doses of 30–60 mg daily, is necessary to cause regression of the early stages of the disease. Established fibrosis will not resolve and in some patients the disease may progress inexorably to respiratory failure in spite of intensive therapy. Farmer's lung is a recognized occupational disease in the UK and sufferers are entitled to compensation depending on their degree of disability.

Humidifier fever

Humidifier fever may present with the typical features of extrinsic allergic alveolitis without any radiographic changes. This disease has occurred in outbreaks in factories in the UK, particularly in printing works. In North America it is more commonly found in office blocks with contaminated air-conditioning systems. The cause remains unknown but probably involves several bacteria or even amoebae.

Humidifier fever is prevented by sterilization of the recirculating water used in the very large humidifying plants in industry.

Drug-induced lung disease

Drugs may produce a wide variety of disorders of the respiratory tract. Pulmonary infiltrates with fibrosis may result from the use of a number of cytotoxic drugs used in the treatment of cancer. The most common cause of these reactions is bleomycin. The pulmonary damage is dose-related, occurring when the total dosage is greater than 450 mg, but will regress in some cases if the drug is stopped. The most sensitive test is a decrease in gas transfer, and therefore gas transfer should be measured repeatedly during treatment with the drug. The use of corticosteroids may help resolution.

Some of the most important drugs affecting the respiratory tract are shown in Table 12.18, together with the types of reaction they produce. The list is not exhaustive; for example, over 20 different drugs are known to produce a systemic lupus erythematosus-like syndrome, sometimes complicated by pulmonary infiltrates and fibrosis. Paraquat ingestion (see p. 879) can cause severe pulmonary oedema and death, and fibrosis develops in many of those who survive.

Radiation damage

Irradiation of the lung during radiotherapy can cause a radiation pneumonitis. Patients complain of breathlessness and a dry cough. Radiation pneumonia results in a restrictive lung defect. Corticosteroids should be given in the acute stage.

Table 12.18
Drug-induced respiratory disease

Disease	Drugs
Asthma ± rhinitis	Penicillins Sulphonamides Cephalosporins Aspirin NSAIDs Tartrazine Iodine-containing contrast media Non-selective β-adrenoreceptor-blocking drugs (e.g. propranolol) Suxamethonium Thiopentone
Diffuse lung injury infiltrate and/or fibrosis	Amiodarone Hexamethonium Nitrofurantoin Paraquat Continuous oxygen Cytotoxic agent (many, particularly busulphan, CCNU, bleomycin)
Pulmonary eosinophilia	Antibiotics Penicillin Tetracycline Sulphonamides NSAIDs Anti-epileptic Phenytoin Carbamazepine Others Chlorpropamide
Opportunistic pulmonary infections	Corticosteroids Azathioprine Other cytotoxic drugs
Respiratory depression	Sedatives Opiates
SLE-like syndrome including pulmonary infiltrates, effusions and fibrosis	Hydralazine Procainamide Isoniazid *p*-Aminosalicylic acid ACE inhibitors

CCNU, chloroethyl-cyclohexyl-nitrosourea (lomustine); NSAIDs, non-steroidal anti-inflammatory drugs; SLE, systemic lupus erythematosus

FURTHER READING

Chan-Yeung M, Muller NL (1997) Cytogenic fibrosing alveolitis. *Lancet* **350**: 651–656.

Newman LS, Rose CS, Maier LA (1997) Sarcoidosis. *New England Journal of Medicine* **336**: 1224–1234.

Savage COS, Harper L, Adu D (1997) Primary systemic vasculitis. *Lancet* **349**: 558–562.

Occupational lung disease

Exposure to dusts, gases, vapours and fumes at work can lead to the development of the following types of lung disease:

- Acute bronchitis and even pulmonary oedema from irritants such as sulphur dioxide, chlorine, ammonia or the oxides of nitrogen
- Pulmonary fibrosis due to mineral dust
- Occupational asthma (see Table 12.13)
- Extrinsic allergic bronchiolar alveolitis (see Table 12.17)
- Bronchial carcinoma due to industrial agents (e.g. asbestos, polycyclic hydrocarbons, radon in mines).

The degree of fibrosis that follows inhalation of mineral dust varies. While iron (siderosis), barium (baritosis) and tin (stannosis) lead to dramatic dense nodular shadowing on the chest X-ray, their effect on lung function and symptoms is minimal. Exposure to silica or asbestos, on the other hand, leads to extensive fibrosis and disability. Coal dust has an intermediate fibrogenic effect and accounts for 90% of all compensated industrial lung diseases in the UK. The term 'pneumoconiosis' means the accumulation of dust in the lungs and the reaction of the tissue to its presence. The term is not wide enough to encompass all occupational lung disease and is now generally used in relation to coal dust and its effects on the lung.

Coal-worker's pneumoconiosis

Improved conditions and contraction of the coal industry in the UK have led to a considerable reduction in the number of cases of pneumoconiosis. The disease is caused by dust particles approximately 2–5 μm in diameter that are retained in the small airways and alveoli of the lung. The incidence of the disease is related to total dust exposure, which is highest at the coal face, particularly if ventilation and dust suppression are poor. Two very different syndromes result from the inhalation of coal.

Simple pneumoconiosis

This simply reflects the deposition of coal dust in the lung. It produces a fine micronodular shadow on the chest X-ray and is by far the most common type of pneumoconiosis. It is graded on the chest X-ray appearance according to standard categories set by the International Labour Office (see below). Considerable dispute remains about the effects of simple pneumoconiosis on respiratory function and symptoms. In many cases the symptoms are due to COPD related to cigarette smoking, but this is not always the case.

Categories of simple pneumoconiosis are as follows:

1. small round opacities definitely present but few in number
2. small round opacities numerous but normal lung markings still visible
3. small round opacities very numerous and normal lung markings partly or totally obscured.

The importance of simple pneumoconiosis is that it may lead to the development of progressive massive fibrosis (PMF) (see below). This virtually never occurs on a background of category 1 simple pneumoconiosis but occurs in 30% of those with category 3. Usually category 2 simple pneumoconiosis, which carries a 7% risk of developing PMF, must be present before benefit may be awarded for disability in the UK.

Progressive massive fibrosis

The lesions in this disease are round fibrotic masses several centimetres in diameter, almost invariably in the upper lobes and sometimes having necrotic central cavities. The pathogenesis of PMF is still not understood, though it seems clear that some fibrogenic promoting factor is present in individuals developing the disease. This was thought to be *M. tuberculosis*, but is probably immune complexes, analogous to the development of large fibrotic nodules in coal miners with rheumatoid arthritis (Caplan's syndrome). The development of both rheumatoid factor and antinuclear factor in the serum of patients with PMF is common, as it is in those suffering from asbestosis and silicosis.

Pathologically there is apical destruction and disruption of the lung, resulting in emphysema and airway damage. Lung function tests show a mixed restrictive and obstructive ventilatory defect with loss of lung volume, irreversible airflow limitation and reduced gas transfer.

The patient with PMF suffers considerable effort dyspnoea, usually with a cough. The sputum can be black. The disease can progress (or even develop) after exposure to coal dust has ceased. Eventually respiratory failure may intervene.

Silicosis

This disease is uncommon though it may still be encountered in workers in foundries where sand used in moulds has to be removed from the metal casts (fettling), in sand blasting, and amongst stonemasons, pottery and ceramic workers.

Silicosis is caused by the inhalation of silica (silicon dioxide). This dust is highly fibrogenic. For example, a coal miner can remain healthy with 30 g of coal dust in his lungs but would be dead if he had inhaled 3 g of silica. Silica seems particularly toxic to alveolar macrophages and readily initiates the fibrogenic mechanism (see Fig 12.42). The chest X-ray appearances and clinical features of the disease are similar to those of PMF. The chest X-ray appearance is distinctive: thin streaks of calcification are seen around the hilar lymph nodes ('eggshell' calcification).

Asbestosis

Asbestos is a mixture of silicates of iron, magnesium, nickel, cadmium and aluminium, and has the unique property of occurring naturally as a fibre. It possesses remarkably resistant properties to heat, acid and alkali, hence its widespread use. Asbestos is mined in southern Africa, Canada and eastern Europe. World production is 4 million tons, of which 90% is chrysotile, 6% crocidolite and 4% amosite in type.

Chrysotile or white asbestos is the softest asbestos fibre. Each fibre is often as long as 2 cm but only a few micrometres thick. It is less fibrogenic than crocidolite.

Crocidolite (blue asbestos) is particularly resistant to chemical destruction. It exists in straight fibres up to 50 μm in length and 1–2 μm in width. It is now known that this type of asbestos is by far the most important in the development of all types of asbestosis and particularly of mesothelioma. This may be due to the fact that it is readily trapped in the lung. Its long, thin shape means that it can be inhaled, but subsequent rotation against the long axis of the smaller airways, particularly in turbulent airflow during expiration, causes the fibres to impact. Crocidolite is also particularly resistant to macrophage and neutrophil enzymic destruction.

Exposure to asbestos occurred particularly in naval shipbuilding yards and in power stations, but its ubiquitous use meant that light exposure was common. Up to 50% of urban dwellers had evidence of asbestos bodies (asbestos fibre covered in protein secretions) in

Table 12.19
The effects of asbestos on the lung

	Exposure	Chest X-ray	Lung function	Symptoms	Outcome
Asbestos bodies	Light	Normal	Normal	None	Evidence of asbestos exposure only
Pleural plaques	Light	Pleural thickening (parietal pleura) and calcification (also in diaphramatic pleura)	Mild restrictive ventilatory defect	Rare, occasional mild effort dyspnoea	No other sequelae
Effusion	First two decades following exposure	Effusion	Restrictive	Pleuritic pain, dyspnoea	Often recurrent
Bilateral diffuse pleural thickening	Light/moderate	Bilateral diffuse thickening (of both parietal and visceral pleura) more than 5 mm thick and extending over more than one quarter of the chest wall	Restrictive ventilatory defect	Effort dyspnoea	May progress in absence of further exposure
Mesothelioma	Light (20–40 year interval from exposure to disease)	Pleural effusion, usually unilateral	Restrictive ventilatory defect	Pleuritic pain, increasing dyspnoea	Median survival 2 years
Asbestosis	Heavy (5–10 year interval from exposure to disease)	Diffuse bilateral streaky shadows, honeycomb lung	Severe restrictive ventilatory defect and reduced gas transfer	Progressive dyspnoea	Poor, progression in some cases after exposure ceases
Asbestos-related carcinoma of the bronchus		The features of asbestosis, bilateral diffuse pleural thickening or bilateral pleural plaques plus those of bronchial carcinoma			Fatal

their lungs at post mortem. Regulations in the UK prevent the use of crocidolite and severely restrict the use of chrysotile, and enforce careful dust control measures. These changes should eventually abolish the problem.

There is an important synergistic relationship between asbestosis and cigarette smoking and the development of bronchial carcinoma, usually adenocarcinoma; the risk is increased fivefold. There is also an increased risk in non-smokers, and it is also present in workers exposed to asbestos who do not have clinically recognized asbestosis but who do have pleural plaques or thickening. Workers will continue to be exposed to blue asbestos in the course of demolition or in the replacement of insulation, and it should be remembered that there is a considerable time lag between exposure and development of the disease, particularly mesothelioma (20–40 years).

The diseases caused by asbestos are summarized in Table 12.19. Bilateral diffuse pleural thickening, asbestosis, mesothelioma and asbestos-related carcinoma of the bronchus are all eligible for industrial injuries benefit in the UK, but account for only one-quarter of the number of cases of compensation compared with coal-worker's pneumoconiosis. Asbestosis is the disease most frequently compensated (900 cases per year).

Asbestosis is defined as fibrosis of the lungs caused by asbestos dust, which may or may not be associated with fibrosis of the parietal or visceral layers of the pleura. It is a progressive disease characterized by breathlessness and accompanied by finger clubbing and bilateral basal end-inspiratory crackles. Fibrosis, not detectable on chest X-ray, may be revealed on CT scan. No treatment is known to alter the progress of the disease, though corticosteroids are often prescribed.

The number of cases of mesothelioma presenting for compensation has increased fivefold since the mid-1980s to over 400 cases per year. Often open lung biopsy is needed to obtain sufficient tissue for diagnosis. No treatment influences the universally fatal outcome. Although pleural effusions are the most common presentation of meso-thelioma, occasionally they may have a benign origin and may regress spontaneously.

Byssinosis

This disease occurs worldwide but is declining rapidly in areas where the numbers of people employed in cotton mills are falling. In the UK the disease is confined to areas of Lancashire and Northern Ireland. The symptoms start on the first day back at work after a break (Monday sickness) with improvement as the week progresses. Tightness in the chest, cough and breathlessness occur within the first hour in dusty areas of the mill, particularly in the blowing and carding rooms where raw cotton is cleaned and the fibres are straightened.

The exact nature of the disease and its aetiology remain disputed. Two important features are that pure cotton does not cause the disease, and that cotton dust has some effect on airflow limitation in all those exposed. Individuals with asthma are particularly badly affected by exposure to cotton dust. The most likely aetiology is endotoxins from bacteria present in the raw cotton causing constriction of the airways of the lung. There are no changes on the chest X-ray and there is considerable dispute as to whether the progressive airflow limitation seen in some patients with the disease is due to the cotton dust or to other effects such as cigarette smoking or coexistent asthma.

Berylliosis

Beryllium–copper alloy has a high tensile strength and is resistant to metal fatigue, high temperature and corrosion. It is used in the aerospace industry, in atomic reactors and in many electrical devices.

Although beryllium is inhaled into the lungs, it causes a systemic poisoning that gives rise to a clinical picture similar to sarcoidosis. The major chronic problem is that of progressive dyspnoea with pulmonary fibrosis. However, strict control of levels in the working atmosphere have made the disease a rarity.

FURTHER READING

Parkes WR (1994) Occupational lung disorders, 3rd edn. Butterworth-Heinemann, Oxford.

Wagner GR (1997) Asbestosis and silicosis. *Lancet* **349**: 1311–1315.

Lung cysts

These may be congenital, bronchogenic cysts or may result from a sequestrated pulmonary segment. Hydatid disease causes fluid-filled cysts. Thin-walled cysts are due to lung abscesses, which are particularly found in staphylococcal pneumonia, tuberculous cavities, septic pulmonary infarction, primary bronchogenic carcinoma, cavitating metastatic neoplasm, or paragonimiasis caused by the lung fluke *Paragonimus westermani*.

Tumours of the respiratory tract

Bronchial carcinoma accounts for 95% of all primary tumours of the lung. Alveolar cell carcinoma accounts for 2% of lung tumours and other less malignant or benign tumours account for the remaining 3%.

Benign tumours

Pulmonary hamartoma

This is the most common benign tumour of the lung and is usually seen on the X-ray as a very well-defined round lesion 1–2 cm in diameter in the periphery of the lung. Growth is extremely slow, but the tumour may reach several centimetres in diameter. Rarely it arises from a major bronchus and causes obstruction.

Bronchial carcinoid

This rare tumour resembles intestinal carcinoid tumour and is locally invasive, eventually spreading to mediastinal lymph nodes and finally to distant organs. It is a highly vascular tumour that projects into the lumen of a major bronchus causing recurrent haemoptysis. It grows slowly and eventually blocks the bronchus, leading to lobar collapse. Rarely, it gives rise to the carcinoid syndrome.

Cylindroma, chondroma and lipoma

These are extremely rare tumours that may grow in the bronchus or trachea, causing obstruction.

Tracheal tumours

Benign tumours include squamous papilloma, leiomyoma, haemangiomas and tumours of neurogenic origin.

Malignant tumours

Tracheal carcinoma

Primary tumours of the trachea are rare – their incidence relative to laryngeal and bronchial tumours is 1:75 and 1:180 respectively. The majority are malignant. These cause severe and rapidly progressive dyspnoea and stridor. Flow–volume curves show typical and dramatic reductions in inspiratory flow (extrathoracic tracheal tumours) (see p. 752). Diagnosis is confirmed by sputum examination and bronchoscopy. Laser treatment provides rapid and effective destruction of tumour with temporary relief of symptoms. Radiotherapy is often given and occasionally surgery may be possible. The prognosis, however, is very poor.

Bronchial carcinoma

This is the most common malignant tumour in the West and is the third most common cause of death in the UK after heart disease and pneumonia. Mortality rates worldwide are highest in Scotland, closely followed by England and Wales. In the UK, 32 000 people die each year from bronchial carcinoma, with a male-to-female ratio of 3.5:1. Although the rising mortality from this disease has levelled off in men, it continues to rise in women, accounting for 1 in 8 of all deaths from malignant disease in women, second only to carcinoma of the breast.

The strength of the association between cigarette smoking and bronchial carcinoma overshadows any other aetiological factors (Table 12.20), but there is a higher incidence of bronchial carcinoma in urban compared with rural areas, even when allowance is made for cigarette smoking. Passive smoking (the inhalation of other people's smoke by non-smokers) increases the risk of bronchial carcinoma by a factor of 1.5. Occupational factors include exposure to asbestos, and an association is also claimed for workers in contact with arsenic, chromium, iron oxide, petroleum products and oils, coal tar, products of coal combustion, and radiation. Tumours associated with occupational factors are mostly adenocarcinomas and appear to be less related to cigarette smoking.

Cell types

Bronchial carcinoma is divided into small-cell carcinoma and non-small-cell carcinoma, a division based on the characteristics of the disease and its response to treatment. Studies of mean doubling times of carcinomas indicate that development from the initial malignant change to presentation takes many years; for adenocarcinoma it takes approximately 15 years, for squamous carcinoma 8 years and for small-cell carcinoma 3 years.

Non-small-cell carcinoma

Squamous or *epidermoid carcinoma* is the most common carcinoma in this group, accounting for approximately 40% of all carcinomas. Most present as obstructive lesions of the bronchus leading to infection. It occasionally cavitates (10%) at presentation but widespread metastases occur relatively late. The cells are usually well differentiated but occasionally anaplastic. Local spread is usually seen.

Large-cell carcinoma represents a less well-differentiated tumour that metastasizes early. It accounts for 25% of all tumours.

Adenocarcinoma arises peripherally from mucous glands in the small bronchi and often produces a subpleural mass. Invasion of the pleura and the mediastinal lymph nodes is common, as are metastases to the brain and bones. Adenocarcinoma accounts for approximately 10% of all

Table 12.20 Death rates from lung cancer (age standardized) per 100 000 according to tobacco consumption in male British doctors

Non-smokers	10	Number of cigarettes per day	
Ex-smokers	43	1–14	78
Continuing smokers		15–24	127
Any tobacco	104	25 or more	251
Pipe/cigar	58		
Cigarettes	140		

bronchial carcinomas and frequently arises in or around scar tissue. It is the most common bronchial carcinoma associated with asbestos and is proportionally more common in non-smokers, in women, in the elderly, and in the Far East.

Alveolar cell carcinoma (bronchiolar carcinoma) accounts for only 1–2% of lung tumours and occurs either as a peripheral solitary nodule or as diffuse nodular lesions of multicentric origin. Occasionally this tumour is associated with expectoration of very large volumes of mucoid sputum.

Small-cell carcinoma

This tumour, often called oat-cell carcinoma, accounts for 20–30% of all lung cancers. It arises from endocrine cells (Kulchitsky cells). These cells are members of the APUD system, which explains why many polypeptide hormones are secreted by these tumours. Some of these polypeptides act in an autocrine fashion: they feed back on the cells and cause cell growth. Small-cell carcinoma is considered to be a systemic disease. Although the tumour is rapidly growing and highly malignant, it is the only one of the bronchial carcinomas that responds to chemotherapy.

CLINICAL FEATURES

The frequencies of the common symptoms of lung cancer on presentation are shown in Table 12.21. Chest pain and discomfort are often described as fullness and pressure in the chest. Sometimes the pain may be pleuritic owing to invasion of the pleura or ribs.

Often there are no abnormal physical signs. Enlarged supraclavicular lymph nodes can be found with small-cell carcinoma. There may be signs of a pleural effusion or of lobar collapse. Signs of an unresolved pneumonia or of associated underlying disease (e.g. diffuse pulmonary fibrosis in asbestosis) may be present.

Direct spread

The tumour may directly involve the pleura and ribs. Carcinoma in the apex of the lung can erode the ribs and involve the lower part of the brachial plexus (C8, T1 and T2), causing severe pain in the shoulder and down the inner surface of the arm (Pancoast's tumour). The sympathetic ganglion can also be involved, producing Horner's syndrome. Further extension may involve the recurrent laryngeal nerve as it passes down the aortic arch, causing unilateral vocal cord paresis with hoarseness and a bovine cough, and rarely the tumour causes spinal cord compression.

Bronchial carcinoma can also directly invade the phrenic nerve, causing paralysis of the diaphragm. It can involve the oesophagus, producing progressive dysphagia, and the pericardium, producing pericardial effusion and malignant dysrhythmias. Superior vena caval obstruction causes early morning headache, facial congestion and oedema involving the upper limbs; the jugular veins are distended, as are the veins on the chest that form a collateral circulation with veins arising from the abdomen.

Table 12.21 The frequency of the common presenting symptoms of bronchial carcinoma

Symptom	Frequency (%)
Cough	41
Chest pain	22
Cough and pain	15
Coughing blood	7
Chest infection	<5
Malaise	<5
Weight loss	<5
Shortness of breath	<5
Hoarseness	<5
Distant spread	<5
No symptoms	<5

Metastatic complications

Bony metastases are common, giving rise to severe pain and pathological fractures. There is frequent involvement of the liver. Secondary deposits in the brain present as a change in personality, epilepsy or as a focal neurological lesion. Secondary deposits occur in the adrenal gland.

Non-metastatic extrapulmonary manifestations

Although approximately 10% of small-cell tumours are thought to produce ectopic hormones at some stage, clinically important extrapulmonary manifestations are relatively rare apart from finger clubbing (Table 12.22).

Hypertrophic pulmonary osteoarthropathy (HPOA) (see p. 500) occurs in approximately 3% of all bronchial carcinomas, particularly squamous-cell carcinomas and adenocarcinomas. Symptoms include joint stiffness and severe pain in the wrists and ankles, sometimes associated with gynaecomastia. X-rays show the characteristic proliferative periostitis at the distal ends of long bones, which have an onion-skin appearance. HPOA is invariably associated with clubbing of the fingers. It may regress after resection of the lung tumour or as a result of vagotomy at thoracotomy.

INVESTIGATIONS

Chest X-ray

This is the most valuable test for bronchial carcinoma. However, it is a relatively insensitive test since the tumour mass needs to be 1–2 cm in size to be recognized reliably. CT scanning can identify small tumour masses but is too time-consuming and expensive to replace the chest X-ray as a screening test.

About 70% of all bronchial carcinomas arise in the hilar region, the rest peripherally in the lung (particularly adenocarcinomas). At the time of clinical presentation the chest X-ray will demonstrate over 90% of carcinomas. A small proportion arise within the main bronchus or trachea or else present with metastatic or non-metastatic complications but with no detectable mass on the chest X-ray.

Table 12.22 Non-metastatic extrapulmonary manifestations of bronchial carcinoma (percentage of all cases)

Metabolic (universal at some stage)
- Loss of weight
- Lassitude
- Anorexia

Endocrine (10%) (usually small-cell carcinoma)
- Ectopic adrenocorticotrophin syndrome
- Syndrome of inappropriate secretion of antidiuretic hormone (SIADH)
- Hypercalcaemia (usually squamous cell carcinoma)
- Rarer: hypoglycaemia, thyrotoxicosis, gynaecomastia

Neurological (2–16%)
- Encephalopathies – including subacute cerebellar degeneration
- Myelopathies – motor neurone disease
- Neuropathies – peripheral sensorimotor neuropathy
- Muscular disorders – polymyopathy, myasthenic syndrome (Eaton–Lambert syndrome)

Vascular and haematological (rare)
- Thrombophlebitis migrans
- Non-bacterial thrombotic endocarditis
- Microcytic and normocytic anaemia
- Disseminated intravascular coagulopathy
- Thrombotic thrombocytopenic purpura
- Haemolytic anaemia

Skeletal
- Clubbing (30%)
- Hypertrophic osteoarthropathy (± gynaecomastia) (3%)

Cutaneous (rare)
- Dermatomyositis
- Acanthosis nigricans
- Herpes zoster

Bronchial carcinoma can appear as round shadows on a chest X-ray (see p. 760). Characteristically the edge of the tumour has a fluffy or spiked appearance, though sometimes it may be entirely smooth with cavitation, particularly when the tumour is epidermoid in type. Carcinoma can also cause collapse of the lung.

Carcinoma causing partial obstruction of a bronchus interrupts the mucociliary escalator, and bacteria are retained within the affected lobe. This gives rise to the so-called secondary pneumonia that is commonly seen on a chest X-ray of a patient presenting with bronchial carcinoma.

The hilar lymph nodes on the side of the tumour are frequently involved in carcinoma of the lung. A large pleural effusion may also be present.

Carcinoma can spread through the lymphatic channels of the lung to give rise to lymphangitis carcinomatosa; this is usually unilateral and associated with striking dyspnoea. The chest X-ray shows streaky shadowing throughout the lung. This appearance may be seen in both lungs, particularly when it is due to metastatic spread, usually from tumours below the diaphragm (the stomach and colon) and from the breast.

Computed tomography

CT is particularly useful for identifying pathological changes in the mediastinum, such as enlarged lymph nodes (see Fig 12.13 on p. 761) or local spread of the tumour, and for identifying secondary spread of carcinoma to the opposite lung by detecting masses too small to be seen on the chest X-ray. Lymph nodes larger than 1 cm are considered pathological, although whether they are due to metastatic tumour, reactive hyperplasia or previous lung disease (e.g. tuberculosis) can only be determined by biopsy. A normal CT scan prior to surgery excludes the need for mediastinoscopy and node biopsy. CT scanning should be extended to include the liver, adrenal glands and the brain to identify distant metastases if present.

Magnetic resonance imaging

MRI is being used increasingly for staging (see p. 761).

Fibreoptic bronchoscopy (see also p. 766)

This technique is used to obtain cytological specimens from peripheral lesions as well as to obtain biopsy evidence of any tumours seen. If the carcinoma involves the first 2 cm of either main bronchus, the tumour is inoperable. Widening and loss of the sharp angle of the carina indicates the presence of enlarged mediastinal lymph nodes, either malignant or reactive. They can be biopsied by passage of a needle through the bronchial wall. Vocal cord paresis on the left indicates involvement of the recurrent laryngeal nerve and inoperability.

Transthoracic fine-needle aspiration biopsy

This involves the direct aspiration through the chest wall of peripheral lung lesions under appropriate X-ray or CT screening. Specimens can be obtained from 75% of peripheral lesions that could not be biopsied transbronchially. Pneumothorax occurs in 25% of patients, occasionally requiring drainage. Mild haemoptysis occurs in 5%. Implantation metastases do not occur.

Other investigations

These include a *full blood count* for the detection of anaemia, *liver biochemistry* for liver involvement, and additional tests for complications.

TREATMENT

Unlike some other cancers, there has been no improvement in survival from carcinoma of the bronchus apart from small-cell cancer (see below). Only 20% of patients are alive one year after diagnosis and only 6–8% after five years (cf. 50% for breast or cervix).

Surgery

The only treatment of any value for non-small-cell cancer of the lung is surgery. Only 20% of all cases are suitable for resection and only 25–30% survive for five years. The mortality of thoracotomy in patients over 65 years with metastatic disease exceeds the expected five-year survival rate and should therefore be avoided.

Preoperative assessment. This requires blood tests and imaging as described above. Because of their common aetiology, COPD is frequently present. An FEV_1 of less than 1.5 L is not compatible with an active life following pneumonectomy, although the surgery itself can be successfully accomplished. This also applies when the gas-transfer test is reduced by 50%.

Radiation therapy for cure

High-dose radiotherapy (6500 rad; 65 Gy) can produce results that are as good as those of surgery in patients who are fit and who have slowly growing squamous carcinoma. It is the treatment of choice if the tumour is inoperable for reasons such as poor lung function. Continuous hyperfractional accelerated radiotherapy (CHART) is showing promising results for non-small-cell lung cancer.

Radiation pneumonitis (defined as an acute infiltrate precisely confined to the radiation area and occurring within three months of radiotherapy) develops in 10–15% of cases. Radiation fibrosis, a fibrotic change occurring within a year or so of radiotherapy and not precisely confined to the radiation area, occurs to some degree in all cases. These complications are usually of little importance.

Symptomatic radiation treatment

Bone pain, haemoptysis and the superior vena cava syndrome respond favourably to irradiation in the short term.

Chemotherapy

Small-cell cancer. Single or combination chemotherapy has resulted in a fivefold increase in median survival from 2 to 10 months. A small number of patients enjoy several years of remission. Good results have been achieved with the combination of mitomycin, ifosfamide and cisplatin (see p. 440). The unwanted effects are greater than with single-agent chemotherapy with etoposide alone, which should be reserved for elderly patients and those with additional medical or physical disabilities.

Non-small-cell lung cancer. Non-small-cell lung cancer (NSCLC) can no longer be regarded as resistent to chemotherapy. Response rates with single-agent treatment with newly introduced drugs exceed 20%. Gemcitabine, a pyramidine antimetabolite, has less toxicity but equivalent antitumour effect to ifosfamide, vindesine and mitomycin C. Combination chemotherapy including cisplatin leads to better response rate in non-operable NSCLC with median survivals of six months and 10–12 months in responding patients. Most patients achieve their best response after two or three courses of treatment. Adjuvant chemotherapy with radiotherapy improves response rate and extends median survival. Preoperative (neoadjuvant) chemotherapy increases by half the number of previously inoperable NSCLC patients who can undergo surgical resection with 30% survival at three years.

Laser therapy, endobronchial irradiation and tracheobronchial stents

These techniques are used in the palliation of inoperable lung cancer. They are used for patients with tracheobronchial narrowing from intraluminal tumour or extrinsic compression causing disabling breathlessness, intractable cough and complications, including infection, haemoptysis and respiratory failure.

A neodymium-Yag (Nd-Yag) laser passed through a fibreoptic brochoscope can be used to vaporize inoperable fungating intraluminal carcinoma involving short segments of trachea or main bronchus. Benign tumours, strictures and vascular lesions can also be treated effectively with immediate relief of symptoms.

Endobronchial irradiation (brachytherapy) is useful for the treatment of both intraluminal tumour and malignant extrinsic compression. A radioactive source is afterloaded into a catheter placed adjacent to the carcinoma under fibreoptic bronchoscope control. Radiation dose falls rapidly with distance from the source, minimizing damage to adjacent normal tissue. Reduction in endoscopically assessed tumour size occurs in 70–95% of cases.

Tracheobronchial stents made of silicone or as expandable metal springs are available for insertion into strictures caused by tumour or from external compression or when there is weakening and collapse of the tracheobronchial wall.

Terminal care (see p. 442)

Patients dying of cancer of the lung need attention to their overall well-being. Palliative care must not be ignored simply because they cannot be cured. Much can be done to make the patient's remaining life symptom-free and as active as possible.

Daily treatment with prednisolone (up to 15 mg daily) may improve appetite. Morphine or diamorphine must be given regularly for pain, either in the form of a sustained-release morphine sulphate tablet twice daily or else as regular elixirs or injections. Many patients benefit from a continuous subcutaneous injection of opiates given by a pump. Candidiasis and other infections in the mouth are common and must be looked for and treated. Patients taking opiates are frequently constipated, so regular laxatives should be prescribed. Short courses of palliative radiotherapy for bone pain, severe cough or haemoptysis are helpful.

Both the patient and the relatives may require counselling, a task that should be shared between nurses, social workers, hospital chaplains and doctors, who make up the palliative care team.

Secondary tumours

Metastases in the lung are very common and usually present as round shadows (1.5–3.0 cm diameter). They may be detected on chest X-ray in patients already diagnosed as having carcinoma. *The primary tumour is usually in the kidney, prostate, breast, bone, gastrointestinal tract, cervix or ovary.*

Metastases nearly always develop in the parenchyma and are often relatively asymptomatic even when the chest X-ray shows extensive pulmonary metastases. It is rare for metastases to develop in the bronchi, when they may present with haemoptysis.

Carcinoma, particularly of the stomach, pancreas and breast, can involve mediastinal glands and spread along the lymphatics of both lungs (lymphangitis carcinomatosa), which can lead to progressive and severe breathlessness. On the chest X-ray, bilateral lymphadenopathy is seen together with streaky basal shadowing fanning out over both lung fields.

Occasionally a pulmonary metastasis may be detected as a *solitary round shadow* on chest X-ray in an asymptomatic patient. The most common primary tumour to do this is a renal carcinoma.

The differential diagnosis includes:

- primary bronchial carcinoma
- tuberculoma
- benign tumour of the lung
- hydatid cyst.

Single pulmonary metastases can be removed surgically but, as CT scans usually show the presence of small metastases undetected on chest X-ray, surgery is seldom performed.

Screening for lung cancer

Screening programmes (yearly chest X-ray, four-monthly sputum cytology) have been tried in high-risk groups but the success rate is minimal, underlining the need for prevention.

FURTHER READING

American Society of Clinical Oncology (1997) Clinical practice guidelines for the treatment of unresectable non-small-cell lung cancer. *Journal of Clinical Oncology* **15**: 2996–3018.

Disorders of the chest wall and pleura

Trauma

Trauma to the thoracic wall can be due to penetrating wounds and can lead to pneumothoraces or haemothoraces.

Rib fractures

Rib fractures are caused by trauma or coughing (particularly in the elderly), and can occur in patients with osteoporosis. Pathological rib fractures are due to metastatic spread from carcinoma of the bronchus, breast, kidney, prostate or thyroid. Ribs can also become involved by a mesothelioma. Fractures may not be readily visible on a PA chest X-ray, so lateral X-rays and oblique views may be necessary.

Pain prevents adequate chest expansion and coughing and this can lead to pneumonia.

Treatment is with adequate analgesia using oral agents or by local infiltration or an intercostal nerve block.

Two fractures in one rib can lead to a flail segment with paradoxical movement, i.e. part of the chest wall moves inwards during inspiration. This can produce inefficient ventilation and may require intermittent positive-pressure ventilation.

Rupture of the trachea or a major bronchus

Rupture of the trachea or even a major bronchus can occur during deceleration injuries, leading to pneumothorax, surgical emphysema, pneumomediastinum and haemoptysis. Surgical emphysema is caused by air leaking into the subcutaneous connective tissue; this can also occur after the insertion of an intercostal drainage tube. A pneumomediastinum occurs when air leaks from the lung inside the parietal pleura and extends along the bronchial walls.

Rupture of the oesophagus

Rupture of the oesophagus from external injury, endoscopic procedures, bougienage or necrotic carcinoma may lead to the serious complication of mediastinitis. This requires vigorous antibacterial chemotherapy.

Lung contusion

This causes widespread fluffy shadows on the chest X-ray owing to intrapulmonary haemorrhage. This may give rise to acute respiratory distress syndrome or shock lung (see p. 856).

Kyphoscoliosis

Kyphoscoliosis is congenital, due to disease of the vertebrae such as tuberculosis or osteomalacia, or due to neuromuscular disease such as Friedreich's ataxia or poliomyelitis. The respiratory effects of severe kyphoscoliosis are often more pronounced than might be expected and respiratory failure and death often occur in the fourth or fifth decade. The abnormality should be corrected at an early stage if possible. Positive airway pressure ventilation delivered through a tightly fitting nasal mask is the treatment of choice for respiratory failure (see p. 854).

Ankylosing spondylitis (see also p. 479)

Limitation of chest wall movement is often well compensated by diaphragmatic movement, and so the respiratory effects of this disease are relatively mild. It is occasionally associated with upper lobe fibrosis of unknown aetiology.

Pectus excavatum and carinatum

Pectus excavatum causes few problems other than embarrassment about the deep vertical furrow in the chest, which can be corrected surgically. The heart is seen to lie well to the left on the chest X-ray. Pectus carinatum (pigeon chest) is often the result of rickets. No treatment is required.

Pleurisy

This is the term used to describe pain arising from any disease of the pleura. The localized inflammation produces sharp localized pain, made worse on deep inspiration, coughing and occasionally on twisting and bending movements. Pleurisy occurs with pneumonia, pulmonary infarct and carcinoma. Rarer causes include rheumatoid arthritis and systemic lupus erythematosus.

Epidemic myalgia (Bornholm disease) is due to infection by Coxsackie B virus. This illness is common in young adults in the late summer and autumn and is characterized by an upper respiratory tract illness followed by pleuritic pain in the chest and upper abdomen with tender muscles. The chest X-ray remains normal and the illness clears within a week.

Pleural effusion

A pleural effusion is an excessive accumulation of fluid in the pleural space. It can be detected on X-ray when 300 mL or more of fluid is present and clinically when 500 mL or more is present. The chest X-ray appearances range from the obliteration of the costophrenic angle to dense homogeneous shadows occupying part or all of the hemithorax. Fluid below the lung (a subpulmonary effusion) can simulate a raised hemidiaphragm. Fluid in the fissures may resemble an intrapulmonary mass. The physical signs are shown in Table 12.2 on p. 757.

DIAGNOSIS

This is by pleural aspiration (see p. 765). The fluid that accumulates may be a transudate or an exudate.

Transudates

Effusions that are transudates can be bilateral. The protein content is less than 30 g L^{-1} and the lactic dehydrogenase is less than 200 IU L^{-1}. Causes include:

- heart failure
- hypoproteinaemia (e.g. nephrotic syndrome)
- constrictive pericarditis
- hypothyroidism
- ovarian tumours producing right-sided pleural effusion – Meigs' syndrome.

Exudates

The protein content of exudates is greater than 30 g L^{-1} and the lactic dehydrogenase is greater than 200 IU L^{-1}. Causes include:

- bacterial pneumonia (common)
- carcinoma of the bronchus and pulmonary infarction – fluid may be blood-stained (common)
- tuberculosis
- connective-tissue disease
- post-myocardial infarction syndrome (rare)
- acute pancreatitis (high amylase content) (rare)
- mesothelioma (rare)
- sarcoidosis (very rare)
- yellow-nail syndrome (effusion due to lymphoedema) (very rare)
- familial Mediterranean fever (rare).

Pleural biopsy (see p. 765) may be necessary if the diagnosis has not been established from the above aspiration. Treatment is of the underlying condition.

MANAGEMENT OF MALIGNANT PLEURAL EFFUSIONS

Malignant pleural effusions that reaccumulate and are symptomatic can be aspirated to *dryness* followed by the instillation of a sclerosing agent such as tetracycline or bleomycin. Effusions should be drained slowly since rapid shift of the mediastinum causes severe pain and occasionally shock. This treatment produces only temporary relief.

Chylothorax

This is due to the accumulation of lymph in the pleural space, usually resulting from leakage from the thoracic duct following trauma or infiltration by carcinoma.

Empyema

This is the presence of pus in the pleural space and can be a complication of pneumonia (see p. 801).

Pneumothorax

'Pneumothorax' means air in the pleural space. It occurs as a result of trauma to the chest or may be spontaneous. Pneumothorax is localized if the visceral pleura has previously undergone adhesion to the parietal pleura, or generalized if the whole hemithorax contains air. Normally the pressure in the pleural space is negative but this is lost once a communication is made with atmospheric pressure; the elastic recoil pressure of the lung then causes it to partially deflate. If the communication between the airways and the pleural space remains (an open pneumothorax), a bronchopleural fistula is created. Once the communication between the lung and the pleural space is obliterated, air will be reabsorbed at a rate of 1.25% of the total radiographic volume of the hemithorax per day. Thus, a 50% collapse of the lung will take 40 days to reabsorb completely once the pneumothorax is closed.

It has been postulated that a valvular mechanism may develop through which air can be sucked during inspiration but not expelled during expiration. The intrapleural pressure remains positive throughout breathing, the lung deflates further, the mediastinum shifts, and venous return to the heart decreases, with increasing respiratory and cardiac embarrassment. This tension pneumothorax is very rare unless the patient is on positive ventilation.

Spontaneous pneumothorax

This usually occurs in young males, the male-to-female ratio being 6:1. It is caused by the rupture of a pleural bleb, usually apical, and is thought to be due to congenital defects in the connective tissue of the alveolar walls. Both lungs are affected with equal frequency. Often these patients are tall and thin.

In patients over 40 years of age, the usual cause is underlying COPD. Rarer causes include bronchial asthma, carcinoma, a lung abscess breaking down and leading to bronchopleural fistula, and severe pulmonary fibrosis with cyst formation.

The sudden onset of unilateral pleuritic pain or increasing breathlessness are the usual presenting features. If the pneumothorax enlarges, the patient becomes more breathless and may develop pallor and tachycardia. There may be few physical signs if the pneumothorax is small.

The characteristic features and management are shown in Fig 12.44. The main aim is to get the patient back to active life as soon as possible.

The procedure for simple aspiration is shown in Practical box 12.6.

Practical

1. Infiltrate 2% lignocaine down to the pleura in the second intercostal space in the mid-clavicular line.
2. Push a 3–4 cm 16 French gauge cannula through the pleura.
3. Connect the cannula to a three-way tap and 50 mL syringe.
4. Aspirate up to 2.5 L of air. Stop if resistance to suction is felt or the patient coughs excessively.
5. Repeat chest X-ray (in exspiration) in the X-ray department.

Practical box 12.6 Simple aspiration

FURTHER READING

Miller AC, Harvey JE (1993) Guidelines for the management of spontaneous pneumothorax. *British Medical Journal* **307**: 114–116.

Disorders of the diaphragm

Diaphragmatic fatigue

The diaphragm can become fatigued if the force of contraction during inspiration exceeds 40% of the force it can develop in a maximal static effort. When this occurs acutely in patients with exacerbations of COPD or CF or in quadriplegics, positive-pressure ventilation is required followed by attempts to increase the strength and endurance of the diaphragm by breathing against a resistance for 30 minutes a day.

Unilateral diaphragmatic paralysis

This is common and symptomless. The affected diaphragm is usually elevated and moves paradoxically on inspiration. A sniff causes the paralysed diaphragm to rise, the unaffected diaphragm to descend. Causes include:

- surgery
- carcinoma of the bronchus with involvement of the phrenic nerve
- neurological, including poliomyelitis, herpes zoster
- trauma to cervical spine, birth injury, subclavian vein puncture
- infection: tuberculosis, syphilis, pneumonia

Bilateral diaphragmatic weakness or paralysis

This causes breathlessness in the supine position and is a cause of sleep apnoea leading to daytime headaches and somnolence. Tidal volume is decreased and respiratory rate increased. Vital capacity is substantially reduced when lying down, and sniffing causes a paradoxical inward movement of the abdominal wall best seen in the supine position. Causes include viral infections, multiple sclerosis, motor neurone disease, poliomyelitis, Guillain–Barré syndrome, quadriplegia after trauma, and rare muscle diseases. Treatment is either diaphragmatic pacing or night-time assisted ventilation.

Complete eventration of the diaphragm

This is a congenital condition (invariably left-sided) in which muscle is replaced by fibrous tissue. It presents as marked elevation of the left hemidiaphragm, sometimes associated with gastrointestinal symptoms. Partial eventration, usually on the right, causes a hump (often anteriorly) on the diaphragmatic shadow on X-ray.

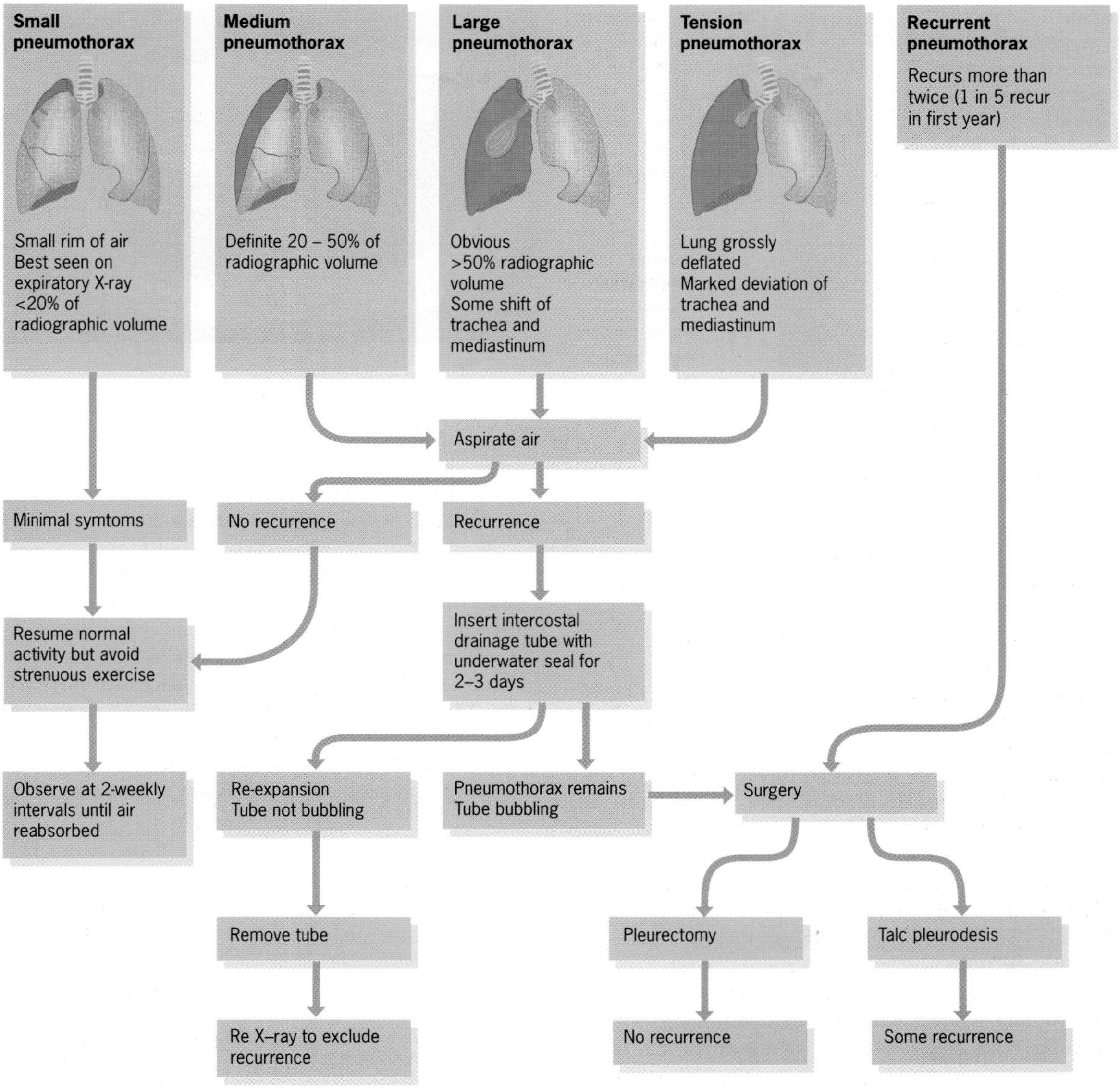

Fig 12.44
Pneumothorax: an algorithm for management

Hernias

These occur through the diaphragm, the most common being through the oesophageal hiatus, but occasionally anteriorly, through the foramen of Morgagni, posterolaterally through the foramen of Bochdalek, or at any site following traumatic tears.

Hiccups

See p. 218.

Mediastinal lesions

The mediastinum is defined as the region between the pleural sacs. It is additionally divided as shown in Fig 12.45. Tumours affecting the mediastinum are rare. Masses are detected very accurately on CT scan (Fig 12.46).

Retrosternal or intrathoracic thyroid

The most common mediastinal tumour is a retrosternal or intrathoracic thyroid, which is nearly always an extension of the thyroid present in the neck. Enlargement of the

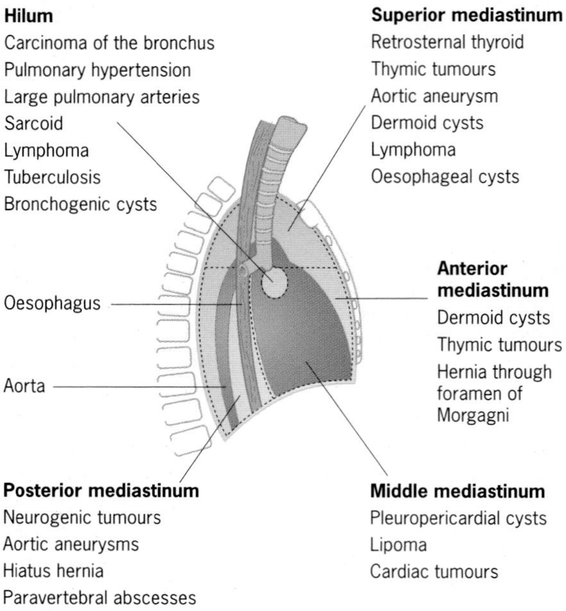

Fig 12.45
Subdivisions of the mediastinum and mass lesions

thyroid by a colloid goitre or malignant disease and, rarely, in thyrotoxicosis causes displacement of the trachea and oesophagus to the opposite side. Symptoms of compression develop insidiously before producing the cardinal feature of dyspnoea. Very occasionally an intrathoracic thyroid may be the cause of dysphagia and, rarely, of hoarseness of the voice and vocal cord paralysis from stretching of the recurrent laryngeal nerve. The treatment is surgical removal.

Thymic tumours

The thymus is large in childhood and occupies the superior and anterior mediastinum. It involutes with age but may be enlarged both by cysts, which are rarely symptomatic, or tumours, which may cause the symptoms

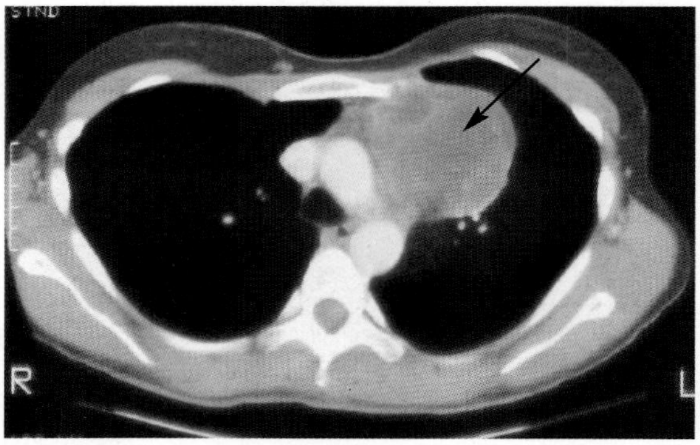

Fig 12.46
CT scan of a dermoid cyst in the mediastinum

of myasthenia gravis or may lead to compression of the trachea or, rarely, the oesophagus. Surgery is the treatment of choice. Approximately half of the patients presenting with a thymic tumour have myasthenia gravis.

Pleuro-pericardial cysts

These cysts, which may be up to 10 cm in diameter, are filled with clear fluid and are usually situated anteriorly in the cardiophrenic angle on the right in 70% of cases. Infection only rarely occurs; malignant change does not occur. The diagnosis is usually made by needle aspiration. No treatment is required, but these patients should be followed up as an increase in cyst size suggests an alternative pathology; surgical excision is then advisable.

FURTHER READING

Cibella F, Cuttitta G, Romano S *et al.* (1997) Evaluation of diaphragmatic fatigue in obstructive sleep apnoea during non-REM sleep. *Thorax* **52**: 731–735.

Karamanoukian HL, O'Toole SJ, Holm BA *et al.* (1997) Making the most out of the least: new insights into congenital diaphragmatic hernia. *Thorax* **52**: 209–212.

Intensive care medicine

13

Intensive care medicine (or 'critical care medicine') is concerned predominantly with the management of patients with acute life-threatening conditions ('the critically ill') in a specialized unit. It also encompasses the resuscitation and transport of those who become acutely ill, or are injured, either elsewhere in the hospital or in the community.

Intensive care units (ICUs) are usually reserved for patients with established or potential organ failure and must therefore provide facilities for the diagnosis, prevention and treatment of multiple organ failure. They are fully equipped with monitoring and technical facilities, including an adjacent laboratory for the rapid determination of blood gases and simple biochemical data such as serum potassium and blood glucose. Patients can receive continuous expert nursing care and the constant attention of appropriately trained medical staff. High dependency units (HDUs) offer a level of care intermediate between that available on the general ward and that provided in an ICU. They provide monitoring and support for patients at risk of developing organ failure, including facilities for short-term ventilatory support and immediate resuscitation. They can also provide a 'step-down' facility for patients being discharged from intensive care (sometimes called a 'progressive care unit'). As well as emergency cases, ICUs and HDUs admit high-risk patients electively after major surgery (Table 13.1).

Teamwork and a multidisciplinary approach is central to the provision of intensive care and is most effective when directed and coordinated by a committed specialist. In the UK about 1–2% of the acute beds in the hospital

Table 13.1
Some common indications for admission to intensive care

Emergency surgical	Elective surgical
Acute intra-abdominal catastrophe	Extensive/prolonged procedure, e.g. oesophagogastrectomy
Ruptured/leaking abdominal aortic aneurysm	Major head and neck surgery
Perforated viscus, especially with faecal soiling of peritoneum (often complicated by septic shock)	Coexisting cardiovascular or respiratory disease
Trauma (often complicated by hypovolaemic and later septic shock)	**Emergency medical**
Multiple injuries	Respiratory failure
Massive blood loss	Exacerbation of chronic obstructive pulmonary disease (COPD)
Severe head injury	Pneumonia (may be complicated by septic shock)

are usually allocated to intensive care, but elsewhere in the developed world the proportion is often much higher.

In all critically ill patients, the immediate objective is to preserve life and prevent, reverse or minimize damage to vital organs such as the brain and the kidneys. This is achieved by supporting cardiovascular and respiratory function in order to maximize perfusion of vital organs and delivery of oxygen to the tissues.

This chapter concentrates on cardiovascular and respiratory problems. Many patients also have failure of other organs such as the kidney and liver; treatment of these is dealt with in more detail in the appropriate chapters. Feeding the critically ill patient is discussed further in Chapter 3.

Oxygen delivery

Oxygen delivery (oxygen flux) is defined as the total amount of oxygen delivered to the tissues per unit time. It is dependent on the volume of blood flowing through the microcirculation per minute (i.e. the total cardiac output, $\dot{Q}_t$) and the amount of oxygen contained in that blood (i.e. the arterial oxygen content, C_aO_2). Oxygen is transported in combination with haemoglobin or dissolved in plasma. The amount combined with haemoglobin is determined by the oxygen capacity of the haemoglobin (usually taken as 1.34 mL of oxygen per gram of haemoglobin) and its percentage saturation with oxygen (SO_2), while the volume dissolved in plasma depends on the partial pressure of oxygen (PO_2). Except when hyperbaric oxygen is administered, the amount of dissolved oxygen in plasma is sufficiently small to be ignored for most practical purposes.

Clinically, however, this global concept of oxygen flux provides little information about the relative flow to individual organs. Furthermore, some organs have high oxygen requirements relative to their blood flow and may become hypoxic even if the overall oxygen flux is apparently adequate.

Cardiac output

Cardiac output is the product of heart rate and stroke volume, and is affected by changes in either (Fig 13.1).

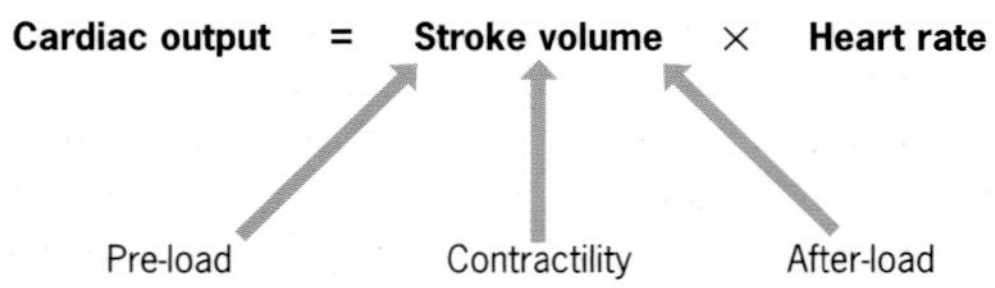

Fig 13.1
The determinants of cardiac output

Heart rate

Increased heart rate

When heart rate increases, the duration of systole remains essentially unchanged, whereas diastole, and thus the time available for ventricular filling, becomes progressively shorter, and the stroke volume eventually falls. In the normal heart this occurs at rates greater than about 160 beats per minute, but in those with cardiac pathology, especially when this restricts ventricular filling (e.g. mitral stenosis), stroke volume may fall at much lower heart rates. Furthermore, tachycardias cause a marked increase in myocardial oxygen consumption and this may precipitate ischaemia in areas of the myocardium that have reduced coronary perfusion.

Decreased heart rate

When the heart rate falls, a point is reached at which the increase in stroke volume is insufficient to compensate for bradycardia and again cardiac output falls. Alterations in heart rate are often caused by disturbances of rhythm (e.g. atrial fibrillation, complete heart block or junctional arrhythmias), in which ventricular filling is not augmented by atrial contraction and stroke volume therefore falls.

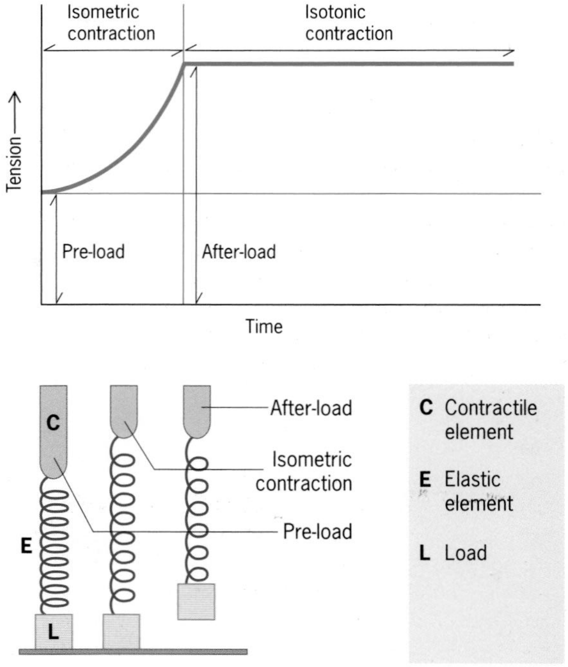

Fig 13.2
The relationship between myocardial tension and contraction. 'Pre-load' is the tension of the myocardial fibres prior to the onset of systole and depends on the degree to which they are passively stretched. During isometric contraction, the tension in the contractile elements increases. The tension required to open the aortic valve and eject blood from the ventricle is 'after-load'

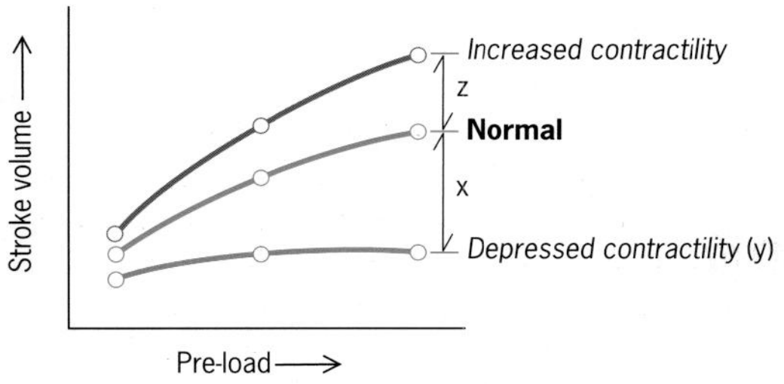

Fig 13.3
Ventricular function (Starling curve). As the pre-load is increased, the stroke volume rises. If the ventricle is overstretched, the stroke volume will fall (x). In myocardial failure, the curve is depressed and flattened (y). Increasing contractility shifts the curve upwards and to the left (z)

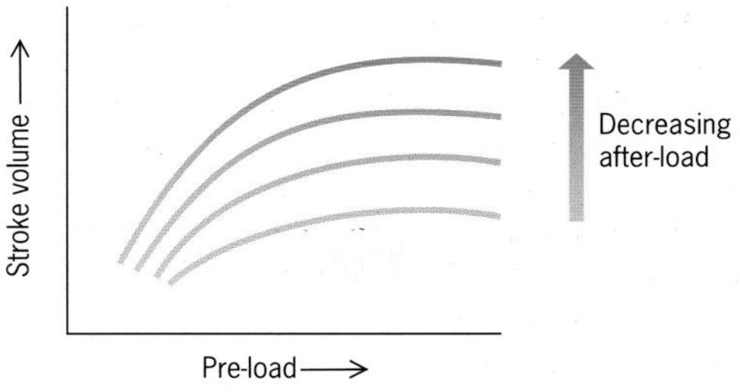

Fig 13.4
The effect of changes in after-load on the ventricular function curve. At any give pre-load, decreasing after-load increases the stroke volume

Stroke volume

Three factors determine the stroke volume: pre-load, myocardial contractility, and after-load (see p. 626).

Pre-load

This is defined as the tension of the myocardial fibres at the end of diastole, just before the onset of ventricular contraction, and is therefore related to the degree of stretch of the fibres (Fig 13.2). As the end-diastolic volume of the ventricle increases, tension in the myocardial fibres is increased and stroke volume rises (Fig 13.3). Myocardial oxygen consumption ($\dot{V}_mO_2$) increases only slightly with an increase in preload and this is therefore the most efficient way of improving cardiac output.

Myocardial contractility

This refers to the ability of the heart to perform work, independent of changes in pre-load and after-load. The state of myocardial contractility determines the response of the ventricles to changes in pre-load and after-load. Contractility is often reduced in intensive care patients, as a result of either pre-existing myocardial damage (e.g. ischaemic heart disease), or the acute disease process itself. Changes in myocardial contractility alter the slope and position of the Starling curve; the resulting worsening ventricular performance is manifested as a depressed, flattened curve (Fig 13.3).

After-load

This is defined as the myocardial wall tension developed during systolic ejection (Fig 13.2). In the case of the left ventricle, the resistance imposed by the aortic valve, the peripheral vascular resistance and the elasticity of the major blood vessels are important determinants of after-load. Ventricular wall tension will also be increased by ventricular dilatation, an increase in intraventricular pressure or a reduction in ventricular wall thickness.

Decreasing the after-load can increase the stroke volume achieved at a given pre-load (Fig 13.4), whilst reducing the myocardial oxygen consumption. The reduction in wall tension may also lead to an increase in coronary blood flow, thereby improving the myocardial oxygen supply/demand ratio. Excessive reductions in after-load will cause hypotension.

Increasing the after-load, on the other hand, can cause a fall in stroke volume and is a potent cause of increased $\dot{V}_mO_2$. Right ventricular after-load is normally negligible because the resistance of the pulmonary circulation is very low.

Oxygenation of the blood

The oxygen content of arterial blood (C_aO_2) is dependent on the amount of haemoglobin present per unit volume of blood, its oxygen capacity and its percentage saturation with oxygen. For this reason, maintenance of an 'adequate' haemoglobin concentration is essential in critically ill patients. Tissue oxygenation is, however, also dependent on blood flow. This is in turn determined not only by the cardiac output and its distribution, but also by the viscosity of the blood. The latter depends largely on the packed cell volume (PCV) and it is generally considered that the optimal balance between oxygen-carrying capacity and tissue flow is achieved at a PCV of approximately 30–35%

Oxyhaemoglobin dissociation curve

The saturation of haemoglobin with oxygen is determined by the partial pressure of oxygen (PO_2) in the blood, the relationship between the two being described by the oxyhaemoglobin dissociation curve (Fig 13.5). The sigmoid shape of this curve is important clinically for a number of reasons:

- Falls in the partial pressure of oxygen in the arterial blood (P_aO_2) may be tolerated provided that the percentage saturation remains above 90%.
- Increasing the P_aO_2 to above normal has only a minimal effect on oxygen content unless hyberbaric oxygen is administered (when the amount of oxygen in solution in plasma becomes significant).
- Once on the steep 'slippery slope' of the curve, a small decrease in P_aO_2 can cause large falls in oxygen content, while increasing P_aO_2 only slightly (e.g. by administering 28% oxygen to a patient with chronic bronchitis) can lead to a useful increase in oxygen saturation.

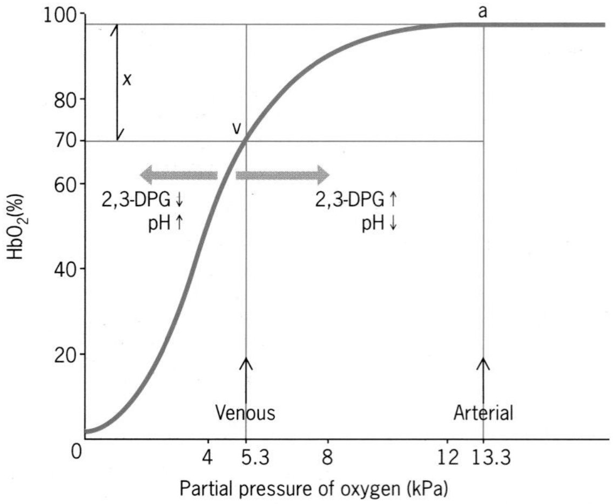

Fig 13.5
The oxyhaemoglobin dissociation curve: a, arterial point; v, venous point; x, arteriovenous oxygen content difference. HbO_2 is the oxygen saturation of haemoglobin. The curve will move to the right in the presence of acidosis (metabolic or respiratory), pyrexia or an increased red cell 2,3-DPG concentration. For a given arteriovenous oxygen content difference, the mixed venous P_{O_2} will then be higher. Furthermore, if the mixed venous P_{O_2} is unchanged, the arteriovenous oxygen content difference increases and more oxygen is off-loaded to the tissues (see p. 357)

The P_aO_2 is in turn influenced by the alveolar oxygen tension (P_AO_2), the efficiency of pulmonary gas exchange, and the partial pressure of oxygen in mixed venous blood ($P_{\bar{v}}O_2$).

Alveolar oxygen tension (P_AO_2)

The partial pressures of inspired gases are shown in Fig 13.6. By the time the inspired gases reach the alveoli they are fully saturated with water vapour at body temperature (37°C) which has a partial pressure of 6.3 kPa (47 mmHg) and contains CO_2 at a partial pressure of approximately 5.3 kPa (40 mmHg). The P_AO_2 is thereby reduced to approximately 13.4 kPa (100 mmHg).

The clinician can influence P_AO_2 by administering oxygen or by increasing the barometric pressure (i.e. administering hyperbaric oxygen). Because of the reciprocal relationship between the partial pressures of oxygen and carbon dioxide in the alveoli, a small increase in P_AO_2 can be produced by lowering the P_ACO_2 (e.g. by using mechanical ventilation).

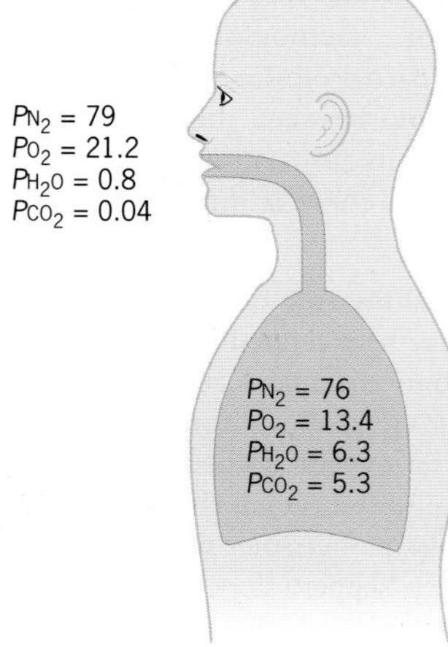

Fig 13.6
The partial pressures of inspired and alveolar gas: values give in kilopascals

Pulmonary gas exchange

In *normal* subjects there is a small alveolar–arterial oxygen difference ($P_{A-a}O_2$). This is due to:

- a small (0.133 kPa, 1 mmHg) pressure gradient across the alveolar membrane
- a small amount of blood (2% of total cardiac output) bypassing the lungs via the bronchial and thebesian veins
- a small ventilation/perfusion mismatch.

Pathologically there are three causes of a $P_{A-a}O_2$ difference, as follows:

Diffusion defect

This is not an important cause of hypoxaemia even in conditions such as fibrosing alveolitis, in which the alveolar capillary membrane is considerably thickened. Certainly carbon dioxide is not affected, as it is more soluble than oxygen.

Right-to-left shunts

In certain congenital cardiac lesions, such as Fallot's tetralogy and when a segment of lung is completely unventilated, a large amount of blood bypasses the lungs and causes arterial hypoxaemia. This hypoxaemia cannot be corrected by administering oxygen to increase the P_AO_2, because blood leaving normal alveoli is already fully saturated and further increases in P_{O_2} will not significantly affect its oxygen content. On the other hand, because of the shape of the carbon dioxide dissociation curve (Fig 13.7), the high P_{CO_2} of the shunted blood can be compensated for by overventilating patent alveoli, thus lowering the CO_2 content of the effluent blood. Indeed, many patients with acute right-to-left shunts

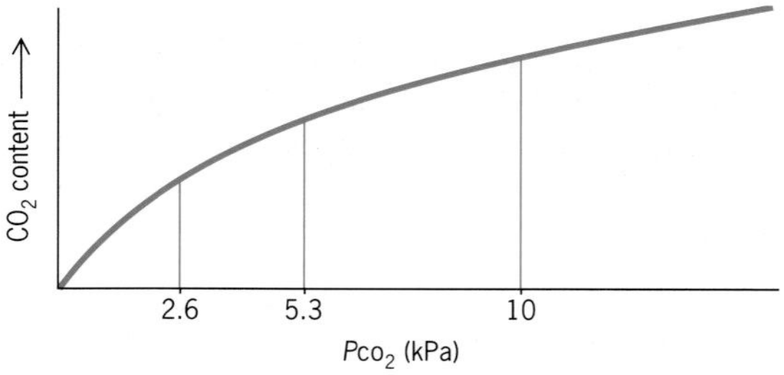

Fig 13.7
The carbon dioxide dissociation curve. Note that in the physiological range the curve is essentially linear

hyperventilate in response to the hypoxia or stimulation of mechanoreceptors in the lung, so that the P_aCO_2 is normal or low.

Ventilation/perfusion mismatch (see Chapter 12)

Diseases of the lung parenchyma result in $\dot{V}/\dot{Q}$ mismatch, producing an increase in alveolar deadspace and hypoxaemia. The increased deadspace can be compensated for by increasing overall ventilation. In contrast to the hypoxia resulting from a true right-to-left shunt (see above), that due to areas of low $\dot{V}/\dot{Q}$ can be partially corrected by administering oxygen and thereby increasing the P_AO_2 even in poorly ventilated areas of lung.

Mixed venous oxygen tension ($P_{\bar{V}}O_2$)

This is the partial pressure of oxygen in pulmonary arterial blood that has been thoroughly mixed during its passage through the heart. If P_aO_2 remains constant, $P_{\bar{V}}O_2$ will fall if more oxygen has to be extracted from each unit volume of blood arriving at the tissues. A fall in $P_{\bar{V}}O_2$ therefore indicates that either oxygen delivery has fallen or that tissue oxygen requirements have increased without a compensatory rise in the cardiac output. If $P_{\bar{V}}O_2$ falls, the effect of a given degree of pulmonary shunting on arterial oxygenation will be exacerbated. Thus, worsening arterial hypoxaemia does not necessarily indicate a deterioration in pulmonary function but may instead reflect a fall in cardiac output and/or a rise in oxygen consumption.

The $P_{\bar{V}}O_2$ is also influenced by the position of the oxyhaemoglobin dissociation curve (see Fig 13.5). Thus, if the arteriovenous oxygen content difference remains constant, a shift of the curve to the right, which occurs with acidosis, hypercarbia, pyrexia and a rise in red cell 2,3-diphosphoglycerate (2,3-DPG) levels, may cause the $P_{\bar{V}}O_2$ to rise. If the $P_{\bar{V}}O_2$ remains unchanged, more oxygen will be unloaded at tissue level. A shift of the curve to the left, on the other hand, will cause a fall in $P_{\bar{V}}O_2$. It might be argued, then, that under certain circumstances an acidosis may be beneficial in terms of tissue oxygenation, provided that it is not severe enough to interfere with cardiac function. It is probable, though, that shifts of the dissociation curve are of little clinical significance.

Acute disturbances of haemodynamic function (shock)

Shock is difficult to define. The term is used to describe acute circulatory failure with inadequate or inappropriately distributed tissue perfusion resulting in generalized cellular hypoxia.

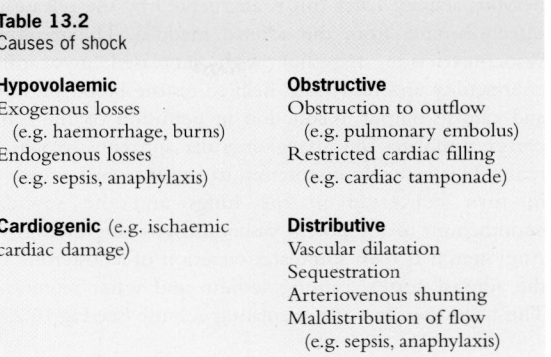

Table 13.2
Causes of shock

Hypovolaemic Exogenous losses (e.g. haemorrhage, burns) Endogenous losses (e.g. sepsis, anaphylaxis)	**Obstructive** Obstruction to outflow (e.g. pulmonary embolus) Restricted cardiac filling (e.g. cardiac tamponade)
Cardiogenic (e.g. ischaemic cardiac damage)	**Distributive** Vascular dilatation Sequestration Arteriovenous shunting Maldistribution of flow (e.g. sepsis, anaphylaxis)

CAUSES OF SHOCK

The causes of shock are shown in Table 13.2. Very often shock can result from a combination of these factors.

Pathophysiology

Sympatho-adrenal response to shock (Fig 13.8)

Hypotension stimulates the baroreceptors, and to a lesser extent the chemoreceptors, causing increased sympathetic

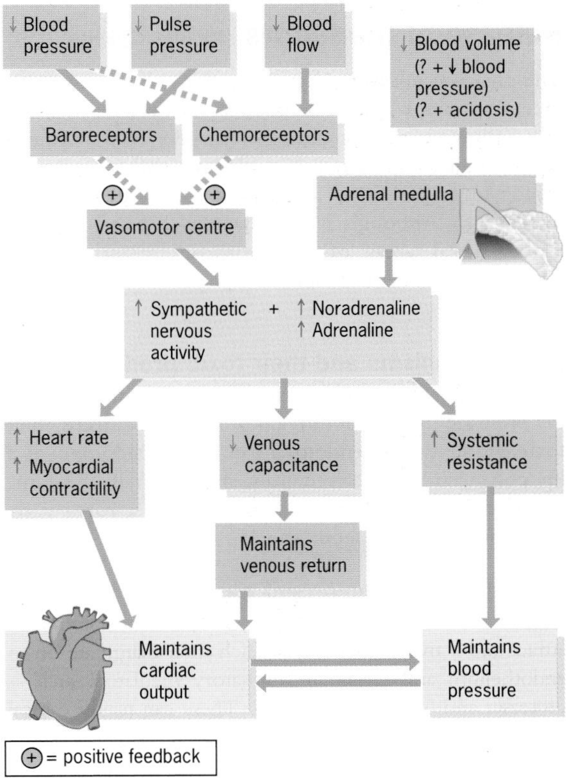

Fig 13.8
The sympatho-adrenal response to shock

nervous activity. Later this is augmented by the release of catecholamines from the adrenal medulla. The resulting vasoconstriction, together with increased myocardial contractility and heart rate, help to restore blood pressure and cardiac output. Reduction in perfusion of the renal cortex stimulates the juxtaglomerular apparatus to release renin. This converts angiotensin to angiotensin I, which is in turn converted in the lungs and the vascular endothelium to the potent vasoconstrictor angiotensin II. Angiotensin II then stimulates secretion of aldosterone by the adrenal cortex, causing sodium and water retention. This helps to restore the circulating volume (see Fig 16.29).

Neuroendocrine response to shock

- There is *release of pituitary hormones* such as adrenocorticotrophic hormone (ACTH), growth hormone (GH), vasopressin (antidiuretic hormone, ADH) and β-endorphin. (Endogenous opioid peptides such as β-endorphin, dynorphin and the enkephalins may be partly responsible for some of the cardiovascular changes.)
- There is *release of cortisol* which causes fluid retention and antagonizes insulin.
- There is *release of glucagon* which raises the blood sugar level.

Release of mediators (see also Chapter 2)

The presence of severe infection (often with bacteraemia or endotoxaemia) or of large areas of devitalized tissue (e.g. following trauma or major surgery) can trigger a massive inflammatory response with systemic activation of leucocytes and release of a variety of potentially damaging 'mediators'. Although clearly beneficial when targeted against local areas of infection or necrotic tissue, dissemination of this response can produce widespread tissue damage.

Micro-organisms and their toxic products

In septic shock, the inflammatory cascade is triggered by the presence in the bloodstream of micro-organisms, their toxic products (e.g. endotoxin) or both. Endotoxin is a lipopolysaccharide derived from the cell wall of Gram-negative bacteria which is thought to be a particularly important trigger of septic shock.

Activation of complement cascade

One of the many functions of the complement system is to attract and activate leucocytes, which then marginate on to endothelium and release inflammatory mediators such as proteases and free oxygen radicals. These can produce local tissue damage. For example, the free radical superoxide (O_2^-) can participate in a number of chemical reactions, yielding hydrogen peroxide (H_2O_2), hydroxyl radicals (OH^-) and peroxynitrite which can damage cell membranes. They also interfere with the functioning of a number of enzyme systems, including mitochondrial enzymes. They activate prostaglandin metabolism, upregulate adhesion molecules (see below), and increase capillary permeability.

Cytokines (see also p. 166)

Macrophage- and lymphocyte-derived cytokines such as the interleukins (ILs) and tumour necrosis factor (TNF) are involved in the pathogenesis of shock. TNF release initiates many of the responses to endotoxin and acts synergistically with IL-1, in part through induction of cyclo-oxygenase, platelet-activating factor (PAF) and nitric oxide synthase (see below). The cytokine network is extremely complex, with many endogenous self-regulating mechanisms. For example, naturally occurring soluble TNF receptors are thought to be shed from cell surfaces during the inflammatory response, binding to TNF and thereby reducing its biological activity. An endogenous inhibitory protein that binds competitively to the IL-1 receptor has also been identified.

In addition to pro-inflammatory mediators such as TNF, anti-inflammatory cytokines, e.g. IL-10, are released. The ratio of IL-10 to TNF has been shown to be related to mortality in septic shock.

Platelet-activating factor

This vasoactive lipid is released from various cell populations, such a leucocytes and macrophages, in shock. Its effects, which are caused both directly and through the secondary release of other mediators, include hypotension, increased vascular permeability and platelet aggregation.

Products of arachidonic acid metabolism

(see Fig 12.32)

Arachidonic acid, derived from the breakdown of membrane phospholipid, is metabolized to form prostaglandins and leukotrienes, which are important inflammatory mediators. Prostaglandins thought to be of importance in shock include:

- *prostacyclin* PGI_2, which is a vasodilator and inhibits platelet aggregation
- *thromboxane* A_2, which causes pulmonary vasoconstriction and activates platelets
- *prostaglandin* $F_{2\alpha}$, which may be responsible for the early phase of pulmonary hypertension commonly seen in experimental septic shock.

Leukotrienes have a variety of effects, including a reduction in cardiac output, vasoconstriction, increased vascular permeability and platelet activation.

Lysosomal enzymes

These are released in response to hypoxia, ischaemia. sepsis and acidosis. As well as being directly cytotoxic, they can cause myocardial depression and coronary vasoconstriction. Furthermore, lysosomal enzymes can convert inactive kininogens, which are usually combined

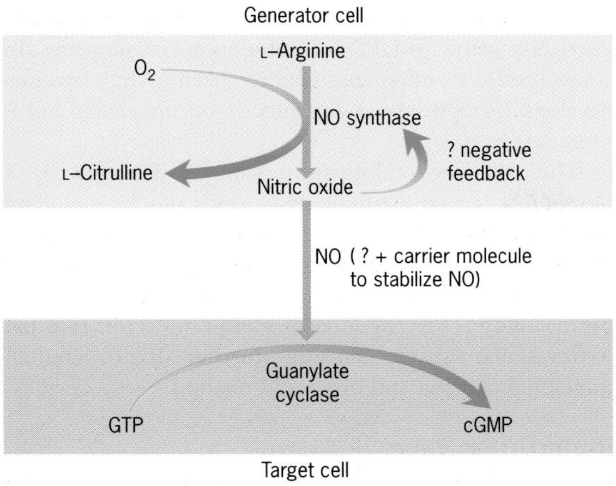

Fig 13.9
Synthesis and biochemical action of nitric oxide

with α_2-globulin, to vasoactive kinins such as bradykinins. These substances cause vasodilatation and increased capillary permeability, as well as myocardial depression. They can also activate clotting mechanisms.

Endothelium-derived vasoactive mediators

Endothelial cells synthesize a number of mediators which contribute to the regulation of blood vessel tone and the fluidity of the blood; these include prostacyclin, endothelin-1 and nitric oxide (NO). Endothelin-1 is a potent vasoconstrictor, which may help to maintain perfusion pressure in cardiogenic and traumatic shock, but its role in shock is not yet well understood. Nitric oxide is synthesized from the terminal guanidino-nitrogen atoms of the amino acid L-arginine under the influence of nitric oxide synthases (NOS). NO inhibits platelet aggregation and adhesion and produces vasodilatation by activating guanylate cyclase in the underlying vascular smooth muscle to form cyclic guanosine monophosphate (cGMP) from guanosine triphosphate (GTP) (Fig 13.9). There is now evidence for the existence of several distinct NOS, as listed below.

- *Constitutive or endothelial NOS (cNOS or eNOS)* present in endothelial cells is responsible for the basal release of NO and is involved in the physiological regulation of vascular tone, blood pressure and tissue perfusion.
- *Inducible NOS (iNOS)* is induced in vascular endothelial smooth muscle cells and monocytes within 4–18 hours of stimulation with certain cytokines, such as TNF, and endotoxin. The resulting prolonged increase in NO formation is now believed to be responsible for the sustained vasodilatation, hypotension and hyporeactivity to adrenergic agonists that characterizes septic shock. This mechanism may also be involved in severe haemorrhage/traumatic shock. The NO generated by macrophages contributes to their role as highly effective killers of intracellular and extracellular pathogens, probably via the production of peroxynitrite.
- *Neuronal NOS (nNOS).* The role of nerves containing nNOS is uncertain but they probably provide neurogenic vasodilator tone. In the central nervous system, nNOS may be an important regulator of local cerebral blood flow as well as fulfilling a number of other physiological functions, such as the acute modulation of neuronal firing behaviour.

Adhesion molecules (see also p. 163)

Adhesion of neutrophils to the vessel wall and subsequent extravascular migration of activated leucocytes is a key component of the sequence of events leading to endothelial injury, tissue damage and organ dysfunction. This process is mediated by inducible intercellular adhesion molecules (ICAMs) found on the surface of leucocytes and endothelial cells. Expression of these molecules can be induced by endotoxin and pro-inflammatory cytokines such as IL-1 and TNF. Several families of molecules are involved in promoting leukocyte–endothelial interaction. The selectins are initial 'capture' molecules and initiate the process of leucocyte rolling on vascular endothelium, whilst members of the immunoglobulin superfamily (ICAM-1 and vascular cell adhesion molecule-1) are involved in the formation of a more secure bond which leads to leucocyte migration into the tissues.

Microcirculatory changes

Since shock is a syndrome caused by inadequate tissue perfusion, the final common pathway for the pathophysiological changes is the microcirculation. In the early stages of septic shock there is:

- vasodilatation
- maldistribution of flow
- arteriovenous shunting
- increased capillary permeability with interstitial oedema.

Although these microvascular abnormalities may partly account for the reduced oxygen extraction often seen in septic shock, there is probably also a *primary defect of cellular oxygen utilization.* Initially, before hypovolaemia supervenes, or when therapeutic replacement of circulating volume has been adequate, *cardiac output is usually high and peripheral resistance is low.* Vasodilatation and increased permeability also occur in anaphylactic shock.

In the initial stages of other forms of shock, and sometimes when hypovolaemia supervenes in sepsis and anaphylaxis, increased sympathetic activity causes constriction of both precapillary arterioles and, to a lesser extent, the postcapillary venules. This helps to maintain the systemic blood pressure. In addition, the hydrostatic pressure within the capillaries falls and fluid is mobilized from the extravascular space into the intravascular compartment. If shock persists, the accumulation of metabolites, such as lactic acid and carbon dioxide, combined with the release of vasoactive substances, causes relaxation of the precapillary sphincters; the postcapillary venules, which are more sensitive to hypoxic damage, become relatively unresponsive to these substances and remain constricted. Blood is therefore sequestered within the dilated capillary bed, and fluid is forced into the extravascular spaces, causing interstitial oedema, haemoconcentration, and an increase in viscosity.

Disseminated intravascular coagulation (DIC)

The reduction in flow through the microcirculation, combined with the increase in viscosity, makes the blood highly coagulable. There is also systemic activation of the clotting cascade and platelet aggregation with clot formation occurring within the capillary bed. Plasminogen is converted to plasmin, which breaks down these clots, liberating fibrin/fibrinogen degradation products (FDPs). The cells that are supplied by capillaries blocked by this process of DIC (see p. 407) inevitably become hypoxic and eventually die. In this way vital organs may suffer serious damage. Finally, because clotting factors and platelets are consumed in DIC, they are unavailable for haemostasis elsewhere and a coagulation defect results – hence the alternative name for DIC is 'consumption coagulopathy'. In some cases a microangiopathic haemolytic anaemia develops. In septic shock this process occurs earlier and is more severe.

The capillary endothelium can be damaged by a number of factors (particularly in septic shock), including DIC, microemboli, release of vasoactive compounds, complement activation, as well as by the adhesion and extravascular migration of leucocytes. Capillary permeability is thereby increased and fluid is lost into the extravascular space, causing further hypovolaemia, interstitial oedema and organ dysfunction.

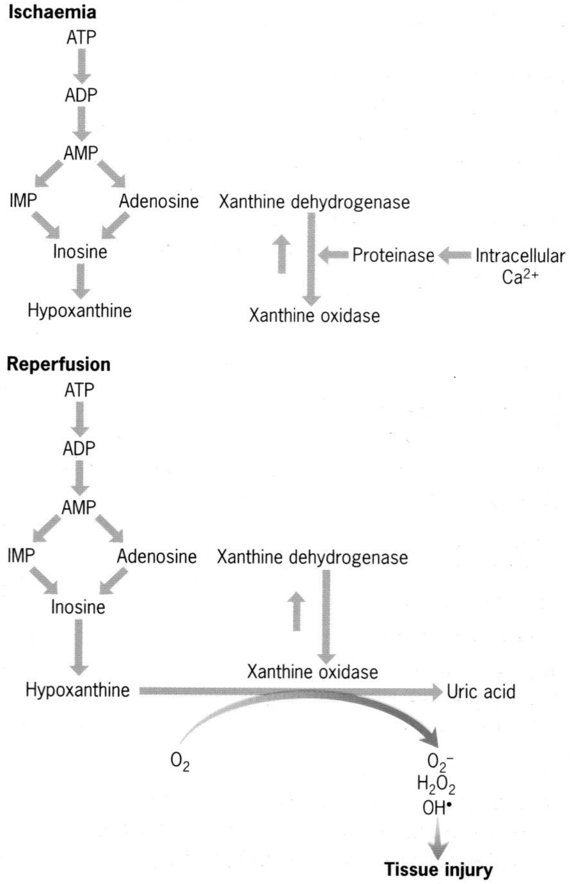

Fig 13.10
Generation of free radicals following ischaemia and reperfusion

Reperfusion injury

If resuscitation is successful and flow through the microcirculation is restored, tissue damage may be exacerbated by activation of phospholipase A2 and the generation of large quantities of oxygen free radicals. During the period of ischaemia, xanthine dehydrogenase is converted to xanthine oxidase and ATP is catabolized to hypoxanthine. When oxygen again becomes available, hypoxanthine is rapidly converted to uric acid under the influence of xanthine oxidase, in the process generating large amounts of free radicals (Fig 13.10). The gut mucosa seems to be especially vulnerable to this 'reperfusion injury'.

Metabolic changes

Gluconeogenesis and triglyceride formation are stimulated by increased glucagon and catecholamine levels, whilst hepatic mobilization of glucose from glycogen is increased. Catecholamines inhibit insulin release and reduce peripheral glucose uptake. Combined with elevated circulating levels of other insulin antagonists such as cortisol, these changes ensure that the majority of shocked patients are hyperglycaemic. Occasionally hypoglycaemia is precipitated by depletion of hepatic glycogen stores and inhibition of gluconeogenesis. Free fatty acid synthesis is also increased, leading to hypertriglyceridaemia.

Muscle proteolysis is initiated to provide energy, and hepatic protein synthesis is preferentially augmented to produce the 'acute phase reactants' (see p. 166). Once the supply of oxygen to the cells is insufficient for continuation of the tricarboxylic acid (TCA) cycle, production of energy in the form of ATP becomes dependent on anaerobic metabolism. Under these circumstances, glucose is metabolized in the normal way to pyruvate, but is then converted to lactate instead of entering the Krebs cycle. The H^+ ions released cause a metabolic acidosis. This pathway is relatively inefficient in terms of energy production. Eventually, because of the reduced availability of ATP, the sodium pump fails, cells swell owing to accumulation of salt and water, and potassium losses increase. In the final stages, release of lysosomal enzymes may contribute to cell death.

Multiple organ dysfunction syndrome – MODS (also known as multiple organ failure – MOF)

In this condition, impaired tissue perfusion, microcirculatory abnormalities, and defective oxygen utilization precipitated by dissemination of the inflammatory response with the systemic release of 'mediators' (see above) can damage vital organs. The most severely ill patients may develop MODS which is almost invariably associated with persistent or recurrent sepsis and a fever. This is partly due to damage to the mucosa of the gastrointestinal tract following severe shock and reperfusion, which allows bacteria or endotoxin within the gut lumen to gain access to the circulation, thereby perpetuating the generalized inflammatory response.

Sequential failure of the organs occurs progressively over weeks, although the pattern of organ dysfunction is variable. In most cases the lungs are the first organs to be affected, with development of the acute respiratory distress syndrome (ARDS) (see below) in association with cardiovascular instability and deteriorating renal function. Secondary pulmonary infection, complicating ARDS, frequently acts as a further stimulus to the inflammatory response. Later, renal failure and liver dysfunction develop (see p. 848). Gastrointestinal failure, with an inability to tolerate enteral feeding and paralytic ileus, is common. Ischaemic colitis, acalculous cholecystitis, pancreatitis and gastrointestinal haemorrhage may also occur. Features of central nervous system dysfunction include impaired consciousness and disorientation, progressing to coma. The metabolic derangement is associated with elevated blood sugar levels, catabolism and wasting. Characteristically, these patients initially have a hyperdynamic circulation with vasodilatation and a high cardiac output, associated with an increased metabolic rate. Eventually, however, cardiovascular collapse supervenes and is the usual terminal event.

The mortality of MODS is extremely high. Factors affecting outcome include the number of organs involved, the duration of organ dysfunction and persistent infection.

TREATMENT OF MODS

This is supportive, and prevention of organ damage in those at risk is therefore crucial. Aggressive early resuscitation is essential, and activation of the inflammatory response must be prevented or minimized by early excision of devitalized tissue and drainage of infection. Preservation of the integrity of the gut mucosal barrier is also necessary by maximizing splanchnic perfusion and by early institution of enteral feeding. Prompt recognition of organ dysfunction and immediate intervention may reverse organ impairment and improve outcome.

Clinical signs of shock

Although many clinical features are common to all types of shock, there are certain important respects in which they differ (Information box 13.1).

Hypovolaemic shock

- Inadequate tissue perfusion:
  - (a) Skin – cold, pale, blue, slow capillary refill
  - (b) Kidneys – oliguria, anuria
  - (c) Brain – confusion and restlessness
- Increased sympathetic tone:
  - (a) Tachycardia, narrowed pulse pressure
  - (b) Sweating

Information

Hypovolaemic shock
Low central venous pressure (CVP) and pulmonary artery occlusion pressure (PAOP)
Low cardiac output
Increased systemic vascular resistance

Cardiogenic shock
Clinical signs usually associated with very low cardiac output
Increased systemic vascular resistance
CVP and PAOP usually high

Cardiac tamponade
Parallel increases in CVP and PAOP
Low cardiac output
Increased systemic vascular resistance

Pulmonary embolism
Low cardiac output
High CVP, high pulmonary artery pressure but low PAOP
Increased systemic vascular resistance

Anaphylaxis
Low systemic vascular resistance
Low CVP and PAOP
High cardiac output

Septic shock
Low systemic vascular resistance
Low CVP and PAOP
Cardiac output usually high
Myocardial depression – low ejection fraction
Stroke volume maintained by ventricular dilatation
Cardiac output increased by tachycardia

Information box 13.1 Haemodynamic changes in shock

(c) Blood pressure – may be maintained initially (despite up to a 25% reduction in circulating volume if the patient is young and fit), but later hypotension supervenes
- Metabolic acidosis – compensatory tachypnoea.

Additional clinical features may occur in the following types of shock.

Cardiogenic shock (see p. 684)

Signs of myocardial failure, e.g. raised jugular venous pressure (JVP), pulsus alternans, 'gallop' rhythm, basal crackles, pulmonary oedema.

Obstructive shock

- Elevated JVP
- Pulsus paradoxus and muffled heart sounds in cardiac tamponade
- Kussmaul's sign (JVP rises on inspiration) in cardiac tamponade
- Signs of pulmonary embolism (if present) (see p. 720).

Anaphylactic shock (see p. 862)

- Signs of profound vasodilatation:
  (a) Warm peripheries
  (b) Low blood pressure
- Erythema, urticaria, angio-oedema, pallor, cyanosis
- Bronchospasm, rhinitis
- Oedema of the face, pharynx and larynx
- Pulmonary oedema
- Hypovolaemia due to capillary leak
- Nausea, vomiting, abdominal cramps, diarrhoea.

Septic shock

- Pyrexia and rigors, or hypothermia (unusual)
- Nausea, vomiting
- Vasodilatation, warm peripheries
- Bounding pulse
- Rapid capillary refill
- Hypotension
- Occasionally signs of cutaneous vasoconstriction
- Other signs:
  (a) Jaundice
  (b) Coma (rare)
  (c) Bleeding due to coagulopathy.

The clinical signs of sepsis are not always associated with bacteraemia and can occur with non-infectious processes such as pancreatitis or severe trauma. In order to avoid confusion, the term 'systemic inflammatory response syndrome' (SIRS) has been suggested to describe the disseminated inflammation that can complicate this diverse range of disorders (Information box 13.2). The usefulness of this terminology has been questioned.

The diagnosis of sepsis is easily missed, particularly in the elderly when the classical signs may not be present. Mild confusion, tachycardia and tachypnoea may be the only clues, sometimes associated with unexplained hypotension, a reduction in urine output, a rising plasma creatinine and glucose intolerance.

Monitoring of patients in shock

Invasive monitoring is unnecessary in straightforward cases, such as a fit young individual with moderate traumatic haemorrhage, but will be required in the more seriously ill patients and in those who fail to respond to initial treatment (see later). Clinical assessment must never be neglected.

Clinical indices of tissue perfusion

Pale, cold skin, delayed capillary refill and the absence of visible veins in the hands and feet indicate poor perfusion. Skin temperature measurements can help clinical evaluation as vasoconstriction is an early compensatory response.

Urinary flow is a sensitive indicator of renal perfusion and haemodynamic performance.

i Information

Systemic inflammatory response syndrome (SIRS)
The systemic inflammatory response to a variety of severe clinical insults. The response is manifested by two or more of the following:

- Temperature >38°C or <36°C
- Heart rate >90 beats/min
- Respiratory rate >20 breaths/min or P_aCO_2 < 4.3 kPa
- White cell count >12 × 10^9/L, <4 × 10^9/L or >10% immature forms

Sepsis
SIRS resulting from documented infection

Severe sepsis
Sepsis associated with organ dysfunction, hypoperfusion or hypotension. Hypoperfusion and perfusion abnormalities may include, but are not limited to, lactic acidosis, oliguria or an acute alteration in mental state

Septic shock
Severe sepsis with hypotension (systolic BP < 90 mmHg or a reduction of >40 mmHg from baseline) in the absence of other causes for hypotension despite adequate fluid resuscitation

(Patients receiving inotropic or vasopressor agents may not be hypotensive when perfusion abnormalities are documented)

Refractory shock
Shock unresponsive to conventional therapy (intravenous fluids and inotropic/vasoactive agents) within one hour

Information box 13.2 Terminology used in sepsis

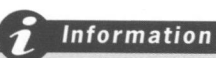

Practical

Technique

1 The arm is supported, with the wrist extended, by an assistant. (Gloves should be worn by the operator.)

2 The radial artery is palpated where it arches over the head of the radius.

3 In conscious patients, local anaesthetic is injected to raise a weal over the artery, taking care not to puncture the vessel or obscure its pulsation.

4 A small skin incision is made over the proposed puncture site.

5 A small parallel-sided cannula (20 gauge for adults, 22 gauge for children) is used in order to allow blood to flow past the cannula. Teflon is less irritant.

6 The cannula is inserted over the point of maximal pulsation and advanced in line with the direction of the vessel at an angle of approximately 30°.

7 'Flashback' of blood into the cannula indicates that the radial artery has been punctured.

8 To ensure that the shoulder of the cannula enters the vessel the needle and cannula are lowered and advanced a few millimetres into the vessel.

9 The cannula is threaded off the needle into the vessel and the needle withdrawn.

10 The cannula is connected to a non-compliant manometer line filled with heparinized saline. This is then connected via a transducer and continuous flush device to an oscilloscope, which records the arterial pressure.

Complications

- Thrombosis
- Loss of arterial pulsation
- Distal ischaemia, e.g. digital necrosis (rare)
- Accidental injection of drugs – can produce vascular occlusion
- Disconnection – leading to hypovolaemia

Practical box 13.1 Radial artery cannulation

Blood pressure

Alterations in blood pressure are often interpreted as reflecting changes in cardiac output. However, if there is vasoconstriction with a high peripheral resistance, the blood pressure may be normal, even when the cardiac output is reduced. Conversely the vasodilated patient may be hypotensive despite a very high cardiac output.

The absolute level of blood pressure is also important, since hypotension may jeopardize perfusion of vital organs. The adequacy of blood pressure in an individual patient must always be assessed in relation to the premorbid value.

Blood pressure is traditionally measured with a sphygmomanometer, but automated instruments can be used. Options are a microphone to detect Korotkoff's sounds, or continuous monitoring with an intra-arterial cannula, usually in the radial artery (Practical box 13.1) (Fig 13.11).

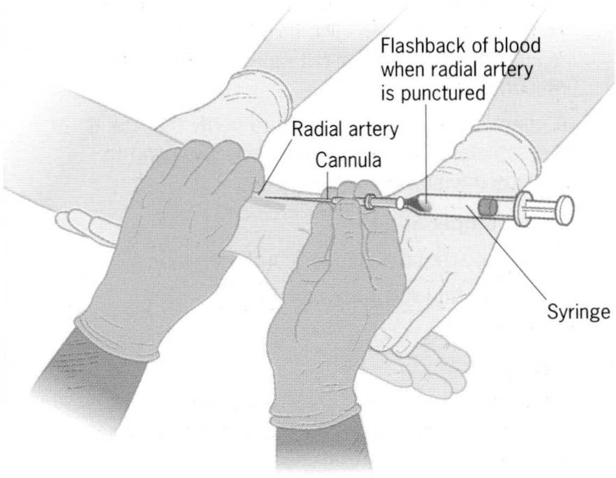

Fig 13.11
Percutaneous cannulation of the radial artery

Central venous pressure (CVP)

This provides a fairly simple method of assessing the adequacy of a patient's circulating volume and the contractile state of the myocardium. The absolute value of the CVP is not as important as its response to a fluid challenge (the infusion of 100–200 mL of fluid over 1–3 min) (Fig 13.12). The hypovolaemic patient will initially respond to transfusion with little or no change in CVP, together with some improvement in cardiovascular function (falling heart rate, rising blood pressure and increased peripheral temperature). As the normovolaemic state is approached, the CVP usually rises slightly and

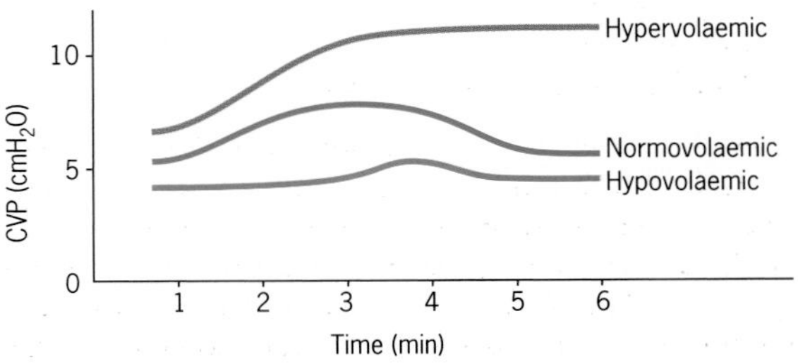

Fig 13.12
The effects of rapid administration of a 'fluid challenge' to patients with a central venous pressure within the normal range. From Sykes MK (1963) Venous pressure as a clinical indication of adequacy of transfusion, *Annals of the Royal College of Surgeons of England* **33**: 185–197

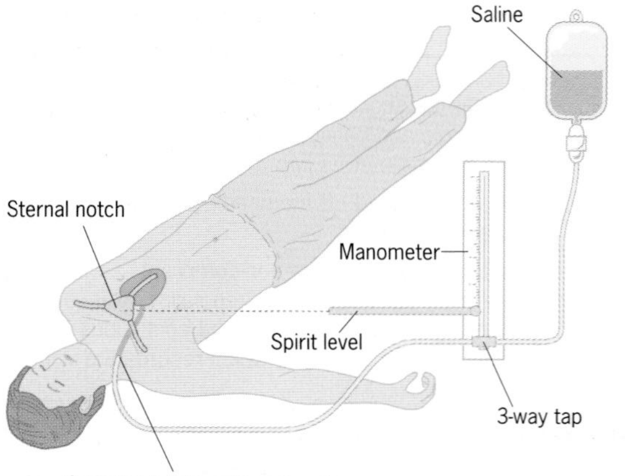

Fig 13.13
Central venous pressure measurement using a manometer system. The reading must be referred to the level of the right atrium (indicated by the axillary fold or, provided the patient is supine, the sternal notch) using a spirit level

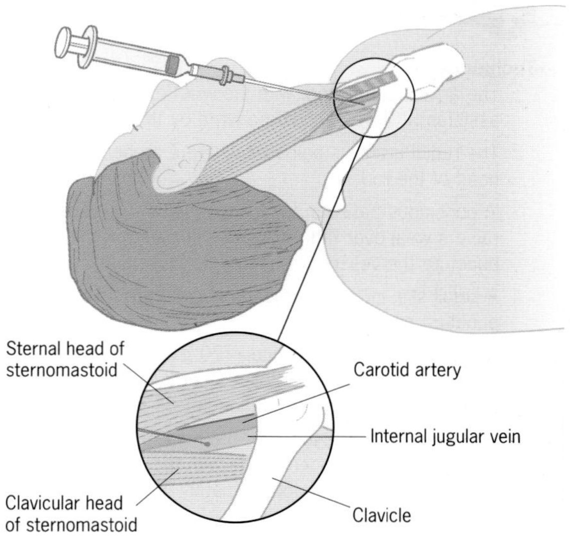

Fig 13.14
Cannulation of the right internal jugular vein

stabilizes, while other cardiovascular values normalize. At this stage, volume replacement should be slowed, or even stopped, in order to avoid overtransfusion (indicated by an abrupt and sustained rise in CVP, often accompanied by some deterioration in the patient's condition). In cardiac failure the venous pressure is usually high; the patient will not respond to volume replacement, which will cause a further, sometimes dramatic, rise in CVP.

The CVP may be read intermittently using a manometer system (Fig 13.13) or continuously using a transducer connected to an oscilloscope, similar to that used for intra-arterial monitoring. It is essential that the pressure recorded always be related to the level of the right atrium. Various landmarks are advocated (e.g. sternal notch with the patient supine, sternal angle or mid-axilla when patient at 45 degrees), but it is largely immaterial which is chosen provided it is used consistently in an individual patient. Pressure measurements should be obtained at end-expiration.

The following are common pitfalls in interpreting CVP results:

Practical

Technique

1. The procedure is explained to the patient.
2. The patient is placed head-down to distend the central veins (this facilitates cannulation and minimizes the risk of air embolism but may exacerbate respiratory distress and is dangerous in those with raised intracranial pressure).
3. The skin is cleaned. Sterile precautions are taken throughout the procedure.
4. Local anaesthetic (1% plain lignocaine) is injected intradermally to raise a weal at the apex of a triangle formed by the two heads of sternomastoid with the clavicle at its base.
5. A small incision is made through the weal.
6. The cannula is inserted through the incision and directed laterally downwards and backwards until the vein is punctured just beneath the skin and deep to the lateral head of sternomastoid.
7. Check that venous blood is easily aspirated using a syringe attached to the cannula.
8. The cannula is threaded off the needle into the vein.
9. The CVP manometer line is connected.
10. If the catheter is in a large vein, venous blood will flow back when the giving-set tap is open and the infusion bottle is on the floor.
11. The CVP is measured. The fluid level in the manometer should then fall rapidly and fluctuate with respiration.
12. A chest X-ray should be taken to verify that the tip of the catheter is in the superior vena cava and to exclude pneumothorax.

Possible complications

- Accidental arterial puncture (carotid or subclavian)
- Damage to thoracic duct on left
- Air embolism
- Pneumothorax
- Thrombosis
- Catheter-related sepsis

Practical box 13.2 Internal jugular vein cannulation

Blocked catheter. This results in a sustained high reading, with a damped waveform which often does not correlate with clinical assessment.

Manometer or transducer wrongly positioned. Failure to level the CVP is a common cause of erroneous readings.

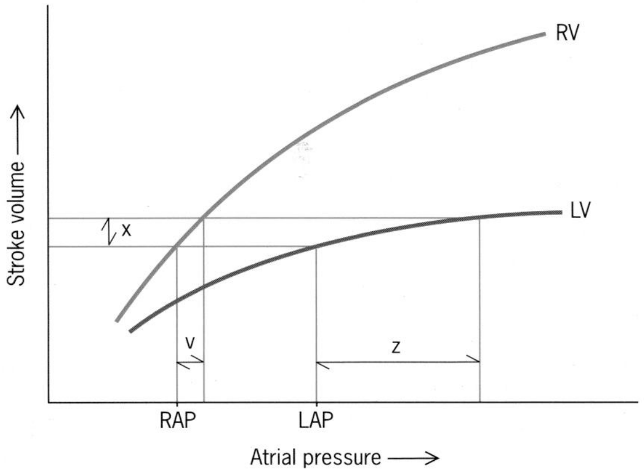

Fig 13.15
Left ventricular (LV) and right ventricular (RV) function curves in a patient with left ventricular dysfunction. Since the stroke volume of the two ventricles must be the same (except perhaps for a few beats during a period of circulatory adjustment), left atrial pressure (LAP) must be higher than right atrial pressure (RAP). Moreover, an increase in stroke volume (*x*) produced by a small rise in RAP (*v*) will be associated with a marked increase in LAP (*z*)

Incorrect calibration. If an electronic transducer and oscilloscope are used, the system should be zeroed and calibrated prior to use, and at regular intervals thereafter.

Catheter tip in right ventricle. If the catheter is advanced too far, an unexpectedly high pressure with pronounced oscillations is recorded. This is easily recognized when the waveform is displayed. The catheter should be positioned in the superior vena cava. It is usually inserted via a percutaneous puncture of a subclavian or internal jugular vein (Practical box 13.2) (Fig 13.14).

Left atrial pressure

In uncomplicated cases, careful interpretation of the CVP is an adequate guide to the filling pressures of both sides of the heart. In many critically ill patients, however, this is not the case and there is a disparity in function between the two ventricles. Most commonly, left ventricular performance is worst, so that the left ventricular function curve is displaced downward and to the right (Fig 13.15). This situation is encountered in some patients with clinically significant ischaemic heart disease and has also been reported in major trauma, sepsis, peritonitis, hepatic failure, valvular heart disease and after cardiac surgery. High right ventricular filling pressures, with normal or low left atrial pressures, are less common but may occur in right ventricular ischaemia and in situations where the

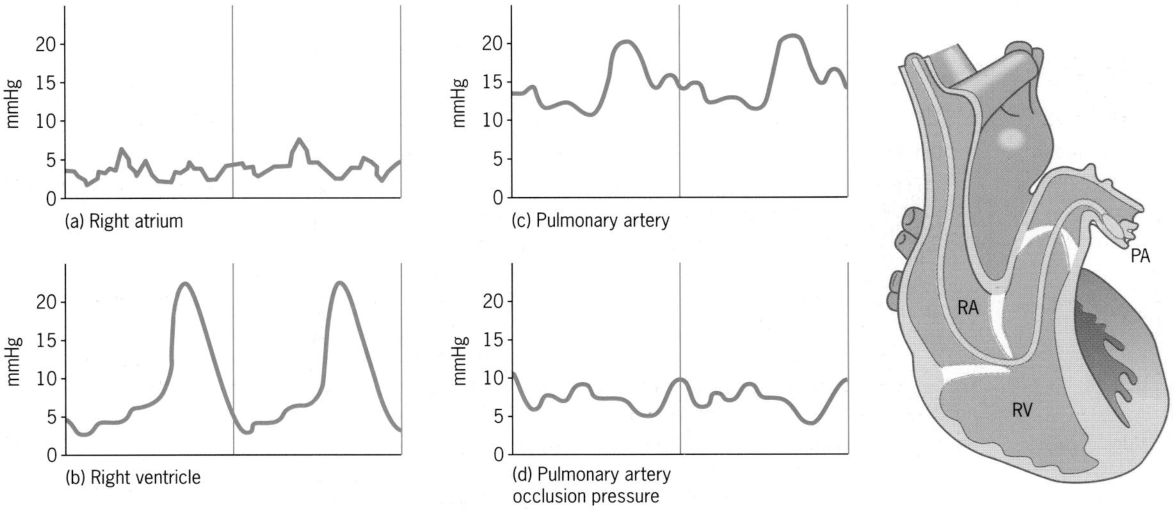

Fig 13.16
Passage of a Swan–Ganz catheter through the chambers of the heart into the 'wedge' position.
(a) Once in the thorax, marked respiratory oscillations are seen. The catheter should be advanced further towards the lower superior vena cava/right atrium, where oscillations become more pronounced. The balloon should then be inflated and the catheter advanced.
(b) When the catheter is in the right ventricle, there is no dicrotic notch and the diastolic pressure is close to zero. The patient should be returned to the horizontal, or slightly head-up, position before advancing the catheter further.
(c) When the catheter reaches the pulmonary artery a dicrotic notch appears and there is elevation of the diastolic pressure. The catheter should be advanced further with the balloon inflated.
(d) Reappearance of a venous waveform indicates that the catheter is 'wedged'. The balloon is deflated to obtain the pulmonary artery pressure. The balloon is inflated intermittently to obtain the pulmonary capillary wedge pressure (also known as pulmonary artery 'wedge' or occlusion pressure).

pulmonary vascular resistance (i.e. right ventricular afterload) is raised, such as in acute respiratory failure and pulmonary embolism.

If there is a disparity in ventricular function after cardiac surgery, then the left atrium can be cannulated directly. If the thorax is not open, however, some other means of determining left ventricular filling pressure must be devised.

PULMONARY ARTERY PRESSURE

A 'balloon flotation catheter' enables prompt and reliable catheterization of the pulmonary artery, without the need for screening, and minimizes the incidence of arrhythmias.

These 'Swan–Ganz' catheters can be inserted centrally or through the femoral vein, or via a vein in the antecubital fossa. Passage of the catheter from the major veins, through the chambers of the heart, into the pulmonary artery and into the wedge position is monitored and guided by the pressure waveforms recorded from the distal lumen (Fig 13.16). A chest X-ray should always be obtained to check the final position of the catheter. Once in place, the balloon is deflated and the pulmonary artery mean, systolic a nd end-diastolic pressures (PAEDP) can be recorded. The pulmonary artery occlusion pressure (PAOP, otherwise known as pulmonary artery wedge pressure PAWP) is measured by reinflating the balloon, thereby propelling the catheter distally until it impacts in a medium-sized pulmonary artery. In this position there is a continous column of fluid between the distal lumen of the catheter and the left atrium, so that PAOP is usually a reflection of left atrial pressure.

The technique is generally safe – the majority of complications are related to user inexperience. Pulmonary artery catheters should preferably be removed within 72 hours, since the incidence of complications then increases progressively (Table 13.3).

Table 13.3
Swan–Ganz catheters: some complications

Complication	Comments
Arrhythmias	Occur during passage of catheter through right ventricle
	Usually benign
	Can often be prevented with lignocaine
Sepsis	Occurs at insertion site
	Bacteraemia or endocarditis may develop
Knotting	Occurs when catheter coils in right ventricle
Valve trauma	Occurs if catheter is withdrawn with balloon inflated, or if valves repeatedly close on the catheter
Thrombosis/embolism	–
Pulmonary infarction	Occurs if catheter remains in 'wedge' position
Pulmonary artery rupture	Usually fatal
	May occur if balloon is inflated when catheter already 'wedged'
Balloon rupture/leak/embolism	Rare

Cardiac output

The only quantitatively accurate methods for measuring cardiac output are invasive. Of these, the thermodilution technique is most commonly used clinically. This uses a modified pulmonary artery catheter with a lumen opening in the right atrium and a thermistor located a few centimetres from its tip. A known volume (usually 10 mL) of ice-cold 5% dextrose is injected as a bolus into the right atrium. This mixes with, and cools, the blood passing through the heart and the transient fall in temperature is continuously recorded by the thermistor in the pulmonary artery. The cardiac output is computed from the total amount of indicator (i.e. cold) injected, divided by the average concentration, i.e. the amount of cooling, and the time taken to pass the thermistor. It is now possible to measure cardiac output continuously using a modified pulmonary artery catheter which transmits low heat energy into the surrounding blood and constructs a 'thermodilution curve'.

In general, pulmonary artery catheters enable the clinician to optimize cardiac output and oxygen delivery, while minimizing the risk of pulmonary oedema. They also allow the rational use of inotropes and vasoactive agents. However their clinical value, and in particular their influence on outcome, is currently a matter of controversy.

Management of shock (see Fig 13.17)

Delays in making the diagnosis and in initiating treatment, as well as inadequate resuscitation, contribute to the development of MOF and must be avoided.

A patent airway must be maintained and oxygen must be given. If necessary, an oropharyngeal airway or an endotracheal tube is inserted. The latter has the advantage of preventing aspiration of gastric contents. *Very rarely* emergency tracheostomy is indicated (see below). Some patients may require mechanical ventilation.

The underlying cause of shock should be corrected – for example, haemorrhage should be controlled or infection eradicated. In patients with septic shock, every effort must be made to identify the souce of infection and isolate the causative organism. As well as a thorough history and clinical examination, X-rays, ultrasonography and CT scanning may be required to locate the origin of the infection. Appropriate samples (urine, sputum, cerebrospinal fluid, pus drained from abscesses) should be sent to the laboratory for microscopy, culture and sensitivities. Several blood cultures should be performed and 'blind' antibiotic therapy (p. 8) should be commenced. If an organism is isolated, the therapy can be adjusted appropriately. The choice of antibiotic depends

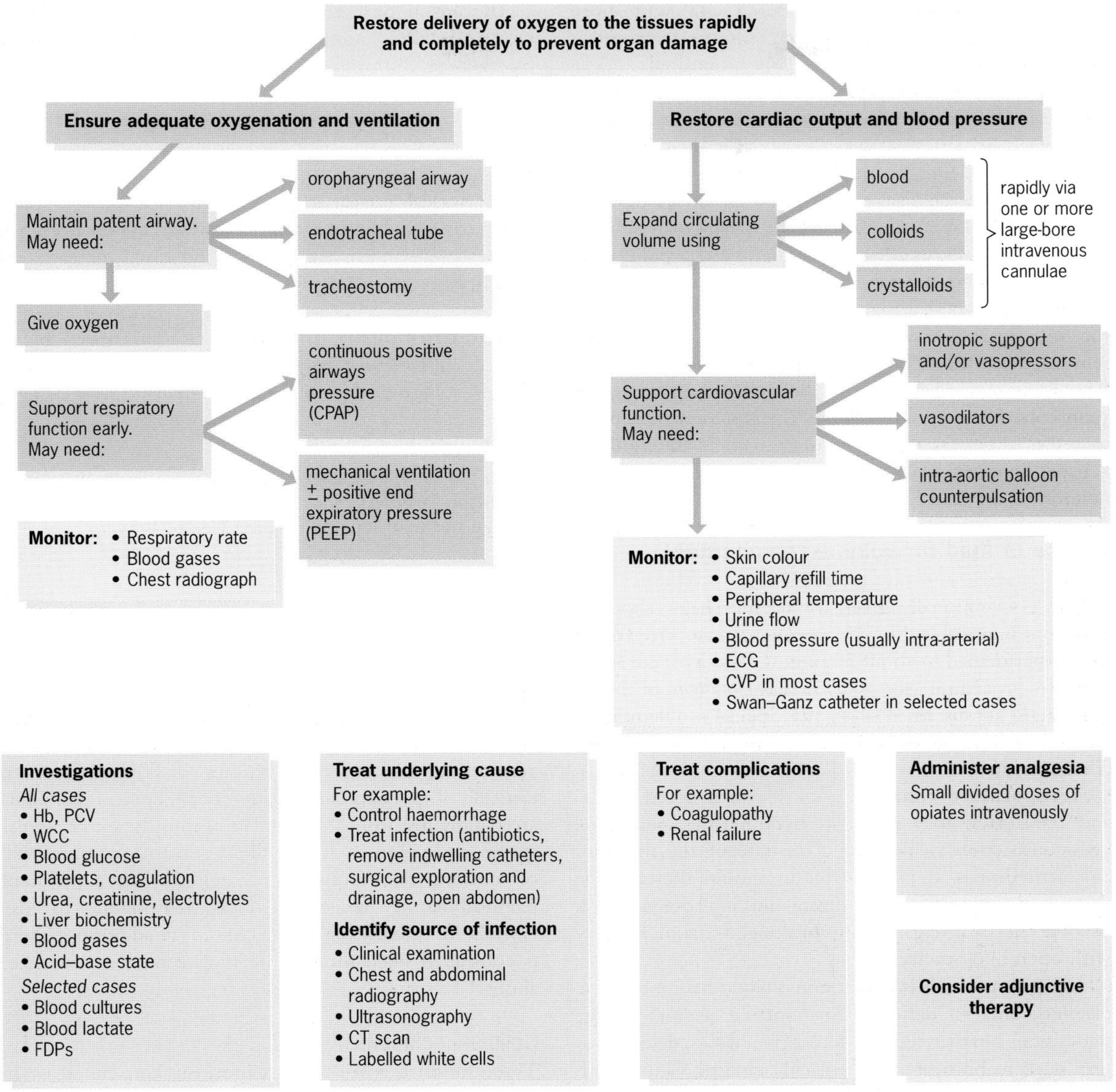

Fig 13.17
Management of shock. Patients require intensive nursing care

on the source of infection as well as on whether it was acquired in hospital or in the community. Abscesses must be drained and infected indwelling catheters removed.

Whatever the aetiology of the haemodynamic abnormality, tissue blood flow must be restored by achieving and maintaining an adequate cardiac output, as well as ensuring that arterial blood pressure is sufficient to maintain perfusion of vital organs.

Preload and volume replacement

Optimizing preload is the most efficient way of increasing cardiac output. Volume replacement is obviously essential in hypovolaemic shock but is also required in anaphylactic and septic shock because of vasodilatation, sequestration of blood and loss of circulating volume due to capillary leak.

In obstructive shock, high filling pressures may be required to maintain an adequate stroke volume. Even in cardiogenic shock, careful volume expansion may, on occasions, lead to a useful increase in cardiac output. On the other hand, patients with severe cardiac failure, in whom ventricular filling pressures may be markedly elevated, often benefit from measures to reduce preload (and afterload) – such as the administration of diuretics and vasodilators (see below).

The circulating volume must be replaced quickly (in minutes not hours) to reduce tissue damage and prevent acute renal failure. Fluid is administered via wide-bore intravenous cannulae to allow large volumes to be given quickly, and the effect is continuously monitored.

Care must be taken to prevent volume overload, which leads to cardiac dilatation, a reduction in stroke volume, and a rise in left atrial pressure with a risk of pulmonary oedema. Pulmonary oedema is more likely in very ill patients because of a low colloid osmotic pressure (usually due to a low serum albumin) and disruption of the alveolar-capillary membrane (e.g. in ARDS). The development of pulmonary oedema can also be influenced by other unquantifiable factors, such as the hydrostatic and oncotic pressures within the intersitial spaces. Since the pulmonary lymphatics remove excess fluid, pulmonary oedema will occur only when this mechanism is overwhelmed or impaired. Left ventricular filling pressures should therefore not be allowed to rise to more than 15–18 mmHg in the critically ill. In general, however, many more patients are undertransfused rather than overtransfused.

Choice of fluid for volume replacement

Blood

This is conventionally given for haemorrhagic shock as soon as it is available. In extreme emergencies, crossmatch can be performed in about 30 minutes and is as safe as the standard procedure (see p. 393). *Complications* of blood transfusion are discussed on p. 393. Special problems arise when large volumes of stored blood are transfused rapidly. These include:

Temperature changes. Bank blood is stored at 4°C and transfusion may result in hypothermia, peripheral venoconstriction (which slows the rate of the infusion) and arrhythmias. If possible blood should therefore be warmed during massive transfusion and in those with risk of hypothermia (e.g. during prolonged major surgery with open body cavity).

Coagulopathy. Essentially, stored blood has no effective platelets and is deficient in clotting factors. Large transfusions can therefore produce a coagulation defect. This may need to be treated by replacing clotting factors with fresh frozen plasma and administering platelet concentrates.

Metabolic acidosis/alkalosis. Stored blood is preserved in citrate/phosphate/dextrose (CPD) solution, and metabolic acidosis attributable solely to blood transfusion is rare and in any case seldom requires correction. A metabolic alkalosis often develops 24–48 hours after a large blood transfusion, probably mainly owing to metabolism of the citrate. This will be exacerbated if any preceding acidosis has been corrected with intravenous sodium bicarbonate.

Hypocalcaemia. Stored blood is anticoagulated with citrate, which binds calcium ions. This can reduce total body ionized calcium levels and cause myocardial depression. This is uncommon in practice, but can be corrected by administering 10 mL of 10% calcium chloride intravenously. Routine treatment with calcium is not recommended.

Increased oxygen affinity. In stored blood, the red cell 2,3-DPG content is reduced, so that the oxyhaemoglobin dissociation curve is shifted to the left. The oxygen affinity of haemoglobin is therefore increased and oxygen unloading is impaired. Red cell levels of 2,3-DPG are substantially restored within 12 hours of transfusion.

Hyperkalaemia. Plasma potassium levels rise progressively as blood is stored. However, hyperkalaemia is rarely a problem as rewarming of the blood increases red cell metabolism – the sodium pump becomes active and potassium levels fall.

Microembolism. Microaggregates in stored blood may be filtered out by the pulmonary capillaries. This process is thought by some to contribute to ARDS.

Red cell concentrates

Nutrient additive solutions – saline, adenine, glucose and mannitol (SAGM) – are available which allow red cell storage in the absence of plasma (see p. 395).

Crystalloid solutions

Blood transfusion carries a risk of disease transmission, as well being expensive. For these reasons, the use of crystalloid solutions, synthetic colloids and plasma for volume replacement is assuming greater importance.

However, although crystalloid solutions such as saline are cheap, convenient to use and free of side-effects, the administration of large volumes of these fluids to critically ill patients should, in general, be avoided. They are rapidly lost from the circulation into the extravascular spaces, and volumes of crystalloid two to four times that of colloid are required to achieve an equivalent haemodynamic response. It is reasonable to use crystalloids initially but to use colloids in addition if there is continued need for volume replacement in excess of about 1 L.

Colloidal solutions

These produce a greater and more sustained increase in plasma volume, with associated improvements in cardiovascular function and oxygen transport. They also increase colloid osmotic pressure.

Polygelatin solutions (Haemaccel, Gelofucin) have an average molecular weight of 35 000, which is iso-osmotic with plasma. They are cheap and do not interfere with crossmatching. Large volumes can be administered, as clinically significant coagulation defects are unusual, and renal function is not impaired. However, because they readily cross the glomerular basement membrane, their half-life in the circulation is approximately 4 hours and they can promote an osmotic diuresis. Allergic reactions occur in up to 10% of cases. These solutions are particularly useful during the acute phase of resuscitation, especially when volume losses are continuing; but in many patients, colloids with a longer half-life will be required later to achieve haemodynamic stability.

Dextrans are polymolecular polysaccharides in either 5% dextrose or normal saline. They are commercially available as low-molecular-weight dextran (dextran 40; mol.wt 40 000) and dextran 70, and have a powerful osmotic effect. They interfere with crossmatching and have a small rate of allergic reactions (0.07–1.1%) which may be extremely violent and life-threatening. Normally a dose of 1.5 g dextran per kilogram of bodyweight should not be exceeded because of the risk of renal damage. In practice, dextrans are rarely used in the UK because of the availability of other agents.

Hydroxyethyl starch (HES) has a mean molecular weight of approximately 450 000 and a half-life of about 12 hours. Volume expansion is equivalent to, or slightly greater than, the volume infused. The incidence of allergic reactions is approximately 0.1%. Although more expensive than gelatins, HES is a valuable volume expander.

Human albumin solution (HAS) is a natural colloid but is not generally used for routine volume replacement, particularly if volume losses are continuing since other cheaper solutions are equally effective in the short term. A few recommend administration of HAS at a later stage in those who are hypoalbuminaemic.

Myocardial contractility and inotropic agents

Myocardial contractility can be impaired by hypoxaemia and hypocalcaemia, as well as by some drugs (e.g. β-blockers, antiarrhythmics and sedatives).

Severe lactic acidosis can depress myocardial contractility and may limit the response to inotropes. Attempted correction of acidosis with intravenous sodium bicarbonate, however, generates additional carbon dioxide which diffuses across cell membranes, producing or exacerbating intracellular acidosis. Other disadvantages of bicarbonate therapy include sodium overload and a left shift of the oxyhaemoglobin dissociation curve. Also, ionized calcium levels may be reduced and, combined with the fall in intracellular pH, may be responsible for impairing myocardial performance. Treatment of lactic acidosis should therefore concentrate on correcting the cause. Bicarbonate should only be administered to corrrect *extreme persistent metabolic acidosis* (pH < 7.0) (see p. 623).

If the signs of shock persist despite adequate volume replacement, and perfusion of vital organs is jeopardized, pressor agents may be administered to improve cardiac output and blood pressure. In some cases inotropic agents are given to redistribute blood flow (e.g. dopamine can be used to increase renal perfusion, dopexamine to improve splanchnic perfusion – see below), and in others inotropic support can be usefully combined with the administration of a vasodilator. It must be remembered that all inotropes increase myocardial oxygen consumption, particularly if a tachycardia develops, and that this can lead to an imbalance between myocardial oxygen supply and demand, with the development or extension of ischaemic areas. For this reason such agents should be used with caution, particularly in cardiogenic shock following myocardial infarction and in those known to have ischaemic heart disease.

Many of the most seriously ill patients become increasingly resistant to the effects of pressor agents, an observation attributed to 'down-regulation' of adrenergic receptors.

All inotropic agents should be administered via a large central vein, and their effects carefully monitored. Some of the currently available inotropes are considered here (see also p. 681 and Table 13.4).

Adrenaline

Adrenaline stimulates both α- and β-adrenergic receptors, but at low doses β effects seem to predominate. This produces a tachycardia, with an increase in cardiac index and a fall in peripheral resistance. At higher doses, α-mediated vasoconstriction develops. If this produces a useful increase in perfusion pressure, urine output may increase and renal failure may be avoided. However, as the dose is further increased, cardiac output may actually fall, accompanied by marked vasoconstriction, tachycardia and a metabolic acidosis. A reduction in renal blood flow then occurs, with oliguria and a risk of acute renal failure. Prolonged high-dose administration may eventually cause peripheral gangrene. For these reasons the minimum effective dose should be used for as short a time as possible. The addition of low-dose dopamine to the regimen may help to preserve urine flow (see below). Despite its disadvantages, adrenaline remains a useful potent inotrope and is used when other agents have failed. When haemodynamic monitoring is not available, adrenaline is probably the agent of choice in septic shock.

Noradrenaline

This is predominantly an α-adrenergic agonist. It can be of value in those with severe hypotension associated with a low systemic resistance, for example in septic shock. There is a risk of producing excessive vasoconstriction with impaired organ perfusion and increased afterload. Noradrenaline administration should normally therefore be accompanied by full haemodynamic monitoring, including determination of cardiac output (see above) and calculation of the peripheral resistance.

Isoprenaline

This β-adrenergic stimulant has both inotropic and chronotropic effects. It reduces peripheral resistance by dilating skin and muscle blood vessels and diverts flow away from vital organs such as the kidneys. The increase in cardiac output produced by isoprenaline is mainly due to the tachycardia, and this, together with the development of arrhythmias, seriously limits its value. There are few indications for isoprenaline in the critically ill adult.

Table 13.4
Receptor actions of sympathomimetic agents

	β_1	β_2	α_1	α_2	DA1	DA2	Dose dependence
Adrenaline							++++
Low dose	++	+	+	±	–	–	
Moderate dose	++	+	++	+	–	–	
High dose	++(+)	+(+)	++++	+++	–	–	
Noradrenaline	++	0	+++	+++	–	–	+++
Isoprenaline	+++	+++	0	0	–	–	0
Dopamine							+++++
Low dose	±	0	±	+	++	+	
Moderate dose	++	+	++	+	++(+)	+	
High dose	+++	++	+++	+	++(+)	+	
Dopexamine	+	+++	0	0	++	+	++
Dobutamine	++	+	±	?	0	0	++

Receptor	**Action**
β_1 – post-synaptic	Positive inotropism and chronotropism Renin release
β_2 – pre-synaptic	Accelerates noradrenaline release
β_2 – post-synaptic	Positive inotropism and chronotropism Vascular dilatation Relaxes bronchial smooth muscle
α_1 – post-synaptic	Constriction of peripheral, renal and coronary vascular smooth muscle Positive inotropism Antidiuretics
α_2 – pre-synaptic	Inhibition of noradrenaline release, vasodilation
α_2 – post-synaptic	Constriction of coronary arteries Promotes salt and water excretion
DA_1 – post-synaptic	Dilates renal, mesenteric and coronary vessels Renal tubular effect (natriuresis, diuresis)
DA_1 – pre-synaptic	Inhibits noradrenaline release

Dopamine

Dopamine is a natural precursor of noradrenaline which acts on β receptors and α receptors, as well as dopaminergic DA_1 and DA_2 receptors.

In *low doses* (e.g. 1–3 $\mu g\ kg^{-1}\ min^{-1}$), dopaminergic vasodilatory receptors in the renal, mesenteric, cerebral and coronary circulations are activated. DA_1 receptors are located on post-synaptic membranes and mediate vasodilation, whilst DA_2 receptors are pre-synaptic and potentiate these vasodilatory effects by preventing the release of noradrenaline. Renal and hepatic flow increase, urine output is improved and it is possible that failure of these vital organs is prevented. The importance of the renal vasodilator effect of dopamine has, however, been questioned and it has been suggested that the increased urine output is largely attributable to the rise in cardiac output, combined with a decrease in aldosterone concentration and inhibition of tubular sodium reabsorption mediated via DA_1 stimulation.

In *moderate doses* (e.g. 3–10 $\mu g\ kg^{-1}\ min^{-1}$), dopamine increases heart rate, myocardial contractility and cardiac output. In some patients the dose of dopamine is limited by β-receptor effects such as tachycardia and arrhythmias.

In *higher doses* (e.g. > 10 $\mu g\ kg^{-1}\ min^{-1}$) the increased noradrenaline produced is associated with vasoconstriction. This increases afterload and raises ventricular filling pressures.

Dopexamine

Dopexamine is an analogue of dopamine which activates β_2 receptors as well as DA_1 and DA_2 receptors. Dopexamine is a very weak positive inotrope, but is a powerful splanchnic vasodilator, reducing afterload and improving blood flow to vital organs, including the kidney. In septic shock, dopexamine can increase cardiac index and heart rate, but causes further reductions in peripheral resistance. It is most useful in those with low cardiac output and peripheral vasoconstriction and has been used as an adjunct to the perioperative management of high-risk patients.

Dobutamine

Dobutamine is closely related to dopamine and has predominantly β_1 activity, although the relative effects of the two agents on heart rate and rhythm are a matter of dispute. Dobutamine has no specific effect on the renal vasculature but urine output often increases as cardiac output and blood pressure improve. It reduces systemic resistance, as well as improving cardiac performance, thereby decreasing afterload and ventricular filling pressures. Dobutamine is therefore useful in patients with cardiogenic shock and cardiac failure. In septic shock, dobutamine increases cardiac output and oxygen delivery.

Enoximone

This agent, active both orally and intravenously, is a phosphodiesterase inhibitor with inotropic and vasodilator properties. Enoximone may, however, cause profound vasodilatation and precipitate or worsen hypotension. It is sometimes useful in the management of acute cardiac failure. Because enoximone acts beyond the β-receptor it may be useful in patients with receptor 'down-regulation' and in those receiving β-blockers.

Summary of inotropic agents

Some still consider dopamine to be the inotrope of choice in most critically ill patients, largely because of its effects on splanchnic blood flow, although others favour dopexamine as a means of increasing cardiac output and organ blood flow. Dobutamine is equally popular and is particularly indicated in patients in whom the vasoconstriction caused by dopamine could be dangerous (i.e. patients with cardic disease and septic patients with fluid overload or myocardial failure). The combination of dobutamine and noradrenaline is currently popular for the management of patients who are shocked with a low systemic resistance. Dobutamine is given to achieve an optimal cardiac output, while noradrenaline is used to restore an adequate blood pressure by reducing vasodilatation. However, this combination can be used safely only when guided by full haemodynamic monitoring. In some vasodilated septic patients with a high cardiac output, noradrenaline is used alone.

Adrenaline, because of its potency, remains a useful agent in patients who are unresponsive to other measures, particularly after cardiac surgery, and is a cheap, effective agent for the management of septic shock.

Diuretic therapy (see p. 604)

Diuretics increase salt and water excretion by the kidneys, thereby decreasing ventricular filling pressure (preload). This is the major form of therapy in sodium retention with fluid overload.

Vasodilator therapy (see p. 680)

In selected cases, afterload reduction may be used to increase stroke volume and decrease myocardial oxygen requirements by reducing the systolic ventricular wall tension. Vasodilatation also decreases heart size and the diastolic ventricular wall tension so that coronary blood flow is improved. The relative magnitude of the falls in preload and afterload depends on the pre-existing haemodynamic disturbance, concurrent volume replacement and the agent selected (see below).

Vasodilator therapy is most beneficial in patients with cardiac failure in whom the ventricular function curve is flat (see Fig 13.4) and falls in preload have only a limited effect on stroke volume. This form of treatment, combined in selected cases with inotropic support, may therefore be useful in cardiogenic shock and in the management of patients with pulmonary oedema associated with low cardiac output. Vasodilators may also be valuable in shocked patients who remain vasoconstricted and oliguric despite restoration of an adequate blood pressure.

Such therapy is potentially dangerous and should be guided by continuous haemodynamic monitoring, including pulmonary artery catheterization or direct measurement of left atrial pressure. The circulating volume must be adequate before treatment is started. Falls in preload should be prevented, except in those with cardiac failure, in order to avoid serious reductions in cardiac output and blood pressure. If diastolic pressure is allowed to fall, coronary blood flow may be jeopardized and, particularly if a reflex tachycardia develops in response to the hypotension, myocardial ischaemia may be precipitated.

Vasodilators acting directly on the vessel wall

These are the agents used most commonly to achieve vasodilatation in the critically ill.

Hydralazine predominantly affects arterial resistance vessels. It therefore reduces afterload and blood pressure, while cardiac output and heart rate usually increase. Hydralazine is usually given as an intravenous bolus to control acute increases in blood pressure, particularly after cardiac surgery.

Sodium nitroprusside (SNP) dilates arterioles and venous capacitance vessels, as well as the pulmonary vasculature by donating nitric oxide. SNP therefore reduces the afterload and preload of both ventricles and can improve cardiac output and the myocardial oxygen supply/demand ratio. On the other hand, it has been suggested that SNP can exacerbate myocardial ischaemia by producing a 'steal' phenomenon in the coronary circulation. The effects of SNP are rapid in onset and spontaneously reversible within a few minutes of discontinuing the infusion. *A large overdose* of SNP can cause cyanide poisoning, with intracellular hypoxia caused by inhibition of cytochrome oxidase, the terminal enzyme of the respiratory chain. This is manifested as a metabolic acidosis and a fall in the arteriovenous oxygen content difference.

Nitroglycerine (NTG) and *isosorbide dinitrate* (ISDN) are both predominantly venodilators. They can therefore cause marked reductions in preload, which may be associated with falls in cardiac output and compensatory vasoconstriction. For the reasons discussed above, they are of most value in those with cardiac failure in whom preload reduction may reduce ventricular wall tension and improve coronary perfusion without adversely affecting cardiac performance. Furthermore, these agents may reverse myocardial ischaemia by increasing and redistributing coronary blood flow. They are therefore often used in preference to SNP in patients with cardiac failure and/or myocardial ischaemia. Both NTG and ISDN reduce pulmonary vascular resistance by donating nitric oxide, an effect that can occasionally be exploited in patients with a low cardiac output secondary to pulmonary hypertension.

α-Adrenergic antagonists

These predominantly dilate arterioles and therefore mainly influence afterload.

Phenoxybenzamine is unsuitable for use in the critically ill because of its slow onset (1–2 hours to maximum effect) and prolonged duration of action (2–3 days).

Phentolamine is very potent with a rapid onset and short duration of action (15–20 min). It can be used for short-term control of blood pressure in a hypertensive crisis, but can produce a marked tachycardia.

Mechanical support of the myocardium

Intra-aortic balloon counterpulsation (IABCP) is the technique used most widely for mechanical support of the failing myocardium. It is discussed on p. 657.

Adjunctive therapy in shock and sepsis

Attempts have been made to identify agents that would prevent the release, or inhibit the effects, of the various mediators released in shock. For example, non-steroidal anti-inflammatory drugs (NSAIDs), which inhibit cyclo-oxygenase, have been used to limit prostaglandin production. Naloxone has been used to block the effects of endogenous opioid peptides. PAF antagonists are available, and monoclonal antibodies to some of the cytokines or their receptors, as well as to endotoxin itself, have been developed and investigated. TNFα monoclonal antibodies, however, do not improve survival in septic shock. In animal studies very large doses of steroids have been shown to reduce mortality in septic shock, but clinical trials in humans have shown that steroids are of no benefit and their administration to such patients is no longer recommended. Currently there is considerable interest in the ability of NO synthase inhibitors to reverse the vasodilatation associated with some forms of circulatory shock. Other approaches have included administration of prostacyclin and removal of mediators by plasma exhange/haemofiltration.

In the future, naturally occurring cytokine antagonists or their soluble receptors may prove useful. At present, however, the role of these various adjunctive therapies in clinical practice remains unclear.

FURTHER READING

Barton R, Cerra FB (1989) The hypermetabolism multiple organ failure syndrome. *Chest* **96**: 1153–1160.

Bone RC (1996) Immunologic dissonance: a continuing evolution in our understanding of the systemic inflammatory response syndrome (SIRS) and the multiple organ dysfunction syndrome (MODS). *Annals of Internal Medicine* **125**: 680–687.

Bone RC, Sprung CL, Sibbald WJ (1992) Definitions for sepsis and organ failure. *Critical Care Medicine* **20**: 724–726.

Forrester JS, Ganz W, Diamond G, McHugh T, Chonette DW, Swan HJC (1972) Thermodilution cardiac output determination with a single flow-directed catheter. *American Heart Journal* **83**: 306–311.

Moncada S, Higgs S (1993) The L-arginine–nitric oxide pathway. *New England Journal of Medicine* **329**: 2002–2012.

Parillo JE (1993) Pathogenetic mechanisms of septic shock. *New England Journal of Medicine* **328**: 1271–1473.

Rudis MI, Basha MA, Zarowitz BJ (1996) Is it time to reposition vasopressors and inotropes in sepsis? *Critical Care Medicine* **24**: 525–532.

Szabo C, Thiememann C (1994) Role of the active oxide in hemorrhagic traumatic and anaphylatic shock and thermal injury. *Shock* **2**:145–155.

Renal failure

Acute renal failure is a common and serious complication of critical illness which adversely affects the prognosis. The importance of preventing renal failure by rapid and effective resuscitation, as well as the avoidance of nephrotoxic drugs (especially NSAIDs), cannot be overemphasized. Shock and sepsis are the most common causes of acute renal failure in the critically ill, but it remains important to diagnose the cause of renal dysfunction and exclude reversible pathology, especially obstruction (see Chapter 9).

Oliguria is usually the first indication of renal impairment and should prompt immediate attempts to optimize cardiovascular function, particularly by expanding the circulating volume and restoring blood pressure to premorbid levels. Low-dose dopamine may be used to enhance renal blood flow and improve urine output, although the efficacy of this agent in preventing or reversing renal impairment is questionable. If these measures fail to reverse oliguria, some recommend administration of diuretics such as frusemide or mannitol. Currently frusemide infusions are most frequently employed (see Chapter 9).

If oliguria persists, it is important to reduce crystalloid intake and review drug doses. Continuous haemofiltration is indicated for fluid overload, electrolyte disturbances (especially hyperkalaemia), severe acidosis and, to a lesser extent, uraemia.

Intermittent haemodialysis has a number of disadvantages in the critically ill. In particular it is frequently complicated by hypotension and it may be difficult to remove sufficient volumes of fluid. Peritoneal dialysis is also frequently unsatisfactory in these patients and is contraindicated in those who have undergone intra-abdominal surgery. The use of continuous haemofiltration, usually with dialysis, is therefore preferred (see Chapter 9).

Respiratory failure

TYPES AND CAUSES

The respiratory system consists of a gas exchanging organ (the lungs) and a ventilatory pump (respiratory muscles/thorax), either or both of which can fail and precipitate respiratory failure. Respiratory failure occurs when pulmonary gas exchange is sufficiently impaired to cause hypoxaemia with or without hypercarbia. In practical terms, respiratory failure is present when the P_aO_2 is <8 kPa (60 mmHg) or the P_aCO_2 is >7 kPa (55 mmHg). It can be divided into:

- **type I** respiratory failure, in which the P_aO_2 is low and the P_aCO_2 is normal or low
- **type II** respiratory failure, in which the P_aO_2 is low and the P_aCO_2 is high.

Type I or '*acute hypoxaemic*' respiratory failure occurs with diseases that damage lung tissue, with hypoxaemia due to right-to-left shunts or $\dot{V}/\dot{Q}$ mismatch. Common causes include pulmonary oedema, pneumonia, ARDS and, in the chronic situation, pulmonary fibrosing alveolitis.

Type II or '*ventilatory failure*' occurs when alveolar ventilation is insufficient to excrete the volume of carbon dioxide being produced by tissue metabolism. Inadequate alveolar ventilation is due to reduced ventilatory effort, inability to overcome an increased resistance to ventilation, failure to compensate for an increase in deadspace and/or carbon dioxide production, or a combination of these factors. The most common cause is chronic obstructive pulmonary disease (COPD). Other causes include chest-wall deformities, respiratory muscle weakness (e.g. Guillain-Barré syndrome) and depression of the respiratory centre.

Deterioration in the mechanical properties of the lungs and/or chest wall increases the work of breathing and the oxygen consumption/carbon dioxide production of the respiratory muscles. The concept that respiratory muscle fatigue (either acute or chronic) is an important factor in the pathogenesis of respiratory failure is controversial.

Monitoring of respiratory failure

A clinical assessment of respiratory distress should be made on the following criteria (those marked with an asterisk may be indicative of respiratory muscle fatigue):

- the use of accessory muscles of respiration
- tachypnoea*
- tachycardia
- sweating
- pulsus paradoxus (rarely present)
- inability to speak
- asynchronous respiration (a discrepancy in the rate of movement of the abdominal and thoracic compartments)*
- paradoxical respiration (abdominal and thoracic compartments move in opposite directions)*
- respiratory alternans (breath-to-breath alteration in the relative contribution of intercostal/accessory muscles and the diaphragm)*.

This can be supplemented by measuring tidal volume and vital capacity. Blood gas analysis should be performed to guide oxygen therapy and to provide an objective assessment of respiratory function. The most sensitive clinical indicator of increasing respiratory difficulty is a rising respiratory rate. Tidal volume is a less sensitive indicator.

Minute ventilation rises initially in acute respiratory failure and falls precipitously only at a late stage when the patient is exhausted. Vital capacity is often a better guide to deterioration and is particularly useful in patients with respiratory inadequacy that is due to neuromuscular problems – such as the Guillain–Barré syndrome, in which the vital capacity decreases as weakness increases.

Pulse oximetry

Lightweight oximeters which measure the changing amount of light transmitted through pulsating arterial blood and provide a continuous, non-invasive assessment of S_aO_2 can be applied to an ear lobe or finger. These devices are reliable, easy to use and do not require calibration, although it is important to appreciate that pulse oximetry is not a very sensitive guide to changes in oxygenation. An S_aO_2 within normal limits in a patient receiving supplemental oxygen in no way excludes the possibility of hypoventilation. Readings may be inaccurate in those with poor peripheral perfusion.

Blood gas analysis

Automation of measurements can give a false impresson of reliability and accuracy and may lead to an uncritical acceptance of the results. Errors can result from malfunctioning of the analyser or incorrect sampling techniques. Care must be taken over the following:

- The sample should be analysed immediately or the syringe should be immersed in iced water (the end having first been sealed with a plastic cap) to prevent the continuing metabolism of white cells causing a reduction in PO_2 and a rise in PCO_2.
- The sample must be adequately anticoagulated to prevent clot formation within the analyser. However, excessive dilution of the blood with heparin, which is acidic, will significantly reduce its pH. Heparin (1000 i.u. mL^{-1}) should just fill the deadspace of the syringe, i.e. approximately 0.1 mL. This will adequately anticoagulate a 2 mL sample.
- Air almost inevitably enters the sample. The gas tensions within these air bubbles will equilibrate with those in the blood, thereby lowering the PCO_2 and usually raising the PO_2 of the sample. However, provided the bubbles are ejected immediately by inverting the syringe and expelling the air that rises to the top of the sample, their effect is insignificant.

Normal values of blood gas analysis are shown in Table 13.5. Interpretation of the results of blood gas analysis can be considered in two separate parts:

- disturbances of acid–base balance
- alterations in oxygenation.

Interpretation of results requires a knowledge of the history, the age of the patient, the inspired oxygen concentration and any other relevant treatment (e.g. the administration of sodium bicarbonate, and the ventilator settings for those on mechanical ventilation).

Disturbances of acid–base balance

The physiology of acid–base control is discussed on p. 616. Acid–base disturbances can be described in relation to the diagram illustrated in Fig 10.9 which shows P_aCO_2 plotted against arterial $[H^+]$.

Both acidosis and alkalosis can occur, each of which may be either metabolic (primarily affecting the bicarbonate component of the system) or respiratory (primarily affecting P_aCO_2). Compensatory changes may also be apparent. In clinical practice, arterial $[H^+]$ values *outside* the range 18–126 nmol L^{-1} (pH 6.9–7.7) are very rarely encountered.

Table 13.5
Blood gas values (normal ranges)

H^+	35–45 nmol L^{-1}	pH 7.35–7.45
PO_2	10–13.3 kPa	(75–100 mmHg)
PCO_2	4.8–6.1 kPa	(36–46 mmHg)
Plasma HCO_3	22–26 mmol L^{-1}	
O_2 saturation	95–100%	

Respiratory acidosis. This is caused by retention of carbon dioxide. The P_aCO_2 and $[H^+]$ rise. A chronically raised P_aCO_2 is compensated by renal retention of bicarbonate and the $[H^+]$ returns towards normal. A constant arterial bicarbonate concentration is then usually established within 5 days. This represents a primary respiratory acidosis with a compensatory metabolic alkalosis (see p. 850). Common causes of respiratory acidosis include ventilatory failure and COPD (type II respiratory failure where there is a high P_aCO_2 and a low P_aO_2 – see Chapter 12).

Respiratory alkalosis. In this case the reverse occurs and there is a fall in P_aCO_2 and $[H^+]$, often with a small reduction in bicarbonate concentration. If hypocarbia persists, some degree of renal compensation may occur, producing a metabolic acidosis, although in practice this is unusual. A respiratory alkalosis is often produced, intentionally or unintentionally, when patients are artificially ventilated; it may also be seen with hypoxaemic (type I) respiratory failure (see Chapter 12), spontaneous hyperventilation and in those living at high altitudes.

Metabolic acidosis (p. 620). This may be due to excessive acid production, most commonly lactic acid during an episode of shock or following cardiac arrest. A metabolic acidosis may also develop in chronic renal failure or in diabetic ketoacidosis. It can also follow the loss of bicarbonate from the gut, for example, or from the kidney in renal tubular acidosis. Respiratory compensation for a metabolic acidosis is usually slightly delayed because the blood–brain barrier initially prevents the respiratory centre from sensing the increased blood $[H^+]$. Following this short delay, however, the patient hyperventilates and 'blows off' carbon dioxide to produce a compensatory respiratory alkalosis. There is a limit to this respiratory compensation, since in practice values for P_aCO_2 less than about 1.4 kPa (11 mmHg) are never achieved. It should also be noted that respiratory compensation cannot occur if the patient's ventilation is controlled or if the respiratory centre is depressed, for example by drugs or head injury.

Metabolic alkalosis. This can be caused by loss of acid, for example from the stomach with nasogastric suction, or in high intestinal obstruction, or excessive administration of absorbable alkali. Overzealous treatment with intravenous sodium bicarbonate is frequently implicated. Respiratory compensation for a metabolic alkalosis is often slight, and it is rare to encounter a P_aCO_2 above 6.5 kPa (50 mmHg), even with severe alkalosis.

Alterations in oxygenation

When interpreting the P_aO_2, remember that it is the oxygen content of the arterial blood that is most important and that this is determined by the percentage saturation of haemoglobin with oxygen. The relationship between the latter and the P_aO_2 is determined by the oxyhaemoglobin dissociation curve. In general, if the saturation is greater than 90%, oxygenation can be considered to be adequate. It must be remembered, however, that on the steep portion of the oxygen dissociation curve small falls in P_aO_2 will cause significant reductions in oxygen content. P_aO_2 is also influenced by factors other than pulmonary function, including alterations in $P_{\bar{v}}O_2$ caused by changes in the metabolic rate and/or cardiac output.

Management of respiratory failure

Conventional management of patients with respiratory failure includes the administration of supplemental oxygen, the control of secretions, the treatment of pulmonary infection, the control of airways obstruction, and measures to limit pulmonary oedema. The load on the respiratory muscles should be reduced by improving lung mechanics and controlling fever. Correction of abnormalities which may lead to respiratory muscle weakness, such as hypophosphataemia and malnutrition, is also important.

Oxygen therapy

Methods of oxygen administration

Oxygen is initially given via a face mask. In the majority of patients (except patients with COPD and chronically elevated P_aCO_2) the concentration of oxygen given is not important and oxygen can therefore be given by a simple face mask or nasal cannulae (Fig 13.18).

With these devices the inspired oxygen concentration varies from about 35% to 55%, with oxygen flow rates of between 6 and 10 L min^{-1}. Nasal cannulae are often preferred because they are less claustrophobic and do not interfere with feeding or speaking, but they can cause ulceration of the nasal or pharyngeal mucosa. Fig 13.18 should be compared with the fixed performance mask shown in Fig 12.26, with which the oxygen concentration can be controlled. It is vital to use this latter type of mask in patients with COPD with chronic type II failure.

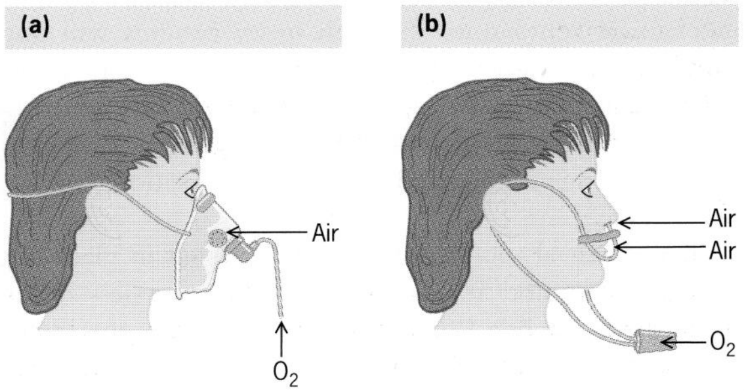

Fig 13.18
Methods of administering supplemental oxygen to the unintubated patient. (a) Simple face mask. **(b)** Nasal cannulae

Oxygen toxicity

Experimentally, mammalian lungs have been shown to be damaged by continuous exposure to high concentrations of oxygen, but oxygen toxicity in humans is less well proven. Nevertheless, it is reasonable to assume that high concentrations of oxygen might damage the lungs, and so the lowest inspired oxygen concentration compatible with adequate arterial oxygenation should be used. Long-term administration of 50% oxygen or less, or of 100% oxygen for less than 24 hours, is probably safe. Dangerous hypoxia should never be tolerated through a fear of oxygen toxicity.

Respiratory support

If, despite the above measures, the patient continues to deteriorate or fails to improve, the institution of some form of respiratory support should be considered. Some of the techniques of respiratory support currently available are shown in Table 13.6.

Negative-pressure ventilation is occasionally employed for long-term ventilation of patients with chronic respiratory failure due to neuromuscular disease or skeletal deformity. The patient's body is enclosed in an airtight 'tank' within which a negative pressure is created intermittently by a separate pump. Cuirass ventilators encase only the thorax.

Table 13.6
Techniques for respiratory support

Technique	Comments
Non-invasive positive pressure ventilation	
Volume mechanical ventilation	Ventilator delivers a set volume for each breath. Patient tolerance poor.
Positive mechanical ventilation	Set pressure but volumes vary
Bilevel positive airway pressure (bilevel PAP)	Inspiratory and expiratory pressures can be set separately. In spontaneous mode responds to patient's own flow rate
Continuous positive airway pressure (CPAP)	Constant pressure but can vary volumes
Invasive positive pressure ventilation	
Intermittent positive-pressure ventilation (IPPV)	May be given with positive end-expiratory pressure (PEEP)
Continuous positive airway pressure (CPAP)	Given via an endotracheal tube
Intermittent mandatory ventilation (IMV)	May be given with PEEP
High-frequency jet ventilation (HFJV)	May be useful in those with lung leak (e.g. bronchopleural fistula)
Low-volume pressure-limited inverse-ratio mechanical ventilation with low-level PEEP	May achieve improved oxygenation whilst minimizing peak airway pressure
Extracorporeal respiratory assistance	Reduces ventilation requirements and 'rests' the lungs

Non-invasive ventilation

This does not require an endotracheal tube and positive pressure ventilation is delivered through a nasal or face mask. Table 13.6 shows the techniques available. Their main use is in acute or chronic respiratory failure and cardiac failure. The patient must be conscious and cooperative for this technique to work well.

Intermittent positive-pressure ventilation (IPPV)

This is achieved by intermittently inflating the lungs with a positive pressure delivered by a ventilator and applied via an endotracheal tube or a tracheostomy.

A number of refinements and modifications of IPPV have been introduced, including IPPV with positive end-expiratory pressure (PEEP), intermittent mandatory ventilation (IMV), and low-volume pressure-limited inverse-ratio ventilation. Other techniques include high-frequency jet ventilation (HFJV) and extracorporeal respiratory assistance. These techniques are discussed later in this chapter.

The rational use of IPPV depends on a clear understanding of its potential beneficial effects, as well as its dangers.

Beneficial effects of IPPV

Improved carbon dioxide elimination. By adjusting the volume of ventilation, the P_aCO_2 can be returned to within normal limits.

Relief from exhaustion. Artificial ventilation removes the work of breathing and relieves the extreme exhaustion that may be present in patients with respiratory failure. In some cases, if ventilation is not instituted, this exhaustion may culminate in respiratory arrest.

Effects on oxygenation. In those with severe pulmonary parenchymal disease, the lungs may be very stiff and the work of breathing is therefore greatly increased. Under these circumstances the institution of IPPV may significantly reduce total body oxygen consumption; consequently $P_{\bar{v}}O_2$ – and thus P_aO_2 – may improve. Because ventilated patients are connected to a leak-free circuit, it is possible to administer high concentrations of oxygen (up to 100%) accurately and to apply a positive end-expiratory pressure. In selected cases the latter may reduce shunting and increase P_aO_2 (see below).

Indications for IPPV

Acute respiratory failure, with signs of severe respiratory distress (e.g. respiratory rate >40 min^{-1}, inability to speak, patient exhausted) persisting despite maximal therapy. Confusion, restlessness, agitation, a decreased conscious level, a rising P_aCO_2 (>8 kPa) and extreme hypoxaemia (<8 kPa) are further indications. Care should be taken before ventilating patients with chronic lung disease as patients previously severely incapacitated will be difficult to wean off the ventilator and also relapse early. The most important criteria are the patient's previous exercise tolerance and ability to lead an independent existence.

Acute ventilatory failure due, for example, to myasthenia gravis or Guillain–Barré syndrome. Artificial ventilation should be instituted when the vital capacity has fallen to 10–15 mL kg^{-1}. This will avoid complications such as atelectasis and infection as well as preventing respiratory arrest. The tidal volume and respiratory rate are relatively insensitive in the above conditions and change late in the course of the disease. A high P_aCO_2 (particularly if rising) is an indication for urgent artificial ventilation.

Other indications include:

- prophylactic postoperative ventilation in poor-risk patients
- head injury – to avoid hypoxia and hypercarbia which increase cerebral blood flow and intracranial pressure, hyperventilation to reduce intracranial pressure
- trauma – chest injury and lung contusion
- severe left ventricular failure with pulmonary oedema
- coma with breathing difficulties, e.g. following drug overdose.

Institution of IPPV

IPPV requires endotracheal intubation. If the patient is conscious the procedure must be fully explained before anaesthesia is induced. The complications of endotracheal intubation are given in Table 13.7.

Intubating patients in severe respiratory failure is an extremely hazardous undertaking and *should only be performed by experienced staff.* In extreme emergencies it may be preferable to ventilate the patient by hand using an oropharyngeal airway, a face mask and a self-inflating bag until experienced help arrives.

The patient is usually hypoxic and hypercarbic, with increased sympathetic activity, and the stimulus of laryngoscopy and intubation can precipitate dangerous arrhythmias and even cardiac arrest. Except in an extreme emergency, therefore, the ECG and oxygen saturation should be monitored, and the patient preoxygenated with 100% oxygen before intubation. If time allows, the circulating volume should be optimized and, if necessary, inotropes commenced before attempting intubation. In some cases it may be appropriate to establish intra-arterial and central venous pressure monitoring before instituting mechanical ventilation, although many patients will not tolerate the supine or head-down position. In some deeply comatose patients, no sedation will be required, but in the majority of patients a short-acting intravenous anaesthetic agent followed by muscle relaxation will be necessary.

Endotracheal tubes can now safely be left in place for several weeks and tracheostomy is therefore less often performed. Tracheostomy may be required for the long-term control of excessive bronchial secretions, particularly in those with a reduced conscious level, and/or to maintain an airway and protect the lungs in those with impaired pharyngeal and laryngeal reflexes.

Table 13.7
Complications of endotracheal intubation

Complication	Comments
Immediate	
Tube in one or other (usually the right) bronchus	Avoid by checking both lungs are being inflated; i.e. both sides of thechest move and air entry is heard on auscultation Obtain X-ray to check position of tube and to exclude lung collapse
Tube is in oesophagus	Gives rise to hypoxia and abdominal distension
Early	
Migration of the tube out of the trachea	
Leaks around the tube	
Obstruction of tube due to kinking or secretions	*A dangerous complication* The patient becomes distressed, cyanosed and has poor chest expansion The following should be performed immediately: • Manual inflation with 100% oxygen • Endotracheal suction • Check position of tube • Deflate cuff • Check tube for 'kinks' If no improvement, ventilate with face mask and then insert new endotracheal tube
Late	
Mucosal oedema and ulceration	
Damage to the crico-arytenoid cartilages	
Tracheal narrowing and fibrosis	

Tracheostomy can be performed surgically, the trachea being opened through the second, third and fourth tracheal rings via a small transverse skin incision, or percutaneously using a guidewire and a series of dilators.

A life-threatening obstruction of the upper respiratory tract that cannot be bypassed with an endotracheal tube should have a cricothyroidotomy, which is safer, quicker and easier to perform than a formal tracheostomy. Percutaneous tracheostomy may also be a useful means of rapidly securing the airway in an emergency. Other indications are head and neck injuries, including burns to the face and upper airway.

Tracheostomy has a mortality rate of up to 3%. Complications of tracheostomy are shown in Table 13.8.

Minitracheostomy involves inserting a small-diameter uncuffed tube percutaneously into the trachea via the cricothyroid membrane using a guidewire. It can be performed under local anaesthesia. This technique facilitates the clearance of copious secretions in those who are unable to cough effectively but can protect their airway.

Table 13.8
Complications of tracheostomy

As for endotracheal intubation (Table 13.7), plus:

Early

Surgical complications
- Pneumothorax
- Haemorrhage

Tube misplaced in pretracheal subcutaneous tissues
Subcutaneous emphysema

Intermediate

Erosion of tracheal cartilages (may cause tracheo-oesophageal fistula)
Erosion of innominate artery (may lead to fatal haemorrhage)
Infection

Late

Tracheal stenosis at level of stoma, cuff or tube tip
Collapse of tracheal rings at level of stoma

Dangers of IPPV

Airway complications. There may be complications with endotracheal intubation or tracheostomy.

Disconnection, failure of gas or power supply, mechanical faults. These are unusual but dangerous. A method of manual ventilation, such as a self-inflating bag, and oxygen must always be available by the bedside.

Cardiovascular complications. The intermittent application of positive pressure to the lungs and thoracic wall impedes venous return and distends alveoli, thereby 'stretching' the pulmonary capillaries and causing a rise in pulmonary vascular resistance. Both these mechanisms can produce a fall in cardiac output.

In *normal subjects*, the fall in cardiac output is prevented by constriction of capacitance vessels, which restores venous return. Hypovolaemia, pre-existing pulmonary hypertension, right ventricular failure and autonomic dysfunction (as may be present in those with Guillain–Barré syndrome, acute spinal cord injury or diabetes) will exacerbate the haemodynamic disturbance. Expansion of the circulating volume, on the other hand, can often restore cardiac output.

In *patients with heart failure*, cardiac output and blood pressure are usually unaffected, or even increased by positive pressure ventilation. Therefore, IPPV should be used without hesitation in patients with cardiogenic pulmonary oedema who have severe respiratory distress and exhaustion.

Respiratory complications. IPPV is frequently complicated by a deterioration in gas exchange due to $\dot{V}/\dot{Q}$ mismatch and collapse of peripheral alveoli. The latter can largely be prevented by using high tidal volumes (10–15 $mL\ kg^{-1}$) and reducing the respiratory rate (usually to 10–12 min^{-1}) to avoid hypocarbia, or by the application of positive end-expiratory pressure (PEEP – see below). Secondary pulmonary infection is a common complication in ventilated patients, and high inflation pressures, with overdistension of compliant alveoli, can disrupt the alveolar–capillary membrane and reduce surfactant activity, leading to 'ventilator-induced lung injury'.

Barotrauma. Overdistention of the lungs during IPPV can rupture alveoli and cause air to dissect centrally along the perivascular sheaths. This pulmonary interstitial air can sometimes be seen on chest X-ray as linear or circular perivascular collections or subpleural blebs. Other complications are pneumothorax, pneumomediastinum, pneumoperitoneum and subcutaneous emphysema. Intra-abdominal air originating from the alveoli is probably always associated with pneumomediastinum. The incidence of barotrauma is greatest in those patients who require high inflation pressures, with or without a positive end-expiratory pressure, and the risk of pneumothorax is increased in those with destructive lung disease (e.g. necrotizing pneumonia, emphysema), asthma or fractured ribs. A tension pneumothorax can be rapidly fatal in ventilated patients with respiratory failure. Suggestive signs include the development or worsening of hypoxia, fighting the ventilator, an unexplained increase in inflation pressure, as well as hypotension and tachycardia, sometimes accompanied by a rising CVP. Examination may reveal unequal chest expansion, mediastinal shift (deviated trachea, displaced apex beat) and a hyperresonant hemithorax. Although, traditionally, breath sounds are diminished over the pneumothorax, this sign can be extremely misleading in ventilated patients. If there is time, the diagnosis can be confirmed by chest X-ray.

Gastrointestinal complications. Initially, many artifically ventilated patients will develop abdominal distension associated with an ileus. The cause is unknown, although the use of non-depolarizing neuromuscular blocking agents and opiates may in part be responsible.

Salt and water retention. IPPV, particularly with PEEP, causes increased ADH secretion and possibly a reduction in circulating levels of atrial natriuretic peptide. Combined with a fall in cardiac output and a reduction in renal blood flow, these can cause salt and water retention. This fluid retention is often particularly noticeable in the lungs.

Positive end-expiratory pressure (PEEP)

A positive airway pressure can be maintained at a chosen level throughout expiration by attaching a threshold resistor valve to the expiratory limb of the circuit. PEEP should be considered if it proves impossible to achieve adequate oxygenation of arterial blood (more than 90% saturation) using conventional positive-pressure ventilation without raising the inspired oxygen concentration to potentially dangerous levels (conventionally 50%). PEEP is not, however, a panacea for all patients who are hypoxic. Indeed, it may often be detrimental, not least because the use of levels of PEEP in excess of 5 cmH_2O is associated with an increased risk of barotrauma. Most recommend that end-expiratory pressures in excess of 15–20 cmH_2O should not be exceeded.

The primary effect of PEEP is to re-expand underventilated lung units, thereby reducing shunts and increasing the P_aO_2. Unfortunately, however, the inevitable rise in mean intrathoracic pressure that follows the application of PEEP may further impede venous return, increase pulmonary vascular resistance and thus reduce cardiac output. This effect is probably least when the lungs are stiff. The fall in cardiac output can be ameliorated by expanding the circulating volume, although in some cases inotropic support may be required. Thus, although arterial oxygenation is often improved by the application of PEEP, a simultaneous fall in cardiac output can lead to a reduction in total oxygen delivery.

OTHER TECHNIQUES FOR RESPIRATORY SUPPORT

Continuous positive airway pressure (CPAP)

The application of CPAP achieves for the spontaneously breathing patient what PEEP does for the ventilated patient. Oxygen and air are delivered under pressure via an endotracheal tube or via a tightly fitting face mask. Not only can this improve oxygenation, but the lungs become less stiff, breathing becomes easier and vital capacity improves.

Intermittent mandatory ventilation (IMV)

This technique allows the patient to breathe spontaneously between the 'mandatory' tidal volumes delivered by the ventilator. It is important that these mandatory breaths are timed to coincide with the patient's own inspiratory effort (synchronized IMV, or SIMV). SIMV can be used with or without PEEP or CPAP. It was originally introduced as a technique for weaning patients from artificial ventilation but is now used extensively as an alternative to conventional IPPV. Spontaneous respiration may be assisted during SIMV by applying a constant preset positive airway pressure, triggered by the patient's spontaneous inspiratory effort, for a given fraction of the inspiratory time or until flow decreases below a specified level ('pressure support'). The level of pressure support can be reduced as the patient improves.

High-frequency jet ventilation (HFJV)

Adequate oxygenation and CO_2 elimination can be achieved by injecting gas into the trachea at rates of up to several thousand breaths per minute. In clinical practice, rates of between 100 and 200 breaths per minute are usually employed. Potential advantages of HFJV are largely related to the low peak airway pressures; for example, the risk of barotrauma and ventilator-induced lung injury may be reduced. Moreover, HFJV can be used to ventilate patients with large air leaks that are due, for example, to a bronchopleural fistula or lung lacerations. The place of HFJV in the management of patients with acute respiratory failure is less clear.

Low-volume pressure-limited inverse-ratio mechanical ventilation

A constant preset inspiratory pressure is delivered for a prescribed time, generating low tidal volumes and reducing peak inspiratory pressure. Respiratory rate is increased in order to achieve adequate CO_2 removal. When combined with a prolonged inspiratory time and low-level PEEP, this technique may provide optimal oxygenation whilst minimizing high peak airway pressures. Hypercarbia is almost inevitable but is generally well-tolerated and should be accepted ('permissive hypercarbia').

Extracorporeal respiratory assistance

Extracorporeal gas exchange can be used to reduce ventilation requirements and 'rest' the lungs. Carbon dioxide is removed using low-flow venovenous bypass through a membrane lung. The combination of preserved pulmonary perfusion and minimum ventilation may reduce barotrauma and provide optimal conditions for lung healing. The precise indications for the use of this demanding technique remain unclear.

Weaning

The respiratory muscles eventually become weak and uncoordinated as they perform no work during conventional mechanical ventilation. Moreoever, there is usually some persisting abnormality of lung function. Thus, in some patients who have been artificially ventiliated for any length of time, spontaneous respiration usually has to be resumed gradually.

Critical illness polyneuropathy

This acquired polyneuropathy has most often been described in association with persistent sepsis and multiple organ dysfunction syndrome (MODS). It is characterized by a primary axonal degeneration involving both motor and, to a lesser extent, sensory nerves. Clinically the initial manifestation is often difficulty in weaning the patient from respiratory support. There is muscle wasting, the limbs are weak and flaccid, and deep tendon reflexes are reduced or absent. Cranial nerves are relatively spared. Nerve conduction studies confirm axonal damage. The cerebrospinal fluid (CSF) protein concentration is normal or minimally elevated. These findings differentiate critical illness neuropathy from Guillain–Barré syndrome, in which nerve conduction studies show evidence of demyelination and CSF protein is usually high (see Chapter 18).

The cause of critical illness polyneuropathy is not known and there is no specific treatment. With resolution of the underlying critical illness, recovery can be expected after 1–6 months, although weaning from respiratory support and rehabilitation are likely to be prolonged.

Critical illness can also be complicated by various abnormalities of muscle, including a severe quadriplegic myopathy.

Criteria for weaning patients from artificial ventilation

Clinical assessment is of paramount importance when deciding whether a patient can be weaned from the ventilator. The patient's consciousness level, psychological state, metabolic function, the effects of drugs, cardiovascular performance and mechanical factors must all be taken into account. Objective criteria are based on an assessment of pulmonary gas exchange (blood gas analysis), lung mechanics and muscular strength.

Techniques for weaning

Patients who have received artificial ventilation for less than 24 hours – for example, elective IPPV after major surgery – can usually resume spontaneous respiration immediately and no weaning process is required. This procedure can also be adopted for those who have been ventilated for longer periods but who clearly fulfil the objective criteria for weaning.

- The *traditional* method of weaning in difficult cases is to allow the patient to breathe entirely spontaneously for a short time, following which IPPV is reinstituted. The periods of spontaneous breathing are gradually increased and the periods of IPPV are reduced. Initially it is usually advisable to ventilate the patient throughout the night. This method can be stressful and tiring for both patients and staff, although some patients do not tolerate SIMV (see below) and the traditional method of weaning may then be necessary.
- SIMV can be used to provide a smoother, more controlled method of weaning. It may also enable weaning to commence at an earlier stage than is possible using the traditional method. The application of inspiratory pressure support is often used in combination with SIMV (see above).
- The application of CPAP can prevent the alveolar collapse, hypoxaemia and fall in compliance that might otherwise occur when patients start to breathe spontaneously. It is therefore often used during weaning with IMV and in spontaneously breathing patients prior to extubation, particularly when they were previously receiving IPPV with PEEP.

Extubation

This should not be considered until patients can cough, swallow, protect their own airway and are sufficiently alert to be cooperative. Patients are assessed on their ability to breathe spontaneously via the endotracheal tube over a period of time. In those who have undergone prolonged artificial ventilation, this period may need to be 24–48 hours, or even longer, while patients ventilated for less than 12–24 hours can often be extubated within 10–15 minutes. During this 'trial of spontaneous respiration' the patient should be observed closely for any signs of respiratory distress.

FURTHER READING

Brochard L, Rauss A, Benito S, et al (1994) Comparison of three methods of gradual withdrawal from ventilatory support during weaning from mechanical ventilation. *American Journal of Respiratory Critical Care Medicine* **150**: 896–903.

Hillberg RE, Johnson DC (1997) Noninvasive ventilation. *New England Journal of Medicine* **337**: 1746–1752.

Acute respiratory distress syndrome

DEFINITION AND CAUSES (see Table 13.9)

Acute respiratory distress syndrome (ARDS) is defined as diffuse pulmonary infiltrates, refractory hypoxaemia, stiff lungs and respiratory distress following a recognized precipitating cause. A PAOP less than 16 mmHg is often included in the definition in an attempt to exclude cardiogenic pulmonary oedema. ARDS can occur as a nonspecific reaction of the lungs to a wide variety of direct and indirect pulmonary insults, including shock (especially septic shock). Hypotension alone is not an important cause of ARDS. By far the commonest predisposing factor is sepsis, and 20–40% of patients with severe sepsis will develop ARDS. Pneumonia is a common complication of ARDS.

Table 13.9
Disorders associated with acute respiratory distress syndrome

Shock	Especially septic shock
Trauma	Lung contusion Fat embolism Blast injury Severe non-thoracic trauma
Infection	Sepsis Pneumonia
Pulmonary aspiration	Gastric contents Near drowning
Inhalation injury	Smoke Corrosive gases
Haematological	Massive blood transfusion Disseminated intravascular coagulation
Obstetric	Amniotic fluid embolism
Drug overdose	Heroin Barbiturates
Miscellaneous	Cardiopulmonary bypass Pancreatitis High altitude

Pathogenesis and pathophysiology of ARDS

ARDS can be considered as the earliest manifestation of a generalized inflammatory response and is therefore frequently associated with the development of MODS.

Non-cardiogenic pulmonary oedema

This is the cardinal feature of ARDS and is the first and clinically most evident sign of a generalized increase in vascular permeability caused by the microcirculatory changes and release of inflammatory mediators described previously (see p. 834). The pulmonary epithelium is also damaged in the early stages of ARDS, reducing surfactant production and lowering the threshold for alveolar flooding.

Pulmonary hypertension

This is a common feature of ARDS. Initially, mechanical obstruction of the pulmonary circulation may occur as a result of vascular compression by interstitial oedema and subsequently oedema of the vessel wall itself. Later, constriction of the pulmonary vasculature may develop in response to increased autonomic nervous activity and circulating substances such as catecholamines, serotonin $PGF_{2\alpha}$, thromboxane and complement. Those vessels supplying alveoli with low oxygen tensions constrict (the 'hypoxic vasoconstrictor response'), diverting pulmonary blood flow to better oxygenated areas of lung, thus limiting the degree of shunt.

Haemorrhagic intra-alveolar exudate

This is rich in platelets, fibrin, fibrinogen and clotting factors; fibrin and fibronectin are deposited along the alveolar ducts with the incorporation of cellular debris. This exudate may inactivate surfactant and stimulate inflammation, as well as promoting hyaline membrane formation.

Fibrosis

Within seven days of the onset of ARDS, formation of a new epithelial lining is under way and activated fibroblasts accumulate in the interstitial spaces. Subsequently, interstitial fibrosis progresses, with loss of elastic tissue and obliteration of the lung vasculature, together with lung destruction and emphysema.

Physiological changes

Shunt and deadspace increase, compliance falls, and there is evidence of airflow limitation. Although the lungs in ARDS are diffusely injured, the pulmonary lesions, when identified as densitites on a CT scan, are predominantly located in dependent regions. This is probably explained by the effects of gravity on the distribution of extravascular lung water and areas of lung collapse.

Clinical presentation of ARDS

The first sign of the development of ARDS is often an unexplained tachypnoea, followed by increasing hypoxaemia, dyspnoea and laboured breathing. Fine crackles are heard throughout both lung fields. Later, the chest X-ray shows bilateral diffuse shadowing, interstitial at first, but subsequently with an alveolar pattern and air bronchograms that may then progress to the picture of complete 'white-out' (Fig 13.19).

Management of ARDS

This is based on treatment of the underlying condition (e.g. eradication of sepsis) and supportive measures. Because conventional methods of mechanical ventilation expose the lung to high airway pressure, especially when combined with high levels of PEEP, it is now widely accepted that techniques of respiratory support which minimize airway pressure (e.g. SIMV and pressure-limited ventilation) should be used in patients with ARDS.

Pulmonary oedema limitation. Pulmonary oedema formation should be limited by minimizing left ventricular filling pressure with fluid restriction, the use of diuretics and, if these measures fail to prevent fluid overload, by haemofiltration. The aim should be to achieve a consistently negative fluid balance. If possible plasma oncotic pressure should be maintained by administering colloidal solutions with a long half-life. In patients with ARDS, however, colloids are unlikely to be retained within the vascular compartment; once they enter the interstitial space, the transvascular oncotic gradient is lost and the main determinants of interstitial oedema formation become the microvascular hydrostatic pressure and lymphatic drainage. There is therefore some controversy concerning the relative merits of colloids or crystalloids for volume replacement in patients likely to develop ARDS, or in whom the condition is established. Cardiovascular support and the reduction of oxygen requirements are also important.

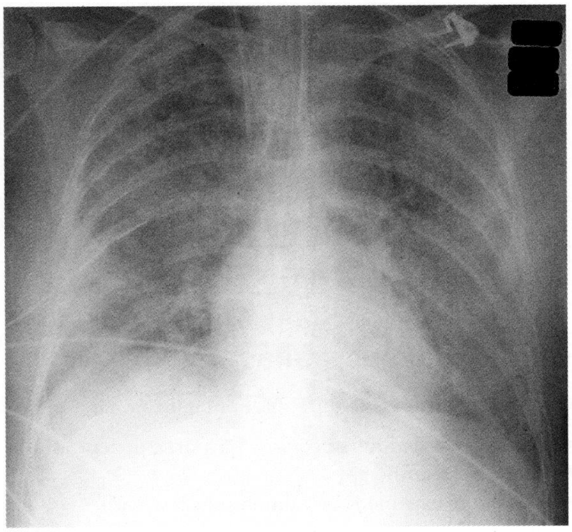

Fig 13.19
Chest radiograph appearances in adult respiratory distress syndrome. Bilateral diffuse alveolar shadowing with air bronchograms and no cardiac enlargement

Body position changes. When the patient is changed from the supine to the prone position, lung densities in the dependent regions are redistributed and gas exchange may improve. Repeated position changes between prone and supine may therefore allow reductions in airway pressures and the inspired oxygen concentration.

High-dose steroids. Administration of high-dose steroids to a patient with established ARDS does not appear to improve outcome, and current evidence suggests that prophylactic administration to those at risk of developing ARDS is of no value. They may, however, be beneficial when administered during the late fibroproliferative phase of ARDS.

Inhaled nitric oxide. This vasodilator, when inhaled, can improve $\dot{V}/\dot{Q}$ matching and oxygenation by increasing perfusion of ventilated lung units, as well as reducing pulmonary hypertension. Its role in the management of ARDS has yet to be established.

Aerosolized prostacylin. This appears to have similar effects to inhaled NO. As with inhaled NO, the response to aerosolized prostacyclin is, however, variable and its effect on outcome is unknown.

Aerosolized surfactant. Surfactant replacement therapy reduces morbidity and mortality in neonatal respiratory distress syndrome and is beneficial in animal models of ARDS. Its role in the management of ARDS is at present unclear.

PROGNOSIS

Despite the treatment outlined, the mortality from established severe ARDS remains high at more than 50% overall, although there is some evidence that mortality rates have fallen over the last decade. Prognosis is very dependent on aetiology. When ARDS occurs in association with septic shock, mortality rates may be as high as 90%, whereas in ARDS associated with fat embolism around 90% may survive. Approximately 40% of uncomplicated cases die, but the mortality rises with increasing age and failure of other organs such as kidneys and liver. Many of those dying with ARDS now do so as a result of MODS and haemodynamic instability rather than impaired gas exchange.

FURTHER READING

Kollef MH, Schoster DP (1995) The acute respiratory distress syndrome. *New England Journal of Medicine* **332**: 27–37.

Brain death

Brain death means 'the irreversible loss of the capacity for consciousness combined with the irreversible loss of the capacity to breathe'. Both these are essentially functions of the brain stem. Death, if thought of in this way, can arise either from causes outside the brain (i.e. respiratory and cardiac arrest) or from causes within the head. With the advent of artificial ventilation it became possible to support such a dead patient temporarily, although in all cases cardiovascular failure eventually supervenes and progresses to asystole.

Before considering a diagnosis of brain stem death it is essential that certain *preconditions* and *exclusions* are fulfilled.

Preconditions

- The patient must be in apnoeic coma (i.e. unresponsive and on a ventilator, with no spontaneous respiratory efforts).
- Irremediable structural brain damage due to a disorder that can cause brain stem death must have been diagnosed with certainty (e.g. head injury, intracranial haemorrhage).

Exclusions

- The possibility that unresponsive apnoea is the result of poison, sedative drugs or neuromuscular blocking agents must be excluded.
- Hypothermia must be excluded as a cause of coma. The central body temperature should be more than 35°C.
- There must be no significant metabolic or endocrine disturbance that could produce or contribute to coma or cause it to persist.
- There should be no profound abnormality of the plasma electrolytes, acid–base balance, or blood glucose levels.

Diagnostic tests for the confirmation of brain death

All brain stem reflexes are absent in brain death.

Tests

The following tests should not be performed in the presence of seizures or abnormal postures.

- The pupils are fixed and unresponsive to bright light. Both direct and consensual light reflexes are absent. The size of the pupils is irrelevant, although most often they will be dilated.
- Corneal reflexes are absent.
- Oculocephalic reflexes are absent: when the head is rotated from side to side, the eyes move with the head and therefore remain stationary relative to the orbit. In a comatose patient whose brain stem is intact, the eyes will rotate relative to the orbit (i.e. doll's eye movements will be present).
- There are no vestibulo-ocular reflexes on caloric testing (see p. 1025).
- There is no motor response within the cranial nerve territory to painful stimuli applied centrally or peripherally. Spinal reflexes may be present.
- There is no gag or cough reflex in response to pharyngeal, laryngeal or tracheal stimulation.
- Spontaneous respiration is absent. The patient should be ventilated with 5% CO_2 in 95% O_2 for 10 minutes and then disconnected from the ventilator for a further 10 minutes. Oxygenation is maintained by insufflation with 100% oxygen at high flow rates via a catheter placed in the endotracheal tube. The patient is observed for any signs of spontaneous respiratory efforts. A blood gas sample should be obtained during this period to ensure that the P_aCO_2 is sufficiently high to stimulate spontaneous respiration (>6.7 kPa (50 mmHg)).

The examination should be performed (and repeated after a few hours) by two doctors of senior status a minimum of 6 hours after the onset of coma or, if due to cardiac arrest, at least 24 hours after restoration of an adequate circulation.

In the UK it is not considered necessary to perform confirmatory tests such as EEG and carotid angiography, as these may be misleading.

In suitable cases, and provided the patient was carrying a donor card and/or the consent of relatives has been obtained, the organs of those in whom brain stem death has been established may be used for transplantation. In all cases in the UK the coroner's consent must be obtained.

FURTHER READING

Pallis C, Harley DH (1996) *ABC of Brain Death*, 2nd edn, BMJ Publishing Group.

General aspects of intensive care

Overall patient management

Critically ill patients require multidisciplinary care with:

- intensive skilled nursing care (1:1 nurse/patient ratio)
- regular physiotherapy
- careful management of pain and distress with analgesics and sedation as necessary
- constant reassurance and support (critically ill patients easily become disorientated and psychologically disturbed)

- nutritional support (enteral nutrition should always be used if possible; see p. 211)
- H_2-receptor antagonists to prevent stress-induced ulceration (they are generally used, but are probably unnecessary in the fed patient)
- TED stockings and subcutaneous heparin to prevent venous thrombosis.
- care of the mouth, prevention of constipation and of pressure sores.

Results, costs and patient selection

For many critically ill patients, intensive care is undoubtedly life-saving and resumption of a normal lifestyle is to be expected. In the most seriously ill patients, however, immediate mortality rates are high, a significant number die soon after discharge from the intensive care unit, and the quality of life for some of those who do survive may be poor. Moreover, intensive care is expensive, particularly for those with the worst prognosis.

Inappropriate use of intensive care facilities has other implications. The patient may experience unnecessary suffering and loss of dignity, while relatives may also have to endure considerable emotional pressures. In some cases treatment may simply prolong the process of dying, or sustain life of dubious quality, and in others the risk of interventions may outweigh the potential benefits.

Both for a humane approach to the management of critically ill patients and to ensure that limited resources are used appropriately, it is therefore important to avoid admitting patients who cannot benefit from intensive care and to limit further aggressive therapy when the prognosis is clearly hopeless. Currently decisions to limit therapy, or not to resuscitate in the event of cardiorespiratory arrest, are made jointly by the medical staff of the unit, the primary physician or surgeon and the nurses, normally in consultation with the patient's family.

Scoring systems

A variety of scoring systems have been developed that can be used to evaluate the severity of a patient's illness. These have included an assessment of the severity of the acute disturbance of physiological function (acute physiology, age, chronic health evaluation – APACHE) and a measure of the therapeutic effort expended on a patient (therapeutic intervention scoring system – TISS). Other systems have been designed for particular categories of patient (e.g. the injury severity score for trauma victims).

The APACHE score is widely applicable and has been extensively validated. It can quantify accurately the severity of illness and predict the overall mortality for large groups of critically ill patients, and is therefore useful when auditing a unit's clinical activity, for comparing results nationally or internationally, and as a means of characterizing groups of patients in clinical studies. Although the APACHE methodology can also be used to estimate individual risks of mortality, no scoring system has yet been devised that can predict with certainty the outcome in an individual patient. *They must not, therefore, be used in isolation as a basis for limiting or discontinuing treatment.*

FURTHER READING

Bion J (1995) Rationing intensive care. *British Medical Journal* **310**: 682–683.

Knaus WA, Wagner DP, Draper EA, et al. (1991) The APACHE III prognostic system: risk prediction of hospital mortality for critically ill hospitalized adults. *Chest* **100**: 1619–1636.

GENERAL FURTHER READING

Hinds CJ, Watson JD (1994) Intensive care: a concise textbook. London, Baillière Tindall.

Adverse drug reactions and poisoning

14

Adverse drug reactions

All drugs which have a proven therapeutic benefit may cause adverse effects. Despite this, a large number of effective drugs produce no adverse effects in the vast majority of patients who take them. This is in part due to the pressures on pharmaceutical companies to produce safe and effective medicines, but is also due to increasingly stringent governmental regulations which regulate the use of new drugs, and organizations which monitor the safety of existing compounds. New drugs are now subjected to a rigorous programme of preclinical and clinical testing before they are licensed for general use (Table 14.1), and are monitored for safety following licensing.

The size of the problem

Overall, approximately 10–20% of hospital inpatients suffer an adverse drug reaction. Up to 5% of hospital admissions are directly due to adverse drug reactions, and about 0.25–0.5% of deaths are attributable to treatment rather than the disease for which the drugs were being used. Unwanted effects of drugs are more common in elderly patients, rising from 3% in 10-–20-year-olds to 20% in patients aged over 80 years. The likelihood of adverse reactions increases sharply with the number of drugs administered (Fig 14.1),

Table 14.1
Evaluation of new drugs

Phase I: Healthy human subjects (usually men) First use in humans Approximately 100 subjects Evaluation of safety and toxicity Pharmacokinetic assessment Sometimes pharmacodynamic assessment	**Phase III: Use in wider patient population** Approximately 2000 patients (often multicentre trials) Efficacy main objective Safety and toxicity also carefully monitored
Phase II: First assessment in patients Approximately 500 subjects Safety and toxicity evaluated Dose range identified Pharmacokinetic and pharmacodynamic monitoring	**Phase IV: Postmarketing surveillance** All patients prescibed the drug are monitored (often very large numbers) Efficacy, safety and toxicity measured Quantification of unusual drug adverse effects Yellow card and Prescription Event monitoring

partly because such patients are likely to be more unwell, provoking a drug–host reaction, and partly because the potential for interaction between drugs increases in a factorial manner with each new drug added to the regimen.

Types of adverse drug reaction

There are two main types of adverse drug reaction:

- dose-dependent (also called type A, augmented, predictable)
- dose-independent (type B, bizzare, unpredictable, idiosyncratic).

Dose-dependent reactions

These often result from the known pharmacological effect of the drug and are increasingly likely as the dose is increased. Good examples of such reactions are gout resulting from treatment with a thiazide diuretic, or bone marrow suppression following therapy with methotrexate. As a general rule, dose-dependent reactions are less serious and rapidly resolve on stopping the drug. However, some dose-dependent reactions such as eighth-nerve damage with aminoglycoside antibiotics, or myocardial damage following doxorubicin therapy, are serious and largely irreversible. They are due to mechanisms that are not completely understood.

Dose-independent reactions

In these reactions there is a large variability between individuals in their susceptibility to an adverse effect; many different mechanisms operate, most of which are not understood. The adverse reactions are often serious and life-threatening; patients should be warned about particular symptoms suggestive of such an adverse reaction.

Percentage of patients with adverse drug reactions

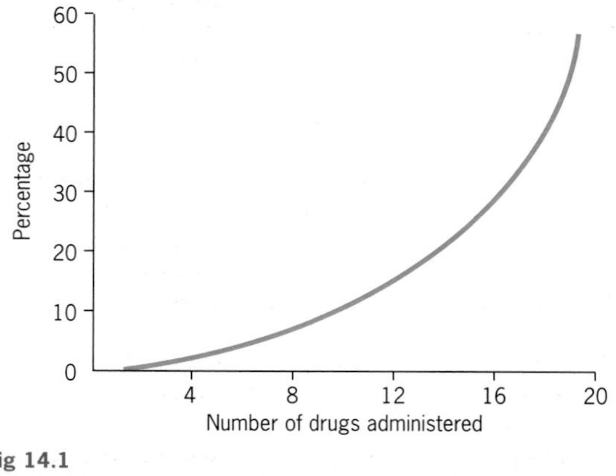

Fig 14.1
The tendency for the number of adverse drug reactions to increase with the number of drugs administered. After Smith JW et al (1966) *Annals of Internal Medicine* **65**: 631

Anaphylactic reactions (type 1 hypersensitivity)

These reactions are most common in patients with a history of anaphylaxis with drugs, foods (such as nuts) or insect stings, and in atopic individuals with a history of asthma and eczema.

Typically, anaphylaxis occurs on the second or third exposure to the drug, and may occur following administration of only very small amounts. The mechanism involves recognition of the drug (or a drug–protein complex) by IgE molecules on the surface of mast cells and subsequent degranulation with release of histamine and other inflammatory mediators.

The onset of the clinical syndrome of anaphylaxis is often dramatic and rapid. Prompt recognition and treatment can be lifesaving (Emergency box 14.1).

Penicillin antibiotics are notorious for causing anaphylaxis, even though the incidence of severe reactions is very low. Other likely causes are radiopaque contrast media, local anaesthetics and streptomycin.

Type II reactions (see also p. 183)

These reactions occur owing to interaction between the drug and a circulating or membrane-bound protein (see drug-induced haemolytic anaemia, p. 385) to cause production of a circulating antibody of the IgG or IgM

! Emergency

Usually follows injections or occasionally insect bites or nut ingestion

Clinical features (rapid and dramatic)
Bronchospasm causing breathlessness
Facial and laryngeal oedema
Hypotension causing dizziness and collapse
Nausea, vomiting and diarrhoea

Treatment

1. Lay the patient down and raise the feet.
2. Ensure the airway is free.
3. Monitor blood pressure.
4. Give (in following order):
   (a) 1.1 mL of 1 in 1000 adrenaline intramuscularly, and repeat after 10–20 minutes **if shock persists**
   (b) antihistamine (such as chlorpheniramine 10 mg) intravenously
   (c) hydrocortisone 100 mg intravenously.
5. **If hypotension persists,** give a rapid intravenous infusion of 1–2 L (colloid is better than crystalloid fluids).
6. **If hypoxia is severe,** oxygen or assisted ventilation may be necessary.

Emergency box 14.1 Anaphylactic shock

class, with subsequent complement activation. The most common target for this type of immune-mediated damage is the haematological system, resulting in Coomb's positive haemolytic anaemia (e.g. with methyldopa and penicillin) or thrombocytopenia (e.g. with quinine). It is likely that some examples of agranulocytosis or marrow aplasia are due to this mechanism of adverse reaction.

Type III (arthus, serum sickness or immune complex) reaction (see also p. 183)

This type of reaction used to occur most commonly following injection of foreign serum to treat infectious diseases (e.g. antitetanus serum). It also occurs with antibiotics such as penicillins, streptomycin and sulphonamides, as well as the antithyroid drugs propylthiouracil and carbimazole. It is thought to be caused by the formation of antibody–antigen complexes which lodge in the small blood vessels of the skin, kidney and joints, and may mimic systemic lupus erythematosus, in which such complexes are also found (see p. 487).

The classic clinical presentation occurs several days following starting therapy and includes fever, urticaria, arthropathy, lymphadenopathy and proteinuria. Eosinophilia is a common and diagnostically useful feature. Other skin rashes, particulary maculopapular in type, are also characteristic.

Type IV reactions (cell-mediated hypersensitivity) (see also p. 183)

The typical example of a type IV reaction is the contact dermatitis which is sometimes produced following application of antibiotic or other topical therapy on the skin. Again it is thought to be due to the formation of hapten–protein complexes which trigger a lymphocytic cellular immune reaction.

Pseudoallergic reactions

These reactions mimic those detailed above, but are not thought to involve immune recognition. Rather they are due to the release of immunological mediators by other mechanisms. They typically occur on first-time exposure to the drug rather than after previous sensitization. Examples of this type of reaction include:

- itching, bronchospasm and vasodilatation following treatment with intravenous morphine
- flushing, urticaria, bronchospasm and even circulatory shock caused by aspirin
- bronchospasm and hypotension caused by *N*-acetylcysteine used in the treatment of paracetamol poisoning – this occurs in approximately 5% of patients and responds to intravenous antihistamines.

Long-term adverse effects of drugs

Adverse effects which occur months or years after institution of a particular drug therapy may not obviously be connected with the agent responsible and will only be discovered by taking a careful drug history. Some of these long-term effects are dose-dependent and can be anticipated (e.g. movement disorders with neuroleptic agents), whereas others are idiosyncratic (e.g. pulmonary fibrosis with amiodarone). Table 14.2 details some of the more common or important long-term effects of drugs.

Carcinogenesis

Certain drugs which damage DNA predispose towards cancer. Many cancers are due to aquired defects in tumour supressor genes which limit cellular division (such as the *p53* gene, see p. 153), or oncogenes, which promote cellular growth. Most cytotoxic chemotherapy relies on its ability to damage DNA. The antitumour effect is achieved by stimulating the transcription of tumour supressor genes in normal cells, resulting in arrested cellular division, leaving tumour cells vulnerable to the effects of DNA damage. Whereas DNA damage is often repairable, cumulative damage due to cytotoxic drugs, environmental factors and genetic predisposition may allow disabling of sufficient regulatory systems to cause uncontrolled proliferation and cancer. Examples include the increase in risk of bladder cancer in patients taking cyclophosphamide, and of leukaemias in patients taking all types of alkylating agents.

Recognition of abnormal cells is one of the important functions of the immune system, and powerful immunosuppressant drugs such as cyclosporin have been linked with an increase in lymphomata (although this does not seem to be as large a problem as once feared).

Cancers of the breast and endometrium are known to be hormone-dependent. There is increasing evidence of a link between oestrogen and breast cancer, in addition to the established association between unopposed oestrogen therapy and endometrial cancer.

Table 14.2
Delayed and long-term adverse effects of drugs

Drug	Effect	Mechanism
Corticosteroids	Osteoporosis	Protein catabolism
Anticonvulsants	Megaloblastic anaemia	Folate antagonism
Amiodarone	Pulmonary fibrosis	Unknown
Neuroleptics	Movement disorders	Probably dopamine antagonism
Thiazide diuretics	Gout	Impaired urate excretion
Methysergide	Retroperitoneal fibrosis	Unknown
Cytotoxic drugs	Malignancy	DNA damage
Analgesics	Tubulointerstitial nephritis	Unknown
Methyldopa	Haemolytic anaemia	Immune stimulation
Hydralazine	SLE	Unknown

Factors predisposing to adverse effects

Prescribing factors

Serious and avoidable toxicity to patients is, and will continue to be, due to error. Common causes include:

- *errors in prescribing*, possibly arising from poor handwriting or doctor inattention (e.g. chlorpromazine instead of chlorpropamide, or milligrammes instead of microgrammes)
- *errors in dispensing*
- *errors in administration* (e.g. extravasation of intra-arterial injection of cytotoxic drugs)
- *wrong or insufficient advice given to the patient* – written information such as steroid cards or anticoagulant cards are very useful to prevent problems.

Drug interactions

Many patients in hospital are prescribed more than one drug. There are a very large number of potential drug interactions, only a handful of which are commonly found to cause serious problems (Table 14.3). Drugs can interact to cause either inhibition or potentiation of the effect of either component of the interaction. Interactions causing adverse effects are due to potentiation, and are conveniently grouped according to pharmaceutic, pharmacokinetic and pharmacodynamic mechanisms.

Pharmaceutic interaction

This is due to interaction between drugs while still outside the body, which leads to inactivation of one or both components. The incompatibility of infusion solutions can lead to precipitation or inactivation of one component. An example is the co-infusion of heparin and hydrocortisone leading to the inactivation of heparin

Pharmacokinetic interactions

These interactions can be subdivided into the familiar categories which describe the pharmacokinetic process – absorption, distribution, metabolism and elimination.

Absorption

Absorption of tetracyclines and iron supplements can be impaired by concurrent administration of calcium, aluminium and magnesium salts. Similarly, the bile salt binding resin cholestyramine will also bind with other drugs such as digoxin and warfarin and inhibit their absorption. Broad-spectrum antibiotics such as amoxycillin interfere with the normal gut bacterial flora which are important in both synthesizing vitamin K (thus causing a potentiation of the effect of warfarin) and the enterohepatic recycling of oestrogen, reducing the contraceptive effectiveness of this hormone.

Table 14.3
Common and potentially serious drug interactions

Drug	Interacting drug	Problem caused
Warfarin	Cimetidine Erythromycin Ciprofloxacin Imidazoles Sulphonamides	Uncontrolled bleeding
Theophylline	Cimetidine Erythromycin Ciprofloxacin	Convulsions Arrhythmias
Digoxin	Amiodarone Verapamil Quinidine Diuretics	Arrhythmias Heart block
β-Blockers	Verapamil Diltiazem	Bradycardia Asystole
Lithium	Thiazide diuretics	Ataxia Convulsions
Azathioprine Mercaptopurine	Allopurinol	Bone marrow failure
Phenytoin	Cimetidine Isoniazid Sulphonamides Imidazoles	Ataxia

Distribution

Displacement of one drug by another from its binding to a plasma protein or tissue can often be demonstrated in a test-tube, but only rarely does this mechanism lead to a clinically significant drug interaction. This is because the increased amount of free (unbound) drug is now available for metabolism or excretion and there is rapid re-establishment of previous unbound concentration of the drug.

The situations where clinically important interactions occur are when there is concomitant inhibition of metabolism or excretion alongside displacement from the binding sites. This appears to be the mechanism explaining the potentially serious interaction between quinidine and digoxin, whereby quinidine both displaces digoxin from its tissue binding site and impairs renal excretion.

Metabolism

Interference with liver metabolism is one of the most common causes of serious drug interactions. Drugs such as rifampicin and phenytoin, as well as alcohol, cause *induction* of cytochrome p450 enzymes, which are responsible for liver metabolism of most drugs, leading to more rapid destruction, reduced plasma concentrations and lack of effect of drugs which are metabolized by these enzymes, and consequent therapeutic failure (Table 14.4).

Serious drug interactions are often due to drugs which *inhibit* liver p450 enzymes. There are a limited number of such drugs, including cimetidine, erythromycin, ciprofloxacin and sodium valproate. Not all these drugs will inhibit all p450 isoenzymes, so such interactions are not entirely predictable. The important interactions in this category are given in Table 14.3. They involve drugs with a low therapeutic ratio, particularly warfarin, theophylline and phenytoin. Theophylline toxicity is commonly caused by co-administration of erythromycin or ciprofloxacin to patients with airflow obstruction and chest infection who are also prescribed theophylline or aminophylline.

Other enzymes responsible for drug metabolism can also be inhibited and result in drug interactions. The administration of the xanthine oxidase inhibitor allopurinol in patients treated with 6-mercaptopurine (6MP) or azathioprine – which is metabolized to 6MP – constitutes a potentially fatal combination as 6MP is itself metabolized by xanthine oxidase.

Monoamine oxidase is responsible for the intercellular degradation of, for example, monoamines, adrenaline, noradrenaline, dopamine and 5-hydroxytryptamine (serotonin). Its inhibition by monoamine oxidase inhibitors (MAOIs) can give rise to serious effects (Fig. 14.2).

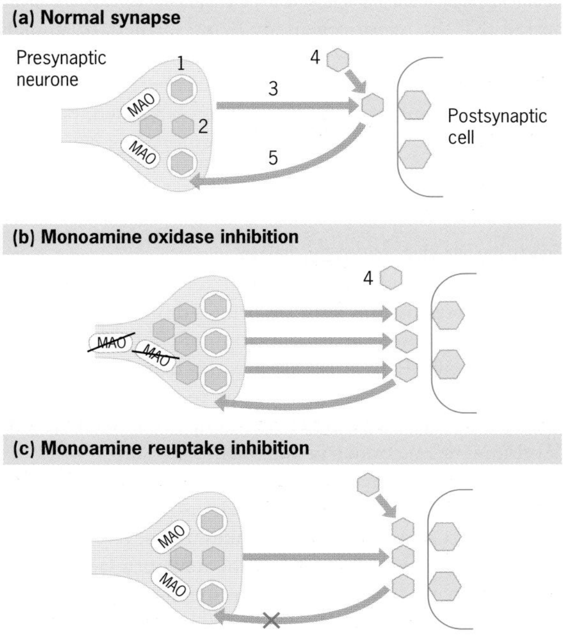

Fig 14.2
Mechanism by which monoamine oxidase inhibitors and monoamine reuptake inhibitors influence indirectly and directly acting sympathomimetic amines.
1. Granular store of catecholamine; 2. free cytoplasmic catecholamine; 3. catecholamine released into synaptic cleft by nerve impulse or indirectly acting amine such as ephedrine or tyramine; 4. exogenously administered, directly acting amine such as noradrenaline; 5. reuptake of catecholamine into the neurone, terminating its action.
(a) Normal synapse; **(b)** monoamine oxidase inhibition leads to increased catecholamine release by nerve impulse and potentiation of the effect, or sympathomimetic amine; **(c)** monoamine reuptake inhibition, e.g. tricyclics, leads to increased effects of transmitter or administered amine

Table 14.4
Cytochrome p450 enzyme-inducing drugs

Alcohol
Carbamazepine
Griseofulvin
Phenobarbitone
Phenytoin
Prednisolone
Rifampicin

Elimination

The inhibition of renal tubular excretion of benzylpencillin by probenecid has been used as a useful drug interaction, to increase the plasma concentration of pencillin. Harmful interactions can also be caused by inhibition of renal tubular transport, as is the case with aspirin and other non-steroidal analgesics reducing methotrexate and lithium excretion. Lithium excretion is also impaired by thiazide diuretics (and to a lesser extent loop diuretics) as a result of increased proximal reabsorption of monovalent cations in response to enhanced distal tubular excretion.

Pharmacodynamic interactions

The body's normal homeostatic mechanisms will often come into play to prevent a potential undesirable effect of a drug. When another drug is added which predisposes to the same unwanted effect by a different mechanism, it is much more likely that the undesired effect will happen. An example of this is the reduction in cardiac output resulting from treatment of angina with verapamil. Heart rate and contractility is maintained by upregulation of the sympathetic supply to the heart. If a β-adrenoreceptor blocker is added, then heart failure or symptomatic bradycardia may result.

A similar example is the profound hypotension that may follow the first dose of an ACE inhibitor in a patient with heart failure who is treated with a high dose of a loop diuretic. Blood pressure is normally maintained in patients on loop diuretics by activation of the renin-angiotensin system, which is suddenly withdrawn when ACE inhibitors are given.

Although the precise mechanisms are less clear, drugs which cause sedation or confusion will often have a synergistic effect. Well-known examples are the combination of alcohol and benzodiazepines, and of opiates and antipsychotics, leading to enhanced sedation.

Toxicity with digoxin is greatly enhanced by reduction in plasma potassium concentration, which is caused most commonly by treatment with loop and thiazide diuretics. Conversely, treatment with potassium-sparing diuretics such as amiloride or triamterene can cause serious toxicity (hyperkalaemia) when co-prescribed with ACE inhibitors.

Pregnancy

Pregnancy poses important problems. Most drugs will diffuse passively across the placenta, and some are transported actively, so the potential benefit of a drug to

Table 14.5
Common adverse effects of drugs in pregnancy

All drugs should be avoided in pregnancy unless benefit clearly outweighs risk

Drug	Effect
ACE inhibitors	Renal damage and oligohydramnios
Retinoic acid derivatives	Multiple gross abnormalities (up to 2 years after stopping)
Alcohol	Fetal alcohol syndrome and growth retardation Withdrawal syndrome in newborn
Aminoglycosides	Vestibular damage (especially streptomycin)
Amiodarone	Neonatal goitre
Warfarin	Bone abnormalities and neonatal haemorrhage
Sedatives, tranquillizers and hypnotics	Sedation or apnoea in neonate
β-Blockers	May cause growth retardation
Carbemazepine	Neural tube defects (may be reduced with folate supplementation)
Antithyroid drugs	Neonatal hypothyroidism
Chloramphenicol	Grey baby syndrome
Glucocorticoids	Neonatal adrenal suppression in high doses
Cytotoxic drugs	Most are potently teratogenic
NSAIDs	Delayed closure of ductus arteriosus
Opiate analgesics	Neonatal depression and withdrawal syndrome
Phenytoin	Hare lip, cleft palate and cardiac abnormalities
Antimalarial drugs	Methaemoglobinaemia and haemolysis in neonate
Stilboestrol	Vaginal carcinoma in offspring
Tetracyclines	Damage to bones and teeth
Valproate	Neural tube defects
Sulphonylureas	Fetal and neonatal hypoglycaemia

NSAIDs, non-steroidal anti-inflammatory drugs

the mother has to be considered in relation to the potential risk to the fetus. Some drugs have been definitely linked to fetal abnormalities (Table 14.5). As a general rule, all drugs should be avoided in pregnancy unless there is a compelling reason for their use.

The safety of most drugs in pregnancy has not been firmly established as the effects may not be apparent for many years after birth. The past use of stilboestrol in pregnant women with threatened abortion has resulted in the development of adenocarcinoma of the vagina in female children in their teens and early twenties. This devastating adverse effect was recognized only because this is normally an extremely rare tumour.

There is the possibility that the use of other drugs in pregnancy predisposes to more common conditions such as diabetes or hypertension. Such associations would not be easily recognized.

Effects on fertilization and implantation

The principal mode of contraceptive action of progestogens is to prevent implantation, which normally occurs 2–3 weeks after fertilization. Intrauterine contraceptive devices have a similar effect. Damage to the embryo before implantation results in failure of implantation and is therefore unlikely to cause fetal abnormalities.

Effects on fetal development

The intrauterine period between two weeks and three months is when the most serious abnormalities of fetal development can be caused by drugs. It is during this period that the major organs are being formed. In animal studies, even one dose of a drug administered at the critical time has been shown to have a major effect. The mechanisms of damage are not yet known, but the molecular basis of differentiation of embryonic cells is an intense area of basic research and is likely to provide new insights in the near future.

Toxicity to the formed fetus

During the second and third trimester of pregnancy, the adverse effects on the fetus of drugs administered to the mother are generally an exaggeration of effects seen in the adult. Exceptions to this rule are the damage to tissues which are still developing such as teeth and bones by tetracycline antibiotics, and the impairment of brain development by coumarin anticoagulants.

Particular care must be taken with drugs given shortly before delivery. Analgesics such as pethidine and tranquillizers such as benzodiazepines may severely impair neonatal respiration. In addition, the newborn lacks many enzymes necessary for the efficient metabolism of drugs.

Breastfeeding

Although most drugs can be detected in breast milk, the dose administered to the infant is generally low. This is because, unless there is concentration of drug by breast tissue, the concentration in milk tends to be similar to that of the maternal plasma. Clearly in this case the final concentration in the infant's plasma is likely to be much less than that in the mother's.

Despite this, it is known that some drugs do cause problems via breastfeeding. Examples are carbimazole, which may affect infant thyroid function, and tetracyclines which are also excreted in milk. As with pregnancy, it is important to avoid all drugs in nursing mothers unless there is a compelling need. A list of drugs excreted in breast milk and known to cause problems is given in an appendix to the *British National Formulary*.

Age

Initial evaluation of the safety and efficacy of drugs is usually carried out in healthy volunteers and patients aged between 18 and 65. For new drugs, in particular, the likelihood of adverse effects are not known in children or the elderly, and information only slowly becomes available through published case reports and monitoring systems (see Table 14.1).

Children

There are several reasons why drugs may have different effects in the young compared with adults.

- Dosage is more difficult to calculate, and formulations are often varied to make oral medicines acceptable to the young. Administration of a precise oral dose is often impossible in babies who spit out unpleasant tasting syrup.
- Absorption of oral drugs may be affected in infants because of reduced gastric acidity.
- Skin absorption of topical drugs and disinfecting agents is particulary enhanced in premature babies, sometimes leading to serious toxicity from steroids, iodine and aminoglycoside antibiotics.
- Adults typically have 20% of their bodyweight as fat, whereas the premature baby may have as little as 1%. This will have a very marked effect to increase plasma concentration of fat-soluble drugs when given on a dose/kg basis.
- The metabolism of certain drugs such as chloramphenicol and theophylline is markedly less rapid in the newborn compared with children and adults. Use of the former has been associated with cardiovascular collapse and 'the grey baby syndrome'.
- Renal excretion of drugs rapidly improves during the first few days of life, making the safe and effective use of aminoglycoside antibiotics, in particular, very difficult.

The elderly

As the proportion of elderly patients rises in industrialized countries, it is becoming more apparent that this group are increasingly likely to suffer adverse effects of drugs. Reasons for this are varied (Table 14.6).

- Patients can be confused and fail to remember the correct dose, especially if many different medicines are prescribed.
- Interactions between drugs is more common in the elderly owing to polypharmacy.
- There may be altered drug absorption, distribution, metabolism and excretion owing to concomitant disease processes.
- Certain drugs have adverse pharmacodynamic effects, particularly exaggerated CNS and cardiovascular effects. For example, patients are much more prone to complain of constipation with drugs which have such adverse effects.
- Non-steroidal anti-inflammatory drugs (NSAIDs) are very commonly prescribed in the elderly and cause a disproportionate number of serious adverse effects in this group of patients.

Table 14.6
Pharmacodynamic adverse effects of drugs in the elderly

Adverse effect	Drugs
Bradycardia	β-blockers Verapamil and diltiazem
Postural hypotension	Organic nitrates Diuretics Tricyclics α-blockers
Glucose intolerance	Diuretics
Bladder function	Diuretics
Bowel function	Verapamil
Temperature regulation	Phenothiazines
Confusion	Tranquillizers Anticonvulsants Antimuscarinics Hypnotics Opiates Anaesthesia

Co-existent disease processes

Diseases can predispose towards adverse drug reactions by two main mechanisms:

- alteration in the pharmacokinetic handling of drugs
- change in the pharmacodynamic profile of drugs.

Pharmacokinetic mechanisms

Alteration in absorption may result from previous gastric surgery or intestinal malabsorption, owing to conditions such as coeliac disease. Infective diarrhoea may decrease transit time sufficiently to impair the absorption of many drugs, including oral contraceptives. Oedema of the gut in patients with severe heart failure has been suggested as a reason for reduced efficacy of oral frusemide in this condition.

Reduced plasma albumin concentration due to poor nutrition or renal or hepatic disease will cause little change in the active unbound fraction of protein-bound drugs, but will cause a reduction in total plasma concentration. This would have little effect were it not for the fact that total, rather than unbound drug, is usually measured when therapeutic drug monitoring is employed, leading to a tendency to overdosing.

Metabolism of many drugs is largely dependent on normal hepatic function and extreme caution must be taken in prescribing to patients with liver failure. In particular, reduced metabolism of opiate analgesics, anticoagulants, anticonvulsant drugs and theophylline may cause serious toxicity. If it is necessary to administer a drug which is metabolized by the liver in a patient with hepatic impairment, then it is important to monitor closely the effect and/or frequently measure plasma concentrations (if such assays are appropriate and available). Reduced metabolism of one drug does not always predict that other drugs which are metabolized by the liver will be similarly affected. Patients with cardiac failure generally have reduced hepatic blood flow and consequently reduced hepatic metabolism of many drugs.

The major route of excretion for most drugs is via the kidneys. In drugs which are not subject to hepatic metabolism, renal excretion is the main factor which determines the concentration of active drug circulating in the plasma. Particular care must be taken with drugs with a low therapeutic ratio which are principally excreted by the kidneys, such as digoxin, lithium and aminoglycoside antibiotics.

Pharmacodynamic mechanisms

It is not surprising that a certain disease will often be exacerbated by a drug which is known to cause this disease as a side-effect. For instance, asthmatics are very sensitive to β-adrenoreceptor blocking drugs and will almost invariably become more wheezy if such agents are inadvertently taken; and those with acne will often encounter a worsening of their skin problem when glucocorticoids are prescribed.

However, patients with liver disease will not necessarily encounter further hepatic damage when antituberculous drugs are given – although, of course, particular caution must be taken in such situations.

Genetic factors

An individual's genetic make-up can profoundly influence the way in which he or she reacts to drugs by pharmacokinetic and pharmacodynamic mechanisms. Susceptibility may be due to a single gene variation or to several genes having an additive effect. With the sequencing of the human genome it is possible that we will realize that many common adverse drug reactions have a genetic basis.

Genetic causes of altered pharmacokinetics

The best known and perhaps the most important genetic cause of altered drug handling is acetylator phenotype. Certain drugs are metabolized by acetylation in the liver and individuals can be classified as slow acetylators or fast acetylators.

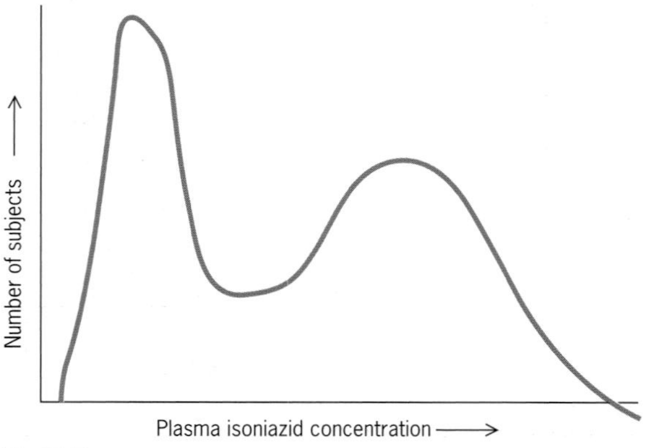

Fig 14.3
Bimodal distribution of acetylator status. Plasma isoniazid concentration shows two distinct groups of subjects. Modified from Evans DAP et al (1960) *British Medical Journal* **2**: 486

Most populations show a distinct bimodal distribution in their acetylator status (Fig 14.3), which is likely to be due to a single gene variation. Those who acetylate slowly will have higher plasma concentrations of drug for any given dose and will tend to develop adverse effects more readily. This is particularly important with the antituberculous drug isoniazid which will cause a polyneuropathy more commonly in patients with slow acetylator status; inhibition of metabolism of the anticonvulsant phenytoin when prescribed concurrently with isoniazid is also more common in slow acetylators. Rapid acetylators may, conversely, be more likely to relapse due to inadequate plasma concentrations of isoniazid. SLE is more likely to develop with procainamide and hydralazine in slow acetylators.

Debrisoquine hydroxylation is also markedly deficient in certain individuals (about 8% of the British population), and such deficiency shows autosomal dominant inheritence. Debrisoquine is rarely used in the treatment of hypertension, not least because almost 10% of patients will have defective metabolism, resulting in enhanced adrenergic blockade with the risk of severe hypotension. The same hydroxylase enzyme is involved in the metabolism of several β-blockers and the antidepressant nortriptyline, although it is not clear whether hydroxylation status predicts adverse effects with these drugs.

The rare failure to metabolize suxamethonium resulting in prolonged muscular paralysis is due to a genetic defect in the production of plasma pseudocholinesterase. The condition is autosomal recessive and affects about 1 in 2500 patients.

Genetic causes of altered pharmacodynamic response

Glucose-6-phosphate-dehydrogenase (G6PD) deficiency is a fairly common X-linked recessive disorder in Mediterranean countries, Africa and the Far East. Individuals with this trait are less able to synthesize NADPH in response to oxidative stress, and are susceptible to red cell haemolysis and methaemo-globinaemia when challenged with certain oxidizing drugs, as well as broad beans. Drugs which are likely to be a problem in G6PD deficiency are given in Table 6.13 Antimalarial drugs, particularly primaquine, can produce severe haemolysis resulting in renal failure.

Table 14.7
Commonly used drugs which may precipitate acute porphyria

A complete list is given in the *British National Formulary*

Barbiturates	Erythromycin
Anticonvulsants	Sulphonamides
Benzodiazepines	Methyldopa
Oral hypoglycaemics	Metoclopramide
Tricyclic antidepressants	Sex steroids
Diuretics	Theophylline
ACE inhibitors	Antihistamines
Flucloxacillin	Calcium-channel blockers
Cephalosporins	

Acute porphyrias (see p. 1004) can be precipitated by a large number of drugs (Table 14.7).

Malignant hyperpyrexia is a rare but potentially fatal condition, where autosomal dominant inheritance can often be shown. General anaesthesia (particularly when halothane or suxamethonium are given) provokes muscular rigidity, hyperpyrexia, sweating, cyanosis, and rapid respiration. Intravenous dantrolene has been advocated as a useful therapy.

Gilbert's syndrome (see p. 298) is exacerbated by oestrogens and improved by low doses of barbiturates, which induce the defective enzyme glucuronyl transferase.

FURTHER READING

Koren G, Pastuszak, Ito S (1998) Drugs in pregnancy. *New England Journal of Medicine* **338**: 1128–1137.

Monitoring the effects of drugs

As a result of genetic or environmental factors (including other drug therapy), the effect of the same dose of drug in different individuals will differ.

The *therapeutic ratio* of a drug is the ratio between the the dose required to produce a toxic effect and the dose required to produce the desired effect (Fig 14.4). For drugs with a low therapeutic ratio – that is, ones with which toxicity occurs at a dose only marginally higher than the therapeutic dose – it is important to try to monitor the effect to establish a safe dose.

Therapeutic drug monitoring

This involves measuring the plasma concentration of a potentially toxic drug and is only useful if:

- there is a reliable and available plasma drug assay
- plasma concentrations correlate well with therapeutic efficacy and toxicity (i.e. the therapeutic range is well-documented).

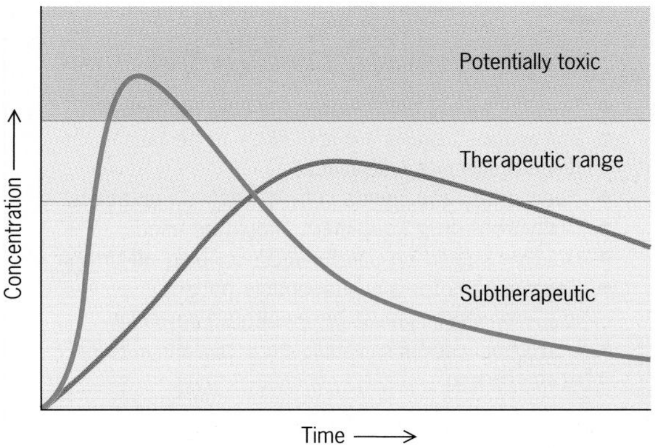

Fig 14.4
Relationships between blood drug concentration, its effect and time after oral administration

Monitoring of the plasma concentration of phenytoin is essential because of saturation kinetics. When the concentration in plasma reaches a certain concentration, the metabolizing enzymes are saturated and the drug is eliminated by zero-order kinetics (Fig 14.5).

Table 14.8 lists the drugs in which therapeutic drug monitoring is routinely employed.

Monitoring of drug effects in individuals

Dosage of other drugs may be adjusted according to their pharmacodynamic effect. A familiar example of this is the use of the *International Normalized Ratio* (INR) for adjusting the dose of warfarin and other coumarin anticoagulants. Other examples are the estimation of circulating thyroid hormone (TSH) concentrations in patients treated with carbimazole, and routine white-cell and platelet counts in patients receiving cytotoxic chemotherapy.

For many drugs (e.g. penicillins) the therapeutic ratio is so high that there is little chance of toxicity with standard doses, so monitoring of plasma concentrations is unnecessary.

Monitoring of adverse drug effects in populations

In order to identify adverse effects of new drugs, or rare adverse effects of established drugs, pharmacoepidemiologists have developed a variety of approaches.

In the UK the *yellow card* system has been useful. This invites clinicians and pharmacists to report to the Committee on Safety of Medicines all definite or

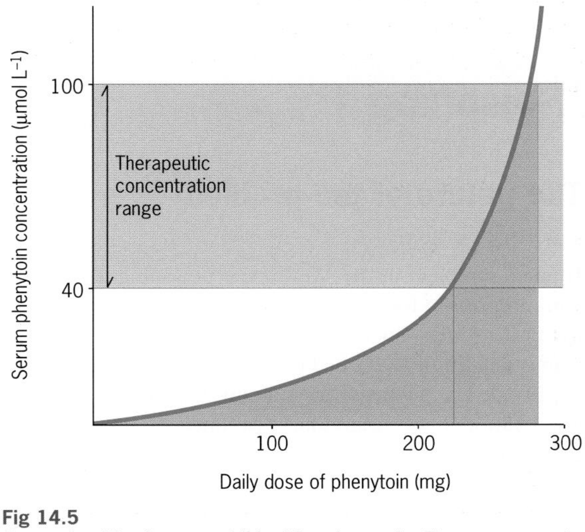

Fig 14.5
Saturation kinetics as exhibited by phenytoin. The measurements were obtained from one patient on several maintenance doses of phenytoin and show a curvilinear relationship between dose and serum concentration. Note the relatively small dose range compatible with a therapeutic concentration

Table 14.8
Drugs for which therapeutic drug monitoring is used.

Drug	Therapeutic plasma concentration range	Toxic levels	Optimum time for sampling after dose (hours)
Carbamazepine	21–42 μmol L^{-1}	> 42 μmol L^{-1}	> 8
Digoxin	1.3–2.6 nmol L^{-1}	> 2.6 nmol L^{-1}	> 8
Gentamicin	Trough < 2 mg L^{-1} Peak 5–10 mg L^{-1}	> 2 mg L^{-1} > 12 mg L^{-1}	6–8 (immediately pre-dose) > 1
Lithium	0.6–1.0 mmol L^{-1}	> 1.5 mmol L^{-1}	> 10
Phenytoin	40–80 μmol L^{-1}	> 80 μmol L^{-1}	> 10
Theophylline	55–110 μmol L^{-1}	> 110 μmol L^{-1}	> 4
Cyclosporin	50–200 μg L^{-1}	> 200 μg L^{-1}	Pre-dose

suspected adverse reactions linked to products newly introduced, as well as serious or unusual reactions to established products. Inevitably the efficacy of such a system is reduced by a low reporting rate, but the yellow card system has uncovered a number of important adverse effects and drug interactions, including thromboembolism in oral contraceptive users, and jaundice with halothane.

Complimentary to this system is *prescription event monitoring*, in which prescriptions for a certain drug are identified at the Prescription Pricing Authority office. A sample of patients or their doctors are then sent a questionnaire to determine if certain adverse effects are occurring at a greater incidence than that found for a comparable drug prescribed for the same clinical indication.

FURTHER READING

Grahame-Smith DG, Aronson JK (1992) Oxford text book of clinical pharmacology and drug therapy, 2nd edn. Oxford University Press, Oxford.

Poisoning

The nature of the problem

(Information box 14.1)

In many hospitals in the West, acute poisoning is the most common reason for acute admission of a young person to a medical ward. Such poisoning is usually by self-administration of prescribed or over-the-counter medicines, or of drugs involved in substance abuse. Sometimes overtreatment of individual patients by a doctor is responsible for poisoning. Occasionally, toxic agents are accidentally ingested or inhaled at home or work or are administered in the pursuit of deliberate harm, Münchausen syndrome by proxy, or financial or sexual crime.

Self-poisoning is commonly a cry for help. These individuals are most often females under the age of 45 and in good or reasonable physical health. They take the overdose in a situation in which they are likely to be found, or with people present. With regard to older people, overdoses are more common with men, usually in the course of a depressive illness or associated with poor physical health. Large amounts of drugs are taken when alone. Such patients often take an overdose where they do not expect to be discovered.

Some 30% of patients admitted with overdose state that they were unaware of the toxic effect of the drug they took. The person often takes whatever drug is easily available at home. Doctors should therefore always prescribe limited amounts of drugs, and it is advisable to keep only small amounts of tablets, preferably foil-wrapped, in the home. Patients should be advised about the potential danger of drugs, which should be kept out of reach of children, preferably in a locked cabinet.

Poisoning in children aged under six months is most commonly iatrogenic and involves overtreatment with digoxin, chloramphenicol or theophylline. Accidental self-poisoning is common in children between eight months and five years. Non-accidental poisoning, substance abuse and deliberate self-harm also occur in children.

Information

Patients usually take what is readiliy available at home.

- Small amounts only of drugs should be bought.
- Foil-wrapped drugs are less likely to be taken.
- Keep drugs in a safe place.
- Keep drugs and liquids in their original containers.
- Child-proof drug containers should be used.
- Doctors should be careful in prescribing **all** drugs.
- Prescriptions for any susceptible patient (e.g. depressed) must be monitored carefully.
- Household products should be kept safely, away from children.

SELF-POISONING KILLS.
All people must be aware of the dangers.

Information box 14.1 Prevention of self-poisoning

The majority of cases (80%) of self-poisoning do not require intensive medical management, but all affected individuals require a sympathetic and caring approach to their problems. Both the patient and the family may require psychiatric help, and the social services should be contacted to help with social and domestic problems.

The number of hospital admissions for self-poisoning is increasing. However, as a result of good supportive care and the reduced availability of barbiturates and coal gas (replaced by natural gas), the mortality of patients has declined and is now well under 1%. Studies of the drugs involved reveal the following facts:

- Acute overdoses usually involve more than one drug.
- Alcohol is the most commonly implicated second 'drug' in mixed self-poisonings – 60% of men and 45% of women consume some alcohol at the same time as the drug.
- There is often a poor correlation between the drug history and the toxicological findings. Therefore, patients' statements about the type and amount of drug ingested should not be relied upon.
- The use of minor tranquillizers and antidepressants is increasing, while barbiturates are now virtually unavailable in the UK.

The extent of the problem

In England and Wales there are over 100 000 hospital admissions each year for self-poisoning, the most common being with benzodiazepines and antidepressants, followed by paracetamol and then aspirin. Deaths from poisoning are gradually declining. Most deaths occur outside hospital, where the most common causes are carbon monoxide poisoning from vehicle exhaust fumes, and faulty appliances that burn natural gas.

Information from other continents is difficult to compare, but in Asia and Africa it seems that poisoning is a significant medical problem, with children being a particularly vulnerable group. In Cairo, over half of the enquiries at the poisons reference centre involve the poisoning of children. The proportion of accidental poisoning in Asia and Africa is higher than in Europe and North America. Snake bite is an important cause of mortality in Asia and Africa.

FURTHER READING

Thomas SHL, Bevan L, Bhattacharyya S et al (1996) Presentation of poisoned patients to accident and emergency departments in the north of England. *Human and Experimental Toxicology* **15**: 466–470.

The approach to the patient

HISTORY

Eighty per cent of adults are conscious on arrival at hospital and the diagnosis of self-poisoning can usually be made easily from the history. In the unconscious patient a history from friends or relatives is helpful, and the diagnosis can often be inferred from tablet bottles or a 'suicide note' brought by the ambulance attendants. It should be emphasized that in any patient with an altered level of consciousness, drug overdose must always be considered in the differential diagnosis.

EXAMINATION

On arrival at hospital the patient must be assessed urgently in the accident and emergency department. The following should be evaluated:

- *Level of consciousness* – a useful practical grading is:
  (I) drowsy but responds to commands
  (II) unconscious but responds to mild stimulation
  (III) unconscious but responds only to maximal painful stimuli (sternal rubbing)
  (IV) unconscious and no response.
  Alternatively the Glasgow Coma Scale should be used (see p. 1043).
- *Respiratory effort and cyanosis*
- *Blood pressure and pulse rate*
- *Pupil size and reaction to light* (NB opiates constrict)
- *Evidence of head injury or drug addiction.*

If the patient is unconscious the following should also be checked:

- *Cough and gag reflex* – present or absent
- *Temperature* – measured with a low-reading rectal thermometer

The physical signs that may aid identification of the agents responsible for poisoning are shown in Fig. 14.6.

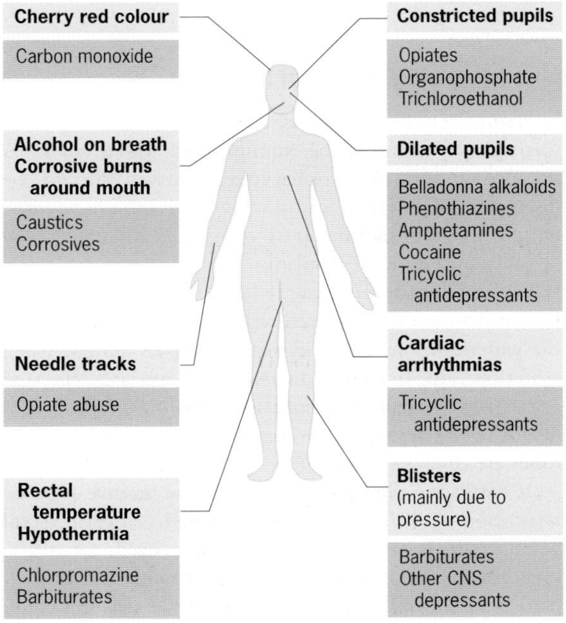

Fig 14.6
Physical signs of poisoning

Principles of management

Most patients with self-poisoning require only general care and support of the vital systems. However, for a few drugs additional therapy is required.

On admission, blood and urine samples should always be taken for the determination of drug levels, as these are invaluable for the management of certain poisons and are helpful in legal disputes. Drug screens of blood and urine are occasionally indicated in the seriously ill, unconscious patient in whom the cause of coma is unknown.

Routine haematological and biochemical investigations, including measurement of arterial blood gases, are of value, particularly in the differential diagnosis of coma.

Care of the unconscious patient (see also p. 1044)

In all cases the patient should be nursed in the lateral position with the lower leg straight and the upper leg flexed; in this position the risk of aspiration is reduced. A clear passage for air should be ensured by the removal of any obstructing object, vomit or dentures, and by backward pressure on the mandible. Nursing care of the mouth and pressure areas should be instituted. Catheterization of the bladder is usually unnecessary as it can be emptied by gentle suprapubic pressure. Insertion of a venous cannula is usual, but administration of intravenous fluids is often unnecessary unless the patient has been unconscious for more than 24 hours.

Respiratory support

If respiratory depression is minimal, oxygen (approximately 60%) should be administered via a mask. A nasopharyngeal or oropharyngeal airway should be inserted, and frequent measurement of minute volume with a Wright spirometer is mandatory to detect any further depression of ventilation.

Loss of the cough or gag reflex is the prime indication for intubation. The gag reflex is assessed by positioning the patient on one side and making him or her gag using a suction tube. In most patients the reflexes are depressed sufficiently to allow intubation without the use of sedatives or relaxants. The complications of endotracheal tubes are discussed on p. 853.

If ventilation is inadequate, intermittent positive-pressure ventilation (IPPV) should be instituted. Arterial blood gas analysis is useful to confirm the need for IPPV. Hypoxaemia is common in the unconscious patient, particularly after the ingestion of opiates and barbiturates, and can easily go undetected without blood gas analysis or pulse oximetry.

Cardiovascular support

Hypotension (blood pressure below 80 mmHg) is a common feature of drug overdose and is caused by the physiological effects listed in Table 14.9. The classic features of shock – tachycardia and pale cold skin – may be present, but vasodilatation may also be seen (e.g. with barbiturate overdose).

In the majority of cases, hypotension is mild and elevation of the feet is the only treatment required. In patients with more severe hypotension, volume expanders such as dextran should be used. In severely hypotensive patients, the measurement of central venous pressure (CVP) is helpful. Urine output (aiming for 0.5 mL kg^{-1} h^{-1}) is also an important longer-term guide to the adequacy of the circulation, as many vasodilated overdosed patients are adequately perfused with a systolic blood pressure of as low as 90–100 mmHg. Some hypotensive patients may need to be catheterized in order to monitor urine output.

If a patient fails to respond to the above measures, more intensive therapy is required (see p. 722).

Arrhythmias are commonly seen with tricyclic antidepressant overdose. All shocked patients should have ECG monitoring. Known arrhythmogenic factors such as hypoxia, acidosis and hypokalaemia should be corrected.

Special problems

Hypothermia

Defined as a rectal temperature of below 35°C, this is a common problem, especially in older patients or those poisoned with chlorpromazine or a similar neuroleptic. Hypothyroidism should always be considered. Hypothermia is compounded by drug-induced vasodilatation and environmental exposure. The patient should be covered with a 'space blanket' and given intravenous and intragastric fluids at normal body temperature. Inspired gases should also be warmed to 37°C.

Rhabdomyolysis

Rhabdomyolysis can occur from pressure necrosis in drug-induced coma, or it may complicate heroin abuse without coma. The risk of renal failure from myoglobinaemia is potentiated by dehydration and acidosis.

Table 14.9
Causes of hypotension after drug overdose

An expanded venous bed due to venous vasodilatation
Hypovolaemia due to inadequate fluid intake in prolonged coma
Institution of intermittent positive-pressure ventilation (IPPV) in an already hypovolaemic patient
Myocardial depression due to the direct effect of the drug, exaggerated by hypoxia, acidosis and hypothermia

Convulsions

These may occur in serious tricyclic antidepressant poisoning, and in antihistamine or phenothiazine poisoning. Diazepam 10 mg i.v. is the standard treatment for fits of any cause. The patient should also receive a loading dose of phenytoin (15 mg kg^{-1}) administered intravenously over fours hours (via a central vein) or more rapidly if fitting is frequent (but not more than 50 mg per minute). A maintenance dose of 100 mg 8-hourly is given if the fits are not immediately controlled. Persistent fits must be controlled rapidly, as they may otherwise result in severe hypoxia, brain damage and laryngeal trauma.

Stress bleeding

Measures to prevent stress ulceration of the stomach should be started on admission in all patients who are unconscious and require intensive care. Administration of antacid by intragastric tube is used, although H_2 antagonists are preferred.

Specific management

Many techniques have been developed to decrease drug absorption and increase drug elimination, but most of these manoeuvres are only helpful with a few drugs. These, as well as antidotes to specific drugs, are described below.

Decreasing drug absorption

Vigorous attempts to empty the gastrointestinal tract are indicated when drugs that cause potentially fatal complications other than coma or respiratory depression have been ingested. Examples of such drugs are aspirin, paracetamol, colchicine, organophosphates, iron salts and tricyclic antidepressants. It is important to remember that the risk of aspiration into the lungs associated with the use of gastric lavage may well cause more problems than the effects of the drugs themselves. Gastric lavage does not remove stomach contents completely.

Gastric lavage (Practical box 14.1)

This procedure is of use only when a large quantity of drug has been taken. The earlier gastric lavage is performed, the greater the amount of drug that is retrieved. It is of little value after four hours except for the drugs shown in Table 14.10. Complications include pulmonary aspiration, rupture of the oesophagus, hypoxia and arrhythmias. Lavage is contraindicated for some poisons, such as corrosives, petrol or paraffin.

Absorbent (Information box 14.2)

This should be administered promptly (within four hours) and in sufficient quantity. Activated charcoal significantly reduces the gastrointestinal absorption of many drugs, but not all. The ratio of charcoal to the amount of poison to be absorbed is about 10:1, so this procedure is most useful when a relatively small dose of a drug is toxic, as with tricyclic antidepressants, aspirin, barbiturates and theophylline, and when emesis, gastric lavage and aspiration are contraindicated. It can be administered by mouth or down a nasogastric tube. The usual dose is 50 g initially and then 50 g every four hours.

Practical

Gastric lavage should be performed by an experienced nurse and doctor.

The main danger is from pulmonary aspiration. It is vital that the tracheobronchial tree be protected, either by an intact cough reflex or by a cuffed endotracheal tube.

1. Position the patient lying on the left side, with the head over the end or side of the bed so that the mouth and throat are at a lower level than the larynx and trachea.
2. Lubricate a wide-bore tube (Jacques' gauge 30) with glycerine or Vaseline and pass it into the stomach.
3. First perform aspiration.
4. Next perform lavage using 300 mL of water at body temperature for the first washing.
5. Repeat the process at least three or four times, using up to 500 mL of water on each occasion.
6. Save an aliquot of the washing in case it is needed for drug analysis.

Practical box 14.1 Technique of gastric lavage

Table 14.10 Drugs for which gastric lavage is useful more than four hours after ingestion

Salicylates
Basic drugs such as quinidine or tricyclic antidepressants, where gastric emptying is delayed
Paracetamol

Induced emesis

Induced emesis may be useful in small children as they are more difficult to lavage. It is rarely used in adults, as only small amounts of drug are recovered.

The emetic of choice is ipecacuanha emetic mixture, Paediatric (BP) (not the undiluted fluid extract). The dose is 10 mL for a child over six months of age. It induces vomiting in over 90% of children within 25 minutes but does not fully empty the stomach. The effect can be terminated with ondansetron.

Other emetics such as apomorphine, saline, copper sulphate and mustard are dangerous and should not be used.

Whole bowel lavage

This technique has been introduced for the treatment of significant poisoning with iron, lithium and other metallic

Information

Cyanide
Iron
Lead
Lithium
Mercury

Organic solvents
Corrosives

Alcohol (ethanol and methanol)
Ethylene glycol

Strong acids and alkalis

Information box 14.2 Substances **not** absorbed by activated charcoal

compounds, slow-release preparations of theophylline and propranolol, and ingested packets of illicit drugs. It has been used when brain damage or a fatal outcome would otherwise be likely. After insertion of a nasogatric tube, isotonic saline is infused at the rate of 0.5 L per hour in children and 2 L per hour in adults, until the rectal effluent is clear.

Contraindications to the use of this technique include ileus, obstruction, perforation and bleeding from the bowel

Skin decontamination

Absorption should be minimized for those poisons which are absorbed through the skin by removal of contaminated clothing and careful washing of the skin with soapy water.

Increasing drug elimination

Alkalinization of urine

This technique is potentially hazardous. Few drugs are excreted in their unchanged form. Its benefits have been shown to be limited to salicylate poisoning, which is discussed below.

Peritoneal dialysis

The use of this technique is limited by its low efficacy, but it may be indicated for patients severely poisoned by ethylene glycol.

Haemodialysis

This technique may be useful for patients with severe poisoning by lithium salts or methyl or ethyl alcohols. Rarely, patients with severe salicylate poisoning (blood salicylate level >700 mg L^{-1} or 5.1 mmol L^{-1}) refractory to urine alkalization may be helped by haemodialysis.

Haemoperfusion

This involves the passage of heparinized blood through devices containing absorbent particles, such as activated charcoal or resins, to which drugs are adsorbed. Its use should be considered in patients severely poisoned with certain drugs (e.g. theophylline, short- and medium-acting barbiturates, and glutethimide) who fail to improve despite the use of adequate supportive measures.

Antagonizing the effects of poisons

These techniques will be considered under the individual drugs. Specific antidotes are available for a small number of drugs. Antidotes act in a number of ways:

- *interaction with the poison to form an inert complex that is then excreted* (e.g. desferrioxamine in iron overdose)
- *acceleration or detoxification of the poison* (e.g. methionine, *N*-acetylcysteine in paracetamol poisoning)
- *prevention of the formation of a more toxic compound* (e.g. ethanol used as a competitive substrate for the metabolizing enzyme to prevent formation of toxic metabolites in methanol poisoning)
- *competition with the poison for essential receptors* (e.g. naloxone in opiate poisoning)
- *blockade of receptors through which the toxic effects are mediated* (e.g. atropine used to block cholinergic receptors in organophosphate poisoning).

FURTHER READING

Manoguerra AS (1997) Gastrointestinal decontamination after poisoning. *Critical Care Clinics* **13**: 709–725.

Specific drug problems

In this section only specific treatment regimens will be discussed. The general principles of management of self-poisoning will always be required.

Analgesics

Analgesic poisoning is common in some areas, accounting for one-third of all cases of self-poisoning admissions to hospital. Salicylate poisoning has decreased over the past decade, while paracetamol poisoning has increased.

Combinations of aspirin or paracetamol and narcotic analgesics such as codeine or dextropropoxyphene are frequently taken. Co-proxamol, a combination of paracetamol and dextropropoxyphene, can cause severe respiratory depression and is a major cause of death.

Accidental poisoning with analgesics has decreased since the introduction of child-resistant bottles.

Aspirin

Acetylsalicylic acid is well absorbed from the stomach and small intestine and is rapidly metabolized to salicylate by the liver and subsequently to salicyluric acid and salicyl phenolic glucuronides, a process that is saturated at therapeutic dosage. At high doses, renal excretion becomes important. Overdosage stimulates the respiratory centre, directly increasing the depth and rate of respiration and thereby producing a respiratory alkalosis. Compensatory mechanisms include renal excretion of bicarbonate and potassium, which results in a metabolic acidosis, and a fall in arterial pH indicates serious poisoning. Salicylates also interfere with carbohydrate, fat and protein metabolism, as well as with oxidative phosphorylation. This gives rise to increased lactate, pyruvate and ketone bodies, all of which contribute to the acidosis.

SYMPTOMS AND SIGNS

Symptoms and signs of aspirin poisoning may be minimal soon after poisoning but later include tinnitus, nausea and vomiting, overbreathing, hyperpyrexia and sweating with a tachycardia. Slow-release tablets may delay the onset of symptoms. Alternatively, the patient may appear completely well, even with high blood levels of salicylate. The ingestion of 10–20 g of aspirin by an adult (or one-tenth of this amount for a child) is likely to cause moderate or severe toxicity.

With severe intoxication (salicylate levels 800–1000 mg L^{-1}; 5.6–7.2 mmol L^{-1}), confusion, delirium, convulsions and coma result. Coma is common in children. It should be remembered that consciousness is not impaired unless the blood salicylate level is very high or, more commonly, another drug has been taken.

Cerebral and pulmonary oedema are serious complications, and may be exacerbated by forced diuresis.

TREATMENT

Aspirin delays gastric emptying, so gastric lavage should be performed up to 12 hours after the ingestion in all but the mildest cases and in severe cases up to 24 hours. Activated charcoal in repeated doses should be given. Aspirin is precipitated by stomach acid and may form a cast of the stomach which can later be absorbed to produce delayed toxicity.

Intravenous fluids and electrolyte supplements may be necessary to correct dehydration and hypokalaemia. Occasionally intramuscular vitamin K is required to correct hypoprothrombinaemia. Making the urine alkaline is also effective in increasing urine salicylate excretion.

Alkalinization of the urine is used if the blood level exceeds 500 mg L^{-1} (3.6 mmol L^{-1}) in adults, 350 mg L^{-1} (2.5 mmol L^{-1}) in children. Increasing the pH of the urine from 7 to 8 increases the renal excretion of salicylic acid by about a factor of 10. In the first hour, 1500 mL of fluid should be given as 500 mL of 5% dextrose, 500 mL of 1.4% sodium bicarbonate, and then 500 mL of 5% dextrose again. Sufficient potassium should be mixed with each 500 mL bag to keep the serum potassium level above 3.5 mmol L^{-1}. The urine pH should be measured regularly (every 15–30 minutes) and further administration of bicarbonate may be needed to keep the urine pH between 7.5 and 8.5. The plasma pH and arterial blood gases should be monitored at least two-hourly to ensure that pH does not rise above 7.6; the plasma electrolytes should also be measured. If facilities are not available for constant observation by medical and nursing staff, alkalinization of the urine is dangerous. Haemodialysis is indicated if the concentration of salicylate exceeds 700 mg L^{-1} (5.1 mmol L^{-1}).

Paracetamol (see also p. 336)

Self-poisoning with paracetamol is now the most common form of poisoning encountered and is responsible for about 45% of all cases in the UK. The outcome can often be fatal. Paracetamol is partly converted to a toxic metabolite, *N*-acetyl-*p*-benzoquinonimine, which is normally inactivated by reduction with glutathione. After a large overdose, glutathione is depleted and the toxic metabolite binds covalently with sulphydryl groups on liver cell membranes, initiating a sequence of changes which leads to hepatocyte necrosis. Marked liver necrosis can occur with as little as 7.5 g (15 tablets), and death with 15 g. Patients who are malnourished, have taken alcohol with the overdose, are alcohol-dependent, are receiving enzyme-inducing drugs (see Table 14.4) or are HIV-positive or with AIDS have lower reserves of glutathione and are more susceptible to liver damage; they should be treated if their plasma concentration is above the high-risk treatment line (Fig. 14.7). The prothrombin time (PTT) or International Normalized Ratio (INR) measured 24 hours after the overdose is the best guide to the severity of liver damage.

The clinical features in the first 24 hours include malaise, nausea and vomiting, but the patient remains fully conscious unless a sedative drug has also been taken. After 24 hours abdominal pain may develop. Most patients recover within 48 hours, but some develop liver failure, which usually becomes apparent in 36–96 hours. Patients who present more than 24 hours after taking paracetamol and who are therefore untreated are at much greater risk of developing liver damage. Acute renal failure due to tubular necrosis can occur, sometimes in the absence of severe liver damage.

MANAGEMENT

Treatment depends on the interval between overdose and presentation and on the plasma concentration of paracetamol (Fig 14.7). Blood for paracetamol level should be taken immediately.

Within four hours of ingestion, gastric lavage is performed in all adults who have taken a single dose of 7.5 g or more, and in children after a single dose of 150 mg kg^{-1} or more.

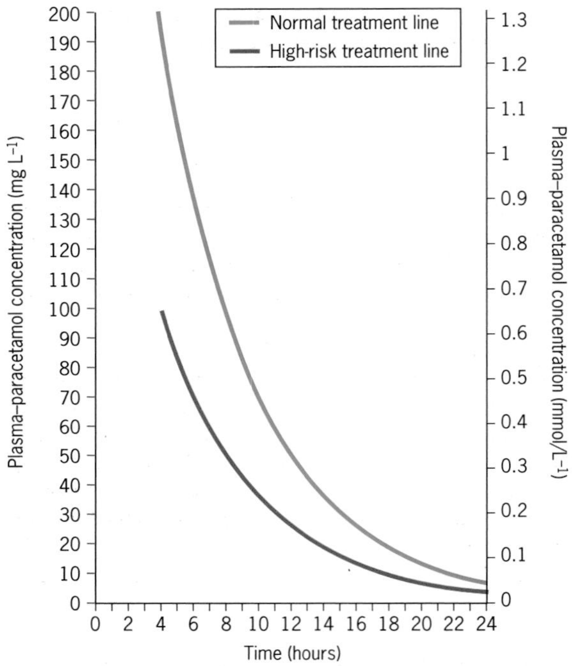

Fig 14.7
Nomogram for paracetamol. From *British National Formulary* 1998, with permission. 'High risk' includes patients who are on enzyme-inducing drugs or who are malnourished

The antidote of choice is *N*-acetylcysteine given intravenously; it provides sulphydryl groups that increase the availability of hepatic glutathione. The decision to give treatment is based on the plasma paracetamol concentration, measured four hours after the overdose, or later by referring to a graph of concentration against time (Fig 14.7). If the concentration is above, on, or even slightly below, the line, treatment should be given. Care must be taken concerning the units in which the results of estimations are reported. If in doubt *N*-acetylcysteine should be given rather than withheld.

Patients taking enzyme-inducing drugs (Table 14.4) should be treated at concentrations of paracetamol half as great as those indicated by the standard treatment graph.

For maximum protective action, treatment should be started within eight hours. If a potentially toxic dose of paracetamol has been taken, treatment must be given at once. Therapy with *N*-acetylcysteine can be stopped if the concentration of paracetamol is subsequently found to be below the treatment line.

N-Acetylcysteine is given as an intravenous infusion diluted with 5% glucose solution with an initial dose of 150 mg kg^{-1} in 200 mL over 15 minutes, followed by 50 mg kg^{-1} in 500 mL over four hours, and then 100 mg kg^{-1} in 1000 mL in the following 16 hours. Occasionally, patients develop a pseudoallergic reaction with wheezing, flushing and hypotension, and if this occurs the infusion should be suspended. Intravenous hydrocortisone and chlorpheniramine should be injected and the infusion restarted at a lower rate when the reaction has subsided.

Oral methionine is an alternative and is significantly cheaper than *N*-acetylcysteine but absorption and efficacy are unreliable if the patient is vomiting. The benefit of methionine in patients presenting late has not been determined. The dose is 2.5 g by mouth every four hours for a total of four doses.

Pregnant women should be treated in the same way as other patients and there is no evidence that either acetylcysteine or methionine are teratogenic or fetotoxic.

Concentrations of paracetamol are not a reliable guide to the value of treatment in patients who present more than 16 hours after ingestion of the drug. The benefit of treatment with acetylcysteine after 24 hours has been established only in patients who have evidence of encephalopathy, but it is worth treating all patients who have taken a potentially dangerous overdose (more than 150 mg kg^{-1}) and who present 16–24 hours later. Treatment can be stopped 24 hours after ingestion if the patient is asymptomatic, if the plasma paracetamol level is below 10 mg L^{-1}, and if the INR is normal.

The risk of severe liver damage is assessed from measurement of the INR, serum creatinine concentration and blood pH. A poor prognosis is indicated by an INR above 3, raised serum creatinine concentration, or a blood pH below 7.3 recorded more than 24 hours after overdose. If any of these abnormalities are present, advice should be sought from a specialist liver or poisons treatment unit.

Further treatment for paracetamol poisoning

- *In patients who present within eight hours of the overdose*, the INR and serum creatinine should be measured about 24 hours after the overdose or when treatment with the antidote is complete. Patients with normal values are not at risk of serious liver damage.
- *In patients presenting after eight hours*, the INR and serum creatinine should be measured after completion of treatment and at 48 hours after overdose. Patients should remain in hospital until it is clear that the tests are not dangerously abnormal and the values are returning towards normal and a decision about psychiatric assessment is made.

A combination of paracetamol and dextropropoxyphene taken in overdose is particularly dangerous as death may occur rapidly from respiratory or cardiac depression, especially when combined with alcohol. Such patients must be monitored carefully and naloxone given intravenously in an initial dose of 0.8–2 mg and repeated at 2–3 minute intervals up to a total of 10 mg if necessary. *N*-Acetylcysteine should be also be given to prevent paracetamol toxicity as above.

In patients who present after 16 hours it is important to maintain fluid and electrolyte balance and glucose levels and to monitor for signs of encephalopathy. Haemorrhage should be treated with fresh frozen plasma. Patients with incipient or established hepatic failure may be candidates for haemoperfusion or liver transplantation. Those who develop severe hepatic damage and then recover do not develop long-term sequelae and can be treated with normal therapeutic doses of paracetamol.

Non-steroidal anti-inflammatory drugs (NSAIDs)

Self-poisoning with NSAIDs has increased, particularly as ibuprofen is available without prescription. Overdoses will produce a variety of effects, including nausea, vomiting, headache, tinnitus and gastrointestinal bleeding. Severe poisoning causes widespread metabolic abnormalities, hepatic and renal damage, and convulsions occur with mefenamic acid.

Treatment is with gastric lavage leaving 50 g activated charcoal in the stomach, oral activated charcoal 50 g every four hours, intravenous H_2 receptor antagonists and diazepam for convulsions.

Opiates

Opiates produce respiratory depression leading to coma. Pin-point pupils are seen. Naloxone 0.8–2 mg i.v. is a competitive antagonist but, as it is short-acting, repeated injections may be required. Recovery may be very abrupt but treatment should be given if there is coma or bradypnoea.

Antimalarials

Overdosage with chloroquine and hydroxychloroquine is hazardous and may cause convulsions and arrhythmias. Quinine is widely used for the treatment of leg cramps but overdosage may result in permanent blindness.

Activated charcoal is used to reduce absorption, and expert advice should be sought from a poisons information centre.

Psychotropic drugs

Benzodiazepines

Benzodiazepines are commonly taken in cases of self-poisoning, accounting for 40% of all drug overdosages in the UK. On their own they are remarkably safe, but they potentiate the CNS-depressant effects of other drugs taken with them, such as barbiturates or ethanol. Benzodiazepines produce drowsiness, ataxia, dysarthria, nystagmus and sometimes coma. Mild hypotension and respiratory depression may occur, especially in patients with chronic lung disease. Most patients recover within 24 hours. Deaths from benzodiazepines alone are rare. Flumazenil, a benzodiazepine antagonist, is useful in the differential diagnosis, but the patient should be monitored carefully as adverse effects occur (e.g. convulsions in patients dependent on benzodiazepines).

Antidepressants

Monoamine oxidase inhibitors (MAOIs)

Self-poisoning with MAOIs is uncommon. Moreover, they have a lower toxicity than tricyclic antidepressants. Symptoms do not usually develop for at least 12 hours after the overdose, when catecholamine levels in the tissues have risen.

The clinical features include CNS overactivity, with agitation, hallucinations and muscle rigidity. Facial grimacing and writhing movements of the limbs and trunk may occur. There is usually dilatation of the pupils, tachycardia, a rising blood pressure and profuse sweating, although hypotension may occur. Muscle tone may be exaggerated and convulsions are common. Hyperpyrexia also occurs.

Gastric lavage is indicated in recent overdose.

Tricyclic antidepressants

Most of the features of self-poisoning with these agents are due to the anticholinergic effects of the drugs. Clinical features include a decrease in the level of consciousness, but deep coma does not usually occur. Convulsions, increased muscle tone, hyperreflexia and extensor plantar responses sometimes occur. The pupils are usually fixed and dilated and there may be ophthalmoplegia and gaze paralysis. Urinary retention may be present. Cardiovascular effects include hypotension and sinus tachycardia. More serious tachyarrhythmias and conduction defects are uncommon and are thought to be due to the quinidine-like action of these drugs. Ventricular arrhythmias are a cause of death in the first few hours following overdose.

If more than 15 tablets have been taken within four hours of admission, or if the patient is unconscious, gastric lavage should be performed, followed by instillation of a single large dose of activated charcoal. Cardiac arrhythmias may need treatment but often this is not necessary. Anti-arrhythmic therapy is often not effective; correction of any accompanying acidosis with sodium bicarbonate and correction of hypoxia are more important. The use of physostigmine has not been shown to improve outcome.

Most patients recover consciousness within 24 hours, while most cardiac abnormalities settle within 12 hours. Electromechnical dissociation may occur and, provided there is no evidence of irreversible brain damage, it is worth performing external cardiac massage for many hours since complete recovery has been reported from such situations.

Amitryptyline and dothiepin may be more toxic than other antidepressants. Antidepressants such as mianserin produce only mild clinical effects, with drowsiness, hypotension and sinus tachycardia, which are less severe than with the other tricyclic antidepressants.

Selective serotonin re-uptake inhibitors (SSRIs)

These are less sedative and have fewer antimuscarinic effects than tricyclic antidepressants. They are safer than other antidepressants in overdosage.

Antipsychotics

Lithium

Self-poisoning with this agent usually occurs in patients on long-term maintenance therapy. It is sometimes accidental owing to:

- impairment of lithium elimination by the kidney through the inadvertent administration of a diuretic
- other factors affecting water and electrolyte balance, such as nausea, vomiting, diarrhoea or exposure to high temperatures.

In acute overdosage there is a delayed onset of symptoms of more than 12 hours owing to the slow entry of lithium into the tissues.

Clinical features include nausea, vomiting, diarrhoea, coarse tremor, apathy and decreased consciousness. There may be restlessness and ataxia with increased muscle tone and rigidity. Electrolyte disturbances, such as hypokalaemia, occur with ECG changes. Acute renal failure is a rare complication. Coma is associated with a bad prognosis.

Serum lithium concentrations correlate poorly with the severity of acute lithium poisoning, but levels in excess of 2 mmol L^{-1} nevertheless can be fatal.

Intravenous fluids are necessary to maintain a good urinary output. Forced diuresis should not be used but peritoneal or haemodialysis may be helpful in severe cases (when levels above 5 mmol L^{-1} are detected).

Phenothiazine

Clinical features include hypotension, hypothermia, CNS and respiratory depression, arrhythmias and dyskinesia. The latter can be treated with benztropine 2 mg i.v., or procyclidine.

Cardiorespiratory drugs

These may be taken deliberately or sometimes accidentally by the elderly, often when one tablet is mistaken for another.

Adrenoceptor blocking drugs

A small overdose of these drugs produces a bradycardia, but a large overdose can produce convulsions, hallucinations, coma, severe bradycardia, hypoglycaemia and hypotension.

Atropine 0.6–1.2 mg i.v. is given. Glucagon in a bolus dose of 50–150 mg kg^{-1} i.v. followed by an infusion of 1–5 mg per hour should be used for severe hypotension. This agent activates adenyl cyclase, promoting formation of cAMP, which is a direct β-stimulant of the heart. If this is unavailable, isoprenaline 2 mg diluted in 500 mL normal saline or 5% dextrose at a rate of 20–40 drops per minute should be given. If bronchospasm is present, salbutamol (i.v. or nebulized) is given.

Digoxin

Self-poisoning with this agent is uncommon, but chronic poisoning in patients taking digoxin is frequent. Clinical features include nausea, vomiting and cardiac arrhythmias, such as heart block and various tachyarrhythmias, including ventricular tachycardia.

Treatment is supportive. Cardiac abnormalities are treated, and hypokalaemia should be corrected.

Digoxin-specific antibody is available for life-threatening overdosage and can be used for severe digitoxin as well as digoxin poisoning.

Theophylline

Overdose causes vomiting, restlessness, agitation, tachycardia and dilated pupils. Convulsions, arrhythmias, gastric haemorrhage and hypokalaemia are seen in severe cases of poisoning.

Gastric lavage is performed and repeated doses of activated charcoal given, with intravenous diazepam to control convulsions. Correction of hypokalaemia may require large doses of potassium.

Other drugs

Self-poisoning by cardiorespiratory drugs is becoming more frequent. Overdose results in an exaggerated pharmacological effect, and treatment should be aimed at counteracting this. For example, an overdose of salbutamol is treated with a β-blocker.

FURTHER READING

Proudfoot AT (1993) Acute poisoning: diagnosis and management, 2nd edn. Butterworth-Heinemann, Oxford.

Household and industrial poisons

Virtually all substances found in the home have been ingested, either by adults because of poorly labelled bottles or accidentally by children. Occasionally household agents are taken deliberately. Many kitchen products contain bleaches (sodium hypochlorite or hydrogen peroxide), acids or alkalis, and the main problem after poisoning with them is their corrosive action on the gut. There is an immediate burning pain in the lips, mouth, throat, retrosternal area and stomach, and ulceration may follow. Vomiting may occur, with blood in severe cases. The major long-term complication is oesophageal stricture.

Poisoning with sodium hypochlorite should be treated with sufficient water or milk to dilute it. Gastric lavage is contraindicated unless very substantial quantities have been taken. Alkalis should not be neutralized.

Some household products contain solvents (e.g. acetone in nail varnish remover and toluene in paints), which may be sniffed accidentally or intentionally (see p. 884).

Paraquat

Over the last few years, accidental poisoning with paraquat has become less common in the developed world and deliberate self-poisoning now accounts for most cases. However, in some developing countries it is the most common single cause of poisoning. Paraquat is found in commonly used brands of weedkiller as an aqueous 20% solution (Gramoxone) or 2.5% solution (Weedol). A dose of 1.5 g may be fatal.

Clinical features include ulcers in the mouth and oesophagus, diarrhoea and vomiting, epistaxis, pulmonary oedema, and later pulmonary fibrosis, respiratory failure and renal failure. Treatment is with gastric lavage with activated charcoal, Fuller's earth or bentonite, and purging with magnesium sulphate can also be used. Haemodialysis or haemoperfusion may be useful in removing the paraquat if started early.

The outcome can be predicted by relating the plasma paraquat concentration to the number of hours that have elapsed since ingestion. It is doubtful whether any treatment affects the outcome.

Carbon monoxide

Carbon monoxide poisoning is a problem worldwide. Domestic gas in the UK (except in Northern Ireland) does not contain carbon monoxide, but the combustion of any fuel gas in the absence of adequate oxygen and ventilation may lead to domestic CO poisoning. The other common sources of carbon monoxide are the exhaust fumes of petrol engines and from certain gas appliances that use propane and butane gases. Methylene chloride, present in many paint strippers, is metabolized to carbon monoxide. The gas is colourless, odourless and tasteless.

Carbon monoxide combines readily with haemoglobin to form carboxyhaemoglobin, thus preventing the formation of oxyhaemoglobin. The clinical features of CO poisoning include mental impairment, nausea, vomiting, headache, hallucinations, fits and drowsiness leading to coma in severe cases. Physical signs are those of tachycardia and tachypnoea in mild-to-moderate toxicity. However, when the carboxyhaemoglobin level reaches 60% the patient may show hypotension, slowing of the pulse and respiration. The classic pink colour of the skin due to the carboxyhaemoglobin is rarely seen before death. Severe toxicity produces widespread effects, including myocardial damage and respiratory distress.

Treatment consists of removing the patient from the carbon monoxide source, and giving as high a concentration of oxygen as possible. Hyperbaric oxygen should be considered if the victim is unconscious or has a blood carboxyhaemoglobin level in excess of 10%.

Disc batteries

Batteries more than 20 mm diameter can lodge in the oesophagus and a chest X-ray should always be performed. Batteries should be removed by endoscopy because they may break open liberating mercury and manganese, which have corrosive effects. Most batteries will pass through the gut in 48 hours but, if they do not and are seen on X-ray to be disintegrating, they should be removed surgically.

Insecticides

Carbamates and organophosphate insecticides are used extensively in the home and agricultural market. They may be ingested accidentally, inhaled, or absorbed through the skin when protective clothing is not worn. These agents are potent inhibitors of cholinesterase and produce an accumulation of acetylcholine. Carbamate poisoning is generally less severe and of shorter duration.

The clinical features are due to the muscarinic and nicotinic effects of acetylcholine. They include nausea, vomiting, hypersalivation, muscle weakness, bronchospasm, and respiratory failure; convulsions may also occur. The plasma cholinesterase activity will be low.

Treatment involves washing any contaminated skin. Atropine 2 mg i.v. is given repeatedly to obtain full atropinization (i.e. the skin becomes flushed and dry, the pupils dilate and tachycardia develops). Pralidoxime mesylate 30 mg kg^{-1} i.v., a cholinesterase reactivator, is used in severe cases but its benefit has not been established.

Chlorphenoxyphenol poisoning may require treatment with alkaline diuresis.

Cyanide

Cyanide is found in a wide range of industrial compounds, such as rodenticide and fertilizers. Hydrogen cyanide is also released from polyurethane foams.

Ingestion or inhalation of this agent produces rapid onset of dizziness and headache, followed by acute shortness of breath, shock and eventual coma. Cyanosis is not present and the skin colour is red. There may be an odour of bitter almonds. Cyanide inhibits cytochrome oxidase, preventing cellular respiration, which leads to hypoxia, metabolic acidosis and frequently death.

Treatment is urgent. Oxygen is given and an intravenous combination of sodium nitrite (300 mg over three minutes) and sodium thiosulphate (12.25 g over 10 minutes). This is followed by 300 mg of dicobalt edetate intravenously over one minute and 300 mg given a minute later if no recovery occurs. Intravenous 50% dextrose 50 mL should also be given after the dicobalt edetate.

Methanol, ethanol and ethylene glycol

These agents are all chiefly metabolized in the liver by alcohol dehydrogenase. In poisoning, there is increased lactate formation, which increases the metabolic acidosis found after methanol ingestion (due to formate) or ethylene glycol ingestion (due to glycoaldehyde and oxalic acid).

Methanol

Minor poisoning with methanol causes headache, breathlessness and photophobia. In severe poisoning there is papilloedema and eventually optic atrophy and blindness.

Poisoning with methanol is treated with gastric lavage and correction of acidosis with bicarbonate infusion. Ethanol infusion and haemodialysis are used to compete with and remove methanol in patients who have taken more than 30 g of the substance and who have a blood level of methanol greater than 500 mg L^{-1} (15.6 mmol L^{-1}). Intravenous folinic acid may prevent ocular toxicity.

Ethanol

Ethanol poisoning produces severe depression of consciousness and hypoglycaemia, fits and apnoeic spells, particularly in children. Poisoning leads to death from respiratory depression much more readily if chlormethiazole, used to assist alcohol withdrawal, is taken concurrently.

Treatment usually consists only of gastric lavage with an endotracheal tube in position. The use of fructose is no longer advised and peritoneal dialysis or haemodialysis is indicated only for very severe cases.

Complications of poisoning with alcohol include aspiration of stomach contents leading to respiratory failure and pneumonia, and acute withdrawal symptoms.

Ethylene glycol

Poisoning with ethylene glycol (antifreeze) causes gastrointestinal upset and neurological involvement, including coma, followed by cardiorespiratory collapse and acute renal failure.

Treatment is by gastric lavage, with correction of the acidosis by means of intravenous sodium bicarbonate and of the hypocalcaemia with intravenous calcium solutions. Ethanol is given orally or intravenously to maintain an ethanol blood level of 1000 mg L^{-1} in severe cases to inhibit the metabolism of ethylene glycol. Haemodialysis is indicated in patients who have taken more than 50 g of ethylene glycol or who have plasma levels above 500 mg L^{-1} (8.1 mmol L^{-1}).

Heavy metals

Mercury

Chronic mercury poisoning causes tremor (hatters' shakes), excessive salivation, scanning speech, anxiety and depression. In the hatters' trade, rabbit fur was stirred in vats of hot mercuric nitrate to make felt, and inhalation of the vapour led to signs of chronic mercury poisoning.

Acute mercury poisoning is seen after the ingestion of mercuric salts (e.g. mercuric chloride), inhalation of mercuric vapours, or the ingestion of mercuric oxide in 'button' batteries. It is treated by induced emesis, lavage and injections of dimercaprol or penicillamine.

Lead

Acute lead poisoning is rare. Chronic lead poisoning, however, commonly occurs.

Occupational lead poisoning

This is a notifiable disease in the UK and work with lead is covered by strict regulations. Most lead poisoning occurs in scrap metal or smelting workers. Blood levels in these workers should be lower than 800 μg L^{-1} (4 mmol L^{-1}).

Domestic lead poisoning

This usually occurs in children owing to the ingestion of old lead-based paint around the home. All toys now have lead-free paint. Chronic ingestion of water from lead pipes and acute accidental ingestion of fluid from car batteries are other frequent causes of lead poisoning.

After absorption, lead interferes with haem and globin synthesis (see p. 364). It also binds to bone, and in patients suffering from chronic exposure small amounts of lead can be found in many tissues.

CLINICAL FEATURES

These include:

- anorexia, nausea and vomiting
- a blue line on the gums
- constipation and severe abdominal colic
- dense metaphyseal bands at the growing end of long bones, particularly the wrist and knee in children (lead lines)
- anaemia, with erythrocytes showing basophil stippling
- peripheral nerve lesions giving wrist drop and foot drop, with muscle involvement

- lead encephalopathy, with eventual seizures and impairment of consciousness.

The diagnosis is made on the basis of the clinical features. The blood level of lead is very variable; levels above 800 g L^{-1} (4 mmol L^{-1}) are toxic.

TREATMENT

It is most important to remove the source of lead intoxication. Sodium calcium edetate (calcium EDTA), D-penicillamine and dimercaprol have all been used for treatment.

Iron

Poisoning with iron tablets is often accidental in children. Symptoms include nausea, vomiting, abdominal pain, diarrhoea and haematemesis due to a direct corrosive effect. In severe cases, hypotension, hepatic damage and coma can occur.

Treatment is urgent and should be commenced even before a serum iron concentration is sent off as an emergency. Administer gastric lavage, and intragastric desferrioxamine 5–10 g and 2 g i.m., followed by a slow intravenous infusion of 15 mg kg^{-1} per hour (maximum 80 mg kg^{-1} in 24 hours).

Arsenic

Acute poisoning with arsenic causes vomiting, abdominal pain and diarrhoea. It is treated with rehydration and dimercaprol. Chronic poisoning causes excess salivation, weakness, anorexia and polyneuritis. There is a 'raindrop' pigmentation of the skin. Arsenic accumulates in the hair and the nails.

FURTHER READING

Van der Hoek W, Konradsen F, Athukorala K *et al.* (1998) Pesticide poisoning: a major health problem in Sri Lanka. *Social Science and Medicine* **46**: 495–504.

Venomous animals

Snakes

The adder (*Vipera berus*) is the only poisonous snake native to the UK. However, a number of dangerous snakes are kept as pets, and worldwide venomous snakes still cause significant mortality. There are three types of venomous snake.

Viperidae

Viperidae have long erectile fangs. They are subdivided into two types:

- viperinae (true vipers, such as Russell's viper (dabora) and the European adder), which are found in all parts of the world except America and the Asian Pacific
- crotalinae (pit-vipers, such as rattlesnakes and the Malayan pit-viper), which are found in Asia and America. They have small heat-sensitive pits between the eyes and the nostrils.

The venom of both of these classes of snake is vasculotoxic.

Elapidae

Elapidae (cobras, mambas, kraits, coral-snakes) are found in all parts of the world except Europe. They have short, unmoving fangs and the venom produces neurotoxic features. Venom from the Asian cobra and the African spitting cobra also produces local tissue necrosis.

Hydrophidae

Hydrophidae (sea-snakes) are found in Asian Pacific coastal waters. They have short fangs and flattened tails. The venom is myotoxic.

CLINICAL FEATURES

Viperidae

Russell's viper is the most important cause of snake-bite mortality in India, Pakistan and Burma. There is local swelling at the site of the bite, which may become massive. Local tissue necrosis may occur, particularly with cobra bites. Evidence of systemic involvement occurs within 30 minutes, including vomiting, evidence of shock and hypotension. Haemorrhage due to incoagulable blood can be fatal.

Elapidae

There is not usually any swelling at the site of the bite, except with Asian cobras and the African spitting cobra – here the bite is painful and is followed by local tissue necrosis. Vomiting occurs first followed by shock and then neurological symptoms and muscle weakness, with paralysis of the respiratory muscles in severe cases. Cardiac muscle can also be involved.

Hydrophidae

Systemic features are muscle involvement, myalgia and myoglobinuria, which can lead to acute renal failure. Cardiac and respiratory paralysis may occur.

MANAGEMENT

A firm pressure bandage should be placed over the bite and the limb immobilized. This greatly delays the spread of the venom.

Arterial tourniquets should not be used and incision or excision of the bite area should not be performed. The type of snake should be identified if possible.

In about 50% of cases no venom has been injected by the bite and antivenoms are not generally indicated (unless systemic effects are present) as they can cause severe allergic reactions. Nevertheless, careful observation for 12–24 hours is necessary and antivenom must always be given when indicated, as the mortality of snake bite is 10–15% with certain snakes.

General supportive measures should be given as necessary, as for all poisoning. These include diazepam for anxiety and intravenous fluids with volume expanders for hypotension. Treatment of acute respiratory, cardiac and renal failure is instituted as necessary.

Specific measures (i.e. antivenoms) can rapidly neutralize venom, but only if an amount in excess of the amount of venom is given. Antivenoms cannot reverse the effects of the venom so they must be given early. They do minimize some of the local effects and may prevent necrosis at the site of the bite. Antivenoms should be administered intravenously by slow infusion, the same dose being given to children and adults.

Allergic reactions are frequent, and adrenaline (1 in 1000 solution) should be available. Antivenoms are usually rapidly effective. In severe cases the antivenom infusion should be continued even with allergic reactions, with subcutaneous injections of adrenaline being given as necessary. Large quantities of antivenom may be required. Some forms of neurotoxicity, such as those induced by the death adder, respond to anticholinesterase therapy with neostigmine and atropine.

Local wounds often require little treatment. If necrosis is present, antibiotics should be given together with initially minimal surgical treatment. Skin grafting may be required later. Antitetanus prophylaxis must be given.

Antivenoms must be kept readily available in all snake-infested areas.

Scorpions

Scorpion stings are a serious problem in the tropics and cause 1000 deaths per year in Mexico. The poison glands are situated in the end of the tail.

Severe pain occurs immediately at the site of puncture, followed by swelling. Signs of systemic involvement include vomiting, respiratory depression and haemorrhage. A firm pressure bandage should be applied to avoid the spread of the neurotoxic venom. Dehydroemetine 1–1.5 mg kg^{-1} should be given intramuscularly or directly into the site of the bite. Corticosteroids may be required in severe cases. Antivenom is available in certain countries.

Spiders

The black widow spider (*Latrodectus mactans*) is found in North America and the tropics and occasionally in Mediterranean countries. The bite quickly becomes painful, and generalized muscle pain, sweating, headache and shock occur owing to absorption of rapidly acting neurotoxins. No systemic treatment is required except in cases of severe systemic toxicity, when specific antivenom should be given where this is available. Intravenous 10% calcium gluconate 10–20 mL may help the muscle spasms.

Loxosceles causes many bites in Central and South America. *L. reclusa*, the brown recluse spider, is also found in the southern USA. Spiders are often found in bedrooms, so that patients are usually bitten at night. There is a burning pain at the site of the bite, followed by a necrotic ulcer in some cases. Systemic effects, which include fever, vomiting and haemolysis, are rare. No treatment is indicated except in severe cases, when an antivenom should be given if available.

Phoneutria nigriventer, the banana spider, and *Atrax robustus*, the Sydney funnel-web spider, can both give nasty bites, which are occasionally fatal.

Insects

Insect stings (e.g. from wasps and bees) and bites (e.g. from ants) produce pain and swelling at the puncture site. Deaths do occur (12 per year in the UK) and are usually due to anaphylaxis, which requires urgent treatment (see p. 862). Patients who have severe local reactions to stings or a mild anaphylactic reaction should carry a Medi-jet syringe for self-administration of adrenaline should a further sting occur. Desensitization can be carried out, but the course is prolonged and often needs to be repeated.

Marine animals

There are many poisonous fish that can be dangerous. They are usually found in tropical waters but cases have been described worldwide. Sting-rays and scorpion fish are two examples that sting by injecting venom through barbed spines. There is immediate severe local pain and swelling, which may be followed by tissue necrosis. Systemic effects include diarrhoea, vomiting, hypotension, cardiac arrhythmias and convulsions. Treatment is supportive. Care should always be taken in waters where these fish are known to be present.

Venomous Coelenterata include jellyfish, sea anemones and the Portuguese man-of-war. The tentacles contain toxin that, following a sting, produces painful wheals at the site of contact. These wheals may become necrotic. Rarely there are systemic side-effects, including abdominal pain, diarrhoea and vomiting, hypotension and convulsions. Treatment consists of removing the tentacles, having first applied acetic acid (vinegar) to them. Alcohol compounds should not be used.

Molluscs

Only the octopus and cone-shells are venomous to humans. The blue-ringed octopus, which is found in

Australia, has saliva which contains the neurotoxin tetrodotoxin. This flows into the wounds from the beak of the octopus and can cause serious systemic effects.

In cone-shells the venom is found in association with their radular teeth. A bite initially produces local numbness, which can then spread over the body and may eventually lead to paralysis.

Seafood poisoning

This can occur with fish and shellfish. In some cases it is attributable to toxins, but most poisonings occur as a result of pathogens such as *Salmonella* or hepatitis A virus. Ichthyosarcotoxic fish contain toxins in their blood, skin and muscle and are the most common cause of poisoning.

Ciguatera

Poisoning occurs chiefly with the reef-dwelling fish from around the Pacific and Caribbean. The fish contain ciguatoxins from the plankton *Gambier discus*. Most cases of poisoning are due to the red snapper, grouper, barracuda and amberjack fish, but many other species may be responsible. The poisonous fish cannot be distinguished from identical fish that do not contain the poison. The toxin is unaffected by cooking.

Symptoms occur from a few minutes to 30 hours after ingestion of the fish. They include numbness and paraesthesia of the lips, abdominal pain, nausea, vomiting and diarrhoea. Visual blurring, photophobia, metallic taste in the mouth, myositis and eventual hypotension and shock can also occur.

Treatment is symptomatic, but symptoms can last for up to two weeks.

Scromboid fish

Fish such as tuna, mackerel and skipjack contain a high degree of histidine. This is decarboxylated by bacteria to histamine and, particularly if the fish are allowed to spoil, large amounts can accumulate in the fish, producing flushing, burning, pruritus, headache, urticaria, nausea, vomiting and bronchospasm 2–3 hours after ingestion.

Treatment is symptomatic. Care should be taken to eat only fresh fish.

Tetrodotoxin-containing puffer-fish are found in both sea and freshwater areas of Asia, India and the Caribbean. Symptoms that follow ingestion are circumoral paraesthesia, malaise and hypotension, with more severe cases producing ataxia and neuromuscular paralysis. The mortality is 50–60%.

Shellfish

Bivalve molluscs (e.g. mussels, oysters, scallops and clams) can acquire the neurotoxin saxitoxin from the dinoflagellate *Gonyaulax*. These protozoa colour the sea red and molluscs should never be taken from such areas. Symptoms are similar to those caused by tetrodotoxin, but are usually less severe. Treatment is symptomatic.

FURTHER READING

Warrell DA (1998) Antivenoms and treatment of snake-bite. *Prescriber's Journal* **38**: 10–18.

Plants

Many plants are known to be poisonous, but in practice it is unusual for severe poisoning to occur. Children are the usual victims. Only two people are known to have died from plant poisoning in the UK since the early 1970s. The most common effects of nettles and poison ivy are dermatitis followed by vomiting. Poisonous plants commonly ingested include hemlock, laburnum, deadly nightshade and green potatoes. Deadly nightshade (*Atropa belladonna*) contains hyoscyamine and hyoscine. When ingested these cause the anticholinergic effects of a dry mouth, nausea and vomiting, eventually leading to blurring of the vision, hallucinations, confusion and hyperpyrexia.

Mushrooms

There are many poisonous mushrooms that can be confused with edible fungi and be eaten by mistake. Nevertheless, apart from transient nausea, vomiting and diarrhoea, which can occur with many species, very severe reactions are rare.

Fatal mushroom poisoning is almost invariably due to *Amanita phalloides* (the death-cap mushroom). This fungus contains phallotoxins and amatoxins, both of which interfere with cell metabolism. Toxicity is increased if the mushrooms are eaten raw, as some toxins are inactivated by heat. In general, the sooner the symptoms occur, the less serious the poisoning, depending on the type of mushroom ingested. Within two hours, nausea, vomiting, diarrhoea and sweating occur. After about six hours, patients complain of headache and dizziness, and severe vomiting occurs at about 12 hours. After 72 hours, the more serious complications of hepatocellular and renal failure may occur, which have a high mortality.

The diagnosis is made by obtaining a careful history, with identification of the mushroom if possible. Amatoxins can be measured in the blood by radioimmunoassay.

Treatment should include gastric aspiration and lavage and general support. There is some evidence that haemodialysis and liver transplantation may be of value.

Other mushrooms that are poisonous include:

- *Amanita muscaria* (fly agaric), which contains a little muscarine and other hallucinogenic substances
- *Coprinus atramentarius* (ink cap), which contains a dehydrogenase inhibitor with a disulfiram-like

effect, producing flushing, swelling, a rash on the face and hands, and cardiovascular effects, particularly after alcohol
- *Amanita pantherina* (false blusher), which produces similar features to deadly nightshade because of its atropine-like effects.

Drug abuse (see also p. 1140)

Solvents

Solvent abuse has become a common problem, particularly in teenagers who inhale volatile organic solvents such as toluene in glues ('glue sniffing'). Many other solvents, such as aerosols (hair lacquer), antifreeze and petrol, can also be misused. Solvents are applied to a piece of cloth or put into a plastic bag and inhaled, often until consciousness is lost. The patient presents either in the acute intoxicated state or as a chronic abuser with excoriation and rashes over the face and a peripheral neuropathy. Sudden death can occur and is probably due to cardiac arrhythmias. Stigmata of solvent abuse include sores or a rash around the nose and mouth and glue on the clothing.

Other drugs

Drug addicts frequently overdose themselves and are commonly admitted to hospital with the signs of opiate injection. Tell-tale injection sites and pin-point pupils are important clues. Naloxone is given in the same dosage as for co-proxamol overdose (see p. 876).

Cannabis

Cannabis is usually smoked and often taken casually. Initially there is euphoria, followed by drowsiness and sleep. Redness of the conjunctivae and pupil dilatation are seen. No specific treatment is required.

Amphetamines

Amphetamines are taken for their stimulatory effect. In overdose there is confusion, delirium, hallucinations and violent behaviour. Cardiac arrhythmias can be a major problem. Treatment is with sedatives, such as diazepam. Forced acid diuresis may be used but is rarely required.

Cocaine

Cocaine can be taken by injection, inhalation or ingestion. It produces excitement, paranoia, euphoria and restlessness. This is followed by delirium, tremor, convulsions, pyrexia, syncope and cardiac arrhythmias, which may cause cardiac failure. Respiratory failure and cerebral haemorrhage may also occur.

Treatment is symptomatic and supportive. There is no specific antidote. β-Blockers should not be used to treat hypertension or tachycardia.

Ecstasy

This drug is also known as MDMA (3,4-methylene-dioxymethamphetamine). It is a semisynthetic hallucinogenic drug whose initial effects are sympathomimetic. It may cause tachyarrhythmias, hyperpyrexia, clonic movements and convulsions, coagulopathy, rhabdomyolysis and renal failure. Treatment consists of gastric lavage, chlorpromazine, α- and β-adrenergic blockade, intravenous fluids and passive cooling.

FURTHER READING

Gerada C, Ashworth M (1997) ABC of mental health: addiction and dependence 1: Illicit drugs. *British Medical Journal* **315**: 297–300.

Poison information services

Information on poisoning can be obtained from the poisons information services at the following telephone numbers:

- Belfast: 01232 240503
- Birmingham: 0121 507 5588
- Cardiff: 01222 709901
- Dublin: 010 837 9964
- Edinburgh: 0131 536 2300
- Leeds: 0131 243 0715
- London: 0171 635 9191
- Newcastle: 0191 232 5131.

Laboratory analysis may help in the diagnosis and management of some cases. Information on the available services can be obtained from the Poisons Information Service in London or the local services in each country.

CHAPTER BIBLIOGRAPHY

Proudfoot AT (1993) Acute poisoning: diagnosis and management, 2nd edn. Butterworth-Heinemann, Oxford.

Hirschfeld RMA, Russell JM (1997) Assessment and treatment of suicidal patients. *New England Journal of Medicine* **337**: 910–915.

Environmental medicine

15

Heat

In health, the core temperature of the body is maintained by the thermoregulatory centre in the hypothalamus at a constant 37°C.

Heat is produced by cellular metabolism, and is lost through the skin by vasodilatation and sweating and in air expired from the lungs. Sweating occurs when the ambient temperature is greater than 32.5°C and during exercise. The evaporation of sweat is the vital mechanism keeping the skin cool and the body temperature down.

Acclimatization

Acclimatization to a hotter climate takes 1–2 weeks. There is a gradual increase in sweating, and the sweat has a lower salt content. This process allows increased evaporation.

Heat cramps

These are painful cramps in the muscles (usually of the legs) after exercise. They often occur in fit young people who are well-acclimatized when they take vigorous exercise in hot weather. The symptoms are thought to be the result of a low extracellular sodium caused by replenishment of water but not salt during prolonged sweating. The cramps respond to salt and water replacement and can be prevented by increasing dietary salt intake.

Heat illness/Heat exhaustion

Anyone in a high environmental temperature, particularly when there is high humidity, who exercises vigorously and wears clothing which inhibits heat loss, is at risk of provoking an elevation in rectal temperature. The symptoms of weakness/exhaustion, dizziness and syncope, with an elevated core temperature, are themselves diagnostic of (and define) heat illness. The elevation of temperature is more important than the water and sodium loss. Heat illness may progress to heat injury, a serious medical emergency.

MANAGEMENT

The patient is removed from the heat and cooled using cold sponging and fans. Oxygen should be given. Blood is taken for liver biochemistry, clotting studies, urea and electrolytes and creatinine kinase. Other causes of hyperpyrexia, e.g. malaria, should be excluded if appropriate.

Oral rehydration with both salt and water (25 g of sodium chloride and 5 L of water) is given in the first 24 hours, with adequate replacements thereafter. In severe heat exhaustion, intravenous fluid is required. Isotonic saline is usually given, depending on the level of sodium in the serum. Careful monitoring is required and any subsequent potassium loss must be corrected.

Heat injury

Heat injury (heat stroke) is an acute life-threatening situation when the body temperature is above 41°C. The patient suffers from headache, nausea, vomiting and weakness. The skin is hot. Sweating is often absent, but this is not invariable, even in severe heat stroke. Neurological involvement leads to confusion, delirium and eventually coma.

Heat injury occurs in hot, humid climates with little cooling wind, even without exercise. Patients are usually unacclimatized; in some, sweating is limited owing to prickly heat (i.e. inflammation of the sweat glands after prolonged exposure to high temperatures). Old age, diabetes, drugs (e.g. anticholinergics, diuretics and phenothiazine) as well as alcohol are all further precipitating factors. The pathogenesis of heat injury is a fall in cardiac output, lactic acidosis and intravascular coagulation.

The diagnosis is clinical. The patient must be removed from the hot area immediately, and then cooled with sponging and ice if available.

Patients should be managed in intensive care and rapid cooling with ice packs started. Fluids may be required but these must be given with care as hypovolaemia is not present in many patients.

Prompt treatment is essential and can lead to a rapid and complete recovery; and delay may be fatal. Prevention is by acclimatization and keeping fit.

COMPLICATIONS

Complications of heat injury include hypovolaemia (shock), intravascular coagulation, cerebral oedema, rhabdomyolysis, and renal and hepatic failure.

Treatment of the complications is described in the appropriate chapters.

Malignant hyperpyrexia

This is discussed on p. 1104.

FURTHER READING

Simon H (1993) Hyperthermia. *New England Journal of Medicine* **329**: 483–487.

Cold

Hypothermia is defined as a fall in the core (i.e. rectal) temperature to below 35°C. It is frequently lethal when the core temperature falls below 32°C.

Frostbite is local cold injury that occurs when tissue freezes.

Hypothermia

Hypothermia occurs in a variety of clinical settings.

In the home environment

Hypothermia may occur in cold climates when there is poor heating, inadequate clothing and poor nutrition. Depressant drugs (e.g. hypnotics), alcohol, hypothyroidism or intercurrent illness also contribute. Hypothermia is commonly seen in the poor and elderly, the latter having a diminished ability to feel cold and often a decrease in the insulating fat layer. Infants and neonates become hypothermic very rapidly at normal room temperature because of their relatively large surface area and lack of subcutaneous fat.

During exposure to extremes of temperature outside

Hypothermia is a prominent cause of death in climbers, skiers, Arctic and Antarctic travellers and in wartime. Wet, cold conditions with windchill, physical exhaustion and inadequate clothing are common contributory factors.

Following immersion in cold water

Dangerous hypothermia can develop after several hours' immersion at temperatures of 15–20°C. Below 12°C the patient's limbs become anaesthetized and paralysed and take some hours to recover after the patient is rescued.

CLINICAL FEATURES

Mild hypothermia (32–35°C) causes shivering and initially a feeling of intense cold. The subject is alert and usually takes appropriate action to rewarm (e.g. huddling, extra clothing or exercise). As the core temperature falls, severe hypothermia (below 32°C) initially causes impairment of judgement (including awareness of the cold) and later leads to altered consciousness and coma. Death follows, usually from ventricular fibrillation.

DIAGNOSIS

If a thermometer is available (which must be the low-reading type), the diagnosis is straightforward. If not, a rapid clinical assessment should be made. The hypothermic patient feels cold to the touch – the abdomen, groin and axillae are cold and clammy. If consciousness is impaired (i.e. if the patient is uncooperative, sleepy or in a coma), the core temperature is almost certainly below 32°C; this is a medical emergency.

SEQUELAE
The pulse rate and volume fall, and respiration becomes shallow and slow. Muscle stiffness develops and the tendon reflexes are depressed. The systemic blood pressure falls. As coma ensues, the pupillary and other brainstem reflexes are lost (the pupils are fixed and may be dilated in severe hypothermia).

Metabolic changes are variable, with either metabolic acidosis or alkalosis occurring. Arterial oxygen tension readings may appear normal since they are measured at room temperature, but these measurements are falsely high as the arterial PO_2 falls 7% for each degree Celcius (°C) fall in temperature.

Ventricular arrhythmias (tachycardia and fibrillation) or asystole are the usual cause of death and may occur during treatment. 'J' waves – rounded waves above the isoelectric line immediately after the QRS complex – are pathognomic of hypothermia. Prolongation of the PR interval, QT interval and QRS complex also occur.

MANAGEMENT
The principles of management of this serious emergency are to rewarm the patient gradually while correcting metabolic abnormalities and treating cardiac arrhythmias. Hypothyroidism must always be looked for (see p. 932).

If the patient is awake, with a temperature above 32°C, rewarming can be achieved by placing the patient in a warm room, using a 'space blanket', and giving warm fluids orally. Outdoors, the same result can be achieved by adding extra clothing, huddling with the subject, and using a warmed sleeping bag. Rewarming may take several hours. Alcohol should be avoided because it may add to confusion, boost confidence factitiously, cause peripheral vasodilatation (and further heat loss), or precipitate hypoglycaemia.

Severe hypothermia
In severe hypothermia, the patient may appear dead. (Hypothermia should always be excluded before brain death is diagnosed.) Warming should take place gradually, aiming at an increase in temperature of 1°C per hour. The patient should be covered with a 'space blanket' and placed in a warm room. Direct surface heat from an electric blanket is also helpful. Any underlying condition should be treated promptly. Drug overdose should always be excluded.

Warmed intravenous fluids are given slowly and metabolic disturbances corrected. Hypothyroidism, if present, should be treated with triiodothyronine 10 μg i.v. 8-hourly. Various methods of artificial rewarming have been suggested – warm humidified air by inhalation, gastric or peritoneal lavage, or haemodialysis – but in practice these are rarely used. The cardiac rhythm should be monitored and arrhythmias corrected.

Careful monitoring of all vital functions is required; appropriate treatment and intensive care are given as necessary.

PREVENTION
Prevention of hypothermia is particularly important in the elderly, who should be advised to try to improve general heating and insulation in the house. Heat should be provided in the bedrooms, and the use of safe electric blankets advised. Financial help will be needed by many patients. Constant supervision should be given during cold spells, when warm food and extra blankets must be provided.

Frostbite

The formation of ice crystals in the skin and superficial tissues begins when the temperature there falls to –3°C; ambient temperatures generally have to be below –6°C for this to occur.

RECOGNITION
Frostbitten tissue is pale, greyish and initially doughy to the touch. Later it freezes hard, when it looks (and feels) like meat taken from a deep freeze. This condition may occur when working or exercising in low temperatures and typically develops without the patient's knowledge. Hands and feet that have 'lost their feeling' are an important feature when the temperature is below –5°C, as frostbite may then develop insidiously.

MANAGEMENT
The frostbitten patient should, if possible, be transported (or walk, even on frostbitten feet), to a place of safety before treatment commences. Warming using the body heat of a companion or by immersion in water at 39–42°C should be continued until obvious thawing occurs. This may be painful. Blisters will form within several days and, depending on the degree of frostbite, a blackened carapace or shell develops as the blisters regress or burst. Dry, non-adherent dressings and strict aseptic precautions are essential. Frostbitten tissues are anaesthetized and are at risk from infection and further trauma. Recovery takes place over many weeks. Surgery may be required, but should be avoided in the early stages, as it is difficult to predict the eventual amount of recovery.

FURTHER READING

Lazar H.L. (1997) Editorial: The treatment of hypothermia. *New England Journal of Medicine* **337**: 1545–1547.

High altitudes

The partial pressure of ambient (and hence alveolar and arterial) oxygen falls in a near-linear relationship to altitude (Fig. 15.1).

Table 15.1
Conditions caused by sustained hypoxia

Condition	Incidence (%)	Usual altitude (m)
Acute mountain sickness	70	3500–4000
Acute pulmonary oedema	2	4000
Acute cerebral oedema	1	4500
Retinal haemorrhage	50	5000
Deterioration	100	5600
Chronic mountain sickness	Rare	4500

Below 3000 m there are few important clinical effects. Commercial aircraft are pressurized to 2750 m and the resulting hypoxia causes breathlessness only in those with severe cardiorespiratory disease. The incidence of thromboembolism is slightly greater in (sedentary) travellers on long flights than in similar population at sea level. Above 3000–3500 m hypoxia causes a spectrum of related clinical syndromes that affect visitors to high altitudes, principally climbers, trekkers, skiers and troops (Table 15.1). These conditions, which often coexist, occur largely during the acclimatization process. This may last some weeks, but enables humans to live (permanently if necessary) at altitudes up to about 5600 m. At greater heights, although humans can survive for days or weeks, deterioration due to chronic hypoxia is inevitable.

It has been demonstrated on several occasions that ascent to the highest of the world's summits is possible without the use of supplementary oxygen. At the summit of Everest (nearly 9000 m) the barometric pressure is 34 kPa (253 mmHg). This enables an acclimatized mountaineer to have an alveolar Po_2 of 4.0–4.7 kPa (30–35 mmHg), which is near the physiological limit of a human being.

Acute mountain sickness (AMS)

This term is used to describe the malaise, nausea, headache and lassitude that are common above 3500 m. Following arrival at this altitude there is usually a latent interval of 6–36 hours before the onset of symptoms. Treatment is rest, with analgesics being given if necessary; recovery is almost invariable.

Prophylactic treatment with the carbonic anhydrase inhibitor acetazolamide is of value in reducing the symptoms of AMS, since these are partly due to the development of alkalosis. Acclimatizing, ascending gradually, is the best prophylaxis.

In a minority of cases, the more serious sequelae of high-altitude pulmonary oedema (HAPO) and high-altitude cerebral oedema (HACO) occur.

High-altitude pulmonary oedema (HAPO)

Predisposing factors include youth, rapidity of ascent, heavy exertion and the presence of mountain sickness. Breathlessness, with frothy bloodstained sputum indicates established HAPO. Unless treated rapidly this leads to cardiorespiratory failure, collapse and death. Milder forms of HAPO are common, presenting with breathlessness that is not severe; it is important to recognize them.

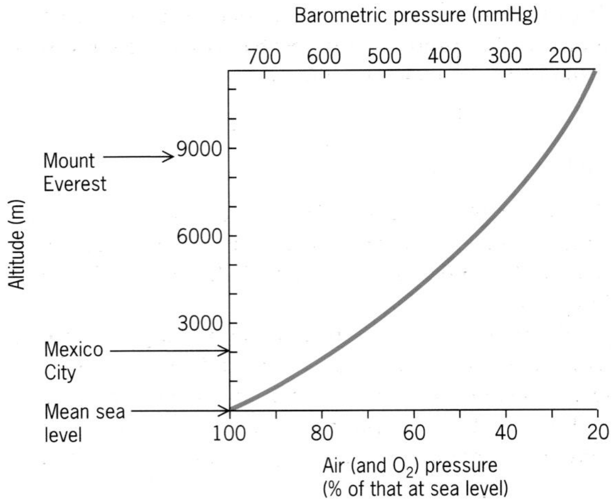

Fig. 15.1
The decrease in oxygen and barometric pressure with increasing altitude

High-altitude cerebral oedema (HACO)

Cerebral oedema is a poorly understood sequel of hypoxia. It is probably the result of the abrupt increase in cerebral blood flow that occurs even at modest altitudes of 3500–4000 m. Headache is usual, and is accompanied by varying disturbances of cerebral function; drowsiness, ataxia, nystagmus and papilloedema are common. Coma and death follow if the condition progresses.

TREATMENT

Any but the milder forms of AMS require urgent treatment. Oxygen should be given if it is available, and descent to a lower altitude should take place as quickly as possible. Nifedipine reduces pulmonary hypertension and is used in the treatment of HAPO. Dexamethasone is effective in reducing brain oedema in HACO. Portable pressure bags, in which the patient is inserted, are helpful in increasing barometric pressure; these have become widely used.

Retinal haemorrhages

Small 'flame' haemorrhages in the nerve fibre layer of the retina are common above 5000 m. They are usually symptomless unless they cover the macula, when there is painless loss of central vision. Recovery is usual.

Deterioration

Prolonged residence at between 5600 and 7000 m leads to a syndrome of weight loss, anorexia and listlessness after several weeks. Above 7500 m, deterioration develops more quickly, although it is possible to survive for a week or more at altitudes over 8000 m.

Chronic mountain sickness

This rare syndrome occurs in long-term residents at high altitudes after several decades. It has been described clearly only in the Andes, but may occur in Tibet and elsewhere in central Asia.

Polycythaemia, drowsiness, cyanosis, finger clubbing, congested cheeks and ear lobes, and right ventricular enlargement occur. The condition is gradually progressive.

By way of contrast, coronary artery disease and hypertension are rare in the native populations of high altitude.

FURTHER READING

Clarke C (1998) High altitude and mountaineering expeditions. In: Warrell D, Anderson S (eds) Expedition medicine. Profile Books and Royal Geographical Society, London, pp. 207–214.

Pollard AJ (1997) The high altitude medicine handbook. Radcliffe Medical Press, Oxford.

UIAA Mountain Medicine Data Centre leaflets available from British Mountaineering Council

Diving

The increases in ambient pressure to which a diver is exposed at various depths are summarized in Table 15.2.

Various methods are used to supply air to the diver. With the simplest (e.g. a snorkel), the limiting factor, which occurs below 0.5 m, is the respiratory effort required to suck air into the lungs. At greater depths this 'forced negative-pressure ventilation' ultimately results in pulmonary capillary damage and haemorrhagic pulmonary oedema. Scuba tanks, the method commonly used for sporting diving down to 50 m, carry compressed air at a pressure balanced with the water pressure.

Divers who work at great depths for commercial purposes or for underwater exploration breathe helium–oxygen or nitrogen–oxygen mixtures delivered by hose from the surface.

A wide variety of complex medical problems may affect divers at all depths. These are summarized below.

Table 15.2
Pressure in relation to sea depth

Sea depth (m)	Absolute pressure (atmospheres)	mmHg
0	1	760
10	2	1520
50	6	4560
90	10	7600

Problems during compression (e.g. descent)

Barotrauma of the middle ear ('squeeze') is the most common disorder in divers. This is caused by an inability to equalize the pressure in the middle ear usually as a result of Eustachian tube blockage. Deafness occurs with eventual rupture of the tympanic membrane, followed by acute vertigo.

Paranasal sinus – sinus barotrauma ('squeeze') – is due to dysfunction of the nasal or paranasal sinus with blockage of the sinus ostea. Pain over the frontal sinus occurs.

Treatment of both conditions consists of decongestants. It can be prevented by avoiding diving when the airways are blocked as occurs with a respiratory tract infection.

Nitrogen narcosis

When compressed air is breathed below 30 m the narcotic effects of nitrogen cause impairment of cerebral function with changes of mood and performance that may be life-threatening. The condition reverses rapidly on ascent.

Nitrogen narcosis is avoided by replacing air with helium–oxygen mixtures, which can enable divers to descend to 700 m.

At these great depths neurological disturbances occur that are believed to be the result of the direct effects of pressure on neurones. Tremor, hemiparesis and psychological changes may occur.

Oxygen narcosis

Pure oxygen cannot be used for diving because oxygen becomes toxic to the lungs when the alveolar oxygen pressure exceeds 1.5 atmospheres absolute (5 m of water) and to the nervous system at around 10 m of water.

In the lungs, linear atelectasis appears and there is endothelial cell damage with exudation and pulmonary oedema. In the nervous system there is initially a feeling of apprehension, nausea and sweating, followed by muscle twitching and generalized convulsions, which may be fatal under water.

Problems during decompression (i.e. ascent)

Breath-hold (shallow-water) diving

Shallow-water swimmers and free divers deliberately hyperventilate prior to a dive to drive off CO_2 in order to lower P_aCO_2 which is the stimulus to breathe. The subsequent breath-hold causes a rise in P_aCO_2 and a fall of P_aO_2 as expected. However, on surfacing, decompression further lowers the P_aO_2 which may cause a loss of consciousness.

Decompression sickness

Decompression sickness ('the bends') occurs in divers on returning to the surface and is caused by the release of inert gases, usually nitrogen or helium, which form bubbles in the tissues as the ambient pressure falls. It occurs only when the diver ascends too rapidly. Decompression tables are available for calculating the time needed to come to the surface safely from any given depth.

The sickness can take a mild form (type 1 'non-neurological bends'), with skin irritation, mottling or joint pain only, or may be more serious (type 2 'bends'), in which a variety of neurological features appear. Patients with type 2 'bends' may develop cortical blindness, hemiparesis, sensory disturbances or cord lesions. If nitrogen bubbles occur in the pulmonary vessels, divers experience retrosternal discomfort, dyspnoea and cough ('the chokes'). These symptoms develop within minutes or hours of a dive.

Treatment is with oxygen. In addition, all but the mildest forms of decompression sickness (i.e. skin mottling alone) require recompression, usually in a pressure chamber.

A long-term problem is aseptic necrosis caused by infarction due to nitrogen bubbles lodging in nutrient arteries supplying bone. It is seen in 5% of deep-sea divers. Neurological damage may also persist.

Lung rupture, pneumothorax and surgical emphysema

These emergencies occur principally when divers 'breath-hold' while making emergency ascents after losing their gas supply. Following lung rupture the patient notes severe dyspnoea, cough and haemoptysis. Pneumothorax and emphysema usually respond to 100% oxygen. Air embolism may occur and should be treated with recompression and hyperbaric oxygen.

FURTHER READING

Bennett P, Elliot D (1993) *The Physiology and Medicine of Diving*, 4th edn. London: WB Saunders.

Melamed Y, Shupak A, Bitterman (1992) Medical problems associated with underwater diving. *New England Journal of Medicine* **326**: 30–36.

Ionizing radiation

Ionizing radiation is either penetrating (X-rays, gamma rays or neutrons) or non-penetrating (alpha or beta particles). Penetrating radiation affects the whole body, while non-penetrating radiation affects only the skin. All radiation effects, however, depend on the type of radiation, the distribution of dose and the dose rate.

Radiation dosage is measured in joules per kilogram ($J\ kg^{-1}$); $1\ J\ kg^{-1}$ is also known as one gray (1 Gy). This is equivalent to 100 rads. Radioactivity is measured in becquerels (Bq); 1 Bq is equal to the amount of radioactive material in which there is one disintegration per second. One curie (Ci) is equal to 3.7×10^{10} Bq.

Radiation differs in the density of ionization it causes. Therefore a dose-equivalent called a sievert (Sv) is used. This is the absorbed dose weighted for the damaging effect of the radiation. The annual background radiation is approximately 2.5 mSv.

Excessive exposure to ionizing radiation occurs following accidents in hospitals, industry, nuclear power plants and strategic nuclear explosions.

Mild acute radiation sickness

Nausea, vomiting and malaise follow doses of approximately 1 Gy (75–125 rad). Lymphopenia occurs within several days, followed 2–3 weeks later by a fall in all white cells and platelets. There is a late risk of leukaemia and solid tumours.

Severe acute radiation sickness

Many systems are affected; the extent of the damage depends on the dose of radiation received. The effects of radiation are summarized in Table 15.3.

Haemopoietic syndrome

Absorption of doses between 2 and 10 Gy (200 and 1000 rad) is followed by early and transient vomiting in some individuals, followed by a period of relative well-being. Lymphocytes are particularly sensitive to radiation damage and severe lymphopenia develops over several days. A decrease in granulocytes and platelets occurs 2–3 weeks later as no new cells are being formed by the damaged marrow. Thrombocytopenia with bleeding develops and frequent overwhelming infections occur, with a very high mortality.

Table 15.3
The effects of radiation

Acute effects	Delayed effects
Haemopoietic syndrome	Infertility
Gastrointestinal syndrome	Teratogenesis
CNS syndrome	Cataract
Radiation dermatitis	Neoplasia
	Acute myeloid leukaemia
	Thyroid
	Salivary glands
	Skin
	Others

Gastrointestinal syndrome

Absorption of doses greater than 6 Gy (600 rad) causes vomiting several hours after exposure. This then stops, only to recur some four days later accompanied by severe diarrhoea. Owing to radiation inhibition of cell division, the villous lining of the intestine becomes denuded. Intractable bloody diarrhoea follows, with dehydration, secondary infection and death.

CNS syndrome

Exposures above 30 Gy (3000 rad) are followed rapidly by nausea, vomiting, disorientation and coma. Death due to severe cerebral oedema follows within 36 hours.

Radiation dermatitis

Skin erythema, purpura, blistering and secondary infection occur. Total loss of body hair is a bad prognostic sign and usually follows an exposure of at least 5 Gy (500 rad).

Late effects of radiation exposure

The survivors of the nuclear bombing of Hiroshima and Nagasaki have provided information on the long-term effects of radiation. The risk of developing acute myeloid leukaemia or cancer, particularly of the skin, thyroid and salivary glands, increases. Infertility, teratogenesis and cataract are also late sequelae of radiation exposure.

TREATMENT

Acute radiation sickness is a medical emergency. Hospitals should be informed immediately of the type and length of exposure so that suitable arrangements can be made to receive the patient. The initial radiation dose absorbed can be reduced by removing clothing contaminated by radioactive materials.

Treatment of radiation sickness is largely supportive and consists of prevention and treatment of infection, haemorrhage and fluid loss. Storage of the patient's white cells and platelets for future use should be considered, if feasible.

Accidental ingestion of, or exposure to, bone-seeking radioisotopes (e.g. strontium-90 and caesium-137) should be treated with chelating agents (e.g. EDTA) and massive doses of oral calcium. Radioiodine contamination should be treated immediately with potassium iodide 133 mg per day. This will block 90% of radioiodine absorption by the thyroid if given immediately before exposure.

Electric shock

Electric shock may produce clinical effects in three ways:

- *Pain and psychological sequelae.* The common 'electric shock' is usually a painful, but harmless, stimulus that is an unpleasant and frightening experience. It produces no lasting neurological damage or cutaneous evidence of damage.
- *Disruption of specific biological processes.* Ventricular fibrillation, muscular contraction and spinal cord damage follow a major shock. These are seen ±typically following a lightning strike.
- *Electrical burns.* These are either superficial burns (e.g. lightning may cause a fern-shaped burn), or necrosis of subcutaneous tissues owing to the heat generated by the electricity.

Smoke

Air pollution is discussed p. 648.

Smoke consists of particles of carbon in hot air and gases. These particles are mainly coated with organic acids and aldehydes. The use of synthetic materials, e.g. polyvinyl chloride, was widespread. On combustion, these materials released other substances, such as carbon monoxide and hydrochloric acid.

Respiratory symptoms may be immediate or delayed. Patients are dyspnoeic and tachypnoeic. Laryngeal stridor may require intubation. Hypoxia and pulmonary oedema can be fatal.

Treatment is to remove the subject from the smoke and give O_2. Intensive care may be required.

Noise

The intensity of sound is expressed in terms of the square of the sound pressure. The bel is a ratio and is equivalent to a 10-fold increase in sound intensity; a decibel (dB) is one-tenth of a bel. Sound is made up of a number of frequencies ranging from 30 hertz (Hz) to 20 kHz, with most being between 1 and 4 kHz. When measuring sound, these different frequencies must be taken into account. In practice a scale known as A-weighted sound is used; sound levels are then reported as dB(A). A hazardous sound source is defined as one with an overall sound pressure greater than 90 dB(A).

Repeated prolonged exposure to loud noise, particularly in the frequency range of 2–6 kHz, causes first temporary and later permanent hearing loss owing to damage to the organ of Corti, with destruction of hair cells and, eventually, the auditory neurones. This is a common occupational problem, not only in industry and the armed forces, but also in the home (e.g. from electric drills and sanders), in sport (e.g. motor racing), and in entertainment (pop stars, their audiences and disc jockeys).

Serious noise-induced hearing loss is almost wholly preventable by personal protection (ear muffs, ear plugs). Little treatment can be offered once deafness becomes established.

Non-auditory effects on health

It has been suggested that excess noise affects the development and reading skills of children. It may also have an effect on some psychiatric disorders.

Drowning and near-drowning

Drowning is a common cause of accidental death, accounting for over 500 000 deaths in 1990 worldwide. Approximately 40% of drownings occur in children under five years of age. Exhaustion, alcohol, drugs and hypothermia all contribute to the overall problem. In addition, drowning can also occur following an epileptic attack or after a myocardial infarct whilst in the water.

'Dry' drowning

Between 10% and 15% of drownings occur without aspiration of water into the lungs. Laryngeal spasm is thought to occur with anoxia occurring due to apnoea.

'Wet' drowning

Aspiration of fresh water affects the pulmonary surfactant, with alveolar collapse and ventilation perfusion mismatch leading to hypoxaemia. Aspiration of hypertonic seawater (5% NaCl) pulls additional fluid into the lungs with further ventilation perfusion mismatch. In practice, however, there is little difference between saltwater and freshwater drowning as in both groups severe hypoxaemia occurs leading to death in some. Severe metabolic acidosis develops in the majority of survivors.

In patients who aspirate more than 22 mL kg^{-1} of water, electrolyte and volume changes do occur, but very few of such patients have survived.

EMERGENCY TREATMENT OF NEAR-DROWNING

It must be remembered that patients can survive for up to 30 minutes under water without suffering brain damage, and if the water is near 0°C this time can be much longer. The exact reasons for this are not clearly understood, but it is probably related to the protective role of the diving reflex. It has been shown experimentally that submersion in water causes a reflex slowing of the pulse and vasoconstriction. In addition, hypothermia decreases oxygen consumption of both the heart and brain.

Patients should be turned to one side and the mouth cleared of any debris. Mouth-to-mouth respiration should be started immediately, together with cardiac resuscitation if this is appropriate (see p. 655).

Mouth-to-mouth resuscitation should always be attempted, even in the absence of a pulse and the presence of fixed dilated pupils, as patients frequently make a dramatic recovery.

All patients should be subsequently admitted to hospital for intensive monitoring. Intensive care therapy may be required, and patients are liable to develop the acute respiratory distress syndrome (ARDS).

PROGNOSIS

The prognosis is good if the patient is fully conscious on admission to hospital but poor if the patient is still in a coma.

FURTHER READING

Modell J H (1993) Drowning. *New England Journal of Medicine* **328**: 253–256.

Ultraviolet light

Ultraviolet (UV) light consists of UVB (wavelength 290–320 nm) and UVA (320–400 nm). Wavelengths of 1200–290 nm are stopped by the Earth's ozone layer.

- UVB causes sunburn (see p. 1171).
- UVA and UVB causes skin ageing and skin cancer.

Sunscreens absorb UV energy but many preparations absorb only UVB. The sun protection factor (SPF) is a guide to the sunscreen's performance, but there is no worldwide standard and often the protective effect is against only UVB. With a normal skin, a water-resistant sunscreen of 8–10 containing *para*-aminobenzoic acid is recommended to avoid sunburn.

Snow blindness This is an exceedingly painful keratoconjunctivitis developing after exposure to a reflection of sunlight from snow. Treatment is with topical steroid eye drops.

Travel

Motion sickness

This common problem, particularly in children, is caused by repetitive stimulation of the labyrinth of the ear. It occurs frequently at sea and in cars, but may occur on horseback or on less usual forms of transport such as camels or elephants. Nausea, sweating, dizziness, vertigo and profuse vomiting occur, accompanied by an irresistible desire to stop moving.

Prophylactic antihistamines or vestibular sedatives (hyoscine or cinnarizine) are of some value.

Jet-lag

Jet-lag, or circadian dyschronism, is the well-known phenomenon in a person changing time-zones, particularly from West to East. Fatigue and insomnia, headache, irritability, poor concentration, and loss of appetite are common. These symptoms last several days.

Pathophysiological mechanisms involved are poorly understood but relate to the body clock, sited within the suprachiasmatic nuclei in the hypothalamus. The body clock is modulated by various Zeitgebers ('time-givers'), such as light and the hormone melatonin.

Management of jet-lag includes its acceptance as a phenomenon causing poor performance, for example in athletes, and waiting for 3–5 days until the symptoms have settled. Various hypnotics are used to combat the insomnia, but their place is disputed. Melatonin by mouth is widely used to reduce the subjective symptoms of jet-lag. It has been shown to increase sleepiness and hasten the adjustment of the body clock. It is not available on prescription.

FURTHER READING

Waterhouse J, Reilly T, Atkinson G (1997) Jet-lag. *Lancet* **350**: 1611–1616.

Building-related illnesses

The term 'building-related illness' is preferable to 'sick building syndrome' as the latter implies a problem with the building itself. More than half the adult workforce in developed countries work in offices. Modern office buildings have a controlled environment with automated heating, ventilation and air-conditioning systems, often without outdoor air.

Specific building-related illness

Legionnaire's disease (see p. 797) is frequently due to contamination of air-conditioned systems. Humidifier fever (p. 816) is also due to contaminated systems, probably by fungi, bacteria and protozoa. Many common viruses are easily transmitted in the enclosed environment (e.g. the common cold, influenza and rarely pulmonary tuberculosis). Allergic disorders (e.g. rhinitis, asthma and dermatitis) also occur owing to exposure to indoor allergens such as dust-mites and plants. Office equipment (e.g. fumes from photocopiers) has also been implicated. Passive smoking (p. 767) is also a problem.

Non-specific building-related illness

A number of vague symptoms such as headache, fatigue and difficulty in concentrating have been reported by workers in office buildings. Although psychological factors may have a role, psychological testing of symptomatic and asymptomatic workers are similar. Temperature, humidity, dust, volatile organic compounds (e.g. paints, solvents) have all been implicated. Maintenance of continuous outdoor air supply and attention to the environment is recommended. However, changes in ventilation have failed to improve the symptoms, which may well be psychosocial in origin.

FURTHER READING

Menzies J, Bourbeau T (1997) Building-related illnesses. *New England Medical Journal* **337**: 1524–1531.

Information

- **High altitudes**: British Mountaineering Council, 177–179 Burton Road, Manchester M20 2BB. Tel: 0161-445-4747; Fax: 0161-445-4500.
- **Diving**: Institute of Naval Medicine, Undersea Medicine Division, Alverstoke, Gosport, Hampshire PO12 2DL. Tel: 01705-768026.
- **Diving emergencies**: Ministry of Defence, Duty Diving Division Medical Officer. Tel: 0831-151 523.

Endocrinology

16

Hormonal activity

Hormones are chemical messengers produced by a variety of specialized secretory cells. They may be transported in the blood to a distant site of action (the classic 'endocrine' effect) or may act directly upon nearby cells ('paracrine' activity). In the hypothalamus, elsewhere in the brain and in the gastrointestinal tract there are many such cells secreting hormones, some of which have true endocrine or paracrine activity, while others behave more like neurotransmitters or neuromodulators. The distinction between neurotransmitters that act across synaptic clefts, intercellular factors acting across gap junctions, classic endocrine and paracrine activity and a variety of other chemical messengers involved in cell regulation – such as cytokines, growth factors and interleukins – is increasingly blurred. Thus, progress in basic cell biology has revealed the biochemical similarities in the messengers, receptors and intracellular post-receptor mechanisms underlying all these aspects of cell function.

Synthesis, storage and release of hormones

Hormones may be of several chemical structures: polypeptide, glycoprotein, steroid or amine. Hormone release is the end-product of a long cascade of intracellular events. In the case of polypeptide hormones, neural or endocrine stimulation of the cell leads to increased transcription from DNA to a specific mRNA, which is in turn translated to the peptide product. This is often in the form of a precursor molecule that may itself be biologically inactive. This 'prohormone' may be further processed before being packaged into granules, in the Golgi apparatus. These granules are then transported to the plasma membrane before release, which is itself regulated by a complex combination of intracellular regulators. Hormone release may be in a brief spurt caused by the sudden stimulation of granules, often induced by an intracellular Ca^{2+}-dependent process, or it may be 'constitutive' (immediate and continuous secretion).

Plasma transport

Most classical hormones are secreted into the systemic circulation where they travel to have effects elsewhere in the body. In contrast, hypothalamic releasing hormones are released into the pituitary portal system so that much higher concentrations of the releasing hormones reach the pituitary than occur in the systemic circulation.

Many hormones are bound to proteins within the circulation. In most cases, only the free (unbound) hormone is available to the tissues and thus biologically active. This binding serves to buffer against very rapid changes in plasma levels of the hormone, and some binding protein interactions may also be involved in the active regulation of hormone action. This principle is important in interpreting many tests of endocrine function, which often measure total rather than free hormone, since binding proteins are frequently altered in disease states. Binding proteins comprise both specific, high-affinity proteins of limited capacity, such as thyroxine-binding globulin (TBG) and other less-specific low-affinity ones, such as prealbumin and albumin. The most important and clinically relevant binding proteins are shown in Table 16.1.

Hormone action and receptors

Hormones act by binding to specific receptors in the target cell, which may be at the cell surface and/or within the cell. Most hormone receptors are proteins with complex tertiary structures, parts of which complement the tertiary structure of the hormone to allow highly specific interactions, while other parts are responsible for the effects of the activated receptor within the cell. Many hormones bind to specific cell-surface receptors where they trigger internal messengers, while others bind to nuclear receptors which interact directly with DNA (Fig 16.1). Cell-surface receptors usually contain hydrophobic sections which span the lipid-rich plasma membrane, while nuclear receptors contain characteristic amino-acid sequences to bind nuclear DNA (e.g. so-called 'zinc fingers', see p. 134) as in the glucocorticoid receptor.

In order to achieve these intracellular effects, hormone receptors interact with a variety of other regulatory factors within the cell membrane, in the cytosol or within the nucleus of the cell. In each case, binding of the hormone to its receptor results in a conformational change in the structure of the receptor which may result in a number of possible outcomes:

- activation of, or modified binding to, other regulatory factors within the cell membrane or cytosol (e.g. binding of transmembrane receptors to the cell-membrane G-proteins, thereby activating the stimulatory or inhibitory effects of the latter on other intracellular mediators)
- activation of enzyme activity in the receptor or its regulatory factors (e.g. receptor adenylate cyclase, other protein kinases, phospholipase C) to generate a variety of intracellular 'second messengers' (e.g. cAMP, cGMP, phosphatidylinositol metabolites, calmodulin) which usually form a complex and branching intracellular cascade of enzyme activation and inhibition and/or mobilization of intracellular stores of ions (primarily calcium)
- dimerization of the receptor, or internalization of some cell-surface receptors
- altered binding of the receptor to DNA or to nuclear transcription factors in order to stimulate or inhibit transcription of one or more genes
- altered activity of cell membrane channels or transporters (e.g. for glucose, potassium or for other ions).

These immediate effects of hormone binding may then cause rapid alterations in cell-membrane ion transport or intracellular calcium concentrations, or slower responses such as DNA, RNA and protein synthesis.

In each case, binding of the hormone to its receptor is the first step in a complex cascade of interrelated intracellular events which eventually lead to the overall effects of that hormone on cellular function. Common 'second messengers' involved in these cascades include cyclic AMP (for adrenocorticotrophic hormone (ACTH), luteinizing hormone (LH), follicle stimulating hormone (FSH) and parathyroid hormone (PTH)), a calcium-phospholipid system (for thyrotrophin releasing hormone (TRH), vasopressin and angiotensin II), tyrosine kinase and other intracellular kinases (for insulin and insulin-like growth factor-1 (IGF-1)) and membrane-bound phosphoinositide pathways.

Some characteristics of hormone systems are shown in Table 16.2.

The sensitivity and/or number of receptors for a hormone are often decreased after prolonged exposure to a high hormone concentration, the receptors thus becoming less sensitive ('down-regulation', e.g. angiotensin II receptors, β-adrenoceptors). The reverse is true when stimulation is absent or minimal, the receptors showing increased numbers or sensitivity ('up-regulation').

Abnormal receptors are an occasional, though rare, cause of endocrine disease (see p. 902), but are being recognized and characterized more frequently owing to advances in molecular endocrinology.

Table 16.1
Plasma hormones with important binding proteins

Hormone	Binding protein(s)
Thyroxine (T_4)	Thyroxine-binding globulin (TBG) Thyroxine-binding prealbumin (TBPA) Albumin
Triiodothyronine (T_3) (less bound than T4)	Thyroxine-binding globulin (TBG) Albumin
Cortisol	Cortisol-binding globulin (CBG)
Testosterone, oestradiol	Sex hormone-binding globulin (SHBG)
Insulin-like growth factor I (IGF-I)	IGF binding proteins (mainly IGF-BP3)

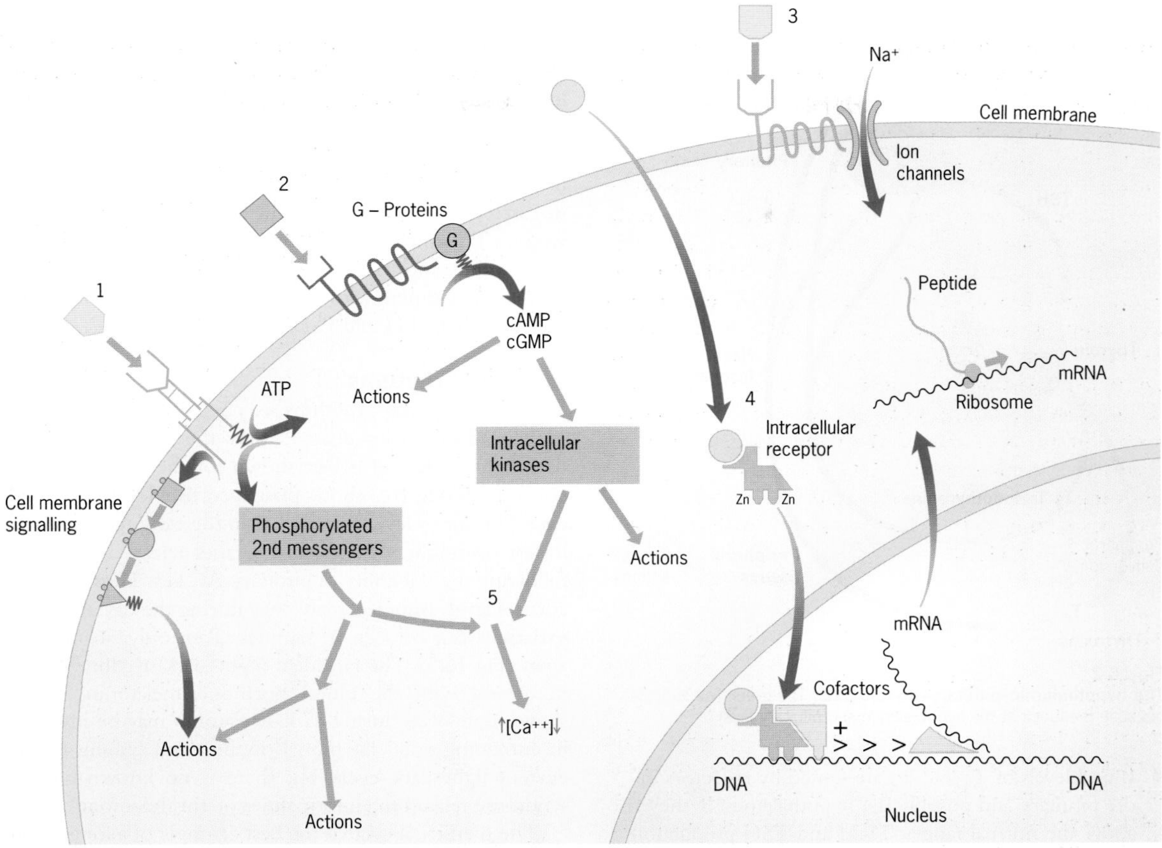

Fig 16.1
Intracellular hormone action Hormones bind to specific receptors on the surface (1,2,3) or in the cytoplasm and nucleus (4) of the cell. Receptor binding may activate cell membrane signalling cascades (1), inherent receptor enzyme activity (1), enzyme activity on cofactors such as G-proteins (2) or cell membrane transport channels (3). Initial effects are followed by an intracellular cascade of activation, inhibition and changes in calcium concentration (5). Nuclear receptors (4) bind with cofactors to DNA to initiate mRNA transcription and protein synthesis.

Control and feedback

Most hormone systems are controlled by some form of feedback; an example is the hypothalamic–pituitary–thyroid axis (Fig. 16.2).

- TRH (thyrotrophin releasing hormone) is secreted in the hypothalamus and travels via the portal system to the pituitary where it stimulates the thyrotrophs to produce thyroid-stimulating hormone (TSH).
- TSH is secreted into the systemic circulation where it stimulates increased thyroidal iodine uptake and thyroxine (T_4) and tri-iodothyronine (T_3) synthesis and release.
- Serum levels of T_3 and T_4 are thus increased by TSH; in addition, the conversion of T_4 to T_3 (the more active hormone) in peripheral tissues is stimulated by TSH.
- T_3 and T_4 then enter cells where they bind to nuclear receptors and promote increased metabolic and cellular activity.

Table 16.2
Characteristics of some different hormone systems

	Peptides and catecholamines	Steroids and thyroid hormones
Protein binding	No	Yes
Changes in plasma concentrations	Rapid changes	Slow fluctuations
Plasma half-life	Short (seconds to minutes)	Long (minutes to days)
Type of receptors	Cell membrane	Intracellular
Mechanism	Activate preformed enzymes	Stimulate protein synthesis
Secretion	Secretory granules Constitutive + bursts	Direct passage rapidly Related to secretion rate
Speed of effect	Rapid (seconds to minutes)	Slow (hours to days)

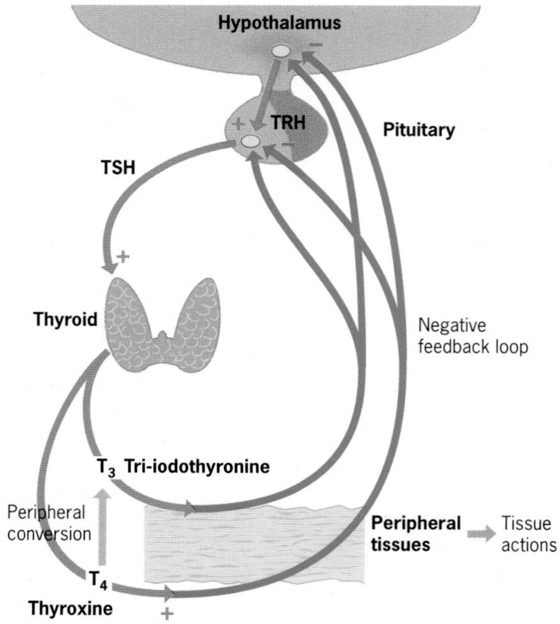

Fig 16.2
The hypothalamic–pituitary–thyroid axis. The green line indicates negative feedback at the hypothalamic and pituitary level

- Blood levels of T_3 and T_4 are sensed by receptors in the pituitary and possibly the hypothalamus. If they rise above the normal ranges, TRH and TSH production is suppressed, leading to reduced T_3 and T_4 secretion.
- Peripheral T_3 and T_4 levels thus fall to normal.
- If, however, T_3 and T_4 levels are low (e.g. after thyroidectomy), increased amounts of TRH and thus TSH are secreted, stimulating the remaining thyroid to produce more T_3 and T_4; blood levels of T_3 and T_4 may be restored to normal, although at the expense of increased TSH drive, reflected by a high TSH level ('compensated euthyroidism').

This is known as a 'negative feedback' system, referring to the effect of T_3 and T_4 on the pituitary and hypothalamus, which represents the most common mechanism for regulation of circulating hormone levels. There are also positive feedback systems, classically seen in the regulation of the normal menstrual cycle.

Patterns of secretion

Hormone secretion may be continuous or intermittent. The former is shown by the thyroid hormones, where T_4 has a half-life of 7–10 days and T_3 of about 6–10 hours. Levels over the day, month and year show little variation.

In contrast, secretion of the gonadotrophins, LH and FSH, is normally pulsatile, with major pulses released every 1–2 hours depending on the phase of the menstrual cycle. Continuous infusion of LH to produce a steady equivalent level does not produce the same result (e.g. ovulation in the female) as the intermittent pulsatility, and may indeed produce down-regulation and amenorrhoea. Thus the long-acting superactive gonadotrophin-releasing hormone (GnRH) analogue, buserelin, produces down-regulation of the GnRH receptors and subsequent very low androgen or oestrogen levels, which are clinically valuable both in carcinoma of the prostate in men and in infertility in women. Pulsatile GnRH administration on the other hand can produce normal menstrual cyclicity, ovulation and fertility in women with hypothalamic amenorrhoea but intact pituitary LH and FSH stores.

Biological rhythms

The most important rhythms are circadian and menstrual.

'Circadian' means changes over the 24 hours of the day–night cycle and is best shown for the glucocorticoid cortisol axis. Fig 16.3 shows plasma cortisol levels measured over 24 hours – levels are highest in the early morning and lowest overnight. Additionally, cortisol release is pulsatile, following the pulsatility of pituitary ACTH. Thus 'normal' cortisol levels (stippled areas) vary during the day and great variations can be seen in samples taken only 30 minutes apart (Fig 16.3). The circadian (light–dark) rhythm is seen in reverse with the pineal hormone, melatonin, which shows high levels during dark. Melatonin may be involved in entraining other hormonal rhythms and systems to the current light–dark cycle, but there is no known clinical syndrome related to abnormalities of this hormone.

The menstrual cycle is the best example of a longer and more complex (28-day) biological rhythm (see p. 911).

Other regulatory factors

- *Stress*. Though difficult to define, 'stress' can produce rapid increases in ACTH and cortisol, growth hormone (GH), prolactin, adrenaline and noradrenaline. These can occur within seconds or minutes.
- *Sleep*. Secretion of GH and prolactin is increased during sleep, especially the rapid eye movement (REM) phase.

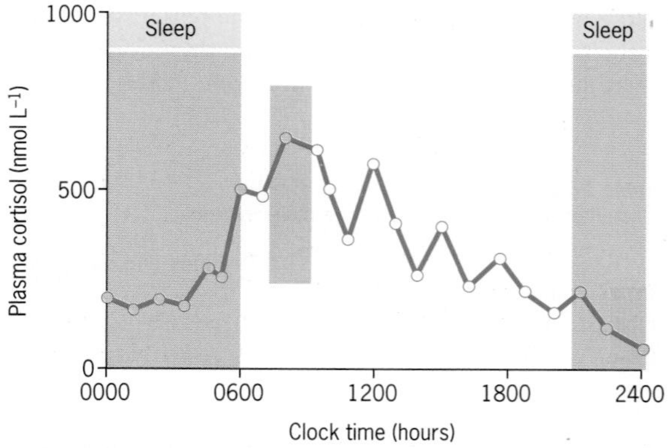

Fig 16.3
Plasma cortisol levels during a 24-hour period. Note both the pulsatility and the shifting baseline. Normal ranges for 0900h and 2400h are shown in the boxes

- *Feeding and fasting*. Many hormones regulate the body's control of energy intake and expenditure and are therefore profoundly influenced by feeding and fasting. Thus, secretion of insulin is increased and growth hormone decreased after ingestion of food, and secretion of a number of hormones is altered during prolonged food deprivation.

All these factors must be considered when attempting to measure hormone levels in normal individuals and in patients with disease. For example, cortisol levels will often be high and fail to suppress during standard tests in a patient who is severely stressed by serious illness, and growth hormone will usually be low in postprandial patients during the daytime.

Testing endocrine function

Ideally, the activity of hormones would be measured at the cellular level, but this is currently impossible. Measurement of hormone levels in body fluids is the normal substitute and is usually an excellent approximation, but it must be remembered that they do not always reflect the current tissue action of the relevant hormone. Most commonly, hormone levels in the blood are measured (or, more technically, levels in plasma or serum), and all references to hormone levels in this chapter refer to blood/plasma levels unless stated otherwise.

Blood levels

Assays for all important hormones are now available. Obviously the time, day and condition of measurement may make great differences to hormone levels. The method and timing of samples will depend upon the characteristics of the endocrine system involved.

Basal levels

Basal levels are especially useful for systems with long half-lives (e.g. T_4 and T_3). These vary little over the short term and random samples are therefore satisfactory.

Basal samples

Basal samples for other hormones may also be satisfactory if interpreted with respect to normal ranges for the time of day/month, diet or posture concerned. Examples are FSH, oestrogen and progesterone (varying with time of month) and renin/aldosterone (varying with sodium intake and posture). For these hormones, all relevant details must be recorded or the results may prove uninterpretable.

Stress-related hormones

Stress-related hormones (e.g. catecholamines, prolactin, GH, ACTH and cortisol) may require samples to be taken via an indwelling needle some time after initial venepuncture; otherwise, high levels may be artefactual.

Urine collections

Collections over 24 hours have the advantage of providing an 'integrated mean' of a day's secretion but are often incomplete or wrongly timed. They also vary with sex and body size or age. Written instructions should be provided for the patient.

Saliva

Saliva is sometimes used for steroid estimations, especially in children.

Stimulation and suppression tests

Stimulation and suppression tests are used when basal levels give equivocal information. In general, stimulation tests are used to confirm suspected deficiency and suppression tests to confirm suspected excess of hormone secretion. These tests are valuable in many instances.

For example, where the secretory capacity of a gland is damaged, maximal stimulation by the trophic hormone will give a diminished output. Thus, in the Synacthen (SYNthetic-ACTH-en) test for adrenal reserve (Fig 16.4(a)), the healthy subject shows a normal response while the subject with primary hypoadrenalism (Addison's disease) demonstrates an impaired cortisol response to ACTH.

A patient with a hormone-producing tumour usually fails to show normal negative feedback. A patient with Cushing's disease (excess pituitary ACTH) will thus fail to suppress ACTH and cortisol production when given a dose of synthetic steroid, in contrast to normal subjects. Fig 16.4(b) shows the response of a normal subject given dexamethasone 1 mg at midnight; cortisol is suppressed the following morning. The subject with Cushing's disease shows inadequate suppression.

The detailed protocol for each test must be followed exactly, since even slight differences in technique will produce variations in results. Details of the most common tests are given in an Appendix (p. 1206).

Measurement of hormone concentrations

Circulating levels of most hormones are very low (10^{-9}–10^{-12} mol L^{-1}) and cannot be measured by simple chemical techniques. Radioimmunoassay (RIA), previously by far the most common technique in endocrine assays, is being rapidly supplanted by immunometric type assays which are increasingly being automated.

All immunoassays rely on highly specific antibodies (polyclonal or now usually monoclonal) which bind specifically to the hormone being measured. This hormone–antibody interaction is measured by use of labelled hormone or antibody during the assay incubation and separation of bound and free fractions, usually employing a solid-phase system. The label was traditionally radioactive (RIA), but now more frequently involves a fluorimetric, colorimetric, chemiluminescent or enzymatic end-point, and does not have the health and safety concerns of radioactivity.

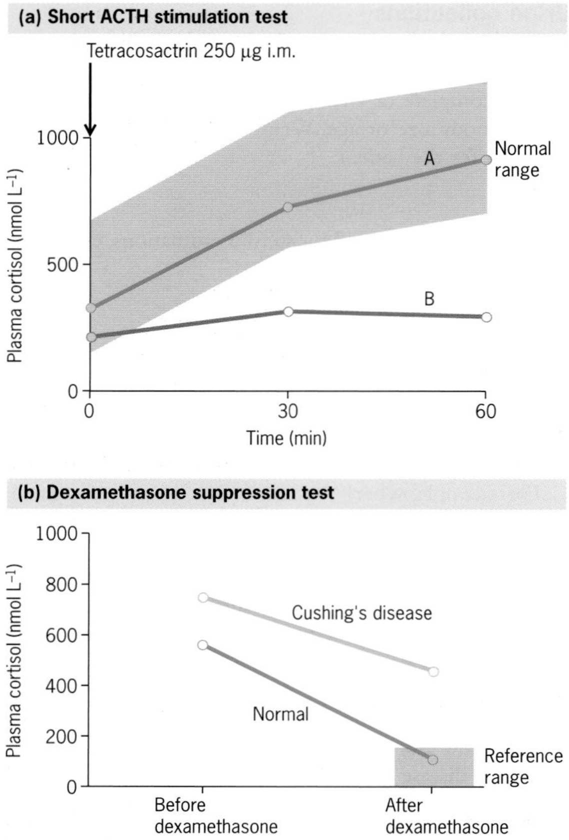

Fig 16.4
Synacthen and dexamethasone tests.
(a) Short ACTH stimulation test showing a normal response in a healthy subject and a decreased response in a patient with Addison's disease
(b) Dexamethasone suppression tests in a normal subject and in a patient with Cushing's disease showing inadequate suppression

Immunoassay is sensitive but has limitations. In particular, the immunological activity of a hormone, as used in developing the antibody, may not necessarily correspond to biological activity. Other measurement techniques include high-pressure liquid chromatography (HPLC).

Endocrine disease: an introduction

See Fig 16.5.

EPIDEMIOLOGY

The most common endocrine disorders, excluding diabetes mellitus (Chapter 17), are:

- *thyroid disorders*, affecting 4–8 new patients per primary care physician each year (the most common problems are thyrotoxicosis, primary hypothyroidism and goitre)
- *subfertility*, affecting 5–10% of all couples, often with an endocrine component, and increasingly treatable
- *menstrual disorders and excessive hair growth in young women*, particularly polycystic ovary syndrome
- *osteoporosis*, especially in postmenopausal women (of increasing clinical importance in an ageing population with fracture of the femur often leading to premature death or disability
- *primary hyperparathyroidism*, affecting about 0.1% of the population.
- *children with short stature or delayed puberty.*

While most other endocrine conditions are very uncommon, they often affect young people and are usually curable or completely controllable with appropriate therapy.

Hormones as therapy

Hormones are also widely used therapeutically:

- The oral contraceptive pill is the choice of perhaps 20–30% of women aged 18–35 years using contraception.
- Hormone replacement therapy (HRT; oestrogens ± progestogens) is increasingly used for postmenopausal women (see p. 913).
- Corticosteroid therapy is widely used in non-endocrine disease such as asthma (see p. 793).

SYMPTOMS

Common endocrine presenting symptoms are shown in Information box 16.1, which demonstrates the many effects that hormonal abnormalities can produce.

Hormones produce widespread effects upon the body; focal symptoms are less common than with other systems. Many endocrine symptoms are diffuse and vague, and the differential diagnosis is often wide.

HISTORY AND EXAMINATION

A detailed history including the past, family and social history should be taken (Information box 16.2).

A full drug history is mandatory as endocrine problems are quite often iatrogenic (Table 16.3).

Physical signs are listed under the relevant systems.

Specific points about endocrine disease

As with other systems, endocrine diseases may be congenital or acquired and can be caused by a variety of pathologies. However, several forms of illness are more common than in other systems.

Autoimmune disease

Organ-specific autoimmune diseases have now been shown for every major endocrine organ (Table 16.4). They are characterized by the presence of specific

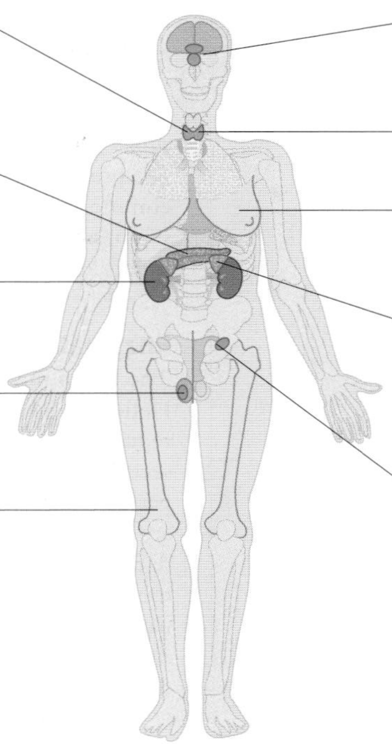

Fig 16.5
The major endocrine organs and common endocrine problems

i **Information**

Body size and shape
Short stature
Tall stature
Excessive weight or weight gain
Loss of weight

'Metabolic' effects
Tiredness
Weakness
Increased appetite
Decreased appetite
Polydipsia/thirst
Polyuria/nocturia
Tremor
Palpitation
Anxiety

Local effects
Swelling in the neck
Carpal tunnel syndrome
Bone or muscle pain
Protrusion of eyes
Visual loss (acuity and/or fields)
Headache

Reproduction/sex
Loss or absence of libido
Impotence
Oligomenorrhoea/amenorrhoea
Subfertility
Galactorrhoea
Gynaecomastia
Delayed puberty
Precocious puberty

Skin
Hirsuties
Hair thinning
Pigmentation
Dry skin
Excess sweating

Information box 16.1
Common presenting complaints in endocrine disease

i **Information**

Past history
Necessary details may include:

- previous pregnancies (ease of conception, postpartum haemorrhage)
- relevant surgery (e.g. thyroidectomy, orchidopexy)
- radiation (e.g. to neck, gonads, thyroid)
- drug exposure (e.g. chemotherapy, sex hormones, oral contraceptives)
- in childhood, developmental milestones and growth.

Family history
Family history of:

- autoimmune disease
- endocrine disease
- essential hypertension
- diabetes.

Family details of:

- height
- weight
- body habitus
- hair growth
- age of sexual development.

Social history

- Detailed records of alcohol intake (e.g. in subfertility, obesity)
- Drug abuse (e.g. cannabis and subfertility)
- Full details of occupation, access to drugs or chemicals
- Diet (e.g. salt, liquorice, iodine).

Information box 16.2
Endocrine disease: past, family and social histories

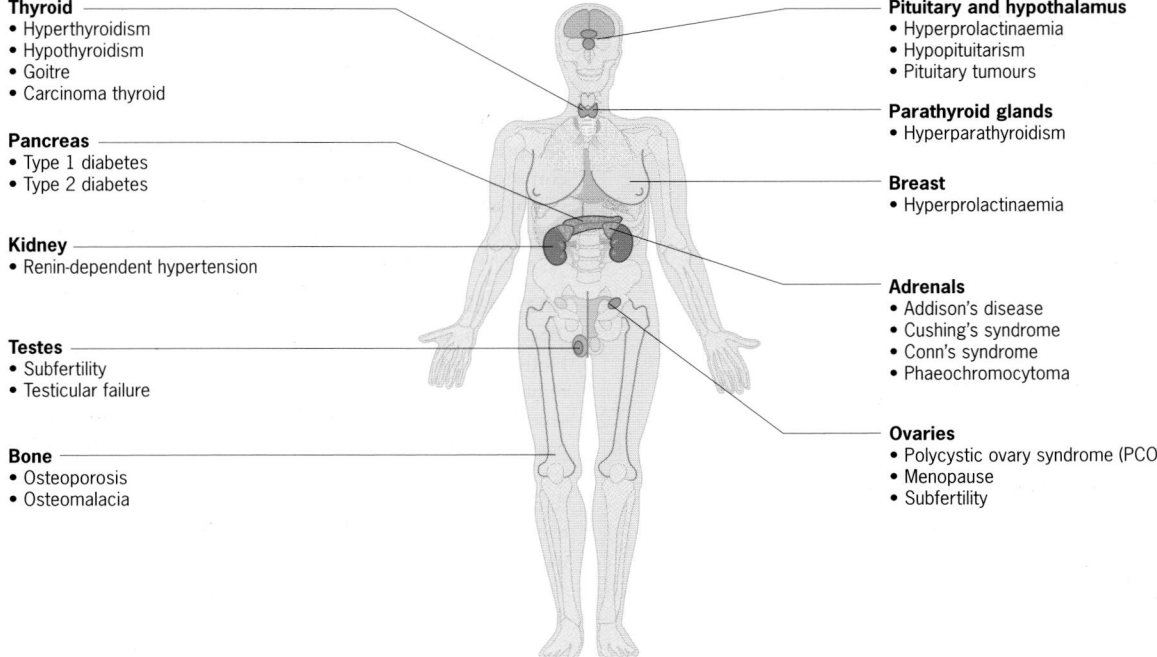

Table 16.3
Drugs and endocrine disease

Drug[a]	Effect
Drugs inducing endocrine disease	
Chlorpromazine Metoclopramide (dopamine agonists) Oestrogens	Increase prolactin, causing galactorrhoea
Iodine Amiodarone	Hyperthyroidism
Lithium Amiodarone	Hypothyroidism
Chlorpropamide	Inappropriate ADH secretion
Ketoconazole Metyrapone, aminoglutethimide	Hypoadrenalism
Drugs simulating endocrine disease	
Sympathomimetics Amphetamines	Mimic thyrotoxicosis or phaeochromocytoma
Liquorice Carbenoxolone	Increase mineralocorticoid activity; mimic aldosteronism
Purgatives	Hypokalaemia
Diuretics	Secondary aldosteronism
ACE inhibitors	Hypoaldosteronism
Drugs affecting hormone binding proteins	
Anticonvulsants	Bind to TBG – decrease total T_4
Oestrogens	Raise TBG and CBG – increase total T_4/cortisol
Exogenous hormones or stimulating agents	
Use, abuse or misuse, by patient or doctor, of the following:	
Steroids	Cushing's syndrome Diabetes
Thyroxine	Thyrotoxicosis factitia
Vitamin D preparations Milk and alkali preparations	Hypercalcaemia
Insulin Sulphonylureas	Hypoglycaemia

[a]Drugs causing gynaecomastia are listed in Table 16.15.
Amiodarone may cause both hypo- or hyperthyroidism.

antibodies in the serum, often present years before clinical symptoms are evident. The conditions are usually more common in women and have a strong genetic component, often with an identical-twin concordance rate of 50% and with HLA associations (see individual diseases). Several of the autoantigens have now been identified

Endocrine tumours

Hormone-secreting tumours occur in all endocrine organs, most commonly pituitary, thyroid and parathyroid. Fortunately, they are more commonly benign than malignant. While often considered to be 'autonomous' – that is, independent of the physiological control mechanisms – many do show evidence of feedback occurring at a higher 'set-point' than normal (e.g. ACTH secretion from a pituitary basophil adenoma).

The molecular basis of some of these tumours is well-understood. Sometimes a very specific mutation of a single gene can be identified, such as the mutations of the *Ret*-proto-oncogene in MEN2 (see p. 956), but more commonly a wide variety of different lesions in tumour suppressor genes, growth factor receptors and other intracellular mediators have been identified.

Enzymatic defects

The biosynthesis of most hormones involves many stages. Deficient or abnormal enzymes can lead to absent or reduced production of the terminal hormone. In general, severe deficiencies present early in life with obvious signs; partial deficiencies usually present later with mild signs or are only evident under stress. An example of an enzyme deficiency is congenital adrenal hyperplasia (CAH). Again the molecular basis is known for several abnormalities, particularly for CAH where the coding gene is on the short arm of chromosome 6, and affected patients have defects such as point mutations or deletions.

Receptor abnormalities

Hormones work by activating cellular receptors. There are rare conditions in which hormone secretion and control are normal but the receptors are defective: thus, if androgen receptors are defective, normal levels of androgen will not produce masculinization (e.g. testicular feminization). There are also a number of rare syndromes of diabetes and insulin resistance from receptor abnormalities (p. 961); other examples include nephrogenic diabetes insipidus, thyroid hormone resistance and pseudohypoparathyroidism.

FURTHER READING

Epidemiology and clinical decision-making. (1997) *Endocrinology and Metabolism Clinics of North America* **26**: 1–3.

Diagnostic evaluation update (1997). *Endocrinology and Metabolism Clinics of North America* **26**: 4.

Davis JR et al (1996) Molecular biology techniques in endocrinology. *Clinical Endocrinology* **45**: 125–133.

Spiegel AM et al (1996) Mutations in G proteins and G-protein-coupled receptors in endocrine disease. *Journal of Clinical Endocrinology and Metabolism* **81**: 2434–2442.

Harris PE et al (1996) Gs protein mutations and the pathogenesis and function of pituitary tumors. *Metabolism* **45** (Suppl 1): 120–122.

Funder JW et al (1996) Mineralocorticoid receptors and glucocorticoid receptors. *Clinical Endocrinology* **45**: 651–656.

Table 16.4
Types of autoimmune disease

Organ and frequency if known	Antibody	Antigen if known	Clinical syndrome
Stimulating			
Thyroid 1 in 100	Thyroid-stimulating immunoglobulin (TSI, TSAb) Thyroid growth immunoglobulin	TSH receptor	Graves' disease, neonatal thyrotoxicosis Goitre
Destructive			
Thyroid 1 in 100	Thyroid microsomal antibody Thyroglobulin	Peroxidase enzyme	Primary hypothyroidism (myxoedema)
Adrenal 1 in 20 000	Adrenal cortex	21-Hydroxylase enzyme	Primary hypoadrenalism (Addison's disease)
Pancreas 1 in 500	Islet cell	GAD (see p. 964)	Type I (insulin-dependent) diabetes
Stomach	Gastric parietal cell Intrinsic factor		Pernicious anaemia
Skin	Melanocyte		Vitiligo
Ovary 1 in 500	Ovary		Primary ovarian failure
Testis	Testis		Primary testicular failure
Parathyroid	Parathyroid chief cell		Primary hypoparathyroidism
Pituitary	Pituitary-specific cells		Selective hypopituitarism (e.g. GH deficiency, hyperprolactinaemia)

Frequencies are approximate and refer to Northern Europe.
GAD, glutamic acid dehydrogenase.
NB Other related diseases include myasthenia gravis and autoimmune liver diseases.

Central control of endocrine function

Anatomy

Many peripheral hormone systems are controlled by the hypothalamus and pituitary. The hypothalamus is sited at the base of the brain around the third ventricle and above the pituitary stalk, which leads down to the pituitary itself, carrying the hypophyseal-pituitary portal blood supply.

The important anatomical relationships of the hypothalamus and pituitary (Fig 16.6) include the optic chiasm just above the pituitary fossa; any expanding lesion from the pituitary or hypothalamus can thus produce visual field defects by pressure on the chiasm. The pituitary is itself encased in a bony box; any lateral, anterior or posterior expansion must cause bony erosion. Upward expansion of the gland through the diaphragma sellae is termed 'suprasellar extension'. Lateral extension of pituitary lesions may involve the vascular and nervous structures in the cavernous sinus and may rarely reach the temporal lobe of the brain.

Embryologically, the anterior pituitary is formed from Rathke's pouch (endodermal) which meets an outpouching of the third ventricular floor which becomes the posterior pituitary.

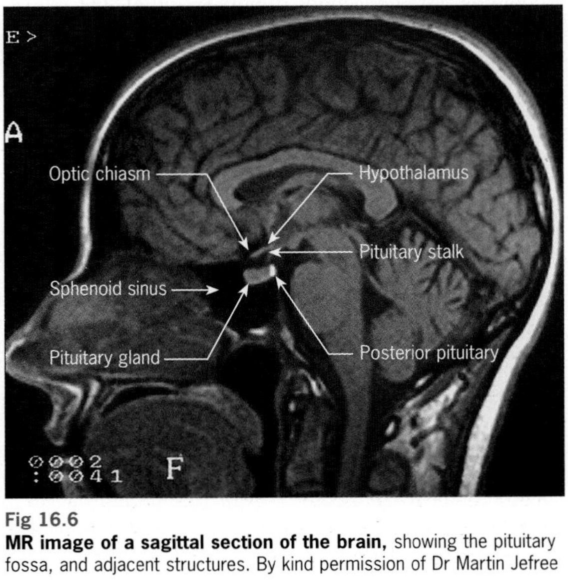

Fig 16.6
MR image of a sagittal section of the brain, showing the pituitary fossa, and adjacent structures. By kind permission of Dr Martin Jefree

Physiology

Hypothalamus

This contains many vital centres for such functions as appetite, thirst, thermal regulation and sleeping/waking. It acts as an integrator of many neural and endocrine inputs to control the release of pituitary hormone releasing factors. Amongst other important influences it plays a role in the circadian rhythm, menstrual cyclicity, and responses to stress, exercise and mood.

From the hypothalamus the portal system runs down the stalk through which releasing factors and hormones are transported to the pituitary.

The hypothalamus also contains large amounts of other neuropeptides such as natriuretic factor, neuropeptide Y and vasoactive intestinal peptide (VIP) that can also alter pituitary hormone secretion.

Synthetic hypothalamic hormones and their antagonists are now available for the testing of many aspects of endocrine function and for treatment.

Anterior pituitary

Hormone secretion is controlled by hypothalamic releasing of inhibitory hormones (Table 16.5 and Fig 16.7). Many hormones are under dual control by both stimulatory and inhibitory hypothalamic factors. Examples are:

- Growth hormone release is *stimulated* by growth-hormone releasing hormone (GHRH) but *inhibited* by somatostatin (growth hormone release inhibitory hormone, GHRIH).
- TSH release is *stimulated* by TRH but partially *inhibited* by somatostatin.

Some hormones have a dual stimulatory control. For example, corticotrophin-releasing factor (CRF) and vasopressin are endogenous stimulators of ACTH release. Uniquely, prolactin is under predominant inhibitory dopaminergic control with some stimulatory TRH control.

Posterior pituitary

This, in contrast, acts merely as a storage organ. Antidiuretic hormone (ADH, vasopressin) and oxytocin, both nonapeptides, are synthesized in the supraoptic and paraventricular nuclei in the anterior hypothalamus. They are then transported along the axon and stored in the posterior pituitary. This means that damage to the stalk or pituitary alone does not prevent synthesis and release of ADH and oxytocin. ADH is discussed on p. 833; oxytocin produces milk ejection and uterine myometrial contraction.

Endorphins and the ACTH families of peptides

Some but not all of the endorphins (ENDogenous mORPHINeS) are derived from part of the ACTH precursor molecule. The prohormone pro-opiomelanocortin undergoes complex processing within the pituitary to produce its major product, ACTH, as well as lipotrophin and some endorphins. Pigmentation in humans is due to ACTH and β-lipotrophin, and not due to α- and β-melanocyte stimulating hormone (MSH) which are not found in humans.

The endorphins have opioid activity and are thought to be mediators of stress-induced analgesia. They have also been found within the gut but their physiological role remains uncertain.

Presentations of hypothalamic and pituitary disease

Pituitary space-occupying lesions and tumours

Pituitary tumours (Table 16.6) are the most common cause of pituitary disease. Problems may be caused by excess hormone secretion, by local effects of a tumour, or as the

Table 16.5
Nomenclature and biochemistry of hypothalamic, pituitary and peripheral hormones

Hypothalamic hormones	Pituitary hormones	Peripheral hormones
Gonadotrophin-releasing hormone (GnRH, LHRH) (*Decapeptide*)	Luteinizing hormone (LH) Follicle-stimulating hormone (FSH) (*Two-chain α, β peptides*)	Oestrogens/androgens (*Steroid ring*)
Prolactin inhibiting factor (PIF – dopamine) (*Amine*)	Prolactin (PRL) (*Single chain peptide*)	–
Growth hormone-releasing hormone (GHRH) (*Peptide*) Somatostatin (GHRIH) (*Cyclic peptide*)	Growth hormone (GH) (*Peptide*)	Insulin-like growth factor I (IGF-1) (*Small peptide*)
Thyrotropin-releasing hormone (TRH) (*Tripeptide*)	Thyroid-stimulating hormone (TSH) (*Two-chain a, β peptide*)	Thyroxine (T_4), tri-iodothyronine (T_3) (*Thyronines*)
Corticotrophin-releasing factor (CRF) (*Single-chain peptide*)	Adrenocorticotrophic hormone (ACTH) (*Single-chain peptide*)	Cortisol (*Steroid ring*)
Vasopressin (antidiuretic hormone; ADH) (*Nonapeptide*)	–	–
Oxytocin (*Nonapeptide*)	–	–

NB: The α chains of LH, FSH and TSH are identical.
GHRIH, growth hormone release inhibitory hormone.

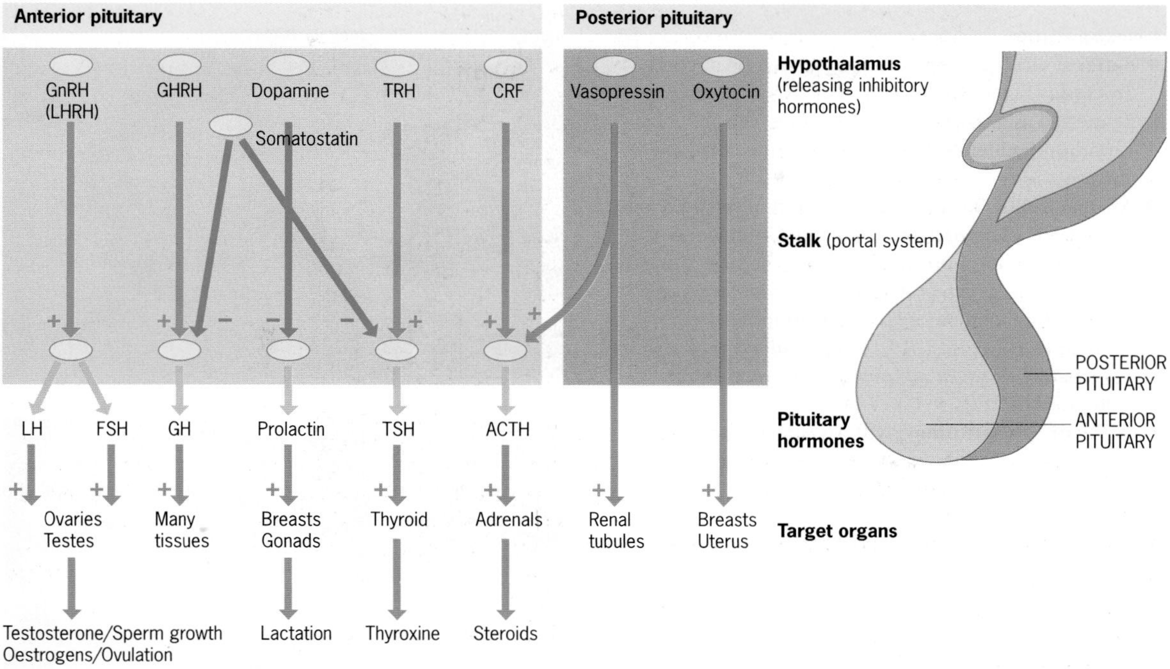

Fig 16.7
Hypothalamic releasing hormones and the pituitary trophic hormones. See the text for abbreviations and an explanation

result of inadequate production of hormone by the remaining normal pituitary – hypopituitarism. The great majority of pituitary tumours are benign pituitary adenomas.

INVESTIGATIONS

The investigation of a possible or proven tumour follows three lines.

Is there a tumour?
If there is, how big is it and what local anatomical effects is it exerting? Pituitary and hypothalamic space-occupying lesions, hormonally active or not, can cause symptoms by infiltration of, or pressure on:

- the visual pathways, with field defects and visual loss
- the cavernous sinus, with III, IV and VI cranial nerve lesions
- bony structures and the meninges surrounding the fossa, causing headache
- hypothalamic centres: altered appetite, obesity, thirst, somnolence/wakefulness or precocious puberty
- the ventricle, causing interruption of cerebrospinal fluid (CSF) flow leading to hydrocephalus
- rarely, the sphenoid sinus with invasion causing CSF rhinorrhoea.

Table 16.6
Characteristics of common pituitary and similar tumours

Tumour or condition	Usual size	Most common clinical presentation
Prolactinoma	Most <10 mm (microprolactinoma)	Galactorrhoea, amenorrhoea, hypogonadism, impotence
	Some >10 mm (macroprolactinoma)	As above plus headaches, visual field defects and hypopituitarism
Acromegaly	Medium→large (>90% of skull X-rays abnormal)	Change in appearance, visual field defects and hypopituitarism
Cushing's disease	Most small (some cases are hyperplasia)	Central obesity, chance observation (local symptoms rare)
Nelson's syndrome	Often large	Post-adrenalectomy, pigmentation, sometimes local symptoms
Non-functioning tumours	Often large	Visual field defects; hypopituitarism; small ones often found at postmortem
Craniopharyngioma	Often very large and cystic (skull X-ray abnormal in >50%; calcification common)	Headaches, visual field defects, growth failure; (50% occur below age 20; about 15% arise from within sella)

Investigations

- **Lateral skull X-ray**. This may show enlargement of the fossa (Fig 16.8). Although an X-ray is now rarely requested as a definitive investigation, this remains a common incidental finding and requires further investigation.
- **Visual fields**. These should be plotted formally by automated computer perimetry or Goldmann perimetry after confrontation at the bedside using a small red pin as target. Common defects are upper-temporal quadrantanopias and bitemporal hemianopias (see p. 1014). Subtle defects may also be revealed by delay or attenuation of visual evoked potentials (VEPs).
- **MRI of the pituitary**. MRI is superior to high-resolution CT scanning with reconstruction (Fig 16.9).

Is there a hormonal excess?

There are three major conditions that may be caused by tumour or hyperplasia:

- GH excess, leading to acromegaly or gigantism – these are usually acidophil adenomas, and a proportion are due to specific G-protein mutations $G_{s\alpha}$ (see p. 126)
- prolactin excess (prolactinoma or hyperprolactinaemia) – histologically, prolactinomas are chromophobe adenomas
- Cushing's disease and Nelson's syndrome (excess ACTH secretion) – basophil adenomas.

Occasional tumours produce both GH and prolactin.

The clinical features of acromegaly and Cushing's disease or hyperprolactinaemia are usually (but not always) obvious, and are discussed below (see pages 928, 946 and 922). Hyperprolactinaemia may be clinically 'silent'. Tumours producing LH, FSH or TSH are very rare.

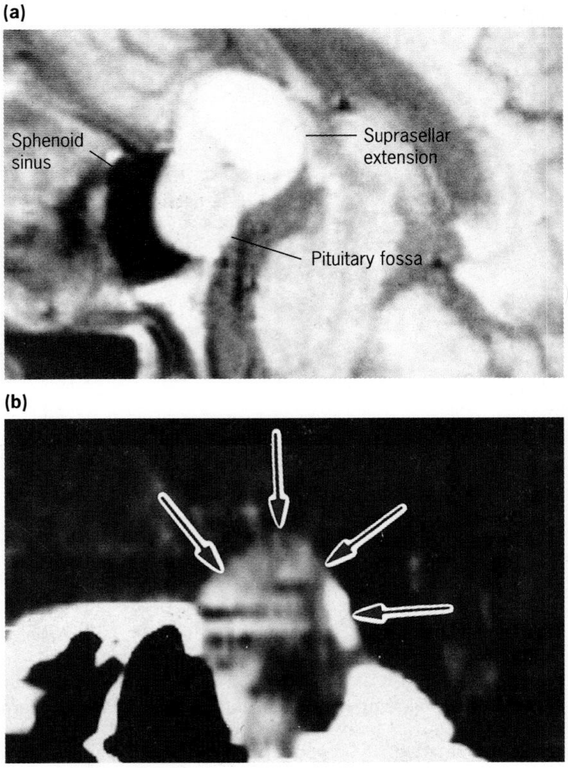

Fig 16.9
(a) MR image of pituitary fossa, showing tumour with suprasellar extension
(b) CT scan (sagittal reconstruction), showing a pituitary tumour with suprasellar extension (arrows show upper border)

Some pituitary tumours cause no clinically apparent hormone excess and are referred to as 'non-functioning' tumours, which are common and usually chromophobe adenomas. Laboratory studies such as immunocytochemistry show that these tumours may often produce LH and FSH or the α subunit of LH, FSH and TSH (see Table 16.5). Studies have shown that pituitary adenomas of all types are usually monoclonal in origin.

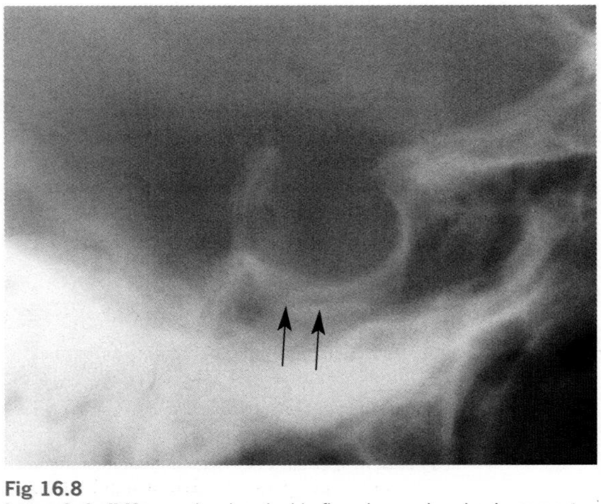

Fig 16.8
Lateral skull X-ray, showing double floor (arrows) and enlargement of the pituitary fossa in a patient with acromegaly

Is there a deficiency of any hormone?

Clinical examination may give clues; thus, short stature in a child with a pituitary tumour is likely to be due to GH deficiency. A slow, lethargic adult with pale skin is likely to be deficient in TSH and/or ACTH. Milder deficiencies may not be obvious, and require specific testing (see Table 16.9).

Differential diagnosis of apparent pituitary adenomas additionally includes craniopharyngioma, or a usually cystic hypothalamic tumour arising from Rathke's pouch that often mimics an intrinsic pituitary lesion. Although presenting at any age, it is the most common tumour in children and is often calcified.

Less common are meningiomas, gliomas, chondromas, pinealomas and carotid artery aneurysms masquerading as tumours. Secondary deposits occasionally present as apparent pituitary tumours, often presenting as diabetes insipidus.

TREATMENT

Treatment depends on the type and size of tumour (Table 16.7) and is discussed in more detail in the relevant sections (acromegaly, see p. 928; prolactinoma, see p. 922). In general, therapy has three aims:

Removal/control of tumour

Surgery via the trans-sphenoidal route is usually the treatment of choice. Large tumours are occasionally removed via the open transfrontal route. Radiotherapy is given if the tumour is incompletely removed.

Radiotherapy may be by an external three-beam technique, stereotactic or rarely via implant of yttrium needles. It is usually employed when surgery is impracticable or incomplete as it rarely abolishes tumour mass. The standard regimen involves a dose of about 45 Gy, given as 20–25 fractions.

Octreotide or dopamine agonists such as bromocriptine sometimes cause shrinkage of specific types of tumour.

Reduction of excess hormone secretion

Reduction is usually obtained by surgical removal but sometimes by medical treatment (e.g. bromocriptine or octreotide alone). Prolactinomas respond with significant tumour shrinkage to dopamine agonists (see p. 922). Acromegaly, however, responds less well (see p. 929). ACTH secretion usually cannot be controlled by medical means.

Replacement of hormone deficiencies

Replacement of hormone deficiencies is detailed in Table 16.10.

Small tumours producing no significant symptoms, pressure or endocrine effects are observed with regular clinical, visual field, imaging and endocrine assessments.

Hypopituitarism

PATHOPHYSIOLOGY

Deficiency of hypothalamic releasing hormones or of pituitary trophic hormones are either selective or multiple. There are, for example, rare isolated deficiencies of LH/FSH and ACTH, some of which may be congenital, autoimmune or idiopathic in nature.

Multiple deficiencies usually result from tumour growth or other destructive lesions. With the latter there is generally a progressive loss of anterior pituitary function in the order shown from left to right in Fig 16.7. GH and gonadotrophins, LH before FSH, are usually first affected. Rather than prolactin deficiency, hyperprolactinaemia occurs relatively early because of loss of tonic inhibitory control by dopamine. TSH and ACTH are usually last to be affected. Panhypopituitarism refers to deficiency of all anterior pituitary hormones; it is most commonly caused by pituitary tumours, surgery or radiotherapy.

Vasopressin and oxytocin secretion will be significantly affected only if the hypothalamus is involved, either by a hypothalamic tumour or by major suprasellar extension of a pituitary lesion.

CAUSES

Disorders causing hypopituitarism are listed in Table 16.8. Pituitary and hypothalamic tumours, and surgical or radiotherapy treatment, are the most common.

Table 16.7
Comparisons of primary treatments for pituitary tumours

Treatment method	Advantages	Disadvantages
Surgical		
Trans-sphenoidal adenomectomy or hypophysectomy	Relatively minor procedure Potentially curative for microadenomas and smaller macroadenomas	Some extrasellar extensions may not be accessible Risk of CSF leakage and meningitis
Trans-frontal	Good access to suprasellar region	Major procedure; danger of frontal lobe damage High chance of subsequent hypopituitarism
Radiotherapy		
External (40–50 Gy)	Non-invasive Reduces recurrence rate after surgery	Slow action, often over many years Not always effective Possible late risk of tumour induction
Stereotactic	Precise administration of high dose to lesion	Long-term follow-up data limited
Yttrium implantation	High local dose	Only ever used in a few centres
Medical		
Dopamine agonist therapy (e.g. bromocriptine)	Non-invasive; reversible	Usually not curative Significant side-effects in minority
Somatostatin analogue therapy (octreotide)	Non-invasive; reversible	Usually not curative; expensive; side-effects

Table 16.8
Causes of hypopituitarism

Congenital Isolated deficiency of pituitary hormones (e.g. Kallmann's syndrome)	**Traumatic** Skull fracture through base Surgery, especially transfrontal
Infective Basal meningitis (e.g. tuberculosis) Encephalitis Syphilis	**Infiltrations** Sarcoidosis Langerhans' cell histiocytosis Hereditary haemochromatosis
Vascular Pituitary apoplexy Sheehan's syndrome (postpartum necrosis) Carotid artery aneurysms	**Others** Radiation damage Fibrosis Chemotherapy Empty sella syndrome
Immunological Pituitary antibodies	**'Functional'** Anorexia nervosa Starvation Emotional deprivation
Neoplastic Pituitary or hypothalamic tumours Craniopharyngioma Meningiomas Gliomas Pinealoma Secondary deposits, especially breast Lymphoma	

CLINICAL FEATURES

Symptoms and signs depend upon the extent of hypothalamic and/or pituitary deficiencies, and mild deficiencies may not lead to any complaint by the patient. Loss of libido, amenorrhoea and impotence are symptoms of gonadotrophin and thus gonadal deficiencies, while hyperprolactinaemia may cause galactorrhoea and hypogonadism. GH deficiency is relatively clinically 'silent' except in children, though recent evidence suggests that it may cause markedly impaired well-being in adults. Secondary hypothyroidism and adrenal failure lead to tiredness, slowness of thought and action, and mild hypotension. Long-standing panhypopituitarism may give the classic picture of pallor with hairlessness ('alabaster skin').

Particular syndromes related to hypopituitarism are considered below.

Kallmann's syndrome

This syndrome is isolated gonadotrophin deficiency, which leads to hypogonadism, usually associated with anosmia (see p. 916). One sex-linked form has been shown to be due to an abnormality of a cell adhesion molecule.

Sheehan's syndrome

This situation, now rare, is pituitary infarction following postpartum haemorrhage.

Pituitary apoplexy

A pituitary tumour may occasionally infarct or haemorrhage into itself. This may produce severe headache sometimes followed by acute life-threatening hypopituitarism.

The 'empty sella' syndrome

An 'empty sella' is sometimes reported on pituitary imaging. This is sometimes due to a defect in the diaphragma and extension of the subarachnoid space (cisternal herniation) or may follow spontaneous infarction of a tumour. All or most of the sella turcica is devoid of apparent pituitary tissue, but, despite this, pituitary function is usually normal, the pituitary being eccentrically placed and flattened against the floor or roof of the fossa.

INVESTIGATIONS

Each axis of the hypothalamic–pituitary system requires separate investigation. However, the presence of normal gonadal function (ovulatory/menstruation or normal libido/erections) suggests that multiple defects of anterior pituitary function are unlikely.

Tests range from the simple basal levels (e.g. T_4 or free T_4 for the thyroid axis), to stimulatory tests for the pituitary, and tests of feedback for the hypothalamus (Table 16.9). The insulin tolerance test is now less widely used, as basal 0900h cortisol levels above 500 nmol L^{-1}, and probably even above 400 nmol L^{-1}, reliably indicate an adequate reserve, while levels below 100 nmol L^{-1} predict an inadequate response. The Synacthen test, though an indirect measure, has been advocated as an adequate indicator of hypothalamic–pituitary–adrenal status, but this remains controversial. Overall the assessment of adrenal reserve is best left in the hands of a specialist endocrinologist.

TREATMENT

Steroid and thyroid hormones are essential for life. Both may be given as oral replacement drugs, aiming to restore the patient to clinical and biochemical normality (Table 16.10). Sex hormone production may be replaced with androgens and oestrogens for symptomatic control; if necessary, human chorionic gonadotrophin (HCG, mainly acting as LH) and purified or biosynthetic gonadotrophins can be given if fertility is desired. Pulsatile GnRH (luteinizing hormone releasing hormone, LHRH) therapy is sometimes used where there is residual pituitary function, but it is expensive and time-consuming.

GH therapy should be given if necessary in the growing child under appropriate specialist supervision. In the adult, GH therapy also produces substantial improvements in body composition, work capacity and psychological well-being in acquired GH deficiency, together with reversal of lipid abnormalities carrying a high cardiovascular risk. Although now licensed for such use in many countries, the long-term safety and efficacy of GH therapy is not yet

Table 16.9
Tests for hypothalamic–pituitary (HP) function

- All hormone levels are measured in plasma unless otherwise stated.
- Tests **shown in bold** are those normally measured on a single basal 0900h sample in the initial assessment of pituitary function.

	Basal investigations			
Axis	**Pituitary hormone**	**End-organ product/function**	**Common dynamic tests**	**Other tests**
Anterior pituitary				
HP-ovarian	**LH** **FSH**	**Oestradiol** Progesterone (day 21 of cycle)		Ovarian ultrasound LHRH test*
HP-testicular	**LH** **FSH**	**Testosterone**		Sperm count LHRH test*
Growth	GH	IGF-1 IGF-BP3	Insulin tolerance test	GH response to sleep, exercise or arginine infusion GHRH test*
Prolactin	**Prolactin**			
HP-thyroid	**TSH**	T_4, **free T_4**, T_3		TRH test*
HP-adrenal	ACTH	**Cortisol**	Insulin tolerance test Short synacthen (tetracosactrin) test	Glucagon test CRH test*
Posterior pituitary				
Thirst and osmoregulation		**Plasma/urine osmolality**	Water deprivation test	Hypertonic saline infusion

* Releasing hormone tests were a traditional part of pituitary function testing, but have been largely replaced by the advent of more reliable assays for basal hormones. They test only the 'readily-releasable pool' of pituitary hormones and normal responses may be seen in hypopituitarism.

fully established, and its cost is £2500–6000 per annum. Two important points should be noted:

- Thyroid replacement should not commence until normal glucocorticoid function has been demonstrated or replacement steroid therapy initiated, as an adrenal 'crisis' may otherwise be precipitated.
- Glucocorticoid deficiency may mask impaired urine concentrating ability, diabetes insipidus only becoming apparent after steroid replacement, the steroids being necessary for excretion of a water load.

Table 16.10
Replacement therapy for hypopituitarism

Axis	**Usual replacement therapies**
Gonadal	
Male	Testosterone intramuscularly, orally, as patch or implant
Female	Cyclical oestrogen/progestogen orally or as patch/implant
Fertility	HCG plus FSH (purified or recombinant) to produce testicular development, spermatogenesis or ovulation Pulsatile LHRH also used
Breast (Prolactin inhibition)	Dopamine agonist as replacement inhibition (e.g. bromocriptine 3–15 mg daily)
Growth	Recombinant human GH used routinely to achieve normal growth in children Also advocated for replacement therapy in adults where GH has effects on muscle mass and well-being
Thyroid	Thyroxine 100–150 μg daily
Adrenal	Hydrocortisone 15–40 mg daily (divided doses) or prednisolone 5–10 mg daily (Normally no need for mineralocorticoid replacement)
Thirst	Desmopressin (DDAVP) 10–20 μg one to three times daily by nasal spray or orally 100–200 μg thrice daily Carbamazepine and thiazides are rarely used in mild diabetes insipidus

Weight, exercise and stress

Anorexia nervosa, the 'slimming disease' commonly affecting young females, is associated with major functional hypopituitarism (see p. 1142). This often presents as amenorrhoea, without which the diagnosis is extremely unlikely. Anorexia is an extreme example, but more marginal degrees of underweight are a cause of secondary amenorrhoea and oligomenorrhoea, and are often unrecognized as a cause of subfertility. Similar effects are seen in female athletes undergoing heavy training with menstrual irregularity that invariably reverts to normal when training stops.

Stress, though difficult to define, also affects endocrine function, especially menstruation. Emotional deprivation in childhood is an important cause of growth retardation and may be mediated by reduced GH secretion.

FURTHER READING

Lamberts SWJ, van der Lely AJ, de Herder WW, Hofland LJ (1996) Drug therapy: octreotide. *New England Journal of Medicine* **334**: 246–254.

Molitch ME, Thorner MO, Wilson C (1997) Therapeutic controversy: management of prolactinomas. *Journal of Endocrinology and Metabolism* **82**: 996–1000.

Reproduction and sex

The normal physiology of the female and male reproductive systems will be considered first, followed by their common disorders. Some relevant terminology is set out in Information box 16.3.

Embryology

Up to eight weeks of gestation the sexes share a common development, with a primitive genital tract including the Wolffian and Müllerian ducts. There are additionally a primitive perineum and primitive gonads.

- In the *presence* of a Y chromosome the potential testis develops while the ovary regresses.
- In the *absence* of a Y chromosome, the potential ovary develops and related ducts form a uterus and the upper vagina.

Production of Müllerian inhibitory factor from the early 'testis' produces atrophy of the Müllerian duct, while, under the influence of testosterone and dihydrotestosterone, the Wolffian duct differentiates into an epididymus, vas deferens, seminal vesicles and prostate. Androgens induce transformation of the perineum to include a penis, penile urethra and scrotum containing the testes, which descend in response to androgenic stimulation. At birth, testicular volume is 0.5–1 mL.

Physiology

The male

An outline of the hypothalamic–pituitary–testicular axis is shown in Fig 16.10.

1. Pulses of LHRH (GnRH) are released from the hypothalamus and stimulate LH and FSH release from the pituitary.
2. LH stimulates testosterone production from Leydig cells of the testis.
3. Testosterone acts systemically to produce male secondary sexual characteristics, anabolism and the maintenance of libido. It also acts locally within the

Information

Menarche	Age at first period
Primary amenorrhoea	Failure to begin spontaneous menstruation by age 16
Secondary amenorrhoea	Absence of menstruation for three months in a woman who has previously had cycles
Oligomenorrhoea	Irregular long cycles; often used for any length of cycle above 32 days
Dyspareunia	Pain or discomfort in the female during intercourse
Libido	Sexual interest or desire; often difficult to assess and is greatly affected by stress, tiredness and psychological factors
Menstruation	Onset of spontaneous (usually regular) uterine bleeding in the female
Impotence	Inability of the male to achieve or sustain an erection adequate for satisfactory intercourse
Azoospermia	Absence of sperm in the ejaculate
Oligospermia	Reduced numbers of sperm in the ejaculate; normal values are disputed
Virilization	Occurrence of male secondary sexual characteristics in the female

Information box 16.3 Definitions in reproductive medicine

testis to aid spermatogenesis. Testosterone circulates largely bound to sex hormone-binding globulin (SHBG) (see p. 896).
4 FSH stimulates the Sertoli cells in the seminiferous tubules to produce mature sperm and the recently characterized feedback glycoprotein hormones, the inhibins (A and B, comprising α and β subunits).
5 Testosterone feeds back on the hypothalamus/pituitary to inhibit LHRH secretion.
6 Inhibin causes feedback on the pituitary to decrease FSH secretion.

The secondary sexual characteristics of the male for which testosterone is necessary are the growth of pubic, axillary and facial hair, enlargement of the external genitalia, deepening of the voice, sebum secretion, muscle growth and frontal balding.

The female

The female situation is more complex (Figs 16.10 and 16.11).

1 In the adult female, higher brain centres impose a menstrual cycle of 28 days upon the activity of hypothalamic GnRH.
2 Pulses of GnRH, at about two-hour intervals, stimulate release of pituitary LH and FSH.
3 LH stimulates ovarian androgen production.
4 FSH stimulates follicular development and aromatase activity (an enzyme required to convert ovarian androgens to oestrogens). FSH also stimulates inhibin from ovarian stromal cells. Inhibin, in turn, inhibits FSH release.
5 Although many follicles are 'recruited' for development in early folliculogenesis, by day 8–10 a 'leading' follicle is selected for development into a mature Graafian follicle.
6 Oestrogens show a double feedback action on the pituitary (Fig 16.10), initially inhibiting gonadotrophin secretion (*negative* feedback), but later high-level exposure results in increased GnRH secretion and increased LH sensitivity to GnRH (*positive* feedback), which leads to the mid-cycle LH surge inducing ovulation from the leading follicle (Fig 16.11).
7 The follicle then differentiates into a corpus luteum, which secretes both progesterone and oestradiol during the second half of the cycle (luteal phase).
8 Oestrogen initially and then progesterone cause uterine endometrial proliferation in preparation for possible implantation; if implantation does not occur, the corpus luteum regresses and progesterone secretion and inhibin levels fall so that the endometrium is shed (menstruation) and allowing increased GnRH and FSH secretion.
9 If implantation and pregnancy follow, human chorionic gonadotrophin (HCG) production from the corpus luteum maintains corpus luteum function until 10–12 weeks of gestation, by which time the placenta will be making sufficient oestrogen and progesterone to support itself.
10 Oestrogen circulates largely bound to SHBG (see p. 896).

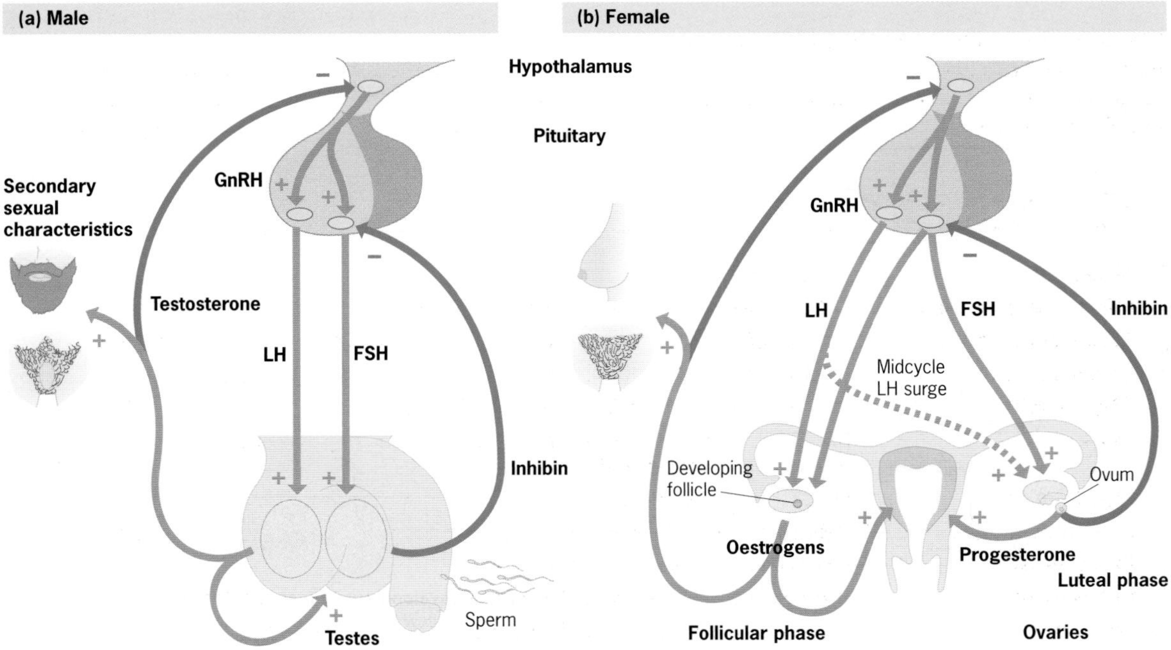

Fig 16.10
Male and female hypothalamic–piuitary–gonadal axes. Note the close parallels. The green lines indicate negative feedback

Oestrogens also induce secondary sexual characteristics, especially development of the breast and nipples, vaginal and vulval growth and pubic hair development. They also induce growth and maturation of the uterus and tubes. They do not, however, usually increase breast size in other circumstances.

Puberty

The mechanisms initiating puberty remain poorly understood but are thought to result from withdrawal of central inhibition of GnRH release. LH and FSH are both low in the prepubertal child.

In early puberty, FSH begins to rise first, initially in nocturnal pulses; this is followed by a rise in LH with a subsequent increase in testosterone/oestrogen levels. The milestones of puberty in the two sexes are shown in Fig 16.12.

In boys, pubertal changes begin at between 10 and 14 years and are complete at between 15 and 17 years. The genitalia develop, testes enlarge and the area of pubic hair increases. Peak height velocity is reached between ages 12 and 17 years during stage 4 of testicular development. Full spermatogenesis occurs comparatively late.

In girls, events start a year earlier. Breast bud enlargement begins at ages 9–13 years and continues to 12–18 years. Pubic hair growth commences at ages 9–14 years and is completed at 12–16 years. Menarche occurs relatively late (age 11–15 years) but peak height velocity is reached much earlier than in boys (age 10–13 years). Growth is completed earlier than in boys.

Precocious puberty

Development of menarche (girls) or secondary sexual characteristics (boys) before the age of nine years is premature.

Idiopathic (true) precocity is most common in girls and very rare in boys. This is a diagnosis of exclusion. With no apparent cause for premature breast or pubic hair development, and an early growth spurt, it may be normal and may run in families. Treatment with long-acting LHRH analogues which cause suppression of gonadotrophin release via down-regulation of the receptor – and therefore reduced sex hormone production – have largely replaced cyproterone acetate, an anti-androgen with progestational activity. LHRH analogues are given by nasal spray, by subcutaneous injection or preferably by implant.

The following are other forms of precocity:

- *Cerebral precocity*. Many causes of hypothalamic disease, especially tumours, present in this way. In boys this must be rigorously excluded.
- *Forbes–Albright syndrome*. This is usually in girls, with precocity, polyostotic fibrous dysplasia and skin pigmentation (café-au-lait).
- *Premature thelarche*. This is early breast development alone, usually transient, at age 2–4 years. It may regress or persist until puberty.
- *Premature adrenarche*. This is early development of pubic hair without significant other changes, usually after age five years and most commonly in girls.

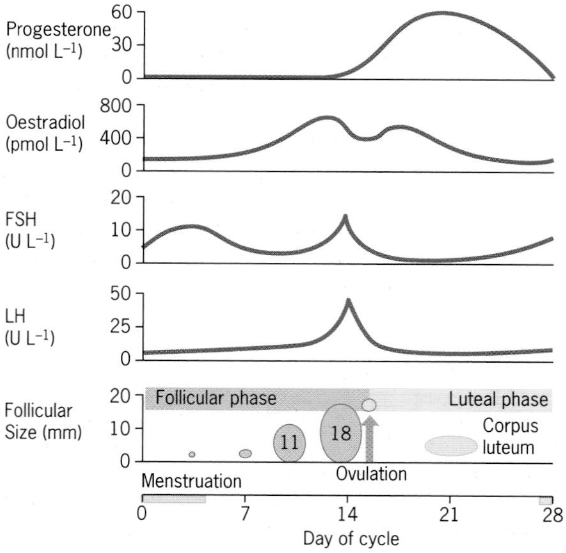

Fig 16.11
Hormonal and follicular changes during the normal menstrual cycle

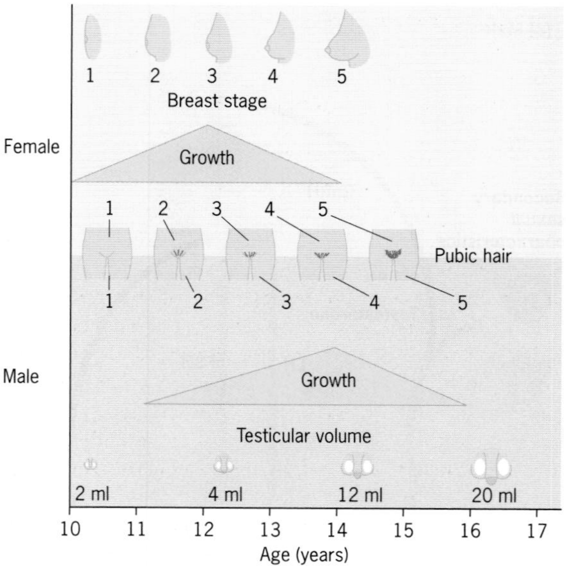

Fig 16.12
The age of development of features of puberty. Stages and testicular size show mean ages and all vary considerably between individuals. The same is true of height spurt, shown here in relation to other data. Numbers 2 to 5 indicate stages of development (see the text)

Delayed puberty

Over 95% of children show signs of pubertal development by age 14 years. In its absence, investigation should begin by age 15 years. Causes of hypogonadism (see below) are clearly relevant but most cases represent constitutional delay.

In *constitutional delay*, pubertal development, bone age and stature are in parallel. A family history may confirm that other family members experienced the same development. Constitutional delay is common in boys but very rare in girls.

In boys, *testicular volume* >5 mL indicates the onset of puberty. A rising serum testosterone is an earlier clue.

In girls, the *breast bud* is the first sign. Ultrasound allows accurate assessment of ovarian and uterine development.

Basal LH/FSH levels may identify the site of a defect, and LHRH tests can indicate the stage of early puberty.

If any progression at all into puberty is evident clinically, investigations are not required. When delay is great and problems are serious (e.g. severe teasing at school), low-dose short-term sex hormone therapy is used. Specialist assessment is advisable.

The menopause

The menopause, or cessation of periods, naturally occurs about the age of 45–55 years. During the late forties, FSH initially, and then LH concentrations begin to rise, probably as follicle supply diminishes. Oestrogen levels fall and the cycle becomes disrupted. Most women notice irregular scanty periods coming on over a variable period, though in some sudden amenorrhoea or menorrhagia occur. Eventually the menopausal pattern of low oestradiol levels with grossly elevated LH and FSH levels (usually >50 and >25 U L^{-1}, respectively) is established. Menopause may also occur surgically, with radiotherapy to the ovaries and with ovarian disease (e.g. premature menopause).

CLINICAL FEATURES AND TREATMENT

Features of oestrogen deficiency are hot flushes (which occur in most women and can be disabling), vaginal dryness and atrophy of the breasts. There may also be vague symptoms of loss of libido, loss of self-esteem, nonspecific aches and pains, irritability, depression, loss of concentration and weight gain. Women show a rapid loss of bone density in the 10 years following the menopause (osteoporosis, see p. 506) and the premenopausal protection from ischaemic heart disease disappears.

Most physicians are now treating symptomatic patients routinely and some recommend the widespread, near universal, use of HRT, though still much less often than in the USA. In treatment, some of the usual hazards of oestrogens apply (see below). However, current evidence suggests that, when given with a progestogen, the benefits of HRT far outweigh the small risks, in all women, unless there are clear contraindications. The overall benefits may be summarized as follows, though randomized trial data are still awaited for some of these conclusions:

- *Symptomatic improvement in many, but not all, menopausal symptoms for the majority of women.* Oestrogen-deficient symptoms respond well to oestrogen replacement, the vaguer symptoms generally, but not always, less well. Vaginal symptoms respond to local oestrogen preparations.
- *Reduction in ischaemic heart disease and cerebrovascular disease mortality*, probably via a direct vascular effect of oestrogen – blood pressure falls in the majority.
- *Protection against fractures of wrist, spine and hip, secondary to osteoporosis* (see Chapter 8), at least where HRT is used before the age of 60 years when loss of bone mass is maximal. This is due to predominant protection of trabecular rather than cancellous bone (p. 507).

Apart from individual risks from oestrogen therapy (e.g. migraine, thrombosis) – and even with these the effect of HRT may not parallel those of the 'pill': the oestrogen dose is much smaller and does not guarantee contraception – the main concerns have been induction of cancer of the uterus or breast. In HRT, oestrogen should be given cyclically with a progestogen (if the uterus is present) to prevent endometrial carcinoma from unopposed oestrogen action. Given with a progestogen, the risk of uterine cancer is not significantly increased, while the data on breast carcinoma are conflicting (current best evidence appears to indicate an increased incidence of breast carcinoma, but no definite increase in breast cancer mortality and a reduction in overall mortality on HRT). There is of course the inconvenience of withdrawal bleeds, unless a hysterectomy has been performed. Bleeding can sometimes be avoided by regimens which include continuous oestrogen and progesterone, but individual patient response is variable. The preferred route of administration has been oral, but oestrogen implants and skin patches are also widely used. The optimal length of treatment with HRT is still controversial, but most physicians who favour the use of HRT would recommend at least 10 years' treatment from the menopause, and some advocate indefinite therapy.

Premature menopause

The most common cause of early menopause in women in their twenties and thirties is ovarian failure, which is usually autoimmune in nature. HRT should be given, as the risk of osteoporosis and premature ischaemic heart disease far outweigh the risks.

The ageing male

In the male there is no sudden 'change of life'. However, there is a progressive loss in sexual function with reduction in morning erections and frequency of intercourse.

The age of onset varies widely, but overall testicular volume diminishes and gonadotrophin levels gradually rise. If premature hypogonadism is present for any reason, replacement testosterone therapy should be given to prevent osteoporosis (see p. 509).

Finasteride, which is an inhibitor of 5α-reductase, is used in benign prostatic hypertrophy. It prevents the conversion of testosterone to dihydrotestosterone which causes local prostatic hyperplasia. It is effective, though somewhat delayed in action (see p. 593).

Physiology of prolactin secretion

The hypothalamic–pituitary control of prolactin secretion is illustrated in Fig 16.13.

It is under tonic dopamine inhibition, while other factors known to increase prolactin secretion (e.g. TRH) are probably of less importance. Prolactin stimulates milk secretion but also reduces gonadal activity. It decreases LHRH pulsatility at the hypothalamic level and, to a lesser extent, blocks the action of LH on the ovary or testis, producing hypogonadism. These actions may be clinically important.

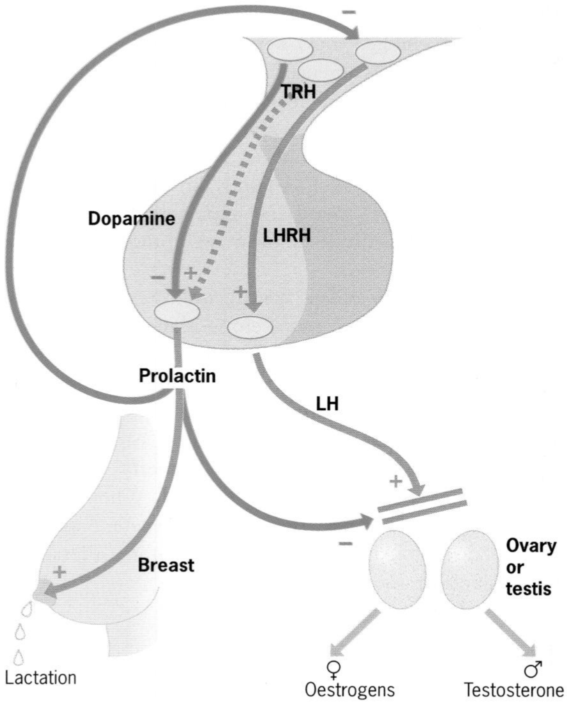

Fig 16.13
The control of prolactin secretion

Clinical features of disorders of sex and reproduction

A detailed history and examination of all systems is required (Information box 16.4).

Tests of gonadal function

The patient and partner are their own best assay for gonadal endocrine function. A man having regular satisfactory intercourse or a woman with regular ovulatory periods is most unlikely to have significant endocrine disease, assuming the history is accurate (check with the partner!). When symptoms are present, much can be deduced by basal measurements of the gonadotrophins, oestrogens/testosterone and prolactin:

- *Low testosterone or oestradiol with high gonadotrophins* indicates primary gonadal disease.
- *Low levels of LH/FSH and of testosterone/oestradiol* imply hypothalamic–pituitary disease.
- *Confirmation of normal female reproductive endocrinology* requires the demonstration of ovulation. This is achieved by measurement of luteal phase serum progesterone and/or by serial ovarian ultrasound in the follicular phase.
- *Complete demonstration of normal male and female function* requires a pregnancy. In the male, in the first instance there should be a healthy sperm count (20–200 × 10^6/mL), good motility (>60% grade I) and few abnormal forms (<20%).
- *Hyperprolactinaemia* can be confirmed or excluded by direct measurement of preferably two to three samples. Levels may increase with stress; ideally, a cannula should be inserted and samples taken through it 30 minutes later.

Information

History
Libido
Potency
Frequency of intercourse
Menstruation – relationship of symptoms to cycle
Breasts (? galactorrhoea)
Hirsuties

Physical signs
Evidence of systemic disease
Secondary sexual characteristics
Genital size (testes, ovaries, uterus)
Clitoromegaly
Breast development, gynaecomastia
Galactorrhoea
Extent/distribution of hair

Information box 16.4 Sexual and menstrual disorders

- *The clomiphene test* examines hypothalamic negative feedback. Clomiphene is a competitive oestrogen antagonist that binds to, but does not activate, oestrogen receptors, thus inducing a rise in gonadotrophin secretion in the normal subject.

More detailed tests are indicated in Table 16.11.

Table 16.11
Tests of gonadal function

Test	Uses/comments
Male	
Basal testosterone	Normal levels exclude hypogonadism
Sperm count	Normal count excludes deficiency Motility and abnormal sperms should be noted
Female	
Basal oestradiol	Normal levels exclude hypogonadism
Luteal phase progesterone (days 18–24 of cycle)	If >30 nmol L^{-1}, suggests ovulation
Ultrasound of ovaries	To confirm ovulation
Both sexes	
Basal LH/FSH	Demonstrates state of feedback system for hormone production (LH) and germ cell production (FSH)
HCG test (testosterone or oestradiol measured)	Response shows potential of ovary or testis; failure demonstrates primary gonadal problem
Clomiphene test (LH and FSH measured)	Tests hypothalamic negative feedback system; clomiphene is oestrogen antagonist
Post-coital test	Demonstrates state of sperm and sperm–mucus interaction
LHRH test (now rarely used)	Shows adequacy (or otherwise) of LH and FSH stores in pituitary

Disorders in the male

Hypogonadism

CLINICAL FEATURES

Male hypogonadism may be a presenting complaint or an incidental finding, such as during investigation for subfertility. The testes may be small and soft. Except with subfertility, the symptoms are usually of androgen deficiency, primarily poor libido, impotence and loss of secondary sexual hair (Table 16.12) rather than deficiency of semen production. Sperm makes up only a very small proportion of seminal fluid volume.

Causes of male hypogonadism are shown in Table 16.13.

INVESTIGATIONS

Testicular disease may be initially apparent but basal levels of testosterone, LH and FSH should be measured. These will allow the distinction between primary gonadal (testicular) failure and hypothalamic–pituitary disease to be made. Biopsy of the testes may be indicated, though this rarely yields a treatable cause.

Table 16.12 Effects of androgens and consequences of androgen deficiency in the male

Physiological effect	Consequences of deficiency
General	
Maintenance of libido	Loss of libido
Deepening of voice	High-pitched voice (if prepubertal)
Frontotemporal balding	Smooth skin
Facial, axillary and limb hair	Decreased hair
Maintenance of erectile and ejaculatory function	Loss of erections/ejaculation
Pubic hair	
Maintenance of male pattern	Thinning and loss of pubic hair
Testes and scrotum	
Maintenance of testicular size/consistency (needs gonadotrophins as well)	Small soft testes
Rugosity of scrotum	Poorly developed penis/scrotum
Stimulation of spermatogenesis	Subfertility
Musculoskeletal	
Epiphyseal fusion	Eunuchoidism (if prepubertal)
Maintenance of muscle bulk	Decreased muscle bulk and power
Maintenance of bone mass	Osteoporosis

Table 16.13
Causes of male hypogonadism

Reduced gonadotrophins (hypothalamic–pituitary disease)
Hypopituitarism
Selective gonadotrophic deficiency (Kallmann's syndrome)
Severe systemic illness
Severe underweight

Hyperprolactinaemia

Primary gonadal disease (congenital)
Anorchia/Leydig cell agenesis
Chromosome abnormality (e.g. Klinefelter's syndrome)
Enzyme defects
5α-reductase deficiency

Primary gonadal disease (acquired)
Testicular torsion
Castration
Local testicular disease
Chemotherapy/radiation toxicity
Renal failure
Cirrhosis/alcohol
Sickle cell disease

Androgen receptor deficiency

Pituitary MRI scan, prolactin levels and other pituitary function tests may be needed. Depending on the causes, semen analysis, chromosomal analysis (e.g. to exclude Klinefelter's syndrome) and bone age estimation are required.

TREATMENT

The cause can rarely be reversed. Replacement therapy should be commenced (Table 16.14). Primary gonadal failure should be treated with androgens. Patients with hypothalamic–pituitary disease are given LH and FSH (purified or synthetic) or pulsatile LHRH if fertility is required; otherwise they should receive androgen replacement.

Special instances of hypogonadism

Cryptorchidism

By the age of five years both testes should be in the scrotum. After that age the germinal epithelium is increasingly at risk, and lack of descent by puberty is associated with infertility. Surgical exploration and orchidopexy are usually undertaken but a short trial of HCG occasionally induces descent: an HCG test with a testosterone response 72 hours later excludes anorchia. Intra-abdominal testes have an increased risk of developing malignancy; if presentation is after puberty, orchidectomy is advised.

Klinefelter's syndrome

Klinefelter's syndrome (seminiferous tubule dysgenesis), a chromosomal disorder (47XXY) affecting 1 in 1000 males, involves both loss of Leydig cells and seminiferous tubular dysgenesis. Patients usually present with poor sexual development, small or undescended testes, gynaecomastia or infertility. They are occasionally mentally retarded. Clinical examination shows small pea-size but firm testes, usually gynaecomastia and often signs of androgen deficiency. Confirmation is by chromosomal analysis. Treatment is androgen replacement therapy, though if the patient is mentally subnormal this should be used carefully. No treatment is possible for the abnormal seminiferous tubules and infertility.

Isolated deficiency of LHRH or LH/FSH

Also known as Kallmann's syndrome or hypogonadotrophic hypogonadism, this is often associated with decreased or absent sense of smell (anosmia), and sometimes with other bony (cleft-palate), renal and cerebral abnormalities (e.g. colour blindness). It is often familial and is usually X-linked; the genetic defect has been identified. Management is that of secondary hypogonadism (see p. 916). Fertility is possible.

Oligospermia or azoospermia

These may be secondary to androgen deficiency and can be corrected by androgen replacement. More often they result from primary testicular diseases in which case they are rarely treatable.

Azoospermia with normal testicular size and low FSH levels suggests a vas deferens block, which is sometimes reversible by surgical intervention.

Lack of libido and impotence

Many patients with impotence have no definable organic cause. A careful history of physical disease, related symptoms, stress and psychological factors, together with drug and alcohol abuse, must be taken. The presence of nocturnal emissions and frequent satisfactory morning erections largely excludes endocrine disease as a cause.

True erectile difficulty may be psychological, neurogenic, vascular, endocrine or related to drugs. *Vascular disease* may be more common than realized and is often associated with vascular problems elsewhere. The *endocrine* causes are those of hypogonadism (see above) and can be excluded by normal testosterone, gonadotrophin and prolactin levels. *Autonomic neuropathy*, most commonly from diabetes mellitus, is a common partial, if not total, identifiable cause (see p. 983). Many drugs can be responsible – cannabis, diuretics, metoclopramide, bethanidine/guanethi-dine, methyldopa and β-blockers all produce impotence.

Psychogenic impotence is frequently a diagnosis of exclusion, though complex tests of penile vasculature and function are now available in some centres.

Apart from cessation of the offending drug, methods of treatment include intracavernosal injections of alprostadil, papaverine or phentolamine, penile implants and vacuum expanders. Recently sildenafil citrate, a phosphodiesterase inhibitor which increases penile blood flow, has been introduced (see p. 984). Specialist advice is essential.

If no organic disease is found, or if there is clear evidence of psychological problems, the couple should receive psychosexual counselling.

Table 16.14
Androgen replacement therapy

Preparation	Dose	Remarks
Testosterone mixed esters	250 mg i.m. every three weeks	Injection can be painful
Testosterone enanthate		Aggression if excessive Usual maintenance therapy dosage
Testosterone propionate	50–100 mg i.m. every 1–2 weeks	Frequent injections needed as half-life is short Good initial therapy
Testosterone undecanoate	80–240 mg daily, orally in divided doses	Variable dose, irregular absorption Expensive
Testosterone transdermal		Convenient but expensive

Mesterolone and methyltestosterone are no longer advised; they are weakly active and can cause cholestasis.

Gynaecomastia

Gynaecomastia is development of breast tissue in the male. Causes are shown in Table 16.15.

Pubertal gynaecomastia occurs in perhaps 50% of normal boys, often asymmetrically. It usually resolves spontaneously within 6–18 months, but after this duration may require surgical removal, as fibrous tissue will have been laid down. The cause is thought to be relative oestrogen excess.

In the older male, gynaecomastia requires a full assessment to exclude potentially serious underlying disease, such as bronchial carcinoma and testicular tumours (e.g. Leydig cell tumour). Drug effects are common (especially digoxin and spironolactone), and once these and significant liver disease are excluded most cases have no definable cause. Surgical removal is occasionally necessary.

Disorders in the female

Hypogonadism

Impaired ovarian function, whether primary or secondary, will lead both to oestrogen deficiency and abnormalities of the menstrual cycle. The latter is very sensitive to disruption, cycles becoming anovulatory and irregular before disappearing altogether. Symptoms will depend on the age at which the failure develops. Thus, before puberty, primary amenorrhoea will occur, possibly with delayed puberty; if after puberty, secondary amenorrhoea and possibly hypogonadism will result.

Oestrogen deficiency

The physiological effects of oestrogens and symptoms/signs of deficiency are shown in Table 16.16.

Amenorrhoea

Absence of periods or markedly irregular infrequent periods (oligomenorrhoea) are a common presentation, often the earliest, of female gonadal disease. Important factors in the clinical assessment of such patients are shown in Information box 16.5.

Pregnancy must always be considered as a possible cause. The possibility of genital tract abnormalities, such as an imperforate hymen, should also be remembered, especially in primary amenorrhoea. Severe illness, even in the absence of weight loss, can lead to amenorrhoea, as can stopping the contraceptive pill.

Polycystic ovary syndrome

Polycystic ovary syndrome is the most common cause of oligomenorrhoea and amenorrhoea in clinical practice and should always be considered in the context of menstrual dysfunction.

Weight-related amenorrhoea

A minimum body weight is necessary for regular menstruation. While anorexia nervosa is the extreme form (see p. 1142), this condition is common and may be seen at weights within the 'normal' range. Many of these subjects may have additional minor endocrine disease (e.g. polycystic ovarian disease), but restoration of bodyweight to above the 50th centile for height is often helpful. Similar problems occur with intensive physical training in athletes and dancers.

Hypothalmic amenorrhoea

Some dispute the existence of this condition, linking all amenorrhoea to low weight or increased stress. A few patients, however, do appear to have defective cycling mechanisms without apparent explanation.

Table 16.15
Causes of gynaecomastia

Physiological	Drugs
Neonatal	Oestrogenic
Pubertal	oestrogens
Old age	digitalis
Hyperthyroidism	cannabis
Liver disease	diamorphine
Oestrogen-producing tumours (testis, adrenal)	Anti-androgens
HCG-producing tumours (testis, lung)	spironolactone
Starvation/refeeding	cimetidine
Carcinoma of breast	cyproterone
	Others
	gonadotrophins
	cytotoxics

Table 16.16
Effects of oestrogens and consequences of oestrogen deficiency

Physiological effect	Consequence of deficiency
Breast	
Development of connective and duct tissue	Small, atrophic breast
Nipple enlargement and areolar pigmentation	
Pubic hair	
Maintenance of female pattern	Thinning and loss of pubic hair
Vulva and vagina	
Vulval growth	Atrophic vulva
Vaginal glandular and epithelial proliferation	Atrophic vagina
Vaginal lubrication	Dry vagina and dyspareunia
Uterus and tubes	
Myometrial and tubal hypertrophy	Small, atrophic uterus and tubes
Endometrial proliferation	Amenorrhoea
Skeletal	
Epiphyseal fusion	Eunuchoidism (if prepubertal)
Maintenance of bone mass	Osteoporosis

Information

History	Examination
? Pregnant	General health
Age of onset	Body shape and skeletal abnormalities
Age of menarche, if any	Weight and height
Sudden or gradual onset	Hirsuties and acne
General health	Evidence of virilization
Weight, absolute and changes in recent past	Maturity of secondary sexual characteristics
Stress (job, lifestyle, exams, relationships)	Galactorrhoea
Excessive exercise	Normality of vagina, cervix and uterus
Drugs	
Hirsuties, acne, virilization	
Headaches/visual symptoms	
Sense of smell	
Past history of pregnancies	
Past history of gynaecological surgery	

Information box 16.5 Clinical assessment of amenorrhoea

Hypothyroidism

Hypothyroidism results in increased TRH which stimulates prolactin secretion.

Miscellaneous

Severe illness, even in the absence of weight loss, after stopping the contraceptive pill.

INVESTIGATIONS

Basal levels of FSH, LH, oestrogen and prolactin allow initial distinction between primary gonadal and hypothalamic-pituitary causes (Table 16.17). Ovarian biopsy may occasionally be necessary to confirm the diagnosis of primary ovarian failure, although elevation of LH and FSH to menopausal levels is usually adequate. Subsequent investigations are shown in Table 16.17.

TREATMENT

Treatment is that of the cause wherever possible (e.g. hypothyroidism, low weight, stress, excessive exercise).

Primary ovarian disease is rarely treatable except in the rare condition of 'resistant' ovary, where high-dose gonadotrophin therapy can occasionally lead to folliculogenesis. Hyperprolactinaemia should be corrected (see below). Polycystic ovarian syndrome is discussed in detail below.

Hirsutism and polycystic ovary syndrome

PATHOPHYSIOLOGY

The extent of normal hair growth varies between individuals, families and races, being more extensive in the Mediterranean and some Asian subcontinent populations. These variations in body hair in the normal population, and the more extensive hair growth seen in patients complaining of hirsutism, appear to represent a continuum from no visible hair to extensive cover with thick dark hair. It is therefore impossible to draw an absolute dividing line between 'normal' and 'abnormal' degrees of facial and body hair in the female. Soft vellous hair is normally present all over the body and this type of hair on the face and elsewhere is 'normal' and is not sex-hormone dependent, nor is hair on the forearm or lower leg. Hair in the beard, moustache, breast, chest, axilla, abdominal midline, pubic and thigh areas is sex-hormone dependent. Any excess in the latter regions is thus usually a mark of increased ovarian or adrenal androgen production.

It has been traditional to divide patients with hirsutism into those with no elevation of serum androgen levels and no other clinical features (usually labelled 'idiopathic hirsutism') and those with an identifiable endocrine imbalance (most commonly polycystic ovary syndrome (PCOS), or rarely other causes). However, in recent years it has become apparent that most patients with 'idiopathic hirsutism' have some radiological or biochemical evidence of PCOS on more detailed investigation, and indeed several studies have demonstrated evidence of mild PCOS in up to 20% of the normal female population. Therefore, in routine clinical practice, the majority of patients with objective signs of androgen-dependent hirsutism will have PCOS, and investigation is mainly required to exclude rarer and more serious causes of virilization.

PCOS, originally known in its severe form as the *Stein–Leventhal syndrome*, is characterized by multiple small cysts within the ovary and by excess androgen production from the ovaries and to a lesser extent from the adrenals, although whether the basic defect is in the ovary, adrenal or pituitary remains unknown. The ovarian 'cysts' represent arrested follicular development. Studies have shown an association of polycystic ovarian syndrome with anovulation and insulin resistance, which may also be associated with hypertension and hyperlipidaemia. The precise mechanisms which link the aetiology of polycystic ovaries, hyperandrogenism, anovulation and insulin resistance remain to be elucidated, but may prove important in the causation of macrovascular disease in women.

Familial or idiopathic hirsutism does occur, but usually involves a distribution of hair growth which is not typically androgenic. Similarly, non-androgen-dependent hair growth occurs with drugs such as phenytoin, diazoxide, minoxidil and cyclosporin. Iatrogenic hirsutism also occurs after treatment with androgens, or more weakly androgenic drugs such as progestagens or danazol.

Rarer, and more serious, endocrine causes of hirsutism and virilization include congenital adrenal hyperplasia (CAH, see p. 948), Cushing's syndrome (p. 946) and virilizing tumours of the ovary and adrenal. All these conditions should be considered in any patient with hirsutism.

A wide variety of ovarian and adrenal steroid hormone products and precursors are androgenic and hypersecretion of androgens from one of both of these endocrine organs is usually found in patients with hirsutism. In addition, oestrogens are converted to androgens in adipose tissue, which represents a further source of androgen excess in obese patients. The response of the hair follicle to circulating androgens also seems to vary between individuals with otherwise identical clinical and biochemical features, and the reason for this variation in end-organ response remains poorly understood. Whatever the underlying pathology, hair has a long growing cycle with spontaneous variations and clinical changes are therefore slow, both as hair develops and as it responds to therapy.

CLINICAL FEATURES

The complaint of hirsutism is common and often accompanied by severe anxiety and social stress. The following are important issues to consider.

The extent and severity of hirsutism

This should be recorded objectively, ideally using a scoring system, to document the problem and to monitor treatment. The method and frequency of physical removal (e.g. shaving, plucking) should also be recorded. Most patients who complain of hirsutism will have an objective excess of hair on examination, but occasionally a normal pattern of hair will be found (and appropriate counselling is then indicated).

Table 16.17
Differential diagnosis and investigation of amenorrhoea

Diagnosis	Biochemical markers	Secondary tests
Ovarian failure		
Ovarian dysgenesis[a]	High FSH	Repeat FSH
Premature ovarian failure[a]	High LH	Karyotype
Steroid biosynthetic defect[a]	Low oestradiol	Laparoscopy/biopsy of ovary
(Ovariectomy)	Normal prolactin	HCG stimulation
(Chemotherapy)		Ultrasound of ovary/uterus
Resistant ovary syndrome		
Polycystic ovarian syndrome[a]		
	Normal/high LH	Serum testosterone/androgens, SHBG
	Normal FSH	Ultrasound of ovary
	Normal/SL: high prolactin	Progesterone challenge
	Variable oestradiol	Laparoscopy and biopsy of ovary
Gonadotrophin failure (see also hypothalamic causes below)		
Hypothalamic–pituitary disease[a]	Low LH	X-ray pituitary fossa
Kallmann's syndrome[a]	Low FSH	Clomiphene test
Anorexia[a]	Low oestradiol	Possibly LHRH test
Weight loss[a]	Normal/low prolactin	Serum thyroxine
General illness[a]		Pituitary MRI if diagnosis unclear
Possible hypothalamic causes		
Hypothalamic cause[a]	Variable LH	Serum thyroxine
Weight gain/loss[a]	Variable FSH	Serum testosterone, SHBG
Exercise-induced amenorrhoea	Normal prolactin	Laparoscopy and biopsy of ovary
Post-pill amenorrhoea	Low/normal oestradiol	Pituitary MRI unless diagnosis clear
Hyperprolactinaemia		
Prolactinoma[a]	High prolactin	Repeat prolactin (if >2000 mU L^{-1} then tumour likely)
Idiopathic hyperprolactinaemia[a]	Normal/low LH	
Hypothyroidism[a]	Normal/low FSH	Serum thyroxine
Polycystic ovarian disease[a]	Normal/low oestradiol	MRI or CT of pituitary
Other endocrine disease		
Hypothyroidism	Variable LH/FSH/oestradiol	Serum thyroxine
Cushing's syndrome	Variable prolactin	Clinically appropriate endocrine and imaging techniques
Androgen excess		
Gonadal tumour	High androgen	Androgen measurement (testosterone, androstenedione)
Uterine/vaginal abnormality		
Imperforate hymen[a]		Examination under anaesthetic
Absent uterus[a]		Ultrasound of pelvis
Lack of endometrium		Progesterone challenge

[a] These conditions may present as primary amenorrhoea.
SHBG, sex hormone binding globulin.

Age and speed of onset
Hirsutism related to PCOS usually begins around the time of the menarche and increases slowly and steadily in the teens and twenties. Rapid progression and prepubertal or late onset suggest a more serious cause.

Accompanying virilization
Hirsutism due to PCOS may be severe and effect all androgen-dependent areas on the face and body. However, more severe virilization (clitoromegaly, frontal balding, male phenotype) implies substantial androgen excess, and usually indicates a rarer cause rather than PCOS

Menstruation
Most patients with hirsutism will have some disturbance of menstruation. The greater the disruption the more likely it is that there is a serious cause.

Weight
Many patients with hirsutism are also overweight or obese. This worsens the underlying androgen excess and insulin resistance and inhibits the response to treatment, and is an indication for appropriate advice on diet and exercise. In severe cases the insulin resistance may have a visible manifestation as acanthosis nigricans on the neck and in the axillae (see Fig 20.22).

PRESENTATION

Typically, PCOS presents with amenorrhoea/oligomenorrhoea, hirsutism and acne, usually beginning shortly after menarche. It is sometimes associated with marked obesity, but weight may be normal. Mild virilization may occur in severe cases. Clinical, biochemical and radiological features of PCOS merge imperceptibly into those of the normal populations, and the incidence of the syndrome will therefore depend on the diagnostic criteria used by the clinician, and indeed by the patient when deciding whether or not to seek medical advice. There is also substantial variation between individuals with similar investigation findings who may present with one or more of the clinical features (menstrual disturbance, hirsutism or acne) alone or in various combinations.

INVESTIGATIONS

A variety of investigations may aid the diagnosis of patients with hirsutism:

- **Serum testosterone** may be elevated in PCOS and is invariably substantially raised in virilizing tumours. Patients with hirsutism and normal testosterone level frequently have low levels of sex hormone binding globulin (SHBG), leading to high free androgen levels. SHBG can be measured in some centres.
- **Other androgens**. Androstenedione and DHEA sulphate (see Fig 16.27) are frequently elevated in PCOS, and even more elevated in congenital adrenal hyperplasia and virilizing tumours.
- **17-α-Hydroxyprogesterone** is elevated in classical CAH (congenital adrenal hyperplasia), but may be apparent in late-onset CAH only after stimulation.
- **Gonadotrophin levels**. LH hypersecretion is a consistent feature of PCOS, but the pulsatile nature of secretion of this hormone means that an increased LH/FSH ratio is not always observed on a random sample.
- **Oestrogen levels**. Oestradiol is usually normal in PCOS, but oestrone levels (which are rarely measured) are elevated due to peripheral conversion. Levels are variable in other causes.
- **Ovarian ultrasound**. The most consistent investigation in PCOS is ovarian ultrasound (Fig 16.14), although a skilled observer is necessary. The typical ultrasonic features are those of a thickened capsule, multiple 3–5 mm cysts and a hyperechogenic stroma. It should also be noted that prolonged hyperandrogenization from any cause may lead to polycystic changes in the ovary. Ultrasound may also reveal virilizing ovarian tumours, although these are often small.
- **Serum prolactin**. Mild hyperprolactinaemia is common in PCOS but rarely exceeds 1500 mU L^{-1}.

If a virilizing tumour is suspected clinically or after investigation, then more complex tests may include dexamethasone suppression tests, CT or MRI of adrenals, and selective venous sampling catheters.

DIFFERENTIAL DIAGNOSIS

Most patients presenting with a combination of hirsutism and menstrual disturbance will be shown to have polycystic ovary syndrome, but the rarer alternative diagnoses should always be born in mind, and excluded with appropriate investigations if suspected. This includes late-onset congenital adrenal hyperplasia (early-onset, raised serum 17-α-OH-progesterone), Cushing's syndrome (look for other clinical features) and virilizing tumours of the ovary or adrenals (severe virilization, markedly elevated serum testosterone).

The extent of investigation will depend on the clinical context. In many cases a single serum testosterone may be sufficient to exclude rare causes. Urine free cortisol should be measured if Cushing's syndrome is a clinical possibility and 17-α-OH-progesterone if early onset or family history suggest congenital adrenal hyperplasia.

TREATMENTS

The underlying cause should be removed in the rare instances where this is possible (e.g. drugs, adrenal or ovarian tumours). Treatment of CAH and Cushing's are discussed on p. 949 and p. 947, respectively. Other therapy depends upon whether the aim is to reduce hirsutism, regularize periods or produce fertility.

Local therapy for hirsutism
Plucking, bleaching, depilatory cream or wax and shaving may all help and are often underused. Waxing is of especial value where the 'bikini area' is causing the concern. Electrolysis is slow and expensive.

Systemic therapy for hirsutism

This always requires a year or more of treatment for maximal benefit, and long-term treatment is frequently required as the problem tends to recur when treatment is stopped. The patient must therefore always be an active participant in the decision to use systemic therapy and must understand the rare risks as well as the benefits.

- *Oestrogens* (e.g. oral contraceptives) suppress ovarian androgen production and reduce free androgens by increasing SHBG levels when these are low. Combined pills, which contain a non-androgenic progestogen (e.g. Dianette or Marvelon), have a theoretical advantage over older combined pills, and will result in a slow improvement in hirsutism in a majority of cases and should normally be used first unless there is a contraindication.
- *Cyproterone acetate* (50–200 mg daily) is an anti-androgen but is also teratogenic and a weak glucocorticoid and progestogen. Given continuously it produces amenorrhoea, and so is normally given for days 1–14 of each cycle. In women of childbearing age, contraception is essential.
- *Prednisolone* given in a reverse circadian manner (5 mg at night, 2.5 mg in the morning) may rarely improve hirsutism in polycystic ovarian syndrome when given alone, though is more effective in restoring regular menstruation.
- *Spironolactone* (200 mg daily) also has anti-androgen activity and can cause useful improvements in hirsutism in selected cases.

While both spironolactone and cyproterone are widely used, it should be noted that neither is licensed in the UK for the treatment of hirsutism, and both are subject to CSM warnings.

Other agents of doubtful efficacy include bromocriptine and cimetidine. Newer agents which remain to be fully evaluated include finasteride and flutamide.

Treatment of menstrual disturbance

Cyclical oestrogen/progestogen will regulate the menstrual cycle and remove the symptom of oligo- or amenorrhoea. This is most frequently an additional benefit of the treatment of hirsutism, but may also be used when menstrual disturbance is the only symptom.

(a)

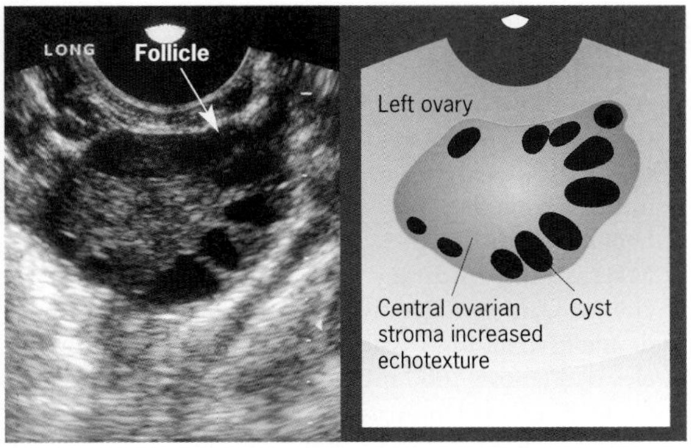

(b)

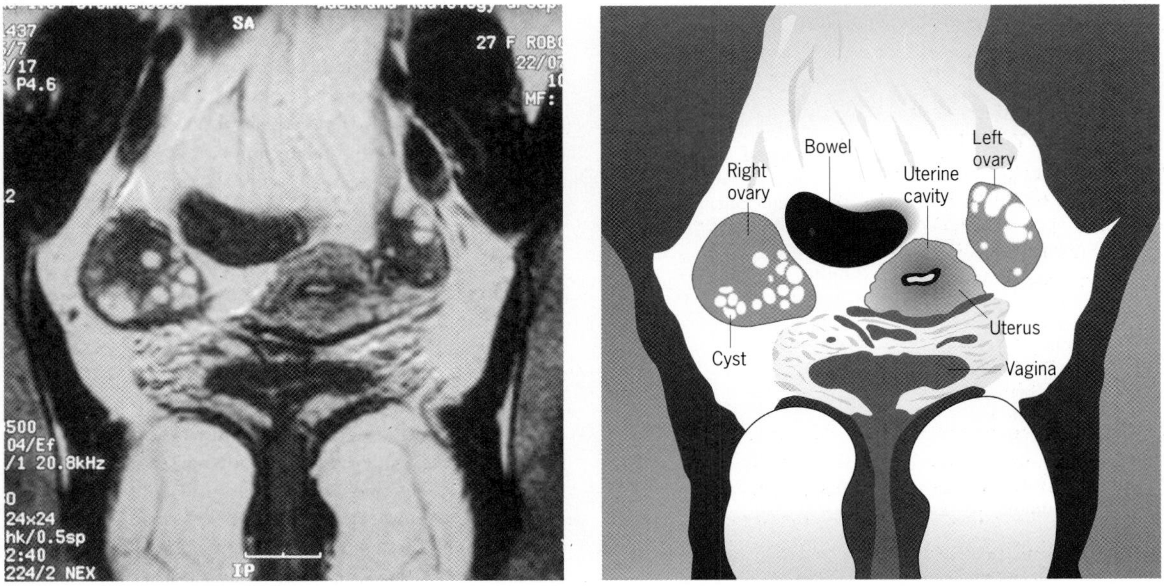

Fig 16.14
Polycystic ovarian syndrome
(a) Longitudinal transvaginal ultrasound of ovary, revealing multiple cysts with central ovarian stroma showing increased echo texture
(b) MR image (coronal) of polycystic ovaries, also showing pelvic anatomy
Reproduced by kind permission of Barbara Hochstein and Geoffrey Cox, Auckland Radiology Group

Treatment for fertility

- Clomiphene 50–200 mg can be given daily on days 2–6 of the cycle (or tamoxifen 10–40 mg daily), sometimes combined with 5000 U of HCG intramuscularly on day 12/13. This can occasionally cause ovarian hyperstimulation and specialist supervision is essential.
- *Reverse the circadian rhythm* with prednisolone (2.5 mg in the morning, 5 mg on retiring) to suppress pituitary production of ACTH upon which adrenal androgens partly depend. Regular ovulatory cycles often ensue. Steroid instruction and a card must be supplied.

More intensive techniques to stimulate ovulation may also be indicated in specialist hands, including *low-dose gonadotrophin therapy*, and ovarian hyperstimulation techniques associated with *in vitro* fertilization.

Wedge resection of the ovary was a traditional therapy which is now rarely required, although ovarian electrodiathermy has gained some popularity in recent years.

Hyperprolactinaemia

Mildly increased prolactin levels (400–600 mU L^{-1}) may be physiological, pathological or secondary to drug therapy (Table 16.18), while higher levels require a diagnosis.

CLINICAL FEATURES

Hyperprolactinaemia stimulates milk production in the breast and inhibits GnRH and gonadotrophin secretion *per se*. It usually presents with:

- galactorrhoea, spontaneous or expressible (60% of cases) (not all patients with galactorrhoea have hyperprolactinaemia, but the other causes are poorly understood – 'normoprolactinaemic galactorrhoea' and duct ectasia)
- oligomenorrhoea or amenorrhoea
- decreased libido in both sexes
- decreased potency in men
- subfertility
- symptoms or signs of oestrogen or androgen deficiency – in the long term osteoporosis may result, especially in women
- delayed or arrested puberty in the peripubertal patient.

Table 16.18
Causes of hyperprolactinaemia

Physiological	**Drug-induced**
Sleep (REM phase)	Dopamine antagonists (e.g. metoclopramide and phenothiazines)
Pregnancy	Oestrogens
Suckling	Opiates
Nipple stimulation	Cimetidine
Stress	Methyldopa
Coitus	Reserpine
Pathological	
Production by tumours	
Prolactinomas	
Occurs in some acromegalics	
Interference with stalk	
Any hypothalamic/ pituitary tumour	
Idiopathic hyperprolactinaemia	
Polycystic ovarian syndrome	
Primary hypothyroidism	
Chest wall injury	
Renal failure	
Liver failure	

Additionally, headaches and/or visual field defects may be present if there is a pituitary tumour (more common in men).

INVESTIGATIONS

At least three prolactin levels should be measured. These tests are appropriate after physiological and drug causes have been excluded.

- **Visual fields** should be checked.
- **Anterior pituitary function** should be assessed if there is any clinical evidence of hypopituitarism or radiological evidence of tumour. Hypothyroidism must be excluded since this is a cause of hyperprolactinaemia.
- **MRI of the pituitary** is necessary if there are clinical features suggestive of a pituitary tumour, and desirable in all cases when prolactin is significantly elevated (above 1000 mU L^{-1}). MRI is more sensitive to small microadenomas than CT, though the latter should be used if MRI is not available.

Macroprolactinoma refers to tumours above 10 mm diameter, *microprolactinoma* to smaller ones. The size of tumour may affect the choice of treatment.

Mean prolactin levels of above 5000 mU L^{-1} in the presence of a macroadenoma, or above 2000 mU L^{-1} in the presence of a microadenoma (or of no radiological abnormality), strongly suggest a prolactinoma (see p. 905).

TREATMENT

Treatment is dependent upon circumstances and facilities. Hyperprolactinaemia should be reduced with a dopamine agonist. Bromocriptine is the best established therapy: initial doses should be small (e.g. 1 mg) and taken with food, or at bedtime. The dose should be gradually increased, usually to 2.5 mg two or three times daily, judged on clinical response and prolactin levels. Maintenance doses are 2.5–15 mg daily in divided doses. Side-effects include nausea and vomiting, dizziness and syncope, constipation and cold peripheries. Newer agents more specific for the D2 dopamine receptor include cabergoline (500 μg once or twice a week) and quinagolide (75–150 μg once daily), both of which are longer-acting and better tolerated and which may become the treatments of choice in due course. If an identifiable adenoma is present this is likely to shrink in size with a dopamine agonist.

Definitive therapy is controversial and will depend upon the size of the tumour, the patient's wishes, including desire for fertility and local expertise and facilities. In many cases it is simply sufficient to continue successful dopamine agonist therapy. *Small tumours* in asymptomatic patients without hypogonadism need only observation.

Trans-sphenoidal surgery often restores normoprolactinaemia in patients with microadenoma in the most skilled hands, but is rarely completely successful with macroadenomas. Some surgeons believe that long-term bromocriptine increases the hardness of the adenoma and makes resection more difficult – but other surgeons dissent from this view.

Radiotherapy is only slowly effective and can sometimes cause eventual hypopituitarism. It is often advocated after medical tumour shrinkage or after surgery in larger tumours, especially where families are complete, but other workers simply advocate continuation of dopamine agonist therapy in responsive cases.

Rarely, tumours enlarge during pregnancy to produce headaches and visual defects. Dopamine agonists should be restarted.

There is some evidence that some *microprolactinomas* do not recur after several years of dopamine agonist therapy in a substantial minority of cases.

Oral contraception

The combined oestrogen–progestogen pill is widely used for contraception and has a low failure rate (<1 per 100 woman-years). 'Pills' contain 20–50 μg of oestrogen, usually ethinyloestradiol, together with a variable amount of one of several progestogens. The mechanism of action is twofold:

- suppression by oestrogen of gonadotrophins, thus preventing follicular development, ovulation and luteinization
- progestogen effects on cervical mucus, making it hostile to sperm, and on tubal motility and the endometrium.

Side-effects of these preparations are shown in Information box 16.6. Most of the serious ones are rare and are less common on modern 20–30 μg oestrogen pills. Evidence suggests that thromboembolism may be slightly more common on 'pills' containing desogestrel and gestodene (approx 30/100 000 woman-years compared with 15/100 000 on older pills and 5/100 000 on no treatment). While some problems require immediate cessation of the pill, the importance of other milder side-effects must be judged against the hazards of pregnancy occurring with inadequate contraception, especially if other effective methods are not practicable or acceptable.

It is clear, however, that the hazards of the combined pill are greater in women aged over 35 years, especially in smokers and those with other risk factors for cardiovascular disease (e.g. hypertension, hyperlipidaemias). The 'mini-pill' (progestogen only) is less effective but is often suitable where oestrogens are contraindicated (Information box 16.6). A progesterone antagonist, mifepristone, has been introduced

Information

General
Weight gain
Loss of libido
Pigmentation (chloasma)
Breast tenderness
Increased growth rate of some malignancies

Cardiovascular
Increased blood pressure[a]
Deep vein thrombosis[a]
Myocardial infarction
Stroke

Gastrointestinal
Nausea and vomiting
Abnormal liver biochemistry[a]
Gallstones increased
Hepatic tumours

Nervous system
Headache
Migraine[a]
Depression[a]

Malignancy
Possible increase in cancer of the breast (but reduced risk of ovarian and endometrial cancer)

Gynaecological
Amenorrhoea
'Spotting'
Cervical erosion

Haematological
Increased clotting tendency

Endocrine/metabolic
Mild impairment of glucose tolerance
Worsened lipid profile, though variable

Drug interactions (reduced contraceptive effect due to enzyme induction)
Antibiotics
Barbiturates
Phenytoin
Carbamazepine
Rifampicin

[a] Common reasons for stopping oral contraceptives.

Information box 16.6 Adverse effects and drug interactions of oral contraceptives (mixed oestrogen–progesterone combinations) which, in combination with a prostaglandin analogue, induces abortion of pregnancy at up to nine weeks' gestation. It prevents progesterone-induced inhi-bition of uterine contraction.

Subfertility

This term, kinder than 'infertility', is defined as the inability of a couple to conceive after one year of unprotected intercourse. Investigation requires the combined skills of gynaecologist, endocrinologist and, ideally, andrologist. Both partners must be considered and every aspect of the physiology critically examined.

CAUSES (Fig 16.15)

A significant proportion of cases have both male and female problems.

Inadequate intercourse, hostile cervical mucus and vaginal factors are uncommon (5%). Fifteen per cent of cases appear to be idiopathic.

Male factors

About 30–40% of couples have a major identifiable male factor. There is some evidence that male sperm counts are declining in many populations. Untreated male hypo-gonadism of any cause (see Table 16.13) is likely to be associated with subfertility.

Female factors

Female tubal problems account for perhaps 20%; a similar proportion have ovulatory disorders. Any cause of oligomenorrhoea or amenorrhoea (see Table 16.17) is likely to be associated with suboptimal ovulation or anovulation.

CLINICAL ASSESSMENT

Both partners should be seen and the following factors checked:

- *The man.* Look for previous testicular damage (e.g. orchitis, trauma), undescended testes, urethral symptoms and venereal problems, local surgery, and use of alcohol and drugs. A semen analysis early in the investigations is essential.
- *The woman.* Look for previous pelvic infection, regularity of periods, previous surgery, alcohol intake and smoking, and adequacy of bodyweight (see p. 910).
- *Together.* Check the frequency and adequacy of intercourse, and the use of lubricants.

Examination should include an assessment of secondary sexual characteristics, body habitus and general health. In men, the size and consistency of the testes are important, plus exclusion of a varicocele. In women, a vaginal examination allows a check on the uterus and ovaries.

Female factors				Joint factors	Male factors		
? Ovulation	? Tubal problems	? Uterine problems	? Cervix Vaginal problems	? Adequate intercourse	? Normal sperm count		
	Patency Function	Anatomy Implantation	Infection Cervical hostility	Frequency Timing Technique	Potency	Vas blockage	Testicular disease

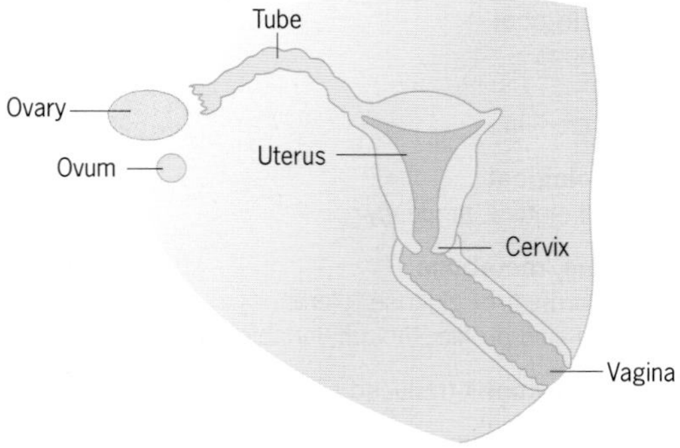

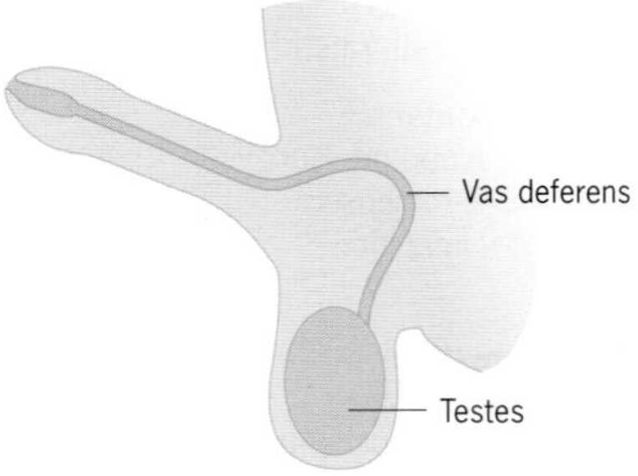

Pelvic ultrasound Serum progesterone	Hysterosalpingogram	Swabs Post-coital test SCMC	Post-coital test History	Sperm count (post-coital test)
Laparoscopy / Egg collection				

Fig 16.15
Major factors involved in subfertility and their investigation. SCMC, sperm–cervical mucus contact test

INVESTIGATIONS

Appropriate tests for particular defects are shown in Fig 16.15.

TREATMENT

Counselling of both partners is essential. Any defect(s) found should be treated if possible. Ovulation can usually be induced by exogenous hormones if simpler measures fail, while *in vitro* fertilization (IVF) and similar techniques are more widely used, especially where there is tubal blockage, oligospermia or 'idiopathic subfertility'. Intracytoplasmic sperm injection (ICSI) appears particularly effective for severe oligospermia and poor sperm function.

Disorders of sexual differentiation

Disorders of sexual differentiation are rare but may affect chromosomal, gonadal, endocrine and phenotypic development (Table 16.19). Such cases always require extensive, multidisciplinary clinical management. An individual's sex can be defined in several ways:

- *Chromosomal sex*. The normal female is 46XX, the normal male 46XY. The Y chromosome confers male sex; if it is not present, development follows female lines.
- *Gonadal sex*. This is obviously determined predominantly by chromosomal sex, but requires normal embryological development.
- *Phenotypic sex*. This describes the normal physical appearance and characteristics of male and female body shape. This in turn is a manifestation of gonadal sex and subsequent sex hormone production.
- *Social sex (gender)*. This is heavily dependent on phenotypic sex and normally assigned on appearance of the external genitalia at birth.
- *Sexual orientation* – heterosexual, homosexual (male/male or female/female) or bisexual (both sexes). Some studies suggest that there may be some element of genetic determination of homosexuality.

FURTHER READING

Bagatell CJ, Bremner WJ (1996) Drug therapy: androgens in men – uses and abuses. *New England Journal of Medicine* **334**: 707–714.

Baird DT (1997) Amenorrhoea. *Lancet* **350**: 275–279.

Franks S (1995) Polycystic ovary syndrome. *New England Journal of Medicine* **333**: 853–861.

Howards SS (1994) Current concepts: treatment of male infertility *New England Journal of Medicine* **332**: 312–317.

Kyel-Mensah AA, Jacobs HS (1995) The investigation of female infertility. *Clinical Endocrinology* **43**: 251–256.

Rittmaster RS (1997) Hirsutism. *Lancet* **349**: 191–195.

Menopause (1997) *Endocrinology and Metabolism Clinics of North America* **27**.

Table 16.19
Disorders of sexual differentiation

Condition	Chromosomes	Gonads	Phenotype	Remarks
Turner's syndrome	45XO	Streak	Female	Often morphological features (e.g. short stature, web neck, coarctation of aorta)
Gonadal dysgenesis	46XY	Streak or minimal testes[a]	Immature female	
Congenital adrenal hyperplasia	46XX	Ovary	Female with variable virilization	Obvious androgen excess
Virilizing tumour	46XX	Ovary	Female with variable virilization	Obvious androgen excess
True hermaphroditism	46XX/XY or mosaic	Testis and ovary	Male or ambiguous	
Klinefelter's syndrome	47XXY	Small testes	Male, often with gynaecomastia	Many are hypogonadal
Testicular feminization	46XY	Testes[a]	Ambiguous or infantile female	Androgen receptor defective
Testicular synthetic defects	46XY	Testes[a]	Cryptorchid, ambiguous	
5α-Reductase deficiency	46XY	Testes	Cryptorchid, ambiguous	Impaired conversion of testosterone to dihydrotestosterone
Anorchia	46XY	Absent	Immature female	

[a]Gonadectomy advised because of high risk of malignancy.

The growth axis

Physiology and control of growth hormone (Fig 16.16)

GH is the pituitary factor responsible for stimulation of body growth in humans. Its secretion is stimulated by GHRH, released into the portal system from the hypothalamus; it is also under inhibitory control by GHRIH (somatostatin). GH stimulates the hepatic production of an intermediate insulin-like growth factor-1 (IGF-1, previously known as somatomedin C) that actually stimulates growth. Plasma levels of IGF-1, however, reflect local growth activity poorly, partly as there are multiple IGF-binding proteins (IGF-BP). The metabolic actions of the system are:

- increasing collagen and protein synthesis
- promoting retention of calcium, phosphorus and nitrogen, necessary substrates for anabolism
- opposing the action of insulin.

GH release is intermittent and mainly nocturnal, especially during REM sleep. The frequency and size of GH pulses increase during the growth spurt of adolescence and decline thereafter. Acute stress and exercise both stimulate GH release while, in the normal subject, hyperglycaemia suppresses it.

IGF-1 may, in addition, play a major role in maintaining neoplastic growth. Recent evidence has shown a relationship between circulating IGF-1 concentrations and breast cancer in pre-menopausal women and prostate cancer in men.

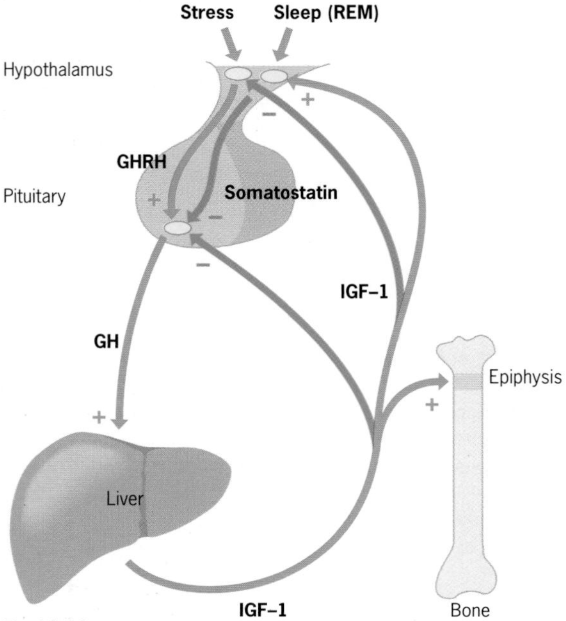

Fig 16.16
The control of growth hormone (GH) and insulin-like growth factor-1 (IGF-1) secretion and action

Normal growth

There are factors other than GH involved in linear growth in the human.

- *Genetic factors*. Children of two short parents will probably be short.
- *Nutritional factors*. Adequate nutrients must be available. Impaired growth can result from inadequate dietary intake or small-bowel disease (e.g. coeliac disease).
- *General health*. Any serious systemic disease in childhood is likely to reduce growth (e.g. renal failure).
- *Intrauterine growth retardation*. These infants often grow poorly in the long term, while infants with simple prematurity usually catch up. There is evidence that low birthweight may predispose to hypertension, diabetes and other health problems in later adult life.
- *Emotional deprivation and psychological factors*. These can impair growth by complex, poorly understood mechanisms, probably involving temporarily decreased GH secretion.

The relevant aspects of history and examination in the assessment of problems are shown in Information box 16.7.

Assessment of growth

Charts showing ranges of height and weight for normal British children are available (Fig 16.17), and other national data are available. Height must be measured very carefully, ideally at the same time of day on the same instrument by the same observer.

Information

History
Pregnancy records
Rate of growth (home/school records, e.g. heights on kitchen door)
Comparison with peers at school and siblings
Change in appearance (old photographs)
Change in shoe/glove/hat size or frequency of 'growing out'
Age of appearance of pubic hair, breasts, menarche

Physical signs
Evidence of systemic disease
Body habitus, size, relative weight, proportions (span versus height)
Skin thickness, interdental separation
facial features
Spade hands/feet
Grading of secondary sexual characteristics

Information box 16.7
Assessment of problems of growth and development

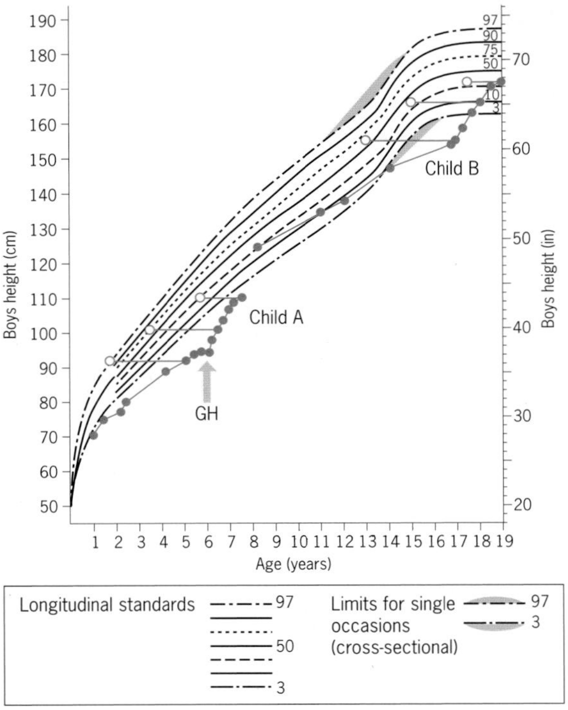

Fig 16.17
A height chart for boys
Child A illustrates the course of a child with hypopituitarism, initially treated with cortisol and thyroxine, but showing growth only after growth hormone treatment
Child B shows the course of a child with constitutional growth delay without treatment. The open circles show the data corrected for bone age. Reproduced by permission of Castlemead Publications

In general, there are three overlapping phases of growth: infantile (0–2 years), which appears largely substrate (food) dependent; childhood (age 2 years to puberty), which is largely GH dependent; and the adolescent 'growth spurt', dependent on GH and sex hormones.

Height velocity is more helpful than current height. It requires at least two measurements some months apart and, ideally, multiple serial measurements. Height velocity is the rate of current growth (cm per year), while already attained height is largely dependent upon previous growth.

Standard deviation scores (SDS) based on the degree of deviation from age–sex norms are widely used by experts – these and growth velocities are far more sensitive than simple charts in assessing growth. Hand-held computer programs also allow calculation of many of these indices.

The approximate future height of a child ('mid-parental height') can be simply predicted from the parental heights. For a *boy*, this is:

[(Maternal height + 13 cm (5 inches) + Paternal height)/2]

and for a *girl*:

[(Paternal height – 13 cm (5 inches) + Maternal height)/2].

Thus, with a father of 180 cm and mother of 155 cm, the predicted heights are 174 cm for a son and 161 cm for a daughter.

Growth failure: short stature

When children or their parents complain of short stature, particular attention should focus on:

- intrauterine growth retardation, weight and gestation at birth
- possible systemic disorder – any system, but especially small-bowel disease
- evidence of skeletal, chromosomal or other congenital abnormalities
- endocrine status – particularly primary hypothyroidism
- dietary intake and use of drugs, especially steroids for asthma
- emotional, psychological, family and school problems.

School, general practitioner, clinic and home records of height and weight should be obtained if possible to allow growth–velocity calculation. If unavailable, such data must be obtained prospectively.

A child with normal growth velocity is unlikely to have significant endocrine disease. However, low growth velocity without apparent systemic cause requires further investigation. Sudden cessation of growth suggests major physical disease; if no gastrointestinal, respiratory, renal or skeletal abnormality is apparent, then a cerebral tumour or hypothyroidism are likeliest.

Consistently slow-growing children require full endocrine assessment.

Features of the more common causes of growth failure are given in Table 16.20.Where constitutional delay is clearly shown and symptoms require intervention, then very low dose sex steroids in 3–6 month courses will usually induce acceleration of growth.

INVESTIGATIONS

Systemic disease having been excluded, the following should be undertaken:

- **Thyroid function tests** – serum TSH and T_4 to exclude hypothyroidism.
- **GH status**. Basal levels are of little value, though urinary GH measurements may prove to be of some value in screening. Overnight repeated sampling is optimal but the GH response to Bovril, exercise, clonidine, arginine and insulin are all used; a normal peak response is >20 mU L^{-1}. The 'gold standard' test has been the insulin tolerance test (ITT), but for safety reasons this should be performed only in specialist centres.
- **Assessment of bone age**. Non-dominant hand and wrist X-rays allow assessment of bone age by comparison with standard charts (Tanner, Greulich and Pyle).

Table 16.20
Clinical features of common causes of short stature

Cause	Family history	Growth pattern, clinical features and puberty	Bone age	Remarks
Constitutional delay	Often present	Slow from birth, immature but appropriate with late but spontaneous puberty	Moderate delay	Often difficult to differentiate from GH deficiency Growth velocity measurement vital
Familial short stature	Positive	Slow from birth, clinically normal with normal puberty	Normal	Need heights of all family members
GH insufficiency	Rare	Slow growth, immature often overweight, delayed puberty	Moderate delay, increasing with time	Early investigation and treatment vital Increased suspicion if child is plump
Primary hypothyroidism	Rare	Slow growth, immature and delayed puberty	Marked delay	Measure TSH, T_4 in all cases of short stature Clear clinical signs not obvious
Small bowel disease	Sometimes	Slow, immature, usually thin for height, delayed puberty	Delayed	Diarrhoea and/or macrocytosis/anaemia Occasionally no GI symptoms

TREATMENT

Systemic illness should be treated. Where there is primary hypothyroidism, start replacement therapy with thyroxine 50–150 μg daily.

For GH insufficiency, human GH (collected from pituitaries) was previously used but was withdrawn as cases of Creutzfeld–Jakob disease were reported. It has been superseded by recombinant GH, which is given as nightly injections in doses of 10–20 U m^{-2} body surface area per week. Treatment is expensive and should be supervised in expert centres.

GH treatment in so-called 'short normal' children has not been shown to produce any worthwhile increase in final height. In Turner's syndrome (see p. 925) large doses of GH are effective in increasing final height and are sometimes combined with oxandrolone, a growth-stimulating synthetic sex steroid. Familial cases of resistance to GH owing to an abnormal GH receptor (Laron-type dwarfism) are well described. They are very rare but may respond to therapy with synthetic IGF-1.

Growth hormone excess: gigantism and acromegaly

GH stimulates skeletal and soft-tissue growth. GH excess therefore produces gigantism in children (if acquired before epiphyseal fusion) and acromegaly in adults.

Tall stature

The most common causes are hereditary (two tall parents!), idiopathic (constitutional) or early development. It can occasionally be due to hyperthyroidism. Other causes include chromosomal abnormalities (e.g. Klinefelter's syndrome, Marfan's syndrome) or metabolic abnormalities. GH excess is a very rare cause and is usually clinically apparent.

Acromegaly

This is due to a pituitary tumour in almost all cases. Hyperplasia due to GHRH excess is rare.

CLINICAL FEATURES

Symptoms and signs of acromegaly are shown in Fig 16.18. One-third of patients present with changes in appearance, one-quarter with visual field defects or headaches; in the remainder the diagnosis is made by an alert observer in another clinic, e.g. diabetic, hypertension, dental, dermatology.

INVESTIGATIONS

- **GH levels** are normally very low (<1 mU L^{-1}) in adults except during stress or as occasional spikes but, unless levels are always below 1 mU L^{-1}, one cannot exclude the diagnosis.
- **Glucose tolerance test** is diagnostic. Acromegalics fail to suppress GH below 1 mU L^{-1} and some show a paradoxical rise; about 25% of acromegalics have a diabetic glucose tolerance test.
- **IGF-1 level** is almost always raised in acromegaly – a single plasma level of IGF-1 reflects mean 24-hour GH levels and is useful in diagnosis. IGFBP-3 level (p. 896) is raised in 80% of cases.
- **Visual field defects** are common.
- **MRI scan of pituitary** – will almost always reveal the pituitary adenoma.
- **Pituitary function** – partial or complete anterior hypopituitarism is common.
- **Prolactin** – mild to moderate hyperprolactinaemia occurs in 30% of patients.

Symptoms

Change in appearance
Increased size of hands/feet
Headaches
Visual deterioration
Tiredness
Weight gain
Amenorrhoea
  oligomenorrhoea
  in women
Galactorrhoea
Impotence or poor libido
Deep voice
Goitre
Breathlessness
Excessive sweating
Pain/tingling in hands
Polyuria/polydipsia
Muscular weakness
Joint pains

Old photographs are
  frequenly useful
Symptoms of
  hypopituitarism may be
  present as well

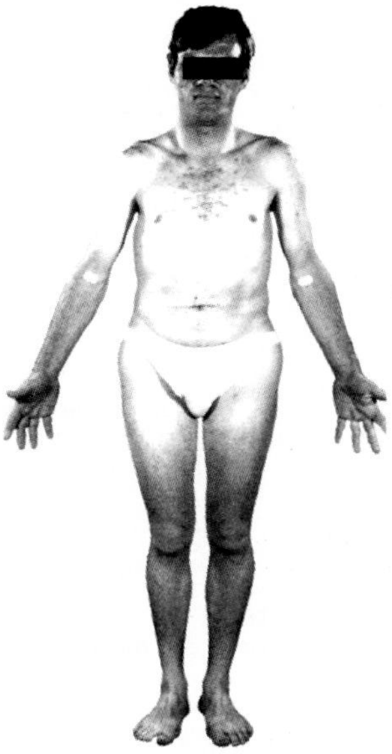

Signs	
Visual field defects	Prominent supraorbital ridge
Broad nose	Prognathism
Large tongue	**Interdental separation**
Goitre	
Gigantism	
Galactorrhoea	Thick greasy skin
Hirsuties	
Carpal tunnel syndrome	**Tight rings**
Spade-like hands and feet	
Proximal myopathy	Heart failure
Arthropathy	Hypertension
	Glycosuria
Oedema	(plus possible signs of hypopituitarism)

Fig 16.18
The signs of acromegaly. Bold type indicates signs of greater discriminant value

MANAGEMENT AND TREATMENT

Untreated acromegaly results in markedly reduced survival with most deaths from heart failure, coronary artery disease and hypertension-related causes. In addition, there appears to be an increase in deaths due to neoplasia, particularly large-bowel tumours. Treatment is therefore indicated in all except the elderly or those with minimal abnormalities. There is now consensus agreement that the aim of therapy should be to achieve a mean growth hormone level below 5 mU L^{-1}, which has been shown to reduce mortality to normal levels. The general pros and cons of surgery, radiotherapy and medical treatment are discussed on p. 907.

Complete cure is often slow, if possible at all. The choice lies between trans-sphenoidal surgery, transfrontal surgery, external radiotherapy, octreotide, and dopamine agonists. Progress can be assessed by mean GH levels and by serial IGF-1 measurements.

When present, hypopituitarism should be corrected (see p. 908) and concurrent diabetes and/or hypertension should be treated conventionally; both usually improve with treatment of the acromegaly.

Surgery

Trans-sphenoidal surgery is generally agreed as the appropriate first-line therapy. It will result in clinical remission in a majority of cases (about 60%) with pituitary micro-adenoma, but in only a minority of those with macroadenoma. Transfrontal surgery is rarely required except for massive macroadenomas.

External radiotherapy

External radiotherapy is normally used after pituitary surgery fails to normalize GH levels rather than as primary therapy. It is often combined with medium-term treatment with octreotide or a dopamine agonist because of the slow biochemical response to radiotherapy, which may take 10 years or more.

Octreotide

Octreotide is a synthetic analogue of somatostatin (GHRIH, p. 926) which is now the treatment of choice in resistant cases, and is employed as a short-term treatment while other modalities become effective. It is conventionally given by subcutaneous injection in doses of 50–200 μg 8-hourly, but a long-acting preparation is also now available. It is generally well tolerated but is associated an increased incidence of gallstones and is extremely expensive.

Dopamine agonists

Dopamine agonists used alone are usually reserved for the elderly and frail. They can be given to shrink tumours prior to definitive therapy or to control symptoms and persisting GH secretion; they are probably most effective in mixed growth-hormone-producing (somatotroph) and prolactin-producing (mammotroph) tumours. The doses are bromocriptine 10–60 mg daily or cabergoline 0.5 mg daily (higher than for prolactinomas) but should be started slowly (see p. 922). They have largely been replaced by octreotide.

FURTHER READING

Le Roith D (1997) Insulin-like growth factors. *New England Journal of Medicine* **336**: 633–640.

Melmed S (1995) Recent advances in pathogenesis, diagnosis and management of acromegaly. *Journal of Clinical Endocrinolgy and Metabolism* **80**: 3395–3402.

Growth and growth disorders (1996) *Endocrinology and Metabolism Clinics of North America* **25**.

The thyroid axis

The metabolic rate of many tissues is controlled by the thyroid hormones, and overactivity and underactivity of the gland pose the most common of all endocrine problems.

Anatomy

The gland consists of two lateral lobes connected by an isthmus. It is closely attached to the thyroid cartilage and to the upper end of the trachea, and thus moves on swallowing. It is often palpable in normal women.

Embryologically it originates from the base of the tongue and descends to the middle of the neck. Remnants of thyroid tissue can sometimes be found at the base of the tongue (lingual thyroid) and along the line of descent. The gland has a rich blood supply from superior and inferior thyroid arteries.

The thyroid consists of follicles lined by cuboidal epithelioid cells. Inside is the colloid, which is an iodinated glycoprotein, thyroglobulin, synthesized by the follicular cells. Each follicle is surrounded by basement membrane, between which are parafollicular cells containing calcitonin-secreting C cells.

Biochemistry

The thyroid hormones, T_4 and T_3, are synthesized within the gland (Fig 16.19).

More T_4 than T_3 is produced, but T_4 is converted in some peripheral tissues (liver, kidney and muscle) to the more active T_3 by 5′-monodeiodination; an alternative 3′-monodeiodination yields the inactive reverse T_3 (rT_3). The latter step occurs particularly in severe non-thyroidal illness (see below).

In plasma, more than 99% of all T_4 and T_3 is bound to hormone-binding proteins (thyroxine-binding globulin, TBG; thyroid-binding prealbumin, TBPA; and albumin). Only free hormone is available for tissue action, where T_3 binds to specific nuclear receptors within the cell. Factors affecting TBG are shown in Table 16.21.

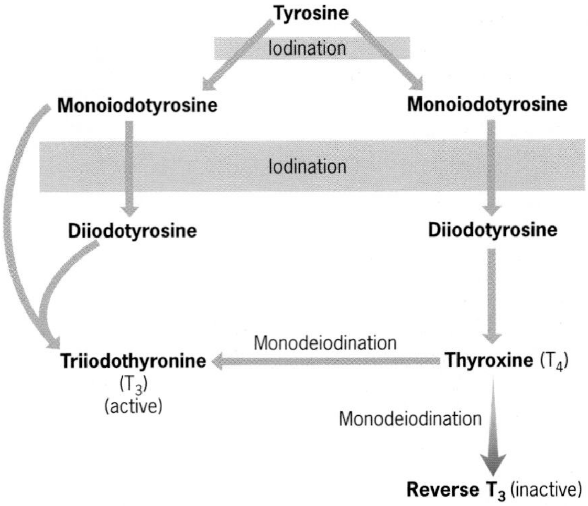

Fig 16.19
Synthesis and metabolism of the thyroid hormones

Table 16.21
Factors affecting thyroxine-binding globulin (TBG) levels

Increased TBG
Hereditary
Pregnancy
Oestrogen therapy
Oral contraceptive use
Hypothyroidism
Phenothiazines
Acute viral hepatitis
Decreased TBG
Hereditary
Androgens
Corticosteroid excess
Thyrotoxicosis
Nephrotic syndrome
Major illness
Malnutrition
Chronic liver disease
Drugs causing altered binding
Non-steroidal anti-inflammatory drugs
Phenytoin

Deficiency

Globally, dietary iodine deficiency is an important cause of thyroid disease as it is an essential requirement for thyroid hormone synthesis. The recommended daily intake of iodine should be at least 140 μg, and dietary supplementation of salt and bread has reduced the number of areas where 'endemic goitre' still occurs (see below).

Physiology of the hypothalamic–pituitary–thyroid axis (see Fig 16.2)

1 TRH is released in the hypothalamus and stimulates release of TSH from the pituitary.

2 TSH stimulates the TSH receptor in the thyroid to increase synthesis of both T_4 and T_3 and also to release stored hormone, producing increased plasma levels of T_4 and T_3.
3 T_3 feeds back on the pituitary and perhaps hypothalamus to reduce TRH and TSH secretion.

Thyroid function tests

Immunoassays for total T_4, free T_4, total T_3, free T_3 and TSH are widely available. There are only minor circadian rhythms, and measurements may be made at any time. Particular uses of the tests are summarized in Table 16.22, with typical findings in common disorders.

TSH measurement
Current assays differentiate between normal and low levels and TSH levels and can thus discriminate between hyperthyroidism, hypothyroidism and euthyroidism. There are pitfalls, however. These are mainly with hypopituitarism, with the 'sick euthyroid' syndrome and with dysthyroid eye disease, all of which may give 'false' (i.e. misleading, not incorrect) low results implying hyperthyroidism. As a single test of thyroid function it is the most sensitive in most circumstances, but many laboratories prefer to perform at least two tests – for example, TSH plus serum T_3 or free T_3 where hyperthyroidism is suspected, TSH plus serum T_4 or free T_4 where hypothyroidism is likely.

'Free' T_4 tests
These attempt to measure only the unbound active hormone. Although not perfect, they are now in routine clinical use in many laboratories. TBG is sometimes measured directly.

TRH test
This has been rendered almost obsolete except for investigation of hypothalamic–pituitary dysfunction.

Problems in interpretation of thyroid function tests

There are three major areas of difficulty.

Serious acute or chronic illness

Thyroid function is affected in several ways, with reduced concentration and affinity of binding proteins, decreased peripheral conversion of T_4 to T_3 with more rT_3 and reduced hypothalamic–pituitary TSH production. Systemically ill patients can therefore have an apparently low total and free T_4 and T_3 with a normal or low basal TSH (the 'sick euthyroid' syndrome). Levels are usually only mildly below normal and are thought to be mediated by interleukins IL-1 and IL-6; the tests should be repeated after resolution of the underlying illness.

Pregnancy and oral contraceptives

These lead to greatly increased TBG levels and thus to high or high-normal total T_4. Free T_4 is usually normal. The normal physiological changes during pregnancy are not fully understood but rarely cause clinical problems, although TSH is often slightly suppressed in the first trimester.

Drugs

Many drugs affect thyroid function tests by interfering with protein binding. The most common are listed in Table 16.21. Basal TSH should be measured.

Antithyroid antibodies

Serum antibodies to the thyroid are common and may be either *destructive* or *stimulating*; both occasionally coexist in the same patient.

Destructive antibodies may be directed against the microsomes or against thyroglobulin; the antigen for thyroid microsomal antibodies is the thyroid peroxidase enzyme. They may be detected by haemagglutination techniques and are found in up to 20% of the normal population, especially older women, but only 10–20% of these develop overt hypothyroidism.

TSH receptor antibodies (TRAb), which are IgG antibodies, can be measured in two ways:

- by the inhibition of binding of TSH to its receptors (TSH-binding inhibitory immunoglobulin, TBII)
- by demonstrating that they stimulate the release of cyclic AMP (thyroid-stimulating immunoglobulin/antibody TSI, TSAb).

Table 16.22
Characteristics of thyroid function tests in common thyroid disorders (the clinically most informative tests in each situation **are shown in bold**)

	TSH ($0.3–3.5\ mU\ L^{-1}$)	Total T_4 ($60–160\ mmol\ L^{-1}$)	Free T_4 ($13–30\ pmol\ L^{-1}$)	T_3 ($1.2–3.1\ nmol\ L^{-1}$)
Thyrotoxicosis	**Suppressed (<0.05 mU L^{-1})**	Increased	**Increased**	**Increased**
Primary hypothyroidism	**Increased (>10 mU L^{-1})**	Low/low-normal	Low/low-normal	Normal or low
TSH deficiency	Low-normal or subnormal	Low/low-normal	**Low/low-normal**	Normal or low
T_3 toxicosis	**Suppressed (<0.05 mU L^{-1})**	Normal	Normal	**Increased**
Compensated euthyroidism	**Slightly increased (5–10 mU L^{-1})**	Normal	**Normal**	Normal

Hypothyroidism

PATHOPHYSIOLOGY

Underactivity of the thyroid may be primary, from disease of the thyroid, or secondary to hypothalamic–pituitary disease (reduced TSH drive) (Table 16.23). It is one of the most common endocrine conditions with a UK prevalence of 1.4% in women, but under 0.1% in men.

Causes of primary hypothyroidism

Atrophic (autoimmune) hypothyroidism

This is the most common cause of hypothyroidism and is associated with microsomal autoantibodies leading to lymphoid infiltration of the gland and eventual atrophy and fibrosis. It is six times more common in females and the incidence increases with age. The condition is associated with other autoimmune disease such as pernicious anaemia. In some instances the condition shows intermittent hypothyroidism with recovery. In some cases antibodies which block the TSH receptor may be involved in the aetiology.

Hashimoto's thyroiditis

This form of autoimmune thyroiditis, again more common in women and most common in late middle age, produces atrophic changes with regeneration, leading to goitre formation. The gland is usually firm and rubbery but may range from soft to hard. Thyroid microsomal antibodies are again present, often in very high titres (>1:100 000). Patients may be hypothyroid or euthyroid, though they may go through an initial toxic phase, 'Hashi toxicity'. Thyroxine therapy may shrink the goitre even when the patient is not hypothyroid, though this may take a long time.

Postpartum thyroiditis

This is usually a transient phenomenon observed following pregnancy and may involve hyperthyroidism, hypothyroidism or the two sequentially. It is believed to result from the modifications to the immune system necessary in pregnancy, and histologically is a lymphocytic thyroiditis. The process is normally self-limiting, but when conventional antibodies are found there is a high chance of this proceeding to permanent hypothyroidism.

Table 16.23
Causes of hypothyroidism

Primary	
Congenital Agenesis Ectopic thyroid remnants	**Post-surgery** **Post-irradiation** Radioactive iodine therapy External neck irradiation
Defects of hormone synthesis Iodine deficiency Dyshormonogenesis Antithyroid drugs Other drugs (e.g. lithium, amiodarone, interferon)	**Infiltration** Tumour **Peripheral resistance to thyroid hormone**
Autoimmune Atrophic thyroiditis Hashimoto's thyroiditis	**Secondary** **Hypopituitarism** Isolated TSH deficiency
Infective Post-subacute thyroiditis	

Iodine deficiency

In mountainous areas (the Alps, Himalayas, South America, Central Africa) dietary iodine deficiency still exists, in some areas as 'endemic goitre' where goitre, occasionally massive, is common. The patients may be euthyroid or hypothyroid depending on the severity of iodine deficiency. The mechanism is thought to be borderline hypothyroidism leading to TSH stimulation and thyroid enlargement in the face of continuing iodine deficiency.

Dyshormonogenesis

This rare condition is due to genetic defects in the synthesis of thyroid hormones; patients develop hypothyroidism with a goitre. One particular familial form is associated with sensorineural deafness (Pendred's syndrome).

CLINICAL FEATURES (Fig 16.20)

Hypothyroidism may produce many symptoms. The classic picture of the slow, dry-haired, thick-skinned, deep-voiced patient with weight gain, cold intolerance, bradycardia and constipation makes the diagnosis easy. The term 'myxoedema' refers to the accumulation of mucopolysaccharide in subcutaneous tissues. Milder symptoms are, however, more common and many cases are detected on biochemical screening.

Special difficulties in diagnosis may arise in certain circumstances:

- *Children with hypothyroidism* may not show classic features but often have a slow growth velocity, poor school performance and sometimes arrest of pubertal development.
- *Young women with hypothyroidism* may not show obvious signs. Hypothyroidism should be excluded in all patients with oligomenorrhoea/amenorrhoea, menorrhagia, infertility or hyperprolactinaemia.
- *The elderly* show many clinical features that are difficult to differentiate from normal ageing.

INVESTIGATION OF PRIMARY HYPOTHYROIDISM

Serum TSH is the investigation of choice; a high TSH level confirms primary hypothyroidism. A low total or free serum T_4 level confirms the hypothyroid state and is especially important if there is any evidence of hypothalamic and pituitary disease, when TSH may be low or normal.

Thyroid and other organ-specific antibodies may be present. Other abnormalities include the following:

- *anaemia*, which is usually normochromic and normocytic in type but may be macrocytic (sometimes

Symptoms

Tiredness/malaise
Weight gain
Anorexia
Cold intolerance
Poor memory
Change in appearance
Depression
Psychosis
Coma
Deafness
Poor libido
Goitre
Puffy eyes
Dry, brittle unmanageable hair
Dry, coarse skin
Arthralgia
Myalgia
Constipation
Menorrhagia or oligomenorrhoea in women

A history from a relative is often revealing
Symptoms of other autoimmune disease may be present

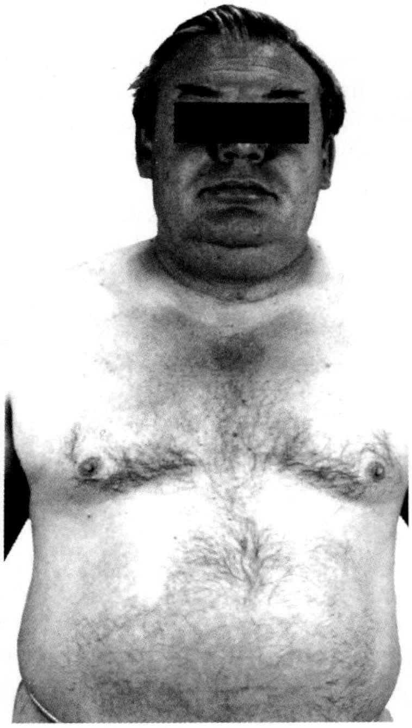

Signs

Mental slowness	Large tongue
Psychosis/dementia	
Ataxia	Periorbital oedema
Poverty of movement	Deep voice
Deafness	(Goitre)
'Peaches and cream' complexion	Dry skin
	Mild obesity
Dry thin hair	
Loss of eyebrows	Myotonia
	Muscular hypertrophy
Hypertension	Proximal myopathy
Hypothermia	Slow-relaxing reflexes
Heart failure	
Bradycardia	Anaemia
Pericardial effusion	
Cold peripheries	
Carpal tunnel syndrome	
Oedema	

Fig 16.20
The signs of hypothyroidism. Bold type indicates signs of greater discriminant value

this is due to associated pernicious anaemia) or microcytic (in women, due to menorrhagia)
- *increased aspartate transferase levels*, from muscle and/or liver
- *increased creatine kinase levels*
- *hypercholesterolaemia*
- *hyponatraemia* due to an increase in ADH and impaired free water clearance.

TREATMENT

Replacement therapy with T_4 is given for life. The starting dose will depend upon the severity of the deficiency and on the age and fitness of the patient, especially cardiac performance. In the young and fit, 100 μg daily is suitable, while 50 μg daily is more appropriate for the small, old or frail. T_3 offers no significant advantage over T_4.

Patients with ischaemic heart disease require even lower initial doses, especially if the hypothyroidism is severe and longstanding. Most physicians would then begin with 25 μg daily and perform serial ECGs, increasing the dose at 3–4 week intervals if angina does not occur or worsen and the ECG does not deteriorate. Some, however, would use T_3 beginning with 2.5 μg 8-hourly, doubling the dose every 48 hours up to 10 μg thrice daily. If progress is satisfactory, T_4 (100 μg daily) is then started and T_3 is discontinued five days later.

Adequacy of replacement should be assessed clinically and by thyroid function tests (TSH and possibly T_4) after at least six weeks on a steady dose; the aim is to restore TSH to well within the normal range. If serum TSH remains high, the dose of T_4 should be increased in 25–50 μg increments and the tests repeated six weeks later. This stepwise progression should be continued until TSH becomes normal, though some physicians believe that complete well-being is only restored in some patients when the T_4 is high-normal and the TSH is slightly suppressed. The usual maintenance dose is 100–150 μg given as a single daily dose; over-replacement may increase the risk of atrial fibrillation in those aged over 60. An annual thyroid function test is recommended.

Clinical improvement on T_4 may not begin for two weeks or more, even though it is quicker on T_3, and full resolution of symptoms may take six months. The importance of lifelong therapy must be emphasized and the possibility of other autoimmune endocrine disease developing, especially Addison's disease, should be considered. During pregnancy about a 50 μg increase in T_4 dosage is often needed to maintain normal TSH levels, probably because of the increased TBG levels.

Borderline hypothyroidism or 'compensated euthyroidism'

Patients are frequently seen with low-normal serum T_4 levels and slightly raised TSH levels. Sometimes this follows surgery or radioactive iodine therapy when it can reasonably be seen as 'compensatory'. Treatment with thyroxine is now normally recommended where the TSH is consistently above 10 mU L^{-1}, or when possible symptoms, thyroid antibodies or lipid abnormalities are present. Where the TSH is only marginally raised, the tests should be repeated 3–6 months later. Conversion to overt hypothyroidism is more common in men or when microsomal antibodies are present.

Myxoedema coma

Although very rare, severe hypothyroidism, especially in the elderly, may present with confusion or even coma.

Hypothermia is often present and the patient may have severe cardiac failure, hypoventilation, hypoglycaemia and hyponatraemia.

The mortality was previously at least 50% and patients require full intensive care. Optimal treatment is controversial and data lacking; most physicians would advise T_3 orally or intravenously in doses of 2.5–5 µg every eight hours, then increasing as above. Large intravenous doses should not be used. Additional measures, though unproven, should include:

- oxygen (by ventilation if necessary)
- monitoring of cardiac output and pressures via a Swan–Ganz catheter
- gradual rewarming
- hydrocortisone 100 mg i.v. 8-hourly
- dextrose infusion to prevent hypoglycaemia.

'Myxoedema madness'

Depression is common in hypothyroidism but occasionally with severe hypothyroidism in the elderly the patient may become frankly demented or psychotic, sometimes with striking delusions. This may occur shortly after starting T_4 replacement.

Screening for hypothyroidism

The incidence of congenital hypothyroidism is approximately 1 in 3500 births. Untreated, severe hypothyroidism leads to permanent neurological and intellectual damage ('cretinism'). Routine screening of the newborn using a blood-spot, as in the Guthrie test, to detect a high TSH level as an indicator of primary hypothyroidism is efficient; cretinism is prevented if T_4 is started within the first few months of life.

Screening of elderly patients for thyroid dysfunction is controversial and not currently recommended. However, patients who have undergone thyroid surgery or received radioiodine should have regular thyroid function tests, as should those receiving lithium or amiodarone therapy.

Goitre (thyroid enlargement)

Goitre is more common in women than in men and may be either physiological or pathological.

CLINICAL FEATURES

Most commonly a goitre is noticed as a cosmetic defect by the patient or by friends or relatives. The majority are painless, but pain or discomfort can occur in acute varieties. Goitres, which may be diffuse or nodular, can produce dysphagia and difficulty in breathing, implying oesophageal or tracheal compression.

Clinical examination should record the size, shape, consistency and mobility of the gland as well as whether its lower margin can be demarcated (thus implying the absence of retrosternal extension). A bruit may be present. Associated lymph nodes should be sought and the tracheal position determined if possible. Examination should never omit an assessment of the patient's clinical thyroid status.

There is a WHO grading of goitre:

- Grade 0 – no palpable or visible goitre
- Grade 1 – palpable goitre
  - 1A: goitre detectable only on palpation
  - 1B: goitre palpable and visible with neck extended
- Grade 2 – goitre visible with neck in normal position
- Grade 3 – large goitre visible from a distance.

Specific enquiry should be made about any medication, especially iodine-containing preparations, and possible exposure to radiation.

ASSESSMENT

There are two major aspects of any goitre: its pathological nature and the patient's thyroid status.

The nature can often be judged clinically. Goitres (Table 16.24) are usually separable into diffuse and nodular types, the causes of which differ.

Particular points of note are:

- *Puberty and pregnancy* may produce a diffuse increase in size of the thyroid.
- *In Graves' disease* (autoimmune hyperthyroidism) the gland is again diffusely enlarged, often somewhat firm and frequently associated with a bruit.

Table 16.24
Goitre

Causes	Types
Physiological	Multinodular goitre
Puberty	Diffuse goitre
Pregnancy	Colloid
Autoimmune	Simple
Graves' disease	Cysts
Hashimoto's disease	Tumours
Thyroiditis	Adenomas
Acute (de Quervain's thyroiditis)	Carcinoma
Chronic fibrotic (Reidel's thyroiditis)	Lymphoma
Iodine deficiency (endemic goitre)	Miscellaneous
Dyshormonogenesis	Sarcoidosis
Goitrogens (e.g. sulphonylureas)	Tuberculosis

- *Acute tenderness* in a diffuse swelling, sometimes with severe pain, is suggestive of an acute viral thyroiditis (de Quervain's). This is usually associated with a systemic viral illness and may produce transient clinical hyperthyroidism with an increase in serum T_4 (see p. 931).
- *Pain* in a goitre may be caused by thyroiditis, bleeding into a cyst or (rarely) a thyroid tumour.
- *Excessive doses of carbimazole or propylthiouracil* will induce goitre.
- *Iodine deficiency and dyshormonogenesis* (see above) can also cause goitre.

Simple goitre

In this instance no clear cause is found for enlargement of the thyroid, which is usually smooth and soft. It may be associated with thyroid growth-stimulating antibodies.

Multiple nodular goitre

Most common is the multinodular goitre, especially in older patients. The patient is usually euthyroid but may be hyperthyroid or borderline with suppressed TSH levels but normal T_4 and T_3. Multinodular goitre is the most common cause of tracheal and/or oesophageal compression and may cause laryngeal nerve palsy. It may also extend retrosternally. The classical 'multinodular goitre' is usually readily apparent clinically, but it should be noted that modern, high-resolution ultrasound frequently reports multiple small nodules in glands which are clinically diffusely enlarged and associated with autoimmune thyroid disease, and there is also a high incidence of these small nodules in the normal population.

Solitary nodular goitre

Such a goite presents a difficult problem of diagnosis. A history of pain, rapid enlargement or associated lymph nodes in such a situation suggests the possibility of thyroid carcinoma. The majority of such nodules are, however, cystic or benign and, indeed, may simply be the largest solitary nodule of a multinodular goitre. Risk factors for malignancy include previous irradiation, longstanding iodine deficiency and occasional familial cases. Solitary toxic nodules (Plummer's syndrome) are quite uncommon and may be associated with T_3 production.

Fibrotic goitre

Fibrotic goitre (Riedel's thyroiditis) is a rare condition, usually producing a 'woody' gland. It is associated with other midline fibrosis and is often difficult to distinguish from carcinoma, being irregular and hard.

Malignancy

Rarely the thyroid is the site of a metastatic deposit or the site of origin of a lymphoma.

INVESTIGATIONS

Clinical findings will dictate appropriate initial tests:

- **Thyroid function tests** – TSH plus T_4 or T_3 (see Table 16.22).
- **Chest and thoracic inlet X-rays** where appropriate to detect tracheal compression and large retrosternal extensions.

Additional investigations

Fine needle aspiration (FNA). In patients with a solitary nodule or a dominant nodule in a multinodular goitre, there is a 5% chance of malignancy; in view of this, FNA should be performed. This can be done in the outpatient clinic. Cytology in expert hands can usually differentiate the suspicious or definitely malignant nodule.

FNA has reduced the need for imaging and will reduce the necessity for surgery, but there is a significant false-negative rate which must be born in mind (and the patient appropriately counselled). Continued observation is required when an isolated thyroid nodule is assumed to be benign without excision.

Ultrasound. Ultrasound with high resolution is a sensitive method for delineating nodules and can demonstrate whether they are cystic or solid. In addition, a multinodular goitre may be demonstrated when only a single nodule is palpable. Unfortunately, even cystic lesions can be malignant and thyroid tumours may arise within a multinodular goitre; therefore FNA is generally required and may be performed under ultrasound control at the same time as the scan.

Thyroid scan. Thyroid scan (^{125}I or ^{131}I) can be useful to distinguish between functioning (hot) or non-functioning (cold) nodules. A hot nodule is rarely malignant; however a cold nodule is malignant in 10% of cases.

TREATMENT

During puberty and pregnancy a goitre associated with euthyroidism rarely requires intervention. If euthyroid, the patient should be reassured that spontaneous resolution is likely. In other situations the patient should be rendered euthyroid. Indications for surgical intervention are:

- *The possibility of malignancy*. A history of rapid growth, pain, cervical lymphadenopathy or previous irradiation to the neck are worrying features. FNA should be performed. Surgery may be necessary if doubt persists.
- *Pressure symptoms on the trachea or, more rarely, oesophagus.* The possibility of retrosternal extension should be excluded.
- *Cosmetic reasons.* A large goitre is often a considerable anxiety to the patient even though functionally and anatomically benign.

Thyroid carcinoma

Types of thyroid carcinoma, their characteristics and treatment are listed in Table 16.25. While not common, these tumours are responsible for 400 deaths annually in the UK. In 90% of cases they present as thyroid nodules (see above), but occasionally with cervical lymphadenopathy (about 5%), or with lung, cerebral, hepatic or bone metastases. Clinically significant metastases to the thyroid are rare.

Carcinomas derived from thyroid epithelium may be papillary or follicular (differentiated) or anaplastic (undifferentiated), while medullary carcinomas (about 5% of all thyroid cancers) arise from the calcitonin-producing C-cells (often part of MEN syndromes). Lymphomas also arise within the thyroid. The pathogenesis of thyroid epithelial carcinomas is not understood except for occasional familial papillary carcinoma and those cases related to previous head-and-neck irradiation or ingestion of radioactive iodine (e.g. post-Chernobyl). These tumours are minimally active hormonally and are extremely rarely associated with hyperthyroidism; over 90%, however, secrete thyroglobulin which can therefore act as a tumour marker. There is a detailed TNM classification.

Papillary and follicular carcinomas

The primary treatment is surgical, normally total thyroidectomy for local disease unless the lesion is small and limited to one lobe. Regional, or more extensive, neck dissection is needed where there is local nodal spread or involvement of local structures. Most of these tumours will take up iodine, and can thus be shown by radioiodine scanning. Such patients after total thyroidectomy may be given a therapeutic radioiodine dose (high dose: 5.5–7.5 GBq), which will be taken up by remaining thyroid tissue or metastatic lesions. Replacement T_4 will subsequently be needed and should be at an adequate dose to suppress TSH completely, as it may otherwise stimulate any residual differentiated carcinoma. Lungs and bone are the most common sites of metastases, while local invasion is often a problem. The measurement of thyroglobulin in plasma is frequently used as a tumour marker for the presence of neoplastic tissue, levels above 10 $\mu g\,L^{-1}$ indicating a high chance of remaining disease.

The prognosis is extremely good when these types of tumour are excised while confined to the thyroid gland, and the specific therapies available lead to a relatively good prognosis even in the presence of metastases at diagnosis. Age below 40 years and papillary tumours do better than those over 40 and with a follicular histology.

Anaplastic carcinomas and lymphoma

These do not respond to radioactive iodine, and external radiotherapy produces only a brief respite.

Medullary carcinoma

Medullary carcinoma, often associated with multiple endocrine neoplasia (MEN, see p. 957), is usually treated by total thyroidectomy. The patient's family should be screened for this and other endocrine neoplastic conditions.

Hyperthyroidism

Hyperthyroidism (thyroid overactivity, thyrotoxicosis) is common, affecting perhaps 2–5% of all females at some time and with a sex ratio of 5:1, most often between ages 20 and 40 years. Nearly all cases (>99%) are caused by intrinsic thyroid disease; a pituitary cause is extremely rare (Table 16.26).

Graves' disease

This is the most common cause of hyperthyroidism/thyrotoxicosis and is due to an autoimmune process. Serum IgG antibodies bind to the thyroid TSH receptor stimulating thyroid hormone production, behaving like TSH. These TSH receptor antibodies can be measured in serum. There is an association with HLA-B8, Dw3 and 50% concordance is seen amongst monozygotic twins with a 5% concordance rate in dizygotic twins.

Yersinia enterocolitica as well as *Escherichia coli* and other Gram-negative organisms contain TSH binding sites. This raises the possibility that the initiating event in the pathogenesis may be an infection with possible 'molecular mimicry' in a genetically susceptible individual, but the precise initiating mechanisms remain unproven in most cases.

Associated with the thyroid disease in many cases are eye changes (see below) and other signs such as vitiligo and pretibial myxoedema. Rarely lymphadenopathy and splenomegaly may occur. Graves' disease is also associated with other autoimmune disorders such as pernicious anaemia and myasthenia gravis.

Table 16.25
Types of thyroid malignancy

Cell type	Frequency	Behaviour	Spread	Prognosis
Papillary	70%	Occurs in young people	Local, sometimes lung/bone secondaries	Good, especially in young
Follicular	20%	More common in females	Metastases to lung/bone	Good if resectable
Anaplastic	<5%	Aggressive	Locally invasive	Very poor
Lymphoma	2%	Variable		Sometimes responsive to radiotherapy
Medullary cell	5%	Often familial	Local and metastases	Poor

Table 16.26
Causes of hyperthyroidism

Common	TSH-secreting tumours (e.g. pituitary)
Graves' disease (autoimmune)	HCG-producing tumours
Solitary toxic nodule/ adenoma	Hyperfunctioning ovarian teratoma (struma ovarii)
Toxic multinodular goitre	
Thyrotoxicosis factitia (secret T_4 consumption)	**Uncommon**
Exogenous iodine	Acute thyroiditis
Drugs – amiodarone	viral
Metastatic differentiated thyroid carcinoma	autoimmune
	post-irradiation

The natural history is one of fluctuation, many patients showing a pattern of alternating relapse and remission; perhaps only 40% of subjects have a single episode. Many patients eventually become hypothyroid.

Other causes of hyperthyroidism/thyrotoxicosis

Toxic solitary adenoma/nodule (Plummer's disease)

This is the cause of about 5% of cases of hyperthyroidism. It does not usually remit after a course of antithyroid drugs.

Toxic multinodular goitre

This commonly occurs in older women. Again, antithyroid drugs are rarely successful in inducing a remission.

De Quervain's thyroiditis

This is transient hyperthyroidism from an acute inflammatory process, probably viral in origin. Apart from the toxicosis there is usually fever, malaise and pain in the neck with tachycardia and local thyroid tenderness. Thyroid function tests show initial hyperthyroidism, the erythrocyte sedimentation rate (ESR) is raised, and thyroid uptake scans show suppression of uptake in the acute phase, though hypothyroidism, usually transient, may then follow after a few weeks. Treatment of the acute phase is with aspirin, using short-term prednisolone in severely symptomatic cases.

Postpartum thyroiditis

This is described on p. 932.

CLINICAL FEATURES OF HYPERTHYROIDISM

The symptoms of hyperthyroidism affect many systems. Symptoms and relevant signs are shown in Fig 16.21.

Symptomatology and signs vary with age and with the underlying aetiology. Important points are:

- *The eye signs, pretibial myxoedema and thyroid acropachy* occur only in Graves' disease. Pretibial myxoedema is an infiltration on the shin, essentially occurring only with eye disease (see below). Thyroid acropachy is very rare and consists of clubbing, swollen fingers and periosteal new bone formation.
- *In the elderly* a frequent presentation is with atrial fibrillation, other tachycardias and/or heart failure, often with few other signs. Thyroid function tests are mandatory in any patient with atrial fibrillation.

Symptoms

Weight loss
Increased appetite
Irritability/behaviour change
Restlessness
Malaise
Muscle weakness
Tremor
Choreoathetosis
Breathlessness
Plapitation
Heat intolerance
Vomiting
Diarrhoea
Eye complaints*
Goitre
Oligomenorrhoea
Loss of libido
Gynaecomastia
Onycholysis
Tall stature (in children)

*Only in Graves' disease

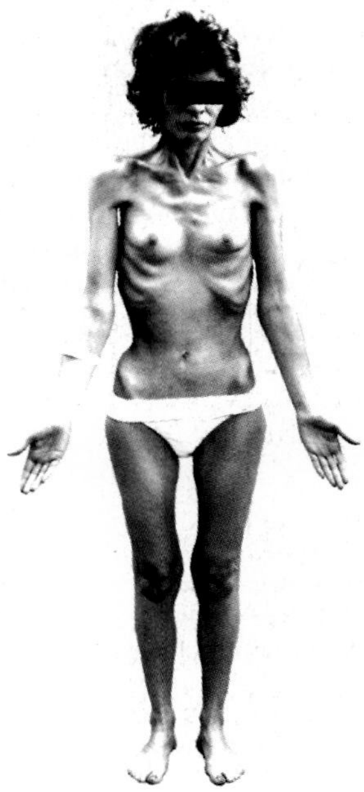

Signs

Irritability	**Exophthalmus**
Psychosis	Lid lag
Hyperkinesis	Conjunctival oedema
Tremor	Ophthalmoplegia
	Goitre, bruit
Systolic hypertension	
Cardiac failure	
Tachycardia or atrial fibrillation	Weight loss
Warm vasodilated peripheries	
	Proximal muscle wasting (shoulder and hips)
Onycholysis	**Proximal myopathy**
Palmar erythema	
Thyroid acropachy	
Pretibial myxoedema	

Fig 16.21
The signs of hyperthyroidism. Bold type indicates signs of greater discriminant value

- *Children* frequently present with excessive height or excessive growth rate, or with behavioural problems such as hyperactivity. They may also show weight gain rather than loss.
- *So-called 'apathetic thyrotoxicosis'* in some elderly patients presents with a clinical picture more like hypothyroidism. There may be very few signs and a high degree of clinical suspicion is essential.

DIFFERENTIAL DIAGNOSIS

Hyperthyroidism is often clinically obvious but treatment should never be instituted without biochemical confirmation.

Differentiation of the mild case from anxiety states may be difficult; useful positive clinical markers are eye signs, a diffuse goitre, proximal myopathy and wasting. The hyperdynamic circulation with warm peripheries seen with hyperthyroidism can be contrasted with the clammy hands of anxiety.

INVESTIGATIONS

Serum TSH is suppressed in hyperthyroidism (<0.1 mU L^{-1}), except for the very rare instances of TSH hypersecretion. Most physicians also like to confirm the diagnosis with a raised serum T_3 or T_4; the former is more sensitive as there are occasional cases of isolated 'T_3 toxicosis'. Microsomal (directed against thyroid peroxidase) and thyroglobulin antibodies are present in most cases of Graves' disease.

TSH receptor antibodies are not measured routinely, but are commonly present: TSI 80% positive, TBII 60–90% in Graves' disease (see p. 936).

TREATMENT

Three possibilities are available: radioiodine, antithyroid drugs, and surgery. Practices and beliefs differ widely within and between countries. Treatment also depends on patient preference and local expertise. This section gives some general guidelines. Patient preference, with informed discussion of the alternatives and long-term sequelae, must be given great weight. Where radioiodine or surgery is chosen, patients need to be rendered euthyroid with antithyroid drugs before their definitive therapy.

Most patients (90%) with hyperthyroidism have a diffuse goitre. Those with large single or multinodular goitres are unlikely to remit after a course of antithyroid drugs. Severe biochemical hyperthyroidism is also less likely to respond.

Radioiodine is now more widely used in the UK as has previously happened elsewhere; theoretical risks of carcinogenesis have not been proven in practice. The range of doses is from about 200 up to 500 MBq, the higher doses having greater 'cure' rates but also more, and quicker, subsequent hypothyroidism. Response usually takes 1–6 months. Radiation safety requirements make it usable only in specialist centres.

Patients with dysthyroid eye disease may show worsening of eye problems after radioiodine, though this association remains controversial and can often be prevented by steroid or early T_4 administration.

Patients who demonstrate poor compliance with drug therapy or medical supervision should probably undergo surgery.

Antithyroid drugs

Carbimazole is most often used in the UK. Occasionally propylthiouracil is also used. Methimazole, the active metabolite of carbimazole, is used in the USA. These drugs inhibit the formation of thyroid hormones and also have minor other actions; carbimazole/methimazole is also an immunosuppressive agent. Initial doses and side-effects are detailed in Table 16.27.

Although thyroid hormone synthesis is reduced very quickly, the long half-life of T_4 (seven days) means that clinical benefit is not apparent for 10–20 days. As many of the manifestations of hyperthyroidism are mediated via the sympathetic system, β-blockers may be used to provide rapid partial symptomatic control; they also decrease peripheral conversion of T_4 to T_3. Drugs preferred are those without intrinsic sympathomimetic activity (Table 16.27). They should not be used alone for hyperthyroidism except when the condition is self-limiting, as in subacute thyroiditis.

Subsequent management is either by gradual dose titration or a 'block and replace' regimen. Neither regime has been shown to be unequivocally superior.

Table 16.27
Drugs used in the treatment of hyperthyroidism

Drug	Usual starting dose	Side-effects	Remarks
Antithyroid drugs			
Carbimazole	10–20 mg 8-hourly	Rash, nausea, vomiting, arthralgia, agranulocytosis (0.1%), jaundice	Active metabolite is methimazole Mild immunosuppressive activity
Propylthiouracil	100–200 mg 8-hourly	Rash, nausea, vomiting agranulocytosis	Additionally blocks conversion of T_4 to T_3
β-Blocker for symptomatic control			
May need higher doses than normal in hyperthyroidism as metabolism is increased			
Propranolol	40–80 mg 6–8 hourly	Avoid in asthma Use with care in heart failure	Use agents without intrinsic sympathomimetic activity as receptors highly sensitive

Gradual dose titration

1 Review after 4–6 weeks and reduce dose of carbimazole depending on clinical state and T_4/T_3 levels. TSH levels may remain suppressed for long periods and are unhelpful at this stage.
2 When clinically and biochemically euthyroid, stop β-blockers.
3 Review after 2–3 months and, if controlled, reduce carbimazole.
4 Gradually reduce dose to 5 mg daily over 6–24 months if hyperthyroidism remains controlled.
5 When the patient is euthyroid on 5 mg daily carbimazole, discontinue.

About 50% of patients will relapse, mostly within the following two years. Long-term antithyroid therapy is then used or surgery or radiotherapy is considered (see below).

Propylthiouracil is used in similar fashion but doses required are tenfold higher and must be given in split doses (50–500 mg daily).

'Block and replace' regimen

With this policy, full doses of antithyroid drugs, usually carbimazole 40 mg daily, are given to suppress the thyroid completely while replacing thyroid activity with 100 μg of thyroxine daily once euthyroidism has been achieved. This is continued usually for 18 months, the claimed advantages being the avoidance of over- or under-treatment and the better use of the immunosuppressive action of carbimazole. This regimen is contraindicated in pregnancy as T_4 crosses the placenta less well than carbimazole.

Toxicity

The major side-effect is agranulocytosis that occurs in approximately 1 in 1000 patients usually within three months of treatment. All patients must be warned to seek immediate medical attention if they develop unexplained fever or sore throat; this is best done with a written sheet. If toxicity occurs on carbimazole, propylthiouracil may be used and vice versa; side-effects are only occasionally repeated on the other drug.

Surgery: subtotal thyroidectomy

Thyroidectomy should be performed only in patients who have previously been rendered euthyroid. Conventional practice is to stop the antithyroid drug 10–14 days before operation and to give potassium iodide (60 mg thrice daily), which reduces the vascularity of the gland.

Particular indications for surgery are:

- patient choice
- a large goitre, which is unlikely to respond to antithyroid medication.

Indications for either surgery or radioiodine are:

- persistent drug side-effects
- poor compliance with drug therapy
- recurrent hyperthyroidism after drugs.

The operation and complications

The operation should be performed only by experienced surgeons to reduce the chance of complications.

- *Early postoperative bleeding* causing tracheal compression and asphyxia is a rare emergency requiring immediate removal of all clips/sutures to allow escape of the blood/haematoma.
- *Laryngeal nerve palsy* occurs in 1%. Vocal chord movement should be checked preoperatively. Mild hoarseness is more common and thyroidectomy is best avoided in professional singers!
- *Transient hypocalcaemia* occurs in up to 10% but with permanent hypoparathyroidism in fewer than 1%.
- *Recurrent hyperthyroidism* occurs in 1–3% within one year, then 1% per year.
- *Hypothyroidism* occurs in about 10% of patients within one year, and this percentage increases with time. It is likeliest if microsomal antibodies are positive. Automated computer thyroid registers with annual TSH screening are used in some regions, and have demonstrated that a high proportion of patients become hypothyroid in the long term.

Radioactive iodine

Iodine-131 in an empirical dose (usually 200–500 MBq) accumulates in the thyroid and destroys the gland by local radiation – though it takes several months to be fully effective. Early discomfort in the neck and immediate worsening of hyperthyroidism are sometimes seen; again patients must be rendered euthyroid before treatment though they have to stop antithyroid drugs at least four days before radioiodine, and not recommence until three days after radioiodine. It is contraindicated in children, in pregnancy and while breast-feeding.

If worsening occurs, the patient should not receive carbimazole for 2–3 days after radioiodine, as it will prevent radioiodine uptake by the gland. They should receive propranolol (Table 16.27) until carbimazole can be restarted if necessary; euthyroidism normally returns in 2–3 months.

Apart from the immediate problems above, a major complication is the progressive incidence of subsequent hypothyroidism affecting the majority of subjects over the following 20 years. Though 75% of patients are rendered euthyroid in the short term, a small proportion remain hyperthyroid; increasing the radioiodine dose reduces recurrence but increases the rate of hypothyroidism. Again, long-term surveillance of thyroid function is necessary with frequent tests in the first year after therapy, and at least annually thereafter.

Special situations in hyperthyroidism

Thyroid crisis

This rare condition, with a mortality of 10%, is a rapid deterioration of hyperthyroidism with hyperpyrexia, severe tachycardia and extreme restlessness. It is usually precipitated by stress, infection, surgery in an unprepared patient, or radioiodine therapy. With careful management it should no longer occur.

Treatment is urgent. Propranolol in full doses is started immediately together with potassium iodide, antithyroid drugs, corticosteroids (which suppress many of the manifestations of hyperthyroidism) and full supportive measures.

Hyperthyroidism in pregnancy and neonatal life

Maternal hyperthyroidism during pregnancy is uncommon and usually mild. Diagnosis can be difficult because of misleading thyroid function tests, although TSH is largely reliable. The pathogenesis is almost always Graves' disease. TSI crosses the placenta to stimulate the fetal thyroid. Carbimazole also crosses the placenta, but T_4 does so poorly so a 'block-and-replace' regimen is contraindicated. The smallest dose of carbimazole necessary is used and the fetus must be monitored (see below). The paediatrician should be informed and the infant checked immediately after birth – overtreatment with carbimazole can cause fetal goitre. Breast-feeding while on usual doses of carbimazole or propylthiouracil appears to be safe.

If necessary (high doses needed, poor patient compliance or drug side-effects), surgery can be performed, preferably in the second trimester. Radioactive iodine is absolutely contraindicated.

The fetus and maternal Graves' disease

Any mother with a history of Graves' disease may have circulating TSI. Even if she has been treated (e.g. by surgery), the immunoglobulin may still be present to stimulate the fetal thyroid, and the fetus can thus become hyperthyroid, while the mother remains euthyroid.

Any such patient should therefore be monitored during pregnancy. Fetal heart rate provides a direct biological assay of thyroid status, and monitoring should be performed at least monthly. Rates above 160 per minute are strongly suggestive of fetal hyperthyroidism and maternal treatment with carbimazole and/or propranolol may be used. To prevent the mother becoming hypothyroid, T_4 may be given as this does not easily cross the placenta. Sympathomimetics, used to prevent premature labour, are contraindicated as they may provoke fatal tachycardia in the fetus.

Hyperthyroidism may also develop in the neonatal period as TSI has a half-life of approximately three weeks. Manifestations in the newborn include irritability, failure to thrive and persisting weight loss, diarrhoea and eye signs. Thyroid function tests are difficult to interpret as neonatal normal ranges vary with age.

Untreated neonatal hyperthyroidism is probably associated with hyperactivity in later childhood.

Thyroid hormone resistance

Thyroid hormone resistance is an inherited condition caused by an abnormality of the thyroid hormone receptor. Mutations to the receptor result in the need for higher levels of thyroid hormones to achieve the same intracellular effect. As a result, the normal feedback control mechanisms (see Fig 16.2 on p. 898) result in high blood levels of thyroxine with a normal TSH in order to maintain a euthyroid state. This has two consequences:

- First, thyroid function tests appear abnormal even when the patient is euthyroid and requires no treatment; this is a particular problem if only T_4 or free T_4 levels are measured and, before sensitive TSH assays were developed, some patients were treated inappropriately for hyperthyroidism.
- Second, different tissues contain different thyroid hormone receptors and, in some families, receptors in certain tissues may have normal activity. In this case the level of thyroid hormones to maintain euthyroidism at pituitary and hypothalamic levels (which controls secretion of TSH) may be higher than that required in other tissues such as heart and bone, so that these tissues may exhibit 'thyrotoxic' effects in spite of a normal serum TSH. This 'partial thyroid hormone resistance' can be very difficult to manage effectively.

Thyroid eye disease

This is also known as dysthyroid eye disease or ophthalmic Graves' disease.

PATHOPHYSIOLOGY

The evidence suggests that the exophthalmos of Graves' disease is due to a specific immune response that causes retro-orbital inflammation with swelling and oedema of the extraocular muscles leading to limitation of movement. This leads to proptosis which can sometimes be unilateral, and increased pressure on the optic nerve may cause optic atrophy. Histology shows a focal oedema and glycosaminoglycan deposition followed by fibrosis. The precise autoantigen which leads to the immune response remains to be identified, but appears to be an antigen in retro-orbital tissue with similar immuno-reactivity to the TSH receptor.

Eye disease, while often associated with Graves' hyperthyroidism, can also occur in patients who may be hyperthyroid, euthyroid or hypothyroid. TSH receptor antibodies are almost invariably found in the serum but their role in the pathogenesis in unclear.

CLINICAL FEATURES

The clinical appearances are characteristic (Fig 16.22). Proptosis and limitation of eye movements (by 'tight' muscles) are direct effects of the inflammation, while conjunctival oedema, lid lag and corneal scarring are secondary to the proptosis and lack of eye cover. The ability to close the eyes completely is important, as otherwise corneal damage may occur. Visual impairment from optic nerve pressure may occur. Eye manifestations often do not parallel the clinical course of Graves' disease – in particular the degree of toxicosis. Only 5–10% of cases threaten sight, but the discomfort and cosmetic problems cause great patient anxiety. A grading system for disease severity is illustrated in Fig 16.22.

INVESTIGATIONS

Few investigations are necessary if the appearances are characteristic and bilateral. TSH and T_3 and T_4 should be measured.

The exophthalmos should be measured to allow progress to be monitored. If appearances or measurements are markedly discrepant in the two eyes, other retro-orbital space-occupying lesions should be considered: CT or MRI of the orbits will exclude other causes and show enlarged muscles and oedema.

TREATMENT

If patients are thyrotoxic this should be normalized, but hypothyroidism must be avoided as this may exacerbate the eye problem: an increased incidence of eye problems after radioiodine treatment probably reflects this. Direct treatment may be either local or systemic, and always requires close liaison between specialist endocrinologist and ophthalmologist:

- *Methylcellulose or hypromellose eyedrops* are given to aid lubrication.
- *Some patients gain relief by sleeping upright.* The eyelids can be taped to ensure closure at night.
- *Systemic steroids* (prednisolone 30–120 mg daily) usually reduce inflammation if more severe symptoms are present. Pulse intravenous methylprednisolone may be more rapidly effective in severe cases.
- *Irradiation of the orbits* (20 Gy in divided doses) is also used in severe instances, with steroid cover.
- *Lateral tarsorrhaphy* will protect the cornea if lids cannot be closed.
- *Surgical decompression* of the orbit(s) is occasionally needed.
- *Corrective eye muscle surgery* may improve diplopia due to muscle changes, but should be deferred until the situation has been stable for six months. Plastic surgery around the eyes may also be of value.

FURTHER READING

Dayan CM, Daniels GH (1996) Medical progress: chronic autoimmune thyroiditis. *New England Journal of Medicine* **335**: 99–107.

Lazarus JH (1997) Hyperthyroidism. *Lancet* **349**: 339–343.

Lindsay RS, Toft AD (1997) Hypothyroidism. *Lancet* **349**: 413–417.

Surks MI, Sievert R (1995) Drug therapy: drugs and thyroid function. *New England Journal of Medicine* **333**: 1688–1694.

Vanderpump MPJ, Ahlqvist JAO, Franklyn JA, Clayton RN (1996) Consensus statement for good practice and audit measures in the management of hypothyroidism and hyperthyroidism. *British Medical Journal* **313**: 539–544.

Thyroid cancer (1995) *Endocrinology and Metabolism Clinics of North America* **24**.

Thyroid cancer (1996) *Endocrinology and Metabolism Clinics of North America* **25**.

The glucocorticoid axis

ADRENAL ANATOMY AND FUNCTION

The human adrenals, weighing only 8–10 g together, comprise an outer cortex with three zones (reticularis, fasciculata and glomerulosa) producing steroids and an inner medulla that synthesizes, stores and secretes catecholamines (see adrenal medulla, p. 955).

The adrenal steroids are grouped into three classes based on their predominant physiological effects.

Glucocorticoids

These are so named after their effects on carbohydrate metabolism. Major actions are listed in Table 16.28.

Mineralocorticoids

Their predominant effect is on the extracellular balance of sodium and potassium in the distal tubule of the kidney. Aldosterone is the predominant mineralocorticoid in humans (about 50%); corticosterone makes a small

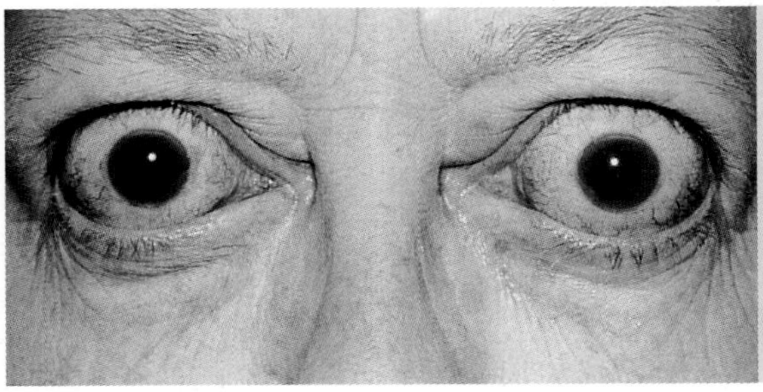

Grade 0	No signs or symptoms
Grade 1	Only signs, no symptoms
Grade 2	Soft tissue involvment
Grade 3	Proptosis (measured with exophthalmometer)
Grade 4	Extraocular muscle involvement
Grade 5	Corneal involvement
Grade 6	Sight loss with optic nerve involvement

Fig 16.22
The signs of thyroid eye disease, and its grading

Table 16.28
The major actions of glucocorticoids

Increased or stimulated	**Decreased or inhibited**
Gluconeogenesis	Protein synthesis
Glycogen deposition	Host response to infection
Protein catabolism	Lymphocyte transformation
Fat deposition	Delayed hypersensitivity
Sodium retention	Circulating lymphocytes
Potassium loss	Circulating eosinophils
Free water clearance	
Uric acid production	
Circulating neutrophils	

Table 16.29 The relative glucocorticoid and mineralocorticoid potency of equal amounts of common natural and synthetic steroids

Steroid	**Glucocorticoid effect**	**Mineralocorticoid effect**
Cortisol (hydrocortisone)[a]	1	1
Prednisolone	4	0.7
Dexamethasone	40	2
Aldosterone	0.1	400
Fludrocortisone	10	400

[a]Cortisol is arbitrarily defined as 1.

contribution. The weak mineralocorticoid activity of cortisol is also important since it is present in considerable excess, but the mineralocorticoid receptor in the kidney is largely protected from this excess by the intrarenal conversion of cortisol to the inactive cortisone by the enzyme 11β-hydroxysteroid dehydrogenase. Aldosterone is produced solely in the zona glomerulosa.

Androgens

Although secreted in considerable quantities, most have only relatively weak intrinsic androgenic activity until metabolized peripherally to testosterone or dihydrotestosterone.

The relative potency of common steroids is shown in Table 16.29.

BIOCHEMISTRY

All steroids have the same basic skeleton (Fig 16.23(b)) and the chemical differences between them are slight. The major biosynthetic pathways are shown in Fig 16.23(a).

PHYSIOLOGY

Glucocorticoid production by the adrenal is under hypothalamic–pituitary control (Fig 16.24). Corticotrophin releasing factors (CRF; the major components of which are corticotrophin releasing hormone and vasopressin) are secreted in the hypothalamus in response to circadian rhythm, stress and other stimuli. CRFs travel down the portal system to stimulate ACTH release from the anterior pituitary corticotrophs. Circulating ACTH stimulates

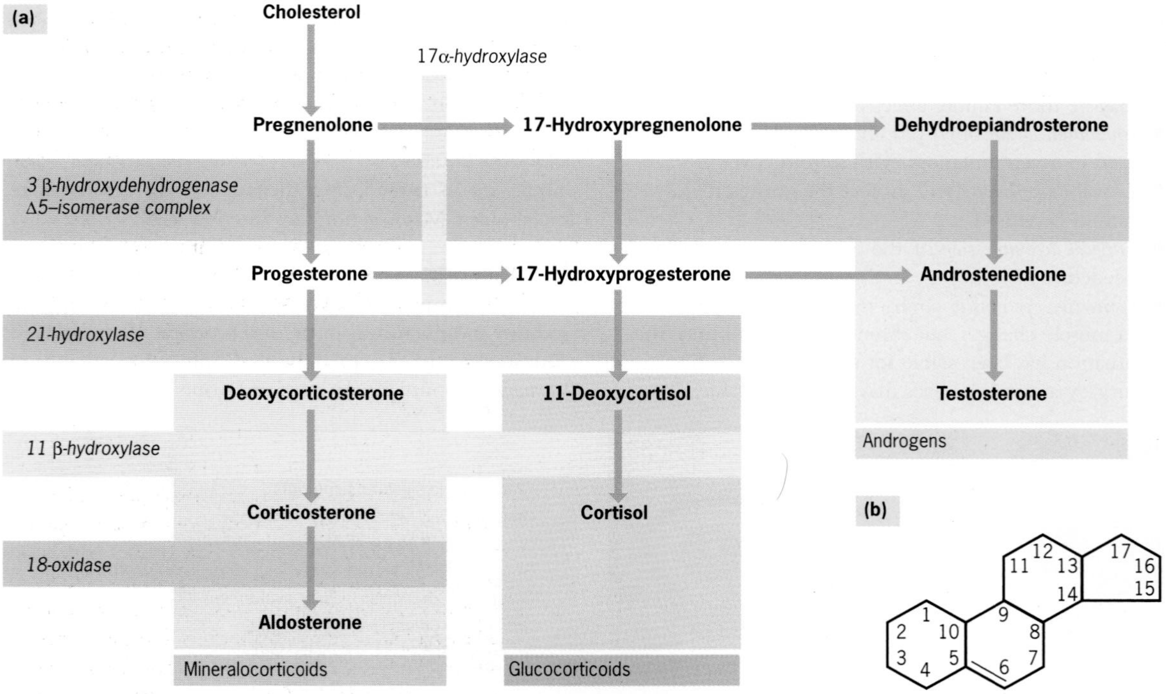

Fig 16.23
(a) The major steroid biosynthetic pathways
(b) The steroid molecule

cortisol production in the adrenal. The cortisol secreted (or any other synthetic corticosteroid administered to the patient) causes negative feedback on the hypothalamus and pituitary to inhibit further CRF/ACTH release. The set-point of this system clearly varies through the day according to the circadian rhythm, and is usually overridden by severe stress.

Following adrenalectomy or other adrenal damage (e.g. Addison's disease), cortisol secretion will be absent or reduced; ACTH levels will therefore rise.

Mineralocorticoid secretion is mainly controlled by the renin–angiotensin system (see p. 953).

INVESTIGATION OF GLUCOCORTICOID ABNORMALITIES

Basal levels

ACTH and cortisol are released episodically and in response to stress. The following precautions are therefore necessary when taking a blood sample:

- Sampling time should be recorded accurately. Conventionally basal levels are obtained at between 0800h and 0900h near the peak of the circadian variation.
- Stress should be minimized.
- Sampling should be delayed for 48 hours after admission if Cushing's syndrome is suspected. Appropriate reference ranges (for time and assay method) should be used.

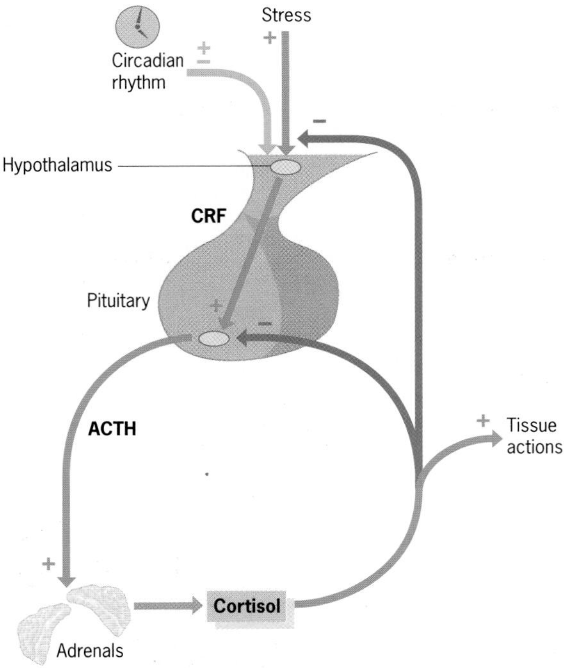

Fig 16.24
Control of the hypothalamic–pituitary–adrenal axis. CRF, corticotrophin-releasing factor

Suppression and stimulation tests are used in suspected excess and deficient cortisol production, respectively.

Dexamethasone suppression tests

Administration of synthetic glucocorticoid to a normal subject produces prompt feedback suppression of CRF and ACTH levels and thus of endogenous cortisol secretion (prednisolone and dexamethasone are not measured by most cortisol assays). Three forms of the test, used in the diagnosis and differential diagnosis of Cushing's syndrome, are available (Table 16.30).

ACTH stimulation tests

Synthetic ACTH (tetracosactrin, which consists of the first 24 amino acids of human ACTH) is given to stimulate adrenal cortisol production. Details are given in Table 16.30 and Fig 16.4(a) on p. 900.

Addison's disease: primary hypoadrenalism

PATHOPHYSIOLOGY AND CAUSES

In this uncommon condition there is destruction of the entire adrenal cortex. Glucocorticoid, mineralocorticoid and sex steroid production are therefore all reduced. This differs from hypothalamic–pituitary disease, in which mineralocorticoid secretion remains largely intact, being predominantly stimulated by angiotensin II.

Adrenal sex steroid production is also largely independent of pituitary action. In Addison's disease reduced cortisol levels lead, through feedback, to increased CRF and ACTH production, the latter being directly responsible for the hyperpigmentation.

Primary hypoadrenalism shows a marked female preponderance and is now most often caused by autoimmune disease (>90%) rather than tuberculosis (<10%). All other causes are rare (Table 16.31). Autoimmune adrenalitis results from the destruction of the adrenal cortex by organ-specific autoantibodies. There are associations with other autoimmune conditions in the polyglandular autoimmune syndromes Types I and II (e.g. type I diabetes mellitus, pernicious anaemia, thyroiditis, hypoparathyroidism, premature ovarian failure).

CLINICAL FEATURES

These are shown in Fig 16.25. The symptomatology of Addison's disease is often vague – nonspecific complaints of weakness, tiredness, weight loss and anorexia predominate.

Pigmentation (dull, slaty, grey-brown) in the mouth (opposite the molars), hand (palmar creases and over joints), face and all flexural regions is the predominant sign in over 90% of cases. It is particularly significant if it occurs in a recent scar. It is caused by the direct action of ACTH on melanocytes.

Postural systolic hypotension, due to hypovolaemia and sodium loss, is present in 80–90% of cases, even if supine blood pressure is normal. Mineralocorticoid deficiency is the cause.

Table 16.30
Details of dexamethasone suppression and ACTH (synacthen) tests in the diagnosis of Cushing's syndrome and Addison's disease

Test and protocol	Measure	Normal test result or positive suppression	Use and explanation
Dexamethasone			
Overnight			
Take 1 mg on going to bed on day 0	Plasma cortisol at 0900h on day 0	Plasma cortisol <100 nmol L^{-1}	Outpatient screening test
'Low-dose'			
0.5 mg 6-hourly			
Eight doses from 0900h on day 0	Plasma cortisol at 0900h on days 0 and +2	Plasma cortisol <50 nmol L^{-1} on second sample	For diagnosis of Cushing's syndrome May not suppress in obesity and depression
'High-dose' used in differential diagnosis			
2 mg 6-hourly Eight doses from 0900h on day 0	Plasma cortisol at 0900h on days 0 and +2 (24 h urinary steroids on days 0 and +2)	Plasma cortisol on day +2 less than 50% of that on day 0 suggests pituitary-dependent disease	Differential diagnosis of Cushing's syndrome Pituitary-dependent disease suppresses in about 90% of cases
ACTH (Synacthen)			
Short			
Tetracosactrin 250 μg i.v. or i.m. at time 0	Plasma cortisol at times 0, +30 minutes	Cortisol at +30 min >600 nmol L^{-1} Rise >330 nmol L^{-1}	To exclude primary adrenal failure
Long			
Depot tetracosactrin 1 mg i.m. at time 0	Plasma cortisol at times 0, +1, +2, +3, +4, +5, +8 and +24 h	Maximum >1000 nmol L^{-1} Rise > 550 nmol L^{-1}	To demonstrate or exclude adrenal suppression

Plasma cortisol values are very dependent upon the assay used – local reference ranges must be consulted.

INVESTIGATIONS

Once Addison's disease is suspected, investigation is urgent. If the patient is seriously ill or very hypotensive, hydrocortisone 100 mg should be given intramuscularly together with intravenous saline. Ideally this should be done immediately after a blood sample is taken for later measurement of plasma cortisol. Alternatively, an ACTH stimulation test can be performed immediately. Full investigation should be delayed until emergency treatment (see below) has improved the patient's condition. Otherwise, tests are as follows:

- **Single cortisol measurements** are of little value, although a random cortisol below 100 nmol L^{-1} during the day is highly suggestive, and a random cortisol >550 nmol L^{-1} makes the diagnosis unlikely (but not impossible).
- **The short ACTH stimulation test** should be performed (see Table 16.30). An absent or impaired cortisol response is seen, confirmed if necessary by a long ACTH stimulation test to exclude adrenal suppression by steroids.
- **A 0900h plasma ACTH level** – a high level (>80 ng L^{-1}) with low or low-normal cortisol confirms primary hypoadrenalism.
- **Electrolytes and urea** classically show hyponatraemia, hyperkalaemia and a high urea, but they can be normal.
- **Blood glucose** may be low, with symptomatic hypoglycaemia.

Table 16.31
Causes of primary hypoadrenalism

Common	Uncommon
Autoimmune disease (approx 90% in UK)	Haemorrhage/infarction
Tuberculosis (<10% in UK)	Meningococcal septicaemia
Surgical removal	Venography
	Infiltration
	Malignant destruction
	Amyloid
	Schilder's disease (adrenal leukodystrophy)

- **Adrenal antibodies** are present in many cases of autoimmune adrenalitis.
- **Chest and abdominal X-rays** may show evidence of tuberculosis and/or calcified adrenals.
- **Serum aldosterone** is reduced with high plasma renin activity.
- **Hypercalcaemia and anaemia** (after rehydration) are sometimes seen. They resolve on treatment.

TREATMENT

Long-term treatment is with replacement glucocorticoid and mineralocorticoid; tuberculosis must be treated if present or suspected. Replacement dosage details are shown in Table 16.32.

Symptoms
Weight loss
Anorexia
Malaise
Weakness
Fever
Depression
Impotence/amenorrhoea
Nausea/Vomiting
Diarrhoea
Confusion
Syncope from postural hypotension
Abdominal pain
Constipation
Myalgia
Joint or back pain

Features of other autoimmune disease (e.g. vitiligo) are quite common

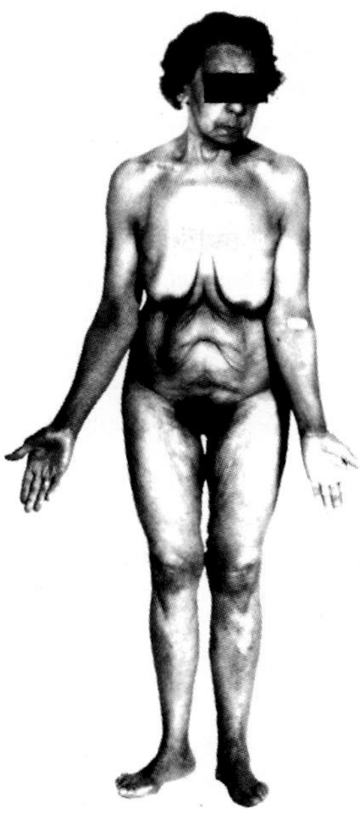

Signs
Buccal pigmentation

Postural hypotension

Pigmentation, especially of new scars
General wasting

Loss of weight
Dehydration

Loss of body hair

(Vitiligo)

Fig 16.25
The signs of primary hypoadrenalism (Addison's disease). Bold type indicates signs of greater discriminant value

Adequacy of glucocorticoid dose is judged by:

- clinical well-being and restoration of normal, but not excessive, weight
- normal cortisol levels during the day while on replacement hydrocortisone (this cannot be used for synthetic steroids).

Fludrocortisone replacement is assessed by:

- restoration of serum electrolytes to normal
- blood pressure response to posture (it should not fall >10 mmHg systolic after 2 minutes standing)
- suppression of plasma renin activity to normal.

Table 16.32 Average replacement steroid dosages for adults with primary hypoadrenalism

Drug	Dose
Glucocorticoid	
Cortisol	20–25 mg daily e.g. 10 mg on waking, 5 mg at 1200h, 5 mg at 1800h
or	
Prednisolone	7.5 mg daily 5 mg on waking, 2.5 mg at 1800h
rarely	
Dexamethasone	0.75 mg daily 0.5 mg on waking, 0.25 mg at 1800h
Mineralocorticoid	
Fludrocortisone	50–400 μg daily

Patient advice

All patients requiring replacement steroids should:

- carry a steroid card
- wear a Medic-Alert bracelet, which gives details of their condition so that emergency replacement therapy can be given if found unconscious
- keep an (up-to-date) ampoule of hydrocortisone at home in case oral therapy is impossible, and the general practitioner has to be called.

Acute hypoadrenalism

The major deficiencies are of salt, steroid and glucose. Assuming normal cardiovascular function, the following procedures are required:

- One litre of normal saline should be given over 30–60 minutes with 100 mg of intravenous hydrocortisone.
- Subsequent saline requirements may be for several litres within 24 hours (assessing with central venous pressure line if necessary) plus hydrocortisone, 100 mg i.m. 6-hourly, until the patient is clinically stable.
- Dextrose should be infused if there is hypoglycaemia.
- Oral replacement medication is then started, initially hydrocortisone about 20 mg 8-hourly or equivalent, reducing to 20–30 mg in divided doses over a few days (Table 16.32).
- Fludrocortisone is unnecessary acutely as the high cortisol doses provide sufficient mineralocorticoid activity – it should be introduced later.

Secondary hypoadrenalism

This may arise from hypothalamic–pituitary disease (inadequate ACTH production) or from long-term steroid therapy leading to hypothalamic–pituitary–adrenal suppression.

Most patients with the former have panhypopituitarism (see p. 907) and need T_4 replacement as well as cortisol; in this case hydrocortisone must be started before T_4.

The most common cause of hypoadrenalism is long-term corticosteroid medication for non-endocrine disease. The hypothalamic–pituitary axis and the adrenal may both be suppressed and the patient may have vague symptoms of feeling unwell. The long ACTH stimulation test should demonstrate a delayed cortisol response. Weaning off steroids is often a long and difficult business.

Cushing's syndrome

Cushing's syndrome is the term used to describe the clinical state of increased free circulating glucocorticoid. It occurs most often following the therapeutic administration of synthetic steroids (see below). All the spontaneous forms of the syndrome are rare.

PATHOPHYSIOLOGY AND CAUSES

Causes of Cushing's syndrome are usually subdivided into two groups (Table 16.33):

- increased circulating ACTH from the pituitary (65% of cases), known as Cushing's disease, or from an 'ectopic', non-pituitary, ACTH-producing tumour elsewhere in the body (10%) with consequential glucocorticoid excess
- a primary excess of endogenous (25% of spontaneous cases) or exogenous glucocorticoid hormone alone, with subsequent (physiological) suppression of ACTH.

CLINICAL FEATURES

The predominant clinical features of Cushing's syndrome are those of glucocorticoid excess and are illustrated in Fig 16.26.

Table 16.33
Causes of Cushing's syndrome

ACTH-dependent disease
Pituitary-dependent (Cushing's disease)
Ectopic ACTH-producing tumours
ACTH administration
Non-ACTH-dependent causes
Adrenal adenomas
Adrenal carcinomas
Glucocorticoid administration
Others
Alcohol-induced pseudo-Cushing's syndrome

- *Pigmentation* occurs only with ACTH-dependent causes.
- A *Cushingoid appearance* can be caused by excess alcohol consumption (pseudo-Cushing's syndrome) – the pathophysiology is poorly understood.
- *Impaired glucose tolerance* or frank diabetes are common, especially in the ectopic ACTH syndrome.
- *Hypokalaemia* due to the mineralocorticoid activity of cortisol is common with ectopic ACTH secretion.

DIAGNOSIS

There are two phases to the investigation:

1 confirmation of the presence or absence of Cushing's syndrome
2 differential diagnosis of its cause (e.g. pituitary, adrenal or ectopic).

Confirmation

Confirmation rests on demonstrating inappropriate cortisol secretion, not suppressed by exogenous glucocorticoids: difficulties occur with obesity and depression where cortisol dynamics are often abnormal. Random cortisol measurements are of no value. Occasional patients are seen with so-called 'cyclical Cushing's' where the abnormalities come and go.

Investigations to confirm the diagnosis include:

- **24-hour urinary free cortisol measurements.** Repeatedly normal values (corrected for body mass) render the diagnosis most unlikely.
- **48-hour low-dose dexamethasone test** (see Table 16.30). Normal individuals suppress plasma cortisol to <50 nmol L^{-1}. Patients with Cushing's syndrome fail to show complete suppression of plasma or urinary cortisol levels (although levels may fall substantially in a few cases). The overnight dexamethasone test is slightly simpler, but has a higher false-positive rate.
- **Circadian rhythm**. After 48 hours in hospital, cortisol samples are taken at 0900h and 2400h (without warning the patient). Normal subjects show a pronounced circadian variation (see Fig 16.3 on p. 898); those with Cushing's syndrome have high midnight cortisol levels (>100 nmol L^{-1}), though the 0900h value may be normal.
- **Other tests**. There are frequent exceptions to the classic responses to diagnostic tests in Cushing's syndrome. If any clinical suspicion of Cushing's remains after preliminary tests then specialist investigations are still indicated. Further tests may include insulin stress test, desmopressin stimulation test and CRF tests.

Differential diagnosis of the cause

This can be extremely difficult. The classical ectopic ACTH syndrome is distinguished by a short history, pigmentation and weight loss, unprovoked hypokalaemia, clinical or chemical diabetes and plasma ACTH levels above 200 ng L^{-1}, but

Symptoms

Weight gain (central)
Change of appearance
Depression
Psychosis
Insomnia
Amenorrhoea/oligomenorrhoea
Poor libido
Thin skin/easy bruising
Hair growth/acne
Muscular weakness
Growth arrest in children
Back pain
Polyuria/polydipsia

Old photographs may be useful
Symptoms of hypopituitarism are rare

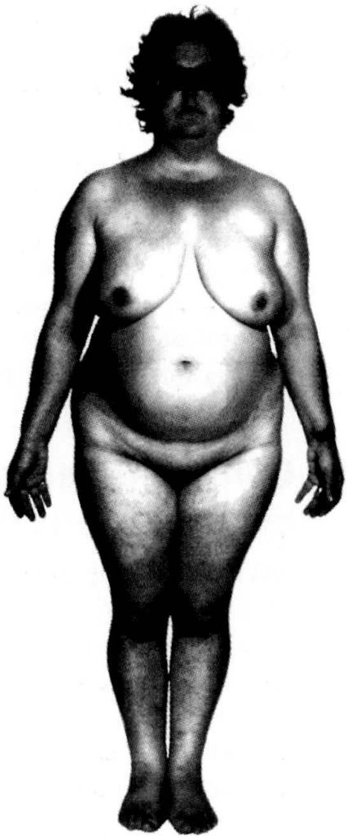

Signs

Depression/psychosis	Frontal balding (female)
Acne, hirsuties	
Thin skin	Moon face
Bruising	**Plethora**
Hypertension	'Buffalo hump'
	Kyphosis
Rib fractures	
Osteoporosis	
Pathological fractures	Centripetal obesity
	Pigmentation
Poor wound healing	
	Striae (purple)
	Sin infections
Proximal muscle wasting	
Proximal myopathy	
	Glycosuria
Oedema	

Fig 16.26
The signs of Cushing's syndrome. Bold type indicates signs of most value in discriminating Cushing's syndrome from simple obesity and hirsuties

many ectopic tumours are benign and mimic pituitary disease closely both clinically and biochemically. Severe hirsutism/virilization suggests an adrenal tumour.

Biochemical and radiological procedures for diagnosis include:

- **Adrenal CT or MRI scan.** Adrenal adenomas and carcinomas causing Cushing's syndrome are relatively large and always detectable by CT scan. Carcinomas are distinguished by large size, irregular outline and signs of infiltration or metastases.
- **Pituitary MRI.** Of less value than the adrenal scan; a pituitary adenoma may be seen but the adenoma is still not visible in a high proportion of cases. Only a minority of tumours of significant size are detected with confidence by pituitary CT.
- **Plasma potassium levels.** All diuretics must be stopped. Hypokalaemia is common with ectopic ACTH secretion.
- **High-dose dexamethasone test** (Table 16.30). Failure of significant plasma cortisol suppression suggests an ectopic source of ACTH or an adrenal tumour.
- **Plasma ACTH levels.** Low or undetectable ACTH levels (<10 ng L^{-1}) on two or more occasions are a reliable indicator of non-ACTH-dependent disease.
- **CRF test.** An exaggerated ACTH and cortisol response to exogenous CRF (with or without vasopressin) suggests pituitary-dependent Cushing's disease, as ectopic sources rarely respond.
- **Chest X-ray** is mandatory to demonstrate a carcinoma of the bronchus or a bronchial carcinoid. Lesions may be very small; if ectopic ACTH is suspected, whole-lung and mediastinal CT scanning should be performed.

Further investigations may involve selective catheterization of the inferior petrosal sinus to measure ACTH for pituitary lesions, or blood samples taken throughout the body in a search for ectopic sources. Bronchoscopy, cytology and regional arteriograms are occasionally necessary. Radiolabelled octreotide (^{111}In octreotide) shows promise in locating ectopic ACTH sites, especially within the thorax where the majority (bronchial or thymic carcinoids) lie.

TREATMENT

Untreated Cushing's syndrome has a very bad prognosis, with death from hypertension, myocardial infarction, infection and heart failure. Whatever the underlying cause, cortisol hypersecretion should be controlled prior to surgery or radiotherapy. Considerable morbidity and mortality is otherwise associated with operating on unprepared patients, especially when abdominal surgery is required. The usual drug is metyrapone, an 11-hydroxylase blocker, which is given in doses of 750 mg to 4 g daily in three to four divided doses. Plasma cortisol should be monitored, aiming to reduce the mean level during the day to 150–300 nmol L^{-1}, equivalent to normal production rates. Ketoconazole and aminoglutethimide are sometimes used.

Choice of treatment depends upon the cause.

Cushing's disease (pituitary-dependent hyperadrenalism)

- *Trans-sphenoidal removal of the tumour*, by an experienced surgeon, is now the treatment of choice. Selective adenomectomy nearly always leaves the patient ACTH-deficient immediately postoperatively, and this is considered a good prognostic sign.
- *External pituitary irradiation* alone is very slow, only effective in 50–60% even after prolonged follow up, and of little value except in those unfit for, or unwilling, to have surgery. Children, however, respond much better to radiotherapy, 80% being cured.
- *Medical therapy to reduce ACTH* (e.g. bromocriptine, cyproheptadine) is rarely effective.
- *Bilateral adrenalectomy* is now an option of last resort, though remains an effective last resort if other measures fail to control the disease. Some centres are performing this laparoscopically.

Other causes

Adrenal adenomas should be resected after achievement of clinical remission with metyrapone or ketoconazole. Contralateral adrenal suppression may last for years.

Adrenal carcinomas are highly aggressive and the prognosis is poor. In general, if there are no widespread metastases, tumour bulk should be reduced surgically. The adrenolytic drug op'DDD (Mitotane) may inhibit growth of the tumour and prolong survival, though can cause nausea and ataxia. Some would also give radiotherapy to the tumour bed after surgery.

Tumours secreting ACTH ectopically should be removed if possible. Otherwise chemotherapy/radiotherapy may be used, depending on the tumour. Control of the Cushing's syndrome with metyrapone, ketoconazole or op'DDD is beneficial for symptoms, and bilateral adrenalectomy may be appropriate to give complete control of the Cushing's syndrome if prognosis from the tumour itself is reasonable.

If the source of ACTH is not clear, cortisol hypersecretion should be controlled with medical therapy until a diagnosis can be made.

Nelson's syndrome

Nelson's syndrome is increased pigmentation (due to high levels of ACTH) associated with an enlarging pituitary tumour which occurs in about 20% of cases after bilateral adrenalectomy for Cushing's disease. The syndrome is rare now that adrenalectomy is an uncommon primary treatment. The incidence of the syndrome may be reduced by pituitary radiotherapy soon after adrenalectomy.

Incidental adrenal tumours ('incidentalomas')

With the advent of abdominal CT, MRI and high resolution ultrasound scanning, unsuspected adrenal masses have been discovered in 1% of scans. These obviously include the adrenal tumours described above, but cysts, myelolipomas and metastases are also seen. Functional tests to exclude secretory activity should be performed (adenomas often secrete cortisol at a low level); if none is found then most authorities recommend removal of large (>4–5 cm) and functional tumours but observation of smaller hormonally inactive lesions.

Congenital adrenal hyperplasia (CAH)

PATHOPHYSIOLOGY

This condition results from an autosomal recessive deficiency of an enzyme in the cortisol synthetic pathways. There are six major types, but most common is 21-hydroxylase deficiency which occurs in about 1 in 15 000 births and which has been shown to be due to defects on chromosome 6 near the HLA-region affecting one of the cytochrome P450 enzymes ($P450_{C21}$).

As a result, cortisol secretion is reduced and feedback leads to increased ACTH secretion to maintain adequate cortisol – this in turn leads to diversion of the steroid precursors into the androgenic steroid pathways (Fig 16.27). Thus, 17-hydroxyprogesterone, androstenedione and testosterone levels are increased, leading to virilization. Aldosterone synthesis may be impaired with resultant salt wasting.

The other forms affect 11-hydroxylase, 17-hydroxylase, 3-hydroxysteroid dehydrogenase (see Fig 16.23(a)) and a cholesterol side-chain cleavage enzyme.

CLINICAL FEATURES

If severe, this presents at birth with sexual ambiguity or adrenal failure (collapse, hypotension, hypoglycaemia), sometimes with a salt-losing state (hypotension, hyponatraemia). In the female, clitoral hypertrophy, urogenital abnormalities and labioscrotal fusion are common, but the syndrome may be unrecognized in the male. Precocious puberty with hirsutism is a later presentation, whereas rare, milder cases only present in adult life, usually accompanied by primary amenorrhoea. Hirsutism developing before menarche is suggestive of CAH.

INVESTIGATIONS

Expert advice is essential in the confirmation and differential diagnosis of $P450_{C21}$ deficiency, and with ambiguous genitalia such advice must be sought urgently before any assignment of gender is made.

- 17-Hydroxyprogesterone levels are increased (Fig 16.27).
- Urinary pregnanetriol excretion is increased.
- Basal ACTH levels are raised.

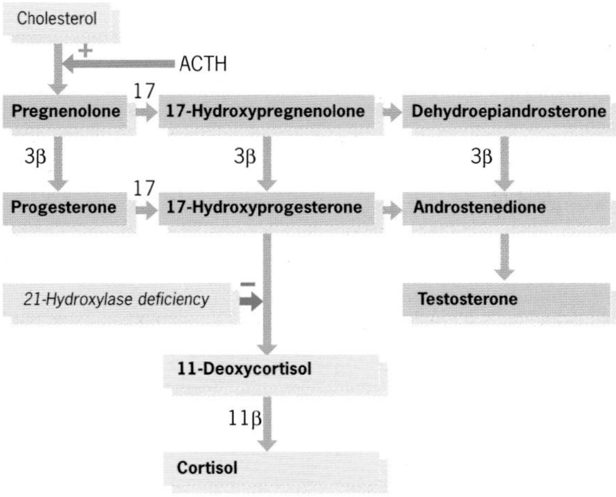

Fig 16.27
Effects of congenital adrenal hyperplasia (21-hydroxylase deficiency) on steroid biosynthesis. Precursors and products present in excess appear in purple boxes. Those present in normal or reduced quantity appear in yellow boxes

TREATMENT

Replacement of glucocorticoid activity, and mineralocorticoid activity if deficient, is as for primary hypoadrenalism (see above). Correct dosage is often difficult to establish in the child but should ensure normal 17-hydroxyprogesterone levels while allowing normal growth; excessive replacement leads to stunting of growth.

Uses and problems of therapeutic steroid therapy

Apart from their use as therapeutic replacement for endocrine deficiency states, synthetic glucocorticoids are widely used for many non-endocrine conditions (Information box 16.8). The mechanisms are believed to involve alteration of cytokine production, in particular through lipocortin I.

Short-term use (e.g. for acute asthma) carries only small risks of significant side-effects except for the simultaneous suppression of immune responses. The danger lies in their continuance, often through medical oversight or patient default. In general, therapy for three weeks or less, or a dose of prednisolone less than 10 mg per day, will not result in significant long-term suppression of the normal adrenal axis.

Long-term therapy with synthetic or natural steroids will, in most respects, mimic endogenous Cushing's syndrome. Exceptions are the relative absence of hirsutism, acne, hypertension and severe sodium retention, as the common synthetic steroids have low androgenic and mineralocorticoid activity.

Excessive doses of steroids may also be absorbed from skin when strong dermatological preparations are used, but inhaled steroids very rarely cause Cushing's syndrome, although they may cause adrenal suppression.

The major hazards are detailed in Information box 16.9. In the long term many are of such severity that the clinical need for high-dose steroids should be continually and critically assessed.

Supervision of steroid therapy

All patients receiving steroids should carry a steroid card. They should be made aware of the following points:

- Long-term steroid therapy must never be stopped suddenly.
- Doses should be reduced very gradually, with most being given in the morning at the time of withdrawal – this minimizes adrenal suppression. Many

Information

Respiratory disease
Asthma
Chronic obstuctive pulmonary disease
Sarcoidosis
Hay fever (usually topical)

Cardiac disease
Post-myocardial infarction syndrome

Renal disease
Some nephrotic syndromes
Some glomerulonephritides

Gastrointestinal disease
Ulcerative colitis
Crohn's disease
Autoimmune hepatitis

Obstetrics
Prevention/treatment of ARDS (see p. 857)

Rheumatological disease
Systemic lupus erythematosus
Polymyalgia rheumatica
Temporal arteritis
Juvenile chronic arthritis
Vasculitides

Neurological disease
Cerebral oedema

Skin disease
Pemphigus, eczema

Tumours
Hodgkin's lymphoma
Other lymphomas

Transplantation
Immunosuppression

Information box 16.8 Common therapeutic uses of glucocorticoids

Information

Physiological
Adrenal and/or pituitary suppression

Pathological
Cardiovascular
Increased blood pressure

Gastrointestinal
Peptic ulceration exacerbation (possibly)
Pancreatitis

Renal
Polyuria
Nocturia

Central nervous
Depression
Euphoria
Psychosis
Insomnia

Endocrine
Weight gain
Glycosuria/hyperglycaemia/diabetes
Impaired growth
Amenorrhoea

Bone and muscle
Osteoporosis
Proximal myopathy and wasting
Aseptic necrosis of the hip
Pathological fractures

Skin
Thinning
Easy bruising

Eyes
Cataracts (including inhaled drug)

Increased susceptibility to infection
(signs and fever are frequently masked)
Septicaemia
Reactivation of TB
Skin (e.g. fungi)

Information box 16.9 Major adverse effects of corticosteroid therapy

authorities believe that 'alternate-day therapy' produces less suppression.

- Doses need to be increased in times of serious intercurrent illness (defined as presence of a fever), accident and stress. Double doses should be taken during these times.
- Other physicians, anaesthetists and dentists must be told about steroid therapy.

Steroids and surgery

Any patient receiving steroids or who has recently received them (within the last 12 months) and may still have adrenal suppression requires careful control of steroid medication around the time of surgery. Details are shown in Table 16.34.

FURTHER READING

Oelkers W (1996) Current concepts: adrenal insufficiency. *New England Journal of Medicine* **335**: 1206–1212.

Orth DN (1995) Cushing's syndrome. *New England Journal of Medicine* **332**: 791–803.

Table 16.34
Steroid cover for operative procedures

Procedure	Premedication	Intra- and postoperative	Resumption of normal maintenance
Simple procedures (e.g. gastroscopy, simple dental extractions)	Hydrocortisone 100 mg i.m.	–	Immediately if no complications and eating normally
Minor surgery (e.g. laparoscopic surgery, veins, hernias)	Hydrocortisone 100 mg i.m.	Hydrocortisone 20 mg orally 6-hourly or 50 mg i.m. every six hours for 24 h if not eating	After 24 h if no complications
Major surgery (e.g. hip replacement, vascular surgery)	Hydrocortisone 100 mg i.m.	Hydrocortisone 50–100 mg i.m. every six hours for 72 h	After 72 h if normal progress and no complications Perhaps double normal dose for next 2–3 days
GI tract surgery or major thoracic surgery (not eating or ventilated)	Hydrocortisone 100 mg i.m.	Hydrocortisone 100 mg i.m. every six hours for 72 h or longer if still unwell	When patient eating normally again Until then higher doses (to 50 mg six-hourly) may be needed

The thirst axis

Thirst and water regulation are largely controlled by vasopressin (antidiuretic hormone; ADH), which is synthesized in the hypothalamus, and then migrates in neurosecretory granules along axonal pathways to the posterior pituitary. Pituitary damage alone without hypothalamic involvement therefore does not lead to ADH deficiency as the hormone can still 'leak' from the damaged end of the intact axon.

At normal concentrations the kidney is the predominant site of action of vasopressin, acting by two receptors known as V1 and V2. Stimulation of the V2 receptors allows the collecting tubule to become permeable to water, thus permitting reabsorption of hypotonic luminal fluid. Vasopressin therefore reduces diuresis and results in overall retention of water. At high concentrations vasopressin also causes vasoconstriction via the V1 receptors.

Changes in plasma osmolality are sensed by osmoreceptors in the anterior hypothalamus. Vasopressin secretion is suppressed at levels below 280 mOsmol kg^{-1}, thus allowing maximal water diuresis. Above this level, plasma vasopressin increases in direct proportion to plasma osmolality. At the upper limit of normal (295 mOsmol kg^{-1}) maximum antidiuresis is achieved and thirst is experienced at about 298 mOsmol kg^{-1} (Fig 16.28).

Other factors affecting vasopressin release are shown in Table 16.35.

Disorders of vasopressin secretion or activity include:

- deficiency as a result of hypothalamic disease ('cranial' diabetes insipidus)
- inappropriate excess of the hormone
- 'nephrogenic' diabetes insipidus – a rare condition in which the renal tubules are insensitive to vasopressin, an example of a receptor abnormality.

While all these are uncommon, they need to be distinguished from the occasional patient with 'primary polydipsia' and those whose renal tubular function has been impaired by electrolyte abnormalities, such as hypokalaemia or hypercalcaemia.

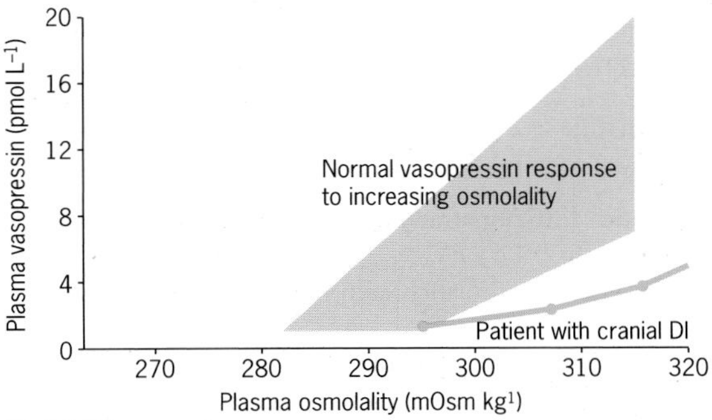

Fig 16.28
Plasma vasopressin response to increasing osmolality in normal subjects and in a patient with DI

Table 16.35
Factors affecting vasopressin release

Increased by:	**Decreased by:**
Increased osmolality	Decreased osmolality
Hypovolaemia	Hypervolaemia
Hypotension	Hypertension
Nausea	Ethanol
Hypothyroidism	α-Adrenergic stimulation
Angiotensin II	
Adrenaline	
Cortisol	
Nicotine	
Antidepressants	

Diabetes insipidus (DI)

CLINICAL FEATURES

Deficiency of vasopressin or insensitivity to its action leads to polyuria, nocturia and compensatory polydipsia. Daily urine output may reach as much as 10–15 L, leading to dehydration that may be very severe if the thirst mechanisms or consciousness are impaired or the patient is denied fluid.

Causes of DI are listed in Table 16.36. The most common is hypothalamic–pituitary surgery, following which transient DI is common, frequently remitting after a few days or weeks. Primary overdrinking (polydipsia) is a common differential diagnosis.

Table 16.36
Causes of diabetes insipidus

Cranial diabetes insipidus	**Nephrogenic diabetes insipidus**
Familial (e.g. DIDMOAD)	Familial (e.g. vasopressin receptor gene, aquaporin-2 gene defect)
Idiopathic	Idiopathic
Tumours	Renal tubular acidosis
Craniopharyngioma	Hypokalaemia
Hypothalamic tumour, e.g. glioma	Hypercalcaemia
Metastases, especially breast	Drugs (e.g. lithium, demethylchlortetracycline (demeclocycline), glibenclamide)
Lymphoma/leukaemia	
Pituitary with suprasellar extension (rare)	
Infections	
Tuberculosis	
Meningitis	
Cerebral abscess	
Infiltrations	
Sarcoidosis	
Langerhan's cell histiocytosis	
Post-surgical	
Trans-frontal	
Trans-sphenoidal	
Post-radiotherapy	
Vascular	
Haemorrhage/thrombosis	
Sheehan's syndrome	
Aneurysm	
Trauma (e.g. head injury)	

Mild temporary nephrogenic DI can occur after prolonged polyuria due to any cause, including cranial DI and primary polydipsia

DI may be masked by simultaneous cortisol deficiency – cortisol replacement allows a water diuresis and DI then becomes apparent.

DIDMOAD syndrome (Wolfram syndrome) is a rare autosomal recessive disorder comprising diabetes insipidus, diabetes mellitus, optic atrophy and deafness. MR scanning may show an absent or poorly developed posterior pituitary.

BIOCHEMISTRY

There may be:

- high or high-normal plasma osmolality with low urine osmolality (in primary polydipsia plasma osmolality tends to be low)
- resultant high or high-normal plasma sodium
- high 24 h urine volumes (less than 2 L excludes need for further investigation)
- failure of urinary concentration with fluid deprivation
- restoration of urinary concentration with vasopressin or an analogue.

The latter two points may be studied with a formal water-deprivation test (see Appendix). In normal subjects, plasma osmolality remains normal while urine osmolality rises above 700 mOsmol kg^{-1}. In DI, plasma osmolality rises while the urine remains dilute, only concentrating after exogenous vasopressin is given (in 'cranial' DI) or not concentrating after vasopressin if nephrogenic DI is present. This test can give equivocal results; measurement of vasopressin during the test is helpful.

TREATMENT

Where there is a reversible underlying cause (e.g. a hypothalamic tumour) this should be treated. Otherwise the synthetic vasopressin analogue desmopressin (DDAVP) is the treatment of choice. It is given intranasally as a spray 10–20 μg once or twice daily, orally as 200 μg thrice daily, or intramuscularly 2–4 μg daily. Response is variable and must be monitored carefully with fluid input/output charts and plasma osmolality measurements.

Alternative agents in mild DI, probably working by sensitizing the renal tubules to endogenous vasopressin, include thiazide diuretics, carbamazepine (200–400 mg daily) or chlorpropamide (200–350 mg daily). These are now rarely used, especially with the risk of hypoglycaemia from chlorpropamide.

Nephrogenic diabetes insipidus

In this condition, renal tubules are resistant to normal or high levels of plasma vasopressin. It may be inherited as a rare sex-linked recessive, with an abnormality in the vasopressin-2 receptor, or as an autosomal post-receptor defect in an ADH-sensitive water channel, called aquaporin-2. More commonly it can be acquired as a result of renal disease, sickle cell disease, drug ingestion (e.g. lithium), hypercalcaemia or hypokalaemia. Wherever possible the cause should be reversed.

Other causes of polyuria and polydipsia

Diabetes mellitus, hypokalaemia and hypercalcaemia are diagnoses to be considered. In the case of diabetes mellitus the cause is an osmotic diuresis secondary to glycosuria which leads to dehydration and an increased perception of thirst owing to hypertonicity of the extracellular fluid.

Primary or hysterical polydipsia

This is a relatively common cause of thirst and polyuria. It is a psychiatric disturbance characterized by the excessive intake of water. Plasma sodium and osmolality fall as a result and the urine produced is appropriately dilute. Vasopressin levels become virtually undetectable. Prolonged primary polydipsia may lead to the phenomenon of 'renal medullary washout', with a fall in the concentrating ability of the kidney.

Characteristically the diagnosis is made by a water-deprivation test. A low plasma osmolality is usual at the start of the test, and since vasopressin secretion and action can be stimulated, the patient's urine becomes concentrated (albeit 'maximum' concentrating ability may be impaired); the initially low urine osmolality gradually increases with the duration of the water deprivation.

Syndrome of inappropriate antidiuretic hormone (SIADH)

CLINICAL FEATURES

Inappropriate secretion of ADH leads to retention of water and hyponatraemia. The presentation is usually vague, with confusion, nausea, irritability and, later, fits and coma. There is no oedema. Mild symptoms usually occur with plasma sodium levels below 125 mmol L^{-1} and serious manifestations are likely below 115 mmol L^{-1}. The elderly may show symptoms with milder abnormalities.

The syndrome must be distinguished from those causing similar dilutional hyponatraemia from excess infusion of dextrose/water solutions or diuretic administration (thiazides or amiloride, see p. 604).

DIAGNOSIS

The usual features are:

- dilutional hyponatraemia due to excessive water retention
- low plasma osmolality with higher 'inappropriate' urine osmolality
- continued urinary sodium excretion >30 mmol L^{-1}
- absence of hypokalaemia (or hypotension)
- normal renal and adrenal and thyroid function.

The causes are listed in Table 16.37.

Table 16.37 Common causes of the syndrome of inappropriate ADH secretion (SIADH)

Tumours	**Metabolic causes**
Small cell carcinoma of lung	Alcohol withdrawal
Prostate	Porphyria
Thymus	
Pancreas	**Drugs**
Lymphomas	Chlorpropamide
	Carbamazepine
Pulmonary lesions	Cyclophosphamide
Pneumonia	Vincristine
Tuberculosis	Phenothiazines
Lung abscess	
CNS causes	
Meningitis	
Tumours	
Head injury	
Subdural haematoma	
Cerebral abscess	
SLE vasculitis	

TREATMENT

The underlying cause should be corrected where possible. Symptomatic relief can be obtained by the following measures:

- Fluid intake should be restricted to 500–1000 mL daily. If tolerated, and complied with, this will correct the biochemical abnormalities in almost every case.
- Plasma osmolality and sodium and bodyweight should be measured frequently.
- If water restriction is poorly tolerated or ineffective, demethylchlortetracycline (600–1200 mg daily) may be given; this inhibits the action of vasopressin on the kidney, causing a reversible form of nephrogenic diabetes insipidus. It may, however, cause photosensitive rashes.
- When the syndrome is very severe, rarely hypertonic saline (300 mmol L^{-1} slowly i.v.) is given and frusemide may be used. These treatments are potentially dangerous and should only be used with extreme caution.

Endocrinology of blood pressure control

The control of blood pressure (BP) is complex involving neural, cardiac, hormonal and many other mechanisms.

BP is dependent upon cardiac output and peripheral resistance. Although cardiac output can be increased in endocrine disease (e.g. hyperthyroidism), the main role of hormonal mechanisms is control of peripheral resistance and of circulating blood volume. The oral contraceptive pill is a common endocrine cause of mild hypertension.

When to investigate for secondary hypertension

Endocrine causes account for less than 5% of all hypertension (Table 16.38). It is impracticable and unnecessary to screen all hypertensive patients for secondary causes. The highest chances of detecting such causes are in:

- subjects under 35 years, especially those without a family history of hypertension
- those with accelerated (malignant) hypertension
- those with indications of renal disease (proteinuria, unequal renal sizes)
- those with hypokalaemia before diuretic therapy
- those resistant to conventional antihypertensive therapy
- those with unusual symptoms (e.g. sweating attacks or weakness).

The renin–angiotensin–aldosterone axis: biochemistry and actions

The renin–angiotensin–aldosterone system is illustrated in Fig 16.29.

Angiotensinogen, an α_2-globulin of hepatic origin, circulates in plasma. The enzyme, *renin*, is secreted by the kidney in response to decreased renal perfusion pressure or flow; it cleaves the decapeptide *angiotensin I* from angiotensinogen. Angiotensin I is inactive but is further cleaved by converting enzyme (present in lung and vascular endothelium) into the active peptide, *angiotensin II*, which has two major actions:

- it causes powerful vasoconstriction (within seconds)
- it stimulates the adrenal zona glomerulosa to increase aldosterone production.

Aldosterone causes sodium retention and urinary potassium loss (hours to days).

Table 16.38
Endocrine causes of hypertension

Excessive renin, and thus angiotensin II, production	**Excessive production of other mineralocorticoids**
Renal artery stenosis	Cushing's syndrome (massive excess of cortisol, a weak mineralocorticoid)
Other local renal disease	Congenital adrenal hyperplasia (in some cases)
Renin-secreting tumours	Tumours producing other mineralocorticoids, e.g. corticosterone
Excessive production of catecholamines	
Phaeochromocytoma	
Excessive GH production	**Exogenous 'mineralocorticoids' or enzyme inhibitors**
Acromegaly	Liquorice ingestion (inhibits 11β–hydroxylase)
Excessive aldosterone production	Abuse of mineralocorticoid preparations
Adrenal adenoma (Conn's syndrome)	
Idiopathic adrenal hyperplasia	
Dexamethasone-suppressible hyperaldosteronism	

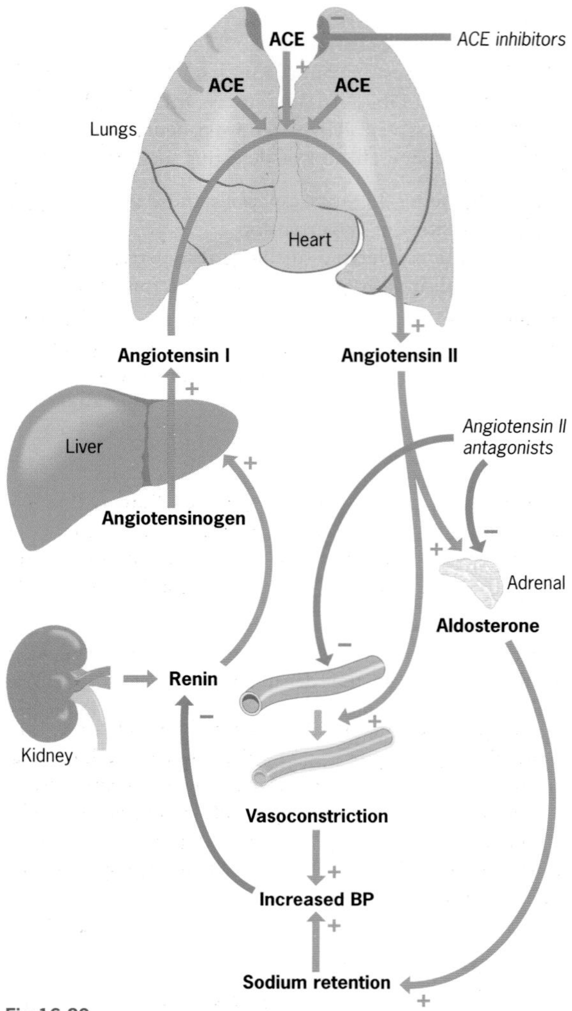

Fig 16.29
The renin–angiotensin–aldosterone system. ACE, angiotensin-converting enzyme. Angiotensin II antagonists act on the adrenals and blood vessels

The vasoconstrictor action of angiotensin II is short term, while the sodium retention induced by aldosterone increases total body sodium and BP in the longer term.

As BP increases and sodium is retained, the stimuli to renin secretion are reduced. Dietary sodium excess will tend to suppress renin secretion, whereas sodium deprivation or urinary sodium loss will increase it.

Atrial and brain natriuretic factors/peptides (ANP and BNP)

Atrial natriuretic peptides, a family of varying length forms, are secreted from atrial granules in response to atrial stretch. They produce marked effects on the kidney, increasing sodium and water excretion and glomerular filtration rate and lowering BP, plasma renin activity and plasma aldosterone (p. 675).

Brain natriuretic peptide is another hormone, found in the ventricle as well as the brain and with moderate sequence homology with ANP; normally its circulating level is much less than for ANP but may exceed it in congestive cardiac failure.

ANP and BNP appear to play a significant role in cardiovascular and fluid homeostasis, but there is no evidence of primary defects in their secretion causing disease. Their plasma levels may, however, reflect accurately the presence and severity of heart failure and thus are useful in defining prognosis and the need for treatment in this situation.

It may prove possible to enhance the action of ANP with agents that both inhibit the endopeptidases that break down ANP and inhibit ACE, as the receptors concerned are similar.

Renin (and angiotensin) dependent hypertension

Many forms of unilateral and bilateral renal diseases are associated with hypertension. The classic example is renal artery stenosis: the major hypertensive effects of this and other situations such as renin-secreting tumours are directly or indirectly due to angiotensin II.

Angiotensin II receptor antagonists (e.g. losartan and irbersartan) have been produced and are effective in hypertension and congestive cardiac failure. They appear to produce much the same effects as angiotensin-converting enzyme inhibitors, though apparently with fewer side-effects (e.g. no cough and less hyperkalaemia). They are a useful alternative.

Renal artery stenosis

This is discussed on p. 554.

Disorders of aldosterone secretion

Primary hyperaldosteronism

PATHOPHYSIOLOGY

This rare condition (<1% of all hypertension) is caused by excess aldosterone production leading to sodium retention, potassium loss and the combination of hypokalaemia and hypertension.

CAUSES (see Table 16.38)

Adrenal adenomas (Conn's syndrome) account for 60% of cases; 30% are due to bilateral adrenal hyperplasia, which may be secondary to excess of a pituitary aldosterone-stimulating factor that is as yet unidentified.

CLINICAL FEATURES

The usual presentation is with hypertension and hypokalaemia (<3.5 mmol L^{-1}), although 20% of patients have initial potassium levels of 3.5–4.2 mmol L^{-1}. The few symptoms are nonspecific; rarely muscle weakness, nocturia and tetany are seen. The hypertension may be severe and associated with renal and retinal damage.

Adenomas, often very small, are more common in young females, while bilateral hyperplasia rarely occurs before age 40 years and is more common in males.

INVESTIGATIONS

The characteristic features are as follows:

- **Hypokalaemia**. A high-salt diet should be given for several days before testing and diuretics must be stopped three weeks before investigation; plasma samples must be separated quickly. Bethanidine or prazosin may be used for temporary control of blood pressure as they do not alter renin or aldosterone secretion.
- **Urinary potassium loss**. Levels over 30 mmol daily during hypokalaemia are inappropriate.
- **Elevated plasma aldosterone levels** that are not suppressed with 0.9% saline infusion (300 mmol over four hours) or fludrocortisone administration.
- **Suppressed plasma renin activity**. β-Blockers and other drugs may interfere with renin activity.

Once a diagnosis of hyperaldosteronism is established, differentiation of adenoma from hyperplasia involves adrenal CT or MRI (not infallible as tumours may be very small), complex biochemical testing including diurnal/postural changes in plasma aldosterone levels (which tend to rise with adenomas between 0900h supine and 1300h erect samples; in contrast they fall with hyperplasia), adrenal scintillation scanning (now rarely needed), and venous catheterization for aldosterone levels.

A rare cause is glucocorticoid (or dexamethasone)-suppressible hyperaldosteronism caused by a chimeric gene on chromosome 8. A fusion gene resulting from an unusual cross-over at meiosis between the genes encoding aldosterone synthase and adrenal 11β-hydroxylase produces aldosterone which is under ACTH control. Treatment with glucocorticoid resolves the problem.

TREATMENT

An adenoma should be removed surgically; BP falls in 70% of patients. Those with hyperplasia should be treated with the aldosterone antagonist spironolactone (100–400 mg daily); side-effects include nausea, rashes and gynaecomastia. Amiloride (10–40 mg daily) is a less effective alternative, used especially as spironolactone in long-term use has been linked with tumour development in animals. Calcium-channel blockers are also effective in controlling the hypertension.

Secondary hyperaldosteronism

This situation arises when there is excess renin (and hence angiotensin II) stimulation of the zona glomerulosa. Common causes are accelerated hypertension and renal artery stenosis, when the patient will be hypertensive. Causes associated with normotension include congestive cardiac failure and cirrhosis, where excess aldosterone production contributes to sodium retention.

Spironolactone is of value in both situations. Angiotensin-converting enzyme inhibitors (e.g. captopril, enalapril or lisinopril), and angiotensin II antagonists (e.g. losartan, irbersartan) are effective in heart failure, both symptomatically and in increasing life expectancy (see p. 680).

Hypoaldosteronism

Except as part of primary hypoadrenalism (Addison's disease, see p. 943), this is very uncommon. Causes include hyporeninaemic hypoaldosteronism, aldosterone biosynthetic defects, and drugs (e.g. ACE inhibitors, heparin).

The adrenal medulla

The major catecholamines, noradrenaline and adrenaline (epinephrine), are produced in the adrenal medulla (Fig 16.30), although most noradrenaline is derived from sympathetic neuronal release. While noradrenaline and adrenaline undoubtedly produce hypertension when infused, they probably play little part in BP regulation in normal humans.

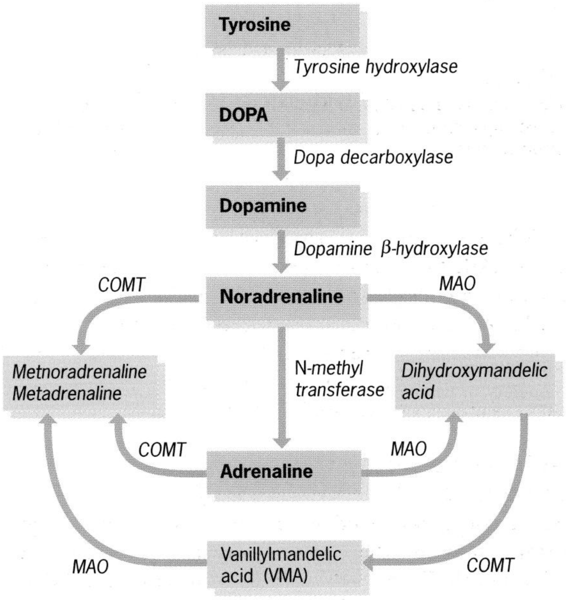

Fig 16.30
The synthesis and metabolism of catecholamines. COMT, catechol-*O*-methyl transferase; MAI, monoamine oxidas

Phaeochromocytoma

Phaeochromocytomas, tumours of the sympathetic nervous system, are very rare (less than 1 in 1000 cases of hypertension). Ninety per cent arise in the adrenal, while 10% occur elsewhere in the sympathetic chain. Twenty-five per cent are multiple and 10% are malignant, though this cannot be determined on simple histological examination. Some are associated with MEN syndromes (see below). Most tumours release both noradrenaline and adrenaline but large tumours produce almost entirely noradrenaline.

CLINICAL FEATURES

The clinical features are those of catecholamine excess and are frequently, but not necessarily, intermittent (Table 16.39). The diagnosis should particularly be considered when cardiovascular instability has been demonstrated, and in severe hypertension in pregnancy.

DIAGNOSIS

The possibility needs to be considered quite frequently in patients with hypertension. Specific tests are:

- **Measurement of urinary metabolites** (preferably metanephrines rather than vanillylmandelic acid (VMA) – Fig 16.30) is a useful *screening* test; normal levels on three 24-hour collections of metanephrines virtually exclude the diagnosis. Many drugs and dietary vanilla interfere with these tests.
- **Plasma and urinary catecholamines** are measured directly.
- **CT scans**, initially of the abdomen, are helpful to localize the tumours which are often large.
- **MRI** usually shows the lesion clearly.
- **Scanning** with [^{131}I]metaiodobenzylguanidine (MIBG) produces specific uptake in sites of sympathetic activity with about 90% success. It is particularly useful with extra-adrenal tumours.

TREATMENT

Tumours should be removed if this is possible; five-year survival is about 95% where not malignant. Medical preoperative and perioperative treatment is vital and includes complete α- and β-blockade with phenoxybenzamine (20–80 mg daily initially in divided doses), then propranolol (120–240 mg daily), plus transfusion of whole blood to re-expand the contracted plasma volume. The α-blockade must precede the β-blockade as worsened hypertension may otherwise result. Labetolol is not recommended. Surgery in the unprepared patient is fraught with dangers of both hypertension and hypotension; expert anaesthesia and an experienced surgeon are both vital and sodium nitroprusside should be available in case sudden severe hypertension develops.

When operation is not possible, combined α- and β-blockade can be used long term. Radionucleotide treatment with MIBG is under investigation.

Patients should be kept under clinical and biochemical review after tumour resection as about 10% recur or develop a further tumour. Catecholamine excretion measurements should be performed at least annually.

Table 16.39
Symptoms and signs of phaeochromocytoma

Symptoms	Signs
Anxiety or panic attacks	Hypertension – intermittent or constant
Palpitations	Tachycardia plus arrhythmias
Tremor	Bradycardia
Sweating	Orthostatic hypotension
Headache	Pallor or flushing
Flushing	Glycosuria
Nausea and/or vomiting	Fever
Weight loss	(Signs of hypertensive damage)
Constipation or diarrhoea	
Raynaud's phenomenon	
Chest pain	
Polyuria/nocturia	

FURTHER READING

Bouloux PM, Fakeeh M (1995) Investigation of phaeochromocytoma. *Clinical Endocrinology* **43**: 657–664.

Goodfriend TL, Elliott ME, Catt KJ (1996) Drug therapy: angiotensin receptors and their antagonists. *New England Journal of Medicine* **334**: 1649–1654.

Gordon RD (1994) Mineralocorticoid hypertension. *Lancet* **344**: 240–243.

Other endocrine disorders

Diseases of many glands

Multiple gland failure (polyglandular autoimmune syndromes)

These are caused by autoimmune disease as detailed in Table 16.4 on p. 903. Most common are the associations of primary hypothyroidism and type 1 diabetes, and either of these with Addison's disease or pernicious anaemia.

Multiple endocrine neoplasia

This is the name given to the simultaneous or metachronous occurrence of tumours involving a number of endocrine glands (Table 16.40). They are inherited in an autosomal dominant manner and are thought to arise from the expression of a recessive oncogenic mutation, some of which have now been isolated.

Affected persons may pass on the mutation to their offspring in the germ cell, but for the disease to become evident a somatic mutation must also occur, such as deletion or loss of a normal homologous chromosome. The defect in MEN 1 is in a novel gene (menin) on the long arm of chromosome 11 which encodes for a 610 amino acid protein. MEN 2a and 2b are caused by mutations of the *Ret*-proto-oncogene on chromosome 10. This gene encodes for a transmembrane glycoprotein receptor, tyrosine kinase. For MEN 2a the mutation is in the extracellular domain, for 2b in the intracellular domain.

Screening unaffected members of a family for the mutation by polymerase chain reaction (PCR) shows that a significant number of affected individuals are unrecognized, especially when screened only by hypercalcaemia, and is more effective than complex endocrine screening. Most neuroendocrine tumours contain somatostatin receptors, and an octreotide scan is useful to detect tumours (see p. 988).

MANAGEMENT

Treatment is surgical.

For type 1, all four parathyroid glands are removed (as all may be involved), followed by vitamin D (1,25-dihydrocalciferol) replacement therapy. Pancreatic tumours are often multiple and recurrence after partial pancreatectomy is invariable. Other tumours are treated surgically if necessary.

Type 2 tumours may also be recurrent or bilateral and a careful follow-up is necessary.

SCREENING

A careful family history should first be taken. If the precise gene mutation has been identified in a particular family, then family members at risk can now be screened directly for the presence of the mutation. In affected individuals, biochemical screening is then required. If initial biochemical screening is negative, this does not exclude later involvement and it may need repeating at regular (1–5 year) intervals.

Screening for type 1

This consists of fasting calcium estimation. If this is elevated, other manifestations of MEN 1 should be sought.

Screening for type 2

- *Medullary carcinoma of thyroid* (MCT) – pentagastrin and calcium infusion test with measurement of calcitonin to pick up 'C' cell hyperplasia; doubling of the calcitonin level is abnormal. Total thyroidectomy may then be indicated to prevent tumour development.
- *Phaeochromocytoma* – metanephrine, catecholamine or VMA estimations.

Ectopic hormone secretion

This terminology refers to hormone synthesis, and normally secretion, from a neoplastic non-endocrine cell, most usually seen in tumours that have some degree of embryological resemblance to specialist endocrine cells. The clinical effects may be those of the hormone produced, with or without manifestations of systemic malignancy. The most common situations seen are the following:

- *Hypercalcaemia of malignant disease*, often from squamous cell tumours of lung and breast, often with bone metastases. Where metastases are not present, most cases are mediated by secretion of PTH-related protein (PTHrP), which has considerable sequence

Table 16.40
Multiple endocrine neoplasia (MEN) syndromes

Organ	Frequency	Tumours/manifestations
Type 1		
Parathyroid	95%	Adenomas/hyperplasia
Pituitary	70%	Adenomas – prolactinoma, ACTH or growth hormone secreting (acromegaly)
Pancreas	50%	Islet cell tumours (secreting insulin, glucagon, somatostatin, VIP, pancreatic polypeptide, growth hormone releasing factor) Zollinger–Ellison syndrome (gastrinoma). Non-functional tumour
Adrenal	40%	Non-functional adenoma
Thyroid	20%	Adenomas – multiple or single
Type 2a		
Adrenal	Most	Phaeochromocytoma (70% bilateral) Cushing's syndrome
Thyroid	Most	Medullary carcinoma (calcitonin producing)
Parathyroid	60%	Hyperplasia
Type 2b		
Type 2a with Marfanoid phenotype and intestinal and visceral ganglioneuromas		

Neuromas also present around lips and tongue.

homology to PTH; a variety of other factors may sometimes be involved, but very rarely PTH itself (see p. 513). Treatment is discussed on p. 514.

- *SIADH* (see p. 952). Again, this is most common from a primary lung tumour.
- *Ectopic ACTH syndrome* (see p. 946). Small-cell carcinoma of the lung, carcinoid tumours and medullary thyroid carcinomas are the most common causes, though many other tumours rarely cause it
- *Production of insulin-like activity* may result in hypoglycaemia (see p. 988).

Endocrine treatment of other malignancies

Endocrine forms of treatment for malignancy have been used for many years; for example oophorectomy for breast cancer and orchidectomy for prostatic malignancy. More acceptable therapies include the anti-oestrogen tamoxifen for breast carcinoma and the LHRH analogues, buserelin and goserelin, for prostatic cancer.

FURTHER READING

Mulligan LM, Ponder BA (1995) Genetic basis of endocrine disease: MEN type 2. *Journal of Clinical Endocrinology and Metabolism* **80**: 1989–1995.

Shreaves R, Jenkins PJ, Wass JAH (eds) (1997) *Clinical Endocrine Oncology.* Oxford: Blackwell Science.

Trump D et al (1996) Clinical studies of MEN type 1. *Quarterly Journal of Medicine* **89**: 653–659.

CHAPTER BIBLIOGRAPHY

Besser GM, Thorner MO (1993) *Atlas of Endocrine Imaging.* London.

Brook CGD (1995) *Clinical Paediatric Endocrinology*, 3rd edn. Oxford: Blackwell Science.

Conn PM, Melmed S (eds) (1997) *Endocrinology: Basic and Clinical Principles.* New Jersey: Humana Press.

Greenspan FS, Gordon J, Strewler MD (eds) (1997) *Basic and Clinical Endocrinology*, 4th edn. Los Altos: Lange Medical.

Grossman, A (ed) (1997) *Clinical Endocrinology*, 2nd edn. Oxford: Blackwell Science.

Diabetes mellitus and other disorders of metabolism

17

Hyperglycaemia: an introduction

Diabetes mellitus is a syndrome characterized by chronic hyperglycaemia that is due to relative insulin deficiency, or resistance, or both. It affects more than 30 million people worldwide. Diabetes is usually irreversible and, although patients can have a reasonably normal lifestyle, its late complications result in reduced life expectancy and considerable uptake of health resources. *Macrovascular* disease leads to an increased prevalence of coronary artery disease, peripheral vascular disease and stroke. *Microvascular* damage causes diabetic retinopathy and nephropathy, and contributes to diabetic neuropathy.

Insulin structure and secretion

Insulin is the key hormone involved in the storage and controlled release within the body of the chemical energy available from food. It is coded for on chromosome 11 and synthesized in the β cells of the pancreatic islets. Insulin consists of A and B chains linked by disulphide bonds.

The synthesis, intracellular processing and secretion of insulin by the β cell is typical of the way that the body produces and manipulates many peptide hormones. The manufacture and release of insulin from the β cell is illustrated in Fig 17.1, and Fig 17.2 illustrates the cellular events triggering the release of insulin-containing granules.

After secretion, insulin enters the portal circulation and is carried to the liver, its prime target organ. About 50% of secreted insulin is extracted and degraded in the liver; the residue is broken down by the kidneys. C-peptide is only partially extracted by the liver (and hence provides a useful index of the rate of insulin secretion), but is mainly degraded by the kidneys.

An outline of glucose metabolism

Blood glucose levels are closely regulated in health and rarely stray outside the range of 3.5–8.0 mmol L^{-1} (63–144 mg dL^{-1}), despite the varying demands of food, fasting and exercise. The principal organ of glucose homeostasis is the liver, which absorbs and stores glucose (as glycogen) in the postabsorptive state and releases it into the circulation between meals to match the rate of glucose utilization by peripheral tissues. The liver also combines 3-carbon molecules derived from breakdown

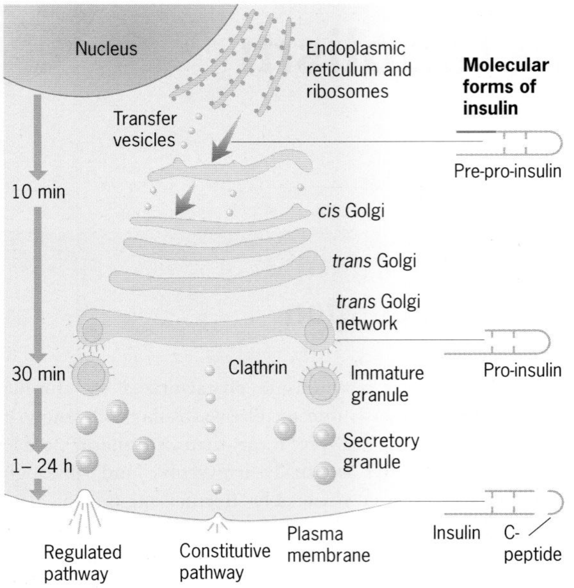

Fig 17.1
Diagrammatic representation of part of a β cell. The ribosomes manufacture pre-pro-insulin from insulin mRNA. The hydrophobic 'pre' portion of pre-pro-insulin allows it to transfer to the Golgi apparatus, and is subsequently enzymatically cleaved off. Pro-insulin is parcelled into secretory granules in the Golgi apparatus. These mature and pass towards the cell membrane where they are stored before release. The pro-insulin molecule folds back on itself and weak disulphide bonds stabilize it. The biochemically inert peptide fragment known as connecting (C) peptide splits off from pro-insulin in the secretory process, leaving insulin as a complex of two linked peptide chains. Equimolar quantities of insulin and C-peptide are released into the circulation. A small amount of insulin is secreted by the β cell directly via the 'constitutive pathway' which bypasses the secretory granules

of fat (glycerol), muscle glycogen (lactate) and protein (e.g. alanine) into the 6-carbon glucose molecule by the process of gluconeogenesis.

Glucose production
About 200 g of glucose is produced and utilized each day. More than 90% is derived from liver glycogen and hepatic gluconeogenesis, and the remainder from renal gluconeogenesis.

Glucose utilization
The brain is the major consumer of glucose. Its requirement is 1 mg kg^{-1} bodyweight per minute, or 100 g daily in a 70 kg man. Glucose uptake by the brain is obligatory and is not dependent on insulin, and the glucose used is oxidized to carbon dioxide and water.

Other tissues, such as muscle and fat, are facultative glucose consumers. The effect of insulin peaks associated with meals is to lower the threshold for glucose entry into cells; at other times, energy requirements are largely met by fatty-acid oxidation. Glucose taken up by muscle is stored as glycogen or broken down to lactate, which re-enters the circulation and becomes an important substrate for hepatic gluconeogenesis. Glucose is used by fat tissue as a source of energy and as a substrate for triglyceride synthesis; lipolysis releases fatty acids from triglyceride together with glycerol, another substrate for hepatic gluconeogenesis.

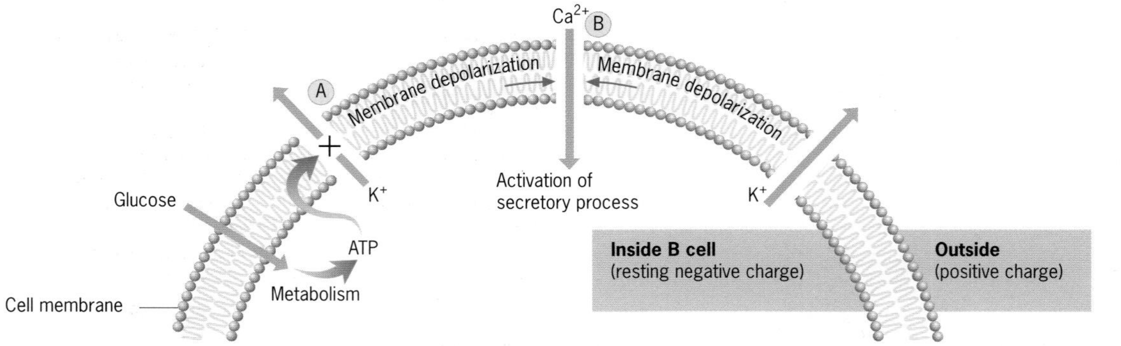

Fig 17.2
Diagrammatic representation of the local forces regulating insulin secretion from β cells. The metabolism of glucose entering the β cell generates ATP. ATP closes potassium channels in the cell membrane (A). The cell membrane depolarizes, allowing calcium ions to enter the cell via calcium selective channels in the membrane (B). The rise in intracellular calcium triggers activation of calcium-dependent phospholipid protein kinase which, via intermediary phosphorylation steps, leads to fusion of the insulin-containing granules with the cell membrane and exocytosis of the insulin-rich granule contents. Similar mechanisms operate to cause hormone-granule secretion in many other endocrine cells

Hormonal regulation

Insulin is the major regulator of intermediary metabolism, although its actions are modified in important respects by other hormones. Dose–response curves for the production and utilization of glucose are shown in Fig 17.3.

At low insulin levels, glucose production is maximal and utilization is minimal; at high insulin levels the situation is reversed. At intermediate plasma insulin levels of 40–50 mU L^{-1}, hepatic glucose production is largely suppressed but peripheral utilization remains low. This observation forms the theoretical basis for the low-dose insulin regimen used to treat diabetic ketoacidosis (see below).

The effect of counter-regulatory hormones (glucagon, adrenaline, cortisol and growth hormone) is to shift both dose–response curves to the right, resulting in greater production of glucose and less utilization for a given level of insulin.

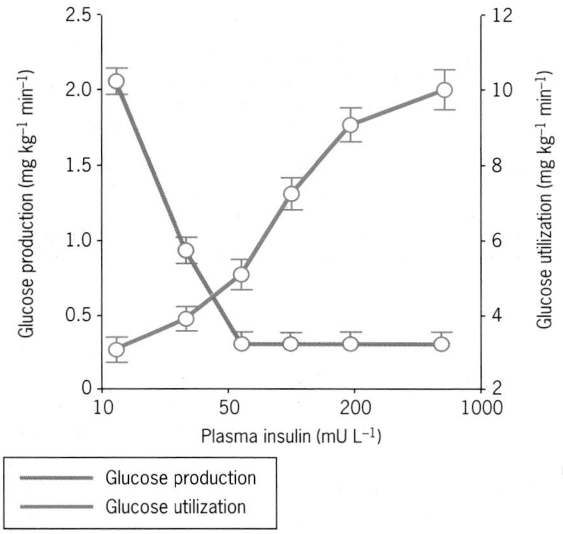

Fig 17.3
The effect of different insulin levels on glucose production and glucose utilization. Hepatic glucose production rises as insulin levels fall. Conversely, peripheral uptake of glucose is promoted at high insulin levels

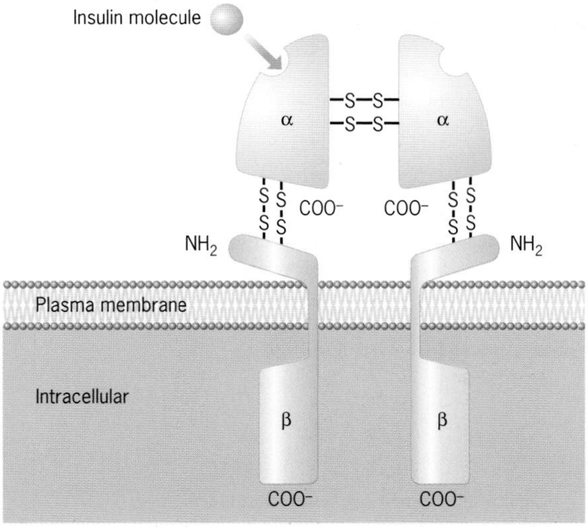

Fig 17.4
The insulin receptor consists of α and β subunits linked by disulphide bridges. The subunits straddle the cell membrane and initiate the intracellular actions of insulin

The insulin receptor

This is a glycoprotein (400 kDa), coded for on the short arm of chromosome 19, which straddles the cell membrane of many cells (Fig 17.4). It consists of a dimer with two α subunits, which include the binding sites for insulin, and two β subunits, which traverse the cell membrane. When insulin binds to the α subunits it induces a conformational change in the β subunits, resulting in activation of tyrosine kinase and initiation of a cascade response involving a number of other intracellular substrates. One consequence of this is migration of the GLUT-4 glucose transporter to the cell surface and increased transport of glucose into the cell. The insulin–receptor complex is then internalized by the cell, insulin is degraded, and the receptor is recycled to the cell surface.

Types of diabetes

Diabetes may be *primary* or *secondary* (Table 17.1). Although secondary diabetes accounts for barely 1–2% of all new cases at presentation, it is important to recognize so that the cause can be treated.

Table 17.1
Causes of secondary diabetes

Liver disease Cirrhosis	**Drug-induced disease** Thiazide diuretics Corticosteroid therapy
Pancreatic disease Cystic fibrosis Chronic pancreatitis Malnutrition-related pancreatic disease Pancreatectomy Hereditary haemochromatosis Carcinoma of the pancreas	**Insulin-receptor abnormalities** Congenital lipodystrophy Acanthosis nigricans **Genetic syndromes** Friedreich's ataxia Myotonic dystrophy
Endocrine disease Cushing's syndrome Acromegaly Thyrotoxicosis Phaeochromocytoma Glucagonoma	

Although insulin-dependent diabetes mellitus (IDDM) and non-insulin-dependent diabetes mellitus (NIDDM) represent two distinct diseases from the epidemiological point of view, clinical distinction can sometimes be difficult. The two diseases should, in clinical terms, be seen as a spectrum, distinct at the two ends but overlapping to some extent in the middle (Table 17.2).

Insulin-dependent diabetes mellitus (type I diabetes)

EPIDEMIOLOGY

Approximately one person in 200 in the UK is treated with insulin, but some of these would be considered to have NIDDM by the criteria shown in Table 17.2. IDDM is most common in populations of European extraction. The incidence rises as one moves north within Europe, with the highest rates in Finland and Scandinavia. The exception is the island of Sardinia, which for unknown reasons has the second highest rate in the world. The frequency of IDDM in various countries is shown in Fig 17.5.

IDDM presents most commonly in childhood, with a peak at 10–13 years of age, but can present at any age. The incidence of IDDM is rising in many parts of the world, and has doubled in Europe over the past 20–30 years.

AETIOLOGY

IDDM results from a slow-burning HLA-linked autoimmune disease process. Genetic susceptibility is polygenic, with the greatest contribution from the HLA region. Autoantibodies directed against pancreatic islet constituents appear in the circulation within the first few years of life, and pre-date clinical onset by many years. Autoantibodies have also been detected in a proportion of older patients, previously thought to have NIDDM, and predict progression to insulin therapy in this group.

Genetic susceptibility

IDDM is not genetically predetermined, but increased susceptibility to the disease may be inherited.

Inheritance

The identical twin of a patient with IDDM has a 30–35% chance of developing the disease. This implies that non-genetic factors must also be involved. The child of an insulin-dependent diabetic patient has an increased chance of developing IDDM. This risk, curiously, is greater with a diabetic father (2.5–5.0%) than with a diabetic mother (1.25–2.5%). If one child in a family has IDDM, each sibling has a 5% risk of developing diabetes. If a sibling is HLA-identical, the risk rises to about 17%.

HLA system. The HLA genes on chromosome 6 are highly polymorphic, and modulate the immune defence system of the body. More than 90% of IDDM patients carry HLA-DR3 and/or DR4, compared with 40% of the general population. The *relative risk* conferred by DR3 is about 7, and by DR4 about 9; but DR3/DR4 heterozygotes have a relative risk of 14, showing an additive effect. In contrast, HLA-DR2 is protective. These associations are due to linkage disequilibrium. In other words, the (as yet unknown) genes causing diabetes tend to be transmitted along with these particular HLA types.

Table 17.2
The spectrum of diabetes: a comparison of insulin-dependent diabetes mellitus and non-insulin-dependent diabetes mellitus

	IDDM (type I)	NIDDM (type II)
Epidemiology	Patients are: Younger Usually lean European extraction (most commonly) Seasonal incidence (↑ spring and autumn) ? Viral aetiology	Patients are: Older Often overweight All racial groups (increasing incidence in immigrants to the UK)
Heredity	HLA-DR3 or DR4 in >90% 30–35% concordance in identical twins	No HLA links Glucokinase gene abnormalities in some families 90% concordance in identical twins
Pathogenesis	Autoimmunity: Islet cell antibody Autoantibodies to insulin, GAD (glutamic acid decarboxylase) and IA-2 (see Fig 17.6) Insulitis Associations with other organ-specific autoimmune diseases Immunosuppression following diagnosis delays β cell destruction	No evidence of immune disturbance
Clinical	Insulin deficiency May develop ketoacidosis Always need insulin	Partial insulin deficiency, insulin resistance May develop non-ketotic hyperosmolar state Sometimes need insulin
Biochemical	Eventual disappearance of C-peptide	C-peptide persists

Even stronger associations have been reported with the DQ region, and substitution of aspartate at position 57 of the HLA-DQ β chain by another amino acid considerably increases susceptibility to IDDM, as do alleles coding for arginine at position 52 on the α chain.

Other gene regions. A genome-wide search for regions conferring susceptibility to or protection against IDDM has been carried out, and more than 15 regions of interest have been identified. These are designated *IDDM1* (HLA locus), *IDDM2* and so on. An intensive search for the genes themselves is under way, and IDDM promises to be among the first complex polygenic disorders to be fully characterized at the gene level.

A DNA region close to the insulin gene on chromosome 11 is designated as *IDDM2* and short, intermediate and long insertions (see p. 144) have been reported. Homozygosity of the short (class I) allele is found in some 80% of patients with IDDM as against 40% of controls.

Autoimmunity and insulin-dependent diabetes mellitus

Several pieces of evidence suggest that autoimmune processes are involved in the pathogenesis of IDDM. These include the HLA associations described above, and associations with other organ-specific autoimmune

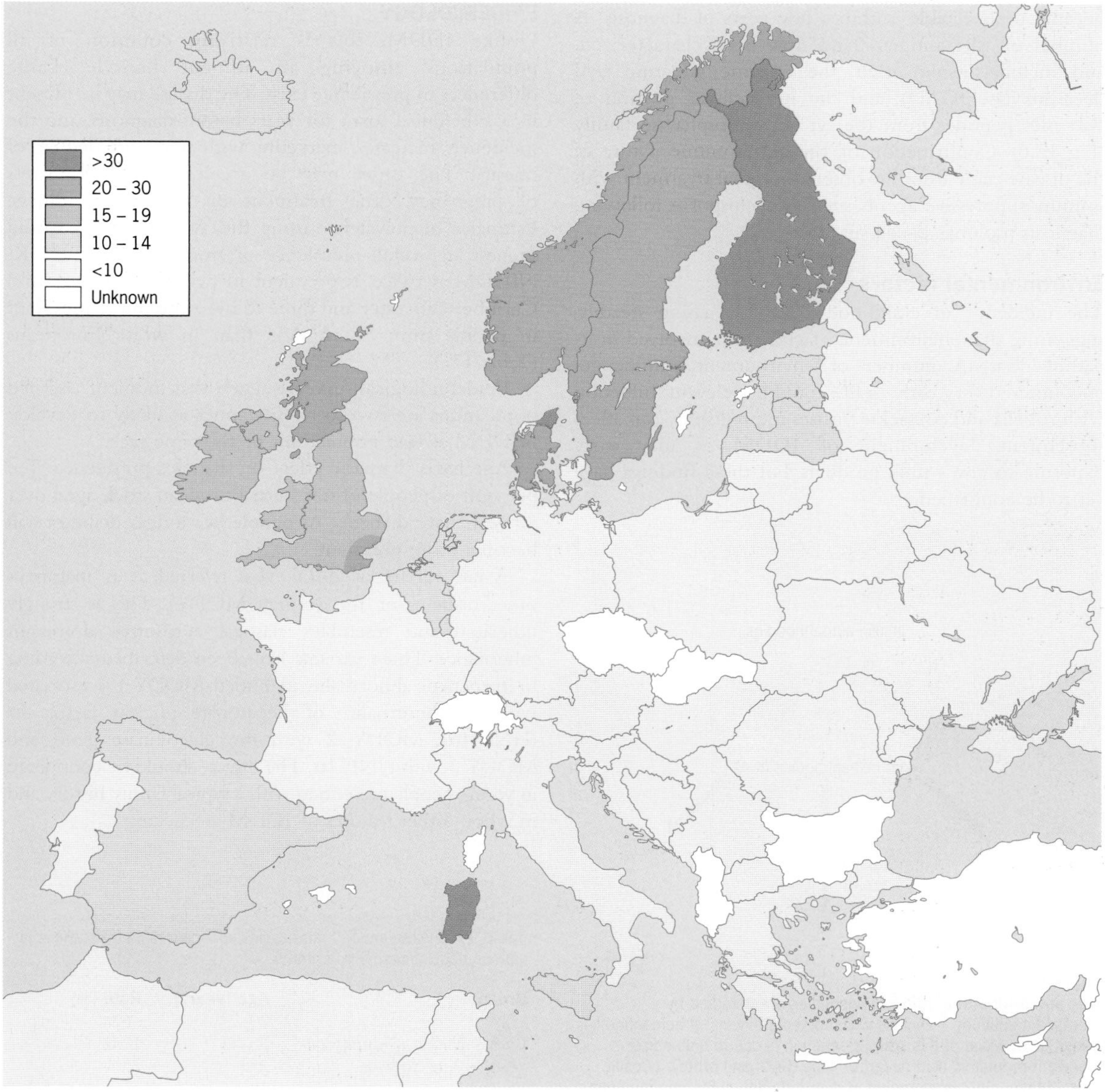

Fig 17.5
Age-standardized incidence rates of IDDM (onset 0–14 years) in Europe, per 100 000 per year.
From Green A, Gale EAM et al (1992) *Lancet* **339**: 905–909

diseases including autoimmune thyroid disease, Addison's disease and pernicious anaemia.

Autopsies of patients who died soon after diagnosis show infiltration of the pancreatic islets by mononuclear cells. This appearance, known as insulitis, resembles that in other autoimmune diseases such as thyroiditis. Increased numbers of activated T lymphocytes are present in the circulation at diagnosis. Autoantibodies directed against islet constituents are also present in some 90% of newly presenting patients. These were first demonstrated by washing serum from newly diagnosed patients across pancreatic sections, and demonstrating the presence of antibodies binding to the islets by immunofluorescence. These were known as *islet cell antibodies* (ICA), and usually became undetectable within a few years of diagnosis. A number of islet antigens have now been characterized, and include insulin itself, the enzyme glutamic acid decarboxylase (GAD), and the intracellular portion of two islet peptides from the tyrosine phosphatase family (Fig 17.6). Confirmation of the autoimmune nature of the disease came from the observation that treatment with immunosuppressive agents such as cyclosporin following diagnosis prolongs β-cell survival.

Environmental factors

The incidence of childhood IDDM is rising steadily, suggesting that environmental factor(s) are involved in its pathogenesis. A number of environmental influences encountered very early in life could be relevant. Infection with rubella and coxsackie viruses in pregnancy can affect subsequent development of IDDM, as may early exposure to cow's milk products, but these findings have yet to be confirmed.

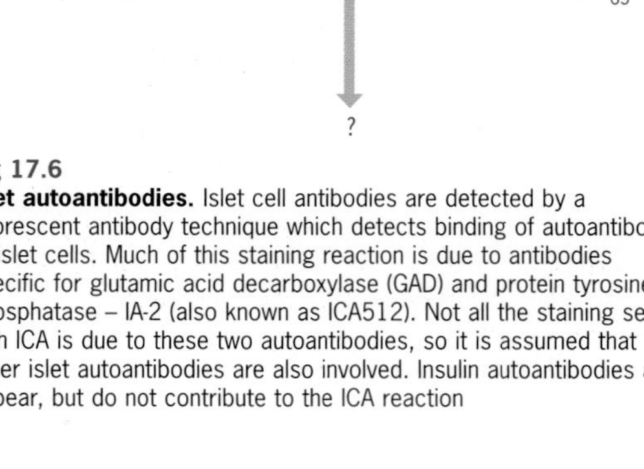

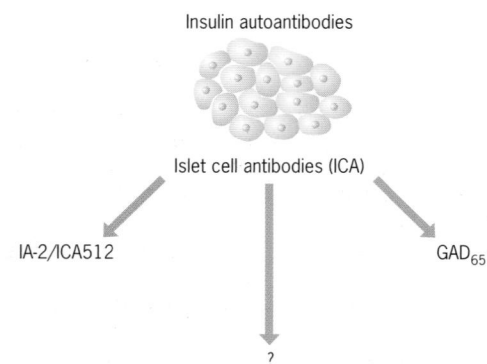

Fig 17.6
Islet autoantibodies. Islet cell antibodies are detected by a fluorescent antibody technique which detects binding of autoantibodies to islet cells. Much of this staining reaction is due to antibodies specific for glutamic acid decarboxylase (GAD) and protein tyrosine phosphatase – IA-2 (also known as ICA512). Not all the staining seen with ICA is due to these two autoantibodies, so it is assumed that other islet autoantibodies are also involved. Insulin autoantibodies also appear, but do not contribute to the ICA reaction

Pre-IDDM

Prospective study of first-degree relatives of children with diabetes has shown that islet autoantibodies appear in the circulation in the first few years of life and many years before diagnosis. Further, they can predict development of the disease, especially when present in combination. The ability to predict the disease has opened the way to possible disease prevention, and large multicentre trials of this type are under way.

Non-insulin-dependent diabetes mellitus (type II diabetes)

EPIDEMIOLOGY

Unlike IDDM, this is relatively common in all populations enjoying an affluent lifestyle. Large differences in prevalence exist. The disease may be present in a subclinical form for years before diagnosis, and the incidence increases markedly with age and degree of obesity. The onset may be accelerated by the stress of pregnancy, drug treatment or intercurrent illness. Estimates of prevalence using the WHO criteria would suggest an overall prevalence of around 2% in the UK. NIDDM is twice as prevalent in people of African and Caribbean ancestry and three to five times more prevalent in people from South Asia than in white Europeans (Table 17.3).

Epidemiological surveys suggest that indolent well-fed populations are two to twenty times as likely to develop NIDDM as lean populations of the same race.

Age has a dramatic effect on diabetes prevalence. Ten per cent of people of northern European stock aged over 70 years have diabetes. As people live longer diabetes will become more prevalent.

A rare variant of NIDDM is referred to as 'maturity-onset diabetes of the young' (MODY). This is strongly inherited and resembles classical autosomal dominant inheritance. Three variants have been described according to the genetic abnormality identified. MODY 1 is associated with an abnormality of hepatocyte nuclear factor 4α (HNF-4α), MODY 2 with the glucokinase gene, and MODY 3 with HNF-1α. The disease should be considered in young people presenting with a typical family history and in whom other features of IDDM are lacking.

Table 17.3 Prevalence of non-insulin-dependent diabetes mellitus in various populations (WHO criteria)

Group	Age (years)	Rate (%)
USA	20–74	6.9
USA – Mexican immigrants	25–65	17.0
USA – Pima Indians	25+	25.5
Malta	15+	7.7
Indonesia	15+	1.7
New Guinea (highlands)	20+	0.0

AETIOLOGY

Genetics

Identical twins of a patient with NIDDM have a greater than 90% chance of developing diabetes and about 25% of other patients have a first-degree relative with NIDDM. These observations suggest a strong genetic component, and it is now clear that NIDDM is a polygenic disorder. A few families show abnormalities of the gene which codes for the enzyme glucokinase on chromosome 7, and other families have been described with abnormalities of genes coding for hepatic nuclear factors 1α and 4α but the genetic defects in most families with NIDDM are as yet unknown. The next decade is likely to see the identification of many of the gene abnormalities which predispose to NIDDM.

Environmental factors: early and late

A strong association has been noted between low weight at birth and at 12 months of age and glucose intolerance later in life, particularly in those who gain excess weight as adults. The concept is that poor nutrition early in life impairs β cell development and function, predisposing to diabetes in later life.

Immunology

There is no evidence of immune involvement in the pathogenesis of NIDDM, but as noted earlier a propor-tion of late-onset patients carry islet autoantibodies – ICA and GAD – at diagnosis, and are more likely to progress to insulin therapy. These presumably represent late-onset IDDM.

Insulin secretion and action

Patients with NIDDM, unlike those with IDDM, retain about 50% of their β-cell mass. Almost all patients show islet amyloid deposition at autopsy, derived from a peptide known as amylin or islet amyloid polypeptide (IAPP) which is co-secreted with insulin. Its role in causation of the disease is uncertain.

Abnormalities of insulin secretion develop early in the course of the disease. Normal subjects have a biphasic insulin response to intravenous glucose. At onset of NIDDM the first-phase insulin response to intravenous glucose is lost, and insulin secretion in response to oral glucose is delayed and exaggerated. The majority of patients manifest reduced insulin secretion relative to the prevailing glucose concentration, and progressive β-cell loss occurs in many patients, although not to the extent seen in IDDM. It is not known whether this is due to 'exhaustion' of surviving β cells or to some independent process of damage. Obesity is present in 80% of patients with NIDDM, but insulin resistance may also be marked in lean individuals.

Impaired glucose tolerance

If an oral glucose tolerance test (Practical box 17.1) is administered at random to a large population, 1–2% will be found to have unsuspected diabetes. A much larger group – 5% or more (depending on the age, race and nutritional state of the population) – fall into an intermediate category referred to as 'impaired glucose tolerance' (IGT). The criteria for this category are given in Practical box 17.1. Follow-up shows that some (2–4% yearly) go on to develop diabetes, but that the abnormality does not progress in the majority. Obesity and lack of regular physical exercise make progression to frank diabetes more likely.

Practical

1. After an overnight fast, 75 g of glucose is taken in 250–350 mL of water.
2. Blood samples are taken in the fasting state and two hours after the glucose has been given.
3. A specific enzymatic glucose assay must be used.

Note: The concentration of glucose measured in plasma is 10% greater than that of whole blood.

Diabetes

This is present when the fasting *blood* glucose is over 6.7 mmol L^{-1} and/or when the 2-hour value is over 10 mmol L^{-1}. Corresponding values for *plasma* glucose are 7.8 mmol L^{-1} and 11.1 mmol L^{-1}.

Impaired glucose tolerance

This is present when the fasting blood glucose is below 6.7 mmol L^{-1} and when the 2-hour value is between 6.7 and 10 mmol L^{-1}. Corresponding values for plasma glucose are 7.8 and 11.1 mmol L^{-1}. Impaired glucose tolerance can only be diagnosed by using the oral glucose tolerance test.

Intermediate sampling times (e.g. 30 min and 60 min) are not needed for the diagnosis of diabetes by WHO criteria. However, simultaneous blood and urine glucose measurements can be used to define a low renal threshold for glucose.

Diabetes can usually be diagnosed on the basis of fasting or random blood glucose measurements (see text). *The glucose tolerance test should be reserved for borderline cases only.*

Note: The American Diabetes Association has proposed changes to the diagnostic criteria for diabetes which suggest the reduction of fasting plasma glucose from 7.8 to 7 mmol L^{-1}. A new catagory of 'impaired fasting glucose' has been introduced, with plasma glucose levels of 6.1–7 mmol L^{-1}. These changes have not as yet been universally adopted.

Practical box 17.1 The oral glucose tolerance test

Classification is complicated by the poor reproducibility of the oral glucose tolerance test and the group is certainly heterogeneous. Some are obese, some have liver disease, and others are on medication that impairs glucose tolerance; individuals in this category have a risk of cardiovascular disease that is twice that of people with normal glucose tolerance, but do not develop the specific microvascular complications of diabetes.

FURTHER READING

Groop LC (1997) Editorial: The molecular genetics of non-insulin-dependent diabetes mellitus. *Journal of Internal Medicine* **241**(2): 95–101.

Yki-Jarvinen H (1997) MODY genes and mutations in hepatocyte nuclear factors. *Lancet* **349**: 516–517.

Clinical presentation of diabetes

Acute and subacute presentations often overlap.

Acute presentation

Young people may present with a brief 2–4 week history and report the classic triad of symptoms:

- *polyuria* – due to the osmotic diuresis that results when blood glucose levels exceed the renal threshold
- *thirst* – due to the resulting loss of fluid and electrolytes
- *weight loss* – due to fluid depletion and the accelerated breakdown of fat and muscle secondary to insulin deficiency.

Ketoacidosis may be the presenting feature if these early symptoms are not recognized and treated.

Subacute presentation

The clinical onset may be over several months, particularly in older patients. Thirst, polyuria and weight loss are usual features, but medical attention is sought for such symptoms as lack of energy, visual blurring (due to glucose-induced changes in refraction), or pruritus vulvae or balanitis that is due to *Candida* infection.

Complications as the presenting feature

These include:

- staphylococcal skin infections
- retinopathy noted during a visit to the optician
- a polyneuropathy causing tingling and numbness in the feet
- impotence
- arterial disease, resulting in myocardial infarction or peripheral gangrene.

Asymptomatic diabetes

Glycosuria or a raised blood glucose may be detected on routine examination (e.g. for insurance purposes) in individuals who have no symptoms of ill-health.

PHYSICAL EXAMINATION

This is often unrewarding in younger patients, but evidence of weight loss and dehydration may be present, and the breath may smell of ketones. Older patients may present with established complications, and the presence of the characteristic retinopathy is diagnostic of diabetes.

Investigation of diabetes

The diagnosis is usually simple. Blood glucose is so closely controlled by the body that even small deviations become important.

- In *symptomatic* patients, a single elevated blood glucose $\geq$ 11.1 mmol L^{-1}, measured by a reliable method, indicates diabetes.
- In *asymptomatic* or *mildly symptomatic* patients, the diagnosis is made on:
  (a) at least one, preferably two, fasting venous *blood* glucose levels above 6.7 mmol L^{-1} (120 mg dL^{-1}) – the equivalent venous plasma level is 7.8 mmol L^{-1} (140 mg dL^{-1}); OR
  (b) at least one, preferably two, random values above 10.0 mmol L^{-1} (180 mg dL^{-1}) in venous whole blood, or 11.1 mmol L^{-1} (200 mg dL^{-1}) in venous plasma.
- A glucose tolerance test (the criteria above are satisfied, and should be reserved for true borderline cases.
- Glycosuria is measured using sensitive glucose-specific dipstick methods. Glycosuria is not diagnostic of diabetes but indicates the need for further investigations. About 1% of the population have renal glycosuria. This is an inherited low renal threshold for glucose, transmitted either as a Mendelian dominant or recessive trait.

Other investigations

No further tests are needed to diagnose diabetes. Other routine investigations include screening the urine for proteinuria, a full blood count, urea and electrolytes, liver biochemistry and a fasting blood sample for cholesterol and triglycerides. The latter test is useful to exclude an associated hyperlipidaemia but should be performed only after blood glucose has been brought under control.

Diabetes may be *secondary* to other conditions (see Table 17.1), may be *precipitated* by underlying illness and be associated with autoimmune disease or hyperlipidaemia. Hypertension is present in one-third of European patients with NIDDM and in 50% of African and Caribbean patients.

Treatment of diabetes

The role of patient education and community care

The care of diabetes is based on self-management by the patient, who is helped and advised by those with specialized knowledge. The quest for improved glycaemic control has made it clear that whatever the technical expertise applied, the outcome depends on willing cooperation by the patient. This in turn depends on an understanding of the risks of diabetes and the potential benefits of glycaemic control and other measures such as maintaining a lean weight, stopping smoking and taking care of the feet.

If accurate information is not supplied, misinformation from friends and other patients will take its place. For this reason, many patients have exaggerated fears of, for example, blindness (less than one patient in 20 is blind after 30 years of diabetes), death during hypoglycaemia (extremely rare), or the risk of passing diabetes on to their children (some 5% of offspring of a person with IDDM develop the condition, whereas about 15% of children of patients with NIDDM develop this form of diabetes).

Organized training programmes involving all healthcare workers, including nurse specialists, dietitians and chiropodists, are now a recognized part of good diabetes care.

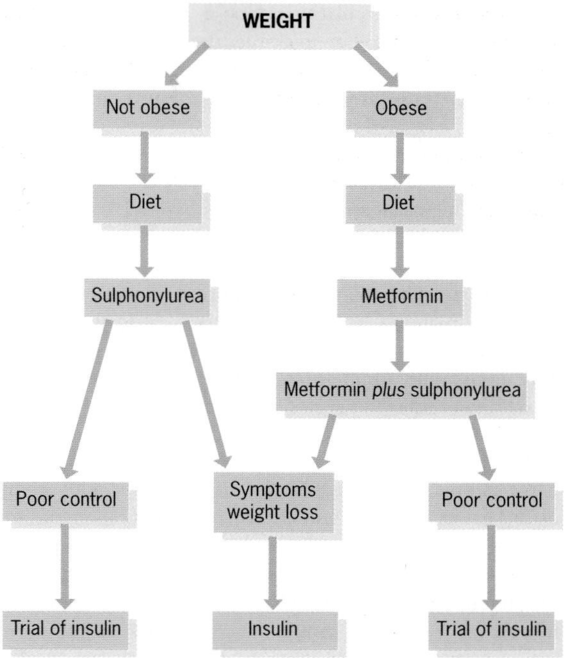

Fig 17.7
Treatment pathway for NIDDM. Diet is the first line of treatment, followed by metformin for the overweight and a sulphonylurea for the lean. Sulphonylureas and insulin should be used with caution in the obese since they predispose to weight gain

Guidelines to therapy

All patients with diabetes require diet therapy. Good glycaemic control is unlikely to be achieved with insulin or oral therapy when diet is neglected, especially when the patient is also overweight.

Regular exercise helps to control weight and reduces cardiovascular risk. Walking instead of using transport, gardening regularly, renting an allotment or getting a dog are all more likely to provide prolonged benefit than buying membership to a gym or 'health club'.

Insulin is always indicated in a patient who has been in ketoacidosis, and is usually indicated in patients who present under the age of 40 years. Insulin is also indicated in older patients following primary or secondary failure of oral therapy (see below). Tablets should be avoided in younger patients and are contraindicated in pregnancy.

In older patients the approach to therapy is empirical. One stepped approach to treatment of non-insulin dependent diabetes is illustrated in Fig 17.7. Diet alone should be tried in the first instance, and dietary knowledge and compliance should always be reassessed with care before proceeding to the next step. This is of particular importance in the obese patient who fails to lose weight.

When diet fails to achieve satisfactory control, thin patients are usually treated with a sulphonylurea drug, and obese patients with a biguanide. Primary failure of treatment occurs when these agents (alone or in combination) never achieve the desired level of control. Other patients may show a good initial response followed by progressive loss of control over the succeeding months or years; this is referred to as 'secondary failure of treatment'.

Since this approach is largely empirical, it is not surprising that practice differs from one country to another. For example, metformin (the only biguanide in common use) is very widely employed in France, tends to be used less in the UK, and has only recently been licensed in the USA. Criteria of control also vary, so that what is classed as primary failure at one centre may be seen as a success in another. The most widespread error in management is procrastination; the patient whose control is inadequate on tablets should start insulin without undue delay.

Diet

The diet for a diabetic patient is in principle no different from the diet considered healthy for the population as a whole.

Carbohydrate

This should consist of unrefined carbohydrate rather than simple sugars such as sucrose. Carbohydrate is absorbed relatively slowly from fibre-rich foods, preventing the rapid swings in circulating glucose seen when refined sugars are ingested. For example, the glucose peak seen after eating an apple is much flatter than that seen after drinking the same amount of carbohydrate as apple juice.

Calories

Calories should be tailored to the needs of the diabetic patient. The total amount of carbohydrate in the diet should provide 50–55% of the total calories, with fat 30–35% and protein 15%.

- An *overweight* patient is started on a reducing diet of approximately 4–6 MJ (1000–1600 kcal) daily.
- A *lean* patient is put on an isocaloric diet.
- Patients who are *underweight* because of untreated diabetes require energy supplementation.

Prescribing a diet

Most people find it extremely difficult to modify their eating habits, and repeated advice and encouragement are needed if this is to be achieved. A diet history is taken, and the diet prescribed should involve the least possible interference with the lifestyle of the patient. Patients on insulin or oral agents should be advised to eat the same amount at the same time each day. Patients on insulin require snacks between meals and at bedtime to buffer the effect of injected insulin. Alcohol is not forbidden, but its energy content should be taken into account. Patients on insulin should be warned to avoid alcoholic binges since these may precipitate severe hypoglycaemia.

Tablet treatment for NIDDM

Diet and lifestyle changes are the key to successful treatment of NIDDM. If satisfactory metabolic control (see 'Measuring control' below) of diabetes is not established by these measures after several weeks, then tablets may be needed in addition. Introduce tablets after an improvement through diet and lifestyle changes has been witnessed by the patient, who may otherwise attribute the improvement to the tablets alone.

Sulphonylureas (Table 17.4)

Properties of the more commonly used sulphonylureas are set out in Table 17.4. Their principal action is to promote insulin secretion in response to glucose and other secretagogues.

Sulphonylureas close ATP-sensitive potassium channels on the β-cell membrane, and the resulting depolarization promotes calcium influx, a signal for insulin release (see Fig 17.2). They were in addition believed to increase insulin sensitivity in peripheral tissues, but this view is now largely discounted. Sulphonylureas are therefore ineffective in patients without a functional β-cell mass and should be avoided in young ketotic patients, who require early insulin therapy, and are contraindicated in pregnancy. Insulin should be substituted during major surgery or severe intercurrent illness.

Table 17.4
Properties of the most commonly used sulphonylureas

Drug	Features
Tolbutamide	Lower maximal efficacy than other sulphonylureas Short half-life – preferable in elderly Largely metabolized by liver – can use in renal impairment
Glibenclamide	Long biological half-life Active metabolites Renal excretion – avoid in renal impairment
Gliclazide	Fairly long biological half-life Largely metabolized by liver – can use in renal impairment More costly
Chlorpropamide	Very long biological half-life Renal excretion – avoid in renal impairment 1–2% develop inappropriate ADH-like syndrome Facial flush with alcohol Very inexpensive – important issue for developing countries

Sulphonylureas should be used with care in patients with liver disease, and only those primarily excreted by the liver should be given to patients with renal impairment. All encourage weight gain and are therefore not drugs of first choice in obese patients. Tolbutamide is the safest drug in the very elderly because of its short duration of action.

Drug interactions and side-effects All sulphonylureas bind to circulating albumin and may be displaced by other drugs, such as sulphonamides, that compete for their binding sites. They interact with warfarin.

Hypoglycaemia is the most common and dangerous side-effect. Because the action of many sulphonylureas persists for more than 24 hours, recurrent or prolonged hypoglycaemia is likely, and hospital admission is advisable. Skin rashes and other sensitivity reactions may rarely occur.

Biguanides

The mechanism of action of metformin remains unclear but it reduces gluconeogenesis, and thus suppresses hepatic glucose output, and it increases insulin sensitivity. Unlike the sulphonylureas it does not induce hypoglycaemia in normal volunteers. It is usually reserved for patients in middle or old age, particularly for the overweight since it does not promote weight gain. It may be given in combination with sulphonylureas when a single agent has proved to be ineffective.

Its side-effects include anorexia, epigastric discomfort and diarrhoea. Lactic acidosis has occurred in patients with severe hepatic or renal disease, and metformin is contraindicated when these are present.

α-Glucosidase inhibitors

One alternative approach to the treatment of overweight patients with NIDDM is to use drugs which inhibit the enzymes involved in the breakdown of carbohydrates in the intestine. Acarbose is a sham sugar that competitively inhibits α-glucosidase enzymes situated on the brush border of the intestine. As a result, dietary carbohydrate is poorly absorbed, and the postprandial rise in blood glucose is reduced. Undigested starch may as a result enter the large intestine where it is broken down by fermentation. Abdominal discomfort, flatulence and diarrhoea can result, and dosage needs careful adjustment to avoid these side-effects. Very little acarbose enters the circulation, since it is mainly inactivated in the gut, but liver dysfunction may rarely occur with high doses.

New drugs for NIDDM

Other drugs shortly to reach the market hold out some promise for the future. These include insulin sensitizers, drugs which reduce insulin resistance by interaction with the PPAR-γ (peroxisome proliferator-activated receptor-γ) a nuclear receptor which regulates genes involved in lipid metabolism. The effect on insulin sensitivity may result from decreased production of non-esterified fatty acids. They thus have the capacity to potentiate the effect of endogenous insulin. One of these, troglitazone, which belongs to the thiazolidinedione group, was briefly used in the UK but has been withdrawn because of severe hepatic reactions. It continues to be used in the USA and Japan. Repaglinide, a benzoic acid derivation which stimulates insulin production at meal times has been given FDA approval for NIDDM patients.

Principles of insulin treatment

Injections

The needles used to inject insulin are very fine and sharp. Even though most injections are virtually painless, patients are understandably apprehensive and treatment begins with a lesson in injection technique. Insulin is either drawn up from the vial into special plastic insulin syringes marked in units (100 U in 1 mL), or is administered by a pen injection device. Injections are given into a pinch on the skin on the thighs, abdomen or upper arm, and the needle is usually inserted to its full length. Most patients starting insulin injection prefer pen devices when given a choice. Both reusable and disposable pen devices are available.

The injection site used should be changed regularly to prevent areas of lipohypertrophy. The rate of insulin absorption depends on local subcutaneous blood flow, and is accelerated by exercise, local massage or a warm environment. Absorption is more rapid from the abdomen than from the arm, and is slowest from the thigh. All these factors can influence the shape of the insulin profile.

All patients need careful training for a life with insulin, but routine hospital admission to begin insulin treatment is unnecessary where facilities exist for community support.

Insulin preparations

Insulin is found in every creature with a backbone, and the central part of the molecule shows few species differences. Small differences in the amino acid sequence may alter the antigenicity of the molecule. Beef insulin differs from human insulin by three amino acids and readily induces antibody formation, whereas pork insulin, which differs by only one amino acid, is relatively non-immunogenic.

However, animal insulins have now largely been replaced by biosynthetic human insulin, which is produced by DNA coding of cultured yeast or bacterial cells to produce proinsulin, with subsequent enzymatic cleavage to insulin. This technology has permitted development of insulin analogues, in which the structure of the insulin molecule is modified in such a way as to modify its pharmacokinetics without altering its biological effect. Human insulin is now standard in most of the West, but animal insulins are still used widely in developing countries. Insulin analogues will be used increasingly in the next few years (see below).

Formulations

Soluble insulin. Soluble insulin forms a clear solution, which is short-acting when injected. Soluble insulin alone should be used in acute situations such as ketoacidosis or surgery.

Prolonged acting insulins. Soluble insulin can also be formulated with protamine or zinc to retard its actions; insulin prepared in this way is cloudy in appearance. Protamine or NPH (neutral protamine Hagedorn) insulin, also known as isophane insulin, can be premixed with soluble insulin to form stable mixtures. A range of these mixtures is available, but the combination of 30% soluble with 70% NPH is the most widely used. Zinc insulins are prepared by precipitation of insulin crystals in the presence of excess zinc. The duration of action of the insulin is proportional to the size of the crystals. Since an excess of zinc is present in the vial, these insulins cannot be premixed with soluble insulin, but both zinc and protamine insulins can be mixed in the syringe with soluble insulin immediately prior to injection.

Insulin analogues. Standard insulin formulations have a number of limitations. The short-acting preparations enter the circulation too slowly, reaching a peak 60–90 minutes after injection, and their effect persists too long after meals. This delay in absorption is due mainly to the fact that soluble insulin forms hexamers, in which six insulin molecules form around a zinc core. These hexamers dissociate relatively slowly following injection. Insulin lispro (Humalog) is an analogue in which reversal of the sequence of two amino acids on the β chain has produced an insulin which dissociates much more rapidly from hexamers, and thus enters the circulation more rapidly than soluble insulin (Fig 17.8). This and similar analogues in development are likely to prove useful in patients on intensified insulin therapy, but their role is not fully defined. Genetically engineered long-acting insulin analogues are also in development and are currently undergoing clinical trials.

Insulin in clinical use

Administration

In normal subjects a sharp increase in insulin occurs after meals; this is superimposed on a constant background of secretion (Fig 17.9). Insulin therapy attempts to reproduce this pattern, but ideal control is usually impossible to achieve for four reasons:

- In normal subjects, insulin is secreted directly into the portal circulation and passes directly to the liver in high concentration; about 50% of the insulin produced by the pancreas is cleared by the liver. In contrast, insulin injected subcutaneously passes into the systemic circulation before passage to the liver. Insulin-treated patients therefore have lower portal levels of insulin and higher systemic levels.
- Subcutaneous soluble insulin takes 60–90 minutes to achieve peak plasma levels, so the onset and offset of action are too slow.
- The absorption of subcutaneous insulin into the circulation is variable. The longer-acting the preparation, the more erratic the absorption.
- Basal insulin levels are constant in the normal state, but injected insulin invariably peaks and declines, with resulting swings in metabolic control.

Individuals vary, and so therapy must be tailored accordingly. One approach to therapy is outlined here.

Young patients
Young people can be started on injections of an intermediate insulin at a dose of 8–10 U twice-daily. Some recovery of endogenous insulin secretion may occur over the first few months (the 'honeymoon period') and the insulin dose may need to be reduced or even stopped for a period. Requirements rise thereafter and a multiple injection regimen is then appropriate for most younger patients. This is flexible and usually highly acceptable.

Patients with NIDDM
There is no consensus for insulin therapy in NIDDM. Twice-daily injections of premixed soluble and isophane insulins (e.g. Mixtard) are widely used and reasonably effective. Combinations of insulin with sulphonylureas or metformin are popular outside the UK. It is increasingly recognized that more aggressive treatment, such as with intensified insulin therapy, will be needed to reduce the risk of late complications.

Multiple injections (Fig 17.10)
If glycaemic control is inadequate with the standard approach, the alternatives are multiple insulin injections or continuous subcutaneous insulin infusion (CSII). Both methods require a planned approach to life, with special attention to diet and exercise and frequent blood-glucose testing.

The introduction of 'pen injection' devices has made this approach much more acceptable to patients. Two variants are shown diagrammatically in Figs 17.10.

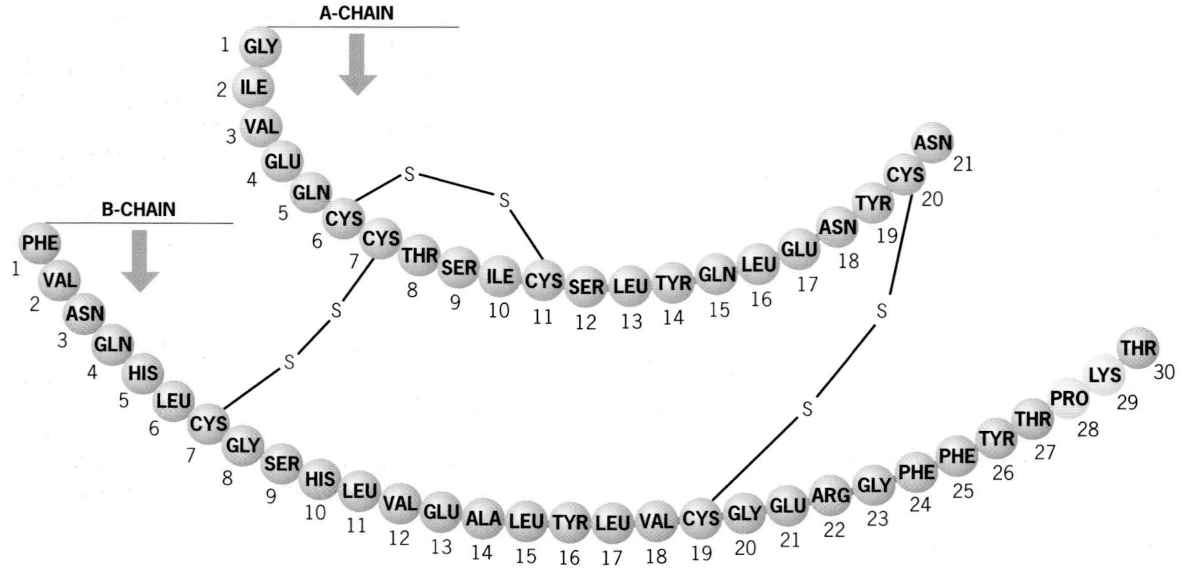

Fig 17.8
Amino acid structure of human insulin. Lispro is an insulin analogue created by reversing the position of the amino acids proline and lysine of positions 28 and 29 of the insulin β chain

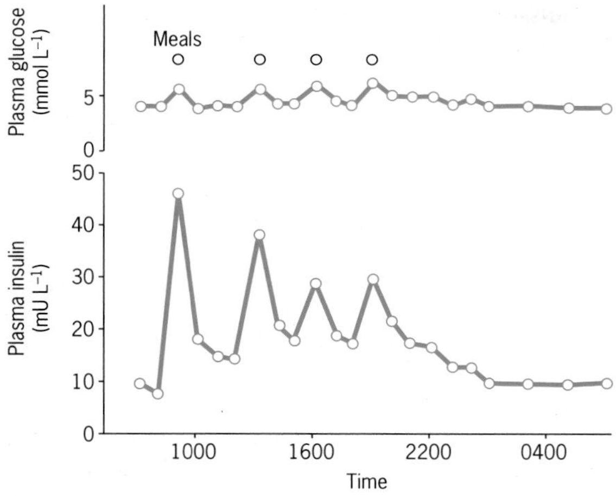

Fig 17.9
Glucose and insulin profiles in normal subjects

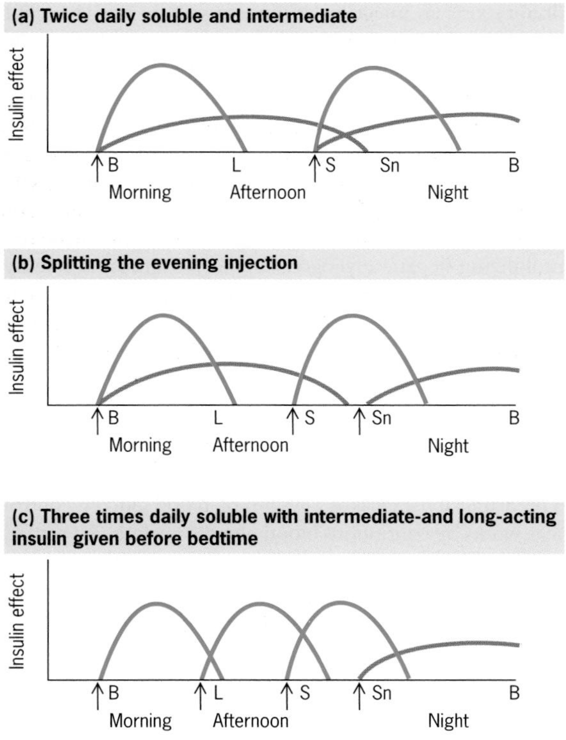

Fig 17.10
Insulin regimens. Profiles of soluble insulins are shown as blue lines and intermediate- or long-acting insulin as purple lines. The arrows indicate when the injections are given. **(a)** Twice-daily soluble and intermediate. **(b)** Splitting the evening injection. **(c)** Thrice-daily soluble with additional intermediate- or long-acting insulin given before bedtime. B, breakfast; L, lunch; S, supper; Sn, snack (bedtime)

Multiple injection regimens and infusion devices have the advantage of flexibility concerning mealtimes, which is of great value to patients with busy jobs, shift workers and those who travel regularly. The amount eaten at each meal can be chosen at mealtime and an appropriate dose of insulin given. With twice-daily regimens, the size and timing of meals is fixed more rigidly.

Infusion devices
CSII (continuous subcutaneous insulin infusion) is delivered by a small pump strapped around the waist that infuses a constant trickle of insulin via a needle in the subcutaneous tissues. Mealtime doses are delivered when the patient touches a button on the side of the pump.

This approach is particularly useful in the overnight period. Disadvantages include the nuisance of being attached to a gadget, skin infections, and the risk of ketoacidosis if the flow of insulin is broken (since these patients have no protective reservoir of depot insulin). Infusion pumps should only be used by specialized centres able to offer a round-the-clock service to their patients.

Social implications

Patients starting on insulin need to inform the driving licence authority and their insurance companies. They are also wise to inform their employers. Certain types of work are unsuitable for insulin-treated patients, including driving heavy goods or public service vehicles, working at heights, piloting an aircraft or working close to dangerous machinery in motion. Certain professions such as the police and the armed forces are barred to all diabetic patients but there are few other limitations, although a considerable amount of ill-informed prejudice exists.

Complications of insulin therapy

At the injection site

Shallow injections result in intradermal insulin delivery and painful, reddened lesions or even scarring. Injection site abscesses occur but are extremely rare.

Local allergic responses sometimes occur early in therapy but usually resolve spontaneously. Generalized allergic responses are exceptionally rare.

Lipodystrophies that may occur include lipoatrophy, a local allergic response now virtually abolished by the use of highly purified insulins, and lipohypertrophy, occurring as a result of overuse of a single injection site with any type of insulin.

Insulin resistance

The most common cause of mild insulin resistance is obesity. Occasional unstable patients require massive insulin doses, often with a fluctuating requirement. There are often associated behavioural problems. Insulin resistance associated with antibodies directed against the insulin receptor has been reported in patients with acanthosis nigricans.

Weight gain

Patients who are non-compliant with their diet and predisposed to weight gain may show progressive weight gain on treatment, especially if the insulin dose is increased inappropriately – insulin makes you feel hungry!

Hypoglycaemia

This is the most common complication of insulin therapy and is a major cause of anxiety for patients and relatives. Symptoms develop when the blood glucose level falls below 3 mmol L^{-1} and typically develop over a few minutes, with most patients experiencing 'adrenergic' features of sweating, tremor and a pounding heart beat. Physical signs include pallor and a cold sweat. Many patients with longstanding diabetes report loss of these warning symptoms and are at a greater risk of progressing to more severe hypoglycaemia. Such patients appear pale, drowsy or detached, signs that their relatives quickly learn to recognize. Behaviour is clumsy or inappropriate, and some become irritable or even aggressive. Others slip rapidly into hypoglycaemic coma. Occasionally, patients develop convulsions during hypoglycaemic coma, especially at night. It is important not to confuse this with idiopathic epilepsy, especially since patients with frequent hypoglycaemia often have abnormalities on the EEG. Another presentation is with a hemiparesis that resolves within a few minutes when glucose is administered.

Hypoglycaemia is a common problem. Virtually all patients experience intermittent symptoms and one in three will go into a coma at some stage in their lives. A small minority suffer attacks that are so frequent and severe as to be virtually disabling.

Hypoglycaemia results from an imbalance between injected insulin and a patient's normal diet, activity and basal insulin requirement. The times of greatest risk are before meals and during the night. Irregular eating habits, unusual exertion and alcohol excess may precipitate episodes; other cases appear to be due simply to variation in insulin absorption.

Hypoglycaemic unawareness. People with diabetes have an impaired ability to counter-regulate glucose levels after hypoglycaemia. The glucagon response is invariably deficient, even though the α cells are preserved and respond normally to other stimuli. The adrenaline response may also fail in patients with a long duration of diabetes, and this is associated with loss of warning symptoms. Recurrent hypoglycaemia may itself induce a state of hypoglycaemia unawareness, and the ability to recognize the condition may sometimes be restored by relaxing control for a few weeks.

Nocturnal hypoglycaemia. Basal insulin requirements fall during the night but increase again from about 4 am onwards, at a time when levels of injected insulin are falling. As a result many patients awake with high blood glucose levels, but find that injecting more insulin at night increases the risk of hypoglycaemia in the early hours of the morning. The problem may be helped by (a) checking that a bedtime snack is taken regularly, (b) taking intermediate insulin at bedtime rather than before supper, and (c) reducing the dose of soluble insulin before supper, since the effects of this persist well into the night.

URGENT TREATMENT OF HYPOGLYCAEMIA

Patients and their families quickly learn to recognize and treat the symptoms of hypoglycaemia.

Mild hypoglycaemia

Any form of rapidly absorbed carbohydrate will relieve the early symptoms, and sufferers should always carry glucose or sweets. Drowsy individuals will be able to take carbohydrate in liquid form (e.g. Lucozade). All patients and their close relatives need careful training about the risks of hypoglycaemia. They should be warned not to take more carbohydrate than necessary, *since this causes a rebound to hyperglycaemia*, and the dangers of alcohol excess and hypoglycaemia while driving need to be emphasized.

Severe hypoglycaemia

The diagnosis of severe hypoglycaemia resulting in confusion or coma is simple and can usually be made on clinical grounds, backed by a bedside blood test. If real doubt exists an injection of glucose will do no harm, but blood should be taken for glucose estimation before the injection is given. Patients should carry a card or wear a bracelet or necklace identifying themselves as diabetic, and these should be looked for in unconscious patients.

Unconscious patients should be given intravenous glucose (25–50 mL of 50% dextrose solution) followed by a flush of normal saline to preserve the vein, or intramuscular glucagon (1 mg). Glucagon acts by mobilizing hepatic glycogen, and works almost as rapidly as glucose. It is simple to administer and can be given at home by relatives. Oral glucose is given to replenish glycogen reserves once the patient revives.

Measuring control

The 'artificial pancreas' is a system of blood glucose control that works by continuous blood glucose analysis. This is fed into a computer, which delivers an appropriate amount of insulin into the circulation. Patients on insulin need to devise their own simplified form of this feedback loop.

Urine tests

Urine tests are simple to perform using dipsticks, and it can usually be assumed that a patient with consistently negative tests and no symptoms of hypoglycaemia is fairly well controlled. Even so, the correlation between urine tests and simultaneous blood glucose is poor for three reasons:

- Changes in urine glucose lag behind changes in blood glucose.
- The mean renal threshold is around 10 mmol L^{-1} but the range is wide (7–13 mmol L^{-1}). The threshold also rises with age.
- Urine tests can give no guidance concerning blood glucose levels below the renal threshold.

Urinary ketones may also be measured by a dipstick test. This is rarely helpful in routine outpatient management, but can be useful in special situations such as with intercurrent infections. Heavy ketonuria can inhibit some dipstick tests for glucose.

Blood glucose testing

This provides the best assessment of day-to-day control. The fasting blood glucose concentration is a useful guide to therapy in NIDDM.

A random blood glucose test (e.g. in the clinic) is of limited value, but patients may easily be taught to provide their own profiles by testing finger-prick blood samples with reagent strips and reading these with the aid of a visual scale or reflectance meter. It has been amply demonstrated that most patients are willing and able to provide reasonably accurate results provided they have been properly taught.

Blood is taken from the side of a fingertip (*not* from the tip, which is densely innervated) using a special lancet (e.g. Monolet), which can be fitted to a spring-loaded device. Patients are asked to take regular profiles (e.g. four daily samples on two days each week) and to note these in a diary or record book. Home blood glucose monitoring is essential for good diabetic control. Patients are encouraged to adjust their insulin dose as appropriate and should ideally be able to obtain advice over the telephone when needed.

Glycosylated haemoglobin (HbA_1 or HbA_{1c}) and fructosamine

Glycosylation of haemoglobin occurs as a two-step reaction, resulting in the formation of a covalent bond between the glucose molecule and the terminal valine of the β chain of the haemoglobin molecule. The rate at which this reaction occurs is related to the prevailing glucose concentration. Glycosylated haemoglobin is expressed as a percentage of the normal haemoglobin (normal range approximately 4–8% depending on the technique of measurement). This test provides an index of the average blood glucose concentration over the life of the haemoglobin molecule (approximately six weeks). The figure will be misleading if the lifespan of the red cell is reduced or if an abnormal haemoglobin or thalassaemia is present. Although the glycosylated haemoglobin test provides a rapid assessment of the level of glycaemic control in a given patient, blood glucose testing is needed before the clinician can know what to do about it.

Glycosylated plasma proteins ('fructosamine') may also be measured as an index of control. Glycosylated albumin is the major component and fructosamine measurement relates to glycaemic control over the preceding 1–3 weeks. The technique is cheaper and quicker to perform than glycosylated haemoglobin measurement and lends itself to automation. It is useful in patients with haemoglobinopathy and in pregnancy (when haemoglobin turnover is changeable). Correlation between the two tests is not strong. This may reflect the greater interindividual variation in plasma proteins than in haemoglobin. It is also less reliable, and measurement of HbA_{1c} is often preferred.

Does good glycaemic control matter?

Studies in experimental animals strongly suggest that improved control is protective and this has been confirmed in humans. The Diabetes Control and Complications Trial (DCCT) in the USA compared standard and intensive insulin therapy in a prospective controlled trial of young patients with IDDM. Even on intensive therapy, mean blood glucose levels were 40% above the non-diabetic range, but this level of control reduced the risk of progression to retinopathy by 60%, nephropathy by 30% and neuropathy by 20% over the seven years of the study.

Near-normoglycaemia should, therefore, be the goal for all young patients with IDDM. The unwanted effects of this policy include weight gain and a 2–3 fold increase in the risk of severe hypoglycaemia. Control should be less strict in those with a history of recurrent severe hypoglycaemia. It remains unclear whether equally stringent standards should be applied in patients with NIDDM, particularly since a protective effect upon progression of macrovascular disease has yet to be clearly demonstrated.

Can established complications be halted or reversed by intensive insulin therapy? Insulin infusion devices have made near-normal blood glucose control possible for closely supervised groups of patients. Studies in patients with established retinopathy have shown that patients with early retinopathy benefit from 2–3 years of intensive therapy, but that patients with more advanced retinal changes generally do not. Retinopathy may show a transient deterioration when strict control is first established. These observations suggest that microvascular lesions are self-perpetuating once a threshold level of damage has been reached.

Is macrovascular disease influenced by control? Patients with impaired glucose tolerance have an increased rate of large vessel disease but rarely develop microvascular lesions. This might be because large arteries are more sensitive to elevated glucose levels, but it has also been suggested that hyperinsulinaemia (present in many patients with NIDDM and a common consequence of insulin treatment) is a cause of accelerated atherogenesis. At present there is little evidence that good glycaemic control protects against arterial disease. A large trial in patients with NIDDM is due to report shortly and should allow this question to be answered.

Regular checks for patients with diabetes

Information box 17.1 is modified from the guidelines set out in *The European Patients' Charter* pulished by the St Vincent Declaration Steering Committee of the WHO. The charter sets out goals for both the healthcare team and the patient.

Information

These items are modified from those set out in *The European Patients' Charter* published by the St Vincent Declaration Steering Committee of the WHO. The charter sets out goals for both the healthcare team and the patient.

Checked at each visit
- Review of self-monitoring results and current treatment.
- Talk about targets and change where necessary.
- Talk about any general or specific problems.
- Continued education.

Checked at least once a year
- Biochemical assessment of metabolic control (e.g. glycosylated Hb test).
- Measure bodyweight.
- Measure blood pressure.
- Measure plasma lipids (except in extreme old age).
- Measure visual acuity.
- Examine state of retina (ophthalmoscope or retinal photo).
- Test urine for proteinuria.
- Test blood for renal function (creatinine).
- Check condition of feet, pulses and neurology.
- Review cardiovascular risk factors.
- Review self-monitoring and injection techniques.
- Review eating habits.

Information box 17.1 Regular checks for patients with diabetes

FURTHER READING

Barnett AH, Owens DR (1997) Insulin analogues. *Lancet* **349**: 47–51.

Ferner RE, Alberti KG (1989) Sulphonylureas in the treatment of non-insulin-dependent diabetes. *Quarterly Journal of Medicine* **73**: 987–995.

Gaster B, Hirsh IB (1998) The effects of improved glycaemic control on complications in type II diabetes. *Archives of Internal Medicine* **158**: 134–140.

Holleman F, Hoekstra JBL (1997) Insulin Lispro. *New England Journal of Medicine* **337**: 176–183.

Petrie J, Small M, Connell J (1997) 'Glitazones', a prospect for non-insulin-dependent diabetes. *Lancet* **349**: 70–71.

St Vincent Declaration Steering Committee of WHO Europe (1991) The European Patient's Charter. *Diabetic Medicine* **8**: 782–783.

Tattersall RB, Gale EA (eds) (1990) *Diabetes Clinical Management*. Edinburgh: Churchill Livingstone.

Diabetic metabolic emergencies

The main terms used are defined in Table 17.5.

Table 17.5
Terms used in uncontrolled diabetes

Ketonuria	Detectable ketone levels in the urine; it should be appreciated that ketonuria occurs in fasted non-diabetics and may be found in relatively well-controlled patients with insulin-dependent diabetes mellitus
Ketosis	Elevated plasma ketone levels in the absence of acidosis
Diabetic ketoacidosis	A metabolic emergency in which hyperglycaemia is associated with a metabolic acidosis due to greatly raised (>5 mmol L^{-1}) ketone levels
Non-ketotic hyperosmolar state	A metabolic emergency in which uncontrolled hyperglycaemia induces a hyperosmolar state in the absence of significant ketosis
Lactic acidosis	A metabolic emergency in which elevated lactate levels induce a metabolic acidosis. In diabetic patients it is rare and associated with biguanide therapy

Diabetic ketoacidosis

Diabetic ketoacidosis is the hallmark of IDDM. Its main *causes* can be grouped as follows:

- previously undiagnosed diabetes
- interruption of insulin therapy
- the stress of intercurrent illness.

The majority of cases reaching hospital could have been *prevented* by earlier diagnosis, better communication between patient and doctor, and better patient education.

The most common error of management is for patients to reduce or omit insulin because they feel unable to eat owing to nausea or vomiting. This is a factor in at least 25% of all hospital admissions. Insulin should never be stopped.

PATHOGENESIS

Ketoacidosis is a state of uncontrolled catabolism associated with insulin deficiency. Insulin deficiency is a necessary precondition since only a modest elevation in insulin levels is sufficient to inhibit hepatic ketogenesis and stable patients do not readily develop ketoacidosis when insulin is withdrawn. Other factors include counter-regulatory hormone excess and fluid depletion. The combination of insulin deficiency with excess of its hormonal antagonists leads to the parallel processes shown in Fig 17.11.

In the absence of insulin, hepatic glucose production accelerates, and peripheral uptake by tissues such as muscle is reduced. Rising glucose levels lead to an osmotic diuresis, loss of fluid and electrolytes, and dehydration. Plasma osmolality rises and renal perfusion falls.

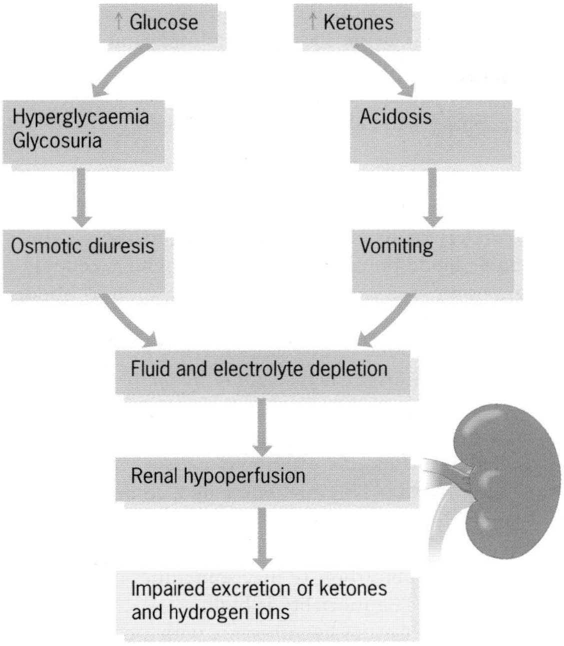

Fig 17.11
Dehydration occurs during ketoacidosis as a consequence of two parallel processes. Hyperglycaemia results in osmotic diuresis, and hyperketonaemia results in acidosis and vomiting. Renal hypoperfusion then occurs and a vicious circle is established as the kidney becomes less able to compensate for the acidosis

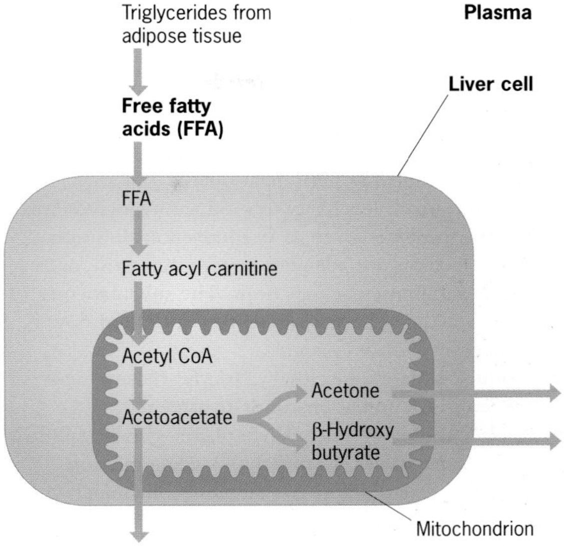

Fig 17.12
Ketogenesis. During insulin deficiency, lipolysis accelerates and free fatty acids taken up by liver cells form the substrate for ketone formation (acetoacetate, acetone and β-hydroxybutyrate) within the mitochondrion

In parallel, rapid lipolysis occurs, leading to elevated circulating free fatty-acid levels. The free fatty acids are broken down to fatty acyl-CoA within the liver cells, and this in turn is converted to ketone bodies within the mitochondria (Fig 17.12).

Accumulation of ketone bodies produces a metabolic acidosis. This is typically associated with nausea and vomiting, leading to further loss of fluid and electrolytes. The excess ketones are excreted in the urine but also appear in the breath, producing a distinctive smell similar to that of acetone. Respiratory compensation for the acidosis leads to hyperventilation, graphically described as 'air hunger'. Progressive dehydration impairs renal excretion of hydrogen ions and ketones, aggravating the acidosis. As the pH falls below 7.0 ($[H^+] > 100$ nmol L^{-1}), pH-dependent enzyme systems in many cells function less effectively. Untreated, severe ketoacidosis is invariably fatal.

CLINICAL FEATURES

The features of ketoacidosis are those of uncontrolled diabetes with acidosis, and include prostration, hyperventilation (Kussmaul respiration), nausea, vomiting and, occasionally, abdominal pain. The latter is sometimes so severe as to cause confusion with a surgical acute abdomen.

Some patients are mentally alert at presentation, but confusion and stupor are common. Up to 5% present in coma. Evidence of marked dehydration is present and the eyeball is lax to pressure in severe cases. Hyperventilation is present but becomes less marked in very severe acidosis owing to respiratory depression. The smell of ketones on the breath allows an instant diagnosis to be made by those able to detect the odour. The skin is dry and the body temperature is often subnormal, even in the presence of infection; in such cases, pyrexia may develop later.

DIAGNOSIS

This is confirmed by demonstrating hyperglycaemia with ketonaemia or heavy ketonuria, and acidosis. No time should be lost and treatment is started as soon as the first blood sample has been taken.

Hyperglycaemia is demonstrated by dipstick, while a blood sample is sent to the laboratory for confirmation. Ketonaemia is confirmed by centrifuging a blood sample and testing the plasma with a dipstick that measures ketones. An arterial blood sample is taken for blood gas analysis.

MANAGEMENT

The principles of management are as follows (Information box 17.2).

- Replace the *fluid losses* with normal saline.
- Replace the *electrolyte losses*. Potassium levels need to be monitored with great care. Patients have a total body potassium deficit although initial plasma levels may not be low. Insulin therapy leads to uptake of potassium by the cells with a consequent fall in plasma K^+ levels. Potassium is therefore given as soon as insulin is started.
- Restore the *acid–base balance*. A patient with healthy kidneys will rapidly compensate for the metabolic acidosis once the circulating volume is restored.

Bicarbonate is seldom necessary and is only considered if the pH is below 7.0 ([H^+] >100 nmol L^{-1}), and is best given as an isotonic (1.26%) solution.
- Replace the *deficient insulin*. Modern treatment is with relatively modest doses of insulin, which lower blood glucose by suppressing hepatic glucose output rather than by stimulating peripheral uptake, and are therefore much less likely to produce hypoglycaemia. Soluble insulin is given as an intravenous infusion where facilities for adequate supervision exist, or as hourly intramuscular injections. The subcutaneous route is avoided because subcutaneous blood flow is reduced in shocked patients.
- Monitor *blood glucose* closely. Hourly measurement is needed in the initial phases of treatment.
- Replace the *energy losses*. When plasma glucose falls to near-normal values (12 mmol L^{-1}), saline infusion should be replaced with 5% dextrose containing 20 mmol L^{-1} of potassium chloride. The insulin infusion rate is reduced and adjusted according to blood glucose.
- Seek the *underlying cause*. Physical examination may reveal a source of infection (e.g. a perianal abscess). Two common markers of infection are misleading: fever is unusual even when infection is present, and polymorpholeucocytosis is present even in the absence of infection. Relevant investigations include a chest X-ray, urine and blood cultures, and an ECG (to exclude myocardial infarction). If infection is suspected, broad-spectrum antibiotics are started once the appropriate cultures have been taken.

Problems of management

- *Hypotension*. This may lead to renal shutdown. Plasma expanders (or whole blood) are therefore given if the systolic blood pressure is below 80 mmHg. A central venous pressure line is useful in this situation. A bladder catheter is inserted if no urine is produced within two hours, but routine catheterization is not necessary.
- *Coma*. The usual principles apply (see p. 1044). It is essential to pass a nasogastric tube to prevent aspiration since gastric stasis is common and carries the risk of aspiration pneumonia if a drowsy patient vomits.
- *Cerebral oedema*. This rare, but feared, complication has mostly been reported in children or young adults. Excessive rehydration and use of hypertonic fluids such as 8.4% bicarbonate may sometimes be responsible. The mortality is high.
- *Hypothermia*. Severe hypothermia with a core temperature below 33°C may occur and may be overlooked unless a rectal temperature is taken with a low-reading thermometer.

Information

Diagnosis
- Hyperglycaemia: measure blood glucose
- Ketonaemia: test plasma with Ketostix/Acetest
- Acidosis: measure blood gases

Investigations
- Blood glucose
- Urea and electrolytes
- Osmolality
- Full blood count
- Blood gases
- Blood and urine culture
- Chest X-ray
- ECG
- Cardiac enzymes

Management
- *Insulin* i.v. 6 U stat, then 6 U hourly by infusion *OR* i.m. 20 U stat, then 6 U hourly by i.m. injection.
- *Fluid replacement*. Normal saline 0.9% (150 mmol each of Na^+ and Cl^- per litre). An average regimen would be 1 L in 30 minutes, then 1 L in one hour, then 1 L in two hours, then 1 L in four hours, and then 1 L in six hours. Add 20 mmol of KCl to each litre.

IF:
- Blood pressure is below 80 mmHg systolic, give 2 U whole blood or plasma expander
- pH below 7.0 ([H^+] > 100 nmol L^{-1}), give 500 mL of sodium bicarbonate 1.26% (150 mmol each of Na^+ and HCO_3^- per litre) plus 10 mmol L^{-1} of KCl. Repeat if necessary to bring pH above 7.0 but monitor carefully.

Special measures
- Broad-spectrum antibiotics if infection is likely
- Bladder catheter if no urine is passed after two hours
- Nasogastric tube if drowsy
- CVP line in elderly or shocked patients
- Consider subcutaneous heparin in the comatose, elderly or obese

Subsequent management
- Monitor glucose hourly for eight hours.
- Monitor electrolytes two-hourly for eight hours.
- Adjust K^+ replacement according to results.
- When blood glucose falls to 10–12 mmol L^{-1}, change infusion fluid to 5% dextrose (1 L plus 20 mmol L^{-1} of KCl) six-hourly. Continue insulin with the dose adjusted according to hourly blood glucose results.

Note: The regimen of fluid replacement set out above is a guideline for patients with severe ketoacidosis. Excessive fluid can precipitate pulmonary and cerebral oedema; inadequate replacement can lead to renal impairment. Infusion must, therefore, be tailored to the individual and monitored carefully throughout treatment.

Information box 17.2 Guidelines for the diagnosis and management of **diabetic ketoacidosis**

- *Late complications.* These include stasis pneumonia and deep-vein thrombosis, and occur especially in the comatose or elderly patient.
- *Complications of therapy.* These include hypoglycaemia and hypokalaemia, due to loss of K^+ in the urine from osmotic diuresis. Overenthusiastic fluid replacement may precipitate pulmonary oedema in the very young or the very old. Hyperchloraemic acidosis may develop in the course of treatment since patients have lost a large variety of negatively charged electrolytes, which are replaced with chloride. The kidneys usually correct this spontaneously within a few days.

Subsequent management

Intravenous fluids and insulin are continued until the patient feels able to eat and keep food down. The drip is then taken down and a similar amount of insulin is given as three or four soluble subcutaneous doses per day until a maintenance regimen can be restarted.

Sliding-scale regimens are often unnecessary and may even delay the establishment of stable blood glucose levels.

The treatment of diabetic ketoacidosis is incomplete without a careful enquiry into the causes of the episode and advice as to how to avoid its recurrence.

Non-ketotic hyperosmolar state

This condition, in which severe hyperglycaemia develops without significant ketosis, is the metabolic emergency characteristic of uncontrolled NIDDM. Patients present in middle or later life, often with previously undiagnosed diabetes. Common precipitating factors include consumption of glucose-rich fluids (e.g. Lucozade), concurrent medication such as thiazide diuretics or steroids, and intercurrent illness.

Non-ketotic coma and ketoacidosis represent two ends of a spectrum rather than two distinct disorders. The biochemical differences (shown in Information box 17.3) may partly be explained as follows:

- *Age.* The extreme dehydration characteristic of non-ketotic coma may be related to age. Old people experience thirst less acutely, and more readily become dehydrated. In addition, the mild renal impairment associated with age results in increased urinary losses of fluid and electrolytes.
- *The degree of insulin deficiency.* This is less severe in non-ketotic coma. Endogenous insulin levels are sufficient to inhibit hepatic ketogenesis, whereas glucose production is unrestrained.

CLINICAL FEATURES

The characteristic clinical features on presentation are dehydration and stupor or coma. Impairment of consciousness is directly related to the degree of hyperosmolality. Evidence of underlying illness such as pneumonia or pyelonephritis may be present, and the hyperosmolar state may predispose to stroke, myocardial infarction or arterial insufficiency in the lower limbs.

Information

Examples of blood values

	Severe ketoacidosis	***Non-ketotic hyperosmolar coma***
Na^+ (mmol L^{-1})	140	155
K^+ (mmol L^{-1})	5	5
Cl^- (mmol L^{-1})	100	110
HCO_3^- (mmol L^{-1})	5	30
Urea (mmol L^{-1})	8	15
Glucose (mmol L^{-1})	30	50
Arterial pH	7.0	7.35

The normal range of **osmolality** is 285–300 mOsmol L^{-1}. It can be measured directly, or can be calculated approximately from the formula:

Osmolality = $2(Na^+ + K^+)$ + glucose + urea.

For example, in the example of severe ketoacidosis given above:

Osmolality = 2(140 + 5) + 30 + 8 = 328 mOsmol L^{-1}

and in the example of non-ketotic hyperosmolar coma:

Osmolality = 2(155 + 5) + 50 + 15 = 385 mOsmol L^{-1}.

The normal **anion gap** is less than 17. It is calculated as $(Na^+ + K^+) - (Cl^- + HCO_3^-)$. In the example of ketoacidosis the anion gap is 40, and in the example of non-ketotic hyperosmolar coma the anion gap is 20. Mild hyperchloraemic acidosis may develop in the course of therapy. This will be shown by a rising plasma chloride and persistence of a low bicarbonate even though the anion gap has returned to normal.

Information box 17.3 Electrolyte changes in **diabetic ketoacidosis** and **non-ketotic hyperosmolar state**

INVESTIGATIONS AND TREATMENT

These are, with some exceptions, according to the guidelines for ketoacidosis. Many patients are extremely sensitive to insulin and the glucose concentration may plummet. The resultant change in osmolality may cause cerebral damage. It is sometimes useful to infuse insulin at a rate of 3 U per hour for the first 2–3 h, increasing to 6 U h^{-1} if glucose is falling too slowly. Normal saline is the standard fluid for replacement. Avoid half-normal saline (0.45%) except in exceptional circumstances, since rapid dilution of the blood may cause more cerebral damage than a few hours of exposure to hypernatraemia.

PROGNOSIS

The reported mortality ranges as high as 20–30%, mainly because of the advanced age of the patients and the frequency of intercurrent illness. Unlike ketoacidosis, non-ketotic hyperglycaemia is not an absolute indication for subsequent insulin therapy, and survivors may do well on diet and oral agents.

Lactic acidosis

Lactic acidosis may occur in diabetic patients on biguanide therapy. The risk in patients taking metformin is extremely low provided that the therapeutic dose is not exceeded and the drug is withheld in patients with advanced hepatic or renal dysfunction.

Patients present with a severe metabolic acidosis, usually without significant hyperglycaemia or ketosis, and treatment is by rehydration and infusion of isotonic 1.26% bicarbonate. The mortality is in excess of 50%.

Complications of diabetes

When insulin was introduced it was assumed that it would provide complete and adequate replacement therapy, just as thyroxine does in hypothyroidism.

Time proved that insulin-treated patients still have a considerably reduced life expectancy. Those diagnosed before the age of 20 years in older studies had only a 60–70% chance of living past the age of 50 years, although there are indications of a steady improvement in survival. The excess deaths are mainly due to diabetic nephropathy, but there is also a considerable excess cardiovascular mortality. Heart disease, peripheral vascular disease and stroke are the major causes of death in patients over the age of 50 years.

Table 17.6
Diabetic risk factors for macrovascular complications

Duration
Increasing age
Systolic hypertension
Hyperinsulinaemia due to insulin resistance associated with obesity and syndrome X
Hyperlipidaemia, particularly hypertriglyceridaemia
Proteinuria (including microalbuminuria)
Other factors are the same as for the general population

Macrovascular complications

(Table 17.6)

Diabetes is a risk factor in the development of atherosclerosis. This risk is related to that of the background population. For example, Japanese diabetics are much less likely to develop atherosclerosis than patients in Europe but are much more likely to develop it than non-diabetic Japanese.

The excess risk to diabetics compared with the general population increases as one moves down the body:

- Stroke is twice as likely.
- Myocardial infarction is 3–5 times as likely and women with diabetes lose their premenopausal protection from coronary artery disease.
- Amputation of a foot for gangrene is 50 times as likely.

Diabetes is additive with other risk factors for large-vessel disease. In other words, the diabetic who smokes or is obese, hypertensive or hyperlipidaemic adds the risks conferred by these conditions to that of diabetes itself.

Insulin resistance

Hyperinsulinaemia that is due to insulin resistance associated with obesity is sometimes known as '*syndrome X*' (confusingly, the same term is used by cardiologists for a rare variant of angina) or the 'metabolic sydrome'. This includes glucose intolerance, hypertension, central obesity and dyslipo-proteinaemia (increased very low density lipoprotein and reduced high-density lipoprotein). It is found in patients with NIDDM and carries a high risk of coronary artery disease.

The cause is unknown. There is an overactivity of the sympathetic nervous system but it is unclear whether this is a primary event or is secondary to insulin resistance.

Microvascular complications

In contrast to macrovascular disease, which is prevalent in the West as a whole, microvascular disease is specific to diabetes. Small blood vessels throughout the body are affected but the disease process is of particular danger in three sites:

- retina
- renal glomerulus
- nerve sheaths.

Diabetic retinopathy, nephropathy and neuropathy tend to manifest 10–20 years after diagnosis in young patients. They present earlier in older patients, probably because these have had unrecognized diabetes for months or even years prior to diagnosis.

Diabetic eye disease

Diabetes can affect the eyes in a number of ways. The most common and characteristic form of involvement is *diabetic retinopathy*. About one in three young people in this patient population is likely to develop visual problems, and in the UK 5% have in the past become blind after 30 years of diabetes. Indeed, diabetes has been the most common cause of blindness in the population as a whole up to the age of 65 years, but its prevalence is falling.

Other forms of eye disease may also occur:

- The *lens* may be affected by reversible osmotic changes in patients with acute hyperglycaemia, causing blurred vision, or by cataracts.
- *New vessel formation* in the iris (rubeosis iridis) may develop as a late complication of diabetic retinopathy and can cause glaucoma.
- *External ocular palsies*, especially of the sixth nerve, can occur (a mononeuritis).

The natural history of retinopathy (Fig 17.13)

Diabetes causes increased thickness of the basement membrane and increased permeability of the retinal capillaries. Aneurysmal dilatation may occur in some vessels while others become occluded. These changes are first detectable by fluorescein angiography: a fluorescent dye is injected into an arm vein and photographed in transit through the retinal vessels. This technique is not necessary to screen effectively for retinal disease. After 20 years of IDDM, almost all patients have some retinopathy, and 60% progress to sight-threatening proliferative retinopathy (Fig 17.14).

Background retinopathy (Fig 17.13b,c)

The first abnormality visible through the ophthalmoscope is the appearance of dot 'haemorrhages', which are actually due to capillary microaneurysms. Leakage of blood into the deeper layers of the retina produces the characteristic 'blot' haemorrhage, while exudates of fluid rich in lipids and protein give rise to hard exudates. These have a bright yellowish white colour and are often irregular in outline with a sharply defined margin.

These changes rarely develop in young patients with a duration of diabetes under 10 years, but by 20 years virtually all eyes will manifest at least the occasional microaneurysm on careful ophthalmoscopy. In contrast, retinopathy may be present at diagnosis or shortly thereafter in older patients.

Background retinopathy does not in itself constitute a threat to vision but may progress to two other distinct forms of retinopathy: maculopathy or proliferative retinopathy. Both are the consequence of damage to retinal blood vessels and resultant retinal ischaemia.

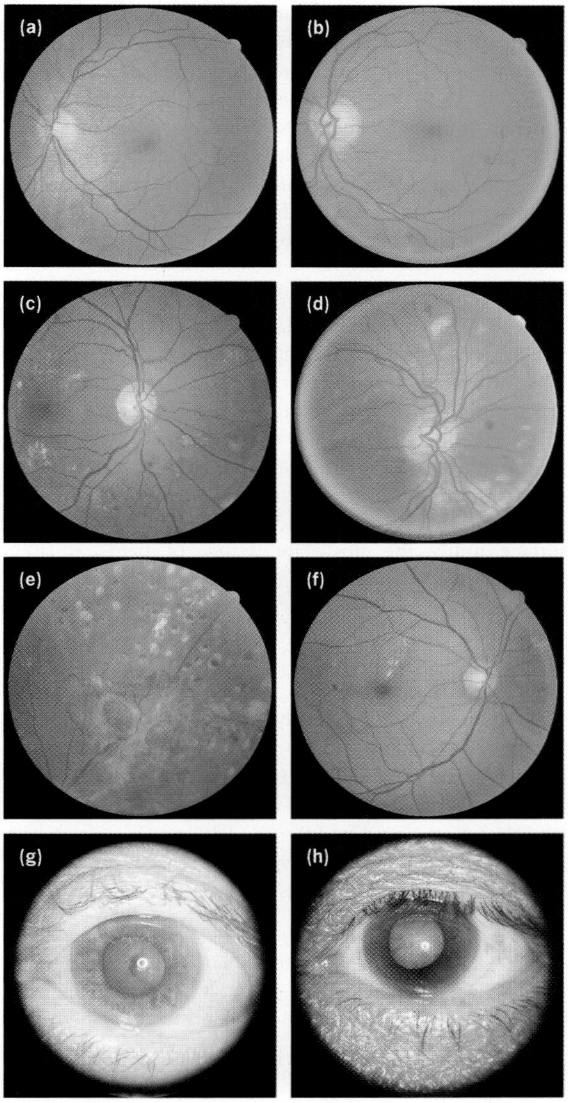

Fig 17.13
Features of diabetic eye disease.
(a) The normal macula (centre) and optic disk
(b) Dot and blot haemorrhages (early background retinopathy)
(c) Hard exudates are present in addition in background retinopathy
(d) Multiple cotton wool spots indicate pre-proliferative retinopathy requiring routine ophthalmic referral
(e) Multiple frond-like new vessels, the hallmark of proliferative retinopathy. White fibrous tissue is forming near the new vessels, a feature of advanced retinopathy (this eye also illustrates multiple xenon arc laser burns superiorly)
(f) Exudates appearing within a disk-width of the macula are a feature of an exudative maculopathy
(g) Central and **(h)** cortical cataracts can be seen against the red reflex with the ophthalmoscope

Diabetic maculopathy

This may lead to blindness in the absence of proliferation and particularly affects the older patient with NIDDM. Macular oedema is the first feature of maculopathy and may in itself result in permanent macular damage if not treated early. The first, and only, sign of this is deteriorating visual acuity and this early condition cannot be diagnosed with standard ophthalmoscopy. This is why it is essential to screen patients with diabetes regularly for changes in visual acuity. In most cases, however, maculopathy does not generate sufficient oedema to cause early loss of acuity. The process may then be detected in its later stages as encroachment of hard exudates and haemorrhages on the macular area. These later changes are easily visible on ophthalmoscopy, but only through fully dilated pupils.

Pre-proliferative retinopathy

Progressive retinal ischaemia leads to further changes which herald proliferative, sight-threatening retinopathy. The earliest sign is the appearance of 'cotton-wool spots', representing oedema resulting from retinal infarcts (Fig. 17.13d). They may also occur in severe hypertensive retinopathy. The term 'soft exudate' is often used synonymously but is best avoided. Cotton-wool spots are greyish white, have indistinct margins and a dull matt surface, unlike the glossy appearance of hard exudates. Venous beading and/or venous loops are other recognized pre-proliferative changes.

Proliferative retinopathy

Hypoxia is thought to be the signal for formation of new vessels. These lie superficially or grow forward into the vitreous, resembling fronds of seaweed. They branch repeatedly, are fragile, bleed easily (because they lack the normal supportive tissue) and may give rise to a fibrous-tissue reaction (Fig. 17.13e).

With advanced retinopathy, haemorrhages can be pre-retinal or into the vitreous. A vitreous haemorrhage presents as a loss of vision in one eye, sometimes noticed on waking, or as a floating shadow affecting the field of vision. Ophthalmoscopy gives the appearance of a featureless, grey haze. Partial recovery of vision is the rule, as the blood is reabsorbed, but repeated bleeds may occur.

Loss of vision may also result from fibrous proliferation associated with new vessel formation. This may give rise to traction bands that contract with the course of time, producing retinal detachment.

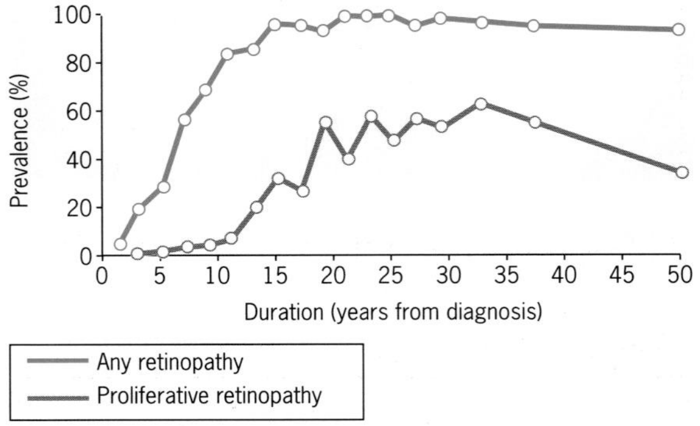

Fig 17.14
Prevalence of retinopathy in relation to duration of the disease in patients with insulin-dependent diabetes mellitus diagnosed under the age of 33 years. Almost all eventually develop background change and 60% progress to proliferative retinopathy. From *Ophthalmology* (1984) **102**: 520

Cataracts

Senile cataracts develop some 10–15 years earlier in diabetic patients than in the remainder of the population.

Juvenile or 'snowflake' cataracts are much less common. These are diffuse, rapidly progressive cataracts associated with very poorly controlled diabetes. They should be distinguished from temporary lens changes that occasionally appear during hyperosmolar states and resolve when the hyperglycaemia is brought under control.

EXAMINATION

Careful systematic examination of the eye is essential. Visual acuity and eye movements are tested, and 15–30 minutes before the eye is examined the pupils are dilated with a mydriatic such as tropicamide 0.5%. Dilating drugs should not be used, however, in patients with a history of glaucoma, except with the advice of an ophthalmologist.

The ophthalmological examination begins at arm's length. At this distance, cataracts are silhouetted against the red reflex of the retina. The ophthalmoscope is advanced until the retina is in focus. The examination begins at the optic disc, moves through each quadrant in turn, and ends with the macula (since this is least comfortable for the patient). The ophthalmoscope is then adjusted to the +10 dioptre lens for examination of the cornea, anterior chamber and lens. The location of abnormalities should always be sketched in the notes for future reference.

MANAGEMENT

There is no specific medical treatment for background retinopathy, but patients are advised not to smoke and hypertension should be treated. Development or progression of retinopathy may be accelerated by rapid improvement in glycaemic control, pregnancy and in those with nephropathy, and these groups need frequent monitoring. All patients with retinopathy should be examined regularly by a diabetologist or ophthalmologist. Early referral to an ophthalmologist is essential in the following circumstances:

- deteriorating visual acuity
- hard exudates encroaching on the macula
- pre-proliferative changes (cotton-wool spots or venous beading)
- new vessel formation.

The ophthalmologist may perform fluorescein angiography to define the extent of the problem. Maculopathy and proliferative retinopathy are often treatable by retinal laser photocoagulation; in the latter condition early effective therapy reduces the risk of visual loss by about 50%. The value of photocoagulation is particularly marked in those with disc (as against peripheral) new vessels. In one trial only 15% of treated, as against 50% of untreated, eyes with disc new vessels progressed to legal blindness. Treatment in this case is by panretinal photocoagulation with 2000–5000 laser burns to each eye. Surgery can be performed to remove vitreous haemorrhages and to treat retinal detachment.

The diabetic kidney

The kidney may be damaged by diabetes in three main ways:

- glomerular damage
- ischaemia resulting from hypertrophy of afferent and efferent arterioles
- ascending infection.

Diabetic glomerulosclerosis

Clinical nephropathy secondary to glomerular disease usually manifests 15–25 years after diagnosis and affects 25–35% of patients diagnosed under the age of 30 years. It is the leading cause of premature death in young diabetic patients. Older patients may also develop nephropathy, but the proportion affected is much smaller. Some centres have reported falling rates of diabetic nephropathy, but this may reflect good-quality local care for diabetes rather than a change in the natural history of the disease itself.

The earliest functional abnormality in the diabetic kidney is renal hypertrophy associated with a raised glomerular filtration rate. This appears soon after diagnosis and is related to poor glycaemic control.

The initial structural lesion in the glomerulus is thickening of the basement membrane. Associated changes may result in disruption of the protein cross-linkages that make the membrane an effective filter. In consequence, there is a progressive leak of large molecules (particularly protein) into the urine. The earliest evidence of this is 'microalbuminuria' – amounts of urinary albumin so small as to be undetectable by dipsticks (see p. 526). Microalbuminuria may be tested for by radioimmunoassay or by using special dipsticks. It is a predictive marker of progression to nephropathy in IDDM, and of increased cardiovascular risk in NIDDM. Microalbuminuria may, after some years, progress to intermittent albuminuria followed by persistent proteinuria. Light-microscopic changes of glomerulosclerosis become manifest; both diffuse and nodular glomerulosclerosis can occur. The latter is sometimes known as the *Kimmelstiel–Wilson lesion*. At a later stage still, the glomerulus is replaced by hyaline material.

At the stage of persistent proteinuria, the plasma creatinine is normal but the average patient is only some 5–10 years from end-stage renal failure. The proteinuria may become so heavy as to induce a transient nephrotic syndrome, with peripheral oedema and hypoalbuminaemia.

Patients with nephropathy typically show a normochromic normocytic anaemia and a raised erythrocyte sedimentation rate (ESR). Hypertension is a common development and may itself damage the kidney still further. A rise in plasma creatinine is a late feature that progresses inevitably to renal failure, although the rate of progression may vary widely between individuals.

The natural history of this process is shown in Fig 17.15. A curious feature is that almost all patients with long-established diabetes have abnormalities on renal biopsy but only a proportion develop the features of a progressive renal disease.

Ischaemic lesions

Arteriolar lesions, with hypertrophy and hyalinization of the vessels, affect both afferent and efferent arterioles. The appearances are similar to those of hypertensive disease but are not necessarily related to the blood pressure in patients with diabetes.

Infective lesions

Urinary tract infections are relatively more common in women with diabetes, but this does not apply to men. Ascending infection may occur because of bladder stasis resulting from autonomic neuropathy, and infections more easily become established in damaged renal tissue. Autopsy material frequently reveals interstitial changes

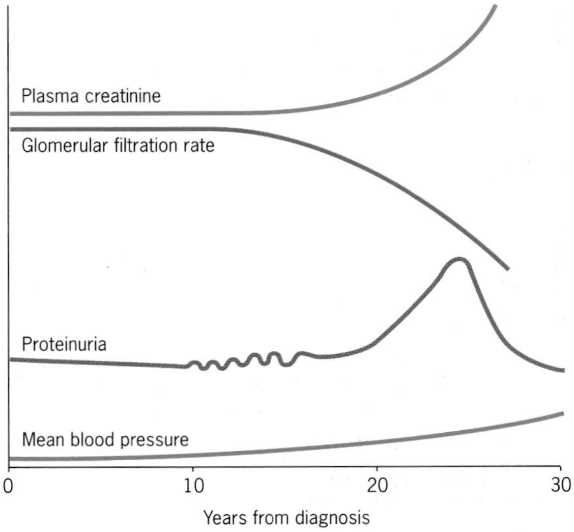

Fig 17.15
Schematic representation of the natural history of nephropathy. The typical onset is 15 years after diagnosis. Intermittent proteinuria leads to persistent proteinuria. In time, the plasma creatinine rises as the glomerular filtration rate falls

suggestive of infection, but ischaemia may produce similar changes and the true frequency of pyelonephritis in diabetes is uncertain.

Untreated infections in diabetics can result in renal papillary necrosis, in which renal papillae are shed in the urine, but this complication is rare.

DIAGNOSIS AND MANAGEMENT

The *urine* of all diabetic patients should be checked regularly for the presence of protein. Many centres also screen for microalbuminuria since there is evidence that meticulous glycaemic control or early antihypertensive treatment at this stage may delay the onset of frank proteinuria.

Once proteinuria is present, other possible causes for this should be considered (see below), but once these are excluded, a presumptive diagnosis of diabetic nephropathy can be made. For practical purposes this implies inevitable progression to end-stage renal failure, although the time course can be markedly slowed by early aggressive antihypertensive therapy.

Clinical suspicion of a non-diabetic cause of nephropathy may be provoked by an atypical history, the absence of diabetic retinopathy (usually but not invariably present with diabetic nephropathy) and the presence of red cell casts in the urine. Renal biopsy should be considered in such cases, but in practice is rarely necessary or helpful. The risk of intravenous urography is increased in diabetes, especially if patients are allowed to become dehydrated prior to the procedure, and a renal ultrasound is preferable but not so informative. A 24-hour urine collection to quantify protein loss and to measure creatinine clearance, and regular measurement of the plasma creatinine level, is performed.

Investigations to detect other treatable causes of nephropathy include urine microscopy and culture, serum protein electrophoresis, serum calcium, serum urate, ESR, and antinuclear factor.

MANAGEMENT

The management of diabetic nephropathy is similar to that of other causes of renal failure, with the following provisos:

- Aggressive treatment of blood pressure with a target below 140/90 mmHg has been shown to slow the rate of deterioration of renal failure considerably. Angiotensin-converting enzyme inhibitors are the drugs of choice (see p. 735). Recent evidence suggests that these drugs should be considered even in normotensive patients with persistent microalbuminuria.
- Oral hypoglycaemic agents partially excreted via the kidney (e.g. chlorpropamide) must be avoided.
- Insulin sensitivity increases and drastic reductions in dosage may be needed.
- Associated diabetic retinopathy tends to progress rapidly and frequent ophthalmic supervision is essential.

Management of end-stage disease is made more difficult by the fact that patients often have other complications of diabetes such as blindness, autonomic neuropathy or peripheral vascular disease. Vascular shunts tend to calcify rapidly and hence chronic ambulatory peritoneal dialysis may be preferable to haemodialysis. The failure rate of renal transplants is somewhat higher than in non-diabetic patients. A segmental pancreatic graft is sometimes performed at the same time as a renal graft. Although pancreatic transplants have a limited viability, owing to progressive fibrosis within the graft, they may give the patient a year or so of freedom from insulin injections.

Diabetic neuropathy

Diabetes can damage peripheral nervous tissue in a number of ways. The vascular hypothesis postulates occlusion of the vasa nervorum as the prime cause. This seems likely in isolated mononeuropathies, but the diffuse symmetrical nature of the common forms of neuropathy implies a metabolic cause. Since hyperglycaemia leads to increased formation of sorbitol and fructose in Schwann cells, accumulation of these sugars may disrupt function and structure.

The earliest functional change in diabetic nerves is delayed nerve conduction velocity; the earliest histological change is segmental demyelination, caused by damage to Schwann cells. In the early stages axons are preserved, implying prospects of recovery, but at a later stage irreversible axonal degeneration develops.

The following varieties of neuropathy may occur (Fig 17.16):

- symmetrical mainly sensory polyneuropathy (distal)
- acute painful neuropathy
- mononeuropathy and mononeuritis multiplex
  (a) cranial nerve lesions
  (b) isolated peripheral nerve lesions
- diabetic amyotrophy
- autonomic neuropathy.

Symmetrical mainly sensory polyneuropathy

This is often unrecognized by the patient in its early stages. Early clinical signs are loss of vibration sense, pain sensation (deep before superficial) and temperature sensation in the feet. At later stages patients may complain of a feeling of 'walking on cotton wool' and can lose their balance when washing the face or walking in the dark owing to impaired proprioception. Involvement of the hands is much less common and results in a 'stocking and glove' sensory loss. Complications include unrecognized trauma, beginning as blistering due to an ill-fitting shoe or a hot water bottle, and leading to ulceration.

Sequelae of neuropathy. Involvement of motor nerves to the small muscles of the feet gives rise to interosseous wasting. Unbalanced traction by the long flexor muscles leads to a characteristic shape of the foot,

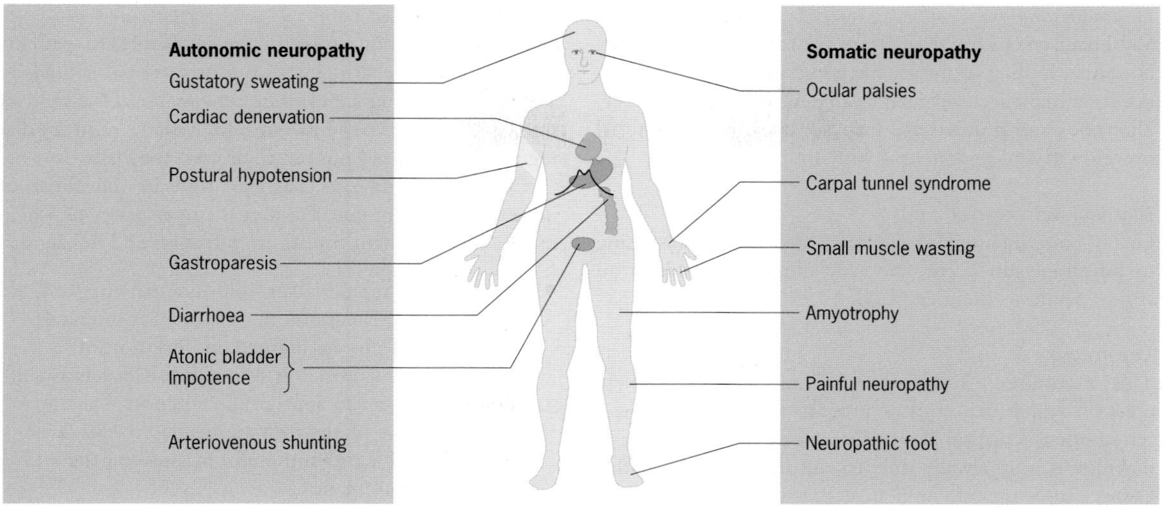

Fig 17.16
The neuropathic man

with a high arch and clawing of the toes, which in turn leads to abnormal distribution of pressure on walking, resulting in callus formation under the first metatarsal head or on the tips of the toes and perforating neuropathic ulceration. Neuropathic arthropathy (Charcot's joints) may sometimes develop in the ankle.

The hands show small-muscle wasting as well as sensory changes, but these signs and symptoms must be differentiated from those of the carpal tunnel syndrome, which occurs with increased frequency in diabetes and may be amenable to surgery.

Acute painful neuropathy

A diffuse, painful neuropathy is less common. The patient describes burning or crawling pains in the feet, shins and anterior thighs. These symptoms are typically worse at night, and pressure from bedclothes may be intolerable. It may present at diagnosis or develop after sudden improvement in glycaemic control (e.g. when insulin is started). It usually remits spontaneously after 3–12 months if good control is maintained. A more chronic form, developing later in the course of the disease, is sometimes resistant to almost all forms of therapy. Neurological assessment is difficult because of the hyperaesthesia experienced by the patient, but muscle wasting is not a feature and objective signs can be minimal.

Mononeuritis and mononeuritis multiplex (multiple mononeuropathy)

Any nerve in the body can be involved in diabetic mononeuritis; the onset is typically abrupt and sometimes painful. Radiculopathy (i.e. involvement of a spinal root) may occur.

Isolated palsies of nerves to the external eye muscles, especially the third and sixth nerves, are more common in diabetes. A characteristic feature of diabetic third nerve lesions is that pupillary reflexes are retained owing to sparing of pupillomotor fibres. Full spontaneous recovery is the rule for most episodes of mononeuritis. Lesions are more likely to occur at common sites for external pressure palsies or nerve entrapment (e.g. the median nerve in the carpal tunnel). The carpal tunnel syndrome (p. 1092) is a common cause for sensory symptoms in the hands in diabetes, but appears to respond less well to decompression.

Diabetic amyotrophy

This condition is usually seen in older men with diabetes. Presentation is with painful wasting, usually asymmetrical, of the quadriceps muscles. The wasting may be very marked and knee reflexes are diminished or absent. The affected area is often extremely tender. Extensor plantar responses sometimes develop and CSF protein content is elevated. Diabetic amyotrophy is usually associated with periods of poor glycaemic control and may be present at diagnosis. It often resolves in time with careful control of the blood glucose.

Autonomic neuropathy

Asymptomatic autonomic disturbances can be demonstrated on laboratory testing in many patients, but symptomatic autonomic neuropathy is rare. It affects both the sympathetic and parasympathetic nervous system and can be disabling.

The cardiovascular system

Vagal neuropathy results in tachycardia at rest and loss of sinus arrhythmia. At a later stage the heart may become denervated (resembling a transplanted heart). Cardiovascular reflexes such as the Valsalva manoeuvre are impaired.

Postural hypotension occurs owing to loss of sympathetic tone to peripheral arterioles. A warm foot with a bounding pulse is sometimes seen in a polyneuropathy as a result of peripheral vasodilatation.

Gastrointestinal tract

Vagal damage can lead to gastroparesis, often asymptomatic, but rarely leading to intractable vomiting. Diarrhoea often occurs at night accompanied by urgency and incontinence. Diarrhoea and steatorrhoea may occur owing to bacterial overgrowth, and treatment is with antibiotics.

Bladder involvement

Loss of tone, incomplete emptying, and stasis (predisposing to infection) can occur, and may ultimately result in an atonic, painless, distended bladder.

Impotence

This is common. The first manifestation is incomplete erection which may in time progress to total impotence; retrograde ejaculation also occurs. However, impotence in diabetes is not always due to autonomic neuropathy. Other causes include anxiety, depression, alcohol excess, drugs, primary or secondary gonadal failure, hypothyroidism, and inadequate vascular supply owing to atheroma in pudendal arteries.

The history and examination should focus on these possible causes, and blood is taken for LH, FSH, testosterone, prolactin and thyroid function. Treatment should ideally include sympathetic counselling of both partners. Some patients may benefit from intracavernous injection of prostaglandin E2 or the use of vacuum devices to produce an erection which is then maintained by slipping a tight rubber band over the base of the penis until intercourse is complete. Sildenafil citrate, a phosphodiesterase type-5 inhibitor, has recently been given FDA approval; it enhances the effects of nitric oxide on smooth muscle and increases penile blood flow.

The diabetic foot

Many amputations in diabetes could be delayed or prevented by more effective patient education and medical supervision. Ischaemia, infection and neuropathy combine to produce tissue necrosis. Although these factors may coexist, it is important to distinguish between the ischaemic and the neuropathic foot (Table 17.7).

Table 17.7 Distinguishing features between ischaemia and neuropathy in the diabetic foot

	Ischaemia	Neuropathy
Symptoms	Claudication Rest pain	Usually painless Sometimes painful neuropathy
Inspection	Dependent rubor Trophic changes	High arch Clawing of toes No trophic changes
Palpation	Cold Pulseless	Warm Bounding pulses
Ulceration	Painful Heels and toes	Painless Plantar

MANAGEMENT

Many diabetic foot problems are avoidable, so patients need to learn the principles of foot care and should be advised concerning appropriate footwear and the risks of smoking. Older patients should visit a chiropodist regularly and should not cut their own toe-nails.

Once tissue damage has occurred in the form of ulceration or gangrene, the aim is preservation of viable tissue. The two main threats are infection and ischaemia.

- *Infection.* This rapidly takes hold in a diabetic foot, and early effective antibiotic treatment is essential. Collections of pus are drained and excision of infected bone is needed if osteomyelitis develops and does not respond to appropriate antibiotic therapy. Regular X-rays of the foot are needed to check on progress. MRI is proving useful in assessing the degree of inflammation.
- *Ischaemia.* The blood flow to the feet is assessed clinically or with the Doppler ultrasound stethoscope. Femoral arteriography may indicate localized areas of occlusion amenable to bypass surgery or angioplasty. Relatively few patients fall into this category, and the risks and benefits of surgical intervention need careful consideration.

Foot problems are the major cause of hospital bed occupancy by diabetic patients. Good liaison between physician, chiropodist and surgeon is essential if this period in hospital is to be used efficiently. When irreversible arterial insufficiency is present, it is often quicker and kinder to opt for an early major amputation rather than subject the patient to a debilitating sequence of conservative procedures.

Infections

There is no evidence that diabetic patients with good glycaemic control are more prone to infection than normal subjects. However, poorly controlled diabetes entails increased susceptibility to the following infections:

- *Skin*
  (a) staphylococcal infections (boils, abscesses, carbuncles)
  (b) mucocutaneous candidiasis
- *Urinary tract*
  (a) urinary tract infections (in women)
  (b) pyelonephritis
  (c) perinephric abscess
- *Lungs*
  (a) staphylococcal and pneumococcal pneumonia
  (b) Gram-negative bacterial pneumonia
  (c) tuberculosis.

One reason why poor control lends to infection is that chemotaxis and phagocytosis by polymorphonuclear leucocytes is impaired because at high blood glucose concentrations neutrophil superoxide generation is impaired. Granulocyte stimulating factor (G-CSF), which increases the release of neutrophils from the bone marrow, is being used in trials.

Conversely, infections may lead to loss of glycaemic control, and are a common cause of ketoacidosis. Insulin-treated patients need to increase their dose by up to 25% in the face of infection, and non-insulin-treated patients may need insulin cover while the infection lasts. Patients should be told never to omit their insulin dose, even if they are nauseated and unable to eat; instead they should test their blood glucose frequently and seek urgent medical advice.

Skin and joints

(see also p. 1178)

Joint contractures in the hands are a common consequence of childhood diabetes. The sign may be demonstrated by asking the patient to join the hands as if in prayer; the metacarpophalangeal and interphalangeal joints cannot be apposed. Thickened, waxy skin can be noted on the backs of the fingers. These features may be due to glycosylation of collagen and are not progressive. The condition is sometimes referred to as diabetic cheiroarthropathy.

Osteopenia in the extremities is also described in IDDM but rarely leads to clinical consequences.

FURTHER READING

Clark CM, Lee DA (1995) Prevention and treatment of the complications of diabetes mellitus. *New England Journal of Medicine* **332**: 1210–1217.

Diabetes and the heart (1997) *Lancet* **350** (Suppl1): 1–32.

Diabetes Control and Complications Trial Research Group (1993) The effect of intensive treatment of diabetes on the development and progression of long-term complications in insulin-dependent diabetes mellitus. *New England Journal of Medicine* **329**: 977–986.

Klein R, Klein BEK (1997) Diabetic eye disease. *Lancet* **350**: 197–204.

Lewis EJ, Hunsicker LG, Bain RP, Rohde RD, for the Collaborative Study Group (1993) The effect of angiotensin-converting enzyme inhibition on diabetic nephropathy. *New England Journal of Medicine* **329**: 1456–1462.

Raine AE, Bilous RW (1996) End-stage renal disease in NIDDM: a consequence of microangiopathy alone? *Diabetologia* **39**: 1673–1675.

Ward JD (1996) Diabetic neuropathy in NIDDM. *Diabetologia* **39**: 1676–1678.

Notes on special situations in diabetes

Surgery

Smooth control of diabetes minimizes the risk of infection and balances the catabolic response to anaesthesia and surgery. The procedure for insulin-treated patients is simple:

- Long-acting and/or intermediate insulin should be stopped the day before surgery, with soluble insulin substituted.
- Whenever possible, diabetic patients should be first on the morning theatre list.
- An infusion of glucose, insulin and potassium is given during surgery. The insulin can be mixed into the glucose solution or administered separately by syringe pump. A standard combination is 16 U of soluble insulin with 10 mmol of KCl in 500 mL of 10% glucose, infused at 100 mL h^{-1}.
- Postoperatively, the infusion is maintained until the patient is able to eat. Other fluids needed in the perioperative period must be given through a separate intravenous line and must not interrupt the glucose/insulin/potassium infusion. Glucose levels are checked every 2–4 hours and potassium levels are monitored. The amount of insulin and potassium in each infusion bag is adjusted either upwards or downwards according to the results of regular monitoring of the blood glucose and serum potassium concentrations.

The same approach is used in the emergency situation, with the exception that a separate variable rate insulin infusion may be needed to bring blood glucose under control before surgery.

Non-insulin-treated patients should stop medication two days before the operation. Patients with mild hyperglycaemia (fasting blood glucose below 8 mmol L^{-1}) can be treated as non-diabetic. Those with higher levels are treated with soluble insulin prior to surgery, and with glucose, insulin and potassium during and after the procedure, as for insulin-treated patients.

Pregnancy and diabetes

Modern management has transformed the outcome of pregnancy in women with diabetes. Forty years ago one pregnancy in three ended with the death of the fetus or neonate. Today, the results in specialized centres approach those of non-diabetic pregnancy. This improvement is due to meticulous glycaemic control and careful medical and obstetric management. When the pregnancy is planned, optimal glycaemic control is sought before conception.

Glycaemic control in pregnancy

The patient should perform daily home blood glucose profiles, recording blood tests before and two hours after meals. The renal threshold falls in pregnancy and urine tests are therefore of little or no value. Insulin requirements rise progressively, and intensified insulin regimens are generally used. The aim is to maintain blood glucose and HbA_{1c} or fructosamine levels within the normal range.

General management

The patient is seen at intervals of two weeks or less at a clinic managed jointly by physician and obstetrician. Circumstances permitting, the aim should be outpatient management with a spontaneous vaginal delivery at term. Retinopathy and nephropathy may deteriorate during pregnancy. Expert fundoscopy and urine testing for protein should be undertaken at booking, at 28 weeks and before delivery.

Obstetric problems associated with diabetes

Poorly controlled diabetes is associated with stillbirth, mechanical problems in the birth canal due to fetal macrosomia, hydramnios, and pre-eclampsia. Ketoacidosis in pregnancy carries a 50% fetal mortality, but maternal hypoglycaemia is relatively well tolerated.

Neonatal problems

Maternal diabetes, especially when poorly controlled, is associated with fetal macrosomia. The infant of a diabetic mother is more susceptible to hyaline membrane disease than non-diabetic infants of similar maturity. In addition, neonatal hypoglycaemia may occur. The mechanism is as follows: maternal glucose crosses the placenta, but insulin does not; the fetal islets hypersecrete to combat maternal hyperglycaemia, and a rebound to hypoglycaemic levels occurs when the umbilical cord is severed.

These complications are due to hyperglycaemia in the third trimester. Poor glycaemic control around the time of conception carries an increased risk of major congenital malformations.

Gestational diabetes

This term refers to glucose intolerance that develops in the course of pregnancy and usually remits following delivery. While it is clear that hyperglycaemia in pregnancy is harmful for the fetus, there is still controversy concerning the best biochemical definition of this, and of the most useful cutoff point for therapy.

The condition is typically asymptomatic and is demonstrated biochemically on the basis of random testing in each trimester and by oral glucose tolerance testing if the plasma glucose concentration is 7 mmol L^{-1} or more. Since the renal threshold for glucose falls during normal pregnancy and glucose tolerance deteriorates, the condition may easily be misdiagnosed.

Treatment is with diet in the first instance, but most patients require insulin cover during the pregnancy. Insulin does not cross the placenta. Oral agents cross the placenta and are thus avoided because of the potential risk to the fetus.

Gestational diabetes has been associated with all the obstetric and neonatal problems described above for pre-existing diabetes, except that there is no increase in the rate of congenital abnormalities. It is likely to recur in subsequent pregnancies. Gestational diabetes is often the harbinger of NIDDM in later life.

Not all diabetes presenting in pregnancy is gestational. True IDDM may develop, and swift diagnosis is essential to prevent the development of ketoacidosis. Hospital admission is required if the patient is symptomatic, or has ketonuria or a markedly elevated blood glucose level.

Brittle diabetes

There is no precise definition for this term, which is used to describe patients with recurrent ketoacidosis and/or recurrent hypoglycaemic coma. Of these, the largest group is made up of those who experience recurrent severe hypoglycaemia.

Recurrent severe hypoglycaemia

This affects 1–3% of insulin-dependent patients. Most are adults who have had diabetes for more than 10 years. By this stage endogenous insulin secretion is negligible in the great majority of patients. Pancreatic α cells are still present in undiminished numbers, but the glucagon response to hypoglycaemia is virtually absent. Long-term patients are thus subject to fluctuating hyperinsulinaemia owing to erratic absorption of insulin from injection sites, and lack a major component of the hormonal defence against hypoglycaemia. In this situation adrenaline secretion becomes vital, but this too may become impaired in the course of diabetes. Loss of adrenaline secretion has been attributed to autonomic neuropathy, but this is unlikely to be the sole cause; central adaptation to recurrent hypoglycaemia may also be a factor.

The following factors may also predispose to recurrent hypoglycaemia:

- *Overtreatment with insulin.* Frequent biochemical hypoglycaemia lowers the glucose level at which symptoms develop. Symptoms often reappear when overall glucose control is relaxed.
- *An unrecognized low renal threshold for glucose.* Attempts to render the urine sugar-free will inevitably produce hypoglycaemia.
- *Excessive insulin doses.* A common error is to increase the *dose* when a patient needs more frequent injections to overcome a problem of *timing.*
- *Endocrine causes.* These include pituitary insufficiency, adrenal insufficiency and premenstrual insulin sensitivity.

- *Alimentary causes.* These include exocrine pancreatic failure and diabetic gastroparesis.
- *Renal failure.* The kidneys are important sites for the clearance of insulin which tends to accumulate if renal function is lost.
- *Patient causes.* Patients may be unintelligent, uncooperative or may manipulate their therapy.

Recurrent ketoacidosis

This usually occurs in adolescents or young adults, and the most severe form is more common in girls. Although metabolic decompensation may develop very rapidly, it is often impossible to pinpoint an underlying abnormality. Many theories exist concerning the causes of this condition, but all agree that it is heterogeneous. The following categories have been suggested:

- *Iatrogenic.* Inappropriate insulin combinations may be a cause of swinging glycaemic control. For example, a once-daily regimen may cause hypoglycaemia during the afternoon or evening and pre-breakfast hyperglycaemia due to insulin deficiency.
- *Intercurrent illness.* Unsuspected infections, including urinary tract infections and tuberculosis, may be present. Thyrotoxicosis can also manifest as unstable glycaemic control.
- *Psychosocial causes.* These certainly form the largest category. It has been suggested that neuroendocrine mechanisms such as catecholamine secretion might mediate the metabolic disturbance. Other patients undoubtedly manipulate their illness, whether consciously or unconsciously.
- *Unknown aetiology.* The most 'brittle' patients of all are usually females aged 15–25 years, often overweight, and typically suffering from amenorrhoea. The insulin requirement is variable but is often high. Sophisticated 'cheating' has been detected in some of these patients, but this should never be assumed without convincing proof.

FURTHER READING

Steel JM, Johnstone FD (1996) Guidelines for the management of insulin-dependent diabetes mellitus in pregnancy. *Drugs* **52**(1): 60–70.

Tattersall RB (1997) Brittle diabetes revisited. *Diabetic Medicine* **14**(2): 99–110.

Hypoglycaemia

Hypoglycaemia develops when hepatic glucose output falls below the rate of glucose uptake by peripheral tissues. Hepatic glucose output may be reduced by:

- the inhibition of hepatic glycogenolysis and gluconeogenesis by insulin
- depletion of hepatic glycogen reserves by malnutrition, fasting, exercise or advanced liver disease
- impaired gluconeogenesis (e.g. following alcohol ingestion).

In the first of these categories, insulin levels are raised, the liver contains adequate glycogen stores, and the hypoglycaemia can be reversed by injection of glucagon. In the other two situations, insulin levels are low and glucagon is ineffective.

Peripheral glucose uptake is accelerated by high insulin levels and by exercise, but these conditions are normally balanced by increased glucose output. Insulin or sulphonylurea therapy for diabetes accounts for the vast majority of cases of severe hypoglycaemia encountered in an accident and emergency department.

The most common symptoms and signs of hypoglycaemia are neurological. The brain consumes about 50% of the total glucose produced by the liver. This high energy requirement is needed to generate ATP used to maintain the potential difference across axonal membranes.

Insulinomas

Insulinomas are pancreatic islet cell tumours that secrete insulin. Most are sporadic but some patients have multiple tumours arising from neural crest tissue (multiple endocrine neoplasia). Some 95% of these tumours are benign. The classic presentation is with fasting hypoglycaemia, but early symptoms may also develop in the late morning or afternoon. Recurrent hypoglycaemia is often present for months or years before the diagnosis is made, and the symptoms may be atypical or even bizarre; the presenting features in one series are given in Table 17.8. Common misdiagnoses include psychiatric disorders, particularly pseudodementia in elderly people, epilepsy and cerebrovascular disease.

DIAGNOSIS

Whipple's triad remains the basis of clinical diagnosis. This is satisfied when:

- symptoms are associated with fasting or exercise
- hypoglycaemia is confirmed during these episodes
- glucose relieves the symptoms.

Table 17.8
Presenting features of insulinoma

Diplopia
Sweating, palpitations, weakness
Confusion or abnormal behaviour
Loss of consciousness
Grand mal seizures

A fourth criterion – demonstration of inappropriately high insulin levels during hypoglycaemia – may usefully be added to these.

The diagnosis is confirmed by the demonstration of hypoglycaemia in association with inappropriate and excessive insulin secretion. Hypoglycaemia is demonstrated by:

- Measurement of *overnight fasting* (16 hours) glucose and insulin levels on three occasions. About 90% of patients with insulinomas will have low glucose and non-suppressed (normal or elevated) insulin levels.
- A prolonged 72-hour *supervised fast* if overnight testing is inconclusive and symptoms persist.

Autonomous insulin secretion is demonstrated by lack of the normal feedback suppression during hypoglycaemia. This may be shown by measuring insulin, C-peptide or proinsulin during a spontaneous episode of hypoglycaemia.

Many patients also have an abnormal (diabetic) glucose tolerance test, but this has no diagnostic value.

TREATMENT

The most effective therapy is surgical excision of the tumour, but insulinomas are often very small and difficult to localize. Many techniques can be used to attempt to localise insulinomas. Sensitivity and specificity vary between centres and between operators. These include highly selective angiography, contrast-enhanced high-resolution CT scanning, scanning with radiolabelled somatostatin (some insulinomas express somatostatin receptors), and endoscopic and intraoperative ultrasound scanning. Venous sampling for the detection of 'hot spots' of high insulin concentration in the various intra-abdominal veins is still used occasionally.

Medical treatment with diazoxide is useful when the insulinoma is malignant, in patients in whom a tumour cannot be located, and in elderly patients with mild symptoms. Symptoms may also remit on treatment with the somatostatin analogue, octreotide.

Hypoglycaemia with other tumours

Hypoglycaemia may develop in the course of advanced neoplasia and cachexia, and has been described in association with many tumour types. Certain massive tumours, especially sarcomas, may produce hypoglycaemia owing to the secretion of insulin-like growth factor 1. True ectopic insulin secretion is extremely rare.

Postprandial hypoglycaemia

If frequent *venous* blood glucose samples are taken following a prolonged glucose tolerance test, about one in four subjects will have at least one value below 3 mmol L^{-1}. The arteriovenous glucose difference is quite marked during this phase, so that very few are truly hypoglycaemic in terms of arterial (or capillary) blood glucose content. Failure to appreciate this simple fact led some authorities to believe that postprandial (or reactive) hypoglycaemia was a potential 'organic' explanation for a variety of complaints that might otherwise have been considered psychosomatic. An epidemic of false 'hypoglycaemia' followed, particularly in the USA. Later work showed a poor correlation between symptoms and biochemical hypoglycaemia. Even so, a number of otherwise normal people occasionally become pale, weak and sweaty at times when meals are due, and report benefit from advice to take regular snacks between meals.

True postprandial hypoglycaemia may develop in the presence of alcohol, which 'primes' the cells to produce an exaggerated insulin response to carbohydrate. The person who substitutes alcoholic beverages for lunch is particularly at risk. Postprandial hypoglycaemia sometimes occurs after gastric surgery, owing to rapid gastric emptying and mismatching of nutrient absorption and insulin secretion. This is referred to as 'dumping' but it is now rarely encountered (see p. 240).

Hepatic and renal causes of hypoglycaemia

The liver can maintain a normal glucose output despite extensive damage, and hepatic hypoglycaemia is uncommon. It is particularly a problem with fulminant hepatic failure.

The kidney has a subsidiary role in glucose production (via gluconeogenesis in the renal cortex), and hypoglycaemia is sometimes a problem in terminal renal failure.

Hereditary fructose intolerance occurs in 1 in 20 000 live births and can cause hypoglycaemia (see p. 999).

Endocrine causes of hypoglycaemia

Endocrine disorders resulting in deficiencies of hormones antagonistic to insulin are rare but well-recognized causes of hypoglycaemia. These include hypopituitarism, isolated adrenocorticotrophic hormone (ACTH) deficiency, and Addison's disease.

Drug-induced hypoglycaemia

Many drugs have been reported to produce isolated cases of hypoglycaemia, but usually only when other predisposing factors are present. The following are among the more important:

- Sulphonylureas may be used in the treatment of diabetes or may be taken by non-diabetics in suicide attempts.
- Quinine may produce severe hypoglycaemia in the course of treatment for falciparum malaria.

- Salicylates may cause hypoglycaemia following accidental ingestion by children, but this complication is very rare in adults.
- Propranolol has been reported to induce hypoglycaemia in the presence of strenuous exercise or starvation.
- Pentamidine may cause hypoglycaemia when used in the treatment of resistant *Pneumocystis* pneumonia in people with AIDS.

Alcohol-induced hypoglycaemia

Alcohol inhibits gluconeogenesis. Alcohol-induced hypoglycaemia was first described in poorly nourished chronic alcoholics but may also present in binge drinkers and in children who have taken relatively small amounts of alcohol, since they have a diminished hepatic glycogen reserve. The clinical presentation is with coma and hypothermia.

Factitious hypoglycaemia

This is a relatively common variant of self-induced disease and is much more common than an insulinoma. Hypoglycaemia is produced by surreptitious self-administration of insulin or sulphonylureas. Many patients in this category have been extensively investigated for an insulinoma. Measurement of C-peptide levels during hypoglycaemia should identify patients who are injecting insulin; sulphonylurea abuse can be detected by chromatography of plasma or urine.

FURTHER READING

Markes V, Teale JD (1996) Investigation of hypoglycaemia. *Clinical Endocrinology* **44**: 133–136.

Disorders of lipid metabolism

Physiology

Lipids are insoluble in water, and are transported in the bloodstream as macromolecular complexes. In these complexes, lipids (principally triglyceride, cholesterol and cholesterol esters) are surrounded by a stabilizing coat of phospholipid. Proteins (called apoproteins) embedded into the surface of these 'lipoprotein' particles exert a stabilizing function and allow the particles to be recognized by receptors in the liver and the peripheral tissues. The structure of a chylomicron (one type of lipoprotein particle) is illustrated in Fig 17.17.

Five principal types of lipoprotein particles are found in the blood (Fig 17.18). They are structurally different and can be separated in the laboratory by their density and electrophoretic mobility. The larger particles give postprandial plasma its cloudy appearance. More than half of all patients aged under 60 with angiographically confirmed coronary artery disease have a lipoprotein disorder.

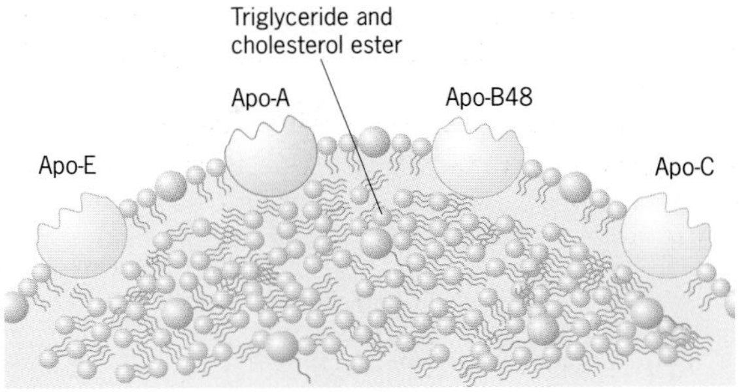

Fig 17.17
Schematic of a chylomicron particle (75–1200 nm) showing apoproteins lying in the surface membrane

The genes for all the major apoproteins and that for the low-density lipoprotein (LDL) receptor have been isolated, sequenced and their chromosomal sites mapped. Production of abnormal apoproteins is known to produce, or predispose to, several types of lipid disorder, and it is likely that others will be discovered.

Chylomicrons

Chylomicrons are synthesized in the small intestine postprandially. They contain triglyceride and a small amount of cholesterol, and provide the main mechanism for transporting the digestion products of dietary fat to the liver and peripheral tissues. Each newly formed chylomicron contains several different apoproteins (B-48, A-I, A-II), and acquires apoproteins C-II and E by transfer from high-density lipoprotein (HDL) particles in the bloodstream. Apoprotein C-II binds to specific receptors in the peripheral tissues and the liver and allows the endothelial enzyme, lipoprotein lipase, to remove triglyceride from the particle. The remaining chylomicron remnant particle, which contains most of the original cholesterol, is taken up by the liver by mechanisms which are not fully understood, possibly mediated by apoprotein E.

Very-low-density lipoprotein (VLDL) particles

These are synthesized and secreted by the liver and contain most of the endogenously synthesized triglyceride and a smaller quantity of cholesterol. Apoprotein B100 is an essential component. Apoproteins C and E are later incorporated into VLDL by transfer from HDL particles. As they pass round the circulation, VLDL particles bind through apoprotein C allowing triglyceride to be progressively removed by lipoprotein lipase. This leaves a particle, now depleted of triglyceride and apoprotein C, called an intermediate-density lipoprotein (IDL) particle.

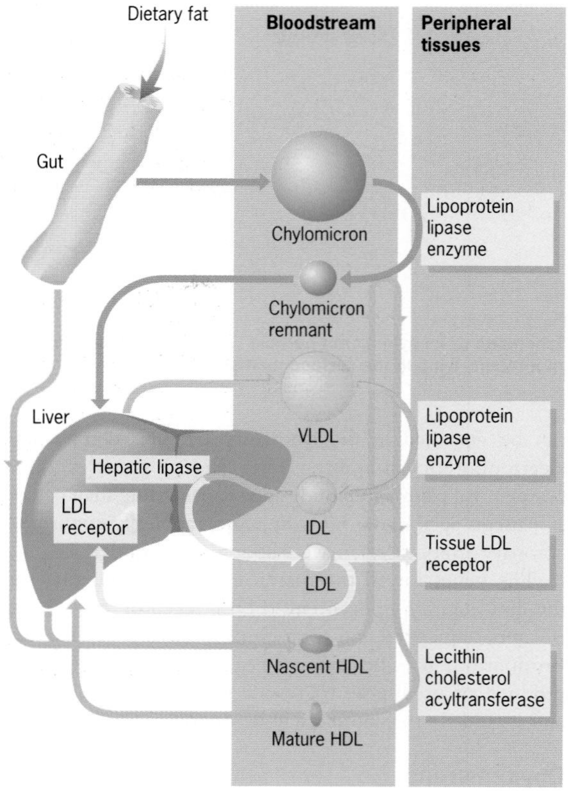

Fig 17.18
Schematic representation of the sites of origin, interaction between, and fate of, the major lipoprotein particles

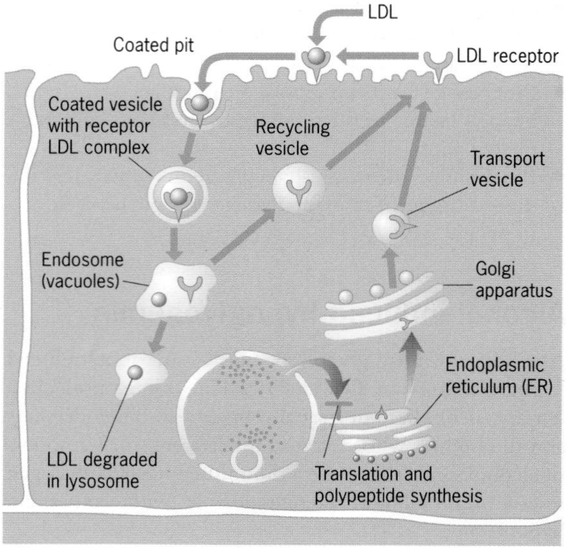

Fig 17.19
Receptor-mediated endocytosis. LDL receptors are formed in the endoplasmic reticulum and transported via the Golgi apparatus to the surface of a hepatocyte. LDLs bind to these receptors, are internalized and taken up by the endosome. The receptor is recycled back to the surface, while the LDL is broken down by the lysosomes, freeing cholesterol needed for membrane synthesis

Intermediate-density lipoprotein particles

These have apoprotein B100 and apoprotein E molecules on the particle surface. Most IDL particles are taken up by liver LDL receptors binding to the apoprotein E on the IDL particle. The particle is then taken up and catabolized. IDL particles that escape clearance this way have further triglyceride removed (by the enzyme hepatic lipase), producing LDL particles.

Low-density lipoprotein particles

LDL particles are the main carrier of cholesterol, and deliver it both to the liver and to peripheral cells. The surface of the LDL particle contains a single apoprotein B100, and also apoprotein E. The apoprotein B100 is the principal ligand for the LDL receptor. This receptor lies within coated pits on the surface of the hepatocyte. Once bound to the receptor, the coated pit invaginates and fuses with liposomes which destroy the LDL particle (Fig 17.19). The number of hepatic LDL receptors regulates the circulating LDL concentration. The circulating LDL concentration is also regulated by controlling the activity of the rate-limiting enzyme in the cholesterol synthetic pathway, hydroxymethylglutaryl coenzyme A (HMG-CoA) reductase. Not all the cholesterol synthesized by the liver is packaged immediately into lipoprotein particles. Some is converted into bile salts. Both bile salts and cholesterol are excreted in the bile: both are then reabsorbed through the terminal ileum and recirculated (enterohepatic circulation).

High-density lipoprotein particles

HDL particles are produced in both the liver and intestine. The nascent particles are disc shaped, seemingly inert and contain E apoproteins. They are modified by acquiring some surface components of chylomicron and VLDL particles as these are broken down into smaller particles. The materials gained by the nascent HDL particles include phospholipids, and the A and C apoproteins. The more mature HDL particles take up cholesterol from cell membranes in the peripheral tissues. As it is taken up the enzyme lecithin-cholesterol acyltransferase (LCAT), activated by the apoprotein A on the particle's surface, esterifies the sequestered cholesterol. The HDL particle is then capable of transporting this cholesterol away from the periphery to the liver (reverse cholesterol transport) where it binds through apoprotein E. HDL particles carry 20–30% of the total quantity of cholesterol in the blood.

Measurement

When a laboratory measures fasting serum lipids, the majority of the total cholesterol concentration consists of LDL particles with a 20–30% contribution from HDL particles. The triglyceride concentration largely reflects the circulating number of VLDL particles, since chylomicrons are not normally present in the fasted state. If the patient is not fasted, the total triglyceride concentration will be raised owing to the presence of triglyceride-rich chylomicrons as well as VLDL particles.

Epidemiology

LDL and total cholesterol

Population studies have repeatedly demonstrated a strong association between both total and LDL cholesterol concentration and coronary heart risk. There is a strong link between mean fat consumption, mean serum cholesterol concentration and the prevalence of coronary heart disease between countries. The exception is France where the cardiovascular risk is only moderate – perhaps owing to high alcohol consumption. Studies of migrants, particularly of Japanese men migrating to Hawaii, have shown that as diet changes, and cholesterol concentrations rise, so does the cardiovascular risk. Such studies show the importance of the environment rather than the genetic make-up of a population.

The Multiple Risk Factor Intervention Trial (MRFIT) screened one-third of a million American men for various cardiovascular risk factors and then followed them for six years. Data from this study have shown that although cardiovascular risk rises progressively as total cholesterol concentration increases (Fig 17.20), the risk increase is modest for individuals with no other cardiovascular risk factors. With each additional risk factor the effect produced by the same difference in cholesterol concentration becomes greatly magnified. The Framingham Study has reproduced these findings in a separate population.

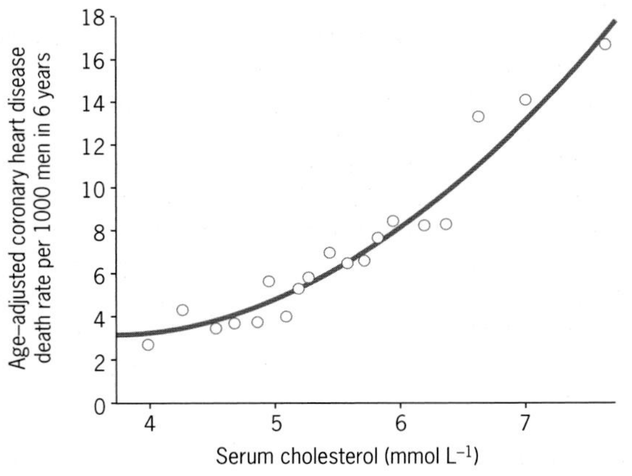

Fig 17.20
The Multiple Risk Factor Intervention Trial: relationship between levels of serum cholesterol and risks of fatal coronary artery disease in a longitudinal study of more than 361 000 men screened for entry into the trial. From Stamler J, Wentworth D, Neaton JD (1986) *Journal of the American Medical Association* **256**: 2823

HDL cholesterol

Epidemiological studies have shown that HDL particles appear to protect against atheroma. This effect may be due to the ability of the particle to transport cholesterol from the peripheral tissues to the liver. HDL particles have important effects on the function of platelets and of the haemostatic cascade. These properties may favourably influence thrombogenesis.

VLDL particles

There is a relatively weak independent link between raised concentrations of (triglyceride-rich) VLDL particles and cardiovascular risk. Very raised triglyceride concentrations (>6 mmol L^{-1}) cause a greatly increased risk of acute pancreatitis and retinal vein thrombosis. Hypertriglyceridaemia tends to occur in association with a reduced HDL concentration. Much of the cardiovascular risk associated with 'hypertriglyceridaemia' turns out on multivariate analysis to be due to the associated low HDL levels and not to the hypertriglyceridaemia itself.

Chylomicrons

Excess chylomicrons do not confer an excess cardiovascular risk, but raise the total plasma triglyceride concentration.

Screening

Most patients with hyperlipidaemia are asymptomatic and have no clinical signs. Many are discovered during the screening of high-risk individuals.

Whose lipids should be measured?

There are great doubts as to whether blanket screening of plasma lipids is warranted. Selective screening of people at high risk of cardiovascular disease should be undertaken, to include those with:

- a family history of coronary heart disease (especially below 50 years of age)
- a family history of lipid disorders
- the presence of a xanthoma
- the presence of xanthelasma or corneal arcus before the age of 40 years
- obesity
- diabetes mellitus
- hypertension
- acute pancreatitis
- those undergoing renal replacement therapy.

Where one family member is known to have a monogenic disorder such as familial hypercholesterolaemia (1 in 500 of the population), siblings and children must have their plasma lipid concentrations measured. It is also worth screening the prospective partners of any patients with this heterozygous monogenic lipid disorder because of the small risk of producing children homozygous for the condition.

Acute severe illnesses such as myocardial infarction can derange plasma lipid concentrations for up to three months. Plasma lipid concentrations should be measured either within 48 hours of an acute myocardial infarction (before derangement has had time to occur) or three months later.

Serum cholesterol concentration does not change significantly after a meal and as a screening test a random blood sample is sufficient. If the total cholesterol concentration is raised above 6.5 mmol L^{-1}, HDL cholesterol, triglyceride, and LDL cholesterol concentrations should be quantitated on a fasting sample. If a test for hypertriglyceridaemia is needed, a fasting blood sample is mandatory.

Secondary hyperlipidaemia

If a lipid disorder has been detected it is vital to carry out a clinical history, examination and simple special investigations to detect causes of secondary hyperlipidaemia (Table 17.9), which may need treatment in their own right. The biochemical tests needed are for thyroid stimulating hormone, fasting blood glucose concentration, urea and electrolyte concentrations, and liver biochemistry.

Table 17.9
Causes of secondary hyperlipidaemia

Hypothyroidism
Diabetes mellitus (when poorly controlled)
Obesity
Renal impairment
Nephrotic syndrome
Dysglobulinaemia
Hepatic dysfunction
Drugs:
Oral contraceptives in susceptible individuals
Retinoids, thiazide diuretics, corticosteroids, opDDD (used in the treatment of Cushing's syndrome)

Classification, clinical features and investigation of primary hyperlipidaemias

As the genetic basis of lipid disorders becomes clearer the genetic classification of Goldstein and colleagues is proving of greater clinical relevance than the Fredrickson (WHO) classification (based on the pattern of lipoproteins found in plasma). The lack of direct correspondence between these two systems of classification can be confusing. For clarity we have used the genetic classification and not the Fredrickson classification. This has the advantage that the genetic disorders may be grouped by the results of simple lipid biochemistry into causes of:

- hypertriglyceridaemia alone
- hypercholesterolaemia alone
- combined hyperlipidaemia.

Hypertriglyceridaemia alone (without hypercholesterolaemia)

The majority of cases appear to be due to multiple genes acting together to produce a modest excess of circulating concentration of VLDL particles, such cases being termed *polygenic hypertriglyceridaemia*. In a proportion of cases there will be a family history of a lipid disorder or its effects (e.g. pancreatitis). Such cases are often classified as *familial hypertriglyceridaemia*. The defect underlying the vast majority of such cases is not understood. The only clinical feature is a history of attacks of pancreatitis or retinal vein thrombosis in some individuals.

Lipoprotein lipase deficiency and apoprotein C-II deficiency

These are rare diseases which produce greatly elevated triglyceride concentrations owing to the persistence of chylomicrons (and not VLDL particles) in the circulation. The chylomicrons persist because the triglyceride within cannot be metabolized if the enzyme lipoprotein lipase is defective or because the triglycerides cannot gain access to the normal enzyme owing to deficiency of the apoprotein C-II on the surface of the chylomicron particles. The disorder is unlikely to be confused clinically with cases of polygenic or familial hypertriglyceridaemia as the patients present in childhood with eruptive xanthomas, lipaemia retinalis and retinal vein thrombosis, pancreatitis and hepatosplenomegaly. If the disorder is not identified in childhood it can present in adults with gross hypertriglyceridaemia resistant to simple measures. The most useful test is to confirm the presence of chylomicrons in fasting plasma stored overnight (chylomicrons float like cream). This is confirmed by plasma electrophoresis or ultracentrifugation. An abnormality of apoprotein C can be deduced if the hypertriglyceridaemia improves temporarily after infusing fresh frozen plasma, and lipoprotein lipase deficiency is likely if it does not.

Hypercholesterolaemia alone (without hypertriglyceridaemia)

The autosomal dominant monogenic disorder of heterozygous familial hypercholesterolaemia is present in 1 in 500 of the normal population. The average primary care physician would therefore be expected to have four such patients on his or her list, but because of clustering within families the prevalence is lower in some lists and much higher in others. There is an increased prevalence in some racial groups (e.g. French Canadians, Finns, South Africans). Surprisingly, most individuals with this disorder remain undetected. Patients may have no physical signs, in which case the diagnosis is made on the presence of very high plasma cholesterol concentrations which are unresponsive to dietary modification and are associated with a typical family history of early cardiovascular disease. Diagnosis can more easily be made if typical clinical features are present. These include xanthomatous thickening of the Achilles tendons and xanthomas over the extensor tendons of the fingers. Xanthelasma may be present, but is not diagnostic of familial hypercholesterolaemia.

The genetic defect of this disorder is the underproduction or malproduction of the LDL cholesterol receptor in the liver (Table 17.10). Over 150 different mutations in the LDL receptor have been described to date. Fifty per cent of men with the disease will die by the age of 60, most from coronary artery disease, if untreated.

Homozygous familial hypercholesterolaemia is very rare indeed. Affected children have no LDL receptors in the liver. They have a hugely elevated LDL cholesterol concentration, and massive deposition of lipid in arterial walls, the aorta and the skin. The natural history is for death from ischaemic heart disease in late childhood or adolescence. Repeated plasmapheresis has been used to remove LDL cholesterol with some success in these patients. Liver transplantation offers the possibility of cure, but the numbers of patients having undergone this procedure is small. The possibility of gene therapy offers a glimmer of hope on the horizon for affected individuals.

Another relatively common single gene disorder causes a mutation in the apoprotein B100 gene. Since LDL particles bind to their clearance receptor in the liver through apoprotein B100, this defect also results in high LDL concentrations in the blood, and a clinical picture which closely resembles classical familial hypercholesterolaemia. The two disorders can be distinguished clearly only by genetic tests. The approach to treatment is the same.

Patients who have raised serum cholesterol concentrations, but do not have familial hypercholesterolaemia, exist in the right-hand tail of the normal distribution of cholesterol concentration, and are deemed to have *polygenic hypercholesterolaemia.* The precise nature of the polygenic variation in plasma cholesterol concentration remains unknown. Variations in the apoprotein E gene (chromosome 19) appear to contribute towards the problem in some individuals in this heterogeneous group.

Combined hyperlipidaemia (hypercholesterolaemia and hypertriglyceridaemia)

The most common patient group is a *polygenic combined hyperlipidaemia.*

Familial combined hyperlipidaemia

This is relatively common, affecting 1 in 200 of the general population. The genetic basis for the disorder has not yet been characterized. It is diagnosed by finding raised cholesterol and triglyceride concentrations in association with a typical family history.

Remnant hyperlipidaemia

This is a rare (1 in 5000) cause of combined hyperlipidaemia. It is due to accumulation of LDL remnant particles and is associated with an extremely high risk of cardiovascular disease. It may be suspected in a patient with raised total cholesterol and triglyceride concentrations by finding xanthomas in the palmar creases (diagnostic) and the presence of tuberous xanthomas typically over the knees and elbows (Fig 17.21). Remnant hyperlipidaemia is almost always due to the inheritance of a variant of the apoprotein E allele (apoprotein E2) together with an aggravating factor such as another primary hyperlipidaemia. When suspected clinically the diagnosis can be confirmed using ultracentrifugation of plasma, or phenotyping apoprotein E.

Table 17.10
The genetic defects underlying the common lipoprotein disorders

Disorder	Affected gene	Chromosome	Frequency
Common disorders			
Heterozygous familial hypercholesterolaemia	LDL receptor	19	1:500
Familial defective apoprotein B	Apo B100	2	1:700
Hypobetalipoproteinaemia	Apo B100	2	1:1000
Familial combined hyperlipidaemia	As yet unknown	As yet unknown	1:200
Familial hypertriglyceridaemia	As yet unknown	As yet unknown	1:500
Some rarer disorders			
Homozygous familial hypercholesterolaemia	LDL receptor	19	1:1 000 000
Lipoprotein lipase deficiency	As yet unknown	As yet unknown	1:1 000 000 (homozygous)
Apolipoprotein CII deficiency	Apo CII	19	40 cases

Management of hyperlipidaemia

Hypertriglyceridaemia (without hypercholesterolaemia)

A serum triglyceride concentration below 2.0 mmol L^{-1} is normal. In the range 2.0–6.0 mmol L^{-1} no specific intervention will be needed unless there are coincident cardiovascular risk factors, and in particular a strong family history of early cardiovascular death. In general, patients should be advised that they have a minor lipid problem, offered advice on weight reduction if obese, and advice on correcting other cardiovascular risk factors.

If the triglyceride concentration is above 6.0 mmol L^{-1} there is a risk of pancreatitis and retinal vein thrombosis. Patients should be advised to reduce their weight if overweight and start a formal lipid-lowering diet (see below). A proportion of individuals with hypertriglyceridaemia have livers which respond to even moderate degrees of alcohol intake by allowing accumulation or excess production of VLDL particles. If hypertriglyceridaemia persists, lipid measurements should be repeated before and after a six-week interval of complete abstinence from alcohol. If a considerable improvement results, lifelong abstinence may prove necessary. Other drugs, including thiazides, oestrogens and glucocorticoids, can have a similar effect to alcohol in susceptible patients.

If the triglyceride concentration remains elevated above 6.0 mmol L^{-1}, despite the above measures, drug therapy is warranted. A fibric acid derivative is the agent of first choice. Nicotinic acid may be used in addition but its side-effects are often a problem. Fish oil capsules (Maxepa) which contain ω-3 long-chain fatty acids are also effective in lowering triglyceride concentrations.

The severe hypertriglyceridaemia associated with the rare disorders of lipoprotein lipase deficiency and apoprotein C-II deficiency may require restriction of dietary fat to 10–20% of total energy intake and the use of special preparations of medium-chain triglycerides in cooking in place of oil or fat. Medium-chain triglycerides are not absorbed via chylomicrons (see p. 249).

Hypercholesterolaemia (without hypertriglyceridaemia)

This can be divided into *primary* prevention and *secondary* prevention (see Information box 17.4). In both groups other risk factors should also be reduced, including stopping smoking, treatment of hypertension, reduction of excessive alcohol consumption and weight.

Primary prevention

Prescribe a lipid-lowering diet. Perimenopausal women should be offered female hormone replacement therapy (HRT) as the risk of cardiovascular disease rises sharply after the menopause and HRT reduces this risk even in normocholesterolaemic women. A small number of women respond adversely to exogenous oestrogens, with a rise in lipids; measurement of the fasting lipid level is therefore necessary shortly after starting treatment.

The level of serum cholesterol at which drug treatment is commenced is shown in Table 17.11.

Individuals with familial hypercholesterolaemia often require treatment with both diet and more than one cholesterol-lowering drug. Concurrent therapy with HMG-CoA reductase inhibitors and fibrates is usually avoided, in view of their overlapping side-effects, but in very severe cases such mixed therapy has been undertaken under very close supervision.

(a)

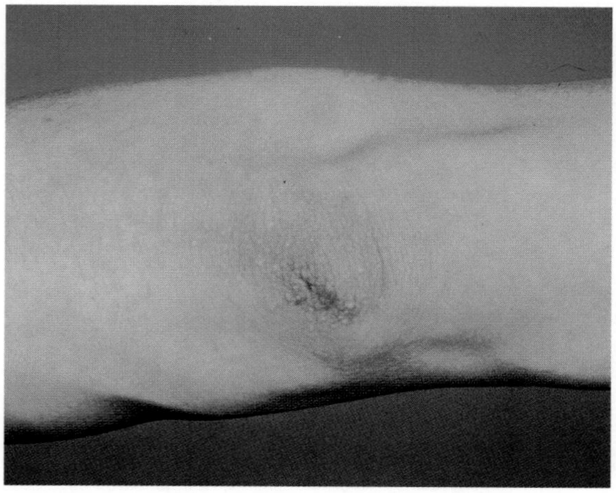

(b)

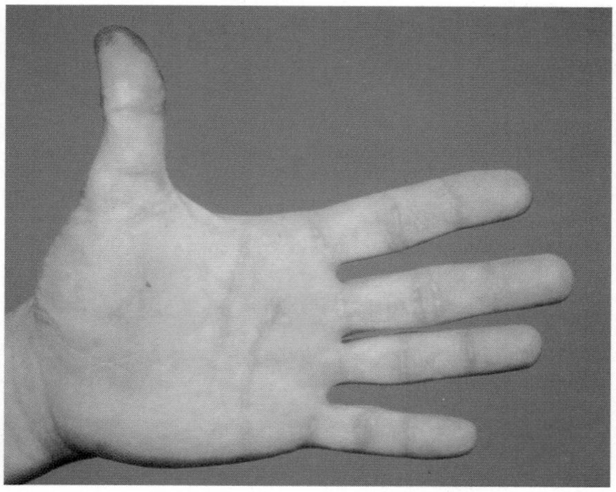

Fig 17.21
Tuberous xanthomata behind the elbow and lipid deposits in the hand creases in a patient with remnant hyperlipidaemia

Secondary prevention

Studies have shown a clear reduction in mortality, and patients should be started on a statin (see below and Table 17.12) at lower serum cholesterol levels than for primary prevention (Table 17.11).

Combined hyperlipidaemia (hypercholesterolaemia and hypertriglyceridaemia)

Treatment is the same for all varieties of combined hyperlipidaemia. For any given cholesterol concentration the hypertriglyceridaemia found in the combined hyperlipidaemias increases the cardiovascular risk considerably. Treatment is aimed at reducing serum cholesterol below 6.5 mmol L^{-1} and triglycerides below 2.0 mmol L^{-1}. Therapy is with diet in the first instance and with drugs if an adequate response has not occurred. Fibric acid derivatives are the treatment of choice since these reduce both cholesterol and triglyceride concentrations, and also have the benefit of raising cardioprotective HDL concentrations. The combination of a fibric acid derivative and bile acid binding resin is of considerable use when a fibrate alone produces an insufficient reduction in LDL cholesterol. Nicotinic acid can be used in addition, although its unwanted effects render it a third-line agent.

Scientific basis of drug treatment of hyperlipidaemia

Fibrates

Fibrates raise HDL concentrations (beneficial) and reduce LDL cholesterol concentrations by 10–15% and are useful in patients with modest hypercholesterolaemia. Gemfibrozil has been demonstrated to reduce the incidence of cardiovascular events in a carefully performed large randomized double-blind placebo-controlled primary prevention trial (the Helsinki Heart Study) of patients with moderate hypercholesterolaemia (Information box 17.4). No similar trials have been carried out to assess the benefit of the other fibrates. Clofibrate is rarely used and is associated with an increased incidence of gallstones.

Bile acid binding resins

These produce an 8–15% reduction in LDL cholesterol concentration. Cholestyramine has been shown to reduce the incidence of cardiovascular events in hypercholesterolaemic patients in a carefully performed randomized double-blind placebo-controlled primary prevention trial (the Lipid Research Clinics Trial). The safety profile of these drugs is good and their long-term safety is established. They are particularly useful when a lipid-lowering agent needs to be given to women of childbearing age. They have a synergistic effect when given with an HMG-CoA reductase inhibitor. This combination can reduce LDL cholesterol concentrations by 50–60%.

HMG-CoA reductase inhibitors (statins)

These reduce LDL cholesterol concentrations by 30–40%. Two large secondary prevention trials – the Scandanavian Simvastatin Survival Study (4S) and the Cholesterol and Rare Events (CARE) trial – and one large primary prevention study, the West of Scotland Coronary Prevention Study (WOSCOPS) have demonstrated clearly the benefits of two drugs, simvastatin and pravastatin, in reducing both mortality and cardiovascular morbidity in hypercholesterolaemic patients, whether they are well or already have had a heart attack or angina (Fig. 17.22). The CARE trial went

Information

Primary prevention trial
Patients are treated before any end organ damage has been discovered.

Secondary prevention trial
Patients who have already sustained end organ damage (e.g. heart attack) are studied.

Information box 17.4 Prevention trials

Table 17.11
Level of serum cholesterol at which drug treatment should be commenced following failure of diet

	Clinical context	Total cholesterol (mmol L^{-1})	LDL cholesterol (mmol L^{-1})
Secondary prevention (see also Fig 17.22(b))	CHD Post CABG angioplasty	>4.8	>3.3
Primary prevention	Genetic, or two of: smoking, diabetes, hypertension	>6.5	>5.0
	Asymptomatic men	>7.8	>6.0
	Postmenopausal women	>7.8	>6.0

CHD, coronary heart disease.
CABG, coronary artery bypass graft surgery.

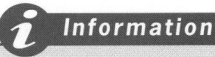

Table 17.12
Drugs used in the management of hyperlipidaemia

Drug	Mechanism of action	Contraindications and adverse reaction	Expected lipid-lowering effect	Long-term safety
Fibric acid derivatives e.g. Gemfibrozil Bezafibrate Fenofibrate Ciprofibrate	Complex and not fully understood 1. Limit substrate availability for hepatic triglyceride synthesis 2. Modulate LDL/ligand interaction 3. Promote action of lipoprotein lipase 4. Stimulate reverse transport of cholesterol	*Contraindications* Severe hepatic or renal impairment, gallbladder disease, pregnancy *Adverse effects* Reversible myositis, nausea, predispose to gallstones, non-specific malaise, impotence	Reduction of LDL cholesterol by 10–15% and triglycerides by 25–35% HDL cholesterol concentrations increase by 0–15% (newer agents often have greater beneficial effect on HDL)	No knowledge of effect on developing foetus Avoid in women of childbearing age Medium-term safety appears good but there is little really long-term experience
Cholesterol binding resins e.g. Cholestyramine Colestipol	Anion exchange resins Bind bile acids in the gut, preventing enterohepatic circulation This promotes liver to convert cholesterol to bile acids Also stimulates formation of hepatic LDL receptors which take up more cholesterol from the circulation	*Adverse effects* Gastrointestinal adverse effects predominate: nausea, flatulence, abdominal bloating, alteration in bowel habit Palatability is a problem for some *Counselling* Other drugs bind to resins and should be taken 1 h before or 4 h afterwards	8–15% reduction in LDL Little or no effect on HDL cholesterol 5–15% rise in triglyceride concentration	Not systemically absorbed Safety profile is good and theoretically resins are of low risk in women of childbearing age Fat-soluble vitamin supplements may be required in children, pregnancy and breast feeding
HMG-CoA reductase inhibitors ('statins') e.g Simvastatin Pravastatin Atorvastatin Cerivastatin Fluvastatin Atorvastatin	Inhibit the rate-limiting step in cholesterol synthesis	*Contraindications* Active liver disease, pregnancy, lactation *Adverse effects* Derangement of liver function tests (recommended to measure liver function before and periodically during treatment) Myositis. Interferes with cyclosporin elimination and raises its blood concentration	30–40% reduction in LDL cholesterol Little effect on triglycerides or HDL cholesterol, except Atorvastatin modestly lowers triglycerides	Undetermined
Nicotinic acid and derivatives e.g. Nicotinic acid Acipimox	Unclear Probably inhibits lipid synthesis in the liver by reducing free fatty acid concentrations owing to an inhibitory effect on lipolysis in fat tissue	*Contraindication* Pregnancy, breast feeding *Adverse effects* Value limited by frequent side-effects: Headache, flushing, dizziness, nausea, malaise, itching, abnormal liver function Glucose intolerance, hyperuricaemia, activation of peptic ulcers, hyper-pigmentation may occur	Reduce LDL and triglycerides by 5–10% Modest HDL increase	Medium-term safety known but marred by the adverse effects listed
ω-3 marine triglycerides	Reduce hepatic VLDL secretion	Occasional nausea and belching	Reduces triglycerides in severe hypertri-glyceridaemia No favourable change in other lipids, and may aggravate hyper-cholesterolaemia in a few patients	No long-term experience

further in showing that cholesterol-lowering therapy using pravastatin reduced the risk of another heart attack in patients with cholesterol concentrations in the upper half of the normal range (4.0–6.0 mmol L^{-1}).

Should all postinfarct patients and hypercholesterolaemic patients be on a lipid-lowering drug? The greater an individual's overall cardiovascular risk, the more the cost/benefit ratio leans towards benefit (see p. 689).

The lipid-lowering diet

Studies have shown that dietitians helping patients to adjust their own diet to meet the nutritional targets set out below produce a better lipid-lowering effect than does the issuing of standard diet sheets and advice from a doctor. The main elements of a lipid-lowering diet are set out below.

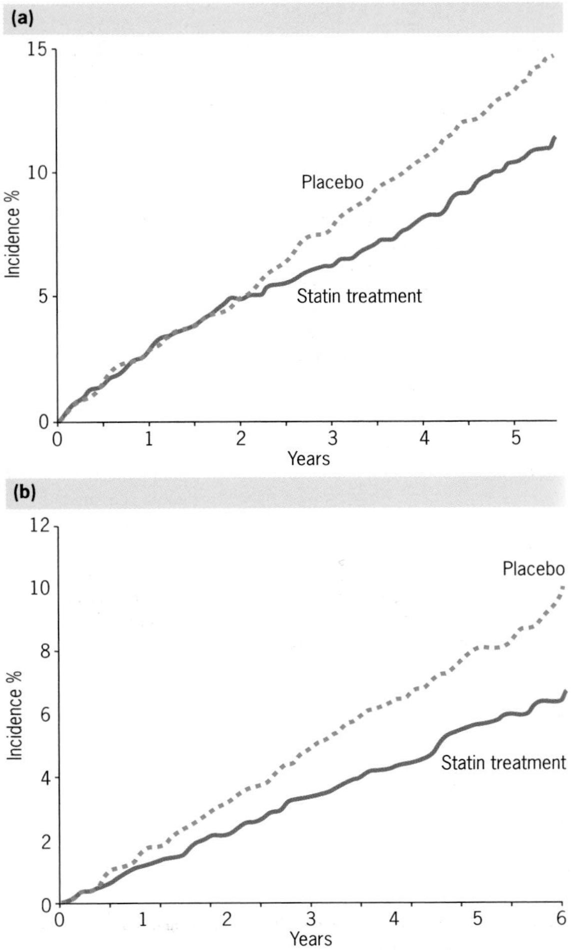

Fig 17.22
Fatal coronary heart disease and non-fatal myocardial infarction according to treatment group in two trials:
(a) WOSCOPS (6595 men studied) and
(b) CARE (4159 studied, predominantly men)

Reduce the total fat intake
Dairy products and meat are the principal sources of saturated fat in the diet. Intake of these products should therefore be reduced, and fish and poultry should be substituted. Visible fat and skin should be removed before cooking and preparing meat dishes. Meat products including sausages and reconstituted meats (such as 'luncheon meat') should be avoided since the concentration of fat is unknown and often high. Baking and grilling of meats reduces the fat content and is preferred to frying. Low-fat or cottage cheese and skimmed or semi-skimmed milk should be substituted for the standard full-fat varieties. Pastries and cakes contain large quantities of fat and should be avoided. The overall aim should be to decrease fat intake such that it is providing approximately 30% of the total energy intake in the diet. Further reduction in fat intake is unacceptable to many patients.

Substitution with monounsaturates and polyunsaturates
Monounsaturated oils, particularly olive oil, and polyunsaturated oils such as sunflower, safflower, corn and soya oil, should be used in cooking instead of saturated fat-rich alternatives.

Reduce the dietary cholesterol intake
Liver, offal and fish roes should be avoided. Although eggs and prawns are rich in cholesterol their total contribution to the body's cholesterol pool is small and they can still be part of a balanced lipid-lowering diet.

Increase the intake of fibre (non-starch polysaccharides, NSPs)
Food high in soluble fibre, such as pulses, legumes, root vegetables, leafy vegetables, and unprocessed cereals, help reduce circulating lipid concentrations. These should be substituted in the diet in the place of higher fat alternatives.

Reduce alcohol consumption
Excess alcohol is an important cause of secondary hyperlipidaemia, and may worsen primary lipid disorders.

Achieve an ideal bodyweight
Treatment of obesity is particularly important in the management of hyperlipidaemia, both because it will exacerbate the lipid disorder itself, and because obesity is an independent cardiovascular risk factor.

Other lipid disorders

Hypolipidaemia

Low lipid levels can be found in severe protein-energy malnutrition. They are also seen occasionally with severe malabsorption and in intestinal lymphangiectasia.

Hypobetalipoproteinaemia (Table 17.10) is a benign familial condition which is being increasingly recognized. The cholesterol levels are in the range 1–3.5 mmol L^{-1}.

Abetalipoproteinaemia

This is described on p. 259.

Familial α-lipoprotein deficiency (Tangier disease)

One of the two HDL apoproteins, apoprotein A-I, is deficient in homozygotes with this very rare disease, so that there is little HDL in plasma. Tangier disease is inherited as an autosomal recessive. The serum cholesterol is low, but serum triglycerides are normal or high. Cholesterol accumulates in reticuloendothelial tissue, although the mechanism is uncertain, producing enlarged and orange-coloured tonsils and hepatosplenomegaly. There are also corneal opacities and a polyneuropathy.

FURTHER READING

Anonymous (1996) Management of hyperlipidaemia. *Drug and Therapeutics Bulletin* **34**(12): 89–93.

Dammerman M, Breslow JL (1995) Genetic basis of lipoprotein disorders. *Circulation* **91**: 505–512.

Farmer JA, Gotto AM (1996) Choosing the right lipid-regulating agent: a guide to selection. *Drugs* **52**: 649–661.

Galton DJ, Krone W (1991) *Hyperlipidaemia in Practice*. London: Gower Medical.

Garber AM, Browner WS, Hulley SB (1996) Cholesterol screening in asymptomatic adults – revisited. *Annals of Internal Medicine* **124**: 518–531.

Grundy SM (1997) Cholesterol and coronary heart disease: the 21st century. *Archives of Internal Medicine* **157**: 1177–1184.

Sacks FM, Pfeffer MA et al (1996) The effect of pravastatin on coronary events after myocardial infarction in patients with average cholesterol levels. *New England Journal of Medicine* **335**: 1001–1009.

Scandanavian Simvastatin Survival Study Group (1994) Randomized trial of cholesterol lowering in 4444 patients with coronary heart disease. *Lancet* **334**: 1383–1389.

Shepherd J, Cobbe SM et al (1995) Prevention of coronary heart disease with pravastatin in men with hypercholesterolaemia. *New England Journal of Medicine* **333**: 1301–1307

Thompson GR (1997) What targets should lipid-modulating therapy achieve to optimize the prevention of coronary heart disease? *Atherosclerosis* **131**: 1–5.

Inborn errors of carbohydrate metabolism

Glycogen storage disease

All mammalian cells can manufacture glycogen, but the main sites of its production are the liver and muscle. Glycogen is a high-molecular-weight glucose polymer. In glycogen storage

Table 17.13
Some glycogen storage diseases

Type	Affected tissue	Enzyme defect	Clinical features	Tissue needed for diagnosis*	Outcome
Liver glycogenoses					
I (Von Gierke)	Liver, intestine, kidney	Glucose-6-phosphatase	Hepatomegaly, hypoglycaemia, stunted growth, obesity, hypotonia	Liver	If patients survive initial hypoglycaemia, prognosis is good; hyperuricaemia is a late complication
III (Forbes)	Liver, muscle (abnormal glycogen structure)	Glycogen debranching enzyme	Like type I	Leucocytes, liver, muscle	Good prognosis but progressive neuropathy and cardiomyopathy
IV (Anderson)	Liver (abnormal glycogen structure)	Branching enzyme	Failure to thrive, hepatomegaly, cirrhosis and its complications	Leucocytes, liver, muscle	Death in first 5 years
VI (Hers)	Liver	Liver phosphorylase or phosphorylase kinase	Hepatomegaly with hypoglycaemia in childhood	Liver	Good
Muscle glycogenoses					
II (Pompé)	Liver, muscle, heart	Lysosomal acid α-glucosidase	Heart failure, cardiomyopathy	Fibroblasts, muscles	Death in first 6 months; juvenile and adult variants seen
V (McArdle)	Muscle only	Phosphorylase	Muscle cramps and myoglobinuria after exercise (in adults)	Muscle	Normal life span; exercise must be avoided
VII (Tarui)	Muscle	Phosphofructokinase	Like type V	Muscle	Like type V

*Tissue obtained is used for the biochemical assay of the enzyme.

disease there is either an abnormality in the molecular structure or an increase in glycogen concentration owing to a specific enzyme defect. Almost all these conditions are autosomal recessive in inheritance and present in infancy, except for McArdle's disease, which presents in adults.

Table 17.13 shows the classification and clinical features of some of these diseases.

Galactosaemia

Galactose is normally converted to glucose. However, a deficiency of the enzyme, galactose-1-phosphate uridyltransferase results in accumulation of galactose-1-phosphate in the blood. This deficiency, inherited as an autosomal recessive, results in hypoglycaemia and acidosis in the neonate. Progressive hepatosplenomegaly, cataracts, renal tubular defects and mental retardation occur.

Treatment is with a galactose-free diet, which, if started early, results in normal development. Untreated patients die within a few days. Prenatal diagnosis and diagnosis of the carrier state are possible by measurement of the level of galactose-1-phosphate in the blood.

Galactokinase deficiency also results in galactosaemia and early cataract formation.

Defects of fructose metabolism

Absorbed fructose is chiefly metabolized in the liver to lactic acid or glucose. Three defects of metabolism in the liver and intestine occur; all are inherited as autosomal recessive traits:

- *Fructosuria* is due to fructokinase deficiency. It is a benign condition.
- *Fructose intolerance* is due to fructose-1-phosphate aldolase deficiency. Fructose-1-phosphate accumulates after fructose ingestion, inhibiting both glycogenolysis and gluconeogenesis, resulting in symptoms of hypoglycaemia. Hepatomegaly and renal tubular defects occur but are reversible on a fructose-free diet. Intelligence is normal and there is an absence of dental caries.
- *Fructose-1,6-diphosphatase deficiency* leads to a failure of gluconeogenesis. Infants present with hypoglycaemia, ketosis and lactic acidosis. Dietary control can lead to normal growth.

Pentosuria

Pentosuria is due to L-xylulose reductase deficiency. It has no clinical significance.

Inborn errors of amino acid metabolism

Inborn errors of amino acid metabolism are chiefly inherited as autosomal recessive conditions. The major ones are shown in Table 17.14.

Amino acid transport defects

Amino acids are filtered by the glomerulus, but 95% of the filtered load is reabsorbed in the proximal convoluted tubule by an active transport mechanism. *Aminoaciduria* results from:

- abnormally high plasma amino acid levels (e.g. phenylketonuria)
- any inherited disorder that damages the tubules secondarily (e.g. galactosaemia)
- tubular reabsorptive defects, either generalized (e.g. Fanconi syndrome) or specific (e.g. cystinuria)
- amino acid transport defects can be congenital or acquired.

Generalized aminoacidurias

Fanconi syndrome

This occurs in a juvenile form (De Toni–Fanconi–Debré syndrome); in adult life it is often acquired through, for example, heavy metal poisoning, drugs or some renal diseases. There is defective tubular reabsorption of:

- most amino acids
- glucose
- urate
- phosphate, resulting in hypophosphataemic rickets
- bicarbonate, with failure to transport hydrogen ions, causing a renal tubular acidosis that then produces a hyperchloraemic acidosis.

Other abnormalities include:

- potassium depletion, primary or secondary to the acidosis
- polyuria
- increased excretion of immunoglobulins and other low-molecular-weight proteins.

Various combinations of the above abnormalities have been described.

The juvenile form begins at the age of 6–9 months, with failure to thrive, vomiting and thirst. The clinical features are as a result of fluid and electrolyte loss and the characteristic vitamin D-resistant rickets.

In the adult, the disease is similar to the juvenile form, but osteomalacia is a major feature.

Treatment of the bone disease is with large doses of vitamin D (e.g. 1–2 mg of 1α-hydroxycholecalciferol with regular blood calcium monitoring). Fluid and electrolyte loss need to be corrected.

Lowe's syndrome (oculocerebrorenal dystrophy)

In this syndrome there is generalized aminoaciduria combined with mental retardation, hypotonia, congenital cataracts and an abnormal skull shape.

Table 17.14
The major inborn errors of amino acid metabolism

Disease	Enzyme defect	Incidence	Biochemical and clinical features	Treatment	Prognosis
Albinism	Tyrosinase	1 in 13 000	Amelanosis: whitish hair, pink–white skin, grey–blue eyes Nystagmus, photophobia, strabismus	Symptomatic	Good
Alkaptonuria	Homogentisic acid oxidase	1 in 100 000	Homogentisic acid polymerizes to produce a black –brown product that is deposited in cartilage and other tissue (ochronosis)	None	Good
Homocystinuria					
Type I	Cystathionine synthetase		Homocystine is excreted in urine Mental handicap Marfan-like syndrome Thrombotic episodes	 – – –	 – – –
Type II	Methylene tetra-hydrofolate reductase		Survivors have mental retardation		Mainly die as neonates
Phenylketonuria	Phenylalanine hydroxylase	1 in 20 000	Brain damage with mental retardation and epilepsy Phenylpyruvate and its derivatives excreted in urine	Diet low in phenylalanine in first few months of life prevents damage	Good but some intellectual impairment
Histidinaemia	Histidase	Very rare	Mental retardation	–	–
'Maple syrup' disease	Branched-chain ketoacid dehydrogenase	Very rare	Failure to thrive Fits, neonatal acidosis and severe cerebral degeneration Valine, isoleucine and their derivatives are excreted in urine A milder form is seen	–	Early death
Oxalosis (hyperoxaluria)	Alanine: glyoxylate amino-transferase	Very rare	Nephrocalcinosis, renal stones, renal failure due to deposition of calcium oxalate Prenatal and early diagnosis now possible	–	Liver transplantation ? gene therapy

There are many other enzyme defects producing, for example, alaninaemia, ammonaemia, argininaemia, citrullinaemia, isovaleric acidaemia, lysinaemia, ornithinaemia or tyrosinaemia.

Specific aminoacidurias

Cystinuria

There is a defective tubular reabsorption and jejunal absorption of cystine and the dibasic amino acids, lysine, ornithine and arginine. Inheritance is either completely or incompletely recessive, so that heterozygotes who have increased excretion of lysine and cystine only can occur. Cystine absorption from the jejunum is impaired but, nevertheless, cystine in peptide form can be absorbed. Cystinuria leads to urinary stones and is responsible for approximately 1–2% of all urinary calculi. The disease often starts in childhood, although most cases present in adult life.

Treatment is with a high fluid intake in order to keep the urinary cystine concentration low. Patients are encouraged to drink up to 3 L over 24 hours and to drink even at night. Penicillamine should be used for patients who cannot keep the cystine concentration of their urine low.

The condition *cystinosis* (see p. 1002) must not be confused with cystinuria.

Hartnup's disease

There is defective tubular reabsorption and jejunal absorption of most neutral amino acids but not their peptides. The resulting tryptophan malabsorption produces nicotinamide deficiency (see p. 203). Patients can be asymptomatic, but others develop evidence of pellagra, with cerebellar ataxia, psychiatric disorders and skin lesions. Treatment is nicotinamide which often brings about considerable improvement.

Tryptophan malabsorption syndrome (blue diaper syndrome)

This is due to an isolated transport defect for tryptophan: the trytophan excreted oxidizes to a blue colour on the baby's diaper.

Familial iminoglycinuria

This occurs when there is defective tubular reabsorption of glycine, proline and hydroxyproline. It seems to have few clinical effects.

Methionine malabsorption syndrome

This is due to failure to absorb and excrete methionine, and results in diarrhoea, vomiting and mental retardation. Patients characteristically have an oast-house smell.

Lysosomal storage diseases

Lysosomal storage diseases are due to inborn errors of metabolism which are mainly inherited in an autosomal recessive manner.

Glucosylceramide lipidoses: Gaucher's disease

This is the most prevalent lysosomal storage disease and is due to a deficiency in glucocerebrosidase, a specialized lysosomal acid β-glucosidase. This results in accumulation of glucosylceramide in the lysosomes of the reticulo-endothelial system, particularly the liver, bone marrow and spleen. Several mutations have been characterized in the glucocerebrosidase gene, the most common being a single base change causing the substitution of arginine to serine; this is seen in 70% of Jewish patients. The typical Gaucher cell, a glucocerebroside-containing reticuloendothelial histiocyte, is found in the bone marrow.

There are three clinical types, the most common presenting in adult life with an insidious onset of hepatosplenomegaly. There is a high incidence in Ashkenazi Jews (1 in 3000 births), and patients have a characteristic pigmentation on exposed parts, particularly the forehead and hands. The clinical spectrum is variable, with patients developing anaemia, evidence of hypersplenism and pathological fractures that are due to bone involvement. Nevertheless, many have a normal lifespan.

Acute Gaucher's disease presents in infancy or childhood with rapid onset of hepatosplenomegaly, with neurological involvement owing to the presence of Gaucher cells in the brain. The outlook is poor.

Some patients with non-neuropathic Gaucher's disease show considerable improvement with infusion of alglucerase (mannose-terminated placental or human recombinant glucocerebrosidase).

Sphingomyelin cholesterol lipidoses: Niemann–Pick disease

The disease is due to a deficiency of lysosomal sphingomyelinase which results in the accumulation of sphingomyelin cholesterol and glycosphingolipids in the reticuloendothelial macrophages of many organs, particularly the liver, spleen, bone marrow and lymph nodes. The disease usually presents within the first six months of life with mental retardation and hepatosplenomegaly. Typical foam cells are found in the marrow, lymph nodes, liver and spleen.

The mucopolysaccharidoses (MPSs)

These are a group of disorders caused by the deficiency of lysosomal enzymes required for the catabolism of glycosaminoglycans (mucopolysaccharides).

The catabolism of dermatan sulphate, heparan sulphate, keratin sulphate or chondroitin sulphate may be affected either singularly or together.

Accumulation of glycosaminoglycans in the lysosomes of various tissues results in the disease. Ten forms of MPS have been described; all are chronic but progressive and a wide spectrum of clinical severity can be seen within a single enzyme defect. The MPS types show many clinical features though in variable amounts, with dysostosis, abnormal facies, poor vision and hearing and joint dysmobility (either stiff or hypermobile) being frequently seen. Mental retardation is present in, for example, Hurler (MPS IH) and San Filippo A (MPS IIIA) types, but normal intelligence and lifespan are seen in Scheie (MPS IS).

The GM2 gangliosidoses

In these conditions there is accumulation of GM_2 gangliosides in the central nervous system and peripheral nerves. It is particularly common (1 in 2000) in Ashkenazi Jews. *Tay-Sachs disease* is the severest form where there is a progressive degeneration of all cerebral function, with fits, epilepsy, dementia and blindness, and death usually occurs before two years of age. The macula has a characteristic cherry spot appearance.

Fabry's disease

This X-linked recessive condition is due to a deficiency of the lysosomal hydrolase α-galactosidase causing an accumulation of glycosphingolipids with terminal α-galactosyl moieties in the lysosomes of various tissues including the liver, kidney, blood vessels and the ganglion cells of the nervous system. The patients present with peripheral nerve involvement, but eventually most patients develop renal problems in adult life.

DIAGNOSIS

Many of the sphingolipidoses can be diagnosed by demonstrating the enzyme deficiency in the appropriate tissue.

Prenatal diagnosis is possible in a number of the conditions by obtaining specimens of amniotic cells. Carrier states can also be identified, so that sensible genetic counselling can be given.

Cystinosis

Cystine accumulates within the lysosomes of most tissues, but particularly the kidneys. This is due to a defect of cystine transport across the lysosomal membrane. There are two cystinosis phenotypes, *nephropathic* and *non-nephropathic*.

The common nephropathic form presents in the first year of life with failure to thrive. This results from the renal tubular Fanconi syndrome caused by cystine deposits in the kidney. Renal damage progresses and visual impairment occurs as the result of cystine deposits in the retina and cornea. Renal transplantation relieves the kidney problems, but cystine accumulation continues to occur.

The nephropathic form can present in older children and in adults, when the condition tends to be less aggressive.

The non-nephropathic form presents in children with visual impairment. The kidneys seem not to be affected.

Amyloidosis

Amyloidosis is a disorder of protein metabolism in which there is an extracellular deposition of pathologic insoluble fibrillar proteins in organs and tissues. Characteristically, the amyloid protein consists of β-pleated sheets that are responsible for its insolubility and resistance to proteolysis.

Amyloidosis can be *acquired* or *inherited*. Classification is based on the nature of the precursor plasma proteins that form the fibrillar deposits. The process for the production of these fibrils appears to be multifactorial and differs amongst the various types of amyloid.

AL amyloidosis

This is a plasma cell dyscrasia, related to multiple myeloma, in which clonal plasma cells in the bone marrow produce immunoglobulins that are amyloidogenic. This may be the outcome of destabilization of light chains owing to substitution of particular amino acids into the light chain variable region. There is a clonal dominance of amyloid light (AL) chains – either the dominant κ or λ isotype – which are excreted in the urine (Bence–Jones proteins). This type of amyloid is often associated with lymphoproliferative disorders, such as myeloma, Waldenström's macroglobulinaemia or non-Hodgkin's lymphoma.

Familial amyloidoses

These are autosomally dominant transmitted diseases where the mutant protein forms amyloid fibrils, starting usually in middle age. The most common form is due to a mutant – transthyretin – which is a tetrameric protein with four identical subunits. It is a transport protein for thyroxine and retinol binding protein and mainly synthesized in the liver. Over 50 amino acid substitutions have been described; for example, a common substitution is that of methionine for valine at position 30 (Met 30) in all racial groups, and alanine for threonine (Ala 60) in the English and Irish. These substitutions destabilize the protein which precipitates following stimulation, and can cause disorders such as familial amyloidotic polyneuropathy (FAP) or cardiomyopathy. Major foci of FAP occur in Portugal, Japan and Sweden.

Other less common variants include mutations of apolipoprotein A-1, gelsolin, fibrinogen Aα and lysosyme.

Reactive systemic (secondary) amyloidoses

These are due to amyloid formed from serum amyloid A (SAA) which is an acute phase protein. It is, therefore, related to chronic inflammatory disorders and chronic infection.

CLINICAL FEATURES

Immunoglobulin light chain-associated (AL) (primary) amyloidosis

The clinical features are related to the organs involved. These include the kidneys (presenting with proteinuria and the nephrotic syndrome) and the heart (presenting with heart failure). Autonomic and sensory neuropathies are relatively common, and carpal tunnel syndrome with weakness and paraesthesia of the hands may be an early feature. Sensory neuropathy is common. There is an absence of central nervous system involvement.

On examination, hepatomegaly and rarely splenomegaly, cardiomyopathy, polyneuropathy and bruising may be seen. Macroglossia occurs in about 20% of cases.

Familial transthyretin-associated (ATTR) amyloidosis

In this condition peripheral sensorimotor and autonomic neuropathy is more common, with symptoms of autonomic dysfunction, diarrhoea and weight loss. Renal disease is less prevalent than with AL amyloidsis. Macroglossia does not occur. Cardiac problems are usually those of con-duction. There may be a family history of unidentified neurological disease.

Other hereditary systemic amyloidoses include other familial amyloid polyneuropathies (e.g. Portuguese, Icelandic, Dutch). There is a familial Creutzfeldt–Jacob disease. In familial Mediterranean fever, renal amyloidosis is a common serious complication.

AA (reactive or secondary) amyloidosis

This depends on the nature of the disorder. Chronic inflammatory disorders include rheumatoid arthritis, inflammatory bowel disease, and untreated familial Mediterranean fever. In developing countries it is still associated with infectious diseases such as tuberculosis, bronchiectasis and osteomyelitis. AA amyloidosis often presents with renal disease, with hepatomegaly and splenomegaly. Macroglossia is not a feature and cardiac involvement is rare.

Cerebral amyloidosis, Alzheimer's disease and transmissable spongiform encephalopathy

The brain is a common site of amyloid deposition, although it is not directly affected in any form of acquired systemic amyloidosis. Intracerebral and cerebrovascular amyloid deposits are seen in Alzheimer's disease. Most cases are sporadic, but hereditary forms caused by mutations have been reported. In hereditary spongiform encephalopathies several amyloid plaques have been seen.

Amyloid deposits are frequently found in the elderly, particularly cerebral deposits of A4 protein. This is also seen in Down's syndrome. Apoprotein E (involved in LDL transport, see p. 990) interacts directly with β-A4 protein in senile plaques and neurofibrillary tangles in the brain. The gene for apoprotein E is on chromosome 19 and may be an important susceptibility factor in the aetiology of Alzheimer's disease.

Local amyloidosis

Deposits of amyloid fibrils of various types can be localized to various organs or tissues (e.g. skin, heart and brain) and amyloid syndrome due to β_2 microglobulin deposition as amyloid fibrils is seen in patients on long-term haemodialysis (see p. 580).

DIAGNOSIS

This is based on clinical suspicion and, if possible, on tissue histology. Amyloid in tissues appears as an amorphous, homogeneous substance that stains pink with haemotoxylin and eosin and stains red with Congo red. It also has a green fluorescence in polarized light. Tissue can be obtained from the rectum or gum. The bone marrow may show plasma cells in primary amyloidosis or a lymphoproliferative disorder. A paraproteinaemia and proteinuria with light chains in the urine may be seen in AL amyloidosis. In secondary or reactive amyloidosis there will be an underlying disorder. Scintigraphy using ^{123}I-labelled serum amyloid P component is useful for the assessment of AL. ATTR and AA amyloidosis, but it is not widely available.

TREATMENT

This is symptomatic or the treatment of the associated disorder. The nephrotic syndrome and congestive cardiac failure require the relevant therapies. Treatment of any inflammatory source or infection should be instituted. Colchicine may help familial Mediterranean fever. Chemotherapy is showing some efficacy in AL amyloidosis. In ATTR amyloidosis where transthyretin is predominantly synthesized in the liver, liver transplantation (when there would be a disappearance of the mutant protein from the blood) is now considered as the definitive therapy.

REFERENCE

Falk RH, Comenzo RL, Skinner M (1997) The systemic amyloidoses *New England Journal of Medicine* **337**: 898–909.

The porphyrias

This heterogeneous group of rare inborn errors of metabolism is caused by abnormalities of enzymes involved in the biosynthesis of haem, resulting in overproduction of the intermediate compounds called 'porphyrins' (Fig 17.23). The porphyrias show extreme genetic heterogeneity. For example, in acute intermittent poprhyria more than 90 mutations have been identified in the porphobilinogen deaminase gene. One mutation has a high prevalence in patients in northern Sweden, suggesting a common ancestor.

Structurally, porphyrins consist of four pyrrole rings. These pyrrole rings are formed from the precursors glycine and succinyl-CoA, which are converted to δ-amino-laevulinic acid (δ-ALA) in a reaction catalysed by the enzyme δ-ALA synthetase. Two molecules of δ-ALA condense to form a pyrrole ring.

Porphyrins can be divided into uroporphyrins, coproporphyrins or protoprophyrins depending on the structure of the side-chain. They are termed type I if the structure is symmetrical and type III if it is

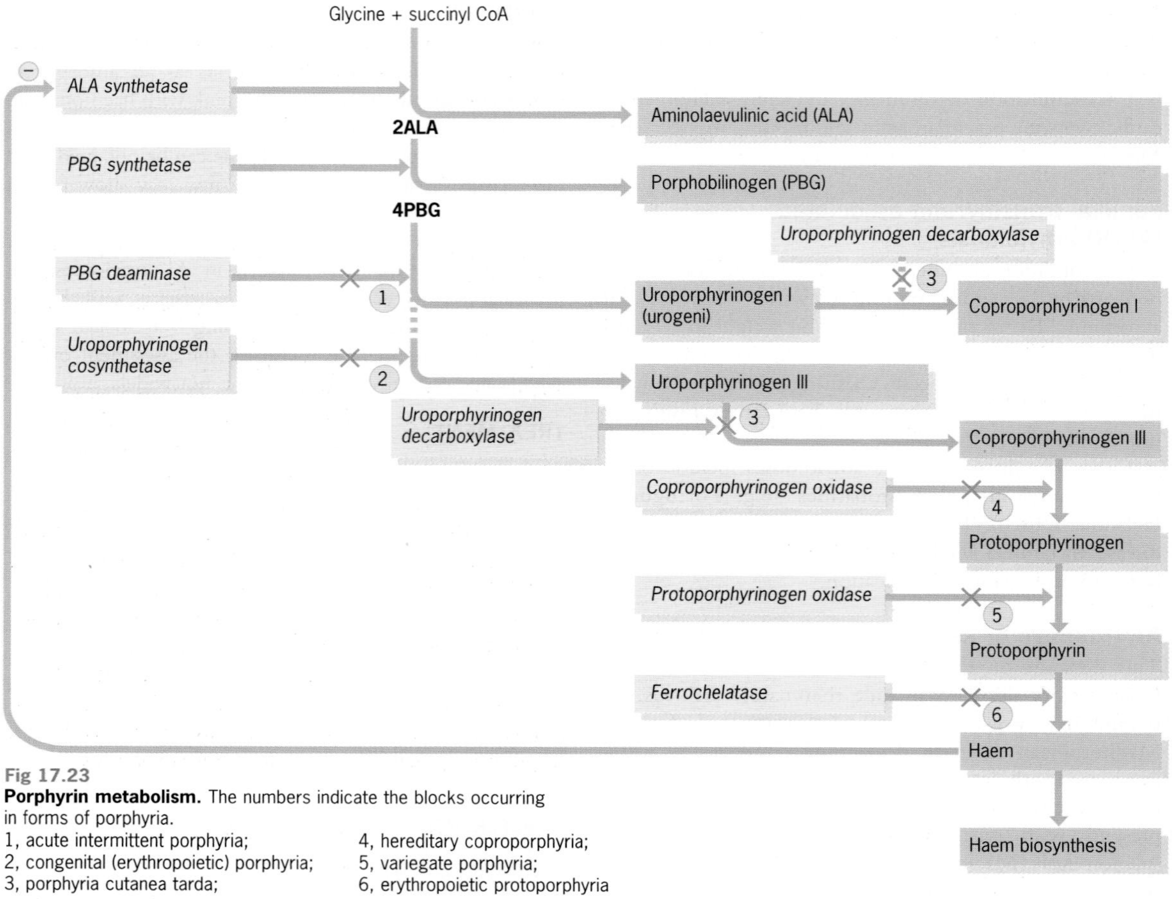

Fig 17.23
Porphyrin metabolism. The numbers indicate the blocks occurring in forms of porphyria.
1, acute intermittent porphyria;
2, congenital (erythropoietic) porphyria;
3, porphyria cutanea tarda;
4, hereditary coproporphyria;
5, variegate porphyria;
6, erythropoietic protoporphyria

asymmetrical. Both uroporphyrins and coproporphyrins can be excreted in the urine.

The sequence of enzymatic changes in the production of haem is shown in Fig 17.23. The chief rate-limiting step is the enzyme δ-ALA synthetase, as an increase in this enzyme results in an overproduction of porphyrins. Haem provides a negative feedback mechanism on this enzyme.

In porphyria the excess production of porphyrins occurs either in the liver (hepatic porphyrias) or in the bone marrow (erythropoietic porphyria), but porphrias can also be classified in terms of clinical presentation as *acute* or *non-acute*. Acute porphyrias usually produce neuropsychiatric problems and are associated with excess production and urinary excretion of δ-ALA and porphobilinogen; these metabolites are not increased in non-acute porphyrias. The second control mechanism is therefore porphobilinogen deaminase (see Fig 17.23); this is depressed or normal in the acute porphyrias and raised in non-acute cases.

A classification of porphyrias is given in Table 17.15.

Table 17.15
The classification of porphyrias

	Hepatic	Erythropoietic
Acute	Acute intermittent porphyria Variegate porphyria Hereditary coproporphyria	
Non-acute	Porphyria cutanea tarda	Congenital porphyria Erythropoietic protoporphyria

Acute intermittent porphyria

This is an autosomal dominant disorder. Presentation is in early adult life, usually around the age of 30 years, and women are affected more than men. It may be precipitated by alcohol and drugs such as barbiturates and oral contraceptives, but a wide range of lipid-soluble drugs have also been incriminated. The abnormality lies at the level of porphobilinogen deaminase in the haem biosynthetic pathway (see Fig 17.23).

DIAGNOSIS

Presentation is with:

- abdominal pain, vomiting and constipation (90%)
- polyneuropathy (motor, but occasionally sensory) (70%)
- hypertension and tachycardia (70%)
- psychiatric disorders (such as depression, anxiety and frank psychosis) (50%).

The diagnosis should be considered whenever there is a combination of these cardinal features or a family history of porphyria.

The urine turns red-brown or red on standing. A classic bedside test for excess porphobilinogen may be performed by adding one volume of urine to one volume of Ehrlich's aldehyde, which produces a pink colour. If excess porphobilinogen is present, the pink colour persists when two volumes of chloroform are added. A negative test does not exclude an attack. A positive test should be confirmed by a specific assay.

Other investigations

- **Blood count.** This is usually normal, with occasional neutrophil leucocytosis.
- **Liver biochemical tests.** There is elevated bilirubin and transferase.
- **Serum urea** is often raised.
- **Faecal and urinary porphyrins** confirm the type of porphyria.

Screening

Family members should be screened to detect latent cases. Urinalysis is not adequate and measurement of erythrocyte porphobilinogen deaminase and ALA synthetase is extremely sensitive.

MANAGEMENT

Management of the acute episodes is largely supportive. A high carbohydrate intake is maintained (this has an indirect effect on porphyrin overproduction), and a narcotic may be given for pain. Intravenous haematin infusion also appears to be of benefit.

Management in the remission period is by avoidance of possible precipitating factors, particularly drugs and alcohol.

Other acute porphyrias

Variegate porphyria

This combines many of the features of acute intermittent porphyria with those of a cutaneous porphyria. A bullous eruption develops on exposure to sunlight owing to the activation of porphyrins deposited on the skin. There is an increased production of protoporphyrinogens owing to an abnormality of protoporphyrinogen oxidase in the haem biosynthetic pathway (see Fig 17.23).

Fluorescence emission spectroscopy of plasma differentiates this from other acute and cutaneous porphyrias.

Hereditary coproporphyria

This is extremely rare and broadly similar in presentation to variegate prophyria. The distinction is based on biochemical analysis.

Porphyria cutanea tarda (cutaneous hepatic porphyria) (see also p. 1178)

This condition, which has a genetic predisposition, presents with a bullous eruption on exposure to sunlight; the eruption heals with scarring. Alcohol is the most common aetiological agent. There is an abnormality in hepatic uroporphyrinogen decarboxylase. Evidence of biochemical or clinical liver disease may also be present. Polychlorinated hydrocarbons have been implicated and porphyria cutanea tarda has been seen in association with benign or malignant tumours of the liver.

The diagnosis depends on demonstration of increased levels of urinary uroporphyrin. Histology of the skin shows subepidermal blisters with perivascular deposition of periodic acid–Schiff-staining material. The serum iron and transferrin saturation are often raised. Liver biopsy shows mild iron overload as well as features of alcoholic liver disease.

Remission can be induced by venesection; this should be repeated if the urinary uroporphyrin rises in the remission phase. Chloroquine may also have a useful role in promoting urinary excretion of uroporphyrins.

Erythropoietic porphyrias

Congenital porphyria

This is extremely rare and is transmitted as an autosomal recessive trait. Its victims show extreme sensitivity to sunlight and develop disfiguring scars. Dystrophy of the nails, blindness due to lenticular scarring, and brownish discolouration of the teeth also occur.

Erythropoietic protoporphyria

This is more common than congenital porphyria and is inherited as an autosomal dominant trait. It presents with irritation and a burning pain in the skin on exposure to sunlight. Hepatic involvement may also occur. Diagnosis is made by fluorescence of the peripheral red blood cells and by increased protoporphyrin in the red cells and stools. Oral β-carotene provides effective protection against solar sensitivity, but the reason for this is not known.

FURTHER READING

Elder GH, Hift RJ, Meissner PN (1997) The acute porphyrias. *Lancet* **349**: 1613–1617.

GENERAL READING

Scriver CR, Beaudet AL, Sly WS, Valle D (1995) *The Metabolic Basis of Inherited Disease*, 7th edn. New York: McGraw-Hill.

Neurological disease

18

The range of neurological conditions seen in the UK is summarized in Table 18.1, showing that clinical neurology is diverse and complex. Specialization within neurology has led to disciplines such as epileptology, neurogenetics and neuro-oncology. Research has provided new information on movement disorders, prion diseases, peripheral nerve and muscle pathology as well as neurological rehabilitation. Advances in imaging have already revolutionized clinical practice, and will continue to do so.

Despite specialization, neurology retains its clinical roots, with clinical diagnosis dependent upon a history and physical signs. The object of this chapter is to provide an outline of practical neurology for anyone working within general and emergency medicine.

Although the subject is concerned primarily with organic diseases, many of which are serious and intractable, neurological symptoms are presenting features of common minor illnesses and psychological conditions, which require interpretation, sympathy and appropriate management.

Neurology in developing countries

Low standards of nutrition, hygiene and education, with widespread economic hardship, contribute to different patterns of disease. Common neurological conditions of the Indian subcontinent, South East Asia and Africa include:

- leprosy
- tuberculosis (meningitis, tuberculoma)
- meningococcal meningitis
- tetanus
- rabies
- cerebral malaria
- multiple vitamin deficiencies
- cysticercosis
- HIV infection
- Japanese encephalitis (Asia).

Of these, only tuberculosis, meningococcal infection and HIV are seen commonly in Europe.

History, symptoms and signs

The *methods* of recording the history and the basic neurological examination are outside the scope of this chapter. Notes should read chronologically and portray

Table 18.1 Neurological diseases: annual UK incidence rates per 100 000 population

Disorder	Rate
Headache (GP consultations)	2200
Herpes zoster	440
Back pain and sciatica	300
Stroke	150
Epilepsy and single seizures	50
Dementia	50
Polyneuropathy	40
Transient ischaemic attacks	30
Bell's palsy	25
Parkinson's disease	20
Alcohol abuse (neurological complications)	20
Meningitis	15
Encephalitis	15
Subarachnoid haemorrhage	15
Metastatic brain tumour	15
Benign brain tumour	10
Primary malignant brain tumour	5
Metastatic cord tumour	5
Trigeminal neuralgia	4
Multiple sclerosis	3
Motor neurone disease	2
All primary muscle disease	1.5
Intracranial abscess	1
Benign spinal cord tumour	1
Huntington's disease	0.4
Myasthenia gravis	0.4

Prevalence rates often differ widely from annual incidence rates: see individual diseases

the story given by the patient, or relative. The interpretation of history, symptoms and findings on examination provides a highly reliable diagnostic approach. Pattern recognition – and hence practical experience – is vital in neurology. The aim in this section is to discuss several common symptoms and findings on examination, and to relate these to the core of functional neuro-anatomy. This is the essence of clinical diagnosis of many neurological diseases, both common and rare.

There are three critical questions in any neurological case:

- What is/are the site(s) of the lesion(s)?
- What is the likely pathology?
- Does the pattern fit with a recognizable disease?

Three common complaints will be discussed briefly here: (a) headaches of various types; (b) difficulty walking and falls; and (c) dizziness, vertigo, blackouts and 'collapse'. Other specific symptoms are mentioned with individual conditions.

Headache

Headache at some time is an almost universal experience, and one of the most common causes of referral in general and neurological practice. It varies from an infrequent and trivial nuisance to a symptom of serious disease.

MECHANISM OF HEADACHE

Pain receptors are found in arteries and veins at the base of the brain and in the meninges. These receptors are also present in extracranial vessels, the muscles of the scalp, neck and face, paranasal sinuses, eyes and teeth. Curiously, the brain itself is almost devoid of pain receptors.

The pain of headache is mediated by mechanical receptors (e.g. in stretching) and chemical receptors (e.g. 5-hydroxytryptamine and histamine stimulation). Nerve impulses are carried centrally via the fifth and ninth cranial nerves and via upper cervical sensory roots.

Although many headaches are benign, the diagnostic issue – and the usual source of concern for patients – is that some headaches are caused by serious intracranial or extracranial disease. The following are some useful clinical pointers.

Chronic (benign) and recurrent headaches

Almost all recurring headaches – band-like, generalized head pains, with a history going back for several years or months – are vaguely ascribed to muscle tension (itself doubtful, because an increase in scalp muscle tension does not occur) and/or migraine (see p. 1081). *Depression* often accompanies recurrent headaches.

In headaches of short duration, sinusitis, glaucoma and migrainous neuralgia should also be considered, but are usually more localized. Accelerated hypertension, with arterial damage and brain swelling, occasionally causes headache (see p. 732). Headaches are not caused by high blood pressure alone.

Eyestrain from minor or major refractive error is an unusual cause of headache, though headaches are frequently attributed to it.

Pressure headaches

Intracranial mass lesions displace and stretch the meninges and the basal vessels. Pain is provoked when these structures are moved physically either by a mass itself or by changes in cerebrospinal fluid (CSF) pressure, such as with coughing. Cerebral oedema, which accumulates around mass lesions, causes further shift. These headaches typically become worse after lying down for some hours, as cerebral oedema increases.

Any headache, however mild, that is present on waking and which is made worse by coughing, straining or sneezing may well be due to a mass lesion. These are often called the 'headaches of raised intracranial pressure', or simply 'pressure headaches'. Vomiting often accompanies them. Such headaches are caused early, over weeks, by a mass in the posterior fossa, because of hydrocephalus (see p. 1079), but over a longer timescale – months or even years – with hemisphere mass lesions.

A rare cause of prostrating headache with weakness of the lower limbs is increase in intracranial pressure with intermittent hydrocephalus caused by an intraventricular tumour.

Headache of subacute onset

The onset and progression of a headache over days or weeks with or without the features of a pressure headache should also always raise the suspicion of an intracranial mass lesion or serious intracranial disease. Encephalitis (see p. 1073), viral meningitis (p. 1071) and chronic meningitis (p. 1071) should also be considered.

Headaches with scalp tenderness

Patches of exquisite tenderness overlying superficial scalp arteries are caused by giant cell arteritis (see p. 494), which occurs almost exclusively in patients aged over 50 years.

Headache following head injury

Subdural haematoma (see p. 1054) must be considered, whether or not the headache is suggestive of a mass lesion. However, the vast majority of post-trauma headaches which last for days, weeks or months – a common problem – are not associated with any serious intracranial cause.

A single episode of severe headache

This common emergency may be caused by one of the following:

- subarachnoid haemorrhage
- migraine
- meningitis (occasionally).

Particular attention should be paid to the suddenness of onset (suggestive of a subarachnoid haemorrhage), neck stiffness and vomiting (e.g. meningeal irritation), and rashes and fever (suggestive of meningitis).

Difficulty walking and falls

A change in the pattern of gait is a common presenting complaint in neurological disease; the main causes are given in Table 18.2. Arthritis and muscle pain also alter the gait, making it stiff and slow. Recognition of the pattern of an abnormal gait is helpful in diagnosis. Falls, especially in the elderly, are a common and important cause of morbidity.

Spasticity

Spasticity (see p. 1029), particularly in extensor muscles, with or without pyramidal weakness causes stiffness and jerkiness of gait, which is maintained on a narrow base.

Table 18.2
Common neurological patterns of difficulty in walking

Spasticity
Parkinson's disease
Cerebellar ataxia
Sensory loss (joint position)
Distal weakness
Proximal weakness
Apraxia of gait

The toes catch level ground, causing wearing down and scuffing of the toes of the shoes. The pace shortens. Clonus may be noticed by the patient as involuntary extensor rhythmic jerking of the legs.

When the problem is predominantly unilateral and weakness is marked, in a hemiparesis, the weaker leg drags stiffly and is circumducted.

Parkinson's disease (see also p. 1062)

Here there is muscular rigidity in both the extensors and the flexors of the limbs. Power remains normal. The gait slows; the pace shortens to a shuffle. The base remains narrow. Falls occur. A stoop is apparent and swinging of the arms is diminished. The gait is festinant (hurried) as small rapid steps are taken. There is particular difficulty in initiating movement and in turning quickly. Sometimes when the patient stops or is halted, rapid, small and unsteady backward steps are taken; this is known as retropulsion.

Cerebellar ataxia (see also p. 1030)

In disease of the lateral lobes of the cerebellum the stance becomes broad-based, unstable and tremulous. *Ataxia* describes this state of imperfect control. The gait tends to veer towards the side of the more affected cerebellar lobe.

In disease confined to the cerebellar vermis, a midline structure, the trunk becomes unsteady without limb ataxia. There is a tendency to fall backwards or sideways – truncal ataxia.

Sensory ataxia

The ataxia of peripheral sensory lesions (e.g. polyneuropathy – see p. 1093) is due to diminution of the sense of joint position – *proprioceptive loss*. The brain cannot perceive accurately the position of the legs. Gait becomes broad-based and high-stepping, or stamping.

The ataxia is made worse by removal of additional sensory input, such as in the dark or when the eyes are closed. This is the basis of the positive Romberg's test: ask the patient to close their eyes while standing, and observe whether or not the person is unstable (while protecting the individual from injury). This was first described in the sensory ataxia of tabes dorsalis (see p. 1074).

Weakness of the lower limbs

With distal weakness the affected leg is lifted over obstacles. When the dorsiflexors of the foot are weak, such as in a common peroneal nerve palsy (see p. 1093), the foot, having been lifted, returns to the ground with a visible and audible slap.

Weakness of proximal lower limb muscles (e.g. in polymyositis or muscular dystrophy) leads to difficulty in rising from the sitting position. Once upright, the patient walks with a waddling gait, the pelvis being ill-supported by each lower limb as it carries the full weight of the body.

Apraxia of gait

With frontal lobe disease (e.g. tumour, hydrocephalus, infarction), the central organization of walking is disturbed. The patient is able to move the legs normally while sitting or lying but cannot walk in an organized way. This is known as *apraxia of gait* – a failure of the skilled movement of walking. Urinary incontinence and a degree of dementia are often present. Apraxia of gait is used to describe various gait disorders seen commonly in the elderly – the shuffling small steps (*marche à petits pas*) of cerebrovascular disease, difficulty initiating walking, and hesitancy of gait in the face of normal leg movements on the examination couch.

Falls

Falls, especially in the elderly, are a major cause of morbidity and a reason for hospital admission, for example following hip or upper limb fracture. Any gait disturbance may lead to falling, but often no precise cause can be found. A multifactorial approach to causation, and to risk factors such as rugs, stairs, footwear and additional aids about the home, is necessary.

Dizziness, vertigo, blackouts and collapse

Dizziness is a word patients use for a wide variety of complaints ranging from a vague feeling of unsteadiness to severe, acute vertigo. It is also frequently used to describe the light-headedness that is felt in anxiety and panic attacks, during palpitations, and in syncope or chronic ill-health. Therefore, the site and real nature of this symptom must be determined.

Vertigo – an illusion of movement – is a more definite symptom. It is usually a sensation of rotation, or tipping in which the patient feels that the surroundings are spinning or moving. It is often accompanied by nausea or vomiting. Vertigo indicates disease of the labyrinth, vestibular pathways or their central connections.

Blackout, like dizziness, is a descriptive term implying either altered consciousness, visual disturbance or falling. Epilepsy, syncope, hypoglycaemia and other conditions must be considered (see p. 1060). However, commonly no sinister cause is found. A careful history, particularly from an eye-witness, is essential.

Collapse is a vague, common term used by patients and relatives. It is not a diagnosis and the possible causes are multiple.

FURTHER READING

Goadsby P, Silberstein SD (1997) *Blue Books of Practical Neurology: Headache*. Oxford: Butterworth–Heinemann.

Hopkins AP (ed) (1988) *Headache: Problems in Diagnosis and Management*. London: WB Saunders.

van Weel C, Vermuelen H, van den Bosch W (1995) Falls: a community perspective. *Lancet* **345**: 1549–1551.

The neurological examination

Clues from the history focus the neurological examination and the findings together frequently identify a recognizable disease.

A short five-part examination (Practical box 18.1)

A very detailed neurological examination is time-consuming and rarely necessary, particularly for patients without a history of neurological disease. A five-part examination is then sufficient.

A full ten-part examination (Practical box 18.2)

When more detail proves necessary, the ten headings shown summarize the essential elements and order of a full examination. Table 18.3 gives the six grades of muscle power proposed by the Medical Reseach Council.

Formulation

It is important to draw together the relevant findings from the history and the examination in a brief *written diagnostic summary*. This will form the basis for investigations, for the transfer of information, and for the patient's management.

FURTHER READING

Aids to Examination of the Nervous System (1996) Baillière Tindall.

Practical

1. **Look at the patient**
   - General demeanour
   - Speech
   - Gait
   - Arm swinging
2. **Examine the head**
   - Fundi
   - Pupils
   - Eye movements
   - Facial movements
   - Tongue
3. **Examine the upper limbs**
   - Posture of outstretched arms
   - Wasting, fasciculation
   - Power, tone
   - Coordination
   - Reflexes
4. **Examine the lower limbs**
   - Power (hip flexion, ankle dorsiflexion)
   - Tone
   - Reflexes
   - Plantar responses
5. **Assess sensation**
   - Ask the patient

Practical box 18.1 Five-part short neurological examination

Practical

1 **State of consciousness, arousal, appearance** (coma)

2 **Mental state, attitude, insight** (see Table 19.1 on p. 1109)

3 **Cognitive function**
Orientation in time and place, recall of recent and distant events (memory, level of intellect, language and speech/cerebral dominance, *other* disorders of skilled function, e.g. apraxia)

4 **Gait and Romberg's test**

5 **Skull shape – circumference, bruits**

6 **Neck stiffness – palpation and auscultation of carotid arteries**

7 **Cranial nerves** (see Table 18.5)

8 **Motor system**
Upper limbs:
Wasting and fasciculation
Posture of arms: drift, rebound, tremor
Tone: spasticity or extrapyramidal rigidity?
Power: MRC 0–5 scale (Table 18.3)
Tendon reflexes: + or ++ normal; +++ increased: 0 absent with reinforcement
Thorax and abdomen:
Respiration
Thoracic and abdominal muscles
Abdominal reflexes
Lower limbs:
Wasting and fasciculation
Tone, power and tendon reflexes
Plantar responses

9 **Coordination and fine movements**

10 **Sensory system**
First, the patient is asked whether or not the feeling in the limbs, face and trunk is entirely normal
Posterior columns:
Vibration (using a 128 Hz tuning fork)
Joint position
Light touch
2-point discrimination (normal: 0.5 cm fingertips, 2 cm soles)
Spinothalamic tracts:
Pain: a split orange-stick *or a sterile pin*
Temperature: hot or cold tubes

If sensation is abnormal, record on a chart the areas involved

Practical box 18.2 Ten-part neurological examination

Table 18.3
Six grades of muscle power (Medical Research Council)

Grade	Definition
5	Normal power
4	Active movement against gravity and resistance
3	Active movement against gravity
2	Active movement with gravity eliminated
1	Flicker of contraction
0	No contraction

Functional neuroanatomy: an introduction

In the next main section, basic and clinically useful neuroanatomy is summarized and illustrated by examples of common neurological conditions. That is followed by a section on the current investigations of clinical neurology (see p. 1037).

The neurone and synapse

The *neurone* is the functional unit of the nervous system. Its cell body and axon terminate in a synapse. The specificity, size and type of each group of neurones varies greatly. For example, an α-motor neurone within the anterior horn of the thoracic spinal cord has an axonal length of over 1 m and innervates between several hundred and 2000 muscle fibres – to form the *motor unit*. By contrast, some spinal or intracerebral internuncial neurones may have an axon under 100 μm in length and terminate solely on another neuronal cell body.

Neurotransmitters

Transmission at synapses is mediated by chemical neurotransmitters. These transmitters are released by action potentials passing down the axon. Transmitters react with receptors on the postsynaptic cell body, increasing ionic permeability and propagating a further action potential. This combination of electrical activity in the axon and chemical release at the synapse is the basis of all neurological function.

Neurotransmitters include acetylcholine, noradrenaline, adrenaline, 5-hydroxytryptamine, γ-aminobutyric acid (GABA), opioid peptides, prostaglandins, histamine, dopamine, glutamate, nitric oxide, neuromelanin and vasoactive intestinal peptide (VIP).

The role of neurotransmitters in pathogenesis continues to be evaluated, but it is thought that a wide variety of acute and chronic neurological disease may be mediated, at least in part, by a final common pathway of neuronal injury involving excessive stimulation of glutamate receptors.

Clinical features of focal lesions: general mechanisms

It is rarely necessary to be familiar with the precise anatomical details and mechanisms described here, but it is important to understand how, in general terms, each part of the nervous system works and how the parts are integrated. We need to be able to recognize, from symptoms and signs, how the rest of the nervous system works without, for example, part of the left frontal lobe, the internal capsule, or the facial nerve; without a cerebellar hemisphere, or a motor root.

Site of lesion	Disorder	L	R
Frontal, either	Intellectual impairment Personality change Urinary incontinence Monoparesis or hemiparesis		
Frontal, left	Broca's aphasia		
Temporo-parietal, left	Acalculia Alexia Agraphia Wernicke's aphasia Right–left disorientation Homonymous field defect		
Temporal, right	Confusional states Failure to recognize faces Homonymous field defect		
Parietal, either	Contralateral sensory loss or neglect Agraphaesthesia Homonymous field defect Neglect of opposite limbs		
Parietal, right	Dressing apraxia Failure to recognize faces		
Parietal, left	Limb apraxia		
Occipital/ occipitoparietal	Visual field defects Visuospatial defects Disturbances of visual recognition		

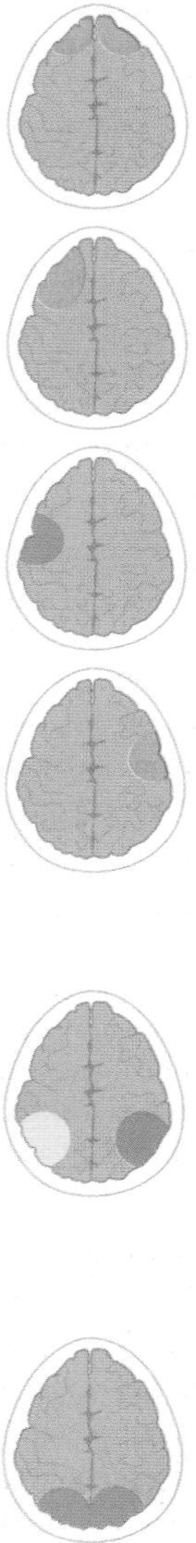

Fig 18.1
Principal features of destructive cortical lesions (right-handed individual)

Focal lesions of the cerebral cortex, and elsewhere in the nervous system cause symptoms and signs by three processes:

- Suppression of function or destruction of neurones and surrounding structures (Fig 18.1). This is the most common process – part of the system is not working normally.
- Synchronous discharge of neurones by irritative lesions which cause partial (focal) seizures that may become generalized (Fig 18.2), or other irritative events
- Displacement of the intracranial contents or spinal cord (see p. 1079) and surrounding oedema.

Localization of function within the cerebral cortex

This subject often causes considerable difficulty. Recent work on neuronal networks and plasticity within the brain has tended to question and expose traditional views relating to highly specific localization of function. However, in practical neurology at the bedside, it is important to understand the main functional divisions of the cerebral cortex, and their roles. The following paragraphs summarize the areas of principal clinical importance in general medicine.

The dominant hemisphere (usually the left)

The concept of cerebral dominance arose with the observation that right-handed stroke (and other) patients with acquired language disorders were found to have

Site of lesion	Effects	L	R
Frontal region	Partial seizures – focal motor seizures of contralateral limbs Conjugate deviation of head and eyes away from the lesion		
Temporal region	Formed visual hallucinations Complex partial seizures Memory disturbances (e.g. *déjà vu*)		
Parietal region	Partial seizures – focal sensory seizures of contralateral limbs		
Parieto-occipital region	Crude visual hallucinations (e.g. shapes in one part of the field)		
Occipital region	Visual disturbances (e.g. flashes)		

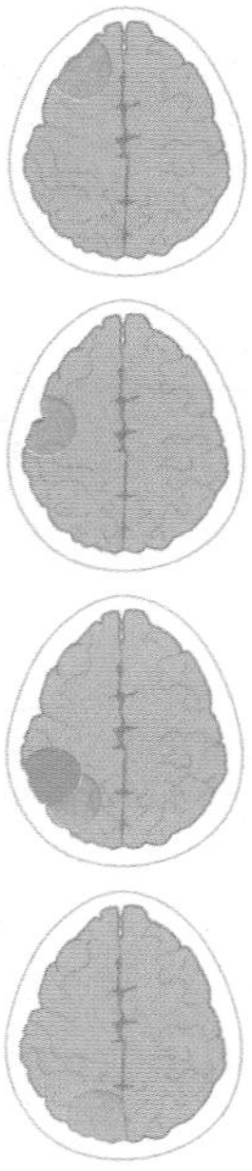

Fig 18.2
Effects of an irritative lesion of the cortex

destructive lesions within the left hemisphere. Almost all right-handed people have language function in the left hemisphere; so do over 70% of those who are apparently left-handed.

Destructive lesions within the left fronto-temporo-parietal region cause disorders of human communication:

- spoken language – *aphasia*, also called *dysphasia*
- writing – *agraphia*
- reading – *acquired alexia*.

Developmental dyslexia describes a condition of delayed and disorganized reading and writing ability in children with normal intelligence.

The non-dominant hemisphere

Disorders in right-handed patients with right hemisphere lesions are more difficult to define but comprise abnormalities of perception of internal and external space. Examples are losing the way in familiar surroundings, failing to put on clothing correctly (*dressing apraxia*), or failure to draw simple shapes – *constructional apraxia*.

Aphasia and dysarthria

Aphasia is the loss of or defect in language and is caused by left fronto-temporo-parietal lesions. *Dysarthria* means disordered articulation. Any lesion that produces paralysis, slowing or incoordination of the muscles of articulation or local discomfort will cause dysarthria. Examples are upper and lower motor neurone lesions of the lower cranial nerves, cerebellar lesions, Parkinson's disease and local lesions of the mouth, larynx, pharynx and tongue. Many aphasic patients are also somewhat dysarthric.

Some varieties of aphasia

Numerous varieties of aphasia have been described. The following are a selection.

Broca's aphasia (expressive aphasia, anterior aphasia)

A lesion in the left frontal lobe causes reduced fluency of speech with comprehension relatively preserved. The patient makes great efforts to initiate speech. Language is reduced to a few disjointed words and there is failure to construct sentences. Patients who recover from this form of aphasia say that they knew what they wanted to say, but could not get the words out.

Wernicke's aphasia (receptive aphasia, posterior aphasia)

A left temporo-parietal lesion leaves language that is fluent but the words themselves are incorrect. This varies from the insertion of a few incorrect or nonexistent words into fluent speech to a profuse outpouring of jargon (that is, rubbish with wholly nonexistent words). Severe jargon aphasia may be so bizarre as to be confused with psychotic behaviour.

Patients who have recovered from Wernicke's aphasia say that when aphasic they found the speech of others like a wholly unintelligible foreign language, and though they knew they were speaking could neither stop themselves nor understand what they said.

Nominal aphasia (anomic aphasia or amnestic aphasia)

This describes difficulty naming familiar objects. When it occurs in a severe and isolated form it is caused by a left posterior temporal/inferior parietal lesion. Naming difficulty is, however, an early sign in all types of aphasia.

Global aphasia (central aphasia)

This is the expressive disturbance characteristic of Broca's aphasia and the loss of comprehension of Wernicke's. The patient can neither speak nor understand language. It is due to widespread damage to the areas concerned with speech and is the most common form of aphasia after a severe left hemisphere infarct. Writing and reading are also affected.

Memory and its disorders (see also p. 1114)

Disorders of memory follow damage to the medial surface of the temporal lobes and their brainstem connections – the hippocampi, fornices and mammillary bodies. Bilateral lesions are necessary to cause amnesia. It is characteristic of all organic disorders of memory that more recent events are recalled poorly, in contrast to the relative preservation of distant memories.

Memory loss is a part of *dementia* of any cause (see p. 1114) but occurs as an isolated specific entity, the *amenstic syndrome*, in a wide variety of clinical situations (Table 18.4).

The essential elements of neuroanatomy

For clinical purposes, and particularly in general medical practice, the extreme complexity of neuroanatomy must be reduced to its essential elements. The following sections cover these as follows:

- the cranial nerves
- systems of motor control:
  (a) the corticospinal or pyramidal system
  (b) the extrapyramidal system
  (c) the cerebellum
  (d) lower motor neurones
  (e) the reflex arc

Table 18.4
Causes of the amnestic syndrome

Alcohol (Wernicke–Korsakoff syndrome)
Head injury (severe)
Anoxia
Posterior cerebral artery occlusion (bilateral)
Herpes simplex encephalitis
Chronic sedative and solvent abuse
Bilateral invasive tumours
Arsenic poisoning
Following hypoglycaemia

- sensory pathways and pain
- control of the bladder and sexual function.

The cranial nerves (see Table 18.5)

I: The olfactory nerve

This sensory nerve arises from olfactory (smell) receptors in the nasal mucosa. Branches pierce the cribriform plate and synapse in the olfactory bulb. The olfactory tract then passes to the olfactory cortex in the anteromedial surface of the temporal lobe.

Loss of the sense of smell (*anosmia*) occurs with head injury and tumours of the olfactory groove (e.g. meningioma, frontal glioma).

The sense of smell is often lost, sometimes permanently, after upper respiratory viral infections. It is diminished in nasal obstruction.

II: The optic nerve and visual system

The visual pathway is shown in Fig 18.3. The lens, which is under the control of the ciliary muscle (see p. 1016), causes the image on the retina to be inverted (**1**). An object in the lower part of the visual field is projected to the upper retina and one in the temporal field to the nasal retina. The photic energy of light, the volume of which is controlled by the pupillary aperture (see p. 1016) is converted to nerve action potentials by the rods and cones and ganglion cells of the retina. Each optic nerve (**2**), sheathed in pia-arachnoid meninges, carries axons from the retinal ganglion cells to the lateral geniculate bodies.

At the optic chiasm (**3**), fibres travelling in the nasal portions of the optic nerves cross, where they join the uncrossed temporal fibres of each optic nerve to form each optic tract. The fibres synapse at the lateral geniculate body. (**4**) One optic tract thus carries fibres from the temporal side of the ipsilateral retina and the nasal side of the contralateral retina. Some optic tract fibres reaching the lateral geniculate bodies pass to the brainstem (see p. 1017) to control refraction (lens) and aperture (pupil).

From the lateral geniculate body, fibres pass in the optic radiation through the parietal and temporal lobes (**5** and **6**) to reach the visual, or calcarine, cortex of the occipital lobe (**7** and **8**). The upper retinae (lower visual fields) project in the optic radiation through the parietal lobes to the upper part of the visual cortex, and the lower retinae (upper fields) through the temporal lobes, beneath the parietal, to the lower visual cortex. Impulses reach the cortex in strictly maintained vertical topographical order (i.e. upper field to lower retina, tract, radiation and cortex, and vice-versa, lower to upper). Within the visual cortex itself there are synaptic connections between groups of cells which detect lines, orientation, shapes, movement, colour, and depth, which are recognized and appreciated by the visual association areas beside it.

Table 18.5
Cranial nerves

No.	Name	Main clinical action
I	Olfactory	Smell
II	Optic	Vision, fields, afferent light reflex
III	Oculomotor	Eyelid elevation, eye elevation, ADduction, depression in ABduction, efferent – to pupil
IV	Trochlear	Eye intorsion, depression in ADduction
V	Trigeminal	Facial and corneal sensation, muscles of mastication
VI	Abducens	Eye ABduction
VII	Facial	Facial movement, taste fibres
VIII	Vestibular	Balance
	Cochlear	Hearing
IX	Glossopharyngeal	Sensation – soft palate, taste fibres
X	Vagus	Palatal movement, vocal cords, cough
XI	Accessory	Head turning, shoulder shrugging
XII	Hypoglossal	Tongue movement

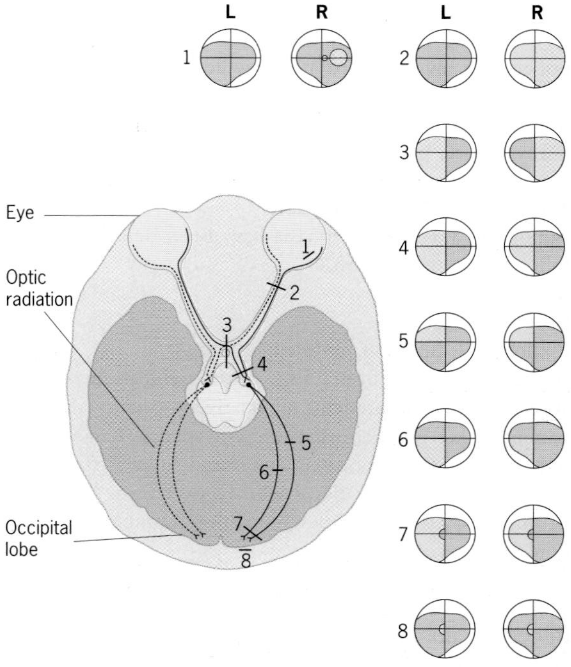

Fig 18.3
The visual pathway. 1, Paracentral scotoma–retinal lesion. 2, Mononuclear field loss–optic nerve lesion. 3, Bitemporal hemianopia–chiasmal lesion. 4, Homonymous hemianopia–optic tract lesion. 5, Homonymous quadrantanopia–temporal lesion. 6, Homonymous quadrantanopia–parietal lesion. 7, Homonymous hemianopia–occipital cortex or optic radiation. 8, Homonymous hemianopia–occipital pole lesion. Blue=lesion; red=normal field

The visual field projected to each optic tract, radiation and cortex is called 'homonymous', to indicate the different (i.e. bilateral) origins of each pathway. (A homonym is the same word used to denote different things.)

Field defects are hemianopic when half the field is affected, by a lesion of the optic tract, radiation or cortex (e.g. left homonymous hemianopia) and quadrantanopic when a quadrant is affected. *Congruous* denotes symmetry and *incongruous* lack of it. Bitemporal defects (damage to crossing nasal fibres) are caused by lesions of the optic chiasm (e.g. pituitary tumour).

Visual acuity

This should be recorded with a Snellen test chart and/or Near Vision Reading Types and corrected for refractive errors with lenses or a pinhole. The normal acuity should be 6/6 to 6/9 in both eyes, and an explanation sought if it is lower than this.

Visual loss is due to:

- ocular causes (e.g. glaucoma, macular degeneration, cataract, retinal detachment, diabetic vascular disease)
- central lesions of the visual neural pathway (e.g. optic nerve lesions, chiasmal compression, tract, radiation or cortical lesions).

Visual field defects

These should be examined by confrontation with white and red headed pins and, if abnormal or in doubt, recorded in detail with a Goldmann (or similar) screen. Examples of field defects at different sites in the visual pathway are shown in Fig 18.3.

Retinal and local eye lesions (site 1)

Lesions of the retina produce either scotomata (small areas of visual loss) or peripheral visual loss (tunnel vision). Common causes are diabetic retinal vascular disease, glaucoma and retinitis pigmentosa. Local lesions of the eye (e.g. cataract) can also cause visual loss.

Optic nerve lesions (site 2)

Unilateral visual loss, commencing as a central or paracentral (off-centre) scotoma, is the hallmark of an optic nerve lesion. A complete lesion of the optic nerve produces total unilateral visual loss with loss of pupillary light reflex (direct and consensual) when the blind eye is illuminated (see afferent pupillary defect, p. 1017).

Causes of optic nerve lesions are given in Table 18.6.

The principal pathological appearances of the visible part of the nerve (the disc) seen on fundoscopy are:

- disc swelling (papilloedema)
- pallor (optic atrophy).

Table 18.6
Principal causes of an optic nerve lesion

Optic and retrobulbar neuritis
Optic nerve compression (e.g. tumour or aneurysm)
Toxic optic neuropathy (e.g. tobacco, ethambutol, methyl alcohol, quinine)
Syphilis
Ischaemic optic neuropathy (e.g. giant cell arteritis)
Hereditary optic neuropathies
Severe anaemia
Vitamin B_{12} deficiency
Trauma
Infective (spread of paranasal sinus infection or orbital cellulitis)
Papilloedema and its causes (see Table 18.7)
Bone disease affecting optic canal (e.g. Paget's)

Papilloedema and optic neuritis

Papilloedema simply means swelling of the papilla – the optic disc. There are many causes (Table 18.7). In all forms of disc oedema there is axonal swelling within the optic nerve, blockage of axonal transport with capillary and venous congestion. Optic neuritis is swelling of the optic nerve owing to inflammation within it.

The earliest ophthalmoscopic signs of disc swelling are pinkness of the disc followed by blurring and heaping up of its margins, the nasal first. There is loss within the disc of the normal, visible, spontaneous pulsation of the retinal veins. The physiological cup becomes obliterated and the disc engorged, with dilatation of its vessels. Small haemorrhages often surround the disc.

Various conditions simulate true disc oedema. Marked hypermetropic (long-sighted) refractive errors make the disc appear pink, distant and ill-defined. Opaque (myelinated) nerve fibres at the disc margin and hyaline bodies (drusen) can be mistaken for disc swelling.

Disc infiltration also causes first a prominent, then a swollen disc, with raised margins (e.g. in leukaemia).

Table 18.7
Causes of optic disc swelling (papilloedema)

Raised intracranial pressure	**Venous occlusion**
Brain tumour, abscess, haematoma, intracranial haemorrhage and SAH, idiopathic intracranial hypertension, hydrocephalus, encephalitis	Cavernous sinus thrombosis Central retinal vein thrombosis/occlusion Orbital mass lesions
	Retinal vascular disease
	Malignant hypertension Vasculitis (e.g. SLE)
Optic nerve disease	**Metabolic causes**
Optic neuritis (e.g. multiple sclerosis) Hereditary optic neuropathy Ischaemic optic neuropathy (e.g. giant cell arteritis) Toxic optic neuropathy (e.g. methanol ingestion) Hypervitaminosis A	Hypercapnia, chronic hypoxia, hypocalcaemia **Disc infiltration** Leukaemia, sarcoidosis, optic nerve glioma

SAH, subarachnoid haemorrhage; SLE, system lupus erythematosus

When there is doubt about disc oedema, fluorescein angiography is diagnostic. Fluorescein injected intravenously leakage is the disc capillaries when there is oedema: leakage is seen and may be photographed.

Early papilloedema from causes other than optic neuritis (see below) often produces few visual symptoms, the patient's complaints being those of the underlying disease. As disc oedema progresses there is enlargement of the blind spot and blurring of the vision. The disc becomes engorged, reducing its arterial blood flow and, in severe papilloedema, infarction of the nerve occurs, often suddenly, causing severe and permanent visual loss.

Optic neuritis

The most common cause of inflammation of the optic nerve is demyelination (e.g. multiple sclerosis). Disc swelling due to optic neuritis is distinguished from other causes of disc oedema by the occurrence of early and severe visual loss.

Retrobulbar neuritis implies that the inflammatory process is within the optic nerve but behind the bulb (i.e. the eye), so that no abnormality may be seen at the disc itself in spite of visual impairment.

Optic atrophy

Optic atrophy means disc pallor, owing to loss of axons, glial proliferation and decreased vascularity which follows a variety of pathological processes, including infarction of the nerve, e.g. thromboembolism, or following papilloedema, inflammation (demyelinating optic neuritis in MS, syphilis), optic nerve compression, previous trauma, toxic and metabolic causes (e.g. vitamin B_{12} deficiency, quinine and methyl alcohol). Optic atrophy is described as consecutive or secondary when it follows papilloedema, of any cause. The degree of visual loss depends upon the underlying pathology.

Lesions of the optic chiasm (site 3)

Bitemporal hemianopic field defects develop when a mass compresses the central part of the chiasm. Common causes are:

- pituitary neoplasm (p. 905)
- craniopharyngioma
- secondary neoplasm.

In any case of bilateral visual failure, chiasmal compression must be considered.

Lesions of the optic tract and optic radiation (sites 4, 5 and 6)

Optic tract lesions (which are rare) cause field defects which are homonymous, hemianopic and often incomplete and incongruous. Optic radiation lesions cause homonymous quadrantanopic defects. Temporal lobe lesions (e.g. tumour or infarction) cause upper quadrantic defects, and parietal lower.

Lesions of the occipital cortex (sites 7 and 8)

Homonymous hemianopic defects are caused by unilateral posterior cerebral artery infarction. The macular region (at the occipital pole) is spared because it has a separate blood supply from the middle cerebral artery: infarction of one occipital pole itself causes a small, congruous, scotomatous, homonymous hemianopia (8).

Widespread bilateral occipital lobe damage by tumour, trauma or infarction causes the syndrome of cortical blindness (Anton's syndrome). The patient is blind but characteristically lacks insight into the degree of visual loss and may even deny it. The pupillary responses are normal (see also p. 1051).

The pupils

Sympathetic impulses in fibres in the nasociliary nerve (which arises from the superior cervical ganglion) cause the pupil to dilate by stimulating the dilator pupillae muscle.

The sympathetic preganglionic fibres to the eye (and face) originate in the hypothalamus, pass uncrossed through the midbrain and lateral medulla, and emerge finally from the spinal cord at T1 (close to the lung apex). Postganglionic fibres begin in the superior cervical ganglion at C2 and form a plexus around the carotid bifurcation. Fibres pass to the pupil in the nasociliary nerve from the part of this plexus surrounding the internal carotid artery. Those fibres to the face (sweating and pilo-erection) arise from the part of the plexus surrounding the external carotid artery. This arrangement is of clinical importance in Horner's syndrome (p. 1017).

Parasympathetic impulses in fibres of the short ciliary nerves, which arise from the ciliary ganglion, stimulate the sphincter muscle of the pupil (sphincter pupillae) causing the pupil to constrict.

A diagram of parasympathetic fibres to and from the eye and the mechanism of the light reflex is shown in Fig 18.4.

The light reflex

Afferent fibres in each optic nerve (1) (some crossing in the chiasm) pass to both lateral geniculate bodies (2) and relay to the Edinger–Westphal nuclei (4) via the pretectal nucleus (3).

Efferent (parasympathetic) fibres from each Edinger–Westphal nucleus pass via the third nerve to the ciliary ganglion (5) and thence to the pupil (6).

Light constricts the pupil of the eye being tested (direct reflex) and the contralateral pupil (consensual reflex).

The convergence reflex

Fixation on a near object requires convergence of the ocular axes and is accompanied by pupillary constriction.

Afferent fibres in each optic nerve, which pass through both lateral geniculate bodies, also relay to the

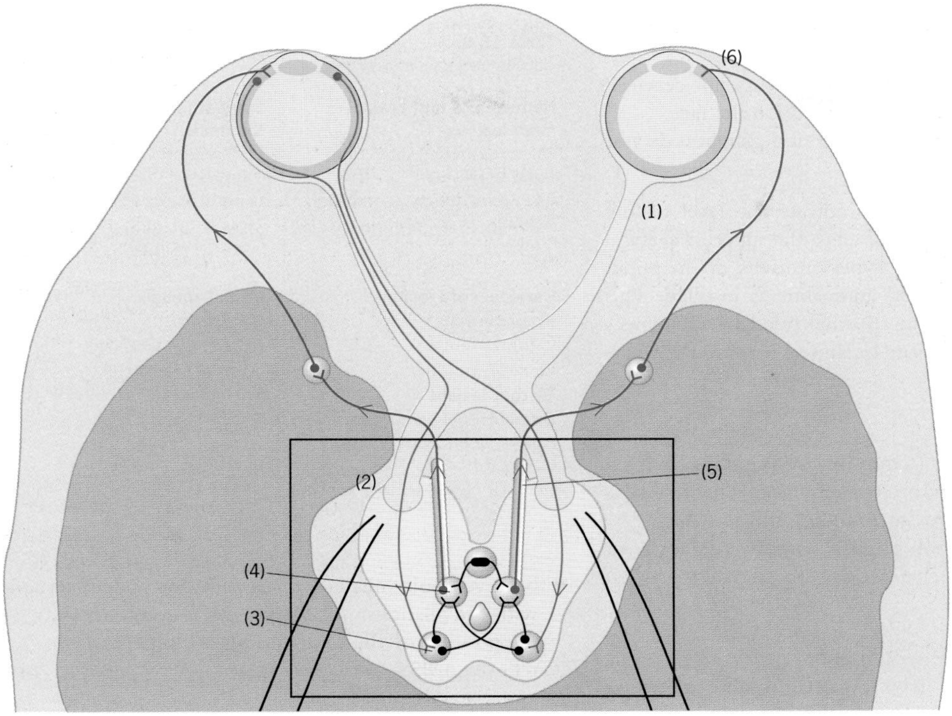

Fig 18.4
Light reflex afferent pathway
A retinal image generates an action potential in the right optic nerve (1). This travels via axons, some of which decussate at the chiasm and pass through the lateral geniculate bodies (2), synapsing at each pretectal nucleus (3).
Light reflex efferent pathway
The action potential is then propagated to each Edinger–Westphal nucleus of III (at 4) and thence via each ciliary ganglion (5) to each pupil (6), which constricts the pupil.

convergence centre. This centre receives 1a spindle afferent fibres from the extraocular muscles – principally the medial recti – which are innervated by the third nerve.

The efferent route is from the convergence centre to the Edinger–Westphal nucleus, ciliary ganglion and pupils. Voluntary or reflex fixation on a near object is thus accompanied by appropriate convergence and pupillary constriction.

A darkened room makes all pupillary abnormalities easier to see.

CLINICAL ABNORMALITIES OF THE PUPILS

Abnormalities of the pupils seen in coma are discussed on p. 1044, and in the brainstem on p. 858.

Physiological changes and changes in old age

A slight difference between the size of the pupils is common (*physiological anisocoria*) at any age. The pupil tends to become small (3–3.5 mm) and irregular in old age (*senile miosis*); anisocoria is more pronounced. A bright light is necessary to demonstrate constriction and the convergence reflex becomes sluggish with ageing..

Afferent pupillary defect. A blind left eye, for example from previous complete section of its optic nerve, has a pupil larger than the right. The features of a left afferent pupillary defect are:

- the left pupil is unreactive to light (i.e. the direct reflex is absent)
- the consensual reflex (constriction of the right pupil when light is shone in the left) is also absent.

Conversely, when light is shone in the intact right eye (which has a normal direct reflex), the left pupil constricts (i.e. the consensual reflex of the right eye is intact).

Relative afferent pupillary defect (RAPD). A relative afferent pupillary defect (RAPD) occurs when there has been incomplete damage to the afferent pupillary pathway (i.e. of one optic nerve relative to the other). This sign can provide evidence of an optic nerve lesion, when there has been apparent complete clinical recovery from, for example, retrobulbar neuritis which occurred many years previously.

- A light shone in the left eye causes both left and right pupils to constrict.
- When a light is shone into the intact right eye, both pupils again constrict (i.e. the right direct and consensual reflexes are intact).
- When the light is then swung to the previously affected left eye, its pupil dilates, relative to its previous state.

The finding of a left RAPD by the *swinging light test*, showing that the consensual reflex is stronger than the direct, indicates residual damage in the afferent pupillary fibres of the left optic nerve.

Horner's syndrome

This collection of signs – of unilateral pupillary constriction with slight relative ptosis and enophthalmos – indicates a lesion of the sympathetic pathway on the same side. The conjunctival vessels are slightly injected. Causes of Horner's syndrome are given in Table 18.8. There is loss of sweating of the same side of the face or body; the extent depending upon the level of the lesion:

- Central lesions affect sweating over the entire half of the head, arm and upper trunk.
- Lesions of the neck proximal to the superior cervical ganglion cause diminished sweating on the face.
- Lesions distal to the superior cervical ganglion do not affect sweating at all.

Pharmacological tests help to indicate the level of the lesion. For example, a lesion distal to the superior cervical ganglion causes denervation hypersensitivity of the pupil, which dilates when 1:1000 adrenaline is instilled. This dose has little effect on the normal pupil or a Horner's pupil from a proximal lesion. In clinical practice the test is of limited value.

Table 18.8
Causes of Horner's syndrome

Hemisphere and brain stem lesions	Sympathetic chain in the neck
Massive cerebral infarction Pontine glioma Lateral medullary syndrome 'Coning' of the temporal lobe	Following thyroid/laryngeal surgery Carotid artery occlusion Neoplastic infiltration Cervical sympathectomy
Cervical cord lesions	**Miscellaneous**
Syringomyelia Cord tumours	Congenital Migrainous neuralgia (usually transient) Isolated and of unknown cause
T1 root lesions	
Bronchial neoplasm (apical) Apical tuberculosis Cervical rib Brachial plexus trauma	

Argyll Robertson pupil

This is a small, irregular (3 mm or less) pupil that is fixed to light, but constricts on convergence. The lesion is believed to be in the area surrounding the aqueduct.

The Argyll Robertson pupil is (almost) diagnostic of neurosyphilis. Similar changes are occasionally seen in diabetes mellitus.

Myotonic pupil (Holmes–Adie pupil)

This is a dilated pupil seen most commonly in young women. It is usually unilateral, and the pupil is often irregular. There is no reaction (or a very slow reaction) to a bright light and also an incomplete constriction to convergence. The condition is due to denervation in the ciliary ganglion, of unknown cause.

The myotonic pupil is of no pathological significance but is often associated with diminished or absent tendon reflexes.

III, IV, VI: The oculomotor, trochlear and abducens nerves

Mechanisms controlling eye movement are:

- central upper motor neurone mechanisms, which drive the normal yoked parallel movements of the eyes (conjugate gaze)
- movements generated by the oculomotor, abducens and trochlear nerves via the extraocular muscles.

Conjugate gaze

Fast voluntary and reflex eye movements originate in each frontal lobe. Fibres pass in the anterior limb of the internal capsule and cross in the pons to end in the centre for lateral gaze (paramedian pontine reticular formation – PPRF, Fig 18.5(a)), which is close to each sixth nerve nucleus. It also receives fibres from:

- the ipsilateral occipital cortex – these pathways are concerned with movements to track or pursue objects within the visual fields
- both vestibular nuclei – these pathways are concerned with the relationship between eye movements and the position of the head and neck (doll's head reflexes, p. 858).

Conjugate lateral eye movements are coordinated by the centre of lateral gaze (PPRF) through the medial longitudinal fasciculus – MLF, Fig 18.5(b)). Fibres from the PPRF pass to both the ipsilateral sixth nerve nucleus and, having crossed the midline, the opposite third nerve nucleus via the MLF. Each sixth nerve nucleus (supplying the lateral rectus) and the opposite third nerve nucleus (supplying the medial rectus and others) are thus linked by the MLF, driving the eyes laterally with parallel axes and with the same velocity.

Abnormalities of conjugate lateral gaze

A destructive lesion of one side of the brain allows lateral gaze to be driven by the intact opposite pathway, as discussed below.

A destructive left frontal lobe lesion (e.g. an infarct) leads to failure of conjugate lateral gaze to the right. In an acute lesion the eyes are often deviated past the midline to the side of the lesion, here to the left, and therefore look towards the normal limbs, as there is usually a contralateral (i.e. right) hemiparesis.

An irritative left frontal lobe lesion (e.g. an epileptic focus), by stimulating the opposite, right, lateral gaze centre (PPRF), drives lateral gaze away from the side of the lesion (i.e. to the right).

A destructive left brainstem lesion involving the PPRF leads to failure of conjugate lateral gaze towards the side of the lesion (i.e. to the left). There is usually a right hemiparesis and lateral gaze is deviated towards the right, the side of the paralysed limbs.

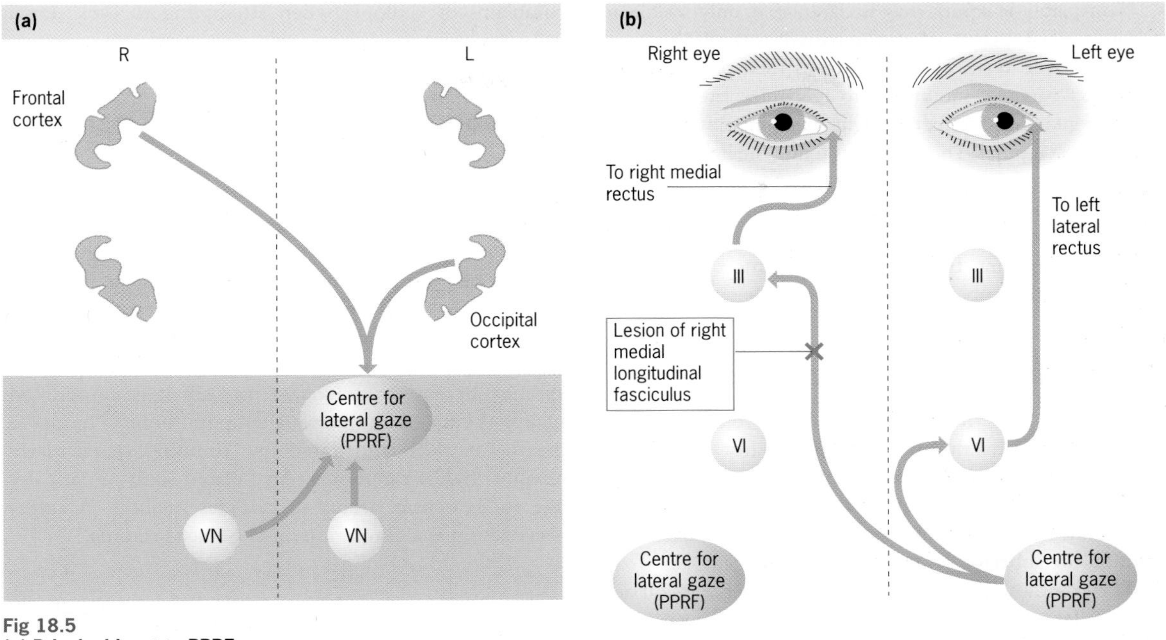

Fig 18.5
(a) Principal input to PPRF
Impulses from the right frontal cortex, the left occipital cortex and both vestibular nuclei (VN) drive the left centre for lateral gaze, or paramedian pontine reticular formation (PPRF).
(b) Principal output from PPRF
Impulses from the PPRF pass via the ipsilateral VIth nerve nucleus to the lateral rectus muscle (ABduction) and via the medial longitudinal fasciculus to the IIIrd nerve nucleus and thus to the opposite medial rectus muscle (ADduction)
X shows lesion with failure of ADduction of right eye

Doll's head reflexes and skew deviation

These are of some diagnostic value in coma (see p. 858).

Internuclear ophthalmoplegia

Internuclear ophthalmoplegia (INO) is one of the more common complex brainstem signs that involve the oculomotor system. It is due to a lesion within the MLF.

The sign is common in multiple sclerosis. When present bilaterally, INO is almost pathognomonic of this disease. Unilateral lesions are also caused by small brainstem infarcts. In a right INO there is a lesion of the right MLF (see Fig 18.5(b)). On attempted left lateral gaze the right eye fails to ADduct. The left eye develops coarse nystagmus in ABduction.

The side of the lesion is on the side of impaired adduction, not on the side of the (obvious, unilateral) nystagmus.

Abnormalities of vertical gaze

A failure of up-gaze is caused by an upper brainstem lesion, such as a supratentorial mass pressing from above, or a tumour of the brainstem (e.g. a pinealoma). When the pupillary convergence reflex fails as well, this combination is called Parinaud's syndrome.

Defective up-gaze also occurs in certain degenerative disorders (e.g. progressive supranuclear palsy).

Some impairment of up-gaze also occurs as part of normal ageing.

Weakness of the extraocular muscles (diplopia)

Diplopia (double vision) indicates weakness of one or more of the extraocular muscles. The causes are:

- a lesion of the third, fourth and/or sixth cranial nerves or nuclei
- disease of the neuromuscular junction (e.g. myasthenia gravis)
- disease of the ocular muscles.

Squint (strabismus)

This describes the appearance of the eyes when the visual axes fail to meet at the fixation point, and is either convergent or divergent.

Paralytic squint. Paralytic or incomitant squint occurs when there is an acquired defect of the movement of an eye – the usual situation in neurological disease. There is a squint (and hence diplopia) maximal in the direction of action of the weak muscle.

Non-paralytic squint. Non-paralytic or concomitant squint describes a squint beginning in childhood in which the angle between the visual axes does not vary when the eyes are moved – the squint remains the same in all directions of gaze. Diplopia is almost never a symptom. The deviating eye (the one that does not fixate) usually has defective vision; this is called *amblyopia ex anopsia*.

Non-paralytic squint may be latent (i.e. only visible at certain times), such as when the patient is tired.

The cover test. The cover test is used principally to assess non-paralytic squint and to recognize latent squint. The patient is asked to fix on a light. The pinpoint reflection is seen in each pupil. The eye that is fixing the light centrally is covered quickly. If the uncovered eye makes any movement to take up central fixation, then a squint must have been present. The test is repeated with the opposite eye. The dominant, fixing eye will not move when the other, squinting, amblyopic eye is covered or uncovered.

The oculomotor (third cranial) nerve

The nucleus of the third nerve lies ventral to the aqueduct in the midbrain. Efferent fibres to four external ocular muscles (superior, inferior and medial recti, and inferior oblique), levator palpebrae superioris and sphincter pupillae (parasympathetic) enter the orbit through the superior orbital fissure.

The common causes of an oculomotor nerve lesion are given in Table 18.9. Signs of a complete third nerve palsy are:

- unilateral complete ptosis
- the eye facing down and out
- a fixed and dilated pupil.

Sparing of the pupil means that parasympathetic fibres which run in a discrete bundle on the superior surface of the nerve remain undamaged, and so the pupil is of normal size and reacts normally. In diabetes, infarction of the third nerve usually spares the pupil.

In a third-nerve palsy the eye can still ABduct (sixth nerve) and rotate inwards or intort (fourth nerve). Preservation of intortion (inward rotation) means that the fourth (trochlear) nerve is intact. In a patient with a right third-nerve palsy, when the attempt is made to converge and look downwards, the conjunctival vessels of the right eye are seen to twist clockwise, indicating that the eye is intorting and the fourth nerve is intact (see below).

The trochlear nerve (fourth cranial)

The trochlear nerve supplies the superior oblique muscle.

An isolated fourth-nerve lesion is a rarity. The head is tilted away from the side of the lesion. The patient complains of diplopia when attempting to look down and away from the affected side.

Table 18.9
Common causes of an oculomotor nerve lesion

Aneursym of the posterior communicating artery
'Coning' of the temporal lobe
Infarction of IIIrd nerve
In diabetes mellitus
Atheroma
Midbrain infarction
Midbrain tumour

The abducens (sixth cranial) nerve

The ABducens nerve supplies the lateral rectus muscle which causes the eye to ABduct.

In a sixth-nerve lesion there is a convergent squint with diplopia maximal on looking to the side of the lesion. The eye cannot be abducted beyond the midline.

There are many causes of a sixth-nerve lesion, as the nerve has a long intracranial course. The nerve can be involved within the brainstem (e.g. MS or pontine glioma). In raised intracranial pressure it is compressed against the tip of the petrous temporal bone. The nerve sheath may be infiltrated by tumours, particularly nasopharyngeal carcinoma. An isolated sixth-nerve palsy due to infarction occurs in diabetes mellitus. A sixth-nerve lesion is a common sequel of head trauma.

Complete external ophthalmoplegia

Complete external ophthalmoplegia describes the immobile eye when III, IV and VI nerves are paralysed by lesions at the orbital apex (e.g. a metastasis) or within the cavernous sinus (e.g. sinus thrombosis).

V: The trigeminal nerve

The trigeminal nerve is large, mainly sensory but contains some motor fibres.

Sensory fibres (Fig 18.6; and see Figs 18.9 and 18.10) from the three divisions – ophthalmic (V_1), maxillary (V_2) and mandibular (V_3) – pass to the trigeminal ganglion at the apex of the petrous temporal bone, within the cavernous sinus. From here central fibres enter the brainstem. Ascending fibres transmitting the sensation of light touch enter the nucleus in the pons. Descending fibres carrying pain and temperature sensation form the spinal tract of the fifth nerve and end in the spinal nucleus in the medulla which extends into the upper cervical cord.

Motor fibres arise in the upper pons and join the mandibular branch to supply the muscles of mastication.

SIGNS OF A TRIGEMINAL NERVE LESION

A complete fifth-nerve lesion causes unilateral sensory loss on the face, tongue and buccal mucosa. When motor fibres are damaged the jaw deviates to the side of the lesion as the mouth is opened.

Diminution of the corneal reflex is an early, and sometimes isolated sign of a fifth-nerve lesion.

Central (brainstem) lesions of the lower trigeminal nuclei (e.g. in syringobulbia, see p. 1086) produce a characteristic circumoral sensory loss.

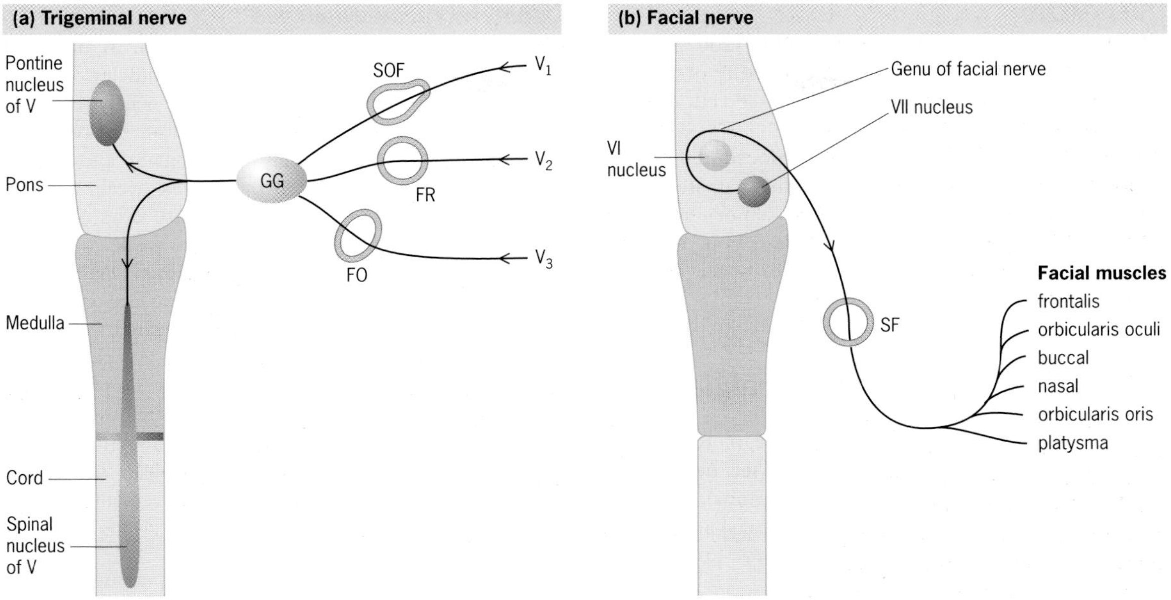

Fig 18.6
Trigeminal and facial nerves
FO, foramen ovale; FR, foramen rotundum; SOF, superior orbital fissure; GG, Gasserian ganglion; SF, stylomastoid foramen

When the spinal tract (or spinal nucleus) alone is involved, the sensory loss is restricted to pain and temperature sensation – i.e. dissociated (see p. 1034).

CAUSES

Within the *brainstem*, lesions involve the fifth nuclei and central connections, e.g.:

brainstem glioma
- multiple sclerosis
- infarction
- syringobulbia.

At the *cerebellopontine angle*, the nerve is compressed by:

- acoustic neuroma
- meningioma
- secondary neoplasm.

As these lesions enlarge, the neighbouring seventh and eighth nerves become involved, producing facial weakness and deafness.

At the *apex of the petrous temporal bone*, spreading infection from the middle-ear, or a secondary tumour, damages the nerve. The combination of this with pain and a sixth-nerve lesion is called Gradenigo's syndrome.

Within the *cavernous sinus*, the trigeminal (Gasserian) ganglion is compressed by:

- aneurysm of the internal carotid artery
- lateral extension of a pituitary neoplasm
- thrombosis of the cavernous sinus
- secondary neoplasm.

The trigeminal ganglion becomes infected in ophthalmic herpes zoster (see p. 1074), the most common lesion of the ganglion itself.

Peripheral branches of the trigeminal nerve are affected by neoplastic infiltration of the skull base.

Trigeminal neuralgia

Trigeminal neuralgia (*tic douloureux*) is a condition of unknown cause, seen most commonly in old age. It is almost always unilateral.

SYMPTOMS

Severe paroxysms of knife-like or electric-shock-like pain, lasting seconds, occur in the distribution of the fifth nerve. The pain tends to commence in the mandibular division (V_3) and spreads upwards to the maxillary (V_2) and to the ophthalmic division (V_1). Spasms occur many times a day.

Each paroxysm is stereotyped, brought on by stimulation of a specific and often tiny trigger zone in the face. Washing, shaving, a cold wind or eating are examples of the trivial stimuli that provoke the intense pain. The face may be screwed up in agony (hence the term *tic* – an involuntary movement).

The pain characteristically does not occur at night. Spontaneous remissions last for months or years before recurrence, which is almost inevitable.

SIGNS

There are no signs of trigeminal nerve dysfunction. The corneal reflex is preserved. Diagnosis is on clinical grounds alone.

TREATMENT

The anticonvulsant carbamazepine 600–1200 mg daily reduces the severity of attacks in the majority of patients. Phenytoin and clonazepam are also used, but are less effective.

If drug therapy fails, surgical procedures (radiofrequency extirpation of the ganglion, neurovascular decompression or sectioning of the sensory root) are useful in difficult cases. Alcohol injection into the trigeminal ganglion or peripheral fifth-nerve branches can also be carried out.

Secondary trigeminal neuralgia

Trigeminal neuralgia occurs in MS (see p. 1069), with lesions of the cerebellopontine angle (see below), and with tumours of the fifth nerve (e.g. neuroma). There are usually physical signs; for example, initially a depressed corneal reflex, progressing to sensory loss in the trigeminal distribution.

Idiopathic trigeminal neuropathy

A chronic and isolated fifth-nerve lesion sometimes develops without apparent cause. When sensory loss is severe, trophic changes (facial scarring and corneal ulceration) occur.

Trigeminal postherpetic neuralgia (see also p. 1074)

Continuous severe burning pain develops in the distribution of one division or more of the trigeminal nerve, but commonly only in the first (ophthalmic) after herpes zoster.

VII: The facial nerve

The facial nerve is largely motor in function, supplying the muscles of facial expression. The nerve carries sensory taste fibres from the anterior two-thirds of the tongue via the *chorda tympani*. It also supplies motor fibres to the stapedius muscle.

The facial nerve (Fig 18.6) arises from the seventh-nerve nucleus in the pons and leaves the skull through the stylomastoid foramen.

Part of each facial nucleus supplying the upper face (principally the frontalis muscle) receives supranuclear fibres from each hemisphere. Therefore in a unilateral upper motor neurone lesion of the facial nerve the upper part of the face is usually not affected.

Unilateral facial weakness

Lower motor neurone (LMN) lesions. A unilateral LMN lesion causes weakness of all the muscles of facial expression on the same side. The face, especially the angle of the mouth, falls, and dribbling occurs from the corner of the mouth. There is weakness of frontalis and of eye closure since the upper facial muscles are weak. Corneal exposure and ulceration occurs if the eye does not close during sleep. The platysma muscle is also weak.

Upper motor neurone (UMN) lesions. UMN lesions cause weakness of the lower part only of the face on the side opposite the lesion. The frontalis muscle is spared; the normal furrowing of the brow is preserved, and eye closure and blinking are not affected.The earliest sign is simply slowing of one side of the face, for example on baring the teeth, or smiling. In UMN lesions, too, there is sometimes relative preservation of spontaneous emotional movement (e.g. smiling) compared with voluntary movement.

CAUSES OF FACIAL WEAKNESS

A common cause of facial weakness is a supranuclear (UMN) lesion (e.g. cerebral infarction), leading to UMN facial weakness and hemiparesis.

Lesions at four lower levels are recognized by the association of LMN facial weakness with other signs.

Within the pons. Here the sixth (abducens) nerve nucleus is encircled by the seventh-nerve fibres. The sixth nucleus is therefore often involved in pontine lesions of the seventh nerve, causing a lateral rectus palsy.

When the neighbouring centre for lateral gaze (PPRF) and corticospinal tract are involved, there is the triple combination of:

- LMN facial weakness
- failure of conjugate lateral gaze (towards the lesion)
- contralateral hemiparesis.

Causes include pontine tumours (e.g. glioma), demyelination and vascular lesions.

The facial nucleus itself is affected unilaterally or bilaterally in poliomyelitis (see p. 1075) and in motor neurone disease (p. 1088); the latter usually causes bilateral weakness.

In the cerebellopontine angle. The fifth, sixth and eighth nerves are affected with the seventh nerve in lesions in the cerebellopontine angle, where they are grouped together. Causes are acoustic neuroma, meningioma and secondary neoplasm.

Within the petrous temporal bone. The geniculate ganglion (a sensory ganglion for taste) lies at the genu of the facial nerve (see Fig 18.6). Fibres join the facial nerve in the chorda tympani and carry taste from the anterior two-thirds of the tongue. The (motor) nerve to the stapedius muscle leaves the facial nerve distal to the genu.

Lesions of the facial nerve within the petrous temporal bone cause the combination of:

- loss of taste on the anterior two-thirds of the tongue
- hyperacusis (unpleasantly loud distortion of noise) owing to paralysis of stapedius muscle.

Causes include:

- Bell's palsy
- trauma
- middle ear infection
- herpes zoster (Ramsay Hunt syndrome, p. 1023)
- tumours (e.g. glomus tumour).

Within the face itself. Branches of the facial nerve which pierce the parotid gland to supply the muscles of facial expression are damaged here by parotid gland tumours, mumps (see p. 64), sarcoidosis (p. 1077) and trauma.

Each nerve is also affected in polyneuritis (e.g. Guillain–Barré syndrome, p. 1093), usually simultaneously.

Weakness of the facial muscles themselves is also seen in primary muscle disease and disease of the neuromuscular junction. Weakness is usually symmetrical. Causes include:

- dystrophia myotonica (p. 1103)
- facio-scapulo-humeral dystrophy (p. 1103)
- myasthenia gravis (p. 1101).

Bell's palsy

This is a common, acute, isolated facial nerve palsy believed to be due to a viral (often herpes simplex) infection that causes swelling of the nerve within the petrous temporal bone.

SYMPTOMS

The patient notices marked unilateral facial weakness, sometimes with loss of taste on the anterior two-thirds of the tongue. Pain behind the ear is common at onset. The diagnosis is made on clinical grounds. No other cranial nerves are involved.

MANAGEMENT AND COURSE

Spontaneous improvement of Bell's palsy usually begins during the second week. Thereafter, recovery continues but this may take 12 months to become complete. Fewer than 10% of patients are left with a severe, unsightly, residual weakness.

Electrophysiological tests (EMG, see p. 1041) are of some help in predicting the outcome. After the third week, the absence of an evoked potential from facial muscle (the nerve is stimulated over the parotid gland) indicates that recovery is unlikely.

Steroids (e.g. prednisolone 60 mg daily, reducing to nil over 10 days) reduce the proportion of patients left with a severe deficit, provided the drugs are given at the onset. Acyclovir is of unproven value but sometimes given.

Suturing of the upper to the lower lid (tarsorraphy) is essential to prevent prolonged corneal exposure if the eye cannot be closed. Adhesive tape to close the eye is an invaluable temporary protective measure.

If there is severe residual paralysis, cosmetic surgery and/or reinnervation (e.g. nerve anastomosis of the lingual to the facial) are sometimes performed after a year has elapsed.

Bell's palsy occasionally recurs and is very rarely bilateral.

Ramsay Hunt syndrome

This is herpes zoster (shingles) of the geniculate ganglion. There is a facial palsy (identical in appearance to Bell's palsy) with herpetic vesicles in the external auditory meatus (which receives a sensory twig from the facial nerve) and sometimes in the soft palate. Deafness may occur. Complete recovery is less likely than in Bell's palsy.

Treatment for shingles should be given (see p. 1155).

Hemifacial spasm

This is an irregular, painless clonic spasm of the facial muscles, usually occurring in middle or old age, and more commonly in women. It varies in severity from a mild inconvenience to a severe and disfiguring condition when it affects all the facial musculature of one side.

The causes are:

- idiopathic
- pressure from vessels in the cerebellopontine angle
- following Bell's palsy
- acoustic neuroma
- Paget's disease of the skull.

SIGNS

There are clonic spasms of the facial muscles on one side. A mild LMN facial weakness is common.

MANAGEMENT

Mild cases require no treatment. In severe cases, various decompressive procedures on the facial nerve in the cerebellopontine angle are sometimes helpful. Local injection of botulinum toxin into facial muscles reduces the movements for some months, and can be repeated. Drugs are of no value.

Myokymia

Facial myokymia describes a rare, continuous, fine, sinuous or wave-like movement of the lower face that is seen in brainstem lesions (e.g. multiple sclerosis, brainstem glioma).

The term myokymia is also used to describe the innocent twitching around the eye that commonly occurs in fatigue.

VIII: The vestibulocochlear nerve

This nerve has two parts – cochlear and vestibular.

Cochlear nerve

Auditory fibres from the spiral organ of Corti in the cochlea pass to the cochlear nuclei in the pons. Fibres from these nuclei cross the midline and pass upwards through the medial lemnisci to the medial geniculate bodies and thence to the temporal gyri.

The symptoms of a cochlear nerve lesion are deafness and tinnitus. The deafness is called 'sensorineural' (or perceptive) deafness. Clinical detection is by tuning fork (256 Hz, not 128 Hz) tests, principally Rinné's test, which distinguishes conductive from sensorineural deafness:

- The contralateral ear is masked (with the examiner's forefinger).
- The vibrating tuning fork is placed adjacent to the external auditory meatus.
- In sensorineural deafness, perception improves when the base of the vibrating tuning fork is placed on the mastoid process, when sound is conducted directly to the ossicular chain through the mastoid process.

In practice, when any neurological cause of deafness is being assessed, pure tone audiometry is carried out.

A second investigation is measurement of auditory evoked potentials which record from scalp electrodes the response from a repetitive click stimulus. The level of the lesion may be detected by abnormalities in the response.

Causes of sensorineural deafness are shown in Table 18.10.

Vestibular nerve

Vestibular fibres from the three semicircular canals, the saccule and the utricle pass to the vestibular nuclei in the pons. Vestibular nerve fibres also pass directly to the cerebellum.

The vestibular nuclei are connected to the cerebellum, nuclei of the ocular muscles and centres for lateral gaze (PPRF), temporal lobes and spinal cord.

The maintenance of balance and posture depends in part upon the interaction of proprioceptive (joint position sense) impulses passing between the neck, spinal muscles and limbs and the vestibular system.

The main symptom of a vestibular lesion is vertigo and loss of balance. Vomiting frequently accompanies acute vertigo of any cause. Nystagmus is the principal physical sign.

Table 18.10
Causes of sensorineural deafness

End organ	Advancing age Occupational acoustic trauma Ménière's disease Drugs (e.g. gentamicin, neomycin)
Eighth-nerve lesions	Acoustic neuroma Cranial trauma Inflammatory lesions: tuberculous meningitis sarcoidosis neurosyphilis Carcinomatous meningitis
Brainstem lesions (rare)	Multiple sclerosis Infarction

Vertigo

Vertigo, the definite illusion of movement of the subject or surroundings, indicates a disturbance of vestibular, eighth nerve, brainstem or, very rarely, cortical function. The principal causes are given in Table 18.11.

Deafness and tinnitus accompanying vertigo indicate that its origin is from the ear or the eighth cranial nerve.

Nystagmus

Nystagmus is a rhythmic oscillation of the eyes. It is a sign of disease of either the ocular or the vestibular system and its connections. Nystagmus is classified, on its appearance, as either *jerk* or *pendular*. For true nystagmus to be present it must be sustained and demonstrable within binocular gaze.

Jerk nystagmus

Jerk nystagmus (the usual nystagmus of neurological disease) has a fast and a slow component to the rhythmic movement. It is seen in vestibular, eighth-nerve, brainstem, cerebellar and (very rarely) cortical lesions.

The direction of the nystagmus is named after the fast component, which can be thought of as a reflex attempt to correct the slower component.

Considerable difficulties exist when attempts are made to use the direction of jerk nystagmus alone as a localizing sign, although it is both a common and valuable indication of abnormality within the vestibular system as a whole. The following are useful diagnostic starting points:

- *Horizontal jerk or rotary jerk nystagmus.* These may be either of peripheral origin (middle ear) or central origin (eighth nerve, brainstem, the cerebellum and their connections). In peripheral lesions, nystagmus is usually acute and transient (minutes or hours) and associated with severe prostrating vertigo; in central lesions it is long-lasting (weeks, months or more).

Table 18.11
Principal causes of vertigo

Ménière's disease
Drugs (e.g. gentamicin, anticonvulsant intoxication)
Toxins (e.g. ethyl alcohol)
'Vestibular neuronitis'
Multiple sclerosis
Migraine
Acute cerebellar lesions
Cerebellopontine angle lesions (e.g. acoustic neuroma)
Partial seizures (temporal lobe focus)
Brainstem ischaemia or infarction
Benign positional vertigo

Vertigo caused by central lesions tends to wane after days or weeks, the nystagmus outlasting it.

- *Vertical jerk nystagmus*. This is caused only by central lesions.
- *Down-beat jerk nystagmus*. This is caused rarely by lesions around the foramen magnum (e.g. meningioma, cerebellar ectopia – p. 1078).

Pendular nystagmus

Pendular movement means movements to and fro which are similar both in velocity and amplitude. Pendular nystagmus is almost always binocular, horizontal and present in all directions of gaze. Its causes are almost invariably ocular, when there is poor visual fixation (e.g. longstanding, severe visual impairment) or as a congenital lesion, when it is sometimes associated with head-nodding. Exceptionally, it occurs in brainstem disease: a fine pendular, jelly-like nystagmus is a sign of a MS brainstem plaque, or brainstem glioma.

Investigations of vestibular lesions

Caloric tests are used to assess function of the labyrinth. These record the evoked nystagmus when first ice cold, then warm, water is run into the external meatus. In the normal caloric test:

- ice cold water in the left ear causes nystagmus with the fast movement to the right
- warm water in the left ear causes nystagmus with the fast movement to the left.

The right ear gives opposite responses. Decreased or absent nystagmus indicates ipsilateral labyrinth, eighth-nerve or brainstem involvement.

Vestibular and auditory lesions – central, VIIIth nerve and end organ

Lesions at six levels can be recognized by the associated abnormalities.

Within the cerebral cortex. Vertigo is occasionally a part of the aura of a partial seizure of temporal lobe origin. Vertigo (see dizziness, see p. 1010) is also a psychological event, for example when experiencing unaccustomed heights.

In cortical lesions, deafness is very rare.

Within the pons. Transient vertigo occurs in basilar migraine (see p. 1082), in syncope, and occasionally in hypoglycaemic attacks; its site of origin is often difficult to ascertain in these conditions.

Vertigo is also common with brainstem demyelinating or vascular lesions that involve the vestibular nuclei and their connections. A sixth- or seventh-nerve lesion, an internuclear ophthalmoplegia or contralateral hemiparesis help localization. Nystagmus is frequently present, while deafness is rare.

Within the cerebellum. Nystagmus, towards the side of a cerebellar mass (e.g. tumour, haemorrhage or infarct) develops. Limb ataxia is usually present. Bilateral cerebellar, or cerebellar connexion disease (e.g. olivo-ponto-cerebellar degeneration) causes bilateral nystagmus. Deafness does not occur.

At the cerebellopontine angle. Sensorineural deafness occurs. Sixth-, seventh- and fifth-nerve lesions develop, followed by cerebellar signs (ipsilateral) and later pyramidal signs (contralateral). Nystagmus is often present.

Causes include acoustic neuroma (see p. 1079), meningioma and secondary neoplasm, carcinomatous meningitis and inflammatory lesions (Table 18.10).

Within the petrous temporal bone. A seventh-nerve lesion accompanies the eighth (see also seventh- and fifth-nerve lesions). Causes include trauma, middle ear infection, secondary neoplasm and Paget's disease of bone.

Within the end organs (cochlear and semi-circular canals). Here the main causes of disease are:

- Ménière's disease
- drugs (e.g. gentamicin)
- noise (acoustic trauma, p. 891)
- middle ear infection
- intrauterine rubella
- congenital syphilis
- mumps
- vestibular neuronitis
- benign positional vertigo
- advancing age.

Ménière's disease

This condition is characterized by recurrent attacks of the three symptoms – vertigo, tinnitus and deafness. It is associated with a dilatation of the endolymph system of unknown cause.

SYMPTOMS

Sudden, unprovoked attacks of vertigo with vomiting and loss of balance last from minutes to hours. Tinnitus and deafness accompany an attack but may be over-shadowed by the degree of vertigo. Attacks are recurrent over months or years. Ultimately deafness develops and vertigo ceases.

SIGNS

Nystagmus often accompanies an attack. Sensorineural deafness is present.

MANAGEMENT

Medical treatment consists of rest, vestibular sedatives (e.g. cinnarizine, betahistine, prochlorperazine), but is unsatisfactory. Each attack is, however, self-limiting.

Recurrent severe attacks may require surgery, such as surgical endolymph drainage, ultrasound destruction of the labyrinth or vestibular nerve section.

Vestibular neuronitis

This common but poorly understood syndrome describes an acute attack of isolated severe vertigo with nystagmus, often with vomiting, but without loss of hearing. It is believed to follow or accompany viral infections that affect the labyrinth or vestibular nerve.

The disturbance lasts for several days or weeks but is self-limiting and rarely recurs. Treatment is with vestibular sedatives. The condition is sometimes followed by benign positional vertigo. Very similar symptoms can be caused by demyelination or vascular lesions within the brainstem, but usually other abnormalities are almost invariably apparent (see above).

Benign positional vertigo and positional nystagmus

Positional vertigo is vertigo precipitated by head movements, usually into a particular position. It may occur when turning in bed or on sitting up. The vertigo is transient, lasting seconds or minutes. The phenomenon fatigues (becomes less severe on repeated movement).

Vertigo can be produced by moving the patient's head suddenly (Hallpike's test). There is a latent interval of a few seconds, followed by nystagmus, which fatigues on repeating the test several times, though repetition is unpleasant for the patient.

The syndrome of benign positional vertigo sometimes follows vestibular neuronitis (see above), head injury or ear infection. It usually lasts for some months. There are no sequelae, although the condition sometimes recurs. Treatment is with vestibular sedatives.

Positional nystagmus (and vertigo) which is immediately apparent on movement (i.e. there is no latent interval) and which persists (it does not fatigue) is occasionally seen with mass lesions of the cerebellum.

IX and X: The glossopharyngeal and vagus nerves

Glossopharyngeal nerve

This mixed nerve, which is largely sensory, arises in the medulla and leaves the skull base through the jugular foramen with the vagus and accessory nerves.

Sensory fibres supply all sensation to the tonsillar fossa and pharynx (the afferent pathway of the gag reflex), and taste to the posterior third of the tongue.

Motor fibres supply the stylopharyngeus muscle, autonomic fibres supply the parotid gland, and a sensory branch supplies the carotid sinus.

Vagus nerve

This mixed nerve, which is largely motor, supplies the striated muscle of the pharynx (efferent pathway of the gag reflex), the larynx (including the vocal cords via the recurrent laryngeal nerves) and the upper oesophagus.There are sensory fibres from the larynx. Parasympathetic fibres supply the heart and abdominal viscera.

Ninth- and tenth-nerve lesions

Isolated single-nerve lesions are most unusual, since disease at the jugular foramen affects both nerves and sometimes the accessory nerve.

A unilateral ninth-nerve lesion causes diminished sensation on the same side of the pharynx. A tenth-nerve palsy produces ipsilateral failure of voluntary and reflex elevation of the soft palate, which is drawn over to the opposite side.

Bilateral combined lesions of the ninth and tenth nerves cause visible weakness of elevation of the palate, depression of palatal sensation and loss of the gag reflex. The vagal recurrent laryngeal branches (see below) are involved. The cough is depressed and the vocal cords are paralysed. The patient complains of difficulty in swallowing, hoarseness, nasal regurgitation and choking (particularly with fluids) – a dangerous situation. *Bulbar palsy* is a general term describing palatal, pharyngeal and tongue weakness of LMN type (see p. 1031).

Ninth- and tenth-nerve lesions often accompany eleventh- and twelfth-nerve lesions. Causes are given in Table 18.12.

Recurrent laryngeal nerve lesions

Paralysis of this important branch of each vagus causes hoarseness (*dysphonia*) and failure of the forceful, explosive part of the cough reflex. There is no visible weakness of the palate but vocal cord paralysis is seen endoscopically. Bilateral acute lesions

Table 18.12
Principal causes of ninth-, tenth-, eleventh- and twelfth-nerve lesions

Within the brainstem
Infarction
Syringobulbia
Motor neurone disease (motor fibres)
Poliomyelitis (motor fibres)
At the skull base (jugular and anterior condylar foramina)
Carcinoma of nasopharynx
Glomus tumour
Neurofibroma
Jugular venous thrombosis (XIIth is spared)
Trauma
Within the neck and nasopharynx
Carcinoma of nasopharynx
Metastases
Polyneuropathy
Trauma

(e.g. postoperatively) are a serious emergency and cause respiratory obstruction.

The left recurrent laryngeal nerve (which loops beneath the aorta) is more commonly damaged than the right.

Causes of recurrent laryngeal nerve lesions include:

- mediastinal primary tumours (e.g. thymoma)
- secondary spread from carcinoma of the bronchus
- aneurysm of the aorta
- trauma or surgery to the neck
- glossopharyngeal neuralgia (rare).

Glossopharyngeal neuralgia describes intensely painful, paroxysmal neuralgic spasms of the pharynx triggered repeatedly by swallowing. There no are physical signs. Treatment of this rare condition is with carbamazepine (see trigeminal neuralgia, p. 1021) or section of the nerve in the pharynx.

XI: The accessory nerve

This motor nerve to the trapezius and sternomastoid muscles arises in the medulla and leaves the skull through the jugular foramen with the ninth and tenth nerves.

A lesion of the eleventh nerve causes weakness of the sternomastoid (rotation of the head and neck to the opposite side) and the trapezius (shoulder shrugging). The principal causes are shown in Table 18.12.

XII: The hypoglossal nerve

The motor nerve to the tongue arises in the medulla and leaves the skull through the anterior condylar foramen.

Twelfth-nerve lesions

An LMN lesion of the twelfth nerve leads to unilateral weakness, wasting and fasciculation of the tongue. When protruded the tongue deviates towards the weaker side. For the principal causes, see Table 18.12.

Bilateral supranuclear (UMN) twelfth-nerve lesions produce slow, limited tongue movements; the tongue is stiff and cannot be protruded far. Fasciculation is absent.

Bulbar palsy

A bulbar palsy describes weakness of LMN type of the muscles whose cranial nerve nuclei lie in the medulla (the bulb). The weakness of the bulbar muscles is caused by disease of lower cranial nerve nuclei (e.g. motor neurone disease), of ninth to twelfth cranial nerves (see Table 18.12), of their neuromuscular junctions (e.g. myasthenia gravis, botulism), or of the muscles themselves (e.g. muscular dystrophies).

Pseudobulbar palsy

The term pseudobulbar palsy describes bilateral supranuclear (UMN) lesions of the lower cranial nuclei producing weakness and poverty of movement of the tongue and pharyngeal muscles. The findings in pseudobulbar palsy are a stiff, slow, spastic tongue (which is not wasted), dysarthria with a stiff, slow, spastic voice which sounds dry and gravelly, and dysphagia. The gag reflex and palatal reflex are preserved. The jaw jerk is exaggerated. Emotional lability (inappropriate laughing or crying) often accompanies pseudobulbar palsy. The principal causes are:

- motor neurone disease, in which there are often both upper UMN and LMN lesions (i.e. elements of both pseudobulbar and bulbar palsy)
- multiple sclerosis, in which it occurs mainly as a late event
- cerebrovascular disease, in which it may occur with multi-infarct dementia
- following severe head injury.

Great difficulty with swallowing, dysarthria and a slow-moving tongue also develop in the late stages of Parkinson's disease. This is aetiologically distinct from both pseudobulbar and bulbar palsy.

Systems of motor control

- The *corticospinal* (or pyramidal) system originates in the cerebral cortex and delivers information to the anterior horn cells of the spinal cord. This system enables purposive, skilled, strong and organized movement to take place, such as grasping and manipulating a key. Defective function within the pathway is recognized by loss of voluntary movement, the pattern of weakness, spasticity, reflex change, and loss of skilled movement. This is seen, for example in a hemiparesis.
- The *extrapyramidal* system facilitates fast, fluid movements, which the corticospinal sytem has generated. Defective function is recognized usually by slowness (bradykinesia), stiffness (rigidity) and/or disorders of movement (rest tremor, chorea and other dyskinesias). Frequently, one sign (e.g. stiffness alone, or chorea alone) will predominate, depending upon the site and nature of the pathology. This makes a single, comprehensive descriptive definition of extrapyramidal disorder difficult.
- The *cerebellum* and its connections have a role in the coordination of smooth movement which has been initiated by the corticospinal system and the

regulation of balance. Cerebellar disease leads to unsteadiness and jerkiness of movement (ataxia), with characterisitic physical signs of past pointing, action tremor and incoordination, but without slowing.

Each motor control system also relies upon connections with the other two, and with sensory input, from the special senses, from proprioception (joint position) and the vestibular system.

The corticospinal or pyramidal system

The corticospinal tracts originate in neurones of the fifth layer of the cortex and terminate at the motor nuclei of the cranial nerves and anterior horn cells of the spinal cord. The nerve fibre pathways of particular importance (Fig 18.7) in clinical diagnosis congregate in the internal capsule and cross in the medulla (the decussation of the pyramids), passing to the contralateral halves of the cord as the crossed lateral corticospinal tracts. This is the pyramidal system, disease of which causes upper motor neurone (UMN) lesions. Pyramidal is simply a descriptive term which draws together the anatomy and physical signs of lesions of this pathway. It is used here interchangably with the term UMN.

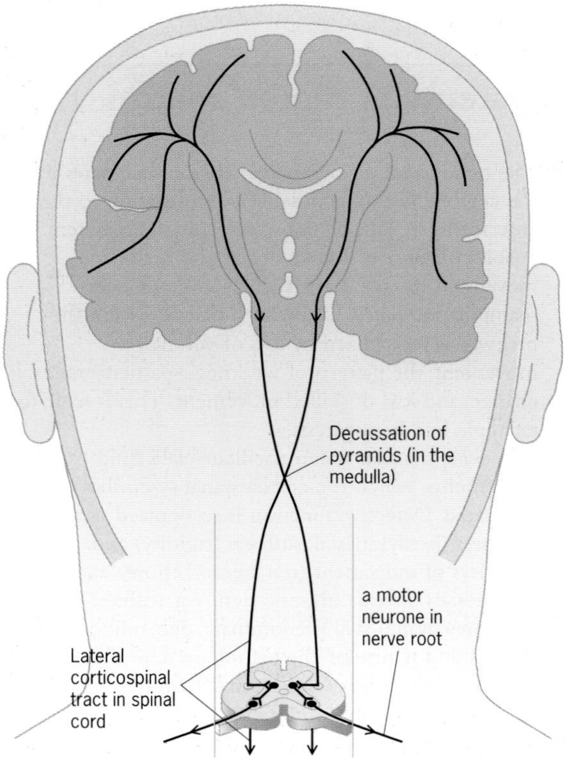

Fig 18.7
Crossed corticospinal or 'pyramidal' tracts

A small proportion of the corticospinal outflow remains uncrossed (the anterior corticospinal tracts), but this does not affect the clinical signs.

Clinical characteristics of pyramidal lesions (see Table 18.13)

It is important to understand that the signs of a pyramidal lesion may be minimal. Weakness, spasticity or changes in superficial reflexes may predominate and the absence of one group of signs does not exclude a UMN lesion.

Drift of the upper limb

In the normal individual the outstretched upper limbs are held symmetrically, even when the eyes are closed. In a pyramidal (UMN) lesion, when both upper limbs are held outstretched, palms uppermost, the affected limb drifts downwards and medially. The forearm tends to pronate and the hand flex slightly at the fingers. This important sign is often the first to occur, sometimes before weakness or reflex changes are evident.

Weakness and loss of skilled movement

A pyramidal (UMN) lesion above the decussation in the medulla (e.g. an infarct in the internal capsule), causes weakness of the opposite limbs; this is a contralateral hemiparesis. In such an acute lesion, this weakness will be immediate and dense – a hemiplegia (see below) – but in partial progressive lesions (e.g. a glioma) there is a characteristic pattern of increasing weakness in the hemiparetic limbs. In the upper limb the flexors remain stronger than the extensors, while in the lower limb the extensors remain stronger than the flexors. In the upper limb the weaker movements are thus shoulder abduction and elbow extension; in the forearm and hand, the wrist and finger extensors and abductors are weaker than their antagonists.

In the lower limb the weaker movements are flexion and abduction of the hip, flexion of the knee, and dorsiflexion and eversion of the ankle.

In addition to weakness, there is loss of skilled movement. For example, fine finger and toe control diminishes.

When the UMN lesion is below the decussation of the pyramids, the hemiparesis is on the same side as the lesion. This situation is unusual.

Table 18.13
Signs of an upper motor neurone lesion

Drift of upper limb
Weakness with a characteristic distribution
Increase in tone of the spastic type
Exaggerated tendon reflexes
An extensor plantar response
Loss of abdominal reflexes
No muscle wasting
Normal electrical excitability of muscle

Increase in tone (spasticity)

An acute lesion of one pyramidal tract (e.g. the internal capsule infarct mentioned above) causes initially a flaccid paralysis, and areflexia. An increase in tone follows within several days owing to loss of the inhibitory effect of the corticospinal pathway and an increase in spinal reflex activity. This increase in tone affects all muscle groups on the affected side but is most easily detected in the stronger muscles. It is characterized by changing resistance to passive movement; the change is sudden – the clasp-knife effect. The tendon reflexes are exaggerated and clonus is often evident.

Changes in superficial reflexes

The normal flexor plantar response becomes extensor. In a severe lesion (e.g. the internal capsule infarct) this extensor response can be elicited from a wide area of the affected limb. As recovery occurs, the area that is sensitive diminishes until only the posterior third of the lateral aspect of the sole is receptive. The stimulus should be unpleasant (an orange-stick is the correct instrument). An extensor plantar is certain when the dorsiflexion of the great toe is accompanied by fanning (abduction) of the other toes.

The abdominal (and cremasteric reflexes) are abolished on the affected side.

Muscle wasting (except from disuse) is not a feature of pyramidal lesions. Muscles remain normally excitable electrically.

Clinical patterns of UMN disorders

Two main patterns of UMN (pyramidal) lesions are recognizable: hemiparesis and paraparesis.

Hemiparesis means weakness of the limbs of one side; it is usually (but not always) caused by a lesion within the brain. *Paraparesis* means weakness of both lower limbs and is characteristically diagnostic (but again, not always) of a spinal cord lesion.

The terms hemiplegia and paraplegia strictly indicate total paralysis, but the terms are often used loosely to describe severe weakness.

Hemiparesis

The level within the corticospinal tract is recognized by various accompanying features.

Motor cortex. Weakness localized to one contralateral limb (monoplegia) or part of a limb (e.g. a weak hand) is characteristic of an isolated lesion of the motor cortex (e.g. a secondary neoplasm). There may be a defect in higher cortical function (e.g. aphasia if the speech area is affected). Focal epilepsy may be present.

Internal capsule. Since all corticospinal fibres are tightly packed in the internal capsule, occupying about 1 cm^2, a small lesion causes a large deficit. For example, an infarct of a small branch of the middle cerebral artery (see p. 1049) causes a sudden, dense, contralateral hemiplegia that includes the face.

Table 18.14
Causes of a spastic paraparesis

Spinal lesions
Spinal cord compression (see Table 18.48)
Multiple sclerosis
Myelitis (e.g. varicella zoster virus)
Motor neurone disease
Subacute combined degeneration of the cord
Syringomyelia
Syphilis
Familial or sporadic paraparesis
Vascular disease of the cord
Non-metastatic manifestation of malignancy
Tropical spastic paraparesis (HTLV-1)
HIV-associated myelopathy
Cerebral lesions[a]
Parasagittal cortical lesions:
Meningioma
Venous sinus thrombosis
Hydrocephalus
Multiple cerebral infarction

[a] All are rare causes of a paraparesis
HTLV-1, human T-cell leukaemia virus

Pons. A pontine lesion (e.g. a plaque of multiple sclerosis) is rarely confined only to the corticospinal tract. As adjacent structures such as the sixth and seventh nuclei, MLF and PPRF (see p. 1018) are involved, there are other localizing signs – VI and VII nerve palsies, intranuclear nuclear ophthalmoplegia (INO) or a lateral gaze palsy, with the contralateral hemiparesis.

Spinal cord. An isolated lesion of a single lateral corticospinal tract within the cord (which is unusual) causes an ipsilateral UMN lesion, the level of which is indicated by a reflex level (e.g. absent biceps jerk), the presence of a Brown–Séquard syndrome or muscle wasting at the level of the lesion (see p. 1034).

Paraparesis (see Table 18.14)

Paraparesis (and tetraparesis, when the four limbs are involved) indicates bilateral damage to the corticospinal tracts. Spinal cord compression (see p. 1085) or other cord disease is the usual cause, but cerebral lesions occasionally can produce paraparesis. Paraparesis, including here tetraparesis, is a feature of many neurological conditions which are recognizable by their clinical features, making this differential diagnosis one of pivotal importance in neurology.

The extrapyramidal system

The extrapyramidal system is a general term for the basal ganglia. In disorders of this system, either or both of two features become apparent in the limbs and axial muscles:

- reduction in speed, known as bradykinesia (slow movement) or akinesia (no movement), with muscle rigidity
- involuntary movements (tremor, chorea, dystonia, hemiballismus, athetosis).

The most common extrapyramidal disorder is Parkinson's disease.

STRUCTURE

The corpus striatum, consisting of the caudate nucleus, globus pallidus and putamen (the latter two forming the lentiform nucleus), lies close to the substantia nigra, thalami and subthalamic nuclei. There are interconnections between these structures and the cerebral cortex, the cerebellum and the reticular formation, the cranial nerve nuclei (particularly the vestibular nerve) and the spinal cord.

FUNCTION AND DYSFUNCTION

The overall function of this complex system is the initiation and modulation of movement. The system modulates cortical motor activity by a series of servo loops, between the cortex and the various structures within the basal ganglia.

It is now clear that in many involuntary movement disorders there are substantial and specific changes in neurotransmitter profile rather than discrete anatomical lesions. As an introduction to this difficult field, neurotransmitter changes in two diseases are considered (Table 18.15).

Therapeutic alteration of the neurotransmitter profile causes characteristic clinical changes. For example:

- In patients with Parkinson's disease, an increase in dopamine activity due to levodopa therapy or dopaminergic agonists such as bromocriptine relieves rigidity. However, in excess (in both normal people and those with Parkinson's disease), levodopa therapy causes chorea.
- In normal subjects, an increase in acetylcholine activity or a decrease in dopamine activity causes rigidity and bradykinesia (parkinsonism). Reserpine (an obsolete hypotensive drug which depletes neurones of dopamine) and phenothiazines or butyrophenones (which block dopaminergic neurones) cause or exacerbate parkinsonism.

Table 18.15 Changes in the major neurotransmitter profile in Parkinson's and Huntington's diseases

Condition	Site	Neurotransmitter
Parkinson's disease	Putamen	Dopamine ↓ 90% Noradrenaline ↓ 60% 5-HT ↓ 60%
	Substantia nigra	Dopamine ↓ 90% GAD + GABA ↓↓
	Cerebral cortex	GAD + GABA ↓↓
Huntington's disease	Corpus striatum	Acetylcholine ↓↓ GABA ↓↓ Dopamine: normal GAD + GABA ↓↓

GABA, γ-amino butyric acid; GAD, glutamic acid decarboxylase, the enzyme responsible for synthesizing GABA; 5-HT, 5-hydroxytryptamine

Extrapyramidal disorders are classified broadly on clinical grounds into the akinetic-rigid syndromes (see p. 1062) in which poverty of movement predominates, and the dyskinesias, in which there are a variety of excessive involuntary movements (p. 1065).

The cerebellum

The third system of motor control is involved with coordination, rather than speed. The cerebellum receives afferent fibres from:

- proprioceptive organs in joints and muscles
- vestibular nuclei
- basal ganglia
- the corticospinal system
- olivary nuclei.

Efferent fibres pass from the cerebellum to:

- each red nucleus
- vestibular nuclei
- basal ganglia
- the corticospinal system.

Each lateral lobe of the cerebellum coordinates movement of the ipsilateral limb. The vermis (a midline structure) is concerned with maintenance of axial (midline) posture and balance.

Cerebellar lesions

Expanding mass lesions within the cerebellum obstruct the aqueduct to produce hydrocephalus, causing severe pressure headaches, vomiting and papilloedema. Coning of the cerebellar tonsils through the foramen magnum and respiratory arrest occur, often within hours. Rarely tonic seizures of the limbs occur with cerebellar masses.

Lateral cerebellar lobes

A lesion within one cerebellar lobe (e.g. a tumour or infarction) causes disruption of the normal sequence of movements (dyssynergia) on the side of the lesion. A collection of specific signs develop.

Posture and gait. The outstretched arm is held still in the early stages of a cerebellar lesion, but there is rebound upward overshoot when the limb is pressed downwards by the examiner and released. Gait is ataxic with a broad base; the patient falters towards the side of the lesion.

Tremor and ataxia. Movement is imprecise in direction, in force and in distance (dysmetria). Rapid alternating movements (tapping, clapping or rotary movements of the hand) are clumsy and disorganized (dysdiadochokinesis). Intention tremor (action tremor, with past-pointing) is seen when the finger-nose-finger and heel-shin tests are performed.

Nystagmus. Coarse horizontal nystagmus (see p. 1024) appears with lateral cerebellar lobe lesions. Its direction is towards the side of the lesion.

Dysarthria. Speech is affected (usually with bilateral lesions). A halting, jerking dysarthria results – the scanning speech of cerebellar lesions.

Other signs. Titubation – rhythmic tremor of the head in either to and fro (yes–yes) movements or rotary (no–no) movements – also occurs, mainly when cerebellar connections are involved (e.g. in essential tremor and MS).

Hypotonia (floppy limbs) and depression of reflexes are also sometimes seen with cerebellar disease, but are usually of little value as localizing signs. Pendular (i.e. slow) reflexes also occur.

Midline cerebellar lesions

Lesions of the cerebellar vermis have a dramatic effect on the equilibrium of the trunk and axial musculature. This truncal ataxia means difficulty in standing and sitting unsupported, with a rolling, broad, ataxic gait.

Lesions of the flocculonodular region cause vertigo, vomiting and ataxia of gait if they extend to the roof of the fourth ventricle.

Table 18.16 summarizes the main causes of cerebellar disease.

Table 18.16
Principal causes of cerebellar syndromes

Tumours	Haemangioblastoma Medulloblastoma Secondary neoplasm Compression by acoustic neuroma
Vascular lesions	Haemorrhage Infarction Arteriovenous malformation
Infection	Abscess HIV Kuru
Developmental	Arnold–Chiari malformation Basilar invagination Cerebral palsy
Toxic and metabolic	Anticonvulsant drugs Chronic alcohol abuse Following carbon monoxide poisoning Lead poisoning Solvent abuse
Inherited	Friedreich's ataxia Ataxia telangiectasia Essential tremor
Miscellaneous	Multiple sclerosis Hydrocephalus Postinfective cerebellar syndrome of childhood Hypothyroidism Non-metastatic manifestation of malignancy Cerebral oedema of chronic hypoxia

Tremor

Tremor is an oscillation, regular and sinusoidal, of a part or parts of the body. Different varieties are outlined below.

Postural tremor

Everyone has a physiological tremor of the outstretched hands at 8–12 Hz. This is increased with anxiety, hyperthyroidism and certain drugs (sympathomimetics, sodium valproate, lithium) or in mercury poisoning. A coarse, postural tremor is seen in chronic alcohol abusers and in benign essential tremor (usually at 5–8 Hz). Postural tremor does not worsen on movement, though it may be more obvious.

Intention tremor

Tremor that is exacerbated by action, with past-pointing and accompanying slowness and incoordination of rapid alternating movement (dysdiadochokinesis), occurs in cerebellar lobe disease and with lesions of cerebellar connections. Titubation (tremor of the head) and nystagmus may be present.

Rest tremor

This is present at rest, is between 4 and 7 Hz and is not made worse by action. It occurs primarily in Parkinson's disease and is sometimes described as pill-rolling between the thumb and index finger.

Other tremors

Tremor is seen following lesions of the red nucleus (e.g. infarction, demyelination) and rarely with frontal lobe lesions.

Lower motor neurone (LMN) lesions

The LMN is the motor pathway from the anterior horn cell (or cranial nerve nucleus) via a peripheral nerve to the motor end plate.

The motor unit consists of a single anterior horn cell, the single fast-conducting motor nerve fibre that leaves the spinal cord via the anterior root, and the group of muscle fibres (100–2000) being supplied via the mixed peripheral nerve. Anterior horn cell activity is modulated by the impulses from:

- the corticospinal tracts
- the extrapyramidal system (basal ganglia and cerebellum)
- afferent fibres from the posterior roots.

SIGNS OF LOWER MOTOR NEURONE LESION

Voluntary muscle depends upon the motor unit for all movement and also for its metabolic integrity. Signs follow rapidly if the LMN is interrupted at any point in

Table 18.17
Signs of a lower motor neurone lesion

Weakness
Wasting
Hypotonia
Reflex loss
Fasciculation
Contractures of muscle
'Trophic' changes in skin and nails

NB: Fibrillation potentials can be detected electromyographically, see p. 1041.

its course (Table 18.17). Muscle wasting appears within three weeks of the development of an LMN lesion. Fasciculation occurs and is due to visible contractions of single motor units. Fibrillation potentials are seen when denervated muscle is sampled electrically (see p. 1041).

CAUSES

Examples of LMN lesions at various levels are:

- cranial nerve nuclei and anterior horn cell – Bell's palsy, motor neurone disease, poliomyelitis
- spinal root – cervical and lumbar disc protrusion, neuralgic amyotrophy (see p. 1097)
- peripheral (or cranial) nerve – nerve trauma or entrapment (see p. 1092), mononeuritis multiplex (see p. 1092).

The spinal reflex arc

The components of the spinal reflex arc are illustrated in Fig 18.8. The stretch reflex is the physiological basis for the tendon reflexes. For example, in the knee jerk, a tap on the patellar tendon activates stretch receptors in the quadriceps. Impulses in first-order sensory neurones pass directly to LMNs (L3 and L4), which activate the quadriceps, causing a contraction.

Loss of a tendon reflex is caused by a lesion anywhere along the spinal reflex path. The reflex lost indicates the level of the lesion (Table 18.18).

Reinforcement

Distraction of the patient's attention, clenching the teeth or pulling of the interlocked fingers increases the activity of the stretch reflex. Such reinforcement manoeuvres should be carried out before a reflex is recorded as absent.

Table 18.18
Spinal levels of tendon reflexes

Spinal level	Reflex
C5–6	Supinator
C5–6	Biceps
C7	Triceps
L3–4	Knee
S1	Ankle

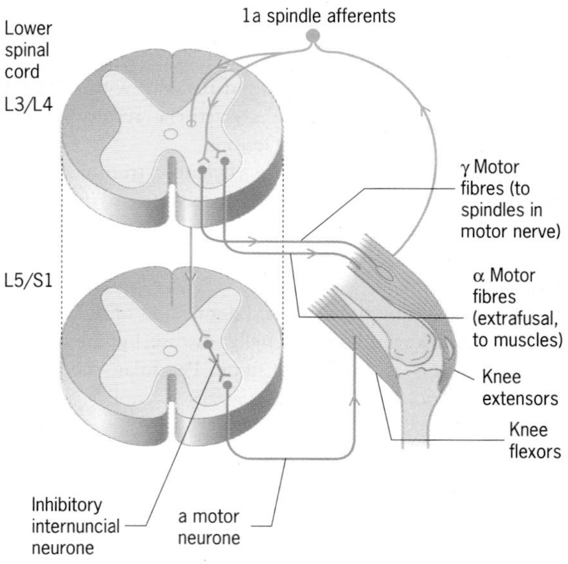

Fig 18.8
The knee jerk: a spinal reflex arc
Sudden stretching of a tendon generates sensory action potentials seen in 1a muscle spindle afferents, which synapse with γ motor fibres (to spindles) and α motor fibres. Motor action potentials thus generated cause muscle contractions

Sensory pathways and pain

Peripheral nerves and spinal roots

Peripheral nerves carry all modalities of sensation from either free or specialized nerve endings to the dorsal root ganglia and thus to the cord. The sensory distribution of the spinal roots (dermatomes) is shown in Fig 18.9.

The spinal cord (Fig 18.10)

Posterior columns

For clinical purposes, axons in the posterior columns whose cell bodies are in the ipsilateral gracile and cuneate nuclei in the medulla carry the sensory modalities of vibration sense, joint position (proprioception), light touch and two-point discrimination. Axons from second-order neurones then cross the midline in the brainstem to form the medial lemniscus and pass to the thalamus.

Spinothalamic tracts

Axons carrying pain and temperature sensation synapse in the dorsal horn of the cord, cross the cord and pass as the spinothalamic tracts to the thalamus and reticular formation.

The sensory cortex

The projection of fibres from the thalamus to the sensory cortex of the parietal region is shown in Fig 18.10. Connections also exist between the thalamus and the motor cortex.

Lesions of the sensory pathways

Paraesthesiae, numbness and pain are the principal symptoms of lesions of the sensory pathways below the level of the thalamus. The quality and distribution of the symptoms suggest the site of the lesion.

Peripheral nerve lesions

The symptoms are felt in the distribution of the affected peripheral nerve (see p. 1092).

Section of a sensory nerve is followed by complete sensory loss. Nerve entrapment (see p. 1092) causes numb-ness, pain and tingling. Tapping the site of compression sometimes causes a sharp, electric-shock-like pain in the distribution of the nerve, such as at the wrist in the carpal tunnel syndrome. This is Tinel's sign.

Neuralgia

Neuralgia refers to local pain of great severity in the distribution of a damaged nerve. Examples are:

- trigeminal neuralgia (p. 1021)
- postherpetic neuralgia (p. 1074)
- causalgia.

Causalgia describes chronic burning pain which sometimes follows nerve section. It is seen occasionally following amputation.

Spinal root lesions

Root pain

The pain of root compression is referred to the myotome supplied by that root, and there is also a tingling discomfort in the dermatome. The pain is made worse by manoeuvres that either stretch the nerve root (e.g. the limitation of straight leg raising in lumbar disc prolapse) or increase the pressure in the spinal subarachnoid space (coughing and straining).

Cervical and lumbar disc protrusions (see p. 1098) are common causes of root lesions.

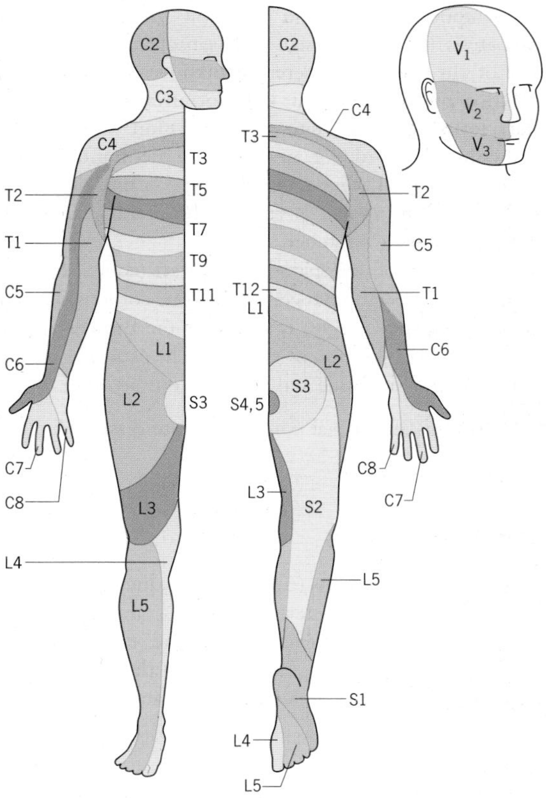

Fig 18.9
Dermatomes of spinal roots and ophthalmic (V_1), maxillary (V_2) and mandibular (V_3) divisions of the trigeminal nerve

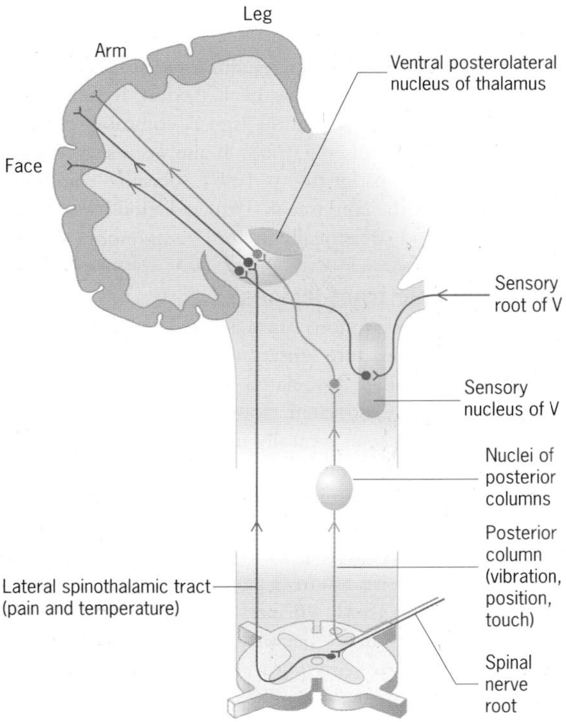

Fig 18.10
Principal sensory pathways
Posterior columns remain uncrossed until the medulla. The spinothalamic tracts cross close to their entry into the spinal cord

Dorsal spinal root lesions

Section of a dorsal root causes loss of all modalities of sensation in the appropriate dermatome (see Fig 18.9). However, the overlap with adjacent dermatomes may make it difficult to detect anaesthesia if only a single root is affected.

Lightning pains. Tabes dorsalis (now a rarity) is a form of neurosyphilis that causes a low-grade inflammation of the dorsal roots and root entry zone of the cord. Its presentation includes irregular, sharp, momentary stabbing pains that involve one or two spots, typically in a calf, thigh or ankle.

Spinal cord lesions

Posterior column lesions

These cause:

- tingling of a limb
- electric-shock-like sensations
- clumsiness
- numbness
- band-like sensations.

These symptoms are often felt vaguely without a clear sensory level on the side of the lesion.

Position sense, vibration sense, light touch and two-point discrimination are lost below the level of the lesion. Loss of position sense produces sensory ataxia (see p. 1009).

Lhermitte's phenomenon

This is an electric-shock-like sensation radiating down the trunk and limbs produced by neck flexion. It indicates a cervical cord lesion. Lhermitte's sign is common in acute exacerbations of MS (see p. 1068). It also occurs in cervical spondylotic myelopathy (see p. 1097), subacute combined degeneration of the cord (see p. 1096), radiation myelopathy (see p. 1087), and occasionally in cord compression.

Spinothalamic tract lesions

Pure spinothalamic lesions cause isolated contralateral loss of pain and temperature sensation below the level of the lesion. This is called dissociated sensory loss – pain and temperature are dissociated from light touch, which is preserved. This is seen typically in syringomyelia.

The spinal level is modified by the lamination of fibres within the spinothalamic tracts. Fibres from the lower spinal roots lie superficially and are therefore damaged first by compressive lesions from outside the cord. As an external compressive lesion (e.g. a midthoracic extradural meningioma; Fig 18.11) enlarges, the spinal sensory level ascends as deeper fibres become involved. Conversely, a central lesion of the cord (e.g. a syrinx, see p. 1086) affects the deeper fibres first.

Symptoms of spinothalamic tract lesions are the absence of pain (resulting in painless burns and minor injuries) or loss of temperature sensation. Perforating ulcers and neuropathic joints (Charcot joints) develop.

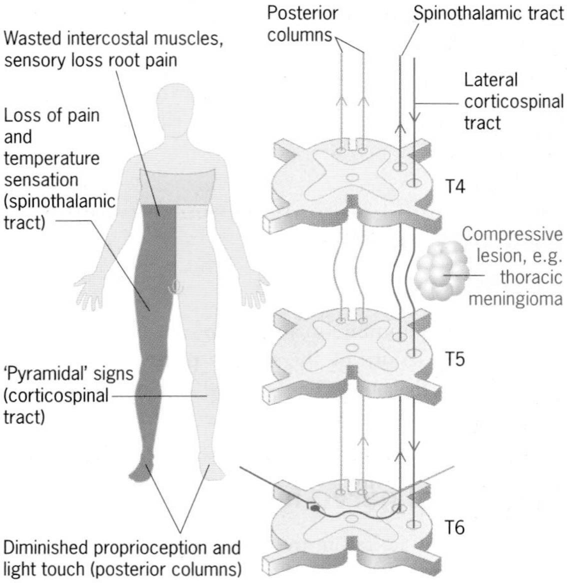

Fig 18.11
Clinical features of spinal cord compression

Spinal cord compression (Fig 18.11)

This important syndrome causes a progressive spastic paraparesis (or tetraparesis) with sensory loss below the level of the lesion. Sphincter disturbance is common.

Root pain is frequent but not invariable. It is felt characteristically at the site of compression. With a lesion of the thoracic cord (e.g. an extradural meningioma), pain radiates in a band around the chest and is made worse by coughing, straining and jarring, as the meningeal sheaths of nerve roots are stretched.

Involvement of one spinothalamic tract (contralateral loss of pain and temperature) together with one corticospinal tract (ipsilateral pyramidal signs) is known as the Brown–Séquard syndrome of hemisection of the cord. The patient complains of numbness on one side and weakness on the other.

- Paraparesis and spinal cord disease are discussed further on p. 1085.

Pontine lesions

Since lesions in the pons (e.g. an MS plaque) lie above the decussation of the posterior columns, and the medial lemniscus and spinothalamic tracts are close together, there is loss of all forms of sensation on the side opposite the lesion. The III, IV, V, VI and VII cranial nerve nuclei are often also involved.

Thalamic lesions

Thalamic pain, sometimes called the thalamic syndrome, is usually caused by a small thalamic infarct. The patient develops a hemiparesis and sensory loss which recovers partially. There remains a constant very severe deep-seated burning pain that affects the paretic limbs. Movement does not change the pain, which continues night and day. Extreme anguish is usual and the secondary depression that follows may lead to suicide.

Thalamic lesions may also produce loss of all modalities of sensation on the opposite side of the body; this is an unusual clinical picture.

Parietal cortex lesions

Sensory loss, neglect of one side and subtle disorders of sensation occur. Pain is not a feature of destructive cortical lesions.

Irritative phenomena (e.g. partial sensory seizures from a glioma) arising in the parietal cortex cause tingling sensations in a limb, or elsewhere.

Pain

Pain is an unpleasant and unique physical and psychological experience. Acute pain serves a biological purpose (e.g. withdrawal of a limb) and causes sympathetic hyperactivity. It is typically self-limiting, when the healing process is complete. Chronic pain (e.g. causalgia, see p. 1033) lasts many months, far longer than the time required for healing.

The physiology of pain

Pain perception is mediated by free nerve endings, the terminations of finely myelinated Aδ and of non-myelinated C fibres. Chemicals released locally as a result of injury either produce pain by direct stimulation or by sensitizing the nerve endings. Aδ fibres give rise to perception of sharp, immediate pain which is followed by slower-onset, duller, more diffuse and prolonged pain mediated by slower-conducting C fibres.

Sensory impulses enter the cord via dorsal spinal roots. Within it, impulses ascend either in each dorsal (posterior) column or in each spinothalamic tract. The cells of the grey matter in the spinal cord are arranged in laminae labelled I to X from dorsal to ventral. A fibres terminate in laminae I and V and excite second-order neurones which send fibres to the contralateral side via the anterior commissure and up the anterolateral column in the direct spinothalamic tract. C fibres mostly terminate in the substantia gelatinosa (laminae II and III). A series of short fibres give rise to long axons which pass through the anterior commissure to the contralateral side and up the spino–reticulo–thalamic tract.

The spinothalamic tracts carry impulses which localize pain. Thalamic pathways to and from the cortex mediate emotional components.

Sympathetic activity increases pain – for example, increasing blood flow in a painful limb.

The gate theory of pain

Gate theory proposes that the entry of afferent impulses is monitored by the cells of the substantia gelatinosa (see above), which acts as a gate determining whether or not sufficient activity penetrates to fire secondary neurones in the dorsal horn. Each gate is dominated by descending influences from the brain that can override spinal cord regulatory mechanisms and alter how far the gate is open.

Endogenous opiates

The endorphin family of peptides have opioid activity and probably account for the very real effects of placebo, stress reducers and acupuncture analgesia. They are neurotransmitters acting at inhibitory synapses via δ, κ and μ receptors.

MANAGEMENT OF CHRONIC PAIN (see also p. 442)

Chronic pain is gravely disabling and distressing, and taxing to treat. Multidisciplinary pain-relief clinics are helpful in providing specific and supportive therapy. Pain control should, however, be part of all doctors' skills.

A *management plan* for intractable pain, when it is often difficult to find the precise cause, has seven components.

Diagnostic

Rigorous attention must be paid to the question of diagnosis, reviewing the history (first hand), the investigations, and radiology. A specific surgical approach may then become apparent (e.g. pain in undiagnosed spinal stenosis, trigeminal neuralgia, glossopharyngeal neuralgia, or discovery of syringomyelia in intractable upper limb pain).

Psychological

Chronic pain influences quality of life and lifestyle. Clinical depression (see p. 1122) is almost universally associated with chronic pain when the underlying pathology is benign, whereas a relative minority of patients suffering pain from secondary cancer are clinically depressed despite the gravity of their disease. Antidepressant drugs and modification of lifestyle are important in improving the quality of life when they are appropriate. Perseverance and compliance with therapy is an invariable issue.

Analgesics

Drugs should be prescribed working up the analgesic ladder (see p. 442). Inadequate pain control following optimal use of one drug group indicates the need to move one rung higher. The prescription should be regular with extra doses as required for breakthrough pain. Medication should be given orally when possible. The degree of pain relief should be reviewed regularly, and self-regulated medication encouraged.

Co-analgesics

Co-analgesics are drugs which have a primary use in conditions other than pain but are also effective, either alone or when added to conventional analgesics. Examples are non-steroidal anti-inflammatory drugs used in bone pain or tricyclic antidepressants and anticonvulsants used in de-afferentation pain (see p. 443). Calcium-channel blockers (nifedipine) improve sympathetically mediated pain, as occurs in, for example, Raynaud's disease. Muscle relaxants, antibiotics and steroids by injection each relieve pain when used in appropriate situations (e.g. severe spasticity, infection, and inflammatory arthropathy, respectively).

Stimulation

Acupuncture, ice, heat, ultrasound, massage, transcutaneous electrical nerve stimulation (TENS) and spinal cord stimulation all achieve analgesia by a gating effect on large myelinated nerve fibres.

Nerve blocks

Pain pathways can be blocked either temporarily by local anaesthetic or permanently with phenol, or with radio-frequency lesions. Examples are:

- somatic blocks
  - (a) peripheral nerve and plexus injections
  - (b) epidural and spinal analgesia
- sympathetic blocks
  - (a) sympathetic ganglia and nerve ending injections
  - (b) central epidural and spinal sympathetic blockade.

Neurosurgery

Highly specialized and sometimes controversial techniques have a place alongside pharmacological remedies. Examples are dorsal rhizotomy, sympathectomy, cordotomy and neurostimulation.

FURTHER READING

Portenoy RK, Kanner RM (eds) (1996) Pain Management: Therapy and Practice. Philadelphia: FA Davis.

Stein C (1995) The control of pain in peripheral tissue by opioids. *New England Journal of Medicine* **332**: 1685–1690.

Control of the bladder and sexual function

Changes in the pattern of micturition and the failure of normal sexual activity are important diagnostic symptoms in sacral, spinal cord and cortical disease.

ESSENTIAL ANATOMY AND FUNCTION

The three efferent LMN pathways to the bladder are shown in Table 18.19.

Afferent fibres (T12-S4) record changes in pressure within the bladder and tactile sensation in the genitalia.

Table 18.19
The three efferent pathways to the bladder and genitalia

Nerve supply	Function
Sympathetic T12–L2	Bladder wall relaxation Internal sphincter contraction Orgasm, ejaculation
Parasympathetic S2–4	Bladder wall contraction Internal sphincter relaxation Penis and clitoris erection/engorgement
Pudendal nerves (Somatic)	External sphincter (skeletal muscle)

When the bladder is distended, continence is maintained by reflex suppression of the parasympathetic outflow, and reciprocal activation of the sympathetic, both being subject to cortical (voluntary) control. Voiding takes place by parasympathetic activation of the detrusor muscle, and relaxation of the internal spincter.

Cortical awareness of bladder fullness is located in the post-central gyrus, parasagittally, while initiation of micturition is in the pre-central gyrus. Voluntary control of micturition is located in the frontal cortex, parasagittally.

Disorders of micturition: incontinence

Three neurological patterns of bladder dysfunction cause urinary incontinence. These may be hard to separate clinically.

Cortical.

- Frontal lesions cause socially inappropriate micturition.
- Pre-central lesions cause difficulty initiating micturition.
- Post-central lesions cause loss of sense of bladder fullness.

Spinal cord. Bilateral UMN lesions (pyramidal tracts) cause frequency of micturition and incontinence. The bladder is small and unusually sensitive to small changes in intravesical pressure (hypertonic bladder). Frontal lobe lesions also sometimes cause a hypertonic bladder.

Lower motor neurone. Sacral lesions (conus medullaris, sacral roots and pelvic nerve lesions, which need to be bilateral) cause a flaccid, atonic bladder, which overflows without warning.

Impotence

Failure of penile erection, engorgement of the clitoris or ejaculation are caused by bilateral upper or lower motor lesions.

The emotional aspects of impotence are discussed no further here, but are of great importance. Depression is a common cause. Endocrine aspects of impotence are discussed on p. 916.

FURTHER READING

Fitzgerald MJT (1996) Neuroanatomy, Basic and Clinical, 3rd edn. Philadelphia: WB Saunders.

Patten J (1996) Neurological Differential Diagnosis, 2nd edn. London: Springer Verlag.

Neurological investigations

The clinically based history and examination, with interpretation of patterns described above, remain reliable diagnostic tools in neurology, despite rapid major advances in noninvasive tests. However, computed tomography (CT), magnetic resonance imaging (MRI), and other techniques have revolutionized the speed and safety of investigations. Despite this ease of modern imaging, expense must be constantly appraised; economy, equity and appropriateness are as important in diagnostic investigations as they are in treatment.

Preliminary routine tests

Examples of results of routine investigations are shown in Table 18.20.

Specific blood tests

Clinical judgement determines more specific tests, used widely in general medicine. Examples are creatine phosphokinase and thyroid function tests in a myopathy, HIV serology where this infection seems likely, B_{12} studies in a polyneuropathy, or a drug screen in unexplained coma. These tests are usually mentioned elsewhere among the conditions described.

Table 18.20
Value of routine investigations in neurology

Test	Yield	Condition
Urinalysis	Glycosuria	Polyneuropathy
	Ketones	Coma
	Bence–Jones protein	Cord compression
Blood picture	↑ MCV	B_{12} deficiency
	↑ ESR	Giant cell arteritis
Blood glucose	Hypoglycaemia	Coma
	Hyperglycaemia	Coma
Serum electrolytes	Hyponatraemia	Coma
	Hypokalaemia	Weakness
Serum calcium	Hypocalcaemia	Tetany, spasms
Serum creatinine phosphokinase	↑	Muscle disease
Chest X-ray	Lytic bone or mass lesion	Bronchial cancer, thymoma

Neuroradiology

Skull and spinal X-rays

Examples of important features are:

- fractures of the skull vault or base
- skull and spinal lesions (e.g. metastases, osteomyelitis, Paget's disease, abnormal skull foramina, fibrous dysplasia)
- enlargement or destruction of the pituitary fossa – intrasellar tumour, raised intracranial pressure
- intracranial calcification – tuberculoma, oligodendroglioma, wall of an aneurysm, cysticercosis
- lateral shift of a calcified pineal – used prior to CT imaging to recognize midline shift.

Spinal films show fractures, congenital bone lesions (e.g. cysts), destructive lesions (infection, metastasis) or degeneration change – spondylosis.

Imaging of the brain and spinal cord

The availability of techniques varies widely both between and within different countries. Brain CT is now widely available worldwide. MRI of both brain and spinal cord is, however, rapidly becoming a standard test, superseding both brain CT, and traditional contrast and CT myelography. These latter tests are nevertheless mentioned below for completeness.

Computed tomography (CT) (see Figs 18.12 and 18.14)

A collimated X-ray beam moves synchronously with its detectors across a slice of brain between 2 mm and 13 mm thick. The transmitted X-irradiation from an element, or pixel, of that slice (< 1 mm^2) is processed by a computer. A numerical value (Hounsfield number) is assigned to its density (air = –1000 units; water = 0; bone = +1000 units).

The difference in X-ray attenuation between bone, brain and CSF makes it possible to distinguish between normal and infarcted tissue, tumour, extravasated blood, or oedema.

Images are enhanced with intravenous contrast media to show areas of increased blood supply and oedema more clearly.

Contrast imaging of the spinal cord (CT myelography) and the cerebral ventricles (ventriculography) is achieved by CT scanning after intrathecal injection of water-soluble contrast media (e.g. metrizamide) at lumbar puncture.

CT is safe apart from occasional systemic reactions to contrast; the irradiation involved is small.

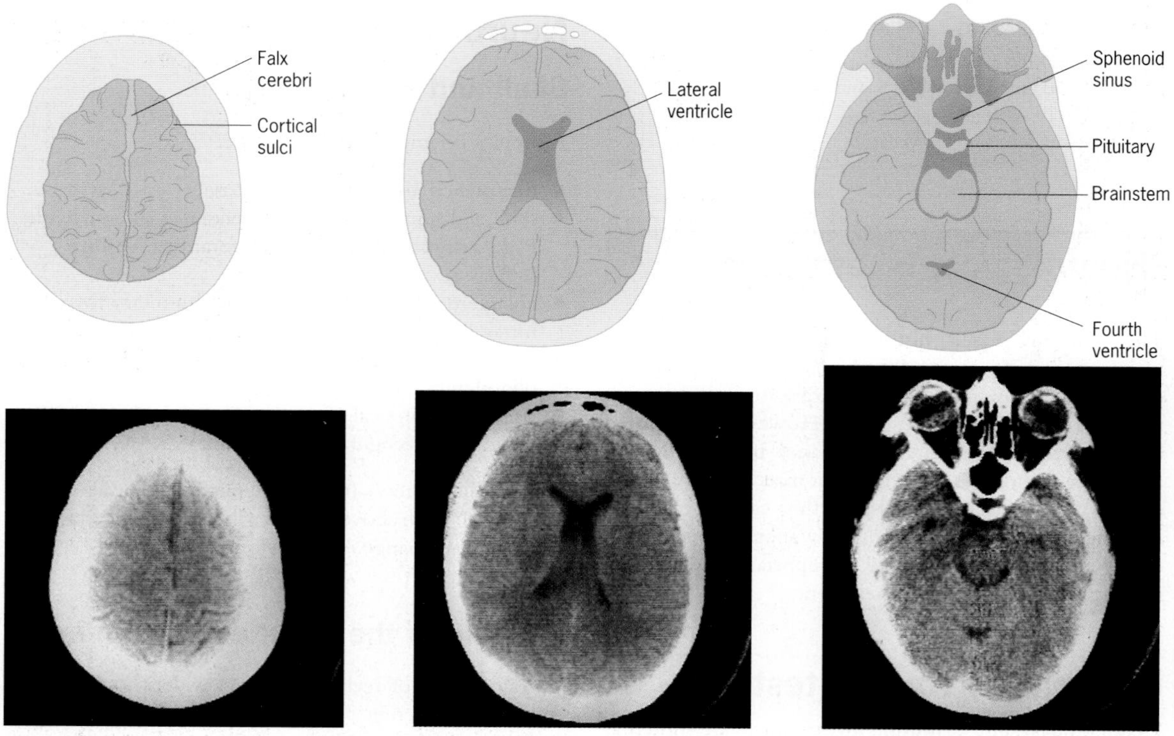

Fig 18.12
Normal CT head scan: transverse section at three different levels

Value of CT

CT scanning demonstrates:

- cerebral tumours
- intracerebral haemorrhage and infarction
- subdural and extradural haematoma
- free blood in the subarachnoid space (SAH, see p. 1053)
- lateral shift of midline structures and displacement/enlargement of the ventricular system
- cerebral atrophy
- pituitary mass lesions
- spinal lesions (with CT myelography).

CT imaging, within its limitations, shows that the brain is anatomically normal, which helps to reassure patients.

Limitations of CT

- Lesions under 1 cm diameter may be missed.
- Lesions with attenuation close to that of bone may be missed if near the skull.
- Lesions with attenuation similar to that of brain are poorly imaged. (e.g. MS plaques, isodense subdural haematoma).
- CT images sometimes miss lesions within the posterior fossa.
- The spinal cord is not imaged directly by CT (contrast is necessary).
- The results are poor when a patient cannot cooperate – a general anaesthetic is occasionally required.

Magnetic resonance imaging (MRI) (see Figs 18.13 and 18.14)

The hydrogen nucleus is a proton whose electrical charge creates a local electrical field. These protons are aligned by a sudden strong magnetic impulse. Protons are then imaged with radiofrequency waves at right angles to their alignment. The protons resonate and spin, then reverting to their normal alignment. As they do so, images are made at different phases of relaxation, known as T1, T2 and other sequences. These sequences are then recorded. From the timings of these sequences, referred to as different weightings, the recorded images are compared with each other. Gadolinium is used as an intravenous contrast medium.

Value of MRI

There are five principal advantages of MRI over CT:

- MRI images distinguish clearly between white matter and grey matter in the brain.
- Spinal cord and nerve roots are imaged directly.
- The resolution of MRI is greater than CT (lesions around 0.5 cm are seen).
- No radiation is involved.
- Magnetic resonance angiography (MRA) images blood vessels without the need for contrast.

Brain tumours, infarction and haemorrhage or haematoma, plaques of MS, the posterior fossa and foramen magnum

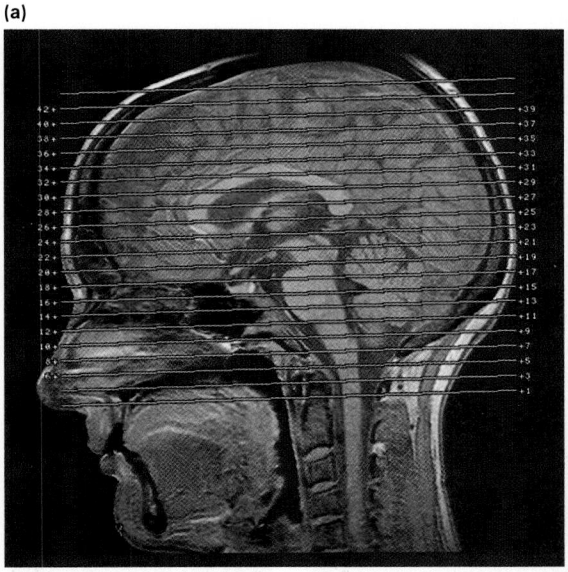

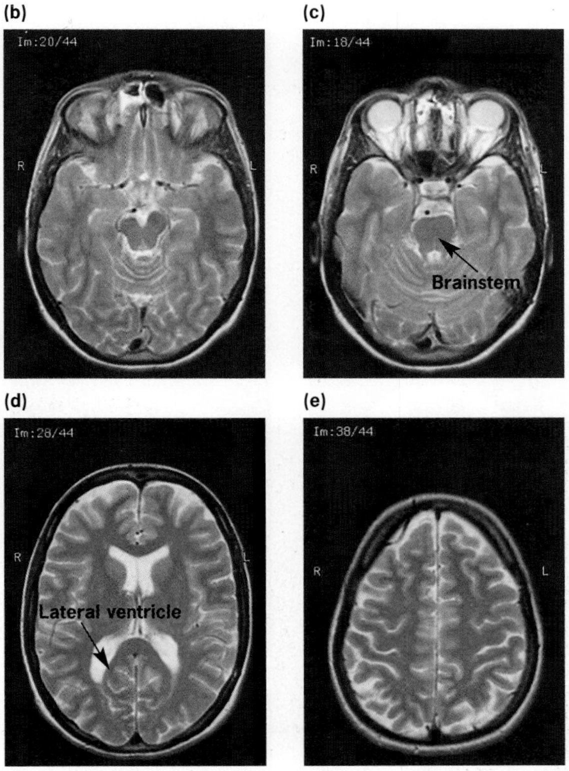

Fig 18.13
Normal brain magnetic resonance images sharing a T1-weighted sagittal section **(a)** of the brain and T2-weighted axial slices **(b–e)**

region are demonstrated well on MRI. In the spinal cord, MRI shows intrinsic and extrinsic tumours, syringomyelia, cord compression and vascular malformations. MRI is rapidly replacing contrast myelography.

Limitations of MRI

The limitations of MRI are principally time, and its costs. Imaging a single region takes about 30 minutes. As with CT, patients do need to cooperate: claustrophobia is an issue within the confined space of an MRI tube. A general anaesthetic may be necessary.

Cerebral and spinal angiography, digital X-ray imaging and myelography

In many centres where MRI is available, these techniques are now becoming obsolete, or greatly restricted in their application. Contrast is injected intra-arterially or intravenously to demonstrate the arterial and venous systems.

Carotid and vertebral arteriography images aneurysms, arteriovenous malformations and venous occlusion. Films of the aortic arch and the carotid and vertebral arteries demonstrate occlusion, stenoses and atheromatous plaques. Spinal angiography images arteriovenous malformations of the cord.

Conventional *percutaneous arteriography* is invasive and requires a general anaesthetic; it should rarely be performed outside a specialist centre. It carries a mortality of around 1% and a 1% risk of stroke.

Digital subtraction angiography (DSA), using a computerized subtraction is superseding traditional angiography. Contrast is injected intravenously or intra-arterially. No anaesthetic is usually necessary.

Myelography, a water-soluble radiopaque dye is injected into the lumbar (or rarely cervical) subarachnoid space and imaged by conventional X-rays or CT. This aids diagnosis of tumours of the spinal cord and other causes of cord compression. *Radiculography* is this examination confined to the lumbosacral region to image nerve roots.

Isotope bone scanning

The radioisotope [^{99m}Tc]-pertechnate is injected intravenously. This is of value in the detection of vertebral and skull lesions (e.g. metastases). Isotope brain scanning for intracranial lesions has been entirely superseded by CT and MRI.

Positron emission tomography (PET)

This research tool maps the function of specific areas of the brain by tracking the uptake and metabolism of radiolabelled compounds.

Electroencephalography (EEG)

The electroencephalogram (Fig 18.15) is recorded from scalp electrodes on 16 channels simultaneously for 10–30 minutes. The main value of the EEG is in diagnosing epilepsy and diffuse brain diseases. *Videotelemetry* combines continuous EEG and video

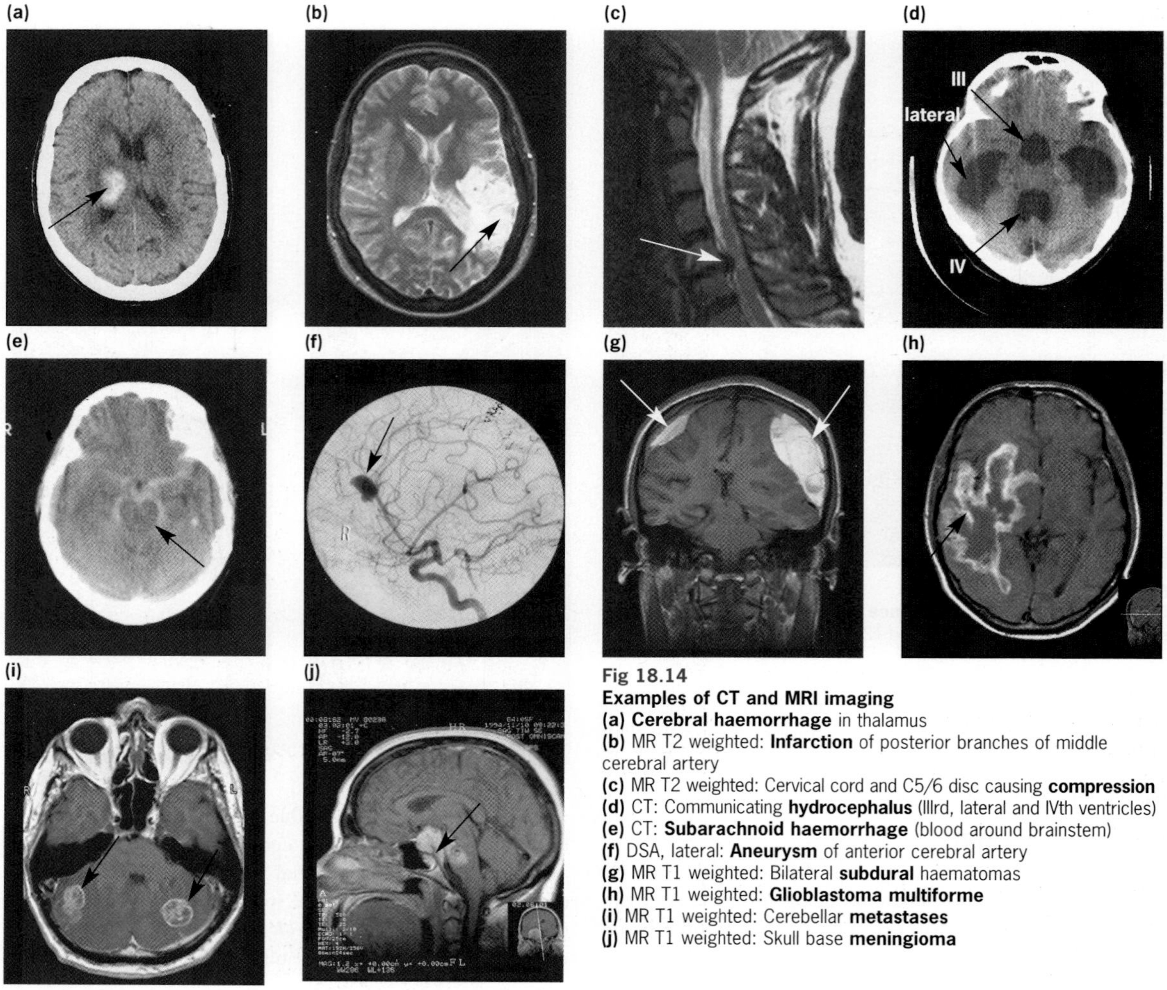

Fig 18.14
Examples of CT and MRI imaging
(a) Cerebral haemorrhage in thalamus
(b) MR T2 weighted: **Infarction** of posterior branches of middle cerebral artery
(c) MR T2 weighted: Cervical cord and C5/6 disc causing **compression**
(d) CT: Communicating **hydrocephalus** (IIIrd, lateral and IVth ventricles)
(e) CT: **Subarachnoid haemorrhage** (blood around brainstem)
(f) DSA, lateral: **Aneurysm** of anterior cerebral artery
(g) MR T1 weighted: Bilateral **subdural** haematomas
(h) MR T1 weighted: **Glioblastoma multiforme**
(i) MR T1 weighted: Cerebellar **metastases**
(j) MR T1 weighted: Skull base **meningioma**

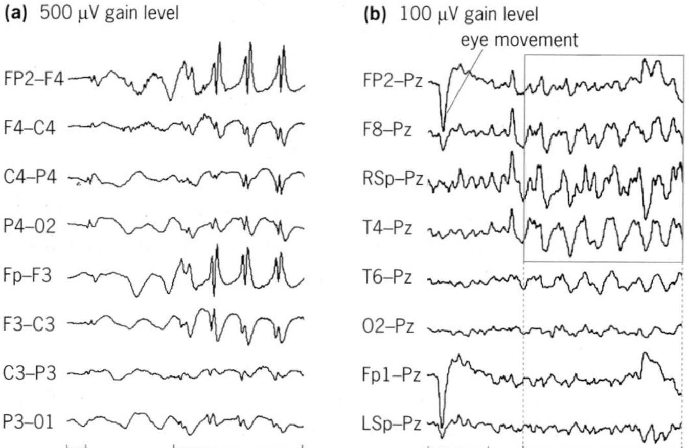

Fig 18.15
Examples of electroencephalogram recordings
(a) Normal activity followed by generalized epileptiform activity in all leads
(b) Normal activity followed by focal activity in the top four leads

recording, and is valuable in the specialist assessment of difficult cases of episodes of disturbed consciousness.

Epilepsy

Spikes, or spike-and-wave abnormalities, are the hallmarks of epilepsy, but it should be emphasized that patients with epilepsy often have a normal EEG between seizures (see p. 1057).

Diffuse brain disorders

Recognizable patterns of slow-wave EEG abnormalities appear in encephalitis, dementia (e.g. Creutzfeld–Jakob disease) and metabolic states (e.g. hypoglycaemia and hepatic coma).

Brain death

The EEG is isoelectric (i.e. flat). This EEG finding is no longer necessary to confirm brain death in the UK (see p. 738).

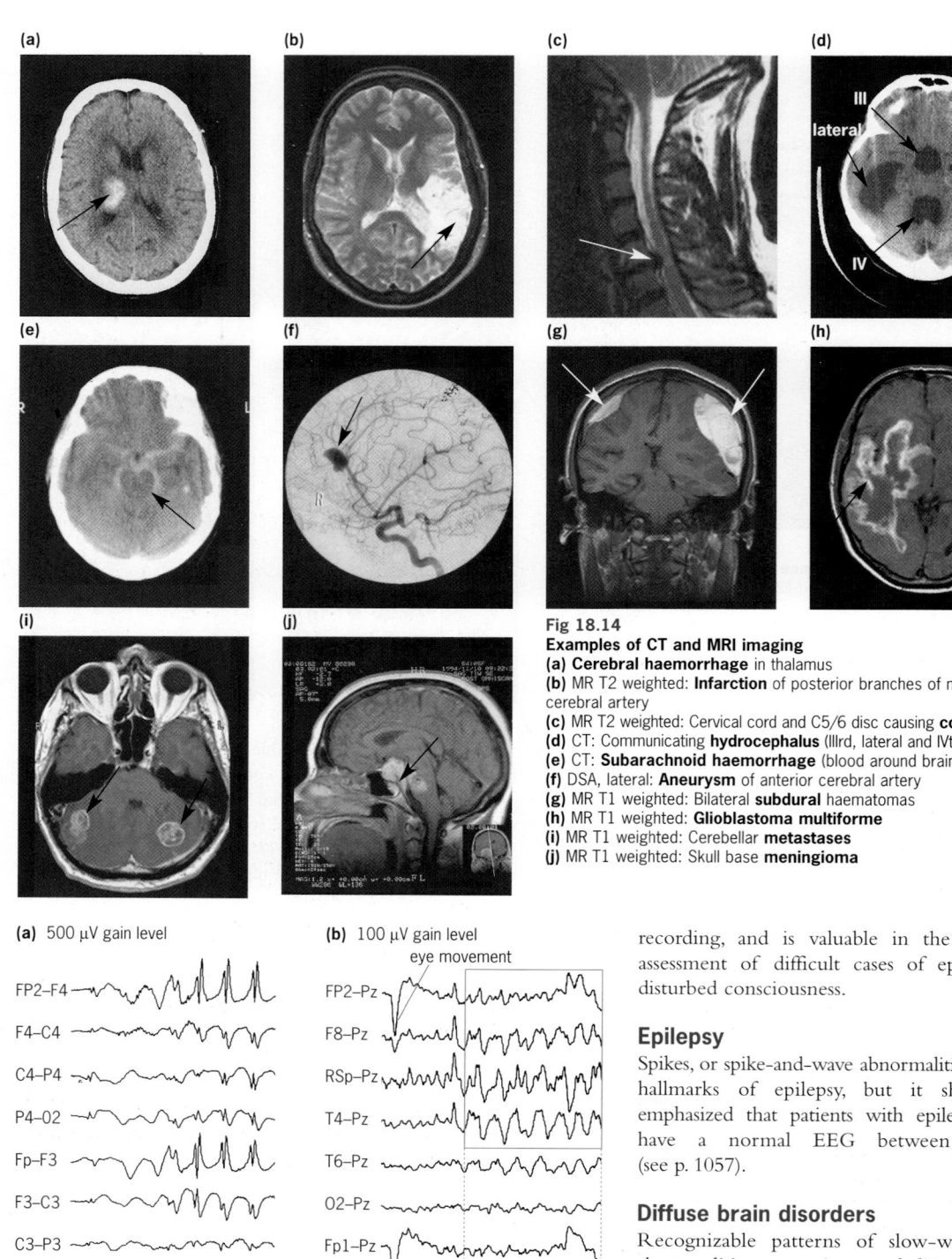

Electromyography and nerve conduction studies

Electromyography

A concentric needle electrode is inserted into voluntary muscle. The amplified recording is viewed on an oscilloscope and heard through a speaker. Three main features can be demonstrated:

- a normal interference pattern
- denervation and reinnervation
- myopathic, myotonic or myasthenic changes (p. 1100).

Peripheral nerve conduction

Four measurements are of principal value in the diagnosis of neuropathies and nerve entrapment:

- mean nerve (motor and sensory) conduction velocity (Fig 18.16)
- distal motor latency
- sensory action potentials
- muscle action potentials.

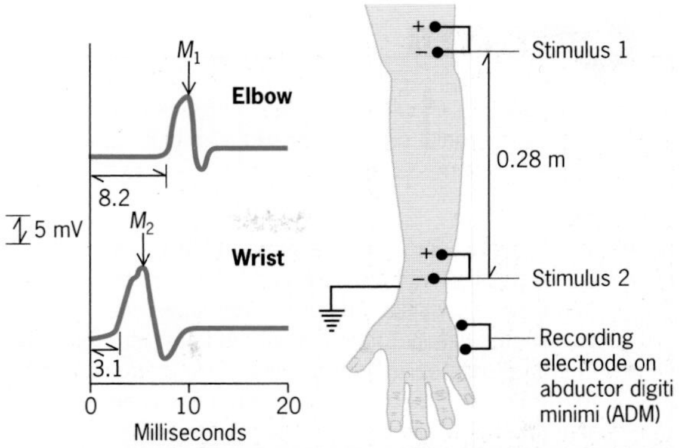

$$\text{Motor conduction velocity (elbow to wrist)} = \frac{0.28}{8.2 - 3.1} \times 1000 = 54.9\ \text{ms}^{-1}$$

Fig 18.16
Measurement of mean (motor) conduction velocity (MCV) in the ulnar nerve
A recording electrode on the abductor digiti minimi records the muscle action potential (*M*) from the ulnar nerve at the elbow (stimulus 1) and at the wrist (stimulus 2). From these values the motor conduction velocity can be calculated:

M_1=muscle action potential (MAP) from stimulus 1
M_2=MAP from stimulus 2
T_1=time from elbow to recording electrode
T_2=time from wrist to recording electrode, in ms (usually measured to onset of *M*)

$$\text{MCV} = \frac{\text{distance in metres}}{T_1 - T_2} \times 1000 = \text{metres per second}$$

Cerebral-evoked potentials

Visual-evoked potentials record the time for a visual stimulus to reach the occipital cortex. Their value is chiefly in documenting previous retrobulbar neuritis (see p. 1016), which leaves a permanent delay in latency despite recovery of vision.

Similar techniques are used for auditory and somatosensory potentials (from the ear or a limb). These are also used during neurosurgery to monitor brain and spinal cord function.

Table 18.21
The normal CSF

Appearance	Crystal clear, colourless
Pressure	60–150 mm of H_2O with patient recumbent
Cell count	5/mm^3 No polymorphs Mononuclear cells only
Protein	0.2–0.4 g L^{-1}
Glucose	⅔ to ½ of blood glucose
IgG	<15% of total CSF protein
Oligoclonal bands	Absent

Examination of the cerebrospinal fluid (CSF) (Table 18.21 and Practical box 18.3)

The indications for lumbar puncture are:

- diagnosis of meningitis and encephalitis
- intrathecal injection of contrast media and drugs
- diagnosis of suspected subarachnoid haemorrhage (sometimes)
- measurement of CSF pressure, e.g. idiopathic intracranial hypertension, p. 1080
- removal of CSF therapeutically, e.g. idiopathic intracranial hypertension
- diagnosis of miscellaneous conditions, e.g. MS, neurosyphilis, sarcoidosis, Behçet's, neoplastic involvement, certain polyneuropathies.

Meticulous attention should focus on microbiological studies in suspected central nervous system infection. Close liaison between clinician and microbiologist is essential. Specific techniques (e.g. polymerase chain reaction to identify meningococci or other bacteria) are sometimes invaluable. Repeated diagnostic CSF examination is often necessary in chronic infections, such as tuberculosis.

Biopsy

Interpretation of brain, muscle and nerve histology requires a specialist neuropathology service.

Brain

Brain biopsy (e.g. of a non-dominant frontal lobe) is undertaken to diagnose inflammatory and degenerative brain diseases. CT-guided stereotactic biopsy of intracranial mass lesions is now a standard procedure. It is

Practical

Lumbar puncture should *not* be performed in the presence of raised intracranial pressure or when an intracranial mass lesion is a possibility.

Technique

- The patient is placed on the edge of the bed in the left lateral position with the knees and chin as close together as possible. The procedure should be explained carefully to the patient, and consent obtained.
- The third and fourth lumbar spines are marked. The fourth lumbar spine usually lies on a line joining the iliac crests.
- Using sterile precautions, 2% lignocaine is injected into the dermis by raising a bleb in either the third or fourth lumbar interspace.
- The special lumbar puncture needle is pushed through the skin in the midline. It is pressed steadily forwards and slightly towards the head, with the head and spine bolstered horizontally with pillows.
- When the needle is felt to penetrate the dura mater, the stylet is withdrawn and a few drops of CSF are allowed to escape.
- The CSF pressure can now be measured by connecting a manometer to the needle. The patient's head must be on the same level as the sacrum. Normal CSF pressure is 60–150 mm H_2O. It rises and falls with respiration and the heart beat, and rises on coughing.
- Specimens of CSF are collected in three sterilized test-tubes and sent to the laboratory. An additional sample in which the sugar level can be measured, together with a simultaneous blood sample for blood sugar measurement, should be taken when relevant (e.g. in meningitis).
- Record the naked-eye appearance of the CSF: clear, cloudy, yellow (xanthochromic), red.
- Patients are usually asked to lie flat after the procedure to avoid a subsequent headache, but this manouevre is probably of little value.
- Analgesics may be required for post-LP headaches.

Contraindications for lumbar puncture

- Suspicion of a mass lesion in the brain or spinal cord. Caudal herniation of the cerebellar tonsils ('coning') may occur if an intracranial mass is present and the pressure below is reduced by removal of CSF. In suspected meningococcal infection, it is usual to avoid LP because of the risk of 'coning' (see p. 1079).
- Any cause of raised intracranial pressure.
- Local infection near the site of puncture.
- Congenital lesions in the lumbosacral region (e.g. meningomyelocele).
- Platelet count below 40×10^9/L and other clotting abnormalities, including anticoagulant drugs.
- Unconscious patients and those with papilloedema must have a CT scan before lumbar puncture.

Notes

- These contraindications are relative. There are circumstances when lumbar puncture is carried out in spite of them.
- The composition of the normal CSF is shown in Table 18.21.

Practical box 18.3 Lumbar puncture

less traumatic and more accurate than traditional biopsy through a skull burr-hole or craniotomy. MRI-guided biopsy and peroperative imaging are developing.

Muscle

Biopsy, with light microscopy, electron microscopy and biochemical analysis where appropriate elucidates diagnosis of inflammatory, metabolic and dystrophic disorders of muscle (see p. 1100).

Peripheral nerve

Biopsy, usually of one sural nerve, at the ankle, aids diagnosis in certain polyneuropathies (e.g. due to vasculitides).

Psychometric assessment

Psychometric testing is valuable for measuring cognitive function. Preservation of *verbal IQ* (a measure of past attainments) in the presence of deterioration of *performance IQ* (a measure of present abilities) is an important indicator of physical impairment of cognitive function, for example following brain injury or in dementia. Low subtest scores (e.g. for block design, various aspects of memory, visual, speech and constructional skills) indicate impaired function of specific regions of the brain.

The main limitation of these techniques is that depression and lack of attention reduces scores. Also, opinions sometimes vary greatly between clinical psychologists about interpretation of agreed numerical values of tests, particularly after brain injury – a matter which limits the clinical value of the tests themselves.

Specialized tests in specific diseases

Certain tests are employed in the diagnosis of individual (and often rare) neurological diseases. Examples are:

- anti-phospholipid antibody and detailed clotting studies in stroke (p. 490)
- antibody to acetylcholine receptor protein in myasthenia gravis (p. 1102)
- serum copper and caeruloplasmin in Wilson's disease (p. 326)

- blood lactate studies (failure to rise on exercise) in McArdle's syndrome
- serum phytanic acid (elevated) in Refsum's disease
- serum long-chain fatty acid (present) in adrenoleucodystrophy
- genetic studies in, for example, Huntington's disease, and hereditary sensorimotor neuropathies (p. 1096).

Unconsciousness and coma

The central reticular formation, which extends from the lower brainstem to the thalamus, influences the state of arousal. Our state of consciousness is the product of complex interactions between parts of the reticular formation itself, cortex and brainstem, and all sensory stimuli reaching them.

Disturbed consciousness: definitions

Each of these terms simply describes a state which is recognizable, either as normal or pathological.

- **Consciousness** means a state of wakefulness in which there is awareness of self and surroundings.
- **Clouding of consciousness** means reduced wakefulness and/or self-awareness, sometimes with confusion; the term is used more in psychiatry than clinical neurology.
- **Confusion** is the state of altered consciousness in which the subject is bewildered and misinterprets their surroundings.
- **Sleep** is a state of normal mental and physical inactivity from which the subject can be roused.
- **Stupor** is an abnormal, sleepy state from which the subject can be aroused by stimuli, applied vigorously or repeatedly. The term is also used to describe various psychiatric states, e.g. catatonic and depressive stupor (see p. 1118).
- **Delirium** is a state of high arousal (seen typically in *delirium tremens*, see p. 1139) in which there is confusion and often visual hallucination.
- **Coma** is a state of unrousable unresponsiveness. The Glasgow Coma Scale for grading coma, particularly in head injury, is shown in Table 18.22

Table 18.22
Glasgow Coma Scale

	Score
Eye opening (*E*)	
Spontaneous	4
To speech	3
To pain	2
No response	1
Motor response (*M*)	
Obeys	6
Localizes	5
Withdraws	4
Flexion	3
Extension	2
No response	1
Verbal response (*V*)	
Orientated	5
Confused conversation	4
Inappropriate words	3
Incomprehensible sounds	2
No response	1

Glasgow Coma Scale = $E + M + V$
(GCS minimum = 3; maximum = 15)

Mechanisms of coma

Altered consciousness is produced by three mechanisms affecting brainstem, reticular formation and cerebral cortex.

- *Diffuse brain dysfunction.* Generalized severe metabolic or toxic disorders (e.g. sedative drugs, uraemia and septicaemia) depress/inhibit overall brain function.
- *Direct effect within the brainstem.* A lesion within the brainstem itself damages/inhibits the reticular activating system.
- *Pressure effect on the brainstem.* A mass lesion within the cerebral hemisphere or cerebellum compresses the brain-stem, inhibiting the ascending reticular activating system.

A single focal hemisphere (or cerebellar) lesion does not produce coma unless it compresses or damages the brainstem. Oedema frequently surrounds a mass lesion, contributing to its effects.

Persistent vegetative state and locked-in syndrome

Other unresponsive states must be distinguished from coma.

- *The persistent vegetative state*, a sequel of, for example, widespread cortical damage after head injury, implies loss of sentient behaviour. The patient perceives little or nothing but lies apparantly awake, breathing spontaneously.
- *The locked-in syndrome* is a state of unresponsiveness due to massive brainstem infarction. The patient has a functioning cerebral cortex, and is thus aware, but cannot move or communicate except by vertical eye movement.
- *Brainstem death* is discussed on p. 858)

Distinction between these states is essential before major issues regarding prognosis, quality of life, and cessation of supportive care can be addressed. The principal features are shown in Table 18.23. Unresponsiveness of psychological origin is also a cause of apparent coma.

Table 18.23 Differentiation of persistent vegetative state from other forms of unresponsiveness (Modified from *Journal of the Royal College of Physicians of London* **30**: 119–121 (1996))

Condition	Vegetative state	Locked-in syndrome	Coma	Brainstem death
Self-awareness	Absent	Present	Absent	Absent
Cyclical eye opening	Present	Present	Absent	Absent
Glasgow Coma Scale	E4, M1–4, V1	E4, M1, V1	E1–2, M1–4, V1–2	E1, M1–2, V1
Motor function	No purposeful movement	Eye movement preserved in the vertical plane and able to blink volitionally	No purposeful movement	None or only reflex spinal movement
Perception of pain	No	Yes	No	No
Respiratory function	Normal	Normal	Depressed or varied	Absent
EEG activity	Polymorphic delta or theta; sometimes slow alpha waves	Normal or minimally abnormal	Polymorphic delta or theta waves; though sometimes silent	Electrocerebral silence or theta waves
Cerebral metabolism	Reduced by 50% or more	Minimally or moderately reduced	Reduced by 50% or more	Absent or greatly reduced
Prognosis	Depends on cause and length	Depends on cause though recovery unlikely	Recovery, vegetative state, or death within 2–4 weeks	No recovery

CAUSES

The principal causes of coma and stupor are shown in Table 18.24. A common cause of coma in UK is self-poisoning. Worldwide, in malarial zones, or in travellers from them, cerebral malaria is a frequent cause.

The unconscious patient

IMMEDIATE ASSESSMENT

Actions which take seconds are essential (Table 18.25).

A history should then be gleaned from relatives, friends, paramedics or the police. Many people with diabetes mellitus, epilepsy or hypoadrenalism, or who take corticosteroids, carry identifying discs or cards.

FURTHER EXAMINATION

- The depth of coma should be assessed and recorded (see Table 18.22).
- A full general and neurological physical examination should then be carried out.

General examination

Many clues may be found.

Temperature

Temperature is raised in infection and hyperpyrexia; it is low in hypothermia. Measure it!

Skin appearance

There may be cyanosis, jaundice, purpura, rashes, pigmentation, injection marks, or trauma.

Skin texture and hydration

The skin is coarse and dry in hypothyroidism.

Table 18.24
Examples of mechanisms of principal causes of coma

Diffuse brain dysfunction
Drug overdose, alcohol
CO poisoning, anaesthetic gases
Hypoglycaemia, hyperglycaemia
Hypoxic/ischaemic brain injury
Hypertensive encephalopathy (p. 732)
Severe uraemia (p. 570)
Hepatocellular failure (p. 322)
Respiratory failure with CO_2 retention (p. 849)
Hypercalcaemia, hypocalcaemia
Hypoadrenalism, hypopituitarism and hypothyroidism (Ch. 16)
Hyponatraemia, hypernatraemia
Metabolic acidosis
Hypothermia, hyperpyrexia
Trauma (following closed head injury)
Epilepsy (following a generalized seizure)
Encephalitis, cerebral malaria, septicaemia
Subarachnoid haemorrhage
Metabolic rarities (e.g. porphyria)
Cerebral oedema from chronic hypoxia (p. 852)

Direct effect within brainstem
Brainstem haemorrhage or infarction
Brainstem neoplasm (e.g. glioma)
Brainstem demyelination
Wernicke–Korsakoff syndrome
Trauma

Pressure effect on brain stem
Hemisphere tumour, infarction, abscess, haematoma, encephalitis or trauma
Cerebellar mass lesions

Table 18.25
The unconscious patient: immediate actions

Examine	Potential action
Airway: clear?	Maintain; intubate?
Pulse: absent?	Cardiopulmonary resuscitation
Pupils: fixed, dilated?	
Head trauma	Observe and investigate
Spinal trauma	Immobilize

Breath
There may be traces of alcohol, ketones (diabetic ketoacidosis), hepatic and uraemic fetor.

Respiration
Depressed but regular respiration occurs in many states of stupor and light coma. As any coma deepens, or in normal deep sleep, there are pauses in regular respiration. The pattern of abnormal respiration is helpful diagnostically:

- *Cheyne–Stokes respiration* (periodic respiration) is alternating hyperpnoea and apnoea. In primary neurological disease this points to bilateral cerebral dysfunction, usually deep in the hemispheres or in the upper brainstem, and is a sign of incipient coning. This respiratory pattern also occurs in metabolic comas, if there is CO_2 retention from pulmonary disease, with chronic hypoxia at high altitude above 3500 m and in normal people during sleep.
- *Kussmaul (acidotic) respiration* is deep, sighing hyperventilation seen principally in diabetic ketoacidosis and uraemia.
- *Central neurogenic (pontine) hyperventilation* describes sustained, rapid, deep breathing seen with pontine lesions. It may be episodic.
- *Ataxic respiration* is the shallow, halting, irregular respiration that occurs when the medullary respiratory centre is damaged. It frequently precedes death.
- *Vomiting, hiccup and excessive yawning* often indicate a lower brainstem lesion in a stuporose patient.

Neurological examination
The following should be noted in coma.

Head, neck and spine
Note trauma, skull burr-holes, cranial bruits, neck stiffness.

Pupils
Record size and reaction to light. The following patterns are seen:

- *Dilatation of one pupil*, which becomes fixed to light, indicates herniation of the uncus of the temporal lobe (coning) which compresses the third nerve. This is a neurosurgical emergency.
- *Horner's syndrome* (ipsilateral pupillary constriction and ptosis, see p. 1017) occurs with lesions of the hypothalamus and also, rarely, in coning.
- *Bilateral mid-point reactive pupils* (i.e. normal pupils) are characteristic in metabolic comas and following most CNS-depressant drugs except opiates.
- *Bilateral light-fixed, dilated pupils* are a cardinal sign of brainstem death. They also occur in deep coma of any cause, but particularly in coma due to barbiturate intoxication or hypothermia.
- *Bilateral pin-point, light-fixed pupils* occur with pontine lesions (e.g. a pontine haemorrhage) that interrupt the sympathetic pathways, or with opiates.
- *Bilateral mid-position light-fixed or slightly dilated light-fixed pupils* (4–6 mm), which are sometimes irregular, are seen when brainstem damage interrupts the light reflex.

Mydriatic drugs administered in coma can confuse diagnosis. Other pupillary changes due to drugs are mentioned on p. 874. Previous pupillary surgery can also sometimes cause diagnostic difficulty.

Fundi
Papilloedema or retinal haemorrhage should be noted.

Ocular movements
In most coma cases the eyes are slightly divergent. Slow, roving, side-to-side eye movements, usually horizontal, are seen in light coma.

Vestibulo-ocular reflexes. Passive head turning produces conjugate ocular deviation away from the direction of induced head rotation (doll's head reflex). This reflex is lost in very deep coma and is absent in brainstem lesions, and thus in brainstem death. Its practical value in coma is somewhat limited.

Calorics. Slow tonic deviation of the eyes towards the irrigated ear is seen when ice-cold water is run into the external auditory meatus; this is known as the caloric or vestibulo-ocular reflex and indicates an intact brainstem. In coma, this test is used mainly in the diagnosis of brainstem death (see p. 858).

Abnormalities of conjugate gaze (see also p. 1018).

- *Sustained conjugate lateral deviation* occurs towards the side of a destructive frontal lesion (the eyes look towards the normal limbs). Rarely, an irritative lesion in one frontal region (e.g. an epileptic focus from a glioma) drives the eyes away from the affected side, so conjugate deviation is away from the side of the lesion. In a pontine, brainstem lesion, when one paramedian pontine reticular formulation (PPRF) itself is damaged (see p. 1018), sustained conjugate lateral deviation occurs away from the side of the lesion, towards the paralysed limbs, because the opposite PPRF is active.
- *Skew deviation* (one eye is deviated upwards and the other down) is rare. It indicates a brainstem or cerebellar lesion.
- *Ocular bobbing* describes sudden, brisk, downward-diving eye movements seen in pontine (or cerebellar) haemorrhage. Other spontaneous eye movements (other than roving eye movements) are distinctly unusual in coma of any cause.

Lateralizing signs. Impairment of consciousness makes it difficult to recognize focal neurological signs. The following should be looked for, all of which indicate the side of a lesion:

- *Response to visual threat* in a stuporose patient. Asymmetry suggests hemianopia.
- *The facial appearance.* Drooping of the weaker side, unilateral dribbling, or blowing in and out of the paralysed cheek is seen.
- *Tone.* Flaccidity or spasticity of the limbs on one side may be the only sign of hemiparesis.
- *Asymmetrical response to painful stimuli.*
- *Asymmetry of plantar responses.* Both are, however, frequently extensor in deep coma of any cause.
- *Asymmetry of tendon reflexes.*
- *Asymmetry of decerebrate and decorticate posturing.*

INVESTIGATIONS

In many instances the explanation for coma is evident from the history and examination (e.g. head injury, cerebral haemorrhage, self-poisoning), and appropriate management follows. If the cause remains unclear, further investigations are required.

Blood and urine

- *Drugs screen* (e.g. salicylates, diazepam, narcotics, amphetamines)
- *Routine biochemistry* (urea, electrolytes, glucose, calcium, liver biochemistry)
- *Metabolic and endocrine studies* (TSH, serum cortisol)
- *Blood cultures*
- *Rarities*, such as cerebral malaria (thick blood film) or porphyria, are often forgotten.

Imaging

CT or MR brain imaging may indicate an otherwise unsuspected mass lesion or intracranial haemorrhage.

CSF examination

Lumbar puncture should be performed in coma only after careful assessment of the possible diagnosis. It is usually contraindicated if an intracranial mass lesion is a possibility. CT is necessary to exclude this. CSF examination is likely to alter therapy only if undiagnosed meningoencephalitis or other identifiable infection is present.

Electrophysiological tests

The EEG is of particular value in the diagnosis of metabolic coma, and encephalitis.

MANAGEMENT

The comatose or stuporose patient – be they in ITU, on a general ward, on a trolley in an A&E department, at home or at the roadside – needs immediate careful nursing, meticulous attention to the airway, and frequent observation to detect changes in vital function.

Longer-term requirements are:

- skin care – turning, removal of rings, avoidance of pressure sores and pressure palsies
- oral hygiene – mouth washes, suction
- eye care – taping of lids, prevention of corneal damage, irrigation
- fluids – intragastric or i.v. fluids
- calories – liquid diet through a fine intragastric tube, 1255 kJ (3000 kcal) daily
- sphincters – catheterization only when essential (Paul's tubing if possible); avoid constipation (evacuate rectum).

FURTHER READING

Posner MJ (1994) Attention: the mechanisms of consciousness. *Proceedings of the National Academy of Sciences USA* **91**: 7398–7403.

The permanent vegetative state (1996) Review *Journal of the Royal College of Physicians* **30:** 119–121.

Cerebrovascular disease and stroke

Stroke is the third most common cause of death in developed countries. The age-adjusted annual death rate from strokes is 116 per 100 000 population in the USA and some 200 per 100 000 in the UK; it is higher in Afro-Caribbean populations than Caucasian. Stroke is uncommon below the age of 40 years and is more common in males. The death rate following a stroke is around 25%.

The incidence of stroke is decreasing in the age range 40–60 years as hypertension is recognized and treated. However, particularly in the elderly population, stroke remains a major cause of morbidity and mortality.

Cerebrovascular disease may comprise:

- thromboembolic infarction
- cerebral and cerebellar haemorrhage
- dissection of carotid and vertebral vessels
- subarachnoid haemorrhage
- subdural and extradural haemorrhage and haematoma
- cortical venous and dural venous sinus thrombosis.

Definitions

- **Stroke**. To the general public, stroke means a weakness, either permanent or transient, of the limbs on one side, often with loss or disturbance of speech. It is defined as a focal neurological deficit due to a vascular lesion. This is usually of rapid onset and, by definition, lasts longer than 24 hours if the patient survives. Hemiplegia due to middle cerebral arterial thromboembolism is a common example.
- **Completed stroke** implies that the neurological deficit has reached its maximum, usually within six hours of onset.
- **Stroke in evolution** describes evolving and deteriorating symptoms and signs, usually during

24 hours from the onset.

- **Minor stroke**. Patients recover without a significant deficit, usually within one week.
- **Transient ischaemic attack** (TIA). This describes a focal deficit, such as a weak limb, aphasia or loss of vision, lasting from a few seconds to 24 hours. There is complete clinical recovery. The attack is usually of sudden onset. TIAs have a tendency to recur, and to herald thromboembolic stroke.

These definitions, although valuable clinically, are somewhat arbitrary. The term 'cerebrovascular accident' should be avoided.

Pathophysiology

Different pathological processes may cause similar clinical events in cerebrovascular disease.

Completed stroke

This is usually caused by one of four principal mechanisms:

- arterial embolism from a distant site and subsequent brain infarction
- atheromatous carotid or vertebral artery occlusion and subsequent brain infarction
- atheromatous arterial thrombosis within a cerebral vessel and subsequent brain infarction
- haemorrhage into the brain.

Less commonly, other processes cause the clinical picture of stroke:

- venous infarction
- dissection of the carotid or vertebral arteries and subsequent cerebral infarction
- air embolism
- multiple sclerosis – a plaque of demyelination
- mass effects of expanding lesions (e.g. brain tumour, abscess, subdural haematoma).

Transient ischaemic attack (TIA)

TIAs are usually caused by the passage of microemboli into the brain, but again other, different mechanisms may produce similar clinical events. For example, TIAs may also be caused by a fall in cerebral perfusion (e.g. due to a cardiac dysrhythmia, postural hypotension or decreased flow through atheromatous carotid and vertebral arteries), but stroke is usually averted by autoregulation. Small areas of brain infarction following thrombosis or even haemorrhage may occasionally cause a clinical TIA. Rarely, brain tumours and subdural haematomas present with episodes indistinguishable from thromboembolic TIAs.

The principal sources of emboli are thrombi and atheromatous plaques within the great vessels, the carotid and vertebral systems, or in the heart. Cardiac thrombi (mural and valvular) follow atrial fibrillation, itself often secondary to valvular disease, or myocardial infarction.

Thromboembolism from vascular disease outside the brain is the cause of 70% of all strokes and 80% of TIAs

Risk factors and primary prevention

The principal accepted risk factors in thromboembolic stroke including TIAs are shown in Table 18.26. There are extreme difficulties of data collection and methodology in apportioning underlying stroke risk factors, and measuring the effects of altering them. The table indicates the probable effects of various interventions.

With regard to primary prevention, the following especially have been shown to reduce stroke incidence:

- treatment of hypertension (the single most important measure)
- cessation of smoking
- an active lifestyle
- moderate consumption of alcohol.
- reduction of LDL-cholesterol with statin therapy (p. 995)

Treatment of diabetes, avoiding obesity, dietary modification (see p. 967) and low-dose aspirin therapy in symptomless populations have all been advocated to reduce stroke risk, but there are still insufficient data. Postmenopausal HRT has so far shown no benefit.

Cerebral and cerebellar haemorrhage

The risk factors for this are hypertension, anticoagulant drugs, bleeding disorders, cerebral aneurysm and, rarely, amyloidosis.

Table 18.26
Risk factors and predisposing causes in cerebrovascular disease

Intervention/risk factor	Effect/findings
Hypertension: treatment	Reduction in stroke risk
Cessation of smoking	Reduction in stroke risk
Alcohol	Decreased stroke risk with moderate consumption
Active lifestyle	Reduction in stroke risk
Treatment of diabetes	Insufficient data
Avoiding obesity	Insufficient data
Diet and dietary modification	Insufficient data
Prophylactic low-dose aspirin	Insufficient data
Post-menopausal HRT	No apparent association
Treatment of high cholesterol	Reduction in stroke risk
High-dose OCPs	Increased stroke risk
Racial origin	Stroke is more common in Afro-Caribbeans in UK
Country of origin	Stroke incidence ratio Portugal:US = 2:1
Family history	Positive weighting of risk
Rarities (e.g. polycythaemia, antiphospholipid syndrome)	Reduction in stroke risk on treatment

OCP, Oral contraceptive pill

Vascular anatomy (Figs 18.17–18.19)

A knowledge of normal arterial anatomy and the likely sites of atheromatous plaques and stenotic lesions helps in an understanding of the main clinical syndromes.

The circle of Willis is supplied by the two internal carotid arteries and by the basilar artery, which is formed by the union of the two vertebral arteries. The distribution of the anterior, middle and posterior cerebral arteries, which supply the cerebrum, is shown in Fig 18.18.

Atheromatous plaques and stenoses in main vessels proximal to the circle of Willis are common at five sites (see Fig 18.19):

- origins of the common carotid arteries
- origins of the internal carotid arteries
- carotid artery syphon – within the cavernous sinus
- subclavian vessels
- origins of vertebral arteries.

Autoregulation

The smooth muscle of small intracerebral arteries responds directly to changes in the pressure gradient across the vessel wall. In the normal situation, constant cerebral blood flow (CBF) is maintained by systolic blood pressures between 80 and 170 mmHg (i.e. CBF is independent of perfusion pressure).

In disease states, CBF autoregulation may fail. The contributory causes are:

- severe hypotension with systolic blood pressure < 75 mmHg
- severe hypertension with systolic blood pressure > 180 mmHg
- increase in blood viscosity – polycythaemia, hyperviscosity
- raised intracranial pressure
- increase in arterial $P\text{CO}_2$ and/or fall in arterial $P\text{O}_2$.

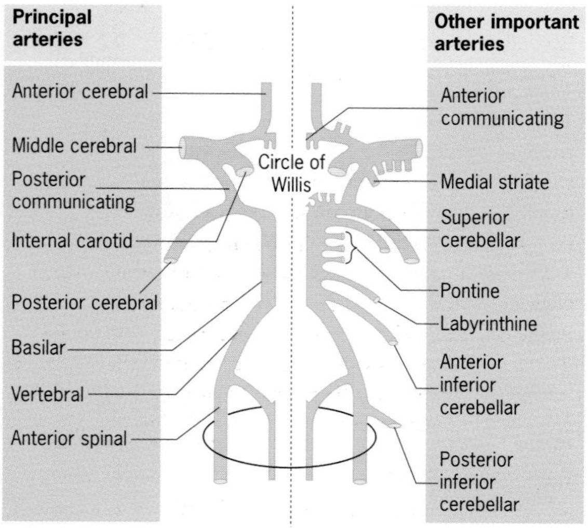

Fig 18.17
Arteries supplying the brain

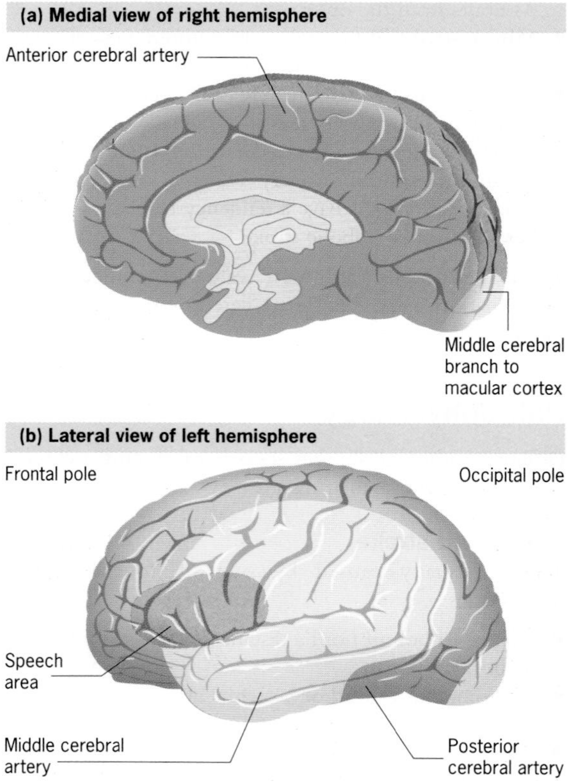

Fig 18.18
Distribution of the three major cerebral arteries

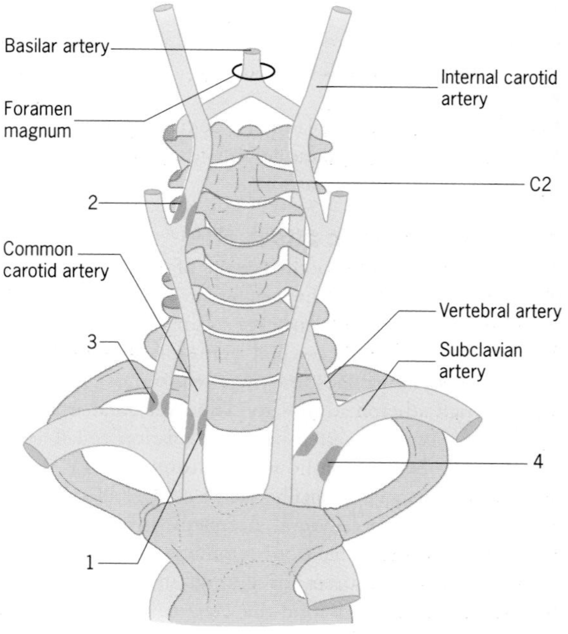

Fig 18.19
Principal sites of atheromatous stenoses in extracerebral arteries. (1. common carotid artery; 2. internal carotid artery; 3. vertebral artery; 4. subclavian artery.)

Transient ischaemic attacks

SYMPTOMS

TIAs cause sudden loss of function in one region of the brain. Symptoms usually reach their peak in seconds and last for minutes or hours (but by definition < 24 hours). The site of the lesion is often suggested by the clinical pattern of the attack.

CLINICAL FEATURES

The clinical features of the principal forms of TIA are given in Table 18.27. Hemiparesis and aphasia are the most com-mon, but two other events will be mentioned briefly here.

Amaurosis fugax

This is a sudden transient loss of vision in one eye. When due to the passage of emboli through the retinal arteries, arterial obstruction is sometimes visible through an ophthal-moscope during an attack. A TIA causing an episode of amaurosis fugax is often the first clinical evidence of internal carotid artery stenosis, which may herald a hemiparesis. Amaurosis fugax also occurs as a benign event in migraine.

Transient global amnesia

Episodes of amnesia with confusion lasting for several hours, occurring principally in people over 65, and in which there is complete recovery, are possibly caused by ischaemia in the posterior cerebral circulation. The exact cause of this striking but unusual event is unknown.

SIGNS

The diagnosis of a TIA is often based solely upon the description of the event. During an attack the loss of function can be seen. Consciousness is usually preserved.

There may be clinical evidence of a source of embolus, such as:

- carotid arterial bruit (stenosis)
- atrial fibrillation or other dysrhythmia
- valvular heart disease or endocarditis
- recent myocardial infarction
- difference in blood pressure between right and left brachial artery (subclavian stenosis).

There may also be evidence of an underlying disease process, e.g.:

- atheroma
- hypertension
- postural hypotension
- bradycardia or low cardiac output
- diabetes mellitus
- rarely, arteritis, polycythaemia
- anti-phospholipid syndrome – recurrrent miscarriage, thrombosis, thrombocytopenia (see p. 490).

Table 18.27
Features of transient ischaemic attacks

Anterior circulation Carotid system	**Posterior circulation Vertebrobasilar system**
Amaurosis fugax	Diplopia, vertigo, vomiting
Aphasia	Choking and dysarthria
Hemiparesis	Ataxia
Hemisensory loss	Hemisensory loss
Hemianopic visual loss	Hemianopic visual loss
	Transient global amnesia
	Tetraparesis
	Loss of consciousness (rare)

DIFFERENTIAL DIAGNOSIS

TIAs must be distinguished, usually on wholly clinical grounds, from transient episodes which have other causes (see p. 1060). Occasionally, events identical to TIAs are produced by mass lesions of the brain.

Focal epilepsy is usually distinguished by the accompanying irritative phenomena (e.g. jerking of the limbs) and characteristically there is a progression of events over minutes. In a TIA the maximum deficit is usually apparent immediately.

Migraine, with a focal prodrome, sometimes causes diagnostic confusion. Headache, common but not invariable in migraine, is rare in a TIA, and in TIAs the visual disturbances typical of migraine are not seen.

PROGNOSIS

A thromboembolic TIA is an important prognostic event. Prospective studies have shown that five years after the TIA:

- 40% of patients will have suffered a stroke
- 25% of patients will have died, usually from heart disease or stroke.

A TIA in the anterior cerebral circulation carries a more serious prognosis than one in the posterior circulation.

INVESTIGATIONS AND MANAGEMENT

These are disussed on p. 1051.

Cerebral infarction

Major cerebral infarction from thromboembolism typically produces a stroke. Some small infarcts may cause TIAs, while others are silent. The clinical picture is thus very variable and depends on the site and extent of the infarct. Diagnosis on clinical grounds of the precise vascular territory involved is often inaccurate. Nevertheless, the general site of major cerebral infarction may be inferred from the pattern of the physical signs (e.g. cortex, internal capsule, brainstem).

CLINICAL FEATURES

The most common stroke is the hemiplegia caused by infarction in the internal capsule following thromboembolism of a branch of the middle cerebral artery. A similar picture is caused by (total) internal carotid occlusion (Fig 18.19). There is weakness of the limbs of the opposite side which develops over seconds, minutes or hours (and occasionally longer).

The signs are those of an acute complete contralateral UMN lesion, including limbs and face. Aphasia is usual when the dominant hemisphere is affected. The affected limbs are at first flaccid and areflexic. Headache is unusual and consciousness is not lost.

After a variable period, usually several days, the reflexes recover and become exaggerated and an extensor plantar response appears. Weakness is maximal at first, and recovers gradually over the course of days, weeks or many months.

Brain infarction following carotid or vertebral artery dissection

This accounts for around one-fifth of strokes below age 40 and is sometimes a sequel of head or neck trauma. Stroke or TIAs occur, often with neck pain, at the site of dissection, with migraine-like symptoms.

Brainstem infarction

Infarction in the brainstem causes complex patterns of dysfunction depending on the site of the lesion and its relationship to the cranial nerve nuclei, long tracts and brainstem connections (Table 18.28).

- *The lateral medullary syndrome*, also called posterior inferior cerebellar artery (PICA) thrombosis, or Wallenberg's syndrome, is the most widely recognized syndrome of brainstem infarction. It is caused by PICA or vertebral artery thromboembolism (Fig 18.20 and Table 18.29). Symptoms include vertigo, vomiting, dysphagia, unsteadiness, and contralateral loss of pain and temperature sensation on the face.
- *Coma* ensues when bilateral brainstem infarction damages the reticular formation.
- *The locked-in syndrome* is caused by upper brainstem infarction (see p. 1043).
- *Pseudobulbar palsy* (see p. 1027) can be caused by brainstem infarction.

Table 18.28
Features of brainstem infarction

Clinical feature	Structure involved
Hemiparesis or tetraparesis	Corticospinal tracts
Sensory loss	Medial lemniscus and spinothalamic tracts
Diplopia	Oculomotor system
Facial numbness	Fifth-nerve nuclei
Facial weakness (lower motor neurone)	Seventh-nerve nucleus
Nystagmus, vertigo	Vestibular connections
Dysphagia, dysarthria	Ninth- and tenth-nerve nuclei
Dysarthria, ataxia, hiccups, vomiting	Brainstem and cerebellar connections
Horner's syndrome	Sympathetic fibres
Altered consciousness	Reticular formation

Table 18.29
Clinical signs in the lateral medullary syndrome

Ipsilateral	Contralateral
Facial numbness (Vth)	Spinothalamic sensory loss
Diplopia (VIth)	Hemiparesis (mild, unusual)
Nystagmus	
Ataxia	
Horner's syndrome	
Ninth- and tenth-nerve lesions	

Other patterns of infarction

Lacunar infarction

Lacunes are small (< 1.5 cm^3) areas of infarction seen on MRI or at autopsy. Hypertension is commonly present. Minor strokes (e.g. pure motor stroke, pure sensory stroke, sudden unilateral ataxia and sudden dysarthria with a clumsy hand) are syndromes caused typically by single lacunar infarcts. Lacunar infarction is often also 'symptomless'.

Hypertensive encephalopathy (see also p. 537)

This describes various neurological sequelae of severe accelerated hypertension with occlusion of small arteries. Severe headaches, TIA, stroke, and rarely subarachnoid haemorrhage occur. Papilloedema may develop, either as part of an ischaemic optic neuropathy or following brain swelling due to multiple acute infarcts.

Multi-infarct dementia (see also p. 1115)

Multiple lacunes or larger infarcts cause the picture of generalized intellectual loss that is seen in patients with advanced cerebrovascular disease. The condition tends to occur with a stepwise progression over months or years with each subsequent infarct. There is dementia, pseudobulbar palsy and a shuffling gait with small steps – the *marche à petits pas*. There may be confusion clinically with idiopathic Parkinson's disease; this has been called

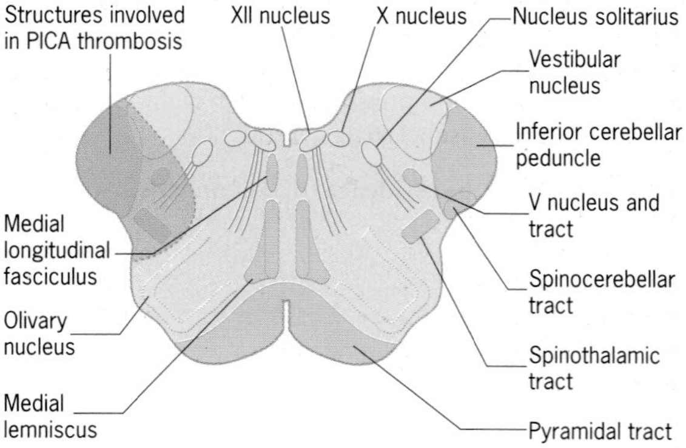

Fig 18.20
Cross-section of medulla showing posterior inferior cerebellar artery (PICA) thrombosis

'atherosclerotic parkinsonism' in the past. Binswanger's disease is a term used to describe low-attenuation areas in cerebral white matter on CT, with dementia, TIAs and stroke episodes in patients who are hypertensive.

Infarction in the visual cortex

Combinations of hemianopic visual loss, cortical blindness and Anton's syndrome follow infarction of the posterior cerebral arteries (see p. 1016), and the middle cerebral branch to the macular cortex (see Fig 18.18).

Weber's syndrome

This consists of an ipsilateral third-nerve paralysis with a contralateral hemiplegia due to a lesion in one half of the midbrain. Paralysis of upward gaze, due to a lesion localized in the region of the red nucleus, is usually present.

Watershed infarction

This describes the multiple cortical infarcts that occur following prolonged periods of very low cerebral perfusion (e.g. from hypotension following massive myocardial infarction or following cardiac bypass surgery). The border zones between the areas supplied by the anterior, middle and posterior cerebral arteries are damaged. A picture of cortical visual loss, memory loss and intellectual impairment is typical.

EXAMINATION

In addition to neurological examination, particular care should be taken to find a possible source of embolus (e.g. carotid bruit, atrial fibrillation, valve lesion or evidence of endocarditis) and to determine whether hypertension or postural hypotension is or has been present. There may be evidence of other emboli or a history of previous TIAs.

The brachial blood pressure should be measured in each arm; a difference of more than 20 mmHg is suggestive of stenosis of a subclavian artery.

IMMEDIATE MANAGEMENT OF STROKE

The initial decision whether to admit a stroke patient to hospital depends upon the clinical state and facilities available at home. Often the practical difficulties of caring for the disabled for what may be a prolonged period determine these immediate decisions. In practice, many TIAs and mild strokes can be managed at home and specialist advice sought when necessary. Patients admitted to stroke units tend to fare better than those admitted to a general ward.

Thrombolytic agents, such as tissue plasminogen activator, have sometimes appeared promising in the immediate treatment of ischaemic stroke but are not in general use.

The management of the unconscious patient is described on p. 1046.

INVESTIGATIONS

The purpose of investigations in both stroke and TIA is to confirm the clinical diagnosis, to look for underlying causes of disease and to direct therapy, either medical or surgical. Internal carotid artery stenosis is the principal surgical target. Preliminary investigations in thromboembolic stroke and TIA with their potential yields are listed in Table 18.30.

Table 18.30
Preliminary investigations in stroke

Test	Yield
Urinalysis, blood glucose	Diabetes mellitus
Haemoglobin, platelets	Polycythaemia
White cell count	Infection
ESR, CRP	Possible artertitis
Serology for syphilis	Possible neurosyphilis
Chest X-ray	Neoplasm
ECG	Recent infarct, dysrhythmia

Blood cultures should be taken if there is any possibility of endocarditis. Autoantibody studies – e.g. antinuclear factor (ANF), double-stranded DNA (dsDNA), cardiolipin antibodies and detailed clotting studies – should be performed in young patients to exclude diseases such as systemic lupus erythematosus (SLE).

Further investigations of TIA and stroke

CT and MR imaging. Imaging will usually demonstrate the site of a lesion and distinguish between a haemorrhage (see p. 1040) and infarction. An infarct appears as an area usually without major mass effect over the succeeding few days. Over 90% of all infarcts are detectable at one week. MRI is more sensitive in detecting infarction than CT. Imaging will also show unexpected mass lesions, such as subdural haematoma, tumour or abscess.

Carotid Doppler and duplex scanning. Ultrasound studies are of value in screening for arterial stenosis and occlusion: in skilled hands they demonstrate accurately the degree of internal carotid artery stenosis.

Angiography. Conventional carotid arteriography, digital subtraction angiography or magnetic resonance angiography is valuable in anterior circulation TIAs to diagnose surgically accessible arterial stenoses, mainly internal carotid artery stenosis.

There is a high probability of finding a carotid stenosis when there is a loud localized carotid bruit in the neck.

The majority of normotensive patients below the age of 75 years with TIA or stroke in the anterior circulation – who recover well – should be considered for vascular imaging, if ultrasound suggests carotid stenosis. In more elderly patients, the risks of the investigation and the relatively poor results of vascular surgery in preventing further stroke usually make further investigation unwise.

Vertebral and arch angiography are rarely performed following posterior circulation TIAs and strokes unless there is a clinical suggestion of subclavian artery disease.

Lumbar puncture. This is no longer a routine investigation in stroke. It is indicated only in special circumstances, such as when blood syphilitic serology is positive.

LONG-TERM MANAGEMENT

Medical therapy

All risk factors (see Table 18.26) should be identified and, if possible, treated. For primary prevention see p. 1047.

Antihypertensive therapy

The control of high blood pressure is the single most important factor in the primary prevention of stroke. Transient hypertension is also often seen in the acute stage of a stroke but hypotensive agents are not immediately necessary. If the hypertension is sustained it needs treatment (see p. 733), but the pressure must be lowered slowly to avoid a sudden fall in cerebral perfusion pressure.

Antiplatelet therapy: soluble aspirin (see also p. 410)

Soluble aspirin (75 mg daily) has been shown to reduce substantially the incidence of further events in patients who have had a TIA or cerebral infarction. Aspirin inhibits cyclo-oxygenase, which converts arachidonic acid to prostaglandins and thromboxanes. The predominant therapeutic effect is to reduce platelet aggregation.

Anticoagulants

Heparin and warfarin should be used when there is atrial fibrillation, other paroxysmal dysrhythmias or when there are certain cardiac valve lesions (uninfected) or cardiomyopathies. Anticoagulants are potentially dangerous in the two weeks following cerebral infarction because of the risk of provoking cerebral haemorrhage. There are still wide differences in clinical practice regarding their use.

Other measures

Polycythaemia should be treated if found (see p. 387). Baclofen (a GABA agonist) is sometimes helpful in the management of severe spasticity following stroke (see p. 1087).

Thrombolysins are currently being evaluated in acute thromboembolic stroke. In the USA the FDA has approved recombinant tissue plasminogen activator for the treatment of ischaemic stroke.

Surgical approaches

Internal carotid endarterectomy

This is considered in TIA or stroke patients who are shown to have internal carotid artery stenosis that narrows the arterial lumen by more than 70%. In these patients, the risk of further TIA/stroke is reduced by approximately 75% following successful surgery. The procedure, however, has a mortality around 3%. It is not currently recommended when internal carotid artery stenosis is less than 70%, or an incidental finding.

Extracranial–intracranial bypass

Anastomosis of the superficial temporal artery (external carotid) through a skull burr-hole to a cortical branch of the middle cerebral artery (internal carotid) was widely used, but as there was no overall benefit, the procedure is now largely obsolete.

REHABILITATION: PHYSIOTHERAPY AND SPEECH THERAPY

Skilled physiotherapy is of particular value in the first few months following the stroke. It is helpful in relieving spasticity, preventing contractures and teaching stroke patients to use walking aids. The benefit of physiotherapy on the longer-term outcome is still inadequately researched.

Speech therapy is recommended following aphasia. The trained therapist has a vital understanding of the problems and frustration of the aphasic patient. It is, however, possible that the spontaneous return of speech itself is hastened as much by normal conversation with a relative as by a therapist.

Both physiotherapy and speech therapy have an undoubted psychological role. Stroke is frequently a devastating event and, particularly when it occurs during working life, radically alters the pattern of the patient's remaining years. Many become unemployable and cannot lead independent lives. The financial consequences are usually considerable. Loss of self-esteem makes secondary depression common.

Following recovery from stroke, various aids and modifications may be necessary at home, for example stair rails, portable lavatories, bath rails, hoists, sliding boards, wheelchairs, tripods, modification of doorways and sleep arrangements, stair lifts and kitchen modifications. Liaison between hospital, occupational therapist and primary care physician to discuss these problems is valuable.

PROGNOSIS

Between one-third and one-half of patients who die do so in the first month following a stroke. This early mortality is lower for thromboembolic infarction (under a quarter) than for intracerebral haemorrhage (around three-quarters). A poor outcome is likely when there is coma, a defect in conjugate gaze and severe hemiplegia. Recurrent strokes are common (10% in the first year) and, in addition, many patients die subsequently from myocardial infarction. Of initial stroke survivors, 30–40% are alive after three years.

Gradual improvement usually follows a stroke, although the patient may be left with a severe residual deficit. Of those who survive a stroke, about one-third return to independent mobility and one-third have severe disability requiring permanent institutional care.

If, in general, there is sufficient language to be intelligible at three weeks, the outlook for recovery of fluent speech is good. Many stroke patients are, however, left with word-finding difficulties.

Intracranial haemorrhage

This group of conditions comprises:

- intracerebral and cerebellar haemorrhage
- subarachnoid haemorrhage
- subdural and extradural haemorrhage and haematoma.

Intracerebral haemorrhage

AETIOLOGY

Intracerebral haemorrhage is the cause of around 30% of strokes. Rupture of microaneurysms (Charcot–Bouchard aneurysms, 0.8–1.0 mm diameter) is the principal cause of primary intracerebral haemorrhage. This occurs typically in patients with hypertension and occurs at well-defined sites – basal ganglia, pons, cerebellum and subcortical white matter. Saccular (berry) aneurysms and arteriovenous malformations also bleed into the brain, but cause principally subarachnoid haemorrhage, rather than intracerebral haemorrhage.

RECOGNITION

Clinically, there is no entirely reliable way of distinguishing between intracerebral haemorrhage and thromboembolic infarction, as both produce a sudden focal deficit. Intracerebral haemorrhage, however, tends to be dramatic and accompanied by a severe headache. It is more likely to cause coma than thromboembolic stroke.

Intracerebral haemorrhage is visualized reliably by imaging almost immediately (cf. infarction, see p. 1040). Intracerebral and intraventricular blood, and blood in the subarachnoid space, are seen.

MANAGEMENT

The general management of haemorrhagic stroke is as for cerebral infarction, although the immediate prognosis is less good. Urgent neurosurgical evacuation of the clot should be considered when an intracerebral haematoma behaves as an expanding mass, causing deepening coma and coning (cerebellar haemorrhage, see below). The outlook in this clinical setting is poor. Antiplatelet drugs, and of course, anticoagulants are contraindicated.

Cerebellar haemorrhage

There is headache and rapid reduction of consciousness with signs of brainstem origin (e.g. nystagmus, ocular palsies). The gaze deviates to the side of the lesion. Skew deviation (see p. 1030) may be present. There are unilateral or bilateral cerebellar signs, if the patient is awake. It is important to recognize cerebellar haemorrhage because it causes acute hydrocephalus. Emergency surgery is usually necessary to remove the haematoma.

Subarachnoid haemorrhage

Subarachnoid haemorrhage (SAH) describes spontaneous rather than traumatic arterial bleeding into the subarachnoid space, and is usually clearly recognizable clinically by its dramatic onset. SAH accounts for 10% of cerebrovascular disease and has an annual incidence of 6 per 100 000.

CAUSES

The causes of SAH are shown in Table 18.31. It is unusual to find any contributing disease.

Saccular (berry) aneurysms

(see Fig 18.14 on p. 1040)

Saccular aneurysms form on the circle of Willis and its adjacent branches. The common sites of aneurysms are:

- the junction of the posterior communicating artery and the internal carotid artery – posterior communicating artery aneurysm
- the junction of the anterior communicating artery and the anterior cerebral artery – anterior communicating artery aneurysm
- the bifurcation of the middle cerebral artery – middle cerebral artery aneurysm.

Other aneurysm sites are on the basilar artery, the PICA, the intracavernous internal carotid artery and the ophthalmic artery. Saccular aneurysms are an incidental finding in 1% of autopsies and may be multiple.

Aneurysms cause symptoms either by spontaneous rupture, when there is usually no preceding history, or by direct pressure on surrounding structures; for example, a posterior communicating artery aneurysm is a cause of a painful third-nerve palsy (see p. 1020).

Arteriovenous malformation (AVM)

This is a lesion of developmental origin, usually within the hemisphere. An AVM may also cause epilepsy, which is often focal. Once an AVM has ruptured to cause SAH there is a tendency to rebleed at a rate of 10% per year.

CLINICAL FEATURES

The onset of SAH is sudden with a devastating headache, often occipital. This is usually followed by vomiting and often by loss of consciousness. The patient remains comatose or drowsy for several hours to several days. Less severe headaches cause diagnostic difficulties (see p. 1081), but SAH is a possible diagnosis in any sudden headache.

Table 18.31
Underlying causes of subarachnoid haemorrhage

Saccular ('berry') aneurysms	70%
Arteriovenous malformation	10%
No lesion found	20%

Rare associations
Bleeding disorders
Mycotic aneurysms (endocarditis)
Acute bacterial meningitis
Brain tumours (e.g. metastatic melanoma)
Arteritis (e.g. systemic lupus erythematosus)
Spinal subarachnoid haemorrhage from a spinal arteriovenous malformation
Coarctation of the aorta
Marfan's syndrome, Ehlers–Danlos syndrome
Polycystic kidneys

On examination, following major SAH there is neck stiffness and a positive Kernig's sign. Papilloedema is sometimes present and accompanied by retinal haemorrhages and subhyaloid haemorrhage (massive retinal haemorrhage tracking beneath the hyaloid membrane). Minor bleeds cause few physical signs, but invariably cause headache.

INVESTIGATIONS

CT imaging is the initial investigation of choice. Subarachnoid or intraventricular blood is usually seen. Lumbar puncture is not necessary if the diagnosis is confirmed by CT, but should be considered when there is doubt. The CSF becomes yellow (xanthochromic) several hours after SAH.

Carotid and vertebral angiography is usually performed in all patients who are potentially fit for surgery – i.e. generally those who are below 65 years and not in coma – to establish the cause and site of the bleeding.

DIFFERENTIAL DIAGNOSIS

SAH must be differentiated from severe migraine. This is sometimes difficult. *Thunderclap headache* is a term used variously to describe either the onset of SAH, or a sudden headache, without obvious migrainous features for which no cause is ever found. The onset of acute bacterial meningitis occasionally causes a very abrupt headache, when a meningeal microabscess ruptures. Subarachnoid bleeding also occasionally occurs at the onset of acute bacterial meningitis.

COMPLICATIONS

Blood clots in the subarachnoid space can lead to obstruction of CSF flow and hydrocephalus. This can be asymptomatic but is a cause of deteriorating conscious level a few days or weeks after the initial bleed. Diagnosis is by CT. Shunting may be required.

Severe spasm of the intracranial arteries sometimes complicates SAH and is a poor prognostic sign.

MANAGEMENT

Nearly half the cases of SAH are either dead or moribund before they reach hospital. Of the remainder, a further 10–20% die in the early weeks in hospital from further bleeding.

Patients who are comatose or who have severe neurological deficits have a poor prognosis. In others, where angiography demonstrates aneurysm, a direct neurosurgical approach to clip the neck of the aneurysm is carried out. In selected cases the results of surgery are excellent. Invasive radiological techniques, such as inserting a fine wire coil into an aneurysm, are being actively pursued. Microembolism and focal radiotherapy are used in cases of AVM. Direct neurosurgical approaches to AVMs are also carried out.

The immediate treatment of patients with SAH is bedrest and supportive measures. Hypertension should be controlled. Dexamethasone is often prescribed, to reduce cerebral oedema; it also is believed to stabilize the blood–brain barrier. Nimodipine, a calcium-channel blocking agent, has been shown to reduce mortality.

All SAH cases should be referred to a specialist centre for a decision about angiography and possible surgery.

Subdural and extradural haemorrhage and haematoma

These conditions are of great neurosurgical importance as both may cause death unless treated promptly.

Subdural haematoma (SDH) (Fig 18.14 on p. 1040)

SDH describes the accumulation of blood in the subdural space following rupture of a vein. It is almost always due to head injury, which may be minor. The interval between injury and symptoms may be days, weeks or months. Chronic, and unsuspected SDH is common in the elderly and in patients with alcohol abuse.

Headache, drowsiness and confusion are common; the symptoms are indolent and often fluctuate. Focal deficits such as hemiparesis or sensory loss develop. Epilepsy occasionally occurs. Stupor and coma gradually ensue.

Extradural haemorrhage (Fig 18.14)

This follows a linear skull vault fracture which tears a branch of the middle meningeal artery. Blood accumulates rapidly over minutes or hours in the extradural space. The most characteristic picture is of a head injury with a brief duration of unconsciousness followed by a lucid interval of recovery. The patient then develops a progressive hemiparesis and stupor, and rapid transtentorial coning, with first an ipsilateral dilated pupil, followed by bilateral fixed dilated pupils, tetraplegia and death.

An acute subdural haemorrhage presents in a similar way.

MANAGEMENT

Suspected extradural or subdural haemorrhage or haematoma is an indication for prompt CT or MR imaging.

Extradural bleeding requires urgent neurosurgery. If performed early, the outlook is excellent. When far from specialist neurosurgical help (e.g. in wartime or at sea), surgical drainage has been lifesaving when the diagnosis has been made on clinical grounds alone.

Subdural bleeding tends to cease spontaneously, and allows more conservative management, sometimes without surgery. Even large subdural collections resolve. Progress can be assessed with serial imaging. Close liason with a neurosurgeon is essential.

Cortical venous thrombosis and dural venous sinus thrombosis

These venous thromboses are unusual complications of skull and paranasal (air) sinus infection, dehydration or severe intercurrent illness. There is also an association with pregnancy and hormonal contraceptive agents, and the antiphospholipid syndrome (p. 490).

Cortical venous thrombosis

The venous infarct caused by the thrombosis leads to focal signs (e.g. hemiparesis) and/or epilepsy. There is often a fever.

Dural venous sinus thromboses

- *Cavernous sinus thrombosis* causes ocular pain, fever, proptosis and chemosis. An external and internal ophthalmoplegia with papilloedema develop.
- *Lateral and sagittal sinus thrombosis* causes raised intracranial pressure with headache, fever papilloedema and often epilepsy.

MANAGEMENT

MR angiography, which is the investigation of choice, shows the occluded sinus or veins. The venous phase of conventional angiography is also diagnostic. Antibiotics, anticonvulsants and anticoagulants are given.

FURTHER READING

Barnett HJM, Eliasziw M, Meldrum H (1995) Drugs and surgery in the prevention of ischaemic stroke. *New England Journal of Medicine* **332**: 238–248.

Bronner LL, Kanter DS, Manson JE (1995) Primary prevention of stroke. *New England Journal of Medicine* **333**: 1392–1400

Bucher HC, Griffith LE, Guyatt GH (1998) Effect of HMG CoA reductase inhibitors on stroke: a meta-analysis of randomized control trials. *Annals of Internal Medicine* **128**: 89–95.

del Zoppo GJ (1995) Acute stroke on the threshold of a therapy? *New England Journal of Medicine* **333**: 1632–1633.

Donnan GA *et al.* (1998) Surgery for prevention of stroke (Commentary on final results of European Carotid Surgery Trial (ECST)).

Editorial (1997) Which prophylactic aspirin? *Drug and Therapeutics Bulletin* **35**: 7–8.

Sandercock P (1998) Transient ischaemic attacks: new treatments, new questions. *Quarterly Journal of Medicine* **91**: 377–380.

Epilepsy and other causes of recurrent loss of consciousness

Epilepsy

An *epileptic seizure* is a convulsion or transient abnormal event experienced by the subject, resulting from a paroxysmal discharge of cerebral neurones. *Epilepsy* is the continuing tendency to have such seizures, even if a long interval separates attacks. A generalized convulsion (i.e. a grand mal fit) is the most common recognized event.

Epilepsy is a common condition. Some 2% of the population have two or more seizures during their lives. In Britain, approximately 65 people suffer from their first seizure each day. Around a quarter of a million people in Britain take anticonvulsants.

MECHANISMS

The spread of electrical activity between cortical neurones is normally restricted. Synchronous discharge of neurones in the normal brain takes place in small groups only; these limited discharges are responsible for the normal rhythms of the EEG.

During a seizure, large groups of neurones are activated repetitively and hypersynchronously. There is failure of inhibitory synaptic contact between neurones. This causes high-voltage spike-and-wave activity on the EEG, the electrophysiological hallmark of epilepsy.

A *partial seizure* is epileptic activity confined to one area of cortex with a recognizable clinical pattern. This activity either remains focal or spreads to generate epileptic activity in both hemispheres – and thus a generalized seizure. This spread is called *secondary generalization of the partial seizure.*

Seizure threshold

Each individual has a threshold for seizure activity. Experimentally some chemicals (e.g. pentylenetetrazol, a gas) induce seizures in all subjects. Individuals who are more likely to have seizures in response to various stimuli, for example flashing lights, are said to have a low seizure threshold. This is a concept, not a measurement.

CLASSIFICATION

Epilepsy is classified by the clinical pattern of seizure (Table 18.32).

- *Generalized* implies abnormal electrical activity which is widespread in the brain.
- *A simple partial seizure* describes a seizure without loss of awareness.
- *A complex partial seizure* describes a seizure with loss of awareness.

Generalized seizure types

Tonic–clonic seizures (grand mal seizures, generalized convulsions)

Following a vague warning, the tonic phase of the seizure commences. The body becomes rigid, for up to a minute. The patient utters a cry and falls, sometimes suffering injury. The tongue is usually bitten. There may be incontinence of urine or faeces.

The clonic phase then begins, a generalized convulsion, with frothing at the mouth and rhythmic jerking of muscles. This lasts from a few seconds to a few minutes. Seizures are usually self-limiting, leaving the patient drowsy, confused or in coma for several hours.

Table 18.32
Classification of epilepsy (International League against Epilepsy)

Generalized seizure types
Absence seizures[a]
(a) Typical absences with 3 Hz spike-and-wave discharge (*petit mal*)
(b) Atypical absences with other EEG changes
Myoclonic seizures
Tonic–clonic seizures (*grand mal*, major convulsions)[a]
Tonic seizures
Akinetic seizures
Partial seizure types
These start by activation of a group of neurones in one part of one hemisphere. They are also called 'focal seizures'
Simple partial seizures (no impairment of consciousness)[a] (e.g. Jacksonian seizures)[a]
Complex partial seizures (with impairment of consciousness)[a]
Partial seizures evolving to tonic–clonic seizures
Apparent generalized tonic–clonic seizures, with EEG but not clinical evidence of focal onset[a]
Unclassifiable seizures
Seizures which do not fit in one of the above categories

[a]Common varieties of epilepsy

Typical absences (petit mal)

This describes a type of generalized epilepsy which almost invariably begins in childhood. Each attack is accompanied by 3 Hz spike-and-wave EEG activity (see Fig 18.15 on p. 1040). The child ceases activity, stares and pales slightly. An attack lasts a few seconds. The eyelids twitch; a few muscle jerks may occur. After an attack, the child resumes normal activity.

Typical absence attacks are never due to acquired lesions such as tumours. They are a developmental abnormality of neuronal control. Children with typical absence attacks may in adult life develop generalized seizures.

Petit mal describes only these 3 Hz seizures, rather than clinically similar absence attacks which are partial seizures.

Other generalized seizure types

Myoclonic seizures are events where there is isolated muscle jerking. Tonic seizures describe events in which stiffening of the body is not followed by convulsive jerking. Atonic seizures describe events where there is sudden loss of tone, with falling and loss of consciousness.

Partial seizure types

Partial seizures (focal seizures)

A partial or focal seizure (which can be either simple or complex, see above) implies that an area of brain (e.g. a temporal lobe) has generated abnormal electrical activity that may spread. The seizure frequently has clinical features that provide evidence of the site of origin.

An *aura* describes the effects of the initial focal electrical events, such as an unusual smell, tingling in a limb or a strange inner feeling which are soon recognized by the patient as a warning of an impending seizure.

Jacksonian, or focal motor seizures

These simple partial seizures originate in the motor cortex. Jerking movements typically begin at the angle of the mouth or in the thumb and index finger, spreading to involve the limbs on the side opposite the epileptic focus. The clinical evidence of this spread of activity is called the march of the seizure. With a frontal lesion, conjugate gaze (see p. 1081) deviates away from the irritative focus. This is called an adversive seizure. Paralysis of the affected limbs may follow a focal motor, or generalized seizure for several hours – a Todd's paralysis.

Temporal lobe seizures

These partial seizures, which are either simple or complex describe feelings of unreality (*jamais vu*) or undue familiarity (*déja vu*) with the surroundings. Absence attacks, vertigo, visual hallucinations (i.e visions or faces) are also examples of temporal lobe seizures.

Many other types of partial seizure occur, such as autonomic disturbances with piloerection, flushing, and overbreathing, strange smells (frontal cortex), sensory disturbances (parietal cortex), crude visual shapes (occipital cortex), or strange sounds (auditory cortex).

AETIOLOGICAL AND PRECIPITATING FACTORS (Table 18.33)

A definite cause for epilepsy is found in under one-quarter of patients.

Genetic predisposition

About 30% of patients with epilepsy have a history of seizures in first-degree relatives. Usually the mode of inheritance is uncertain; a low seizure threshold appears to run in some families. Generalized typical absence seizures (petit mal) are sometimes inherited as an autosomal dominant trait with variable penetrance.

Developmental anomalies

Primary generalized epilepsies (e.g. petit mal) are due to developmental abnormalities of neuronal control. It is

Table 18.33
Aetiological and precipitating factors in epilepsy

Genetic predisposition
Developmental abnormalities
Trauma and surgery
Pyrexia in children
Intracranial mass lesions
Cerebral infarction
Drugs, e.g. lidocaine, alcohol and drug withdrawal
Encephalitis
Metabolic abnormalities, e.g. porphyria, hypocalcaemia
Degenerative brain disorders
Photosensitivity and auditory stimuli

uncertain whether these are anatomical, because of abnormal synaptic connections, or due to anomalies in neurotransmitter distribution, release and control.

Ectopic dysfunctional areas of cerebral cortex and hamartomas are other examples of abnormalities present at birth which can cause seizures at some time, even commencing in adult life.

Trauma and surgery

Perinatal trauma (causing cerebral contusion and haemorrhage) and fetal anoxia are common causes of seizures in childhood. Hypoxic damage to the hippocampi (mesial temporal sclerosis) is another cause of epilepsy.

Brain injury is sometimes followed by epilepsy within the first week (early epilepsy) or many months or years later (late epilepsy). To cause epilepsy, the injury must (almost always) be sufficient to cause coma. The presence of early epilepsy, a depressed skull fracture, penetrating brain injury, cerebral contusion, dural tear or intracranial haematoma increases the incidence of late post-traumatic epilepsy.

Surgery to the cerebral hemispheres is followed by seizures in about 10% of patients.

Pyrexia

Convulsions sometimes occur when children under five years have high fevers (febrile convulsions). In the majority there is no tendency for the seizures to recur in adult life.

Intracranial mass lesions

Mass lesions affecting the cerebral cortex can cause epilepsy – either partial or secondary generalized seizures. If the onset of seizures is in adult life, the chance of an unsuspected mass lesion such as a tumour being present is around 3%.

Hydrocephalus, of any cause, lowers the threshold for seizures.

Vascular

Seizures can occasionally follow cerebral infarction, especially in the elderly.

Drugs, alcohol and drug withdrawal

Phenothiazines, monoamine oxidase inhibitors, tricyclic antidepressants, amphetamines, lignocaine and nalidixic acid can sometimes provoke fits either in overdose or in therapeutic doses in individuals with a low seizure threshold.

Chronic alcohol abuse is a common cause of seizures. These occur either while drinking heavily or during periods of withdrawal. Alcohol-induced hypoglycaemia also provokes attacks (see p. 989).

Withdrawal of anticonvulsant drugs (especially phenobarbitone) and withdrawal of benzodiazepines may provoke seizures.

Encephalitis and other inflammatory conditions of the brain

Seizures are frequently the presenting feature of encephalitis, chronic meningitis (e.g. tuberculosis), cerebral abscess, cortical venous thrombosis and neurosyphilis.

Metabolic abnormalities

Seizures are seen with the following metabolic abnormalities:

- hypocalcaemia
- hypoglycaemia
- hyponatraemia
- acute hypoxia
- porphyria
- uraemia
- hepato-cellular failure.

Degenerative brain disorders

Seizures can occur in Alzheimer's disease and in many rarer degenerative diseases. Epilepsy is three times more common in patients with multiple sclerosis than in the general population.

Photosensitive and other types of reflex epilepsy

Seizures are occasionally precipitated by flashing lights or a flickering television screen. This photosensitivity can be seen on the occipital recording of the EEG. Very rarely other stimuli (e.g. music) provoke attacks.

DIAGNOSIS AND INVESTIGATIONS

The history from a witness is of prime importance.

EEG

The EEG remains the single most useful test in the diagnosis of epilepsy, though the test has limitations. It should be performed after a first fit.

- *During a seizure* the EEG is almost invariably abnormal, because epileptic activity reaches the surface of the brain.
- *EEG evidence of seizure activity* is shown typically by a cortical spike focus (e.g. in a temporal lobe) or by generalized spike-and-wave activity.
- *3 Hz spike-and-wave activity* occurs only and specifically in petit mal, the generalized epilepsy of childhood (see Fig 18.15 on p. 1040). This is always present during an attack and is frequently seen in the interictal intervals (i.e. between attacks).
- *A normal EEG between attacks* does not exclude epilepsy. Many people suffering from epilepsy have normal interictal EEG activity. In addition, an abnormal interictal EEG does not prove that a particular attack was epileptic.
- *EEG videotelemetry* adds value to the conventional EEG in the study of attacks whose nature is uncertain (see pseudoseizures, p. 1061).

CT and/or MR imaging

The trend in developed countries is towards full imaging of all new cases of epilepsy. In practice, CT is a reasonable screening test in adults, to diagnose unsuspected mass lesions. MRI is used for detailed study, when for example neurosurgical treatment is being considered.

Other investigations

Routine investigations (blood picture, serum biochemistry including calcium, chest X-ray) indicate an underlying metabolic or other cause. Such tests are normal in idiopathic epilepsy.

TREATMENT

Emergency measures

The emergency treatment of a seizure is simply to ensure that the patient comes to as little harm as possible, and that the airway is maintained both in a prolonged seizure and in postictal coma. Wooden mouth gags, tongue forceps and physical restraint frequently cause injury.

Most seizures last only minutes, and end spontaneously. A prolonged seizure – longer than three minutes – or repeated seizures outside hospital are best treated with rectal diazepam (10 mg), or intravenous diazepam.

If there is any suspicion of hypoglycaemia, blood should be taken for the measurement of glucose, and intravenous glucose should be given.

Long-term anticonvulsant drugs

Anticonvulsant drugs are indicated in recurrent seizures when there is a firm clinical diagnosis. Their use carries the stigma of the diagnosis of epilepsy. Acceptance by the patient is essential, and their understanding of potential unwanted effects. Opinions differ as to whether treatment is necessary following the first attack.

For both partial and generalized seizures, monotherapy with a first-line anticonvulsant drug (Table 18.34) is used with increasing doses until seizure control is achieved. If this is not possible, a further first-line drug is given, or a second-line drug is added.

Ethosuximide is also used as a first-line drug in children with petit mal. Primidone, the benzodiazepines clonazepam and clobazam, and acetazolamide are also used as second-line drugs.

Table 18.34
Anticonvulsant drugs

First-line drugs	Second-line drugs
Sodium valproate	Lamotrigine
Carbamazepine	Vigabatrin
Phenytoin	Gabapentin
	Topiramate
	Phenobarbitone
Ethosuximide	Primidone
(for petit mal)	Clobazam
	Acetazolamide

Table 18.35
Doses and therapeutic levels of anticonvulsant drugs

Drug	Adult daily dose (mg)	Therapeutic level ($\mu mol\ L^{-1}$)
Phenytoin	300	40–80
Carbamazepine	200 × 3	20–50[a]
Sodium valproate	200 × 3	200–700[a]

[a]Poorly defined

There are differences in practice about the most appropriate drugs for each particular variety of seizure.

Drug levels for most anticonvulsants can be monitored. In the case of phenytoin the serum therapeutic level is well-defined and this should be monitored in the majority of patients (Table 18.35). The therapeutic serum levels of other anticonvulsants are less well-defined and routine estimations are not usually performed, unless compliance or toxicity are issues.

Unwanted effects of drugs. Intoxication with all anticonvulsants causes a syndrome of ataxia, nystagmus and dysarthria.

Chronic administration of phenytoin can cause gum hypertrophy, hypertrichosis, osteomalacia, folate deficiency, polyneuropathy and encephalopathy. A wide range of potential unwanted effects are known. Some of the serious idiosyncratic (i.e. non-dose-related) side-effects are noted in Table 18.36.

Pregnancy, hormonal contraception and anticonvulsants

The overall risk of birth defects in mothers who take an anticonvulsant is around 5%, higher than in the general population. Counselling before conception is essential. Some women choose to withdraw from anticonvulsants prior to becoming pregnant. If drugs are continued, monotherapy with a first-line drug is advisable with folic acid (5 mg a day) supplement. Vitamin K 20 mg orally should also be prescribed daily to the mother during the week prior to delivery, to prevent neonatal haemorrhage, caused by inhibition of vitamin K transplacental transport.

Table 18.36
Some idiosyncratic unwanted effects of anticonvulsant drugs

Drug	Non-dose-related side-effects
Phenytoin	Rashes
	Blood dyscrasias
	Lymphadenopathy
	Systemic lupus erythematosus
Carbamazepine	Rashes
	Blood dyscrasias, particularly severe leucopenia
Sodium valproate	Anorexia
	Hair loss
	Liver damage
Lamotrigine	Stevens–Johnson syndrome
Vigabatrin	Retinal damage (visual field constriction)
	Psychological change

Anticonvulsants which induce enzymes (carbamazepine, phenytoin and phenobarbitone) reduce the efficacy of the contraceptive pill. A combined contraceptive pill containing at least 50 μg of oestrogen should be used, or an IUCD or barrier methods of contraception.

Drug withdrawal

Epilepsy, when controlled, may stay in remission. Drug withdrawal is sometimes possible, and the question often raised by patients. Withdrawal is only achieved successfully in less than 50% of cases where it is attempted. Recurrence of seizures following drug withdrawal can cause considerable difficulty if, for example the individual's driving licence has been regained. The British Driving Licensing Authority (DVLA Swansea) recommend that patients do not drive during reduction of doses and for six months following stopping anticonvulsants. Careful discussion and a full explanation is necessary. Withdrawal should not usually be considered until the patient has been free of all fits for at least two years.

Status epilepticus

This describes seizures which follow each other without recovery of consciousness. Status epilepticus is a medical emergency with a mortality of 10–15% with death from cardiorespiratory failure. Over 50% of episodes occur in patients without a history of epilepsy. Several treatment regimes are available.

Immediate intravenous injection of diazepam 10–20 mg is given at 0.5 mL per minute (2.5 mg per 30 s), and repeated once. Rectal diazepam, or rectal paraldehyde, are given if the intravenous route is not immediately accessible. Intravenous lorazepam, clonazepam and chlormethiazole are also used. Full ventilatory support must be available when status is treated because all these drugs cause respiratory depression. A loading dose of phenytoin 15 mg kg^{-1} at a rate of not more than 50 mg per minute, followed by maintenance dosage, is then given to prevent recurrent fits. If status persists for more than 90 minutes, and is unresponsive to therapy, anaesthesia with thiopentone or propofol is used, with assisted ventilation.

Focal status epilepticus describes the condition in partial seizures. In absence status, for example, status is non-convulsive – the patient is in a distant, stuporose state. *Epilepsy partialis continua* is continuous seizure activity involving part of the body, such as a finger or a limb, without loss of consciousness. This is often due to a cortical neoplasm or, in the elderly, a cortical infarct.

Neurosurgical treatment

Several surgical approaches are available in epilepsy. The most important is amputation of the anterior temporal lobe (usually of the non-dominant side) in those with partial seizures or partial seizures that are secondarily generalized. Indications for surgery include poor control on drug therapy and a clearly defined focus of abnormal electrical activity, for example mesial temporal sclerosis in the hippocampus. In appropriate cases (under 1% of all patients with epilepsy) selected in a specialist centre this surgical treatment is highly effective.

The social consequences of epilepsy

The great majority of patients with epilepsy are managed by a general practitioner or as an outpatient, and have infrequent seizures that alter the pattern of their lives relatively little. In a very small minority who have exceedingly frequent seizures, treatment in hospital or even residential care is necessary.

There remains, however, a considerable social stigma attached to the word epilepsy, an important fact to be considered when the nature of attacks is uncertain. Employers are reluctant to accept people with epilepsy.

Both adults and children with epilepsy should be encouraged to lead lives as unrestricted as reasonably possible, though with simple, sensible provisos such as avoiding swimming alone and dangerous sports such as rock-climbing or solo canoeing. Domestic issues are also important, such as that a bathroom or lavatory door should perhaps remain unlocked.

Driving and epilepsy

Complex regulations apply. A central feature is that it is illegal to drive a motor vehicle if any form of seizure or any episode of unexplained loss of consciousness has taken place during the previous year. There is variation between different countries.

In the UK those who have suffered from epilepsy cannot legally hold an ordinary (Group 1) driving licence (to drive a car or motorcycle) unless they satisfy the following legal criteria whether on or off treatment. The regulations state:

- A person who has suffered an epileptic attack *whilst awake* must refrain from driving for one year from the date of the attack before a driving licence may be issued.
- A person who has suffered a single epileptic attack *whilst asleep* must also refrain from driving for one year from the date of that attack, unless they have had attacks exclusively whilst asleep over a period of three years and no awake attacks, i.e. *attacks occurring exclusively in sleep must be shown to have occurred over a three-year period.*
- In any event, the driving of a vehicle by such a person should not be likely to cause danger to the public.

The UK regulations for Group 2 drivers (vocational and for truck drivers) are far stricter. Persons with a history of seizures must meet all the following three criteria:

- They must have been free of epileptic attacks for at least the last ten years.
- They must not have taken anticonvulsant medication during this ten-year period.
- They do not have a continuing liability to epileptic seizures.

Strict regulations also exist for potential aircraft pilots, sea captains, divers and other similar activities. The correct diagnosis of an attack at any age is therefore of major social and legal importance. It is an essential requirement of a doctor to inform patients of these regulations. In the UK the patient should then write to the licensing authorities.

Other causes of recurrent attacks of disturbed consciousness and falls (Table 18.37)

Episodes of transient disturbance of consciousness and falls are common clinical problems. It is usually possible to distinguish between a fit (i.e. a seizure), a faint (i.e. syncope), and other types of attack from the history given by the patient and the account of an eyewitness. The term 'collapse' is non-diagnostic and should be avoided. The precise cause of falls in the elderly, with their important sequelae such as a femoral fracture, often remains ill-defined, despite consideration of some the conditions described below. Falls without loss of awareness are common in Parkinson's disease, sometimes before other features become obvious.

Syncope, vasovagal attacks and related disorders (see also p. 631)

Sudden reflex bradycardia and peripheral and splanchnic vasodilatation leading to loss of consciousness occurs commonly in response to prolonged standing, fear, venesection or pain. This is also known as neurocardiogenic syncope. Syncope almost never occurs in the recumbent posture. The subject falls to the ground and is unconscious for less than two minutes. Recovery is rapid. A few jerking movements are uncommon, but can occur. Incontinence of urine is exceptional.

This is the *simple faint* which the majority of the population suffer at some time, particularly in childhood, in youth or in pregnancy. Syncope occurs with severe anaemia, of any cause, at any age.

Table 18.37
Causes of attacks of disturbed consciousness and falling

Syncope (situational or vasovagal) 'Fainting' Cough Effort Micturition Carotid sinus	Cardiac arrhythmias Postural hypotension
	Hypoglycaemia Hypocalcaemia
Epilepsy Narcolepsy and cataplexy	Vertigo Drop attacks
Transient ischaemic attacks	Hydrocephalus
Psychogenic attacks Panic attacks Hyperventilation	Acute dystonic reactions (drugs)
Night terrors } in children Breath holding } in children Choking	

Syncope occurs *after micturition in men*, particularly at night, and in either sex when the venous return to the heart is obstructed by breath-holding and severe coughing.

Postural hypotension causing syncope occurs in patients with impaired autonomic reflexes (e.g. in the elderly), in autonomic neuropathy, or with ganglion-blocking drugs used in hypertension, with phenothiazines, levodopa or tricyclic antidepressants. The tilt test will show hypotension as the patient is raised to the vertical and is useful in diagnosis (see p. 646).

Transient cerebral ischaemia in the posterior cerebral circulation is also a cause of episodes of loss of consciousness.

The rare syndrome of *carotid sinus syncope* is due to excessive sensitivity of the sinus to external pressure. This tends to occur in elderly patients who lose consciousness after touching the neck.

Cardiac arrhythmias (cardiac syncope, Stokes–Adams attacks; see p. 631) are important causes of recurrent episodes of loss of consciousness, particularly in the elderly. There is sometimes a preceding warning of palpitation (either fast or slow). The loss of consciousness is sudden and accompanied by pallor. Exceptionally, there are convulsive movements – anoxic convulsions. Flushing may be seen as the patient recovers. The usual cardiac arrhythmias that cause loss of consciousness are paroxysmal bradycardias (e.g. in complete heart block), or ventricular dysrhythmias. Supraventricular tachycardias are unusual causes of loss of consciousness.

Effort syncope (syncope on exertion) is of cardiac origin and occurs in aortic stenosis and hypertrophic obstructive cardiomyopathy.

Drop attacks are very sudden wholly unexpected episodes of weakness of the lower limbs with falling but without loss of consciousness, largely in women over 60 years. They are believed to be due to sudden changes in tone in the lower limbs, presumably of brainstem origin. They used to be regarded as forms of TIA, from which they are distinct, as other vascular events do not follow them.

INVESTIGATIONS

Syncope and related conditions where cerebral blood flow is impaired can usually be distinguished from epilepsy on the clinical history alone. A witness account is extremely valuable: persistent jerking movements, incontinence and post-episode confusion and amnesia are very suggestive of a fit, not a faint.

Cardiac monitoring is used to detect dysrhythmia. Tilt testing (see p. 646) is useful in neurocardiogenic syncope.

MANAGEMENT

The immediate management of syncope, or impending syncope, is to lie the patient down, to elevate the lower limbs and to record the pulse. In the rare circumstances where cerebral blood flow cannot be restored (e.g. propped upright in a dentist's chair), syncope may be followed by cerebral infarction.

Other conditions

Panic attacks, night terrors, psychogenic attacks (pseudoseizures) and hyperventilation

Panic attacks are usually associated with an autonomic disturbance, such as tachycardia, sweating and piloerection. Consciousness is usually preserved. Hyperventilation (see below) is common.

Night terrors are sudden episodes seen in children who awake as if from a dream in a state of terror.

Psychogenic attacks cause considerable difficulty in diagnosis.

Pseudoseizures are attacks resembling grand mal fits. Usually there are bizzare limb movements, but on occasion there is extreme difficulty in separating pseudoseizures from epilepsy. EEG videotelemetry is valuable. Apparent status epilepticus can be caused by pseudoseizures.

Hyperventilation causing alkalosis leads to a feeling of light-headedness, sometimes accompanied by circumoral and peripheral tingling and tetany – for example, carpopedal spasm (see p. 515). Occasionally there is loss of consciousness.

Hypoglycaemia (see also p. 987)

Hypoglycaemia causes attacks in which the patient either feels unwell or loses consciousness, sometimes with a convulsion. There is often some warning, with hunger, shaking and sweating. Prompt recovery occurs with intravenous (or oral) glucose. Prolonged hypoglycaemia causes widespread cerebral damage.

Hypoglycaemic attacks unrelated to diabetes are rare (see p. 987). Most patients who feel unwell after fasting or in the early morning have no serious organic disease.

Hypocalcaemia (see also p. 515)

A grand mal fit may accompany hypocalcaemia, as the seizure threshold is lowered.

Vertigo

Acute episodes of vertigo can be severe enough to cause prostration: consciousness is sometimes lost for a few seconds.

Choking

Choking causes sudden loss of speech, with intense coughing and laryngeal spasm, followed by hypoxia, when larygeal obstruction is partial. When a large food bolus completely blocks the larynx, the person becomes blue and speechless, grasping their throat. Death occurs if this obstruction is not relieved promptly.

Immediate treatment of this emergency is to encircle the abdomen from behind with both arms and to compress the lower chest and abdomen hard to eject the food bolus (Heimlich manoeuvre, see p. 774). The force of gravity – holding the person upside down – is also useful where possible.

Drug reactions

Acute dystonic reactions (oculogyric crises, see p. 1065) sometimes cause diagnostic difficulty, being mistaken for epilepsy. Consciousness is preserved.

Sleep and its disturbances

Sleep is required on a regular basis. It is thought that its role involves the laying down of recent memory, and refreshing both cognitive and emotional equilibrium. Complex pathways between the cortex and reticular formation are involved in the production and maintenance of sleep. During normal sleep, there are periods of deep sleep associated with rapid eye movement (REM). Dreaming occurs during REM sleep.

In insomnia, sleep is fitful. Less time than usual is spent in REM sleep. In old age, sleep requirement falls to as little as four hours a night. Fitful sleep, particularly with early morning waking, is a common indicator of depression (see p. 1122). In practice, insomnia itself is rarely a feature of serious organic neurological disease. In the elderly, nocturnal confusion and/or nightmares are often caused by drugs (e.g. levodopa in Parkinson's disease), and by organic brain disease such as dementia.

Sleep apnoea

In pathological sleep apnoea, the normal short periods of apnoea seen during REM sleep become unduly prolonged. This occurs occasionally with brainstem lesions, often as a pre-terminal event but more commonly with upper airways obstruction, when it is accompanied by snoring. The latter is particularly important in patients with chronic obstructive airways disease, who may become severely hypoxic during sleep apnoea (see p. 781). This sleep apnoea syndrome is also a cause of excessive daytime drowsiness.

Narcolepsy and cataplexy

Narcoleptic attacks are periods of irresistible sleep – excessive daytime drowsiness – in inappropriate circumstances. Episodes tend to occur when there is little distraction, after meals, while travelling in a vehicle, but sometimes without obvious cause. Genetically, narcolepsy is strongly associated with HLA-DR2 and HLA-DQl antigens.

Cataplexy is sudden loss of tone in the lower limbs – falling with preservation of consciousness. Attacks are set off by sudden surprise or emotion.

The two conditions sometimes coexist and are accompanied by vivid hypnagogic hallucinations (i.e. on falling asleep), hypnopompic hallucinations (i.e. on waking), with sleep paralysis – a frightening inability to move whilst drowsy. The EEG remains normal during and between attacks.

TREATMENT

Treatment is with methylphenidate, dexamphetamine and other amphetamine-like drugs, or small doses of tricyclic antidepressants, particularly clomipramine.

FURTHER READING

Ashton CA (1997) Management of insomnia. *Prescribers' Journal* **37**: 1–10.

British National Formulary, current edition.

Cleland PG (1996) Management of pre-existing disorders in pregnancy. *Prescribers' Journal* **36**: 102–109.

Dichter MA, Brodie MJ (1996) New antiepileptic drugs. *New England Journal of Medicine* **334**: 1583–1589.

DVLC Swansea (1998) *At a Glance Guide to the Current Medical Standards of Fitness to Drive.*

Lowenstein DH, Alldredge BK (1998) Status epilepticus. *New England Journal of Medicine* **338**: 970–976.

van Weel et al (1995) Falls: a community care perspective. *Lancet* **345**: 1549–1551.

Parkinson's disease and other movement disorders

Disorders of movement can be classified broadly into akinetic–rigid syndromes, where there is loss of movement with increase in muscle tone, and dyskinesias, where there are added movements outside voluntary control. Both are due to disorders of neurotransmitters of the extrapyramidal system.

Parkinson's disease is much the most common of these conditions. A classification of movement disorders is given in Table 18.38.

Table 18.38
A classification of movement disorders

Akinetic–rigid syndromes
Idiopathic Parkinson's disease
Drug-induced parkinsonism (e.g. phenothiazines)
MPTP-induced parkinsonism
Postencephalitic parkinsonism
Parkinsonism-plus
Childhood akinetic–rigid syndrome
Dyskinesias
Essential tremor
Chorea
Hemiballismus
Myoclonus
Tic or 'habit spasms'
Torsion dystonias

MPTP, 1-methyl-4-phenyl-1,2,3,6-tetrahydropyridine

Akinetic–rigid syndromes

Idiopathic Parkinson's disease

In 1817, James Parkinson, a physician in Hoxton, London, published a monograph *The Shaking Palsy*, describing the clinical appearance of these patients. The disease is common and worldwide, with prevalence increasing sharply with age to about 1 in 200 in those over 70 years. The condition is clinically distinct from other parkinsonian syndromes.

There are few real clues as to its cause. The relatively uniform worldwide prevalence of the disease would suggest that an environmental agent is not responsible. Some factors possibly involved are the following.

Nicotine. Some epidemiological studies suggest the curious and unexplained fact that the disease is less prevalent in tobacco smokers than in lifelong abstainers.

MPTP. Minute doses of the pyridine compound, methylphenyltetrahydropyridine (MPTP) cause a severe parkinsonian syndrome. Any significance between this and idiopathic Parkinson's disease is unclear. The suggestion has been made that environmental MPTP-like herbicides might be relevant.

Encephalitis lethargica. Survivors of encephalitis lethargica (see p. 1065), which is presumed to be a viral disease, develop parkinsonism. However, it is not thought that the idiopathic disease is related to this or to another infective agent.

Genetic factors. The condition is not usually inherited, though there is occasional clustering in families. It is postulated that a failure of dopamine synthesis, genetically programmed, could be responsible.

PATHOLOGY

In the pars compacta of the *substantia nigra* there is progressive cell degeneration and the appearance of eosinophilic inclusion bodies (Lewy bodies). Degeneration also occurs in other brainstem nuclei. Biochemically there is loss of dopamine (and melanin) in the striatum that correlates well with the areas of cell loss and also with the degree of akinesia. The underlying cause of the progressive changes in neurotransmitter profile (see p. 1030) remains obscure.

CLINICAL FEATURES

There is the combination of tremor, rigidity and akinesia, together with important changes in posture.

Symptoms

The most common symptoms are tremor and slowness of movement. Patients also complain that the limbs feel stiff and ache and that fine movements are difficult. The slowness of movement causes the characteristic symptoms of difficulty in rising from a chair or getting into or out of bed. Writing becomes small (micrographia) and spidery, with a tendency to tail off at the end of a line. Other evidence of the disease often comes from relatives who have noted slowness and an impassive facial expression. The disease is almost always more prominent on one side.

Signs

The diagnosis is often made immediately from the overall appearance of the patient.

Tremor

This is a characteristic 4–7 Hz rest tremor that is usually decreased by action and increased by emotion. Pill-rolling movements between the thumb and forefinger are seen.

Rigidity

Stiffness of the limbs develops that can be felt throughout the range of movement and is equal in opposing groups of muscles, in contrast to the selective increase in tone found in spasticity. This lead pipe-like rigidity is often more marked on one side and is also present in the neck and axial muscles, where it is difficult to examine.

The rigidity is usually more easily felt when a joint is moved slowly and gently. Simultaneous active movement of the opposite limb increases the tone of the side under examination. When combined with tremor, the smooth plasticity of the increase in tone is broken up into a jerky resistance to passive movement, a phenomenon known as cogwheeling, or cogging.

Akinesia

Poverty and slowing of movement (bradykinesia) is an additional handicap, distinct from rigidity. There is difficulty in initiating movement. Rapid fine finger movements, such as piano-playing, become indistinct, slow and tremulous. The immobility of the face gives a mask-like facies with the appearance of depression. The frequency of spontaneous blinking is reduced, producing a serpentine stare.

Postural changes

A stoop is characteristic and the gait is shuffling, festinant and with poor arm swinging. The posture is sometimes called 'simian' to describe the ape-like forward flexion, immobility of the arms and lack of facial expression. The patient sits with the trunk bent forward and motionless, without gesture or animation, while the limbs are tremulous. Balance is impaired, but despite this the gait remains on a narrow base. Falls are common as the usual corrective righting reflexes fail, the sufferer falling stiffly, like a falling tree.

Speech

Speech is at first monotonous, progressing to a characteristic tremulous slurring dysarthria, owing to the combination of akinesia, tremor and rigidity. Dribbling is frequent, and dysphagia develops as the disease worsens.

Power remains normal until advanced akinesia makes its assessment difficult. There is no sensory loss. Patients often complain of discomfort in the limbs and joints. The reflexes become brisk; their asymmetry follows the increase in tone. The plantar responses remain flexor.

Cognitive function is preserved, at least early in the condition. Dementia sometimes develops in the late stages.

Gastrointestinal and other symptoms

These include heartburn, dysphagia, constipation and weight loss. Urinary difficulties are common, especially in men. The skin is greasy and sweating is excessive.

Natural history

Parkinson's disease progresses over a period of years, beginning as a mild inconvenience but slowly overtaking the patient. Remissions are unknown except for rare and remarkable short-lived periods of release. These tend to occur at times of great emotion, fear or excitement, when the sufferer is released for seconds or minutes and able to move quickly.

The rate of progression is very variable, with a benign form running over several decades. Usually the course is over 10–15 years, with death resulting from bronchopneumonia.

DIFFERENTIAL DIAGNOSIS

There is no laboratory test for the disease. The diagnosis is made by recognizing the clinical pattern. Imaging is unhelpful. The condition must be distinguished from other akinetic–rigid syndromes. Hypothyroidism and depression also cause slowing of movement.

Certain diffuse or multifocal brain diseases cause some features of parkinsonism, particularly the slowing, rigidity and tremor seen in idiopathic Parkinson's. Examples are Alzheimer's disease, multi-infarct dementia, and the sequelae of repeated head injury (e.g. in boxers, see p. 1114), or the late effects of severe hypoxia or carbon monoxide poisoning.

TREATMENT

Older treatments with anticholinergic drugs altered the disease little, and frequently caused mental confusion. Of these, benzhexol is still used in mild cases and as an adjunct to other therapy. Amantadine, originally introduced as an antiviral agent, is also sometimes helpful.

Levodopa

Levodopa is combined with an aromatic amino acid decarboxylase inhibitor – benserazide (co-beneldopa, as Madopar) or carbidopa (co-careldopa, as Sinemet). The drugs are interchangeable. This combined therapy reduces the peripheral side-effects, principally nausea, of levodopa alone and its metabolites. L-Dopa undergoes *O*-methylation by catechol-*O*-methyltransferase (COMT), inhibitors of which will shortly be available, allowing lower doses of L-dopa to be used.

Treatment is commenced gradually (co-beneldopa 125 mg or co-careldopa 110 mg, one tablet three times daily) and increased until either an adequate improvement has taken place or side-effects limit further increase in dose.

The great majority of patients with idiopathic Parkinson's disease (but not other parkinsonian syndromes) improve initially with levodopa. The response in severe, previously untreated disease is sometimes dramatic.

Unwanted effects of levodopa therapy

Nausea and vomiting within an hour of treatment are the most common symptoms of the dose being too large. Confusion and visual hallucinations also occur with excessive doses. Chorea occurs in acute overdose.

There are difficult issues with long-term levodopa and therapy should not be started until necessary. Sometimes the drug becomes ineffective, even with increasing doses. As the disease progresses, the patient suffers from episodes of severe immobility, known as freezing, and falls. Fluctuation in the response to levodopa also develops, its effect apparently turning on and off. Dopa-induced dyskesias, chorea and dystonic movements appear. The duration of action of the drug shrinks, with dyskinesia becoming prominent at the end of the duration of action of the dose of levodopa ('end-of-dose dyskinesia').

The treated patient begins to suffer not only from Parkinson's disease but also from a chronic levodopa-induced syndrome, fluctuating between dopa-induced dyskinesias and severe and sometimes sudden immobility ('on-off syndrome').

Levodopa therapy does not appear to alter the natural progression of the disease itself. After five years' treatment, around half the patients with Parkinson's are suffering from minor or major unwanted effects of therapy. These more distressing problems are difficult and often largely insoluble. Approaches to treatment of these complications include the following:

- The interval between levodopa doses is shortened; individual doses may need to be increased.
- Selegiline, a type B monoamine oxidase inhibitor, inhibits the catabolism of dopamine in the brain. This sometimes has the effect of smoothing out the response to levodopa. It has been suggested that there is an increased morbidity from cardiovascular disease in patients taking selegiline, but this remains unproven.
- Oral dopaminergic agonists (see below) are used, to add, or replace existing levodopa therapy.
- Apomorphine, a directly acting dopinergic agonist, given by daily subcutaneous infusion, is probably the best method of smoothing out the fluctuations in response. Skilled nursing help is required to train patients and their relatives to administer the drug. An unusual side-effect of apomorphine is severe haemolytic anaemia.
- Drug holidays – periods of drug withdrawal – are sometimes helpful. They require close supervision since severe rigidity and akinesia follow the withdrawal of levodopa.

Dopaminergic agonists

Bromocriptine, lysuride, pergolide are directly acting dopaminergic agonists, acting principally on D_1 and D_2 receptors, and also on other receptors D_{3-5}. Additional drugs are being marketed. These are used as an alternative or an addition to levodopa therapy.

Dopaminergic agonists are in general less effective in treating the symptoms of Parkinson's disease, but are associated with fewer late unwanted dyskinetic effects.

There is much variation in clinical practice between the different regimes of levodopa and dopaminergic agonists, either singly or in combination. Some neurologists tend to use dopaminergic agonists as a primary treatment, before levodopa. There is a trend towards delaying the start of drug treatment until this is clinically essential.

Other agents

Antioxidant compounds such as vitamins C and E possibly help the progression of the condition and are sometimes prescribed. Their role is uncertain.

Neurosurgery

Stereotactic placement of small lesions, usually unilaterally in the ventrolateral nucleus of the thalamus or globus pallidus, was used widely before the advent of levodopa. When successful the procedures still provide effective, if temporary improvement in severe tremor.

Attempts to transplant fetal or autologous dopamine-containing adrenal medulla to the cerebral ventricles or basal ganglia, though technically feasible, have not produced any major clinical improvement in the majority of patients with Parkinson's disease despite some early promise, and compelling laboratory studies in rats with MPTP-induced parkinsonism. Experimental studies continue.

Physiotherapy and physical aids

Skilled and determined physiotherapy can improve the gait and help the patient to overcome particular problems. Practical guidance is of value about:

- clothing – avoiding zips, fiddly buttons and lace-up shoes.
- cutlery – using built-up handles.
- chairs – high, upright chairs are easier to rise from than deep, comfortable armchairs
- rails – should be fitted near the lavatory and bath
- shoes – should be easy to put on and have smooth soles
- flooring – patients complain that their feet sometimes stick to carpets and rugs, so they prefer to walk on vinyl or linoleum.

Walking aids are often a hindrance in the early stages, but later a frame or a tripod may be helpful. All attempts must be made to prevent falls, the effects of which may be catastrophic in these patients.

Psychiatric aspects

Depression is common in Parkinson's disease as the symptoms become worse and unresponsive to treatment. It is particularly difficult to treat, since type A monoamine oxidase inhibitor antidepressants (e.g. phenelzine) are *absolutely contraindicated* with levodopa, and tricyclic antidepressants (e.g. amitriptyline) have extrapyramidal side-effects.

All antiparkinsonian drugs, especially in high doses, can bring on confusion particularly with nocturnal visual hallucinations, which may exacerbate any cognitive impairment.

Drug-induced parkinsonism

Reserpine (a drug once used in the treatment of hypertension), phenothiazines and butyrophenones induce a parkinsonian syndrome, with slowness and rigidity but usually little tremor. Methyldopa and tricyclic antidepressants also cause some slowing of movement. These unwanted effects tend not to progress. They respond poorly, if at all, to levodopa and usually disappear when the drug causing them is stopped.

Other movement disorders due to neuroleptic drugs

Neuroleptic drugs (i.e. phenothiazines and butyrophenones) also produce other varieties of movement disorder. Three are described here.

- *Akathisia*. This is a restless, repetitive and irresistible need to move.
- *Acute dystonic reactions*. These sometimes follow, dramatically and unpredictably, single doses of neuroleptics, and related drugs used as antiemetics or vestibular sedatives (such as prochlorperazine and metoclopramide). Spasmodic torticollis, trismus and oculogyric crises (i.e. episodes of sustained upward gaze) occur. These acute dystonias respond promptly to the intravenous injection of an anticholinergic drug such as benztropine (1–2 mg) or procyclidine 5–10 mg. Both the offending drug, and all drugs from the same group, should be avoided subsequently.
- *Chronic tardive dyskinesias*. These disabling disorders consist of mouthing and smacking of the lips, grimaces with contortion of the face and neck. They tend to occur several years after commencing neuroleptic therapy and may be made temporarily worse when the dose of the drug is reduced. Improvement occurs in fewer than half the cases if the neuroleptic can be stopped.

Postencephalitic parkinsonism

An epidemic of encephalitis lethargica, a condition of unknown cause, last occurred between 1918 and 1930. This disease causes an encephalitis which evolves over several weeks, with intense sleepiness as a prominent feature, and sometimes psychosis. Some of the survivors left in its wake remained permanently disabled by a severe parkinsonian syndrome with dystonic movement disorders. Levodopa produced a dramatic but temporary improvement in some of these survivors. Occasional sporadic cases of the disease are seen.

MPTP-induced parkinsonism

MPTP (1-methyl-4-phenyl-1,2,3,6-tetrahydropyridine) is an impurity produced inadvertently when opiates are synthesized illicitly. A severe and largely irreversible parkinsonian syndrome follows ingestion of minute quantities of MPTP. The relevance of this to idiopathic Parkinson's disease is not clear.

Parkinsonism-plus

This term describes rare disorders in which there is parkinsonism and evidence of a separate pathology. Progressive supranuclear palsy is the most common disorder, and consists of axial rigidity, dementia and signs of parkinsonism together with a striking inability to move the eyes vertically or laterally.

Other examples of parkinsonism-plus are the rare multiple system atrophies, such as olivopontocerebellar degeneration and primary autonomic failure (Shy–Drager syndrome).

Akinetic–rigid syndromes in children

A group of extremely rare disorders cause an akinetic–rigid syndrome primarily in those under 20 years of age. The most important are Wilson's disease and athetoid cerebral palsy.

Wilson's disease

This is a rare and treatable disorder of copper metabolism that is inherited as an autosomal recessive. There is deposition of copper in the brain, particularly in the basal ganglia, in the cornea and in the liver (see p. 326), where it causes cirrhosis. It is most important that all young patients with cirrhosis are screened for this condition, as the neurological damage is irreversible unless early treatment is instituted.

Children with the disease have an akinetic–rigid syndrome and/or dyskinesias followed by progressive intellectual impairment.

Diagnosis and treatment with the chelating agent penicillamine is mentioned on p. 327.

Athetoid cerebral palsy

Writhing movements of the limbs, sometimes with dystonia, are seen in cerebral palsy following kernicterus. The dystonia tends to progress. The condition is now much less common following the prophylactic treatment of rhesus haemolytic disease.

Dyskinesias

Benign essential tremor

This common condition, often inherited as an autosomal dominant trait, causes tremor at 5–8 Hz that is usually worse in the upper limbs. The head is often tremulous (titubation) and also the trunk. Pathologically there is patchy neuronal loss in the cerebellum and cerebellar connections. Tremor is seen when the hands adopt a posture, such as holding a glass or a spoon. Oscillations are not usually present at rest nor do they worsen on movement.

Essential tremor may be seen at any age but occurs most frequently in the elderly. It is slowly progressive but rarely produces a severe disability. Writing is shaky and untidy but there is no micrographia. Anxiety exacerbates the tremor, sometimes dramatically.

Treatment is often unnecessary. Many of those affected are reassured to find they do not have Parkinson's disease, with which the condition is often confused.

Small doses of alcohol and β-adrenergic blockers such as propranolol often reduce the tremor. The anticonvulsant primidone also helps some patients. Sympathomimetics (e.g. salbutamol) make the tremor worse.

The tremor is usually postural, although in some cases it occurs at rest, as in Parkinson's disease or with action, as in cerebellar disease.

Chorea

Chorea consists of jerky, quasi-purposive and sometimes explosive fidgety movements, following each other but flitting from one part of the body to another. The principal causes of chorea are listed in Table 18.39; the most common conditions are outlined below.

Huntington's disease

Relentlessly progressive chorea and dementia in middle life are the hallmarks of this inherited disease.

The prevalence of the disease is about 5 in 100 000. It occurs worldwide. Inheritance is as an autosomal dominant trait with full penetrance; the children of an affected parent have a 50% chance of inheriting the disease. The family history of the disease in previous generations is often concealed, either by design or default. A mutation has been identified at the distal short arm of chromosome 4 with an abnormal sequence of randomly repeated trinucleotides (p. 147). The expansion of a CAG-repeat sequence in DNA results in the translation of an extended glutamine sequence in the protein product of the gene (called *huntingtin*). This protein is ubiquitously expressed but its function is as yet unknown.

Table 18.39
Causes of chorea

Huntington's disease
Sydenham's chorea
Benign hereditary chorea
Abetalipoproteinaemia (see p. 259) with chorea
Chorea associated with:
- Drugs – phenytoin, levodopa, alcohol
- Thyrotoxicosis, pregnancy and oral contraceptive pill
- Systemic lupus erythematosus
- Polycythaemia vera
- Encephalitis lethargica
- Stroke (basal ganglia)
- Rarities (tumour, trauma, subdural haematoma, carbon monoxide poisoning)

Pathology

There is cerebral atrophy with marked loss of small neurones in the caudate nucleus and putamen. Three changes in neurotransmitters occur:

- reduction in the enzymes synthesizing acetylcholine (choline acetyl transferase) and GADA in the striatum
- depletion of GABA, angiotensin-converting enzyme and met-enkephalin in the substantia nigra
- high somatostatin levels in the corpus striatum.

These changes may be secondary to the cell damage. In contrast to Parkinson's disease, dopamine and tyrosine hydroxylase activity are normal.

Management and course

Other causes of chorea should be considered and investigated. Imaging in Huntington's, if it is possible with the chorea, shows atrophy of the caudate nucleus.

There is steady progression, of both the dementia and chorea. No treatment arrests the disease, although phenothiazines (e.g. sulpiride) may reduce the chorea, by causing drug-induced parkinsonism. Tetrabenazine helps to control the movements. Death usually occurs between 10 and 20 years after the onset.

Mutation analysis, which is accurate and specific, is available for presymptomatic testing of family members. This raises ethical problems: centres performing these tests have a common protocol for counselling.

Sydenham's chorea (St Vitus' dance)

This is a postinfective chorea occurring largely in children and young adults. Fewer than half the cases follow within three months of rheumatic fever (see p. 699). It may recur, or appear, in adult life during pregnancy as chorea gravidarum or in those taking hormonal contraceptives. In each case there is a diffuse mild encephalitis.

The onset of the chorea is usually gradual over a few weeks. Irritability, emotional lability, and inattentiveness herald the onset of fidgety movements, which are sometimes predominantly unilateral. A minority of patients become confused. Although rheumatic heart disease is sometimes found, the patient usually does not have a fever or other features of rheumatic fever. The antistreptolysin-O (ASO) titre and ESR are sometimes normal. Patients may require sedation but recovery occurs spontaneously within weeks or months. Phenoxymethyl penicillin should be given until the age of 20, to prevent rheumatic heart disease.

Hemiballismus

Hemiballismus (also called hemiballism) describes violent swinging movements of one side of the body caused usually by infarction or haemorrhage in the contralateral subthalamic nucleus.

Myoclonus

Myoclonus is the sudden, involuntary jerking of a single muscle or a group of muscles. It occurs in a wide range of disorders and is sometimes provoked by a sudden stimulus such as a loud noise.

Benign essential myoclonus

Nocturnal myoclonus – sudden jerking of a limb or the body on falling asleep – is extremely common and not pathological.

Paramyoclonus multiplex describes widespread, random muscle jerking usually occurring in adolescence. Fits do not occur.

Myoclonus in epilepsy

Muscle jerking is a feature of many different forms of epilepsy.

Progressive myoclonic epilepsies

These very rare conditions include various familial and metabolic disorders where myoclonus accompanies a progressive encephalopathy. An example is Lafora body disease, a syndrome of myoclonus, epilepsy and dementia, with mucopolysaccharide inclusion bodies in neurones, liver cells and intestinal mucosa.

Static myoclonic encephalopathy

Non-progressive myoclonus is sometimes seen following recovery from a severe brain insult such as severe cerebral anoxia after cardiac arrest.

Tics

Repetitive twitching movements of the face, neck or hand are part of our normal motor gestures. Patients or their relatives seek advice about them when they become too frequent or irritating. Simple transient tics (e.g. sniffing or a particular facial grimace) are common in childhood, but may persist into adult life. The borderland between normal and pathological is vague.

Gilles de la Tourette syndrome

This rare syndrome is the occurrence of multiple tics accompanied by explosive barking and grunting utterances of sexual obscenities and gestures. The condition develops in childhood or adolescence, more commonly in males, and is lifelong. It is an organic basal ganglia disorder, of unknown cause. Treatment with haloperidol is sometimes helpful.

Torsion dystonias

Dystonia means a movement caused by a prolonged muscular contraction – part of the body is thrown into spasm. A brief explanatory classification of these unusual conditions is given in Table 18.40. Their cause is largely unknown, but they are classified as organic diseases of the basal ganglia.

Dystonia musculorum deformans

This rare and very distressing disease is usually inherited. There are various modes of transmission. Dystonic spasms of the limbs affecting gait and posture commence in childhood, and progress, spreading to all parts of the body over one to four decades. Cognitive function is largely not impaired. Spontaneous remissions very occasionally occur.

Spasmodic torticollis

Dystonic spasms gradually develop around the neck, usually in the third to fifth decade. These cause the head to turn (torticollis) or to be drawn backwards (retrocollis) or forwards (antecollis). Minor dystonic movements often also affect the trunk or limbs. A curious feature in some patients is a single trigger area, often situated on the jaw. A gentle touch with a fingertip at this one site relieves the involuntary movement, temporarily.

Torticollis may remit but many cases remain for life.

Writer's cramp

This is a specific inability to perform a previously highly developed skilled movement, especially writing, owing to a curious dystonic posturing. It occurs particularly in those who spend many hours each day writing, and is thus seen less frequently now than in former years. Other skilled functions of the hand are normal and there are no other neurological signs. Prolonged rest sometimes seems to help the condition. It can, however, become a major disability.

Blepharospasm and oromandibular dystonia

These related conditions consist of spasms of forced blinking or involuntary movement of the mouth and tongue (e.g. lip-smacking and protrusion of the tongue and jaw). Speech may be affected.

TREATMENT

All dystonic movement disorders are particularly difficult to improve with drugs. Butyrophenones (e.g. haloperidol and sulpiride) and anticholinergics (e.g. benzhexol) are sometimes helpful. Botulinum toxin carefully sited by injection can help, temporarily, blepharospasm, torticollis and writer's

Table 18.40
A classification of dystonias

Generalized dystonia
Dystonia musculorum deformans
Drug-induced dystonia (e.g. metoclopramide)
Symptomatic dystonia (e.g. after encephalitis lethargica or in Wilson's disease)
Paroxysmal dystonia (very rare, familial, with marked fluctuation)

Focal dystonia
Spasmodic torticollis
Writer's cramp
Oromandibular dystonia
Blepharospasm
Hemiplegic dystonia (e.g. following stroke)

cramp. Neurosurgical approaches to treatment, principally stereotactic thalamotomy for torticollis, or neurostimulation bring some temporary alleviation in selected cases.

FURTHER READING

Marsden CD, Fahn S (eds) (1987) Movement Disorders. London: Butterworths.

Multiple sclerosis (MS)

PREVALENCE

MS is a common disease of unknown cause in which there are multiple plaques of demyelination within the brain and spinal cord. These are disseminated in time and place, hence the old name *disseminated sclerosis*. There is a genetic predisposition but an acquired defect in the oligodendroglial cells that produce myelin is believed to be responsible.

The most common age of onset is between 20 and 45 years, the disease being more common in women. In the UK, MS causes disability of varying degree in over 50 000 people.

The disease occurs worldwide, but the prevalence varies widely, being directly proportional to the distance from the equator. At latitudes of 50 to 65 degrees north, roughly from southern England to Iceland, the prevalence is 60–100 per 100 000 people; at latitudes less than 30 degrees north the prevalence is less than 10 per 100 000; and at the equator it is a rarity. In the southern hemisphere the trend is similar, with progressive increase in prevalence away from the equator.

AETIOLOGY

The cause of the disease is unknown.

Familial incidence, HLA linkage and migration

First-degree relatives of a patient have an increased chance of developing MS, although there is no clear-cut pattern of inheritance. There is an increased concordance amongst monozygotic twins.

In Caucasians in northern Europe and the USA, there is a positive association between MS and antigens HLA-A3, B7, D2 and DR2.

Immigrants from low to high prevalence zones (e.g. from near the equator to northern Europe) acquire the prevalence of the country of their destination, provided they arrive before the age of 10 years.

Infection

Although efforts to transmit MS experimentally have been uniformly unsuccessful, there is an abnormal immune response in MS patients, with an increase in the titres of serum and CSF antibodies to many common viruses, particularly measles.

It has been suggested that certain epidemic transmissible zoonoses, such as scrapie, the demyelinating disease in sheep, have some similarities to MS. Human T-cell leukaemia virus 1 (HTLV-1) infection in humans causes tropical spastic paraparesis (see p. 1029), an example of a viral demyelinating disease. There are, however, no definite links between MS and any known infective illness.

Diet

It has been suggested that MS is related to the consumption of large quantities of animal fats. Surveys in Norway have shown that MS is distinctly uncommon in coastal fishing communities compared with agri-cultural areas. However, the role of diet is particularly difficult to evaluate.

PATHOLOGY (see Fig 18.21)

The essential features are plaques of demyelination, initially 2–10 mm in size. These lesions are perivenular and have a predilection for the following sites within the brain and spinal cord:

- optic nerves
- periventricular region
- brainstem and its cerebellar connections
- cervical spinal cord – corticospinal tracts and posterior columns.

Plaques rarely destroy large groups of neighbouring anterior horn cells in the spinal cord – so that focal muscle wasting is unusual. Demyelination in MS never occurs in the myelin sheaths of peripheral nerves. The mechanism of relapse and remission of symptoms is unclear.

CLINICAL FEATURES

No single group of signs or symptoms is entirely diagnostic of MS. Despite this, the disease is often recognizable on clinical grounds. There are two principal patterns:

- relapsing and remitting MS with lesions occurring in different parts of the CNS at different times
- chronic progressive MS (some 30% of cases).

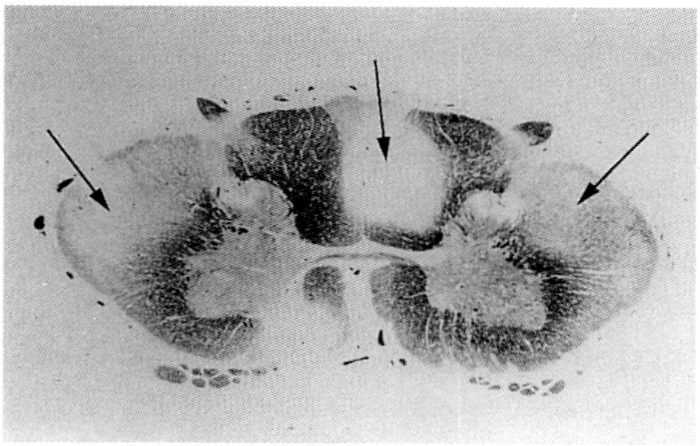

Fig 18.21
Multiple sclerosis
Cross-section of the spinal cord showing demyelination (arrows) in the posterior column and lateral corticospinal tracts. (Courtesy of Professor WI Macdonald)

Three characteristic and common presentations of relapsing and remitting MS are described below.

Optic neuropathy (ON)

Symptoms

The patient complains of blurring of vision in one eye, over hours or days, varying from a sensation of looking through frosted glass to more severe unilateral visual loss, but rarely complete blindness. Mild ocular pain is usual. Recovery occurs, typically within one or two months. Bilateral ON occasionally occurs.

Signs

The optic disc appearance depends upon the site of the plaque within the optic nerve. When the lesion is in the nerve head there is disc swelling (optic neuritis). If the lesion is several millimetres behind the disc there are often no ophthalmoscopic features – 'the doctor sees nothing and the patient sees nothing'. This is retrobulbar neuritis.

Worsening of vision in ON during a fever, in hot weather or after exercise is known as Uthoff's phenomenon – central conduction is slowed by an increase in local body temperature.

Disc swelling from optic neuritis causes early and measurable visual acuity loss, thus distinguishing it from disc swelling from raised intracranial pressure. Such papilloedema causes late and sudden visual loss when it occurs at all.

A relative afferent pupillary defect (see p. 1017) is often present from the early stages. This may persist after recovery.

Late sequelae

There are usually no residual symptoms, but small scotomata and defects in colour vision can be demonstrated. Following the attack, disc pallor appears (optic atrophy), first in the temporal region. The visual evoked responses (VER) remain abnormal (see below).

Brainstem demyelination

An acute episode affecting the brainstem causes diplopia, vertigo, facial numbness and/or weakness or dysphagia. Pyramidal signs in the limbs occur when the corticospinal tracts are involved.

A typical picture is sudden diplopia and vertigo with nystagmus, but without tinnitus or deafness. This lasts for some weeks before recovery. Diplopia in MS is the result of many different lesions – a sixth-nerve lesion and internuclear ophthalmoplegia (INO) are two examples.

Spinal cord lesion

A spastic paraparesis developing over days or weeks (see p. 1029) is the typical result of a plaque of demyelination in the cervical or thoracic cord. There is difficulty in walking and sensory disturbance. Lhermitte's sign may be present (see p. 1034). Urinary symptoms are common.

Unusual presentations

Epilepsy occurs more commonly in MS patients than in the general population. So, too, does trigeminal neuralgia (see p. 1021). Tonic spasms or brief spasms of a limb are other unusual symptoms of this disease. Dementia or organic psychosis is occasionally a feature of early MS.

In an isolated neurological event it is often impossible to be sure, even with MR imaging, whether or not a lesion is due to demyelination. The pattern of subsequent lesions allows the clinical diagnosis to be made. Remissions may last for several or more years; their length is unpredictable.

End-stage multiple sclerosis

In the later stages of the disease the patient is severely disabled with a combination of spastic tetraparesis, ataxia, optic atrophy, nystagmus, brainstem signs (e.g. bilateral INO), pseudobulbar palsy, and incontinence of urine. Dementia is common. Death follows from uraemia and/or bronchopneumonia.

DIFFERENTIAL DIAGNOSIS

Few other neurological diseases of young people follow a similar relapsing and remitting course. Thromboembolism causes events with more sudden onset. Other degenerative conditions, such as Friedreich's ataxia, are gradually progressive, without remissions.

Initially individual plaques (e.g. in the optic nerve, brainstem or cord) may cause diagnostic difficulty; they must be distinguished from compressive, inflammatory, mass or vascular lesions.

CNS sarcoidosis, SLE and Behçet's syndrome may mimic the pattern of relapsing MS. Adrenoleucodystrophy (a disorder of saturated fatty acid deposition in lipid-containing tissues) can cause a paraparesis with signs compatible with chronic progressive MS.

INVESTIGATIONS

MRI of the brain and spinal cord is the first-line investigation where it is available. Multiple plaques are visible, principally in the periventricular region (Fig 18.22), brainstem, and cervical cord. Lesions are rarely visible on CT. Examination of peripheral blood, urine and plain X-rays is unhelpful.

With diagnostic MR images and a compatible clinical picture, CSF examination is often unnecessary but would show, in 80% of cases, oligoclonal IgG bands indicating immunoglobulin production within the CNS in response to an unknown antigen, and a raised mononuclear cell count of 5–60 cells/mm^3.

Electrophysiological tests

Delay in the visual-evoked response (VER) follows optic neuropathy. As some ON attacks are subclinical, a delayed VER can provide evidence of a previous lesion within the CNS in, for example, an undiagnosed and apparently solitary spinal cord lesion.

Brainstem and somatosensory evoked potentials become delayed when these pathways have been damaged.

Peripheral nerve studies are normal. EEG recordings are unhelpful.

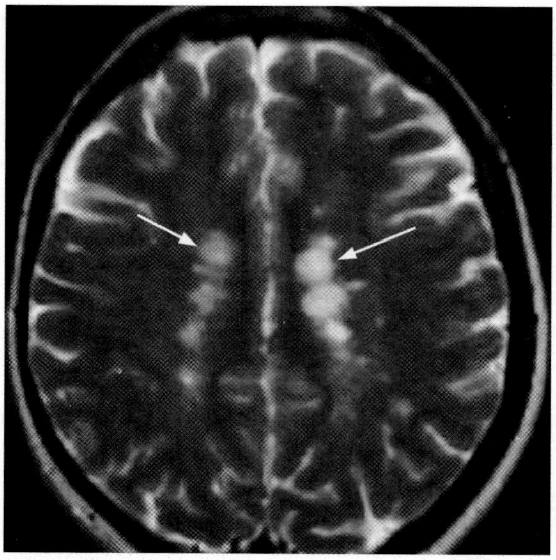

Fig 18.22
Multiple areas of high signal (arrows) on T2-weighted images in the periventricular white matter in a patient with multiple sclerosis

MANAGEMENT AND PROGNOSIS

Once diagnosed, practical decisions need to be taken about employment, home and plans for the future in the face of a potentially disabling disease for which there is no curative treatment. It is essential to inform patients of the diagnosis when it is certain.

There is no method of predicting the course of MS but there is wide variation in its severity. Many MS patients continue to live self-sufficient, productive lives while others are gravely disabled.

Straightforward advice, tempered with reassurance of the benign course of many cases of MS, is important. The MS Society, a national UK charity, and others have helpful literature.

Therapy

Many forms of treatment have been suggested for MS, among them cryotherapy, pyrotherapy, radiotherapy, various vaccines, purified TB protein derivative (PPD), transfer factor, electrical stimulation, gluten-free diets, sunflower seed oil, arsenicals and hyperbaric oxygen. None has been shown to improve outcome.

- Short courses of ACTH and corticosteroids, such as i.v. methylprednisolone for several days, are used widely in relapses and do sometimes reduce their severity. They do not influence long-term outcome.
- Immunosuppressants (azathioprine, cyclophosphamide) are also used, but there is little agreement about their value.
- β-Interferon has been used for patients with relapsing remitting disease (characterized by at least two recurrences of neurological dysfunction over the preceding three years) without evidence of progression of disability. β-Interferon, by self-administered injection, reduces the relapse rate by a third and prevents an increase in the number of lesions seen on MRI over time. Long-term outcome, in terms of decreased disability, has not been shown to be altered. For side effects see p. 311. Cost–benefit analyses are a source of serious concern, because the treatment is prolonged and expensive.
- Other new therapies, including copolymer-1 and glatiramer acetate, are being evaluated.

In any chronic neurological disease, treatment of intercurrent infections is important. Urinary infection frequently exacerbates the symptoms.

Physiotherapy is of particular value in reducing the pain and discomfort of spasticity, particularly when there are flexor spasms of the lower limbs. Muscle relaxants (e.g. baclofen, benzodiazepines and dantrolene) are also sometimes helpful. Prevention of pressure sores is vital.

General measures in chronic neurological disease

There is much that can be done for a patient with any chronic disabling disease. Practical advice at work, on walking aids, wheelchairs, car conversions, alterations to houses and gardens is required. Support in a wide range of areas from fear and reactive depression to the sexual difficulties of the disabled is also helpful. Liaison between medical practitioners, physiotherapists, occupational therapists and social workers is helpful.

FURTHER READING

Rudick RA *et al.* (1997) Management of multiple sclerosis. *New England Journal of Medicine* **337**: 1604–1611.

β-Interferon in MS (1998) *Drug and Therapeutics Bulletin* **36**: 7–8.

Infective and inflammatory disease

Meningitis

Meningitis means inflammation of the meninges. It may be caused by:

- bacteria
- viruses
- fungi
- other organisms
- malignant cells
- drugs and contrast media
- blood (following SAH).

The word 'meningitis' usually describes inflammation owing to infective agents (Table 18.41). Micro-organisms reach the meninges either by direct extension from the

Table 18.41
Infective causes of meningitis in the UK

Bacteria	
Neisseria meningitidis[a]	
Streptococcus pneumoniae[a]	
Staphylococcus aureus	
Listeria monocytogenes	
Gram-negative bacilli	
Mycobacterium tuberculosis	
Treponema pallidum	
Viruses	
Enteroviruses	
Echo	
Coxsackie	
Polio	
Mumps	
Herpes simplex	
HIV	
Epstein–Barr virus	
Fungi	
Cryptococcus neoformans	
Candida	
(*Coccidioides immitis*, *Histoplasma capsulatum*, *Blastomyces dermatitidis* in USA)	

[a]These organisms account for 70% of acute bacterial meningitis outside the neonatal period. A wide variety of infective agents are responsible for the remaining 30% of cases. *Haemophilus influenzae b* has been eliminated as a cause in the UK by immunization

ears, nasopharynx, a cranial injury or congenital meningeal defect, or by spread via the bloodstream.

Immunocompromised patients (HIV and those taking cytotoxic drugs) are at an increased risk of meningeal infection by unusual organisms.

PATHOLOGY

In acute bacterial meningitis, the pia-arachnoid is congested with polymorphs. A layer of pus forms that may organize to form adhesions, causing cranial nerve palsies and hydrocephalus.

In chronic infection (e.g. TB), the brain is covered in a viscous greyish green exudate with numerous meningeal tubercles. Adhesions are typically seen. Cerebral oedema is common in any bacterial meningitis.

In viral meningitis there is a predominantly lymphocytic inflammatory reaction in the CSF without pus formation or adhesions. There is no cerebral oedema unless viral encephalitis develops.

CLINICAL FEATURES

The meningitic syndrome

This means the triad of headache, neck stiffness and fever. Photophobia and vomiting are often present.

In acute bacterial infection, there is intense malaise, fever, rigors, severe headache, photophobia and vomiting, developing within hours or minutes. The patient is irritable and often prefers to lie still. Neck stiffness and a positive Kernig's sign appear within hours.

Table 18.42
Clinical clues in meningitis

Clinical feature	Probable cause
Petechial rash	Meningococcal infection
Skull fracture Ear disease Congenital CNS lesion	Pneumococcal infection
Immunocompromised patients	HIV opportunistic infection
Rash or pleurodynia	Enterovirus infection
International travel	Poliomyelitis Malaria
Occupational history (working with drains, canals, polluted river water), recreational swimming: prostration, myalgia, conjunctivitis and jaundice	Leptospirosis

In less severe cases (e.g. many viral meningitides) there are often few other signs, but fatal bacterial infection may also be indolent, with a deceptively mild onset. Clinical severity itself is diagnostically unreliable.

In uncomplicated meningitis, consciousness is not impaired, although the patient with a high fever may be delirious. Progressive drowsiness, lateralizing signs and cranial nerve lesions indicate complications such as venous sinus thrombosis (see p. 1054), severe cerebral oedema or hydrocephalus, or an alternative diagnosis such as cerebral abscess (see p. 1077) or encephalitis (p. 1073). Papilloedema may develop in any of these complications.

Specific varieties of meningitis

Features readily visible on examination, such as rashes, or the presence of middle ear or paranasal sinus infection, point to a diagnosis (Table 18.42).

Acute bacterial meningitis

The onset is typically sudden, with rigors and a high fever. A petechial rash, often sparse, is strong evidence of meningococcal meningitis. Septicaemia may present with acute septicaemic shock. *Haemophilus influenzae type b* infection has been virtually eliminated in developed countries by immunization.

Viral meningitis

This is almost always a benign, self-limiting condition lasting 4–10 days. Headache may follow for some weeks but there are no serious sequelae.

Chronic meningitis

Tuberculosis or cryptococcal meningitis commences with vague headache, lassitude, anorexia and vomiting. Meningitic signs may take some weeks to develop. Drowsiness, focal signs and seizures are common. Syphilis, sarcoidosis and Behçet's syndrome can also cause chronic meningitis. In some cases a cause is never found.

Malignant meningitis

Malignant cells can cause a subacute or chronic non-infective meningitic process. A meningitic syndrome, cranial nerve palsies, paraparesis and root lesions are seen, often in complex and fluctuating patterns. The CSF cell count is raised, with high protein and low glucose. Treatment is with intrathecal cytotoxic agents, but the prognosis is poor.

DIFFERENTIAL DIAGNOSIS

It may be difficult to distinguish between the sudden headache of subarachnoid haemorrhage, migraine and acute meningitis. Meningitis should be considered seriously in anyone with a sudden headache, and anyone with headache and fever. Neck stiffness should be assessed carefully – it may not be obvious. Chronic meningitis sometimes resembles an intracranial mass lesion, with headache, epilepsy and focal signs. Cerebral malaria can mimic bacterial meningitis.

MANAGEMENT

The recognition and immediate treatment of acute bacterial meningitis is vital. The condition is lethal, and even with optimal care the mortality is around 15%. In this acute illness, minutes save lives.

When meningococcal meningitis is diagnosed clinically by the petechial rash, immediate parenteral antibiotic treatment should be given before any investigations. Lumbar puncture is usually contraindiciated if the clinical diagnosis is meningococcal disease, because coning of the cerebellar tonsils may follow – the organism is found by blood culture. If a presumptive diagnosis of the organism can be made (e.g. pneumococcus is likely when there is sinus infection or skull fracture), treatment should also be started immediately. A scheme for the immediate antibiotic treatment in acute bacterial meningitis is given in Table 18.43. Antibiotic resistance is a concern and vancomycin has been recommended.

Thereafter, if there is any suspicion of an intracranial mass lesion, an immediate CT scan should be carried out.

Table 18.43
Antibiotics and acute bacterial meningitis

Organism	Antibiotic	Alternative
Unknown pyogenic	Cefotaxime	Benzylpenicillin and chloramphenicol
Meningococcus	Benzylpenicillin	Cefotaxime
Pneumococcus	Cefotaxime	Penicillin
Haemophilus	Cefotaxime	Chloramphenicol

Immediate lumbar puncture should follow, if this is deemed safe. Typical changes in the CSF are shown in Table 18.44. CSF pressure is characteristically elevated. Blood should be taken for cultures and glucose level as well as for routine tests. Chest and skull films should be taken if possible.

Gram-staining of the CSF demonstrates organisms (e.g. Gram-positive intracellular diplococci – pneumococcus; Gram-negative cocci – meningococcus). Ziehl–Nielsen stain demonstrates acid-fast bacilli (tuberculosis), though these organisms are rarely numerous. Indian ink stains fungi.

It cannot be emphasized enough that meticulous attention should focus on microbiological studies in suspected CNS infection. Close liaison between clinician and microbiologist is essential. Specific techniques (e.g. polymerase chain reaction to identify meningococci or other bacteria) are sometimes invaluable. Repeated diagnostic CSF examination is often necessary in chronic infection such as TB or fungi. Syphilitic serology should always be carried out.

The clinical picture and CSF examination should thus allow a presumptive diagnosis of the cause of meningitis to be made within several hours. Patients with impaired consciousness should be nursed as described on p. 1046.

It is often possible to distinguish between viral, pyogenic, tuberculous and other organisms from the clinical setting and immediate examination of the CSF. If bacterial meningitis is diagnosed, discussion with the microbiologist should extend to the choice of antibiotics, drug resistance, recent infections in the locality, and questions of barrier nursing and prophylaxis.

In bacterial meningitis in children, dexamethasone is also given as this reduces the frequency of complications, particularly deafness.

Tuberculous meningitis is treated for at least nine months with antituberculous drugs; rifampicin, isoniazid and pyrazinamide is the usual combination (p. 804).

Intrathecal antibiotics are no longer given in meningitis.

Local infection (e.g. an infected paranasal sinus) should be treated, surgically if necessary. Surgical repair of depressed skull fracture or meningeal tear may be required.

Prophylaxis

Meningococcal infection condition should be notified to local public health authorities, and advice sought about immunization and prophylaxis of contacts with rifampicin. A vaccine is available against serogroup A and C meningococci.

Table 18.44
Typical changes in the CSF in meningitis

	Normal	Viral	Pyogenic	Tuberculosis
Appearance	Crystal-clear	Clear/turbid	Turbid/purulent	Turbid/viscous
Mononuclear cells	<5 mm^3	10–100 mm^3	<50 mm^3	100–300 mm^3
Polymorph cells	Nil	Nil[a]	200–300/mm^3	0–200/mm^3
Protein	0.2–0.4 g L^{-1}	0.4–0.8 g L^{-1}	0.5–2.0 g L^{-1}	0.5–3.0 g L^{-1}
Glucose	⅔ > ½ blood glucose	> ½ blood glucose	< ½ blood glucose	< ⅓ blood glucose

[a]Some polymorph cells may be seen in the early stages of viral meningitis and encephalitis

Recurrent pneumococcal meningitis, such as when there is a CSF leak following skull fracture, can be prevented by a polyvalent vaccine.

DIFFERENTIAL DIAGNOSIS OF CSF PLEOCYTOSIS

Difficulties occur in meningitis when a raised, often mixed (lymphocyte and polymorph, i.e. pleocytic) picture is found but no infecting organism. The conditions listed in Table 18.45 should be considered.

Table 18.45
Causes of CSF pleocytosis

Partially treated bacterial meningitis	Cerebral venous or arterial infection
Viral meningitis	Following subarachnoid haemorrhage
Tuberculosis or fungal infection	Encephalitis, including HIV
Neoplastic meningitis	Rare causes (e.g. cerebral malaria, sarcoidosis, Behçet's syndrome, Lyme disease)
Parameningeal foci (e.g. paranasal sinus)	
Syphilis	
Intracranial abscess	

Encephalitis

Encephalitis is inflammation of brain parenchyma. The word usually implies viral infection by a wide variety of viruses, though brain inflammation is also a complication of bacterial and fungal meningitis.

Acute viral encephalitis

In many cases a viral aetiology is presumed but not confirmed serologically or by culture. The usual organisms cultured from cases of viral encephalitis in adults in the UK are herpes simplex, Echo, Coxsackie, mumps and Epstein–Barr viruses. Adenovirus, varicella zoster, influenza, measles and other viruses are rarer causes. Rabies (see p. 64) is also a variety of viral encephalitis.

Epidemic and endemic viral encephalitides occur in many parts of the world, for example:

- Japanese encephalitis in SE Asia
- Ross River fever in Australia
- California encephalitis in the USA
- Omsk haemorrhagic fever in Russia
- Tick-borne flavivirus encephalitis in Sweden and Central Europe.

CLINICAL FEATURES

Many of these infections cause a mild self-limiting illness. In a minority there is a more serious disease. Fever, headache, mood change and drowsiness develop over several hours to several days and are accompanied by focal signs, seizures and coma. Death, or severe lasting brain injury, ensues. Herpes simplex virus (HSV-1) accounts for many of these severe infections in Britain. The mortality remains around 20% even with treatment. In South East Asia, Japanese arbovirus encephalalitis is more usual, causing a serious illness with higher mortality than herpes simplex.

DIFFERENTIAL DIAGNOSIS

This includes:

- bacterial meningitis with cerebral oedema and/or cerebral venous thrombosis
- cerebral abscess
- acute disseminated encephalomyelitis (see below)
- cerebral malaria
- toxic confusional states in febrile illnesses and in septicaemia.

INVESTIGATIONS

CT and MR imaging show diffuse areas of oedema, often in the temporal lobes. The EEG, which is useful in doubtful cases, shows characteristic slow-wave changes. A normal EEG is exceptional in encephalitis. The CSF shows cells typical of a viral aetiology (see Table 18.44). Specific viral blood and CSF serology is helpful.

Brain biopsy is now seldom performed.

TREATMENT

Suspected herpes simplex encephalitis is immediately treated with intravenous acyclovir, the active form of which inhibits DNA synthesis. Phosphorylation of this drug is dependent upon the presence of viral thymidine kinase; thus the drug is specific for herpesvirus infections. If the patient is in coma the outlook is poor whether or not drugs are given.

Supportive measures are required for comatose patients. Seizures are treated with anticonvulsants.

Prophylactic immunization is possible against Japanese encephalitis and sometimes advised for travellers to endemic areas in South East Asia.

Acute disseminated encephalomyelitis (ADE)

This follows many common viral infections (e.g. measles, varicella zoster, mumps and rubella) and rarely after immunization against rabies, influenza or pertussis. The clinical syndrome is often similar to acute viral encephalitis, with added focal brainstem and/or spinal cord lesions due to demyelination (see MS, p. 1068), but in which viral particles are not usually present. These foci are seen on T2 weighted MR images. The prognosis is variable. Mild cases recover completely, but in severe cases (those in coma) mortality is around 25% and the survivors often have permanent brain damage. Treatment is supportive, with steroids and anticonvulsants.

Myelitis

Myelitis means inflammation of the spinal cord causing paraparesis or tetraparesis. It occurs with varicella zoster or as part of a postinfective encephalomyelitis (ADE). Poliomyelitis is a specific enterovirus infection of anterior horn cells (see p. 56).

Transverse myelitis is discussed on p. 1087.

Herpes zoster (shingles)

This is a recrudescence of infection with varicella zoster virus within the dorsal root ganglia, the original infection having been acquired in an attack of chickenpox many years previously. The virus causing chickenpox and shingles is identical.

CLINICAL FEATURES

The skin changes of shingles of dorsal root ganglia are described on p. 1154.

In the cranial nerves, herpes zoster has a predilection for the fifth and seventh nerves. Ophthalmic herpes is infection of the first division of the fifth nerve and may lead to corneal scarring and secondary panophthalmitis. Geniculate herpes (the geniculate ganglion of the facial nerve), or Ramsay Hunt syndrome (see p. 1013), leads to facial palsy accompanied by vesicles on the pinna, external auditory meatus and fauces.

The local complications of shingles are secondary bacterial infection, very rarely purpura and necrosis in the affected segment (*purpura fulminans*), generalized herpes zoster, and postherpetic neuralgia.

A myelitis, meningo-encephalitis or motor radiculopathy (usually lumbar or brachial) are also caused by varicella zoster.

Treatment with acyclovir is described on p. 1155.

Postherpetic neuralgia

Postherpetic neuralgia is pain in the zone of the previous eruption; it occurs in some 10% of patients (often elderly). It is a burning, continuous pain responding poorly to all analgesics. An associated depression is almost universal. Treatment is unsatisfactory but there is a trend towards gradual recovery over two years.

Neurosyphilis

Syphilis is described on p. 101. Tertiary neurosyphilis described below is now rare. A wide variety of syndromes can occur, sometimes in mixed forms.

Asymptomatic neurosyphilis

This term describes positive CSF serology without signs.

Meningovascular syphilis

This causes:

- subacute meningitis often with cranial nerve palsies and papilloedema
- a gumma, which is a localized, chronic, expanding intracranial mass causing epilepsy, raised pressure and focal signs (e.g. hemiparesis)
- paraparesis caused by a spinal meningovasculitis.

Tabes dorsalis

This is a complex syndrome in which demyelination occurs in the dorsal roots. Many of the features are due to de-afferentation. The elements of tabes are:

- lightning pains (p. 1034)
- ataxia, stamping gait, loss of reflexes, widespread sensory loss and some muscle wasting
- neuropathic joints (Charcot's joints)
- Argyll Robertson pupils (p. 1018)
- ptosis and optic atrophy.

General paralysis of the insane (GPI)

The grandiose title describes madness and weakness. The dementia is, however, often similar to that of Alzheimer's disease (see p. 1114). Progressive cognitive decline, brisk reflexes, extensor plantar reflexes and tremor occur. Death follows within three years of the onset. Argyll Robertson pupils are usual. Seizures may occur.

Other forms of neurosyphilis

In congenital neurosyphilis (acquired *in utero*), there are features of both tabes dorsalis and GPI in childhood; this is known as *tabo-paresis*.

In secondary syphilis, a self-limiting meningeal reaction occurs that may be symptomless or may cause a subacute meningitis.

TREATMENT

Benzylpenicillin 1 g daily by injection for 10 days in primary infection eliminates the risk of future tertiary syphilis. Established neurological disease can be arrested but not usually reversed with penicillin. Parenteral penicillin for 2–3 weeks is given for all forms of neurosyphilis. Allergic reactions (Jarisch–Herxheimer reactions) may occur; high-dose steroid cover is usually given with penicillin to reduce their severity.

HIV infection and the nervous system

Individuals with HIV infection frequently present with or develop neurological disease, primarily infective and complex, which requires speedy and expert treatment. In addition, HIV-infected patients have a high rate of cerebrovascular disease. A wide variety of clinical patterns occur.

Brain and meningeal disease

Meningitis

Acute aseptic meningitis is believed to be a primary HIV infection. Spontaneous recovery is usual.

Chronic meningitis may occur with HIV itself, fungi (e.g. *Cryptococcus neoformans* or *Aspergillus*), tuberculosis, *Listeria monocytogenes*, *Escherichia coli* or other organisms. Successful treatment is difficult.

Diffuse encephalopathies

The HIV-dementia complex. This is a diffuse, progressive, usually fatal HIV-related dementia, sometimes associated with a cerebellar syndrome. It is thought to be due to cerebral HIV infection.

Encephalitis and brain abscess. Cytomegalovirus, herpes simplex, toxoplasma and other organisms cause a severe and often fatal encephalitis. Multiple brain abscesses are common.

CNS lymphoma and progressive multifocal leucoencephalopathy. These are progressive late complications of HIV infection. They are usually fatal.

Spinal cord disease

Paraparesis occurs in HIV patients in the following clinical settings:

- acute HIV transverse myelitis, a primary HIV myelitis (spontaneous recovery is usual)
- myelopathy due to infection, such as with herpes simplex, zoster or cytomegalovirus
- CNS lymphoma (tumour masses cause cord compression or malignant meningitis).

Peripheral nerve disease

Three principal patterns of HIV-related neuropathy occur:

- mononeuropathy (e.g. a common peroneal nerve lesion)
- mononeuritis multiplex (p. 1093)
- polyneuropathy (p. 1093).

MANAGEMENT OF HIV

This is discussed on p. 120.

Other nervous system infections

The nervous system is involved in many infective diseases. Some of the more important conditions are mentioned below.

Rabies (see also p. 64)

Rabies is transmitted to humans from infected animals via penetrating wounds. Rabies virus multiplies in the wound and migrates via peripheral nerves and dorsal root ganglia to the CNS. A fatal encephalitis follows.

Tetanus (see also p. 25)

Tetanus can follow even a trivial wound. There is liberation of a powerful toxin that travels within motor nerves to reach the CNS. Here toxin binds irreversibly with certain sialic acid-containing gangliosides, blocking inhibition of spinal reflexes. Severe muscular spasms follow.

Botulism (see also p. 27)

Paralytic symptoms of botulism are caused by presynaptic block in neuromuscular transmission.

Lyme disease (see also p. 47)

Involvement of the nervous system produces a radiculopathy and/or paraparesis with inflammatory CSF.

Leprosy (see also p. 41)

The infected nerves (in leprosy, called 'nerves of predeliction') become thickened, palpable and then visible. These are:

- the ulnar nerve at the elbow
- the median nerve and superficial branch of the radial at the wrist
- the greater auricular nerve at the posterior border of the sternomastoid
- the lateral popliteal nerve at the fibula head
- the posterior tibial nerve behind the medial malleolus
- the sural, superficial peroneal and supraorbital nerves.

Varying degrees of nerve thickening occur in the different forms of leprosy. Marked generalized nerve thickening is seen in leprosy of borderline-lepromatous type. A single thickened nerve, or no nerve thickening at all, is seen in tuberculoid leprosy. In all forms of this chronic disease it is persistent progressive sensory loss which leads to tissue damage and deformities. Clinically, the leprosy should be borne in mind when anyone who has resided in an endemic area presents with:

- a chronic anaesthetic patch on the skin, often hypopigmented (see Fig 1.22)
- a thickened peripheral nerve, with pain in its distribution, with or without skin lesions.

Poliomyelitis (see also p. 56)

When the nervous system is affected in this enterovirus infection, there is first a meningeal rection (a mild meningitis). Virus then invades spinal anterior horn cells and cranial nerve motor neurones to cause paralysis. Many infections are subclinical, but in a minority there is serious paralytic disease affecting limb muscles, respiratory and bulbar muscles often in a patchy and asymmetrical way. Sensation is not affected.

Creutzfeld–Jakob disease (CJD): sporadic and iatrogenic forms

This is a slowly progressive dementia developing usually after 50 years of age characterized pathologically by spongiform changes in the brain. It occurs worldwide and is transmitted by an agent resistant to many of the usual sterilization processes. CJD is one example of prion (a proteinaceous infectious particle) disease. CJD cases are usually single (sporadic CJD). Infection is also known to pass from surgical specimens and autopsy material (e.g. corneal grafts) to recipients, and from human pituitary glands to those treated with human growth hormone (iatrogenic CJD). Iatrogenic CJD has a long incubation period, sometimes up to five years. Death is invariable usually within six months of onset, in both iatrogenic and sporadic forms. No treatment alters the course of the disease.

The pathology of CJD is very similar to bovine spongiform encephalopathy (BSE) of cattle, which was recognized first in Britain in the early 1980s.

CJD: incidence, familial forms and new variant CJD (nvCJD)

Sporadic CJD occurred in Britain with a variable annual incidence between 1985 and 1997 of 20 to 55 cases. The numbers have not been rising. The incidence of iatrogenic CJD is lower, between none and 5 cases annually in the same period. Familial CJD cases, 0–4 annually in Britain, are associated with mutations of the prion protein (*PrP*) gene. An even rarer form, the Gerstmann–Straüssler–Scheinker syndrome, is an inherited autosomal recessive condition, typified by chronic progressive ataxia and terminal dementia, with duration 2–10 years.

A new variant of CJD (nvCJD) was noted in Britain in 1995. By December 1996 some 15 cases had been reported. These nvCJD cases were younger than sporadic cases, some in their 20s. Early symptoms are neuropsychiatric, followed by ataxia, and dementia with myoclonus or chorea. This nvCJD, still uniformly fatal, has a longer course than the sporadic form, of up to several years. The appearance of nvCJD has given rise to speculation that there has been, in Britain, transmission from the animal to human food chain, with infection from BSE-infected cattle to humans (p. 66). A common source of infection, for both man and cattle, is an alternative explanation.

Kuru

This dementia and cerebellar ataxia, classified as a prion disease, occurs in the highlands of New Guinea. It is believed to have been spread by ritual cannibalism. Spongiform change occurs in the brain, very similar to that in CJD.

Progressive multifocal leucoencephalopathy (see also p. 55)

Opportunistic CNS infection with the papovaviruses JC and SV-40 (and others) occurs in immunocompromised and HIV-positive patients. Multifocal viral demyelinating hemisphere lesions develop. Death occurs after one or more years.

Other infections

Other examples of infection involving the nervous system are summarized in Table 18.46. See also individual viral infections in Chapter 1.

Miscellaneous inflammatory conditions

Subacute sclerosing panencephalitis (SSPE)

Persistence of measles antigen in the CNS is believed to cause this rare late sequel of measles. Progressive mental deterioration, fits, myoclonus and pyramidal signs develop, usually in a child. Diagnosis is confirmed by the high measles antibody titre in blood and CSF. Measles immunization protects against SSPE, which is now almost unknown in the UK.

Table 18.46
Miscellaneous CNS infections

Organism	Disease	CNS manifestation
Rickettsia	Typhus Scrub typhus Rocky mountain spotted fever	Meningoencephalitis
Plasmodium falciparum	Malaria	Meningoencephalitis
Toxoplasma gondii	Toxoplasmosis	Meningoencephalitis (e.g. in AIDS)
Naegleria fowleri (a freshwater amoeba)		Meningoencephalitis
Entamoeba histolytica	Amoebiasis	Brain abscess
Trypanosoma rhodesiense *Trypanosoma gambiense*	Trypanosomiasis	Subacute encephalitis
Echinococcus granulosus	Hydatid disease	Intracranial cysts
Taenia solium	Cysticercosis	Multiple intracranial cysts
Schistosoma mansoni	Schistosomiasis	Encephalopathy Cord lesions
Strongyloides stercoralis	Strongyloidiasis	Meningoencephalitis

Progressive rubella encephalitis

Some 10 years after primary infection, this syndrome, which is rarer than SSPE, causes progressive mental impairment, fits, optic atrophy, cerebellar and pyramidal signs. Antibody to rubella viral antigen is produced locally within the CNS. This condition has not been noted following rubella immunization.

Reye's syndrome (see also p. 335)

This is a severe encephalitic illness, usually of children, accompanied by fatty infiltration of the liver and hypoglycaemia. A viral cause has been postulated but other factors, including aspirin therapy, have also been implicated.

Mollaret's meningitis

This describes recurrent episodes of aseptic meningitis (i.e. where no bacterial cause is found) over many years. A recurrent viral infection is postulated. Attacks are sometimes terminated and prevented by the antimitotic agent, colchicine.

Vogt–Koyanagi–Harada syndrome

This obscure recurrent inflammatory disease of cells of neural crest origin causes uveitis, meningoencephalitis, vitiligo, deafness and alopecia.

Myalgic encephalomyelitis (ME, epidemic neuromyasthenia, chronic fatigue syndrome, see also p. 1112)

Headache, fever, lassitude, torpor, myalgia and depression sometimes follow viral infections, such as hepatitis, infectious mononucleosis, or Coxsackie infections. It is particularly difficult to distinguish between organic and psychological elements. There is wide variation of opinion about causation.

Neurosarcoidosis

Sarcoid lesions within the nervous system, occurring either with or without systemic sarcoidosis, cause chronic meningoencephalitis, spinal cord disease, cranial nerve palsies, particularly bilateral seventh nerve lesions, polyneuropathy, and myopathy (see p. 805).

Behçet's syndrome (see also p. 497)

Behçet's three principal features are recurrent oral and/or genital ulceration, inflammatory ocular disease and neurological syndromes. Brainstem and cord lesions, aseptic meningitis (meningitic symptoms with cells in the CSF for which no infective agent is found), encephalitis and cerebral venous thrombosis occur, in less than a third of cases.

Abscesses within the nervous system

Brain abscess (see Fig 18.23)

A focal area of bacterial infection within the cerebrum or cerebellum causes an expanding mass lesion (see p. 1079). The typical infective agents are *Streptococcus milleri*, *Bacteroides* species and staphylococci. Mixed bacterial infections are common. Multiple abscesses develop, particularly in HIV-positive patients. Fungi also cause brain abscesses. A parameningeal infective focus (e.g. ear, nose, paranasal sinus, skull fracture) or a distant source of infection (e.g. lung, heart, abdomen) may be present. Frequently, however, no cause is found. The incidence of brain abscess is less than 10% of all brain tumours in the UK.

CLINICAL FEATURES

Headache, focal signs (e.g. hemiparesis, aphasia, hemianopia), epilepsy and raised intracranial pressure occur. Fever, leucocytosis and raised ESR are usual but are not invariable. The presentation may thus be very similar to a cerebral tumour. The symptoms may also be indolent, developing over weeks, particularly in the cerebral hemispheres. Cerebellar abscesses tend to develop more acutely, producing hydrocephalus.

MANAGEMENT

Urgent imaging is essential. The search for a local focus of infection should include a detailed examination of the skull, ears and paranasal sinuses, and distant foci, such as the heart and abdomen should be considered. Lumbar puncture is contraindicated in suspected brain abscess before imaging, and rarely gives diagnostically useful information if an abscess has been shown to be present.

Treatment should be carried out with liaison between neurosurgeon and microbiologist. Surgical decompression may be necessary if parenteral antibiotics are unsuccessful. Despite treatment, the mortality of brain abscess remains high, at around 25%. Epilepsy is common in survivors.

Brain tuberculoma

Tubercle bacilli cause chronic caseating intracranial granulomas, tuberculomas, which are the most common

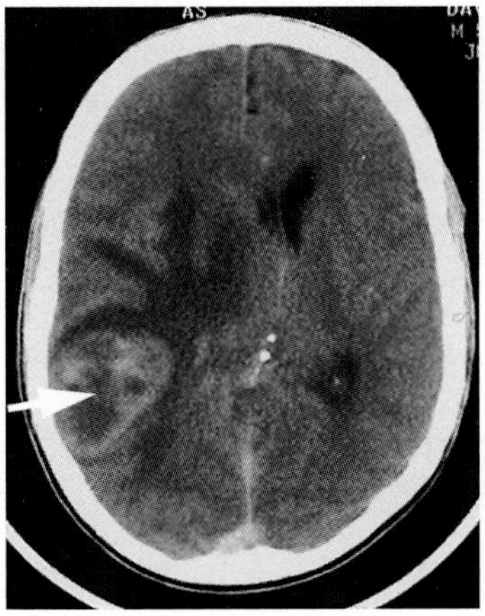

Fig 18.23
Parietal lobe abscess

single intracranial masses in areas such as India where tuberculosis is common. Brain tuberculomas either present as mass lesions or develop in the course of tuberculous meningitis. Tuberculomas can also be symptomless and are visible on imaging as areas of intracranial calcification many years later. Spinal cord tuberculomas also occur.

Subdural empyema and intracranial epidural abscess

A subdural empyema is a collection of pus in the subdural space, usually secondary to local skull or middle ear infection. The features are similar to those of a cerebral abscess. Imaging indicates the site of the collection.

In an epidural abscess, a thin layer of pus tracks along the intracranial epidural space, causing sequential cranial nerve lesions, typically without evidence of raised pressure. There is usually evidence of local infection, such as in the middle ear. CT imaging is sometimes normal in this situation, as the layer of pus is 1–3 mm thick. MRI is the test of choice.

Drainage is required for these abscesses, and appropriate antibiotics.

Spinal epidural abscess

Staphylococcus aureus is the usual organizm responsible, reaching the spine via the bloodstream, possibly from a boil. There is fever and usually back pain followed by paraparesis and/or root lesions. Emergency imaging and antibiotics are essential. Surgical decompression is often necessary.

FURTHER READING

Chronic Fatigue Syndrome: Report of the Joint Working Group of the Royal College of Physicians, Psychiatrists and General Practitioners (1996). London: Royal College of Physicians.

Memorandum on Leprosy (August 1997). London: HMSO.

Salisbury DM, Begg NT (1996) *Immunization Against Infectious Disease*. London: HMSO.

Will RG, Ironside JW, Zeidler M, et al (1996) A new variant of Creutzfeldt–Jacob disease in the UK. *Lancet* **347**: 921–925.

Meningococcal Infection: Meningitis and septicaemia. *Communicable Disease Report Review* (1997) **7**: 3–4. Public Health Laboratory Service.

Intracranial tumours

Primary intracranial tumours account for some 10% of all neoplasms. The most common tumours are outlined in Table 18.47. See also Fig 18.14 on p. 1040.

Differences between overall annual incidence rates (Table 18.1) and presentation as clinical problems (Table 18.47) are accounted for by the fact that small symptomless meningiomas are commonly found at postmortem. In general medical practice in the UK, metastases are the most common intracranial tumours.

Gliomas

These malignant, intrinsic tumours originate in neuroglia, usually within the cerebral hemispheres. Their cause is unknown. Glioma is occasionally associated with neurofibromatosis.

Primary intracranial malignant tumours virtually never metastasize outside the CNS. They tend to spread only by direct extension.

Astrocytomas

These gliomas arise from astrocytes. They are classified into grades I–IV, depending on histology. Grade I astrocytomas grow slowly over many years, while grade IV tumours cause death within several months.

Cystic astrocytomas occur in childhood, usually within the cerebellum. They are relatively benign.

Oligodendrogliomas

These gliomas arise from oligodendroglia and grow slowly, usually over several decades. Calcification is common.

Meningiomas (see Fig 18.14)

These benign tumours arise from the arachnoid membrane and may grow to a large size, usually over years. When close to the skull they erode bone. They often occur along the intracranial venous sinuses, which they may invade. They are rare below the tentorium. Sites of predilection are the parasagittal region, sphenoidal ridge, subfrontal region and skull base.

Table 18.47 Relative frequency of common intracranial tumours on the basis of clinical presentation

Tumour	Approximate relative frequency
Metastases	**50%**
Bronchus	
Breast	
Stomach	
Prostate	
Thyroid	
Kidney	
Primary malignant (glioma)	**35%**
Astrocytoma	
Oligodendroglioma	
Benign	**15%**
Meningioma	
Neurofibroma	

Neurofibromas (Schwannomas)

These solid benign tumours arise from Schwann cells and occur principally in the cerebellopontine angle, where they arise from the eighth nerve sheath (see p. 1025).

Other neoplasms

Other less common neoplasms include:

- cerebellar haemangioblastoma
- ependymoma of the fourth ventricle
- colloid cyst of the third ventricle
- pinealoma
- chordoma of the skull base
- glomus tumour – a vascular neoplasm of the jugular bulb
- medulloblastoma – a cerebellar tumour of childhood
- craniopharyngioma (p. 908)
- cerebral lymphoma.

Pituitary tumours

These are discussed on p. 904.

CLINICAL FEATURES

Mass lesions within the cranium produce symptoms and signs by three mechanisms:

- by direct mass effect on surrounding structures, which are either destroyed or suffer impairment of function from infiltration, pressure or cerebral oedema
- by secondary effects of raised intracranial pressure and shift of intracranial contents (e.g. papilloedema, vomiting, headache)
- by provoking either generalized or partial seizures.

Although neoplasms, either secondary or primary, are the most common mass lesions in the UK, cerebral abscess, tuberculoma, subdural and intracranial haematoma can also produce symptoms and signs that are clinically indistinguishable.

Direct effects of mass lesions

The hallmark of a direct effect of a mass lesion is local progressive deterioration of function. Tumours can occur anywhere within the brain, but three examples are given below:

- A *left frontal meningioma* (see Fig 18.14) caused a frontal lobe syndrome – a vague disturbance of personality, apathy and impairment of intellectual function over several years. When the speech area became affected, expressive aphasia developed. As the corticospinal pathway became involved, a progressive right hemiparesis developed. As the mass enlarged further, pressure headaches and papilloedema followed.
- A *right parietal lobe glioma* involving the fibres of the optic radiation caused a left homonymous field defect. Cortical sensory loss in the left limbs and a left hemiparesis followed over three months. Partial seizures causing episodes of tingling of the left limbs developed.
- A *left eighth-nerve sheath neurofibroma* (an *acoustic neuroma* or *Schwannoma*) growing in the cerebellopontine angle over three years caused progressive perceptive deafness (VIII), vertigo (VIII), numbness of the left side of the face (V) and facial weakness (VII), followed by cerebellar ataxia on the same side, as the cerebellar connections were compressed. Papilloedema was a late sequel.

With a hemisphere tumour, epilepsy and the direct effects commonly bring the patient to seek medical attention initially. The rate of tumour progression varies greatly, from a few days or weeks in a highly malignant glioma, to several years in the case of a slowly enlarging mass, such as a meningioma. Cerebral oedema surrounds mass lesions: it is difficult on clinical grounds to distinguish its effect from that of the mass itself.

Secondary effects and shift of intracranial contents

The secondary effect of a mass, the raised intracranial pressure causing the triad of headache, vomiting and papilloedema, is an important, though relatively unusual, presentation of a mass lesion. These symptoms usually imply obstruction to CSF pathways. Typically this picture is produced early by posterior fossa masses (which obstruct the aqueduct and fourth ventricle to produce hydrocephalus) but later with lesions above the tentorium.

Shift of the intracranial contents produces symptoms and signs that coexist with the direct effects of an expanding mass:

- *Distortion of the upper brainstem*, as midline structures are displaced either caudally or laterally by a hemisphere mass (see Fig 18.14 on p. 1040), causing impairment of consciousness.
- *Compression of the medulla*, by herniation of the cerebellar tonsils caudally through the foramen magnum – an example of coning – causes impairment of consciousness, respiratory depression, bradycardia, decerebrate posturing and death.
- *False localizing signs*, which are false only because they do not point directly to the site of the mass.

Three examples of the false localizing signs are:

- A *sixth-nerve lesion*, first on the side of a mass and later bilaterally, is caused as the nerve during its long intracranial course is compressed by expanded brain.
- A *third-nerve lesion* develops as the uncus of the temporal lobe herniates caudally, compressing the third nerve against the petroclinoid ligament. The first sign is ipsilateral dilatation of the pupil as parasympathetic fibres are compressed.
- *Hemiparesis* on the same side as a hemisphere tumour (i.e. the side you would not expect) is produced by compression of the contralateral cerebral peduncle within the brainstem on the free edge of the tentorium.

These false localizing signs, though rare, are of importance in clinical neurology and neurosurgery because their appearance indicates that shift of brain has occurred.

Seizures

Partial seizures, simple or complex, which may evolve to generalized tonic–clonic seizures, are characteristic features of many hemisphere masses, whether malignant or benign. Their clinical site of origin is of localizing value (see p. 1057).

INVESTIGATIONS

Imaging is the investigation of choice when a tumour is suspected.

CT and MR imaging

It is important to emphasize that imaging indicates only the site of a mass and not its absolute nature. Cerebral abscess, cerebral infarction, benign and malignant tumours have characteristic, but not entirely diagnostic, appearances. Contrast enhancement adds to the discriminating ability of imaging.

EEG

The EEG is rarely of major importance in the study of mass lesions. One exception is in cerebral abscess, where characteristic marked focal slow waves are seen.

Technetium brain scan

This investigation is only of value in the diagnosis of destructive skull vault or skull base lesions.

Skull films (see also p. 1037)

In hemisphere lesions, plain films are of little screening value, except where the vault lesions are present. In pituitary and parasellar lesions they give important information about changes in the dorsum sellae and clinoid processes.

Routine tests

Since the proportion of cerebral tumours that prove to be metastases is high, routine tests such as a chest X-ray are of value.

More specialized neuroradiology

Angiography and volumetric MRI are occasionally used to define the blood supply or changing size of a mass.

Lumbar puncture

Lumbar puncture is *contraindicated* when the differential diagnosis includes any mass lesion. Examination of CSF rarely yields diagnostically useful information in this situation, and the procedure may be followed by immediate herniation of the cerebellar tonsils. It should be carried out only after imaging, if at all.

Biopsy

Stereotactic biopsy via a skull burr-hole is usually carried out to diagnose histologically a hemisphere maligancy. Open exploration at craniotomy is usually carried out when a meningioma is suspected.

MANAGEMENT

Cerebral oedema surrounding a tumour is rapidly reduced by corticosteroids; intravenous dexamethasone is used in an emergency. Intravenous mannitol is used as an osmotic diuretic to reduce cerebral oedema. Epilepsy is treated with anticonvulsants.

Whilst complete surgical removal of a brain tumour is an objective, it is not always possible, nor is surgery always necessary. Follow-up with serial imaging is sometimes preferable initially. At surgical exploration, some but not all benign tumours can be removed in their entirety (e.g. some parasagittal meningiomas). With a brain malignancy it is usually impossible to remove the entire infiltrating mass; this is the most common situation. Biopsy and debulking is carried out.

Within the posterior fossa, tumour removal is often necessary because of the effects of raised pressure or the imminent danger of coning. However, overall mortality for posterior fossa exploration remains around 10%. An isolated posterior fossa metastasis can sometimes be excised successfully, with prolonged survival thereafter.

Radiotherapy is usually carried out for gliomas and for radiosensitive metastases. Chemotherapy has little real value in the majority of primary or secondary brain tumours. With all malignant brain tumours the overall outlook is poor, with less than 50% survival at two years. Difficult issues surround the management of these patients.

Idiopathic intracranial hypertension (benign intracranial hypertension)

This syndrome, once called *pseudotumor cerebri*, is included under brain tumours because marked papilloedema occurs. There is neither a mass lesion nor an increase in ventricular size. The condition occurs mainly in obese young women with vague menstrual irregularities. Headaches and visual blurring (caused by severe papilloedema) are common. A sixth-nerve palsy may be present, as a false localizing sign. The CSF pressure is elevated; the constituents are normal. Imaging is normal. Steroid therapy is sometimes thought to be a cause and many other drugs have occasionally been implicated. Other causes of papilloedema should be excluded. Sagittal sinus thrombosis sometimes causes a similar picture.

The condition is benign only in that it is not fatal. Infarction of the optic nerve occurs, with consequent visual loss when papilloedema is severe and longstanding. Thiazide diuretics and acetazolamide appear to reduce the intracranial pressure in this condition. Weight reduction is important. Surgical decompression or shunting is sometimes necessary.

Hydrocephalus

Hydrocephalus means an excessive volume of CSF within the cranium. In practice the term hydrocephalus describes different syndromes in which there is, or has been, obstruction to CSF outflow with consequent high pressure and dilatation of the cerebral ventricles. Rarely, increase in CSF production also occurs.

Infantile hydrocephalus

Enlargement of the head in infancy is diagnosed in about 1 in 2000 live births. There are several recognized causes:

- *Arnold–Chiari malformation*. There is elongation of the medulla. Abnormal cerebellar tonsils descend into the cervical canal. Associated spina bifida is common. Syringomyelia may develop (see p. 1086).
- *Dandy–Walker syndrome*. There is cerebellar hypoplasia and obstruction to the outflow foramina of the fourth ventricle.
- *Stenosis of the aqueduct of Sylvius* (see Fig 18.14 on p. 1040). This is either congenital or acquired following neonatal meningitis or haemorrhage.

Hydrocephalus in adult life

Whilst hydrocephalus may remain symptomless, and be an unsuspected finding on brain imaging, infantile hydrocephalus can become apparent in adult life. The features are various combinations of headache, cognitive impairment, vomiting, papilloedema, ataxia and bilateral pyramidal signs. Hydrocephalus may develop in other circumstances.

- *Tumours of the posterior fossa and brainstem* can obstruct the aqueduct or fourth ventricular outflow.
- *Following subarachnoid haemorrhage, head injury or meningitis* (particularly tuberculous), hydrocephalus is sometimes a transient phenomenon.
- *A colloid cyst of the third ventricle* causes enlargement of the lateral ventricles, headache and papilloedema. These rare intraventricular tumours also sometimes produce intermittent hydrocephalus, recurrent prostrating headaches with episodes of weakness of the lower limbs.
- *Papilloma of the choroid plexus*, an extremely rare neoplasm, secretes CSF.

TREATMENT

Ventriculoatrial or ventriculoperitoneal shunting may be necessary when hydrocephalus is progressive or causes symptoms. Neurosurgical removal of tumours should be carried out where appropriate, sometimes urgently.

Normal pressure hydrocephalus

This rare syndrome describes enlarged cerebral ventricles without cortical atrophy, with dementia, urinary incontinence and gait apraxia, usually in the elderly. The CSF pressure is characteristically normal, and so are CFS constituents. It is thought that this is a result of previous episodes of high pressure, of unknown cause. Shunting seldom helps the condition.

FURTHER READING

Davies E, Clarke C, Hopkins A (1996) Malignant cerebral glioma. *British Medical Journal* **313**: 1507–1512.

Headache, migraine and facial pain

Tension headache

The vast majority of chronic and recurrent headaches are believed, on no good evidence, to be due to tension within the scalp muscles. What is certain is that they are, in terms of pathology, innocent. Tight band sensations, pressure behind the eyes, and throbbing and bursting sensations are common.

There may be obvious precipitating factors such as worry, noise, concentrated visual effort or fumes. Depression is also a frequent underlying cause. Tension headaches are often attributed to cervical spondylosis, refractive errors or high blood pressure; the evidence for these is poor. Similar headaches also follow head injuries, which may be minor.

There are no abnormal physical signs other than tenderness and tension in the nuchal and scalp muscles.

MANAGEMENT

This involves:

- firm reassurance
- avoiding the causes
- analgesics
- physical treatments – massage, icepacks, relaxation
- antidepressants – when indicated.

Imaging is occasionally needed to confirm the benign nature of the problem.

Migraine

Migraine is defined as recurrent headaches associated with visual and gastrointestinal disturbance. The borderline between migraine and tension headaches is vague. Over 10% of any population sampled admit to these symptoms.

MECHANISMS

The precise mechanism of migraine is unknown. The headache, often throbbing, is due to vasodilatation or oedema of blood vessels, with stimulation of nerve endings near affected extracranial and meningeal arteries. The release of vasoactive substances such as nitric oxide are thought to play a role. In addition, the serum level of 5-hydroxytryptamine rises at the onset of the prodromal symptoms and falls during the headache.

Cerebral symptoms and signs, such as tingling of limbs, aphasia and weakness, are caused by focal depression of cortical function.

Definite precipitating factors are unusual. Some patients complain of symptoms at times of relaxation ('weekend migraine'). Others find that chocolate (high in phenylethylamine) and cheese (high in tyramine) precipitate attacks. Migraine is common around puberty, at the menopause and premenstrually, and sometimes increases in severity or frequency with hormonal contraceptives, in pregnancy and with the development of hypertension.

There is no reason to suppose that the development of migraine is suggestive of any major intracranial lesion. However, since migraine is such a common symptom complex, an intracranial mass lesion and migraine sometimes both occur in the same patient by coincidence.

Rarely, migraine follows a head injury, which can be minor.

CLINICAL PATTERNS

There are several patterns of migraine, the attacks varying from intermittent headaches indistinguishable from tension headaches to discrete episodes that mimic thromboembolic cerebral ischaemia. The distinction between the variants is somewhat artificial.

Migraine can be separated into phases:

- occasionally, a feeling of well-being prior to the attack
- prodromal symptoms
- headache and associated symptoms.

Migraine with aura (classical migraine)

Prodromal symptoms are usually visual and are related to depression of visual cortical function, or retinal function. There are unilateral patchy scotomata (when the retina is affected) or cortical hemianopic symptoms. Teichopsia (flashes) and fortification spectra (jagged lines resembling battlements) are common.

Transient aphasia sometimes occurs, together with tingling, numbness or vague weakness of one side. The patient feels nauseated.

The prodrome lasts from 15 minutes to an hour or more. Headache then follows. This is occasionally hemicranial (i.e. splitting the head) but often begins locally and becomes generalized. Nausea increases and vomiting follows. The patient is irritable and prefers to be in a darkened room. The superficial temporal artery is engorged and pulsating.

After several hours the attack ceases. There is sometimes a diuresis towards the end of an attack. Sleep often follows.

Migraine without aura (common migraine)

This is the usual variety of migraine. Prodromal visual symptoms are vague. There is recurrent headache accompanied by nausea and malaise.

Basilar migraine

The prodromal symptoms are circumoral tingling, numbness of the tongue, vertigo, diplopia, transient visual disturbance or complete blindness, syncope, dysarthria and ataxia. These occur either in isolation or progress to a migrainous headache.

Hemiplegic migraine

This is a rarity in which classical migraine is accompanied by hemiparesis. Recovery occurs within 24 hours. Exceptionally, cerebral infarction occurs.

Ophthalmoplegic migraine

This is a third-nerve, or exceptionally a sixth-nerve, palsy occurring in a migraine attack. The condition is rare and is difficult to distinguish from other causes of a third-nerve palsy (see p. 1020) without investigation.

Facioplegic migraine

This rarity is unilateral facial weakness occurring during a migraine attack.

DIFFERENTIAL DIAGNOSIS

The sudden onset of headache may be similar to meningitis or SAH.

The hemiplegic, visual and hemisensory symptoms must be distinguished from thromboembolic TIAs (see p. 1049). In TIAs the maximum deficit is present immediately and headache is unusual.

Unilateral tingling or numbness should be distinguished from sensory epilepsy (partial seizures). In the latter a distinct march of symptoms is usual.

MANAGEMENT

General measures include:

- reassurance and relief of anxiety
- avoidance of precipitating dietary factors, which is rarely helpful.

Patients taking a hormonal contraceptive may benefit from a change in brand, or stopping the drug. Severe hemiplegic symptoms are an indication for stopping these drugs.

During an attack. Paracetamol or other simple analgesics should be given, with an antiemetic such as metoclopramide if necessary.

In some 30% of cases where there are recurrent severe attacks, the 5-hydroxytryptamine ($5HT_1$) agonist, sumatriptan, is of value either by self-administered subcutaneous injection, orally, or by inhaler. Zolmitriptan and naratriptan are similar drugs available orally. Ergotamine tartrate (1–2 mg orally or rectally, 360 μg by inhaler or 0.25–0.5 mg by injection) is sometimes, though not often, helpful if given early in an attack. Ergotamine, sumatriptan and zolmitriptan should not be used in patients with a history of vascular disease.

Prophylaxis. It is particularly difficult to discern the true, as opposed to placebo, effects of prophylactic drugs in migraine. When drugs are necessary, the following are used:

- pizotifen (a 5-hydroxytryptamine antagonist) 0.5 mg at night for several days, increasing to 1.5 mg at night – common side-effects are slight weight gain and drowsiness
- propranolol 10 mg three times daily, increasing to 40–80 mg three times daily
- methysergide (a 5-hydroxytryptamine antagonist) 2–6 mg daily – an occasional side-effect is retroperitoneal fibrosis, which precludes its use for longer than six months.
- amitriptyline in small doses at night: 10–30 mg at night is sometimes helpful.

Facial pain

The face is richly supplied with pain-sensitive structures – the teeth, gums, sinuses, temporomandibular joints, jaw and eyes – disease of which causes facial pain. Facial pain is also caused by some specific neurological conditions; these are mentioned below.

Trigeminal neuralgia (see p. 1021), trigeminal nerve lesions (p. 1020) and postherpetic neuralgia (p. 1074) are described elsewhere.

Cluster headache (migrainous neuralgia, Horton's neuralgia)

This condition, which is distinct from migraine despite its name, causes recurrent bouts of excruciating pain that wake the patient at night and are centred around one eye. It affects adults, commmencing in the third and fourth decades and is more common in men. Alcohol sometimes precipitates an attack.

The pain rises to a crescendo over half an hour and lasts for several hours. Vomiting occurs. One side of the face and one nostril feel congested. A transient ipsilateral Horner's syndrome is common during the attack.

Despite the very severe pain there are no serious sequelae. Attacks recur at intervals over several years but tend to disappear over the age of 55. Treatment of the attack with analgesics is unhelpful. Prophylactic drugs for migraine are of little value. Lithium carbonate (400–1200 mg daily) sometimes has a dramatic effect in preventing attacks: the drug level should be monitored carefully. Inhalation of oxygen sometimes helps abort an attack.

Atypical facial pain

Facial pain for which no cause can be found is seen in the elderly, mainly in women. It is believed to be a somatic equivalent of depression. Tricyclic antidepressants are sometimes helpful.

Other causes of facial pain

Facial pain occurs in variants of migraine and in giant cell arteritis (see below).

Giant cell arteritis (cranial arteritis, temporal arteritis, see also p. 494)

This important condition is a granulomatous arteritis of unknown aetiology occurring chiefly in those over the age of 60 years and affecting in particular the extradural arteries. Other forms of arteritis, such as SLE and polyarteritis nodosa, can occasionally present with similar features. Giant cell arteritis is closely related to polymyalgia rheumatica and these can occur in the same patient.

CLINICAL FEATURES

Headache

Headache is almost invariable in giant cell arteritis. Pain is felt over the inflamed superficial, temporal or occipital arteries. Touching the skin over the inflamed vessel (e.g. combing the hair) causes pain. Arterial pulsation is soon lost and the artery becomes hard, tortuous and thickened. The skin over the vessels may become red. Rarely, gangrenous patches appear in the scalp.

Facial pain

Pain in the face, jaw and mouth occurs in giant cell arteritis and is caused by inflammation of the facial, maxillary and lingual branches of the external carotid artery. Pain is characteristically worse on eating (jaw claudication). Opening the mouth and protruding the tongue is difficult. A painful, ischaemic tongue occurs rarely.

Visual problems

Visual loss owing to inflammation and occlusion of the ciliary and/or central retinal artery occurs in 25% of cases of untreated giant cell arteritis. The patient complains of sudden uniocular visual loss, either partial or complete, which is painless. Amaurosis fugax (see p. 1049) may precede total visual loss, which is usually permanent, if the transient loss of vision lasts more than an hour.

When the ciliary vessels are inflamed, an ischaemic optic neuropathy causes the disc to become swollen and pale; the retinal branch vessels usually remain normal. When the central retinal artery is occluded, there is sudden unilateral blindness, pallor of the disc and visible retinal ischaemia.

Systemic features

Generalized muscle pains, proximal limb girdle pain and tenderness, without joint effusion – i.e. polymyalgia rheumatica (see p. 494) – occur in under half the cases. Weight loss, sweating and malaise are also often present.

Rare complications

Brainstem ischaemia, cortical blindness, ischaemic neuropathy of peripheral or cranial nerves, and involvement of the aorta, coronary, renal and mesenteric arteries are sometimes seen.

INVESTIGATIONS

The ESR is greatly elevated, 60–100 mm h^{-1} being common, although very rarely the ESR is normal. CRP and plasma α_2-globulins are raised and the albumin is occasionally reduced. Normochromic normocytic anaemia develops.

The diagnosis should be confirmed by biopsy of a superficial temporal artery. A 1 cm (or greater) segment should be excised because characteristic granulomatous changes within the arterial wall (lymphocytes, plasma cells, multinucleate giant cells, destruction of the internal elastic lamina) is patchy.

TREATMENT

The diagnosis should be established without delay because of the risk of blindness. High doses of steroids (prednisolone, initially 60–100 mg daily) should be started immediately in a patient with typical features even before the biopsy. The dose is reduced as the ESR falls. A usual feature of giant cell arteritis is that the headache subsides within hours of the first large dose of steroid. It is usually possible to stop steroid treatment after some months to several years.

FURTHER READING

Ferrari MD (1998) Migraine. *Lancet* **351**: 1043–1051.

Goadsby P, Silberstein SD (1997) *Headache: Problems in Diagnosis and Management*. Oxford: Butterworth–Heinemann.

Traumatic brain injury

In most western countries there are about 250 hospital admissions annually following head injury, per 100 000 population. Traumatic brain injury (TBI) is the preferred term. Per 100 000, 10 people die annually; 10–15 are transferred to a neurosurgical unit, of which the majority require rehabilitation for a prolonged period of 1–9 months. The prevalence of survivors with a major persisting handicap is of the order of a 100 per 100 000. Road traffic accidents and alcohol abuse are the principal aetiological factors in this major cause of morbidity and mortality.

Skull fractures

Linear skull fracture of the vault or base is one indication of the severity of injury, but is itself not necessarily associated with any neurological sequelae. Healing takes place and surgical intervention is usually unnecessary.

Depressed skull fracture of the vault is followed by a high incidence of post-traumatic epilepsy. Surgical elevation and debridement are usually necessary.

The principal local complications of skull fracture are:

- *meningeal artery rupture*, causing an extradural haematoma (p. 1054)
- *dural vein tears*, leading to subdural haematoma (p. 1054) or CSF rhinorrhoea/otorrhoea with the risk of meningitis.

Mechanisms of brain damage

Older classifications attempted to separate concussion (i.e. transient coma followed by complete clinical recovery) from brain contusion (prolonged coma, with brain damage and focal signs). Pathological support for this division is poor. The mechanisms of traumatic brain injury are complex and interrelated. They involve:

- axonal and neuronal damage, from shearing and rotational stresses on decellerating brain, often at sites distant from the impact (*contracoup effect*)
- axonal and neuronal damage from direct trauma
- brain oedema
- raised intracranial pressure
- brain hypoxia
- brain ischaemia.

CLINICAL COURSE

In a mild TBI a patient is first stunned or dazed for a few seconds or minutes. Loss of consciousness is transient and following this the patient is alert, and there is little or no post-traumatic amnesia. The period of loss of con-sciousness and particularly post-traumatic amnesia (PTA) indicates severity. PTA over 24 hours indicates severe brain injury. The Glasgow Coma Scale (GCS, see p. 1043) is used to record the degree of coma and brain injury and indicates prognosis. A low GCS score below 5/15 at 24 hours implies a severe injury, and 50% of such patients die or remain in a persistent vegetative state (see p. 1043). Prolonged coma of up to several weeks is, however, sometimes followed by good recovery.

Recovery may take many weeks or months, depending on the severity of the injury. During the first few weeks patients are often intermittently restless and/or lethargic and have focal neurological deficits, such as hemiparesis or aphasia. Gradually patients become more aware of their surroundings, but despite being awake, may remain in a state of post-traumatic amnesia, being unable to lay down any memory of current events. This sometimes lasts several weeks, and may not be obvious clinically. PTA is the best predictor of outcome. Two weeks' PTA predicts that an organic cognitive deficit is inevitable, although a return to unsupported paid work is possible. This is impossible after two weeks' PTA.

Late sequelae

Sequelae of TBI are major causes of morbidity and have important social and medicolegal consequences. They include:

- *Incomplete and prolonged recovery*. These are patients left with impairment of higher cerebral function, hemiparesis and other deficits.
- *Post-traumatic epilepsy* (p. 1057).
- *Chronic traumatic encephalopathy*, which follows repeated (and often minor) injuries. This 'punch drunk' syndrome is cognitive impairment with extrapyramidal and pyramidal signs. It is seen principally in professional boxers.
- *The post-traumatic syndrome*, which describes the vague complaints of headache, dizziness and malaise that follow even minor head injuries. Depression is prominent. Symptoms may be prolonged.
- *Benign positional vertigo* (p. 1026).
- *Chronic subdural haematoma* (p. 1054).
- *Hydrocephalus* (p. 1081).

IMMEDIATE MANAGEMENT AND REHABILITATION

Attention to the airway of is primary importance. If there is coma, depressed fracture or the suspicion of an intracranial haematoma, discussion with a neurosurgical unit and prompt imaging are essential. Assisted ventilation may be required. Monitoring of intracranial pressure (with an intracranial bolt) is valuable. Patients with head injury require skilled, prolonged and energetic supportive therapy. Care of the unconscious patient is described on p. 1046.

TBI survivors with severe physical and cognitive deficits require rehabilitation in a specialized unit. Treatment includes not only intensive physiotherapy but also care from a multidisciplinary team, with both physical and psychological skills. Many patients have specific cognitive problems, such as amnesia, neglect, disordered attention and motivation, behavioural problems, such as temper dyscontrol, or emotional problems, such as post-traumatic stress disorder, depression or grief reactions. Both patients and their families need long-term support.

FURTHER READING

Editorial (1997) Best practice in traumatic brain injury. *Lancet* **349**: 1041–1042.

Greenwood RJ, McMillan TM (1993) Models of rehabilitation programmes for the brain-injured adult. 1: Current provision. *Clinical Rehabilitation* **7**: 248–283.

Diseases of the spinal cord

The cord extends from C1 (i.e. its junction with the medulla) to the vertebral body of L1 where it is called the conus medullaris.

The blood supply is via the anterior spinal artery and a plexus on the posterior cord. This network is supplied by the vertebral arteries, the thyrocervical trunk and several branches from the lumbar and intercostal vessels.

Spinal cord compression (Table 18.48)

The principal features of cord compression are of radicular *pain* at the site of compression, *spastic paraparesis or tetraparesis*, and *sensory loss* which rises to the level of compression.

For example, in compression at the level of T6 a band of pain radiates around the chest wall and is characteristically worse on coughing or straining. A spastic paraparesis develops over many months, days or hours, depending upon the underlying pathology. Numbness commencing distally in the lower limbs rises to the level of compression, known as the sensory level. Sphincter disturbance develops, principally retention of urine and loss of bladder control.

Compression of the cord is a potential medical emergency. It is sometimes difficult to distinguish chronic cord compression from other causes of paraparesis and tetraparesis on clinical grounds alone. This is principally because pain at the site of compression and the sensory level may be absent.

Spinal cord neoplasms (Table 18.49)

Extramedullary tumours, both extradural and intradural, cause cord compression gradually over weeks to months, with local or referred root pain and a sensory level (see p. 1034).

Intramedullary tumours (e.g. glioma) typically have a very slowly progressive course over many years. Sensory disturbances similar to syringomyelia may appear (see p. 1086).

Table 18.48
Causes of spinal cord compression

Spinal cord neoplasms (see Table 18.49)	Epidural haemorrhage
Disc and vertebral lesions Trauma Chronic degenerative	Rarities Paget's disease, scoliosis and vertebral anomalies Epithelial, endothelial and parasitic cysts Aneurysmal bone cyst Vertebral angioma Haematomyelia, arachnoiditis Osteoporosis with fracture Arteriovenous malformation
Inflammatory Epidural abscess Tuberculosis Granuloma	
Vertebral neoplasms Metastases Myeloma	

Table 18.49
Principal spinal cord neoplasms

Extradural	
Metastases	
	Bronchus
	Breast
	Prostate
	Lymphoma
	Thyroid
	Melanoma
Extramedullary	
Meningioma	
Neurofibroma	
Ependymoma	
Intramedullary	
Glioma	
Ependymoma	
Haemangioblastoma	
Lipoma	
Arteriovenous malformation	
Teratoma	

Disc and vertebral lesions

Central cervical disc protrusion and thoracic disc protrusion causing cord compression are considered on p. 1098.

Spinal epidural abscess

This is described on p. 1078.

Epidural haemorrhage and haematoma

These are rare sequelae of anticoagulant therapy, bleeding disorders and trauma. A rapidly progressive cord lesion develops.

Tuberculosis

Spinal tuberculosis is a frequent cause of cord compression in countries where tuberculosis is common (e.g. India, Pakistan, Bangladesh and Africa). It is also seen in patients with HIV infection. There is destruction of vertebral bodies and disc spaces, with spread of infection along the extradural space. Cord compression and paraparesis follow, known as Pott's paraplegia.

MANAGEMENT

Early recognition of cord compression is vital. Plain spinal films show degenerative bone disease and destruction of vertebrae by infection or neoplasm. Routine tests (e.g. chest X-ray) may indicate a primary neoplasm or infection.

MRI identifies most lesions and, where it is available, has entirely replaced contrast myelography. Surgical exploration is frequently necessary and, if this is not performed sufficiently early, irreversible cord damage may follow. The results following the early removal of benign tumours are excellent.

Other causes of paraparesis

Paraparesis, including here tetraparesis, is a presenting or evolving feature of many neurological conditions which are recognizable by their clinical patterns, making the differential diagnosis of fundamental importance in practical neurology. These diseases are shown in Table 18.14 on p. 1029, and most are mentioned elsewhere in this chapter.

Syringomyelia and syringobulbia

A fluid-filled cavity, the syrinx within the cervical spinal cord (syringomyelia), sometimes extending into the thoracic cord, and into the brainstem (syringobulbia) is the essential feature.

AETIOLOGY AND MECHANISM

Classical syringomyelia is associated with the Arnold–Chairi malformation (see p. 1089). Bony anomalies at the foramen magnum, spina bifida (p. 1089), arachnoiditis, hydrocephalus (p. 1081) and intrinsic cord tumours (e.g. glioma and ependymoma) are sometimes also followed by syrinx formation, and its subsequent enlargement. It is believed that in the presence of an anatomical abnormality at the foramen magnum, the normal pulsatile CSF pressure waves are transmitted to the soft fragile tissues of the cervical cord and brainstem, with secondary cavity formation. The syrinx is in continuity with the central canal of the cord. Cord trauma can be followed by cavity formation, which is usually not progressive.

PATHOLOGICAL ANATOMY

The expanding cavity within the cervical cord gradually destroys spinothalamic neurones, anterior horn cells, lateral corticospinal tracts, and trigeminal nuclei, sympathetic trunk, ninth-, tenth-, eleventh- and twelfth-nerve nuclei and the vestibular system if the cavity extends in to the medulla.

CLINICAL FEATURES

Patients with classical syringomyelia associated with the Arnold–Chiari malformation usually develop symptoms at the age of 20–30 years. Pain in the upper limbs exacerbated by exertion or coughing is typical. Spinothalamic sensory loss (of pain and temperature) in the upper limbs leads to painless upper-limb burns, and trophic changes. Difficulty in walking with paraparesis develops. The following are signs of a cavity in the cervical region:

- *Areas of dissociated sensory loss*, i.e. spinothalamic loss but not light touch. These may develop into bizarre patterns over upper limbs and trunk.
- *Loss of upper limb reflexes.*

- *Wasting* of the small muscles of the hand and forearm.
- *Spastic paraparesis*. This may initially be mild and symptomless.
- *Neuropathic joints*, trophic skin changes (scars, nail dystrophy) and ulcers.
- *Brainstem signs*. When the cavity extends upwards through the foramen magnum into the brainstem (syringobulbia), there is atrophy and fasciculation of the tongue, bulbar palsy, nystagmus, Horner's syndrome, hearing loss and impairment of facial sensation.

COURSE, INVESTIGATION AND MANAGEMENT

Syringomyelia is gradually progressive over several decades. Sudden deterioration sometimes follows minor trauma, or apparently spontaneously.

MR imaging demonstrates the intrinsic cavity and herniation of the cerebellar tonsils through the foramen magnum. Myelography, which sometimes causes deterioration, is an alternative investigation.

There is no curative treatment for classical syringomyelia. Surgical decompression of the foramen magnum sometimes reduces the rate of deterioration.

Metabolic and toxic cord disease

Vitamin deficiency (p. 366)

Subacute combined degeneration of the cord resulting from vitamin B_{12} deficiency is the most important example of metabolic disease causing spinal cord damage.

Cord lesions may also be seen in severe malnutrition, when they are probably due to multiple B-vitamin deficiencies.

Lathyrism

This curiosity is an endemic, spastic paraparesis of central India caused by the toxin β-(*N*)-oxalylaminoalanine. It occurs when excessive quantities of a drought-resistant pulse, *Lathyrus sativa*, are consumed.

Transverse myelitis

This broad and somewhat vague term is used to describe acute inflammation of the cord and paraplegia or paraparesis occurring with viral infections, MS and other inflammatory and vascular disorders – for example syphilis, radiation myelopathy, or anterior spinal artery occlusion. MRI or myelography is usually required to exclude cord compression.

Anterior spinal artery occlusion

Cord infarction, causing an acute paraplegia or tetraplegia, or paresis occurs in many thrombotic or embolic vascular diseases – for example, endocarditis, severe hypotension, atheroma, diabetes mellitus, syphilis, polyarteritis nodosa. Infarction sometimes occurs during surgery to the posterior mediastinum, or follows dissection of the aorta and trauma. It occasionally occurs as an isolated event.

Radiation myelopathy

A mild paraparesis and sensory loss sometimes develops within several weeks to a year of radiotherapy if the cord has been damaged. Particular care is usually taken to shield the cord during radiotherapy.

Management of paraplegia

General considerations

The general health and morale of the patient should be considered carefully and regularly. Any intercurrent infection, possibly urinary or respiratory, is potentially dangerous and should be recognized and treated early. Chronic renal failure is the single most common cause of death in paraplegia.

The patient who becomes paraplegic from any cause needs skilled and prolonged nursing care. Particular problems are discussed below.

Bladder

Catheterization is usually necessary initially. Many patients manage to self-catheterize, or a reflex bladder emptying develops, which is initiated by abdominal pressure exerted by the patient. Free urinary drainage is essential to avoid the complications of urinary stasis – infection, renal and bladder calculi.

Bowel

Constipation and faecal impaction must be avoided. Manual evacuation is necessary following acute paraplegia, but reflex rectal emptying later develops.

Skin care

The risk of pressure sores is great. Meticulous attention must be paid to cleanliness and to turning the patient every two hours. The sacrum, iliac crests, greater trochanters, heels and malleoli should be inspected frequently. Ripple mattresses and water beds are useful.

If pressure sores develop, plastic surgical repair should be considered. Pressure palsies (e.g. of ulnar nerves) must be avoided.

Lower limbs

In the paralysed limbs, passive physiotherapy helps to prevent contractures. Severe spasticity, with spasms either in flexion or extension, may be helped by baclofen, diazepam or dantrolene sodium.

Rehabilitation

Many patients with traumatic paraplegia or tetraplegia return to full or partial self-sufficiency and a wheelchair existence. Specialist advice from a skilled rehabilitation unit is necessary. Lightweight, specially adapted wheelchairs are available. The patients have demanding practical, psychological and social needs but with guidance and help can often return to an active role in society.

Degenerative neuronal diseases

The term 'degenerative' underlines the present lack of understanding of the aetiology of this group of progressive diseases of the nervous system.

Motor neurone disease (MND)

In this disease there is progressive degeneration of lower and upper motor neurones (LMNs, UMNs) in the spinal cord, in the somatic motor nuclei of the cranial nerves and within the cortex. The condition is sporadic and of entirely unknown cause. Though not familial, the gene locus for the condition is on chromosome 21. Presumably the relentless degeneration of motor nerve cells is programmed genetically. The prevalence is about 6 in 100 000, with a slight male predominance. The onset is in middle life. The sensory system is not involved.

CLINICAL FEATURES

Three patterns have been noted:

- progressive muscular atrophy
- amyotrophic lateral sclerosis
- progressive bulbar palsy.

Although useful as a means of recognizing the disease, these are not distinct aetiological or pathological variants; the three merge later in the course of the condition.

Progressive muscular atrophy

Wasting beginning often in the small muscles of one hand spreads inexorably throughout the arm. Although it may begin unilaterally, wasting soon follows on the opposite side.

Fasciculation is common. It is due to the spontaneous firing of abnormally large motor units formed by the branching fibres of surviving axons that are striving to innervate muscle fibres that have lost their nerve supply. Cramps may occur but pain does not.

The physical signs are of wasting and weakness, with fasciculation that is often widespread. Tendon reflexes are lost when the reflex arc is interrupted, by anterior horn cell loss, but are preserved or exaggerated when there is loss of corticospinal motor neurones.

Amyotrophic lateral sclerosis (ALS)

Lateral sclerosis means disease of the lateral corticospinal tracts (i.e. one cause of spastic paraparesis). Amyotrophy means simply atrophy of muscle, which would be unusual in most other forms of spastic tetraparesis or paraparesis. The clinical picture is of a progressive spastic tetraparesis or paraparesis with added lower motor neurone signs and fasciculation. ALS is the term usually given to motor neurone disease in the USA.

Progressive bulbar palsy

Here the brunt of the disease falls initially upon the lower cranial nerve nuclei and their supranuclear connections. Dysarthria, dysphagia, nasal regurgitation of fluids and choking are common symptoms. For reasons unknown, this form of MND is more common in women than in men. The characteristic features are of a bulbar and pseudobulbar palsy, (see p. 1027), with a mixture of UMN and LMN signs in the lower cranial nerves – for example, a wasted fibrillating tongue with a spastic weak palate.

The ocular movements are not affected, in all forms of MND. There are never cerebellar or extrapyramidal signs. Awareness is preserved and dementia unusual. Sphincter disturbance occurs late, if at all.

DIAGNOSIS

There are no specific diagnostic tests and the diagnosis is made on clinical grounds, by exclusion of other conditions, and compatible neurophysiological studies (EMG and nerve conduction). Cervical radiculopathy and myelopathy and the rare (almost extinct) syphilitic cervical pachymeningitis sometimes cause diagnostic difficulty. Motor neuropathies and spinal muscular atrophies also sometimes mimic the progressive muscular atrophy form of MND, but their course is more prolonged. Bulbar myasthenia gravis may sometimes appear similar in the early stages.

Denervation is confirmed by electromyography, which characteristically shows chronic partial denervation with preserved motor conduction velocity. The CSF constituents are usually normal; the protein may be slightly raised.

COURSE AND MANAGEMENT

Remission is unknown. The disease progresses, spreading gradually and causes death, often from bronchopneumonia. Survival for more than three years is most unusual, although there are rare variants of the condition in which patients survive for a decade or longer.

No treatment has been shown to influence the outcome of MND, although riluzole, a glutamate antagonist, has been shown to slow progression slightly, particularly in patients with disease of bulbar onset. Contentious issues surround the cost-effectiveness of this expensive drug. Management of patients with MND, who are often well-informed and aware of the outlook, is particularly difficult.

Spinal muscular atrophies

These are rare genetically determined disorders of the motor neurone that give rise to slowly progressive, usually symmetrical, muscle wasting and weakness. An acute infantile type (Werdnig–Hoffman disease), a chronic childhood type (Kugelberg–Wielander disease) and adult forms are recognized. Clinically these conditions may be confused with muscular dystrophies (see p. 1102), hereditary neuropathies or MND.

Dementia

This is a diffuse deterioration in brain neuronal function produced by a number of pathological processes. The most common is Alzheimer's disease. Dementia is discussed on p. 1114.

FURTHER READING

Riluzolf for ALS (1997) *Drugs and Therapeutics Bulletin* **35**: 11–12.

Serratrice G, Munsat T (1995) Pathogenesis and Therapy of ALS. Lippincott–Raven.

Congenital and inherited diseases

Cerebral palsy

This term describes disorders apparent at birth or in childhood due to brain damage in the neonatal period leading to non-progressive deficits.

Mental retardation, varying from severe intellectual impairment to mild learning disorders, is common in all forms of cerebral palsy, but severe physical disability is not necessarily associated with a severe defect in higher cerebral function.

The precise cause of brain damage in an individual child may be difficult to determine. The following are responsible:

- hypoxia *in utero* and/or during parturition
- neonatal cerebral haemorrhage and/or infarction
- trauma, during parturition or in the neonatal period
- prolonged convulsions or coma – febrile convulsions, severe hypoglycaemia in infancy
- kernicterus.

CLINICAL FEATURES

Failure to achieve normal developmental milestones is often the earliest feature of cerebral palsy. More specific motor syndromes become apparent later in childhood or, rarely, in adult life.

Spastic diplegia

This is spasticity (predominantly of the lower limbs) with scissoring of the gait.

Athetoid cerebral palsy

This is described on p. 1065.

Infantile hemiparesis

Hemiparesis may be noted at birth or during childhood. Hemiatrophy of the limbs, and atrophy of the contralateral hemisphere, is usual. Seizures are common.

Congenital ataxia

This is incoordination and hypotonia of the trunk and limbs.

Dysraphism

Failure of normal fusion of the fetal neural tube leads to this group of congenital anomalies. Folate deficiency during pregnancy is a contributary factor.

Anencephaly

Anencephaly is absence of the brain and cranial vault, and is incompatible with life.

Meningo-encephalocele

This is an extrusion of brain and meninges through a midline skull defect that varies from a minor protrusion to a massive defect.

Spina bifida

In spina bifida there is failure of fusion of the neural tube, usually in the lumbosacral region. Several varieties occur.

Spina bifida occulta

This is failure of fusion of the vertebral arch only. There are rarely neurological abnormalities and a bony anomaly is seen on X-ray. It occurs in 3% of the population. A dimple or a tuft of hair may overlie the lesion, commonly in the lumbar region.

Meningomyelocele and myelocele with spina bifida

Meningomyelocele consists of elements of the cord and lumbosacral roots contained within a meningeal sac that herniates through a defect in the vertebrae. In severe cases the lower limbs and sphincters are paralysed. The defect is visible in the lumbosacral region at birth. Meningocele is a meningeal defect alone.

Basilar impression of the skull (platybasia)

This is usually a congenital anomaly in which there is invagination of the foramen magnum and skull base upwards. The lower cranial nerves, medulla, upper cervical cord and roots are affected. It is often associated with the *Arnold–Chiari malformation*, in which aberrant cerebellar tissue extends through the foramen magnum. The condition also develops in Paget's disease and rarely in osteomalacia. The clinical features are spastic tetraparesis with cerebellar and lower brainstem signs.

Neuroectodermal syndromes

These are disorders in which organs derived from ectoderm show a tendency to form tumours and hamartomas, with lesions in the skin, eye and nervous system.

Neurofibromatosis (von Recklinghausen's disease)

This is characterized by multiple skin neurofibromas and pigmentation. The neurofibromas arise from the neurilemmal sheath. One new case occurs in every 3000 live births. The mode of inheritance is autosomal dominant.

CLINICAL FEATURES (see also p. 1177)

Clinically neurofibromatosis can be divided into type 1 (or peripheral type) and type 2 (bilateral acoustic neuromas or central type). The predisposing gene for type 1 has been localized to chromosome 17 and for type 2 to the long arm of chromosome 22. The main application for these genetic markers will be for antenatal diagnosis and genetic counselling, although the severity of the disease itself will not be predictable. A wide variety of abnormalities occur.

Skin neurofibromas

Subcutaneous, soft, sometimes pedunculated, tumours appear. They may be multiple.

Skin pigmentation

Multiple *café-au-lait* patches – pale brown macules 1–20 cm diameter – are found. Isolated patches are common in the normal population, but more than five patches is suggestive of neurofibromatosis.

Neural tumours

Many neural tumours occur more frequently in von Recklinghausen's disease than in the general population, including:

- cutaneous neurofibroma
- eighth-nerve sheath neurofibroma
- spinal cord and nerve root neurofibroma
- meningioma
- glioma (including optic nerve glioma)
- plexiform neuroma (massive cutaneous overgrowth).

Rarely, the benign tumours undergo sarcomatous change.

Associated abnormalities

These include:

- scoliosis
- orbital haemangioma
- local gigantism of a limb
- phaeochromocytoma and ganglioneuroma
- renal artery stenosis
- pulmonary fibrosis
- obstructive cardiomyopathy
- fibrous dysplasia of bone.

TREATMENT

Surgery may be necessary for cosmetic reasons. Tumours causing pressure within the nervous system require excision, if this is feasible.

Tuberose sclerosis (epiloia)

This is a rare autosomal dominant condition whose principal features are adenoma sebaceum, epilepsy and mental retardation (often severe).

Adenoma sebaceum

These are reddish nodules (angiofibromas) that develop on the cheeks in childhood.

Other lesions

Other lesions include shagreen patches, amelanotic naevi, retinal phakomas (glial masses), renal tumours, glial overgrowth in brain and gliomas. Cardiac rhabdomyomas, hamartomas of lung and kidney, and polycystic kidneys may also occur.

Sturge–Weber syndrome (encephalofacial angiomatosis)

There is an extensive port-wine naevus on one side of the face (usually in the distribution of a division of the fifth nerve) and a leptomeningeal angioma. Epilepsy is common. Familial occurrence is exceptional.

von Hippel–Lindau syndrome (retinocerebellar angiomatosis)

This is the occurrence in families (dominant inheritance with variable penetrance) of retinal and cerebellar haemangioblastomas or, less commonly, haemangioblastomas of the cord and cerebrum. Renal, adrenal and pancreatic tumours (and haemangioblastomas) may also be found. Polycythaemia sometimes occurs.

There are numerous other disorders which can be classified with these conditions – for example, ataxia telangiectasia (see p. 182) and Osler–Weber–Rendu syndrome (p. 402).

Spinocerebellar degenerations

The classification of this large group of rare inherited disorders is complex. Three conditions will be mentioned here.

Friedreich's ataxia

This is a progressive degeneration of dorsal root ganglia, spinocerebellar tracts, corticospinal tracts and Purkinje cells of the cerebellum. It is due to an abnormal sequence of DNA triple nucleotide repeats in the gene for fraxatin, a protein of unknown function. Difficulty in walking occurs around the age of 12 years and is progressive. Death is usual before the age of 40. The clinical findings are:

- ataxia of gait and trunk
- nystagmus (in 25%)
- dysarthria
- absent joint position and vibration sense in lower limbs
- absent reflexes in lower limbs
- optic atrophy (in 30%)
- pes cavus
- cardiomyopathy.

Hereditary spastic paraparesis

Isolated progressive paraparesis runs in some families. The inheritance is variable. Additional features including cerebellar signs, pes cavus, wasted hands and optic atrophy are sometimes seen. The conditions are usually mild and progress slowly over many years.

Ataxia telangiectasia (see also p. 182)

This is a rare, autosomal recessive condition that produces a progressive ataxic syndrome in childhood and early adult life. There is striking telangiectasia of the conjunctiva, nose, ears and skin creases. There are also defects in cell-mediated immunity and antibody production. A defect in DNA repair has been demonstrated. Death is usual by the third decade, either from infection or from the development of lymphoreticular malignancy.

Genetically determined neuropathies

These are discussed on p. 1096.

FURTHER READING

Bonn A (1997) Anticipating the future by counting DNA triplet repeats. *Lancet* **349**: 782.

Lesions of peripheral nerves

The various nerve fibre types within a peripheral nerve are shown in Table 18.50. All are myelinated except the C fibres, which carry impulses from pain receptors.

Table 18.50
Fibre types in peripheral nerves

Type	Fibre diameter (mm)	Conduction velocity (m s^{-1})	Function
Aα	10–18	90	Primary spindle afferents α Motor neurones
Aγ	4–8	30	γ Afferents; motor to muscle spindles
Aδ	2–6	30	Fast pain
C	1–2	<1	Slow pain and temperature afferents Autonomic postganglionic

Mechanisms of damage to peripheral nerves

The peripheral nerve consists of two principal cellular structures – the axon, with its anterior horn cell, and the myelin sheath, which is produced by Schwann cells between each node of Ranvier. Blood supply is via *vasa nervorum*. Six principal mechanisms, some of which may coexist, cause malfunction of the nerve as a whole:

- demyelination
- axonal degeneration
- Wallerian degeneration
- compression
- infarction
- infiltration.

Demyelination

When the Schwann cell is damaged, the myelin sheath is disrupted, causing marked slowing of nerve conduction. This occurs in the Guillain–Barré syndrome, in the neuropathy which follows diphtheria, and in hereditary sensorimotor neuropathies, where there are defects in myelin production.

Axonal degeneration

Here the primary lesion affects the axon, which dies back from the periphery. Conduction velocity tends to remain normal because axonal continuity is maintained in surviving fibres. Axonal degeneration occurs typically in toxic neuropathies.

Wallerian degeneration

This describes changes following section of a nerve. The axon and the distal myelin sheath degenerate, over the course of several weeks.

Compression

This causes focal, also called segmental demyelination at the point of compression with disruption of the myelin sheath. This occurs typically in entrapment neuropathies such as the carpal tunnel syndrome.

Infarction

Microinfarction of vessels supplying the nerve occurs in arteritis, such as polyarteritis nodosa, and in diabetes. Wallerian degeneration occurs distal to the focal area of ischaemia.

Infiltration

Peripheral nerves are infiltrated by inflammatory cells in sarcoidosis or leprosy, or by malignant cells.

Nerve regeneration

Regeneration occurs either by remyelination, when recovering Schwann cells spin new myelin sheaths around the axon, or by axonal growth down the nerve sheath and axonal sprouting from the stump. Axonal growth takes place at a rate of up to 1 mm daily. In a chronic polyneuropathy, sprouts from terminal axons of normal motor axons reinnervate denervated muscle fibres; giant polyphasic units are then seen on electromyography.

Definitions

- *Neuropathy* means a pathological process affecting a peripheral nerve or nerves.
- *Mononeuropathy* is a process affecting a single nerve.
- *Mononeuritis multiplex* (multiple mononeuropathy) is a process affecting several or multiple nerves.
- *Polyneuropathy* is a diffuse, symmetrical disease process, usually progressing proximally. It is either acute, subacute or chronic and the course progressive, relapsing or towards recovery. Polyneuropathy may be motor, sensory, sensorimotor (i.e. mixed) or autonomic. Polyneuropathies are classified broadly into demyelinating and axonal types, depending upon which principal pathological process predominates. It is often not possible to separate these varieties clinically.
- *Radiculopathy* means a disease process affecting the nerve roots.

Mononeuropathies

Peripheral nerve compression or entrapment (Table 18.51)

Damage to a nerve by compression is either acute (e.g. due to a tourniquet or other sustained pressure) or chronic, such as in entrapment neuropathy. In both, demyelination predominates, but some axonal degeneration occurs.

Table 18.51
Nerve compression and entrapment

Nerve	Site of entrapment or compression
Median	Carpal tunnel
Ulnar	Cubital tunnel
Radial	Spiral groove of humerus
Posterior interosseous	Supinator muscle
Lateral cutaneous of thigh ('meralgia paraesthetica')	Inguinal ligament
Common peroneal	Neck of fibula
Posterior tibial	Flexor retinaculum (tarsal tunnel)

Acute compression usually affects nerves which are exposed anatomically (e.g. the common peroneal nerve at the head of the fibula). Entrapment develops where a nerve passes through relatively tight anatomical passages (e.g. the carpal tunnel).

These conditions are diagnosed largely from the clinical features. Diagnosis is confirmed by nerve conduction studies and electromyography. The most common conditions are mentioned below. All are more common in people with diabetes. In countries where leprosy is prevalent, such as in India, this disease is a cause of an apparently isolated nerve lesion, which, if seen in the UK, would be likely to be caused by compression or entrapment.

Carpal tunnel syndrome (p. 456)

This is the common condition of median nerve compression at the wrist. Many cases are idiopathic, but this entrapment neuropathy is sometimes seen in:

- hypothyroidism
- diabetes mellitus
- pregnancy and obesity
- rheumatoid arthritis
- acromegaly.

There is nocturnal tingling and pain in the hand (and sometimes forearm) followed by weakness of the thenar muscles. Wasting of abductor pollicis brevis develops, with sensory loss of the palm and radial three-and-a-half fingers. Tinel's sign may be positive, i.e. tapping on the carpal tunnel will reproduce the pain.

Treatment with a splint at night or a local steroid injection in the wrist gives temporary relief. When the condition occurs in pregnancy, owing to fluid retention, it is often self-limiting. Surgical decompression of the carpel tunnel is a simple and definitive treatment.

Ulnar nerve compression

This typically occurs at the elbow, where the nerve is compressed in the cubital tunnel. It follows fracture of the ulna or prolonged or recurrent pressure on the nerve at this site.

Wasting of the ulnar-innervated muscles develops (hypothenar muscles and interossei) together with sensory loss in the ulnar one-and-a-half fingers.

Decompression and transposition of the nerve at the elbow may be necessary.

The deep, solely motor, branch of the ulnar nerve may be damaged in the palm by recurrent pressure from tools, e.g. a screwdriver, crutches or cycle handlebars.

Radial nerve compression

The radial nerve is compressed acutely against the humerus, such as when the arm is draped over a hard chair for several hours ('Saturday night palsy'). Wrist drop and weakness of finger extension and of brachioradialis follow. Recovery is usual within 1–3 months.

Meralgia paraesthetica

Entrapment of the lateral cutaneous nerve of the thigh beneath the inguinal ligament causes burning, tingling and numbness on the anterolateral aspect of the thigh. Many patients are obese; weight reduction helps to relieve the symptoms. Division of the inguinal ligament is not usually effective.

Common peroneal nerve palsy

When the common peroneal (lateral popliteal) nerve is compressed against the head of the fibula, following prolonged squatting, wearing a plaster cast, prolonged bedrest or coma, there is foot drop and weakness of ankle eversion. Frequently no cause is found. A patch of numbness on the anterolateral border of the shin or dorsum of the foot develops. Recovery is usual, though not invariable, within several months.

Mononeuritis multiplex (multiple mononeuropathy)

Mononeuritis multiplex occurs in:

- diabetes mellitus
- leprosy (still the most common worldwide cause)
- vasculitis
- sarcoidosis
- amyloidosis
- malignancy
- neurofibromatosis
- HIV infection.

Diagnosis is largely clinical, supported by electrical studies. Several nerves become affected, for example sequential involvement of an ulnar nerve, a lateral popliteal and radial, over the course of some weeks. When mononeuritis multiplex is symmetrical, there may be difficulties separating it clinically from polyneuropathy. Treatment is that of the underlying disease.

Polyneuropathies

Many toxins and disease processes are known to be associated with polyneuropathy (see below), though the cause of the majority of cases remains undetermined. The most common presentation is a chronic or subacute sensorimotor neuropathy. A classification of polyneuropathy is given in Table 18.52.

Table 18.52
Varieties of polyneuropathy

Guillain–Barré syndrome (acute postinfective polyneuropathy)
Chronic inflammatory demyelinating polyneuropathy
Diphtheritic polyneuropathy
Idiopathic sensorimotor neuropathy
Drugs, toxic, metabolic and vitamin deficiency neuropathies
Polyneuropathy in cancer
Polyenuropathy associated with systemic disease and vasculitis
POEMS syndrome
Autonomic neuropathy
Hereditary sensorimotor neuropathies

Guillain–Barré syndrome (acute inflammatory or postinfective polyneuropathy)

CLINICAL FEATURES

This demyelinating neuropathy, which is the most common recognizable acute neuropathy, has an autoallergic basis. It follows 1–3 weeks after infection that is often trivial, and rarely identified. *Campylobacter* infection is, however, a recognized cause of GBS. The patient complains of weakness of distal limb muscles and/or distal numbness. This ascends over several days or over a period up to three weeks. In mild cases there is little disability, before spontaneous recovery begins, but in some 20% of cases the respiratory and facial muscles are affected and the patient may become paralysed.

Weakness, areflexia and sensory loss are found in an ascending pattern from the fingers and toes.

Autonomic features (see below) are sometimes seen. There is a rare proximal form of the condition that initially affects the ocular muscles and in which ataxia is found (Miller–Fisher syndrome).

DIAGNOSIS

This is established on clinical grounds and is confirmed by nerve conduction studies, which show the slowing of conduction, prolonged distal motor latency and/or conduction block seen in demyelinating neuropathies. The CSF contains a normal cell count and sugar level but the protein is frequently raised to 1–3 $g\ L^{-1}$.

The differential diagnosis includes other paralytic illnesses such as poliomyelitis, botulism or primary muscle disease.

COURSE AND MANAGEMENT

In the untreated case, recovery begins to take place after the initial period of progression of up to three weeks. However by this time, paralysis may be so severe as to require assisted ventilation. It is essential, even in the early stages, that particular attention be paid to measuring ventilatory function (vital capacity, blood gases) repeatedly and recognizing the development of weakness of bulbar muscles. Prolonged assisted ventilation may be necessary. Subcutaneous heparin should be given to reduce the risk of venous thrombosis.

High-dosage intravenous γ-globulin reduces the duration and severity and should be given to all patients. Serum of patients should be screened for IgA deficiency before γ-globulin is given – severe allergic reactions due to IgG antibodies may occur if this congenital deficiency is present.

Plasmapheresis is also of proven benefit in shortening the period of disability. Corticosteroids have been used to treat the Guillain–Barré syndrome but are not of proven value in improving the outcome.

Recovery, though gradual over many months, is usual but may be incomplete.

Chronic inflammatory demyelinating polyneuropathy (CIDP)

This condition, recognized in the 1980s, is a polyneuropathy which develops over weeks or months, usually with a relapsing and remitting course. CSF protein is raised and segmental demyelination is seen in peripheral nerves, with Schwann cells arranged in lamellae resembling an onion skin – hence the pathological term, onion bulbs. The neuropathy responds to steroids and to γ-globulin, which is used in exacerbations. There is particular interest in this neuropathy because, in some cases, plaques resembling MS lesions are seen on MRI, in both the brain and spinal cord.

The outlook is variable, but many cases, with steroid therapy run a benign course over many years. Recovery occasionally occurs.

There are several other varieties of this condition – the classical demyelinating form, an axonal form, and mononeuritis multiplex.

Diphtheritic neuropathy

Demyelinating neuropathy is caused by the exotoxin of *Corynebacterium diphtheriae* (see p. 24). Palatal weakness followed by pupillary paralysis and a sensorimotor neuropathy occur several weeks after faucial infection. The condition is now rare in countries where immunization against diphtheria is practised efficiently.

Idiopathic chronic sensorimotor neuropathy

The patient complains of a progressive symmetrical numbness and tingling in the hands and feet, which spreads proximally in a glove and stocking distribution. There is distal weakness, which also ascends. Rarely the cranial nerves are affected. Tendon reflexes involving affected nerves are lost. The symptoms may progress over many months, remain static or remit at any stage. Autonomic features are sometimes seen.

Table 18.53
Toxic, metabolic and vitamin deficiency neuropathies

Metabolic	**Toxic**
Diabetes mellitus	Drugs
Uraemia	Alcohol
Hepatic disease	Industrial toxins, e.g. lead
Thyroid disease	
Porphyria	**Vitamin deficiency**
Amyloid disease	B_1 (thiamin)
Malignancy	B_6 (pyridoxine)
Refsum's disease	Nicotinic acid
	B_{12}

Investigation (nerve conduction studies and electromyography) shows either axonal degeneration or demyelination, or features of both these processes. Peripheral nerve biopsy is also helpful in classifying these cases, some of which are diagnosed as chronic inflammatory demyelinating polyneuropathy (see above).

Cranial polyneuropathy

This describes simultaneous or sequential cranial nerve lesions, which occur in malignant infiltration, particularly with lymphomas, and in sarcoidosis

Metabolic, toxic and vitamin-deficiency neuropathies

The most common of these neuropathies are shown in Table 18.53. All are due to impairment of normal metabolism of the axon, myelin or both.

Metabolic neuropathies

Diabetes mellitus

Several varieties of neuropathy occur in diabetes mellitus:

- symmetrical sensory polyneuropathy
- acute painful neuropathy
- mononeuropathy and multiple mononeuropathy:
  cranial nerve lesions
  isolated peripheral nerve lesions (e.g. median)
- diabetic amyotrophy
- autonomic neuropathy.

These are discussed in more detail on see p. 982.

Uraemia

Progressive sensorimotor neuropathy occurs in chronic uraemia. The response to dialysis is variable but the neuropathy usually improves after renal transplantation.

Thyroid disease

A mild chronic sensorimotor neuropathy is sometimes seen in both hyperthyroidism and hypothyroidism (see pp. 937 and 932). Myopathy also occurs in hyperthyroidism (p. 937).

Porphyria

Acute intermittent porphyria is a rare metabolic disorder (see p. 1003) in which there are episodes of a severe, mainly proximal, neuropathy, sometimes associated with abdominal pain, confusion and later coma. Alcohol and barbiturates may precipitate attacks.

Amyloidosis

This is described on p. 1002. Either a polyneuropathy or a multineuritis multiplex occurs.

Refsum's disease

This is a rare condition inherited as an autosomal recessive trait. There is a sensorimotor polyneuropathy with ataxia, retinal damage and deafness. It is due to a defect in the metabolism of phytanic acid.

Toxic neuropathies

Alcohol

A polyneuropathy, mainly in the lower limbs, occurs with chronic excess alcohol. Calf pain is common. Thiamine is usually given as treatment, but the response is variable, even with complete abstention. A recurrence or progression of the neuropathy occurs if even small amounts of alcohol are consumed.

Drugs

Many drugs have been reported to be associated with a polyneuropathy. The more important are shown in Table 18.54.

Industrial toxins

A wide variety of industrial toxins have been shown to cause polyneuropathy:

- *Lead poisoning* causes a motor neuropathy.
- *Acrylamide* (plastics industry), *trichlorethylene* (a solvent), *hexane* and other *fat-soluble hydrocarbons* (e.g. those inhaled in glue-sniffing) (see p. 1140) cause a progressive mixed polyneuropathy.
- *Arsenic and thallium* cause a polyneuropathy which is initially sensory.

Vitamin-deficiency neuropathies

Vitamin deficiencies are an important cause of nervous system disease because they are largely preventable and potentially reversible if treated early – and inexorably progressive if not. Deficiency states occur in malnutrition, when they are commonly multiple.

Thiamin (vitamin B_1)

Dietary deficiency causes the clinical syndrome of beriberi (see p. 202). The principal features are polyneuropathy and cardiac failure. It also leads to an amnesic syndrome (Wernicke–Korsakoff psychosis); alcohol abuse is the most common contributing cause in Western countries. Other neurological consequences of alcohol are summarized in Table 18.55.

Wernicke–Korsakoff syndrome

This important thiamine-responsive syndrome associated typically with chronic alcohol abuse is an acute or gradual encephalopathy. The typical triad comprises ocular signs, ataxia and a confusional state, but the condition occurs in partial forms. It is due to ischaemic damage to the brainstem and its connections owing to thiamin dietary deficiency, alcohol or other causes, such as anorexia nervosa. Clinical features include:

- *Ocular signs*. Nystagmus, bilateral lateral rectus palsies, conjugate gaze palsies, fixed pupils and, rarely, papilloedema are found.
- *Ataxia*. There is a broad-based gait, cerebellar signs in the limbs and vestibular paralysis – absent response to caloric stimulation.
- *Confusion*. Apathy, decreased awareness or restlessness, an amnestic syndrome, stupor and coma occur.
- *Hypothermia and hypotension*. These are due to hypothalamic damage and are rare findings.

The condition is underdiagnosed. Erythrocyte transketolase activity is reduced but is of limited practical value as a test because the measurement is rarely available.

Thiamine should be given parenterally if the diagnosis is in question. The drug is harmless; the condition is not. Untreated, Wernicke–Korsakoff syndrome commonly leads to a severe irreversible amnestic state (see Table 18.4 on p. 1013) and residual brainstem signs.

Table 18.54
Drug-related neuropathies

Drug	Neuropathy	Mode/site of action
Phenytoin Chloramphenicol Procarbazine	Sensory	Axon
Isoniazid	Sensory	Pyridoxine metabolism
Dapsone Gold Amphotericin	Motor	Axon
Nitrofurantoin Vincristine Chlorambucil Disulfiram Cisplatin	Sensorimotor	Axon
Perhexiline (not available in UK)	Sensorimotor	Myelin

Table 18.55
Effects of ethyl alcohol

Acute intoxication Disturbance of balance, gait and speech Coma Head injury and its sequelae	Epilepsy (3–10%) Acute intoxication Alcohol withdrawal Hypoglycaemia
Alcohol withdrawal 'Morning shakes' Tremor of arms and legs Delirium tremens	Cerebellar degeneration Cerebral infarction Cerebral atrophy Dementia Central pontine myelinolysis
Thiamin deficiency Polyneuropathy Wernicke–Korsakoff syndrome	Marchiafava–Bignami syndrome (a rare degeneration of the corpus callosum)

Pyridoxine (vitamin B_6)

Deficiency causes a mainly sensory neuropathy. In practical terms it is seen during isoniazid therapy for tuberculosis in those who acetylate the drug slowly. Prophylactic pyridoxine 10 mg daily is usually given with isoniazid.

Vitamin B_{12} (cobalamin)

Deficiency causes disease of the brain, spinal cord and peripheral nerves.

Subacute combined degeneration of the cord

This syndrome of combined spinal cord and peripheral nerve damage is a sequel of addisonian pernicious anaemia and rarely other causes of vitamin B_{12} deficiency (see p. 366).

The patient complains initially of numbness and tingling of the extremities. The signs are of distal sensory loss, particularly posterior column, with absent ankle jerks, owing to the neuropathy, combined with evidence of cord disease – exaggerated knee jerks, extensor plantar responses. Optic atrophy and retinal haemorrhage may occur. In the later stages sphincter disturbance, severe generalized weakness and dementia are seen. Exceptionally dementia is seen in the early stages of the condition. Without treatment the disease is fatal within five years.

Macrocytosis with megaloblastic changes in the bone marrow are invariable in subacute combined degeneration of the cord. Treatment with parenteral B_{12} reverses the peripheral nerve damage but has little effect on the CNS signs (i.e. spinal cord and brain).

Hereditary sensorimotor neuropathies (HMSN)

These disorders are classified within a large and complex group – the hereditary motor and sensory neuropathies (HMSN).

Peroneal muscular atrophy

Peroneal muscular atrophy, or Charcot–Marie–Tooth (CMT) disease, describes a common clinical syndrome in which there is distal limb wasting and weakness that slowly progresses over many years, mostly in the legs, with variable loss of sensation and reflexes. There are several, genetically determined causes. In advanced disease, distal wasting below the knees is so marked that the legs are said to resemble inverted champagne bottles. Mild cases have only pes cavus and clawing of the toes. This may pass unnoticed.

Three principal genetic variants forms of CMT are recognized:

- HMSN type I – a demyelinating neuropathy
- HMSN type II – an axonal neuropathy
- distal spinal muscular atrophy.

Both autosomal dominant and recessive inheritance is seen in different families. In HMSN type I with dominant inheritance – the most common form – linkage has been demonstrated for the locus on the long arm of chromosome 1.

Optic atrophy, deafness, retinitis pigmentosa and spastic paraparesis are sometimes seen in variants of these conditions.

HMSN type III

This was formerly known as the hypertrophic neuropathy of Déjérine–Sottas. It is an autosomal recessive demyelinating sensory neuropathy of childhood leading to severe incapacity during adolescence. It is notable because the CSF protein may be greatly elevated to 10 g L^{-1} or more, and the CSF pathways are obstructed by greatly hypertrophied nerve roots.

Other polyneuropathies

Neuropathy in cancer

Polyneuropathy is seen as a non-metastatic manifestation of malignancy.

Polyneuropathy occurs in myeloma and other dysproteinaemic states, probably owing to impaired perfusion of nerve trunks or to demyelination associated with allergic reactions within peripheral nerves.

Individual nerves are sometimes infiltrated with metastatic malignant cells.

Neuropathies with systemic diseases and vasculitis

Neuropathy occurs in SLE (see p. 489), polyarteritis nodosa (p. 495), Churg–Strauss syndrome (p. 810), rheumatoid disease (p. 475), sarcoidosis and giant cell arteritis (p. 494). Both multiple mononeuropathy and symmetrical sensorimotor polyneuropathy are seen in these conditions.

The POEMS syndrome

This rare eponymous condition is characterized by a chronic inflammatory demyelinating Polyneuropathy, Organomegaly (hepatomegaly 50%), Endocrinopathy (gynaecomastia and atrophic testes), an M protein band on electrophoresis with less than 5% of plasma cells in the bone marrow, and Skin hyperpigmentation.

Autonomic neuropathy

Autonomic neuropathy causes postural hypotension, retention of urine, impotence, diarrhoea (or occasionally constipation), diminished sweating, impaired pupillary responses and cardiac arrhythmia. This situation develops in diabetes mellitus, in amyloidosis and in the Guillain–Barré syndrome.

Many varieties of neuropathy affect autonomic function to a mild, and often subclinical, degree. Occasionally, when there is damage to small myelinated and non-myelinated B and C fibres, the clinical features of the autonomic neuropathy predominate. This is particularly so in diabetes.

Plexus and nerve root lesions

The common conditions that cause these lesions are summarized in Table 18.56. The more important are mentioned below.

Cervical rib (thoracic outlet syndrome)

A fibrous band or cervical rib extending from the tip of the transverse process of C7 to the first rib stretches the lower roots of the brachial plexus (C8 and T1). There is pain along the ulnar border of the forearm, and sensory loss initially in the distribution of T1 with wasting of the thenar muscles, principally the abductor pollicis brevis muscle. Horner's syndrome may occur. The rib or band can be excised.

In some patients the rib or band causes subclavian artery or venous occlusion. The neurological and vascular problems rarely occur together. The term 'thoracic outlet syndrome' is also used, rather vaguely, to describe upper limb symptoms presumed to be due to plexus or nerve root traction or compression.

Neuralgic amyotrophy

This is a clinically distinct condition in which severe pain in the muscles of the shoulder, developing over hours or several days, is followed by wasting, usually of the infraspinatus, supraspinatus, deltoid and serratus anterior muscles, a demyelinating brachial plexus neuropathy. The cause is unknown but, since the condition follows viral infection or immunization in some cases, an allergic basis is postulated.

Recovery of the wasted muscles occurs over some months.

Malignant infiltration

Metastatic disease of nerve roots of the brachial or lumbosacral plexus causes a painful radiculopathy.

Table 18.56
Principal causes of plexus and nerve root lesions

Plexus
Trauma
Malignant infiltration
Cervical rib
Neuralgic amyotrophy
Nerve root
Trauma
Herpes zoster
Meningeal inflammation (e.g. syphilis, arachnoiditis)
Tumours (neurofibroma, metastases)
Cervical and lumbar spondylosis

A common example is an apical bronchial neoplasm (Pancoast's tumour) that causes a T1 lesion and involves the sympathetic outflow. There is wasting of the small muscles of the hand, pain and sensory loss in areas supplied by T1 with ipsilateral Horner's syndrome. This condition also occasionally occurs in apical tuberculosis.

Cervical and lumbar spondylosis (see Tables 8.4 and 8.7)

Spondylosis describes the degenerative changes within vertebrae and intervertebral discs that occur during ageing or secondarily to trauma or rheumatoid disease. Several, often related, factors are important in producing signs and symptoms, including:

- osteophytes – local overgrowth of bone into spurs or bars
- congenital narrowing of the spinal canal
- intervertebral disc degeneration with posterior or lateral disc protrusion
- ischaemic changes in the cord and nerve roots.

Changes on plain X-rays are common in the mid and lower cervical and lower lumbar region in the normal population and correlate poorly with symptoms and signs. Narrowing of the disc space, osteophytes, narrowing of exit foramina, and narrowing of the spinal canal are seen. Unsuspected malignancy or osteomyelits may also be shown.

The most common clinical syndromes will be described. In all these syndromes MRI is the investigation of choice, if available, replacing myelography/radiculography.

Lateral cervical disc protrusion (see Fig 18.24)

The patient complains of pain in the upper limb. A C7 protrusion is the most common lesion. There is root pain, which radiates into the C7 myotome (triceps, deep to scapular and extensor aspect of forearm), with a sensory disturbance, tingling, numbness in the C7 dermatome.

In a C7 root lesion there is:

- weakness and wasting of triceps, wrist and finger extensors
- loss of the triceps jerk
- sensory loss in the C7 dermatome.

Although the initial pain is often very severe, most cases recover with rest and analgesics. It is usual to immobilize the neck in a collar. In cases where recovery is delayed, disc protrusion with root compression is seen on MRI or myelography and surgical root decompression usually performed.

Lateral lumbar disc protrusion

The L5 and S1 roots are commonly compressed by lateral prolapse of the L4–L5 and L5–S1 discs, respectively. There is low back pain and sciatica (pain radiating down the

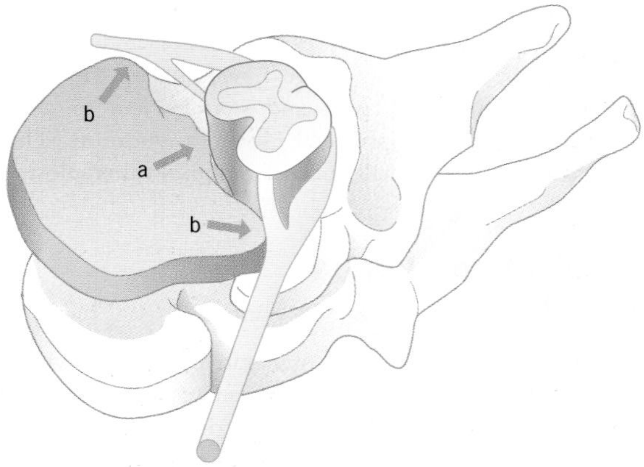

Fig 18.24
Central and lateral cervical disc protrusion
(a) Central disc protrusion compressing spinal cord
(b) Lateral disc protrusion compressing nerve root

buttock and lower limb). The onset is typically acute. It sometimes follows lifting a heavy weight, bending or minor injury. When the pain follows such an event, it is tempting to ascribe the condition entirely to it. However, lateral lumbar disc protrusion is commonly apparently spontaneous, and lifting or injury are usually only precipitating events in an established and inevitable process.

Straight leg raising is limited. There is loss of reflexes (e.g. ankle jerk in a complete S1 root lesion) and weakness of plantar flexion (S1). Sensory loss is found in the affected dermatome.

Most cases of sciatica resolve with rest and analgesics. In the minority, MRI or myelography is necessary and laminectomy is indicated when a root lesion is shown.

Acute low back pain

Acute low back pain is an extremely common problem. Most cases are of disc origin (discogenic) or the pain arises from the facet joints. It is unusual that it causes clinically important nerve root compression. Bedrest for back pain, and rest on hard boards, has long been advocated. However, recent studies suggest that patients should be recommended to be as active as possible and to seek manipulative treatment.

Central disc protrusion (p. 1034)

Central cervical disc protrusion (cervical myelopathy)

Posterior disc protrusion (Fig 18.23), which is common at C4–C5, C5–C6 and C6–C7 levels, causes spinal cord compression. Congenital narrowing of the canal, osteophytic bars and ischaemia are contributory factors.

The patient complains of difficulty in walking. Frequently there are no symptoms in the neck. A spastic paraparesis (or tetraparesis) is found, with variable sensory loss. A reflex level in the upper limbs and evidence of lateral disc protrusion may coexist. MRI or myelography is necessary to demonstrate the level and extent of cord compression.

Manipulation of the neck should be avoided, and a collar should be fitted.

Cervical laminectomy or anterior fusion of the vertebral bodies with removal of the disc may be necessary when the cord compression is severe or progressive. The results of surgery are often disappointing. Complete recovery of the pyramidal signs is unusual, although progression may be halted.

Thoracic disc protrusion

Central protrusion of a thoracic disc is a rare cause of paraparesis.

Central lumbosacral disc protrusion

A central disc protrusion causes a lesion of the cauda equina (cauda equina syndrome) with back pain, bilateral weakness of the lower limbs, sacral numbness, retention of urine, impotence and areflexia. Many nerve roots are involved. The onset is either acute (a cause of an acute flaccid paraparesis) or chronic, when intermittent claudication occurs. The condition should be suspected immediately if a patient with back pain develops retention of urine or sacral numbness. Urgent MRI or myelography followed by surgical decompression is indicated for this emergency.

Neoplasms in the lumbosacral region cause a similar picture.

Spinal stenosis

Narrowing of the spinal canal is developmental and frequently symptomless.

Congenital narrowing of the cervical canal predisposes the cervical cord to damage from minor disc protrusion.

In the lumbar region, further narrowing of the canal by a disc protrusion is a cause of root pain, or the syndrome of buttock and lower limb claudication. As the patient walks, nerve roots become hyperaemic and swell. This causes buttock and lower limb pain with numbness.

Surgical decompression is required in these conditions.

FURTHER READING

Royal College of General Practitioners (1996) *The Management of Acute Low Back Pain.* London: RCGP.

Non-metastatic manifestations of malignancy

Many neurological syndromes may accompany malignancy in the absence of metastases. Clinical pictures include:

- sensorimotor neuropathy (p. 1096)
- mononeuritis multiplex (p. 1093)

- cranial polyneuropathy (p. 1094)
- Lambert–Eaton myasthenic myopathic syndrome (LEMS, p. 1102)
- motor neurone disease variants (p. 1088)
- spastic paraparesis (p. 1085)
- cerebellar syndrome (p. 1030)
- dementia and encephalopathy (p. 1114)
- progressive multifocal leucoencephalopathy (p. 1075).

The mechanism of the above remains obscure. The clinical importance is that the neurological syndrome sometimes precedes clinical recognition of the neoplasm, which is often a small cell carcinoma of the bronchus or a lymphoma. The neurological signs may recede if the tumour is resected or treated.

Diseases of voluntary muscle

Definitions

- *Myopathy* is a general term to describe disease of voluntary muscle.
- *Myositis* indicates inflammation, while *muscular dystrophy* describes inherited disorders with progressive weakness.
- *Myotonia* is the sustained contraction and slow relaxation seen in dystrophia myotonica, and other myotonias.
- *Channelopathy* is a term used to describe disorders of the ion channels within skeletal muscle cells.

Weakness is the predominant feature of primary muscle disease. Its distribution and pattern is of diagnostic importance. A classification of muscle disease is given in Table 18.57. Only the more common conditions are mentioned below.

Table 18.57
Classification of muscle disease

Acquired myopathies	Genetically determined myopathies
Inflammatory myopathy	**Muscular dystrophies**
Polymyositis	Duchenne muscular dystrophy
Alone	Facio-scapulo-humeral dystrophy
With skin lesions (dermatomyositis)	Limb girdle dystrophy
With collagen disease	**Myotonias**
With malignancy	Dystrophia myotonica
Viral, bacterial and parasitic infection	Myotonia congenita
Sarcoidosis	**Channelopathies (periodic paralyses)**
Metabolic and endocrine myopathy	Hypokalaemic periodic paralysis
Corticosteriods/Cushing's syndrome	Hyperkalaemic periodic paralysis
Thyroid disease	Normokalaemic periodic paralysis
Calcium metabolism disorders	**Specific metabolic myopathies** (e.g.)
Hypokalaemia	Myophosphorylase deficiency
Ethanol	Other defects of glycogen and fatty acid metabolism
Drugs	Mitochondrial disease (ragged red muscle fibres)
Myasthenic disorders	Malignant hyperpyrexia
Myasthenia gravis	
Lambert–Eaton myasthenic–myopathic syndrome (LEMS)	

PATHOPHYSIOLOGY

Muscle fibres are affected by:

- acute inflammation and fibre necrosis (e.g. polymyositis, infection)
- chronic degeneration of muscle fibres (e.g. Duchenne muscular dystrophy)
- infiltration by inflammatory tissue (e.g. sarcoidosis)
- fibre hypertrophy and regeneration
- complex immune, ion-channel and mitochondrial disorders.

Examples of the latter are:

- In myasthenia gravis, antibodies to postsynaptic membrane acetylcholine receptor protein cause blocking of neuromuscular transmission.
- In Lambert–Eaton myasthenic–myopathic syndrome (LEMS), antibodies to muscle calcium-channel components are found.
- In myotonias, defective chloride-ion membrane conductance is associated with delayed muscle relaxation.
- In myophosphorylase deficiency (McArdle's syndrome), the enzyme defects in the glycolytic pathway causes weakness after exercise.
- In mitochondrial disease, various enzyme defects in the ATP pathway cause muscle weakness.

INVESTIGATIONS

Diagnosis is made by the recognition of a clinical pattern in many muscle diseases. The distribution of weakness, wasting or hypertrophy, and the consistency of the muscles should be noted.

Serum muscle enzymes

Serum creatine phosphokinase (and aldolase) is greatly elevated in many dystrophies (e.g. Duchenne muscular dystrophy) and in inflammatory disorders of muscle, particularly polymyositis. These enzymes are normal in myasthenia gravis and LEMS, and usually remain normal in myotonias and chronic partial denervation.

Electromyography

When a muscle is weak the normal interference pattern is reduced. Changes in the interference pattern indicate the following:

- *Myopathy*. Short-duration spiky polyphasic muscle action potentials are seen. Spontaneous fibrillation is occasionally recorded.
- *Denervation*. Fibrillation potentials of about 1 ms in duration and 50–200 μV in amplitude are seen, and are evidence of reinnervation.
- *Myotonic discharges*. These consist of high-frequency activity that varies repeatedly to cause a characteristic whining sound on the loudspeaker. These are diagnostic of myotonias.
- *Decrement and increment*. In myasthenia gravis, a characteristic decrement in the evoked muscle action potential follows stimulation of the motor nerve. The reverse is seen (i.e. an increment in repetitive response) in the rare Lambert–Eaton myasthenic-myopathic syndrome (LEMS, see p. 1102), which accompanies small cell carcinoma of the bronchus.

Muscle biopsy

Histology of muscle fibre types (type 1, slow; type 2, fast), denervation, inflammation, dystrophic changes and muscle histochemistry is obtained by muscle biopsy. Electron microscopy is sometimes necessary.

In chronic partial denervation, fibre type grouping (i.e. groups of atrophic fibres of the same fibre type) is seen. Hypertrophic fibres also occur. In acute denervation, small angulated fibres are seen scattered randomly between normal fibres. In dystrophies and myositis, the muscle fibres are diffusely abnormal, the nuclei become central, and invasion by inflammatory cells and/or necrosis occurs.

Considerable experience is required to assess these changes accurately.

Imaging

MR images of muscle show characteristic changes in some cases of inflammatory muscle disease.

Inflammatory myopathies

Polymyositis

This group of disorders is characterized by non-suppurative inflammation of skeletal muscle. The muscles are weak and usually painful. In many cases there are skin changes (dermatomyositis, see p. 1175) or other connective tissue diseases (see p. 487).

CLINICAL FEATURES

Isolated polymyositis is a rare disease, most common in the fourth and fifth decades. Symptoms are of difficulty in rising from a chair, climbing stairs or lifting. Weakness is typically proximal (see Box 8.12). The weak muscles ache and are sometimes tender and indurated. The course of the disease is variable, from a mild condition to a severe progressive disability. If the disease progresses, widespread weakness and wasting develop, with dysphagia, respiratory muscle weakness and cardiac involvement.

INVESTIGATIONS

Preliminary investigations show a raised ESR and a mild normochromic normocytic anaemia. ANF is sometimes positive. The serum creatine phosphokinase is usually greatly elevated. EMG shows myopathic changes. Occasionally fibrillation potentials occur and cause diagnostic difficulty. Muscle biopsy shows inflammatory changes with infiltration of the muscle by mononuclear cells.

DIFFERENTIAL DIAGNOSIS

Muscular dystrophies rarely progress as rapidly as polymyositis and there is no muscle pain. Pseudohypertrophy, which occurs in some dystrophies, does not occur in polymyositis. There is no family history.

Motor neurone disease is always eventually accompanied by upper motor neurone signs, and prominent fasciculation is common.

TREATMENT

Corticosteroids with azathioprine or cyclophosphamide reduce symptoms in about 75% of cases. Only rarely does the disease progress to cause death.

Viral, bacterial and parasitic infection

Muscle tissue is involved in many infections. These are outlined in Table 18.58.

Myopathy in sarcoidosis and rheumatoid disease

In sarcoidosis, a subacute myopathy sometimes occurs, either with limb muscle swelling and induration, or with

Table 18.58
Muscle involvement in infections

Myalgia	Influenza viruses
Bornholm's disease	Cocksackie B5
Acute polymyositis, with myoglobinuria	Cocksackie B6, Echo 9
Acute suppurative (tropical) myositis	*Staphylococcus* spp.
Gas gangrene (clostridial myositis)	*Clostridium perfringens*
Necrotizing myositis	*Streptococcus* spp.
Tuberculous myositis (rare)	*Mycobacterium tuberculosis*
Trichinosis	*Trichinella spiralis*
Cysticercosis	*Taenia solium* (larval form)
Hydatid disease	*Echinococcus granulosus*
Toxoplasma myositis	*Toxoplasma gondii*
Sarcosporidiosis	*Sarcocystis lindemanni*
Chagas' disease	*Trypanosoma cruzi*
Actinomycosis	*Actinomyces* spp.

wasting. This is usually in the course of pulmonary sarcoidosis, but occasionally is an isolated phenomenon. Sarcoid nodules in muscle are seen on biopsy. Treatment is with steroids.

In rheumatoid disease, a rare localized nodular myositis causes painful swelling of limb, trunk and facial muscles.

Metabolic and endocrine myopathies

Corticosteroids and Cushing's syndrome

Proximal muscle weakness occurs with prolonged high-dose steroid therapy, particularly with 9α-fluorinated steroids such as dexamethasone and triamcinolone and in Cushing's syndrome. Selective type-2 fibre atrophy is seen on muscle biopsy.

Thyroid disease (see also p. 812)

Several specific muscle diseases occur. Thyrotoxicosis is sometimes accompanied by a severe proximal myopathy. There is also an association between thyrotoxicosis and myasthenia gravis, and between thyrotoxicosis and hypokalaemic periodic paralysis. Both associations are seen more frequently in South East Asia.

In ophthalmic Graves' disease, there is swelling and lymphocytic infiltration of the extraocular muscles (see p. 940).

Hypothyroidism is sometimes associated with muscle pain and stiffness, resembling myotonia. A true proximal myopathy also occurs.

Disorders of calcium metabolism

Proximal myopathy develops in hypocalcaemia and rickets and osteomalacia of any cause (see p. 510).

Hypokalaemia

Acute hypokalaemia (e.g. in diuretic therapy) causes a severe flaccid paralysis that is reversed by correcting the electrolyte disturbance. (See also periodic paralysis, p. 1104.)

Chronic mild hypokalaemia (also commonly caused by diuretics) gives rise to a mild, mainly proximal, weakness.

Alcohol excess

Severe myopathy with muscle pain, necrosis and myoglobinuria occurs in acute alcoholic excess. A similar syndrome occurs in diamorphine and amphetamine addicts. A subacute proximal myopathy occurs with chronic alcohol abuse.

Drugs

Many drug-induced muscle disorders have been described (Table 18.59). All are rare, and most respond to drug withdrawal.

Neuromuscular junction disorders

Myasthenia gravis

This acquired condition is characterized by weakness and fatiguability of proximal limb, ocular and bulbar muscles. The heart is not affected. The prevalence is about 4 in 100 000. It is twice as common in women as in men, with a peak incidence around the age of 30 years.

The cause is unknown. IgG antibodies to acetylcholine receptor protein are found. Immune complexes (IgG and complement) are deposited at the postsynaptic membranes, causing interference with and later destruction of the acetylcholine receptor.

Thymic hyperplasia is found in 70% of myasthenic patients below the age of 40 years. In 10% of patients a thymic tumour is found, the incidence increasing with age; antibodies to striated muscle can be demonstrated in these patients. Young patients without a thymoma have an increased association with HLA-B8, and DR3.

There is an association between myasthenia gravis and thyroid disease, rheumatoid disease, pernicious anaemia and SLE. Myasthenia gravis is sometimes caused by D-penicillamine treatment in rheumatoid disease.

CLINICAL FEATURES

Fatiguability is the single most important feature. The proximal limb muscles, the extraocular muscles, and the muscles of mastication, speech and facial expression are those commonly affected in the early stages. Respiratory difficulties may occur.

Complex extraocular palsies, ptosis and a typical fluctuating proximal weakness are found. The reflexes are initially preserved but may be fatiguable. Muscle wasting is sometimes seen late in the disease.

INVESTIGATIONS

The clinical picture of fluctuating weakness may be diagnostic. Early symptoms of weakness and fatigue are frequently dismissed by attending doctors.

Table 18.59
Drug-induced muscle disorders

Disorder	Drugs responsible
Subacute proximal myopathy	Diamorphine Clofibrate Chloroquine Lithium Quinine
Myasthenic syndromes	D-Penicillamine Lithium Propranolol
Malignant hyperpyrexia	Psychotropic drugs General anaesthetics

Tensilon (edrophonium) test

Edrophonium 10 mg (an anticholinesterase) is injected intravenously as a bolus after a test dose of 1–2 mg. Improvement in weakness occurs within seconds and lasts for 2–3 minutes when the test is positive. To be certain it is wise to have an observer present and to perform a control test using an injection of saline.

Occasionally the test itself causes bronchial constriction and syncope. It should therefore not be carried out where there are no facilities for resuscitation.

Serum acetylcholine receptor antibodies

These disease-specific IgG antibodies are present in 90% of cases of generalized myasthenia gravis. The antibodies are found in no other condition. In pure ocular myasthenia they are usually undetectable.

Nerve stimulation

There is a characteristic decrement in the evoked muscle action potential following continued stimulation of the motor nerve.

Other tests

Preliminary tests may show a thymoma on chest X-ray that can be confirmed by mediastinal imaging. Small thymomas are seen only with CT or MR imaging.

Routine peripheral blood studies are normal – the ESR is not raised, and the CPK normal. Autoantibodies to striated muscle, intrinsic factor or thyroid may be found. Rheumatoid factor and antinuclear antibody tests may be positive.

Muscle biopsy is usually not performed but ultrastructural abnormalities can be seen.

COURSE AND MANAGEMENT

The severity of myasthenia gravis fluctuates but most cases have a protracted course. It is important to recognize respiratory impairment, dysphagia and nasal regurgitation; emergency assisted ventilation may be required in myasthenic crises. Simple monitoring tests, such as the duration the arm can be held outstretched, and the vital capacity, are useful.

Exacerbations are usually unpredictable and unprovoked but may be brought on by infections, by aminoglycosides or other drugs. Enemas (magnesium sulphate) may provoke severe weakness.

TREATMENT

Oral anticholinesterases

Pyridostigmine (60 mg tablet) is the most widely used drug. Its duration of action is 3–4 hours. The dose (usually 4–16 tablets daily) is determined by the patient's response. This drug prolongs the action of acetylcholine by inhibiting the action of the enzyme cholinesterase. Overdose of anticholinesterase causes severe weakness (a cholinergic crisis).

Colic and diarrhoea may occur with anticholinesterases. Oral atropine 0.5 mg with each dose helps to reduce this.

Although anticholinesterases are of value in treating the weakness, they do not alter the natural history of the disease.

Thymectomy

Thymectomy offers long-term benefit, though the reason is uncertain. It improves the prognosis, particularly in patients below 40 years with positive receptor antibodies and in those who have had the disease for less than 10 years.

Following thymectomy, some 60% of non-thymoma cases improve. If a thymoma is present, surgery is necessary to remove a potentially malignant tumour, but in this setting it is less usual for the myasthenia to improve.

Immunosuppressant drugs

Corticosteroids are used when there is an incomplete response to anticholinesterases. There is improvement in 70% of cases, although this may be preceded by an initial relapse. Azothiaprine is often used in addition.

Plasmapheresis and immunoglobulin

During exacerbations of myasthenia these interventions are of value.

Lambert–Eaton myasthenic–myopathic syndrome (LEMS)

This is a rare non-metastatic manifestation of small cell carcinoma of the bronchus. There is defective acetylcholine release at the neuromuscular junction. Proximal muscle weakness, sometimes involving the ocular and bulbar muscles, is found, with absent reflexes. Weakness tends to improve after a few minutes' muscular contraction, and absent reflexes return, unlike in myasthenia gravis, where reflexes tend to be normal initially, but become depressed as fatiguability develops. Diagnosis is confirmed by EMG and repetitive stimulation.

Antibodies to calcium-channel components are found in some cases. 3,4-Aminopyridine is used in treatment, with variable effect.

Other rare myasthenic syndromes exist, for example congenital myasthenia.

Muscular dystrophies

These are progressive, genetically determined disorders of skeletal and sometimes cardiac muscle. The classification and molecular genetics of these conditions is complex.

Duchenne muscular dystrophy (DMD)

This is inherited as an X-linked recessive disorder, but one-third of cases arise by spontaneous mutation. It occurs in 1 in 3000 male infants. The DMD locus has been localized to the Xp21 region of the X chromosome and the disease is characterized by the absence of the gene product – the protein dystrophin, which is a rod-shaped cytoskeletal muscle protein. DMD is usually obvious by the fourth year, and causes death by the age of 20 years.

Dystrophin is essential for the stability of the cell membrane and, when deficient, leads to a reduction in the three glycoproteins (now called α, β and γ-sarcoglycan) which link dystrophin to laminin in the cell membrane.

Becker's muscular dystrophy which is a milder but disabling condition developing in young adults is due to mutation in the same gene, with, again, abnormalities in dystrophin.

CLINICAL FEATURES

The boy with Duchenne dystrophy is noticed to have difficulty in running and in rising to an erect position from the floor, when he has to use the hands to climb up his legs (Gowers' sign). There is initially a proximal limb weakness with pseudohypertrophy of the calves. The myocardium is affected. The boy becomes severely disabled by the age of 10 years.

INVESTIGATIONS

The diagnosis is often made on clinical grounds alone. The creatine phosphokinase is grossly elevated (100–200 times the normal level). Muscle biopsy shows characteristic variation in fibre size, fibre necrosis, regeneration and replacement by fat, and on immunochemical staining an absence of dystrophin. The electromyogram shows a myopathic pattern.

MANAGEMENT

There is no curative treatment. Passive physiotherapy helps to prevent contractures in the later stages of the disease.

Carrier detection. A female with an affected brother has a 50% chance of carrying the gene. In carrier females, 70% have a raised creatine phosphokinase level and the remainder usually have electromyographic abnormalities or changes on biopsy. Accurate carrier and prenatal diagnosis can be made using cDNA probes that are co-inherited with the DMD locus.

Genetic advice explaining the inheritance of the condition and counselling about abortion should be given. Determination of the fetal sex by amniocentesis and selective abortion of a male fetus is sometimes carried out. Many proven carrier females choose not to have offspring.

Table 18.60
Limb-girdle and facioscapulohumeral dystrophies

	Limb-girdle	Facioscapulo-humeral
Inheritance	Autosomal recessive	Autosomal dominant
Onset	10–20 years	10–40 years
Muscles affected	Shoulder and pelvic girdle	Face, shoulder and pelvis
Progress	Severe diability within 20–25 years	Normal life expectancy slow progression
Pseudohypertrophy	Rare	Very rare

Limb girdle and facioscapulohumeral dystrophy

These less severe but disabling dystrophies are summarized in Table 18.60. There are many other varieties of muscular dystrophy. Most are associated with a sarcoglycan deficiency. Genes for various limb girdle muscular dystrophies (LGMD) have been located on many chromosomes and code for various proteins, e.g. calpain. The rare autosomal dominant LGMD is now called type I. All the recessive varieties are called type II and these are further subdivided depending on the deficiency, e.g. LGMD2A (calpain III deficiency), LGMD2C (γ-sarcoglycan deficiency).

Myotonias

These conditions are characterized by myotonia – continued muscle contraction after the cessation of voluntary effort. The electromyogram is characteristic (see p. 1041). The myotonias are important because patients tolerate general anaesthetics poorly. The two most common of these conditions are mentioned below. Since there is defective chloride-ion membrane conductance in the skeletal muscle cell, these conditions are also classified as channelopathies (see below).

Dystrophia myotonica

This autosomal dominant condition is an example of a gene disorder with triple repeat mutations (see p. 147). It causes progressive distal muscle weakness, with ptosis, weakness and thinning of the face and sternomastoids. Myotonia is usually present. The muscle disease is part of a larger syndrome comprising:

- cataracts
- frontal baldness
- intellectual impairment (mild)
- cardiomyopathy and conduction defects
- small pituitary fossa and hypogonadism
- glucose intolerance
- low serum IgG.

The onset of obvious clinical disease is usually between the ages of 20 and 50 years. The condition is gradually progressive and there appears to be a correlation between disease severity, age at onset and the approximate size of the triple repeat mutations. Phenytoin or procainamide sometimes helps the myotonia slightly.

Myotonia congenita (Thomsen's disease)

This is an autosomal dominant disorder. An isolated myotonia, usually mild, occurs in childhood and persists throughout life. The myotonia is accentuated by rest and by cold. Diffuse muscle hypertrophy occurs – the patient appears to have well-developed muscles.

Channelopathies

These are rare ion-channel disorders characterized by intermittent flaccid muscle weakness and alterations in serum potassium (see also myotonias, above).

Hypokalaemic periodic paralysis

This condition, usually inherited as an autosomal dominant trait, is characterized by generalized weakness, including the speech and bulbar muscles that often starts after a heavy carbohydrate meal or after a period of rest after exertion. Attacks last for several hours. It is often first noted in the teenage years and tends to remit after the age of 35 years. The serum potassium is usually below 3.0 mmol L^{-1} in an attack. The weakness responds to the administration of potassium chloride.

Similar weakness also occurs in hypokalaemia due to diuretics, and may occur during thyrotoxicosis.

Hyperkalaemic periodic paralysis

This condition, usually inherited as an autosomal dominant trait, is characterized by sudden attacks of weakness that are sometimes precipitated by exercise. Attacks start in childhood and tend to remit after the age of 20 years. They last from 30 minutes to two hours. Myotonia may occur. The serum potassium is raised. The attacks can be terminated by giving intravenous calcium gluconate or chloride.

A very rare normokalaemic, sodium-responsive periodic paralysis also occurs.

Specific metabolic myopathies

This is a large complex group of rare, genetically determined muscle diseases. Three of these conditions will be mentioned here.

Myophosphorylase deficiency (McArdle's syndrome)

This is an autosomal recessive disorder in which there is a lack of skeletal muscle myophosphorylase. The disorder causes easy fatiguability and severe cramp on exercise, with myoglobinuria.

The normal rise in venous lactate during ischaemic exercise does not occur, so this forms the basis of a test for the condition.

Malignant hyperpyrexia

Widespread skeletal muscle rigidity and hyperpyrexia developing as a sequel to general anaesthesia is due to a genetic defect in the calcium-release channel of the sarcoplasmic reticulum. Sudden death during or after anaesthesia may occur in this rare condition, which is sometimes inherited as an autosomal dominant trait. Dantrolene is useful in controlling the rigidity.

Mitochondrial diseases

These comprise a complex group of disorders involving muscle, peripheral nerves and the central nervous system. They are characterized by morphological and biochemical abnormalities in mitochondria, with unusual genetic characteristics, for example maternal inheritance. Clinically the spectrum of disease is large, ranging from optic atrophy to myopathies, neuropathies and encephalopathy. MELAS (mitochondrial encephalomyopathy, lactic acidosis, stroke-like episodes) is one well recognized form. Chronic progressive ophthalmoplegia (CPEO) is another, and MERRF describes the occurrence of myoclonic epilepsy and 'ragged red' muscle fibres on biopsy. Further developments in this complex field continue.

FURTHER READING

Ackerman MJ, Clapham DE (1997) Ion channels – basic science and clinical disease. *New England Journal of Medicine* **336**: 1575–1586.

Dubowitz V (1997) The muscular dystrophies – clarity or chaos? *New England Journal of Medicine* **336**: 650–651.

Fadic R, Johns DR (1996) Clinical spectrum of mitochondrial diseases. *Seminars in Neurology* **16**: 11–20.

Poulton J (1996) New genetics of mitochondrial DNA diseases. *British Journal of Medicine* **55**: 712–716.

Psychological medicine

19

Introduction and general aspects

Psychiatry is the branch of medicine that is concerned with the study and treatment of disorders of mental function. A substantial proportion of patients seen by a doctor suffer from psychiatric illness rather than organic disease. Some of these psychiatric problems occur as a consequence of individual social circumstances that may be difficult to alter. Physical and psychiatric disorders often coincide because:

- Patients with psychiatric problems can present with physical manifestations (e.g. abdominal pain in the irritable bowel syndrome).
- Chronic or severe physical ill-health can result in a psychiatric disorder (e.g. depression in the setting of chronic pain).
- Psychiatric symptoms can be part of a physical disease complex (e.g. depression in hypothyroidism).
- Patients with established psychiatric disorders can also develop physical disease.

For these reasons, the psychological aspects of disease cannot be the exclusive preserve of psychiatrists but must be the concern of all doctors.

Epidemiology (see Information box 19.1)

The prevalence of psychiatric ill-health among adults living in private households in the UK is about 14%. Most at some stage consult their family doctor. The majority of the illnesses are minor mood disorders, taking the form of various combinations of depression and anxiety, and about two-thirds are short-lived in nature and clear within six months. However, about 5% of primary care consultations involve patients suffering from major depression requiring energetic treatment. The major psychoses – schizophrenia and manic-depressive illness – are much less common in this setting. The general hospital physician and surgeon will tend to see psychiatric disorders that are associated with physical disease or caused by certain physical treatments, as well as disorders related to alcohol and other forms of drug use and abuse.

About 25% of all those referred to psychiatric departments are aged 65 years and over; this includes patients with disorders such as depression and confusional states, which may be reversible, and dementias, which usually are not. It has been estimated that in England and

Information

- 14% of adults have a neurotic health problem. Women are more likely to suffer this type of problem than men.
- The most common neurotic symptoms are fatigue, sleep problems, irritability and worry.
- The most prevalent neurotic disorder is mixed anxiety and depressive disorder followed by generalized anxiety disorder. The prevalence of all neurotic disorder is higher among women than men.
- The overall rates of alcohol and drug dependence are 4.7% and 2.2% respectively. Men are three times more likely than women to have alcohol dependence and twice as likely to be drug dependent.
- Alcohol and drug dependence are most prevalent among young adults, particularly young men aged 16–24.

Information box 19.1 Psychiatric morbidity among adults in the UK

Wales about half a million people over 65 years suffer from moderate or severe dementia, and about one-quarter of these are aged 85 years or more.

Transcultural psychiatry

There are important similarities and differences in the way that psychiatric ill-health presents in different societies and ethnic groups. Biological factors in mental illness are similar across cultural boundaries whereas psychological and social factors will vary. For example, research carried out by the World Health Organization has demonstrated that the core symptoms of schizophrenia are found in patients from a wide variety of societies, suggesting a biological factor operating independent of cultural factors. Other conditions in which psychosocial rather than biological factors appear to play a key role, such as hypochondriacal states, anxiety and anorexia nervosa, do appear to vary in prevalence and presentation across cultures.

Community psychiatry

During the nineteenth century the rise of psychiatry resulted in a remarkable growth in mental asylums. Today these mental hospitals are being closed and patients are being discharged to community-based facilities, such as hostels, supervised accommodation and rehabilitation facilities. This community care has led to the integration of psychiatry into the community, but there is considerable worry that chronic psychiatric patients end up sleeping rough or occupying low-grade accommodation. The closure of mental hospitals should always be accompanied by the simultaneous development of community facilities linked to a hospital inpatient service, but this has not always been the case.

The psychiatric interview

The interview is of prime importance in making a psychiatric diagnosis:

- It is a technique for obtaining information.
- It serves as a standard situation in which to assess the patient's emotions and attitudes.
- The first interview serves to establish an understanding with the patient that will be the basis of any subsequent therapeutic relationship.

The psychiatric history

The history records data from several sources. These include the patient's complaints, recent and remote past history, and his or her present life situation up to the time of referral or admission. The history consists of:

- **Reason for referral** – a brief statement of why and how the patient came to the attention of the doctor.
- **Complaints** – as reported by the patient.
- **Present illness** – a detailed account of the illness from the earliest time at which a change was noted until the patient came to the attention of the doctor, and the degree to which the illness is recognized by the patient (insight).
- **Family history** – focusing on the family atmosphere in the patient's childhood, early stresses (including death or separation) and the occurrence of mental illness in family members.
- **Personal history** – a short biography that covers childhood and school, jobs held and lost, marriage and divorce, children, and the present housing, social and financial situation.
- **Personality** – consisting of a person's attitudes and beliefs, moral values and standards, leisure activities and interests, and usual reaction to stress and setback.
- **Medical history** – including health during childhood, menstrual and sexual history, previous mental health, and the use and abuse of alcohol, tobacco and drugs.

Supplementary information should be obtained from a close relative or friend who can provide corroboration and additional details.

Symptoms and signs of a psychiatric disorder

Appearance and general behaviour

Facial appearance, posture and movement provide information about a patient's mood. Patients with retarded depression sit with shoulders hunched, immobile, and with the gaze directed at the floor. Agitated depressives are often tremulous and restless, adjusting their clothing and pacing up and down. Manic patients are often overactive and disinhibited.

Certain uncommon disorders of behaviour are encountered, mainly in schizophrenia. These include the following:

- **Stereotypy** is repetition of movements that do not appear to have a purpose. The movement may be repeated in a regular sequence (e.g. rocking backwards and forwards).
- **Mannerisms** are repeated movements that *appear* to have some functional significance (e.g. saluting).
- **Negativism** is when patients do the opposite of what is asked and actively resist efforts to persuade them to comply.
- **Echopraxia** is when patients automatically imitate the interviewer's movements despite being asked not to do this.

Speech

Disorders of thinking are usually recognized from the patient's speech.

Disorders of the stream of thought

These are abnormalities in the amount and speed of the thoughts experienced. At one extreme there is *pressure of thought*, in which ideas arise in remarkable abundance and variety and pass rapidly through the mind. *Poverty of thought* is the opposite experience, when there appears to be a lack or absence of any thoughts whatsoever and patients report their minds to be blank or starved of ideas. Pressure of thought characteristically occurs in mania, and poverty of thought in depression; either may be experienced in schizophrenia. The *stream of thought* can also be suddenly interrupted. Minor degrees of this phenomenon are not uncommon in normal people, especially when they are tired or tense.

Severe *thought blocking*, in which there is a particularly abrupt and complete interruption of the stream of thought, strongly suggests schizophrenia. Patients often describe the experience as a sudden and complete emptying of their minds and may interpret the experience in an unusual way (e.g. as having had their thoughts removed by some alien person, presence or machine).

Disorders of the form of thought

- **Flight of ideas** – The patient's thoughts and speech move quickly from one topic to another, such that one train of thought is not completed before another appears. It is often accompanied by clang associations (the tendency to use two or more words with a similar sound), punning (the use of one word with two or more different meanings), rhyming, and responding to distracting cues in the immediate surroundings. Flight of ideas is characteristic of mania.
- **Perseveration** – This is the persistent and inappropriate repetition of the same thoughts or actions. It is often associated with dementia but can occur in other conditions.
- **Loosening of associations** – This is manifested by a loss of the normal structure of thinking. The most striking impression is an extreme lack of clarity. There are several forms. Knight's move or derailment denotes transition from one topic to another, either between sentences or within a sentence, with no logical relationship between the two topics and no evidence of flight of ideas as described above. When this abnormality is extreme and disrupts not merely the connections between sentences but also the finer grammatical structure of speech, it is termed 'word salad' or 'verbigeration'. One effect of loosened associations is sometimes termed 'talking past the point'; the patient always seems to get near to talking about the matter in hand but never quite gets there.

Mood

The terms *affect*, *emotion*, *feeling* and *mood* refer to the current frame of mind, the predominant feelings of the moment. While the terms affect and mood tend to be used interchangeably, affect is more accurately used to describe a short-term emotional state, mood to describe a more sustained one.

In psychiatric disorders, mood may be altered in three ways:

- Its nature may be changed.
- It may fluctuate more than usual.
- It may be inconsistent either with the patient's thoughts and actions or with occurrences in the patient's immediate environment.

Changes in the nature of mood

Changes in the nature of mood may be towards depression, anxiety or elation.

- **Depression** may mean the symptom of feeling sad, melancholic or low in spirits; or it may mean the syndrome of depression as characterized by low mood, lack of enjoyment, reduced energy and changes in appetite, sleep and libido.
- **Anxiety** is a common symptom of worry or apprehension that is often accompanied by physical symptoms such as palpitations, trembling, butterflies in the stomach and hyperventilation.
- **Anxiety and depression** can occur separately or together and may be associated with an obvious cause or may appear to arise without reason.
- **Elation** refers to a subjective feeling of high spirits, vitality and even ecstasy, which may or may not be accompanied by exuberant behaviour, increased energy and overactivity.

- **Phobia** is an intense fear of a specific object, activity or situation coupled with a wish to avoid it. The fear is irrational in that it is out of all proportion to the real danger. The patient recognizes that it is an exaggerated fear but finds it difficult to control. Objects that provoke such fear include insects, spiders and other animals (e.g. dogs, cats and horses) or natural phenomena such as lightning or the dark. Situations that provoke phobic reactions include open spaces (agoraphobia), closed spaces such as lifts and underground trains (claustrophobia), high places, and crowds.

Changes in the fluctuation of mood

These may result in a total loss of emotion or an inability to experience pleasure. The former is termed *apathy*. When the normal variation of mood is reduced rather than lost, the mood is described as *blunted*. Emotions that are changeable in a rapid, abrupt and excessive way are termed *labile* emotions.

Inconsistent or inappropriate mood

This occurs when the normal emotional expression of the person fails to match their thoughts and actions. For example, a patient may laugh when describing the death of a close and loved relative. Such incongruity needs to be distinguished from laughter that indicates that someone is ill at ease when talking about a distressing subject.

Changes of mood are found in a variety of psychiatric disorders, including depression, mania, anxiety, organic psychoses and schizophrenia.

Thought content

Thought content refers to the worries and preoccupations manifested by the patient and elicited at interview. Abnormal beliefs and experiences are, of course, part of the thought content, but are regarded as sufficiently important to be discussed separately (see below).

- **An obsession** is a recurrent, persistent thought, impulse or image that enters the mind despite the individual's effort to resist it. The individual recognizes that the obsession is self-generated and is not implanted by anyone nor arises from elsewhere.
- **A compulsion** is a repetitive and seemingly purposeful action performed in a stereotyped way, referred to as a *compulsive ritual*. Compulsions are accompanied by a subjective sense that they must be carried out and by an urge to resist. Common obsessions concern dirt, contamination, orderliness and dread of illness, while corresponding compulsions would be repeated hand-washings and checkings.

Insight

This is the degree to which a person recognizes that he or she is ill.

Abnormal beliefs and interpretations of events

The main form of abnormal belief is the delusion (Information box 19.2).

- Delusions can be **primary** or **autochthonous** – they appear suddenly and with full conviction but without any preceding or related mental events. For example, a patient on being offered a cup of tea suddenly believes that this indicates that the Martians have landed.
- Delusions can be **secondary** – derived from some preceding morbid experience, such as a depressed mood or an auditory hallucination.

Delusions are classified according to their content, and include persecutory delusions (also called paranoid delusions), delusions of reference, guilt, worthlessness or nihilism, religious delusions, and delusions of grandeur, jealousy or control. These are further defined when discussed in relation to specific conditions.

Particular delusions concerning thought control can occur. Patients who have *delusions of thought insertion* believe that some of their thoughts are not their own but have been implanted by some outside force or agency. The same or other patients may believe that thoughts are taken out of their minds by external forces or agencies (*thought withdrawal*), while in *delusions of thought broadcasting* patients believe that their unspoken thoughts are known to other people through radio, television, telepathy or in some other way. Feelings and actions may also be interpreted by the individual as being under the influence or control of some external, usually alien, power. Such passivity experiences, occurring in the absence of clear-cut brain diseases, are regarded as diagnostic of schizophrenia. Patients may merely assert that their behaviour is controlled from without and may be unable to give any further explanation. This is usually described as an *experience of passivity*. Patients may develop secondary delusions that explain this alien control as a result of witchcraft, hypnosis, radio waves, television – so-called *delusions of passivity*. The disturbances of thought control discussed above are examples of passivity experiences involving the thought processes.

i Information

Delusion is defined as an abnormal belief arising from distorted judgements and that is:

- held with absolute conviction
- not amenable to reason or modifiable by experience
- not shared by those of a common cultural or social background
- experienced as a self-evident truth of great personal significance
- false.

Information box 19.2 Delusion

Delusions should be distinguished from overvalued ideas – deeply held personal convictions that are understandable when the individual's background is known. *Ideas of reference* that fall short of delusions are held by people who are particularly self-conscious. Such individuals cannot help feeling that people take particular notice of them in public places, pass comment about them and/or observe things about them that they would prefer were ignored. Such a feeling is not delusional in that individuals who experience it realize that it originates within themselves and that they are no more noticeable or noteworthy than anyone else, but nevertheless cannot dismiss the feeling.

Abnormal experiences referred to the environment, body or self

- **Illusions** are misperceptions of external stimuli and are most likely to occur when the general level of sensory stimulation is reduced.
- **Hallucinations** are perceptions that are experienced in the absence of any external stimulus to the sense organs in the outside world, and are not within one's mind as in imagery (Information box 19.3). Normal people occasionally experience hallucinations, mainly auditory in type, particularly when tired and during the transition between sleeping and waking. Hallucinations can be *elementary* (e.g. bangs, whistles) *or complex* (e.g. faces, voices, music), and may be auditory, visual, tactile, gustatory, olfactory or of deep sensation.
- **Depersonalization** is a change in self-awareness such that the person feels unreal. In this state the person feels detached or remote from self-experience and unable to feel emotion. The individual is aware, however, of the subjective nature of this alteration.
- **Derealization** is the feeling that the external environment has become unreal and/or remote. Both this and depersonalization can occur in healthy people when they are tired, after sensory deprivation and when using hallucinogenic drugs, and also occur in certain conditions such as anxiety, depression, schizophrenia and temporal lobe epilepsy.

i Information

Hallucination is defined as a thorough conviction of a sensation when no external object to excite or provoke such a sensation is present. It is:

- a false perception and not a distortion
- perceived as inhabiting objective space
- perceived as having qualities of normal perception
- perceived alongside normal perceptions
- independent of the individual's will.

Information box 19.3 Hallucination

Cognitive state (see Table 19.1)

There are four processes involved in normal memory:

- **Registration** is the ability to add new material to the existing memory stores.
- **Retention** is the ability to retain the memory.
- **Recall** is the ability to bring it back into awareness.
- **Recognition** is the feeling of familiarity indicating that a particular person, event or object has been encountered before.

Some patients describe the recognition of a situation, person or event as having been encountered before when it is in fact novel – the so-called *déjà vu* experience. Others report the reverse experience (*jamais vu*) when there is failure to recognize a situation, person or event that has been encountered before. *Déjà vu* experiences occur in healthy people as well as in anxiety states. Both types of experience can occur in epilepsy (see p. 1056).

Patients with Wernicke–Korsakoff syndrome (p. 1095), who have extreme difficulty in remembering recent and past events, sometimes report remembering past events that have not actually taken place; this is known as *confabulation*. Failure of memory is termed *amnesia*.

Consciousness can be defined as the awareness of the self and the environment. Attention, concentration and memory are impaired and orientation is disturbed in any condition in which a disorder of consciousness occurs. This subject is considered on p. 1043.

Table 19.1
Assessment of cognitive functions

Function	Questions
Orientation	What is the time/day/month/year? Where are you? What is this place? Whom do you recognize?
Concentration	Repeat months of the year backwards Take 7 serially from 100 (serial 7s) Repeat a span of digits (e.g. 5-figure: 43701; 6-figure: 732156)
Memory	
Short-term	Recall test name and address after 2 and 5 minutes
Medium/ long-term	Current affairs (e.g. name of the prime minister, occupant of the throne, events in the news) Dates of World War II
Intelligence	Simple arithmetic sums Meanings of words Meanings of proverbs Ability to read and write
Higher cortical function	Spatial awareness – drawing 3D objects Naming of objects Right–left discrimination (touch your left ear with your right hand)

Defence mechanisms

These are a series of subconscious mental processes. The individual is unaware of employing them, although may become aware of such motives through self-analysis or demonstration by another person. The defence mechanisms described below are among the most commonly used and are useful in understanding many aspects of behaviour.

- **Repression** is the exclusion from awareness of memories, emotions and/or impulses that would cause anxiety and distress if allowed to enter consciousness.
- **Denial**, a related concept, is believed to be employed when patients behave as though unaware of something that they might reasonably be expected to know. One example would be a patient who, despite being told that a close relative has died, continues to behave as though the relative were still alive.
- **Regression** is the unconscious adoption of patterns of behaviour appropriate to an earlier stage of development. It is often seen in ill people who become childlike and highly dependent in relation to their doctor and nursing care.
- **Projection** involves the unconscious attribution to another person of thoughts or feelings that are in fact one's own.
- **Reaction formation** refers to the unconscious adoption of behaviour opposite to that which reflects the individual's true feelings and intentions.
- **Displacement** involves the transferring of emotion from a situation or object with which it is properly associated to another that gives less distress.
- **Rationalization** refers to the unconscious process whereby a false but acceptable explanation is provided for behaviour that in fact has other, much less acceptable, origins.
- **Sublimation** refers to the unconscious diversion of unacceptable outlets into acceptable outlets.
- **Identification** refers to the unconscious process of taking on some of the characteristics or behaviours of another person, often to reduce the pain of separation or loss.

Summary of symptoms and signs

When the full psychiatric history is taken and the patient's mental state has been assessed, it is important to provide a concise assessment of the case which is termed a *formulation*. In addition to summarizing the essential features, the formulation includes a differential diagnosis, a discussion of possible causal factors, identification of outstanding issues to be clarified, and an outline of further investigations needed. It concludes with a concise plan of treatment and a statement of the likely prognosis.

Causes of a psychiatric disorder

A single psychiatric disorder may result from several causes.

Predisposing factors

These are factors, often operating from early life, that determine a person's vulnerability to psychological distress. Such causes include:

- genetic endowment
- environment *in utero*
- personality
- childhood trauma.

There is evidence for a strong genetic factor in the psychoses, and a weaker genetic factor in the neurotic disorders. Intrauterine disturbances may result in minor organic damage to the brain and central nervous system, which in turn may render the individual liable to develop a serious mental disorder in later life in response to particular kinds of stress.

Personality results from the interaction of genetic endowment, uterine development, early childhood experience and various physical, psychological and social influences manifesting themselves up to and including adolescence. Certain personalities are believed to be particularly prone to develop certain disorders. For example, individuals who manifest certain obsessional traits as part of their personality have an increased risk of developing depressive and obsessional illnesses whereas anxious, apprehensive individuals are prone to develop a variety of neurotic disorders. When taking the history, particular care should be taken to assess whether the individual's personality was well developed and mature prior to the development of the illness, as this will be a major factor in determining the outcome of treatment and the prognosis.

Precipitating factors

These are factors that occur shortly before the onset of a disorder and that appear to have caused it. They may be physical, psychological or social in nature. Whether they produce a disorder depends partly on their severity and partly on the presence of predisposing factors.

- **Physical** precipitating factors include physical diseases (e.g. hypothyroidism, tumours, metabolic disorders) or drugs (e.g. steroids) and alcohol.
- **Psychological** factors include loss of self-esteem owing to a setback or misfortune such as marital infidelity or financial disaster.
- **Social** factors include moving house, job difficulties and family disturbances.

Occasionally, the same factor can act in more than one way. A head injury can induce psychological disturbances either through physical changes in the central nervous system or through the stress it provokes in the individual, while marital breakdown may lead to over-indulgence in alcohol with secondary impairment of mental processes and psychiatric illness.

Perpetuating factors

These are factors that prolong the course of a disorder after it has occurred. For example, some psychiatric disorders lead to secondary demoralization. A medical student who suffers a depressive illness may well find it difficult to accept the diagnosis, may feel weak and flawed, and may withdraw from social activities. Such a response could prolong the original disorder.

Psychiatric aspects of physical disease

Psychological and physical symptoms commonly occur together; surveys have shown that they tend to cluster in some people, while others remain relatively free from illnesses. The most common presentation of psychiatric ill-health in physically ill patients is as mood disorders or acute organic mental disorders. The relationship between psychological and physical symptoms may be understood in one of three ways:

- Psychological distress and disorder can provoke and precipitate physical disease.
- Physical distress and disease can cause psychological ill-health (Table 19.2), as can the medication given for the disease.
- Physical and psychological symptoms and disorders coexist because both are common, particularly in the elderly.

Physically ill patients often respond to their illness by feeling depressed, anxious, angry and/or unable to cope. Such reactions are very often transient and require little in the way of management other than recognition, reassurance and support. Sometimes, however, they persist after the acute stage of the physical illness has passed. Certain factors also increase the risk of a psychiatric disorder occurring in the setting of physical disease (Table 19.3). Treatment is the same as for physically healthy, psychiatrically ill patients, but care must be taken to avoid drug interactions when prescribing psychotropic drugs.

Pain

Pain is one symptom that can be thought of as both physical and psychological. It is the most common medical symptom, can cause considerable psychological distress, and can arise from psychological disturbance. The main sites of psychologically determined pain are the head, the neck, the lower back, the abdomen and the genitalia.

Table 19.2
Psychiatric symptoms commonly associated with physical disease

Symptom	Examples of physical disease
Depression	Carcinoma Infection Thyroid disorders Adrenal disorders Diabetes mellitus
Anxiety	Hyperthyroidism Phaeochromocytoma Hypoglycaemia Partial seizures Alcohol/drug withdrawal
Irritability	Head injury Premenstrual tension Early dementia Hypoglycaemia
Fatigue	Anaemia Sleep disorders Infections Carcinoma
Behavioural disturbance	Epilepsy Toxic confusional states Dementia Porphyria Hypoglycaemia

Psychologically determined pain is often continuous for lengthy periods and responds poorly to analgesics. It is often described by the patient as waxing and waning in response to emotional stress and, despite its severity, does not necessarily wake the patient from sleep. A particularly dramatic form of chronic, atypical pain is facial pain, and antidepressant therapy has been found to be effective in up to 50% of such patients. Another common painful condition in which depression is often present but is masked by the physical symptoms is the irritable bowel syndrome (p. 280).

Table 19.3
Factors increasing the risk of psychiatric illness in physically ill patients

Patient	Physical illness
Previous history of psychiatric illness	Carcinoma
History of difficulty in coping with stress	Endocrine disorders
Disturbed personal, family or social circumstances	Infections
	Metabolic disorders
	Head injury
	Mutilating surgery
Setting	**Physical treatment**
Intensive care units	Drugs (e.g. steroids)
Coronary care units	Radiotherapy
Renal dialysis units	

Chronic fatigue syndrome

The cardinal symptoms are fatigue, poor concentration, fever, lymphadenopathy, impaired memory, irritability, alteration in sleep and muscular aches occurring for a minimum of six months. This syndrome, previously known as myalgic encephalomyelitis (ME), Icelandic disease or Royal Free Hospital disease, has been attributed to an infection, usually viral. Suspect viruses include the enteroviruses and the Epstein–Barr virus. There is, however, no good evidence of any infective cause of this condition at present and laboratory investigations are normal. Those fatigue states which clearly do follow on a viral infection are classified as *post-viral fatigue states*.

The characteristic symptom of chronic fatigue syndrome is abnormal muscle fatigue on exercise with very slow recovery from exercising to the point of exhaustion. There is often an associated depression. Treatment involves a pragmatic approach to rehabilitation using behavioural techniques to gradually and consistently increase activity (graded exercise), reduce avoidance behaviour and improve confidence and illness control. Cognitive techniques are used to assist patients to re-evaluate their understanding of illness, combat depression and anxiety, and look for underlying thoughts and assumptions that may contribute to disability. The serotonin reuptake inhibitor group of antidepressants (p. 1125) may well have a specific effect on energy.

Classification of psychiatric disorders

The concept of mental illness is complicated. The diagnosis is only made when:

- there is a recognizable disturbance in one or more psychological functions (e.g. perception, emotion, thought)
- the disturbance is not under the comprehensive control of the individual concerned
- the disturbance usually – though not invariably – causes distress to the affected individual
- the disturbance usually – though not invariably – requires expert, professional assessment and treatment for recovery.

Particular problems in psychiatry are posed by such conditions as sexual disorders, drug and alcohol dependence, and personality disorders.

In 1994, the fourth edition of the *Diagnostic and Statistical Manual* of the American Psychiatric Association (DSM-IV) was published to provide clear descriptions of diagnostic categories in order to enable clinicians and investigators to diagnose, communicate about, study and treat people with various mental disorders. This scheme has *five axes*.

I Psychiatric syndromes, clinical syndromes
II Personality disorders, mental retardation
III General medical conditions
IV Psychosocial and environmental problems
V Overall level of functioning

Another system – the *International Classification of Diseases and Related Health Problems* (ICD-10) – includes a detailed classification of 300 psychiatric and behavioural disorders. It is published by the World Health Organization and is currently in its tenth edition. The traditional division between neurosis and psychosis, evident in earlier editions, has been discarded, although the terms are still used. Instead of following the neurotic–psychotic dichotomy, the disorders are now arranged in groups according to major common themes (e.g. mood disorders, schizophrenia, disorders of adult personality and behaviour, and marked psychomotor retardation). This makes for increased convenience of use.

A classification of psychiatric disorders derived from ICD-10 is shown in Table 19.4, and this is the classification used in the main in this chapter.

Psychosis

This is the term usually applied to a psychiatric disorder that significantly impairs insight, involves a substantial break with reality, exercises a major impact on the individual's personality and functioning, and which may require specialized, inpatient treatment. Certain symptoms that by definition involve an impairment of reality – such as delusions, hallucinations and formal thought disorder – are often termed *psychotic symptoms*.

Neurosis

This is the term applied to psychiatric disorders in which psychotic symptoms and features are absent, the patient's personality is relatively undamaged, and contact with reality is unimpaired. Neuroses can be thought of as exaggerated forms of the normal reactions to stressful events. Anxiety, depression, irritability and physical symptoms lacking an organic cause are experienced by many people in response to stressful circumstances and events.

Table 19.4
International classification of psychiatric disorders (ICD-10)

Organic disorders [F00–F09]
Mental and behavioural disorders due to psychoactive substance use [F10–F19]
Schizophrenia and delusional disorders [F20–F29]
Mood (affective) disorders [F30–F39]
Neurotic, stress-related and somatoform disorders [F40–F49]
Behavioural syndromes [F50–F59]
Disorders of adult personality and behaviour [F60–F69]
Mental retardation [F70–F79]

The three-character F codes refer to the diagnostic categories of the latest edition (the 10th) of the *International Classification of Diseases*, produced by the World Health Organization

FURTHER READING

Americal Psychiatric Association. *Diagnostic and Statistical Manual of Mental Disorders* (DSM–IV). Washington, DC: APA, 1994.

Royal College of Physicians/Royal College of Psychiatrists. *The Psychological Care of Medical Patients: Recognition of Need and Service Provision.* London, 1995.

Editorial on chronic fatigue syndrome. *Journal of the Royal College of Physicians*, November/December 1996: 497.

World Health Organization. *International Classification of Diseases and Related Health Problems* (ICD–10). Geneva: WHO, 1992.

Folstein MF, Folstein SE, McHugh PR (1995) 'Mini-mental state'; a practical method of grading the cognitive state of patients for the clinician. *Journal of Psychiatric Research* **12**: 189–198

Organic mental disorders [F00–F09]

Organic brain disorders result from structural pathology, as in senile dementia, or from disturbed central nervous system (CNS) function, as in fever-induced delirium. A classification of organic mental disorders is shown in Table 19.5. They do not include mental and behavioural disorders due to alcohol and abuse of drugs, which are classified separately (see Table 19.4)

Delirium

Delirium, also termed *toxic confusional state*, is an acute or subacute condition in which impairment of consciousness is accompanied by abnormalities of perception and mood. The impairment of consciousness can range from mild befuddlement to serious disorientation and confusion. The degree of impairment classically fluctuates, so that there are intermittent lucid periods. Confusion is usually worse at night. During the acute phase, thought and speech are incoherent, memory is impaired and misperceptions occur. Transient hallucinations, usually visual, and delusions may occur and, as a consequence, the patient may be frightened, suspicious, restless and uncooperative. A large number of diseases may be accompanied by delirium, particularly in elderly patients. Some causes of delirium are listed in Table 19.6. Delirium usually clears within a few days as the underlying illness resolves. If the delirium runs a subacute course, more permanent disorders of cognition, memory or personality may occur.

Table 19.5
Classification of organic mental disorders [F00–F09]

Dementia
Organic amnesic syndrome
Delirium
Personality/behavioural disorders due to organic factors
Organic mood (affective disorders)

INVESTIGATION AND TREATMENT

Investigation and treatment of the underlying physical disease should be undertaken. The patient should be carefully nursed and rehydrated. Pain relief should be adequate and sedation provided if necessary. If a high fever is present, the temperature should be reduced with fans, ice-packs and antipyretic drugs. All current drug therapy should be reviewed and, where possible, stopped. Benzodiazepines are the drugs of choice in the management of minor restlessness, but in severe delirium haloperidol is probably a more effective choice, the daily dose usually ranging between 10 and 60 mg. If necessary, the first dose of 2–10 mg can be administered intramuscularly.

MANAGEMENT OF THE DISTURBED OR VIOLENT PATIENT

Psychotic, organically impaired and intoxicated patients may be frightened, aggressive, confused and difficult to manage. It is important that those involved in their acute management refrain from threatening behaviour, appear in control (even if they do not feel it!), and avoid being drawn into a confrontation.

When evaluating a disturbed patient in the emergency department, a crucial question is: Could this behaviour be the result of an organic disturbance? Organic psychiatric disorders, particularly those associated with drugs and alcohol, are important causes of behavioural and thought disturbances in emergency clinic attenders. Some organic disorders such as poisoning, meningitis and hypoxia can initially show signs and symptoms of psychosis and may be life-threatening

Table 19.6
Causes of delirium

Systemic infection
Any infection, particularly with high fever (e.g. malaria, septicaemia)

Metabolic disturbance
Hepatic failure
Renal failure
Disorders of electrolyte balance
Hypoxia

Vitamin deficiency
Thiamine (Wernicke–Korsakoff syndrome, beri beri)
Nicotinic acid (pellagra)
Vitamin B_{12}

Endocrine disease
Hypoglycaemia
Cushing's syndrome

Intracranial causes
Trauma
Tumour
Abscess
Subarachnoid haemorrhage
Epilepsy

Drug intoxication
Anticonvulsant
Anticholinergic
Anxiolytic/hypnotic
Opiates
Industrial poisons, e.g. DDT, trichloroethylene

Drug/alcohol withdrawal

Postoperative states

DDT, dichlorodiphenyltrichloroethane

Treatment of the disturbed patient is with chlorpromazine in doses of 25–50 mg orally; i.m. haloperidol 2–10 mg, causes less hypotension and is an alternative.

Dementia

Dementia is a syndrome due to disease of the brain in which there is a disturbance of multiple higher cortical functions, including memory, thinking, orientation, comprehension, calculation, learning capacity, language and judgement. However, consciousness is not clouded. There is often an associated deterioration in emotional control, social behaviour and motivation. Presenile dementia and early-onset dementia are terms used for patients under 70 years of age and senile dementia for older patients; there is, however, no clinical difference.

About 25% of the elderly population suffer from a psychiatric disability, mainly anxiety and depression. However, dementia affects about 10% of those aged over 65 years and 20% of those over 80 years of age – a total of 650 thousand people in England and Wales.

The causes of dementia are shown in Table 19.7. Seventy per cent are due to Alzheimer's disease (AD).

Differential diagnosis
This includes a depressive disorder which may exhibit many of the features of an early dementia, especially memory impairment, slowed thinking, and lack of spontaneity; delirium; mild or moderate retardation; iatrogenic mental disorders due to medication (see Table 19.9).

Table 19.7
Causes of dementia

Degenerative	**Traumatic**
Alzheimer's disease	Post-head injury
Pick's disease	Punch drunk syndrome (boxers)
Huntington's disease	**Intracranial space occupying lesions**
Parkinson's disease	Subdural haematoma
Normal pressure hydrocephalus	Tumours
Vascular	**Anoxic**
Cerebrovascular disease (see Table 19.8)	Cardiac arrest
Cranial arteritis	Respiratory failure
Metabolic	Carbon monoxide poisoning
Uraemia, renal dialysis	**Infections**
Liver failure	Encephalitis of any cause
Remote effects of carcinoma	Creutzfeld–Jacob disease
Toxic	HIV infection
Alcohol	Syphilis
Occupational exposure (e.g. chemicals)	**Endocrine**
Heavy metals (e.g. lead)	Hypothyroidism
Vitamin deficiency	Hypocalcaemia
B_{12}	
Thiamin	

Alzheimer's disease [F00]

This is a primary degenerative brain disease of unknown aetiology that is insidious in onset followed by gradual deterioration and then death in about ten years. The onset can be in middle adult life or even earlier (of presenile onset) but the incidence is higher in later life. Patients particularly at risk of developing Alzheimer's disease are those who have a family history, who have sustained a head injury, or have Down's syndrome.

Clinical features of Alzheimer's disease
The cardinal clinical deficits include:

- impaired ability to learn new information or to recall previously learned information
- a decline in language function and, in particular, increased difficulty with names and understanding what is being said
- apraxia – an impaired ability to carry out motor activities despite intact motor function
- agnosia – the failure to recognize or identify objects despite intact sensory function
- impairment of executive functioning – planning, organizing, sequencing, abstracting.

Behavioural changes are common, including wandering, agitation and aggression. Paranoia with persecutory delusions occurs in up to 50% of patients. Depressive symptoms are also common, but severe depression is not usual.

Pathophysiology of Alzheimer's disease
Neuropathological changes include neuronal reduction, neurofibrillary tangles, senile neuritic plaques and a variable amyloid angiopathy. These changes are particularly seen in the hippocampus, substantia innominata, locus ceruleus and the tempoparietal and frontal cortices. Neurofibrillary tangles are found within the cell body and are made up of paired helical filaments containing the microtubular associated protein, tau. Ubiquitin is found in association with the neurofibrillary tangles. Lewy bodies, eosinophilic cytoplasmic inclusions in neurones, are also seen in some cases. Granulovacuolar degeneration is seen in the hippocampus. Senile plaques, consisting of a central core of amyloid, develop progressively. Aggregation of amyloid appears to be a central event. The gene for the precursor protein of amyloid is localized close to the defect on chromosome 21, causing familial Alzheimer's disease.

Neurochemical changes occur, including a marked reduction in the enzyme choline acetyltransferase, in acetylcholine itself, and in other neurotransmitters and neuromodulators.

The apolipoprotein E gene is present in the general population in three alleles, ε2, ε3 and ε4. Genetic linkage studies have shown that the ε4 allele is commonly seen in patients with Alzheimer's disease, whereas the ε2 allele is under-represented. It has been suggested that the

Table 19.8
Types of vascular dementia

Dementia type	Vessels involved	Clinical features
Multi-infarct	ACA, MCA, PCA	Aphasia, amnesia, apraxia, agnosia
Strategic infarct		
Angular gyrus syndrome	MCA (Left inf. parietal branch)	Anosmia, agraphia, alexia, acalculia, right/left disorientation, finger agnosia, constructional deficit
Thalamic	Thalamoperforant arteries	Amnesia, executive dysfunction apathy
Lacunar state	Lenticulostriate	Psychomotor slowing, memory disturbance, executive dysfunction, apathy
Binswanger's	Medullary arteries of white matter	Psychomotor slowing, memory disturbance, executive dysfunction, apathy
Mixed vascular	Large and small cerebral arteries	Evidence of cortical and subcortical dysfunction

ACA, anterior cerebral artery; MCA, middle cerebral artery; PCA, posterior communicating artery.

accumulation of β-amyloid protein is more extensive in subjects with the ε4 allele than in those without it, whereas the presence of allele ε2 may be associated with less amyloid protein. The great majority of cases of AD are sporadic and are of late onset. Early-onset AD is inherited as an autosomal dominant disorder with mutations on chromosome 14 or 21.

Increased free radicle formation and *impaired anti-oxidant defences* may play a role in the neurodegenerative process. There is a 25–35% reduction in the free radicle defence enzyme superoxide dismutase in the frontal cortex and hippocampus. Anti-oxidant therapy is suggested for treatment (see below).

Vascular dementia (multi-infarct dementia) [F01]

This is the second most common cause of dementia and is distinguished from Alzheimer's disease by its history of onset, clinical features and subsequent course. There is usually a history of transient ischaemic attacks with brief impairment of consciousness, fleeting pareses or visual loss. The dementia may follow a succession of acute cerebrovascular accidents or, less commonly, a single major stroke. Vessel occlusion is the most common cause of vascular dementia, and this may produce a variety of cognitive deficits depending on the site of the ischaemic damage. Five major vascular dementia syndromes have been recognized (Table 19.8). Multi-infarct dementia results from involvement of several vessels supplying the cerebral cortex and subcortical structures and is typically associated with signs of cortical dysfunction.

Dementia in other disease [F02]

Dementia occurs due to, or suspected of being due to, other disorders including Creutzfeldt–Jakob disease, Huntington's disease, Parkinson's disease and HIV infection.

In *Pick's disease*, a progressive dementia occurs, commencing in middle life and characterized by slowly progressing changes of social and personal deterioration. This is followed by impairment of intellect, memory and language functions. The characteristic neuropathological change is that of selective atrophy of the frontal and temporal lobes with silver-staining cytoplasmic inclusion bodies (Pick's bodies). There are no senile plaques or neurofibrillary tangles in excess of that seen in normal ageing, and this distinguishes Pick's disease from Alzheimer's.

Patients who manifest both cognitive deficits and depressive symptoms may have either dementia of depression (so-called depressive 'pseudodementia') or dementia with depression (Table 19.9). Patients with pseudodementia show memory loss and executive dysfunction and often have a previous history of depression or a family history of mood disorder. Successful treatment of the mood disorder results in restoration of intellectual function.

DIAGNOSIS OF DEMENTIA

The presence of dementia is usually diagnosed clinically (see p. 1109), but it can be confirmed by psychometric testing (e.g. the Wechsler scale). A careful history and examination is essential. The history must also be taken from someone who has known the patient for a long time. Secondary causes (Table 19.7) are infrequent, but must be excluded as some causes are potentially reversible. Investigations should include blood tests and radiology (Information box 19.4)

i Information

Blood tests
- Full blood count
- Urea and electrolytes
- Blood glucose
- Liver biochemistry
- Serum calcium
- Vitamin B_{12}
- TSH, T4, T3
- Syphilis serology
- HIV antibodies

Radiology
- Chest X-ray
- CT or MRI scan to confirm the presence of cortical atrophy and to exclude other lesions, such as a brain tumour

Information box 19.4 Diagnosis of dementia

Table 19.9
Clinical features of delirium, dementia and acute affective psychosis

Feature	Delirium	Dementia	Acute affective psychosis
Onset	Sudden	Insidious	Sudden
24-h course	Fluctuating	Stable	Stable
Consciousness	Reduced	Clear	Clear
Attention	Globally impaired	Globally impaired	Variably affected
Cognition	Globally impaired	Globally impaired	May be selectively impaired
Hallucinations	Usually visual	Often absent	Mainly auditory
Delusions	Fleeting, poorly systematized	Often absent	Sustained, systematized
Orientation	Usually impaired	Often impaired	May be impaired
Psychomotor	Increased, reduced or shifting	Often normal	Varies from retardation to hyperactivity
Speech	Often slow, rapid or incoherent perseveration	Difficulty finding words	Normal, slow or rapid
Involuntary movements	Often asterixis or coarse tremor	Often absent	Usually absent
Physical illness or drug toxicity	One or both are present	Often absent	Usually absent

After Lipowski ZJ (1989) *New England Journal of Medicine* **320**:578–581

MANAGEMENT OF DEMENTIAS

There are five aspects to the management of dementia:

- treating any underlying disorder (Table 19.7)
- treating the cognitive deficit in selected patients with AD
- ameliorating associated behavioural disturbances
- reducing the consequences of disability
- addressing the needs of the caregiver.

Vascular dementia patients are usually treated with aspirin to forestall further strokes. Depression is treated with antidepressants or ECT. Patients with Parkinson's disease and dementia often show motor – though rarely cognitive – improvement with selegiline and dopaminergic drugs.

The cognitive deficit of Alzheimer's disease in some patients shows a response to tacrine (not yet available in the UK). This drug inhibits cholinesterase and produces an improvement in intellectual function in 33–50% of patients who can tolerate the higher doses. Patients who respond to the drug usually improve to the level of function present 6–12 months previously. However, tacrine is potentially hepatotoxic and aminotransferase levels must be monitored weekly for the first six months. Tacrine therapy requires that a patient has a well-established diagnosis of AD, normal liver function and a caregiver willing to give the drug four times daily and to ensure that liver biochemistry is tested as required.

The first drug to be licensed in the UK for the treatment of AD is the acetylcholinesterase inhibitor, donepezil. Its benefits appear modest, but it is easily administered and its side-effect profile is favourable. α-Tocopherol (vitamin E), a potent anti-oxidant, and selegiline, a monoamine oxidase B inhibitor which also facilitates catecholaminergic activity, have shown encouraging results in one study with a delay in functional deterioration. HRT in postmenopausal women and NSAIDS have shown protective effects against developing AD.

Organic amnestic syndrome [F04]

This is characterized by a marked impairment of memory occurring in clear consciousness and not as part of a delirium or dementia. Long-term memory is affected but the typical feature is impairment of short-term memory. Often the patient is blandly unconcerned and commonly displays confabulation. One of the most common causes is severe thiamin deficiency secondary to chronic alcohol abuse (this is classified separately in ICD-10 as F10, see p. 1135) but other, less common causes are shown in Table 18.4.

Personality/behavioural disorders due to organic factors

Organic delusional disorder

The organic delusional disorder is characterized by a mental state dominated by delusions that are often accompanied by a persistent and distressing misperception of the environment, sometimes referred to as *delusional tone*. The delusions are very often persecutory but may also be hypochondriacal, pathologically jealous, grandiose or erotic.

Organic affective disorders

Organic affective disorders consist of marked mood changes that result from organic brain damage. There are depressive and manic phases, often occurring suddenly, or there may be a persistently dysphoric state. There is no significant intellectual loss, delusions or hallucinations, and a family history of an affective disorder is uncommon.

FURTHER READING

Cummings JL (1995) Dementia: the failing brain. *Lancet* **345**: 1481–1484.

Donaldson C, Tarrier N, Burns A (1997) The impact of the symptoms of dementia on caregivers. *British Journal of Psychiatry* **170**: 62–66.

Drachman DA, Leber P (1997) Editorial: Treatment of Alzheimer's disease. *New England Journal of Medicine* **336**: 1245–1249.

Schizophrenia [F20–F29]

The group of illnesses conventionally referred to as 'schizophrenia' is diverse in nature and covers a broad range of cognitive, emotional and behavioural disturbances. The term schizophrenia was coined by the Swiss psychiatrist Eugen Bleuler in 1908 as a 'rending (disconnection) or splitting of the psychic functions'. The normal integration of emotional and cognitive functions is ruptured in schizophrenia. The annual prevalence of the condition is 2–4 per 1000. The lifetime risk of contracting schizophrenia is 1%, but for first-degree relatives of sufferers it is 12%. High rates have been reported in Slovenia and among the Tamils of South India.

CAUSES

No one cause has been identified to date. A number of possible causes have been implicated and are the subject of research.

Genetic factors

Adoption studies and twin studies have revealed a 40% risk for children of two affected parents and a 50% risk for the monozygotic twin of an affected individual. Studies suggesting a linkage between a schizophrenia susceptability gene and markers on chromosome 5 have not been established. However, a linkage has been found in patients and family members between a neurophysiological deficit and a dinucleotide polymorphism at chromosome 15q 13–14.

Dopamine

Although the pathophysiology of schizophrenia has not been delineated, drug development has been heavily influenced by the hypothesis that certain dopamine pathways are overactive. Evidence for dopamine overactivity includes the capacity for antipsychotic drugs to block dopamine receptors *in vivo* and *in vitro* and the fact that the clinical efficacy of antipsychotic drugs is, in general, highly correlated with their ability to block dopamine D_2 and D_1 receptors. Dopamine agonists, such as amphetamine, exacerbate schizophrenia. Postmortem studies show increased dopamine binding sites in the brains of affected patients.

Serotonin

An abnormality in the 5-HT (serotonin) system has been suggested as there are relatively consistent findings of altered 5-HT receptor densities and 5-HT metabolism in the brain. Furthermore, atypical antipsychotics such as clozapine, risperidone and olanzepine (see below) have a high affinity for serotonin receptors. Recently, it has been shown that a 5-HT receptor gene (5-$HT_{2\alpha}$-receptor) or a locus in linkage disequilibrium to it confers susceptibility to schizophrenia.

Brain damage

This is implicated in some forms of schizophrenia. The possible role of damage *in utero* from long-acting viruses is still being explored. In a subgroup of patients with schizophrenia, enlargement of the ventricles and widening of the cerebral fissures and sulci have been shown on CT scans.

Psychological theories

These suggest that schizophrenics have an impaired ability to handle the amount and speed of incoming perceptual stimuli and/or that some schizophrenics have a left hemisphere limbic dysfunction. A popular social theory suggests that disturbances in family relationships or communication are the cause, but the evidence is poor. Studies of so-called expressed *emotion* suggest that schizophrenic patients are particularly vulnerable to highly expressed emotions, and such family atmospheres increase the chances of relapse in treated patients as do intensive psychotherapy and social demands.

Environmental factors

Schizophrenia is more common in those born in the winter and early spring, suggesting an environmental factor, possibly a virus.

CLINICAL FEATURES

The illness can begin at any age but is rare before puberty. The peak age of onset is in late adolescence and the early twenties. The overall gender incidence is about equal. The symptoms that have been considered as diagnostic of the condition have been termed *first-rank symptoms* and were described by the German psychiatrist Kurt Schneider. They consist of:

- auditory hallucinations – patients hear their own thoughts spoken aloud and/or hear one or several voices referring to themselves in the third person or referring to them by name, and/or hear voices commenting on their behaviour
- thought withdrawal, insertion and interruption
- thought broadcasting

- delusional perceptions
- external control of emotions
- somatic passivity and feelings – patients believe that thoughts or acts are due to the influence of others.

The World Health Organization's International Pilot Study of Schizophrenia has shown that the presence of any one of these symptoms, in the absence of physical disease, is highly discriminating for the diagnosis in a variety of countries and cultures. Other symptoms of acute schizophrenia include behavioural disturbances, thought disorder, hallucinations, delusions and mood abnormalities. Schizophrenia is sometimes divided into the so-called 'positive' and 'negative' types:

- Positive schizophrenia is characterized by acute onset, prominent delusions and hallucinations, normal brain structure and function, a biochemical disorder involving dopaminergic transmission, good response to neuroleptics, and better outcome.
- Negative schizophrenia is characterized by a slow, insidious onset, a relative absence of acute symptoms, the presence of apathy, social withdrawal, lack of motivation, underlying brain structure abnormalities, and poor neuroleptic response.

It is still customary to divide schizophrenia into a number of subtypes even though many patients present with symptoms and behaviours belonging to more than one subtype. The main subtypes are as follows.

Paranoid schizophrenia

This is the most common presentation of schizophrenia throughout the world. It usually has a later age of onset and a more insidious course than other subtypes. Delusions, persecutory in nature, dominate the clinical picture, together with hallucinatory voices that often threaten the patient. 'Negative' symptoms such as blunting of affect and impaired drive are much less common and appearance and behaviour are usually well-preserved and normal.

Simple schizophrenia

This is characterized by the insidious deterioration of the personality from early in adolescence. 'Positive' symptoms such as delusions and hallucinations are often absent or difficult to elicit. There is a slow but remorseless withdrawal from social interaction, an increasing eccentricity of manner, and an inability to meet personal and social demands. The characteristic 'negative' symptoms develop without being preceded by any overt 'positive' symptoms. With increasing social deterioration vagrancy commonly ensues.

Hebephrenic schizophrenia

In this type, delusions and hallucinations are often fleeting and fragmentary and the clinical picture is dominated by a markedly shallow and inappropriate mood. Like simple schizophrenia, this type usually develops in late adolescence. Thought processes are often disturbed and disorganized and speech rambling and incoherent. Commonly there is inappropriate giggling, grimaces, mannerisms, hypochondriacal complaints and an aimless and purposeless behaviour.

Catatonic schizophrenia

For reasons that are unclear, this form of schizophrenia is now rarely seen in developed countries although reportedly it is common elsewhere. The central feature is a marked psychomotor disturbance which alternates between hyperkinesis and stupor or between automatic obedience and marked negativism. Stereotyped movements and fixed postures may be maintained for a long period, while episodes of violent agitation also feature. Hallucinations and delusions are usually conspicuous.

Chronic schizophrenia

This is characterized by thought disorder and the so-called negative symptoms of underactivity, lack of drive, social withdrawal and emotional emptiness. Motor disturbances can occur but they are extremely rare. Such disorders are often described as catatonic and include stupor, excitement, mannerisms, stereotypies and automatic obedience. Delusions in chronic schizophrenia are often held with little emotional response (the so-called *systematized* delusions) and may be encapsulated from the rest of the patient's beliefs and behaviour.

DIFFERENTIAL DIAGNOSIS

Schizophrenia must be distinguished from:

- organic mental disorders
- mood (affective) disorders
- personality disorders.

The most important organic disorders, particularly in young patients, are drug-induced psychoses and temporal-lobe epilepsy. Some of the drugs that can produce psychosis are listed in Table 19.10.

In older patients, any acute brain syndrome as well as dementia can present in a schizophrenia-like manner. A helpful diagnostic point is that clouding of consciousness

Table 19.10
Some drugs causing psychosis

Glucocorticoids
Anticholinergic agents
Sympathomimetic central stimulants
Phenytoin
Carbamazepine
Lithium
Disulfiram
Cardiac glycosides
Hallucinogens (e.g. LSD, mescaline, ecstasy)
Amantadine
L-Dopa
Indomethacin

LSD, lysergic acid diethylamide

and disturbances of memory do not occur in schizophrenia, and visual hallucinations are unusual.

Mood (affective) disorders present with a more sustained disturbance of mood and any delusions and hallucinations that are detected are usually understandable in terms of the mood disturbance. First-rank symptoms are not normally a feature of affective disorders. Differentiating insidiously arising schizophrenia from a personality disorder in a young person can be exceptionally difficult and the passage of time may be needed for the condition to be clarified.

The term 'schizoaffective' is often used to describe a clinical presentation in which clear-cut mood (affective) and schizophrenic symptoms coexist.

COURSE AND PROGNOSIS

The prognosis of schizophrenia is highly variable (Table 19.11). The patient's psychosocial environment appears important. In an understimulating environment negative symptoms worsen, whereas in an excessively stimulating environment positive symptoms may emerge or worsen. Some patients suffer only acute episodes that leave them relatively unimpaired; others insidiously develop chiefly negative symptoms. The most common presentation and course is an initial acute episode of floridly positive symptoms followed by the emergence and persistence of negative symptoms.

A review of treatment studies suggests that 15–25% of schizophrenics recover completely, about 70% will have relapses and may develop mild to moderate negative symptoms, while about 10% will become seriously disabled.

TREATMENT

The best results are obtained by combining drug and social treatments.

Drug treatment: antipsychotic (neuroleptic) drugs

These act by blocking the D_1 and D_2 groups of dopamine receptors, so reducing psychomotor excitement and controlling many of the symptoms of schizophrenia without causing disinhibition, confusion or sleep. Such drugs are most effective against acutely occurring, positive symptoms and least effective in the management of chronic, negative symptoms. Complete control of positive symptoms can take up to three months and premature discontinuation of treatment can result in prompt relapse. Until the superiority of clozapine (see below) was demonstrated in patients who had not responded adequately to other drugs, antipsychotic drugs were thought to be interchangeable in terms of efficacy.

As antipsychotic drugs block both D_1 and D_2 dopamine receptors, they usually produce extrapyramidal side-effects. This limits their use in the maintenance therapy of many patients. They also block adrenergic and cholinergic receptors and thereby cause a number of unwanted effects (Table 19.12). An infrequent but potentially dangerous unwanted effect is the neuroleptic malignant syndrome (Information box 19.5).

In patients manifesting good prognostic features and responding well to drugs, treatment may be discontinued under supervision after several months. Poor-prognosis schizophrenia, on the other hand, usually requires regular maintenance therapy for many months or even years.

Pregnancy. Data on the potential teratogenicity of antipsychotic (neuroleptic) medications are still limited. The disadvantages of not treating an acute psychosis or mania during pregnancy have to be balanced against possible developmental risks to the fetus. Acuteness and severity of symptoms, past response and state of gestation must all be considered, although it is generally agreed that the more potent butyrophenones (e.g. haloperidol) are safer than the phenothiazines. Subsequent management decisions on dosage will depend primarily on the ability to avoid side-effects, since the antiparkinsonian agents are still believed to be teratogenic and should be avoided.

Antipsychotic drugs available

Phenothiazines are the group of neuroleptics used most extensively. Chlorpromazine (100–1000 mg daily) is the drug of choice when a more sedating drug is required. Trifluoperazine is used when sedation is undesirable. Fluphenazine decanoate is used as a long-term prophylactic to prevent relapse as a depot injection (25–100 mg i.m.

Table 19.11
Prognostic factors of schizophrenia

	Good factors	**Bad factors**
Premorbid state	No family history of schizophrenia	Family history of schizophrenia
	Stable personality	Withdrawn, solitary, eccentric personality
	Warm personal relationships	Poor work record; poverty of relationships
	Stable home relationships	Stormy domestic situation
Features of illness	Identifiable precipitating factor or life event	No obvious triggering factor or life event
	Acute onset	Insidious onset
	Few first-rank symptoms	Many first-rank symptoms
	Disturbance of mood	No mood disturbance
	Initiative, interest and motivation maintained	Blunting of emotional responses; initiative, motivation and interest impaired
	Prompt treatment	Treatment delayed

every 1–4 weeks). Promazine or thioridazine are useful in the elderly when it is desirable to reduce the risk of extrapyramidal and anticholinergic side-effects.

The *butyrophenones* (e.g. haloperidol 2–30 mg daily, droperi-dol) are also powerful antipsychotics used in the treatment of acute schizophrenia and mania. They are highly likely to cause extrapyramidal side-effects but are much less sedating than the phenothiazines.

Substituted benzamides (e.g. sulpiride 200 mg daily) are highly selective D_2 receptor antagonists and are less likely to produce extrapyramidal disorders. They are used to control florid positive symptoms.

'Atypical antipsychotics' '

Clozapine is used in patients with intractable schizophrenia (approximately 20% of patients) who have failed to respond to at least two conventional antipsychotic drugs. This drug is a dibenzodiazepine with a relative high affinity for D_1 compared with D_2 dopamine receptors, and muscarinic and α-adrenergic receptors. It also blocks 5-HT_2 and 5-HT_1 receptors. Clozapine has been shown to exercise a dramatic therapeutic effect on positive and negative symptoms, cognitive function and quality of life and is increasingly being used in treatment-resistant schizophrenic patients, that is, those patients who are not responsive to or intolerant of conventional neuroleptics. However, this drug is expensive and produces severe agranulocytosis in 1–2% of patients. Therefore it can only be prescribed to registered patients by doctors and pharmacists registered with the Clozaril patient-monitoring service. The starting dose is 25 mg per day with a maintenance dose of 150–300 mg daily. White cell counts should be monitored weekly for 18 weeks and then two-weekly for the length of treatment. In addition to its antipsychotic actions, clozapine may also help reduce aggressive and hostile behaviour and the risk of suicide.

Table 19.12
Unwanted effects of neuroleptic drugs

Common effects	Rare effects
Extrapyramidal	**Hypersensitivity**
Acute dystonia*	Cholestatic jaundice
Parkinsonism	Leucopenia
Akathisia	Skin reactions
Tardive dyskinesia	
Autonomic	**Others**
Hypotension	Precipitation of glaucoma
Failure of ejaculation	Galactorrhoea
	Amenorrhoea
Anticholinergic	Cardiac arrhythmias
Dry mouth	Seizures
Urinary retention	Retinal degeneration (with thioridazine in high doses)
Constipation	
Blurred vision	
Metabolic	
Weight gain	

*Treated by i.m. procyclidine

Risperidone is a benzisoxazole derivative with combined dopamine D_2-receptor and serotonin 5-HT_2-receptor-blocking properties. The superiority of this drug to existing agents for routine treatment or its similarity to clozapine for refractory patients is still being determined. Dosage ranges from 6 to 16 mg per day. The drug is not markedly sedative and the overall incidence and severity of extrapyramidal side effects is lower than with more conventional antipsychotics.

Olanzepine is another new receptor-targeted atypical antipsychotic to appear. It has affinity for 5-HT_2, D_1, D_2 and muscarinic receptor sites. Clinical studies indicate its effectiveness in ameliorating negative as well as positive symptoms and its lower incidence of extrapyramidal side-effects. Early indications suggest that there is better compliance with the drug which may be related to its lower side-effect profile and its once-daily dosage of 5–10 mg.

Sertindole is also available. It is associated with QT interval prolongation. Its place in therapy is being evaluated.

Psychological treatment

This consists of reassurance, support and a good doctor–patient relationship. Psychotherapy of an intensive or exploratory kind is contraindicated.

Social treatment

Social treatment involves attention being paid to the patient's environment and social functioning. Patients with any degree of residual impairment and negative symptoms usually require rehabilitation in a structured

i Information

Neuroleptic malignant syndrome occurs in 0.2% of patients on neuroleptic drugs, particularly potent dopaminergic antagonists such as haloperidol.

Symptoms appear a few days to a few weeks after initiation of therapy and consist of:

- hyperthermia
- muscle rigidity
- autonomic instability (tachycardia, labile BP, pallor)
- fluctuating level of consciousness.

Investigations show:

- ↑ creatine phosphokinase
- ↑ WCC
- abnormal liver biochemistry.

Treatment can be:

- *Specific*
  bromocriptine – to enhance dopaminergic accuracy
  dantrolene – to reduce muscle tone
- *Nonspecific*
  general management including temperature reduction.

Information box 19.5 Neuroleptic malignant syndrome

work and social environment. Parents and relatives need advice concerning the optimum amount of emotional and social stimulation to be provided for the patient. Some patients can manage a normal job, whereas others require a sheltered workshop. A very small number of severely disabled patients require long-term residential medical and nursing care.

As with most psychiatric conditions, the treatment of schizophrenia is multidisciplinary. In addition to the active involvement of psychiatrists and psychiatric nurses, other professionals including psychologists, psychiatric social workers, community psychiatric nurses, occupational therapists and counsellors play important therapeutic roles. This is particularly true in the case of the major psychoses. While psychiatrists and psychiatric nurses are crucially involved in the hospital management of such conditions, community psychiatric nurses play important roles in maintaining patients within the community. Psychologists, in addition to their skills in assessing the psychological status of patients, deliver cognitive, behavioural and other forms of therapy while occupational therapists work within hospital and community settings to assess and improve patient's social and occupational skills.

FURTHER READING

Eaton WW, Thara R, Federman B, Melton B, Liang K-Y (1995): Structure and course of positive and negative symptoms in schizophreina. *Archives of General Psychiatry* **52**: 127–134.

Kane J (1996) Drug therapy: schizophrenia. *New England Journal of Medicine* **334**(1): 34–41.

Kennedy JL (1996) Schizophrenia genetics: the quest for an anchor. *American Journal of Psychiatry* **153**: 1513–1514.

Mood (affective) disorders [F30–F39]

The central and common feature of these disorders is an abnormality of mood, either depressed or elated or both. Mood is best considered in terms of a continuum ranging from severe depression at one extreme to severe mania at the other, with the normal, stable mood at the centre (Fig 19.1). Manic-depressive disorders are divided into bipolar manic-depression, in which patients suffer attacks of both depression and mania, and unipolar disorders, in which there is either mania alone or, more commonly, depression alone. DSM-IV further differentiates manic disorders into so-called 'bipolar I', which encompasses mania of a severity usually requiring hospitalization, and 'bipolar II', which describes milder mania or hypomania which rarely requires hospitalization. The term 'secondary mania' describes manic symptoms or a syndrome that is seen in various organic conditions.

First-degree relatives of patients suffering from bipolar illness have an increased risk of manic-depressive illness but not those of patients with unipolar illness.

Depression is classically divided into *endogenous depression* and *reactive depression*, although the validity of this distinction is doubtful.

Principal criteria of endogenous depression

- Pervasive and unresponsive depression
- Early morning waking
- Diurnal variation of mood (worse in the morning)
- Profoundly depressive ideas (e.g. guilt, suicidal feelings)
- The lack of an obvious precipitating cause
- A stable premorbid personality.

Principal criteria of reactive depression

- A fluctuating depression responsive to environmental change
- Self-pity rather than self-blame
- A clear precipitating cause
- A vulnerable or predisposed personality
- Absence of the criteria of endogenous depression.

A mixture of both types is a more common presentation than a pure form of either.

Dysthymia

This term is used to describe a depression lasting for at least two years and characterized by depressed mood, sleep and appetite disturbances, fatigue, loss of self-esteem, disturbances of concentration and a feeling of discouragement. The point prevalence of dysthymia in the general population has been estimated at 3.1%.

CLINICAL FEATURES

The clinical features of *mania* reflect a marked elevation of mood (Table 19.13). The term 'hypomania' refers to a

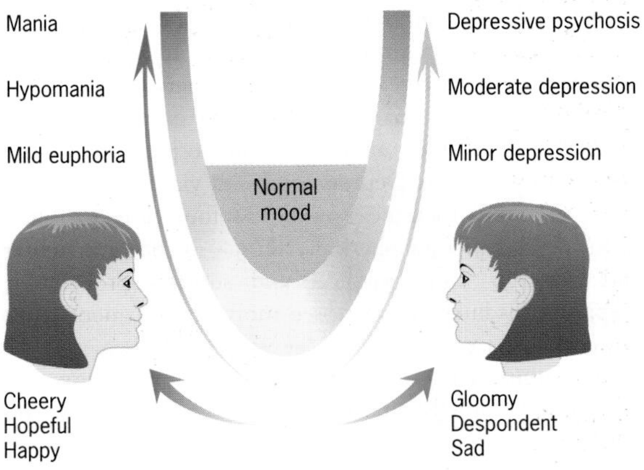

Fig 19.1
Continuum of normal and abnormal mood

Table 19.13
Clinical features of mania

Characteristic	Clinical appearance
Mood	Elevated, infectious, labile
Talk	Fast, pressurized, flight of ideas, punning, rhyming
Energy	Excessive, restless, distractable
Ideation	Grandiose, self-confident, delusions of wealth, power, influence or of religious significance, persecutory delusions
Cognition	Formal testing difficult, disturbance of retrieval of memories
Physical	Insomnia, mild to moderate weight loss
Behaviour	Disinhibition, increased sexual interest, excessive drinking or spending
Hallucinations	Fleeting auditory or, more rarely, visual

Table 19.14
Clinical features of depression

Characteristic	Clinical appearance
Mood	Depressed, miserable, unhappy
Talk	Impoverished, slow, monotonous, incomplete
Energy	Lacking, retarded (in some cases agitation), apathetic
Ideation	Feelings of futility, guilt, self-reproach, unworthiness, hypochondriacal preoccupations, worrying, suicidal thoughts, delusions of guilt, nihilism, persecution
Cognition	Verbal memory impaired, pseudo-dementia in elderly patients
Physical	Early waking, appetite and weight loss, constipation, loss of libido, impotence, fatigue, bodily aches and pains
Behaviour	Retardation or agitation, poverty of movement and expression
Hallucinations	Auditory – often abusive, hostile, critical

mild form of mania characterized by euphoria, overactivity and disinhibition. It can be difficult to distinguish this from simple exuberance, enthusiasm and good humour.

At the opposite pole of the affective continuum, major *depressive illness* is also characterized by disturbances of mood, talk, energy and ideation (Table 19.14). The mood may be described by the patient in physical terms, such as: like a weight in the head, a tightness of the chest, or a feeling of almost physical pain. Depressed patients describe the world as grey, themselves as lacking a zest for living, and their bodies as devoid of pleasure and feeling. Anxiety is common, obsessional symptoms may emerge and, in the severer forms, delusions of guilt, persecution and of bodily disease are not uncommon. In severe depression, apparent organic impairment, detectable on cognitive testing, can result in disorientation. Seasonal affective disorder is characterized by recurrent episodes of depression occurring during the winter months. Such depression can be successfully treated with supplementary exposure to artificial full spectrum light delivered on a daily basis.

Depression is a common experience. It occurs in the setting of physical disease, social stress, personal problems and life crises. As many as one-third of patients with physical disease, either at home or in hospital, have some degree of depression. Depressed patients view themselves as more sick, visit their doctors almost four times as often as the non-depressed physically ill, stay in hospital longer and undergo more medical and surgical procedures. Depression is linked to increased mortality in patients with physical illness, especially in those with heart disease.

It is important to distinguish the more severe and potentially life-threatening major form, requiring energetic treatment, from the less severe minor form which, with simple support, sympathy and reassurance, usually lifts (Table 19.15). It is also important to avoid the pitfall of not treating a treatable depression just because it seems an 'understandable' reaction to serious illness or difficult circumstances. This is particularly likely to happen if the patient is elderly or severely or even terminally ill.

AETIOLOGY

Possible factors involved in the aetiology of mood (affective) disorders are shown in Table 19.16. In addition, depression in adult women has recently been linked in some instances to a history of sexual abuse experienced in childhood. Estimates of the prevalence of childhood sexual abuse vary but there is a consensus to the effect that it is common, serious, and infrequently reported. The abuser is usually known to the child and preadolescent girls are at greatest risk. The severity of the abuse may be related to the development of psychiatric ill-health in adult life. Other negative outcomes of abuse in childhood include a decline in socioeconomic status, increased sexual problems and difficulties in intimate relationships. More information is needed concerning the long-term outcome of survivors of childhood sexual abuse and the results of intervention, as well as more specific information about different types of abuse, the relationship with the perpetrator and the context in which the abuse occurred.

DIFFERENTIAL DIAGNOSIS

This is shown in Table 19.17.

Occasionally, doctors are called upon to distinguish between normal grief following a separation or bereavement, and depressive illness. A number of symptoms that commonly occur in depressive illness also follow bereavement, most notably sleep disturbance, appetite and weight loss, and tearfulness. However, a number of distinguishing features can usually be identified (Table 19.18).

Table 19.15
Depression: features that help distinguish major from minor depression

Characteristic	Minor	Major
Mood	Transiently low Responsive to environment	Persistently low Unresponsive to environment
Behaviour	Capable of being lifted out of gloom and sadness	Persistently agitated and/or retarded
Suicidal feelings	Fleeting	Persistent
Delusions	Absent	Often present
Physical symptoms	Vague aches and pains, some appetite and sleep loss	Persistent bowel changes, appetite and weight loss, sleep disturbance and early waking
Hallucinations	Absent	Occasionally present

Table 19.16
Possible aetiological factors involved in affective disorders

Biological

Genetic

10–15% of first-degree relatives have an affective disorder (risk in community is 1–2%)
68% of monozygotic twins reared together or apart are concordant for manic-depressive disorder
23% of dizyotic twins are concordant
Possible links with genetic markers

Biochemical

Imbalance in neurotransmitters (e.g. monoamine neurotransmitters are depleted in depression, but increased in mania)
Loss of diurnal rhythm of plasma cortisol in depression
Hormonal factors (e.g. depression is more common after childbirth, in premenstrual phase, with use of oral contraceptives, the menopause and post-hysterectomy)
Electrolytes – intracellular sodium is high in affective disorders

Psychological

Maternal deprivation

Psychoanalysis initially suggested that loss of maternal affection in early life and any significant loss in early childhood predisposes individuals to affective disorder in later life

Learned helplessness

Experimental animals put in a position where they cannot escape or control punishing stimuli develop a behavioural syndrome that resembles depression in humans. It has led to the suggestion that a similar mechanism is at work in humans

Social

Stressful events

An excess of life events is found in the months before the onset of depression. Life events include bereavement, loss of a job, moving house, marriage and going on vacation

Vulnerability factors

In women, it has been claimed that certain factors render them vulnerable to becoming depressed. These include lack of a job outside the home, the presence of three or more young children in the family, and lack of a confiding, intimate relationship

Two conditions presenting in women and characterized by disturbance of mood may well be related to manic-depressive disorders. These are the premenstrual syndrome and puerperal affective disorders. Despite the fact that the linking of the menopause with depression is pervasive in lay and medical discourse, there is no substantial scientific evidence to support the view that a natural menopause causes depression.

The premenstrual syndrome

Symptoms consist of irritability, depression and tension during the 7–10 day premenstrual period. These symptoms are often accompanied by breast tenderness, a subjective feeling of weight gain and bloatedness, and headache, and are usually dramatically relieved with the onset of the period. Women who suffer from affective disorders may be more prone to experience premenstrual symptoms and to have exacerbations of their psychiatric disorder during the premenstrual phase.

The cause or causes of the premenstrual syndrome remain unclear, and the various treatments proposed, which include the use of vitamin B_6 (p. 204), diuretics, progesterone, oral contraceptives, oil of evening primrose and oestrogen implants, remain empirical.

Puerperal affective disorders [F53]

It has been shown that childbirth has the highest relative risk of any factor so far measured in psychiatry – considerably higher than adverse events or physical illness in depression. In postpartum women, affective disorders occur. Such disturbances are usually divided into maternity blues, postpartum (puerperal) psychosis, and chronic depression, although other rarer conditions can occur including mother–infant relationship disorders, child abuse and infanticide. 'Maternity blues' is used to describe the brief episodes of emotional lability, irritability and tearfulness that occur in about 50% of women 2–3 days postpartum and that resolve spontaneously in a few days. 'Postpartum psychosis' occurs once in every 500–1000 births. Over 80% of cases are affective in type and the onset is usually within the first two weeks following delivery. In addition to the classical features of an affective psychosis,

Table 19.17
Affective disorders – differential diagnosis

Mania	
Drug-induced psychosis	Amphetamines, cannabis or steroids
Acute schizophrenia	Other classical (i.e. first-rank) schizophrenic symptoms usually present or eventually emerge
Dementia	Global cognitive impairment may present with euphoria and irritability; in mania, any cognitive impairment improves with treatment
Hyperthyroidism	Check TSH
Depression	
Systemic physical disease	Malignancy Hypothyroidism Hyperparathyroidism Cushing's syndrome Vitamin and mineral disorders Infection and postinfection Neurological disease (e.g. multiple sclerosis, Parkinson's disease) Collagen disorders Cerebral ischaemia Congestive heart failure Porphyria
Drug-induced depression	Corticosteroids
Hormones	Oestrogen Progesterone
Hypotensive agents	Reserpine Methyldopa Clonidine
Antiparkinsonian drugs	Levodopa Amantadine hydrochloride
Anticancer drugs	Vincristine Vinblastine
Psychiatric disorders	Schizophrenia Alcohol abuse Drug abuse Anxiety neurosis Dementia (see Table 19.7)

disorientation and confusion are often noted. Severely depressed patients may have delusional ideas that the child is deformed, evil or otherwise affected in some way, and such false ideas may lead to attempts to kill the child and to suicide. The response to speedy treatment is generally good. The recurrence rate for a depressive illness in a subsequent puerperium is 15–20%.

Less severe depressive disorders occur during the first postpartum year in 10–20% of mothers. Depression after childbirth is clinically similar to any other depression. Most patients recover after a few months. Social and psychological factors are important but the underlying aetiological factor is unknown.

TREATMENT

The treatment of affective disorders involves physical, psychological and social therapies. Hospitalization is usually required in the case of severely depressed, potentially suicidal patients and in mania. In general, neither severe depression nor mania respond to psychotherapy, and both require energetic physical treatment. Simple support, reassurance, sympathy and the opportunity to express distress and negative feelings are often sufficient to bring about relief of minor depressive episodes.

Drugs in the treatment of depression

Tricyclic and related antidepressants

These are the drugs used most frequently. Imipramine and amitriptyline are the two used most commonly, but many related compounds have been introduced, some having fewer autonomic and cardiotoxic effects. Imipramine and amitriptyline are given by mouth in initial doses of 25–75 mg daily, building up over a week to 150–200 mg daily. The full therapeutic impact can take up to 2–3 weeks to occur. These drugs potentiate the action of monoamines, noradrenaline and serotonin by inhibiting their reuptake into nerve terminals (see Fig 14.2). Other tricyclics in

Table 19.18
Bereavement reaction versus depressive illness following bereavement (morbid grief reaction)

Characteristic	Normal bereavement	Depressive illness
Onset	Immediately follows loss	Delay for weeks or months
Duration	Lasts weeks rather than months	Persists for weeks/months/years
Pattern	Person slowly accepts loss and adjusts accordingly	Patient denies loss and refuses to accept implications
Grief	Expressed openly	Difficulty in expressing grief
Guilt	Mild regret in early stages	Marked guilt often present

Table 19.19
Unwanted effects of tricyclic antidepressants

Anticholinergic effects Dry mouth Constipation Tremor Blurred vision Urinary retention Postural hypotension	**Convulsant activity** Lowered seizure threshold **Other effects** Weight gain Sedation Mania Agranulocytosis (mianserin)
Cardiac effects ECG changes Arrhythmias	

common use include nortriptyline, doxepin, mianserin, clomipramine, lofepramine and trazodone. Tricyclic antidepressants have a number of side-effects (Table 19.19). In patients with established cardiac disease, mianserin, dothiepin or trazodone are preferred over the more cardiotoxic compounds.

Serotonin reuptake inhibitors and related drugs

Fluvoxamine, fluoxetine, paroxetine and sertraline appear to produce less troublesome side-effects and a speedier onset of therapeutic effect. These drugs appear to act by way of selective inhibition of serotonin reuptake only (rather than of both noradrenaline and serotonin) within the synaptic cleft and are thus termed 'selective serotonin reuptake inhibitors' or SSRIs. While there is still argument as to their superiority as antidepressants over the more established tricyclics, and concern about their cost, they are becoming popular (fluoxetine is now one of the most commonly prescribed antidepressants in the USA) because of their lower rate of serious side-effects. The most common side-effects include nausea, headache, agitation and restlessness, insomnia and diarrhoea. A less common but troublesome toxic effect is the so-called 'serotonin syndrome'. This occurs coincident with the addition of or increase in a known serotonergic agent to an established medication regimen. It is characterized by uncontrollable shivering, incoordination, restlessness, initial involuntary contractions followed by myoclonic-like movements in the legs, hyper-reflexia, agitation and diarrhoea. Fever and oculogyric crises can also occur. The SSRI should be discontinued and a non-selective serotonin receptor antagonist such as methysergide, cyproheptadine or alternatively propranolol administered.

Venlafaxine is a potent blocker of both 5HT and noradrenaline reuptake (SNRI). It has negligible affinity for other neurotransmitter receptor sites and so produces less sedation and fewer anticholinergic effects.

Noradrenaline reuptake inhibitors

Reboxetine is a selective inhibitor of noradrenaline reuptake (NARI) only.

Monoamine oxidase inhibitors (MAOIs)

These act by inhibiting the intracellular enzymes monoamine oxidase A and B, leading to an increase of noradrenaline, dopamine and 5-hydroxytryptamine in the brain. There are two types:

- hydrazine derivatives, such as isocarboxazid, phenelzine (potentially hepatotoxic)
- amphetamine-related, such as tranylcypromine (potentially addictive).

The most widely used is phenelzine, which is given in doses of 30–60 mg daily. The onset of action of MAOIs is within 24–48 hours. Unwanted effects include increased appetite and weight gain and difficulty in sleeping. MAOIs also produce hypertensive reactions with foods containing tyramine or dopamine and therefore a restricted diet is prescribed. These amines are normally broken down in the gut mucosa and the liver. Tyramine is present in cheese, pickled herrings, yeast extract, certain red wines, and any food – such as game – that has undergone partial decomposition. Dopa is present in broad beans. This tyramine reaction is treated with intravenous phentolamine. MAOIs interact with drugs such as pethidine (see p. 865) and can also occasionally cause liver damage. Particular caution should be taken when changing from an MAOI to a tricyclic or vice versa; it is safest to allow a two-week drug-free interval between the two types of drug.

MAOIs which only inhibit monoamine oxidase A are more readily reversible – hence their description as reversible inhibitors of monoamine oxidase A (RIMA). An example is moclobemide 300 mg daily. These drugs appear to have fewer side-effects, work rapidly and constitute a low risk in overdose. At present, patients prescribed such antidepressants are advised that they can eat a broad diet but they should be careful to avoid excessive amounts of food rich in tyramine.

MAOIs are used in depressions that present with marked anxiety and obsessional or hypochondriacal features, and that lack marked biological symptoms characteristic of severe depression.

Antidepressant therapy in pregnancy

Drug therapy must be avoided if possible and psychotherapy should always be tried initially. If this is ineffective the risks of drug therapy should be balanced against no treatment which can affect fetal progress and the future mother–child relationship.

Tricyclic antidepressants are generally believed to be safe in pregnancy, with no proven statistical increase in the role of congenital malformations in fetuses exposed to them. However, occasionally their anticholinergic side effects produce jitteriness, sucking problems and hyperexcitability in the newborn. Postpartum plasma levels of babies breast fed by treated mothers are negligible.

SSRIs (e.g. fluoxetine) are not teratogenic but, nevertheless, manufacturers advise against their use in pregnancy.

MAOIs should be avoided during pregnancy because of the possibility of a hypertensive reaction in the mother.

Electroconvulsive therapy (ECT) for depression

This is the most rapidly acting of the available physical treatments of depression. It can be the treatment of first choice in those cases where:

- the patient is dangerously suicidal
- a delay in treatment represents a serious risk to health
- the patient is refusing food and drink
- the patient is in a depressive stupor.

The treatment involves the passage of an electric current, usually 80 V for a duration of 100–300 ms, across two electrodes applied to the anterior temporal areas of the scalp. Before the treatment is given, the patient is anaesthetized (usually by means of thiopental 125–150 mg) and receives a muscle relaxant (usually suxamethonium 30–50 mg). A modified convulsion is produced. A course of 6–8 treatments over three weeks has been shown to be superior to placebo treatment in severe depression characterized by retardation and delusions.

ECT is sometimes used in the management of acute schizophrenia, but the evidence of its effectiveness in this condition is less clear.

ECT is a controversial treatment, yet it is remarkably safe and free of serious side-effects. Serious complications are rare. However, post-ictal, short-term retrograde amnesia and a temporary defect in new learning can occur, but these are short-lived effects. The mode of action of ECT in depressive illness is unclear.

Physical treatment of mania

Acute attacks

The main physical treatment in mania is the use of neuroleptic drugs such as chlorpromazine, haloperidol and pimozide. Doses similar to those used in schizophrenia are used. Excitement and overactivity are usually reduced within days, but elation, grandiosity and associated delusions often take longer to respond. If improvement does not occur rapidly, larger doses of haloperidol (up to 120 mg daily) may be required. First attacks of mania usually require treatment for up to three months. Subsequent attacks, especially if they occur rapidly on cessation of treatment, may need drugs for at least a year after hypomanic features have disappeared. Carbamazepine is also used (see below).

Prophylaxis

Prevention of relapse is the major therapeutic challenge in the overall management of bipolar affective disorder. Most patients relapse at least once, many several times. As a rule, any patient who has experienced more than two episodes of affective disorder (either major depression or mania) within a five-year period is a candidate for prophylaxis with a mood-stabilizing drug. Lithium (carbonate or citrate) is the main agent used for prophylaxis in patients with repeated episodes of mania and/or depression. It is rapidly absorbed into the gastrointestinal tract and more than 95% is excreted by the kidneys; small amounts are found in the saliva, sweat and breast milk. Renal clearance of lithium correlates with renal creatinine clearance. In the body it substitutes for sodium and potassium ions and thus can exercise profound effects on a number of metabolic processes.

Lithium takes 10 days to take effect. Its mode of action is unknown. Poor responses to lithium are associated with a negative family history, an unstable premorbid personality, and a rapid cycling pattern of illness.

Patients should be screened for thyroid and renal disease before starting on lithium. Lithium interferes with thyroid function and can produce frank hypothyroidism; however, subclinical hypothyroidism, as judged by a raised plasma level of TSH, is more common, occurring in 5–35% of patients on long-term lithium prophylaxis. The therapeutic range for prophylaxis is 0.5–1.0 mmol L^{-1}. Lithium levels should be checked every 3–4 months, along with regular thyroid and renal function tests.

Other side-effects of lithium include:

- gastrointestinal symptoms (6%)
- a fine tremor (15%)
- polyuria and polydipsia (owing to inhibition of the antidiuretic hormone (ADH)-sensitive adenylate cyclase in the distal tubule of the nephron, and hence a rise in plasma ADH)
- weight gain, mainly through increased appetite.

Toxic symptoms begin to occur when the serum concentration exceeds 1.5 mmol L^{-1}. These include drowsiness, blurred vision, a coarse tremor, ataxia and dysarthria. Such symptoms progress to delirium and convulsions, and coma and death can occur. Long-term effects include non-toxic goitre, hypothyroidism and nephrogenic diabetes insipidus.

As a rule, lithium is not advised during pregnancy, particularly in the first trimester, because of an increased risk of fetal malformation involving the cardiovascular system (Ebstein's anomaly). Between 25% and 30% of women with a history of bipolar disorder relapse within two weeks of delivery. Restarting lithium within 24 hours of delivery (if the mother is prepared to forgo breast feeding) markedly reduces the risk of relapse.

Carbamazepine is used both in prophylaxis and in the treatment of manic states. Some patients who do not respond to lithium may respond to carbamazepine. In patients who relapse on lithium and in those prone to rapid cycling, the combination of carbamazepine and lithium may be more effective than either given alone. For antimanic treatment, dosage in the initial stage of treatment will be 200 mg once a day for two days, followed by 200 mg twice daily for two days, then 200 mg thrice daily. Rarely dosage may have to be increased to a maximum of 1200 mg daily. The usual prophylactic dosage is 600 mg daily. Carbamazepine can be teratogenic but folic acid supplements during pregnancy can protect against this.

Valproate has also been shown to be useful in the prevention of manic episodes in bipolar patients and appears particularly effective in patients with a rapid cycling pattern of illness.

Social treatment of mood (affective) disorders

Many patients with depression, particularly of the milder form, have associated social problems. Assistance with such social problems can make a significant contribution to clinical recovery. Other social interventions include the provision of group support, social clubs, occupational therapy and training to cope with particularly stressful situations. Successful management of a bipolar disorder requires a well-informed patient who has a social network primed to recognize the early symptoms of an episode and to seek help for the patient who often lacks insight into the condition. Educational programmes, self-help groups and informed and supportive family members have been shown to be important factors in improving treatment compliance and response.

Psychological treatment of mood (affective) disorders

Psychological treatments in affective disorders can be divided into supportive, dynamic and cognitive.

Supportive therapy, involving sympathy, reassurance and information, should be part of every patient's treatment

Dynamic psychotherapy (see p. 1133) has a limited value in the treatment of affective disorders. In general, its use is restricted to the less severe cases.

Cognitive therapy is a behavioural form of therapy that combines behavioural tasks with questioning and arguments designed to alter some of the ideas that are common among depressed patients and that appear to prolong their depression. Among these are negative interpretations of events and maladaptive assumptions (e.g. assuming that because friends do not telephone they no longer care). In treatment, the patient is required to record such ideas and examine the evidence for and against them. Patients are also encouraged to undertake some of the pleasurable activities they gave up when they became depressed. There is some evidence that the effects of cognitive therapy are about the same as those of antidepressant drugs in the treatment of mild to moderate depression.

COURSE AND PROGNOSIS

Between two-thirds and three-quarters of patients admitted with a major depressive illness will suffer at least one relapse requiring hospital admission. The number of less severe relapses is even higher. It has been estimated that 15–20% of depressives never fully recover. It may take those who do recover 4–18 months before they can expect to regain full social functioning.

Virtually all manic patients recover and the main problem is the prevention of relapse. Estimates of the proportion of patients who have only a single episode of mania vary widely between 1% and 50%! Subsequent depressive disorder is common in manic patients who relapse. Between 5% and 10% of manic-depressive sufferers develop a chronic disability that may follow the first episode. Between 5% and 10% become long-term hospital inpatients and an additional 25% have persistent affective symptoms that are disabling to some degree. The continuation of antidepressant therapy for up to six months after recovery from a depressive episode does reduce the probability of recurrence, while the use of lithium carbonate and carbamazepine as prophylactic therapy to prevent recurrence of bipolar manic-depressive swings is widely recommended.

FURTHER READING

Brockington I (1996) *Motherhood and Mental Health.* Oxford: Oxford University Press.

Daly I (1997) Mania. *Lancet* **349**: 1157–1160.

Goodwin FK, Jamison KR (1990) *Manic Depressive Illness.* Oxford: Oxford University Press.

Hay AG, Scott AIF (1994) Electroconvulsive therapy and brain damage. *British Journal of Psychiatry* **164**: 120–121.

Suicide and attempted suicide (deliberate self-harm) (see also p. 870)

Suicide accounts for 2% of male and 1% of female deaths in England and Wales each year, equivalent to a rate of 8 per 100 000. The rate increases with age, peaking for women in their sixties and for men in their seventies.

Suicide is the second most common cause of mortality in 15–34 year olds, and rates in young men are increasing alarmingly. In contrast, suicide rates have declined markedly in older men and in women of all ages. Between 11% and 17% of people who have suffered a severe depressive disorder at any time will eventually commit suicide. Suicide rates in schizophrenia sufferers are likewise high, being 20–50 times the rate in the general population; 20–40% of people with schizophrenia make suicide attempts, and 9–13% are successful. A Finnish study suggests that the suicide rate is higher in women who have sustained a miscarriage or undergone an induced abortion, whereas it is significantly reduced in women who are pregnant. The highest rates of suicide have been reported in Hungary (40 per 100 000), while the lowest are those of Spain (3.9 per 100 000) and Greece (2.8 per 100 000), but such variations may reflect differences in reporting as much as genuine differences. Factors that increase the risk of suicide are indicated in Table 19.20.

A distinction must be drawn between those who attempt suicide – deliberate self-harm (DSH) – and those who succeed (suicides). In this regard the following points should be considered:

Table 19.20
Factors that increase the risk of suicide

Living alone
Immigrant status
Recent bereavement, separation or divorce
Recent loss of a job or retirement
Living in a socially disorganized area
Male sex
Older age
Family history of affective disorder, suicide or alcohol abuse
Previous history of affective disorder, alcohol or drug abuse
Previous suicide attempt
Addiction to alcohol or drugs
Severe depression or early dementia
Incapacitating, painful physical illness

- The majority of cases of DSH occur in people under 35 years of age.
- The majority of suicides occur in people over 60 years of age.
- In men, suicides are most common, while DSH is more common in women.
- Suicides are more common in older men, but rates in young men are rising fast throughout the UK and Western Europe
- Suicides in women are slowly falling in the UK.
- Approximately 90% of cases of DSH involve self-poisoning.
- A formal psychiatric disorder is unusual in DSH.

There is, however, overlap between the DSH and suicide groups. Between 1% and 2% of people who attempt suicide will kill themselves in the year following their original attempt. In the UK, over 100 000 suicide attempts are made each year, and the overwhelming majority of these are seen and treated within accident and emergency departments.

The guidelines given in Information box 19.6 for the assessment of such patients will help ensure that the risk factors relating to suicide are covered. Indications for referral to a psychiatrist before discharge from hospital are also given.

In general, it is worth trying to interview a family member or other close associate and check these points with him or her. Requests for immediate re-prescription or discharge should be denied, except in cases of essential medication (e.g. for epileptics). In such cases, however, only three days' supply of medication should be given, and the patient should be requested to report to their general practitioner or to their psychiatric outpatient clinic for further supplies.

FURTHER READING

Henry JA (1996) Suicide risk and antidepressant treatment. *Journal of Psychopharmacology* **19**: 39–40.

Mann JJ, Arango V (1992) Integration of neurobiology and psychopathology in a unified model of suicidal behaviour. *Journal of Clinical Psychopharmacology* **12**: 2–7.

Neurotic, stress-related and somatoform disorders [F40–F49]

These disorders constitute the largest portion of psychiatric disorders, accounting for 50% of admissions to psychiatric hospitals, 75% of patients seen in psychiatric

Information

Questions to ask
- Was there a clear precipitant/cause for the attempt?
- What was the patient's state of mind at the time?
- Was the act premeditated or impulsive?
- Did the patient leave a suicide note?
- Had the patient taken pains not to be discovered?
- Did the patient make the attempt in familiar or strange surroundings (i.e. at home or away from home)?
- What are the patient's feelings about the attempt now? Would they do it again?
- Was the patient under the influence of alcohol or drugs?

Other relevant factors
- Has the precipitant or crisis resolved?
- Is there continuing suicidal intent?
- Does the patient have any psychiatric symptoms?
- What is the patient's social support system?
- Has the patient inflicted self-harm before?
- Has anyone in the family ever taken their life?
- Does the patient have a physical illness?

Indications for referral to a psychiatrist
Absolute indications include:
- Clinical depression
- Psychotic illness of any kind
- Clearly preplanned suicidal attempts which were not intended to be discovered
- Persistent suicidal intent (the more detailed the plans, the more serious the risk)
- A violent method used.

Other common indications include:
- Alcohol and drug abusers
- Older patients over 45 years, especially if male, and young adolescents
- Those with a family history of suicide in first-degree relatives
- Those with serious (especially incurable) physical disease
- Those living alone or otherwise unsupported
- Those in whom there is a major unresolved crisis
- Persistent suicide attemptors
- Any patients who give you cause for concern.

Information box 19.6 Guidelines for the assessment of patients with deliberate self-harm outpatient clinics, and over 90% of the psychiatric disorders seen and managed by general practitioners. There is an overlap between neuroses and personality disorders (see p. 1144), although in general they can be distinguished.

The neuroses are defined below. Personality disorders are deeply ingrained maladaptive patterns of behaviour generally recognizable by the time of adolescence and often becoming less obvious in middle or old age. The personality is abnormal either in the balance of its components, its quality or expression, or in its total aspect, and this deviation has an adverse effect upon the individual or on society.

Anxiety disorder [F41]

This is a condition in which anxiety dominates the clinical symptoms.

CLINICAL FEATURES

The patient looks worried, has a tense posture, restless behaviour, a pale skin, and sweaty hands, feet and axillae. The physical and psychological symptoms (Table 19.21) result from either overactivity of the sympathetic nervous system or increased tension in the skeletal muscles. Sleep is disturbed: the patient has difficulty in getting to sleep because of worry and restlessness, and when asleep wakes intermittently and may have unpleasant dreams. Another feature is the *hyperventilation syndrome* (Information box 19.7).

Sometimes anxious patients have the conviction that they suffer from heart disease. The conviction is accompanied by palpitations, fatigue, breathlessness and inframammary pain. The terms 'cardiac neurosis', 'effort syndrome' and 'neurocirculatory asthenia' used to be applied to the disorder. β-Blockers are sometimes useful in controlling these symptoms.

Types of anxiety

Anxiety may be divided into the following categories:

- *A more or less continuous state of anxiety* that fluctuates to some extent in response to environmental circumstances.
- *Panic attacks*, which are sudden and unpredictable attacks of anxiety that are usually accompanied by severe physical symptoms.
- *Phobic anxiety*, which is anxiety triggered by a single stimulus or set of stimuli that are predictable and that normally cause no particular concern to others (e.g. agoraphobia, claustrophobia, social phobia).
- *An anxious personality* – an individual who has a lifelong tendency to experience tension and anxiety, and to have a worrisome attitude towards life and a constant anticipation of setback and stress.

AETIOLOGY

Genetic factors. Anxiety neurosis occurs in 15% of relatives of affected patients, compared with 3% of the general population. The genetic role is less important in phobic anxiety.

Table 19.21
Physical and psychological symptoms of anxiety

Physical symptoms	**Nervous system**
Gastrointestinal	Tinnitus
Dry mouth	Blurred vision
Difficulty in swallowing	Dizziness
Epigastric discomfort	Headache
Flatulence	Sleep disturbance
'Diarrhoea' (usually frequency)	
	Psychological symptoms
Respiratory	Apprehension and fear
Feeling of chest constriction	Irritability
Difficulty in inhaling	Difficulty in concentrating
Overbreathing	Distractability
	Restlessness
Cardiovascular	Sensitivity to noise
Palpitations	Depression
Awareness of missed beats	Depersonalization
Feeling of pain over heart	Obsessional symptoms
Genitourinary	
Increased frequency	
Failure of erection	
Lack of libido	

Information

Features
Panic attacks – fear, terror and impending doom – accompanied by some or all of the following:
- dyspnoea
- palpitations
- chest pain or discomfort
- choking sensation
- dizziness
- paraesthesiae
- sweating
- carpopedal spasms.

Cause
Overbreathing leading to a decrease in P_aCO_2 and an increase in arterial pH.

Diagnosis
A provocation test – voluntary overbreathing for 2–3 minutes – provokes similar symptoms; rebreathing from a paper bag relieves them.

Management
- Explanation and reassurance is given.
- The patient is trained in relaxation techniques and slow breathing.
- The patient is asked to breathe into a closed paper bag.

Information box 19.7 The hyperventilation syndrome

Table 19.22
Anxiety neurosis – the differential diagnosis

Psychiatric disorder	Physical disorder
Depressive illness	Hyperthyroidism
Schizophrenia	Hypoglycaemia
Presenile dementia	Phaeochromocytoma
Alcohol dependence	
Drug dependence	
Benzodiazepine withdrawal	

Table 19.23
Withdrawal syndrome with benzodiazepines

Insomnia
Anxiety
Tremulousness
Muscle twitchings
Perceptual distortions
Frank convulsions

Psychodynamic theory. This is a theoretical explanation that suggests that anxiety neurosis reflects overwhelming stress, anxiety and difficulties in the child–parent relationship in early childhood or even at birth. Psychoanalysts also interpret phobic neurosis as an unconscious avoidance of unacknowledged feelings of temptation (usually sexual), the phobia representing a displacement of the real fear (e.g. the agoraphobic patient is really afraid of the feelings of temptation aroused when meeting people in the street).

Learning theory. This regards anxiety as a fear response that has been attached to another stimulus through conditioning.

DIFFERENTIAL DIAGNOSIS

This is given in Table 19.22.

TREATMENT

Psychological treatment of anxiety neurosis

For many people with brief episodes of anxiety neurosis, a discussion with a doctor involving explanation and reassurance concerning the nature of physical symptoms of anxiety is usually sufficient. Relaxation training can be as effective as drugs in relieving mild or moderate anxiety. Such an approach uses an elaborate system of exercises designed to bring about relaxation of individual groups of skeletal muscles and to regulate breathing. A further development is anxiety management training, which involves two stages. In the first stage, verbal cues and mental imagery are used to arouse anxiety. In the second stage, the patient is trained to reduce this anxiety by relaxation, distraction and reassuring self-statements. Both of these approaches are forms of behaviour therapy.

The term 'behaviour therapy' is applied to psychological treatments derived from experimental psychology and intended to change symptoms and behaviour. A variety of such treatments, including desensitization, flooding and programmed practice, are now used in the management of anxiety, phobias and obsessions. Non-behavioural treatments include individual and group-based psychotherapy.

Drugs in the treatment of anxiety neurosis

Drugs used in the treatment of anxiety can be divided into two groups: those that act primarily on the central nervous system, and those that block peripheral autonomic receptors. The main group of centrally acting anxiolytic drugs are the benzodiazepines. They appear to bind to specific receptors on neuronal cell membranes, producing a facilitation of the effects of the inhibitory transmitter γ-aminobutyric acid (GABA). Diazepam (5 mg twice daily, up to 10 mg thrice daily in severe cases) and nitrazepam have relatively long half-lives (20–40 hours) and are more suitable as antianxiety drugs than as hypnotic drugs. Oxazepam, temazepam and lorazepam have shorter half-lives and may be used as hypnotics.

Overdosage, which may be accidental or deliberate, produces drowsiness, sleep, confusion, incoordination, ataxia, diplopia and dysarthria. Physical as well as psychological dependence has been described, and convulsions have occurred on withdrawal of such drugs after long-term administration. The withdrawal syndrome (Table 19.23) is particularly severe when high doses have been given (e.g. 30 mg of diazepam daily or more). Tolerance can occur with repeated doses and can lead to an escalation of dosage. Thus, if a benzodiazepine drug is prescribed for anxiety, it should be given in as low a dose and for as short a time as possible (for not more than 3–4 weeks). A withdrawal programme includes changing therapy to diazepam followed by a very gradual reduction in dosage.

Many of the symptoms of anxiety are due to an increased release of adrenaline and noradrenaline from the adrenal medulla and the sympathetic nerves. Thus, adrenergic blocking drugs such as propranolol (20–40 mg two or three times daily) are effective in reducing symptoms such as palpitations, tremor and tachycardia.

Obsessive–compulsive disorder [F42]

Obsessive–compulsive disorder (OCD) is characterized by obsessional thinking and compulsive behaviour (see p. 1108) together with varying degrees of anxiety, depression and depersonalization. It account for some 2% of referrals to psychiatrists and has a prevalence in the general population of about 1 in 1000.

CLINICAL FEATURES

The obsessions and compulsions are so persistent and intrusive that they greatly impede the patient's functioning and cause considerable distress. There is a constant need to check that things have been done correctly, and no amount of reassurance can remove the small amount of doubt that persists – the so-called *folie de doute*. Some rituals are derived from superstitions, such as repetitive actions done a required number of times, with the need to start again at the very beginning if interrupted. When severe, obsessional neuroses last for many years and are very resistant to treatment. However, obsessional symptoms commonly appear in the setting of other disorders, most notably anxiety neurosis, depression, schizophrenia and organic mental disorders, and disappear rapidly with the resolution of such disorders.

Minor variants of morbid obsessional symptoms can be noted fairly frequently in people who are not regarded as ill or in need of treatment. The mildest grade is that of obsessional personality traits such as over-conscientiousness, tidiness, punctuality and other attitudes and behaviours indicating a strong tendency towards rigidity, conformity and inflexibility. Such individuals are perfectionists, have a poor tolerance of shortcomings in others, and take pride in their high standards. When such traits are so marked that they override and dominate other aspects of the personality, in the absence of clear-cut obsessional thinking and compulsive rituals, the picture becomes that of an obsessional compulsive personality (see p. 1144).

AETIOLOGY

Genetic factors. Obsessional neuroses are found in 5–7% of the parents of obsessional patients. Such a finding may, of course, reflect environmental as well as genetic causes.

Organic factors. OCD is associated with a number of neurological disorders involving dysfunction of the striatum, including Parkinson's disease, Sydenham's chorea, and Huntington's chorea. Onset of OCD has occurred following head trauma.

Neuroimaging data suggest that abnormalities exist in the frontal lobe and basal ganglia (Fig 19.2). Hyperactivity of the orbitofrontal cortex has been a consistent finding in more than a decade of brain imaging research on OCD patients. The PET images shown here are from the initial report of this finding by a research group at the University of California at Los Angeles. Pharmacological and neuroendocrinological research suggest that there may be abnormalities in serotonin function in patients with OCD. Placebo-controlled studies show therapeutic benefits from agents mediating selective 5-HT reuptake inhibition, including clomipramine, fluvoxamine, sertraline, fluoxetine and paroxetine. Antidepressants which do not exert a potent effect on 5-HT are not effective in OCD. The possibility of abnormalities within the dopaminergic and cholinergic systems has also been raised.

Dynamic factors. Freud suggested that symptoms result from repressed impulses of an aggressive or sexual nature. He also suggested that they occur as a result of regression to the anal stage of development – an idea consistent with the obsessional patient's frequent concern over excretory functions and dirt.

Learning theory. This suggests that obsessional rituals are the equivalent of avoidance responses.

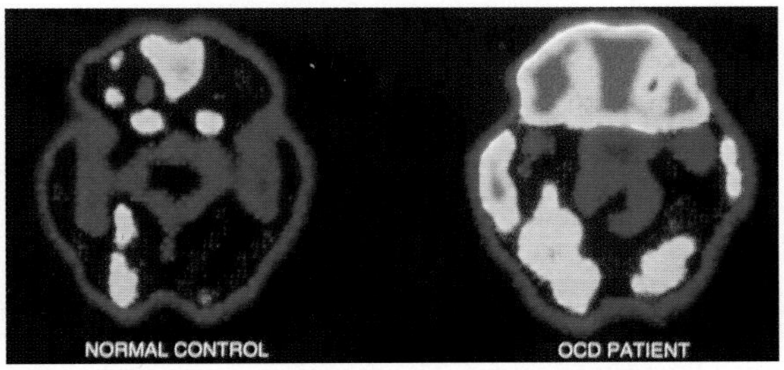

Fig 19.2
PET images of (left) a normal patient and (right) an OCD patient. The right image shows the hyperactivity of the orbitofrontal cortex which is a consistent finding in this condition

However, anxiety actually increases rather than falls after some rituals, which is against such a theory.

TREATMENT

Psychological treatment

A form of behaviour therapy that is particularly effective in the treatment of obsessional rituals is *response prevention*. Patients are instructed not to carry out their rituals; initially there is a rise in distress but with persistence both the rituals and the distress diminish. Patients are encouraged to practise keeping them under control while returning to situations that normally make them worse.

Another approach, known as *modelling*, involves demonstrating to the patient what is required and encouraging the patient to follow this example. In the case of hand-washing rituals, this might involve holding an allegedly contaminated object and carrying out other activities without washing, the patient being encouraged to follow suit. When obsessional thoughts accompany rituals, thought stopping is advocated. In this procedure the patient is taught to arrest the obsessional thought by arranging a sudden intrusion (e.g. snapping an elastic band, clicking the fingers).

Physical treatment of OCD

Anxiolytic drugs provide short-term symptomatic relief. Selective serotonin reuptake inhibitors (SSRIs) have been shown to be effective in reducing OCD symptoms, but the doses required are usually some 50–100% higher than those customarily found to be effective in depression. Positive correlations between reduced severity of OCD and decreased orbitofrontal and caudate metabolism following behavioural and SSRI treatments have been demonstrated in a number of recent studies.

Psychosurgery

Psychosurgery is sometimes recommended in cases of severe obsessional neurosis. The development of stereotactic techniques has led to the replacement of the earlier, crude leucotomies with more precise surgical interventions such as subcaudate tractotomy and limbic leucotomy, with lesions placed in the cingulate area and the ventromedial quadrant of the frontal lobe. These are undertaken to relieve patients of obsessional symptoms unresponsive to other treatments. Psychosurgery is now performed only in specialist centres, and formal and detailed consent requirements are laid down in England and Wales in the Mental Health Act 1983.

PROGNOSIS

Two-thirds of cases improve within a year. The remainder run a fluctuating course. The prognosis is worse when the personality is obsessional and the symptoms are severe.

Dissociative (conversion) disorders [F44]

Until recently these disorders were known as 'hysteria'; but because the word hysteria is used in everyday language to denote extravagant behaviour, that term is now inappropriate. These are mental disorders in which there are symptoms and signs of disease with three characteristics:

- They occur in the absence of physical pathology.
- They are produced unconsciously.
- They are not caused by overactivity of the sympathetic nervous system.

The lifetime prevalence has been estimated at 3–6 per 1000 in women, with a lower incidence in men. Most cases begin before the age of 35 years and it occurs rarely after 40 years. However, dissociative symptoms commonly occur after this age as part of some other disorder.

CLINICAL FEATURES

The various symptoms are usually divided into dissociative and conversion categories (Table 19.24). The term *dissociative* indicates the seeming dissociation between different mental activities, and covers such phenomena as amnesia, fugues, somnambulism and multiple personality. The term *conversion* derives from Freud's theory that mental energy can be converted into certain physical symptoms. Such symptoms include paralysis, fits, sensory loss, aphonia, blindness, deafness, disorders of gait and abdominal pain.

Table 19.24
Common dissociative/conversion symptoms

Mental	Physical
Amnesia	Paralysis
Fugue	Disorders of gait
Pseudodementia	Tremor
Ganser syndrome	Aphonia
Somnabulism	Mutism
Multiple personality	Sensory symptoms
Psychosis	Repeated vomiting
	Globus hystericus
	Hysterical fits
	Dermatitis artifacta
	Blindness
	Deafness

The main characteristics of these symptoms include the following:

- They are not produced wilfully or deliberately.
- They often reflect a patient's ideas about illness.
- They may imitate symptoms of a relative/friend who has been ill.
- There are obvious discrepancies between these symptoms and signs and those of an organic disease.
- The symptoms usually confer some advantage on the patient (so-called secondary gain).
- They are often accompanied by less than the expected amount of emotional distress (*belle indifference*).

Dissociative amnesia commences suddenly. Patients are unable to recall long periods of their lives and may even deny any knowledge of their previous life or personal identity. A proportion who present thus have concurrent physical disease, especially epilepsy, multiple sclerosis or the effects of head injury. In a dissociative fugue, patients not only lose their memory but wander away from their usual surroundings, and when found deny all memory of their whereabouts during this wandering. Apart from dissociation, fugue states are associated with epilepsy, depression and alcohol abuse.

Dissociative pseudo-dementia involves a memory loss and behaviour that initially suggest severe and generalized intellectual deterioration. Simple tests are answered wrongly but in such a way as to suggest that the correct answer is in the patient's mind. The *Ganser syndrome* is a rare condition composed of four features:

- the giving of approximate answers (i.e. almost correct)
- physical or mental symptoms of dissociative disorder
- hallucinations
- clouding of consciousness.

The relationship of somnambulism, or sleep-walking, to other dissociative disorders is unclear, but its similarity to the condition arising through hypnosis suggests that it may be a form of dissociation.

In multiple personality, there are rapid alterations between two patterns of behaviour, each of which is forgotten by the patient when the other is present. Each personality appears to be a complex and integrated set of emotional responses. The condition is rare.

A variation of dissociation is the epidemic or so-called 'mass hysteria', seen mainly in institutions for girls or young women, in which the combined effects of suggestion and shared anxiety produce explosive outbreaks of sickness or other disturbed behaviour. Another variant is *Briquet's syndrome*, which is said only to occur in women, follows an intractable course, runs in families, and involves multiple somatic symptoms occurring in several different bodily systems for which no organic cause is found.

AETIOLOGY

Genetic factors. Studies have been inconclusive, but reported rates in relatives of affected patients do appear higher than in the general population.

Psychodynamic factors. Central to the theory of psychoanalysis is the view that dissociaton is the result of emotionally charged ideas lodged in the unconscious at some point in the past. Symptoms are explained as the combined effects of repression and the conversion of psychic energy into physical channels.

Organic disease. Dissociative (conversion) disorders are sometimes associated with physical disease. However, it also quite clearly occurs in the absence of such pathology.

DIFFERENTIAL DIAGNOSIS

An erroneous diagnosis of dissociative (conversion) disorder may be made for a number of reasons.

Undetected physical disease. The symptoms may be those of a physical disease not yet detected. For example, globus hystericus (see p. 226) may actually be difficulty in swallowing secondary to an oesophageal cancer.

Undetected brain disease. A tumour in the frontal lobe, or early dementia, for example, may in some way produce dissociative symptoms.

Physical disease. Physical disease may provide a nonspecific stimulus to dissociative elaboration or an exaggeration of symptoms by a somewhat dramatic or histrionic patient. True physical disease must be excluded. The distinction between conversion and malingering (i.e. the conscious pretence of illness) should be considered but is difficult to make.

TREATMENT

Psychological treatment for dissociative disorders

Psychotherapy of a psychodynamic kind often uncovers striking memories of early childhood sexual experiences and other problems relevant to the patient's presenting condition. Psychodynamic psychotherapy is derived from psychoanalysis and is based on a number of key analytical concepts. These include Freud's ideas about psychosexual development, mechanisms of defence (including repression, projection and denial), free association as the method of recall, and the therapeutic techniques of interpretation, including that of transference, defences and dreams. Such therapy usually involves once-weekly 50-minute sessions, the length of treatment varying between three months and two years. The long-term aim of such therapy is twofold: symptom relief and personality change. Psychodynamic psychotherapy is classically indicated in the treatment of the neuroses and personality disorders, but to date there is a lack of convincing evidence concerning its superiority over other forms of treatment.

Simpler forms of psychotherapy involving more straightforward reassurance and explanation, greater involvement of the therapist in the actual sessions, and the elimination of factors that appear to reinforce symptoms, are as effective and probably more so than the more complex and time-consuming forms. Group psychotherapy involving 6–8 patients, which facilitates the development of confidence, the recollection of painful experiences and the growth of social and interpersonal skills, is also useful in a number of neurotic and personality disorders, although its usefulness in dissociative disorders is doubtful.

Abreaction brought about by hypnosis or by intravenous injections of small amounts of amylobarbitone with or without amphetamine may produce a dramatic, if short-lived, recovery. In the abreactive state, the patient is encouraged to relive the stressful events that provoked the disorder and to express the accompanying emotions; i.e. to abreact. Such an approach has been useful in the treatment of acute dissociative neuroses in wartime, but appears to be of much less value in civilian life.

Drug treatment for dissociative disorders

Drugs have no part to play in dissociative disorders unless the symptoms are secondary to a depressive illness or anxiety neurosis requiring treatment.

PROGNOSIS

Most cases of recent onset recover quickly. Those that last longer than a year are likely to persist for a very long time.

Somatoform disorders [F45]

This category of disorder includes those patients who repeatedly present with physical symptoms and complaints. They have had repeated negative findings on many medical investigations and much medical reassurance that the symptoms and complaints do not have a demonstrable physical cause. Such physical disorders as are present do not explain the nature and severity of the patient's distress and preoccupation with ill-health. The patient is usually exceedingly reluctant to accept a psychological and/or social explanation for the symptoms even when such a link seems obvious and rational. Some patients can be quite attention-seeking and complain about the medical care and attention they have received previously. The main types of disorder are described below.

Hypochondriacal disorder

The conspicuous feature is a preoccupation with an underlying and progressive serious disease process and its consequences. Commonly patients are preoccupied with the possibility that they suffer from cancer, AIDS, thyroid disease or some other serious and often life-threatening condition. Characteristically, such patients repeatedly request laboratory and other investigations to prove they are ill or reassure them that they are well, but such reassurance rarely lasts long before another cycle of worry and request begins. The symptoms of hypochondriasis occur in a variety of psychiatric disorders, particularly major depressive disorder and anxiety disorder. They may also coexist with actual physical disease but the diagnostic point is that the patient's concern is quite disproportionate and unjustified.

Somatization disorder

Somatizing patients classically complain of a variety of physical symptoms and usually have a lengthy history of contact with medical services. They commonly are in receipt of multiple medical and sometimes surgical interventions with little or no relief. Abdominal pain, nausea, regurgitation, flatulence, atypical chest pain, dizziness, backache and abnormal skin sensations are among the most common complaints, but symptoms may be referred to almost any part or bodily system. The course of the disorder is chronic and is often associated with long-standing family, marital and/or occupational problems. It often starts quite early in life, is more common in women than in men, and is associated with dependence upon or abuse of prescribed medication, usually sedatives and analgesics.

Persistent somatoform pain disorder

The patient complains of persistent, distressing and severe pain which cannot be explained fully by any underlying physical pathology and is inconsistent with anatomical patterns of innervation. The pain commonly occurs in association with psychosocial problems or emotional distress. Common sites for such pain include the face and jaw, the abdomen and the back. The pain may enable the sufferer to avoid certain activities or situations and may earn much sympathy, particularly from family, friends and workmates.

MANAGEMENT

From the outset it is important not to become embroiled in arguments concerning causation with somatizing patients. It is foolish to tell these patients that 'there is nothing wrong with you' when clearly there is, although there is no established physical pathology. Management consists of appropriate reassurance that no serious disease has been uncovered, together with a sensitive exploration of possible psychological and social difficulties. These factors may play an aggravating and/or perpetuating role in the physical complaint or worry under discussion. Repeated investigations should be discouraged and medication avoided. It is vital that all members of the staff involved with the patient and important family members be encouraged to adopt the same approach to the patient's problems – such patients are often adept at exploiting medical and family disagreements. Graded exercise programmes and other behavioural approaches to the control of physical symptoms can be effective. In some cases of somatoform pain disorder, a trial of antidepressant medication can prove helpful.

Acute stress reaction [F43]

Acute stress reactions occur in individuals without any other apparent psychiatric disorder, in response to exceptional physical and/or psychological stress. While severe, such reactions usually subside within hours or days. The stress may be an overwhelming traumatic experience (e.g. accident, battle, physical assault, rape) or an unusually sudden change in the social circumstances of the individual, such as multiple bereavement. Individual vulnerability and coping capacity play a role in the occurrence and severity of acute stress reactions, as evidenced by the fact that not all people exposed to exceptional stress develop symptoms. These symptoms show considerable variation but usually include an initial state of 'daze' with some constriction of the field of consciousness and narrowing of attention, inability to comprehend stimuli, and disorientation. This state may be followed either by further withdrawal from the surrounding situation to the extent of a dissociative stupor or by agitation and overactivity. Autonomic signs of panic anxiety, including tachycardia, sweating and hyperventilation, are commonly present. The symptoms usually appear within minutes of the impact of the stressful stimulus and disappear within 2–3 days.

Post-traumatic stress disorder (PTSD)

This arises as a delayed and/or protracted response to a stressful event or situation of an exceptionally threatening nature and likely to cause pervasive distress in almost anyone. Causes include natural or human disasters, war, serious accident, witnessing the violent death of others, being the victim of sexual abuse, rape, torture, terrorism or hostage-taking. Predisposing factors such as personality traits or previous history of psychiatric illness may lower the threshold for the development of the syndrome or may aggravate its course. They are, however, neither necessary nor sufficient to explain its occurrence. Typical symptoms of PTSD include:

- 'flashbacks' – the repeated reliving of the trauma in the form of intrusive memories or dreams
- intense distress at exposure to events that symbolize or resemble an aspect of the traumatic event, including anniversaries of the trauma
- avoidance of activities and situations reminiscent of the trauma
- emotional blunting or 'numbness'
- a sense of detachment from other people
- autonomic hyperarousal with hypervigilance, an enhanced startle reaction and insomnia
- marked anxiety and depression and, occasionally, suicidal ideation.

The course is fluctuating but recovery can be expected in the majority of cases. In a small proportion of cases the condition may show a chronic course over many years and a transition to an enduring personality change. Treatment involves exploration of memories of the traumatic event, relief of associated symptoms, and counselling.

FURTHER READING

Hales RE, Zatazick DF (1997) What is PTSD? *American Journal of Psychiatry* **154**: 143–145.

Royal College of Physicians/Royal College of Psychiatrists (1995) *The Psychological Care of Medical Patients: Recognition of Need and Service Provision*. London: RCPhys/RCPsych.

Alcohol abuse and dependence [F10]

There are a number of different types of alcohol abuse, and a wide range of physical, social and psychological problems are associated with excessive drinking. Much attention is devoted to the syndrome of alcohol dependence, but doctors should be concerned with the health problems caused by alcohol abuse whether or not such abuse is related to actual physiological dependence on alcohol. The term 'alcoholism' is a confusing one with off-putting connotations of vagrancy, 'meths' drinking and social disintegration. It has been replaced by the term 'alcohol dependence syndrome', which has seven essential elements:

- There is a compulsive need to drink.
- There is a stereotyped pattern of drinking. Whereas 'ordinary' drinkers vary their weekly pattern, addicted drinkers drink at regular intervals to avoid or relieve withdrawal symptoms.
- Drinking takes primacy over other activities.
- Tolerance to alcohol is altered. The dependent drinker is usually unaffected by blood alcohol levels that would incapacitate an 'ordinary' drinker. Increasing tolerance is an important sign of increasing dependence. In the later stages of dependence, tolerance falls.
- Repeated withdrawal symptoms occur some 8–12 hours after cessation of drinking or after a sharp fall in blood alcohol in people who have been drinking heavily for many years. Symptoms characteristically appear on waking as a result of the fall in the blood alcohol level during sleep.
- There may be relief drinking. Many dependent drinkers take a drink early in the morning to stave off withdrawal symptoms. In most cultures, early morning drinking is diagnostic of alcohol dependence.
- Severely dependent drinkers who drink again after a period of abstinence are likely to relapse quickly and return to their old addictive pattern.

The problem drinker is one who causes or experiences physical, psychological and/or social harm as a consequence of drinking alcohol. Many problem drinkers, while heavy drinkers, are not physiologically addicted to alcohol. Heavy drinkers are those who drink significantly more in terms of quantity and/or frequency than the average drinker. Binge drinkers are those who drink excessively in short bouts, usually 24–48 hours long, separated by often quite lengthy periods of abstinence. Their overall monthly or weekly alcohol intake may be relatively modest. The interrelationship between these types of drinking is shown in Fig 19.3.

Extent of the problem

A conservative estimate is that there are at least 300 000 people in the UK with alcohol-related problems. A survey on drinking in England and Wales found that 5% of men and 2% of women reported alcohol-related problems. People with serious drinking problems have an increased risk of dying that is between two and three times greater than that of members of the general population of the same age and sex. Approximately one in five male admissions to acute medical wards are directly or indirectly due to alcohol. Between 33% and 40% of accident and emergency attenders have blood alcohol concentrations above the present UK legal limit for driving. Up to one in five seemingly healthy men attending health screening programmes are found to have biochemical evidence of heavy alcohol consumption, though they are a selected population coming mainly from the upper social classes. Of the 2000 patients on the practice list of the average general practitioner, about 100 will be heavy drinkers, 40 will be problem drinkers, and 10 will be physically dependent on alcohol.

Over the past 40 years, the alcohol consumption of the average British adult has increased considerably (from 5.2 L of absolute alcohol per year in 1950 to 8.5 L in 1991). There has been a downward trend since 1989. Over a similar period, admissions to psychiatric hospitals for treatment of alcohol problems have increased more than 25-fold, cirrhosis rates have doubled, and drunkenness offences have risen from 60 thousand to over 100 thousand per year.

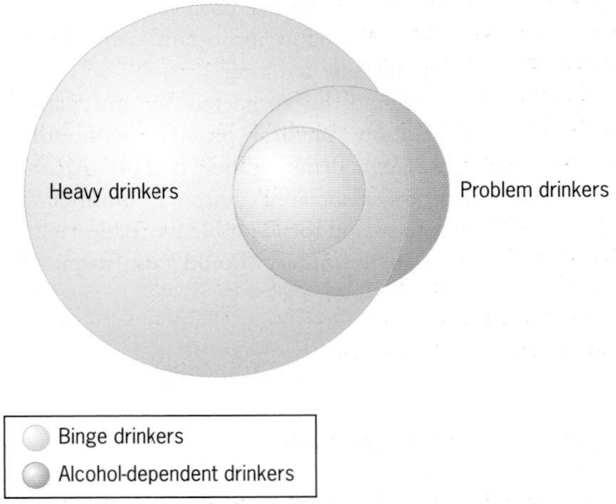

Fig 19.3
The terminology of drinking

Table 19.25 Approximate correlation between blood alcohol level and behavioural/motor impairment

Rising blood alcohol (mg dL^{-1})	Expected effect
20–99	Impaired coordination, euphoria
100–199	Ataxia, poor judgement, labile mood
200–299	Marked ataxia and slurred speech; poor judgement, labile mood, nausea and vomiting
300–399	Stage 1 anaesthesia, memory lapse, labile mood
400+	Respiratory failure, coma, death

Table 19.26
Common alcohol-related psychological and social problems

Psychological	Social
Depression	Marital and sexual difficulties
Anxiety and phobias	Family problems
Memory disturbances	Child abuse
Personality disturbances	Employment problems
Delirium tremens	Financial difficulties
Attempted suicide	Accidents at home, on the roads, at work
Pathological jealousy	Delinquency and crime
	Homelessness

Table 19.25 provides an approximate estimate of what can be expected in an average individual in the way of behavioural impairment resulting from a particular blood alcohol level. For each of these values, the level of impairment at falling blood alcohol concentrations is usually less than the effects observed with rising concentrations. The usual drink contains about 8–12 g of absolute alcohol and raises the blood alcohol concentration by about 15–20 mg dL^{-1}, the amount that is metabolized in one hour.

DETECTION

Many doctors still fail to recognize the heavy drinker and even the problem drinker. Greater awareness is urgently needed to allow intervention at a stage when something can still be achieved, and to provide better statistics. Alcohol abuse and depression co-occur far more commonly than would be expected. Alcoholic subjects with a coexisting depression exhibit heavier alcohol abuse, more severe physical damage and greater liability to both psychotropic drug abuse and overdose behaviour than non-depressed alcoholics. Alcohol abuse is also significantly associated with personality disorder and schizophrenia. Women with alcohol-related problems – a growing problem in most Western societies – suffer especially from low self-esteem and feelings of shame and guilt. Broken relationships, sexual problems and sexual abuse have all been reported as important contributory factors to women's problem drinking.

Alcohol abuse should be suspected in any patient presenting one or more physical problems commonly associated with excessive drinking (see p. 214). Alcohol abuse may also be associated with a number of psychological symptoms and social problems (Table 19.26).

Certain features in the *history* should raise suspicion, most notably:

- absenteeism from work
- frequent attendances for unexplained dyspepsia or gastrointestinal bleeds
- hospital admissions for accidents of all kinds
- fits, 'turns' or falls.

Certain *signs* may be helpful, if present, in detecting alcohol abuse in patients. These include:

- plethoric face with/without telangiectases
- bloodshot conjunctivae
- smell of stale alcohol
- facial appearance resembling Cushing's syndrome
- marked tremor
- signs of alcohol-related diseases.

Guidelines

The patient's frequency of drinking and quantity drunk on typical occasions should be established. Alcohol consumption can be assessed on the basis of units of alcohol. One standard unit of alcohol is equivalent to 8 g of absolute alcohol (see p. 214).

- Drinking up to 20 units of alcohol a week for men and 13 units for women carries no long-term health risk. There is suggestive evidence that alcohol consumption of 1–2 units a day may actually reduce the risk of coronary heart disease (CHD), particularly in men under 35 years and in premenopausal women. The fall in the risk of CHD seems to be mediated largely by alcohol-induced increases in high-density lipoprotein cholesterol concentrations.
- There is unlikely to be any long-term health damage with 21–36 units (men) and 14–24 units (women), provided the drinking is spread throughout the week.
- Beyond 36 units a week in men and 24 units a week in women, damage to health becomes increasingly likely.
- Drinking above 50 units a week in men (35 units in women) is currently regarded as a definitive health hazard.

'At risk' factors

- Marital difficulties may conceal heavy drinking or may be used to justify it.
- Alcohol abusers have twice as many days off work as their more sober colleagues.
- There may be an affected relative – 25% of the male relatives of alcohol abusers have similar problems.
- High-risk occupations include company directors, salesmen, doctors, journalists, publicans and seamen.
- There may be associated physical and mental conditions, such as depression.

Table 19.27
Comparison of different laboratory tests for the diagnosis of alcohol abuse

	Normal range	Available in routine clinical practice	Abnormal after 60 g daily	Normalization after withdrawal of alcohol	False positive
γ-GT	< 50 U L^{-1} (males) < 32 UL^{-1} (females)	++	> 21 days	14–60 days	Liver diseases Anticonvulsant therapy Other drugs Nicotine abuse Diabetes mellitus
MCV	< 95 fL	++	> 42 days	60–90 days	Folate deficiency B_{12} deficiency Liver diseases Nicotine abuse
CDT	< 20 U L^{-1} (males) < 26 U L^{-1} (females)	+	14–21 days	10–14 days	Liver cirrhosis Genetic liver Diseases Pregnancy Iron deficiency
HDL-cholesterol	< 50 mg L^{-1} < 0.5 mmol L^{-1}	+	14–28 days	10–30 days	Jogging Underweight

CDT, carbohydrate-deficient transferrin

Markers

Laboratory parameters indicating alcohol abuse are often called *markers*. They can be categorized as genetic/biological (trait) markers and diagnostic (state) markers.

Genetic markers are indicators of a higher risk or vulnerability for the development of alcoholism even in non-drinking subjects. The risk varies with respect to the degree of expression. Dopamine-2 receptor allele A1, alcohol dehydrogenase subtypes and monoamine oxidase B activity are suggested as genetic markers of alcohol dependance but they are not specific.

The currently available *diagnostic markers* (Table 19.27) identify only recent alcohol abuse. They have very different time ranges in which they can show increased alcohol consumption.

Laboratory parameters indicating alcohol abuse can be required in very different situations: intoxication, denial of abuse and forensic or legal purposes.

- **γ-Glutamyl transpeptidase** (γ-GT). Elevated serum γ-GT activity is observed in about 75% of patients hospitalized for alcohol abuse; in outpatients and heavy drinkers, the prevalence reaches 90%. Acute alcohol consumption does not lead to abnormal levels, but regular, moderate drinkers often have a slight elevation of the γ-GT. Levels return to normal with abstention from alcohol.
- **Mean corpuscular volume** (MCV). A level of more than 95 fL is found in about 60% of alcohol abusers. The response to abstinence is a return to normal over a period of about two months.
- **Carbohydrate-deficient transferrin (CDT) and HDL-cholesterol**. These identify only recent alcohol abuse. They can be useful in diagnosing relapse which is being denied by formerly abstinent alcohol abusers.
- **Blood alcohol**. This is a useful sign in anyone suspected of, but who denies, drinking. Most people have no detectable alcohol in their blood in the middle of the day.
- **Urinary alcohol**. A value exceeding 120 mg dL^{-1} is suggestive of chronic alcohol abuse, and a value over 200 mg dL^{-1} (44 mmol L^{-1}) is said to be diagnostic.

Alcohol dependence syndrome

The dependence syndrome is introduced by both DSM-IV and ICD-10 as a cluster of cognitive, behavioural and physiological symptoms. DSM-IV describes 'a pattern of repeated self-administration that usually results in tolerance, withdrawal and compulsive drug-taking behaviour', the essential element of which is the continued use of the substance despite significant substance-related problems. ICD-10 introduces as key elements of the syndrome the high priority given to substance use over other behaviours, and the strong desire felt by the individual to take the substance. A diagnosis of dependence can be applied to all classes of substances including alcohol, opiates, cocaine, other stimulants, barbiturates, benzodiazepines and hallucinogens and nicotine. This is especially relevant as individuals presenting for treatment are increasingly using more than one drug or are substituting one drug for another. The same criteria apply to all substances, but some will be less relevant to some classes or are rarely applicable at all (e.g. withdrawal symptoms are not specified for hallucinogens).

The alcohol dependence syndrome is usually very much easier to identify than problem-related drinking. Fig 19.4 outlines the main characteristics of the syndrome but these do not necessarily present in any particular order. Symptoms of alcohol dependence in a typical order of occurrence are shown in Table 19.28. Diagnostic criteria for alcohol withdrawal syndrome are shown in Table 19.29.

Table 19.28
Symptoms of alcohol dependence

Unable to keep a drink limit	Trembling after drinking the day before
Difficulty in avoiding getting drunk	Morning retching and vomiting
Spending a considerable time drinking	Sweating excessively at night
Missing meals	Withdrawal fits
Memory lapses, blackouts	Morning drinking
Restless without drink	Increased tolerance
Organizing day around drink	Hallucinations, frank delirium tremens

Table 19.29
Diagnostic criteria for alcohol withdrawal syndrome: ICD-10 [F10.3]

Any **three** of the following:

Tremor of outstretched hands, tongue or eyelids
Sweating
Nausea, retching or vomiting
Tachycardia or hypertension
Anxiety
Psychomotor agitation
Headache
Insomnia
Malaise or weakness
Transient visual, tactile or auditory
Hallucinations or illusions
Grand mal convulsions

COURSE OF THE ALCOHOL DEPENDENCE SYNDROME

The course of the syndrome comprises three linked stages. The first stage is heavy social drinking – the ingestion of between three and five standard drinks (units) of alcohol a day for several years. This stage can continue asymptomatically for a lifetime or, because of a change of circumstances or peer group, it can revert to a more moderate pattern of drinking or can progress to the second stage of alcohol abuse. This stage is usually associated with frequent ingestion of more than eight drinks a day, and there are associated medical, legal, social and/or occupational complications. About half of such abusers either return to asymptomatic (controlled) drinking or achieve stable abstinence. In a small number of cases, such alcohol abuse can persist intermittently for decades with minor morbidity and become milder with time. About 25% of all cases of alcohol abuse will lead to chronic alcohol dependence, withdrawal symptoms and the eventual need for detoxification. This last stage most commonly ends in social incapacity and death or abstinence.

Evidence suggests that alcohol-dependent drinkers do not develop their dependence after a few drinks but that the disorder requires up to 10 years of heavy drinking to evolve (3–4 years in women). In some individuals who use alcohol to alter consciousness, obliterate conscience and defy social canons, dependence and apparent loss of control may appear in only a few months to a few years.

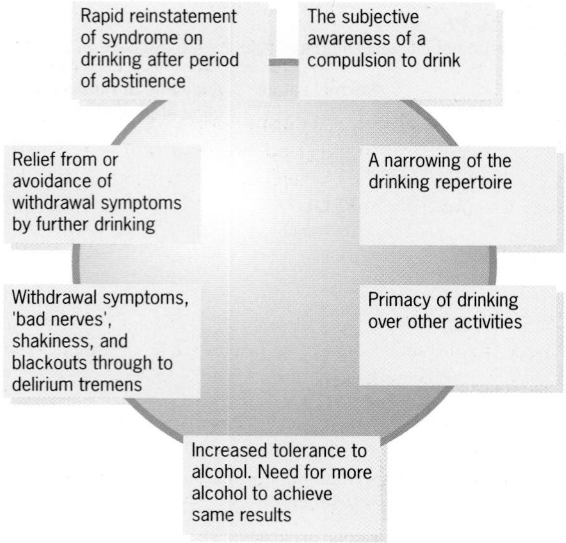

Fig 19.4
Elements of the alcohol dependence syndrome

Delirium tremens (DTs) [F10.4]

Delirium tremens is the most serious withdrawal state and occurs 1–5 days after alcohol (or barbiturate) withdrawal. Patients are disorientated, agitated, and have a marked tremor and visual hallucinations (e.g. 'pink elephants').

Signs include sweating, tachycardia, tachypnoea and pyrexia. Additional signs include dehydration, infection, hepatic disease or the Wernicke–Korsakoff syndrome. If delirium tremens is not treated promptly, death can occur.

CAUSES

Genetic factors. Sons of alcohol-dependent people who are adopted by other families are four times more likely to develop drinking problems than are the adopted sons of non-alcohol abusers (see p. 1136).

Environmental factors. A Boston follow-up study showed that one in ten boys who grew up in a household where neither parent abused alcohol subsequently became alcohol dependent, compared with one in four of those reared by alcohol-abusing fathers and one in three of those reared by alcohol-abusing mothers.

Biochemical factors. Several factors have been suggested, including abnormalities in alcohol dehydrogenase, neurotransmitter substances and brain amino acids, such as GABA. To date, there is no conclusive evidence that these or other biochemical factors play a causal role.

Personality. Follow-up studies have failed to identify any trait or tendency that significantly distinguishes those who subsequently abuse alcohol from those who do not.

Psychiatric illness. This is not a common cause of addictive drinking but it is a treatable one. Some depressed patients drink excessively in the hope of raising their mood. Patients with anxiety states or phobias are also at risk.

Excess consumption in society. The idea has grown that rates of alcohol dependence and alcohol-related problems correspond to the general level of alcohol consumption in society and, in turn, to factors that may control overall consumption – including price, licensing laws, the number and nature of sales outlets, and the customs and moral beliefs of society concerning the use and abuse of alcohol.

TREATMENT

Psychological treatment of problem drinking

Successful identification at an early stage constitutes an important treatment in its own right. It should lead to:

- the provision of information concerning safe drinking levels
- a recommendation to cut down where indicated
- simple support and advice concerning associated problems.

Such an approach has been found to be as effective as more expensive and specialized forms of psychotherapy in the treatment of moderate to heavy non-addictive drinking. With addictive drinking, the most favoured psychological treatment is group therapy, which involves identification, confession, emotional arousal, the implantation of new ideas, and the long-term support by fellow-members of the group. Family and marital therapy involving both the alcohol abuser and spouse may also be important.

Behaviour therapies involving teaching patients how to drink in a more controlled way are the subject of much study.

Drugs in the treatment of problem drinking

Addicted drinkers often experience considerable difficulty when they attempt to reduce or stop their drinking. Withdrawal symptoms are a particular problem and delirium tremens needs urgent treatment (Table 19.30). Drugs that show cross-tolerance for alcohol, such as *diazepam* or *chlormethiazole*, may be used in a regimen that involves a steady reduction over 5–7 days. A useful chlormethiazole regimen is 9–12 capsules on the first day, 6–8 on the second day and 4–6 on the third day.

However, long-term treatment with drugs should not be prescribed in those patients who continue to abuse alcohol. Many alcohol abusers add dependence on diazepam or chlormethiazole to their problems.

Drugs such as *disulfiram* (Antabuse) react with alcohol to cause very unpleasant acetaldehyde intoxication and histamine release. A daily maintenance dose of such a drug means that an alcohol-dependent drinker must wait until the disulfiram is eliminated from the body before drinking safely. Such drugs, therefore, can provide a 'chemical fence' around the drinker for at least 24 hours. Disulfiram implants have been developed that have a treatment life of six months. As yet there is doubt as to whether their benefit is psychological rather than pharmacological.

Recently there have been claims concerning the effectiveness of *acamprosate* (calcium bisacetylhomotaurinate) in maintaining abstinence in alcohol-dependent patients. Acamprosate lowers neuronal excitability by reducing the postsynaptic efficacy of excitatory amino acid (EAA) neurotransmitters and, possibly, by enhancing GABAergic inhibition; it has been shown to attenuate postsynaptic activity of EAA agonists in neocortical neurons. The responsiveness to excitatory amino acids is thought to encourage 'craving', the profound desire for and preoccupation with alcohol experienced by alcoholics in various stages of abstinence. The daily dose of acamprosate is 1–2 g.

Other drug treatments aimed at reducing 'craving' and hence relapse include the serotonin reuptake inhibitors, the opioid antagonist naltrexone, as well as lithium. It has been suggested that some alcoholics drink in order to enhance deficient brain levels of serotonin.

Table 19.30
Management of delirium tremens

The patient should be hospitalized

- Chlormethiazole 9–12 capsules (each capsule contains 192 mg) for 24 hours, then reduced over 5 days

or

- Diazepam 4–100 mg for 2 days then reduced

Any dehydration should be corrected
Any electrolyte imbalance should be corrected
Any systemic infection should be treated
B vitamins should be given parenterally

Chlormethiazole i.v. should be avoided, if possible

OUTCOME

Whereas in the case of non-dependent heavy drinkers the goal of normal drinking within safe limits can be a very reasonable one, the alcohol-dependent drinker must be persuaded to abstain. Abstention, particularly after many years of drinking, is a difficult goal and not surprisingly many fail in the attempt. Research suggests that 40–50% of alcohol-dependent drinkers are abstinent or drinking very much less up to two years following intervention. Specialized treatment units, psychiatric treatment, group therapy and attendance at meetings of Alcoholics Anony-mous – the self-help organization that provides members with a social structure to fill the gap previously occupied by drinking – are all potential elements in the attempt to keep the alcohol-dependent individual abstinent and healthy. To date, however, there is little convincing evidence that highly expensive, time-consuming and specialized modes of treatment are superior in their efficacy to straightforward advice, support, encourage-ment and monitoring.

FURTHER READING

Helzer JE, Canino GJ (1992) *Alcoholism in North America, Europe and Asia*. Oxford: Oxford University Press.

Schuckit MA, Hesselbrock V (1994) Alcohol dependence and anxiety disorders: what is the relationship? *America Journal of Psychiatry* **151**: 1723–1734.

Hall W, Zador D (1997) The alcohol withdrawal syndrome. *Lancet* **349**: 1897–1900.

Drug abuse and dependence [F10–F19]

In addition to alcohol and nicotine, there are a number of psychotropic substances that are used for their effects on mood and other mental functions (Table 19.31).

CAUSES OF DRUG ABUSE

There is no single cause of drug abuse and/or dependence. Three factors appear important:

- the availability of drugs
- a vulnerable personality
- social pressures, particularly from peers.

Once regular drug-taking is established, pharmacological factors are particularly important in determining dependence.

Solvents

Adolescents engage in glue-sniffing for the intoxicating effects produced by the solvents inhaled. The glue is sniffed directly from tubes, plastic bags or smears on pieces of cloth. Tolerance develops over weeks or months. Intoxication is characterized by euphoria, excitement, a floating sensation, dizziness, slurred speech, and ataxia. Acute intoxication can cause amnesia and visual hallucinations. The habit is dangerous because:

- inhaled vomit can lead to asphyxiation
- there is a risk of tissue damage, including damage to bone marrow, brain, liver and kidneys which can prove fatal
- acute intoxication can result in aggressive and impulsive behaviour.

Table 19.31
Commonly used drugs of abuse and dependence

Stimulants	**Narcotics**
Methylphenidate	Morphine
Phenmetrazine	Heroin
Phencyclidine ('angel dust')	Codeine
Cocaine	Pethidine
Amphetamine derivates	Methadone
Hallucinogens	**Hypnotics**
Cannabis preparations	Barbiturates
Solvents	Benzodiazepines
LSD	
Mescaline	
Ecstasy	

LSD, lysergic acid diethylamide

Amphetamines and related substances

These have temporary stimulant and euphoriant effects that are followed by depression, anxiety and irritability. Psychological rather than true physical dependence is the rule. In addition to restlessness, over talkativeness and over-activity, amphetamines can produce a paranoid psychosis indistinguishable from acute paranoid schizophrenia. Ecstasy is another amphetamine derivative (see below).

Cocaine

Cocaine is a central nervous system stimulant (with similar effects to amphetamines) derived from *Erythroxylon coca* trees grown in the Andes. In purified form it may be taken by mouth, sniffed or injected. If cocaine hydrochloride is converted to its base ('crack') it can be smoked. This is an effective way of obtaining an intense stimulating effect and free-basing has become common. Compulsive use and dependence are thought to occur more frequently among users who are free-basing. Dependent users take large doses and alternate between the withdrawal phenomena of depression, tremor and muscle pains, and the hyperarousal produced by increasing doses. Prolonged use of high doses produces irritability, restlessness, paranoid ideation and occasionally convulsions. Persistent sniffing of the drug can cause perforation of the nasal septum.

Cocaine binds strongly to the dopamine-reuptake transporter and is a classic blocker of such reuptake after normal neuronal activity. Because of this blocking effect, dopamine remains at high concentrations in the synapse and continues to affect adjacent neurons, producing the characteristic cocaine 'high'.

There are no specific pharmacological treatments for cocaine intoxication because the behavioural symptoms and signs, such as psychomotor agitation or retardation, may be diametrically opposite to the physiological ones, such as elevated or lowered blood pressure. A number of medications, including antidepressants, opioid antagonists, dopamimetic drugs such as bromocriptine, and carbamazepine have been used in abuse and dependence but none is considered to be highly effective.

Hallucinogenic drugs

Hallucinogenic drugs such as lysergic acid diethylamide (LSD), cannabis and mescaline produce distortions and intensifications of sensory perceptions as well as frank hallucinations.

Cannabis

Cannabis is a drug widely used in some subcultures. It is derived from the plant *Cannabis sativa.* It is not thought to cause physical dependence. The drug, when smoked, seems to exaggerate the pre-existing mood, be it depression, euphoria or anxiety. There is no definite withdrawal syndrome or tolerance. There is disagreement over whether it can produce a psychosis (see below).

Ecstasy

'Ecstasy' is the street name for 3,4-methylenedioxy-methamphetamine (MDMA), a psychoactive phenyliso-propylamine, synthesized in Germany early in this century. It is a psychodelic drug which is often used as a 'dance' drug. It has a brief duration of action (4–6 hours) and is usually ingested in a dose of 75–150 mg orally. There is anxiety concerning the possibility of MDMA causing permanent brain damage, and deaths have been reported from hyperpyrexia, collapse and dehydration at 'rave' parties. Acute renal and liver failure can occur.

Hypnotics

Other drugs of dependence include barbiturates and benzodiazepines. Discontinuing treatment with benzo-diazepines may cause withdrawal symptoms such as anxiety, restlessness, tachycardia and sensory disturbances (see Table 19.32). For this reason, withdrawal should be supervised and gradual.

Narcotics

Physical dependence occurs with morphine, heroin and codeine as well as with synthetic and semisynthetic narcotic analgesics such as methadone and pethidine. These substances display cross-tolerance – the withdrawal effects of one are reduced by administration of one of the others. The psychological effect of such substances is of a calm, slightly euphoric mood associated with freedom from physical discomfort and a flattening of emotional response. This is believed to be due to the attachment of morphine and its analogues to receptor sites in the CNS normally occupied by endorphins. Tolerance to this group of drugs is rapidly developed and marked. Following abstinence it is rapidly lost. The abstinence syndrome consists of a constellation of signs and symptoms (Table 19.32) that reach peak intensity on the second or third day after the last dose of the opiate. These rapidly subside over the next seven days. Withdrawal is dangerous in patients with heart disease, tuberculosis or other chronic debilitating conditions.

Narcotic addicts are reported to have a high mortality rate owing to acute illness associated with drug abuse. Heart disease (including infective endocarditis), tuberculosis and glomerulonephritis are common causes of death, while tetanus, malaria and acute viral hepatitis B are also causally related to addiction.

TREATMENT OF CHRONIC ABUSE AND OVERDOSE

Blood and urine screening for toxic substances are required in circumstances where drug abuse is suspected (Table 19.33).

The treatment of chronic dependence is usually directed towards helping the addict to live without drugs. Some who cannot manage such a regimen may be maintained on oral methadone. In the UK, only specially licensed doctors may legally prescribe heroin and cocaine to an addict for maintenance treatment of addiction.

The treatment of a narcotic drug overdose requires immediate action. If opioid overdose is suspected, naloxone given intravenously (see p. 877) can be life-saving and diagnostic. There should be an immediate recovery of consciousness or a lightening of the comatose state if the offending agent is an opioid. Care must be taken, however, as opiate antagonists can precipitate violent abstinence symptoms. A constant infusion of naloxone hydrochloride may be required in methadone overdose.

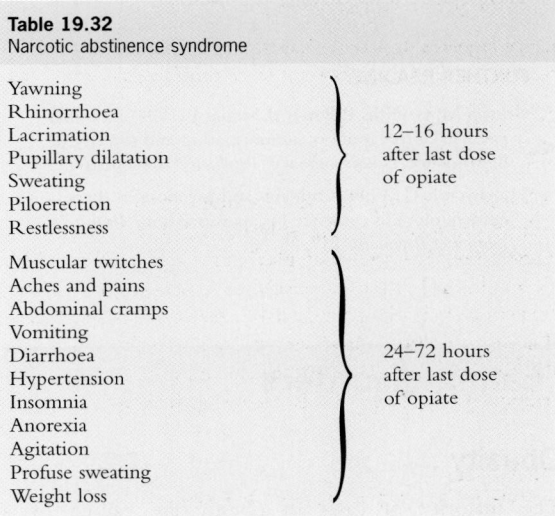

Table 19.32
Narcotic abstinence syndrome

Yawning Rhinorrhoea Lacrimation Pupillary dilatation Sweating Piloerection Restlessness	12–16 hours after last dose of opiate
Muscular twitches Aches and pains Abdominal cramps Vomiting Diarrhoea Hypertension Insomnia Anorexia Agitation Profuse sweating Weight loss	24–72 hours after last dose of opiate

Table 19.33 Length of time urine toxicology screens are likely to remain positive after abstinence

Substance	Usual time positive
Amphetamines	48 hours
Barbiturates	
Short-acting	24 hours
Long-acting	7+ days
Benzodiazepines	3+ days
Cannabinols	5+ days
Cocaine	3+ days
Codeine	48 hours
Morphine	48 hours

Substance-induced psychotic disorder

This is characterized by a cluster of phenomena that occur during or immediately after psychoactive drug use and which include vivid hallucinations (usually auditory, but often in more than one sensory modality), misidentifications, delusions and/or ideas of reference (often of a paranoid or persecutory nature), psychomotor disturbances (excitement or stupor) and an abnormal affect. ICD-10 requires that the condition occurs within two weeks and usually within 48 hours of drug use and that it should persist for more than 48 hours but not more than six months. Drug-induced psychoses have been reported following amphetamine, cocaine, hallucinogen and opiate use.

While cannabis use can result in a 'bad trip', characterized by acute anxiety, depression or hallucinations, there is no convincing data that a persistent psychosis can result. Psychoses occurring after long-term cannabis use have no characteristic psychopathology or unique mode of onset and it remains unclear as to whether these clinical pictures are related to the cannabis itself. However, there is evidence that cannabis smoking increases the risk of developing schizophrenia in individuals so predisposed, and may aggravate the condition once it has manifested itself.

FURTHER READING

Gossop M, Griffiths P, Powis B, Strang J (1994) Cocaine: patterns of use, route of administration and severity of dependence. *British Journal of Psychiatry* **164**: 660–665.

Thornycroft G (1990) Cannabis and psychosis: is there epidemiological evidence for an association? *British Journal of Psychiatry* **157**: 25–33.

Eating disorders

Obesity (see p. 207)

The majority of cases of obesity are caused by a combination of constitutional and social factors that encourage overeating. It is relatively infrequent for psychological causes to be involved. However, even when obesity is not due to definite psychological causes, it may itself produce a psychological reaction of depression and tension, particularly if attempts by the patient to lose weight are repeatedly ineffective.

TREATMENT

Behavioural methods of treatment that make use of positive rewards for weight loss or for behaviour likely to lead to a reduction of weight have been attempted, but their efficacy is doubtful.

Anorexia nervosa

The main clinical criteria for diagnosis are:

- a bodyweight more than 15% below the standard weight, or a Body Mass Index (BMI) below 17.5 (DSM-IV)
- an intense wish to be thin
- a morbid fear of fatness
- amenorrhoea in women.

Clinical features may include:

- onset usually in adolescence
- a previous history of chubbiness or fatness
- a relentless pursuit of low bodyweight
- usually a distorted image of own body size
- the patient generally eats little
- particular avoidance of carbohydrates
- vomiting, excessive exercise and purging
- amenorrhoea – an early symptom; in 20% it precedes weight loss
- binge eating
- usually a marked lack of sexual interest
- lanugo.

The physical consequences of anorexia include sensitivity to cold, constipation, hypotension and bradycardia. In most cases, amenorrhoea is secondary to the weight loss. Vomiting and abuse of purgatives may lead to hypokalaemia and alkalosis.

PREVALENCE

Case register data suggest a rate of 1–10 per 100 000 females aged between 15 and 34 years. Surveys have suggested a prevalence rate of 1–2% among schoolgirls and university students. However, many more young women have amenorrhoea accompanied by less weight loss than the 15% required for the diagnosis. The condition is much less common among men. The onset in women is usually at between 16 and 17 years of age and it seldom occurs after the age of 30 years.

AETIOLOGY

Biological factors

Genetic. Six to ten per cent of siblings of affected girls suffer from anorexia nervosa. There is an increased concordance amongst monozygotic twins, suggesting a genetic predisposition.

Hormonal. There could be a disturbance of hypothalamic function:

- Amenorrhoea can precede weight loss in 20% of sufferers.
- Hormonal disturbances include low luteinizing hormone levels with impaired response to luteinizing hormone releasing hormone and to clomiphene. However, such findings could be due to the effect of prolonged fasting, as they resolve after weight gain.

Psychological factors

Individual. Patients usually have:

- a disturbance of body image
- dietary problems in early life.

Anorexia has often been seen as an escape from the emotional problems of adolescence and a regression into childhood. Recent studies suggest that survivors of childhood sexual abuse are particularly at risk of developing an eating disorder, usually anorexia nervosa, in adolescence. The implication of such findings is that therapists should enquire about and address the eating behaviours of patients with a history of sexual abuse and be aware of the possible history of childhood sexual abuse in patients presenting with eating disorders.

Family. The specific pattern of relationships described is characterized by:

- overprotectiveness
- rigidity
- lack of conflict resolution.

Anorexia serves to prevent dissension in families. However, evidence in favour of such patterns is conflicting.

Social. There is a higher prevalence in higher social classes, and a high rate in certain occupational groups (e.g. ballet students and nurses) and in societies where cultural value is placed on thinness.

COURSE AND PROGNOSIS

The condition runs a fluctuating course, with exacerbations and partial remissions. Long-term follow-up suggests that about two-thirds of patients maintain normal weight and that the remaining one-third are split between those who are moderately underweight and those who are seriously underweight. Indicators of a poor outcome include:

- a long initial illness
- severe weight loss
- bulimia (see below), vomiting or purging
- difficulties in relationships.

Suicide has been reported in 2–5% of patients with chronic anorexia nervosa. More than one-third have recurrent affective illness, and various family, genetic and endocrine studies have found associations between eating disorders and depression.

TREATMENT

Treatment can be conducted on an outpatient basis. However, if the weight loss is severe it is accompanied by marked physical symptoms of lassitude, dizziness and weakness and/or electrolyte and vitamin disturbances; hospital admission may then be unavoidable. Rarely the patient's weight loss may be so severe as to be life-threatening. If the patient cannot be persuaded to enter hospital, compulsory admission may have to be used. Treatment goals include:

- establishing a good relationship with the patient
- restoring the weight to a level between the ideal bodyweight and the patient's idea of what her weight should be
- the provision of a balanced diet of at least 3000 calories in three to four meals per day
- the elimination of purgative and/or laxative use and vomiting.

Treatment can be conducted on behavioural or dynamic psychotherapeutic lines or on a combination of both. The usual behavioural approach is to remove privileges on the patient's admission and to restore them gradually as rewards for weight gain. Intense psychoanalytically derived psychotherapy is not helpful. Family therapy, involving the exploration of problems in family relationships and their modification through counselling, is used; however, evidence that it is superior to simple supportive psychotherapy is lacking.

Bulimia nervosa

This refers to episodes of uncontrolled excessive eating, which are also termed 'binges'. There is a preoccupation with food and a habitual adoption of certain behaviours that can be understood as the patient's attempts to avoid the fattening effects of periodic binges. These behaviours include:

- self-induced vomiting
- laxative abuse
- misuse of drugs – diuretics, thyroid extract or anorectics.

Additional clinical features include:

- physical complications of vomiting:
  (a) cardiac arrhythmias
  (b) renal impairment – consequences of low K^+
  (c) muscular paralysis
  (d) tetany – from hypokalaemic alkalosis
  (e) swollen salivary glands – from vomiting
  (f) eroded dental enamel
- associated psychiatric disorders:
  (a) depression in reaction to vomiting
  (b) alcohol dependence
- fluctuations in bodyweight
- menstrual function – periods irregular but amenorrhoea rare
- personality – neurotic traits present premorbidly.

The prevalence of bulimia in community studies is high; it affects between 5% and 30% of girls attending high schools, colleges or universities in the USA. Bulimia is often associated with anorexia nervosa. The prognosis is uncertain.

TREATMENT

It is not yet clear what is the most effective form of treatment. Admission to hospital with careful control over eating has been advocated, while a behavioural approach involving careful diary-keeping regarding eating and making patients responsible for control is under extensive study. In this approach, patients attempt to identify and avoid any environmental stimuli or emotional changes that regularly precede the desire to binge. Results of this approach are promising.

FURTHER READING

Dancyger IF, Garfinkel PE (1995) The relationship of partial syndrome eating disorders to anorexia nervosa and bulimia nervosa. *Psychological Medicine* **25**: 1019–1025.

Walters E, Kendler K (1995) Anorexia nervosa and anorexic-like symptoms in a population-based female twin study. *American Journal of Psychiatry* **152**: 64–71.

Disorders of adult personality and behaviour [F60–F69]

These disorders comprise deeply ingrained and enduring patterns of behaviour which manifest themselves as inflexible responses to a broad range of personal and social situations. Personality disorders differ from personality changes in their timing and the mode of their appearance. They are developmental conditions which appear in childhood or adolescence and continue into adult life. They are not secondary to another psychiatric disorder or brain disease, although they may precede or coexist with other disorders. Personality change, in contrast, is acquired, usually in adult life, following severe or prolonged stress, extreme environmental deprivation, serious psychiatric disorder or brain injury or disease.

Personality disorders are usually subdivided according to clusters of traits that correspond to the most frequent or obvious behavioural manifestations. The main categories of personality disorder are described below.

Paranoid. A paranoid personality is characterized by extreme sensitiveness, suspiciousness, litigiousness, a tendency to excessive self-importance, and a preoccupation with unsubstantiated conspiratorial explanations of events.

Schizoid. A schizoid personality is characterized by emotional coldness and detachment, a limited capacity to express emotions, indifference to praise or criticism, an almost invariable preference for solitary activities, lack of close friendships, and a marked insensitivity to prevailing social norms and conventions.

Dissocial. A dissocial personality is characterized by a callous unconcern for the feelings of others, an incapacity to maintain enduring relationships, a very low tolerance of frustration, an incapacity to experience guilt and to profit from experience, and a marked proneness to rationalize and blame others.

Histrionic. A histrionic personality is characterized by self-dramatization, theatricality, suggestibility, shallow and labile emotions, a continual seeking for excitement and appreciation by others, an inappropriate seductiveness in appearance or behaviour, and an overconcern with physical attractiveness.

Anankastic (obsessive-compulsive). Such a personality is characterized by feelings of excessive doubt and caution, preoccupation with details, rules, lists, order, perfectionism, excessive conscientiousness, scrupulousness, excessive pedantry, rigidity and stubborness, and intrusion of unwelcome thoughts or impulses.

Dependent. A dependent personality is characterized by the following: a tendency to encourage or allow others to make most of one's personal life decisions, subordination of one's needs to others on whom one is dependent, unwillingness to make demands on others, feelings of helplessness and exaggerated fears of inability to care for oneself, a preoccupation with fears of being abandoned by a person with whom one has a close relationship, and a limited capacity to make everyday decisions without an excessive amount of advice and reassurance from others.

Many individuals with disturbed personalities do not fit neatly into such categories, but manifest a mixture of features.

MANAGEMENT

In making a diagnosis of a personality disorder it is necessary to establish that it has been present since adolescence. Any additional psychiatric disorder should be looked for and treated as necessary. Organic causes, such as epilepsy, may need treatment. Supervision and support, group therapy and other forms of psychotherapy are sometimes useful.

FURTHER READING

Swanson MC, Bland RC, Newman SC (1994) Antisocial personality disorder. *Acta Psychiatrica Scandinavica* **376**: 63–70.

Sexual dysfunction not caused by organic disorder or disease [F52]

Sexual disorders can be divided into sexual dysfunctions, sexual deviations, and gender role disorders (Table 19.34). In ICD-10 these are classified under Disorders of Adult Personality and Behaviour.

Sexual dysfunction

Sexual dysfunction in men refers to repeated inability to achieve normal sexual intercourse, whereas in women it

Table 19.34
Classification of sexual disorders

Sexual dysfunction	Sexual deviations	Disorders of the gender role
Affecting sexual desire	Variations of the sexual 'object'	Transsexualism
Low libido	Fetishism	
Impaired sexual arousal	Transvestism	
Erectile impotence	Paedophilia	
Failure of arousal in women	Bestiality	
Affecting orgasm	Necrophilia	
Premature ejaculation	**Variations of the sexual act**	
Retarded ejaculation	Exhibitionism	
Orgasmic dysfunction in women	Voyeurism	
	Sadism	
	Masochism	
	Frotteurism	

refers to a repeatedly unsatisfactory quality of sexual satisfaction. Problems of sexual dysfunction can usefully be classified into those affecting sexual desire, those affecting sexual arousal, and those affecting orgasm. Among men presenting for treatment of sexual dysfunction, impotence is the most frequent complaint. The prevalence of premature ejaculation is low, while ejaculatory failure is rare.

Sexual drive is affected by constitutional factors, ignorance of sexual technique, anxiety about sexual performance, medical conditions and certain drugs (Tables 19.35 and 19.36).

The treatment of sexual dysfunction involves careful assessment, the participation (where appropriate) of the patient's partner, and specific therapeutic techniques, including relaxation, behavioural training and supportive counselling (see p. 925).

Sexual deviation

Nowadays, sexual deviations are more likely to be regarded as unusual forms of behaviour than as illnesses. Doctors are only likely to be involved when the behaviour involves breaking the law (e.g. paedophilia or bestiality) and when there is a question of an associated mental or physical disorder. Homosexuality was formerly classified as an illness but it is now an accepted alternative sexual lifestyle.

Transvestism is a form of sexual deviation in which individuals, usually men, dress in clothes of the opposite sex. The cross-dressing may either be a symptom of some other sexual deviation or may be employed as a means of fetishistic sexual excitement. It usually begins at about puberty and the transvestite experiences sexual excitement and may masturbate when indulging in this behaviour. The overwhelming majority of cross-dressers believe that they are of the correct gender, in contrast to transsexuals (see below).

Table 19.35
Medical conditions affecting sexual performance

Endocrine	**Renal**
Diabetes mellitus	Renal failure
Hyperthyroidism	**Neurological**
Hypothyroidism	Neuropathy
Cardiovascular	Spinal cord lesions
Angina pectoris	**Musculoskeletal**
Previous myocardial infarction	Arthritis
Disorders of peripheral circulation	**Respiratory**
Hepatic	Asthma
Cirrhosis, particularly alcohol-related	COPD

Gender role disorders [F64]

Transsexualism involves a disturbance in sexual identity. The criteria for establishing sexual identity are described on p. 925.

In transsexualism, there is no evidence as yet of abnormality in the chromosomal or phenotypic sex; social sex conforms to biological sex. There is, however, a severe disturbance in psychosexual differentiation. A person's gender identity refers to the individual's sense of masculinity or femininity as distinct from sex. It is thought to arise from a biological component (prenatal endocrine influences), psychological imprinting and social conditioning. Disturbances in these three areas have

Table 19.36
Drugs adversely affecting sexual arousal

Male arousal	Female arousal
Alcohol	Alcohol
Benzodiazepines	CNS depressants
Neuroleptics	Oral combined contraceptives
Cimetidine	Methyldopa
Narcotic analgesics	Clonidine
Methyldopa	
Clonidine	
Spironolactone	
Antihistamines	

Alcohol increases the desire but diminishes the performance

variously been blamed for the cause of transsexualism. The four key features of transsexualism are:

- a sense of belonging to the opposite sex and of having been born into the wrong sex
- a sense of estrangement from one's own body – all manifestations of anatomical sexual identification are regarded as repugnant
- a strong desire to resemble physically the opposite sex and seek treatment, including surgery, towards this end
- a wish to be accepted in the community as belonging to the opposite sex.

For males, treatment includes hormone administration (oestrogen is used to produce some breast enlargement and fat deposition around hips and thighs) and, if surgery is to be recommended, a period of living as a woman as a trial beforehand. In the case of female transsexuals, treatment involves surgery and the use of methyltestosterone.

FURTHER READING

Halaris A (ed) (1997) Sexual dysfunction. In: *Baillière's Clinical Psychiatry: International Practice and Research*, Vol 3. London: Baillière Tindall.

Psychiatry and the law

At the heart of the relationship between psychiatry and the law is the issue of *responsibility*. Mental disorder, by virtue of its severity and/or quality, may impair individuals' responsibility for their thinking and actions. The law in most Western countries provides for the compulsory admission and/or treatment of mentally disordered persons for their own protection and/or the protection of others and for mitigation in the case of mentally disordered individuals who commit a criminal offence.

In England and Wales the law relating to the care and control of the mentally ill has evolved out of common law. The Act of Parliament that is crucially involved is the Mental Health Act 1983. This Act is concerned not merely with provisions governing the compulsory admission and treatment of mentally disordered persons, but also with patients' rights, appeals tribunals and the overall supervision of the use of compulsory powers. The Act is divided into a number of sections, each of which deals with a different aspect of the process. The Mental Health (Scotland) Act 1984 and the Mental Health (Northern Ireland) Order 1986 contain clauses broadly similar to those in England and Wales.

Apart from one provision of the National Assistance Act 1948, the Mental Health Act 1983 is the only method whereby individuals can legally be deprived of their liberty without having committed a crime or being suspected of committing a crime. It is, therefore, very important that doctors understand the seriousness of their responsibility and the details of the legislation.

There are three conditions that need to be met before an appropriate compulsory section form is signed. The patient must be:

- suffering from a defined mental disorder
- at risk to his/her and/or other people's health or safety
- unwilling to accept hospitalization voluntarily.

The reasons why there is no alternative approach to the treatment suggested for the patient should be outlined.

Sexual deviance or alcohol/drug dependence are not mental disorders, but otherwise the definition of mental disorder is broad and includes:

- mental illness
- mental impairment
- severe mental impairment
- psychopathy.

Any registered medical practitioner may sign a medical recommendation under the Act, but the added signature of a specialist psychiatrist approved under Section 12 is needed for compulsory orders lasting for more than 72 hours. Unless the patient is already in hospital, the nearest relative or an approved mental health social

Table 19.37
Important sections of the Mental Health Act 1983

Section	Duration	Signatures required	Purpose
2	28 days	Two doctors (one approved) plus nearest relative or social worker	Assessment and treatment
3	6 months	Two doctors (one approved) plus nearest relative or social worker	Treatment
4	72 hours	One doctor plus relative or social worker	Emergency admission
5(2)	72 hours	Doctor in charge of patient's care	Emergency detention of a patient already in hospital
5(4)	6 hours	Nurse (RMN)	Emergency detention of a patient already in hospital
136	72 hours	Police officer	Psychiatric assessment of those in public places thought by police to be mentally ill and in need of a place of safety

worker is also required to sign the application form. Important sections of the Act are detailed in Table 19.37.

Sections 4, 5(2), 5(4) and 136 cannot be extended by repetition. They must be converted to a Section 2 or 3 if prolonged detention is necessary. Likewise, Section 2 should be converted to a Section 3 if required. Patients on the longer orders (2 and 3) can appeal to a Mental Health Review Tribunal.

The Act also deals with consent to treatment, guardianship, mentally abnormal offenders and hazardous treatments. A Mental Health Act Commission supervises the Act, provides second opinions and regularly visits hospitals. Although much of the process of detention against one's will is formalized, there is no liability for a doctor who acts in good faith with a patient's best interests at heart. Clearly written medical notes, accepted forms of treatment and common sense remain the basis of good practice.

FURTHER READING

Duggan C (ed) (1997) Assessing risk in the mentally disordered. *British Journal of Psychiatry* **170** (Suppl 32).

Dermatology

20

Skin diseases have a high prevalence throughout the world. In developing countries infectious diseases such as tuberculosis, leprosy and onchocerciasis are common, whereas in developed countries inflammatory disorders such as eczema and acne are more common. Skin disorders can be inherited (e.g. Ehlers–Danlos syndrome), be a part of normal development (e.g. acne vulgaris), or may present as part of a systemic disorder (e.g. systemic lupus erythematosus).

Approximately 25% of the UK population will develop a skin problem, and although self-medication is common, skin disease still accounts for up to 10% of the workload of family doctors. The common reasons for this are: itching or pain, which can interfere with people's ability to function normally or to sleep; rashes, which cause anxiety, depression and lack of self-confidence and can lead to social isolation if obviously visible; and an inability to work, because certain dermatoses (such as allergic hand eczema in a builder or hairdresser) can interfere with or even prevent working.

Rarely skin disease can be fatal. Examples are malignant melanoma, toxic epidermal necrolysis and pemphigus.

Structure and functions of the skin

The skin consists of four distinct layers: the epidermis, the basement membrane zone, the dermis and the subcutaneous layer (Fig 20.1). The functions are summarized in Information box 20.1.

The epidermis

The epidermis is a stratified epithelium of ectodermal origin that arises from dividing basal keratinocytes. The lower cells (basal layer) produce a variety of keratin filaments and desmosomal connections – the so-called 'cytoskeleton'. This confers strength to the epidermis and prevents it shedding off. Higher up in the granular layer, complex lipids are secreted by the keratinocytes and these form into intercellular lipid bilayers which act as a semipermeable skin barrier. The upper cells (stratum corneum) lose their nuclei and become surrounded by a tough impermeable 'envelope' of various proteins (loricrin, involucrin and filaggrin and keratin). Changes in lipid metabolism, protein expression in the outer layers allow normal shedding of keratinocytes.

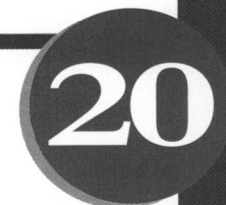

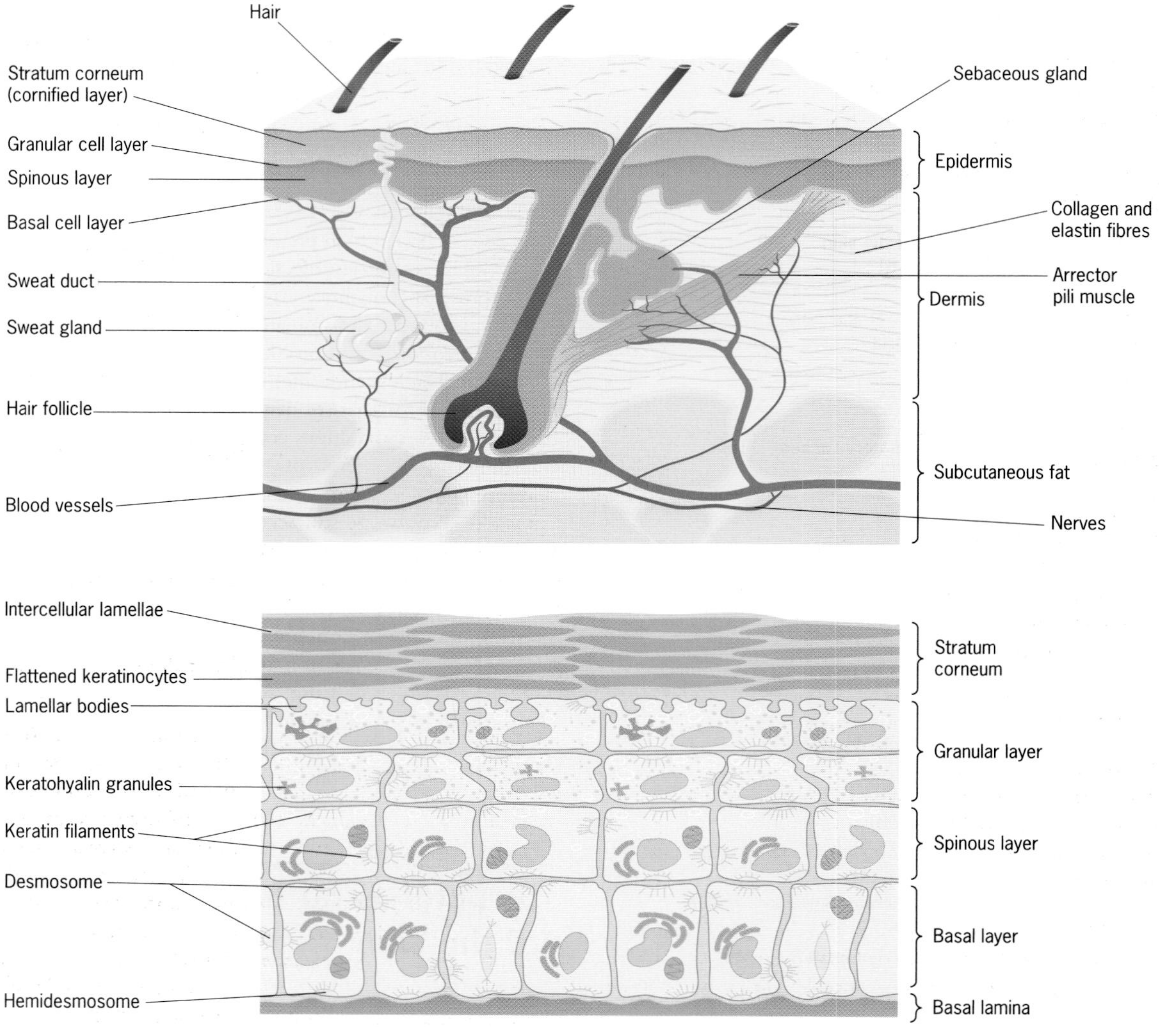

Fig 20.1
The structure of the skin

It has recently been recognized that the keratinocytes can secrete a variety of cytokines (e.g. interleukins, interferon, tumour necrosis factor alpha) in response to tissue injury or in certain skin diseases. These play a role in immune function, cutaneous inflammation and tissue repair.

Information

- Physical barrier against friction and shearing forces
- Protective barrier to infection
- Prevention of excessive water loss or absorption
- Ultraviolet induced synthesis of vitamin D
- Temperature regulation
- Sensation (pain, touch and temperature)
- Antigen presentation/immunological reactions/wound healing
- Protection from ultraviolet irradiation

Information box 20.1 Functions of the skin

Other cells on the epidermis

Melanocytes are found in the basal layer and secrete the pigment melanin. These protect against ultraviolet irradiation. Racial differences are due to variation in melanin production, not melanocyte numbers.

Merkel cells are also found in the basal layer and probably originate from the neural crest. They are numerous on finger-tips and in the oral cavity and play a role in sensation.

Langerhans cells are dendritic cells found in the suprabasal layer. They derive from the bone-marrow and act as antigen-presenting cells.

Basement membrane zone (see Fig 20.26)

The basement membrane zone is a complex proteinaceous structure consisting of type IV and VII collagen, hemidesmosomal proteins, integrins and laminin. Inherited or autoimmune induced deficiencies of these proteins can cause skin fragility and a variety of blistering diseases (see p 1179).

The dermis

The dermis is of mesodermal origin and contains blood and lymphatic vessels, nerves, muscle, appendages (e.g. sweat glands, sebaceous glands and hair follicles) and a variety of immune cells such as mast cells and lymphocytes. It is a matrix of collagen and elastin in a ground substance.

The sweat glands

- *Eccrine* sweat glands are found throughout the skin except the mucosal surfaces.
- *Apocrine* sweat glands are found in the axillae, anogenital area and scalp and do not function until puberty.

The sweat glands and vasculature are important in temperature control.

Sebaceous glands

These are inactive until puberty. They are responsible for secreting sebum or grease onto the skin surface (via the hair follicle) and are found in high number on the face and scalp.

Nerves

The skin is richly innervated. These fibres allow sensation of touch, pain, itch, vibration and change in temperature.

Hair

Hairs arise from a downgrowth of epidermal keratinocytes into the dermis. The hair shaft has an inner and outer root sheath, a cortex and sometimes a medulla. The lower portion of the hair follicle consists of an expanded bulb (which also contains melanocytes) surrounding a richly innervated and vascularized dermal papilla. The hair regrows from the bulb after shedding. There are three types of hair:

- *terminal* – medullated coarse hair (e.g. scalp, beard, pubic)
- *vellus* – non-medullated fine downy hairs seen on the face of women and in prepubertal children
- *lanugo* – non-medullated soft hair on newborns (most marked in premature babies) and occasionally in people with anorexia nervosa.

All hair follicles follow a growth cycle: anagen (growth phase), catagen (involution phase), and telogen (shedding phase). At any one time most hairs (> 90%) will be in the anagen phase, which is typically 3–5 years for scalp hair.

Nails

Nails are tough plates of hardened keratin which arise from the nail matrix (just visible as the moon-shaped lunula) under the nailfold. It takes six months for a finger-nail to grow out fully and one year for a toe-nail.

The subcutaneous layer

The subcutaneous layer consists predominantly of adipose tissue as well as blood vessels and nerves. This layer provides insulation and acts as a lipid store.

Approach to the patient

The *history* should aim to elicit the following points:

- the time course of the rash
- the distribution of lesions
- symptoms (e.g. itch or pain)
- family history (especially of atopy and psoriasis)
- drug/allergy history
- past medical history
- provocating factors (e.g. sunlight or diet)
- previous skin treatments.

Examination entails looking *and* feeling a rash (for terminology, see Table 20.1). It should include an assessment of nails, hair, and mucosal surfaces, even if these are recorded as unaffected. The following terms are used to describe distribution: flexural, extensor, acral (hands and feet), symmetrical, localized, widespread, facial, unilateral, linear, centripetal (trunk more than limbs), annular and reticulate (lacey network or mesh like).

With regard to *investigations*, clinical acumen remains the most useful tool in dermatology, but a variety of tests are useful in confirming a diagnosis (Table 20.2).

FURTHER READING

Montagna W, Kligman AM, Carlisle KS (1992) *Atlas of Normal Human Skin*. New York: Springer Verlag.

Infections

Bacterial infections

The skin's normal bacterial flora prevents colonization by pathogenic organisms. A break in epidermal integrity by trauma, leg ulcers, fungal infections (e.g. athlete's foot) or abnormal scaling of the skin (e.g. in eczema) can allow entry of bacteria. If reinfection occurs this may be due to asymptomatic nasal carriage of bacteria or the presence of other infected close contacts.

Table 20.1
Morphological description of skin lesions

Atrophy	Thinning of the skin
Bulla	Large fluid-filled blister
Crusted	Dried serum or exudate on the skin
Ecchymosis	Large confluent area of purpura ('bruise')
Erosion	Denuded area of skin (partial epidermal loss)
Excoriation	Scratch mark
Lichenified	Thickened epidermis with prominent normal skin markings
Macule	Flat, circumscribed non-palpable lesion
Nodule	Large papule (>0.5 cm)
Papule	Small palpable, circumscribed lesion (<0.5 cm)
Petechia	Pinpoint-sized macule of blood in the skin
Plaque	Large flat-topped, palpable lesion
Purpura	Larger macule or papule of blood in the skin which does not blanch on pressure
Pustule	Yellowish white pus-filled lesion
Scaly	Visible flaking and shedding of surface skin
Telangiectasia	Abnormal visible dilation of blood vessels
Ulcer	Deeper denuded area of skin (full epidermal and dermal loss)
Vesicle	Small fluid-filled blister
Weal	Itchy raised 'nettle rash'-like swelling due to dermal oedema

Table 20.2
Investigations used in skin disorders

Test	Use	Clinical example
Skin swabs	Bacterial culture	Impetigo
Blister fluid	Electron-microscopy and viral culture	Herpes simplex
Skin scrapes	Fungal culture Microscopy	Tinea pedis Scabies
Nail sampling	Fungal culture	Onychomycosis
Wood's light	Fungal fluorescence	Scalp ringworm Erythrasma
Blood tests	Serology	Streptococcal cellulitis
	Autoantibodies HLA typing DNA characterization	Discoid lupus erythematosus Dermatitis herpetiformis Epidermolysis bullosa
Skin biopsy	Histology Immunohisto-chemistry Immunofluorescence	General diagnosis Cutaneous lymphoma Immunobullous disease
	Culture	Mycobacteria/fungi
Patch tests	Allergic contact eczema	Hand eczema
Urine	Biochemistry	Diabetes mellitus

Impetigo

Impetigo is a highly infectious skin disease most common in children (Fig 20.2). It presents as weeping, exudative areas with a typical honey-coloured crust on the surface. It is spread by direct contact. The term 'Scrum pox' is impetigo spread between rugby players. Occasionally this infection can cause blistering ('bullous impetigo') due to bacterial toxins. *Staphylococcus aureus* is implicated in over 90% of cases but, rarely, group A *Streptococcus* can be responsible. Therefore skin swabs should always be taken.

TREATMENT

Localized disease is treated with topical fusidic acid (three times daily) and the antiseptic povidone iodine for one week. Extensive disease is treated with oral antibiotics for 7–10 days (flucloxacillin 500 mg four times daily for *Staphylococcus*; penicillin V 500 mg four times daily for *Streptococcus*). Other close contacts should be examined and children should avoid school for one week after starting therapy. If impetigo appears resistant to treatment or is recurrent, take nasal swabs and check other family members. Nasal mupirocin (thrice daily for one week) may be useful to eradicate nasal carriage.

Cellulitis (erysipelas)

Cellulitis presents as a hot, sometimes tender area of confluent erythema of the skin. It often affects the lower leg causing an upwards-spreading erythema. It may also be seen affecting one side of the face. Patients are often unwell with a high temperature. It is usually caused by a *Streptococcus*. There may be an obvious portal of entry for infection such as a recent abrasion or a venous leg ulcer. The web spaces of the toes should be examined for evidence of fungal infection. Skin swabs are usually unhelpful. Confirmation of infection is best done serologically by streptococcal titres.

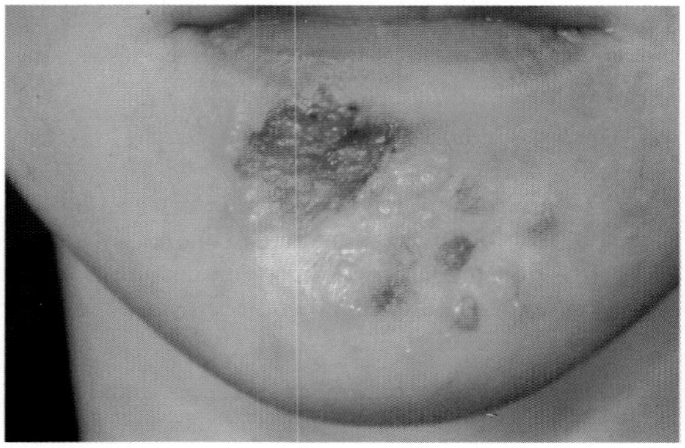

Fig 20.2
Crusted blistering lesions of impetigo

TREATMENT

Treatment is with penicillin V or erythromycin (both 500 mg four times daily). If disease is advanced, intravenous therapy is given for 3–5 days, followed by 1–2 weeks of oral therapy. It is also important to treat any identifiable underlying cause. If cellulitis is recurrent, antibiotic prophylaxis (e.g. penicillin V 500 mg twice daily) should be given.

Ecthyma

Ecthyma is also an infection due to *Streptococcus* or *Staphylococcus aureus* or occasionally both. It presents as chronic, well-demarcated, ulcerative lesions sometimes with an exudative crust. It is more common in developing countries, being associated with poor nutrition and hygeine. It is rare in the UK but is seen more commonly in intravenous drug abusers and people with HIV infection.

TREATMENT

Treatment is with 10–14 days of penicillin V and flucloxacillin (both 500 mg four times daily).

Erythrasma

Erythrasma is caused by *Corynebacterium minutissimum*. It usually presents as an orange-brown flexural rash, and is often seen in the axillae or toe web spaces (Fig 20.3). It is frequently misdiagnosed as a fungal infection. The rash shows a dramatic coral pink fluorescence under Wood's (ultraviolet) light.

TREATMENT

It responds well to oral erythromycin 500 mg four times daily for 10 days.

Folliculitis

Folliculitis is an inflammation of the hair follicle. It presents as itchy or tender papules and pustules. *Staphylococcus aureus* is frequently implicated. It is more common in humid climates and when occlusive clothes are worn. A variant occurs in the beard area (called 'sycosis barbae') which is more common in Afro-Caribbeans. This is probably caused by the ability of shaved hair to grow back into the skin, especially if the hair is naturally curly.

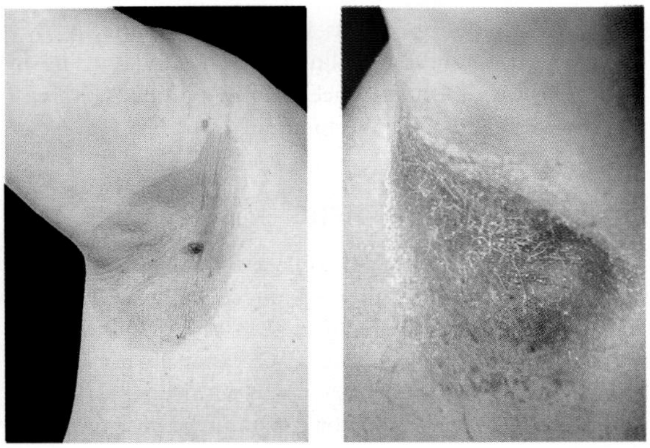

Fig 20.3
Erythrasma of the axilla, showing pink fluorescence under a Wood's lamp

Extensive, itchy folliculitis of the upper trunk and limbs should alert one to the possibility of underlying HIV infection.

TREATMENT

Treatment is with topical antiseptics, topical antibiotics (e.g. fucidin) or oral antibiotics (e.g. flucloxacillin 500 mg or erythromycin 500 mg both four times daily for 2–4 weeks).

Boils (furuncles)

Boils are a rather deep-seated infection of the skin often caused by *Staphylococcus*. They can cause painful red swellings. Boils are more common in teenagers and are often recurrent. Recurrent boils may also occur rarely in diabetes mellitus or in immunosuppression. Large boils are sometimes called 'carbuncles'.

TREATMENT

Treatment is with oral antibiotics (e.g. erythromycin 500 mg four times daily for 10–14 days) and occasionally by incision and drainage. Antiseptics such as povidone iodine, chlorhexidine (as soap) and a bath oil (e.g. Oilatum plus™) can be useful in prophylaxis.

Hidradenitis suppurativa

This is a rare condition characterized by a painful, discharging, chronic inflammation of the skin at sites rich in apocrine glands (axillae, groins, natal cleft). The cause is unknown, but it is more common in females and within some families it appears to be inherited in an autosomal dominant fashion. Clinically it presents after puberty with papules, nodules and abcesses which often progress to cysts and sinus formation. With time, scarring may arise. The condition follows a chronic relapsing/remitting course.

TREATMENT

Treatment is very difficult, but antibiotics, oral retinoids and Dianette™ (2 mg cyproterone acetate + 35 μg ethinyloestradiol in females only) have been tried. They should be used as for acne vulgaris (p. 1169). Severe recalcitrant cases have been treated occasionally with surgery and skin grafting.

Pitted keratolysis

This is a superficial infection of the horny layer of the skin caused by a corynebacterium. It frequently involves the soles of the forefoot and appears as numerous small punched-out circular lesions of a rather macerated skin (e.g. as seen after prolonged immersion). There may be an associated hyperhidrosis of the feet and a prominent odour.

TREATMENT
Topical antibiotics (e.g. fucidic acid or clindamycin, applied thrice daily for 2–4 weeks) and topical anti-sweating lotions are effective therapies.

Erysipeloid

This is a very rare infection due to *Erysipelothrix insidiosa.* It is seen in people who handle raw meat (especially pork) and fish. The organism gains entry through breaks in the skin. It presents as a spreading, well-demarcated purplish-red lesion usually on the fingers, hands or forearms. There are no systemic symptoms.

TREATMENT
Treatment is with penicillin V or oxytetracycline (both 500 mg four times daily for 7–10 days).

Mycobacterial infections

Leprosy (Hansen's disease) (p. 41)

Leprosy usually involves the skin and the clinical features depend on the body's immune response to the organism *Mycobacterium leprae.*

Indeterminate leprosy is the most common clinical type, especially in children. This presents as hypopigmented or erythematous circular macules with occasional mild anaesthesia and scaling. This may resolve spontaneously or progress to one of the other types. Biopsy reveals a perineural granulomatous infiltrate and scant acid-fast bacilli.

Tuberculoid leprosy presents with a few hypopigmented or erythematous plaques with an active erythematous, raised rim. Lesions are usually markedly anaesthetic, dry and hairless, reflecting the nerve damage. Nerves may be enlarged and palpable. Biopsy shows a granulomatous infiltrate centred on nerves but no organisms.

Lepromatous leprosy presents with multiple inflammatory papules, plaques and nodules. Loss of the eyebrows ('madarosis') and nasal stuffiness are common. Skin thickening and severe disfigurement may follow. Anaesthesia is much less prominent. Biopsy shows numerous acid-fast bacilli.

Diagnosis and treatment are discussed on p. 43.

Skin manifestations of tuberculosis

Tuberculosis can occasionally cause skin manifestations.

- *Lupus vulgaris* usually arises as a post-primary infection. It often presents on the head or neck with red-brown nodules which look like apple jelly when pressed with a glass slide. They heal with scarring and new lesions slowly spread out to form a chronic solitary erythematous plaque. Chronic lesions are at high risk of developing squamous cell carcinoma.
- *Tuberculosis verrucosa cutis* arises in people who are partially immune to tuberculosis but who suffer a further direct inoculation in the skin. It presents as warty lesions on a 'cold' erythematous base.
- *Scrofuloderma* arises when an infected lymph node spreads to the skin causing ulceration, scarring and discharge (see p. 40).
- *The tuberculides* are a group of rashes caused by an immune manifestation of tuberculosis rather than direct infection. Erythema nodosum is the most common and is discussed on p. 1173. Erythema induratum ('Bazin's disease') produces similar deep red nodules but these are usually found on the calves rather than the shins.

Atypical mycobacteria

Atypical mycobacteria (non-tuberculous) can occasionally infect the skin. *Mycobacterium marinum* is found in fish tanks and occasionally swimming pools. It can gain access via a break in the skin and then causes deep granulomatous nodules, often in a linear fashion.

Viral infections

Viral exanthem

This is probably the most common type of viral-induced rash which presents clinically as a widespread nonspecific erythematous maculopapular rash, often in the prodromal phase of illness. It probably arises owing to circulating immune complexes of antibody and viral antigen localizing to dermal blood vessels. The rash can be caused by many different viruses (e.g. echovirus, parvovirus, human herpes virus-6, Epstein–Barr virus; see p. 57) and so is rarely diagnostic. The rash will resolve spontaneously in 7–10 days.

Slapped cheek syndrome (erythema infectiosum, Fifth disease)

This affects children and is caused by parvovirus B19 (see p. 55). It is a mild viral illness which is followed by an intense erythema on the cheeks ('slapped cheeks') and a reticulate erythema on the upper arm.

Herpes simplex virus (see also p. 51)

Herpes simplex virus (HSV) occurs as two genomic subtypes. HSV type 1 is spread by direct contact and droplet infection. Most people are affected in early childhood but the infection is usually subclinical. Occasionally it can cause a self-limiting pyrexial primary illness with either clusters of painful blisters on the face or a painful gingivostomatitis. Once infected, cell-mediated immunity develops. In some individuals this response is poor and they may get recurrent attacks of HSV, often manifest as cold sores. Immunosuppression can also cause a recrudescence of HSV. HSV can also autoinoculate into sites of trauma and present as painful blisters/pustules. For example, they may be seen on the fingers of health-care workers ('herpetic whitlow').

HSV type 2 infections occur mainly after puberty and usually affect the genital area. Infections are often symptomatic and transmitted sexually. However, HSV type 1 can also be found in the genital area arising from orogenital contact.

Other rare complications of HSV infection include corneal ulceration, acute encephalitis, eczema herpeticum (see p. 115), chronic perianal ulceration in AIDS patients and erythema multiforme.

TREATMENT

Acylovir is used topically and systemically for both primary and recurrent infection of the skin and mucous membranes. Oral acyclovir 200 mg five times a day is given. Penciclovir is used as a cream for herpes labialis.

Varicella zoster virus

Varicella zoster virus (VZV) causes the common childhood infection called chickenpox . It is discussed on p. 52. It also causes herpes zoster.

HERPES ZOSTER

'Shingles' results from a reactivation of the herpes zoster virus (VZV). It may be preceded by a prodromal phase of tingling or pain which is then followed by a painful and tender blistering eruption in a dermatomal distribution (Fig 20.4). The blisters occur in crops, may become pustular and then crust over. The rash lasts 2–4 weeks and is usually more severe in the elderly. Occasionally more than one dermatome is involved.

Complications of shingles include severe, persistent pain (post-herpetic neuralgia), ocular disease (if the ophthalmic nerve is involved), and rarely motor neuropathy.

TREATMENT

Treatment of herpes zoster requires adequate analgesia, and antibiotics if secondary bacterial infection is present. Oral acyclovir (800 mg, five times daily for seven days) helps shorten the attack if given early in the illness. High-dose intravenous acyclovir is needed for immuno-suppressed patients. It remains unclear how useful acyclovir therapy is in preventing prolonged post-herpetic neuralgia.

Human papilloma virus

Human papilloma virus (HPV) is responsible for the common cutaneous infection of 'viral warts'. There are more than 70 subtypes as detected by DNA hybridization. All can cause overgrowth of differentiated squamous epithelium.

Common warts are papular lesions with a coarse, roughened surface, often seen on the hands and feet, but also on other sites. Small black dots (bleeding points) are often seen within the lesion (Fig 20.5). Children and adolescents are usually affected. Spread is by direct contact and is also associated with trauma.

Plantar warts (verrucae) is the term used for lesions on the soles of the feet. They often appear flat ('inward growing') although they have the same papillomatous surface change and black dots are often revealed if the skin is pared down (unlike callosities). Warts may be painful or tender if they are over pressure points or around nailfolds.

Filiform warts occur on the face, at the nasal vestibule or around the mouth, or on the neck. They are elongated, with a horny cap.

Plane warts are much less common and are caused by certain HPV subtypes. They are clinically different and appear as very small, flesh-coloured or pigmented, flat-topped lesions (best seen with side-on lighting) with little in the way of surface change and no black dots within them. They are usually multiple and are frequently found on the face or the backs of the hands.

Anogenital warts are usually seen in adults and are normally transmitted by sexual contact. They are rare in

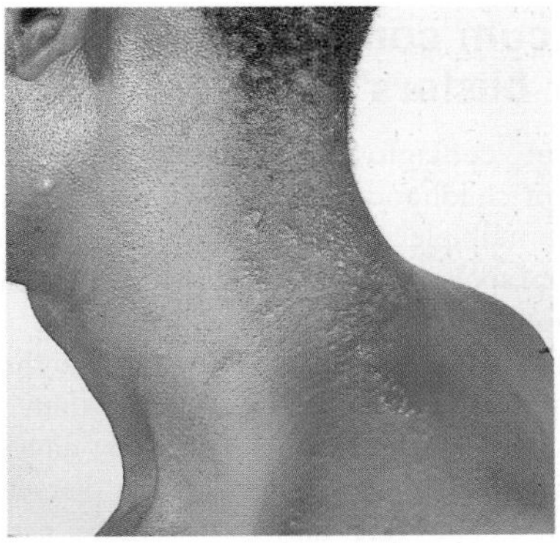

Fig 20.4
Herpes zoster in an African. Courtesy of Dr P Matondo, Lusaka, Zambia

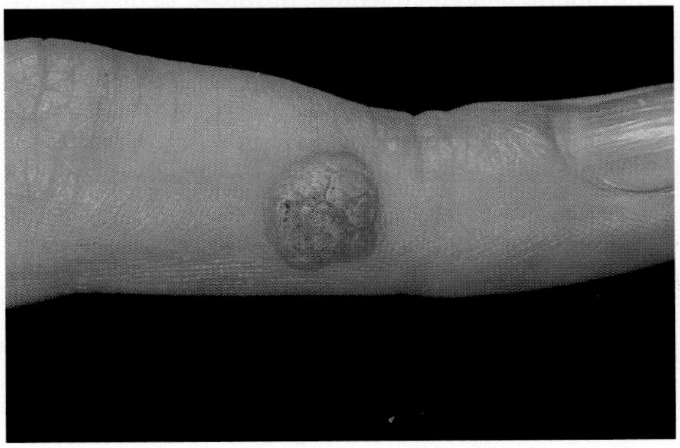

Fig 20.5
Viral wart

childhood and whilst child sex abuse should be delicately discussed, it should be remembered they may well have been transmitted through non-sexual contact. HPV subtypes 16 and 18 are potentially oncogenic and are associated with cervical and anal carcinomas.

TREATMENT

Common warts on the skin are surprisingly difficult to treat effectively but they almost always resolve spontaneously after months to years (with no scarring), presumably due to cell-mediated immune recognition. When they do resolve, they tend to do so rapidly within a few days.

Regular use of a topical keratolytic agent (e.g. 2–10% salicylic acid) over many months with weekly paring of the lesion helps speed up resolution in some patients and remains the mainstay of treatment. A course of cryotherapy (freezing) can also help. Cautery, surgery, carbon dioxide laser, α-interferon injection and bleomycin injection have all been used with variable success. These treatments may be very painful and can cause permanent scarring.

Genital warts (see p. 104) are usually treated with either cryotherapy, trichloracetic acid or topical podophyllin. Patients with genital warts (and their sexual partners) must be screened for other sexually transmitted diseases.

Molluscum contagiosum ('water blisters')

Molluscum contagiosum is a common cutaneous infection of childhood caused by a pox virus. Clinically, lesions are multiple small (1–3 mm) translucent papules which often appear to look like fluid-filled vesicles but are in fact solid. Individual lesions may have a central depression called a punctum. They exhibit the Köbner phenomenon (p. 1165). They can occur at any body site including the genitalia. Transmission is by direct contact. Occasionally lesions may be up to 1 cm diameter ('giant molluscum'). They are said to be more extensive in children with atopic eczema, which may just reflect that scratching aids their spread.

They usually continue to occur in crops over 6–12 months and rarely require treatment as they resolve spontaneously. Any form of localized trauma, including scratching, helps speed up resolution and cryotherapy may be considered in an older child. Molluscum in an adult, especially if giant, should raise the underlying possibility of immunosuppression, especially HIV infection.

Orf

Orf is a disease of sheep (and occasionally goats) due to a pox virus infection. It causes a vesicular and pustular rash around the mouths of young lambs. People who come into contact with the affected fluid may develop lesions on the hands. Clinically they appear as 1–2 cm reddish papules with a surrounding erythema which usually become pustular. The lesion(s) resolves spontaneously after 4–6 weeks and immunity lasts lifelong. Occasionally orf is complicated by erythema multiforme (see p. 1174).

Fungal infections

Fungi are primitive, saprophytic organisms found throughout our environment. Fungal skin disease (mycoses) has a high prevalence in humans with 'thrush' and 'athletes foot' being two of the most common examples. In the immunosuppressed, mycoses can be widespread and life-threatening. There are three groups of pathogenic fungi that commonly affect the outer layer of skin or keratinizing epithelium: dermatophytes, *Candida albicans* and pityrosporum.

Dermatophyte infection

By definition, dermatophytes cause a 'ringworm' type of rash. The three main genera responsible are *Trichophyton*, *Microsporum* and *Epidermophyton*. These organisms are identified by microscopy and culture of skin, hair or nail samples. The clinical appearance of mycoses depends in part on the organism involved, the site affected and the host reaction. All are spread by direct contact from other humans or from infected animals. The use of communal showers and swimming baths and the sharing of towels or sportswear aids indirect fomite transmission.

Tinea corporis

Ringworm of the body usually presents as slightly itchy, asymmetrical, scaly patches which show central clearing and an advancing, scaly, raised edge. Occasionally vesicles or pustules may be seen in the edge. Central clearing is not a universal feature and it is recommended that all asymmetrical scaly lesions should be scraped for fungus. Ringworm of the face (tinea faciei) often arises after the use of topical steroids. It tends to be more erythematous and less scaly than trunk lesions and it may become itchy after sun exposure.

Tinea cruris

Ringworm of the groin is extremely common world-wide. Early on the lesions appear as well demarcated red plaques with an arc-like border extending down the upper thigh (Fig 20.6). Central clearing may appear and a few pustules or vesicles may be seen if inflammation is intense. Satellite lesions, suggestive of *Candida*, are not present.

Tinea pedis

Athletes foot may be confined to the toe clefts where the skin looks white, macerated and fissured. It may also be more diffuse, usually causing a diffuse scaly erythema of the soles spreading on to the sides of the foot. Annular lesions are rarely present leading to frequent misdiagnosis. There may be an associated hyperhidrosis and fungal involvement of one or more toe-nails. In severe infection a strong inflammatory reaction can occur causing pustules or blistering and this often leads to a misdiagnosis of pompholyx-type eczema.

Tinea manuum

Ringworm of the hands presents with a diffuse erythematous scaling of the palms with variable skin peeling and thickening. Annular lesions are rare at this site.

Tinea capitis

Ringworm of the scalp is an increasing problem for developed countries. Fungus may confine itself to within the hair shaft (endothrix) or spread out over the hair surface (ectothrix). The latter can cause fluorescence under a Wood's lamp (ultraviolet light). Scalp ringworm is spread by close contact (especially in schools and households) and may also be spread indirectly by hairdressers. The number of new cases has risen enormously in the large cities in developed countries. Increase in travel and immigration has allowed the spread of different pathogenic fungi (e.g. *Trichophyton tonsurans* from Central America, *T. violaceum* from India and Pakistan) into new countries where overcrowding and poor social conditions have allowed spread. The majority of UK cases are currently due to *T. tonsurans* (which does not show fluorescence).

Tinea capitis is much more common in children, especially those of African origin whose scalp and hair seems more susceptible to fungal invasion. The clinical appearance of scalp ringworm is highly variable making underdiagnosis a very real problem. At mildest there may be some diffuse scaling with no hair loss – similar to dandruff. The more typical appearance is of circular scaly patches in the scalp with associated alopecia and broken hairs. As the host's immune response increases, a few pustules may appear and an exudate may be present. At worst, a full blown 'kerion' develops; a boggy swollen mass with copious quantities of discharging pus and exudate accompanied by severe alopecia. This is still poorly recognized and inappropriately treated with antibiotics and attempted surgical drainage.

Extensive infection is occasionally accompanied by a widespread papulopustular rash on the trunk. This is a so-called 'Id reaction' and probably relates to the host immune response to the fungus. It seems more common in African children. It resolves when the fungal infection is treated.

Tinea unguium

Ringworm of the nails is increasingly common with age and frequently ignored as it is often asymptomatic. Clinically this presents as asymmetrical whitening (or yellowish black discoloration) of one or more nails which usually starts at the distal or lateral edge before spreading throughout the nail (Fig 20.7). The nail-plate appears thickened. Crumbly white material appears under the nail-plate and this is the best specimen to obtain for mycology sampling. The nail-plate may become destroyed with advanced disease.

'Tinea incognito'

This is the term used to describe a fungal skin infection that has been modified by therapy with a topical steroid. The clinical appearance is variable but may show a non-specific erythema with little in the way of scaling or a few reddish nodules. The history of the rash improving with treatment (owing to the suppression of inflammation) but worsening and spreading every time it is stopped is typical. Skin scrapings for mycology or even a biopsy should confirm the diagnosis.

TREATMENT

Treatment of localized ringworm of the body or flexures may be successful with topical antifungal creams (clotrimazole, miconazole, terbinafine or amorolfine) applied thrice daily for 1–2 weeks). More widespread infection, including tinea pedis, tinea mannum and tinea capitis, requires oral antifungal therapy. Itraconazole (100 mg daily) and terbinafine (250 mg daily) are the most effective drugs used for periods of 1–3 months, but are not currently licensed for use in children. Tinea unguium is the most resistant to treatment. Itraconazole (100 mg daily)

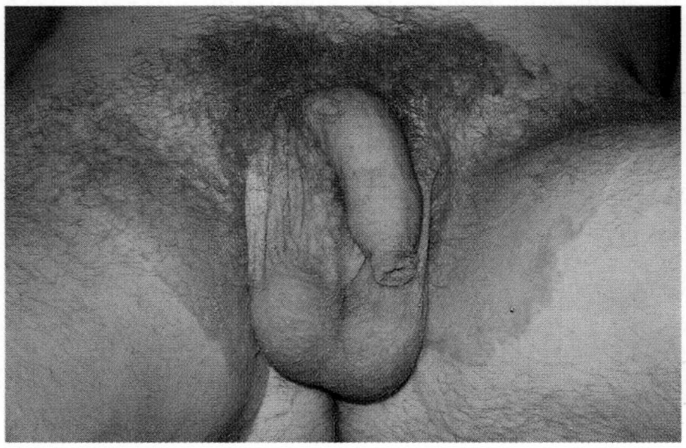

Fig 20.6
Tinea cruris

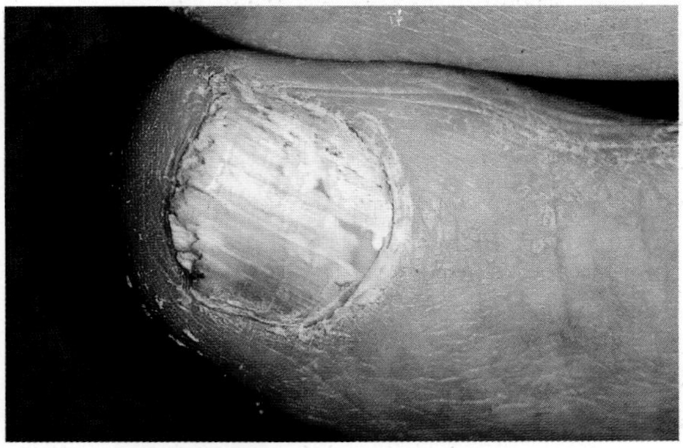

Fig 20.7
White crumbling dystrophy of a toe-nail due to dermatophyte infection

and terbinafine (250 mg daily) are more effective than griseofulvin but need to be given for three months in the case of toe-nail infections, and even then will cure only up to about 80% of cases. Griseofulvin is still used in children for scalp ringworm (10–20 mg kg^{-1} per day for 8 weeks).

Candida albicans (see also p. 67)

Candida albicans is a yeast that is sometimes found as part of the body's flora, especially in the gastrointestinal tract. It is an opportunist infection in a suitable warm moist environment, such as in nappy rash (see p. 1192) or intertrigo in obese individuals (Fig 20.8).

The flexural areas affected are red with a rather ragged peeling edge that may contain a few small pustules. Small circular areas of erythema or small papules and pustules may be seen in front of the advancing edge (satellite lesions). *Candida* may also affect the moist interdigital clefts of the toes, mimicking tinea pedis, and the finger web spaces or damaged skin around the nail-folds ('chronic paronychia') in people who have their hands immersed frequently in water (e.g. cleaners, nurses). Nail infection may mimic tinea unguium. It can infect mucosal surfaces of the mouth or genital tract, particularly in patients taking broad-spectrum antibiotics (owing to suppression of protective bacterial flora) or in immunosuppressed patients. Clinically superficial white or creamy pseudomembranous plaques appear which can be scraped off leaving raw areas underneath.

TREATMENT

Treatment is aimed at removing any underlying predisposing factor, and applying topical antifungal creams such as clotrimazole or miconazole (or the equivalent as mouth lozenges/pessaries). *Candida* nail infections require systemic antifungal therapy with an imidazole such as itraconazole (100 mg daily for three months). Recurrent candidiasis is relatively common especially in women. Diabetes mellitus should always be excluded. Repeated topical treatment or an oral imidazole may be needed.

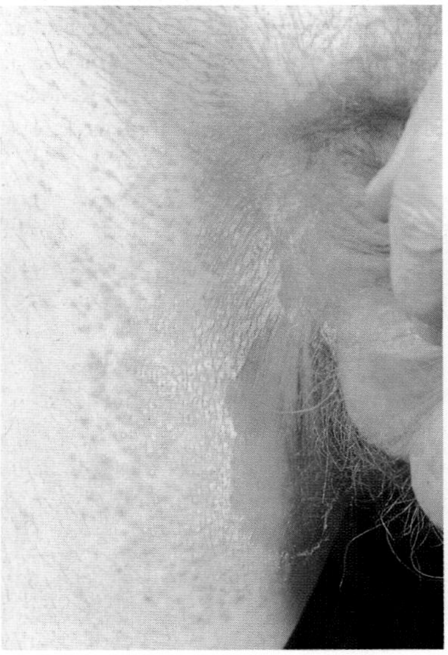

Fig 20.8
Intertrigo with satellite lesions typical of candidiasis

Pityrosporum

This yeast occurs as part of the normal flora of human skin. Colonization is prominent in the scalp, flexures and upper trunk. There are two morphological variants called *Pityrosporum ovale* and *P. orbiculare*, and the mycelial form of this yeast is called *Malassezia furfur*. *Pityrosporum* can overgrow in some individuals and has been implicated in three dermatoses:

- pityriasis versicolor
- seborrhoeic dermatitis (see p. 1163)
- pityrosporum folliculitis.

PITYRIASIS VERSICOLOR

This is a relatively common condition of young adults caused by infection with *Pityrosporum*. In Caucasians it presents most commonly on the trunk with reddish brown scaly macules which are asymptomatic. In black-skinned individuals (or in whites who are sun-tanned) it more commonly presents as macular areas of hypopigmentation. Inappropriate use of topical steroids tends to spread the rash. Diagnosis can be confirmed by skin scrapings or Wood's light examination (yellow fluorescence).

Treatment

Treatment is with selenium sulphide shampoo (applied to the body and removed after 30 minutes, and repeated daily for one week) or a topical imidazole cream (twice daily for 10 days). Oral itraconazole (100 mg twice daily for one week) can be used for resistant cases. The pigmentation takes months to recover even after successful treatment. The condition may recur but can be retreated.

PITYROSPORUM FOLLICULITIS

This is common in young adult males and characterized by small itchy papules and pustules on the upper back which are centred on hair follicles. It is more common in people with Down's syndrome.

Treatment

Pityrosporum folliculitis responds well to ketoconazole shampoo or a topical imidazole cream (twice daily for two weeks).

Infestations

Scabies

Scabies is an intensely itchy rash caused by the mite *Sarcoptes scabiei*. It can affect all races and people of any social class. It is most common in children and young adults but can affect any age group.

Scabies is spread by prolonged close contact such as within households or institutions, and by sexual contact. It presents clinically with itchy red papules (or occasionally vesicles and pustules) which can occur anywhere in the skin but rarely on the face, except in neonates. The distribution of lesions is often suggestive of the diagnosis (Fig 20.9). Sites of predeliction are between the web spaces of the fingers and toes, on the palms and soles, around the wrists and axillae, on the male genitalia, and around the nipples and umbilicus.

The pathognomonic sign is of linear or curved skin burrows but these are not always present. The pruritus is normally worse at night. Excoriations and secondary bacterial infection may complicate the rash. Scabies can be confirmed by taking skin scrapings of a lesion and examining a potassium hydroxide preparation for the mite and/or its eggs by microscopy.

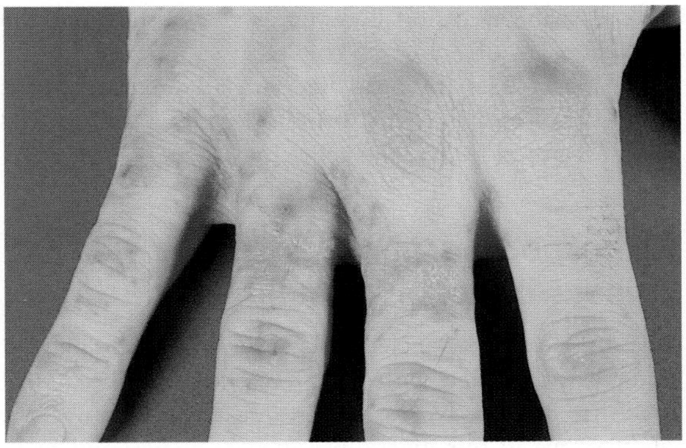

Fig 20.9
Scabies Itchy papules and pustules centred on the web spaces of the hand

TREATMENT

Treatment involves application of a topical scabicide (e.g. malathion or 5% permethrin to the whole body and washed off after 24 hours). There appears to be little if any resistance to permethrin currently. For the treatment to be successful the following factors should be noted:

- All the skin below the neck should be treated, including the genitalia, palms and soles, and under the nails. Treat the head and neck regions in infants (up to age two years).
- All close contacts should be treated at the same time even if asymptomatic.
- Reapply scabicide to the hands if they are washed during the treatment period.
- Patients should be warned that the pruritus may persist for up to four weeks after successful treatment. Adjunctive treatment with crotamiton cream, an emollient or a mild topical steroid is helpful.
- A patient information leaflet about therapy helps improve compliance.

Crusted scabies (Norwegian scabies)

Crusted scabies is a clinical variant that occurs in immunosuppressed individuals where huge numbers of mites are carried in the skin. The patient is extremely infectious after relatively minimal contact, which is unfortunate as the diagnosis is often delayed. Clinically this presents as hyperkeratotic crusted lesions especially on the hands and feet. Itch is often absent or minimal. Lesions may progress such that the patient has a widespread erythema with irregular crusted plaques. It can therefore mimic eczema or psoriasis.

Treatment is with careful barrier nursing, repeated applications of a scabicide. In resistant cases oral ivermectin (200 $\mu g\ kg^{-1}$ – one dose) may be given but this is an unlicensed use.

Lice infection

Lice are blood sucking ectoparasites that can affect man in three ways.

Head lice (pediculosis capitis)

Head lice is a common infection world-wide, affecting predominantly children and being more common in females. Spread is by direct contact and encouraged by overcrowding. It usually presents with itch or scalp excoriations. Occasionally erythematous papules on the neck may be seen. Diagnosis can be confirmed by the presence of eggs ('nits') seen tightly bound to the hair shaft. Adult lice may be seen rarely in heavy infection. School nurses and parents are usually adept at this.

Treatment varies in different areas depending on local policy and resistance patterns. Malathion, phenothrin and permethrin applications are the most commonly used. Treatment is usually repeated after seven days and metal nit combs may help remove the eggs. Some areas in the UK have given up with specific anti-lice treatments but have a policy of treating schools and family members with regular nit-combing, shampooing and conditioning of the hair.

Body lice (pediculosis corporis)

Body lice is a disease of poverty and neglect. It is rarely seen in developed countries except in homeless individuals and vagrants. It is spread by direct contact or sharing infested clothing. The lice and eggs are rarely seen on the patient but are commonly found on the clothing. It presents with itch, excoriations and sometimes post-inflammatory hyperpigmentation of the skin.

Treatment consists of malathion or permethrin for the patient and high-temperature washing and drying of clothing.

Pubic lice (phthiriasis pubis, crabs)

Pubic lice are transmitted by direct contact, usually sexual. It presents with itching, especially at night. Lice can be seen near the base of the hair with eggs somewhat further up the shaft. Occasionally eyebrows, eyelashes and the beard area are affected.

Treatment is as for head lice, but all sexual contacts should be treated and other sexually transmitted diseases should be screened for.

Arthropod-borne diseases ('insect bites' or papular urticaria)

These depend on contact with an animal (e.g. dog, cat, bird) that is infested with a flea (*Cheyletiella*). The animal itself may be itchy with scaly and thickened skin. The flea can also live in soft furnishings such as carpets and beds, even after the animal has been removed. Bites present as itchy urticated lesions which are often grouped in clusters. They may cause blisters. The legs are most commonly affected. It is not unusual for an individual to react badly to bites when other family members seem unaffected. Anti-flea treatment of the animal and furnishings is required.

FURTHER READING

Mandell GL, Douglas RG, Bennett JE (eds) (1995) *Principles and Practice of Infectious Diseases*, 4th edn. New York: Churchill Livingstone.

Papulo-squamous/ inflammatory rashes

Eczema

The term 'eczema' (Greek for 'boiling') describes an acutely inflamed weeping skin with vesicles. It is synonymous with the term 'dermatitis' and the two words are interchangeable.

In the developed world eczema accounts for a large proportion of skin disease, both in hospitals and in the community. It is estimated that 10% of people have some form of eczema at any one time, and up to 40% of the population will have an episode of eczema during their lifetime.

All eczemas have some features in common and there is a spectrum of clinical presentation from acute through to chronic. Vesicles or bullae may appear in the acute stage if inflammation is intense. In subacute eczema the skin can be erythematous, dry and flaky, oedematous, and crusted (especially if secondarily infected). Chronic persistent eczema is characterized by thickened or lichenified skin. Eczema is nearly always itchy. Histologically, 'eczematous change' refers to a collection of fluid in the epidermis between the keratinocytes ('spongiosis') and an upper dermal perivascular infiltrate of lymphohistiocytic cells. In more chronic disease there is marked thickening of the epidermis ('acanthosis').

Atopic eczema

This type of eczema (often called 'endogenous eczema') occurs in individuals who are 'atopic' (see p. 786). It is common, occurring in up to 5% of the UK population. It is more common in early life, occurring at some stage during childhood in up to 10% of all children.

AETIOLOGY

The exact pathophysiology is not fully understood. There is undoubtedly a strong hereditary component, but the condition appears to be both polygenetic and influenced by environmental factors. A positive family history of atopic disease is often present: there is a 90% concordance in monozygotic twins but only 20% in dizygotic twins. Genetic studies in atopy have so far shown linkage to three different loci. Linkage has been demonstrated between atopy and the β-subunit of the high-affinity IgE receptor on mast cells (on chromosome 11q13), but this site does not demonstrate linkage with familial atopic eczema. Polymorphisms in the mast cell chymase gene have also been associated with atopic eczema – thus genetic heterogeneity is likely. It may be that certain genes are more important in developing eczema rather than asthma, and other genes may be important in determining the severity of the disorder or the age of onset. If one parent has atopic disease the risk for a child of developing eczema is about 20–30%. If both parents have atopic eczema the risk is greater than 50%.

Exacerbating factors

Strong detergents, chemicals and even woollen clothes can be irritant and exacerbate eczema. Infection either in the skin or systemically can also lead to a deterioration, possibly by a superantigen effect. Teething is another factor in young children. Severe anxiety or stress appears to exacerbate eczema in some individuals. Cat and dog fur can certainly make eczema worse, possibly by both allergic and irritant mechanisms. The role of the house dust mite and diet is less clear-cut. There is some evidence that food allergens may play a role in triggering atopic eczema and that dairy products may be important in exacerbating eczema in infants under 12 months of age.

In general, however, it is a misconception to think of atopic eczema as an allergy. In fact children with atopic eczema have a lower risk of developing allergic contact eczema. Exacerbating factors are not necessarily allergens.

CLINICAL FEATURES

Atopic eczema can present as a number of distinct morphological variants. The most common presentation is of itchy erythematous scaly patches especially in the flexures such as in front of the elbows and ankles, behind the knees and around the neck (Fig 20.10). In infants, eczema often starts on the face before spreading to the body. Very acute lesions may weep or exude and can show small vesicles. Scratching can produce excoriations and repeated rubbing produces skin thickening (lichenification) with exaggerated skin markings.

In patients with pigmented skin, eczema often shows a reverse pattern of extensor involvement. Also the eczema may be papular or follicular in nature and lichenification is common. A final problem in pigmented skin is of post-inflammatory hyper- or hypopigmentation which is often very slow to fade after control of the eczema.

Associated features

Involvement of the nail-bed may produce pitting and ridging of the nails. In some atopic individuals the skin of the upper arms and thighs may feel roughened owing to follicular hyperkeratosis ('keratosis pilaris'). The palms may show very prominent skin creases ('hyperlinear palms'). There may be an associated dry 'fish-like' scaling of the skin which is non-inflammatory and often prominent on the lower legs ('ichthyosis vulgaris').

COMPLICATIONS

Broken skin commonly becomes secondarily infected by bacteria, usually *Staphylococcus aureus*, although streptococci can colonize eczema especially in macerated flexural areas such as the neck and groin. Clinically this infection may appear as crusted, weeping impetigo-like lesions. Occasionally *Pseudomonas* can be grown from skin swabs, but this does not seem to cause a clinical problem. Cutaneous viral infections (e.g. viral warts and molluscum) are often widespread in atopic eczema and are probably spread by scratching. HSV can cause a widespread eruption called eczema herpeticum (Kaposi's varicelliform eruption). This can occasionally be a very severe infection and has rarely caused death. It appears as multiple small blisters or punched-out crusted lesions associated with malaise and pyrexia, and needs rapid treatment with oral acyclovir. Intravenous acyclovir may need to be used if the infection is severe. Ocular complications of atopic eczema include conjunctival irritation and less commonly keratoconjunctivitis and catarct. Retarded growth may be seen in children with chronic severe eczema; it is usually due to the disease itself and not the use of topical steroids.

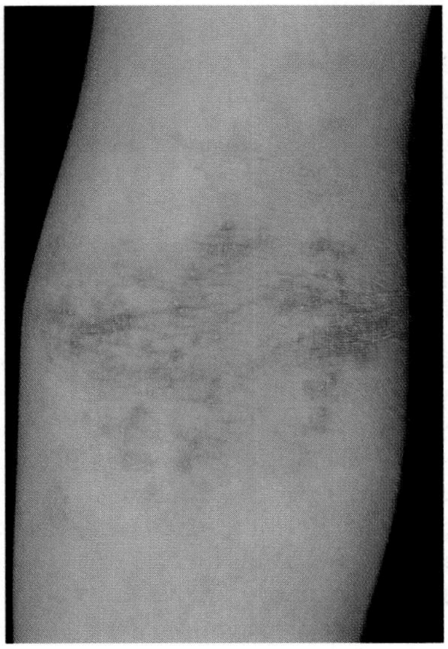

Fig 20.10
Flexural eczema

INVESTIGATIONS

The diagnosis of atopic eczema is normally clinical. Atopy is characterized by high serum IgE levels or high specific IgE levels to certain ingested or inhaled antigens. The latter can be tested by radio-immunoabsorbent assay (RAST tests) of blood, or indirectly by skin-prick testing (p. 766). A peripheral blood eosinophilia may also be seen.

PROGNOSIS

The vast majority of children with early-onset atopic eczema will improve spontaneously and 'clear' before the teenage years, 50% being clear by the age of 6. A few will get a recurrence as adults, even if just as hand eczema. However, if the onset of eczema is late in childhood or in adulthood, the disorder follows a more chronic remitting/relapsing course.

TREATMENT

General measures

These include avoiding known irritants (especially soaps or furry animals), wearing cotton clothes, and not getting too hot. Manipulating the diet (e.g. a dairy-free diet) has not shown significant benefit except in a few children under 12 months. Any change in diet should be done under supervision, especially with growing children who may need supple-ments such as calcium.

Topical therapies

Topical therapies (see p. 1194) are sufficient to control atopic eczema in most people and the following 'triple' combination often helps:

- topical steroid twice daily when needed
- emollient frequently (see Table 20.14)
- bath oil (e.g. Oilatum or balneum) and soap substitute (e.g. aqueous cream).

Written information or a practical demonstration of how to apply these treatments improves compliance.

Use of topical steroids. Unjustified fear of the dangers of topical steroids has often led to undertreatment of eczema. Provided that steroid preparations of appropriate strength are used for the right body site, these compounds can be used quite safely on a long-term *intermittent* basis. Topical steroids can be divided into four groups depending on their potency (Table 20.3).

The following guidelines should be followed to allow their safe use in common chronic inflammatory skin conditions.

- The face should be treated with mild steroids.
- In adults the body should be treated with either mild, moderately potent or diluted potent steroids.
- Potent steroids may be used for short courses (7–10 days).
- Young children should be treated with mild and moderately potent steroids on the body.
- Treatment of the palms and soles (but not the dorsal surfaces) may require potent or very potent steroids as the skin is much thicker.
- Regular use of emollients may lessen the need for steroid use.
- Only use steroids on inflamed skin. Do not use as an emollient.
- 'Apply sparingly' means use sufficient to leave a glistening surface to the skin after application.
- Use weaker steroid preparations in flexures (e.g. the groin, and under breasts) as apposition of the skin at these sites tends to occlude the treatment and increase absorption.

Antibiotics

These are needed for bacterial infection and are usually given orally for 7–10 days. Flucloxacillin (500 mg four times daily) is effective against *Staphylococcus*, and penicillin V (500 mg four times daily) acts against *Streptococcus*. Erythromicin (500 mg four times daily) is useful if there is allergy to penicillin. Topical antiseptics may be useful in cases of recurrent infection but they can be irritant. They are usually added to the bath water rather than directly on to the skin. Combination topical steroid/antibiotic creams can also be used.

Sedating antihistamines

These are useful at nighttime but probably help by their sedative properties rather than by their antihistamine activity.

Paste bandaging

Paste bandaging can be useful for resistant or lichenified eczema of the limbs. It helps absorption of treatment and acts as a barrier to prevent scratching.

Table 20.3
Classification of topical steroids by potency

Very potent	0.05% clobetasol proprionate 0.3% diflucortolone valerate
Potent	0.1% betamethasone valerate 0.025% fluocinolone acetonide
Diluted potent	0.025% betamethasone valerate 0.00625% fluocinolone acetonide
Moderately potent	0.05% clobetasone butyrate 0.05% alclometasone diproprionate
Mild	2. 5% hydrocortisone 1% hydrocortisone

Second-line agents

These may be considered in severe non-responsive cases, especially if the eczema is significantly interfering with an individual's life (e.g. sleeping, schoolwork or job). Ultraviolet phototherapy (see p. 1171), prednisolone (doses up to 30 mg daily), cyclosporin (3–5 mg kg^{-1} daily) and azathioprine (50–100 mg daily) (p. 1179) can all be effective treatments. However, they all have side-effects and the risk/benefit ratio must be openly discussed with the patient before they are used.

Use of cyclosporin. Cyclosporin is a selective immuno-suppressant that inhibits interleukin-2 production. A large number of other drugs interact with cyclosporin (e.g. eryth-romycin, NSAIDS) and should be avoided. Renal damage and hypertension are the two most serious side-effects, so blood pressure and serum creatinine should be measured every six weeks. Creatinine clearance should be measured yearly in people on long-term therapy. Renal damage becomes increasingly common with time and tends to be dose-dependent. Hypertrichosis, paraesthesia and nausea are less serious side-effects. Pregnancy should be avoided.

Discoid eczema (nummular eczema)

Discoid eczema is a morphological variant of eczema characterized by well-demarcated scaly patches especially on the limbs, and this can be confused sometimes with psoriasis. It is more common in adults and can occur in both atopic and non-atopic individuals. It tends to follow an acute/subacute course rather than a chronic pattern. There is often an infective aetiology (*Staphylococcus aureus*).

Hand eczema

Eczema may be confined to the hands (and feet). It can present with:

- itchy vesicles of the palm and along the sides of the fingers or occasionally with larger blisters called 'pompholyx' (Fig 20.11)
- a diffuse erythematous scaling and hyperkeratosis of the palms
- a scaling and peeling most marked at the finger tips.

Hand eczema is not unusual in atopics but more frequently occurs in non-atopic individuals and a cause is not always found. A history of contact with irritants (e.g. detergents, chemicals) and an occupational history should be sought, especially in finger-tip eczema. Patch testing for specific allergic or contact eczema should always be considered as up to 10% of individuals with hand eczema will show a positive test. Finally, look for evidence of fungal infection as this can occasionally induce a secondary pompholyx of the hands or feet (a so-called 'Id reaction').

Seborrhoeic eczema

There is some evidence that the yeast *Pityrosporum ovale* (also called *Malassezia furfur* in its hyphal form) is important and it may act as an 'antigenic drive' to produce the characteristic inflammation and scaling of seborrhoeic eczema. The condition is more common in parkinsonism as well as in HIV disease.

CLINICAL FEATURES

Seborrhoeic eczema affects body sites rich in sebaceous glands, although these do not appear to be important in its cause. Three age groups are affected.

- *In childhood* it is common and presents in the first few months of life as 'cradle cap' in most babies. This may be in part due to the affect of maternal androgens on infant sebaceous glands. Yellowish, greasy, thick crusts are seen on the scalp. A more widespread erythematous, scaly rash can be seen over the trunk, especially affecting the nappy area. Unlike atopic eczema, the child is normally unbothered as there is little associated pruritus. The rash normally improves spontaneously after a few weeks.
- *In young adults* (especially males) it occurs in 1–3% of the population. The rash is more persistent and presents as an erythematous scaling along the sides of the nose (Fig 20.12), in the eyebrows, around the eyes and extending into the scalp (which shows marked dandruff). It may affect the skin over the sternum and of the glans penis. A blepharitis may also be present.
- *In elderly people* seborrhoeic eczema can be more severe and progress to involve large areas of the body and even cause erythroderma.

TREATMENT

The treatment is suppressive rather than curative. A combination of a mild steroid ointment (e.g. 1% hydrocortisone applied twice daily) and a topical antifungal cream (e.g. miconazole cream applied twice daily) will help to control the eruption. 2% sulphur or 2% salicylic acid can be added to help control resistant cases. Ketoconazole shampoo and arachis oil are useful for the scalp. Emollients and a soap substitute are useful adjuncts.

Contact and irritant eczema

Eczema can be caused by a variety of environmental agents (exogenous eczema). One may suspect this if the eczema is in an unusual or localized distribution (Fig 20.13), especially if there is no personal or family history of atopic disease. A history of an exacerbation of eczema at the workplace is also suggestive. This can happen by two mechanisms: direct irritation or an allergic reaction (type IV delayed hypersensitivity). A detailed history about occupation, hobbies, cosmetic products, clothing and contact with chemicals is necessary.

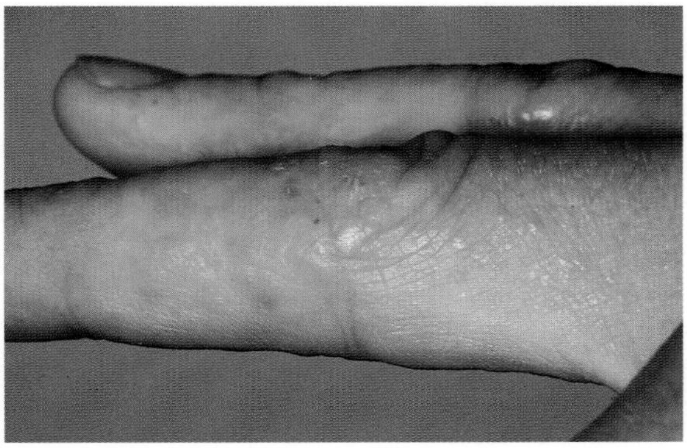

Fig 20.11
Pompholyx eczema (Courtesy of Dr A Bewley, London)

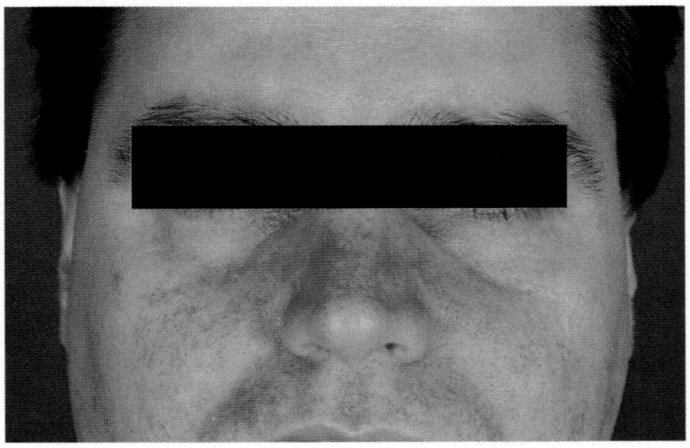

Fig 20.12
Seborrhoeic eczema affecting the sides of the nose

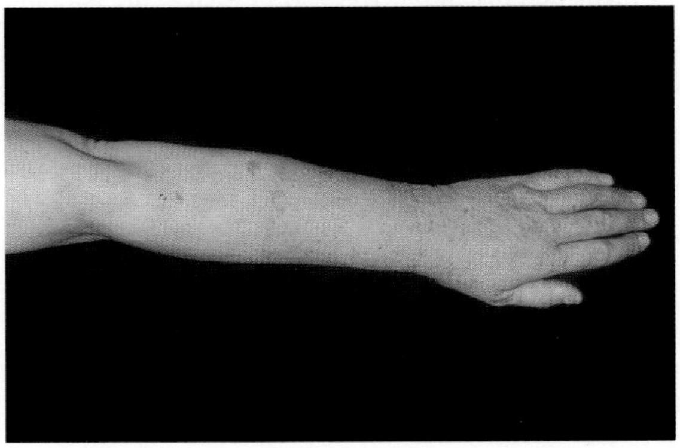

Fig 20.13
Contact eczema (allergy to latex in rubber gloves)

Irritant eczema can occur in any individual. It often occurs on the hands after repeated exposures to irritants such as detergents, soaps or bleach. It is therefore common in housewives, cleaners, hairdressers, mechanics and nurses.

Contact eczema occurs after repeated exposure to a chemical substance but only in those people who are susceptible to develop an allergic reaction. It is common, occurring in up to 4% of some populations. Many substances can cause this type of reaction, but the most common culprits are nickel (in costume jewellery and buckles), chromate (in cement), latex (in surgical gloves), perfume (in cosmetics and air fresheners), and plants (such as primula or compositae). The most important point is to take a good history and, if suspicious, patch testing should be arranged to prove any allergy.

TREATMENT

Treatment is as for atopic eczema as well as strict avoidance of any causative agent. This may also involve the wearing of protective clothing such as gloves, or in extreme cases (such as with chromate sensitivity in builders) even changing occupation or hobbies.

Venous eczema (varicose eczema, gravitational eczema)

This type of eczema occurs on the lower legs and is caused by chronic venous hypertension (usually of more than two years' duration) (see p. 1185). The exact cause remains unknown, but it has been suggested that venous hypertension causes endothelial hyperplasia and extravasation of red and white blood cells, which in turn causes inflammation, purpura and pigmentation.

CLINICAL FEATURES

Venous eczema tends to occur in older people, especially women. It usually appears on the lower legs around the ankles. There may be a past history of venous thrombosis or previous surgery for varicose veins. Brownish pigmentation (haemosiderin) may be seen in the skin, and a venous leg ulcer or varicose veins may be present.

Superimposed contact eczema is common in venous eczema patients, especially when there have been chronic venous leg ulcers. This is usually due to an allergic reaction to topical therapies or skin dressings. Patch testing should always be done in cases resistant to treatment.

Treatment should include emollients and a moderately potent topical steroid, but the most important part of therapy is the use of support stockings or compression bandages, which together with leg elevation help reverse the underlying venous hypertension.

Asteatotic eczema (winter eczema, eczema craquelé, senile eczema)

This is a dry plate-like cracking of the skin with a red, eczematous component which occurs in elderly people. It occurs predominantly on the lower legs and the backs of the hands, especially in winter. The exact cause is unknown, but the repeated use of soaps in the elderly is undoubtedly of importance. The loss of the stratum corneum lipids with age may also be of some relevance. Rarely asteatotic eczema can be the presenting sign of myxoedema or can follow the commencement of diuretic therapy.

TREATMENT

Avoiding soaps and the regular use of emollients and bath oils should be encouraged. Humidifying centrally heated rooms may help. If the skin is very inflamed, a mild topical steroid can be used. Finally, some advocate the regular use of oral evening primrose oil.

Photosensitive eczema

This is discussed on p. 1172.

Nodular prurigo/lichen simplex (neurodermatitis)

These two terms are applied to a pattern of cutaneous response to scratching or rubbing in the absence of an underlying dermatosis. They are more common in Asians and also in African and oriental patients.

Lichen simplex appears as thickened, scaly and hyper-pigmented areas of lichenification (Fig 20.14). It starts with intense itching that becomes tender with increased rubbing or scratching. It is rare before adolescence and is more common in females. Common sites are the nape of the neck, the lateral calfs, the upper thighs, the upper back and the scrotum or vulva, but any accessible site can be affected.

Nodular prurigo is a different pattern of cutaneous response to scratching, rubbing or picking. It is a chronic unremitting condition which is often resistant to treatment. Individual, itchy papules and domed nodules appear, especially on the upper trunk and the extensor surfaces of the limbs. They show significant surface damage from scratching.

These two conditions overlap with some patients showing mixed features. Atopic individuals seem predisposed to develop these conditions (in the absence of obviously active eczema). However, they can occur in non-atopics. Emotional stress appears to be a contributory factor in many of these patients.

The diagnosis is made by exclusion of other pathologies and may require a skin biopsy. General medical causes of pruritus should be excluded (see p. 1171). In the elderly, nodular prurigo may be an early sign of bullous pemphi-goid, before the more typical blistering phase has appeared.

TREATMENT

Treatment is often difficult as symptoms can be intractable. Very potent topical steroids (e.g. 0.05% clobetasol proprionate) with occlusive tar bandaging may sometimes help. Intralesional steroids can also be useful. For resistant cases (especially of prurigo lesions), phototherapy (see p. 1171) and even cyclosporin (3–5 mg kg^{-1} daily) can be considered, but the risk/benefit ratio must be discussed with the patient as these therapies are potentially toxic.

Psoriasis

Psoriasis is a common papulo-squamous disorder affecting 2% of the population and is characterized by well demarcated, red scaly plaques. The skin becomes inflamed and hyperproliferates to about ten times the normal rate. It affects males and females equally and can affect all races. The age of onset occurs in two peaks. Early onset (age 16–22) is more common and is often associated with a positive family history. Late-onset disease peaks at age 55–60 years.

AETIOLOGY

The condition appears to be polygenic but is also dependent on certain environmental triggers. To date, three genetic regions (on chromosomes 6p21, 17q and 4q) have been shown to be of importance in psoriasis, but it is likely that more genetic loci are involved. Infection (group A *Streptococcus*), drugs (e.g. lithium), ultraviolet light, alcohol abuse and possibly stress may be important triggers or exacerbating factors in certain individuals. The exact aetiology is unknown, but there is an increasing body of evidence suggesting that psoriasis is a T-lymphocyte driven disorder with a possible altered response from the keratinocyte.

- Group A streptococcal sore throats can set off guttate psoriasis (see below), possibly by immune cross-reactivity or by a superantigen mechanism.
- There is an association between psoriasis and HLA-Cw6.
- One of the earliest histological changes in a new psoriatic lesion is the infiltration of $CD4^+$ T-cells and the maintenance of the lesion appears to depend on $CD8^+$ T-cells.
- Certain immunosuppressive therapies (e.g. cyclosporin) which act on T helper cells are useful in treating psoriasis.
- Many alterations in cell kinetics have been demonstrated. There is an increase in eicosanoids as well as cyclic AMP and GMP. Cytokines including the interleukins and growth factors (TGFα and -β) are also expressed in the lesions. However, none of these have been shown to have a definite role in the pathogenesis.
- The immune dysfunction seen in patients with AIDS may be associated with a deterioration of their psoriasis.

PATHOLOGY

Skin biopsy shows acanthosis and parakeratosis, reflecting the increase in skin turnover. The granular layer is often absent. Polymorphonuclear abcesses may be seen in the upper epidermis. The epidermal rete ridges appear elongated and clubbed as they fold down into the dermis. Dermal changes include capillary dilation surrounded by a mixed neutro-philic and lymphohistiocytic perivascular infiltrate.

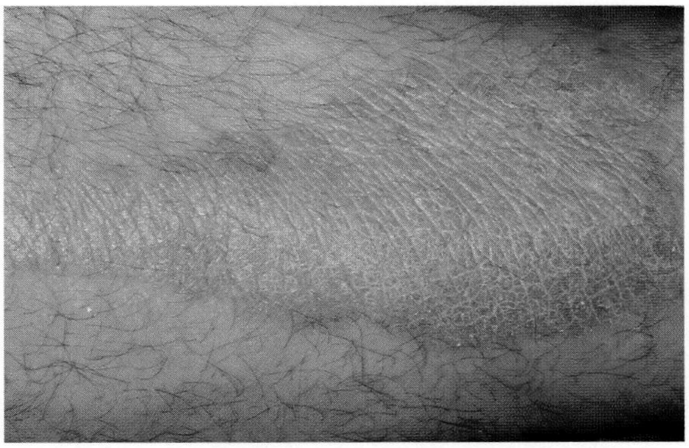

Fig 20.14
Lichen simplex from chronic rubbing

CLINICAL FEATURES

Psoriasis can present in different clinical patterns but they may overlap between the different forms. It should be remembered that certain drugs can make psoriasis worse – notably lithium, antimalarials and rarely β-blockers.

Chronic plaque psoriasis

This is the 'common' type of psoriasis. It is characterized by pinkish red scaly plaques especially on extensor surfaces such as knees (Fig 20.15a) and elbows. The lower back, ears and scalp are also commonly involved. New plaques of psoriasis may occur at sites of skin trauma – the so-called Köbner phenomenon. The lesions can become itchy or sore.

Flexural psoriasis

This tends to occur in later life. It is characterized by well-demarcated, red glazed plaques confined to flexures such as the groin, natal cleft and sub-mammary area. As these sites are apposed there is rarely any scaling. In the absence of psoriasis elsewhere the rash is often misdiagnosed as candida intertrigo, but the latter will normally show satellite lesions.

Guttate psoriasis

'Raindrop like' psoriasis is a variant most commonly seen in children and young adults (Fig 20.15b). An explosive eruption of very small circular or oval plaques appears over the trunk about two weeks after a streptococcal sore throat. It usually resolves spontaneously over 1–2 months even without treatment (see below).

Erythrodermic and pustular psoriasis

These are the most severe types of psoriasis, reflecting a widespread intense inflammation of the skin. They can occur together ('Von Zumbusch' psoriasis) and may be associated with malaise, pyrexia and circulatory disturbance. This form can be life-threatening. The pustules are not infected but are sterile collections of inflammatory cells. There is also a more localized variant of pustular psoriasis that confines itself to the hands and feet but is not associated with severe systemic symptoms.

(a)

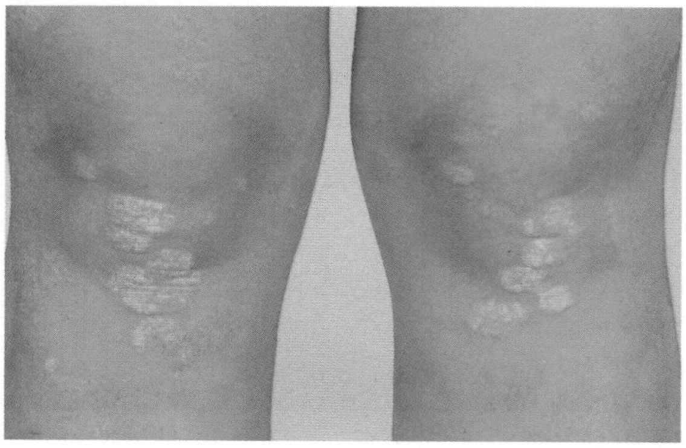

(b)

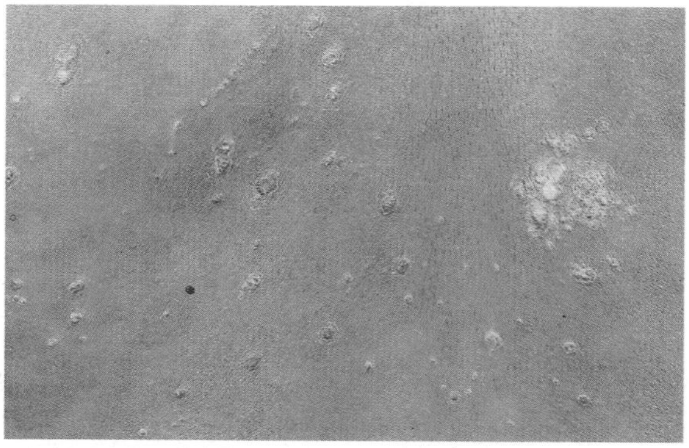

Fig 20.15
(a) Psoriasis of the knees
(b) Guttate psoriasis in an African. Courtesy of Dr P Matondo, Lusaka, Zambia

Associated features

Nails. Up to 50% of individuals with psoriasis develop nail changes (Fig 20.16) and rarely these can precede the onset of skin disease. There are five types of nail change: (a) pitting of the nail-plate, (b) distal separation of the nail-plate (onycholysis), (c) yellow-brown discoloration, (d) subungual hyperkeratosis, and (e) rarely a damaged nail matrix and lost nail-plate. Treatment of nail dystrophy is very difficult.

Arthritis. Up to 5% of patients develop psoriatic arthritis and most of these will have nail changes (p. 480). Five patterns are recognized: (a) distal interphalangeal arthritis, (b) peripheral mono- or oligoarthritis, (c) symmetrical 'rheumatoid arthritis pattern' but seronegative, (d) spondylitis or sacro-iliitis (especially if HLA-B27 positive), and (e) rarely, arthritis mutilans causing destruction and resorption of bone leading to telescoping of affected digits.

PROGNOSIS

Most individuals who develop chronic plaque psoriasis will have the condition lifelong. It fluctuates in severity and there are no available tests to predict outcome. Guttate psoriasis resolves spontaneously and in up to a third of individuals does not recur. However, two-thirds will go on to get recurrent guttate attacks or will progress to chronic plaque psoriasis.

TREATMENT

This is concerned with control rather than cure. It should be tailored to the patient's wishes and not just to the doctor's assessment of disease severity. Most patients can be improved with topical therapies. Mild-to-moderate topical steroids, calcipotriol (a synthetic vitamin D_3 analogue) and purified coal tar are the most popular. Salicylic acid can be a useful adjunct. All should be applied twice daily to palpable lesions. Once lesions have flattened therapy can be discontinued. Dithranol can also be helpful but it causes staining of the skin and clothing and it may prove difficult to use at home on a regular basis. It is normally applied for 20–60 minutes and then washed off. It must be applied carefully to the lesions as it causes irritation to normal skin. Dithranol is more likely to induce remission than other topical therapies.

Topical therapies are sometimes used in combination with UVB or PUVA. The 'Goeckerman regime' consists of tar and UVB; the 'Ingram's regime' consists of dithranol and UVB.

Guttate psoriasis is usually treated with topical therapies and/or UVB phototherapy.

Management of erythroderma resulting from psoriasis requires specific systemic therapy as well as general supportive measures (see p. 1173).

Phototherapy (UVB and PUVA) or systemic therapy (such as methotrexate, acitretin, cyclosporin or hydroxyurea) is used for disabling skin psoriasis, erythrodermic or pustular psoriasis, and psoriatic arthritis. All these treatments must be monitored for toxicity.

Use of methotrexate. Methotrexate is normally given once weekly. Some patients experience severe nausea on the day they take it. Pregnancy should be avoided. Some patients are allergic to methotrexate and develop a pyrexia and mouth ulceration. Regular blood tests need to be done to monitor for bone marrow suppression and liver damage. Alcohol must be avoided as

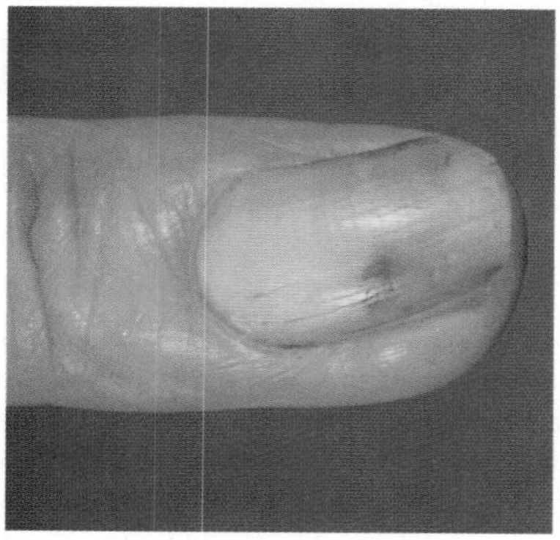

Fig 20.16
Yellowish brown discoloration and distal nail-plate separation (onycholysis) due to psoriasis

this increases the risk of hepatotoxicity. NSAIDs should also be avoided. Long-term users will need a liver biopsy every 2–3 years to accurately monitor for hepatic damage.

Urticaria

Urticaria (hives, 'nettle rash') is a common skin condition characterized by the acute development of itchy weals or swellings in the skin due to leaky dermal vessels (Fig 20.17).

AETIOLOGY

The final event in pathogenesis appears to involve degranulation of cutaneous mast cells which releases a number of inflammatory mediators (including histamine) which in turn make the dermal capillaries leaky. In most cases the underlying cause is unknown. Occasionally urticaria is secondary to viral or parasitic infection, drug reactions (e.g. aspirin or penicillin allergy), food allergy (e.g. to strawberries, food colourings or seafood), or rarely systemic lupus erythematosus. There is evidence for an autoimmune aetiology in some of the 'idiopathic' cases as certain individuals develop autoantibodies against the high-affinity IgE receptor α subunit of the mast cell. Urticaria is more common in atopic individuals and usually presents in children and young adults.

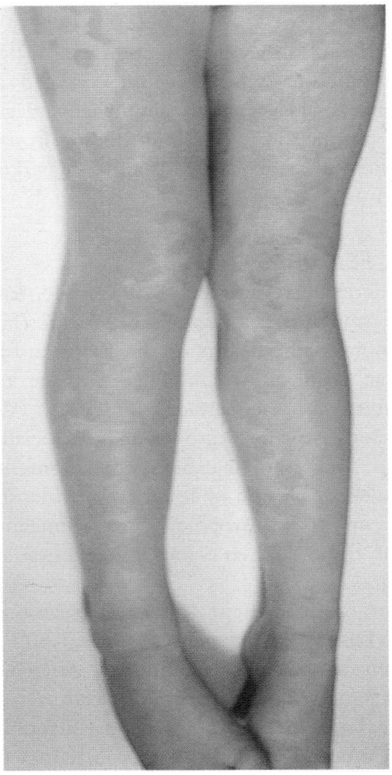

Fig 20.17
Extensive urticaria of the legs

CLINICAL FEATURES

The history is of cutaneous swellings or weals developing acutely over a few minutes. They can occur anywhere on the skin and last between minutes and hours before resolving spontaneously. Lesions are intensely itchy and show no surface change or scaling. Lesions are normally erythematous, but if they are very acutely swollen they may appear flesh-coloured or whitish and people often mistake them for blisters. Severe urticaria with subcutaneous involvement can present as soft tissue swelling (angio-oedema) especially around the eyes, the lips and the hands. This can be very alarming to the patient. It can also be dangerous if mucosal areas such as the mouth and larynx are involved, but fortunately this is very rare.

Physical urticarias

Occasionally urticaria can be caused by physical stimuli such as cold (cold urticaria), deep pressure (delayed pressure urticaria), stress or heat (cholinergic urticaria), sunlight (solar urticaria – see p. 1172), water (aquagenic urticaria) or chemicals such as latex (contact urticaria).

Cholinergic urticaria is one of the most common physical urticarias and has rather different clinical lesions from the other forms. Small itchy papules rather than weals appear on the upper trunk and arms after exercise or anxiety.

Pressure can cause two types of urticaria. *Delayed pressure urticaria* is rare and occurs as deep swellings some hours after pressure is removed (e.g. on the soles of the feet or under a tight belt). More superficial pressure can cause *dermographism* which is relatively common. This presents as urticated weals occurring a few minutes after application of pressure. Even scratching or rubbing will bring up linear weals in dermographic individuals.

INVESTIGATIONS

A careful history is the most important factor in diagnosing urticaria. Routine investigations are probably not justifed unless the history suggests one of the underlying causes listed above. The physical urticarias should be reproducible by applying the relevant stimulus.

TREATMENT

Any identifiable underlying cause should be treated appropriately. Patients should avoid salicylates and opiates as they can degranulate mast cells. Oral antihistamines (H_1 blockers) are the most important part of treating the idiopathic cases. Therapy should be started with regular use of a non-sedating antihistamine (e.g. cetirizine 10 mg daily or loratadine 10 mg daily). If control proves difficult, addition of a sedating antihistamine or an H_2 blocker may be helpful. Dietary manipulation (e.g. additive- and colouring-free diets) may help a small proportion of patients with chronic urticaria but it is generally unrewarding. Angio-oedema of the mouth and throat may require urgent treatment with intravenous steroids and subcutaneous adrenaline (see Emergency box 14.1).

PROGNOSIS

Most cases of 'idiopathic' urticaria last a few weeks to months before disappearing spontaneously. The majority of these will be controlled with an antihistamine. A small percentage of people go on to develop chronic urticaria which can last for several months or years. The physical urticarias (especially cholinergic urticaria) are more persistent, often lasting for years and they are often resistant to therapy.

Urticarial vasculitis

This is a variant of urticaria and should be suspected if individual urticarial lesions last longer than 24 hours and leave bruising behind after resolution. The diagnosis is confirmed by skin biopsy. A full vasculitis screen should be carried out for an underlying cause (see p. 496). Treatment is with oral dapsone (50–100 mg daily) or immunosuppressants.

Hereditary angio-oedema

This is an extremely rare autosomal dominant condition due to an inherited deficiency of C1-esterase inhibitor, a component of the complement system. The defect may be due to either reduced function or reduced absolute levels. Serum C2 and C4 levels are normally low but C3 is normal. Rarely this condition is acquired and associated with lymphoma and this type also shows low C1 esterase inhibitor levels.

CLINICAL FEATURES

It presents with attacks of non-itchy cutaneous angio-oedema (but no urticaria) which may last up to 72 hours. It may also present with recurrent abdominal pain (due to intestinal oedema) and there may be a family history of suddden death (due to laryngeal involvement). A nonspecific erythematous rash may precede an attack of angio-oedema but urticaria is not a feature.

TREATMENT

In the acute setting, treatment is with C1 esterase inhibitor concentrates and fresh frozen plasma. Adrenaline and steroids are often ineffective. Maintenance treatment with the anabolic steroid stanozolol (or danazol) stimulates an increase in hepatic synthesis of C1 esterase inhibitor but this should not be used in children.

Pityriasis rosea

Pityriasis rosea is a self-limiting rash seen in adolescents and young adults. The cause is unknown but it is thought to be a viral or post-viral rash. There is an increased incidence in spring and autumn and outbreaks may occur in institutions. The herpesvirus HHV type 7 has recently been implicated.

CLINICAL FEATURES

The rash consists of circular or oval pink macules with a collarette of scale and is more prominent on the trunk than the limbs. The long axis of the oval lesions tends to run along dermatomal lines, giving a 'Christmas tree' pattern on the back. The rash may be preceded by a large solitary patch with peripheral scaling ('herald patch') and this is most commonly found on the trunk. The rash is usually asymptomatic and spontaneously resolves over 4–8 weeks.

TREATMENT

Treatment is not normally required, but 0.5% menthol in aqueous cream may help relieve itching. In persistent cases UVB may be helpful.

Lichen planus

Lichen planus is a pruritic inflammatory dermatosis that is commonly associated with mucosal involvement and rarely with nail dystrophy and scarring alopecia. The cause is unknown, but it has been postulated that a T-cell driven immune mechanism is important. This stems from the fact that an almost identical rash can be caused by certain drugs (e.g. gold, levamisole, penicillamine or antimalarials) or by graft-versus-host disease.

PATHOLOGY

A mixed lymphohistiocytic infiltrate is seen at the dermo-epidermal junction, which becomes ragged and saw-toothed. The basal layer shows a liquefactive degeneration with the production of colloid bodies in the upper dermis. There may be acanthosis and a hyperkeratosis of the epidermis.

CLINICAL FEATURES

The rash is characterized by small, purple, flat-topped, polygonal papules that are intensely pruritic (Fig 20.18). It is common on the flexors of the wrists and the lower legs but can occur anywhere. There may be a fine lacy white pattern on the surface of lesions (Wickham's striae). Lesions may fuse into plaques, especially on the lower legs and in Africans. Hyperpigmentation is common after resolution of lesions, especially in patients with pigmented skin. Atrophic, hypertrophic and annular variants can occur. Lichen planus lesions often localize to scratch marks.

If lesions occur in the scalp they may cause a scarring alopecia. Mucosal involvement is seen in 50% of cases. The mouth is the most commonly affected, but the anogenital region can be involved. It can present as lacy white streaks, white plaques or as ulceration. The prominent mucosal symptom is of pain rather than itch. Nails may be dystrophic and can be lost altogether (with scarring and 'wing' formation) in severe disease.

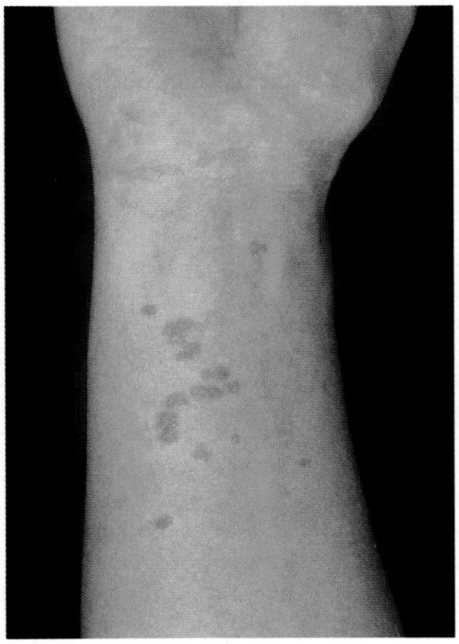

Fig 20.18
Lichen planus

PROGNOSIS

The condition often clears by two years but can recur at intervals. The hypertrophic and atrophic variants, and mucosal disease are more persistent, lasting years. Ulcerative mucosal disease is premalignant.

TREATMENT

This requires the use of potent topical steroids (0.05% clobetasol proprionate) and occasionally oral prednisolone (30 mg daily for 2–4 weeks). Occlusion of topical treatments can be helpful. Resistant cases may respond to PUVA, oral retinoids (0.5 mg kg^{-1} daily) or azathioprine (50–100 mg daily).

Granuloma annulare

Granuloma annulare is a dermatosis predominantly of children and young adults. It is characterized by clusters of small dermal papules (with no surface change) that often form into rings or part of a ring. They are common on the dorsal surface of the hands and feet. They are flesh coloured or slightly erythematous and are usually asymptomatic. As they heal the centre becomes dusky and altered in texture. A deep form, which is tender, exists in children. Diffuse granuloma annulare may be associated with diabetes mellitus.

The pathology shows a granulomatous dermal infiltrate with foci of degeneration of collagen (necrobiosis). Spontaneous resolution often occurs but cryotherapy or triamcinolone injection may help localized disease.

FURTHER READING

Atherton DJ (1994) *Eczema in Childhood: The Facts.* Oxford: Oxford University Press.

Coleman R et al (1997) Genetic studies of atopy and atopic dermatitis. *British Journal of Dermatology* **136**: 1–5.

Drago F et al (1997) Human herpesvirus 7 in pityriasis rosea. *Lancet* **349**: 1367–1368.

Greaves MW (1995). Chronic urticaria. *New England Journal of Medicine* **332**: 1767–1772.

Greaves MW, Weinstein GD (1995) Treatment of psoriasis. *New England Journal of Medicine* **332**: 581–587.

Rees JL et al (1997) Psoriasis. *Journal of the Royal College of Physicians of London* **31**: 238–240.

Facial rashes

Facial rashes often cause diagnostic confusion, but a close examination of the clinical signs should help differentiate the underlying cause (Table 20.4). All facial rashes, by virtue of their visibility, can cause significant distress to the patient and this should never be underestimated.

Acne vulgaris

Acne is a common facial rash occurring in adolescence and rarely in early and mid-adult life. The cause is multifactorial, but the blockage of pilosebaceous units with surrounding inflammation is the main pathological process and this can occur owing to a number of different factors (Fig 20.19).

CLINICAL FEATURES

Acne appears in areas rich in sebaceous glands, such as the face, back and sternal area. The three cardinal features are open comedones (blackheads) or closed comedones (whiteheads), inflammatory papules, and pustules. The skin may be very greasy (seborrhoea). Rupture of the inflamed lesions may lead to deep-seated dermal inflammation and nodulocystic lesions, which are more likely to cause facial scarring. A premenstrual exacerbation of acne is sometimes

Table 20.4
Differential diagnosis of facial rashes

Acne vulgaris	Perioral dermatitis
Rosacea	Photosensitivity
Seborrhoeic eczema	Sarcoidosis
Atopic eczema	Chronic discoid lupus erythematosus
Contact eczema	Systemic lupus erythematosus
Dermatomyositis	Subacute cutaneous lupus erythematosus

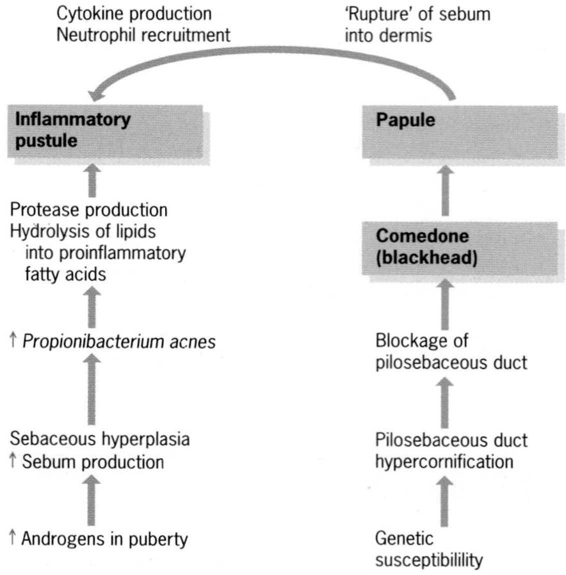

Fig 20.19
Pathophysiology of acne vulgaris

noticed. There is a tendency for spontaneous improvement over a number of years, but acne can persist unabated into adult life.

A number of clinical variants exist:

- *Infantile acne*. Facial acne is occasionally seen in infants and is sometimes cystic. It is thought to be due to the influence of maternal androgens and resolves spontaneously.
- *Steroid acne*. Acne may occur secondary to corticosteroid therapy or Cushing's syndrome. Comedones and cysts are rare in this variant, but involvement of the back and shoulders (rather than the face) is common. Clinically the rash often appears as a pustular folliculitis.
- *Oil acne*. This is an industrial disease seen in workers who have prolonged contact with oils or other hydrocarbons and is common on the legs and other exposure sites.
- *Acne fulminans*. This is a rare variant seen most commonly in young male adolescents. Severe necrotic and crusted acne lesions appear associated with malaise, pyrexia, arthralgia and bone pain (due to sterile bone cysts). It requires urgent treatment with oral prednisolone (30–40 mg daily) and analgesics, followed by a course of oral isotretinoin (see below).
- '*Follicular occlusion triad*'. This is a rare disorder most commonly seen in Africans. It is characterized by the presence of severe nodulocystic acne, dissecting cellulitis of the scalp (see p. 1191) and hidradenitis suppurativa (p. 1153). It has been suggested that this is caused by a problem of follicular occlusion rather than having an infective aetiology.

TREATMENT

Treatment is aimed at decreasing sebum production, decreasing bacteria, normalizing duct keratinization or decreasing inflammation.

Regular washing with acne soaps should be encouraged to remove excess grease (normal soaps can be comedogenic), and 'picking' should be discouraged.

First-line therapy

Mild acne can respond to a variety of topical agents such as antibiotics (tetracycline, clindamycin), keratolytics (benzoyl peroxide) or topical retinoids. If these fail, second-line agents should be added.

Second-line therapy

- *Low-dose oral antibiotic therapy* often helps but must be given for at least 4–6 months. Examples are oxytetracycline 500 mg twice daily, minocycline 100 mg daily, erythromycin 500 mg twice daily, or trimethoprim 100 mg twice daily.
- An extra second-line treatment ('cyproterone acetate 2 mg/ethinyloestradiol 35 μg' *Dianette*™) can be considered in females if there are no contraindications to oral contraception. This acts as a normal combined contraceptive but has anti-androgen activity. It may take 6–8 months to have its maximum effect.
- *UVB phototherapy* can be helpful but is rarely used now owing to the development of retinoid drugs (see below).

Third-line therapy

Third-line treatment with a retinoid drug should be given if:

- the above measures fail
- there is nodulocystic acne with scarring
- there is severe psychological disturbance.

Use of retinoids (isotretinoin or acitretin). Retinoids are synthetic vitamin A analogues that affect cell growth and differentiation. They are very teratogenic.

Isotretinoin is a 'hospital-only drug' in most countries owing to its teratogenicity and is restricted to use by dermatologists. A pregnancy test is advisable prior to its use in fertile women. It is given as a four-month course at a dose of 1 mg kg^{-1} daily. Over 90% of individuals will respond to this therapy and 65% of people will obtain a long-term 'cure'. Patients must avoid pregnancy during therapy and for one month after stopping isotretinoin (but for two years after stopping acitiretin as it is very lipophilic). Both drugs cause drying of the skin, especially of the lips. Hair thinning and exercise-induced myalgia are not uncommon. Blood count, liver biochemistry and fasting lipids need to be monitored during therapy.

Rosacea

Rosacea (acne rosacea) is a common inflammatory rash predominantly affecting the face. The onset is usually in middle age and it is more common in women. It often causes significant psychological distress.

The cause is unknown. Theories have suggested an underlying problem in vasomotor stability of blood vessels or a role of the skin mite *Demodex*, but there is little evidence to confirm these speculations.

CLINICAL FEATURES

The cardinal features are of facial flushing, inflammatory papules and pustules affecting the nose forehead and cheeks. The flushing may precede the other signs by some years. There are no comedones. Additional features may include dilated blood vessels (telangiectasia), inflammation of the eyelid margins (blepharitis), keratitis and sebaceous gland hypertrophy, especially of the nose. The latter is more common in men and can cause a disfiguring enlargement of the nose called rhinophyma. The flushing may be exacerbated by alcohol, hot drinks, sunlight and changes in ambient temperature. Prolonged use of topical steroids can exacerbate or trigger the condition. As the disease progresses the flushing may be replaced by a permanent erythema.

TREATMENT

This is suppressive rather than curative. Long-term use of topical 0.075% metronidazole gel is helpful. Avoid topical steroids. A three-month course of oral tetracycline (500 mg twice daily) is also helpful. Oral metronidazole (400 mg twice daily) or oral isotretinoin (0.5–1 mg kg^{-1} daily) is occasionally given in resistant cases (p. 1170). The papules and pustules tend to respond best to therapy, but repeat courses may be necessary. The flushing and erythema are often resistant to treatment; cosmetic camouflage can be helpful. Rhinophyma can be treated with plastic surgery or by carbon dioxide laser.

Perioral dermatitis

Perioral dermatitis is a common rash found around the mouth, especially in young females. The exact cause is unknown, but it often has an iatrogenic component.

CLINICAL FEATURES

Perioral dermatitis presents with erythema, scaling, papules and occasionally pustules around the mouth. It usually spares a halo of skin immediately adjacent to the lips.

TREATMENT

There is frequently a history of initial improvement after use of topical steroids followed by an exacerbation despite continued use (as also seen in rosacea). Treatment in this case involves stopping topical steroids, although they may have to be withdrawn slowly to prevent too severe a rebound after withdrawal. The mainstay of treatment is with a 3–4 month course of oxytetracycline or erythromycin (both 500 mg twice daily).

FURTHER READING

Cunliffe WJ (1989) *Acne*. London: Martin Dunitz.

Plewig G, Kligman AM (1993) *Acne and Rosacea*, 2nd edn. Berlin: Springer Verlag.

Munro CS (1997) Acne. *Journal of the Royal College of Physicians* **31**: 360–363.

Leyden JJ (1997) Therapy for acne vulgaris. *New England Journal of Medicine* **336**: 1156–1162.

Photodermatology

Sunlight – light in the ultraviolet (UV) part of the spectrum – combines short, medium and long wavelengths (UVC, UVB and UCA respectively). Both UVB and UVA can penetrate the atmosphere and reach the human skin. This light energy is potentially mutagenic and carcinogenic, but it can also can suppress cutaneous inflammation. Thus, UV irradiation can both *cause* skin disease and be used to *treat* it.

Photosensitive rashes usually appear on sites exposed to the sun's rays, such as the face, the anterior 'V' of the chest, the ears and the backs of the hands. Certain 'protected' areas are characteristically spared, such as under the chin or the upper eyelid and between the finger webs. Porphyria, drug sensitivity and lupus erythematosus should be excluded in all photosensitive patients.

Photosensitive rashes may be divided into photoexacerbated rashes and the idiopathic photodermatoses (Table 20.5). The former are discussed on pp. 204, 488 and 1005.

THERAPIES AND PREVENTION

Phototherapy

UVB and UVA are used in the treatment of inflammatory dermatoses. They have a suppressive effect on cutaneous inflammation, and there is increasing evidence that they can suppress systemic immunoreactivity to some degree. However, both types can cause skin ageing and predispose to skin malignancy if excessive doses are used. This is more of a problem in white-skinned individuals. Unaffected regions of skin and high-risk areas such as the scrotum can be screened during phototherapy.

UVB is more likely to cause burning of the skin, but it is less carcinogenic than UVA. It is used in the treatment of eczema and psoriasis (especially in children) and is usually given three times a week for 6–10 weeks. Eye protection is necessary during therapy.

Table 20.5
Differential diagnosis of photosensitive rashes

Photoexacerbated/provoked rashes	
Systemic disease	SLE, CDLE, SCLE (p. 488)
Metabolic disease	Porphyrias (p. 1003 and p. 1178) Pellagra (p. 203)
Drugs	Thiazides, phenothiazines, tetracyclines, amiodarone
Plant phototoxins	Phytophotodermatitis (photosensitivity induced by contact of the skin with certain plants, e.g. celery, hogweed, rue
Skin disease	Rosacea Rarely, atopic eczema, psoriasis, lichen planus (these normally improve in sunlight)
Idiopathic photodermatoses	
Polymorphic light eruption	
Chronic actinic dermatitis	
Solar urticaria	

CDLE, chronic discoid lupus erythematosus;
SCLE, subacute cutaneous lupus erythematosus.

UVA therapy is relatively ineffective on its own, so it is used in conjunction with a photosensitizer ('psoralen') – hence the term 'PUVA'. The psoralen can be given either by mouth or applied to the skin in bathwater. PUVA is given twice weekly, and eye protection must been worn *for the whole of the treatment day* as the psoralen sensitizes the retina. It is more effective than UVB but is limited by its carcinogenic potential. A maximum dose is given over a lifetime depending on skin type (1000 J, or 200 sessions approximately). It is used for many conditions including psoriasis, eczema, cutaneous T-cell lymphoma, some photosensitive dermatoses and vitiligo.

Sunbeds, as used for skin tanning, emit predominantly UVA light and are therefore rarely effective in treating skin disease. If used frequently there may be an increased incidence of carcinoma.

Sunblocks (sunscreens)

There are two broad classes of 'sunblock' cream: they either absorb UV light (e.g. aminobenzoic acid or methoxycinnamate) or reflect it (e.g. titanium dioxide). Most modern creams protect against UVB and UVA to varying degrees.

UVB protection is graded by the 'sun protection factor' (SPF): an SPF of 15 implies that a person can spend 15 times as long in the sun before burning. However, SPFs above 15 appear to confer little extra protection. There is no standardized way of assessing efficiency against UVA.

Some sunscreens (especially aminobenzoates) may rarely cause photosenstive rashes. This can be proven by photopatch testing.

Idiopathic photodermatoses

Polymorphic light eruption

This is the most common photosensitive eruption in temperate regions, affecting up to 10–20% of the population. It is most common in young women. In many it is mild and often goes undiagnosed. An itchy rash appears some hours after sun exposure, strictly confined to the exposed sites. Lesions may be papules, vesicles or plaques. They can last for several hours or several days. The condition starts in the springtime and often improves during the summer owing to skin 'hardening'.

TREATMENT

Avoidance of sunlight and the use of sunblocks is helpful in mild cases. Otherwise, 'desensitization' with low-dose PUVA in the springtime may be required.

Chronic actinic dermatitis (photosensitive eczema, actinic reticuloid)

This is a relatively rare type of eczema occurring in a photosensitive distribution over the face, neck and hands. It typically affects middle-aged or elderly males. There may be a pre-existing eczema, so the subsequent development of photosensitivity is often missed. This is further confounded by the fact that the eczema will usually spread to affect skin not exposed to sunlight, and in fact the patient can become erythrodermic. The skin has typical features of eczema but there is often marked skin thickening. Histology is often atypical and can look almost like lymphoma. The diagnosis can be confirmed by specialist monochromator light-testing. The most severe cases can be exacerbated even by artificial lighting, as these patients can become exquisitely photosensitive.

TREATMENT

This consists of strict avoidance of sunlight, and the use of high-factor sunblocks and the screening of house and car windows. Topical steroids and emollients are useful in milder cases. Oral prednisolone may be needed, and azathioprine (100–200 mg daily) should be considered for long-term suppression. Low-dose PUVA under steroid cover may help with 'desensitization'.

Solar urticaria

This is very rare. Itchy urticarial lesions occur within minutes of sun exposure and characteristically settle within 1–2 hours. Sun avoidance, sunblocks, H_1 antihistamines and low-dose PUVA are all used in treatment.

FURTHER READING

Harber LC, Bickers DR (1989) *Photosensitivity Diseases*, 2nd edn. Toronto: BC Decker.

Erythroderma

Erythroderma, meaning 'red skin', refers to the clinical state of inflammation or redness of all (or nearly all) of the skin. It is sometimes called *exfoliative dermatitis*, but dermatitis is not always present. It is most common in males and later in life. Patients often complain of their skin feeling 'tight' as well as itchy. Longstanding erythroderma is often associated with hair loss, ectropion of the eyelids and even nail-shedding. Systemic symptoms are common, such as malaise, pyrexia, widespread lymphadenopathy and possibly serious circulatory disturbance. Erythroderma can occasionally lead to death, so it should be regarded as a medical 'emergency'.

AETIOLOGY

There are a number of underlying causes (Table 20.6). A careful history should be sought, paying particular attention to previous skin disease and any drug history. Examination should look specifically for pustules and nail changes suggestive of psoriasis. A skin biopsy may further help to elucidate the cause, especially of cutaneous lymphoma. Newer techniques such as T-cell receptor gene rearrangement studies (looking for evidence of clonal T-cell expansion in the skin) are also useful in the diagnosis of lymphoma.

A number of cases defy an exact diagnosis. Lymph node biopsy should be considered if lymphoma is suspected. In non-malignant disease, lymph nodes normally show nonspecific, reactive (dermatopathic) changes.

COMPLICATIONS

Since the skin is one of the largest organs of the body, perhaps it is not surprising that inflammation of the whole organ can cause metabolic and haemodynamic problems. Examples are:

- high-output cardiac failure from increased blood flow
- hypothermia from heat loss
- fluid loss by transpiration
- hypoalbuminaemia
- increased basal metabolic rate
- 'capillary leak syndrome'.

Capillary leak syndrome is the most severe complication and has been responsible for a fatal outcome in some cases of psoriasis, although this is extremely rare. It is thought that the inflamed skin releases large quantities of cytokines that cause a generalized vascular leakage. This can cause cutaneous oedema, but more worryingly it can also cause leaky vessels in the lungs, resulting in adult respiratory distress syndrome.

Table 20.6
Causes of erythroderma

Common
Atopic eczema
Psoriasis
Drugs (e.g. sulphonamides, gold)
Chronic actinic dermatitis/seborrhoeic dermatitis
Idiopathic
Rare
Cutaneous T-cell lymphoma (Sézary syndrome) (p. 1184)
Malignancy (especially leukaemias)
Pemphigus foliaceus
Pityriasis rubra pilaris (a hereditary disorder of keratinization)
HIV infection
Toxic shock syndrome (p. 21)

TREATMENT

Treatment of erythroderma is best initiated in hospital. Patients must be kept very warm (with space blankets and heaters) and put on fluid balance charts. Their vital signs should be monitored regularly. Changes in electrolytes, albumin and circulatory status must be corrected. Swabs should be taken to detect secondary skin infections.

The skin condition is treated with bedrest and either a bland emollient or a mild topical steroid. All unessential drugs should be stopped. Where known, the underlying cause should be treated appropriately. The use of systemic steroid therapy for erythroderma remains controversial in view of possible side-effects.

Advanced capillary leak syndrome will often require specialized haemodynamic management in an intensive care unit.

FURTHER READING

Champion RH, Burton JL, Ebling FJG (eds) (1998) *Textbook of Dermatology*, 6th edn. Oxford: Blackwell Scientific.

Cutaneous signs of systemic disease

Some dermatoses are associated with a variety of underlying systemic diseases. Furthermore some medical conditions may present with cutaneous features.

Erythema nodosum

Erythema nodosum has a number of underlying causes (Table 20.7). It presents as painful or tender dusky blue-red nodules, commonly over the shins or lower limbs, which fade over 2–3 weeks to leave a bruised appearance (see Fig 20.36). It is most common in young adults, especially females. It can be associated with arthralgia, malaise and fever. Inflammation occurs in the dermis and the subcutaneous layer (panniculitis).

TREATMENT

Treatment is of the symptoms, with non-steroidal anti-inflammatory drugs and bedrest, as the condition resolves spontaneously. The underlying cause should be treated appropriately. In very persistent cases, oral dapsone (100 mg daily) or colchicine (500 mg twice daily) can be useful. Oral steroids are sometimes necessary.

Erythema multiforme

Erythema multiforme is a hypersensitivity rash of acute onset, frequently caused by infection or drugs. A cell-mediated cutaneous lymphocytotoxic response is present. Clinically the lesions can be erythematous, polycyclic, annular or show concentric rings called 'target lesions' (Fig 20.20). Frank blistering is not uncommon. The rash tends to be symmetrical and commonly affects the limbs – especially the hands and feet, where palms and soles may be involved. Occasionally there is severe mucosal involvement leading to necrotic ulcers of the mouth and genitalia, and a conjuntivitis ('erythema multiforme major'). This is also called *Stevens Johnson Syndrome*, which is now thought to be a form of toxic epidermal necrolysis (see p. 1190).

Erythema multiforme usually resolves in 2–4 weeks. The cause is not found in 50% of cases. Causes include:

- herpes simplex virus (the most common identifiable cause)
- other viral infections (e.g. EBV, Orf disease)
- drugs (e.g. sulphonamide, barbituates)
- *Mycoplasma* infection
- connective tissue disease (e.g. SLE, classical polyarteritis nodosa)
- HIV infection
- Wegener's granulomatosus
- carcinoma, lymphoma.

Rarely, recurrent erythema multiforme can occur and this is triggered by herpes simplex infection in at least 80% of cases.

Table 20.7
Causes of erythema nodosum

Streptococcal infection*
Drugs* (e.g. sulphonamides, oral contraceptive)
Sarcoidosis*
Idiopathic*
Yersinia infection
Fungal infection (histoplasmosis, blastomycosis)
Tuberculosis
Leprosy
Inflammatory bowel disease
Chlamydia infection

* Common causes in the UK.

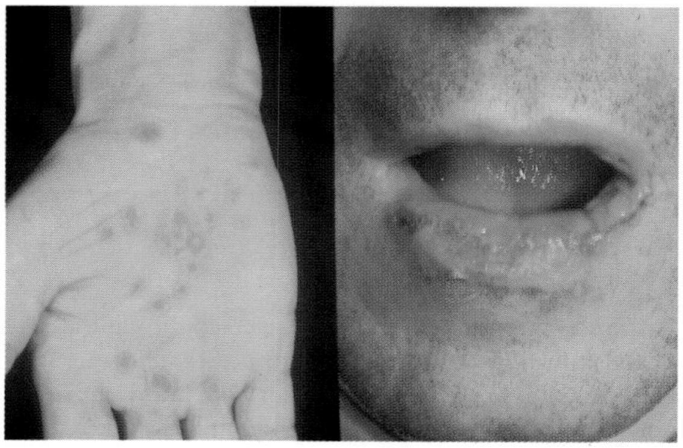

Fig 20.20
Erythema multiforme major – target lesions of the palm with mucosal involvement

TREATMENT

This is symptomatic and involves treating the underlying cause. Some advocate the use of oral steroids in severe disease but this remains controversial. Recurrent erythema multiforme can be treated with prophylactic oral acyclovir (200 mg twice daily) even if no cause has been found, as 80% are viral in origin. In resistant cases, azathioprine (50–100 mg daily) is used.

Pyoderma gangrenosum

Pyoderma gangrenosum is a condition of unknown aetiology that presents with erythematous nodules or pustules which frequently ulcerate (Fig 20.21). The ulcers can be large and grow at an alarming speed. The ulcer has a typical bluish black ('gangrenous') undermined edge and a purulent surface ('pyoderma'). There may be an associated pyrexia and malaise.

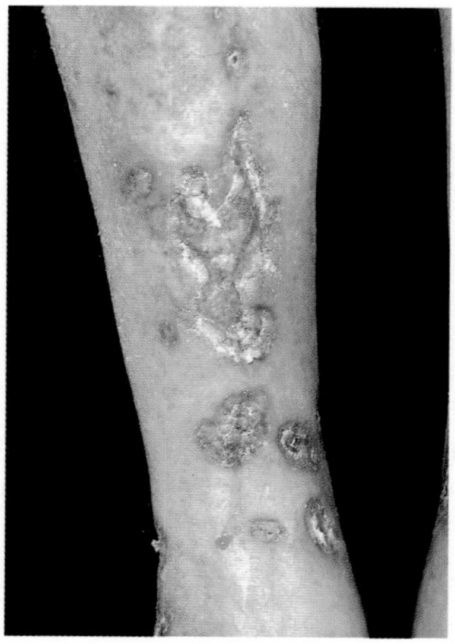

Fig 20.21
Ulcerative lesions of pyoderma gangrenosum

Biopsy through the ulcer edge shows an intense neutrophilic infiltrate and occasionally a vasculitis, but the diagnosis depends mostly on the clinical appearance. The main causes are:

- inflammatory bowel disease
- rheumatoid arthritis
- myeloma, monoclonal gammopathy, leukaemia, lymphoma
- liver disease (e.g. primary biliary cirrhosis)
- idiopathic (>20% in some series).

TREATMENT

This is with very potent topical steroids and/or high-dose oral steroids to prevent rapidly progressive ulceration. Oral dapsone and minocycline may help. Other immunosuppressants, such as cyclosporin, are useful in resistant cases. The underlying cause should be treated appropriately.

Acanthosis nigricans

Acanthosis nigricans presents as thickened, hyperpigmented skin predominantly of the flexures (Fig 20.22). It can appear warty or velvety when advanced. In early life it is seen in obese individuals who have very high levels of insulin owing to insulin resistance. In older people it normally reflects an underlying malignancy (especially gastrointestinal tumours), but it has been described with the polycystic ovary syndrome.

TREATMENT

Oral retinoids (0.5 mg kg^{-1} daily) may help (p. 1170). Any underlying malignancy should be treated appropriately.

Dermatomyositis (see also p. 492)

Dermatomyositis is a rare disease affecting skin and muscle, with an associated vasculitis. The cause is unknown but there is some evidence of immune dysfunction as immune complexes are often detected and T-lymphocytes cytotoxic to muscle cells may be present.

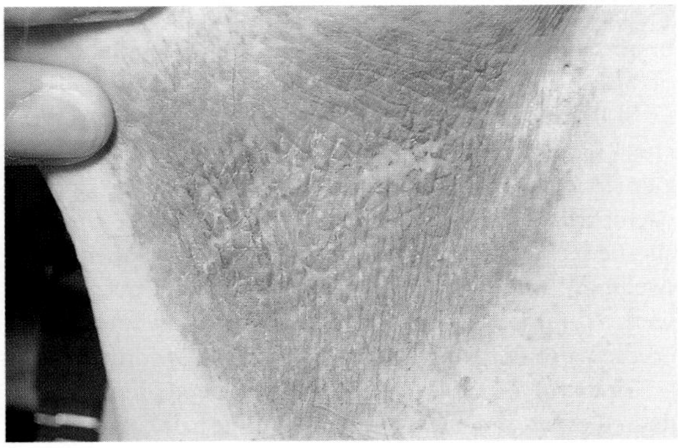

Fig 20.22
Acanthosis nigricans of the axilla

The rash is distinctive. Facial erythema and a magenta rash around the eyes with associated oedema are often present. Bluish red nodules or plaques may be present over the knuckles and extensor surfaces. The nail-folds are frequently ragged with dilated capillaries. The diagnosis is made from the clinical appearance, muscle biopsy, EMG and a serum creatine phosphokinase. Skin biopsy is not diagnostic.

There is a childhood form which usually occurs before the age of 10 years and which eventually resolves. This type is often associated with calcinosis in the skin and can cause significant long-term functional problems with weak muscles and contractures. Life-threatening bowel infarction can also occur in the childhood form. The adult form usually occurs after the age of 40. Some are associated with an underlying malignancy whereas others appear to reflect a 'connective tissue disease'. This latter group may overlap with scleroderma and lupus erythematosus.

TREATMENT

Treatment is with steroids and other immunsuppressants such as cyclosporin and azathioprine (see p. 858). Malignant disease should be treated appropriately, when present.

Scleroderma (see also p. 490)

The term 'scleroderma' refers to a thickening or hardening of the skin owing to abnormal dermal collagen. It is not a diagnostic entity in itself. Systemic sclerosis and morphoea both show sclerodermatous changes but are separate conditions.

Systemic sclerosis has cutaneous and systemic features (see p. 491). The early skin changes are of Raynaud's phenomenon and a puffy oedema of the hands and feet. This progresses to stiff fibrotic skin which feels tightly bound to deeper structures. There is a loss of finger pulps and tapering of the digits (sclerodactyly). Joint contractures may occur. Telangiectasia, pigmentation, calcinosis and ischaemic skin ulceration may also occur. Furrows may form around the mouth (which is often small) and wrinkles tend to disappear from the forehead. A rather fixed facial expression appears with time. All of the skin may be affected, but changes are often most marked on the hands, feet and the face. Similar cutaneous changes may be seen in the CREST syndrome and in the overlap syndrome (p. 493).

Morphoea is confined to the skin and usually presents in children or young adults. It is more common in females and the cause is unknown. Lesions are usually on the trunk and appear as bluish red plaques which progress to induration and then central white atrophy. A linear variant exists in childhood which is more severe as it can cause atrophy of underlying deep tissues and thus can cause unequal limb growth or cause scarring alopecia.

Rarely, sclerodermatous skin changes may be seen in chronic Lyme disease (acrodermatitis chronica atrophicans), chronic graft-versus-host disease, poly (vinyl chloride) disease, eosinophilic myalgia syndrome (due to tryptophan therapy) and bleomycin therapy.

Lupus erythematosus

There are three clinical variants to this disease, but some patients may show features of more than one type:

- chronic discoid lupus erythematosus (CDLE)
- subacute cutaneous lupus erythematosus (SCLE)
- systemic lupus erythematosus (SLE).

The aetiology is unknown but is presumably a reflection of some abnormality in immune function as variable autoantibodies may be found in all types. Very rarely it can be induced by certain drugs such as phenothiazines, hydrallazine, methyldopa, isoniazid, tetracycline and penicillin.

Chronic discoid lupus erythematosus (CDLE)

Skin biopsy shows a dense, patchy, dermal lymphohistiocytic infiltrate which often is centred around appendages. Epidermal basal layer damage, follicular plugging and hyperkeratosis may be present. Direct immunofluorescence studies of lesional skin may show the presence of IgM and C3 at the dermoepidermal junction ('lupus band').

CDLE is the most common type of lupus erythematosus seen by dermatologists and more frequently affects females. Clinically it presents with fixed erythematous, scaly, atrophic plaques with telangiectasia, especially on the face or other sun-exposed sites (Fig 20.23). Follicular plugging may be apparent. Scalp involvement may lead to a scarring alopecia. It may be triggered and exacerbated by UV exposure. A few patients may also suffer with Raynaud's phenomenon or unusual chilblain-like lesions (chilblain lupus). Approximately 5% of cases will go on to develop SLE but this is more common in children.

Serum antinuclear factor (ANF) is positive in 30% of cases.

TREATMENT

First-line therapy is with sunscreens and potent topical steroids. Certain oral antimalarials (hydroxychloroquine 100–200 mg twice daily and mepacrine 100 mg daily) can prove very useful and are generally safe for long-term intermittent use. Oral prednisolone is beneficial but its use is limited by its side-effect profile. Azathioprine, retinoids and cyclosporin can be useful in resistant cases.

PROGNOSIS

The disease is usually chronic although it may fluctuate in severity. CDLE remains confined to the skin in most patients and it will eventually go into remission in up to 50% of cases (after many years).

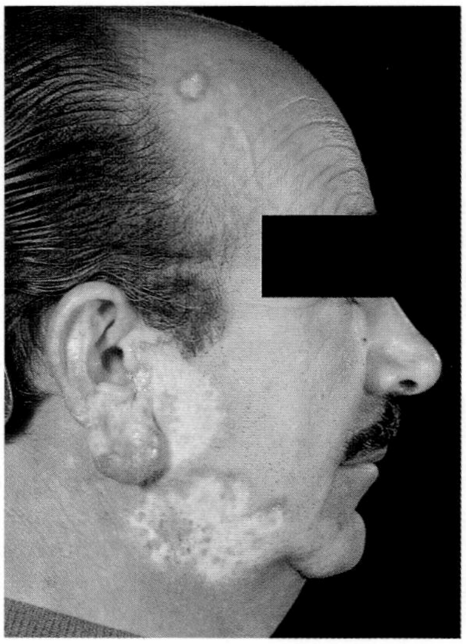

Fig 20.23
Chronic discoid lupus erythematosus, showing scaling, atrophy and hypopigmentation

Subacute cutaneous lupus erythematosus (SCLE)

SCLE is a rare cutaneous variant of lupus erythematosus. It presents with widespread indurated, sometimes urticated erythematous lesions, often on the upper trunk. The lesions can also be annular. Photosensitivity is often a prominent feature. Complications, such as arthralgia and mouth ulceration, are seen but significant organ involvement is rare. ANF and extractable nuclear antibodies (anti-Ro and anti-La) are usually positive (see p. 489).

Treatment is with oral dapsone, antimalarials or systemic immunosuppression (prednisolone and cyclosporin).

Systemic lupus erythematosus (SLE) (see also p. 487)

SLE is a severe multisystem disorder and is much more common in females and in certain races such as Afro-Caribbeans. In many ways the cutaneous involvement is one of the minor problems of this disease but it is important to recognize as it may be the presenting feature of SLE.

SLE may present with a macular erythema over the cheeks, nose and forehead ('butterfly rash' – Fig 20.24). Palmar erythema, dilated nail-fold capillaries, splinter haemorrhages and digital infarcts of the finger-tips may also be seen but are not always noticed by the patient. Joint swellings, livedo reticularis and purpura are occasionally seen. Rarely SLE can be complicated by an atypical erythema multiforme-like rash ('Rowell's syndrome').

Treatment of SLE (see p. 489) is dependent on the degree of systemic involvement and is usually managed by rheumatologists. The cutaneous manifestations of SLE may respond to treatments as for SCLE.

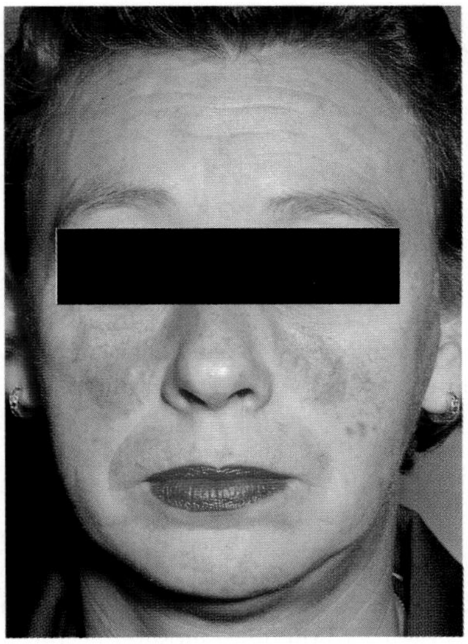

Fig 20.24
Systemic lupus erythematosus 'butterfly' rash

Pruritus

The mechanisms of pruritus are poorly understood. Histamine, tachykinins (e.g. substance P) and cytokines (e.g. interleukin-2) may play a role peripherally in the skin. The major nerve pathways for itch and the influence of the central nervous system are not well-characterized, but opioid μ-receptor dependent processes can regulate the perception and intensity of itch.

Pruritus (see lichen simplex, nodular prurigo) in the absence of a demonstrable rash can be caused by a number of medical problems (Table 20.8).

Asteatotic eczema and cholinergic urticaria are common causes of pruritus where the rash is often missed. The terms 'idiopathic pruritus' or 'senile' pruritus probably overlap with asteatotic eczema and this is common in the elderly.

Treatment involves avoiding soaps, and symptomatic measures (as for asteatotic eczema). Phototherapy may help intractable cases. Underlying medical problems should be treated appropriately.

Table 20.8
Medical conditions associated with pruritus

Iron-deficiency anaemia
Internal malignancy (especially lymphoma)
Diabetes mellitus
Chronic renal failure
Chronic liver disease (especially primary biliary cirrhosis, hereditary haemochromatosis)
Thyroid disease
HIV infection
Polycythaemia vera

Sarcoidosis (see also p. 806)

Sarcoidosis is a multisystem granulomatous disorder of unknown aetiology. It may present as reddish brown dermal papules and nodules especially around the eyelid margins and the rim of the nostrils. More polymorphic lesions (papules nodules and plaques) may appear on the body. It is most common in Afro-Caribbeans where it is often accompanied by hypo- or hyperpigmentation. Rarely it can present with a bluish red infiltrate or swelling especially of the nose or ears, called lupus pernio (Fig 20.25). Both these types of lesion can be seen anywhere on the body but are common on the face. Erythema nodosum (see p. 1173) can also occur, usually on the shins, and is seen in 30% of patients with acute-onset sarcoidosis. Erythema nodosum is an immunological reaction and is not due to sarcoid tissue infiltration. Swollen fingers from a dactylitis may also be present. Whilst sarcoidosis may be confined to the skin, all patients should be investigated for evidence of systemic disease (see p. 808).

Treatment of cutaneous lesions (excluding erythema nodosum) includes very potent topical steroids (0.05% clobetasol proprionate), intralesional steroids, oral steroids and occasionally methotrexate or antimalarials.

Neurofibromatosis type 1 (Von Recklinghausen's disease)

(see also p. 1090)

Type 1 neurofibromatosis is an autosomal dominant condition which often presents in childhood with a variety of cutaneous features. Many cases are new mutations in the NF1 gene. Early signs include *café au lait*

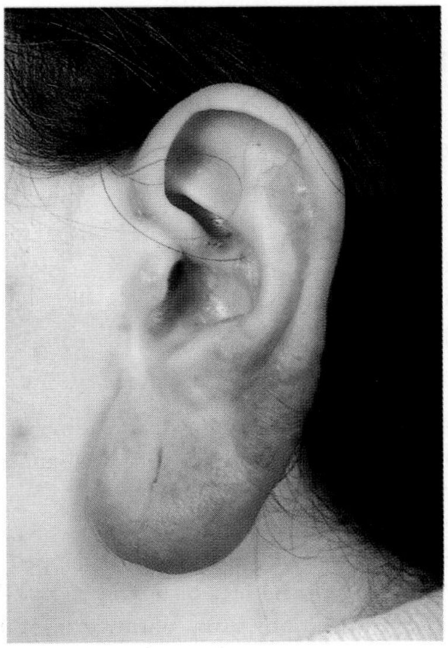

Fig 20.25
Lupus pernio of the ear (sarcoidosis)

spots (brown macules, greater than 2.5 cm diameter and more than five lesions) and axillary freckling. Lisch nodules (hyperpigmented iris hamartomas) may be seen in the eyes by slit lamp examination. Later on, fleshy skin tags and deeper soft tumours (neurofibromas) appear and they may progress to completely cover the skin, causing significant cosmetic disability. Rarely a number of endocrine disorders may be associated, including phaeochromocytoma, acromegaly and Addison's disease.

Tuberous sclerosis (epiloia)

Tuberous sclerosis is an autosomal dominant condition of variable severity which may not present until later childhood. The defect has been localized to chromosome 9q34. It is characterized by a variety of hamartomatous growths. The three cardinal features are (a) mental retardation, (b) epilepsy, and (c) cutaneous abnormalities – but not all have to be present. The skin signs include:

- adenoma sebaceum (reddish papules/fibromas around the nose)
- periungual fibroma (nodules arising from the nail-bed)
- shagreen patches (firm, flesh-coloured plaques on the trunk)
- ash-leaf hypopigmentation (pale macules best seen with UV light)
- forehead plaque (indurated flesh-coloured patch)
- *café au lait* patches.

Later in life, internal hamartomas can arise in the heart, kidney, retina and CNS. Parents of a suspected case should be examined carefully under UV light as they may have a forme fruste of the condition which can manifest just as hypopigmented patches. This would have genetic implications for future offspring.

Diabetes mellitus (see also p. 985)

Diabetes mellitus can have a number of cutaneous features. Complications of diabetes itself include:

- fungal infection (e.g. candidiasis)
- bacterial infections (e.g. recurrent boils)
- xanthomas
- arterial disease (ulcers, gangrene)
- neuropathic ulcers.

Specific dermatoses of diabetes include

- necrobiosis lipoidica (a patch of spreading erythema over the shin which becomes yellowish and atrophic in the centre and may ulcerate)
- diffuse granuloma annulare (p. 1169)
- diabetic dermopathy (red-brown flat-topped papules)
- blisters (usually on the feet or hands)
- diabetic stiff skin (tight waxy skin over the fingers with limitation of joint movement owing to thickened collagen – also called cheiroarthropathy).

Chronic liver disease (see also p. 297)

Chronic liver disease may present with jaundice, palmar erythema, spider naevi, white nails, hyperpigmentation and pruritus.

Porphyria cutanea tarda (see p. 1005) is a rare genetic disorder associated with liver disease, usually due to excessive alcohol consumption or hepatitis C infection. It presents clinically on exposed skin with sun-induced blisters, skin fragility, scarring, and hypertrichosis. Treatment is with repeated venesection and/or very-low-dose chloroquine, plus an avoidance of alcohol.

Chronic renal failure (see also p. 572)

Chronic renal failure is commonly associated with intractable pruritus. Longstanding renal transplant patients often suffer with recurrent viral warts and squamous cell carcinomas owing to the immunosuppression.

Thyroid disease (see also p. 930)

Hypothyroidism may cause dry, firm, gelatinous (myxoedematous) skin with diffuse hair thinning and a loss of the outer third of the eyebrows. Hyperthyroidism may be associated with warm, sweaty skin and a diffuse alopecia. Grave's disease is rarely associated with thyroid acropachy ('clubbing' with underlying bone changes) and pretibial myxoedema (a red-brown infiltration on the shins which can become lumpy and tender).

Cushing's syndrome (see also p. 946)

Cushing's syndrome can cause hirsutism, a moon face, a buffalo hump, stretchmarks (striae) and a pustular folliculitis (often called steroid acne) of the skin.

Hyperlipidaemias (see also p. 992)

Hyperlipidaemias can present with xanthomas which are abnormal collections of lipid in the skin. All patients with xanthomas should be investigated for hyperlipidaemia, although the most common type called xanthelasma (yellow plaques around the eyes) are usually associated with normal lipids. There are a number of other clinical variants of xanthomas such as (i) tuberous xanthoma (firm orange-yellow nodules and plaques on extensor surfaces), (ii) tendon xanthoma (firm subcutaneous swellings attached to tendons), (iii) plane xanthoma (orange-yellow macules often affecting palmar creases), and (iv) eruptive xanthoma (numerous small yellowish papules commonly on the buttocks).

Cutaneous amyloid

Cutaneous amyloid can be confined to the skin or be part of systemic disease (see p. 1002). Macular amyloid is a

Table 20.9
Non-metastatic cutaneous manifestations of underlying malignancy

Dermatosis	Tumour
Dermatomyositis	Lung, GI tract, GU tract
Acanthosis nigricans	GI tract, lung, liver
Paget's disease (localized patch of eczema around the nipple)	Ductal breast carcinoma
Erythroderma	Lymphoma/leukaemia
Tylosis (thickened palms/soles)	Oesophageal carcinoma
Ichthyosis (dry flaking of skin)	Lymphoma
Erythema gyratum repens (concentric rings of erythema which change rapidly)	Lung, breast
Necrolytic migratory erythema (burning geographic and spreading annular areas of erythema)	Glucagonoma

common purely cutaneous variant seen in Asians. It is characterized by itchy brown rippled macules on the upper back.

Systemic amyloid may be associated with reddish brown papules, nodules or plaques especially around the eyes, the flexural areas and mucosal surfaces. Distinctive periorbital bruising and macroglossia may also be present.

Systemic malignant disease

Certain rashes may be a non-metastatic manifestation of an underlying malignancy (Table 20.9). Rarely tumours can metastasize to the skin where they normally present as papules or nodules which may proceed to ulceration.

FURTHER READING

Braverman IM (ed) (1997) *Skin Signs of Systemic Disease*, 3rd edn. Philadelphia: WB Saunders.

Fitzpatrick TB, Eisen AZ, Wolff K, Freedberg IM, Austen KF (eds) (1998) *Dermatology in General Medicine*, 5th edn. New York: McGraw-Hill.

Lovell CR, Maddison PJ, Campion GV (1990) *The Skin in Rheumatic Disease*. London: Chapman & Hall.

Bullous disease

Primary blistering diseases of the skin are rare. A variety of skin proteins are important in holding the skin together. Inherited abnormalities or immune damage of these proteins causes abnormal cell separation, inflammation, fluid accumulation and blistering (Fig 20.26). The level of blistering is important in determining the clinical picture as well as the prognosis. Therefore skin biopsy for light and electron microscopy, together with immunfluorescence (IMF) studies, is paramount in diagnosis. However, remember that the most common causes of skin blistering are chickenpox, herpes, impetigo, pompholyx eczema and insect bite reactions, although these are often localized.

Immunobullous disease

Pemphigus vulgaris

Pemphigus vulgaris is a potentially fatal blistering disease occurring in all races, but it is more common in Ashkenazy Jews and possibly in people from the Indian subcontinent. Onset is usually in middle age and both sexes are affected equally. Prior to the development of oral steroids this condition was frequently fatal. The development of autoantibodies against desmosomal proteins (dsg 3) are pathogenic in this disease and they can be measured as markers of disease activity. Rarely the disease can be drug-induced (e.g. by penicillamine or captopril).

Skin biopsy shows a superficial intraepidermal split with acantholysis (separation of individual cells). The level of the split varies and can be subdivided into two types. In pemphigus vulgaris the split is just above the basal layer, and in pemphigus foliaceus there is a superficial epidermal split. Both direct IMF of the skin and indirect IMF using the patient's serum show intercellular staining of IgG within the epidermis.

CLINICAL FEATURES

Mucosal involvement (especially oral ulceration) is common and may be the presenting sign in up to 50% of cases. This is then followed by the appearance of flaccid blisters, particularly involving the trunk. They tend to be sore rather than itchy. Blistering usually becomes widespread but they rapidly denude; thus pemphigus often presents with erythematous, weeping erosions. Blisters can be extended with gentle sliding pressure (Nikolsky's sign). Flexural lesions often have a vegetating appearance.

TREATMENT

This is with very high-dose oral prednisolone (60–100 mg daily) or pulsed methylprednisolone and this may need to be lifelong. Therefore other immunosuppressants such as azathioprine (or occasionally cyclophosphamide or cyclosporin) are used as steroid-sparing agents. Intravenous immunoglobulin infusions can be useful in resistant cases.

Whilst treatment is normally effective, up to 20% of patients may succumb either due to complications of the disease or more commonly from side-effects of the treatment.

Use of azathioprine. Azathioprine can cause bone marrow suppression and very occasionally a hepatitis. Therefore blood counts and liver biochemistry should be monitored regularly during therapy (every six weeks). Long-term use with other immunosuppressants causes a slightly increased risk of malignancy, especially of the skin.

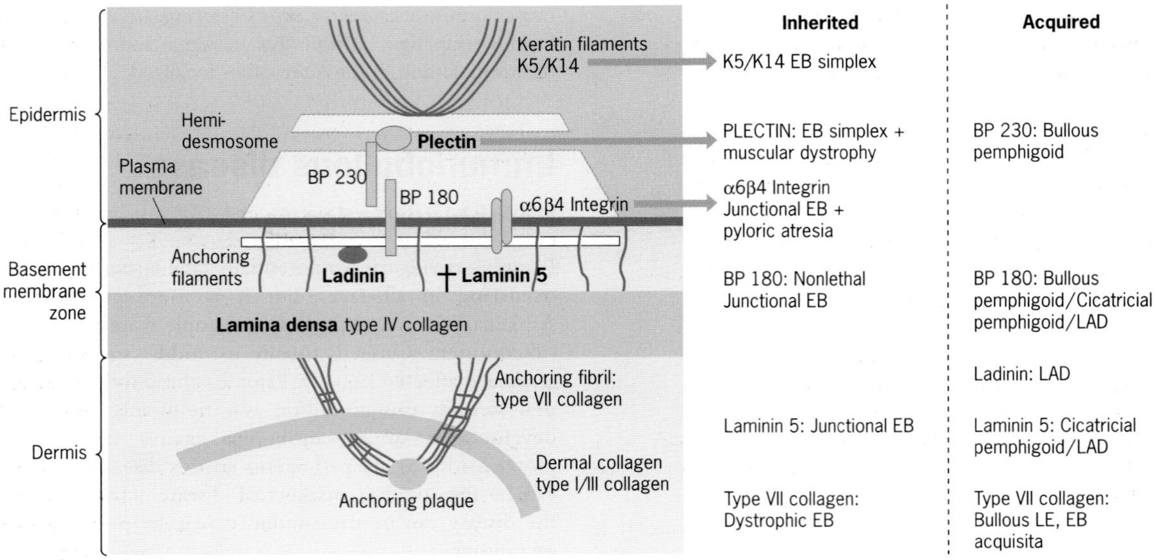

Fig 20.26
Section of the basement membrane zone, showing the structural sites of damage in bullous disorders
LAD, linear IgA disease; EB, epidermolysis bullosa

Bullous pemphigoid

Bullous pemphigoid is more common than pemphigus. It presents in later life (usually over the age of 60 years) and mucosal involvement is rarer. Autoantibodies against a 230 kDa or 180 kDa hemidesmosomal protein ('bullous pemphigoid antigens 1 and 2') play an aetiological role.

Skin biopsy shows a deeper blister (than in pemphigus) owing to a subepidermal split through the basement membrane. Direct and indirect IMF studies show linear staining of IgG along the basement membrane.

CLINICAL FEATURES

Large tense bullae appear anywhere on the skin (Fig 20.27) but often involve limbs, hands and feet. They may be centred on an erythematous or urticated background and they can be haemorrhagic. Pemphigoid can be very itchy. Mucosal ulceration is uncommon but can cause scarring (cicatricial pemphigoid).

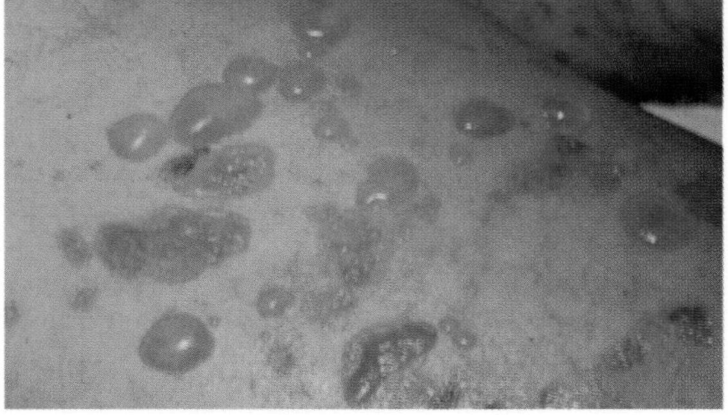

Fig 20.27
Bullous pemphigoid

TREATMENT

This is with high-dose oral prednisolone (30–60 mg daily) and steroid-sparing agents such as azathioprine. In general, disease control is easier than with pemphigus. Often treatment can be withdrawn after 2–3 years. However, pemphigoid treatment often causes side-effects, especially as most pateints are elderly. Occasionally localized disease can be controlled with potent topical steroids or oral dapsone.

Dermatitis herpetiformis (see also p. 256)

Dermatitis herpetiformis is a rare blistering disorder associated with gluten sensitive enteropathy (coeliac disease) and occasionally other organ-specific autoimmune disorders. The HLA associations (B8, DRw3, DQw2 in 80–90% of cases) and immunological findings (endomysial, reticulin and gliadin autoantibodies may be present in serum) are similar to coeliac disease.

Skin biopsy shows a subepidermal blister with neutrophil microabcesses in the dermal papillae. Direct Immunofluorescence studies of uninvolved skin shows IgA in the dermal papillae and patchy granular IgA along the basement membrane. The jejunal mucosa shows variable changes but sub-total villous atrophy is uncommon (see p. 256).

CLINICAL FEATURES

Dermatitis herpetiformis is most common in males and can present at any age but is most likely to appear for the first time in young adult life. It presents with intensely small, itchy blisters of the skin. The lesions have a predilection for the elbows, extensor forearms, scalp and buttocks. The tops of the blisters are usually scratched off; thus crusted erosions are often seen at presentation. Remissions and exacerbations are common.

TREATMENT

This should always be with a gluten-free diet (GFD). Control of the skin disease can be obtained with oral dapsone (50–200 mg daily) or sulphonamides. If a strict GFD is adhered to, oral medication can often be withdrawn after two years. The GFD will need to be lifelong. It protects against the rare complication of small bowel lymphoma.

Use of dapsone. Dapsone frequently causes a mild dose-related haemolytic anaemia (which is usually well-tolerated), but the haemolysis can be devastating if there is G6PD deficiency. Liver damage, a polyneuropathy and aplastic anaemia also occur rarely, so regular monitoring of a blood count and liver biochemistry is needed.

Linear IgA disease (chronic bullous dermatosis of childhood)

Linear IgA disease (LAD) is a further subepidermal blistering disorder of adults and children. Pathogenic autoantibodies can bind to a variety of basement membrane proteins including ladinin, BP 180 antigen and laminin 5. It is the most common immunobullous disease seen in children.

Clinically it can present with circular clusters of blisters, a pemphigoid type of blistering or a dermatitis herpetiformis picture. Mucosal involvement of the mouth, vulva and eyes is not uncommon and can cause scarring. Direct IMF studies of skin show linear IgA deposition along the basement membrane.

Treatment is with oral dapsone (50–200 mg daily) or sulphonamides. Many patients show spontaneous resolution after 3–6 years.

Mechanobullous disease (epidermolysis bullosa, 'EB')

Mechanobullous disorders are due to inherited abnormalities in structurally important skin proteins which lead to 'skin fragility'. The resultant blistering tends to arise secondary to trauma and often appears at or shortly after birth. These conditions can be a mild inconvenience, severely disabling or fatal, but fortunately they are very rare. There are three groups of disorders, in which the fundamental gene/protein abnormalities have been characterized. This enables prenatal amniocentesis diagnosis.

Epidermolysis bullosa simplex is a group of autosomal dominant genodermatoses characterized by 'superficial' blistering owing to mutations of cytoskeleton proteins within the basal layer of the epidermis, e.g. mutations of keratin 5 (chromosome 12q) or keratin 14 (chromosome 17q). Most forms of EB simplex show mild disease with intermittent blistering of the hands and feet, especially in hot weather. The teeth and nails are normal and scarring is absent.

Epidermolysis bullosa dystrophica is a group of genodermatoses characterized by 'deeper' blistering associated with scarring and milia formation. The level of split is deep within the basement membrane and is due to mutations in the gene causing a loss of collagen VII in the anchoring fibrils. Nails, mucosae and even the larynx are often involved. The autosomal dominant variety is milder but the autosomal recessive type produces severe disease with disabling scarring, fusion of digits, joint contractures and dysphagia. Life expectancy is significantly reduced. Repeated scarring can result in the development of multiple squamous cell carcinomas.

Junctional epidermolysis bullosa is the most severe form characterized by a split in the lamina lucida of the basement membrane. It is due to mutations in various proteins, mainly laminin 5 but also $\alpha_6\beta_4$ integrin. It presents at birth with widespread blistering and areas of absent skin. Erosions of the central face and hoarseness from laryngeal involvement are common. Nail and teeth abnormalities are also common. Both a lethal and a rarer non-lethal form of junctional EB exist and they show an autosomal recessive inheritance.

INVESTIGATION AND TREATMENT

Investigation and treatment of EB should be carried out in a specialist centre. Diagnosis at birth on clinical grounds is difficult and should be avoided. Exact diagnosis depends on ultrastructural analysis of induced blisters in the skin and immunohistochemistry. Only then can prognosis and genetic counselling be given accurately to parents. Prenatal diagnosis is available for the more severe forms of EB.

FURTHER READING

Wojnarowska F, Briggaman RA (eds) (1990) *Management of Blistering Disease.* London: Chapman & Hall.

Wakelin SH, Black MM (1997) The autoimmune bullous diseases. *Journal of the Royal College of Physicians of London* **31**: 364–368.

Fine JD (1995) Managment of acquired bullous skin disease. *New England Journal of Medicine* **333**: 1475.

Skin tumours

Benign cutaneous tumours

Melanocytic naevi (moles)

Moles are a benign overgrowth of melanocytes that are common in white-skinned people. They appear in childhood and increase in number and size during adolescence and early adult life. They often start as flat brown macules with proliferation of melanocytes at the dermoepidermal junction (junctional naevi). The melanocytes continue to proliferate and grow down into the dermis (compound naevi) which causes an elevation of the mole above the skin surface. The pigmentation is usually even and the border regular. They eventually mature into a dermal naevus (cellular naevus) often with a loss of pigment.

Blue naevus is an acquired asymptomatic blue-looking mole. It is due to a proliferation of melanocytes deep in the mid-dermis.

Basal cell papilloma (seborrhoeic wart)

This is a common benign overgrowth of the basal cell layer of the epidermis. The lesion can be flesh-coloured, brown or even black and often has a greasy appearance. The surface is irregular and warty and the lesions appear very superficial as though stuck on to the skin (Fig 20.28). Tiny keratin cysts may be seen on the surface. They can be treated with cryotherapy or curettage.

Dermatofibroma (histiocytoma)

Dermatofibromas appear as firm, elevated pigmented nodules which may feel like a button in the skin. A peripheral ring of pigmentation is sometimes seen. They are often found on the leg and are most common in females. There may be a preceding history of trauma or insect bite. The lesion consists of histiocytes, blood vessels and varying degrees of fibrosis. If symptomatic, excision is required.

Epidermoid cyst (previously 'sebaceous cyst')

Epidermoid cysts present as cystic swellings of the skin with a central punctum. They contain 'cheesy' keratin rather than sebum; thus the old term 'sebaceous cyst' should be avoided. These cysts occasionally rupture, causing significant dermal inflammation which is not infected.

Pilar cyst (trichilemmal cyst)

Pilar cysts are smooth cysts without a punctum, usually found on the scalp. They may be multiple and familial.

Keratoacanthoma

Keratoacanthomas are rapidly growing epidermal tumours which develop central necrosis and ulceration (Fig 20.29). They occur on sun-exposed skin in later life and can grow up to 2–3 cm across. Whilst they may resolve spontaneously over a few months, they are best excised both to exclude a squamous cell carcinoma (which they can mimic) and to improve the cosmetic outcome.

Pyogenic granuloma (granuloma telangiectaticum)

Pyogenic granulomas are a benign overgrowth of blood vessels. They present as rapidly growing pinkish red nodules which are friable and readily bleed. They may follow trauma and are often found on the fingers and lips. They are best excised to exclude an amelanotic malignant melanoma.

Cherry angioma (Campbell de Morgan spots)

These are benign angiokeratomas that appear as tiny pin-point red papules, especially on the trunk, and increase with age. No treatment is required.

Potentially pre-malignant cutaneous tumours

Solar keratoses (actinic keratoses)

These frequently develop later in life in white-skinned people who have had significant sun exposure. They appear on exposed skin as erythematous silver-scaly papules or patches with a conical surface and a red base (Fig 20.30). The background skin is often inelastic and wrinkled and may show flat brown macules ('liver spots' or lentigos), reflecting diffuse solar damage. A small proportion of these keratoses can transform into squamous cell carcinoma but only after many years.

Treatment of the lesions is with cryotherapy or topical 5-fluorouracil cream.

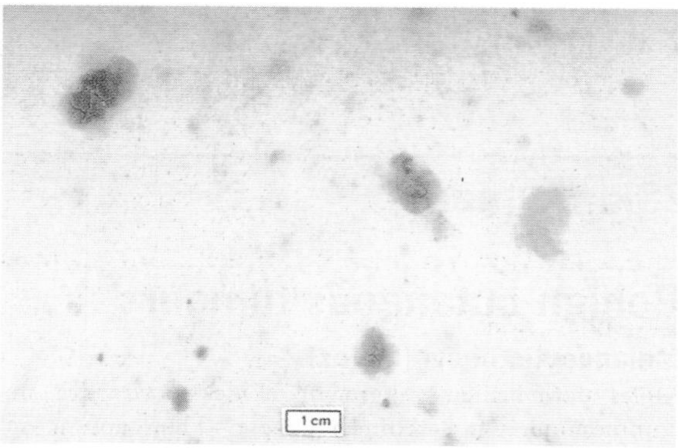

Fig 20.28
Basal cell papilloma

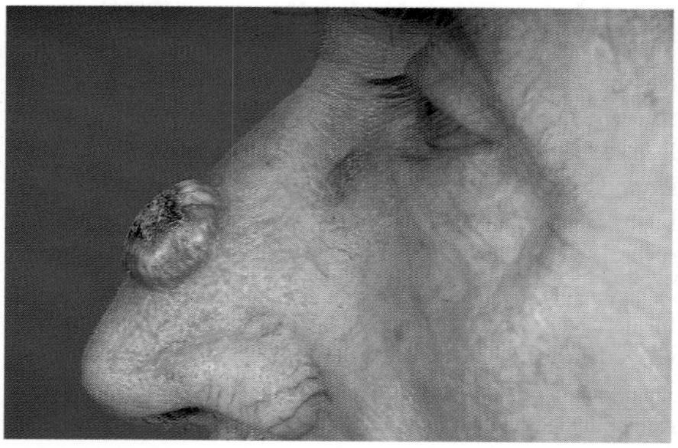

Fig 20.29
Keratoacanthoma

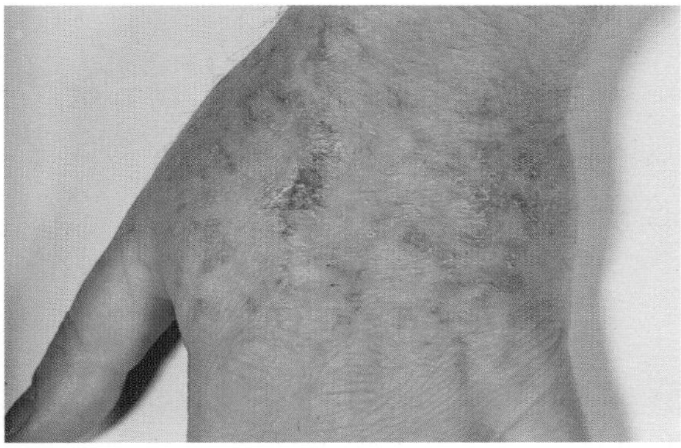

Fig 20.30
Solar keratoses

Bowen's disease

This is a form of intraepidermal carcinoma-in-situ which rarely can become invasive. It presents on exposed skin as an isolated scaly red patch or plaque looking rather like psoriasis, although it has a rather irregular edge. The lesions do not clear but slowly increase in size over the years.

Treatment is with topical 5-fluorouracil, cryotherapy or curettage.

Atypical mole syndrome (dysplastic naevus syndrome)

This is often familial. A large number of melanocytic naevi begin to appear in childhood, even on unexposed sites. Individual lesions may be large with irregular pigmentation and border, and histologically they may look atypical but not frankly malignant. Individuals with this condition have an increased risk of developing malignant melanoma. They should have their moles photographed and be regularly reviewed. Suspicious lesions should be excised.

Giant congenital melanocytic naevi

These are very large moles present at birth. They show an increase risk of developing malignant melanoma. Excision should be considered if it is possible.

Lentigo maligna

This is a slow-growing macular area of pigmentation seen in elderly people, commonly on the face. The border and pigmentation are often irregular. Some people regard this lesion as a melanoma-in-situ. There is an increased risk of developing invasive malignant melanoma. Treatment is by excision if necessary.

Malignant cutaneous tumours

Basal cell carcinoma (rodent ulcer)

Basal cell carcinomas are the most common malignant skin tumour and most relate to excessive sun exposure. They are common later in life on exposed sites although

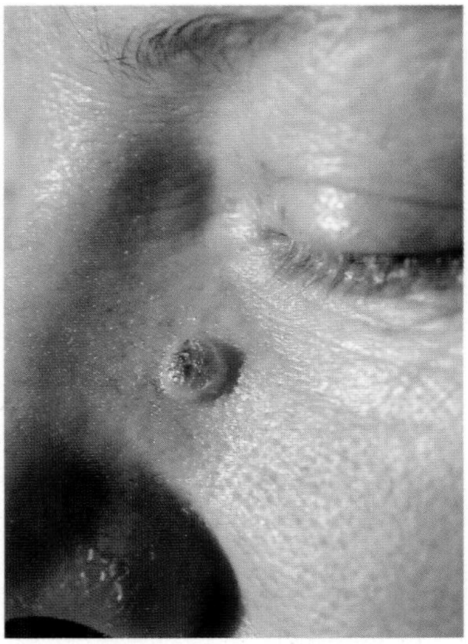

Fig 20.31
Ulcerating basal cell carcinoma

rare on the ear. They can present as a slow-growing papule or nodule (or rarely be cystic) which may go on to ulcerate (Fig 20.31). Telangiectasia over the tumour or a skin-coloured jelly-like 'pearly edge' may be seen. A flat, diffuse superfical form exists ('morphoeic'). The lesion will grow slowly and erode structures if untreated, but these tumours almost never metastisize.

TREATMENT

Treatment is usually with surgical excision, although radiotherapy can be useful for large superficial forms. Curettage is occasionally used in older patients, although not for central facial lesions as they often recur. Very superficial lesions may be treated with cryotherapy, and follow-up is advised.

Squamous cell carcinoma

Squamous cell carcinoma is a somewhat more aggressive skin tumour which can metastasize. Most relate to sun exposure and they can arise in pre-existing solar keratoses or Bowen's disease. They can also arise as a result of chronic inflammation such as in lupus vulgaris. Rarely multiple tumours may arise owing to arsenic ingestion in early life. Multiple tumours also occur in people who have had prolonged periods of immunsuppression, such as renal transplant patients where certain human papilloma virus subtypes may be important in malignant transformation.

They present clinically as fairly rapidly growing nodules which often ulcerate (Fig 20.32). Examination of regional lymph nodes is essential. They are most common on sun-exposed sites in later life. One should have a high index of suspicion for ulcerated lesions on the lower lip or ear.

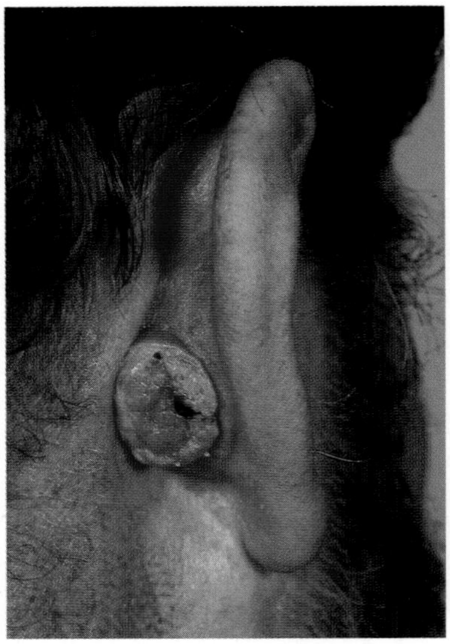

Fig 20.32
Squamous cell carcinoma

TREATMENT
Treatment is with excision or radiotherapy. Curettage should be avoided.

Malignant melanoma

Malignant melanoma is the most serious form of skin cancer as metastasis can occur early, and it causes a number of deaths even in young people. As with other types of skin cancer the incidence is continuing to increase, probably owing to excessive exposure to sunlight. The history of childhood sun exposure and sun burning appears to be particularly important in the development of malignant melanoma. Other risk factors include atypical mole syndrome, giant congenital melanocytic naevi, lentigo maligna and a positive family history of malignant melanoma.

Malignant melanoma is more common in later life but many young adults are also affected. It should always be suspected in rapidly growing or bleeding pigmented lesions. The ABCD criteria (Asymmetry, Border irregularity, Colour variegation, Diameter >6 mm) further help in assessing pigmented lesions. A halo of erythema or the appearance of satellite lesions should also alert the examiner. Clinical diagnois of melanoma is not always easy, but examination with epiluminescence microscopy can further help to distinguish benign from malignant lesions.

Four clinical types exist:

- *Lentigo maligna melanoma* is where a patch of lentigo maligna develops a papule or nodule, signalling invasive tumour.
- *Superficial spreading malignant melanoma* is a large, flat, irregularly pigmented lesion which grows laterally before vertical invasion develops.

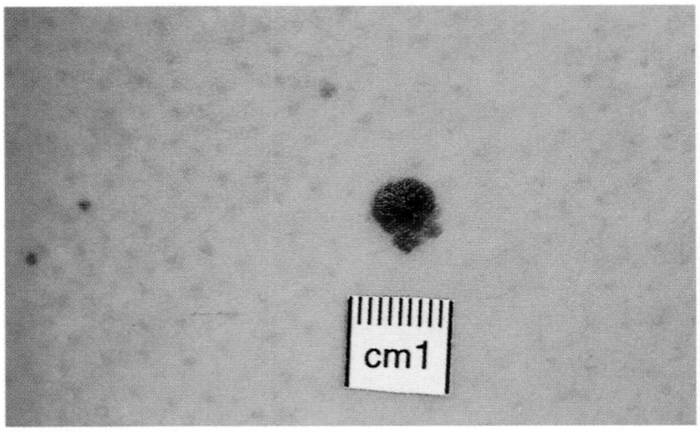

Fig 20.33
Nodular malignant melanoma

- *Nodular malignant melanoma* (Fig 20.33) is the most aggressive type. It presents as rapidly growing pigmented nodules which bleed or ulcerate. Rarely they are amelanotic.
- *Acral lentiginous malignant melanomas* arise as pigmented lesions on the palm, sole or under the nail and they usually present late.

TREATMENT
Treatment consists of urgent wide excision of the lesion. Histological analysis will determine the depth of invasion and the thickness of the tumour. These two factors are important in predicting the prognosis and five-year survival. Excision and histological interpretation should be done only by experts to ensure optimum treatment and assessment of prognosis. Metastatic disease is best managed by an oncologist and can involve surgery to lymph nodes, radiotherapy, immunotherapy and chemotherapy.

The role of governments and medical personnel in public health education to discourage sunbathing and to use sunscreens is of the utmost importance in skin cancer prevention.

Cutaneous T-cell lymphoma (mycosis fungoides)

This is a rare type of skin tumour which often follows a relatively benign course. It presents insidiously with scaly patches and plaques which can look eczematous or psoriasiform. Lesions often appear initially on the buttocks. These lesions may come and go or remain persistent over many years. Patients may well die of unrelated causes. Skin biopsy confirms the diagnosis, showing invasion by atypical lymphocytes. T-cell receptor gene rearrangement studies show that there is often a monoclonal expansion of lymphocytes in the skin.

Occasionally the disease can progress to a cutaneous nodular or tumour stage which may be accompanied by systemic organ involvement. In elderly males the disease may progress rarely to an erythrodermic variant accompanied by lymphadenopathy and peripheral blood involvement ('Sézary syndrome').

TREATMENT

Early disease can be left untreated or be treated with topical steroids or PUVA. More advanced disease may require radiotherapy, chemotherapy, immunotherapy or electron-beam therapy.

Kaposi's sarcoma

This is a tumour of vascular and lymphatic endothelium that presents as purplish nodules and plaques. The 'classic'or 'sporadic' form (as described by Kaposi) occurs in elderly males, especially Jews from eastern Europe. It presents as slow-growing purple tumours on the foot and lower leg which rarely cause any significant problems. The 'endemic' form occurs in males from central Africa and shows more widespread cutaneous involvement as well as lymph node (or occasionally systemic) involvement. Oedema is a prominent feature. Kaposi's sarcoma is also a marker of 'underlying immunosuppression' of any cause but is most common in homosexual patients with HIV infection (see p. 118). Lesions are widespread and often affect the skin, bowel, oral cavity and lungs. Recent research has shown that all three types have a strong association with herpes virus type 8, but other factors must be involved as herpes type 8 occurs in up to 25% of the population of the USA.

TREATMENT

Treatment of advanced Kaposi's sarcoma is with radiotherapy, immunotherapy or chemotherapy.

FURTHER READING

Rees J (1997) Skin cancer. *Journal of the Royal College of Physicians of London* **31**: 246.

Goldberg LH (1996) Malignant tumours. *Lancet* **347**: 663–667.

Marks R (1997) Squamous cell carcinoma. *Lancet* **347**: 735–738.

Rees JL (1997) Skin cancer. In: Scriver CR, Beaudet AL, Sly WS, Valle D (eds), *The Metabolic and Molecular Basis of Inherited Disease*. New York: McGraw-Hill.

Mackie RM (1996) *Skin Cancer*, 2nd edn. London: Martin Dunitz.

White G (1997) *Levene's Color Atlas of Dermatology*, 2nd edn. London: Mosby–Wolfe.

Disorders of blood vessels/lymphatics

Leg ulcers

Leg ulcers are common in the West and can have many causes (Table 20.10). Venous ulcers are the most common type in developing countries.

Table 20.10
Causes of leg ulceration

Venous insufficiency Arterial insufficiency Neuropathic (e.g. diabetes, leprosy) Neoplastic (e.g. squamous or basal cell carcinoma) Vasculitis (e.g. rheumatoid arthritis, SLE, pyoderma gangrenosum)	Infection (e.g. ecthyma, tuberculosis, deep mycoses, tropical ulcer, syphilis, yaws) Haematological (e.g. sickle cell disease, spherocytosis) Other (e.g. necrobiosis lipoidica, trauma, artefact)

Venous ulcers are the result of sustained venous hypertension in the superficial veins, owing to incompetent valves in the deep or perforating veins, or to previous deep vein thrombosis. This increased pressure causes extravasation of fibrinogen through the capillary walls, giving rise to perivascular fibrin deposition, which leads to poor oxygenation of the surrounding skin.

Venous ulcers are common in later life and cause a significant drain on health-care budgets as they are often chronic and recurrent; they affect 1% of the population over the age of 70 years. They are most commonly found on the lower leg in a triangle above the ankles, and may be associated with:

- venous eczema (p. 1164)
- brown pigmentation from haemosiderin
- varicose veins
- lipodermatosclerosis (the combination of induration, reddish brown pigmentation and inflammation)
- scarring white atrophy with telangiectasia (atrophie blanche).

The most important part of treatment is high-compression bandaging and leg elevation to try to decrease the venous hypertension. Doppler studies should always be done before bandaging, to exclude arterial disease. 'Four-layer bandaging' is increasingly popular as this provides high levels of graduated compression up the leg. The choice of ulcer dressing is less important, but one should be chosen to keep the ulcer moist and free of slough and exudate. Up to 80% of ulcers can be healed within 26 weeks. Slower-healing rates occur in patients with decreased mobility and if the ulcers are very large, present for longer than six months or are bilateral. Diuretics are sometimes helpful to reduce the oedema. Antibiotics are necessary only for overt infection.

Venous leg ulcers can be very painful so adequate analgaesia should be given, including opiates if required. Split-thickness skin grafting may be considered in resistant cases. Lifelong support stockings should be worn after healing.

Underlying venous disease is best investigated with duplex ultrasound or plethysmography. Surgery for purely superficial venous disease can occsasionally be useful for ulcer healing but, in general, venous surgery is unhelpful.

Pressure sores (decubitus ulcers)

These occur in elderly, immobile, unconscious or paralysed patients. They are due to skin ischaemia from sustained pressure over a bony joint, most commonly the heel and sacrum. Normal individuals feel the pain of continued pressure, and even during sleep movement takes place to change position continually.

The majority of pressure sores occur in hospital. Seventy per cent appear in the first two weeks of hospitalization, and 70% are in orthopaedic patients, especially those on traction. Between 20% and 30% of pressure sores occur in the community.

Eighty per cent of patients with deep ulcers involving the subcutaneous tissue die in the first four months.

Altered sensation of the skin increases the risk of ulceration, and patients with diseases that affect the circulation and tissue nutrition also are predisposed (e.g. rheumatoid arthritis, diabetes mellitus, peripheral vascular disease). General illness, anaemia, malnutrition and oedema may affect skin breakdown.

Other precipitating factors include anaesthesia, surgery, sedation, dehydration, urinary incontinence or faecal impaction.

The early sign of red/blue discoloration of the skin can lead rapidly to ulcers in 1–2 hours. Leaving patients on hard accident and emergency trolleys, or sitting them in chairs for prolonged periods, must be avoided.

MANAGEMENT

General measures should include identifying at-risk patients. Those with non-fading marking of the skin on pressure sites need immediate attention. The following are used in management:

- bedrest with pillows to keep pressure off bony areas (e.g. pelvis and heels)
- regular turning, but avoid pressure on hips
- fleece over lower one-third of bed for heels
- roto cushions for patients in wheelchairs
- treatment of general condition
- special mattresses and beds to relieve pressure areas
- topical treatment – keep ulcer clean and moist (many topical therapies are harmful)
- pain relief (may need diamorphine)
- plastic surgery.

Arterial ulcers

Arterial ulcers may present as punched-out, painful ischaemic ulcers higher up the leg or on the feet. There may be a history of claudication, hypertension, angina or smoking. Clinically the leg may be cold and show pallor. Absent peripheral pulses, arterial bruits and loss of hair may be present. Doppler ultrasound studies will confirm arterial disease and digital subtraction angiography will further delineate the extent and site of the disease.

Treatment depends on keeping the ulcer clean and covered, adequate analgaesia and vascular reconstruction if appropriate.

Neuropathic ulcers

Neuropathic ulcers tend to be seen over pressure areas of the feet, such as the metatarsal heads, owing to repeated trauma. These are most commonly seen in diabetics as a result of polyneuropathy. In developing countries leprosy is a common cause.

Treatment consists of keeping the ulcer clean and removing pressure or trauma from the affected area. Diabetics should pay particular attention to footcare and correctly fitting shoes.

Vasculitis (see also p. 493)

Vasculitis is the term applied to an inflammatory disorder of blood vessels which causes endothelial damage. It can be confirmed by skin biopsy. The classification used here (Table 20.11) depends more on the site of the vessel involved than on its size. An alternative classification, depending on size, is shown in Tables 8.19 and 8.20.

The cutaneous features are of haemorrhagic papules, pustules, nodules or plaques which may erode and ulcerate. These purpuric lesions do not blanche with pressure. Occasionally a fixed livedo reticularis pattern may appear which does not disappear on warming. Pyrexia and arthralgia are common associations even in the absence of significant systemic involvement. Other clinical features depend on the underlying cause.

Table 20.11
A classification of vasculitis

Necrotizing venulitis
Septic vasculitis (*Streptococcus*, hepatitis B, dental abscess)
Allergic 'leucocytoclastic' vasculitis (including Henoch–Schönlein purpura)
Connective tissue disease (e.g. SLE, rheumatoid arthritis)
Urticarial vasculitis
Necrotizing arteritis
Polyarteritis nodosa (classic and microscopic variants)
Granulomatous vasculitis
Wegener's granulomatosis
Churg–Strauss disease
Giant cell arteritis
'Occlusion'
Cryoglobulinaemia (lymphoma, hepatitis C)
Dysproteinaemia (Waldenström's macroglobulinaemia)
Anti-phospholipid syndrome

The most common cutaneous vasculitis is leucocytoclastic vasculitis which usually appears on the lower legs as a symmetrical palpable purpura. It is rarely associated with systemic involvement. This can be caused by drugs or infection but often no cause is found. Whilst it often settles spontaneously, treatment with analgesia, support stockings, dapsone or prednisolone may be needed to control the pain and to heal any ulceration.

Klippel–Trenauney–Weber syndrome

This refers to a rare condition in which there is an extensive vascular malformation of a limb with both deep and superficial involvement. There is a mixture of capillary and cavernous haemangiomas. There may be an underlying arteriovenous malformation which can cause faster growth of the affected limb. The growth may also be increased by local production of growth factors in the affected limb.

Lymphatics

Lymphoedema

Lymphoedema refers to a chronic non-pitting oedema due to lymphatic insufficiency. It is most commonly seen affecting the legs and tends to progress with age. The legs can become enormous and prevent wearing of normal shoes. Chronic disease may cause a secondary 'cobblestone' thickening of the skin. Lymphoedema can be primary (and present early in life) due to an inherited deficiency of lymphatic vessels (e.g. Milroys disease) or can be secondary due to obstruction of lymphatic vessels (e.g. filarial infection or malignant disease).

Treatment is with compression stockings and physical massage. If there is recurrent cellulitis, long-term antibiotics are advisable as each episode of cellulitis will further damage the lymph vessels. Surgery should be avoided.

Lymphangioma circumscriptum

This is a rare hamartoma of lymphatic tissue. It usually presents in childhood with multiple small vesicles in the skin which weep lymphatic fluid and sometimes blood. They reflect deeper vessel involvement so surgery should be avoided. Cryotherapy or CO_2 laser treatment may help the superficial lesions.

FURTHER READING

Jeanette CJ, Falk RJ (1997) Small vessel vasculitis. *New England Journal of Medicine* **337**: 1512–1523.

Disorders of collagen and elastic tissue

Lichen sclerosus et atrophicus

Lichen sclerosus et atrophicus is an inflammatory dermatosis that occurs in all age groups and particulary affects the anogenital region. It is more common in females. It presents with atrophic ivory-white macules with a well-defined edge on the vulva, glans penis, foreskin or perianal skin. Telangiectasia may be seen over the surface. Occasionally lesions involve the shaft of the penis and the urethral meatus. Lesions are often itchy but may be sore at times. Longstanding vulval lesions may be associated with fissuring and a marked loss of architecture, especially of the clitoral hood and the labium minora, which may become fused. Early lesions in young girls may present as haemorrhagic blisters and these are occasionally mistaken as signs of sexual abuse. Involvement of the foreskin can cause phimosis, and urethral disease may interfere with micturition. Perianal lesions may fissure and cause constipation.

Lichen sclerosus can affect non-genital skin, but this is most common in females and clinically it may show rather more hyperkeratosis and follicular plugging than is seen in the anogenital region.

If the clinical picture is unclear, diagnosis may require biopsy to exclude genital lichen planus and extramammary Paget's disease. Vulval scarring can also occur with cicatricial pemphigoid (a localized variant of pemphigoid affecting mucosal surfaces), so occasionally immunofluorescence studies may be needed.

Treatment with very potent topical steroids helps control the symptoms. Hydroxychloroquine (200 mg twice daily) helps resistant cases. The condition may burn itself out after many years, especially in children. There is a risk of developing squamous cell carcinoma in longstanding lesions.

Ehlers–Danlos syndrome (see also p. 518)

Ehlers–Danlos syndrome can be subdivided into at least ten variants. They are all inherited disorders causing abnormalities in collagen of the skin, joints and blood vessels. Clinically this causes increased elasticity of the skin, hypermobile joints and fragile blood vessels, causing easy bruising. The skin is velvety to the touch and hyperextensible, but recoils normally on stretching. It is easily injured and heals slowly with scarring like tissue-paper. Pseudotumours may occur over elbows and knees, consisting mainly of fat, but calcification can occur.

Pseudoxanthoma elasticum

Pseudoxanthoma elasticum is a rare group of disorders characterized by abnormalities in collagen and elastic tissue affecting the skin, eye and blood vessels. The skin may be loose, lax and wrinkled. It can look yellowish and papular ('plucked chicken skin') and tends to lose its elastic recoil. Skin changes are best seen in the flexures, especially the sides of the neck. Non-cutaneous features include recurrent gastrointestinal bleeding, early myocardial infarction, claudication and angioid streaks on the retina reflecting disruption of vascular elastic tissue.

Marfan's syndrome (see also p. 518)

Marfan's syndrome is an autosomal dominant disorder of connective tissue. The basic genetic defect is a mutation in the extracellular matrix glycoprotein fibrillin. The syndrome is characterized by tall stature and long thin digits (arachnodactyly). The arm span can exceed the height of the patient and a high arched palate may be present. Lax ligaments result in frequent dislocation of joints. Inguinal and femoral hernias are common. Pulmonary changes include emphysema, diaphragmatic hernia and spontaneous pneumothorax. Degeneration of the media of blood vessels can lead to cardiovascular complications such as aortic and mitral incompetence and aortic aneurysm, and this is a common cause of death in these patients. Dislocation of the ocular lens is common. Skin changes are usually absent but striae may develop. Patients with homocystinuria (see Table 17.14) have similar features.

Striae

Striae are visible linear scars caused by dermal collagen damage and stretching. Histologically a thinned epidermis overlies parallel bundles of fine collagen. They occur commonly over the abdomen and breasts in pregnancy, but also occur on the thighs and trunk in rapidly growing adolescents as well as in some obese individuals. They are also seen in Cushing's syndrome and with corticosteroid therapy. Striae are initially reddish blue but fade to white atrophic marks. Puberty-related striae normally disappear completely.

Keloid scars

Keloid scars are characterized by smooth hard nodules caused by excessive collagen production. They may occur spontaneously or follow skin trauma/surgery, and they are often itchy. They tend to affect young adults and are much commoner in Africans. Sites of predilection include the shoulder, upper back and chest, earlobes and the chin. Unlike hypertrophic scars (which fade within 12 months) keloids are persistent and may continue to enlarge. Treatment is with triamcinolone injection, compression with silica gels or surgery, but the latter must be followed by steroid injection or superficial radiotherapy or it may make the problem worse.

FURTHER READING

Leibowitch M, Staughton R, Neill S, Bowen S, Marwood R (1995) *An Atlas of Vulval Disease*. London: Martin Dunitz.

Royce PM, Steinmann B (eds) (1993) *Connective Tissue and its Heritable Disorders*. New York: Wiley–Liss.

Disorders of pigmentation

Hypopigmentation

Vitiligo

Vitiligo is a common disorder of depigmentation which probably has an autoimmune aetiology. Sufferers often have relatives with other organ-specific autoimmune disorders. It presents in childhood or early adult life with well-demarcated macules of complete pigment loss. There is no history of preceding inflammation. Patients are very susceptible to sunburn. Lesions are often symmetrical and frequently involve the face, hands and genitalia (Fig 20.34). The hair can also depigment. Trauma may induce new lesions. Spontaneous repigmentation can occur and often starts around hair follicles, giving a speckled appearance. However, repigmentation is rare if a lesion has persisted for more than a year. The psychological consequences of vitiligo can be devastating, especially in Asian or African people.

Treatment is very unsatisfactory and has no impact on the long-term outcome. Sunblocks should be used to prevent burning. Potent topical steroids or PUVA therapy may help some individuals. If vitiligo is almost universal, depigmentation may be considered as a treatment. Finally, referral to a specialist camouflage clinic can be useful.

Post-inflammatory hypopigmentation

This is probably one of the most common causes of pale skin. It is much more common in people with pigmented skin. It may be seen as a consequence of eczema, acne or psoriasis and may even be the reason for individuals presenting to a doctor. Provided the skin disease is controlled the pigmentation will recover slowly after many months. Post-inflammatory hyperpigmentation can also occur.

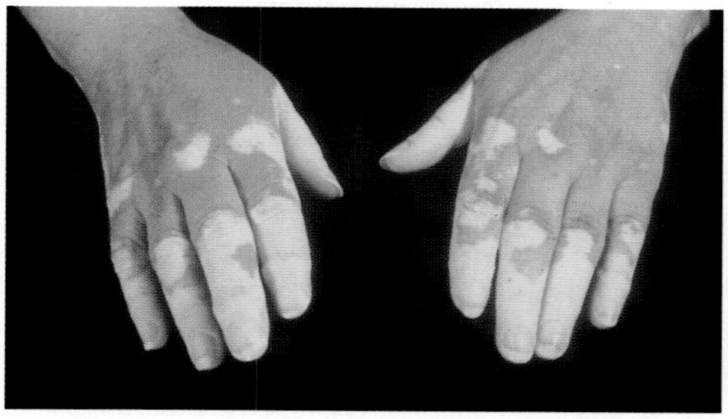

Fig 20.34
Vitiligo of the hands

Oculocutaneous albinism

This is a group of rare autosomal recessive disorders affecting the pigmentation of skin, hair and eyes. It can affect all races. Melanocytes are in normal number but have abnormal function. Clinically it presents with universal pale skin, white or yellow hair and a pinkish iris. Photophobia, nystagmus and a squint are also present in most cases.

Treatment involves obsessive protection against sunlight to avoid sunburning and the development of skin cancer.

Idiopathic guttate hypomelanosis

This occurs most commonly in African people and is of unknown aetiology. It presents with small (2–4 mm) asymptomatic porcelain-white macules, often on skin exposed to sunlight. The borders are often sharply defined and angular. There is no effective treatment.

Leprosy (see also p. 41)

Both tuberculoid leprosy and indeterminate leprosy can present with anaesthetic patches of depigmentation and should always be considered in people from endemic regions.

Hyperpigmentation

Freckles (ephelides)

These appear in childhood as small brown macules after sun exposure. They fade in the winter months.

Lentigos

These are a more permanent macule of pigmentation similar to freckles but they tend to persist in the winter. Solar lentigos (also called 'liver spots') occur in older people on exposed skin owing to actinic damage.

Chloasma

These are brown macules often seen symmetrically over the cheeks and forehead and are most common in women. It can occur spontaneously but it is also associated with pregnancy and the oral contraceptive pill.

Metabolic/endocrine effects

A generalized skin darkening can occur with chronic liver disease, especially hereditary haemochromatosis. It is also sometimes seen in Cushing's syndrome, Addison's disease (more marked in palmar creases and buccal mucosa) and Nelson's syndrome.

Peutz–Jegher syndrome (p. 260)

This presents with brown macules of the lips and perioral region. It is associated with gastrointestinal polyposis, which virtually never becomes malignant.

Urticaria pigmentosa (cutaneous mastocytosis)

This presents most commonly with multiple pigmented macules in children. These lesions tend to become red, itchy and urticated if they are rubbed (Darier's sign). Occasionally lesions may blister and in the rare congenital form of the disease the skin may become thickened and leathery. Skin biopsy shows an excess of mast cells in the skin. Occasionally systemic symptoms are present such as wheeze, flushing, syncope or diarrhoea, reflecting extensive mast cell degranulation from the skin. Anaphylaxis occurs very rarely and may be precipitated by mast cell degranulators such as aspirin or opiates. The condition resolves spontaneously after some years in children but is persistent in adults.

Rarely there may be infiltration of internal organs with mast cells (*systemic mastocytosis*), especially in adult disease. This can involve any organ but especially the bone (where it can cause severe pain), gastrointestinal tract, liver and spleen. There is a risk of developing leukaemia if the bone marrow is heavily infiltrated.

FURTHER READING

Levine N (ed) (1993) *Pigmentation and Pigmentary Disorders.* Florida: CRC Press.

Drug-induced rashes

Drugs can be toxic and teratogenic but they can also cause problems through allergic reactions. This frequently presents in the skin where just about any type of skin rash can arise (Table 20.12), although a widespread symmetrical maculopapular rash is the most common type (Fig 20.35).

Table 20.12
Morphological types of drug rashes and some common causes

Maculopapular	Penicillins
Urticaria	Penicillins, aspirin
Vasculitis	Gold, hydralazine
Fixed drug rash	Phenolphthalein in laxatives, tetracyclines, paracetamol
Pigmentation	Minocycline (black), amiodarone (slate grey)
Lupus erythematosus	Penicillamine, isoniazid
Photosensitivity	Thiazides, chlopromazine, sulphonamides, amiodarone
Pustular	Carbamazepine
Erythema nodosum	Sulphonamides, oral contraceptives
Erythema multiforme	Barbiturates
Acneiform	Corticosteroids
Lichenoid	Chloroquine, thiazides, gold
Psoriasiform	Methyldopa, gold
Toxic epidermal necrolysis	Penicillins, cotrimoxazole, carbamazepine, NSAIDs
Pemphigus	Penicillamine, ACE inhibitors
Erythroderma	Gold, sulphonylureas, allopurinol

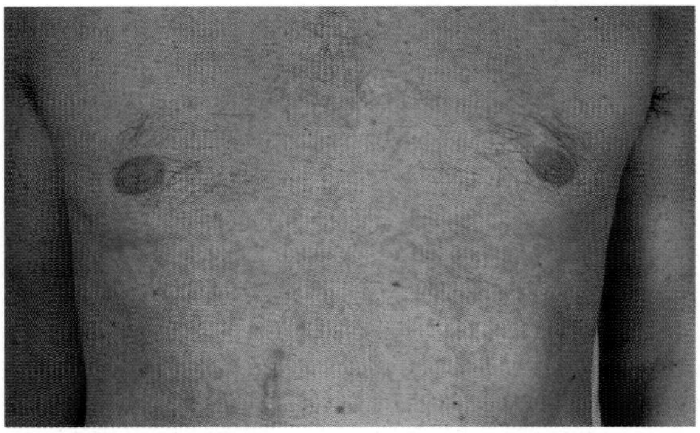

Fig 20.35
Morbilliform drug rash, due to penicillin allergy

'Fixed drug eruptions' may occur where a rash evolves and resolves at a specific site. The rash is reproduced at exactly the same site after a repeated exposure.

Taking a thorough history is of much greater value than any laboratory investigations in assessing drug reactions. A drug cause for any skin condition should always be suspected. The use of prick-testing and patch-testing is rarely helpful and not without risk. Drug allergy can be proven only by rechallenging, but this is rarely justified as it carries some risks. Rechallenging is occasionally justified for antituberculosis drugs or antiretroviral drugs, but it should be carried out as an inpatient as there is a risk of anaphylaxis. Certain individuals (e.g. those with HIV infection) are more susceptible to drug rashes (Fig 20.36).

Most rashes will settle spontaneously once the offending agent is removed. The two most serious types of drug rash are *erythroderma* (see p. 1173) and toxic *epidermal necrolysis*. The latter is characterized by a widespread subepidermal blistering and sloughing of most of the skin. The internal epithelial surfaces (lung, bladder, gastrointestinal tract) are also involved. Multiorgan failure and sepsis often occurs. Toxic epidermal necrolysis can be fatal even after drug withdrawal and intensive care support.

There is no specific treatment, but cyclosporin is currently under assessment. A milder variant exists called *Stevens Johnson syndrome* where the damage is restricted to the skin and mucosal surfaces.

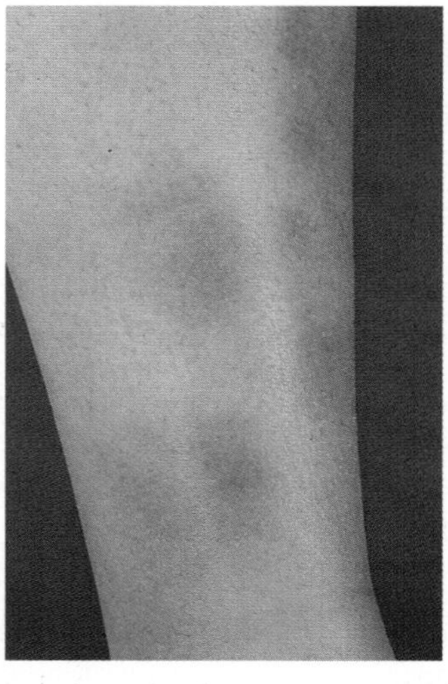

Fig 20.36
Erythema nodosum in a patient on cotrimoxazole with HIV

FURTHER READING

Breathnach SM, Hintner H (1992) *Adverse Drug Reactions and the Skin*. Oxford: Blackwell Scientific.

Becker DS (1998) Toxic epidermal necrolysis. *Lancet* **351**: 1417–1420.

Disorders of nails

Psoriasis and fungal nail infection are the most common causes of nail dystrophy and are discussed on p. 1157 and p. 1166).

- *Nail pitting* can be caused by psoriasis, alopecia areata and atopic eczema. A few pits can be present due to trauma.
- *Onycholysis* (distal nail-plate separation) is caused by psoriasis, thyrotoxicosis, following trauma and rarely is due to a photosensitive reaction to drugs such as tetracyclines.
- *Koilonychia* (thin spoon-shaped nails) can be caused by iron-deficiency anaemia or rarely is congenital.
- *Leuconychia* (white nails) is seen in hypoalbuminaemia. A striate congenital leuconychia exists.
- *Beau's lines* (transverse lines) appear as solitary depressions which grow out slowly over many months. They arise from a severe illness or shock which causes a temporary arrest in nail growth.
- *Yellow-nail syndrome* is a rare disorder of lymphatic drainage. It presents with thickened, slow-growing, yellow nails which may be associated with pleural effusions, bronchiectasis and lymphoedema of the legs.
- *Onychogryphosis* is a gross thickening of the nail which is seen in later life, especially in the great toe-nail. There is often a history of preceding trauma. Both psoriasis and fungal infection can also cause nail thickening.
- *Nail-patella syndrome* is an autosomal dominant condition which presents with triangular rather than half-moon shaped lunulae, especially of the thumb and forefingers. The nail-plates may be small or dystrophic. The patellae are hypoplastic or absent. Other skeletal anomalies may be present, and renal impairment (glomerulonephritis) occurs in up to 30% of individuals.
- *Longitudinal brown streaks* (melanonychia) may be seen as a normal variant in black-skinned patients. In a white patient it may reflect an underlying subungual melanoma.
- *Clubbing* is discussed on p. 758.

Table 20.13
Causes of alopecia

Scarring alopecia	Non-scarring alopecia
Discoid lupus erythematosus	Androgenic alopecia
Kerion (tinea capitis)	Telogen effluvium
Lichen planus	Alopecia areata
Dissecting cellulitis	Trichotillomania (self-induced hair-pulling)
X-irradiation	Tinea capitis
Idiopathic ('pseudopelade')	Traction alopecia
	Metabolic (iron deficiency, hypothyroidism)
	Drug (e.g. heparin, isotretinoin, chemotherapy)

FURTHER READING

Baran R, Dawber RPR (eds) (1994) *Diseases of the Nails and their Management*, 2nd edn. Oxford: Blackwell Scientific.

Disorders of hair

Hair loss

Hair loss can be due to a disorder of the hair follicle in which the scalp skin looks normal (non-scarring alopecia) or due to a disorder within the scalp skin that causes permanent loss of the follicle (scarring or cicatricial alopecia). This latter form causes shiny atrophic bald areas in the scalp which are devoid of follicular openings. There are many causes of alopecia to consider (Table 20.13)

Androgenic alopecia

Androgenic alopecia (male pattern baldness) is the most common type of non-scarring hair loss and depends on genetic factors and an abnormal sensitivity to androgens. It presents in young men with frontal receding followed by thinning of the crown, and there is often a positive family history. It also occurs in females but tends to occur at a later age, be milder and show little in the way of frontal recession. If acne and menstrual disturbance are also present one should consider polycystic ovary syndrome and other endocrine disorders of androgens.

Treatment

Treatment may not be required. Topical 2% minoxidil lotion can help in up to a third of cases but must be used lifelong to maintain the benefit. The cosmetic improvement is, however, seldom perfect. In females, anti-androgen therapy (e.g. cyproterone acetate or spironolactone) may help some individuals. Low-dose oral finasteride is currently under trial in males in the USA.

Alopecia areata

Alopecia areata may be regarded as an immune mediated type of hair loss. It may be associated with other organ-specific autoimmune diseases. It presents in childhood or young adults with complete circles of baldness. These may regrow to be followed by new patches of hair loss. The presence of broken exclamation mark hairs (narrow at the scalp/wider and more pigmented at the tip) at the edge of a bald area is diagnostic. Regrowth may initially be with white hairs and often occurs slowly over months. Occasionally all the scalp hair is lost (alopecia totalis) and rarely all body hair is lost (alopecia universalis). The nails may be pitted or roughened.

Treatment

Treatment is poor and has no effect on the long-term progression. Potent topical or injected steroids may be of limited use. Wigs can be provided for severe cases and patient support groups are often beneficial.

Traction alopecia

This refers to the 'mechanical damage' type of hair loss that arises from pulling the hair back into a bun or tight plaiting. It is more common in Africans.

Telogen effluvium

Telogen effluvium refers to the pattern of diffuse hair loss that occurs some three months after pregnancy or a severe illness. It occurs because the 'stress' puts all the hairs into the telogen phase of hair shedding at the same time. The hair fully recovers and the normal staggered hair growth/hair shedding cycle resumes.

Dissecting cellulitis

This is a chronic folliculitis affecting predominantly young black males. It presents with papules and pustules over the occipital region of the scalp with hair loss. If severe, the back of the scalp becomes a boggy swelling (disharging pus) with areas of scarring alopecia. It can be complicated by keloid scar formation (acne keloidalis nuchae).

Treatment

Treatment is difficult as antibiotics are rarely useful except in acute inflammatory episodes. Prolonged courses of isotretinoin can help, and deep surgical excision with grafting can be used in recalcitrant cases.

Increased hair growth

Hirsutism (p. 918)

Hirsutism refers to the male pattern of hair growth seen in females. The racial variation in hair growth must be considered. Certain races (e.g. Mediterranean and Asian) have more male pattern hair growth than northern European females. This is not due to excess androgens but may reflect a genetically determined altered sensitivity to them. If acne and menstrual disturbance are present one should consider a full endocrine assesment. Hirsutism can cause severe psychological distress to some individuals.

Treatment involves physical methods such as bleaching, waxing, electrolysis and ruby laser therapy. Antiandrogen therapy is occasionally helpful.

Hypertrichosis

Hypertrichosis refers to the state of excessive hair growth at any site and occurs in both sexes. It can be seen in anorexia nervosa, porphyria cutanea tarda, and underlying malignancy. It is also caused by certain drugs (e.g. cyclosporin, minoxidil).

FURTHER READING

Dawber R, Van Neste D (1995) *Hair and Scalp Disorders.* London: Martin Dunitz.

Birth marks/neonatal rashes

Strawberry naevus (cavernous haemangioma)

Strawberry naevus affects up to 1% of infants. It presents at, or shortly after, birth as a single red lumpy nodule that grows rapidly for the first few months. Multiple lesions can be present. They will resolve spontaneously with good cosmetic appearance, but this may take up to seven years for complete resolution. Occasionally plastic surgery is needed after resolution to remove residual slack skin. Reassurance of parents is usually all that is required.

Treatment is indicated if:

- the lesion interferes with feeding or vision
- the lesion ulcerates and bleeds frequently
- there is a large lesion on the lip or the tip of the nose, as they resolve slowly and often only partially (such visible lesions lead to teasing at school)
- the lesion is associated with high-output cardiac failure from shunting of large volumes of blood
- the lesion consumes platelets and/or clotting factors causing potentially life-threatening haemorrhage ('Kasabach–Merritt syndrome').

The latter two complications are very rare and tend to occur only in large lesions with significant deep vessel involvement.

Treatment modalities include intralesional or oral corticosteroids, surgery (for selected lesions), tunable dye laser (for treating ulceration) and embolization (for life-threatening events only).

Port-wine stain (naevus flammeus)

Port-wine stain is also called a capillary haemangioma, but strictly speaking it is not a haemangioma but is just an abnormal dilation of dermal capillaries. It presents at birth as a flat red macular area and is commonly found on the face. It does not improve spontaneously and it may become thickened with time. If the lesion is found in the disribution of the first division of the trigemminal nerve it may be associated with ipsilateral meningeal vascular anomalies which can cause epilepsy and even hemiplegia (Sturge–Weber syndrome). If a port-wine stain involves the skin near the eye, glaucoma is a risk and ophthalmic assessment is mandatory.

Treatment of port-wine stains is ideally with the tunable dye laser.

Milia

'Milk spots' are small follicular epidermal cysts. They are small pinhead white papules commonly found on the face of infants. They resolve spontaneously.

Mongolian blue spot

This appears in infants as a deep blue-grey bruise-like area over the sacrum or back and is occasionally mistaken as a sign of child abuse. It is due to deep dermal melanocytes. It is very common in Mongoloids (East Asians), less common in Africans and rare in Caucasians. It has usually disappeared by the age of seven years.

Toxic erythema of the newborn (erythema neonatorum)

Toxic erythema of the newborn is a term used to describe a common transient blotchy maculopapular rash in newborns. The rash is occasionally pustular but the child is not toxic or unwell. It disappears within a few days, spontaneously.

Nappy rash ('diaper dermatitis')

This is an irritant eczema caused by occlusion of faeces and urine against the skin. It is almost universal in babies. The flexures are usually spared, which is a useful differentiating feature from seborrhoeic and atopic eczema. Satellite lesions around the edge may indicate a superimposed *Candida* infection.

Treatment involves frequent changing of the nappy and regular application of a barrier cream.

Acrodermatitis enteropathica (p. 206)

This is caused by a rare inherited deficiency of zinc absorption. It presents 4–6 weeks after weaning, or earlier in bottle-fed babies. There is an erythematous, sometimes blistering, rash around the perineum, mouth, hands and feet. It is associated with photophobia, diarrhoea and alopecia.

Treatment is with oral zinc, which seems to override the poor absorption. The response is rapid.

FURTHER READING

Hurwitz S (1993) *Clinical Pediatric Dermatology*, 2nd edn. Philadelphia: WB Saunders.

Weinberg S, Prose NS, Kristal L (1998) *Colour Atlas of Pediatric Dermatology*, 3rd edn. New York: McGraw Hill.

Human immunodeficiency virus and the skin (p. 116)

HIV infection commonly causes significant dermatological problems. A rash may even be the presenting feature of underlying HIV infection. It is estimated that 90% of HIV-positive patients will suffer with a mucocutaneous disorder during the illness. It is also estimated that up to 30% of people with AIDS will suffer from three different dermatoses. These rashes can often be clinically atypical and difficult to diagnose. One must have a low threshold for skin biopsy and skin culture. On top of this many of the skin problems are resistant to standard treatments. The dermatoses may be arbitarily divided into six groups:

Cutaneous infection and opportunistic infection

Not surprisingly, infections are increased owing to the HIV-induced immune deficiency. Molluscum contagiosum are particularly common, especially on the face. They are often multiple and of a 'giant' size measuring over 1 cm across. Molluscum are rarely seen in adults and they can be the presenting feature of HIV. Other viral infections such as extensive ulcerative herpes or widespread viral warts may be seen. Bacterial infections (e.g. staphylococcal boils) and fungal infections (e.g. ringworm and *Candida*) are also common. Recalcitrant and recurrent oropharyngeal candidiasis is a particular problem.

Opportunistic infections such as cutaneous cytomegalovirus (pustules or necrotic ulcers), sporotrichosis (linear nodules) or cryptococcus (red papules, psoriasiform or molluscum-like lesions) can pose diagnostic difficulties, stressing the need for skin biopsy and culture.

Inflammatory dermatoses

Inflammatory dermatoses show an increased incidence with HIV infection, probably owing to an immune dysfunction or imbalance rather than as a consequence of immune suppression. Severe seborrhoeic eczema is very common and may be a presenting sign of HIV. Other types of eczema, psoriasis, ichthyosis (dry scaly skin), nodular prurigo and pruritus are all common in HIV infection and can be very severe. Granuloma annulare and lichen planus are probably increased in incidence. The treatment of these conditions is difficult as oral immunosuppressive therapies (e.g. prednisolone, cyclosporin) are best avoided. Topical therapies and phototherapy seem relatively safe. Oral retinoids are useful in the management of psoriasis. Antiretroviral therapy (reverse transcriptase inhibitors and protease inhibitors) often helps these conditions, presumably due to a restoration of immune function.

'Autoimmune dermatoses'

Bullous pemphigoid, thrombocytopenic purpura, and vitiligo seem to be increased in incidence. The polyclonal stimulation of B-lymphocytes by HIV and the resulting abnormal antibody production may be important in their aetiology. Erythroderma is sometimes seen in HIV disease where skin biopsy suggests a 'graft-versus-host disease' mechanism. This presumably reflects a severe underlying immune dysfunction.

Drug rashes

Adverse drug rashes are much more common in patients with HIV infection. Reactions to cotrimoxazole and dapsone (used in *Pneumocystis carinii* pneumonia prophylaxis) appear particularly common. Drug rashes may be severe, resulting in erythroderma or toxic epidermal necrolysis.

Cutaneous tumours

Kaposi's sarcoma (see p. 1185) may present with purplish nodules and plaques in the skin and on the oral and genital mucosa. It is much more common in homosexuals with HIV than in other groups. Basal and squamous cell carcinomas and benign melanocytic naevi are also increased in incidence, presumably reflecting a loss of immune surveillance.

'Specific' HIV dermatoses

Papular pruritic eruption of HIV (itchy folliculitis)

This is common as CD4 counts decline. The previously described staphylococcal folliculitis, eosinophilic folliculitis, pityrosporum folliculitis, and demodex mite folliculitis are probably all part of a spectrum. The authors prefer the unifying term 'papular pruritic eruption' of HIV. It presents with intensely itchy papules centred on hair follicles and occurring over the upper trunk and upper arms. Individual lesions frequently have the top scratched off, leaving a crateriform appearance.

The aetiology is unknown but may reflect a hypersensitivity reaction as high IgE and eosinophil counts may be present.

Treatment with oral minocyclin, topical steroids and emollients may help. Phototherapy is useful in resistant cases.

Oral hairy leucoplakia

This is characterized by white plaques with vertical ridging on the sides of the tongue. Unlike with oral *Candida*, the lesions cannot be peeled off to leave raw areas underneath. It was first recognized in HIV disease but can rarely occur in other forms of immunsuppression. It is thought to be due to co-infection with Epstein–Barr virus.

Treatment with acyclovir, gancyclovir or foscarnet may help.

FURTHER READING

Penneys NS (1995) *Skin Manifestations of AIDS*, 2nd edn. London: Martin Dunitz.

Dermatoses of pregnancy

There are a number of minor skin changes during pregnancy. There is an increase in spider naevi, melanocytic naevi, skin tags and chloasma. The abdomen shows mid-line pigmentation (linea nigra) and striae (stretch marks). There are, however, four less common skin problems associated with pregnancy.

Polymorphic eruption of pregnancy (PEP)

This rash tends to appear in the last trimester of a first pregnancy in 1 in 160 cases. It is of unknown aetiology and recurs only rarely in subsequent pregnancies. It presents with very itchy urticated papules and plaques and occasionally small vesicles. Lesions usually start on the abdomen and striae but may spread to the upper arms and thighs. The umbilicus may be spared. PEP is more common in twin pregnancies.

The rash is not associated with any maternal or fetal risk. *Treatment* is with reassurance, bland emollients and mild topical steroids. The rash disappears after childbirth.

Prurigo of pregnancy

This affects 1 in 300 pregnancies. It usually starts on the abdomen in the third trimester but may persist for some months after delivery. Clustered excoriated papules (prurigo-like lesions) occur on the abdomen and extensor surfaces of the limbs. The cause is unknown but pregnancy-related itch (pruritus gravidarum) may be due to cholestasis (p. 333). Rarely liver biochemical tests are abnormal and urinary HCG levels may be elevated. It can recur in subsequent pregnancies. Some authors believe the condition is associated with an increase in fetal mortality, but this remains controversial.

Treatment is with topical steroids and oral antihistamines.

Pruritic folliculitis of pregnancy

This may occur in the second or third trimester of pregnancy and is characterized by an itchy folliculitis which looks similar to steroid-induced 'acne'.

Treatment with topical benzoyl peroxide and hydrocortisone cream help relieve the symptoms.

Pemphigoid gestationis (herpes gestationis)

This is the rarest of the pregnancy related rashes (1 in 60 000). The immune changes of pregnancy appear to set off pemphigoid. It is characterized by an itchy blistering urticated eruption starting on the abdomen but may become widespread. Large bullae may be present. Unlike PEP it can occur early, starting in the second or even first trimester of pregnancy and the umbilicus is often involved. It tends to recur in subsequent pregnancies and at an earlier stage. Diagnosis is confirmed by immunfluorescence studies.

A transient bullous eruption occurs in 5% of infants, presumably due to transplacental passage of the offending antibody. There is no increase in fetal mortality, but there is an increased incidence of prematurity and low birthweight, which is probably due to the autoantibody causing placental insufficiency. Therefore, it seems sensible to keep such pregnancies closely monitored and to advise on hospital rather than home delivery.

Treatment of mild cases is with potent topical steroids, but most cases will require oral corticosteroids. The steroid dose may need to be increased after delivery as there is often a post-partum flare-up of the disease. The rash can be set off again by the oral contraceptive pill, which should be avoided.

FURTHER READING

Holmes RC et al (1983) The specific dermatoses of pregnancy. *Journal of the American Academy of Dermatology* **8**: 405–412.

Principles of topical therapy

Dermatology is unique in having such direct accessibility to the affected organ. This allows the use of topical treatments which can avoid certain systemic side-effects.

A topical therapy consists of an *active ingredient*, an appropriate *vehicle* or *base* to deliver this, and often a *preservative* or *stabilizer* to maintain the product's shelf-life. It is important to find a cosmetically acceptable product and to instruct patients about correct usage. Without this, compliance tends to be poor. Perfumed or scented products should be avoided.

Table 20.14
Emollients commonly used in the UK

Greasy emollients	Lighter creams
Diprobase ointment*	E45 cream*
Oily cream	Diprobase cream*
Unguentum Merck*	Aveeno cream*
50:50 white soft paraffin/liquid paraffin	Aqueous cream

*Trade names

Bases and their uses

Creams

These are a semisolid mixture of oil and water held together by an emulsifying agent. They need to have added preservatives such as parabens. They are 'lighter' and rub in more easily than ointments. They have a high cosmetic acceptibility and are useful for topical treatments of the face and hands. Aqueous cream is a particularly useful as a soap substitute.

Ointments

Ointments are semisolid and contain no water, being based usually on oils or greases such as polyethylene glycol (water-soluble) or paraffin (fatty). They feel greasy or sticky to the touch. Ointments are the best treatment for dry, flaky skin disorders as they are good at hydrating the stratum corneum and they deliver an active ingredient (e.g. a steroid) more effectively.

If a patient dislikes the greasy nature of an ointment, a cream is better than no treatment at all, but creams are less effective and do have to be used more frequently. A compromise may be to use a cream on the face and an ointment elsewhere (Table 20.14).

Lotions

These are based on a liquid vehicle such as water or alcohol. They are usually volatile and rapid evaporation promotes a cooling effect on the skin. Lotions are useful for weeping skin conditions and are ideal for scalp dermatoses. The cooling effect can be a useful antipruritic. Alcohol-based lotions should be avoided on broken skin as they cause stinging.

Gels

Gels are semisolid preparations of high-molecular-weight polymers. They are non-greasy and liquefy on contact with the skin. They are useful for treating the scalp.

Pastes

Pastes contain a high percentage (>40%) of powder in an ointment base. They are thick and stiff and difficult to remove from the skin. They are useful when a treatment needs to be applied precisely to a skin lesion without it smearing on to surrounding normal skin. An example is dithranol in Lassar's paste (used on plaques of psoriasis), as dithranol will burn the surrounding normal skin.

Safety of topical steroids

Provided that preparations of appropriate strength are used for the body site being treated, these compounds can be used safely on a long-term intermittent basis (see p. 1161). If potent steroids are misused they will cause skin atrophy, manifested as striae, wrinkling, fragility and telangiectasia.

Problems with topical therapies

- *Systemic absorption* may occur if large areas of inflamed skin are treated topically, especially if the treatment is occluded with bandages or polyurethane films. Neonates are particularly susceptible to this owing to the relative increase in body surface area to volume.
- *Contact allergy* is not uncommon and may be suspected by unusually resistant disease or by apparent worsening of a condition after application of a substance. It is more common with creams as it is often the result of allergy to the preservative or emulsifying agent. Allergy can also be due to the active ingredient itself (e.g. neomycin or hydrocortisone).
- *Folliculitis* can occur owing to blockage of hair follicles. Creams and ointments should be applied to the skin in the same direction as hair growth to try to prevent this blockage. It is a particular problem with the use of ointments in hot weather (especially if under occlusive bandages) and a lighter cream may be more appropriate at this time.

CHAPTER BIBLIOGRAPHY

Champion RH, Burton JL, Ebling FJG (eds) (1998) *Textbook of Dermatology*, 6th edn. Oxford: Blackwell Scientific.

Hunter JAA, Savin JA, Dahl MV (1995) *Clinical Dermatology*. Oxford: Blackwell Scientific.

Weedon D (ed) (1997) *Skin Pathology*. London: Churchill Livingstone.

UK PATIENT SUPPORT GROUPS

DEBRA (Dystrophic Epidermolysis Bullosa Research Association): DEBRA House, 13 Wellington Business Park, Duke's Ride, Crowthorne, Berkshire RG11 6LS.

Hairline International: 1668 High Street, Knowle, West Midlands B93 0LY.

National Eczema Society: 163 Eversholt Street, London NW1 1BU.

Psoriasis Association: Milton House, 7 Milton Street, Northampton NN2 7JG.

Psoriatic Arthropathy Support Group: D. Chandler, PO Box 111, St. Albans, Hertfordshire AL1 3JQ.

Vitiligo Society: 19 Fitzroy Square, London W1P 5HQ.

Appendices

British National Formulary (BNF) – name changes

Drugs mentioned in this book are given their non-proprietary (generic) names as published in the BNF. The BNF is published on behalf of the British Medical Association and the Royal Pharmaceutical Society of Great Britain. We recognize that other countries have their own list of non-proprietary titles and that the World Health Organisation also publishes a list. This means that different names exist for the same drug, and great care should be taken when prescribing, particularly when this book is used outside the UK. In this book all drugs have been given the UK name.

A directive, 97/27/EEC, has recently been published giving recommended International Non-proprietary Names (rINN). Many of the UK approved names are identical with rINN. List 1 below shows drugs where both names will be required to appear on manufacturer's labels for at least 5 years. List 2 shows those drugs where the rINN will be required to appear exclusively. In this edition of *Clinical Medicine* the UK name has most commonly been used.

List 1
Both names to appear

UK name	rINN
adrenaline	epinephrine
amethocaine	tetracaine
bendrofluazide	bendroflumethiazide
benzhexol	trihexyphenidyl
chlorpheniramine	chlorphenamine
dicyclomine	dicycloverine
dothiepin	dosulepin
flurandrenolone	fludroxycortide
frusemide	furosemide
mitozantrone	mitoxantrone
mustine	chlormethine
noradrenaline	norepinephrine
oxpentifylline	pentoxifylline
procaine penicillin	procaine benzylpenicillin
salcatonin	calcitonin (salmon)
thymoxamine	moxisylyte
trimeprazine	alimemazine

List 2
rINN to appear exclusively

UK name	rINN
amoxycillin	amoxicillin
amphetamine	amfetamine
amylobarbitone	amobarbital
amylobarbitone sodium	amobarbital sodium
beclomethasone	beclometasone
benorylate	benorilate
bethanidine	betanidine
busulphan	busulfan
butobarbitone	butobarbital
cephalexin	cefalexin
cephamandole nafate	cefamandole nafate
cephazolin	cefazolin
cephradine	cefradine
chloral betaine	cloral betaine
chlorbutol	chlorobutanol
chlormethiazole	clomethiazole
chlorthalidone	chlortalidone
cholecalciferol	colecalciferol
cholestyramine	colestyramine
clomiphene	clomifene
colistin sulphomethate sodium	colistimethate sodium
corticotrophin	corticotropin
danthron	dantron
desoxymethasone	desoximetasone
dexamphetamine	dexamfetamine
dienoestrol	dienestrol
dimethicone(s)	dimeticone
dimethyl sulphoxide	dimethyl sulfoxide
doxycycline hydrochloride (hemihydrate hemiethanolate)	doxycycline hyclate
ethacrynic acid	etacrynic acid
ethamsylate	etamsylate
ethinyloestradiol	etinylestradiol
ethynodiol	etynodiol
flumethasone	flumetasone
flupenthixol	flupentixol
guaiphenesin	guaifenesin
hexamine hippurate	methenamine hippurate
hydroxyprogesterone hexanoate	hydroxyprogesterone caproate
hydroxyurea	hydroxycarbamide
indomethacin	indometacin
lignocaine	lidocaine
lysuride	lisuride
methohexitone	methohexital
methotrimeprazine	levomepromazine
methyl cysteine	mecysteine
methylene blue	methylthioninium chloride
methylphenobarbitone	methylphenobarbital
nicoumalone	acenocoumarol
oestradiol	estradiol
oestriol	estriol
oestrone	estrone
oxethazaine	oxetacaine
oxyphenisatin	oxyphenisatine
pentaerythritol tetranitrate	pentaerithrityl tetranitrate
phenobarbitone	phenobarbital
pipothiazine	pipotiazine
polyhexanide	polihexanide
potassium clorazepate	dipotassium clorazepate
pramoxine	pramocaine
prothionamide	protionamide
quinalbarbitone	secobarbital
riboflavine	riboflavin
sodium calciumedetate	sodium calcium edetate
sodium cromoglycate	sodium cromoglicate
sodium ironedetate	sodium feredetate
sodium picosulphate	sodium picosulfate
sorbitan monostearate	sorbitan stearate
stilboestrol	diethylstilbestrol
sulphacetamide	sulfacetamide
sulphadiazine	sulfadiazine
sulphadimidine	sulfadimidine
sulphaguanidine	sulfaguanidine
sulphamethoxazole	sulfamethoxazole
sulphasalazine	sulfasalazine
sulphathiazole	sulfathiazole
sulphinpyrazone	sulfinpyrazone
tetracosactrin	tetracosactide
thiabendazole	tiabendazole
thioguanine	tioguanine
thiopentone	thiopental
thyroxine sodium	levothyroxine sodium
urofollitrophin	urofollitropin
vitamin A	retinol

Reproduced with permission from the *British National Formulary* 1998.

Dietary advice

The following are general guidelines. Any patient requiring a therapeutic diet should receive individual advice from a state-registered dietitian.

These diets were compiled by the dietitians at St Bartholomew's and the Royal London Hospitals, co-ordinated by Liz Rogers and Barbara Engel.

Diabetes mellitus

All newly diagnosed patients with diabetes should be referred to a dietitian. The basic principles of the diet for diabetes are given below. These are based on the British Diabetic Association's guidelines for the dietary management of diabetes for the 1990s.

The diet is based around the broad principles of healthy eating.

Carbohydrate should make up about half the total dietary energy intake, the majority coming from complex sources (high-fibre foods and starchy foods in general).

Foods with a high sugar content, e.g. sweets, preserves, cakes, puddings, should be avoided generally, but it is recognized that up to 25 g daily of added sugar (sucrose) can be incorporated into a low-fat, high-fibre diet. 'Sugary' soft drinks (ordinary fruit squashes, cordials and fizzy drinks) should be avoided and replaced with sugar-free 'diet' drinks. Large volumes of pure (unsweetened) fruit juices should also be avoided. Low-calorie/sugar-free products sweetened with non-nutritive sweeteners (e.g. saccharin, aspartame, acesulfame K) are acceptable and may be useful in the diet.

Commercial 'diabetic' foods should be avoided.

Dietary fibre (non-starch polysaccharides) intake should be increased, concentrating on soluble fibre (pulses, oats, fruits and vegetables). High-fibre foods may also promote satiety and assist weight loss. Non-starch polysaccharides (NSP) should be incorporated into an overall high-carbohydrate diet; 18 g NSP daily is recommended.

Fat in the diet should be reduced to 30–35% of total energy intake. Of this, 10% should be from saturated fat, with the remainder coming from both polyunsaturated and monounsaturated fat sources.

Protein intake should be 10–15% of energy intake, i.e. not exceed normal intake.

Salt should be limited to <6 g (100 mmol) daily if normotensive; 3 g (50 mmol) daily if hypertensive. (In practice this may be difficult to achieve.)

Alcohol taken in moderation is acceptable. Sweet alcoholic beverages and high-alcohol beers should be avoided.

Insulin-dependent diabetes mellitus (Type I)

Carbohydrate distributed evenly throughout the day to include between-meal and bedtime snacks helps minimize fluctuations in blood glucose concentrations. In practice a regular intake of food is used to prevent hypoglycaemia.

Carbohydrate exchange lists are rarely used. However, an understanding of the carbohydrate content of foods remains necessary. Many centres are beginning to discuss the 'glycaemic index' (GI) of foods with patients, encouraging them to choose more of the lower GI (more slowly absorbed) carbohydrate foods in order to achieve better post-prandial blood glucose control. These foods include pulses, oats, pasta and granary breads.

It should be remembered that patients will have to be instructed how to maintain their carbohydrate intake during illness, cope with their diet while travelling, and adjust their intake prior to exercise.

Non-insulin-dependent diabetes mellitus (Type II)

Obesity is a problem in 75% of patients with type II diabetes. Reduction of energy intake and regular exercise are the main aims for the overweight patient.

Reduction in fat intake may be relatively more important in type II to help reduce the incidence of cardiovascular disease and aid weight loss.

Food should be evenly distributed throughout the day at mealtimes, snacks not being necessary for the overweight patient. Patients taking certain oral hypoglycaemic agents may need to have between-meal snacks to prevent hypoglycaemia.

Gluten-free diet

This diet is used for the treatment of coeliac disease and dermatitis herpetiformis. It involves the exclusion of wheat, rye and barley. Current evidence suggests that oats do not cause intestinal damage.

Any food containing gluten, either as an obvious constituent (e.g. flour, bread) or as a 'hidden' ingredient (e.g. in stock cubes, dessert mixes), must be avoided.

It is not always possible to tell from the list of ingredients on a food label whether or not a manufactured food is gluten free. To help with this problem, the Coeliac Society produces a comprehensive list of manufactured foods which are gluten free. In the UK patients prescribed a gluten-free diet are advised to join the Society.

The Coeliac Society
PO Box 220
High Wycombe
Bucks HP11 2HY

A selection of foods included in a gluten-free (GF) diet includes:

- GF bread*, GF crispbread*, GF pasta*
- GF flour*, soya flour, potato flour, pea flour, rice flour
- Soya bran, rice bran
- GF biscuits*, GF cakes
- Breakfast cereals – corn or rice based
- Rice, tapioca, sago, arrowroot, buckwheat, millet, maize
- Fresh or frozen meat, poultry, offal
- Plain fresh or frozen fish, fish canned in oil
- Eggs, plain cheeses
- Milk, cream, butter, margarine, oils
- Plain fresh, frozen or tinned vegetables and potatoes
- Tinned fruit in syrup or natural juice, fresh or frozen fruit
- Nuts
- Tea, coffee, fruit juices, fruit squash, most fizzy drinks
- Sugar, syrup, honey, jam, marmalade, jelly
- Herbs, plain spices, vinegar, salt, pepper.

* Products prescribable in the UK for coeliac disease and dermatitis herpetiformis.

In addition, any home-made items, e.g. soups or sauces, made with GF ingredients are suitable.

Sodium-restricted diets

'No added salt' diet

This limits sodium intake to about 100 mmol a day, in the absence of other dietary restrictions.

A small amount of salt may be used in cooking, but none should be used at the table. The following foods contain considerable amounts of sodium and should be *avoided*:

- Cheese
- Bacon, ham, sausages, salt beef and other salted meats
- Smoked fish and smoked meats
- Tinned meat, tinned fish, meat and fish pâtés and pastes
- Stock cubes, meat extracts, vegetable extracts, such as 'Oxo', 'Bovril', 'Marmite'
- Soya sauce and other liquid seasonings
- Salted nuts and crisps.

Most ready-made meals and convenience foods are relatively high in sodium and their use needs to be limited. This can make even this level of sodium restriction difficult to achieve for some patients.

40 mmol sodium diet

This is used in the treatment of ascites or severe oedema associated with salt and water retention. It is used in conjunction with diuretics.

In addition to avoiding the high-salt foods listed above, the following restrictions apply:

- No salt to be used in cooking or at the table
- Salt-free butter or margarine should be used
- Milk should be restricted to about 300 ml daily
- Bread: about 4 slices ordinary bread daily; extra bread must be salt free
- Breakfast cereals that are free from added salt are recommended.

Patients are advised that 'salt substitutes' should only be used under medical supervision.

Weight-reducing diet

Energy restriction is achieved by reducing fat, alcohol and sugar, while maintaining a relatively high intake of starchy carbohydrate foods, in particular fibre-containing types. Wholegrain cereals and high-fibre breads are encouraged. The principles of a healthy diet are used as a basis for the advice.

This diet is suitable for people with diabetes who are obese.

The following meal plan would not be used prescriptively, but is given here as an example of the type of plan discussed.

Sample meal plan

Breakfast

- *Small* cupful of breakfast cereal or porridge with low-fat milk, no sugar
- Bread or toast with a little low-fat spread or reduced-sugar jam or marmalade

Snack meal

- *Small* helping of lean meat, poultry, fish, eggs, low-fat cheese or portion of baked beans
- Salad vegetables
- Bread or crispbreads
- Fresh fruit or 'diet' yoghurt

Main meal

- *Small* helping of lean meat, poultry, fish, eggs, low-fat cheese or pulses
- Large helping of vegetables and/or side salad
- Potatoes, boiled rice, pasta or bread
- Fruit, fresh or tinned in natural juice

Low-fat milk (skimmed or semi-skimmed) is recommended for use in tea, coffee and on cereals. Artificial sweeteners may be used if necessary. Suitable drinks include sugar-free squashes and fizzy drinks, soda water, and mineral water.

The most common area of misunderstanding concerns fats. In particular, there is a widespread belief that oils and other fats of vegetable origin are 'less fattening' than butter and other animal fats. Clear advice about the importance of reducing total dietary fat intake is essential.

Advice about including ready-made meals and convenience foods is often needed.

Limit

- *All* high-fat foods: butter, margarines, oils, fried foods, cream, mayonnaise, salad dressing, full-fat cheeses, pastry, dumplings, avocado, nuts and crisps.
- High-sugar foods: sweets, chocolate, honey, sweet biscuits, cakes, puddings, ordinary fruit squash and fizzy drinks.

Alcohol

Patients are told that alcohol is high in calories and usually advised to drink as little as possible while trying to lose weight.

Cholesterol-lowering diet

This diet involves reducing intakes of both saturated and total fat. Moderate use of appropriate polyunsaturated or monounsaturated oils/fats is advised unless the patient is overweight. (Overweight patients would be given a suitably modified reducing diet.)

Healthy eating principles form the basis of the advice.

Patients are advised to eat more fruit and vegetables and starchy foods, and it is explained that these should form the basis of their meals.

Low-fat milks and yoghurts are encouraged as a calcium source.

Foods high in soluble fibre are encouraged. These include beans, lentils and other pulses, oats – and fruits and vegetables generally.

It may be necessary to limit dietary cholesterol.

Sample meal plan

Breakfast

- Fruit or fruit juice
- Cereal or porridge with low-fat milk
- Bread with polyunsaturated (or monounsaturated) margarine or low-fat spread
- Jam, marmalade or honey.

Snack meal

- Sandwich or salad with *lean* meat, chicken, fish, egg or low-fat cheese
- Bread or crispbreads with tinned fish or low-fat cheese or baked beans on toast
- Fresh fruit or low-fat yoghurt/fromage frais.

Main meal

- *Lean* meat, poultry, fish, low-fat cheese or pulses
- Large helping of vegetables and/or salad
- Pasta, rice, bread, potatoes (including chips – cooked in appropriate oil – occasionally)
- Fruit or other low-fat dessert or pudding made with low-fat milk.

Foods to avoid include the following sources of saturated fat:

- Butter, lard, suet, cooking fats, other 'hard' margarines, coconut oil, coconut cream
- Full-fat cheeses, whole milk, cream, yoghurt made with whole milk
- Duck, goose, sausages, pâté, luncheon meat, salami-type sausages and other fatty meats
- Ice creams
- Ordinary pastries, pies and cakes.

Other high-fat foods would usually be 'limited', for example:

- Mayonnaise, conventional salad creams
- Crisps and other savoury snacks
- Many puddings and desserts.

The moderate use of unsaturated fats and oils for cooking, baking etc. is discussed.

Cholesterol- and triglyceride-lowering diet

In addition to the advice given above, sugar and foods with a high sugar content are limited.

Complex carbohydrates are encouraged, including starchy foods with a high-fibre content.

Oily fish may be recommended.

Alcohol intake should be restricted.

For overweight patients a modified reducing diet is used.

Diets in renal disease

Restricted protein diet

Early dietary intervention and frequent review of all patients with progressing renal failure by an appropriately trained dietitian has four important goals:

- To prevent malnutrition
- To potentially retard the progression of renal disease
- To prevent uraemic toxicity and the adverse effects of alterations in vitamin, mineral and lipid metabolism
- To improve quality of life.

There is no consensus of opinion regarding when, or even if, to start a low-protein diet. However, in the absence of factors which prevent adaptation to a reduced protein intake, such as infection and catabolism, it is beneficial to discourage a high-protein diet and the recommended intake can fall between 0.6 and 1.0 g protein per kilogram ideal weight. A reduced protein intake will also reduce the intake of phosphate, which will aid the control of bone disease. The lower the protein intake, the more attention must be paid to ensuring adequate energy, vitamin and mineral intake.

Protein 0.6–1.0 g protein per kilogram ideal body weight (IBW) daily.

Energy 30–35 kcal/kg (energy requirements can be calculated using standard formulas: carbohydrate 'energy' supplements may need to be prescribed). The balance of carbohydrate to fat should follow the COMA (Committee on Medical Aspects of Food Policy) recommendations for Healthy Eating.

Sodium 80–100 mmol/d (unless a salt waster) if hypertensive.

Potassium No more than 1mmol/kg IBW if plasma potassium exceeds normal range. Otherwise Healthy Eating recommendations apply, i.e. 5 portions fruit and vegetables a day.

Phosphate No more than 0.5 mmol/kg IBW/day if the plasma phosphate is >1.5 mmol/L.

Sample meal plan for 0.8 g protein per kilogram IBW per day

For a 70 kg person, moderately active, not overweight or hypertensive

Protein 56g 60% high biological value to meet essential amino acid requirements) 36g HBV (high biological value) + 20g LBV (low biological value).

Energy 2100–2500 kcal.

B vitamins, folate, vitamin C, zinc, iron and calcium intakes and biochemistry will need monitoring regularly.

Breakfast

- 2–3 slices of bread (higher fibre varieties are recommended)
- jam, honey, marmalade.

Lunch

- 25g meat or 40g fish
- 2 slices of bread
- 1 portion of vegetable
- 1 portion of fruit.

Evening meal

- 100g meat or 150g fish
- 300g potato or 200g rice
- 1–2 portion vegetables
- 1 portion fruit.

Daily

175 ml milk, 2–3 additional slices of bread can be taken between meals; fats and oils should be used sparingly; supplements may be required as described above. A small amount of salt can be added to the cooking water but do not add at the table. See 'no added salt' for further restrictions. Tea, squashes and fizzy drinks are suitable.

N.B. Regular monitoring is required: biochemistry, food intake, anthropometrics, urinary urea nitrogen.

Nephrotic syndrome

Protein 0.8–1.0 g/kg ideal body weight (IBW) daily. (0.8g protein per kilogram IBW plus 1g for every gram protein lost in the urine).

Energy Energy requirements can be calculated using standard formulas. The balance of carbohydrates to fat should follow the COMA (Committee on Medical Aspects of Food Policy) recommendations for Healthy Eating, i.e. a predominance of complex carbohydrates and minimum use of fat (see cholesterol-reducing diet).

Sodium 80–100 mmol/d.

Vitamins and minerals Some vitamins and minerals are protein bound. Therefore, proteinuria may also result in increased losses of these nutrients.

Sample meal plan for 1.0 g protein per kilogram IBW per day

Breakfast

- 2–3 slices of bread (higher fibre varieties are recommended)
- jam, honey, marmalade.

Lunch

- 50g meat or 80g fish
- 4 slices of bread
- 1 portion vegetable
- 1 portion fruit.

Evening meal

- 100g meat or 150g fish
- 300g potato or 200g rice
- 1–2 portion vegetables
- 1 portion fruit.

Daily

300 ml milk; 2–3 additional slices of bread can be taken between meals; fats and oils should be used sparingly; supplements may be required as described above. A small amount of salt can be added to the cooking water but do not add at the table. See 'no added salt' for further restrictions. Tea, squashes and fizzy drinks are suitable.

Kidney stone diet

The nutritional factors which affect the formation of kidney stones are: calcium, protein, oxalate, fluid, salt, vitamin C and vitamin D. Severe calcium restriction results in negative calcium balance which may lead to osteoporosis. In addition, a lower calcium intake may allow greater absorption and hence urinary excretion of oxalate (Curhan et al 1993). A high-protein intake will increase the excretion of calcium and other stone-forming substances, such as uric acid. Calcium excretion is proportional to sodium excretion/intake.

The recommended diet contains 1g protein per kilogram IBW, <100 mmol sodium, RNI* calcium, 2.5–3 litres fluid; avoid oxalate- and purine-rich foods; avoid supplements of vitamin D and vitamin C above the RNI (Goldfarb 1994; Juneja 1992).

Oxalate-rich foods	rhubarb, gooseberries, blackberries, strawberries, beetroot, spinach, okra, sweet potato, parsley, leek, celery, chocolate, cocoa, nuts, seeds, wheatgerm.
Purine-rich foods	offal, seafood, oily fish, game, meat and yeast extracts.

* Recommended Nutrient Intake:
700 mg/d adult men and women
1200 mg/d for lactating women and post-menopausal women (Smith et al 1992).

FURTHER READING

Curhan G et al (1993) A prospective study of dietary calcium and other nutrients and the risk of symptomatic kidney stones. *New England Journal of Medicine* **328**: 833–838.

Goldfarb S (1994) Diet and nephrolithiasis. *Annual Review of Medicine* **45**: 235–243.

Juneja V (1992) Idiopathic calcium oxalate lithiasis in a recurrent stone forming patient. *Journal of Renal Nutrition* **2**: 165–170.

Smith C L et al (1992) Dietary factors in calcium nephrolithiasis. *Journal of Renal Nutrition* **2**: 146–153.

Normal values

These normal values were compiled by Ruth Halliday SRN and were modified by Katherine Woodward RGN and Therese Taylor RGN and, for this edition, by Anne Smart RGN, St Bartholomew's Hospital. Values vary from one laboratory to another. Please check with your own laboratory.

Haematology

Haemoglobin	
Male	14.0–17.7 g dL^{-1}
Female	12.0–16.0 g dL^{-1}
Mean corpuscular haemoglobin (MCH)	27–33 pg
Mean corpuscular haemoglobin concentration (MCHC)	32–35 g dL^{-1}
Mean corpuscular volume (MCV)	80–96 fL
Packed cell volume (PCV)	
Male	0.42–0.53 L L^{-1}
Female	0.36–0.45 L L^{-1}
White cell count (WCC)	4–11 × 10^9/litre
Basophil granulocytes	<0.01–0.1 × 10^9/litre
Eosinophil granulocytes	0.04–0.4 × 10^9/litre
Lymphocytes	1.5–4.0 × 10^9/litre
Monocytes	0.2–0.8 × 10^9/litre
Neutrophil granulocytes	2.0–7.5 × 10^9/litre
Total blood volume	60–80 ml kg^{-1}
Plasma volume	40–50 ml kg^{-1}
Platelet count	150–400 × 10^9/litre
Serum B_{12}	160–925 ng L^{-1} (150–675 pmol L^{-1})
Serum folate	4–18 μg L^{-1} (5-63 nmol L^{-1})

Red cell folate	160–640 μg L^{-1}
Red cell mass	
Male	25–35 ml kg^{-1}
Female	20–30 ml kg^{-1}
Reticulocyte count	0.5–2.5% of red cells (50–100 × 10^9/litre)
Erythrocyte sedimentation rate (ESR)	<20 mm in 1 hour

Coagulation

Bleeding time (Ivy method)	2–7 min
Partial thromboplastin time (PTTK)	24–31 s
Prothrombin time	12–16 s
International Normalized Ratio (INR)	1

Biochemistry

Acid phosphatase	1–5 U L^{-1}
Alanine aminotransferase (ALT)	5–40 U L^{-1}
Albumin	36–53 g L^{-1}
Alkaline phosphatase	25–115 U L^{-1}
Amylase	<220 U L^{-1}
Angiotensin-converting enzyme	10–70 U L^{-1}
α_1-Antitrypsin	1.1–2.1 g L^{-1}
Aspartate aminotransferase (AST)	7–40 U L^{-1}
Bicarbonate	22–30 mmol L^{-1}
Bilirubin	<17 μmol L^{-1} (0.3–1.5 mg dL^{-1})
Caeruloplasmin	0.20–0.61 L^{-1}
Calcium	2.20–2.67 mmol L^{-1} (8.5–10.5 mg dL^{-1})
Chloride	95–106 mmol L^{-1}
Cholinesterase	2.25–7.0 U L^{-1}
Copper	11–20 μmol L^{-1} (100–200 mg dL^{-1})
C-reactive protein	<10 mg L^{-1}
Creatinine	0.06–0.12 mmol L^{-1} (0.6–1.5 mg dL^{-1})
Creatine kinase (CPK)	
Female	24–170 U L^{-1}
Male	24–195 U L^{-1}
CK-MB fraction	25 U L^{-1} (<60% of total activity)
C3	0.55–1.20 g L^{-1}
C4	0.20–0.50 g L^{-1}
Ferritin	
Female	6–110 μg L^{-1}
Male	20–260 μg L^{-1}
Post menopausal	12–230 μg L^{-1}
α-Fetoprotein	<10 k U L^{-1}
Glucose (fasting)	4.5–5.6 mmol L^{-1} (70–110 mg dL^{-1})
Fructosamine	up to 285 μmol L^{-1}
γ-Glutamyl transpeptidase (γ-GT)	
Male	11–50 U L^{-1}
Female	7–32 U L^{-1}
Glycosylated haemoglobin (HbA_{1c})	3.8–8.5%

Hydroxybutyric dehydrogenase (HBD)	40–150 U L^{-1}
Immunoglobulins (11 years and over)	
IgA	0.8–4 g L^{-1}
IgG	7.0–18.0 g L^{-1}
IgM	0.4–2.5 g L^{-1}
Iron	13–32 μmol L^{-1} (50–150 μg dL^{-1})
Iron binding capacity (total) (TIBC)	42–80 μmol L^{-1} (250–410 μg dL^{-1})
Lactate dehydrogenase	240–460 U L^{-1}
Lead	<0.7 μmol L^{-1}
Magnesium	0.7–1.1 mmol L^{-1}
β_2-Microglobulin	1.0–3.0 mg L^{-1}
Osmolality	280–296 mosmol kg^{-1}
Phosphate	0.8–1.5 mmol L^{-1}
Potassium	3.5–5.0 mmol L^{-1}
Prostate-specific antigen	up to 4.0 μg L^{-1}
Protein (total)	62–80 g L^{-1}
Sodium	135–146 mmol L^{-1}
Urate	0.18–0.42 mmol L^{-1} (3.0–7.0 mg dL^{-1})
Urea	2.5–6.7 mmol L^{-1} (8–25 mg dL^{-1})
Vitamin A	0.5–2.01 μmol L^{-1}
Vitamin D	
25-hydroxy	37–200 nmol L^{-1} (0.15–0.80 ng L^{-1})
1,25-dihydroxy	60–108 pmol L^{-1} (0.24–0.45 pg L^{-1})
Zinc	7–18 μmol L^{-1}

Lipids and lipoproteins

Cholesterol	3.5–6.5 mmol L^{-1} (ideal <5.2 mmol L^{-1})
HDL cholesterol	
Male	0.95–2.15 mmol L^{-1}
Female	0.70–2.00 mmol L^{-1}
Lipids (total)	4.0–10.0 g L^{-1}
Lipoproteins	
VLDL	0.128–0.645 mmol L^{-1}
LDL	1.55–4.4 mmol L^{-1}
HDL	
Male	0.70–2.1 mmol L^{-1}
Female	0.50–1.70 mmol L^{-1}
Non-esterified fatty acids	
Male	0.19–0.78 mmol L^{-1}
Female	0.06–0.9 mmol L^{-1}
Phospholipid	2.9–5.2 mmol L^{-1}
Triglycerides	
Male	0.70–2.1 mmol L^{-1}
Female	0.50–1.70 mmol L^{-1}

Blood gases (arterial)

$Pa\text{CO}_2$	4.8–6.1 kPa (36–46 mmHg)
$Pa\text{O}_2$	10–13.3 kPa (75–100 mmHg)
$[H^+]$	35–45 nmol L^{-1}
pH	7.35–7.45
Bicarbonate	24–28 mmol L^{-1}

Urine values

Calcium	7.5 mmol daily or less (<300 mg daily)
Copper	0.2–1.0 μmol daily
Creatinine	0.13–0.22 mmol per kilogram body weight, daily
5-Hydroxyindole acetic acid	<75 μmol daily; amounts lower in females than males
Protein (quantitative)	<0.15 g per 24 hours

Tests in endocrinology

These tests were compiled by Dr Paul Drury, Medical Director, Auckland Diabetes Centre, Auckland, New Zealand and updated by Anne Smart.

General

Different laboratories will have slightly different reference ranges for many of these tests, and even slightly different protocols. *Always* consult your own laboratory before performing complex, expensive and inconvenient tests. Also check what specimen is required (e.g. serum, plasma, acidified urine) and whether any special handling is required (e.g. freezing).

The recent introduction of multichannel endocrine analysers by a number of different manufacturers increases the need for reference to local laboratory ranges and guidelines.

Date, time and sampling conditions (plus date of last menstrual period where appropriate) should always be noted on the request form as they are critical for interpretation.

Gonadal axis

Basal levels

Basal levels are often sufficient to indicate the site of the problem; they may also indicate the stage of the menstrual cycle or of puberty.

The international standard for LH may change during the currency of this book with resultant changes in reference ranges - please check your own laboratory for their new values.

Adult male

Testosterone	10–35 mmol L^{-1}
Luteinizing hormone (LH)	1–10 U L^{-1}
Follicle-stimulating hormone (FSH)	1–7 U L^{-1}

Adult Female

	Follicular	Mid-cycle	Luteal	Post-menopausal
LH (U L^{-1})	2.5–10	25–70	1–13	>30
FSH (U L^{-1})	2.5–10	25–70	0.3–21	>30
Oestradiol (pmol L^{-1})	<110	500–1100	300–750	<150
Progesterone (nmol L^{-1})	<10	–	>30	<6
Testosterone (nmol L^{-1})			1–3.5	

LHRH test

100 μg of luteinizing hormone releasing hormone (LHRH) is given intravenously into an indwelling catheter at time 0; samples are taken at time 0, +20 and + 60 min for LH and FSH. Normal responses are:

	20 min	60 min
Female (follicular phase)		
LH (U L^{-1})	15–42	12–35
FSH (U L^{-1})	1–11	1–25
Male		
LH (U L^{-1})	13–58	11–48
FSH (U L^{-1})	1–7	1–5

Sperm counts/seminal fluid analysis

Volume	2–6 mL
Density	>20–200 × 10^6 mL^{-1}
Motility	>60% motile

Full assessment of normal and abnormal forms is needed for fertility work.

Prolactin

Stress can affect prolactin levels. To establish a definite abnormality several samples should be taken, ideally through an indwelling venous catheter.

Normal levels are below 400mU L^{-1} in most laboratories. The significance of minor increases (400–600 mU L^{-1}) is disputed. Levels of 2000–5000 mU L^{-1} are strongly suggestive of prolactinoma but can occur with other tumours/stalk disconnection.

Growth axis

Basal levels

Growth hormone (GH) release is episodic; however, an undetectable or very low level (<1mUL^{-1}) on a random sample excludes acromegaly.

Acromegaly

In normal subjects, GH levels are suppressed to below 1–2 mU L^{-1} during an oral glucose tolerance test (for details see Chapter 17).

GH deficiency

In children, exercise and arginine are often used to stimulate GH secretion; a level above 20 mU L^{-1} is a normal response. The insulin tolerance test is, however, the optimal test for adults and children.

The insulin tolerance test should only be used for children when essential and must only be performed in expert centres with considerable expertise and constant medical supervision.

Insulin tolerance test for GH reserve

After an overnight fast, a rapid-acting human insulin is administered at 0900 via an indwelling intravenous catheter. The dose is usually 0.15 u kg^{-1} body weight but should be 0.1u kg^{-1} for hypopituitarism and 0.2–0.3u kg^{-1} in cases of insulin resistance (e.g. acromegaly, Cushing's syndrome). Clinical hypoglycaemia and a blood glucose <2.2 mmol L^{-1} should be produced; if not, repeat the dose at 45 min. Samples are collected at 0, +30, +45, +60, + 90 and +120 min. A normal response for GH is >20 mUL^{-1}. A large breakfast should be given afterwards.

The test should not be used in patients with epilepsy, heart disease or profound hypopituitarism – a normal ECG and a cortisol result >100 mmol L^{-1} should be seen before the test. Syringes loaded with 50% dextrose and hydrocortisone must always be available during the test.

This test is also used to measure ACTH reserve (see below).

Thyroid axis

Basal levels

Levels of the thyroid hormones vary very little by hour or day unless patients are acutely ill; basal levels thus usually suffice.

Total serum thyroxine (T_4)	58–174 mmol L^{-1}
Free serum thyroxine (fT_4)	10–22 pmol L^{-1}
Total serum tri-iodothyronine (T_3)	1.07–3.18 nmol L^{-1}
Free serum tri-iodothyronine (fT_3)	5–10 pmol L^{-1}
Thyroid-stimulating hormone (TSH)	0.3–4.0 mU L^{-1}

TRH test – now much less used

200 µg of thyrotropin-releasing hormone (TRH) is given via an indwelling intravenous catheter at time 0 after a basal sample is collected; subsequent samples are taken at +20 and +60 min. Normal responses (levels of TSH) are:

0 min	0.3–3.5 mU L^{-1}
20 min	3.4–20 mU L^{-1}
60 min	<20 min level
Increment	>20 mU L^{-1}

An excessive response indicates hypothryoidism; an inadequate one indicates either primary hyperthyroidism or pituitary disease.

Adrenal axis

All cortisol values here refer to specific assay methods, e.g. radioimmunoassay, and not to fluorimetry.

Basal levels

Adrenocorticotrophic hormone (ACTH) and cortisol levels vary episodically and with a circadian rhythm; single timed values are thus of limited use except at 0900 exactly, the peak of the circadian rhythm, when cortisol values are predictive of response to a stimulatory test:

0900 cortisol < 100 nmol L^{-1}
highly predictive of adrenal/pituitary failure

0900 cortisol > 500 nmo L^{-1}
highly predictive of intact adrenal/pituitary axis

Intermediate values are essentially of little value.

Reference ranges

	0900 h	2400 h (must be asleep)
Cortisol (nmol L^{-1})	180–700	<100
ACTH (ng L^{-1})	10–80	<10

Intravenous synacthen test

This is now frequently used as a safer and easier surrogate for the insulin tolerance test, though it tests only adrenal reserve. A basal cortisol sample is taken at 0 min, followed by intravenous Synacthen 250 μg, and a further sample taken at +30 min. A cortisol value ≥550 nmol L^{-1} is normal.

Short ACTH stimulation test

This test is used to exclude Addison's disease. After taking a first sample for cortisol, 0.25 mg of tetracosactrin is given at time 0. Further samples are taken at +30 and +60 min. Normal values are:

30 min	550–1160 nmol L^{-1}
60 min	690–1290 nmol L^{-1}
Increment	330–850 nmol L^{-1}

Dexamethasone suppression tests

These are used to excluded Cushing's syndrome. They are described on p. 946

Insulin tolerance test – for ACTH reserve

This can be used to measure ACTH reserve; details and precautions are given under investigation of GH reserve. It should only be performed where an 0900 cortisol is ≥100 nmol L^{-1}.

A normal response to adequate hypoglycaemia (≤ 2.2 mmol L^{-1}) is a peak cortisol level ≥550 nmol L^{-1}; most authorities also require an increment of >180 nmol L^{-1}.

Endocrinology of blood pressure and thirst

Blood pressure

Plasma renin activity (PRA) varies very widely according to method – your own laboratory should be consulted.

Aldosterone (and PRA) should be measured after at least 30 min recumbency and, possibly, after 4 hours ambulation. Normal values are:

Lying	130–400 pmol L^{-1}
Standing	330–830 pmol L^{-1}

Thirst

As a screening test, early morning plasma and urine osmolalities are measured. Normal values are:

Plasma	275–290 mosmol kg^{-1}
Urine	Above 600 mosmol kg^{-1} suggests good concentration

Plasma and urine osmolalities must be interpreted together. Further study requires a water deprivation test.

Water deprivation test

Start at 0800–0830 after free fluid intake overnight. Light breakfast; no caffeine or smoking.

Dehydration for 8 hours; dry food only permitted (no access to fluids). Plasma osmolality measured hourly. Urine osmolality and volume measured hourly. Body weight measured hourly; *consider* stopping test if weight loss >3% of body weight.

After 8 hours give 2 μg desmopressin i.m.; continue urine collections hourly (2–4 hours usually sufficient). Patient may drink but intake over 12 hours restricted to 1.5 times the volume excreted in dehydration period.

The normal person will maintain normal plasma osmolality while concentrating urine >800 mosmol kg^{-1} during dehydration, unenhanced by desmospressin. In cranial diabetes insipidus (DI) urine will fail to concentrate during dehydration while plasma osmolality rises; this will be corrected by desmopressin with a urine osmolality >800 mosmol kg^{-1}. Those with nephrogenic DI behave as cranial DI initially but do not concentrate urine after desmopressin, while those with psychogenic polydipsia respond generally normally. Overlaps are, however, not infrequent.

Weight and height charts

Guidelines for body weight

Values given are weights without clothes.

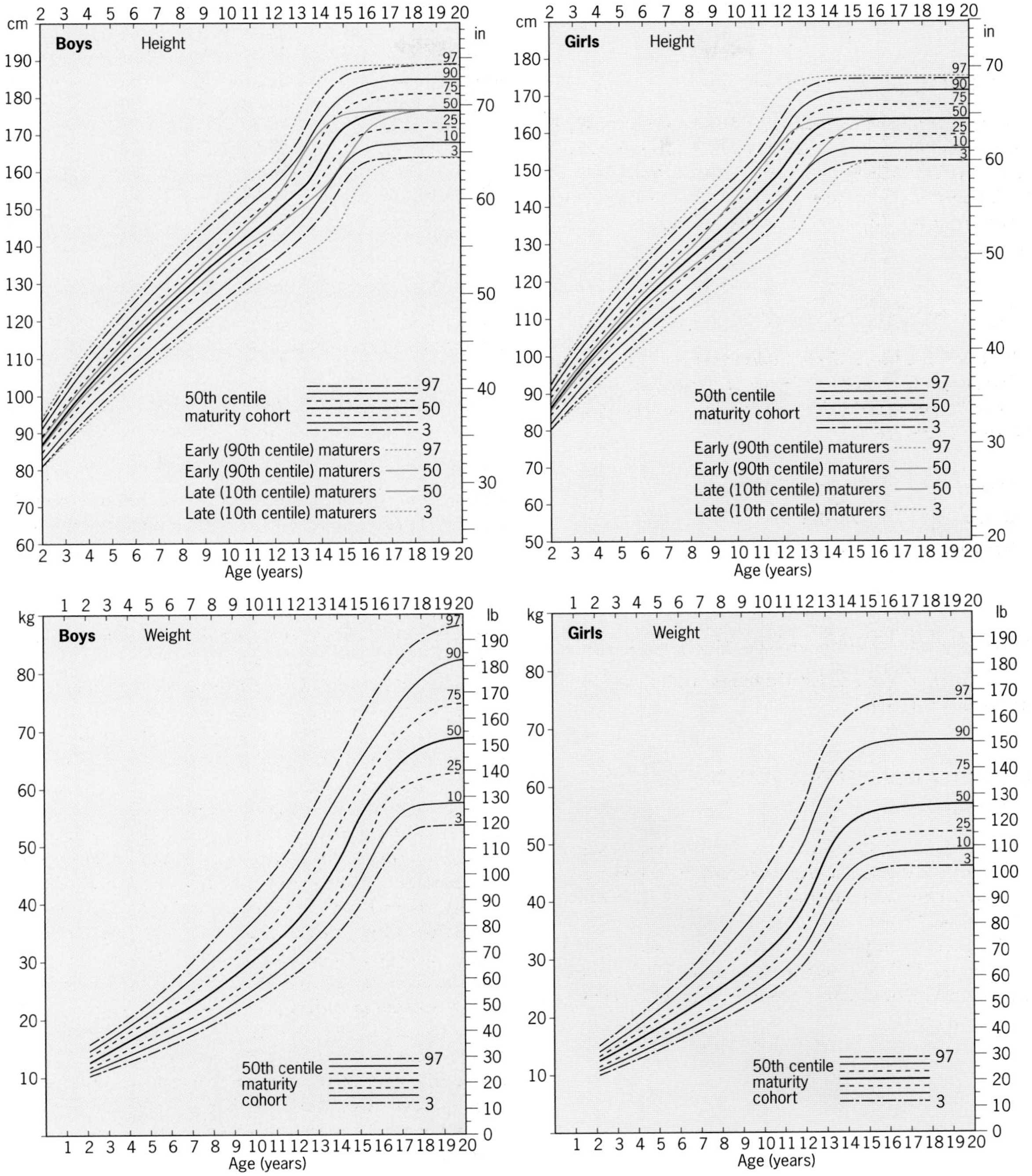

Fig. A.1
Weight and height charts. Based on Buckler-Tanner (1995) charts, reference 11B and 12B, reproduced by permission of Castlemead Publications

Measurements of height and weight

	Men (kg)			Women (kg)		
Height (m)	*Acceptable average*	*Acceptable weight range*	*Obese*[a]	*Acceptable average*	*Acceptable weight range*	*Obese*[a]
1.45				46.0	42–53	64
1.48				46.5	42–54	65
1.50				47.0	43–55	66
1.52				48.5	44–57	68
1.54				49.5	44–58	70
1.56				50.4	45–58	70
1.58	55.8	51–64	77	51.3	46–59	71
1.60	57.6	52–65	78	52.6	48–61	73
1.62	58.6	53–66	79	54.0	49–62	74
1.64	59.6	54–67	80	55.4	50–64	77
1.66	60.6	55–69	83	56.8	51–65	78
1.68	61.7	56–71	85	58.1	52–66	79
1.70	63.5	58–73	88	60.0	53–67	80
1.72	65.0	59–74	89	61.3	55–69	83
1.74	66.5	60–75	90	62.6	56–70	84
1.76	68.0	62–77	92	64.0	58–72	86
1.78	69.4	64–79	95	65.3	59–74	89
1.80	71.0	65–80	96			
1.82	72.6	66–82	98			
1.84	74.2	67–84	101			
1.86	75.8	69–86	103			
1.88	77.6	71–88	106			
1.90	79.3	73–90	108			
1.92	81.0	75–93	112			
Body mass index[b]	22.0	20.1–25.0	30.0	20.8	18.7–23.8	28.6

[a] Value and above for all entries.
[b] Body mass index = weight (kg)/height^2 (m).
From Bray GA (ed) (1979) *Obesity in America*. Proceedings of the 2nd Fogarty International Center Conference on Obesity, No. 79. Washington: US DHEW.

Index

Note

Page numbers in **bold** refer to major discussions in the text, and usually include aspects such as epidemiology, clinical features, diagnosis, pathology and treatment.

Page numbers in *italics* refer to pages on which tables/information boxes are to be found.

vs denotes differential diagnosis.

Abbreviations used in subentries include:

CMV Cytomegalovirus
GFR glomerular filtration rate
IPPV Intermittent positive pressure ventilation
HIV Human immunodeficiency virus
SLE Systemic lupus erythematosus

Other abbreviations are to be found in the index.

A

B

C

D

E

F

G

I

J

K

L

M

N

P

Q

R

T

U

V

W

X

Y

Z